# Surgery of the Chest

# *Surgery of*
# the
# *Chest*

Volume

## II

## SIXTH EDITION

### David C. Sabiston, Jr., M.D.
James B. Duke Professor of Surgery
Duke University School of Medicine
Chief of Staff
Duke University Medical Center
Durham, North Carolina

### Frank C. Spencer, M.D.
George David Stewart Professor
Chairman, Department of Surgery
New York University School of Medicine
New York, New York

**W.B. SAUNDERS COMPANY**
*A Division of Harcourt Brace & Company*
Philadelphia    London    Toronto    Montreal    Sydney    Tokyo

**W.B. SAUNDERS COMPANY**
*A Division of Harcourt Brace & Company*

The Curtis Center
Independence Square West
Philadelphia, Pennsylvania 19106

**Library of Congress Cataloging-in-Publication Data**

Surgery of the chest / [edited by] David C. Sabiston, Jr., Frank C.
Spencer.—6th ed.
p. cm.

Includes bibliographical references and index.

ISBN 0-7216-5271-9

1. Chest—Surgery.    I. Sabiston, David C.
II. Spencer, Frank Cole.
[DNLM: 1. Thoracic Surgery. WF 980 S961 1995]

RD536.G48   1995

617.5′4059—dc20

DNLM/DLC                                                94-22780

SURGERY OF THE CHEST                              ISBN 0-7216-5271-9

Last digit is the print number:    9   8   7   6   5   4   3   2   1

# Contributors

**Alon S. Aharon, M.D.**
Department of Surgery Resident, Cardiothoracic Division, University of California at Los Angeles Medical Center, Los Angeles, California
*Congenital Malformations of the Mitral Valve*

**Robert W. Anderson, M.D.**
The David C. Sabiston Professor and Chairman, Department of Surgery, Duke University Medical Center; Duke University Hospital, Durham, North Carolina
*Shock and Circulatory Collapse*

**Mark P. Anstadt, M.D.**
Resident in Chief in General Surgery, Duke University Medical Center, Durham, North Carolina
*Assisted Circulation*

**Erle H. Austin III, M.D.**
Professor of Surgery, University of Louisiana, Department of Surgery; Chief, Pediatric Cardiac Surgery, Kosair Children's Hospital, Louisville, Kentucky
*Pulmonary Atresia with Intact Ventricular Septum; Univentricular Heart*

**John A. Bartlett, M.D.**
Assistant Professor of Medicine, Duke University Medical Center, Durham, North Carolina
*Thoracic Disorders in the Immunocompromised Host*

**Thomas M. Bashore, M.D.**
Professor of Medicine; Director, Fellowship Training Program, Associate Director, Duke Heart Center, Duke University Medical Center, Durham, North Carolina
*Cardiac Catheterization, Angiography, and Interventional Techniques in Valvular and Congenital Heart Disease; Coronary Arteriography*

**Harvey W. Bender, Jr., M.D.**
Professor of Surgery, Vanderbilt University, School of Medicine; Chairman, Department of Cardiac and Thoracic Surgery, Vanderbilt University Medical Center, Nashville, Tennessee
*Major Anomalies of Pulmonary and Thoracic Systemic Veins*

**Arthur D. Boyd, M.D.**
Professor of Surgery, New York University School of Medicine; Attending Surgeon, Tisch Hospital of the New York University Medical Center; Attending Surgeon, Bellevue Hospital Center; Attending Surgeon, Manhattan Veterans Administration Center, New York, New York
*Endoscopy: Bronchoscopy and Esophagoscopy; Tracheal Intubation and Mechanical Ventilation: The Surgeon's Viewpoint*

Robert M. Califf, M.D.

Associate Professor of Medicine, Duke University; Director, Coronary Care Unit; Director, Clinical Epidemiology and Biostatistics, Duke University Medical Center, Durham, North Carolina
*Fibrinolytic Therapy in the Management of Acute Myocardial Infarction*

David N. Campbell, M.D.

Associate Professor of Surgery, University of Colorado, Health Services Center, Denver, Colorado
*Thrombosis and Thromboembolism of Prosthetic Cardiac Valves and Extracardiac Prostheses*

Aldo R. Castañeda, M.D., Ph.D.

Director, The Aldo Castañeda Institute for Congenital Heart Disease, Clinique de Genolier, Genolier, Switzerland
*Anatomic Correction of Transposition of the Great Arteries at the Arterial Level*

Jessie Chai, M.D.

Brigham and Women's Hospital, Boston, Massachusetts
*Role of Computed Tomographic Scans in Cardiovascular Diagnosis*

Robbin G. Cohen, M.D.

Assistant Professor of Surgery, Division of Cardiothoracic Surgery, Department of Surgery, University of Southern California School of Medicine; University of Southern California University Hospital; University of Southern California—Kenneth Norris Jr. Cancer Hospital; LAC University of Southern California Hospital, Los Angeles, California
*The Pleura*

Lawrence H. Cohn, M.D.

Professor of Surgery, Harvard Medical School; Chief, Division of Cardiac Surgery, Brigham and Women's Hospital, Boston, Massachusetts
*Thoracic Aortic Aneurysms and Aortic Dissection*

Stephen B. Colvin, M.D.

Associate Professor of Surgery, New York University Medical School; Director, Cardiac Surgical Residency and Pediatric Cardiac Surgery, New York Medical Center, New York, New York
*Atrial Septal Defects, Atrioventricular Canal Defects, and Total Anomalous Pulmonary Venous Return; Acquired Disease of the Mitral Valve; Bypass Grafting for Coronary Artery Disease*

Joel D. Cooper, M.D.

Joseph C. Bancroft Professor of Surgery; Head, Section of General Thoracic Surgery, Division of Cardiothoracic Surgery, Washington University School of Medicine, Barnes Hospital, St. Louis, Missouri
*Lung Transplantation*

James L. Cox, M.D.

Evarts A. Graham Professor of Surgery, Washington University School of Medicine; Professor of Surgery, Chief, Division of Cardiothoracic Surgery, Barnes Hospital at Washington University School of Medicine, St. Louis, Missouri
*The Surgical Management of Cardiac Arrhythmias*

Fred A. Crawford, Jr., M.D.

Professor and Chairman, Department of Surgery, Medical University of South Carolina, Charleston, South Carolina
*Thoracic Incisions*

Ronald D. Curran, M.D.
Fellow, Cardiovascular and Thoracic Surgery, Northwestern University Medical School, Chicago, Illinois
*Shock and Circulatory Collapse*

Thomas A. D'Amico, M.D.
Fellow in Cardiothoracic Surgery, Duke University Medical Center, Durham, North Carolina
*Carcinoma of the Lung; Benign Tumors of the Lung and Bronchial Adenomas; Immunology and Immunotherapy of Carcinoma of the Lung; Surgical Management of Pulmonary Metastases; Kawasaki's Disease*

Gordon K. Danielson, M.D.
Roberts Professor of Surgery, Mayo Medical School and Graduate School of Medicine; Consultant, Cardiothoracic Surgery, Mayo Clinic/Foundation, Rochester, Minnesota
*Atrioventricular Canal; Ebstein's Anomaly*

Charles J. Davidson, M.D.
Associate Professor of Medicine, Northwestern University Medical School; Chief, Cardiac Catheterization Laboratories, Northwestern Memorial Hospital, Chicago, Illinois
*Cardiac Catheterization, Angiography, and Interventional Techniques in Valvular and Congenital Heart Disease; Coronary Arteriography*

R. Duane Davis, Jr., M.D.
Assistant Professor of Surgery, Duke University School of Medicine, Durham, North Carolina
*The Mediastinum*

Tom R. DeMeester, M.D.
Professor and Chairman, Department of Surgery, University of Southern California School of Medicine, Los Angeles, California
*The Pleura*

Roberto M. Di Donato, M.D.
Professor of Clinical Surgery, Professor of Clinical Pediatrics, University of Medicine and Dentistry of New Jersey; Director, Division of Pediatric Cardiothoracic Surgery, Children's Hospital of New Jersey, United Hospitals Medical Center, Newark, New Jersey
*Anatomic Correction of Transposition of the Great Arteries at the Arterial Level*

J. Michael DiMaio, M.D.
Chief Resident in Surgery, Duke University Medical Center, Durham, North Carolina
*Thoracic Disorders in the Immunocompromised Host*

James M. Douglas, Jr., M.D.
Director of Cardiovascular Surgery, St. Joseph Hospital, Bellingham, Washington
*The Pericardium; Thoracoscopic Surgery*

John J. Downes, M.D.
Professor of Anesthesia and Pediatrics at the University of Pennsylvania; Department of Anesthesia and Critical Care Medicine, Children's Hospital of Philadelphia, Philadelphia, Pennsylvania
*Respiratory Support in Infants*

André Duranceau, M.D.
Professor of Surgery, Faculté de Médecine, Université de Montreal; Division of Thoracic Surgery, Hôtel-Dieu de Montréal, Montréal, Québec, Canada
*Disorders of the Esophagus in the Adult*

**L. Henry Edmunds, Jr., M.D.**
Julian Johnson Professor of Cardiothoracic Surgery, University of Pennsylvania; Staff, Division of Cardiothoracic Surgery, Hospital of the University of Pennsylvania, Philadelphia, Pennsylvania
*Respiratory Support in Infants*

**T. Bruce Ferguson, Jr., M.D.**
Associate Professor of Surgery, Division of Cardiothoracic Surgery, Washington University School of Medicine; Associate Surgeon, Barnes Hospital, St. Louis, Missouri
*Congenital Lesions of the Lung and Emphysema*

**Thomas B. Ferguson, M.D.**
Emeritus Professor of Surgery, Washington University School of Medicine at Barnes Hospital, St. Louis, Missouri
*Congenital Lesions of the Lung and Emphysema*

**Gregory P. Fontana, M.D.**
Assistant Clinical Professor, University of California at Los Angeles School of Medicine, Division of Cardiothoracic Surgery, Department of Surgery; Attending Cardiothoracic Surgeon, Cedars-Sinai Medical Center, Department of Cardiothoracic Surgery, Los Angeles, California
*Acute Pulmonary Embolism*

**Robert M. Freedom, M.D., F.R.C.P.(C.), F.A.C.C.**
Professor of Paediatrics (Cardiology) and Pathology, University of Toronto, Faculty of Medicine; Head, Division of Cardiology, The Hospital for Sick Children, Toronto, Ontario, Canada
*The Mustard Procedure*

**David A. Fullerton, M.D.**
Assistant Professor, Department of Surgery, University of Colorado; Chief, Cardiothoracic Surgery, Veterans Administration Medical Center; Surgeon, Denver Children's Hospital, Denver, Colorado
*Prosthetic Valve Endocarditis*

**Aubrey C. Galloway, M.D.**
Associate Professor of Surgery, New York University Medical School; Director of Surgical Research, New York University Medical Center, New York, New York
*Atrial Septal Defects, Atrioventricular Canal Defects, and Total Anomalous Pulmonary Venous Return; Acquired Disease of the Mitral Valve; Bypass Grafting for Coronary Artery Disease*

**William A. Gay, Jr., M.D.**
Professor, Department of Surgery, Washington University School of Medicine; Attending Surgeon, Cardiothoracic Surgery, Barnes Hospital, St. Louis, Missouri
*Cardiac Transplantation*

**J. William Gaynor, M.D.**
Assistant Professor of Surgery, Pediatric Cardiothoracic Surgery, Children's Hospital of Philadelphia, Philadelphia, Pennsylvania
*Patent Ductus Arteriosus, Coarctation of the Aorta, Aortopulmonary Window, and Anomalies of the Aortic Arch; Pulmonary Atresia or Stenosis with Intact Ventricular Septum*

**Brian Ginsberg, M.D., B.Ch.**
Assistant Professor of Anesthesiology, Duke University Medical Center, Durham, North Carolina
*Acute Pain Management After Surgical Procedures*

**Donald D. Glower, Jr., M.D.**
Associate Professor of Surgery, Duke University, Durham, North Carolina
*Acquired Aortic Valve Disease*

**William J. Greeley, M.D.**
Division Chief, Division of Pediatric Anesthesia and Critical Care Medicine; Associate Professor of Anesthesiology; Associate Professor of Pediatrics, Duke University Medical Center, Durham, North Carolina
*Anesthesia and Supportive Care for Cardiothoracic Surgery*

**Katherine Grichnik, M.D.**
Assistant Professor of Anesthesiology, Duke University Medical School; Assistant Professor of Anesthesiology, Duke University Medical Center, Durham, North Carolina
*Anesthesia and Supportive Care for Cardiothoracic Surgery; Acute Pain Management After Surgical Procedures*

**Hermes C. Grillo, A.B., M.D.**
Professor of Surgery, Harvard Medical School; Visiting Surgeon, Thoracic Surgery, Massachusetts General Hospital, Boston, Massachusetts
*Congenital Lesions, Neoplasms, Inflammation, Infections, Injuries, and Other Lesions of the Trachea*

**Michael A. Grosso, M.D.**
Assistant Professor of Cardiothoracic Surgery, University of Medicine and Dentistry of New Jersey, Cooper Hospital/University Medical Center, Camden, New Jersey
*Left Ventricular Aneurysm*

**Frederick L. Grover, M.D.**
Professor of Surgery; Head, Division of Cardiothoracic Surgery, University of Colorado Health Sciences Center; Chief, Surgical Service, Veterans Administration Medical Center, Denver, Colorado
*Prosthetic Valve Endocarditis; Thrombosis and Thromboembolism of Prosthetic Cardiac Valves and Extracardiac Prostheses*

**John R. Guyton, M.D.**
Associate Professor of Medicine; Assistant Professor of Pathology, Duke University Medical Center, Durham, North Carolina
*Dietary and Pharmacologic Management of Atherosclerosis*

**John W. Hammon, Jr., M.D.**
Professor of Cardiothoracic Surgery, Bowman Gray School of Medicine of Wake Forest University; Attending Cardiothoracic Surgeon, Medical Center of Bowman Gray School of Medicine and North Carolina Baptist Hospital, Winston-Salem, North Carolina
*Major Anomalies of Pulmonary and Thoracic Systemic Veins*

**John R. Handy, Jr., M.D.**
Assistant Professor of Surgery, Medical University of South Carolina College of Medicine, Charleston, North Carolina
*Tricuspid Atresia*

**Alden H. Harken, M.D.**
Staff Surgeon, Veterans Administration Hospital; Professor and Chairman, Department of Surgery; Staff Surgeon, Cardiovascular Surgery, University of Colorado; Staff Surgeon, Rose Medical Center, Denver, Colorado
*Left Ventricular Aneurysm*

**J. Kevin Harrison, M.D.**

Assistant Professor of Medicine; Assistant Director, Diagnostic and Interventional Catheterization Laboratories, Duke University Medical Center, Durham, North Carolina

*Cardiac Catheterization, Angiography, and Interventional Techniques in Valvular and Congenital Heart Disease; Coronary Arteriography*

**Lucius D. Hill, M.D.**

Clinical Professor of Surgery, University of Washington, Seattle, Washington

*The Nissen Fundoplication; The Hill Repair; Paraesophageal Hernia*

**William L. Holman, M.D.**

Associate Professor in Surgery, University of Alabama at Birmingham; Associate Professor in Surgery, Veterans Administration Medical Center, Birmingham, Alabama

*Aneurysms of the Sinuses of Valsalva*

**O. Wayne Isom, M.D.**

Professor of Cardiothoracic Surgery, Cornell University Medical College; Cardiothoracic Surgeon-in-Chief, The New Hospital, New York, New York

*Aortic Grafts and Prostheses; Occlusive Disease of Branches of the Aorta*

**Robert H. Jones, M.D.**

Mary and Deryl Hart Professor of Surgery; Associate Professor of Radiology, Duke University School of Medicine; Duke University Medical Center, Durham, North Carolina

*Radionuclide Imaging in Cardiac Surgery*

**Allen B. Kaiser, M.D.**

Professor of Medicine, Vanderbilt University School of Medicine; Vice-Chairman, Department of Medicine, Vanderbilt University Medical Center, Nashville, Tennessee

*Use of Antibiotics in Cardiac and Thoracic Surgery*

**Robert B. Karp, M.D.**

Professor of Surgery, University of Chicago, Chicago, Illinois

*Acquired Disease of the Tricuspid Valve*

**James K. Kirklin, M.D.**

Professor of Surgery, University of Alabama at Birmingham, School of Medicine; Professor and Surgeon, University of Alabama at Birmingham, Hospitals and Clinics, Birmingham, Alabama

*Cardiopulmonary Bypass for Cardiac Surgery; Surgical Treatment of Ventricular Septal Defect*

**Joseph A. Kisslo, M.D.**

Professor, Division of Cardiology, Department of Medicine; Director, Echocardiography, Duke University Medical Center, Durham, North Carolina

*Ultrasound Applications in Cardiac Surgery: Echocardiography*

**John M. Kratz, M.D.**

Professor of Surgery, Medical University of South Carolina, Charleston, South Carolina

*Thoracic Incisions*

**Marino Labinaz, M.D., F.R.C.P.(C.)**

Assistant Professor of Medicine (Cardiology), University of Ottawa, Heart Institute, Ottawa, Ontario, Canada

*Percutaneous Transluminal Coronary Angioplasty*

### Edwin Lafontaine, M.D., F.R.C.S.(C.)
Assistant Professor of Surgery, Department of Surgery, University of Montreal; Attending Surgeon, Department of Surgery, Hospital Hôtel-Dieu, Montreal, Quebec, Canada
*The Pleura*

### Hillel Laks, M.D.
Professor and Chief, Cardiothoracic Surgery Department, University of California at Los Angeles Medical Center, Los Angeles, California
*Congenital Malformations of the Mitral Valve*

### Kevin P. Landolfo, M.D.
Assistant Professor of Surgery, Duke University Medical Center, Durham, North Carolina
*Postoperative Care in Cardiac Surgery; Congenital Deformities of the Chest Wall; Postinfarction Rupture of the Papillary Muscles and Ischemic Mitral Insufficiency*

### Bruce Leone, M.D.
Associate Professor of Anesthesiology; Assistant Professor of Medicine; Chairman, Duke University Animal Care and Use Committee; Director, Anesthesiology Cardiopulmonary Research Laboratory, Duke University Medical Center, Durham, North Carolina
*Anesthesia and Supportive Care for Cardiothoracic Surgery*

### John Leslie, M.D.
Clinical Professor of Anesthesiology, Duke University Medical School; Staff Attending, Duke University Medical Center; Staff Anesthesiologist, The Duke Heart Center, Durham, North Carolina
*Anesthesia and Supportive Care for Cardiothoracic Surgery*

### Gary K. Lofland, M.D.
Clinical Professor of Surgery, Georgetown University, Washington, District of Columbia; Director, Columbia/HCA Congenital Heart Center; HCA Henrico Doctors' Hospital, Richmond, Virginia
*Truncus Arteriosus*

### Floyd D. Loop, M.D.
Chairman, Board of Governors and Executive Vice President, The Cleveland Clinic Foundation, Cleveland, Ohio
*Repeat Coronary Artery Bypass Grafting for Myocardial Ischemia*

### James E. Lowe, M.D.
Professor of Surgery; Associate Professor of Pathology, Attending Surgeon, Cardiothoracic Surgery, Duke University Medical Center, Durham, North Carolina
*Bronchoplastic Techniques in the Surgical Management of Benign and Malignant Pulmonary Lesions; Cardiac Pacemakers and Implantable Cardioverter-Defibrillators; Congenital Malformations of the Coronary Circulation; Prinzmetal's Variant Angina and Other Syndromes Associated with Coronary Artery Spasm; Assisted Circulation*

### Philip D. Lumb, M.B.B.S., F.C.C.M.
Professor of Anesthesiology; Professor of Surgery; Chairman, Department of Anesthesiology, Albany Medical College; Anesthesiologist-in-Chief, Co-Director, Surgical Intensive Care Unit, Albany Medical Center Hospital, Albany, New York
*Perioperative Pulmonary Physiology*

### H. Kim Lyerly, M.D.
Associate Professor of Surgery; Assistant Professor of Pathology, Duke University Medical Center, Durham, North Carolina
*Thoracic Disorders in the Immunocompromised Host; Pulmonary Arteriovenous Fistulas*

Neil R. MacIntyre, M.D.
   Associate Professor of Medicine; Medical Director, Respiratory Care Services, Duke
   University Medical Center, Durham, North Carolina
   *Tracheal Intubation and Assisted Ventilation: The Anesthesiologist's Viewpoint*

David C. McGiffin, M.D.
   Associate Professor of Surgery, University of Alabama at Birmingham, Birmingham,
   Alabama
   *Cardiopulmonary Bypass for Cardiac Surgery*

Eli Milgalter, M.D.
   Division of Cardiothoracic Surgery, Hadassah Hospital, Jerusalem, Israel
   *Congenital Malformations of the Mitral Valve*

Jon F. Moran, M.D.
   Division of Cardiac Surgery, Department of Surgery, School of Medicine, East Carolina
   University, Greenville, North Carolina
   *Surgical Treatment of Pulmonary Tuberculosis*

James J. Morris, M.D.
   Associate Professor of Surgery, Mayo Medical School; Consultant, Cardiovascular
   Surgery, Mayo Clinic; Associate, Department of Physiology, Mayo Graduate School of
   Medicine, Mayo Clinic, Rochester, Minnesota
   *Utilization of Autologous Arterial Grafts for Coronary Artery Bypass*

Kurt D. Newman, M.D.
   Associate Professor of Surgery and Pediatrics, George Washington University School
   of Medicine; Senior Attending Surgeon, Children's National Medical Center, Washington, District of Columbia
   *Surgery of the Esophagus in Infants and Children*

William I. Norwood, M.D., Ph.D.
   The Aldo Castañeda Institute, Chief of Surgery, Clinique de Genolier, Genolier, Swit-
   zerland
   *Hypoplastic Left Heart Syndrome*

H. Newland Oldham, Jr., M.D.
   Professor of Surgery, Duke University Medical School; Professor of Surgery, Duke
   University Medical Center, Durham, North Carolina
   *The Mediastinum*

Mark B. Orringer, M.D.
   Professor and Head, Section of Thoracic Surgery, University of Michigan Medical
   School, Ann Arbor, Michigan
   *Short Esophagus and Reflux Stricture*

A. D. Pacifico, M.D.
   John W. Kirklin Professor of Surgery, University of Alabama at Birmingham, School
   of Medicine; Director, Division of Cardiothoracic Surgery, Vice Chairman, Department
   of Surgery, University of Alabama at Birmingham, Hospitals and Clinics, Birmingham,
   Alabama
   *Surgical Treatment of Ventricular Septal Defect; The Senning Procedure for Transposition of
   the Great Vessels*

Peter C. Pairolero, M.D.
   Chair, Department of Surgery; Professor, Mayo Medical School, Mayo Graduate School
   of Medicine, Rochester, Minnesota
   *Surgical Management of Neoplasms of the Chest Wall*

G. Alexander Patterson, M.D.
  Professor of Cardiothoracic Surgery, Department of Surgery, Washington University School of Medicine, St. Louis, Missouri
  *Lung Transplantation*

Robert B. Peyton, M.D.
  Carolina Cardiovascular Surgical Associates, P.A., Wake Heart Center, Rex Hospital, Raleigh, North Carolina
  *Aortic Grafts and Prostheses; Occlusive Disease of Branches of the Aorta*

Harry R. Phillips III, M.D.
  Associate Professor, Division of Cardiology, Department of Medicine; Co-Director, Interventional Cardiovascular Program, Duke University Medical Center, Durham, North Carolina
  *Percutaneous Transluminal Coronary Angioplasty*

William S. Pierce, M.D.
  College of Medicine, The Pennsylvania State University; Professor of Surgery, University Hospital, The Milton S. Hershey Medical Center, Hershey, Pennsylvania
  *The Artificial Heart*

Francisco J. Puga, M.D., F.A.C.S., F.A.C.C.
  Professor of Surgery, Mayo Medical School and Graduate School of Medicine; Consultant, Cardiothoracic Surgery, Mayo Clinic/Mayo Foundation, Rochester, Minnesota
  *Atrioventricular Canal*

Judson Randolph, M.D.
  Professor of Surgery, Meharry Medical College; Attending Surgeon, Metropolitan Nashville General Hospital, Nashville, Tennessee
  *Surgery of the Esophagus in Infants and Children*

J. Scott Rankin, M.D.
  Clinical Associate Professor, Department of Cardiac and Thoracic Surgery, Vanderbilt University Medical Center; Attending Surgeon, St. Thomas Hospital, Nashville, Tennessee
  *Cardiopulmonary Resuscitation; Physiology of Coronary Blood Flow, Myocardial Function, and Intraoperative Myocardial Protection; Utilization of Autologous Arterial Grafts for Coronary Artery Bypass; Postinfarction Ventricular Septal Defect*

Russell C. Raphaely, M.D.
  Professor of Anesthesia and Pediatrics, University of Pennsylvania School of Medicine; Associate Director, Department of Anesthesiology and Critical Care Medicine; Director, Division of Critical Care Medicine, Children's Hospital of Philadelphia, Philadelphia, Pennsylvania
  *Respiratory Support in Infants*

Maruf A. Razzuk, B.Sc., M.D.
  Professor in Thoracic and Cardiovascular Surgery, University of Texas Southwestern Medical School; Baylor University Medical Center, Dallas, Texas
  *Thoracic Outlet Syndrome*

Bruce A. Reitz, M.D.
  Professor and Chairman, Department of Cardiothoracic Surgery, Stanford University School of Medicine, Stanford; Chief of the Pediatric Cardiac Surgical Services, Lucile Salter Packard Children's Hospital at Stanford; Chief of the Cardiac Surgical Service, Stanford Health Services, Palo Alto, California
  *Clinical Heart-Lung Transplantation*

**J. G. Reves, M.D.**
Professor and Chairman, Department of Anesthesiology; Director, The Duke Heart
Center, Duke University Medical Center, Durham, North Carolina
*Anesthesia and Supportive Care for Cardiothoracic Surgery*

**Greg H. Ribakove, M.D.**
Assistant Professor of Surgery; Attending Cardiac Surgeon, New York University
Medical Center, New York, New York
*Tracheal Intubation and Mechanical Ventilation: The Surgeon's Viewpoint*

**William C. Roberts, M.D.**
Executive Director, Baylor Cardiovascular Institute; Dean, A. Webb Roberts Center for
Continuing Education, Baylor University Medical Center, Dallas, Texas
*Pathology of Coronary Atherosclerosis*

**Bradley M. Rodgers, M.D.**
Professor of Surgery and Pediatrics; Chief, Pediatric Surgery, University of Virginia
Health Sciences Center, Charlottesville, Virginia
*Management of Infants and Children Undergoing Thoracic Surgery*

**David C. Sabiston, Jr., M.D.**
James B. Duke Professor of Surgery, Duke University School of Medicine; Chief of
Staff, Duke University Medical Center, Durham, North Carolina
*Congenital Deformities of the Chest Wall; The Mediastinum; Carcinoma of the Lung; Bron-
choplastic Techniques in the Surgical Management of Benign and Malignant Pulmonary
Lesions; Benign Tumors of the Lung and Bronchial Adenomas; Immunology and Immunother-
apy of Carcinoma of the Lung; Surgical Management of Pulmonary Metastases; Acute
Pulmonary Embolism; Chronic Pulmonary Embolism; Pulmonary Arteriovenous Fistulas;
Patent Ductus Arteriosus, Coarctation of the Aorta, Aortopulmonary Window, and Anomalies
of the Aortic Arch; Physiology of Coronary Blood Flow, Myocardial Function, and Intraoperative Myocardial Protection; Congenital Malformations of the Coronary Circulation; Tumors of
the Heart*

**Robert M. Sade, M.D.**
Professor of Surgery, Medical University of South Carolina, Charleston, South Carolina
*Tricuspid Atresia*

**Mark W. Sebastian, M.D.**
Department of Surgery, Duke University Medical Center, Durham, North Carolina
*Chronic Pulmonary Embolism; Benign and Malignant Tumors of the Esophagus*

**David B. Skinner, M.D.**
Professor of Surgery, Cornell University Medical College; Attending Surgeon, Presi-
dent/Chief Executive Officer, The Society of the New York Hospital, New York,
New York
*The Condition: Clinical Manifestations and Diagnosis; The Belsey Mark IV Antireflux Repair*

**Robert N. Sladen, M.B., Ch.B., M.R.C.P.(U.K.), F.R.C.P.(C.)**
Associate Professor of Anesthesiology, Associate Professor of Surgery, Assistant Pro-
fessor of Cell Biology, Duke University School of Medicine; Vice-Chair, Department
of Anesthesiology, Co-Director, Surgical Intensive Care Unit, Duke University Medical
Center, Durham, North Carolina
*Tracheal Intubation and Mechanical Ventilation: The Anesthesiologist's Viewpoint*

**Peter K. Smith, A.B., B.M.E, M.D.**
Professor of Surgery; Associate Professor of Biomedical Engineering, Duke University
Medical Center; Division Chief, Thoracic and Cardiovascular Surgery; Medical Direc-

tor, Cardiac Acute Care Unit; Director, Core Cardiac Physiology Laboratory, Duke University Medical Center, Durham, North Carolina
*Preoperative Assessment of Pulmonary Function: Quantitative Evaluation of Ventilation and Blood Gas Exchange; Postoperative Care in Cardiac Surgery; Computer Applications in Cardiothoracic Surgery; Ultrasound Applications in Cardiac Surgery: Echocardiography*

### Peter Snopkowski, M.D.
Resident in Surgery, Ryan Hill Research Foundation, Seattle, Washington
*The Hill Repair*

### Robert J. Sparaco, B.S., J.D., R.R.T.
Associate Professor, Department of Allied Health Sciences, Nassau Community College, Garden City; Educational Coordinator, Respiratory Care Department, Tisch Hospital of New York University Medical Center, New York, New York
*Tracheal Intubation and Mechanical Ventilation: The Surgeon's Viewpoint*

### Frank C. Spencer, M.D.
George David Stewart Professor and Chairman, Department of Surgery, New York University Medical Center, New York, New York
*Atrial Septal Defects, Atrioventricular Canal Defects, and Total Anomalous Pulmonary Venous Return; Acquired Disease of the Mitral Valve; Bypass Grafting for Coronary Artery Disease*

### Charles E. Spritzer, M.D.
Associate Professor; Director, Body Magnetic Resonance Section; Co-Director, Magnetic Resonance Imaging, Duke University Medical Center, Durham, North Carolina
*Role of Computed Tomographic Scans in Cardiovascular Diagnosis; Role of Magnetic Resonance Imaging in Cardiovascular Diagnosis*

### Richard S. Stack, M.D., F.A.C.C.
Associate Professor of Medicine; Director, Interventional Cardiovascular Program, Duke University Medical Center, Durham, North Carolina
*Percutaneous Transluminal Coronary Angioplasty*

### James M. Steven, M.D.
Assistant Professor of Anesthesia and Pediatrics, University of Pennsylvania School of Medicine; Associate Anesthesiologist, Children's Hospital of Philadelphia, Philadelphia, Pennsylvania
*Respiratory Support in Infants*

### John H. Stevens, M.D.
Chief Resident, Department of Cardiothoracic Surgery, Stanford University School of Medicine, Stanford, California
*Clinical Heart-Lung Transplantation*

### Bret W. Stolp, M.D., Ph.D.
Assistant Professor, Department of Anesthesiology; Associate, Department of Cell Biology, Duke University Medical Center, Durham, North Carolina
*Tracheal Intubation and Assisted Ventilation: The Anesthesiologist's Viewpoint*

### Mark Tedder, M.D.
Cardiothoracic Surgery Fellow, Duke University Medical Center, Durham, North Carolina
*Bronchoplastic Techniques in the Surgical Management of Benign and Malignant Pulmonary Lesions*

George A. Trusler, M.D., F.R.C.S.(C.)
Professor Emeritus, Department of Surgery, University of Toronto; Senior Surgeon, Cardiovascular Surgery Division, Hospital for Sick Children, Toronto, Ontario, Canada
*The Mustard Procedure*

Ross M. Ungerleider, M.D.
Professor of General and Thoracic Surgery; Associate Professor of Pediatrics; Chief, Pediatric Cardiac Surgery, Duke University Medical Center, Durham, North Carolina
*Tetralogy of Fallot; Pulmonary Atresia or Stenosis with Intact Ventricular Septum; Congenital Aortic Stenosis*

Harold C. Urschel, Jr., A.B., M.D.
Professor of Thoracic and Cardiovascular Surgery, University of Texas Health Science Center at Dallas (Southwestern Medical School); Baylor University Medical Center, Dallas, Texas
*Thoracic Outlet Syndrome*

Peter Van Trigt III, M.D.
Professor of Surgery, Surgical Director, Cardiopulmonary Transplantation, Duke University Medical Center, Durham, North Carolina
*Lung Infections and Diffuse Interstitial Lung Disease; Diaphragm and Diaphragmatic Pacing; Tumors of the Heart*

Andrew S. Wechsler, M.D.
Stuart McGuire Professor and Chairman, Department of Surgery; Professor of Physiology, Virginia Commonwealth University Medical College of Virginia; Chairman of Surgery, Medical College of Virginia Hospitals, Richmond, Virginia
*Surgical Management of Myasthenia Gravis*

J. Marcus Wharton, M.D.
Associate Professor of Medicine; Director, Clinical Cardiac Electrophysiology, Duke University Medical Center, Durham, North Carolina
*Cardiac Pacemakers and Implantable Cardioverter-Defibrillators*

David H. Wisner, M.D.
Associate Professor, Department of Surgery, University of California at Davis, Sacramento, California
*Trauma to the Chest*

Walter G. Wolfe, M.D.
Attending Cardiothoracic Surgeon; Professor of Surgery, Duke University Medical Center, Durham, North Carolina
*Preoperative Assessment of Pulmonary Function: Quantitative Evaluation of Ventilation and Blood Gas Exchange; Benign and Malignant Tumors of the Esophagus*

# Preface

It is astonishing to reflect on the wide number of advances made in cardiac and thoracic surgery since the last edition of *Surgery of the Chest* was published in 1990. Many changes have occurred that have led to improved diagnostic techniques and therapeutic procedures for a host of disorders.

As advances occur, it is important to add new subjects and contributors to this work. In the Sixth Edition of *Surgery of the Chest,* there are 40 new authors and additional subjects. Drs. Robert N. Sladen, Bret Stolp, and Neil R. MacIntyre have added a completely new chapter on "Tracheal Intubation and Assisted Ventilation: The Anesthesiologist's Viewpoint" and a new co-author, Dr. Greg H. Ribakove, has been added to the chapter on "Tracheal Intubation and Mechanical Ventilation: The Surgeon's Viewpoint." Drs. Katherine Grichnik and Bruce Leone are new authors of the chapter on "Anesthesia and Supportive Care for Cardiothoracic Surgery." Drs. Brian Ginsberg and Katherine Grichnik have contributed a new chapter on "Acute Pain Management After Surgical Procedures." Dr. Ronald D. Curran is also a new author with Dr. Robert W. Anderson of an extensively revised and updated chapter on "Shock and Circulatory Collapse." Dr. Kevin P. Landolfo has been added as an author of "Postoperative Care in Cardiac Surgery" and Dr. James M. Steven for the chapter on "Respiratory Support in Infants." The chapter on "Trauma to the Chest" has been completely rewritten by Dr. David H. Wisner, and Dr. Kevin P. Landolfo has been added to the authorship of "Congenital Deformities of the Chest Wall," as has Dr. Robbin G. Cohen to the chapter on "The Pleura." Dr. Thomas A. D'Amico is a new author for the chapter on "Carcinoma of the Lung" and Dr. Mark Tedder on the chapter "Bronchoplastic Techniques in the Surgical Management of Benign and Malignant Pulmonary Lesions." Drs. Thomas A. D'Amico and David C. Sabiston, Jr., have completely rewritten the chapters on "Benign Tumors of the Lung and Bronchial Adenomas," "Immunology and Immunotherapy of Carcinoma of the Lung," and "Surgical Management of Pulmonary Metastases." Dr. J. Michael DiMaio has been added as one of the authors of "Thoracic Disorders in the Immunocompromised Host." Dr. Gregory P. Fontana is a new co-author of the chapter "Pulmonary Embolism," and Dr. Mark W. Sebastian is a co-author of the chapter on "Chronic Pulmonary Embolism." The chapter on "Benign and Malignant Tumors of the Esophagus" has been completely rewritten by Drs. Walter G. Wolfe and Mark W. Sebastian, as has the chapter on "Disorders of the Esophagus in the Adult" by Dr. André Duranceau. Dr. Lucius D. Hill has rewritten the chapter on "The Nissen Fundoplication" and, with Dr. Peter Snopkowski, has redone "The Hill Repair." Dr. J. Kevin Harrison has been added as an author of "Cardiac Catheterization, Angiography, and Interventional Techniques in Valvular and Congenital Heart Disease." New authors for the chapter on "Percutaneous Transluminal Coronary Angioplasty" are Drs. Marino Labinaz and Harry R. Phillips.

Many advances have been made in "Fibrinolytic Therapy in the Management of Acute Myocardial Infarction" and this chapter has been completely revised by Dr. Robert M. Califf. Similarly, the chapters on the "Role of Computed Tomographic Scans in Cardiovascular Diagnosis" and the "Role of Magnetic Resonance Imaging in Cardiovascular Diagnosis" have been completely rewritten by a new author, Dr. Charles E. Spritzer. Dr. David C. McGiffin has been added as an author to the chapter on "Cardiopulmonary Bypass for Cardiac Surgery." The chapter on "The Pericardium" has been rewritten by Dr. James M. Douglas, Jr., and Drs. Aubrey C. Galloway and Stephen B. Colvin have been added as authors of the chapter on "Atrial Septal Defects, Atrioventricular Canal Defects, and Total Anomalous Pulmonary Venous Return." A completely new chapter, "Pulmonary Atresia or Stenosis with Intact Ventricular Septum," has been written by Drs. Ross M. Ungerleider and J. William Gaynor. Dr. Alon S. Aharon is a new co-author of the chapter on "Congenital Malformations of the Mitral Valve." Completely new chapters have been written by Dr. Erle H. Austin III on "Pulmonary Atresia with Intact Ventricular Septum" and "Univentricular Heart." Dr. John R. Handy, Jr., has been added as an author of the chapter on "Tricuspid Atresia" and Drs. Aubrey C. Galloway and Stephen B. Colvin have been added as co-authors of the chapter on "Acquired Disease of the Mitral Valve." Totally new chapters have been written on "Prosthetic Valve Endocarditis" by Drs. David A. Fullerton and Frederick L. Grover and on "Thrombosis and Thromboembolism of Prosthetic Cardiac Valves and Extracardiac Prostheses" by Drs. David N. Campbell and Frederick L. Grover. Dr. Donald G. Glower is the new author of "Acquired Aortic Valve Disease." Dr. J. Marcus Wharton is the new co-author of "Cardiac Pacemakers and Implantable Cardioverter-Defibrillators." In the chapter on "Coronary Arteriography," Dr. J. Kevin Harrison has been added as a co-author, and Drs. Aubrey C. Galloway and Stephen B. Colvin are additional authors on "Bypass Grafting for Coronary Artery Disease." An additional author, Dr. James J. Morris, has been added on "Utilization of Autologous Arterial Grafts for Coronary Artery Bypass." Dr. Michael A. Grosso has been added as a co-author of the chapter on "Left Ventricular Aneurysm," and Dr. Kevin P. Landolfo has written a new chapter on "Postinfarction Rupture of the Papillary Muscles and Ischemic Mitral Insufficiency." Dr. J. Scott Rankin has added a new chapter on "Postinfarction Ventricular Septal Defect," and Drs. Mark P. Anstadt and James E. Lowe have written the new chapter on "Assisted Circulation."

Since the last edition, the role of "Dietary and Pharmacologic Management of Atherosclerosis" has received increasing attention, especially in relationship to reducing the severity of atherosclerosis. This subject chapter has been completely rewritten by Dr. John R. Guyton. For the chapter on "Lung Transplantation," Dr. Joel D. Cooper has added his colleague Dr. G. Alexander Patterson as a co-author, and Dr. John H. Stevens is the new co-author of "Clinical Heart-Lung Transplantation."

For this edition of *Surgery of the Chest,* a companion *Atlas of Cardiothoracic Surgery* is now available in its first edition, published by W. B. Saunders. This atlas is a comprehensive text of cardiac and thoracic surgical procedures. Included are more than 700 illustrations of correction of congenital deformities of the sternum, tracheal and bronchial procedures, the thoracic outlet syndrome, and surgical procedures involving the mediastinum and diaphragm. Neoplasms of the chest wall and thoracic sympathectomy are covered and thoroughly illustrated. The text contains a host of pulmonary procedures for benign and malignant lesions. There is an extensive section on *thoracoscopic* surgery, which is increasingly utilized in a variety of thoracic procedures. Surgical procedures for acquired heart disease are covered in detail, and congenital lesions of the heart are illustrated with the various procedures indicated for their correction. An extensive chapter describes cardiac neoplasms and their surgical management, and cardiac and pulmonary transplantation are extensively illustrated. Coronary bypass procedures are illustrated by multiple drawings describing various alternative techniques that can be utilized. This *Atlas* is a comprehensive one, including all the surgical techniques currently used in cardiac and thoracic surgery.

This edition of *Surgery of the Chest* is viewed as an essentially unabridged work designed to be a reference resource for the pathogenesis, pathologic features, diagnosis, and treatment of all cardiac and thoracic disorders.

DAVID C. SABISTON, JR.
FRANK C. SPENCER

# Contents

# VOLUME I

# VOLUME II

# Surgery of the Chest

# 30 Surgical Management of Myasthenia Gravis

Andrew S. Wechsler

Myasthenia gravis is a disorder of neuromuscular transmission that is characterized by weakness and fatigue of voluntary muscles. It is now reasonably established to be due to an autoimmune attack directed against the postsynaptic nicotinic acetylcholine (ACh) receptors of voluntary muscles. Many detailed accounts of the clinical picture were recorded before this century. The similarity of the clinical features of myasthenia gravis to those resulting from curare poisoning and the beneficial effect of prostigmine, shown by Mary Walker in 1934, focused attention on impaired neuromuscular transmission as the basis of the disorder.

Interactions between quanta of ACh released from the presynaptic terminal at the neuromuscular junction and acetylcholine receptors (AChR) on the postsynaptic membrane determine the likelihood of muscular contraction. The excessive number of potential interactions beyond that necessary to provide for maximal muscle contraction is referred to as the "safety factor" for neuromuscular transmission. Elmqvist and associates (1964) showed that patients with myasthenia gravis had reduced miniature end-plate potential amplitudes, reflecting fewer interactions between ACh and AChR and thus a reduced safety factor. Initially, this was thought to be due to inadequate release of ACh. More recent studies using specific neurotoxins (prepared from snake venom) have shown a reduction in the number of AChR in patients with myasthenia gravis, which has been suggested by histologic and electron microscopic studies. In 1960, Simpson proposed that myasthenia gravis was due to an autoimmune disorder. The recognition by Patrick and Lindstrom in 1973 of an experimental allergic myasthenia gravis after immunization of rabbits with purified AChR and the detection of specific AChR antibodies in 90% of patients with myasthenia gravis support this hypothesis.

A relationship between myasthenia gravis and the thymus gland has been appreciated since at least 1901. In 1912, Sauerbruch removed an enlarged thymus gland from a patient with myasthenia gravis whose condition subsequently improved. In 1939, Blalock removed an enlarged thymus from a young woman with generalized myasthenia gravis. Encouraged by her response, in 1941, he made the important demonstration that removal of nontumorous thymus glands could lead to clinical improvement in patients with myasthenia gravis. His success stimulated subsequent investigators to examine the role of thymectomy in the treatment of myasthenia gravis. Although the role of the thymus gland in myasthenia gravis is incompletely defined, numerous reports suggest that thymectomy is an effective therapy. Studies in the author's clinic have shown that the use of thymectomy as the sole method of treatment produces dramatic clinical improvement in many patients and suggests that a specific thymic factor contributes to the development of clinical weakness in myasthenia gravis.

## CLINICAL FEATURES

Myasthenia gravis has a prevalence in the population of 1 : 75,000. There is a biphasic mode of distribution, with a tendency for populations of young women and elderly men to be affected. Women are involved twice as often as men, and in younger patients this ratio is increased to 4.5 : 1. The mean age of onset of symptoms is 26 years. Men tend to be affected at a later age and tend to have a higher incidence of thymoma. A genetic predisposition to develop myasthenia gravis is suggested by a high incidence of specific human leukocyte antigens (HLA).

Weakness and fatigue with activity are the hallmarks of myasthenia gravis (Fig. 30–1). Almost any muscle group in the body may be involved, and fluctuation daily in strength and even from hour to hour is common. Individual muscle groups may be selectively involved. Weakness tends to be more pronounced as the day progresses and after exercise. It may develop gradually or rapidly, and recovery may be total or incomplete. The ocular muscles, the most frequently affected muscle group, are the presenting feature in 50 to 60% of patients with myasthenia gravis and they are ultimately involved in 90% of patients. This is most often manifested by ptosis and diplopia and may be exaggerated by repetitive testing or sustained exercise. Ptosis may fluctuate during the course of the examination, and Cogan's sign (a downward fall of the levator palpebrae superioris after upward gaze) may be shown. Weakness of the orbicularis oculi is a frequent accompanying feature of ocular muscle involvement. Other cranial nerves may also be affected, which leads to potentially fatal complications such as dysphagia and respiratory distress. Impaired chewing, dysarthria, and nasal speech are

1100

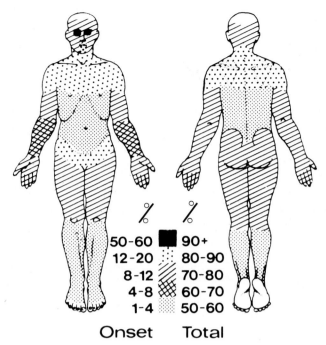

| % | % |
|---|---|
| 50-60 ■ | 90+ |
| 12-20 | 80-90 |
| 8-12 | 70-80 |
| 4-8 | 60-70 |
| 1-4 | 50-60 |

Onset    Total

**FIGURE 30–1.** Involvement of muscle groups in patients with myasthenia gravis at time of onset *(left column)* and during course of illness *(right column)*. (From Simpson, J. A.: Myasthenia gravis and myasthenic syndromes. *In* Walton, J. N. [ed]: Disorders of Voluntary Muscle. 4th ed. Edinburgh, Churchill Livingstone, 1978, pp. 585–624.)

particularly common in patients with late-onset myasthenia gravis. Facial weakness with a transverse smile and involuntary grimace may develop. The tongue may become atrophic with a characteristic triple furrow. Weakness of the flexor or extensor muscles of the neck may require that patients support their heads with their hands.

In the extremities, there is generally symmetric weakness, involving proximal muscles more than distal groups and the arms more than the legs. This pattern varies considerably, and in a specific patient, there may be asymmetric involvement, with any muscle group or even an isolated muscle being affected. The deep tendon reflexes tend to be preserved but may temporarily disappear with repetitive stimulation. The results of sensory examination are within normal limits, although patients may complain of nonspecific sensations. Autonomic system involvement with pupillary changes, bladder disturbances, and increased sweating have all been described but are uncommon.

The onset of symptoms may be insidious or sudden, spontaneous or precipitated by emotional stress, exercise, allergies, vaccinations, or pregnancy. Myasthenia gravis may also become manifest as prolonged weakness after the use of relaxant drugs and anesthesia during surgical therapy. Symptoms may be confined to the ocular muscles, but more than 80% of patients develop generalized weakness within 1 year of the onset of ocular disturbances. Grading systems to monitor clinical status are handicapped by diffi-

culty in quantifying muscular strength and the variation that occurs in myasthenic patients, particularly after exposure to heat, exercise, stress, and drugs that interfere with neuromuscular transmission. The most widely used scale is the Osserman classification, which is given in Table 30–1. This is a clinical classification that is limited by its failure to consider dependency on medication or to reflect subtle clinical improvement, creating difficulty in monitoring response to treatment.

The incidence of spontaneous remission, without drug or other therapy, is not known but is thought to be uncommon and short-lasting and to occur in patients primarily with ocular involvement. The ultimate course cannot be predicted with certainty, and many variations, including spontaneous remission in patients with long-standing disease or sudden deterioration in patients who have been asymptomatic for many years, have been recorded. A fixed myopathy late in the course of the disorder with permanent muscle weakness has been described. The author has been concerned that this may be due to chronic anticholinesterase administration, but it has also been recorded in patients who have not received such medication.

Transient neonatal myasthenia gravis has been reported in infants of mothers with myasthenia gravis. Symptoms usually include diffuse weakness, impaired crying and sucking, poor swallowing, and, occasionally, feeble respiration. Symptoms are self-limited and generally resolve within 6 weeks. There are no clinical consequences as long as the initial symptoms are recognized and managed appropriately. Passive transfer of immunoglobulin across the placenta (presumably anti-AChR antibodies) is thought to be responsible. Interestingly, there is little correlation between the clinical status of the infant and that of the mother, despite comparable AChR antibody titers, supporting the hypothesis that host factors contribute to the development of clinical weakness.

Congenital myasthenia gravis that is more common in males has been described; it is often familial, but the mother is usually unaffected. The clinical configuration is usually not severe, and improvement occurs after 6 to 10 years of symptoms. Drugs and thymectomy are generally not effective. It has been postulated that a delay in the maturation of the neuromuscular apparatus causes a prolonged reduction of the safety factor for neuromuscular transmission. Another congenital myasthenic syndrome, due to a reduction of acetylcholinesterase in the subneural apparatus of the end-plate, has also been described. These patients do not have AChR antibodies and do not respond to anticholinesterase medications.

The myasthenic or Eaton-Lambert syndrome consists of weakness and fatigability of proximal muscles, particularly in the lower extremities. Ocular and bulbar involvement is mild or absent. Deep tendon reflexes tend to be depressed or absent, and there is a characteristic electrophysiologic abnormality on the electromyogram. This syndrome is usually seen in

**■ Table 30–1.** MODIFIED CLINICAL CLASSIFICATION OF PATIENTS WITH MYASTHENIA GRAVIS

**Group I**

*Ocular Myasthenia*

Ocular muscles are involved, with ptosis and diplopia. Its form is very mild; no mortality occurs.

**Group II**

A. *Mild Generalized*

Onset is slow and frequently ocular, gradually spreading to skeletal and bulbar muscles. Respiratory system is not involved. Response to drug therapy is good. Mortality is low.

B. *Moderate Generalized*

Onset is gradual with frequent ocular presentations, progressing to more severe generalized involvement of the skeletal and bulbar muscles. Dysarthria, dysphagia, and difficult mastication are more prevalent than in mild generalized myasthenia gravis. Respiratory muscles are not involved. Response to drug therapy is less satisfactory; patients' activities are restricted, but mortality is low.

C. *Severe Generalized*

1. *Acute fulminating.* Onset of severe bulbar and skeletal muscle weakness is rapid with early involvement of respiratory muscles. Progress is normally complete within 6 months. Percentage of thymomas is highest in this group. Response to drug therapy is less satisfactory, and patients' activities are restricted, but mortality is low.
2. *Late severe.* Severe myasthenia gravis develops at least 2 years after most of Group I or Group II symptoms. Progression of myasthenia gravis may be either gradual or sudden. The second highest percentage of thymomas occurs in this group. The response to drug therapy is poor, and the prognosis is poor.

association with an underlying oat-cell carcinoma of the lung and may antedate recognition of the tumor. Less frequently, it occurs with other chronic disease states. The condition is due to the release of decreased quanta of ACh from nerve endings. Anticholinesterase drugs are less effective than they are in myasthenia gravis. Agents that facilitate the release of ACh from the presynaptic nerve terminal, such as guanidine, calcium, or 4-aminopyridine, may be helpful.

In general, the diagnosis of myasthenia gravis is not difficult to make if it is considered. Hysteria, thyroid disease, neuromyopathies, and other myasthenic conditions are occasionally mistaken for myasthenia gravis, but a Tensilon test, single-fiber electromyography, and determination of AChR antibody levels allow a definitive diagnosis in most patients.

## Associated Conditions

Various conditions have been associated with myasthenia gravis. Many of these, such as rheumatoid arthritis, systemic lupus erythematosus, polymyositis, Sjögren's syndrome, and ulcerative colitis, are thought to be autoimmune. An association with vitamin $B_{12}$ deficiency, thyroid disorders, diabetes mellitus, parathyroid disease, adrenal disorders, and vitiligo has been described as part of a polyglandular failure syndrome. These may be predetermined genetically, based on their linkage with histocompatibility antigens, particularly HLA-A1, HLA-B8, and HLA-Dw3. These may constitute genetic risk factors for autoimmune diseases by which a specific exposure triggers an abnormal immune response in a patient with a particular haplotype. This theory is supported

by studies of monozygotic twins in which only one of the twins has been affected.

Thyroid dysfunction has been reported in 5% of patients with myasthenia gravis, and the overall incidence may be much higher. It may sometimes be difficult to distinguish features of thyroid disease from those of myasthenia gravis, because each can cause proximal muscle weakness and ocular disturbances. These conditions appear to be distinct, however, because it has been shown that increased quantities of thyroid hormone per se do not cause myasthenia gravis and that the relationship is more likely to be immunologic or genetic than hormonal. All forms of thyroid disease, including goiter, myxedema, Graves' disease, and Hashimoto's thyroiditis, have been associated with myasthenia gravis.

## Thymic Abnormalities

Disorders of the thymus gland are found in 75 to 85% of patients with myasthenia gravis, and new staining techniques suggest that this incidence may be even higher. Ten to 15% of patients with myasthenia gravis have thymomas. In most cases, these are benign, well-defined, encapsulated lesions that may be cystic or calcified. They are generally composed of epithelial or lymphoid cells. However, two-thirds of thymomas have no association with myasthenia gravis and contain mainly spindle cells. Malignancy is usually defined by tumor infiltration into surrounding tissue such as pleura and pericardium rather than by changes in the histologic pattern. As many as 43% of thymomas were malignant in one series. However, in the author's experience, malignancy is a rare occurrence, perhaps reflecting the tendency to perform thymectomy earlier in the course of myasthenia gravis. Thymomas have not been described in children and are generally not seen before the age of 30 years. They are more common in male patients. High-quality computed tomography (CT) of the mediastinum can detect almost all thymomas (Fig. 30–2). The author has occasionally seen false-positive CT results but has not failed to recognize a thymoma by CT in the study in which all patients with myasthenia gravis have undergone thymectomy, regardless of the interpretation of the CT.

Lymphoid hyperplasia of both the cortex and medulla is found in the thymus gland of most young patients with myasthenia gravis. The number of germinal centers may increase, but this is not unique to myasthenia gravis, and its significance is uncertain. Attempts to relate the numbers of germinal centers to the duration and severity of the disease and the response to treatment have been inconclusive. The T-cell composition of the thymus gland, in terms of both numbers and subsets, is generally normal. However, there is an increased number of B cells in the thymus glands of patients with myasthenia gravis.

Patients with late-onset myasthenia gravis (after the age of 55 years) most often have an atrophic involuted thymus gland. Occasionally, these can be recognized on CT by the existence of relatively low density (presumably fat) throughout the anterior mediastinum punctuated by dots of high density (presumably thymic tissue). Evidence suggests that an atrophic thymus gland may still be immunologically active, and thymic cells may be identified within the anterior mediastinal fat. This consideration is important with respect to the role of thymectomy in these patients. They have relative lymphopenia in the peripheral blood consisting primarily of a reduction in T lymphocytes and 3A1+ and OKT4+ T-cell subsets. These changes are rapidly reversed after the removal of the "involuted" thymus gland.

## DIAGNOSTIC STUDIES

### Pharmacologic Agents

Anticholinesterase agents block the hydrolysis of ACh in the synaptic cleft, prolonging its action and increasing the likelihood of an interaction between ACh and the postsynaptic AChR. The result is an increase in the miniature end-plate potential and in the safety factor for neuromuscular transmission. These agents may reverse or improve the clinical and electrical abnormalities in myasthenia gravis. The most widely used anticholinesterase agent for diagnosis is edrophonium (Tensilon). This drug is short-acting and improves clinical or electrical abnormalities in 95% of patients with myasthenia gravis. Its use is widespread, and before more sophisticated laboratory evaluations, a positive response was central to the definition of myasthenia gravis. The response in individual patients differs from dramatic improvement, confirming the diagnosis, to subtle or no change. The ocular muscles are least sensitive to this drug and occasionally make it difficult to diagnose cases of myasthenia gravis confined to the ocular muscles. However, failure to respond to edrophonium does not exclude myasthenia gravis. It is recommended that the test be done at the end of the day or after exercise, when the patient's weakness is maximal.

Two to 10 mg of edrophonium are administered intravenously. The initial 2 mg may detect hypersensitivity so that the possibility of enhancing cholinergic weakness in patients receiving anticholinesterase medications may be avoided. Facilities to treat anaphylactic and respiratory complications should be available. A positive response generally develops within 30 to 60 seconds and lasts for approximately 1 to 5 minutes. It has been the author's practice to do the edrophonium test in a triple-blind fashion with saline and nicotinic acid as control agents. Edrophonium generally causes a light-headed, hot sensation associated with lacrimation and flushing that patients may learn to recognize. Nicotinic acid reproduces some of these features without influencing neuromuscular transmission and thus serves as a suitable control substance.

Long-lasting anticholinesterase agents may be used when responses are too transient to record by standard bedside techniques. These agents have a longer latency and duration. Neostigmine may be used in a dose of 1.5 mg administered intramuscularly. Improvement is seen within 10 to 30 minutes and lasts up to 4 hours. When the response is still equivocal, a long-term trial of orally administered anticholinesterase agents over several weeks can be considered.

Patients with myasthenia gravis are highly sensitive

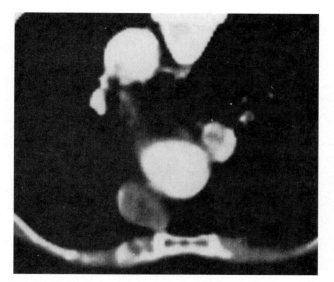

**FIGURE 30–2.** Computed tomography (CT) scan from a patient with a thymoma. The anterior mediastinal mass is easily visualized. With increasing experience, this test has become progressively more helpful in separating patients with thymomas from those with normal thymus glands and has even been able to identify islands of functioning thymus tissue within generally atrophic glands.

to the neuromuscular blocking effect of curare and curare-like drugs. This heightened sensitivity has previously been used as a test to confirm the diagnosis. One-tenth of a curarizing dose may cause the patient to become significantly weak. An anesthetist must be present at this test because of the risk of respiratory decompensation and, consequently, this test is now rarely used.

An abnormal "dual response" after administration of decamethonium has been described, consisting of brief depolarization after a longer period of curare-like competitive block. Although interesting pharmacologically, this test is no longer used in practice.

## Electrophysiologic Studies

The hallmark of myasthenia gravis is failure of neuromuscular transmission, which is characterized electrically by a reduction in the amplitude of the miniature end-plate potential. In 1895, Jolly recognized that faradic stimulation of a peripheral nerve causes muscle fatigue. He recognized that, in patients with myasthenia gravis, supramaximal repetitive stimulation of the nerve led to a gradual decrease of the evoked action potential without a change in antidromic conduction. The Jolly test consists of repetitive stimulation of a peripheral nerve. In normal patients, the safety margin is large enough that repeated stimulations can be tolerated to a rate of 40 to 50 per second. In patients with myasthenia gravis, abnormal diminution begins at stimulation rates of 2 to 3 per second, particularly if these are done after tetanic contractions of muscle or the regional administration of curare. This test has the advantage of being simple and inexpensive but, unfortunately, it is not particularly sensitive. Changes are not detected in more than 50% of patients with myasthenia gravis, particularly in the early stages.

The development of single-fiber electromyography has provided a more sensitive method of detecting impaired neuromuscular transmission. A single-fiber needle electrode is placed between two muscle fibers innervated by the same motor unit. The variation in the latency between the two action potentials is referred to as jitter (Fig. 30–3). The variation of neuromuscular transmission in myasthenia gravis leads to increased jitter or blocking of one of the action potentials in severe cases. Jitter measurements are abnormal in 95% of patients with myasthenia gravis if multiple muscle groups are studied. In patients with purely ocular symptoms, the frontalis or levator palpebrae superioris muscle should be examined. Jitter measurements must be analyzed in light of the clinical picture, because abnormalities can be seen in disorders other than myasthenia gravis. Because jitter is a function of the amplitude of the miniature end-plate potential, this test can be used to monitor the clinical course of patients with myasthenia gravis. Although it has the advantage of being sensitive in the early detection of myasthenia gravis, it requires expensive complex machinery and neurophysiologic expertise.

Stapedial reflex decay has been used as a diagnostic study in myasthenia gravis. Preliminary results indicate a high sensitivity in patients with ocular dysfunction, but results are less encouraging in patients with generalized weakness.

## Serum Antibodies

Numerous nonspecific antibodies have been described in patients with myasthenia gravis. These include antistriational, antinuclear, antithyroid, antigastric, antispermatogenic, and antineuronal antibodies.

The isolation of specific neurotoxins from the venom of elapid snakes such as cobras and kraits allowed the recognition of specific serum anti-AChR

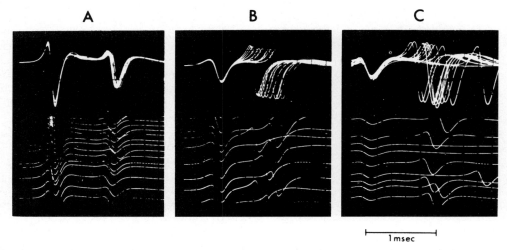

**FIGURE 30–3.** Electromyographic jitter recordings; traces are superimposed on top line. *A*, Normal jitter. Note the constant latency between the two muscle action potentials. *B*, Increased jitter but without impulse blocking in a patient with myasthenia gravis. *C*, Increased jitter with occasional blocking in a patient with severe myasthenia gravis. (*A–C*, From Stalberg, E., Trontel, J. V., and Schwartz, M. S.: Single muscle fiber recording of jitter phenomenon in patients with myasthenia gravis and in members of their families. Ann. N. Y. Acad. Sci., 274:189, 1976.)

antibodies. Alpha-bungarotoxin, a specific neurotoxin from the banded krait, has been found to bind specifically and irreversibly to the active site of the AChR. This toxin can be used to measure the number of receptors, to purify receptors, and to assay for serum AChR antibody. The assay consists of the reaction between test serum and AChR antigen derived from human muscle that has been incubated with $^{125}$I-labeled alpha-bungarotoxin. If serum AChR antibodies are present, they bind to the AChR and form a complex with the $^{125}$I-labeled alpha-bungarotoxin, which is bound to an adjacent site on the receptor. Antihuman globulin then precipitates this complex, and the radioactivity in the precipitant allows for an estimation of the quantitative AChR antibody level. Serum AChR antibodies are present in 90% of patients with myasthenia gravis. These antibodies are highly specific for myasthenia gravis and have been found otherwise only after administration of penicillamine or inoculation with snake venom, but in no other disease state. Furthermore, AChR released from damaged muscle does not evoke the development of AChR antibodies. AChR antibody levels do not directly correlate with the clinical status of patients with myasthenia gravis, but patients with purely ocular disease tend to have the lowest antibody titers.

## PATHOGENESIS

Considerable evidence has accumulated since the original hypothesis by Simpson (1960) to support the concept that myasthenia gravis is an autoimmune disorder involving the postsynaptic nicotinic AChR. Histologically, the postsynaptic membrane is simplified and disorganized (Fig. 30–4). Alpha-bungarotoxin binding studies have shown quantitative reduction in the amount of AChR correlating with the reduction in the amplitude of the miniature end-plate action potential and the clinical severity of the condition. The detection of specific AChR antibodies in the serum of approximately 90% of patients with myasthenia gravis has focused attention on this antibody in the pathogenesis of myasthenia gravis. It has been postulated that these antibodies induce clinical weakness by reducing the number of functioning AChR, thus impairing neuromuscular transmission. Mechanisms proposed include (1) accelerated degradation of AChR on the postsynaptic membrane, (2) immunopharmacologic blockade in which the antibody hinders interactions between ACh and the AChR, (3) modulation or accelerated internalization with intracellular degradation of the AChR-AChR antibody complex, and (4) reduced synthesis of AChR.

Passive transfer of serum, more specifically immunoglobulin (Ig) G from patients with myasthenia gravis to experimental animals, can induce a myasthenic syndrome characterized by clinical, electrical, and pharmacologic features similar to those of human myasthenia gravis. This syndrome may also be caused by specific monoclonal AChR antibodies. Passive transfer among animal species has been shown.

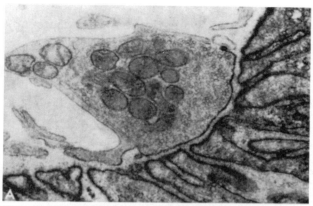

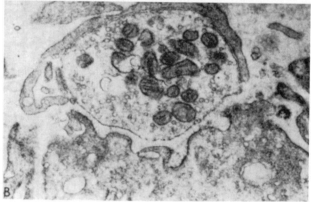

FIGURE 30–4. Neuromuscular junction with acetylcholine receptors (AChR) stained by peroxidase-labeled alpha-bungarotoxin technique. *A*, Normal neuromuscular junction with normal quantity of AChR. *B*, Neuromuscular junction in a patient with moderately severe myasthenia gravis. Note the disorganization and destruction of the postsynaptic membrane, with reduction in staining for AChR. (*A* and *B*, Courtesy of A. G. Engel.)

Furthermore, IgG from patients with myasthenia gravis accelerates the degradation of AChR in myotube tissue culture. In human myasthenia gravis, plasmapheresis and steroids lead to clinical benefit in association with a reduction in the serum AChR antibody titer. The removal of thoracic duct lymph containing immunoglobulin also produces clinical improvement, and the readministration of this material causes rapid clinical deterioration. These observations support the hypothesis that AChR antibodies contribute to and may be the major mechanism responsible for receptor damage in myasthenia gravis.

Nevertheless, it is by no means clear that the AChR antibody is the sole factor responsible for clinical weakness. In studies at Duke University in which all patients were treated with thymectomy as the sole type of therapy and in which all drugs, including anticholinesterase agents, were avoided, dramatic clinical benefit was seen in most patients without a reduction in the AChR antibody titer. There was no direct correlation between the serum AChR antibody level and the clinical status of individual patients. The author and his colleagues hypothesized that a thymic factor was essential to the development of clinical weakness in myasthenia gravis. This is supported by the development of transient neonatal myasthenia gravis in the infant of an asymptomatic thymectomized mother, with comparable levels and bioactivity of AChR antibody in each. Although steroids and plasmapheresis provide dramatic clinical improvement in many patients, the corresponding reduction in AChR antibody titer may be an independent phenomenon. It is presumptive to assume that this reduction is essential for clinical improvement, and clearly, more than AChR antibodies are removed by plasmapheresis. Furthermore, the reduction in the AChR antibody titer after plasmapheresis is often short-lived, whereas clinical benefit may persist for weeks or months.

Different AChR antibodies that react to different sites on the AChR have been identified, and it is possible that the current techniques fail to identify the specific subset that would better correlate with the clinical status of patients with myasthenia gravis. Furthermore, serum AChR antibody titers may not accurately reflect antibody activity at the neuromuscular junction. In the Duke drug-free group, no patient's antibody titer converted to negative after thymectomy, despite clinical improvement, and when antibody titers did fall, they did so gradually over a period of years rather than in direct correlation with the clinical status.

In an elegant series of experiments, Engel and associates (1977) showed deposits of IgG and C3 complement on segments of the postsynaptic membrane in the distribution of the AChR and on fragments of degenerating junctional folds in the synaptic space

(Fig. 30–5). More severely affected myasthenic patients bind relatively smaller amounts of IgG and C3 complement, presumably because there are fewer residual AChR. The presence of C3 complement indicates activation of the complement reaction. Subsequent activation of the major or alternate pathway could then set the stage for a complement-mediated lysis of the membrane.

Sahashi and associates (1980), by using an immunoperoxidase method, showed the presence of the C9 terminal and lytic complement component at the postsynaptic junctional folds and in debris within the synaptic clefts in the same basic distribution as C3 complement. Once again, there was an inverse relationship between the structural integrity of the junctional folds and the abundance of C9. The areas of involvement were discrete and widely separated, supporting the concept of an autoimmune attack. C3 complement does not necessarily cause membrane damage and may be found over long portions of junctional membrane. Activation to C9, however, causes irreversible damage to the membrane. Demonstration of C9 over only short portions of junctional folds and in abundance in the degenerated material of the synaptic cleft supports the role of the complement-mediated lysis as the mechanism of membrane damage in myasthenia gravis. This differs from other conditions such as Duchenne's muscular dystrophy in which degeneration of junctional folds occurs in the absence of IgG or C9 complement. It is possible that the AChR antibody marks the receptor for complement-mediated lysis, and some current evidence

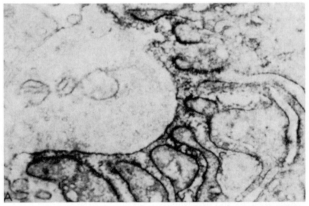
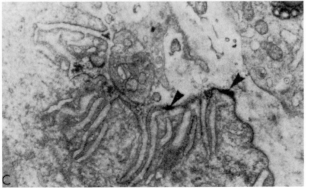
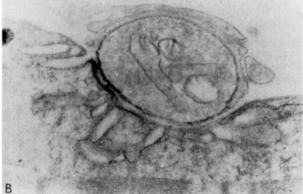

FIGURE 30–5. *A*, Ultrastructural localization of IgG in a patient with mild myasthenia gravis. Note the relative preservation of the postsynaptic region. *B*, Ultrastructural localization of C3 on postsynaptic membrane of a patient with myasthenia gravis. *C*, Ultrastructural localization of C9 at end-plates and on debris in synaptic folds in a patient with myasthenia gravis. *Arrows* indicate intense reaction for C9 over short segments of postsynaptic membrane. (*B*, From Engel, A. G., Lambert, E. H., and Howard, F. M., Jr.: Immune complexes [IgG and C3] at the motor end plate in myasthenia gravis. Mayo Clin. Proc., *52*:267, 1977; *C*, From Sahashi, K., Engel, A. G., Lambert, E. H., and Howard, F. M., Jr.: Ultrastructural localization of the terminal and lytic 9th complement component [C9] at the motor end-plate in myasthenia gravis. J. Neuropathol. Exp. Neurol., *39*:160–172, 1980, Fig. 4-A, p. 166.)

suggests that the thymus gland may activate the alternate complement pathway and may facilitate this reaction.

Although most attention has been focused on humoral immune mechanisms, cell-mediated immune mechanisms have not been excluded from the pathogenesis of myasthenia gravis. Studies in the author's laboratories have shown a reduction in the number of peripheral blood T cells in patients with late-onset myasthenia gravis. This reduction consists primarily of T-cell subsets 3A1[+] and OKT4[+], and these changes normalize rapidly after thymectomy. Lymphocyte transformation has been described in several laboratories after exposure of peripheral blood and thymic lymphocytes to purified AChR antigen. This stimulation index has also been reported to be reduced after thymectomy. Alterations in mixed lymphocyte reactions and autologous lymphocyte reactions have been observed and are currently being studied. Although not a consistent finding, lymphorrhages, which are small groups of lymphocytes within muscle, are occasionally detected. All of these changes suggest that a cell-mediated mechanism has some role in the pathogenesis of myasthenia gravis, but its importance has not yet been defined. The possibility of multiple mechanisms and heterogeneous populations of patients must be considered.

## Experimental Allergic Myasthenia Gravis

Using snake venom such as alpha-bungarotoxin, Patrick and Lindstrom (1973) were able to isolate AChR from homogenized muscle. Purified receptor was then injected into rabbits in an effort to provoke specific AChR antibodies. Several weeks after this immunization, the rabbits became weak and died. The weakness had clinical, electrical, and pharmacologic features resembling those of human myasthenia gravis, and this disorder is now known as experimental autoimmune myasthenia gravis. It is thought to be the result of AChR antibodies generated by immunization with AChR cross-reacting with the rabbits' own AChR, leading to impaired neuromuscular transmission. Histologic changes seen at the neuromuscular junction are similar to those seen in human patients, and passive transfer of serum or lymphocytes from these animals can induce the disease when injected into normal animals. An acute state occurs approximately 1 week after immunization and is characterized by severe muscle weakness and a cellular invasion of the neuromuscular junction with breakdown of the postsynaptic membrane and AChR. Approximately 3 weeks after immunization, a chronic stage develops in association with a rising AChR antibody titer. The postsynaptic membrane becomes decreased in area and simplified, with a consequent reduction in the total number of AChR. The chronic phase of experimental autoimmune myasthenia gravis is almost identical to that in the human disorder, but the experimental autoimmune condition differs from human myasthenia gravis in that the acute transient phase is not seen in human patients. This may reflect a differing nature of the immunizing event, with the human patient not being exposed to a massive bolus of antigen at one time, or differences in host response. It has also been suggested that the acute phase may be related to the adjuvant rather than the AChR.

Significantly, experimental autoimmune myasthenia gravis does not develop in animals that have been thymectomized before immunization. A thymic factor may be essential to the development of clinical weakness in this condition. Furthermore, C3 complement deficiency also attenuates the clinical and electrical features of experimental autoimmune myasthenia gravis and supports the hypothesis that complement-mediated lysis may be the mechanism leading to membrane damage.

## Role of the Thymus Gland

A relationship between the thymus gland and myasthenia gravis has been appreciated since the beginning of the 20th century. Seventy to 80% of patients with myasthenia gravis undergo pathologic changes in their thymus gland, and for 50 years thymectomy has been known to influence the clinical course of myasthenia gravis. It is therefore not surprising that thymic factors have been suggested to have a role in the pathogenesis of myasthenia gravis. The exact role of the thymus gland must still be defined, however. There are cells within the thymus gland (myoid cells) that have a striking similarity to embryonic muscle cells. These cells contain AChR on their surface and react with AChR antibodies. The thymic cells in culture can produce AChR antibody, and radiated thymic cells that have been thus rendered functionally inactive can augment the production of AChR antibody from peripheral lymphocytes. The thymus gland has a major part in lymphocyte maturation and is capable of influencing almost all humoral and cellular immune reactions. It has been proposed that an initiating event, possibly viral, induces "thymitis." Because of the unique location of myoid cells in immediate proximity to maturing lymphocytes, an autoimmune reaction may develop directed against the AChR on myoid cells that later cross-reacts with AChR at the neuromuscular junction. The altered thymus gland might also generate a population of killer T cells, which destroy the neuromuscular junction, or a population of helper cells, which stimulate the production of AChR antibody by peripheral lymphocytes. More recently, it has been suggested that thymic factors may also have a role in activating the complement pathway leading to membrane lysis. The association of myasthenia gravis with other autoimmune disorders, particularly the polyglandular failure syndrome, suggests that the immunologic attack may be more widely directed than to the AChR alone in some patients. The relationship with HLA in some patients with myasthenia gravis also suggests that there is a genetically predisposed population of patients whose immunologic tolerance may be altered in such a manner that a specific exposure produces altered immunologic responses.

The mechanism by which thymectomy leads to clinical benefit has not yet been elucidated. It has been shown that thymectomy influences cell-mediated immunity and peripheral T-cell counts in patients with late-onset myasthenia gravis, but the clinical relevance of this finding is not established. Thymectomy may serve to remove a source of (1) AChR antigen, (2) AChR antibody production, (3) sensitized killer T cells directed against the neuromuscular junction, (4) sensitized helper T cells that facilitate the production of AChR antibody by peripheral lymphocytes, and (5) a putative thymic factor that may activate the complement pathway leading to complement-mediated lysis at antibody-labeled receptor sites. It is also possible that thymectomy acts by multiple or unknown mechanisms.

Failure of thymectomy to induce clinical remission might be due to (1) incomplete thymectomy, (2) permanent irreparable damage to the neuromuscular junction, (3) a thymic influence exerted by extra-thymic populations of lymphocytes within the spleen, lymph nodes, and so on that are unaffected by thymectomy, (4) the influence of long-lived peripheral T cells, and (5) heterogeneous disease mechanisms by which the thymic influence differs in individual patients.

## TREATMENT

Numerous methods of treatment have been used in the management of myasthenia gravis. Variations in the natural history and the lack of prospective control studies of the different treatment modalities prevent an absolute determination of the preferred form of treatment for a particular patient at the present time. Furthermore, it has been suggested that the natural history of myasthenia gravis as it is seen today follows a more benign course than that seen in previous decades. Improvement in supportive measures and surgical technique may contribute to the improved statistics on patients, independent of the specific therapy chosen. The large number of variables to be controlled and physician bias favoring one form of therapy over another make it unlikely that a controlled study can be effected, and at least for the present, some judgment is required in instituting therapy.

I favor total thymectomy as early as possible after the development of generalized weakness. Drugs are avoided and used only when necessary rather than as a routine part of treatment. All patients are managed according to a prospective standardized treatment protocol to minimize variables and to avoid a physician bias. In my practice, after a mean follow-up of 25.5 months, 87% of patients were free from generalized weakness, and 61% required no medication. The protocol does not compare thymectomy with other forms of treatment, but the excellent results and the possibility of avoiding additional medications lead

me to prefer this form of treatment in patients with generalized myasthenia gravis. Before a more detailed discussion of thymectomy, the advantages and disadvantages of the major forms of treatment currently being used are considered. In each case, drugs that interfere with neuromuscular transmission (Table 30–2) should be avoided or used cautiously, because they may lead to a deterioration in the myasthenic status.

## Medical Treatment

**Anticholinesterase Agents.** Anticholinesterase agents have been a standard form of medical treatment for myasthenia gravis since their introduction in the mid-1930s. They act by preventing the hydrolysis of ACh and increase the likelihood of interactions between ACh and the AChR. The safety margin for neuromuscular transmission is thus increased, providing temporary improvement in the clinical and electrical features of myasthenia gravis. These agents may produce considerable improvement with restoration of muscle strength. However, this response is only symptomatic, and these drugs in and of themselves do not lead to remission. Side effects of anticholinesterase drugs include abdominal colic, diarrhea, nausea, salivation, and lacrimation as a result of smooth muscle and glandular stimulation. These symptoms may be controlled by atropine. This is not recommended, however, because the symptoms may forewarn the patient and physician of developing "cholinergic crisis." Cholinergic crisis is the result of excessive stimulation of AChR with prolonged depolarization of receptors and consequent muscle weakness not directly related to myasthenia gravis. Cholinergic weakness can be differentiated from myasthenic weakness by administration of a test dose of Tensilon, because symptoms fail to respond or deteriorate after the administration of additional anticholinesterase medication. Treatment

■ **Table 30–2.** DRUGS THAT INTERFERE WITH NEUROMUSCULAR TRANSMISSION UNDER EXPERIMENTAL CONDITIONS

| Antibiotics | Psychotropics |
|---|---|
| Amikacin | Amitriptyline |
| Paramycin | Amphetamines |
| Polymyxin A | Droperidol |
| Sisomicin | Haloperidol |
| Viomycin | Imipramine |
| | Paraldehyde |
| **Antiarrhythmics** | Trichloroethanol |
| Ajmaline | |
| | **Others** |
| **Antirheumatics** | Amantadine |
| Colchicine | Diphenhydramine |
| | Emetine |
| | Pindolol |
| **Anticonvulsants** | Sotalol |
| Ethosuximide | |

consists of discontinuation of anticholinesterase agents and appropriate support measures.

Neostigmine (Prostigmin) and pyridostigmine (Mestinon) are the most commonly used anticholinesterase agents. Neostigmine is available in 15-mg tablets, which are usually administered every 4 hours or more frequently when required. There is usually a 30-minute delay before maximal efficacy, and the optimal dosage is determined by trial and error. Parenteral administration of 0.5 mg is equivalent to 15 mg administered orally. Pyridostigmine is the more popular medication because it is thought to have a smoother effect and to be longer-acting, with a less abrupt loss of efficacy. Sixty milligrams of pyridostigmine is equivalent to 15 mg of neostigmine, and the time-release form of 180 mg is available for more prolonged use, such as at night.

Despite the popularity of these agents, the author has preferred not to use them whenever possible. The symptomatic benefits that they provide may delay the introduction of early thymectomy, which is believed to be the preferred form of therapy. These agents increase bronchial and oropharyngeal secretions, which may lead to respiratory complications, particularly at the time of operation. Furthermore, after thymectomy, there appears to be an increased sensitivity to anticholinesterase medications, which may lead to cholinergic weakness, complicating the postoperative management. Thus, anticholinesterase agents have been avoided in patients with thymectomy without an evident loss of clinical efficacy and with what appears to be a smoother operative and postoperative course.

Evidence in experimental animals indicates that chronic exposure to anticholinesterase agents independently leads to AChR damage and electron microscopic alterations identical to those seen in myasthenia gravis. Although there is no proof that a similar phenomenon occurs in human patients, there has been the concern that long-term use of these agents may lead to a fixed myopathic state unrelated to the myasthenia.

**Corticosteroids.** Many studies have shown the beneficial effect of corticosteroids in patients with myasthenia gravis. The clinical response may be dramatic with total remission of symptoms, but it is important to appreciate that the introduction of steroids may be associated with a transient clinical deterioration (usually between the fourth and eighth days), and it is recommended that they be initiated in the hospital setting, where provisions for respiratory assistance are available. Prednisone has been most widely used, beginning with a dosage of 60 to 80 mg/day. Once an adequate response is obtained, patients are changed to an alternate-day dosage schedule, and the medication is gradually tapered as clinically appropriate. When an alternate-day dosage of 60 mg of prednisone has been reached, it is recommended that reductions in dosage should not exceed 5 mg every other day, no more frequently than once every other month, to minimize the risk of inducing myasthenic crisis.

Although many use steroids as a primary mode of therapy, particularly for patients with late-onset myasthenia gravis, the author prefers to use them only in patients who cannot or will not undergo thymectomy or in patients who have had a clinically unsatisfactory response to thymectomy. Corticosteroids have also been used in a low-dose alternate-day schedule for patients with ocular myasthenia gravis or with residual ocular dysfunction after thymectomy. Corticosteroids have been used to prepare patients for thymectomy, but the same can now be accomplished with plasmapheresis without the risk of clinical deterioration or the difficulty in withdrawing steroid medication.

The mechanism of action of corticosteroids is not understood. Most attention has focused on immunosuppression. Several groups have reported a reduction in the AChR antibody titer that correlates with clinical improvement in patients with myasthenia gravis, raising the possibility that suppression of immunoglobulin is responsible for clinical benefit. However, studies of thymectomy as the sole treatment modality have failed to confirm a direct correlation between the clinical status of patients with myasthenia gravis and the AChR antibody titer. Although these studies suggest that an essential thymic factor contributes to the development of clinical weakness, the possibility exists that steroids and thymectomy act by different mechanisms. Steroids may have a thymolytic effect, although it is noteworthy that they may be effective in patients who have already undergone thymectomy. A direct effect on neuromuscular transmission has also been suggested by the transient deterioration during the off day reported by patients on an alternate-day steroid schedule.

Once steroids have been initiated, they may be difficult to discontinue. Although the dosage may be substantially reduced, in many patients steroids have to be maintained indefinitely. Aside from the risk of clinical deterioration related to dosage change, there are many side effects associated with sustained administration of steroids. These side effects include cataracts, psychosis, gastrointestinal bleeding, carbohydrate intolerance, hypertension, obesity, osteoporosis, growth failure in the juvenile population, and decreased resistance to infection. In one large series, as many as 50% of patients developed cushingoid features. Although the benefit of the steroids is not questioned, prospective control studies showing that they are superior to other forms of therapy such as thymectomy do not exist, and the author prefers to use these drugs only when necessary rather than routinely in an effort to avoid these potential complications.

**Plasmapheresis.** Plasmapheresis is a technique that permits the selective removal of plasma or plasma components by a centrifugal method. The remaining red blood cells are then suspended in a solution such as lactated Ringer's solution and reintroduced to the patient. The procedure, which is easy to accomplish, produces a rapid transient clinical improvement in patients with myasthenia gravis and has proved to be a valuable method. The author has used plasmapheresis primarily to optimize the medical status of patients before thymectomy. One to 3 liters of plasma is removed per run on alternate days until the maximal clinical benefit has been obtained (usually four to six runs). This clinical improvement facilitates the perioperative period while avoiding the need for additional medications. Except for occasional hypotension during the first or second run, plasmapheresis is generally well tolerated. Hypocalcemia and hypoalbuminemia may result from repeated runs and need to be identified and treated appropriately. To minimize the risk of bleeding and infection due to removal of clotting factors or immunoglobulins, surgical intervention is not recommended within 48 hours of the last run of plasmapheresis.

Plasmapheresis has been used in some centers as a primary therapeutic modality. Because plasmapheresis produces only temporary clinical benefit, immunosuppressive drugs must be used as well to obtain a stable clinical improvement, and it has not been established that plasmapheresis increases the likelihood of clinical remission compared with the use of immunosuppressive drugs alone. The author has used this form of treatment only in patients whose symptoms are refractory to thymectomy or who have suffered acute deterioration after thymectomy.

The mechanism of action of plasmapheresis is presumably related to the removal of a specific plasma factor. The serum AChR antibody has been implicated because levels are dramatically reduced at the time of plasmapheresis in conjunction with clinical improvement. Clinical benefit, however, may persist for substantially longer periods than the AChR antibody remains depressed, and some patients respond to plasmapheresis who have no detectable serum antiAChR antibodies. It must be emphasized that more than serum immunoglobulins are removed at the time of plasmapheresis, and the removal of additional factors may contribute to the improvement after plasmapheresis.

**Immunosuppressive Agents.** The evidence supporting an immunologic basis for myasthenia gravis and the response to plasmapheresis and thoracic duct drainage have fostered an interest in immunosuppressive drugs. Generally, these drugs have been used in patients who are refractory to more conventional therapies such as thymectomy or steroids. Azathioprine has been most widely used in a dose of 1.5 to 3 mg/kg. There is a latency period of 6 to 12 weeks before the onset of benefit, and maximal effect may not be obtained for 1 year or longer. European physicians have a wide experience with this drug and report favorable responses in most of their patients, although serious complications such as marrow suppression, gastrointestinal bleeding, decreased resistance to infection, and death have been reported. The possibility of delayed side effects such as the development of malignancies must also be considered. Generally, the medication is well tolerated, although severe nausea, vomiting, and diarrhea have restricted its use in some patients. More potent cytotoxic drugs, such

as cyclophosphamide, have not been widely studied, but there are occasional reports of benefit.

Immunosuppressant drugs may be more effective when combined with plasmapheresis, such as those described earlier. Antilymphocyte serum, antithymocyte serum, and splenic radiation have all been tried and have been reported to have some effectiveness in refractory cases of myasthenia gravis. Clearer delineation of the humoral or cellular immune mechanism directed against the AChR may allow more specific immunosuppression. Trials of monoclonal antibodies directed against the putative etiologic agents may be seen in the future.

## Surgical Treatment

### Thymectomy

Evidence suggesting the central role of the thymus gland in myasthenia gravis combined with the deficiencies of medical management has resulted in the increasing application of thymectomy in the management of myasthenia gravis. At Duke University Medical Center, thymectomy is used as the primary mode of therapy for myasthenia gravis. Patients with myasthenia gravis are considered for thymectomy as soon as possible after the development of generalized weakness. Plasmapheresis is used to optimize medical status before thymectomy if patients show significant weakness. Patients referred on anticholinesterase agents have these agents slowly withdrawn during plasmapheresis. It is rare to identify patients who cannot be withdrawn from anticholinesterase agents with plasmapheresis, and as a result, patients come to the operating suite without these supportive pharmacologic agents and consequently undergo a less complex perioperative course.

Patients receiving corticosteroids are maintained on them throughout the perioperative period to prevent adrenal insufficiency; after this period, attempts are made to gradually lower the dosage as tolerated.

Thymectomy should be done in an institution with an experienced treatment team. There must be a close working relationship among the neurologist, the anesthesiologist, the surgeon, and the intensive care unit personnel. When thymectomy is done under these conditions, the operative mortality rate should be below 1%, and death should occur only in high-risk patients with profound clinical weakness. Preoperative sedation may be given, but doses should be less than in patients without myasthenia gravis. Atropine is avoided. Most anesthesiologists use short-acting barbiturates for induction of anesthesia and maintain anesthesia with an inhalation agent. Succinyl chloride and curare are rarely necessary and are best avoided. Patients who have experienced significant respiratory difficulty or profound weakness before operation are generally managed with nasotracheal intubation, because it is more comfortable if ventilator support is required. When early extubation is anticipated, orotracheal intubation is used, which has the advantages of speed and avoidance of nasal mucosal trauma.

**Surgical Anatomy of the Thymus Gland.** Knowledge of the surgical anatomy of the thymus gland begins with an understanding of its embryonic differentiation. Human thymic primordium arises primarily from the third branchial pouch in close association with the inferior parathyroid gland, which affixes to the posterior side of the thyroid gland, whereas the thymus descends into the thorax. A portion of the thymic primordium may also develop from the fourth branchial pouch in association with the superior parathyroid gland. In the branchial complex stage, the pharyngobranchial duct closes and the communication between the pharynx and the thymus is loosened. Ultimately, the lobes of the thymus separate from the parathyroid glands and descend into the thorax. Controversy remains regarding ectopic portions of the thymus gland found in the neck, cephalad to the main body of the thymus gland. This thymic tissue may derive from the fourth branchial pouch along with parathyroid tissue. An alternative postulate suggests that this thymic tissue originates from the third branchial pouch but breaks off during its descent into the thorax. This complex migratory pattern of the thymus gland is thought to be responsible for the finding of ectopic thymic tissue in locations such as the left main bronchus, the parenchyma of the lung, the posterior mediastinum, and the hilum of the lung. This is shown in Figure 30–6A, which shows the branchial complex stage in which thymus is identified in close approximation to the cervical sinus and originating from the third branchial cleft before its descent into the thorax and before the formation of the gland from ectodermal cells surrounding the cervical sinus.

In the definitive form stage (Fig. 30–6B), a separation of thymic tissue has occurred after migration of the thymic tissue from the third branchial cleft inferiorly, and residual thymus is identified superiorly in proximity to the superior parathyroid gland.

After the thymus gland has migrated into the inferior mediastinum, it relates to the major mediastinal structures (Fig. 30–7). It overlies the pericardium and great vessels at the base of the heart and is close to the left innominate vein. The thymus gland has an H-shaped configuration, with variable fusion of the right and left lobes at about the midportion of the gland. The superior poles of the gland are thinner than the inferior poles. The upper portion of the gland attenuates into the thyrothymic ligament, which connects the thymus gland to the thyroid gland. There are many variations in the regional anatomy of the thymus gland. It may lie posterior or anterior to the left innominate vein, and the superior pole of the gland may extend along the pretracheal fascia into the root of the neck. At the lateral extent of the gland, there is a fine capsule that separates it from the pleura and the parapleural mediastinal fat that lies proximal to the phrenic nerve. The arterial supply to the thymus gland comes from the internal mammary arteries via their pericardiophrenic branches. Venous drainage is through one or two large veins that drain into the anterior aspect of the left innominate vein. When the thymus gland lies posterior to the left innominate vein, drainage may be into the posterior portion of that vein. The thymus gland is largest relative to body size within the first or second year of life, when it may attain as much as 50% of its ultimate weight.

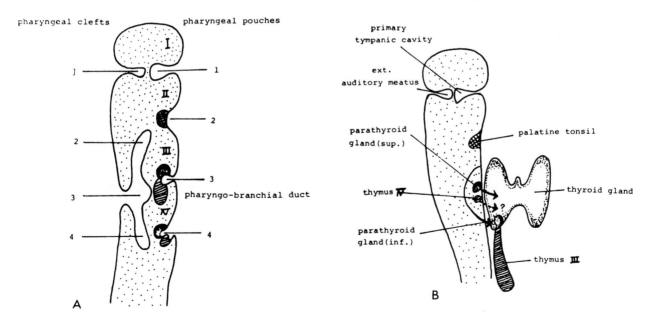

**FIGURE 30–6.** A, Primordial stage showing early development of the thymus gland in the vicinity of the pharyngobranchial duct and from the third branchial pouch. B, Definitive form showing later embryonic development of the thymus gland. By this stage, the close association of the thymus gland to the thyroid gland superiorly is shown as well as the overlapping anatomic areas for location of the parathyroid gland. Some minor controversy still exists regarding some contribution to thymic development from the fourth branchial pouch. (A and B, From Langman, J.: Medical Embryology. 2nd ed. Baltimore, Williams & Wilkins Co., copyright © 1969.)

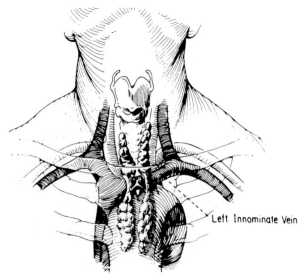

**FIGURE 30–7.** Location of the "normal" thymus gland in relation to other major intrathoracic structures. Of particular importance is the relationship of the thymus gland to the innominate vein. The draining veins from the thymus to the innominate vein are occasionally inconstant and may be a source of bleeding if not identified and carefully ligated. Occasionally, the thymus gland runs behind the innominate vein in proximity to the innominate artery. Various amounts of thymic fusion make the innominate vein more or less visible in the course of the dissection. (From Kark, A. E., and Kirschner, P. A.: Total thymectomy by the transcervical approach. Br. J. Surg., *58*:321, 1971.)

The mass of the gland is usually greatest at the time of puberty and weighs 25 to 50 g. After puberty, there is gradual replacement of the densely packed lymphocyte architecture of the gland by adipose tissue, and in late life, thymic remnants may be detected only microscopically. Normally, there is a distinct thymic capsule that allows its separation from surrounding mediastinal and cervical structures.

Two contributions to the literature have further enhanced our understanding of the surgical anatomy of the thymus gland. Jaretzki has emphasized variations in the location of the thymic gland at its cervical extent. In Figure 30–8, taken from his article, important relationships of the thymus to the recurrent laryngeal nerve as indicated by the arrow are shown. Number 1 identifies the usual location of the thymus gland with a narrow further cervical extension that is either isthmus or a retrothyroid extension. Number 2 demonstrates a separate retrothyroid lobe. Number 3 demonstrates a lateral cervical lobe, and Number 4 demonstrates variable locations of the parathyroid glands. Another important location of thymic tissue was identified by Fukai and is illustrated in Figure 30–9. In an autopsy study, he identified thymic tissue present in the anterior mediastinal fat about one-half of the time and demonstrated the surprising presence of thymic tissue in the retrocarinal fat in 7% of patients. This somewhat unusual location of thymic tissue supports further the general notion that thymic tissue may be in most mediastinal fat but is much less common in fat appearing in the posterior medias-

tinum. This was evident in Fukai's series in which he was unable to demonstrate thymic tissue in the preaortic fat.

Some representative anatomic thymus configurations are shown in Figure 30–10. The degree of fusion and the extent of upper pole development vary to a great extent.

**Surgical Technique.** Various surgical techniques are available for thymectomy. The particular choice of technique varies as dictated by the personal preference of the surgeon and his or her beliefs concerning the pathogenesis of myasthenia and the role of thymectomy in the treatment of myasthenia gravis. Thymic tissue has been documented to be a normal component of perithymic fat, and if a diligent search for this tissue is made, it can be found approximately 75% of the time. Thymic tissue is frequently located in multiple sites within the anterior mediastinum,

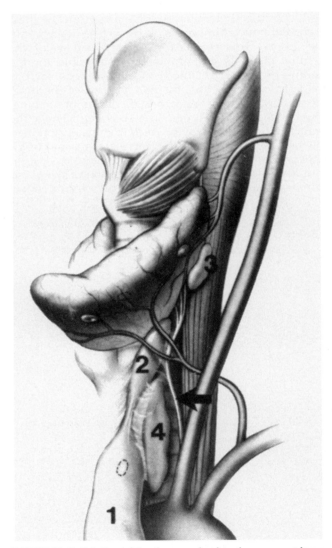

**FIGURE 30–8.** Relation of the thymus gland to the recurrent laryngeal nerve and other important neck structures in the vicinity of the thymus gland. (From Jaretzki, A., III, and Wolff, M.: "Maximal" thymectomy from myasthenia gravis. J. Thorac. Cardiovasc. Surg., *96*:711–716, 1988.)

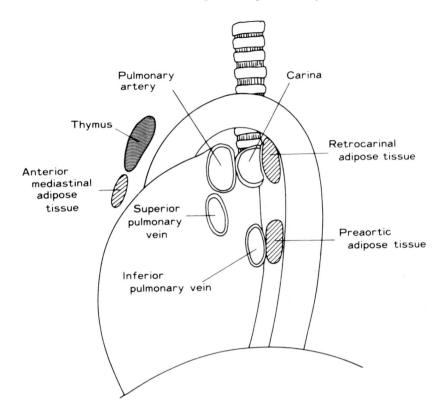

**FIGURE 30–9.** Location of adipose tissue sampled for the presence of thymic remnants. Only the adipose tissue from the posterior mediastinal site failed to disclose any evidence of thymus gland components. (From Fukai, I., Funato, Y., Mizuno, T., et al.: Distribution of thymic tissue in the mediastinal adipose tissue. J. Thorac. Cardiovasc. Surg., *101*:1099–1102, 1991.)

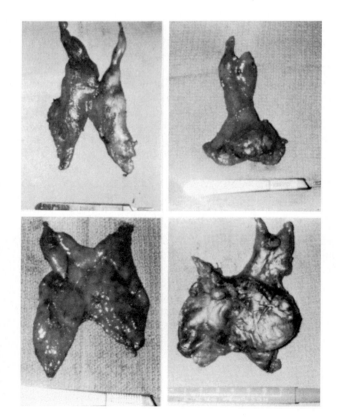

**FIGURE 30–10.** Operative specimens showing the broad range of anatomic variation in the normal thymus gland. The figure at the upper left represents the generally described H configuration. Other figures show greater fusion between the right and the left portions of the gland, disproportionate development of the lower poles compared with the upper poles of the gland, and disproportionate development of one upper pole compared with the other pole. The number of upper poles varies, and careful anatomic dissection is required for complete removal of the gland.

and thus the median sternotomy approach for thymectomy is preferred because it allows the most complete approach for total removal of thymic tissue. Surgical approaches for thymectomy include the following:

1. Transcervical thymectomy
2. Median sternotomy
3. Partial median sternotomy
4. Median sternotomy plus cervical incision

The technique of cervical thymectomy was initially described by Crotti in 1938, was reintroduced by Crile, and was extended by Kark and Kirschner. The technique is preferred by some surgeons because of the cosmetic incision, low morbidity, and minimal stay in the hospital. It has been advocated to be particularly useful in patients with significant respiratory distress and who have not undergone tracheostomy. When cervical thymectomy is performed, the patient is prepared and draped for a median sternotomy in the event of the occurrence of an intrathoracic complication requiring exploration or an unanticipated problem in removing the gland. The procedure is initiated by making a curvilinear incision approximately 2 cm above the supersternal notch and then extending this incision to the level of the strap muscles. After retraction of the strap muscles, the cervical fascia covering the thymus gland is entered, and the manubrium can be raised anteriorly. Special retractors have been devised that allow anterior traction to be placed on the sternum to facilitate the dissection. The thymus is mobilized from the innominate vein, and its venous attachment is divided between silver clips (Fig. 30–11). By traction on the upper pole of the gland, it is possible to continue mobilization, and the arterial supply to the gland is then divided by using electrocautery. Resection is generally limited to that portion of the gland enclosed within the thymic capsule. If the wound is dry, drainage is generally not necessary. Inadvertent pleural entry can be treated by hyperinflation of the lungs as the deep tissue planes are closed. If the wound is not entirely free from bleeding at termination of the procedure, a small drainage catheter can be introduced into the superior mediastinum for several hours to a day to collect any residual blood. Advocates of this procedure generally cite remission rates for their patients comparable with those using the trans-sternal approach, although patients are usually preselected and the studies are neither standardized nor controlled. Further residual mediastinal thymic tissue has been found in up to 60% of patients after transcervical sternotomy. Recurrent myasthenia associated with significant amounts of residual thymic tissue and even thymomas have been reported after transcervical thymectomy. Although it is an aesthetically pleasing and technically feasible procedure, transcervical thymectomy achieves a less complete thymectomy than trans-sternal thymectomy. Although the importance of total thymectomy is unknown, there is concern that incomplete removal of

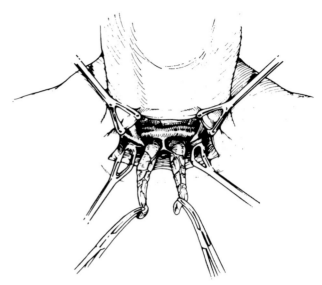

**FIGURE 30–11.** Transcervical thymectomy. The patient's head is at the upper portion of the picture, and the figure shows the surgeon's view after retraction of the upper poles of the thymus gland to expose the venous drainage into the innominate vein. The use of specially constructed sternal retractors facilitates this procedure that generally results in removal of a good operative specimen, which is defined by the capsule of the gland. Thymic tissue in the mediastinum is more difficult to visualize and remove with this technique. (From Kark, A. E., and Kirschner, P. A.: Total thymectomy by the transcervical approach. Br. J. Surg., *58*:321, 1971.)

the thymus may be associated with a higher recurrence rate of myasthenia gravis.

The initial concern with median sternotomy for thymectomy is related to impaired pulmonary mechanics after a major chest incision. Splinting of the chest, damage to the phrenic nerves, mediastinal infection, a higher pain medication requirement, a cosmetically less appealing incision, and postoperative pulmonary complications such as atelectasis and pneumonia have all been cited as disadvantages to the trans-sternal approach. Several factors have changed this situation. Patients are referred for thymectomy earlier in the course of their disease and tend to be less ill. Medical status can usually be improved by plasmapheresis before thymectomy so that even patients having respiratory difficulty come to thymectomy with good ventilatory potential. The better clinical state of patients before thymectomy has allowed early mobilization and has reduced the incidence of pulmonary complications after the procedure. For patients requiring tracheostomy, an incision can be used that is anatomically separated from the tracheostomy stoma and that minimizes the risk of contamination and mediastinal sepsis.

A composite drawing constructed from the work of Jaretzki and associates (1977), who did a careful anatomic and histologic examination of the mediastinal and cervical regions at the time of thymectomy, is shown in Figure 30–12. The normal location of the thymus gland is shown along with the variety of other locations for thymic tissue that were noted.

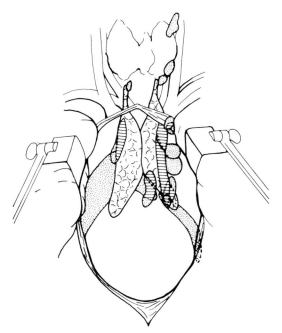

FIGURE 30–12. "Classic" location of the thymus gland. Based on the work of Jaretzki and associates (1977), the location of other thymic tissue is shown in the *stippled* or *lined areas*. Of particular importance is the location of thymic tissue deep in the lateral mediastinum and superiorly in relation to the thyroid gland, frequently not in continuity with the remainder of the thymus gland.

The wide range of locations of thymic tissue in the mediastinum emphasizes the need for good exposure of both the mediastinal contents and the cervical extent of the thymus gland if thymectomy is to be attempted. This exposure can be obtained with a median sternotomy. In men, a short vertical skin incision can be made and can be mobilized adequately cephalad and caudad to allow median sternotomy, sternal separation, and adequate cervical exposure by retraction of the skin. In women, a median sternotomy with excellent exposure of the superior extent of the thymus gland and the lower cervical region can be obtained by using supramammary or inframammary incisions that leave a cosmetically excellent scar. In these approaches, a curvilinear incision is made just over the breast and is extended inferiorly in the midline (supramammary incision) or beneath the breasts (inframammary incision).

By using skin hooks and electrocautery, it is possible to establish a bloodless plane of dissection that allows elevation of the anterior chest wall to well above the suprasternal notch superiorly and to the xiphoid inferiorly. The sternotomy is then done by using a saw and by taking care to remain in the midline of the sternum. This approach affords an excellent visualization of the thymus gland and its vascular attachments and is a cosmetically acceptable incision (Fig. 30–13). It also allows extensive removal of perithymic tissue and mediastinal fat.

The pleural reflections onto the thymus gland are pushed gently to the sides by blunt dissection. A plane is then established between the inferior aspect

of the thymus gland and the anterior aspect of the pericardium. Starting in the midline and working toward the pleural spaces, the surgeon frees each lobe of the inferior thymus gland from its superficial pericardial attachments. As the gland gradually assumes form, gentle traction separates it from the pleura. Efforts are made not to enter the pleural space, but if this occurs it is not a significant complication. As the dissection proceeds cephalad, the thymus gland is retracted superiorly to identify the thymic vein or veins on the posterior surface of the gland as they enter the left innominate vein. These veins are divided between silver clips, and the gland is separated from the innominate vein. Each of the superior poles of the thymus gland is then dissected from the surrounding fascial tissue until it is identified as an attenuated fibrous cord. Both fibrous cords are transected, and the thymus is removed. This technique is shown in Figure 30–14.

Placement of a warm cotton pad in the anterior mediastinum for a few moments generally creates excellent hemostasis, after which a No. 28 chest tube is positioned in the mediastinum and the sternum is reapproximated. If the pleural space has been entered, the tip of the chest tube may be advanced into that pleural space, but a separate pleural drainage catheter is almost never necessary. Postoperative bleeding is usually minimal, and the tube can be removed several hours after the operation. The sternotomy wound is closed in layers, with a subcuticular skin closure.

**Modification of Thymectomy for Thymoma.** When the thymus gland appears to be unusually firm or adheres to any of the surrounding structures, the surgeon should strongly suspect a thymoma. This may not have been appreciated in the preoperative assessment, even if CT of the mediastinum was done.

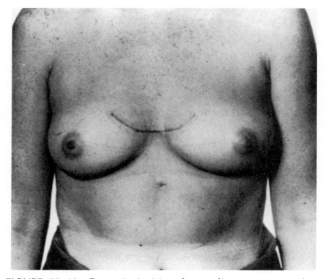

FIGURE 30–13. Cosmetic incision for median sternotomy in a young woman. The incision can be placed just on the superior surface of the breast as shown here, or it can be placed entirely in the inframammary region. In either case, the incision leaves an acceptable scar, and the resultant dissection allows excellent visualization of both the intrathoracic and the cervical thymus gland.

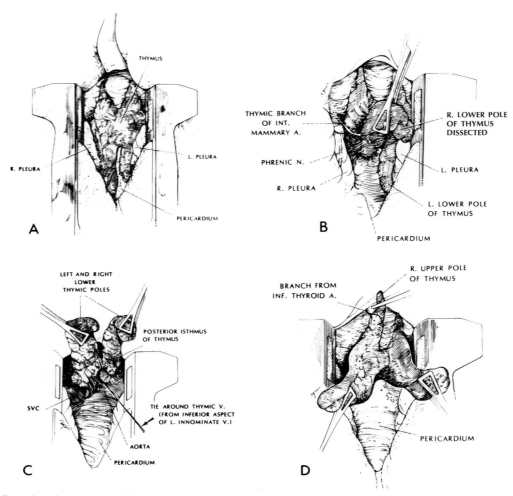

**FIGURE 30–14.** Procedure for removal of the thymus gland by using a median sternotomy. *A–D,* The important steps for safe and complete removal of the thymus gland. (*A–D,* From Wilkins, E. W.: Thymectomy. *In* Cohn, L. H. [ed]: Modern Techniques in Surgery. Cardiac/Thoracic Surgery. Mt. Kisco, NY, Futura, 1979.)

If a thymoma is present, infiltration into surrounding structures must be searched for carefully, because this is the major criterion for malignancy. Because there may be recurrences even after removal of a benign thymoma, a complete and careful dissection of the tumor mass is required. Care should be taken to avoid injury to the phrenic nerve; however, if it is incorporated within the tumor mass and complete resection is otherwise impossible, it may be sacrificed. Extensive involvement of the left innominate vein or of the internal surface of the pericardium is an ominous prognostic sign, and complete resection may not be possible. If a malignancy is suspected, however, an aggressive attempt at removal of the tumor is warranted, and removal of a portion of the pericardium, the left innominate vein, one of the phrenic nerves, and the pleural reflections should be done. Total surgical extirpation offers the best chance for long-term cure in cases of malignant thymoma. If removal of the tumor is impossible, radiation therapy is generally used, and the field can be better defined by marking the peripheral extent of tumor involvement with sur-

gical clips. Frozen-tissue biopsies are of little help in diagnosing malignant thymomas because the determination of malignancy is primarily from the biologic behavior of the tumor. Biopsy may, however, disclose the presence of cell types other than thymomas.

**Postoperative Care.** After thymectomy, the patient is returned to the intensive care unit to be observed by the physician and nursing team. The effects of the anesthetic agents are allowed to dissipate while the patient is supported with a ventilator, usually using intermittent mandatory ventilation at low-rate settings. The decision of when to extubate the patient is based mainly on the preoperative condition. In patients with disease of relatively short duration and mild symptoms, extubation is considered several hours after operation. Patients with more severe myasthenia gravis may require intubation for longer periods. Extubation is done when the patient is alert and shows a satisfactory vital capacity. The patient should be able to generate inspiratory negative pressure greater than 20 cm $H_2O$. After extubation, frequent measurements of vital capacity should be obtained by using a bedside digital spirometer. Patients must be watched carefully, because deterioration of ventilatory status may occur several days postoperatively. Preoperative preparation reduces the likelihood of prolonged intubation or subsequent ventilatory deterioration. The patient may be ambulated the morning after operation and, in most cases, is prepared for discharge within a few days.

**Results of Thymectomy.** Improvement after thymectomy has been reported in 57 to 86% of patients, and permanent remission in 20 to 36%. This clinical improvement may be delayed from 3 to 5 years from the time of operation. Analysis of these data is hampered by differences in patients selected for operation, timing of thymectomy, choice of route, underlying pathologic conditions, and perioperative care. Furthermore, even without treatment, spontaneous remission may occasionally occur. There are no prospective controlled studies that allow comparison of the results of thymectomy versus medical therapy versus the natural history of myasthenia gravis in a particular population. Nonetheless, a review of most published articles did not find any reported series in which patients treated medically fared better than those treated surgically. A retrospective, controlled, matched, computerized study (Fig. 30–15) favored thymectomy over medical therapy with respect to remission and survival (Buckingham et al., 1976). It is difficult to determine which patients with delayed improvement after thymectomy might have experienced spontaneous remission without therapy. Although the data are confusing, it is the impression of most groups that the greatest chance for permanent remission is seen after thymectomy. In general, patients with nonthymomatous myasthenia gravis have better remission rates and long-term survival rates

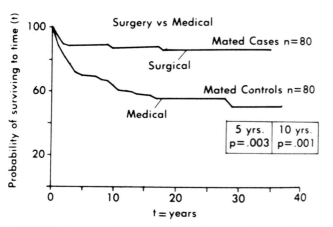

**FIGURE 30–15.** A matched, computerized, retrospective analysis of medical versus surgical management in myasthenia gravis. This work done at the Mayo Clinic provides the longest comparative follow-up for patients treated both medically and surgically in which the patients were matched for severity of disease as well as for their personal characteristics. The improved survival in the surgical group of patients was statistically significant at both 5 and 10 years, and this difference was maintained with additional passage of time. (From Buckingham, J. M., Howard, F. M., Bernatz, P. E., et al.: The value of thymectomy in myasthenia gravis: A computer-assisted matched study. Ann. Surg., *184*:453, 1976.)

than those with thymomatous myasthenia gravis (Papatestas et al., 1971).

Only 10% of patients with a noninvasive thymoma are reported to have remission. When the tumor is invasive, remission is less likely, and more than 50% of patients die within 5 years. Most of these deaths occur in the first year after operation and are related to myasthenic complications. Because the primary feature of malignancy in thymoma is local invasion, the argument for early thymectomy has been advanced in an attempt to avoid infiltration of surrounding tissues. This approach may produce a lower percentage of malignant thymomas. The present ability to perform thymectomy safely and to potentially avoid long-term drug side effects leads many experts to consider thymectomy as the treatment of choice for myasthenia gravis.

A prospective management plan for patients with myasthenia gravis was established at Duke University Medical Center. All patients with evidence of generalized myasthenia gravis, regardless of severity, underwent thymectomy. Preoperative plasmapheresis was used to optimize medical status if necessary. Efforts were made to use thymectomy as the sole treatment modality and to use medications only if necessary rather than by routine. The results were most gratifying and are indicated in Table 30–3. Thymectomy was not withheld because of age, and good results were obtained in all age groups with all types of thymic pathology. Residual myasthenic symptoms have been confined mainly to the ocular muscles. Forty-six of 47 patients improved after thymectomy compared with their prethymectomy, preplasmapheresis state (mean follow-up 25.5 months). Thirty patients were functionally intact and free of generalized weakness at normal levels of activity. Nine patients had only residual ocular dysfunction. Thus, 83% of patients were free of significant generalized weakness. Most patients required no medication. Before thymectomy, AChR antibody titers generally correlated with the severity of the myasthenia. Postoperatively, there was no direct relationship between AChR antibody titer and clinical status, because AChR antibody levels did not change significantly, but there was dramatic clinical improvement in the patients.

Because the early results were encouraging, the series was continued and a second group of patients was analyzed (Olanow et al., 1987) in which 55 patients were treated for myasthenia gravis by using thymectomy as the primary therapy. None of these 55 patients were receiving long-term medical management for myasthenia gravis at the time of entry into the study, and all patients were prepared for operation individually by using plasmapheresis as the interim treatment modality when indicated. None of the patients had isolated ocular myasthenia, and patients with long-standing myasthenia thought to have a fixed neurologic deficit were excluded. Clinical status was assessed by using the modified Osserman grading system that was described earlier, and all patients were followed for at least 1 year. The mean follow-up for the group was 39.3 months.

■ **Table 30–3.** CLINICAL STATUS OF PATIENTS UNDERGOING THYMECTOMY FOR TREATMENT OF MYASTHENIA GRAVIS IN THE DUKE MEDICAL CENTER SERIES

| | Before Thymectomy | | No. of Patients After Thymectomy | | | | | |
|---|---|---|---|---|---|---|---|---|
| Clinical State | No. of Patients | No. Receiving Medication | Normal | I | IIA | IIB | IIC | Died |
| IIA | 28 | 21 | 24 | 4 | | | | |
| IIB | 9 | 8 | 4 | 2 | 3 | | | |
| IIC | 10 | 10 | 2 | 3 | 3 | 1 | | 1 |
| Number of patients receiving antimyasthenia drugs after thymectomy according to post-thymectomy clinical state | | | 1 | 1 | 3 | 1 | | |

Sixty-four per cent of the patients (35 of 55) were asymptomatic and had no functional neurologic deficit. Sixteen per cent (9 patients) had residual ocular dysfunction, but no generalized weakness. Thus, 80% of the patients (44 of 55) were free of generalized weakness an average of 39.3 months after thymectomy. Ten patients continued to have mild generalized weakness, but none had residual bulbar dysfunction. Ninety-two per cent of the patients (50 of 55) improved by at least one stage compared with their prethymectomy, preplasma exchange baseline status. Seventy-one per cent of patients (39 of 55) improved by two or more stages. Four patients did not improve, and there was one death related to management of an acute exacerbation with high-dose steroids, later development of a cushingoid state, and later pulmonary embolism. Thymic pathology included thymic hyperplasia, atrial thymic involution, thymoma, and thymic cysts. Improvement in patients was the rule regardless of the underlying thymic pathology. After thymectomy, drug therapy was avoided whenever possible. Fifty-five per cent of the patients (30 of 55) were not taking medication. Twenty-two per cent of the patients (12 of 55) required chronic prednisone therapy for generalized myasthenic symptoms, and an additional 24% of patients (13 of 55) received low doses of prednisone every other day for management of ocular symptoms.

By using thymectomy as primary treatment for generalized myasthenia gravis, 92% of patients enrolled in the series improved and 80% were free of generalized weakness at the time of latest medical follow-up (mean of 39.3 months). Fifty-five per cent of patients received no medical therapy, and 38% never received medical therapy in the course of their treatment. Particularly important for surgeons is the awareness that early use of thymectomy and avoidance of medical management avoided perioperative problems associated with the use of corticosteroid therapy. Specifically, slow wound healing, difficult postoperative management, and occasional postoperative deterioration were all avoided.

Previous series relating thymectomy to symptoms of myasthenia gravis have focused on the occurrence of pathology in the thymus gland and have considered involution to be an absence of pathology, but a normal consequence of aging. Evaluation of patients with late-onset myasthenia gravis, regardless of the mode of therapy, at our institution showed that 10 of 11 patients had atrophic involuted thymus glands. Contrary to initial reports, there is accumulating evidence of immunologic competence even with atrophic involuted thymus glands. Thymic epithelial cells interspersed within anterior mediastinal fat stain for $alpha_1$-thymosin, which is an immunopotentiating peptide. Moreover, studies at Duke University have shown reduced numbers of peripheral blood T-cell subsets $3A1^+$ and $OKT4^+$ compared with age-matched control subjects and patients with hyperplastic thymus glands. After thymectomy, these changes are corrected (Haynes et al., 1983).

Commitment to median sternotomy is still a consequence of the author's belief that thymectomy may exert its beneficial effect by removal of a thymic factor leading to acceleration of the complement cascade that produces a complement-mediated lysis of the AChR previously marked by ACh antibodies (Olanow et al., 1981).

There has not been a prospective randomized study that compares the effects of thymectomy with the effects of other forms of management for myasthenia gravis. The Duke Medical Center study is unique in its use of thymectomy as the primary mode of therapy for all patients once they enter the program. It is difficult to compare these results with other thymectomy series, because in some institutions thymectomy is used only when medical management for treatment of myasthenia gravis has failed or when thymoma is suspected. Because of the strict treatment protocol in the Duke series, no physician bias with regard to which patient should have thymectomy entered into the treatment decision. Rather than pursuing medical management, every effort was made to avoid the use of antimyasthenic medications. Optimization of the clinical state was by plasmapheresis without immunosuppression rather than with drug therapy when necessary. All thymectomies were done in a standardized manner, were radical in nature, and were done by the same surgeon. This approach showed that in most patients, thymectomy alone could produce dramatic and sustained clinical improvement without the need for additional medications. Moreover, reduction in the AChR antibody titer was not essential for clinical improvement. These observations support the hypothesis that a factor elaborated by or in the thymus gland has a role in AChR destruction. Further studies to identify, isolate, and characterize a putative thymic factor are necessary, because the identification of such a "thymic factor" could lead to special techniques for its removal or neutralization.

Cooper and associates described their results with transcervical thymectomy and compared these results with those reported both in the Duke experience and in a series by Jaretzki and associates favoring "maximal" thymectomy. With a relatively short-term follow-up of 1 year, the results with transcervical thymectomy were alleged comparable with both those in the Duke series and with the more radical resection performed in the Jaretzki and co-workers series. Unfortunately, comparison between the series was difficult. There were differences in patient age, the medical approach to treatment, and perioperative drug treatment. In a meta-analysis, Jaretzki and co-workers reviewed 18 reports from the literature and evaluated the remission percentage in each of these. Jaretzki and associates used a strict definition of remission, and the results of their analysis are reproduced in Figure 30–16. These data may be misinterpreted because of the wide variability of the patient populations studied. Remission rates from thymectomy in sternal and extended sternal approaches to thymectomy have generally been better when performed early in the course of the disease, as may be surmised by comparing these results with results from two Italian series, in which remission rates of 30% were common following thymectomy but in which patient populations were at a more advanced stage of their illness.

Because data continue to emerge relating the effects of thymectomy to the course of myasthenia gravis, it appears to be particularly important that thymectomy should be as complete as possible. Assessment of long-term data should not be confused by uncertainty regarding the presence of residual thymic tissue.

## Algorithms for Management of Patients with Myasthenia Gravis

Because of success with the ongoing treatment plans discussed in this chapter, a summary for the diagnosis and management of patients with myasthenia gravis is provided here.

As outlined in Figure 30–17, when a patient with myasthenic symptoms is examined, the first portion of the evaluation is a diagnostic phase, starting with a careful history and physical examination. One of the primary goals at this time is to determine whether the patient has myasthenia gravis or weakness associated with another clinical condition. The diagnosis of true myasthenia gravis is made by a combination of history, physical examination, and appropriate laboratory tests. The response to Tensilon, the Jolly and jitter tests, and determination of the level of the AChR antibodies usually identify the disease correctly in more than 95% of cases. The patient is then placed in a subgroup according to functional classification, and careful distinction is made as to whether the patient has ocular or generalized myasthenia gravis. Many patients who seek the attention of a physician because of ocular symptoms have generalized myasthenia gravis but are unaware of it. Because the method of treatment for each type differs at this time, it is important to make this differentiation. Various laboratory tests are designed to determine whether there are associated conditions in addition to the clinical myasthenia gravis, and when present, these conditions are specifically treated. Radiographic studies are used to detect the presence of a thymoma.

Once the diagnosis of generalized myasthenia has been made, the therapeutic phase is entered, which is shown in Figure 30–18. In patients who are thought to have isolated ocular myasthenia, a conservative treatment program is initiated, generally by using low-dose corticosteroids on alternate days. These pa-

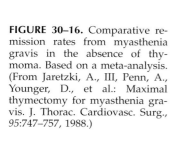

FIGURE 30–16. Comparative remission rates from myasthenia gravis in the absence of thymoma. Based on a meta-analysis. (From Jaretzki, A., III, Penn, A., Younger, D., et al.: Maximal thymectomy for myasthenia gravis. J. Thorac. Cardiovasc. Surg., 95:747–757, 1988.)

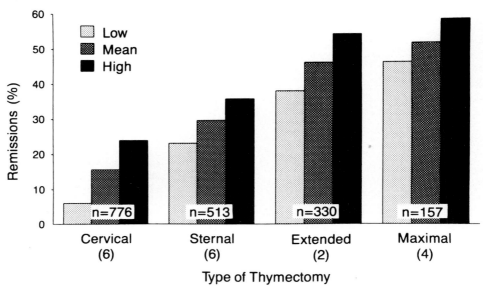

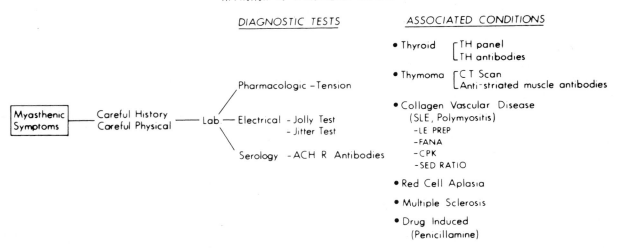

FIGURE 30–17. An algorithm for evaluating patients with myasthenia gravis. Identification of associated conditions is important for optimal management of patients with myasthenia gravis. (ACH R = acetylcholine receptor; CPK = creatine phosphokinase; CT = computed tomography; FANA = fluorescent antinuclear antibody; LE PREP = lupus erythematosus preparation; SED = sedimentation; TH = thyroid hormone.)

tients are followed carefully, because most develop generalized weakness and are then treated similarly to patients who initially present with generalized myasthenia gravis. In the author's clinic, the primary treatment mode is thymectomy. For patients who are weak or who become weak when pharmacologic treatment is withdrawn, plasmapheresis is used to prepare the patient for thymectomy. If the patient's general condition is good, if weakness is not severe, and if there are no other contraindications, thymectomy is then performed as the primary treatment. For

those few patients with specific contraindications or who oppose surgery, medical therapy is used.

This overall treatment plan minimizes or avoids the systemic complications of pharmacologic management of myasthenia gravis. Thymectomy as the primary therapy for myasthenia gravis yields remission in most patients and allows reduced pharmacologic requirements in patients with residual symptoms after thymectomy.

Despite the appeal of the approach outlined in this chapter, it is important to recognize that these views

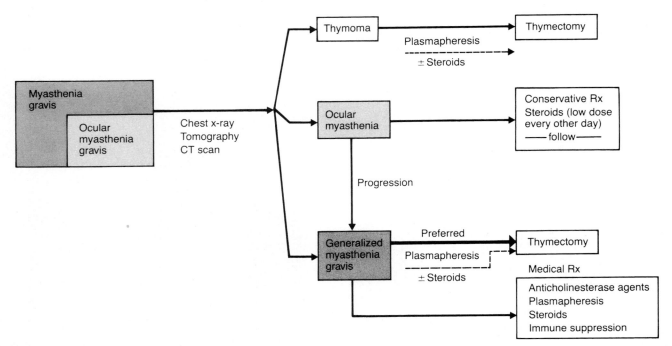

FIGURE 30–18. Therapeutic phase in the treatment of myasthenia gravis. The decision that isolated ocular myasthenia gravis exists is made only if careful single-fiber testing of peripheral muscles is entirely normal.

are not widely held among neurologists. Myasthenia gravis unassociated with thymoma is a disease with a high spontaneous remission rate and unpredictable long-term response to medication, and many of the recommendations for treatment are based on historic series containing sicker patients than are seen today as recognition of the entity has improved. In a consensus poll of 49 neurologists (Lanska, 1990), all actively involved in the management of patients with myasthenia, most favored thymectomy for patients with severe disease or after other modalities had failed. Most of the neurologists supported the view presented in this article that ocular myasthenia is not an indication for thymectomy. Of the 49 neurologists responding, only 3 favored thymectomy as primary therapy in the absence of radiologic evidence of thymoma. The need for a prospectively randomized study remains and would be an extraordinarily important contribution to the future management of patients with myasthenia gravis.

## SELECTED BIBLIOGRAPHY

Blalock, A., Mason, M. F., Morgan, H. J., and Riven, S. S.: Myasthenia gravis and tumors of the thymic region. Ann. Surg., 110:544, 1939.

Blalock and colleagues report the first successful removal of a thymic tumor for the treatment of myasthenia gravis. They use this case as the impetus for reviewing the literature and provide an excellent summary of the rationale for surgical extirpation of the thymus gland in the treatment of myasthenia gravis. The comments from the audience at the end of the manuscript are well worth reading.

Drachman, D. B.: Myasthenia gravis. N. Engl. J. Med., 298:136, 186, 1978.

This is a broad review of myasthenia gravis in which the disease process is discussed from the basic concepts of neuromuscular transmission to specific therapy. It is a good reference for the reader interested in pursuing certain areas of the subject in greater depth. It differs slightly from the views presented in this chapter in that treatment depends more on medical therapy, and indications for thymectomy are more conservative.

Jaretzki, A., Bethea, M., Wolff, M., et al.: A rational approach to total thymectomy in the treatment of myasthenia gravis. Ann. Thorac. Surg., 24:120, 1977.

This article is important for physicians interested in the surgical technique of thymectomy. The authors explore the completeness of thymectomy done by transcervical, median sternotomy, and combined transcervical and median sternotomy routes in a group of their own patients. There are extremely well-done anatomic drawings that show some of the atypical thymus gland locations encountered in the course of their clinical experience. There is also an excellent discussion that includes comments by proponents of other techniques of thymectomy and the reasons behind their arguments.

Lindstrom, J. M., Lennon, V. A., Seybold, M. E., et al.: Experimental autoimmune myasthenia gravis and myasthenia gravis: Biochemical and immuno-chemical aspects. Ann. N. Y. Acad. Sci., 274:254, 1976.

This is a well-presented and comprehensive review of experimental work dealing with immune mechanisms in myasthenia gravis. It provides an excellent background for the understanding of current therapies designed to interfere with humoral and cell-mediated immunity.

Olanow, C. W., Wechsler, A. S., and Roses, A. D.: A prospective study of thymectomy and serum acetylcholine receptor antibodies in myasthenia gravis. Ann. Surg., 196:113, 1982.

This study, done at Duke University Medical Center, is unique in that every patient admitted with the diagnosis of myasthenia gravis was treated in accordance with a strict clinical protocol. For most patients, thymectomy was used as the primary and frequently the only method of therapy. High remission rates were reported with minimal reliance on drug therapy.

## BIBLIOGRAPHY

Abdou, N. I., Lisak, R. P., Sweiman, B., et al.: The thymus in myasthenia gravis: Evidence for altered cell populations. N. Engl. J. Med., 291:1271, 1974.

Abramsky, O., Aharonov, A., Teitelbaum, D., et al.: Myasthenia gravis and acetylcholine receptor: Effect of steroids in clinical course and cellular immune response to acetylcholine receptor. Arch. Neurol., 32:684, 1975.

Appel, S. H., Almon, R. R., and Levy, N.: Acetylcholine receptor antibodies in myasthenia gravis. N. Engl. J. Med., 293:760, 1975.

Argov, Z., and Mastaglia, F. L.: Disorders of neuro-muscular transmission caused by drugs. N. Engl. J. Med., 301:409, 1979.

Beghi, E., Antozzi, C., Batocchi, A. P., et al.: Prognosis of myasthenia gravis: A multicenter follow-up study of 844 patients. J. Neurol. Sci., 106:213–220, 1991.

Castleman, B.: The pathology of the thymus gland in myasthenia gravis. Ann. N. Y. Acad. Sci., 135:496, 1966.

Chang, C. C., Chen, T. F., and Chuang, S.-T.: Influence of chronic neostigmine treatment on the number of acetylcholine receptors and the release of acetylcholine from the rat diaphragm. J. Physiol., 230:613, 1973.

Cooper, J. D., Al-Jilaihawa, A. N., Pearson, F. G., et al.: An improved technique to facilitate transcervical thymectomy for myasthenia gravis. Ann. Thorac. Surg., 45:242–247, 1988.

Dau, P. C., Lindstrom, J. M., Cassel, C. K., et al.: Plasmapheresis and immunosuppressive drug therapy in myasthenia gravis. N. Engl. J. Med., 294:1134, 1977.

Drachman, D. B.: Myasthenia gravis. N. Engl. J. Med., 298:136, 186, 1978.

Drachman, D. B., Kao, I., Pestronk, A., et al.: Myasthenia gravis as a receptor disorder. Ann. N. Y. Acad. Sci., 274:226, 1976.

Durelli, L., Maggi, G., Casadio, C., et al.: Actuarial analysis of the occurrence of remissions following thymectomy for myasthenia gravis in 400 patients. J. Neurol. Neurosurg. Psychiatry, 54:406, 1991.

Early thymectomy for myasthenia gravis [Editorial]. Br. Med. J., 3:262, 1975.

Emeryk, B., and Strugalska, M. H.: Evaluation of results of thymectomy in myasthenia gravis. J. Neurol., 211:155, 1976.

Engel, A. G., Lambert, E. H., and Howard, F. M., Jr.: Immune complexes (IgG and C3) at the motor end plate in myasthenia gravis. Mayo Clin. Proc., 52:267, 1977.

Frambrough, D. M., Drachman, D. B., and Satyamurti, S.: Neuromuscular junction in myasthenia gravis: Deceased acetylcholine receptors. Science, 182:293, 1973.

Fukai, I., Funato, Y., Mizuno, T., et al.: Distribution of thymic tissue in the mediastinal adipose tissue. J. Thorac. Cardiovasc. Surg., 101:1099–1102, 1991.

Genkins, G., Papatestas, A. E., Horowitz, S. H., et al.: Studies in myasthenia gravis. Early thymectomy: Electrophysiologic and pathologic correlations. Am. J. Med., 58:517, 1975.

Goldman, A. J., Hermann, C., Jr., Keesey, J. C., et al.: Myasthenia gravis and invasive thymoma: A 20-year experience. Neurology, 25:1021, 1975.

Haynes, B. F., Harden, E. A., Olanow, C. W., et al.: Effective thymectomy on peripheral lymphocytes subsets in myasthenia gravis: Selective effect on T-cells in patients with thymic atrophy. J. Immunol., 131:773, 1983.

Jaretzki, A., Bethea, M., Wolff, M., et al.: A rational approach to total thymectomy in the treatment of myasthenia gravis. Ann. Thorac. Surg., 24:120, 1977.

Jaretzki, A., III, Penn, A. S., Younger, D. S., et al.: "Maximal" thymectomy for myasthenia gravis. J. Thorac. Cardiovasc. Surg., 95:747–757, 1988.

Jaretzki, A., III, and Wolff, M.: "Maximal" thymectomy for myasthenia gravis. J. Thorac. Cardiovasc. Surg., 96:711–716, 1988.

Koelle, G. B.: Anticholinesterase agents. In Goodman, L. S., and Gilman, A. (eds): The Pharmacological Basis of Therapeutics. 5th ed. New York, Macmillan, 1975, pp. 445–466.

Langman, J.: Medical Embryology. Baltimore, Williams & Wilkins, 1969.

Lanska, D. J.: Indications for thymectomy in myasthenia gravis. Neurology, 40:1828–1829, 1990.

Legg, M. A., and Brady, W. J.: Pathology and clinical behavior of thymomas: A survey of 51 cases. Cancer, 18:1131, 1965.

Lindstrom, J. M., Lennon, V. A., Seybold, M. E., et al.: Experimental autoimmune myasthenia gravis and myasthenia gravis: Biochemical and immuno-chemical aspects: Ann. N. Y. Acad. Sci., 274:254, 1976.

Matell, G., Bergstrom, K., Franksson, C., et al.: Effects of some immuno-suppressive procedures on myasthenia gravis. Ann. N. Y. Acad. Sci., 274:659, 1976.

Mittag, T., Kornfeld, P., Tormay, A., et al.: Detection of antiacetylcholine receptor factors in serum and thymus from patients with myasthenia gravis. N. Engl. J. Med., 294:691, 1976.

Mulder, D. G., Hermann, C., and Buckberg, G. D.: Effect of thymectomy in patients with myasthenia gravis: A sixteen year experience. Am. J. Surg., 128:202, 1974.

Namba, T., Brown, S. B., and Grob, D.: Neonatal myasthenia gravis: Report of two cases and review of the literature. Pediatrics, 45:488, 1970.

Olanow, C. W., Wechsler, A. S., and Roses, A. D.: A prospective study of thymectomy and serum acetylcholine receptor antibodies in myasthenia gravis. Ann. Surg., 196:113, 1982.

Olanow, C. W., Wechsler, A. S., Sirotkin-Roses, M., et al.: Thymectomy as primary therapy in myasthenia gravis. Ann. N. Y. Acad. Sci., 505:595, 1987.

Papatestas, A. E., Alpert, L. I., Osserman, K. E., et al.: Studies in myasthenia gravis. Effects of thymectomy: Results on 185 patients with nonthymomatous and thymomatous myasthenia gravis, 1941–1969. Am. J. Med., 50:465, 1971.

Papatestas, A. E., Genkins, G., Horowitz, S. H., et al.: Thymectomy in myasthenia gravis: Pathologic, clinical and electrophysiologic correlations. Ann. N. Y. Acad. Sci., 274:555, 1976.

Patrick, J., and Lindstrom, J.: Autoimmune response to acetylcholinase receptor. Science, 180:871, 1973.

Pinching, A. J., Peters, D. K., and Newsom, D. J.: Remission of myasthenia gravis following plasma-exchange. Lancet, 2:1373, 1976.

Roses, A. D., Olanow, C. W., McAdams, M. W., and Lane, R. J. M.: There is no direct correlation between serum antiacetylcholine receptor and antibody levels and the clinical status of individual patients with myasthenia gravis. Neurology, 31:220, 1981.

Rowland, L. P.: Controversies about the treatment of myasthenia gravis. J. Neurol. Neurosurg. Psychiatry, 43:644, 1980.

Sahashi, K., Engel, A. G., Lambert, E. H., and Howard, F. M.: Ultrastructural localization of the terminal and lytic 9th complement component (C9) at the motor end plate in myasthenia gravis. J. Neuropathol. Exp. Neurol., 39:160, 1980.

Simpson, J. A.: Myasthenia gravis: A new hypothesis. Scot. Med. J., 5:419, 1960.

Stalberg, E., Trontel, J. V., and Schwartz, M. S.: Single muscle fiber recording of jitter phenomenon in patients with myasthenia gravis and in members of their families. Ann. N. Y. Acad. Sci., 274:189, 1976.

van der Geld, H. W. R., and Strauss, A. J. L.: Myasthenia gravis: Immunological relationship between striated muscle and thymus. Lancet, 1:57, 1966.

Wechsler, A. S., and Olanow, C. W.: Myasthenia gravis. Surg. Clin. North Am., 60:946, 1980.

# 31

# Special Diagnostic and Therapeutic Procedures in Cardiac Surgery

■ **I Cardiac Catheterization, Angiography, and Interventional Techniques in Valvular and Congenital Heart Disease**

Thomas M. Bashore, J. Kevin Harrison, and Charles J. Davidson

## HISTORICAL ASPECTS

Modern cardiac catheterization and angiography, like many advances in science, owes its origin and maturation to the merging of technologic advances on several fronts. The roots of cardiac catheterization lie in the development of x-ray equipment, contrast media, appropriate catheters, and a safe method of cannulating the vascular system.

Roentgen's discovery of the x-ray in 1895 quickly led to a surge of articles describing its use. The first angiogram (of a hand) was reported by Haschek and Lindenthol (1896), and in the same year Williams (1896) noted the pulsatile action of the heart on a newly developed fluoroscopic screen. X-ray motion pictures required the development of the motion picture concept and improved x-ray techniques. This advancement was highlighted by the development of a 16mm cine camera in 1937 (Stewart et al., 1937) and a modern roll-film changer in 1953 (Rigler and Watson, 1953). Developmental changes continue today; the future will see routine use of computerized digital storage of x-ray information and a gradual shift from a cine-film-based medium to a computer-based system.

Paralleling the development of appropriate x-ray techniques was the discovery that the vascular system could be invaded safely using catheter systems. In 1929, the first human catheterization was performed by Forssmann in a classic story of medical intrigue (Forssmann, 1931, 1974; Warren, 1980). When Forssmann described his plan to pass a urethral catheter from his arm to his right atrium, his supervisors intervened and refused to give him permission to do so. Enlisting the assistance of a nurse, he manipulated her into believing that he would use her for the first attempt at catheterization. She allowed him access to the venesection instruments in the surgical suite. After securing her, under the pretext that the local anesthesia might cause her to collapse, he inserted the urethral catheter into his own arm and then walked to the basement, where an x-ray film was taken to show the catheter in his heart.

Others gradually realized the merit in Forssmann's adventure. Activity increased in the 1940s stimulated by the work of Cournand and Richards at Bellevue Hospital in New York (Cournand, 1978). In 1956, Forssmann, Cournand, and Richards received the Nobel Prize in medicine for their pioneering efforts.

Many other investigators contributed to the early development of cardiac catheterization. Brannon and associates (1948) described findings in a patient with an atrial septal defect. The pulmonary capillary wedge pressure was identified in the laboratory of Dexter and colleagues (Hellems et al., 1949).

Though Zimmerman and co-workers (1950) described the first left-sided heart catheterization in humans, left-sided heart catheterization continued to pose a formidable challenge, and numerous approaches were tried. These attempts included left atrial puncture during bronchoscopy (Facquet et al., 1952), a posterior transthoracic approach (Bjork et al., 1953), a suprasternal method (Radner, 1954), a left-sided subcostal technique (Brock et al., 1956), and puncture of the interatrial septum (Cope, 1959). The breakthrough in this area occurred when Seldinger described a method of percutaneous needle puncture with catheter exchange over a guidewire (Seldinger, 1953)—a modification of which is in general use today. Thus, retrograde left-sided heart catheterization became the standard.

Visualization of the coronary arteries posed problems and required innovative approaches. Radner (1945) is generally credited with first visualizing the coronary arteries in humans with contrast media (using a needle inserted from the manubrium), and in 1962, Sones and Shirey described a practical method of selectively cannulating those arteries using a cutdown for isolation of the brachial artery. By using the percutaneous femoral approach, Ricketts and Abrams (1962) suggested that a preformed catheter might be used. These were subsequently modified by Judkins

1123

(1967) and by Amplatz and associates (1967); the Judkins technique is the most widely used today. Other modifications, such as that by Schoonmaker and King (1974), are occasionally used in certain laboratories.

The next advance in catheter design came in 1970, when balloon-tip, flow-directed catheters that could be inserted without fluoroscopy were introduced (Swan et al., 1970). The 1980s saw a resurgence in catheter design and innovation with the advent of interventional cardiac catheter techniques. Newer catheter design has allowed the routine acquisition of myocardial biopsies (Mason, 1978), the performance of coronary angioplasty (Gruntzig et al., 1979), and the performance of percutaneous valvuloplasty (Cribier et al., 1986). Investigators now can use laser technology to "vaporize" coronary artery plaques (Sanborn et al., 1987), "Roto-Rooter" atherectomy devices to drill open obstructed vessels (Perez et al., 1988), and intraluminal stents to maintain patency of vessels (Sigwart et al., 1987).

The final step in the maturation of modern cardiac catheterization procedures was accomplished with the development of a safe x-ray contrast agent. Forssmann (1931) showed that a bolus of sodium iodomethamate (Uroselectan B) could be injected in the right atrium and cause only dizziness. Other attempts to obtain x-ray contrast included such notable methods as using buckshot, air, bismuth and oil, potassium iodide, and so on (Miller, 1984), and have mercifully been abandoned. In the 1950s, the development of a safe, triiodinated benzoic acid contrast medium allowed a substantial reduction in contrast reactions and improved absorbance of the x-ray photons. Newer nonionic and low ionic contrast media that have been shown to be even safer than diatrizoate compounds (Bettman et al., 1984), which had been the standard, were introduced in the 1980s and are now standard.

## INDICATIONS FOR DIAGNOSTIC CARDIAC CATHETERIZATION

Diagnostic cardiac catheterization is indicated in almost all adult patients who are to undergo cardiac operative therapy (with few exceptions). The operating room is not the proper setting for diagnosing the severity of valvular or coronary lesions, because visual inspection or palpation cannot be expected to define disease severity adequately and reliably.

As with any diagnostic procedure, the decision to recommend cardiac catheterization is based on an appropriate risk/benefit ratio. Generally, diagnostic cardiac catheterization is recommended whenever it is clinically important to define the presence or severity of a suspected cardiac lesion. Because the mortality rate from cardiac catheterization is approximately 0.1% in most laboratories, few patients cannot be studied safely in an active laboratory.

The indications for cardiac catheterization are changing and are likely to continue to evolve. The trend during the last 10 years in the United States has been in two broad directions: At one extreme, many seriously ill and hemodynamically unstable patients are being studied during acute myocardial ischemia. At the other end of the spectrum, more and more studies are being done in an outpatient setting. The result has been the expansion of traditional indications for cardiac catheterization to include both critically ill patients and ambulatory patients.

Cardiac catheterization should be considered a diagnostic test for use with other, complementary diagnostic tests in cardiology. For example, although coronary angiography is still the basis for defining the presence and severity of coronary disease (despite the substantial inaccuracy and variation of visual estimates of the severity of disease) (Marcus et al., 1988), the role of pharmacologic or exercise stress in defining the functional significance of anatomic lesions should not be overlooked when making clinical decisions. Cardiac catheterization in valvular or congenital heart disease is, likewise, best done with full knowledge of the echocardiographic and any other functional information. In this manner, catheterization can be directed, simplified, and shortened by not obtaining redundant anatomic information.

Identification and description of *coronary artery disease* are the most common indications for cardiac catheterization in adults. The information is crucial to the care of patients with various chest pain syndromes. In addition, dynamic coronary vascular lesions (e.g., spasm, thrombosis) may be identified, and the consequences of coronary heart disease (e.g., the presence of ischemic valvular regurgitation or left ventricular aneurysm formation may be defined). In this era of active catheter intervention in coronary disease, patients may be studied during myocardial infarction or soon after acute myocardial injury. The aggressiveness of individual centers in approaching these patients depends on local facilities and treatment philosophies as well as the availability of appropriate therapy and surgical support. In the thrombolytic era, it is clear that most patients can be studied later following intravenous thrombolytics. The "open artery" hypothesis still remains a goal, though, and studies using primary angioplasty are underway. The open artery hypothesis assumes that mortality and morbidity will be reduced if perfusion is restored to the infarcted myocardial bed. It is now clear that most patients who receive thrombolytics are best studied only if symptoms recur or a functional test confirms ongoing ischemic jeopardy after acute myocardial infarction.

In patients with *myocardial disease,* cardiac catheterization may provide useful information. Besides identifying the etiologic role of coronary disease in patients with cardiomyopathy, cardiac catheterization permits detection of active myocarditis by analysis of the endomyocardial biopsy, quantification of the severity of both diastolic and systolic dysfunction, differentiation of myocardial restriction from pericardial constriction, assessment of the extent of valvular regurgitation, and observation of the cardiovascular response to acute pharmacologic intervention.

■ **Table 31–1.** COMPLICATIONS OF CARDIAC CATHETERIZATION

| | Overall Complications | | | Coronary Angiography | |
|---|---|---|---|---|---|
| | *Cooperative Study 1968\** | *SCA Registry 1982†* | *SCA Registry 1989‡* | *Adams Survey 1973§* | *CASS Study 1979‖* |
| Number of patients | 12,367 | 53,581 | 222,553 | 46,904 | 7553 |
| Death | 0.75% | 0.14% | 0.10% | 0.45% | 0.2% |
| Myocardial infarction | NA | 0.07% | 0.06% | 0.61% | 0.25% |
| Stroke | 0.2% | 0.07% | 0.07% | 0.23% | 0.03% |
| Vascular | 0.3% | 0.56% | 0.46% | NA | 0.7% |
| Arrhythmias | 1.3% | 0.56% | 0.47% | 0.77% | 0.63% |

*Key:* SCA = Society of Cardiac Angiography; CASS = Collaborative Study of Coronary Artery Surgery.
\*Data from Braunwald and Swan, 1968.
†Data from Kennedy, 1982.
‡Data from Johnson et al., 1989.
§Data from Adams et al., 1973.
‖Data from Davis et al., 1979.

In patients with *valvular heart disease,* cardiac catheterization provides data to confirm and complement noninvasive echocardiography and Doppler studies. We believe that patients with valvular heart disease should rarely undergo cardiac surgical procedures in the absence of catheterization data, despite dissenting opinions (St. John Sutton, 1981). We agree with Roberts' (1982) and Rahimtoola's (1982) opinion that the risk/benefit ratio of preoperative cardiac catheterization in these patients is weighted heavily in favor of performing the procedure. Catheterization may be unnecessary in some clinical situations, such as patients with an atrial myxoma or young patients with endocarditis, acute mitral regurgitation, or acute aortic insufficiency. Nevertheless, additional confirmation of the severity of the valvular lesion, identification of associated coronary disease, quantification of the hemodynamic consequences of the valvular lesions, and occasionally the acute hemodynamic response to pharmacologic therapy all provide useful preoperative information that allows a safer and more directed surgical approach.

Finally, the role of cardiac catheterization in certain *congenital disease* states is less well defined, with the steady improvement in the accuracy and reliability of echo-Doppler techniques and the maturation of color-flow Doppler and cardiac magnetic resonance imaging (MRI). Because gross cardiac anatomy can generally be well defined by echocardiographic methods, catheterization need only by done if certain hemodynamic information (e.g., shunt size or pulmonary vascular resistance) is important to the surgical procedure or if catheter interventional methods are contemplated. Angiography remains the best study for peripheral pulmonary artery lesions or coronary anomalies. In children, it is particularly important that catheterization information be obtained in combination with the noninvasive data to avoid acquiring redundant or insufficient data.

## COMPLICATIONS ASSOCIATED WITH CARDIAC CATHETERIZATION

The overall risks of cardiac catheterization are difficult to define because of wide discrepancies in the methods used to collect this information and because of the recent advances in the procedure itself (such as the introduction of nonionic radiographic contrast or the use of the percutaneous brachial artery approach rather than brachial artery cutdown). For the purpose of this discussion, several large multicenter trials, the American Heart Association's Cooperative Study on cardiac catheterization (Braunwald and Swan, 1968), and the Society of Cardiac Angiography's Registry (Johnson et al., 1989; Kennedy, 1982) are considered representative. Two studies evaluating the specific risk of coronary angiography are also available: a survey by Adams and associates (1973) of 46,904 patients and the report from the Collaborative Study of Coronary Artery Surgery that included 7553 prospectively studied patients reported in 1979 (Davis et al., 1979). The major complications reported in each of these studies are shown in Table 31–1.

Death rates from cardiac catheterization range from 0.14 to 0.75%, depending on the population of patients and the era. The Registry report analyzed the characteristics of patients at highest risk for death, and these data are summarized in Table 31–2. The

■ **Table 31–2.** HIGH-RISK PROFILE FOR MORTALITY FROM CARDIAC CATHETERIZATION

| Parameter | % |
|---|---|
| Overall mortality | 0.14 |
| Age | |
|   <1 year | 1.75 |
|   >60 years | 0.25 |
| Coronary disease | |
|   One-vessel disease | 0.03 |
|   Three-vessel disease | 0.16 |
|   Left main disease | 0.86 |
| Heart failure | |
|   NYHA FC I or II | 0.02 |
|   NYHA FC III | 0.12 |
|   NYHA FC IV | 0.67 |
| Valvular disease | |
|   All valvular disease patients | 0.28 |
|   Mitral disease | 0.34 |
|   Aortic disease | 0.19 |

*Key:* NYHA = New York Heart Association; FC = functional class.

highest-risk patients in the adult population are those with significant disease in the left main coronary artery and poor left ventricular function. In addition, the extremes of age and the presence of associated valvular disease increase the observed risk of mortality during cardiac catheterization.

The risk of myocardial infarction varies from 0.06 to 0.07%, cerebrovascular accidents from 0.03 to 0.2%, and significant bradyarrhythmias or tachyarrhythmias from 0.56 to 1.3%. Reports of local arterial problems have varied widely, and most series suggest a slightly higher incidence of complications when the brachial approach is used. Women appear more likely to incur vascular complications than men (Bourassa and Noble, 1976). Local complications include thrombosis, subcutaneous hematoma formation (occasionally extensive), recurrent bleeding, pseudoaneurysm formation, and, rarely, cellutitis or phlebitis. Systemic reactions vary from mild vasovagal responses to severe vagal discharges that lead to cardiac arrest. Hypotension may also result from various mechanisms that include the vasodepressor vagal response, vasodilation occurring after ionic contrast ventriculography, diuresis during the catheterization procedure, cardiac tamponade due to myocardial or coronary laceration, myocardial infarction, or an acute anaphylactoid reaction to the contrast media. Less common complications include precipitation of pulmonary edema, showering of cholesterol emboli (trash foot), and injury (dissection) of the coronary or pulmonary arteries.

After the procedure, diuresis from the radiographic contrast load and subsequent hypotension are common. Liberal use of fluids usually restores the blood pressure. Reactions to protamine sulfate can also occur if it is used to reverse the effects of heparin, and pulmonary emboli have been reported as a late sequela.

Controversy exists concerning the optimal vascular access approach (femoral or brachial) and whether heparin should be used routinely. It is also unclear whether there is a minimal number of catheterization procedures that each physician must do to maintain proficiency (Fisher, 1983), but 100 to 150 procedures each year should be considered minimal for diagnostic procedures. The safety and efficacy of free-standing cardiac catheterization laboratories in nontraditional settings such as mobile laboratories or free-standing laboratories are being scrutinized carefully. It is clear that supervised mobile settings can be operated safely, but free-standing units have yet to demonstrate that oversight is adequate to ensure efficacy and safety, and they are generally not recommended.

A final unresolved controversy concerns the use of nonionic versus ionic contrast media. Using ionic contrast media, several reviews have suggested an overall contrast-related toxicity in 1.4 to 2.26% of cases (Fareed et al., 1984; Shehadi, 1982). Ionic contrast produces various adverse hemodynamic and electrophysiologic effects during coronary angiography. Most of these adverse events are clearly related to the osmolality, sodium content, and calcium binding characteristics of the ionic contrast solutions. In addition, myocardial depression, peripheral vasodilation, and increased coronary flow results (Fischer and Thomson, 1978). Nonionic contrast agents clearly reduce acute adverse hemodynamic and electrophysiologic reactions (Bashore et al., 1988; Higgins et al., 1980), experimentally may reduce nephrotoxicity in patients at highest risk and appear to release less histamine from mast cells, and potentially reduce allergic reactions (Humes et al., 1988; Salem et al., 1986). Clinical studies completed at Duke University Medical Center suggest no advantage of nonionic over ionic agents in preventing nephrotoxicity in patients with normal renal function (Davidson et al., 1988; Schwab et al., 1989), but others have suggested a modest advantage in patients with elevated serum creatinine (especially in association with diabetes mellitus (Manske et al., 1990). The question of some inherent thrombogenicity of nonionic agents has also been raised (Grollman et al., 1988) and may relate to the formation of "thin" fibrin in the clot (Granger et al., 1992). The difference in costs between ionic and nonionic media is substantial (ionic being 15- to 20-fold less expensive), which makes the routine use of nonionic contrast controversial, especially as we move to a managed care environment, where costs are a greater issue than patient comfort (ACC Cardiovascular Imaging Committee, 1993).

## BASIC CATHETER TECHNIQUES

Most cardiac catheterization procedures in the United States are now done by the femoral approach, with a minority done via the brachial artery. The relevant basic concepts are described later (for further details, see Chapter 54).

The brachial (Sones) approach can be done either by cutdown or by percutaneous insertion of the catheter system in the brachial artery (Pepine et al., 1984). Adjunctive systemic heparin is generally also used in most laboratories. A catheter is then passed either directly into the artery or through a sheath placed in the vessel, and the catheter is advanced to the aortic root and eventually to the coronary arteries and left ventricle. Different catheters can be used to cannulate each coronary ostium as well as to obtain pressure data from the left ventricle by retrograde insertion across the aortic valve. Left ventriculography is done by power injection of the left ventricle with radiographic contrast; coronary angiography is usually done by hand injection of contrast. The Sones technique allows good catheter control but requires greater operator skill, and when an antecubital dissection is required to expose the artery, vascular repair is required at the end of the procedure. The preformed catheters traditionally used for the femoral approach have been used with the brachial approach, with good results.

The Judkins approach is less traumatic, allows the operator to be further removed from the x-ray source (reducing operator exposure), and is done through a percutaneous needle puncture of the femoral artery. After insertion of a guidewire through the entry needle, either a sheath and then a catheter or the catheter alone is placed in the femoral vessel. The catheter is then advanced to the heart. Left-sided heart catheterization generally uses three preformed catheters—one for each coronary artery and a pigtail catheter with multiple side holes for left-sided ventriculography. Surgical repair of the vessel is not required, and the coronary catheters generally seek the coronary ostia with minimal manipulation, requiring less skill on the part of the physician performing the catheterization. A single-catheter system from the femoral artery is also used in a few institutions (Schoonmaker and King, 1974).

Because some patients have severe iliac or aortic vascular disease that prohibits the femoral approach, cardiologists should have experience with both the Judkins and the Sones techniques. The familiarity the physician has with one procedure or the other appears to be a greater determinant of the risks of the brachial versus femoral approach than does the access site alone (Johnson, 1989).

Transseptal left-sided heart catheterization (O'Keefe et al., 1985) has become infrequent in many cardiac catheterization laboratories. However, with the growing popularity of some prosthetic valves in the aortic position (i.e., the disk valves such as the St. Jude valve) that cannot safely be crossed retrogradely at catheterization, and with the emergence of percutaneous balloon mitral commissurotomy as a viable option to surgical commissurotomy, the transseptal procedure has become more widely used. The transseptal catheter is a short, curved catheter with a tapered tip and side holes. In one approach, it is placed in the right atrium over a 70-cm curved Brockenbrough needle inserted through the catheter until it is just inside the catheter tip. Techniques vary, but in general the catheter-needle combination is manipulated into the fossa ovalis while atrial pressure is continuously monitored. Mere advancement of the catheter system against the fossa ovalis often causes the catheter-needle apparatus to enter the left atrium. If this does not occur, the needle tip is abruptly advanced several millimeters out the distal catheter tip into the left atrium. Further manipulations advance the catheter into the left ventricle, and left ventricular pressures and angiograms are obtained. The mitral gradient (left atrium vs. left ventricle) can be obtained or pulmonary veins can be injected as necessary. The major risk of transseptal catheterization lies in inadvertent puncture of atrial structures, such as the atrial free wall or coronary sinus, or entry into the aortic root.

Right ventricular endomyocardial biopsy is readily done with little risk (Mason, 1978). Both an internal jugular and a femoral vein approach are available. From the neck, the bioptome is usually directed without a sheath while the intracardiac electrogram is monitored. From the leg, the bioptome is guided with an appropriate guiding sheath to sample the interventricular septum. Approximately 1 mg of tissue is obtained with each biopsy. Multiple biopsy samples can be obtained at one setting. In experienced centers, biopsies can be obtained using echocardiography rather than fluoroscopy. Finally, catheterization of the coronary sinus can be achieved with some difficulty from brachial, subclavian, or femoral access sites. Coronary sinus flow and metabolism studies as well as oxygen content can be assessed (Baim et al., 1982) and may be useful after interventions. The coronary sinus may also provide a "back door" to the coronary circulation through which supportive therapy may be delivered to ischemic myocardium.

## BASIC FUNCTION OF THE X-RAY SYSTEM

High-quality cine film is essential for appropriate assessment of angiographic catheterization results. Details of such filming are available from other sources (Curry et al., 1984). A basic understanding is useful, though, for every physician who wishes to examine the results of cardiac catheterization. A brief overview of this area is now provided.

The major components of the cardiac catheterization x-ray system are shown schematically in Fig. 31–1. This schematic ignores the complex interrelated electronics, switching devices, collimators, and so on

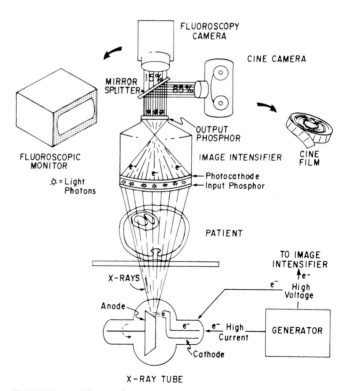

FIGURE 31–1. *The cinefluoroscopy system.* The current from the generator powers the image intensifier and x-ray tube. Electrons *(e⁻)* flow through the x-ray tube cathode, and then "jump" to bombard the anode, where they are converted to x-rays. X-rays pass through the patient to the face of the image intensifier. From here they are converted to light, then back to electrons. These electrons are then accelerated to the output phosphor where an image is visible. The x-ray–enhanced image is then picked up by the fluoroscopy camera or reflected to the cine camera.

required to eventually produce an x-ray image. It concentrates on the practical aspects of how electrons are converted to x-rays and how these x-rays eventually produce a visual outline of the cardiac structures.

The story begins in the generator. Two types of current are produced by the generator: one high in voltage (the "strength" of the current) and one high in amperage (the number of electrons). The x-ray tube is a vacuum tube within which reside a cathode and an anode. The cathode is a coil through which the high-amperage current from the generator is passed. High voltage (25,000 volts) is then applied across the x-ray tube, causing electrons in the cathode to "jump" over to the anode and release x-rays. By slanting of the anode's surface, the resultant x-ray beam can be directed out of the x-ray tube and subsequently through the patient to the image intensifier. The system is inefficient, and only one x-ray is produced for each 100 electrons.

As the x-rays pass from the x-ray tube toward the image intensifier, they diverge. The patient absorbs some of the x-rays, some reach the image intensifier, and the remainder are scattered. Extensive measures to ensure protection from this scatter radiation are rigorously practiced in all laboratories. The various tissues absorb x-rays in a differential manner, and this variable penetration eventually results in certain body structures being outlined on the final image. Radiographic contrast containing iodine is used in all angiography specifically because the iodine atom absorbs these x-ray photons so well.

The x-rays that reach the face of the image intensifier produce a faint image. The image intensifier strengthens this image by two methods: by a minification or shrinking of the size of the image and by electronic enhancement of the image by accelerating electrons through the intensifier (using the high voltage from the generator). The face of the image intensifier is covered by an input phosphor that converts the x-ray photon energy to light, which then travels a minuscule distance before it meets a photocathode. When light strikes the photocathode, an electron is produced. The high-voltage field then accelerates these electrons toward the output phosphor, where they are converted back to light. The result is a visible x-ray image. The image on the output phosphor can be viewed with the eye.

The light next passes through a mirror splitter placed in the output path from the image intensifier. Differential silvering of the mirror allows a certain amount of light to pass through to the fluoroscopic video camera (usually about 15%), while the remainder of the image is reflected to the 35mm cine camera. When cine film is to be recorded, the operator activates the cine camera by a foot switch, and film exposure begins (usually at speeds of 30 to 60 frames per second). The cine film is developed in a manner similar to the 35mm film development process.

The final step in viewing the film is the cine projector. Because the eye can detect flicker at framing rates less than 50 frames per second, and because most cardiac catheterization laboratories expose film at 30 frames per second, flicker would be routinely seen in reviewing cine film. To avoid flicker during cine review, the cine projector projects each frame twice, thus misleading the eye and brain into perceiving that the true filming rate is double the actual. The result is a flicker-free image.

In the 1990s, many changes are occurring in this entire system. Some of those changes are imminent, but others are under active development at many sites around the world. There is a gradual trend away from x-ray systems that produce only cine film to those that produce computerized digital images or enhanced video data. The advantages are numerous but include flicker-free images even at very low frame rates, the ability to use less x-ray exposure, the ability to immediately access the image data without waiting for film processing, the ability to improve the images even after the catheterization study is completed, and the opportunity to apply quantitative computer algorithms to the image data. Thus, one can obtain quantitative and qualitative information in addition to the visual observations. This revolution requires a storage medium different from cine film, however, and that transition is still one of the major obstacles to the widespread application of routine digital angiographic systems. A cooperative venture between manufacturers and physicians has produced an agreement to store digital images in a common format (DICOM 3 standard). A computer medium to transfer film data between laboratories will soon become available (rewritable CD-ROM). As large, mass-storage devices are developed, cine film will no longer be used, and all-digital imaging laboratories will become commonplace in the next decade. This will allow networking of the image data and improve access considerably.

## HEMODYNAMIC MEASUREMENTS

### Pressure Measurement

#### Methods

One of the major goals of cardiac catheterization is to record the pressure waveforms and their magnitude from various vascular structures. Although this may superficially appear readily obtainable, there are some important errors inherent in the measurement of these data that should be recognized to avoid overdependence on small variations in the values obtained.

Any pressure data obtained from inside vascular organs reflects the sum of the pressures not only in the chamber being analyzed but also in the contiguous structures around that chamber. For example, because the heart is in the pericardium and both structures are surrounded by the lungs, changes in either pulmonary or pericardial pressure can be expected to alter intracardiac pressure. Likewise, ventricular interaction causes the pressure of one ventricle to affect the pressure in the other. Physiologic variations such as simple respiration also affect all of the pressure data. The "hard" numbers reported from cardiac catheterization thus reflect only the average data at an arbitrary point in time. This does not imply that the data are incorrect, but rather that they represent only an average value considering the expected normal physiologic variation. Some pathologic states and conditions obviously affect these values to an even greater degree.

Sources of error in the measurement of pressures include the routine use of fluid-filled catheters; poor zeroing practices (in which the transducer diaphragm is not placed at midchest); air, kinking, or other obstructions in the tubing between the catheter and the diaphragm (resulting in damping of the pressure); and, perhaps most common, catheter whip artifact as the fluid-filled catheter tip is flexed inside the beating heart or great vessels. In addition, end-hole catheter pressure data may not be the same as side-hole pressure data, particularly in areas of streaming or high velocity. In small vessels or valvular orifices, the catheters themselves may also become partially obstructive.

Although micromanometer-tip catheters greatly reduce many of these errors, they have been impractical in most clinical situations. Therefore, pressure data from fluid-filled systems must be interpreted with the appreciation of the inherent pitfalls in the actual data derived. When data do not agree with the clinical situation, it is wise to reexamine the pressure data to ensure that none of the mentioned artifacts are present.

### Normal Pressure Waveforms

Normal waveforms must be appreciated if the effects of pathologic states are to be understood. Subtle alterations in pressure waveforms can affect the detection and quantitation of certain myocardial, valvular, and pericardial disease states.

The range and average for normal right-sided and left-sided heart pressures are outlined in Table 31–3. Whenever fluid is compressed within a chamber or added to the chamber, the pressure rises; conversely, whenever fluid is lost from a chamber or the chamber expands (goes into diastole), the pressure falls. This simple construct can explain all of the various waveforms noted. Normal waveforms are outlined in Figures 31–2 and 31–3.

The *right atrial pressure waveform* consists of two major positive deflections that are called A and V waves. The A wave is due to atrial systolic contraction and follows electrical activation of the atria (represented by the P wave of the electrocardiogram). When atrial contraction occurs, the tricuspid valve is open. The height of the A wave thus reflects not only the vigor of the atrial contraction but also the resistance presented by the diastolic right ventricle. The height of the A wave increases when there is poor compliance of the right ventricle. Ventricular systole begins immediately after atrial contraction. The pressure rise in the right ventricle closes the tricuspid valve, causing protrusion of the valve into the right atrium, reducing right atrial volume slightly and causing the C wave. As right ventricular contraction continues, the tricuspid annulus is pulled into the body of the

**■ Table 31–3.** NORMAL PRESSURES IN THE HEART AND VASCULATURE

|  | Range (mm Hg) | Average (mm Hg) |
|---|---|---|
| *Cardiac Chambers* | | |
| Right atrium | | |
|   a wave | 3–7 | 6 |
|   v wave | 2–7 | 5 |
|   Mean | 1–5 | 3 |
| Right ventricle | | |
|   Peak systolic | 17–30 | 26 |
|   End-diastolic | 1–7 | 5 |
| Pulmonary artery | | |
|   Peak systolic | 17–30 | 25 |
|   End-diastolic | 5–13 | 9 |
|   Mean | 9–19 | 15 |
| Pulmonary capillary wedge | | |
|   Mean | 5–13 | 9 |
| Left atrium | | |
|   a wave | 4–16 | 10 |
|   v wave | 3–12 | 8 |
|   Mean | 6–21 | 13 |
| *Vasculature* | | |
| Aorta | | |
|   Peak systolic | 85–140 | 125 |
|   End-diastolic | 60–90 | 70 |
|   Mean | 70–105 | 80 |
| Right brachial | | |
|   Peak systolic | 90–140 | 130 |
|   End-diastolic | 60–90 | 70 |
|   Mean | 70–105 | 85 |
| Left brachial | | |
|   Peak systolic | 85–140 | 125 |
|   End-diastolic | 60–90 | 70 |
|   Mean | 70–105 | 83 |
| Femoral artery | | |
|   Peak systolic | 95–150 | 135 |
|   End-diastolic | 60–90 | 70 |
|   Mean | 75–115 | 90 |

right ventricle, and the atrium concurrently goes into diastole. This combination reduces right atrial pressure, the X descent. Atrial filling occurs during late ventricular systole and causes a gradual rise in atrial pressure, which peaks at the V wave. The tricuspid valve then opens and atrial pressure falls (the Y descent). The atrium and ventricle once again function as a common chamber, and atrial and ventricular diastolic pressures eventually equalize during the remainder of diastole. The magnitude of the atrial V wave is indirectly related to atrial compliance and directly related to the amount of blood returning to the atrium from the periphery.

The *left atrial pressure waveform* is similar to the right atrial waveform except that the V wave is usually higher than the A wave. This occurs because the left atrium is a thicker-walled chamber, is in a relatively confined space, and is restricted posteriorly by the four pulmonary veins. Conversely, the right atrium is readily decompressed by the inferior and superior venae cavae. Indeed, when left atrial compliance is poor and atrial flow is high, a large left atrial V wave can be noted even in the absence of mitral valve regurgitation (Fuchs et al., 1982).

The *pulmonary artery wedge pressure waveform* is similar to that of the left atrial pressure, but it is usually

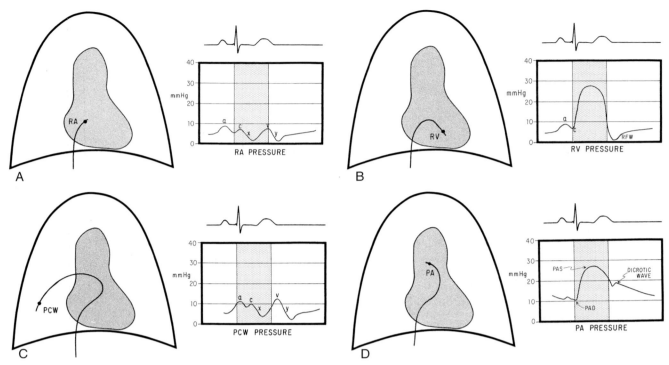

**FIGURE 31–2.** *Normal pressure waveforms during right-sided heart catheterization.* Each frame illustrates an anteroposterior schematic view of the catheter position (as seen during fluroscopy) along with the characteristic pressure waveform obtained via the catheter in that location. *A,* Right atrium (RA). *B,* Right ventricle (RV). *C,* Pulmonary capillary wedge (PCW)—note the temporal delay in the pressure waveform. *D,* Pulmonary artery (PA). See text for explanation of a, c, v waves and x, y descents. (PAS and PAD = pulmonary artery systolic and diastolic pressures, respectively; RFW = rapid-filling wave.)

dampened, and there is a delay in transmission of this waveform through the pulmonary capillary vessels. In particular disease states, and occasionally after procedures such as mitral valve replacement, the pulmonary artery wedge pressure may not accurately reflect left atrial pressure (Schoenfeld et al., 1985).

The diastolic phases of the *right* and *left ventricular pressures* differ primarily only in the magnitude of the waveforms. The ventricular diastolic pressure is characterized by a rapid initial decline followed by a brief rapid-filling phase and then a longer slow-filling phase. At the most negative point, early in the ventricular diastolic pressure tracing, almost half of ventricular filling has already occurred. After the rapid-filling wave, about 25% of the ventricular filling occurs during the slow-filling period in mid-diastole. A final 15 to 25% enters the ventricle during atrial systolic contraction (Rankin et al., 1988). The rise in pressure during atrial systole is referred to as the ventricular A wave, and the pressure crossing at the end of the A wave and the rise in the ventricular pressure is called the C point. This point is generally chosen as the ventricular end-diastolic pressure. When the C point is not well seen, the peak of the R wave from the simultaneous electrocardiogram is used to define end-diastole.

The *pulmonary artery pressure waveform* reflects the systolic right ventricular pressure. When right ventricular pressure declines, the pulmonary pressure falls until the pulmonary valve closes. A notch or incisura is then evident. The high compliance (low

resistance) in the pulmonary circuit often causes this incisura to be delayed (referred to as *hangout*). A small dicrotic wave is usually seen and is followed by a slow fall in the pulmonary diastolic pressure until the initiation of ventricular systole again. A small systolic pressure gradient normally exists between the right ventricle and pulmonary artery. Right atrial contraction occasionally produces a small pressure deformation just before the minimal pulmonary artery pressure. This is reflected as a wave in the pulmonary artery pressure tracing.

Arterial resistance is determined by the smaller arteries (<1,000 μm), the arterioles (20 to 200 μm), and the capillaries. An abrupt change in resistance occurs over a short path between the peripheral arteries and veins. The systolic *aortic pulse* is a composite of waves that results from forward flow (the percussion wave), a reflected wave from upper-extremity resistance (the tidal wave), and a reflected wave from lower-body resistance after aortic valve closure (the dicrotic wave) (O'Rourke, 1982). As blood moves from the central aorta toward the periphery, the height of the pulse pressure increases because there is less elastic tissue in the descending aorta and because the wavefront approaches the areas of the resistance vessels at the periphery. The reflected wave thus summates with the forward wavefront, and the height of the pressure wave increases toward the periphery (McDonald and Taylor, 1959; O'Rourke, 1967). Therefore, central aortic pressure may not be equal to the peripheral pressure. In addition, the relatively direct ejection of blood into

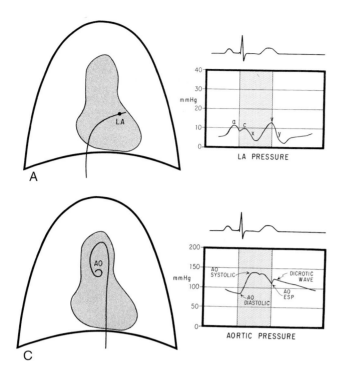

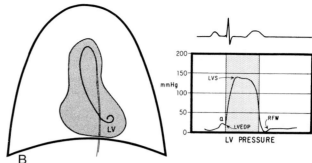

**FIGURE 31–3.** *Normal left-sided pressure waveforms* showing catheter position yielding the pressure data from that location, similar to Figure 31–2. *A,* Left atrium (LA). *B,* Left ventricle (LV). *C,* Aorta (AO). (See text for explanation of a, c, v waves and x, y descents.) (LVS and LVEDP = left ventricular systolic and end-diastolic pressures, respectively; RFW = rapid-filling wave, AO ESP = aortic end-systolic pressure.)

the right subclavian artery often makes the systolic pressure in the right brachial artery slightly higher than that of the left brachial artery. Representative pressure recordings from the ascending aorta to the femoral artery are shown in Figure 31–4.

Mean arterial pressure is calculated traditionally as the pressure at one-third of the value between diastole and systolic pressure (because the shape of the pressure waveform is approximately triangular). Although these mean pressure calculations are reason-

ably accurate in the peripheral circulation, the actual mean pressure may be closer to midway between systolic and diastolic pressure in the central aorta. In gross terms, the difference between systolic and diastolic pressure, or pulse pressure, reflects both stroke volume and arterial cushioning (compliance), whereas the mean pressure more closely represents conduit function (peripheral resistance). With aging, both the pulse pressure and the mean arterial pressure normally rise (see Fig. 31–4).

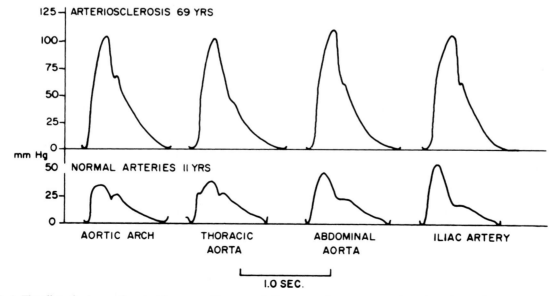

**FIGURE 31–4.** *The effect of aging on the arterial pressure.* The normal discrepancy between central aortic and peripheral pressure lessens with age. (From O'Rourke, M. F.: Wave reflections. *In* O'Rourke, M. F. [ed]: Arterial Function in Health and Disease. New York, Churchill Livingstone, 1982.)

■ **Table 31–4.** VASCULAR RESISTANCE UNITS—NORMAL VALUES

| Measurement | Absolute Units dyn · sec · cm$^{-5}$ | Wood Units mm Hg · min · liters$^{-1}$ |
|---|---|---|
| Total pulmonary resistance | 205 ± 51 | 2.5 ± 1.0 |
| Pulmonary vascular resistance | 67 ± 30 | 1 ± 0.5 |
| Systemic vascular resistance | 1170 ± 270 | 15 ± 3.5 |

## Vascular Resistance Measurement

With the analogy of Ohm's law to vascular flow, resistance calculations have proved clinically useful. Normal values are shown in Table 31–4, and the general equations are shown in Figure 31–5.

To determine the resistance across any particular vascular bed, one must know the mean pressures just proximal and distal to the bed and the flow through the vascular bed. Pulmonary vascular resistance thus uses the mean pulmonary pressure, the mean pulmonary capillary wedge pressure, and the cardiac output. Systemic vascular resistance can be defined with the mean systemic pressure and the mean right atrial pressure; if the right atrial pressure is unknown, it can be dropped, and the result is called total peripheral resistance. Resistance in the pulmonary circuit not only can be affected by pressure and flow but also may vary with the "critical closing pressure" of the pulmonary vasculature (McGregor and Sniderman, 1985). The zones of the lung from which the pulmonary capillary wedge pressure is measured may also vary slightly.

To describe the arterial system accurately, one should consider arterial compliance and the blood viscosity in a frequency-dependent model. Impedance calculations relate pressure to flow as a function of frequency. The relationship between pressure and flow cannot be readily obtained clinically, nor is this relationship readily apparent by inspecting either the pressure curve or the flow contour. Impedance measurements, therefore, have not been widely adopted because of the difficulty in obtaining the simultaneous pressure and flow data required.

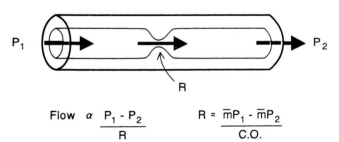

$$\text{Flow} \ \alpha \ \frac{P_1 - P_2}{R} \qquad R = \frac{\overline{m}P_1 - \overline{m}P_2}{\text{C.O.}}$$

**FIGURE 31–5.** *Calculation of peripheral resistance.* Flow is proportional to the difference in pressures (P) from one end of the "pipe" to the other and is inversely related to the resistance (R). Resistance measurements require knowledge of mean (static) pressures ($\overline{m}$P) and flow (cardiac output [C.O.]).

## Cardiac Output Measurements: Indicator-Dilution Measures

There is no accurate way to measure cardiac output in vivo, but one can base cardiac output estimates on various assumptions. Generally, the two major methods clinically used for the measurement of cardiac output are the Fick method and thermodilution method. Cardiac output is often normalized for the patient's size according to the body surface area and is expressed as cardiac index. This assumption, like many "facts" in medicine, is open to question, but it has generally proven useful clinically.

The indicator-dilution method has been used to measure cardiac output since its introduction by Stewart (1897), with modifications by Hamilton and associates (1932). The basic equation, commonly referred to as the Stewart-Hamilton equation, is shown below:

Cardiac output (l/min) =
$$\frac{\text{amount of indicator injected (mg)} \times 60 \text{ sec/min}}{\text{mean indicator concentration (mg/ml)} \times \text{curve duration}}$$

The assumption is that the injection of a certain amount of an indicator into the circulation appears and then disappears from any downstream point in a manner commensurate with the cardiac output. For example, if the indicator rapidly appears at a particular point downstream and washes out quickly, the assumption is that the cardiac output is high. Although sites may vary, the site of injection is usually a systemic vein on the right side of the heart, and the site of sampling is generally a systemic artery. The normal curve itself has an initial rapid upstroke followed by a slower downstroke and eventually the appearance of recirculation of the tracer. In reality, this recirculation creates some uncertainty at the end of the curve, and assumptions are made to correct for this distortion. Because the indicator concentration declines exponentially in the absence of recirculation, the initial data points from the descending limb are used to extrapolate the area under the ascending and descending limbs. The results, therefore, assume that the ascending and descending limbs form a triangular shape. The base of this triangle then represents the total curve duration, and the mean area of the triangle is assumed to be a function of the mean indicator concentration. Both of these can be used to determine the cardiac output by using the Stewart-Hamilton equation. A representative curve is shown in Figure 31–6.

There are several sources of error in this particular approach. When indocyanine green dye is used, fresh preparations are necessary because the dye is unstable over time and can be affected by light. The exact amount of dye is also critical to the performance of the study, and this must be accurately measured, generally in a tuberculin syringe, and rapidly injected as a single bolus. The indicator, when injected, must also mix well before reaching the sampling site, and the dilution curve must have an exponential decay

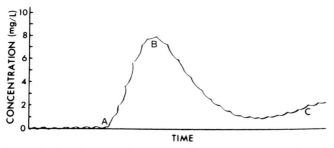

**FIGURE 31–6.** *Representative normal indicator-dilution curve.* The indocyanine green dye is injected on the right side of the heart and sampled on the left side of the circulation. The dye is first detected at A and initially peaks at B. After washout, recirculation of the dye around the body occurs and the density is noted at C. (From Grossman, W.: Blood flow measurement: The cardiac output. *In* Grossman, W. [ed]: Cardiac Catheterization and Angiography. 3rd ed. Philadelphia, Lea & Febiger, 1986.)

over time to allow extrapolation. Extrapolation is particularly significant if, for example, there is severe valvular regurgitation or a low-output state in which the washout of the indicator is so prolonged that recirculation begins well before there has been an adequate decline in the indicator curve. Thus, the green dye method is inaccurate in patients with regurgitant lesions or low cardiac output states. Intracardiac shunts may also greatly affect the shape of the curve.

### Thermodilution Techniques

The rather tedious and time-consuming indicator-dilution techniques have been replaced by the thermodilution techniques. The popularity of the Swan-Ganz catheter has greatly expanded the ability to obtain thermodilution cardiac outputs in many clinical settings.

The thermodilution procedure requires the injection of a bolus of cool liquid (saline or dextrose) into the proximal port of the catheter. The resultant change in temperature due to the cool liquid is measured by a thermistor mounted in the distal end of the catheter. The change in temperature can be plotted versus time in a manner similar to the dye-dilution method described (wherein the indicator is now the cooler temperature). The cardiac output is then calculated by a rather complex equation that considers the temperature of the injectate and the temperature of the blood together with the volume and the specific gravity. In addition, certain calibration factors are used. The basic concept is that the cardiac output is inversely related to the area under a thermodilution curve plotted as temperature versus time. The smaller the area, the higher the cardiac output.

The thermodilution method has several advantages. Not only does it obviate the need to withdraw blood or perform an arterial puncture, it is affected less by recirculation. Perhaps its greatest advantage is the rapid display of results via computer. Computers use the washout rate of the downslope of the curve to obtain a decay constant. This method allows recon-

struction of the triangular-shaped curve and the area under the curve. With knowledge of the injectate volume, temperature, and specific gravity, as well as the blood temperature and its specific gravity, plus the area under the curve, one can calculate cardiac output.

Thermodilution cardiac outputs are susceptible to problems like those of indicator-dilution methods using green dye. Because the data represent right-sided heart output, tricuspid regurgitation can be a particular problem as the bolus of saline is subsequently broken up. Thermodilution tends to overestimate the cardiac output in states of low cardiac output because the loss of the cold temperature to the surrounding cardiac structures reduces the total area under the curve. This creates a falsely high cardiac output value. Other problems include fluctuations in blood temperature during respiratory or cardiac cycles and the warming of the injectate before its injection into the catheter.

From a practical viewpoint, thermodilution cardiac outputs have become standard. Their range can be relatively broad, however, and small changes should not be overinterpreted. It is estimated that, overall, cardiac output data can only be defined to ±15% (Grondelle et al., 1983).

### Fick Cardiac Output Principle

The Fick principle, first espoused by Adolph Fick (1870), assumes that the rate at which oxygen is consumed is a function of the rate of blood flow times the rate of oxygen pickup by the red blood cells. The basic assumptions are shown schematically in Figure 31–7. In simple terms, it is assumed that the same number of red blood cells that enter the lung leave the lung. If one knows how many oxygen molecules were attached to the red blood cells entering the lung,

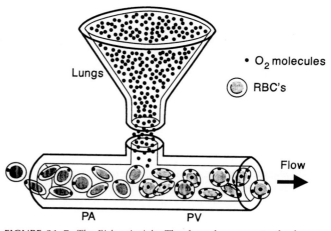

**FIGURE 31–7.** *The Fick principle.* The funnel represents the lungs. As the red blood cells (RBCs) pass through the lungs, oxygen (black dots) is picked up. The cardiac output is determined by knowing the hemoglobin and oxygen saturation in the pulmonary artery (PA), the oxygen consumption per minute (the amount being picked up by the red cells), and the oxygen saturation in the pulmonary veins (PV). The rate of flow = oxygen consumption/A-Vo₂ difference.

how many oxygen molecules were attached to the red blood cells leaving the lung, and how much oxygen was consumed during travel through the lung, then one can determine the rate of flow of these red blood cells as they passed through the lung. This can be expressed in the following terms:

$$\text{Cardiac output (l/min)} = \frac{O_2 \text{ consumption (ml/min)}}{\text{A-Vo}_2 \text{ difference (vol\%)} \times 10}$$

Measurements must be done in steady state. Automated methods can accurately determine the oxygen content within the blood samples; the more difficult measurement is that of the oxygen consumption. Van Slyke's method was traditionally used in the past; in it, expiratory gas samples are collected in a large bag over a particular period. By measuring the oxygen consumption within the bag and by knowing the amount of room air oxygen, one could determine the amount of oxygen consumed per volume over time. Newer devices now measure oxygen consumption polargraphically: expired oxygen can be quantitated by noting the change in electrical current between a gold cathode and silver anode embedded in a potassium chloride gel. These devices can be connected to the patient via a plastic hood or a mouthpiece and tubing.

The Fick method suffers primarily from the vagaries of obtaining accurate oxygen consumption measurements and the inability to obtain a steady state under certain conditions. It requires considerable time and effort on the part of the catheterization laboratory to obtain the appropriate data. Most laboratories use an "assumed" Fick method in which oxygen consumption is assumed on the basis of the patient's age, sex, and body surface area or is estimated using body surface area (125 ml/m²). This method may err greatly if the patient is seriously ill. The advantage of the Fick method is that it is most accurate in patients with low cardiac output and thus provides better data than thermodilution does in these situations. It is also independent of the factors that affect curve shape (discussed earlier), which may introduce errors when using thermodilution or indicator-dilution methods. Variability is ±10%; this may be even higher when only an assumed oxygen consumption is available.

## SHUNT DETERMINATIONS

### Oximetric Method

Various techniques are now available to assist in the determination of intracardiac shunts. In most cases, intracardiac shunting is suspected before catheterization is done. Because routine right-sided heart catheterizations are becoming less common, the opportunity to detect small left-to-right shunts at catheterization has declined. The increased use of echocardiography, however, has clearly allowed the cardiac catheterization procedure to be more focused, which compensates for this loss. Shunts can be measured both noninvasively and invasively by various meth-

ods. In the invasive laboratory, shunts are most commonly measured by noting the presence of saturated blood in chambers supplied by the venous system (the oximetric method). A left-to-right shunt can be located and detected if a significant "step-up" in blood oxygen saturation or contents is observed in one of the right-sided heart chambers (Antman et al., 1980; Dexter et al., 1947). Also, the continuous registration of oxygen saturation is now possible with a fiberoptic catheter.

Before blood oxygen level can accurately measure abnormal shunting, however, a review of the normal chamber saturations is important. The inferior vena cava oxygen content is essentially always higher than the superior vena cava oxygen content, because the kidneys use substantially less oxygen relative to their blood flow than do the other organs. Renal vein oxygen saturation is therefore high. As blood returns to the right atrium from the inferior vena cava, it is directed toward the interatrial septum by the eustachian valve, which creates turbulence and nonuniform mixing. In addition, small amounts of blood with very low oxygen saturation flow into the right atrium from the coronary sinus. Thus, the right atrium receives three different sources of blood with quite different oxygen saturations. For this reason, a great deal of physiologic variability in oxygen saturation is seen in the right atrium, and it is important to appreciate that random right atrial blood samples may vary considerably. More complete mixing occurs as blood enters the right ventricle and then the pulmonary artery. Therefore, mixed venous saturation is most accurately measured in the pulmonary artery. As expected from the physiologic variability noted, the maximal allowable step-up in oxygen content varies considerably from one chamber to another in the right side of the heart. This variability makes it more difficult to detect a small shunt at the atrial level than at the ventricular or pulmonary artery level. In fact, assuming a systemic cardiac index of 3 l/min/m², oximetry cannot accurately detect a shunt of less than 1.5:1 at the atrial level, whereas the smallest detectable shunt at the ventricular or great vessel level is 1.3:1. Fortunately, from a clinical standpoint, most important shunts are much greater than this.

To detect a shunt, one must obtain the oxygen saturation of blood just before it enters the chamber receiving the shunt and note the amount of oxygen step-up that occurs in the chamber. This creates the most difficulty when assessing left-to-right flow into the right atrium, because, as noted above, the vessels supplying the right atrium (the *superior vena cava* [SVC], *inferior vena cava* [IVC], and *coronary sinus* [CS]) each contain differing amounts of oxygen saturation. For this reason, several formulas have been devised to determine the mixed venous saturation at the level of the superior vena cava and inferior vena cava. The most common formula used (Flamm et al., 1969) is as follows:

Mixed venous oxygen content =

$$\frac{3 \text{ (SVC O}_2 \text{ content)} + 1 \text{ (IVC O}_2 \text{ content)}}{4}$$

■ **Table 31–5.** MINIMAL VARIATION IN OXYGEN CONTENT AND SATURATION AMONG RIGHT-SIDED HEART STRUCTURES TO DETECT A SHUNT

| Shunt | Step-up Sites | Minimal Change in Oxygen Content (Vol %) | Minimal Change in Oxygen Saturation Changes (%) |
|---|---|---|---|
| Patent ductus arteriosus | Right ventricle to pulmonary artery | 0.5 | 5 |
| Ventricular septal defect | Right atrium to right ventricle | 0.9 | 7 |
| Atrial septal defect | Mixed venous to right atrium | 1.9 | 11 |

Right atrial content should be the average of the high, low, and mid right atrial oxygen content; right ventricular oxygen content should be the average of the inflow and outflow right ventricular content. When these data are obtained, the presence or absence of a shunt can be defined (Table 31–5).

To determine the size of a left-to-right shunt, both pulmonary blood flow and the systemic blood flow determinations are required. The flow across any bed in the body can be defined by measuring the A-V$O_2$ difference across the bed and the oxygen consumption used.

*Pulmonary blood flow* (PBF) is equal to oxygen consumption divided by the saturation difference across the pulmonary bed (pulmonary venous minus pulmonary arterial). Similarly, *systemic blood flow* (SBF) is defined by the oxygen consumption divided by the systemic arterial oxygen minus mixed venous oxygen (the saturation difference across the systemic bed). These equations are shown below:

$$SBF = \frac{O_2 \text{ consumption}}{SA_{O_2} - MV_{O_2} \text{ (vol\%)} \times 10}$$

$$PBF = \frac{O_2 \text{ consumption}}{P\overline{V}_{O_2} - PA_{O_2} \text{ (vol\%)} \times 10}$$

A left-to-right shunt will cause the pulmonary blood flow to be higher than the systemic blood flow. To measure the shunt magnitude, a new term *effective pulmonary blood flow* (EPBF) must be understood. The effective pulmonary blood flow is defined as the fraction of mixed venous return received by the lungs without contamination by shunt flow. In the absence of a shunt, the effective pulmonary blood flow, the systemic blood flow, and the pulmonary blood flow are all equal.

In the presence of a left-to-right shunt, however, pulmonary blood flow is equal to the effective pulmonary blood flow plus the left-to-right shunt flow. The effective pulmonary blood flow is defined from the Fick equation as the oxygen consumption divided by the pulmonary venous oxygen content minus the mixed venous oxygen content:

$$EPBF = \frac{O_2 \text{ consumption (ml/min)}}{P\overline{V}_{O_2} - MV_{O_2} \text{ (vol\%)} \times 10}$$

The magnitude of a left-to-right shunt can therefore be defined as the pulmonary blood flow minus the effective pulmonary blood flow; the blood samples

used for an atrial septal defect are shown in Figure 31–8. Note that saturations are measured from the chamber just before the shunt origin and on either side of the shunt destination.

This calculation is similarly applicable to right-to-left shunts. In a right-to-left shunt, the shunt flow is added to the pulmonary blood flow to obtain total systemic blood flow. As in the previous example, a right-to-left shunt at the atrial level requires oxygen saturation from the chamber just before the shunt (the mixed venous) and from the chamber just before and after the shunt (the pulmonary venous and left ventricular or systemic arterial), respectively. The method of calculating a right-to-left shunt at the atrial level is thus shown in Figure 31–9. By using similar logic, shunts at any level (ventricular, great vessel) can be determined. These same equations can be used to determine bidirectional shunts.

### Indicator-Dilution Method

Indicator-dilution methods to detect shunts are more sensitive than oximetric methods but suffer from various limitations. There is a growing trend away from indicator-dilution methods in catheterization laboratories, so lack of familiarity also presents a great disadvantage. An indicator such as indocyanine

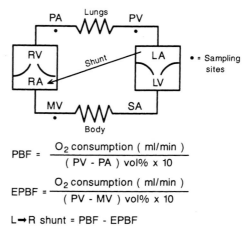

$$PBF = \frac{O_2 \text{ consumption ( ml/min )}}{( PV - PA ) \text{ vol\%} \times 10}$$

$$EPBF = \frac{O_2 \text{ consumption ( ml/min )}}{( PV - MV ) \text{ vol\%} \times 10}$$

L→R shunt = PBF − EPBF

**FIGURE 31–8.** *Use of oxygen saturations to calculate a left-to-right shunt at the atrial level.* Assuming an atrial septal defect with left-to-right shunt (L → R shunt), the sampling sites required are those just before the origin of the shunt (the pulmonary vein [PV]), and those before and after the shunt destination (the mixed venous [MV] and pulmonary artery [PA]). The left-to-right shunt plus the effective pulmonary blood flow (EPBF) combine to determine the pulmonary blood flow (PBF). (SA = systemic arterial.)

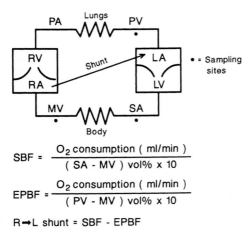

$$SBF = \frac{O_2 \text{ consumption ( ml/min )}}{( SA - MV ) \text{ vol\% x 10}}$$

$$EPBF = \frac{O_2 \text{ consumption ( ml/min )}}{( PV - MV ) \text{ vol\% x 10}}$$

$$R \rightarrow L \text{ shunt} = SBF - EPBF$$

**FIGURE 31–9.** *Use of oxygen saturation to calculate a right-to-left shunt.* Just as in Figure 31–8, the saturations required are those before the shunt origin (mixed venous [MV]) and those before and after the shunt destination (pulmonary vein [PV] and systemic artery [SA]). The systemic blood flow (SBF) is equal to the shunt flow plus the effective pulmonary blood flow (EPBF). (See text for explanation). (LA = left atrium; LV = left ventricle; RA = right atrium; RV = right ventricle.)

green dye is injected into one chamber while a densitometer is used to sample another chamber. The density of dye over time is then displayed. Indicator-dilution methods are used more for qualitative than for quantitative detection of shunt presence, but both diagnosis and quantitation can be obtained by using these procedures.

To detect a left-to-right shunt, a bolus can be injected into the venous system, and sampling is performed in the arterial system. The first wavefront of dye is then observed, with a second wavefront normally appearing only after the sample has circulated throughout the body. If there is a left-to-right intracardiac shunt, the first wavefront of indicator to the brachial artery will be soon followed by a second wavefront because the dye recirculates through the shunt. This is *early recirculation*. If a right-to-left shunt is present, some dye will cross the shunt and appear in advance of the major bolus. The location of a shunt can be precisely located by various sites of injection and sampling. Examples of left-to-right and right-to-left shunt tracings are shown in Figure 31–10.

## CALCULATION OF STENOTIC VALVE ORIFICE AREAS

### Determination of Significant Valvular Stenosis

A normal cardiac valve offers little obstruction to forward flow. Abnormal leaflet structure or leaflet injury can impede flow. By using a fundamental hydraulic formula, Gorlin and Gorlin (1951) developed a method of determining the valvular orifice area. This method required knowledge only of the flow across the valve and the pressure gradient that occurs

as a result of the stenosis. The basic formula was based on Torricelli's law:

$$\text{Effective orifice area} = \frac{\text{flow}}{\text{constant} \times 44.3 \times \sqrt{\text{mean gradient}}}$$

Gorlin and Gorlin observed that different constants corrected the resulting data compared with measurements obtained at autopsy. In the equation, flow is expressed in terms of the volume of blood traversing the valve when the valve is open. For atrioventricular valves, diastolic flow intervals are used; for semilunar valves, systolic flow intervals are used. The time in each minute that flow is occurring is obtained by measuring the diastolic filling period or the systolic ejection period and multiplying by the heart rate. For mitral stenosis, the diastolic filling period is defined from mitral valve opening to mitral valve closure. For aortic stenosis, the systolic ejection period is defined from aortic valve opening to closure. To convert cardiac output measurements to flow during these diastolic or systolic intervals, the cardiac output is divided by the heart rate times either the diastolic filling period or the systolic ejection period, respectively. The final equation is therefore defined as follows:

$$\text{Valve area} = \frac{\text{CO}/(\text{DFP or SEP}) (\text{HR})}{44.3 \times \text{constant} \times \sqrt{\text{mean gradient}}}$$

where CO = cardiac output, DFP = diastolic filling period, SEP = systolic ejection period, HR = heart rate, and 44.3 is a gravitation correction coefficient

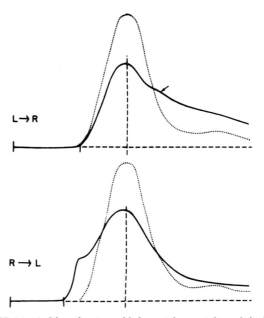

**FIGURE 31–10.** Identification of left-to-right or right-to-left shunts using indicator-dilution methods. The *broken line* represents a normal forward curve after injection of indocyanine green in the right side of the heart and sampling in the brachial artery. If a left-to-right shunt is present (*upper panel*), the onset of the curve is normal, and recirculation of the dye appears prematurely (*arrow*). If a right-to-left shunt is present, the dye that bypassed the lung will appear prematurely in the brachial artery (*lower panel*).

that also corrects for energy loss as pressure is converted to kinetic or velocity energy.

Gorlin and Gorlin validated the constant to be used for the mitral valve in 11 patients, and the maximal discrepancy observed varied by only 0.2 cm² compared with the calculated values when the constant 0.85 was used. For the aortic valve, a constant of 1.0 was used. Because there is no general clinical agreement about what constitutes a significant effective orifice area in tricuspid or pulmonic valvular stenosis, pressure gradients alone, rather than valve areas, are usually reported for these right-sided valves.

The normal *mitral valve* (MV) orifice area in adults is generally considered to be 4 to 5 cm². Symptoms in mitral stenosis directly reflect left atrial pressure and pulmonary venous hypertension. The previous formula is rearranged as follows:

$$\text{MV gradient} \propto \frac{\text{cardiac output}}{\text{diastolic filling period}}$$

Thus, the mitral valve gradient should rise with any high flow state or with any condition that shortens the diastolic filling period (e.g., during tachycardia). Because tachycardia tends to shorten diastolic filling time more than systolic ejection time, toleration of tachycardia is particularly poor in patients with mitral stenosis.

The relationship among the mitral gradient, the cardiac output, and the calculated mitral valve effective orifice area is nonlinear, and is shown in Figure 31–11. When the orifice area declines to about 1.5 cm², it becomes progressively more difficult to increase flow (cardiac output) without causing high mitral valve gradients. This is generally considered the threshold for intervening in mitral valve stenosis. Conversely, a small increase in the mitral valve area of severely stenotic valves (such as might occur after commissurotomy) creates a large reduction in the pressure gradient.

The normal aortic valve area is considered to be 2.6 to 3.5 cm² in adults. As with the mitral valve, the aortic valve gradient is proportional to cardiac output and is inversely proportional to the systolic ejection period.

$$\text{Aortic gradient} \propto \frac{\text{cardiac output}}{\text{systolic ejection period}}$$

Because the systolic ejection period declines less than the diastolic filling period with tachycardia, patients with aortic stenosis are more susceptible to cardiac output demands (e.g., exercise) than they are to tachycardia alone. The relationship among gradient, flow, and the aortic valve area is shown in Figure 31–12. As with mitral stenosis, the aortic gradient depends on both the aortic valve effective orifice area and the cardiac output. At an aortic valve area of 0.8 cm² or less, the aortic gradient rises disproportionately to the increase in cardiac output; this level is usually

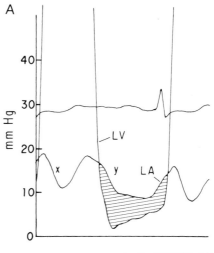

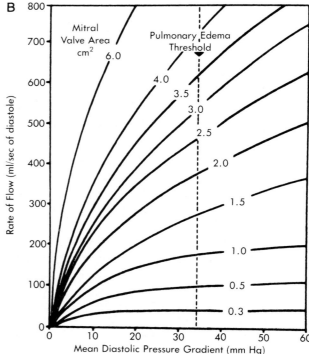

**FIGURE 31–11.** *The mitral gradient and the relationship of gradient to flow and valve area. A,* The gradient between the left atrium (LA) and left ventricle (LV) in diastole in mitral stenosis. *B,* The dependence of the mitral gradient on both flow and the mitral valve area. (*A,* Adapted from Wallace, A. G.: Pathophysiology of cardiovascular disease. *In* Smith, L. H., and Thier, O. S. [eds]: Pathophysiology: The Biological Principles of Disease: The International Textbook of Medicine. Philadelphia, W. B. Saunders, 1981; *B,* From Schlant, R. C.: Altered cardiovascular function of rheumatic heart disease and other acquired valvular disease. *In* Hurst, J. W. [ed]: The Heart. 3rd ed. New York, McGraw-Hill, 1974.)

considered the threshold for intervention in patients with aortic stenosis.

## Errors in Using Valvular Effective Orifice Area Measurements

Many potential errors are associated with the use of catheterization-derived valvular orifice area estimates

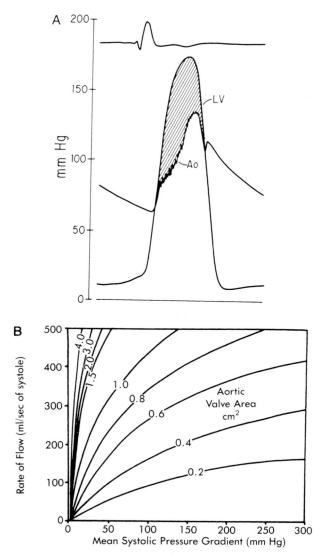

**FIGURE 31–12.** *The aortic gradient and the relationship of gradient, flow, and valve area. A,* The gradient between the aorta (Ao) and the left ventricle (LV). *B,* The gradient between the aorta and the LV. (*A,* Adapted from Wallace, A. G.: Pathophysiology of cardiovascular disease. *In* Smith, L. H., and Thier, O. S. [eds]: Pathophysiology: The Biological Principles of Disease: The International Textbook of Medicine. Philadelphia, W. B. Saunders, 1981; *B,* From Schlant, R. C.: Altered cardiovascular function of rheumatic heart disease and other acquired valvular disease. *In* Hurst, J. W. [ed]: The Heart. 3rd ed. New York, McGraw-Hill, 1974.)

(Carabello, 1987; Gorlin, 1987). These errors relate both to the difficulty in measuring the variables in Gorlin's equation and to a fundamental concern about the validity of this approach to estimate the orifice size. This concern also applies to prosthetic valve area estimations (Cannon et al., 1988).

The valvular orifice size estimate depends on accurate determination of cardiac output. This may be difficult at low-output states. If valvular regurgitation is present, the angiographically determined cardiac output must be used, because the formula depends on determining flow occurring across the valve of interest. If both aortic regurgitation and mitral regur-

gitation are present, neither the mitral nor the aortic valve area can be assessed accurately, because flow across a single valve cannot be determined.

Problems in calculating the effective orifice area of the mitral valve also include the use of pulmonary capillary wedge pressure to substitute for left atrial pressure, calibration errors, and difficulty in defining the beginning and the end of the diastolic filling period. Estimation of the effective orifice area of the aortic valve is subject to the same cardiac output errors as estimation of the mitral valve area. In aortic insufficiency, the total flow across the aortic valve can be estimated by using angiographic rather than Fick or thermodilution cardiac output. If mitral and aortic regurgitation are present, the aortic valve area cannot be determined. Additionally, because most catheterization laboratories use peripheral arterial pressure rather than central aortic pressure to define the aortic gradient, the delay between the onset of the peripheral waveform and the left ventricular pressure rise requires temporal realignment of the pressure data. A substantial difference in the height of the systolic pressure contour when the central aortic and peripheral arterial pressures are compared (see Fig. 31–3) also creates errors. If a discrepancy exists, the central aortic pressure can be determined by inserting a second catheter (preferred) or by use of a "pull-back" gradient. The catheter itself may also reduce the true valvular orifice area sufficiently to artifactually increase the gradient. Indeed, a rise in peripheral pressure has been observed with the removal of the catheter from the orifice of patients with aortic valve areas smaller than 0.5 cm² (Carabello et al., 1979).

The dependence of Gorlin's formula on cardiac output has been examined in patients with aortic stenosis, and the results have been particularly disturbing when one considers the importance placed on these "hard" numbers. Use of inotropic agents such as dopamine (Casale et al., 1988) or isoproterenol (McCristin et al., 1988) to increase cardiac output substantially changes the calculated aortic valve areas. These results may be related to increased lifting of the heavily burdened calcific valve or to other inherent errors in the correction factor used in the in-vivo state. The dependence of the calculations of valve area on forward flow has been confirmed by Cannon and associates (1985); the "constant" used in the formula was a linear function of the square root of the mean pressure gradient and was in fact not a constant at all. This is particularly a problem in low cardiac output states in which, for instance, in aortic stenosis, a small gradient may be observed, but the calculated aortic valve area may be well under the 0.8 cm² threshold. If the cardiac output is less than 3 l/min, the Gorlin formula predicts a smaller aortic valve area than may actually be present.

## Alternative Measures of the Effective Orifice Area of Stenotic Valves

Despite the dependence of valve gradients on flow, some institutions still rely solely on gradients to determine operability in most patients. For example, an aortic peak-to-peak gradient of 50 mm Hg or more or a mean mitral gradient of 15 mm Hg has been assumed to imply serious valvular stenosis and the need for operation. Similarly, a mean gradient of 5 mm Hg across the tricuspid and 50 mm Hg peak-to-peak gradient across the pulmonic valve is considered to indicate significant valvular stenosis.

Because of the concerns with Gorlin's formula, other attempts to define the effective orifice area have been proposed. Hakki (1981) suggested a simplified formula that clinically appeared to be effective:

$$\text{Valve area} = \frac{\text{cardiac output (l/min)}}{\sqrt{\text{mean pressure gradient (mm Hg)}}}$$

At normal heart rates, the effect of the systolic ejection period or the diastolic period was noted to be a relative constant; thus, this function was eliminated from the equation. The validity of this approach at higher heart rates was assessed by Angel and colleagues (1985); an empiric constant was added, depending on whether the heart rate was less than 75 beats per minute for mitral stenosis and more than 90 beats per minute for aortic stenosis. Rather than assume a given constant, Cannon and associates (1985) proposed the following:

$$\text{Valve area} = \frac{\text{flow (ml/sec)}}{K' \times \sqrt{\text{mean gradient} + C}}$$

where the valve orifice area is assumed to be inversely proportional to the actual mean gradient and $K'$ and $C$ are constants that vary with the valve being studied. The acceptance of these alternative methods of estimating the orifice area of stenotic valves awaits the test of time.

## ANGIOGRAPHIC DATA ANALYSIS

### Angiographic Left Ventricular Volume Determination

Measurement of the volume of blood in the cardiac chambers and the relationship with disease states and with overall cardiac function have obvious clinical relevance. The major problems in determining cardiac volume lie with the difficulty of appropriately modeling the cardiac chambers to a mathematically usable configuration (Dodge et al., 1962). This is particularly true for cardiac chambers other than the left ventricle.

Several methods have been used to measure left ventricular volumes, but most laboratories use an area-length determination (Dodge and Sheehan, 1983). Adequate opacification of the left ventricle without arrhythmia is required. The area-length method assumes that the left ventricle is shaped like a football (prolated ellipsoid). With knowledge of the corrected area of the silhouette and length, one can derive the volumes by using the formula:

$$V = \frac{4}{3}\pi \times \frac{D(1)}{2} \times \frac{D(2)}{2} \times \frac{L}{2}$$

where $D(1)$ = minor diameter in one view (*anteroposterior* or *right anterior oblique*) and $D(2)$ = minor diameter in the orthogonal view (*lateral* or *left anterior oblique*) and $L$ = long axis length. For biplane ventriculography, $D(1)$ and $D(2)$ are directly determined; for single-plane ventriculography, $D(1)$ is assumed to be equal to $D(2)$. The minor axes are calculated with knowledge of the planimetered area of the left ventricular contour and $L$ and by using the following equation:

$$D = \frac{4A}{\pi L}$$

where $A$ = area of the projected image obtained by planimetry. Substituting this $D$ into the formula for volume means that all of the necessary data can be derived from the area and the length calculations (thus the area-length name).

Because x-rays diverge as they emerge from the x-ray tube and travel to the image intensifier, a magnification correction factor must be determined to calculate the true area and length. This is generally obtained by measuring a known quantity (e.g., ball, bar, catheter markers, grid) at the level of the mid-ventricle or by using various other geometric methods.

When these corrections are made, however, there still remains an offset between actual and calculated ventricular volumes. In the authors' laboratories, each x-ray suite has this offset determined by linear regression analysis of 20 human heart casts of known volume. This regression is slightly different for each x-ray room. In laboratories that are not equipped for this technique, the regression equation obtained by Kennedy and associates (1970) has generally proved to be satisfactory.

Angiographic volumes suffer greatly from many limitations, including the basic assumption that the shape of the left ventricular chamber is that of a prolated ellipsoid. Segmental wall motion abnormalities present particular problems. Errors in defining the silhouette of the left ventricle, errors in defining the appropriate correction factors, and the effects of arrhythmias all contribute to make the variation of these data as great as ±15 to 20%. Alternative methods, such as use of Simpson's rule, have not been proven to be more accurate. Representative normal values are shown in Table 31–6 (Graham et al., 1971; Sandler and Dodge, 1968; Wynne et al., 1978).

### Ejection Fraction Determination

From a practical clinical standpoint, the major advantage of the ability to measure left ventricular volume has been the derivation of the most commonly used ejection phase index, the ejection fraction. Despite depending heavily on afterload and modestly on preload, the ejection fraction remains the single

■ **Table 31–6.** NORMAL LEFT VENTRICULAR VOLUMES AND EJECTION FRACTION DETERMINATIONS IN ADULTS AND CHILDREN

| Patients | End-Diastolic Volume (ml/m²) | End-Systolic Volume (ml/m²) | Ejection Fraction (%) |
|---|---|---|---|
| Adults | 72 ± 15 | 20 ± 8 | 0.72 ± 0.08 |
| Children | | | |
| <2 years | 42 ± 10 | NA | 0.68 ± 0.05 |
| >2 years | 73 ± 11 | NA | 0.63 ± 0.05 |

most useful systolic performance characteristic derived at cardiac catheterization. The *ejection fraction* (EF) is simply the ratio of *stroke volume* (SV) to *end-diastolic volume* (EDV):

$$EF = \frac{EDV - ESV}{EDV} = \frac{SV}{EDV}$$

Because volumetric correction factors cancel each other in this ratio, errors in determining the correction factor for ventricular volumes become irrelevant in the ejection fraction determination. In most laboratories, a normal ejection fraction is defined as ≥ 55%. Minor variability is noted between biplane and single-plane methods and between groups who use a *right anterior oblique* and *left anterior oblique* view compared with those who use an anteroposterior and lateral view. Each laboratory should establish its own normal values.

## Assessment of Valvular Regurgitation

### Regurgitant Fraction

The regurgitant fraction can be estimated by combining knowledge of forward cardiac output (from the thermodilution or Fick output determinations) and the angiographic output. If there is a single regurgitant valve, the difference between the angiographic stroke volume and the forward stroke volume can be defined as the regurgitant stroke volume by the following formula, and *regurgitant fraction* (RF) can be determined:

$$RF = \frac{\text{angiographic SV} - \text{forward SV}}{\text{angiographic SV}}$$

$$= \frac{\text{regurgitant SV}}{\text{angiographic SV}}$$

This formula incorporates many assumptions: that both the angiographic and forward cardiac output are correct, that heart rates are similar, that the hemodynamic state has not changed between the times the two measurements were made, and that only one valve is regurgitant. Because of these vagaries, the ratio provides only a gross estimate of the degree of valvular regurgitation.

### Visual Assessment of Valvular Regurgitation

Valvular regurgitation is commonly assessed angiographically by visual estimation. When contrast is injected into the chamber distal to the regurgitant lesion, the amount of regurgitation into the proximal chamber can be assessed. The resultant opacity of the proximal chamber depends on the size and contractile properties of the proximal chamber as well as the regurgitant volume. For example, a large, dilated proximal chamber appears less opacified by regurgitant contrast than a small chamber, despite a similar regurgitant volume. The basic classification of the degree of regurgitation was originally outlined by Sellers and associates (1964) and is essentially unchanged:

| | |
|---|---|
| + | Minimal regurgitant jet. Clears rapidly from proximal chamber with each systole. |
| + + | Moderate opacification of proximal chamber, clearing with subsequent systoles. |
| + + + | Intense opacification of proximal chamber becoming equal to that of the distal chamber. |
| + + + + | Intense opacification of proximal chamber becoming more dense than the distal chamber. Opacification often persists over the entire series of images obtained. |

In chronic mitral or tricuspid regurgitation, the atria often are greatly enlarged. In tricuspid regurgitation, contrast may be observed to pulsate into the inferior vena cava during ventricular systole.

## Regional Wall-Motion Analysis

Adequate definitions of regional contractility have assumed greater importance with the advent of interventional procedures (coronary artery bypass or angioplasty) for patients with coronary artery disease. Both visual (qualitative) and quantitative methods have been applied.

### Visual Interpretation of Segmental Wall Motion

Of five basic forms of segmental asynergy originally proposed by Herman and associates (1967), the following definitions have emerged in common use (Fig. 31–13):

| | |
|---|---|
| *Normal* | No abnormality |
| *Hypokinesia* | A mild-to-moderate reduction in contraction with preservation of some degree of contractile wall motion |
| *Akinesia* | Total absence of wall motion |
| *Dyskinesia* | Paradoxic systolic expansion of the ventricular wall |

In most laboratories, regional wall motion is as-

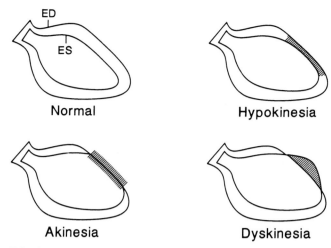

**FIGURE 31–13.** *Regional definitions of wall-motion abnormalities.* The end-diastolic (ED) and end-systolic (ES) contours and the severity of regional wall motion are defined as shown.

sessed in three areas in the right anterior oblique or anteroposterior views (anterior, apical, inferior) and three areas of the lateral or left anterior oblique view (septal, apical, posterolateral). These regions are arbitrary, and several alternative divisions of the left ventricular silhouette are also used today.

Aneurysmal dilatation is difficult to define angiographically, but some guidelines are helpful (Cabin and Roberts, 1980). An aneurysm is probable if there is a diastolic bulge in the left ventricular contour, discrete separation between the involved segment and the adjacent myocardium, and loss of trabeculation within the aneurysmal sac. The coronary artery supplying the aneurysmal area is usually poorly visualized or not visualized on selective injection. A false aneurysm or pseudoaneurysm may be present if a discrete area (neck) is seen between the aneurysmal sac and the remainder of the left ventricle in both systole and diastole. Pseudoaneurysms represent myocardial rupture with the formation of a localized pocket walled off by the pericardium. The narrow neck represents the area of myocardial rupture between the normal left ventricular cavity and the pseudoaneurysm. Thrombus formation is a frequent observation in aneurysms.

Visual estimates of the severity of wall motion abnormalities are highly subjective. The precise delineations of various segments, the variability in wall motion even during one systole (tardokinesia is defined as normal but delayed contractility), the influence of chamber size, cardiac rotation, and systolic motion of the aortic and mitral valves all complicate visual analysis. In addition, the thin left ventricular apex increases wall stress at the apex, and because most of the stroke volume is due to short-axis rather than long-axis shortening, the apex is particularly difficult to assess. Asynchrony in relaxation also is occasionally present (segmental early relaxation) (Gaasch et al., 1985), but it is rarely reported.

### Quantitative Segmental Wall-Motion Analysis

To circumvent some of the difficulties with the visual interpretation of regional contraction abnormalities, various quantitative methods have been proposed. Each method requires certain inherent assumptions, and each has been variably accepted. In all of these methods, the end-systolic silhouette is superimposed on the end-diastolic silhouette, and segmental areas are then defined.

In the hemiaxial method, the end-systolic and diastolic silhouettes are realigned by several methods, including aligning the aortic valve plane and the long axis of each contour and then constructing perpendicular chords to the long axis. Individual chordal shortening can then be described. The radial method assumes that the ventricle contracts toward some predefined point. Chord lengths toward this point are then drawn, and chordal shortening is described. A variation of these methods uses the reduction of the areas enclosed by these hemiaxial or radial lines.

Sheehan and colleagues (1986) validated a centerline approach in which there was no realignment of the end-systolic or end-diastolic contours. The distance between the outer edges of these silhouettes is simply divided in half (the centerline), and 100 chords are drawn perpendicularly to this centerline. After the data for the end-diastolic contour length are normalized, a plot of each chord motion is displayed. When patient data are compared with a group of normal control ventriculograms, the motion of each chord can be defined in terms of standard deviations from the norm. Often, selected chords (e.g., the worst 50% of chords in an infarct area) are meaned, and a single mean standard deviation number is reported. At Duke University Medical Center, a modification of this program is used clinically, and with more extensive analysis of the data it is also used for serial research studies (Fig. 31–14).

## REPRESENTATIVE CLINICAL DATA

The following paragraphs briefly describe representative cardiac catheterization data for different disease states and are intended only to discuss pertinent hemodynamic observations.

### Valvular Disease

#### Valvular Aortic Stenosis

Obstruction of the left ventricular outflow tract may occur at the level of the aortic valve, above the valve (supravalvular stenosis), or below the valve (subvalvular stenosis). These stenoses can be observed angiographically, and pressure gradients can be obtained. Valvular aortic stenosis is more common in men and rarely occurs as an isolated lesion in rheumatic disease. It is usually congenital or degenerative. Various degrees of commissural fusion, cusp malformation, and calcium deposition are seen in adult patients with

DUKE CENTERLINE WALL MOTION

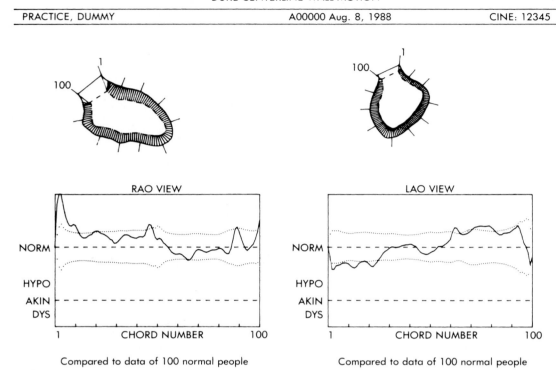

PRACTICE, DUMMY                          A00000 Aug. 8, 1988                          CINE: 12345

**FIGURE 31–14.** *Duke centerline wall-motion program.* This method of displaying regional wall motion quantitatively is a modification of that originally reported by Sheehan and associates (1986). The *upper part* of the figure outlines the end-diastolic (ED) and end-systolic (ES) silhouettes in the right anterior oblique (RAO) *(left)* and left anterior oblique (LAO) *(right)* views. The *hatched area* represents each of 100 chords drawn perpendicular to a centerline between the ED and the ES contours. In the *bottom panels,* the normal (NORM) area is defined for each chord (within 1 standard deviation). Similarly, the areas of hypokinesia (HYPO), akinesia (AKIN), and dyskinesia (DYS) are plotted. Each chord motion relative to that observed in 100 normal patients is then shown.

aortic stenosis. Acquired aortic stenosis may be seen in rheumatic heart disease, in rheumatoid arthritis, in ochronosis, and with amyloid infiltration. Most adults with aortic stenosis have either a bicuspid aortic valve or tricuspid valves with "degenerative" calcific deposits that stiffen and literally weigh the leaflets down. Turbulent blood flow across the leaflet repeatedly injures the leaflet surface. Thus, leaflet injury initiates further injury and provides the substrate for calcium deposition, fibroblastic ingrowth, and scar formation. These processes stiffen the leaflet and narrow the effective orifice. With obstruction to outflow, left ventricular pressures rise and left ventricular wall thickness increases to reduce wall stress:

$$\text{Wall stress} \propto \frac{\text{pressure} \times \text{radius}}{\text{wall thickness}}$$

Hypertrophy may become severe in pressure-overloaded states and is usually concentric. The resultant hypertrophy lowers wall stress and maintains the ejection fraction. Hypertrophy, however, increases diastolic stiffness, and symptoms of congestive failure and angina can result from the hypertrophic response despite preserved ventricular systolic performance. Atrial contraction becomes particularly important in an effort to fill these stiff ventricles, and the left ventricular A wave may become prominent. Cardiac out-

put at rest is usually normal, although it may fail to increase appropriately during exercise. The ejection fraction, which may remain normal for many years, may decline as the "afterload mismatch" presented by the stenotic valve and high wall stress becomes dominant (Ross, 1976; Selzer, 1987). Because the ejection fraction and wall stress are inversely related (Gunther and Grossman, 1979), the reduction in ejection fraction noted in some patients with severe aortic stenosis may be a function only of high wall stress rather than true myocardial dysfunction. Consequently, dramatic increases in ejection fraction may be observed after relief of the outflow obstruction when aortic valve replacement is performed.

The hypertrophy accompanying aortic stenosis is responsible for the congestive symptoms due to abnormal chamber stiffness, and although coronary flow per milligram of tissue is normal, the increased mass may alter transmural coronary flow, reduce coronary flow reserve (Marcus et al., 1982), and cause angina. Coronary arterial lesions of marginal significance under normal conditions may limit flow in the presence of such high coronary flow; this phenomenon makes it difficult at times to opacify coronary arteries adequately during angiography in patients with aortic stenosis. In general, an effective orifice of 0.8 cm$^2$ or less and a peak systolic gradient greater than 50 mm Hg in the presence of a normal cardiac output are considered thresholds for performing surgery in symptomatic patients. In patients with aortic stenosis, diastolic stiffness usually produces congestive symptoms before systolic function deteriorates. Therefore, surgery should be done for symptoms.

### Aortic Regurgitation

Although most adult patients with aortic stenosis have either bicuspid aortic valves or a degenerative calcific process, the causes of aortic regurgitation are more varied. Aortic regurgitation may result from a dilated aortic root (e.g., in Marfan's syndrome, Ehlers-Danlos syndrome, annuloaortic ectasia, cystic medial necrosis, hypertension, pseudoxanthoma elasticum), from primary aortic cusp involvement (e.g., endocarditis, rheumatic disease, alkylosing spondylitis, rheumatoid arthritis, sinus of Valsalva'a aneurysm), from aortitis (e.g., syphilis, giant-cell arteritis), or from loss of commissural support (e.g., trauma, ventricular septal defect, aortic dissection).

Whatever the cause, the associated hemodynamics are directly related to the acuteness of the process. In *acute aortic regurgitation,* the left ventricle has had inadequate time to adapt to the sudden insult from the regurgitant volume. Diastolic left ventricular pressure increases dramatically (Morganroth et al., 1977) and may prematurely close the mitral valve in mid or late diastole. This "preclosure" can be readily observed through echocardiography. Because stroke volume declines, the systemic pulse pressure may be narrow. To compensate for this, heart rates are often high. Because there may be little gradient between the aortic diastolic and left ventricular diastolic pressures, an aortic regurgitant murmur may not be audible, and the turbulance observed by Doppler color-flow echocardiographic imaging may be minimal. The patient is usually acutely ill. Representative hemodynamics are shown in Figure 31–15.

Compared with acute aortic regurgitation, the hemodynamics of *chronic aortic regurgitation* differ greatly. In chronic aortic regurgitation, the left ventricle hypertrophies and dilates over time. This gradual wall thickening in response to the dilated left ventricle maintains normal wall stresses in accordance with Laplace's equation (Grossman et al., 1975). The left ventricular chamber may greatly enlarge, and the ejection fraction may remain in the normal range for a long time. Although some have used a decline in exercise ejection fraction as a harbinger of impending myocardial failure (Kawanishi et al., 1986), the meaning of the exercise ejection fraction is complicated because of the shortened diastole (and less aortic regurgitation per beat) that occurs during stress testing.

The pulse pressure is usually wide, and the left ventricular end-diastolic pressure is almost normal. When myocardial failure ensues, the resting ejection fraction falls and the end-systolic volume rises. As contractility falls, the end-systolic volume rises; this is the most important value to follow serially. Systolic wall tension increases late in the course, and afterload mismatch occurs as a result of inadequate hypertrophy (Ricci, 1982). Forward stroke volume ultimately declines. End-diastolic wall stress may then rise, and this can be estimated approximately by the echo end-diastolic radius/wall thickness ratio (Gaasch et al., 1978). With the fall in stroke volume and rise in end-diastolic volume, the end-systolic volume appears to be the most sensitive indicator of both operative mortality and postoperative improvement after aortic valve replacement (Borow et al., 1980). Patients with aortic insufficiency should undergo operation if any symptoms emerge or if the end-systolic volumes increase (even if no symptoms are present).

### Mitral Stenosis

Mitral stenosis predominantly occurs secondary to rheumatic fever, although congenital forms (e.g., mitral arcade or parachute mitral valve) and other acquired forms (e.g., carcinoid, lupus, rheumatoid arthritis, amyloid, tumor) are less commonly encountered. As the affected population has gotten older, mitral annular calcification has become a more prevalent cause.

When the normal mitral orifice (4 to 6 cm$^2$) is reduced, a gradient occurs between the left atrium and the left ventricle in diastole. Severe mitral stenosis is present when valve area is less than 1.5 to 1 cm$^2$. Atrial contraction helps to fill the left ventricle and can represent up to 30% of the gradient across the valve (Stott et al., 1970). With left ventricular filling reduced, the left ventricular end-diastolic volumes are often low or normal, and left ventricular mass is consequently normal or slightly reduced. A mild degree of global ventricular dysfunction may then result. In addition, scarring of the submitral apparatus and papillary muscle may create regional wall-motion abnormalities (Colle et al., 1983). With exercise, symptoms in mitral stenosis are primarily related to the rise in the mitral gradient and not to exercise-induced left ventricular dysfunction (Johnson and Kostuk, 1986). The left atrial (pulmonary capillary wedge) pressure shows a prominent A wave and a blunted Y descent as left ventricular filling from the left atrium is inhibited by the valvular stenosis (see Fig. 31–11).

Pulmonary hypertension eventually occurs not only from the elevated left atrial pressure, but also from arteriolar constriction and obliterative changes in the pulmonary vascular bed. There may be a reversible component to pulmonary hypertension (Halperin et al., 1985), and pressures usually fall rapidly after relief of the mitral valvular obstruction (Foltz et al., 1984). Pulmonary compliance is often reduced, pulmonary blood flow is redistributed from the base to apex, and abnormal pulmonary function test results are observed. There is a poor correlation between the results of commissurotomy and symptoms, and restenosis may not always be present when symptoms recur after operation (Higgs et al., 1970).

### Mitral Regurgitation

Normal function of the mitral valve apparatus involves the proper alignment and coaptation of the

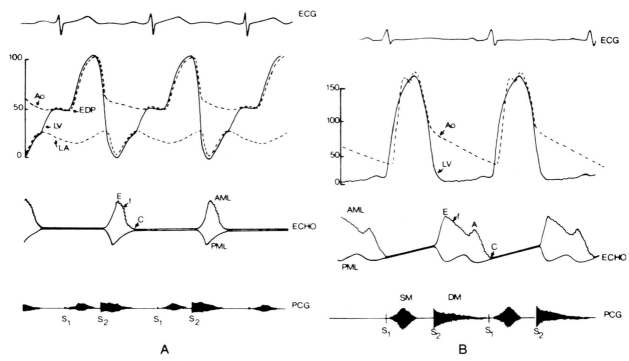

**FIGURE 31–15.** *The hemodynamics of acute and chronic aortic regurgitation. A,* Acute aortic regurgitation (AR) results in a sharp increase in the left ventricular end-diastolic pressure (LVEDP), a normal aortic (Ao) pulse pressure, elevated left atrial (LA) pressures, premature closure of the mitral valve (C) on the echocardiogram (ECHO), and a relatively short and often soft diastolic murmur (DM) on phonocardiogram (PCG). *B,* Chronic AR. In this situation, the LVEDP may be normal, the aortic pulse pressure is wide with a reduced aortic diastolic pressure, the mitral valve closes normally with the onset of left ventricle (LV) systole, and the AR murmur is obvious. (E = E point; f = f point of mitral valve opening; A = A wave; SM = systolic murmur; AML = anterior mitral leaflet; PML = posterior mitral leaflet.) (*A* and *B,* From Morganroth, J., Perloff, J. K., Zeldis, S. M., and Dunkman, W. B.: Acute severe aortic regurgitation. Ann. Intern. Med., *87:*225, 1977.)

mitral leaflets. It requires appropriate function of the mitral annulus, the chordae tendineae, and the papillary muscles. Mitral regurgitation results whenever any component of this apparatus is dysfunctional.

The consequences of mitral regurgitation are due to both the magnitude and the acuteness of the process. With *acute mitral regurgitation,* the left atrium is unable to accept the increased volume, markedly elevating left atrial pressure. A large V wave can then be seen in the pulmonary capillary wedge tracing and may even be reflected into the pulmonary arterial pressure (Fig. 31–16). In *chronic mitral regurgitation,* the left atrium has usually enlarged over time and is able to absorb the effect of the regurgitant volume without greatly raising the left atrial and pulmonary pressures.

Pathophysiologically, acute mitral regurgitation reduces the systolic workload on the left ventricle and allows it to empty more completely, increasing the measured ejection fraction. Over time, the left ventricular end-diastolic volume gradually increases, and myocardial failure eventually ensues.

The "afterload sink" provided by the left atrium may maintain ejection fraction in the relatively normal range for a long time, however, which creates a dilemma in the timing of the operation in this situation. As with aortic regurgitation, the end-systolic volume or stress/volume ratio may provide the most useful information regarding operative outcome

(Borow et al., 1980; Carabello et al., 1981). Patients with chronic mitral regurgitation who experience even mild symptoms (Class II) should probably undergo surgery if exercise hemodynamics suggest inadequate compensation with stress or if resting left ventricular end-systolic volumes are increased. When the resting ejection fraction begins to decline, one must assume that myocardial dysfunction is well under way.

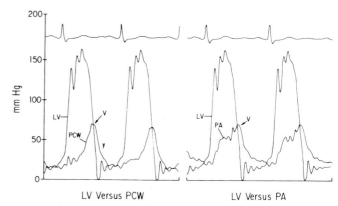

**FIGURE 31–16.** *Mitral regurgitation and poor left atrial compliance.* The left ventricular (LV) pressure versus the pulmonary capillary wedge (PCW) pressure is shown on the *left.* A large regurgitant v wave is evident. This marked v wave is transmitted through the pulmonary bed to the pulmonary arterial (PA) tracing and is seen to be superimposed in the *right panel.*

### Right-Sided Heart Valvular Lesions

**Tricuspid Stenosis.** Tricuspid stenosis is generally the result of rheumatic heart disease or congenital atresia, although other causes (e.g., tumor, vegetations, carcinoid) may be etiologic. As the right atrial outflow obstruction increases, right atrial pressures rise, the Y descent becomes blunted, and the A wave increases dramatically. A mean gradient in diastole of 5 mm Hg is considered significant. Most patients with tricuspid stenosis have other associated rheumatic valvular disease (usually mitral stenosis). Tricuspid regurgitation frequently accompanies tricuspid stenosis. Surgical approaches such as commissurotomy are infrequently effective, and valve replacement (often with a porcine heterograft) is required (Cobanoglu and Starr, 1986).

**Tricuspid Regurgitation.** The tricuspid valve apparatus differs in many ways from the mitral valve apparatus. In addition to three large leaflets, numerous chordae attach to a variety of small papillary muscles and to the right ventricular endocardium directly. Papillary muscle dysfunction therefore is rarely a cause of tricuspid regurgitation, compared with mitral regurgitation. Tricuspid annular dilation may prevent adequate valvular coaptation (Come and Riley, 1985) and is the most common cause of tricuspid regurgitation—usually as a result of right ventricular dilatation from any of a number of causes. Various other diseases, both rheumatic and nonrheumatic, can affect the tricuspid leaflet primarily.

Right atrial pressure and the right ventricular end-diastolic pressure are usually increased in tricuspid regurgitation. As the condition worsens, the right atrial V wave occurs earlier in ventricular systole and gradually obliterates the X descent (C-V wave) as the regurgitation fills the atrium during ventricular systole. Severe tricuspid regurgitation causes "ventricularization" of the right atrium. Right atrial pressures may then lose the characteristic changes with respiration; in fact, an actual rise may occur during inspiration (Cha and Gooch, 1983)—the Kussmaul sign.

When the right ventricular systolic pressure is greater than 40 to 45 mm Hg, one may assume that tricupsid regurgitation is functional (i.e., due to the elevated right ventricular pressure) rather than intrinsic disease of the valve itself. Right ventriculography is useful, although the right ventricular catheter may hold the valve open during injection and artificially create some tricuspid regurgitation. Contrast injected into the right ventricle is seen jetting into the right atrium; with proper positioning, the contrast may also be seen pulsating into the inferior vena cava or hepatic veins during ventricular systole in patients with severe tricuspid regurgitation. Various catheters and techniques (e.g., low injection rates) have been used to minimize catheter-induced tricuspid regurgitation during right-sided ventriculography (Ubago et al., 1981).

Tricuspid valvular prolapse may occasionally be seen on angiography by the billowing of the tricuspid leaflets. In Ebstein's anomaly, the tricuspid valve ring is displaced toward the right ventricular apex and there is atrialization of a portion of the right ventricle. Simultaneous pressure recording and intracardiac electrocardiography demonstrate that a catheter can be placed into a hemodynamic right atrium, yet record a right ventricular electrogram.

**Pulmonic Valve Disease.** Most pulmonic stenosis occurs as a result of a congenitally abnormal pulmonic valve. Rarely, acquired forms (such as rheumatic diseases, carcinoid tumors, or compression by contiguous structures) may obstruct the pulmonic outflow at the valvular level.

Pulmonic regurgitation is usually a result of dilation of the pulmonic annulus. Dilation can result from pulmonary hypertension or can be secondary to idiopathic pulmonary dilatation. Less frequent causes are collagen vascular diseases (e.g., Marfan's syndrome) and endocarditis. Surgical trauma to the valve causing pulmonic regurgitation may occur during repair of right-sided heart lesions (e.g., repair of tetralogy of Fallot). Other valvular lesions have been reported with congenitally malformed pulmonic leaflets—often in association with tetralogy of Fallot or ventricular septal defect. The use of pulmonary artery catheters has also been reported to cause pulmonic regurgitation in rare instances (O'Toole et al., 1979).

Pulmonic stenosis is diagnosed by the simultaneous measurement of right ventricular and pulmonary artery pressures. A 50 mm Hg peak-to-peak gradient is usually considered significant, and repair (balloon dilatation) is recommended. The right ventricle is often greatly hypertrophied, and subpulmonic infundibular hypertrophy may be especially prominent, causing infundibular obstruction to right ventricular outflow as well. After sudden relief of valvular pulmonary outflow obstruction (e.g., with balloon valvuloplasty), the right ventricle may eject rigorously and fail to fill adequately on subsequent beats—the "suicide right ventricle phenomenon."

Pulmonic regurgitation is difficult to define by using commonly employed catheter techniques. When pulmonary systolic pressure is greater than 70 mm Hg, the pulmonary artery is often dilated. A Graham Steell murmur of pulmonic regurgitation results. Intracardiac phonocardiography documents the presence of pulmonic regurgitation, although echo-Doppler methods are clearly superior. Pulmonary arteriography reveals pulmonic regurgitation, but catheter-induced valvular regurgitation makes the degree of regurgitation difficult to assess. Surgical intervention is rarely required, because the right ventricle is designed for volume work and rarely fails as a result of pulmonic regurgitation alone (Emery et al., 1979). When pulmonic insufficiency is associated with a hypertrophied right ventricle (as in postoperative tetralogy of Fallot), pulmonic valve replacement has become more common.

### Prosthetic Valve Assessment

All prosthetic valves are inherently obstructive, and some gradient can normally be detected across all of them. The effective orifice area and resultant pressure gradients across prosthetic valves can be approximated by in vitro studies using a pulse duplicator (Gabby and Kresh, 1985). When mean effective orifice areas are evaluated for small prostheses at a common output (5 l/min) values from 1.2 to 1.9 cm² are common. Medium-sized prostheses have effective orifice areas in the range of 1.7 to 2.8 cm², and large prostheses range from 1.9 to 3.4 cm². These prostheses carry mean gradients of 10 to 30 mm Hg for small, 5 to 19 mm Hg for medium, and 3 to 8 mm Hg for large valves.

The translation of in vitro data to the clinical setting is difficult at best, but the prosthetic valve type and size are major factors in determining the potential degree of inherent stenosis. The determined effective orifice area depends on output, and Gorlin's formula may lead to interpretive bias (Cannon et al., 1988).

At catheterization, the ball valves and tissue valves usually can be crossed in a retrograde manner without hemodynamic embarrassment. This is not true of disk valves (e.g., the St. Jude or the Björk-Shiley valves) because the disk valves are held open by the crossing catheter. In addition, the catheter may become entrapped within the disk valve prosthesis. Gradient measurement with an aortic disk prosthesis in place must be accomplished by left ventricular pressure recording using a catheter placed transseptally into the left ventricle. Ventriculography is accomplished using the same catheter.

Aortic prostheses are inherently more obstructive than mitral prostheses because of the smaller ring diameters. Resting hemodynamics may also fail to reflect the gradient potential observed during exercise. In patients with mitral valve replacement, removal of the papillary muscles may also contribute to left ventricular dysfunction (Kazama et al., 1986); newer attempts to preserve the native valve by valve repair are promising (Carpentier et al., 1980). Preservation of the posterior leaflet and associated chordae is also becoming more widespread.

The inherent stenotic nature of most prosthetic valves limits valve replacement for stenotic lesions to severe valvular stenosis. Valvular replacement for mild to moderate stenosis may make no effective hemodynamic change.

The fluoroscopic image for each prosthetic valve is unique to the device implanted and has been reviewed (Mehlman, 1988). Motion of the prosthetic valve ring in and out of the direction of flow should be considered normal, whereas motion perpendicular to the direction of flow may imply valvular dysfunction. The acceptable tilt for most prosthetic aortic valves is less than 12 to 15 degrees (White et al., 1973).

A few comments regarding each prosthesis may be useful. Further details may be found in other sources (Morse et al., 1985). The evaluation of caged ball valves should include poppet motion and configuration, the clearance between the ball and the struts or the ring, and the evenness of the stroke. The sewing ring of Starr-Edwards' valves may normally tilt from

2 to 6 degrees in the aortic position and from 5 to 21 degrees in the mitral position (White et al., 1973).

The hinged or tilting monocuspid valves, exemplified by the Björk-Shiley prosthesis, should close completely against the sewing ring to rule out thrombosis. Fractures have been reported at the junction of the small struts and the sewing ring in these valves, and this area should be closely evaluated. The base should tilt less than 6 degrees in the aortic and less than 10 degrees in the mitral position, and the opening angle should be 60 degrees (Heystraten and Paalman, 1981). Either low forward flow or thrombosis can affect the maximal opening angle.

Caged-disk prostheses, such as the Beall valve, are now used less commonly. The disk should be parallel to the suture ring at end-diastole and end-systole, although some cocking movement is seen normally. Disk sticking or cocking at end-diastole or end-systole is distinctly abnormal. Over time, disk shrinkage can occur and is noted by defining the disk-to-suture ring ratio. An abnormal ratio is less than 0.85 (Carlson et al., 1981).

Bileaflet prostheses, such as the St. Jude's valve, are difficult to evaluate because the base ring is not radiopaque. When closed, the leaflets, which are radiopaque when viewed on end, meet the base at a 30- to 35-degree angle and open to an 85-degree angle. Valve orientation varies, and angulated views are usually required to observe the leaflets. In the aortic position, left anterior oblique view with some angulation is often the best position for observing the thin lines of the leaflets in profile. The Duromedic bileaflet valve has an opaque base ring and is more readily assessed with fluoroscopy.

The fluoroscopic evaluation of heterografts is often difficult, although tilting of the base can be observed. Calcification may occasionally be seen, indicating degenerative changes within the leaflets. The large struts of the Carpentier-Edwards porcine or pericardial valves or the Ionescu-Shiley bovine pericardial valves are readily seen; however, only the metal supporting ring is opaque in the Hancock porcine valve.

## Cardiomyopathies

Primary cardiac muscle disorders are now generally classified according to anatomic, hemodynamic, and functional features. Dilated (formerly congestive) cardiomyopathies are characterized by a dilated left ventricle (or right ventricle) chamber with large end-diastolic volumes. Hypertrophy that should be present to reduce wall stress is not always achieved, and wall thickness is usually inappropriately normal or thin. Contractile performance is poor. Hypertrophic cardiomyopathies have inappropriately increased left ventricular hypertrophy with normal left ventricular diastolic volume and either normal or hypercontractile systolic function. Restrictive cardiomyopathies have normal or almost normal systolic function, usually normal or mildly increased left ventricular end-diastolic volumes, and often greatly raised left ventricular end-diastolic pressures. Restrictive cardiomyopathies are primarily due to infiltrative processes. Restrictive myocardial disease almost always affects the left ventricle more than the right ventricle, and this distribution aids in differentiating restrictive hemodynamics from constrictive pericarditis.

The cause cannot be defined in most cases of *dilated cardiomyopathy,* and the condition likely reflects the final result of myocardial injury from a host of potential causes. Possible causes include infective myocarditis (usually viral), ischemic disease, collagen vascular diseases, thyroid disease, hemochromatosis, toxic agents (such as alcohol, cancer chemotherapeutic agents), chronic volume overload (atrioventricular shunts, sickle cell anemia), radiation, transplant rejection, genetic associations (such as Friedreich's ataxia). Dilated cardiomyopathy has been described in the postpartum period and can be associated with myocarditis, obesity, and other endocrine disorders (Johnson and Palacios, 1982).

At catheterization, besides defining the severity of the systolic and diastolic dysfunction and excluding coronary artery disease as causative, myocardial biopsies now can be done routinely. Myocardial biopsies can identify cardiac transplant rejection, myocarditis, sarcoidosis, amyloidosis, chemotherapy toxicity (due to high-dose cyclophosphamide [Cytoxan] or doxorubicin [Adriamycin]), hemochromatosis, carcinoid, endocardial fibroelastosis, glycogen storage disease, or tumor (Laser et al., 1985).

Left ventriculography shows diffuse hypocontractility, although regional differences in the degree of wall motion abnormality occur frequently. Left ventricular thrombi can occasionally be identified.

In the normal left ventricle, the short-axis dimension at end-diastole is about one-half the long axis, and approximately 85% of the stroke volume ejected is due to short-axis shortening. In dilated cardiomyopathies, the short-axis and long-axis diameters have almost equal dimensions (Krevlen et al., 1980). Teleologically, the thin left ventricular apex has greater wall stress (based on Laplace's equation), and as left ventricular systolic function declines, the left ventricle is therefore expected to dilate more in the short-axis than in the long-axis dimension—thus becoming more spherical as failure occurs. A spherical left ventricular shape is common in dilated cardiomyopathies. The dilated left ventricular chamber is also associated with a dilated mitral annulus and malalignment of the mitral apparatus; therefore, mitral regurgitation of varying severity often is present.

*Hypertrophic cardiomyopathy* is generally considered a genetic disorder (Clark et al., 1973; Rosenzweig et al., 1991). It is now clear that certain genetic markers are associated with its presence in selected families. Because outflow obstruction of various degrees may be present, the terms *idiopathic hypertrophic subaortic stenosis* and *hypertrophic obstructive cardiomyopathy* are often used to describe this condition. Hypertrophy may not be confined to the septum, however, and an apical form is also encountered. The unique dynamic nature of the left ventricular outflow obstruction ob-

served has attracted the attention of most diagnosticians, but although outflow tract obstruction may be hemodynamically interesting, the major symptoms experienced by the patient are due to the high ventricular filling pressures. Diastolic dysfunction produces symptoms of angina and congestive heart failure due to coronary underperfusion and pulmonary congestion. The magnitude of the outflow tract gradient has not been shown to correlate with either symptoms or survival.

The classic hemodynamic findings in hypertrophic cardiomyopathy include increased left ventricular end-diastolic pressure caused by both increased ventricular stiffness and reduced active relaxation (Hanrath et al., 1980). Mitral regurgitation is relatively common, and the combination of mitral regurgitation and increased left ventricular end-diastolic pressure increases pulmonary pressures. Right ventricular outflow tract obstruction occasionally is noted. The subaortic jet may damage the aortic leaflets and can also cause aortic insufficiency over time.

The most notable feature of hypertrophic cardiomyopathy is the dynamic nature of the left ventricular outflow gradient. Any maneuver that decreases left ventricular afterload, reduces left ventricular volume, or increases inotropy causes an increased left ventricular outflow gradient. The converse of this is also true. At catheterization, the dynamic nature of the systolic gradient can be demonstrated by the Valsalva maneuver, amyl nitrite, or isoproterenol (Fig. 31–17). Careful analysis of the outflow gradient reveals a subaortic chamber with no left ventricular-to-aortic pressure gradient (Fig. 31–18). The aortic systolic pressure in the beat following a single premature ventricular contraction would be expected to increase in normal patients, whereas it may decrease in patients with hypertrophic cardiomyopathy (an observation usually known as Brockenbrough's sign) (Brockenbrough et al., 1961) (Fig. 31–19).

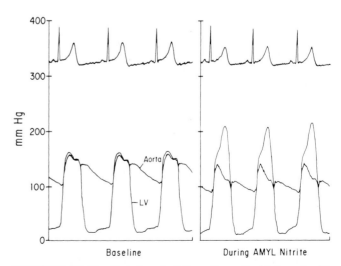

**FIGURE 31–17.** *The effect of amyl nitrite on the gradient in hypertrophic cardiomyopathy. At baseline, little gradient is present, although slight notching of the aortic contour is noted. With amyl nitrite, the aortic pressure falls, the left ventricular (LV) pressure rises, and the LV outflow tract gradient is increased.*

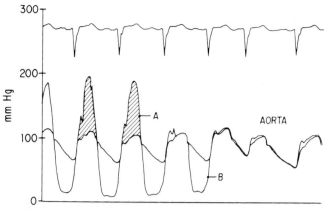

**FIGURE 31–18.** *Left ventricle (LV) pressure during pullback from LV to the aorta in hypertrophic cardiomyopathy.* By using a double-micromanometer catheter, the aortic tracing remains unchanged as the LV tracing shows a subaortic gradient (A), then no subaortic gradient (B). Despite the loss of an outflow tract gradient, the distal pressure still reflects LV pressure, confirming no valvular gradient.

The rapid emptying of the left ventricle creates a prominent percussion wave in the aortic tracing, and the early cessation of forward flow causes an initial decline and then a second, rounded tidal wave (the spike and dome configuration). The rapid ejection of blood from the ventricle through the narrowed outflow tract causes the anterior mitral leaflet to be drawn anteriorly toward the ventricular septum during systole (systolic anterior motion). The role of the mitral valve in the creation of the outflow gradient is still controversial (Murgo et al., 1980; Wigle et al., 1985), because maximal obstruction occurs when the ventricle is essentially empty.

An angiogram indicates obvious left ventricular hypertrophy, and regional accentuation in the degree of hypertrophy (septal, midventricular, or apical) is

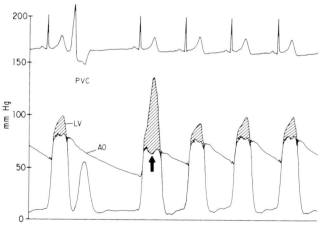

**FIGURE 31–19.** *Brockenbrough's phenomenon in hypertrophic cardiomyopathy.* After premature ventricular contraction (PVC), the left ventricular (LV) pressure gradient rises dramatically, but the aortic (AO) pulse pressure actually is less than the baseline pulse pressure. In addition, the "spike and dome" contour in the aortic pulse *(arrow)* becomes evident on the post-PVC beat.

observable. An "empty ventricle" is sometimes present, with almost complete expulsion of blood by late systole. Systolic anterior motion of the mitral valve can be observed in the cranial left anterior oblique view in many patients. Mitral regurgitation varies in severity, and aortic regurgitation is occasionally present as well. Coronary angiography may also demonstrate septal perforator compression (Pichard et al., 1979). Ventricular dilatation may develop if myocardial infarction occurs. Myocardial infarction has been reported in these patients despite normal epicardial coronary vessels (Maron et al., 1979).

Outflow tract obstruction under basal conditions is not required for the diagnosis of hypertrophic cardiomyopathy. Indeed, Maron and associates (1987) estimate that only about 25% of patients have an outflow gradient without provocation.

*Restrictive cardiomyopathies,* due to infiltrative processes, are uncommon. Differentiation from constrictive pericarditis may be difficult, but some guidelines are useful. In most patients with restrictive cardiomyopathies, diastolic pressures in the left ventricle are higher than in the right ventricle when the pressures are simultaneously tracked (Tyberg et al., 1981). A difference of greater than 5 mm Hg is common. The abnormal left ventricular end-diastolic pressure often elevates pulmonary pressure above 50 mm Hg (an uncommon finding in constriction) (Grossman, 1986). Although early diastolic filling is excessively rapid in constrictive pericarditis, early filling may be blunted as a result of abnormal active relaxation in restrictive cardiomyopathy. Systolic performance (ejection fraction) may be normal or only slightly reduced in restrictive disease. Echocardiography, computed tomography, or magnetic resonance imaging may help to exclude pericardial disease.

Right ventricular pressure tracings during acute right ventricular infarction at times show a dip and plateau pattern similar to that of constrictive pericarditis (Lorell et al., 1979), which in effect mimics a form of right ventricular restriction. This pattern may be due to dilation of the right ventricle to the extent that the normal pericardium becomes physiologically constrictive (Goldstein et al., 1982). Acute dilation of any of the cardiac chambers, which may occur in tricuspid or mitral regurgitation (Bartle and Hermann, 1967), can also produce this dip and plateau pattern.

## Pericardial Disease

One can conceptually visualize the pericardium as a balloon or sac. The heart can then be viewed as an organ pushed into the side of this sac. The visceral pericardium represents the portion of the sac that covers the heart, and the parietal pericardium represents the remainder of the sac. The normal pericardium contains less than 50 ml of fluid produced by serosal cells that line the pericardium (Roberts and Spray, 1976). Lymphatics drain along the epicardial surface and eventually to the mediastinum and right-sided heart cavities (Miller et al., 1971).

The functions of the pericardium have been described as mechanical, membranous, and ligamentous (Spodick, 1983). Diseases of the pericardium restrict diastolic filling of the heart. Cardiac tamponade compresses the ventricles and prevents filling in both early and late diastole. Constrictive pericarditis is characterized by rapid early filling of the left ventricle with sudden cessation of filling at mid and late diastole. Mixed disorders (effusive constrictive) also exist.

Pericardial disorders are relatively common in the postoperative period after cardiac surgery. Pericardial tamponade and the postpericardiotomy syndrome are the most common complications that follow open heart procedures (Engle et al., 1978). Other etiologies that cause pericarditis are numerous, and include infections that mimic a form of right ventricular restriction. The degree of intrapericardial pressure that occurs when fluid accumulates is a function of the compliance of the pericardium, the size of the heart within the pericardium, the volume of the pericardial fluid, and the rapidity with which the fluid accumulates. After about 150 ml of fluid accumulates in a normal pericardium, the intrapericardial pressure rises exponentially as a function of increasing pericardial volume, and pericardial tamponade may occur. The rise in intrapericardial pressure prevents right ventricular filling and eliminates the Y descent in the right atrial tracing. Inspiratory changes are usually normal, with a normal fall in right atrial pressure during inspiration (i.e., no Kussmaul's sign). The inspiratory increase in right atrial and right ventricular filling, together with normal pooling of blood in the lungs, reduces left ventricular filling with inspiration. Left ventricular stroke volume thus declines during inspiration and causes systemic blood pressure to fall by more than 10 mm Hg (pulsus paradoxus). The high intrapericardial pressures also elevate and equalize end-diastolic right atrial, right ventricular, left ventricular, and pulmonary capillary wedge pressures (within 5 mm Hg of each other). The exception is when there is preexisting left ventricular diastolic dysfunction (Reddy et al., 1978). The failure to transport blood from the right side of the heart to the left side of the heart produces normal or only modestly raised pulmonary artery pressures. Consequently, pulse pressure in the pulmonary artery and aorta may be narrow.

Angiography is rarely necessary in cardiac tamponade. Right atrial angiography in the anteroposterior view may reveal a thickened right atrial silhouette outside the right atrial angiographic border, confirming pericardial thickening or fluid. Echocardiography is clearly the most sensitive and useful diagnostic test to confirm pericardial fluid. Pericardiocentesis is easily done and is useful from both a diagnostic and a therapeutic standpoint.

*Pericardial constriction* occurs when the two pericardial layers (parietal and visceral) fuse from scar formation. The potential etiologies of constrictive pericarditis are extensive. Idiopathic causes, viral infections, uremia, neoplasm, radiation, rheumatic disorders, and cardiac surgical intervention have replaced tuberculosis as the leading causes of constriction (Lorell and Braunwald, 1988). Fibrin and thrombus accumulation in the pericardium may produce a picture of constrictive pericarditis rapidly after heart operations (Cohen and Greenberg, 1979).

When the pericardium scars and fuses together, it acts physiologically like a cement vault. The heart within this vault can fill rapidly only in early diastole. As the heart fills, it expands against the walls of the vault, and the filling ceases. The high atrial pressures before antrioventricular valve opening create a large early diastolic gradient and rapid early flow into the ventricles (the rapid Y descent). The sudden cessation of inflow and the abrupt rise in ventricular diastolic pressure create a dip and plateau pattern in ventricular diastole. In severe constriction, normal inspiratory changes do not occur, and the right atrial pressure may even rise (Kussmaul's sign). Representative hemodynamics are shown in Figures 31–20 and 31–21. This failure to fill the right side of the heart with inspiration differs from that observed in tamponade, and thus pulsus paradoxus is unusual in constrictive pericarditis. Pulmonary pressures are usually normal or only minimally increased, and the right ventricular diastolic pressure is usually greater than one-third of the right ventricular systolic pressure. The hemodynamics can be confused with those in restrictive cardiomyopathy or those in severe atrioventricular valvular regurgitation, as noted earlier, since any time there is "more heart than pericardium," constriction physiology may be observed.

Mixed effusive-constrictive physiology is also occasionally noted and becomes evident when constrictive hemodynamics persist after pericardiocentesis (Mann et al., 1978). In addition, some suggest that an occult pericardial constriction exists that can be identified by rapid volume loading in certain patients with normal baseline hemodynamics (Bush et al., 1977).

Angiography is rarely useful in pericardial constriction. Coronary angiography may reveal pericardial scarring that can compress or impede coronary flow (Navetta et al., 1988). Pericardial thickening can be seen by right atrial injection and by observing the right atrial lateral wall thickness. When this is done, a slow, jerky pattern of forward flow of radiographic contrast is often observed due to the limited portion of the cardiac cycle (early diastole) when ventricular filling can occur. Pericardial calcium may also be noted by fluoroscopy, and it usually spares the left ventricular apex (as opposed to left ventricular aneurysmal calcification).

## Congenital Heart Disease

An outline of representative data in patients with congenital heart disease is beyond the scope of this discussion. Several brief comments are pertinent, however.

Techniques for catheterization of infants and chil-

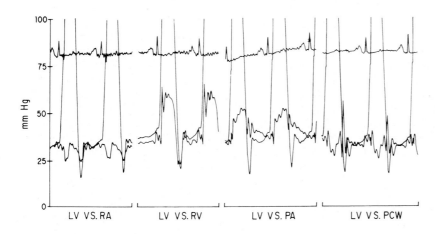

**FIGURE 31–20.** *Equalization of diastolic pressures in constrictive pericarditis.* When the left ventricular pressure (LV) is tracked versus the right atrial (RA), right ventricular (RV), pulmonary artery (PA), and pulmonary capillary wedge (PCW) pressures, all the diastolic pressures are similar. Note that the RV diastolic is half the RV systolic in the *second panel* and that all the diastolic pressures are greatly elevated.

dren vary widely with the age of the child. The catheterization should be guided by the results of careful echo-Doppler examinations to prevent acquisition of redundant information. If the infant is less than 1 week old, an umbilical artery is generally catheterized for pressure monitoring. Venous access is usually easiest to achieve using the femoral vein, although the umbilical vein may be an option in neonates. The atrial septum may be readily crossed, and left-sided heart catheterization is done through the patent foramen ovale. In children over 1 year of age, the femoral approach is routinely used in most laboratories. Various sedatives are used at the time of the procedure, depending on the child's age and whether cyanosis is present.

Cardiac catheterization in neonates carries a higher risk than in older children or in adults (Stanger et al., 1974). Urgent catheterization is generally done in cyanotic neonates, because interventional procedures (e.g., atrial septostomy) or the use of prostaglandin $E_1$ infusions to maintain a patent ductus arteriosus can be life-saving. A discussion of newer interventional procedures for patients with congenital heart

disease is included in the section on valvuloplasty and other invasive therapeutic procedures.

## PERCUTANEOUS BALLOON VALVULOPLASTY AND OTHER INTERVENTIONAL TECHNIQUES

Coronary angioplasty and other percutaneous interventional techniques for the treatment of coronary artery disease are described in Part II of this chapter. Interventional catheterization procedures currently are employed in selected patients with congenital and valvular heart disease. Rashkind and Miller (1966) initiated the use of balloon catheter techniques for patients with congenital heart disease, reporting 31 children with transposition of the great vessels in whom catheter balloon atrioseptostomy was performed (Rashkind and Miller, 1968). Since then, the field of catheter intervention has grown considerably, and its application has been broadened to include aortic coarctation (Lock et al., 1983a; Morrow et al., 1988), obstructed intracardiac baffles (Lloyd et al.,

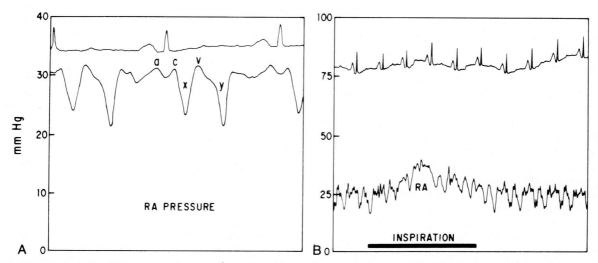

**FIGURE 31–21.** *Representative right atrial (RA) tracings in constrictive pericarditis. A,* The rapid x and y descents and the "square root" sign in diastole. *B,* Inspiration results in a rise in the RA pressure. The rise or lack of fall in the RA pressure with inspiration is referred to as *Kussmaul's sign.*

1987; Lock et al., 1984; Pelikan et al., 1988), and stenosed pulmonary veins (Driscoll et al., 1982) and arteries (Lock et al., 1983b). Catheter methods have also been used to insert devices to close atrial septal defects (King et al., 1976) and to close patent ductus arteriosus (Portsmann et al., 1967; Rashkind and Tait, 1985), arteriovenous fistulas (Terry et al., 1983), and even ventricular septal defects (Lock et al., 1988). Although a great deal must still be learned, these therapeutic catheterization procedures have steadily grown to significant caseloads for many busy pediatric cardiac catheterization laboratories (Lock et al., 1986).

More recently, the procedures have been applied in adult cardiac catheterization laboratories (Rahimtoola, 1987). The Food and Drug Administration has concluded that percutaneous valvuloplasty for pulmonic valve stenosis and mitral stenosis is an appropriate clinical option. Aortic valvuloplasty in adults has also been approved, although its use is much more limited.

Sembh and associates (1979) generally are acknowledged to have been the first surgeons to successfully perform balloon dilation of the pulmonic valve in a patient with pulmonary stenosis and severe tricuspid regurgitation. The procedure was initially accomplished by pulling an inflated balloon catheter back through the affected pulmonic valve. Kan and associates (1982) and Pepine and colleagues (1982) reported the procedure in isolated pulmonic stenosis. The number of reports has grown substantially since that time, and the technique has become widely used and accepted.

In 1984, the first attempts at percutaneous balloon valvuloplasty as therapy for adults with mitral stenosis and aortic stenosis were reported. Inoue and associates (1984) described successful dilation of mitral stenosis in six patients with a transseptal approach, using a single specially designed balloon catheter. In 1984, Lababidi and colleagues (1984) performed percutaneous aortic valvuloplasty in 23 children and young adults. These successes were followed by numerous other reports in young patients, most notably from Lock and associates (1985) and Al Zaibag and colleagues (1986) in rheumatic mitral stenosis and Rupprath and Neuhaus (1985) in aortic stenosis.

McKay and associates (1986) and Palacios and colleagues (1986b) were the first physicians to report the successful application of percutaneous balloon valvuloplasty in adult patients with calcific mitral stenosis. In 1986, Cribier and co-workers described three elderly patients who had calcific aortic stenosis and in whom the procedure was successful.

Follow-up results in patients with pulmonic or mitral stenosis are extremely encouraging. Early restenosis is evident in calcific aortic stenosis, however, and severely limits the use of balloon aortic valvuloplasty procedures in adults. The high rate of restenosis in elderly patients after aortic valvuloplasty is particularly frustrating, because this population also experiences the highest morbidity and mortality rates from open heart surgical procedures (Edmunds et al., 1988).

## Balloon Septostomy

Interventional percutaneous therapies for patients with congenital heart disease began in 1968 with the description of percutaneous transcatheter balloon septostomy of the atrial septum for infants with transposition of the great vessels. This procedure remains in wide use today. A catheter is inserted via either the internal jugular vein or the femoral vein into the right atrium and across the foramen ovale into the left atrial chamber. The balloon catheter is then inflated, with a mixture of contrast and saline to a diameter of 10 to 15 mm. The balloon is then withdrawn abruptly through the atrial septum to enlarge the defect in the atrial septum. Percutaneous blade septostomy is a modification of this technique for use in infants and children with thicker, more resistant atrial septums. A specially designed catheter, with a retractable blade, is placed in the left atrium. The blade is exposed and the catheter is then withdrawn into the right atrium, creating a slice in the atrial septum. Multiple angulated passes are generally made, often followed by balloon dilatation. These procedures increase atrial mixing, improving cardiac output and systemic oxygenation in these infants, allowing critically ill infants to survive to surgical correction. Currently, arterial switch is performed even in infancy. These patients, palliated with balloon septostomy, may undergo complete repair with arterial switch before discharge from the hospital.

## Balloon Pulmonic Valvuloplasty

Pulmonic valvuloplasty is usually performed using the percutaneous right femoral venous approach (Fig. 31–22). A pulmonary artery catheter is replaced by a guidewire, and the balloon catheter is positioned across the pulmonic valve over this wire. Balloon sizes have evolved over time, and most physicians now prefer oversized balloons, because both animal (Ring et al., 1984) and clinical (Radtke et al., 1987) data suggest that maximal dilation about 30% greater than the pulmonic valve annulus improves the acute hemodynamic results. Balloons that inflate to 1.2 to 1.4 times the pulmonary annulus size, as assessed by echocardiography or angiography, are used. Either a double-balloon technique (Ali Khan et al., 1986) or a specially designed trefoil balloon catheter (Meier et al., 1986) is frequently required in adults. If the iliac vein is obstructed, an axillary approach can be used (Sideris et al., 1988).

The immediate and long-term results from pulmonic valvuloplasty have been impressive. This procedure is equally effective in children and in adults with valvular pulmonic stenosis. Pulmonary valve gradients in excess of 50 mm Hg are generally considered sufficient to warrant intervention. "Typical" results that have been reported are summarized in Table 31–7 (Ali Kahn et al., 1986; Cooke et al., 1987; Griffith et al., 1982; Kan et al., 1982, 1984; Marantz et al., 1988; Meier et al., 1986; Pepine et al., 1982; Radtke et al.,

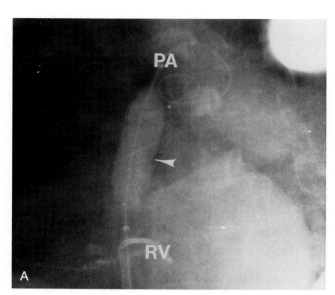
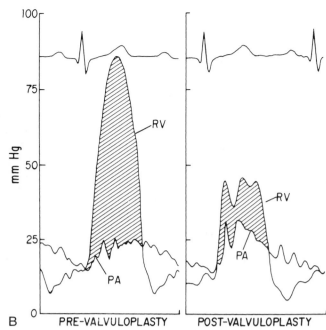

**FIGURE 31–22.** *Pulmonic valvuloplasty. A,* Radiograph, lateral projection, showing a single balloon inflated across the pulmonary valve *(arrowhead).* The tip of the wire-directed catheter is coiled in the pulmonary artery (PA). A second catheter, for pressure measurement, is seen in the right ventricle (RV). *B,* The markedly elevated RV systolic pressure and distorted, "damped" PA pressure change dramatically acutely after balloon pulmonary valvuloplasty (pressure gradient *shaded*).

1987; Rao et al., 1988; Rocchini et al., 1984; Sembh et al., 1979). Immediate hemodynamic data may underestimate the final pulmonic gradient if transient right ventricular dysfunction occurred during the procedure, but such data would overestimate the final gradient if subpulmonic obstruction transiently increased. Either of these situations may effect acute changes. Significant subpulmonic obstruction can occur immediately after the procedure, but fortunately this usually responds to beta-blocker therapy (Rao et al., 1988). This infundibular obstruction regresses over time after either pulmonary valvotomy (Engle, 1958; Griffith, 1982) or balloon valvuloplasty (Rao et al., 1988; Sullivan et al., 1986). If dysplasia of the pulmonic valve is present, balloon dilation appears to

be less effective, although larger balloon sizes may provide satisfactory results with these valves as well (DiSessa et al., 1987; Marantz et al., 1988). The true incidence of pulmonic regurgitation after pulmonic valvuloplasty ranges from 0 to 74%, depending on the methods used for assessment. Echo-Doppler studies suggest that pulmonic insufficiency of at least a mild degree is a frequent consequence of the procedure. Pulmonary insufficiency created by balloon dilation does not cause any short-term adverse effects. Long-term follow-up data will be required to see whether this will have any late adverse effect on right ventricular function or clinical outcome.

Follow-up data up to several years have shown a very low rate of recurrent pulmonary valve stenosis. This is especially true if the final gradient at the end of the procedure is 30 mm Hg or less. The uncommon finding of significant stenosis in follow-up often represents an inadequate acute result rather than true valvular restenosis.

## Balloon Valvuloplasty for Congenital Aortic and Mitral Valve Stenosis

Although percutaneous balloon valvuloplasty for congenital pulmonic stenosis is extremely effective and has become the initial procedure of choice for this disorder, the results following dilation of congenital aortic and mitral valve stenosis are less uniform. Balloon valvuloplasty for congenital bicuspid aortic stenosis in infants and children provides effective palliation and may thereby delay the need for eventual

■ **Table 31–7.** "TYPICAL" IMMEDIATE HEMODYNAMIC RESULTS AFTER PERCUTANEOUS VALVULOPLASTY PROCEDURES

| Procedure and Measure | Before | After |
|---|---|---|
| Pulmonic valvuloplasty | | |
|   Peak right ventricular pressure (mm Hg) | 100 | 50 |
|   Peak gradient (mm Hg) | 80 | 30 |
|   Cardiac index (l/min/m$^2$) | 3 | 3 |
| Mitral valvuloplasty | | |
|   Mean mitral gradient (mm Hg) | 17 | 7 |
|   Mitral valve area (cm$^2$) | 1 | 2.2 |
|   Cardiac index (l/min/m$^2$) | 2.5 | 3 |
| Aortic valvuloplasty | | |
|   Mean aortic gradient (mm Hg) | 75 | 35 |
|   Aortic valve area (cm$^2$) | 0.6 | 0.9 |
|   Cardiac index (l/min/m$^2$) | 2 | 2.2 |

valve replacement (Choy et al., 1987; Sholler et al., 1988). The most frequent limitation of this technique is the creation of aortic insufficiency. The procedure is usually done via the antegrade transseptal approach. This avoids the use of large sheaths and catheters in the arterial system and thus avoids the risk of severe arterial injury in these infants and young children. Single- or double-balloon catheter techniques have been described (Beekman et al., 1988), positioning the balloon(s) across the aortic valve from the femoral vein via a transseptal approach.

Conversely, congenital mitral stenosis is rarely amenable to balloon dilatation (Alday and Juaneda, 1987; Kyeselis et al., 1986). Unlike rheumatic mitral valve stenosis, commissural fusion is uncommon in these children. The stenosis results primarily from abnormal valvular architecture, chordal fusion, or abnormal chordal attachments. The parachute-type mitral valve (single papillary muscle), for example, produces fusion of the subvalvular apparatus that is not improved by balloon dilatation. Severe acute mitral regurgitation often results from attempted dilatation of these valves. Its use remains under investigation.

## Percutaneous Treatment of Coarctation of the Aorta

Controversy continues regarding the optimal treatment for coarctation of the aorta (Khalilullah et al., 1987). Balloon angioplasty of the aorta is not technically difficult; the controversial issues relate more to the risk of the procedure and its long-term complications. Balloon angioplasty of the aorta may create large intimal tears that may extend into the deeper layers of the aortic wall (Harrison et al., 1990b). In the extreme case, this may lead to aortic rupture and death. Although acute aortic rupture is rare with this procedure, the deep intimal and medial injury resulting from balloon dilatation coupled with long-term aortic pressure may cause late aneurysm formation at the site of the balloon dilatation. Thus, although balloon angioplasty of coarctation can effectively reduce the degree of stenosis, the long-term results of this form of treatment and its success rate in comparison with surgical repair remain incompletely defined. Initial enthusiasm for treatment of the adult patient with coarctation has declined, although some still feel that balloon angioplasty may have a role in late recoarctation following initial surgical therapy (Saul et al., 1987).

## Balloon Angioplasty and Intravascular Stents for Venous and Pulmonary Artery Stenosis

Congenital stenosis of the systemic and pulmonary veins and branch stenosis of the pulmonary arteries have posed difficult problems in management. Surgical attempts to correct these stenoses have been disappointing. Many stenoses in the distal segments of the pulmonary arteries are inaccessible to the surgeon. In addition, venous stenoses are often quite difficult to correct with surgery and have been fraught with problems of postoperative venous thrombosis. Many venous stenoses and stenoses in the pulmonary arteries are now approachable via catheterization (Ali et al., 1987; Dodds et al., 1994). Patients with pulmonary artery stenoses related to left-to-right shunts that are native or surgically corrected (e.g., patients with previous systemic-to-pulmonary artery shunts for tetralogy of Fallot) now can be relieved with percutaneous dilatation techniques (Hoekenga et al., 1987). The pulmonary artery has tremendous elasticity, and gross overdilation of these vessels, up to 2 to 3 times the normal vessel's diameter, is often required. Despite even this degree of overdilation, recoil is not infrequent, leading to only moderate improvement of the stenosis severity even immediately following balloon dilatation. For this reason, metallic intervascular stents to date have been employed successfully in these areas. The most effective of these stents to date have been the balloon-expandable Palmaz-Schatz stents (Johnson and Johnson, New Brunswick, NJ) (O'Laughlin et al., 1993). These stents are preloaded onto an angioplasty balloon and delivered to the site of the stenosis through a long intravascular sheath (Mullins sheath, Cook Inc., Bloomington, MA). This approach prevents the stent from being dislodged while it is inserted to the site of the stenosis. Once in place, the long sheath can be withdrawn, leaving the stent exposed at the stenotic area. The stent is then expanded with the balloon angioplasty catheter, which embeds it in the vessel wall. Subsequent balloon inflations are performed to achieve the diameter of the normal vessel.

Potential complications from stent use include vessel rupture, hemoptysis, and improper stent deployment or embolization. In addition, relief of pulmonary arterial stenoses may infrequently cause transient localized pulmonary edema in the stented segment of lung. This is due to the high pulmonary flow in these areas. This problem resolves over several days with conservative supportive management. Because of the large caliber of the pulmonary arteries and the high flow through these areas, restenosis and thrombosis of pulmonary arterial stents have not been significant.

## Closure Devices

Various closure devices are now available or under investigation for closure of intravascular shunts and even intracardiac defects. The simplest of these devices are the metallic intravascular coils. These coils can be used to occlude vessels. For example, patients with Eisenmenger's syndrome may develop large systemic-to-pulmonary artery collaterals. These friable vessels may rupture and cause severe, life-threatening hemoptysis. Once the vessel is selectively cannulated, the metallic coil is inserted through the catheter into the vessel, causing thrombosis. Each metallic coil contains Dacron mesh attached to the wire, promoting thrombosis. This simple technique can be life-saving in cases of severe hemoptysis.

The closure of intracardiac defects is more complex, and no device is currently available for widespread use. Several devices are under investigation. The earliest of these is the Rashkind device for closure of patent ductus (Fig. 31–23). This is a double umbrella-type device that is inserted via a catheter across the ductus. The distal end of the umbrella is allowed to expand, and then the device is withdrawn back into the ductus. The proximal end of the umbrella is then allowed to expand, trapping the device within the ductus and closing it. Similar devices are now under investigation for closure of atrial septal defects as well as muscular ventricular septal defects (Figs. 31–24 and 31–25). These devices hold great promise for nonoperative closure of these congenital defects.

## Balloon Mitral Commissurotomy

Percutaneous balloon mitral commissurotomy (also called balloon mitral valvotomy or valvuloplasty) is an effective alternative to surgical treatment in se-

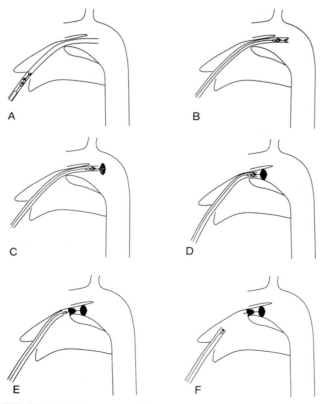

**FIGURE 31–23.** *Percutaneous closure of patent ductus arteriosus (PDA). A,* Long sheath positioned across PDA. *B,* Double-umbrella device positioned within sheath. *C,* Distal umbrella deployed by advancing device. *D,* Sheath/device assembly withdrawn into ductus. *E,* Sheath withdrawn to display proximal umbrella. *F,* Device release within PDA. *(A–F,* From Rashkind, W. J., and Tait, M. S.: Interventional cardiac catheterization in congenital heart disease. *In* Schroeder, J. S. [ed]: Invasive cardiology. Cardiac Clin., 15:303, 1985.)

lected cases of rheumatic mitral valve stenosis. This procedure was first described in 1984 and has recently been approved by a Food and Drug Administration advisory panel as appropriate therapy for treatment of mitral stenosis. Although the acute procedural success of this procedure has been confirmed in many patients, optimal patient selection for this procedure and the long-term outcome of the procedure continue to be defined.

Balloon mitral commissurotomy may be accomplished with one or two polyethylene balloons (McKay et al., 1987), a system used most frequently in the United States, or with the single latex Inoue balloon catheter (Al Zaibag et al., 1986; Inoue et al., 1993) (Fig. 31–26). The latter technique is gaining increasing popularity because of its simplicity, decreased procedural time, and lower operative risk. In addition, a retrograde technique using a specialized balloon catheter system to cross the mitral valve from the left ventricular side has been described. Representative results of balloon mitral commissurotomy are shown in Table 31–7 (Babic et al., 1988; Chen et al., 1988; DeUbago et al., 1987; McKay et al., 1987, 1988; Palacios et al., 1987). Balloon commissurotomy usually decreases the mean valvular gradient by about 50% and roughly doubles the mitral valve area, often to valve areas that exceed 1.5 cm².

These acute hemodynamic improvements have been associated with marked clinical improvement in follow-up. Most patients achieve and remain in functional Class I or II for at least the current duration of follow-up available (5 years). Patient selection for balloon commissurotomy depends largely on mitral valve morphology as assessed by echocardiography. Early investigators examined the prognostic value of multiple echocardiographic and clinical variables in patients undergoing balloon mitral commissurotomy. They devised a semiquantitative echocardiographic scoring system consisting of four components: leaflet mobility, leaflet thickening, valvular calcification, and the degree of subvalvular thickening. These individual components were scored on a scale from 0 to 4, and individual component scores were added to yield a total valve score. These investigators found that a total echo score less than 8 predicted a successful acute hemodynamic result with balloon commissurotomy. Other investigators, however, have recently shown a poor correlation comparing this echo scoring system and results, especially in series using the Inoue balloon. Assessment of the presence or absence of commissural fusion in the short axis view may prove to be more useful in this regard, because splitting of commissures is the mechanism of improvement in mitral stenosis with balloon dilatation (Reid et al., 1987).

Echocardiography remains an important component of the preprocedural assessment of patients with mitral stenosis. In our institution we obtain both transthoracic and *transesophageal echocardiograms* (TEEs) immediately before performing balloon mitral commissurotomy. In particular, the TEE has become important in excluding patients with left atrial

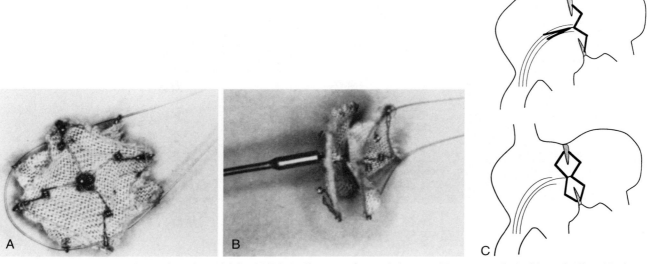

**FIGURE 31–24.** *Percutaneous closure of atrial septal defect (ASD).* A, Close-up of wire skeleton and Dacron mesh double-umbrella ASD closure device. B, Side view of device attached to delivery catheter. C, Illustration of device deployment facilitated by the use of a long sheath.

thrombi and in reducing procedurally related embolic complications. Left atrial thrombi are an absolute contraindication to balloon commissurotomy, because the balloon catheter may dislodge the thrombus and cause systemic embolization. Transthoracic echocardiography is often better than the TEE in determining the degree of subvalvular thickening, an area often inadequately visualized by the TEE. Thus, the two studies complement each other in the preprocedural assessment of the patient. Currently, patients with symptomatic mitral valve stenosis and mitral valve area of less than 1.5 cm² whose valves appear pliable without significant valvular calcification are considered good candidates for balloon commissurotomy.

The presence of greater than 2+ mitral regurgitation or left atrial thrombi are contraindications to the procedure. These criteria are similar to those for surgical commissurotomy.

With the double-balloon technique, transseptal catheterization of the left atrium is performed via the right femoral vein. After transseptal catheterization, a wire is directed across the mitral valve and coiled near the left ventricular apex. The interatrial septum is dilated with a 6- or 8-mm balloon catheter, and a double-lumen sheath is then positioned across the mitral valve over the guidewire. A second guidewire is then placed near the left ventricular apex. Separate balloon catheters are positioned side by side over

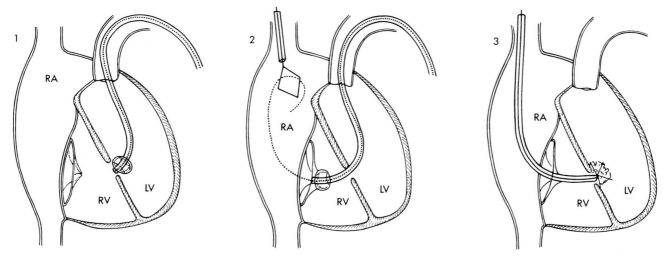

**FIGURE 31–25.** *Transcatheter closure of ventricular septal defect (VSD).* 1, A balloon-tip catheter is shown transversing the VSD from the left ventricle (LV). 2, A wire is introduced through the balloon-tip catheter and is snared by a catheter in the right atrium (RA). The RA wire is then pulled through to the LV, and the guiding catheter with the umbrella prosthesis is inserted into the LV. 3, The distal umbrella is then allowed to open and is pulled back against the septum. (RV = right ventricle.) (1–3, From Lock J. E., Block, P. C., McKay, R. G., et al.: Transcatheter closure of ventricular septal defects. Circulation, 78:361, 1988. By permission of the American Heart Association, Inc.)

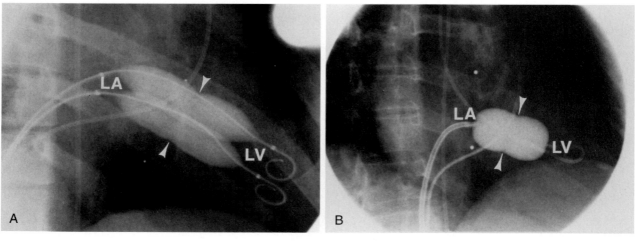

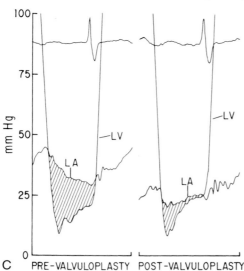

**FIGURE 31–26.** *Balloon mitral commissurotomy.* Radiograph in right anterior oblique projection illustrating the double-balloon *(A)* and the Inoue balloon *(B)* techniques. Position of the mitral valve shown by *arrowheads. C,* A representative hemodynamic result is shown. (LA = left atrium, LV = left ventricle.)

each guidewire and manipulated into position across the mitral valve. The balloons are then simultaneously hand-inflated until the "waists" in the balloons disappear (see Fig. 31–23).

The Inoue balloon catheter system has several advantages over the polyethlyene double-balloon technique. The Inoue balloon catheter has a curved inner-steering wire that facilitates placement of the balloon through the stenotic mitral valve, eliminating the need for a guidewire. Once transseptal catheterization of the left atrium is performed, a rigid No. 14 French dilator is used to dilate the interatrial septum. The Inoue balloon catheter is then placed across the inter-atrial septum into the left atrium. An inner-stretching tube is employed that stiffens and thins the balloon portion of the catheter to present a low-profile device for insertion and removal across the interatrial septum. Once in the left atrium, this stretching tube is removed and the balloon catheter is directed through the stenotic mitral valve orifice using the curved, torqueable steering stylette. Once across the mitral valve, the distal portion of the balloon is inflated on the ventricular side of the valve. The balloon is then withdrawn slightly into the mitral valve annulus, and

further hand-inflation of the contrast saline mixture inflates the proximal portion of the balloon, seating the "waist" of the balloon in the mitral annulus. Final inflation of the balloon dilates the mitral valve annulus and commissures. Stepwise inflation of the valve is possible with this catheter simply by injecting calibrated amounts of the contrast saline mixture to achieve specific balloon diameters. This eliminates the need for multiple catheter exchanges.

Although percutaneous balloon mitral commissurotomy has been very successful, this complex percutaneous procedure is associated with significant morbidity and mortality (Harrison et al., 1994). In the early (1987–1989) NHLBI Registry, the procedure-related mortality rate was 1.6%, and the 30-day mortality rate was 3.2% with the double-balloon techniques. Embolic events were encountered in 2.2% of patients. Severe mitral regurgitation (defined as greater than or equal to 3+ mitral regurgitation) was encountered in 3.3% of patients. Cardiac perforation occurred in 27 of these 738 patients. Left ventricular perforation, due to the left ventricular guidewires and balloon catheters (required with the double-balloon technique), was responsible for most of the procedure-related deaths (5 of the 12 deaths). The M-Heart Registry analysis of the double-balloon technique confirmed left ventricular perforation as the complication most likely to cause procedure-related mortality. In addition, the double-balloon technique in these studies was associated with an atrial septal defect rate (> 1.5:1 left-to-right shunt) in 9.6% of patients. In contrast, severe complications were less frequent in the North American Inoue Registry. The procedure-related mortality rate was 0.1%, and the 30-day mortality rate was 0.6%. Central nervous system emboli occurred in only 1% of patients; cardiac perforation was encountered in 1% as well. None of the cardiac perforations involved the left ventricle, and none required emergency surgery or caused death. Atrial septal defects with this low-profile single catheter were less common as well, occurring in 2.5%. Increased mitral regurgitation (two or more grades), however, was not infrequent, occurring in 10.5% of patients using the Inoue balloon catheter.

Although long-term data on the results of balloon mitral commissurotomy remain incomplete, several studies examining data out to 5 years look very encouraging. Restenosis has been a very infrequent problem, and the overwhelming majority of patients remain improved in New York Heart Association Functional Class I or II. Several studies have compared surgical commissurotomy with percutaneous balloon commisurotomy. The acute, 6-month, and 1-year results of these studies have shown similar efficacy of the surgical and balloon commissurotomy techniques (Mullin et al., 1972).

## Percutaneous Balloon Valvuloplasty for Aortic Stenosis

Although percutaneous balloon aortic valvuloplasty has been a suitable palliative option to delay surgery for many children with bicuspid aortic stenosis, this procedure has been largely ineffective for adults with calcified aortic valves. Aortic stenosis in children is primarily due to bicuspid aortic valves with commissural fusion. The standard surgical approach to these patients has been open surgical valvotomy with sharp dissection of the commissures to reduce the degree of stenosis. Similar improvements in the severity of aortic stenosis can be achieved through percutaneous balloon valvuloplasty in infants and children. In 200 patients with congenital aortic stenosis in Children's Hospital in Boston, gradient reduction of greater than 50% has been achieved in 88% of children. Severe aortic regurgitation requiring valve replacement has been an infrequent complication, occurring in less than 2% of patients. There have been no deaths or strokes, and restenosis has occurred in less than 5%, with follow-up extending to 6 years.

Surgical aortic commissurotomy and valve repair for adults with calcific aortic stenosis (Bailey et al., 1956; Hsieh et al., 1986) using mechanical or ultrasonic débridement (Harken et al., 1958; King et al.,

1986; Leithe et al., 1991; Worley et al., 1988) have failed because of a high rate of early restenosis or the creation of significant aortic regurgitation. Similarly, percutaneous balloon aortic valvuloplasty for adults with calcific aortic stenosis, though it generated early enthusiasm, has been associated with disappointing mid- and long-term results.

The procedure was initially described in 1986 (Cribier et al., 1986) and was promoted as an alternative to surgery for elderly patients with aortic stenosis (Cribier et al., 1987; Davidson et al., 1987; Safian et al., 1988). These patients often have co-morbidity and are at high risk for morbidity and mortality following aortic valve replacement. In adults, balloon aortic valvuloplasty usually is performed using a retrograde approach via the femoral artery (Fig. 31–27). Large arterial sheaths (No. 10 to 14 French) are required. Several techniques have been described (Block et al., 1987; Dorros et al., 1987; Isner et al., 1987), ranging from using a single balloon to using up to three balloon catheters simultaneously to dilate the valve. With the balloon(s) positioned retrogradely across the aortic valve, the stenotic valve is dilated by hand-inflation of a contrast-saline mixture. The actual technique used to dilate the valve, however, has little bearing on the acute hemodynamic results. The aortic valve gradient usually improves modestly immediately following balloon aortic valvuloplasty. This improvement is associated with about a 30% increase in aortic valve area but uncommonly results in absolute valve areas of 1.0 cm$^2$ or more. This leaves many patients with at least moderately severe aortic stenosis (Robicsek and Harbold, 1987).

The complication rate due to the balloon aortic valvuloplasty procedure is also significant (NHLBI Balloon Valvuloplasty Registry, 1991). Fifty-seven per cent of elderly patients enrolled in the NHLBI registry experienced at least one complication during the procedure or within the following 24 hours. The most frequent complication was bleeding and vascular damage due to the large arterial sheaths required in these elderly patients. Surprisingly, worsening aortic insufficiency was a rare event. A serious complication before discharge from the hospital occurred in 31%, and the procedure-related mortality rate approached 5% (Bashore et al., 1991).

Although clinical improvement often follows balloon aortic valvuloplasty, this clinical response is almost always short-lived (Davidson et al., 1990; Litvack et al., 1988; Otto et al., 1994). Restenosis of the aortic valve frequently follows balloon aortic valvuloplasty. By 6 months, 75% of patients demonstrate hemodynamic restenosis of the aortic valve (Harrison et al., 1990a). Clinical follow-up of these patients has shown a poor long-term prognosis consistent with the follow-up hemodynamic observations. At 6 months following balloon aortic valvuloplasty, 60% of patients had recurrent symptoms, and by 1 year, the survival rate was only 50%. The 3-year survival rate in our series of 165 patients was only 7% (Lieberman et al., 1994). Follow-up studies of these patients reveals that left ventricular function, rather than the

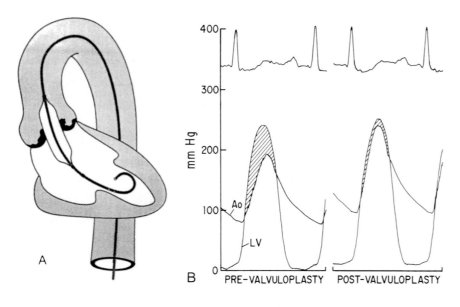

400

300

mm Hg

200

Ao

100

LV

0

A

B    PRE-VALVULOPLASTY    POST-VALVULOPLASTY

**FIGURE 31–27.** *Aortic valvuloplasty. A,* The single-balloon technique is shown with the inflated balloon retrograde across the aortic valve. *B,* A representative hemodynamic result is shown.

severity of the valvular stenosis, most significantly affects clinical outcome and prognosis (Davidson et al., 1991). In addition, selected patients who were originally felt to be nonoperative candidates but who developed recurrent symptoms following balloon aortic valvuloplasty did surprisingly well after aortic valve replacement. In this very-high-risk group, a low mortality rate (about 10%) and excellent 3-year survival rates of approaching 85% were reported (Lieberman et al., 1994).

Thus, although balloon aortic valvuloplasty may be appropriate for children with pliable bicuspid aortic stenosis, very few indications for percutaneous balloon valvuloplasty exist for adults with calcific aortic stenosis. The high incidence of restenosis at 6 months, the poor long-term outcome, and the high complication rate should limit balloon aortic valvuloplasty to severely symptomatic elderly patients with calcific aortic stenosis and normal left ventricular function who are not candidates for surgical aortic valve replacement for other reasons. Advanced age, by itself, is not a contraindication to aortic valve replacement.

## SELECTED BIBLIOGRAPHY

Carabello, B. A.: Advances in the hemodynamic assessment of stenotic cardiac valves. J. Am. Coll. Cardiol., 10:912, 1987.

This review summarizes the concepts related to Gorlin's formula. It reviews the use of this formula and suggests how it might be changed. This article is followed by a response by Gorlin that is positive regarding the practical use of this formula for the determination of valve area.

Marcus, M. L., Skorton, D. J., Johnson, R. R., et al.: Visual estimates of percent diameter coronary stenosis: "A battered gold standard." J. Am. Coll. Cardiol., 11:882, 1988.

This review focuses on the difficulties in using the percentage of stenosis in assessing the severity of coronary disease. It is brief and summarizes the vagaries in the use of visual data regarding coronary stenoses. The editorial is followed by a response by Gould commenting on functional tests that are currently available for the assessment of coronary stenoses.

Mehlman, D. J.: A pictorial and radiographic guide for identification of prosthetic heart valves. Prog. Cardiovasc. Dis., 30:441, 1988.

The author summarizes the radiographic appearance of prosthetic heart valves and provides a useful review of this area. This reference guide is excellent for the identification of the prosthetic heart valve devices.

Perry, S. B., Keane, J. D., and Lock, J. E.: Interventional catheterization in pediatric congenital and acquired heart disease. Am. J. Cardiol., 61:1090, 1988.

This article presents the present status of catheter-directed therapy in pediatric congenital and acquired disease. Although it again focuses on a single institution's experience, it is well referenced and provides a concise summary of this area.

Sheehan, F. H., Bolson, E. L., Dodge, H. T., et al.: Advantages and applications of the centerline method for characterizing regional ventricular function. Circulation, 74:293, 1986.

The centerline method for determining regional ventricular function is described. This particular method has become popular because it allows the regional function to be analyzed statistically in a readily achievable manner.

Wigle, E. D., Sasson, Z., Henderson, M. A., et al.: Hypertrophic cardiomyopathy. The importance of the site and the extent of hypertrophy: A review. Prog. Cardiovasc. Dis., 28:1, 1985.

This is a clinically relevant and complete review of hypertrophic cardiomyopathy. It discusses in depth many of the controversies regarding the disease process.

## BIBLIOGRAPHY

Adams, D. F., Fraser, D. B., and Abrams, H. L.: The complications of coronary arteriography. Circulation, 48:609, 1973.

ACC Cardiovascular Imaging Committee: Use of nonionic or low-osmolar contrast agents in cardiovascular procedures. J. Am. Coll. Cardiol., 21:269, 1993.

Alday, L. E., and Juaneda, E.: Percutaneous balloon dilatation in congenital mitral stenosis. Br. Heart J., 57:479, 1987.

Ali, M. K., Ewer, M. S., Balakrishnan, P. B., et al.: Balloon angioplasty for superior vena cava obstruction. Ann. Intern. Med., 107:856, 1987.

Ali Khan, M. A., Yousef, S. A., and Mullins, C. E.: Percutaneous transluminal balloon pulmonary valvuloplasty for relief of pulmonary valve stenosis with special reference to double-balloon technique. Am. Heart J., 112:158, 1986.

Al Zaibag, M., Kasab, S. A., Ribeiro, P. A., and Fagih, M. R.: Percutaneous double balloon mitral valvotomy for the rheumatic mitral valve stenosis. Lancet, 1:757, 1986.

Amplatz, K., Formanek, G., Stanger, P., and Wilson, W.: Mechanics of selective coronary artery catheterization via femoral approach. Radiology, 89:1040, 1967.

Angel, J., Soler-Soler, J., Anivarro, I., and Domingo, E.: Hemodynamic evaluation of stenotic cardiac valves. II: Modification of the simplified valve formula for mitral and aortic valve area calculation. Cathet. Cardiovasc. Diagn., 11:127, 1985.

Antman, E. M., Marsh, J. D., Green, L. H., and Grossman, W.: Blood oxygen measurements in the assessment of intracardiac left to right shunts: A critical appraisal of methodology. Am. J. Cardiol., 46:265, 1980.

Babic, V. V., Dorros, G., Pejcic, P., et al.: Percutaneous mitral valvuloplasty: Retrograde transarterial double balloon technique utilizing the trans-septal approach. Cathet. Cardiovasc. Diagn., 14:229, 1988.

Babic, V. V., Pejcic, P., Djurisic, Z., et al.: Percutaneous transarterial balloon valvuloplasty for mitral valve stenosis. Am. J. Cardiol., 57:1101, 1986.

Bailey, C. P., Bulton, H. E., Nichols, H. T., et al.: The surgical treatment of aortic stenosis. J. Thorac. Surg., 31:375, 1956.

Baim, D. S., Rothman, M. T., and Harrison, D. C.: Simultaneous measurement of coronary venous flow and oxygen saturation during transient alterations in myocardial oxygen supply and demand. Am. J. Cardiol., 49:743, 1982.

Bartle, S. H., and Hermann, H. J.: Acute mitral regurgitation in man: Hemodynamic evidence and observations indicating an early role for the pericardium. Circulation, 36:839, 1967.

Bashore T. M., Davidson C. J., Berman, A. D., et al.: Acute and 30-day outcome in 674 patients following balloon aortic valvuloplasty. Circulation, 84:2383, 1991.

Bashore, T. M., Davidson, C. J., Mark, D. B., et al.: Iopamidol use in the cardiac catheterization laboratory: A retrospective analysis of 3,313 patients. Cardiology, 5(Suppl.):6, 1988.

Beekman, R. H., Rocchini, A. P., Crowley, D. C., et al.: Comparison of single and double balloon valvuloplasty in children with aortic stenosis. J. Am. Coll. Cardiol., 12:480, 1988.

Bettman, M. A., Bourdillon, P. D., Barry, W. H., et al.: Contrast agents for cardiac angiography: Effects of a nonionic agent vs. a standard ionic agent. Radiology, 153:583, 1984.

Björk, V. O., Balstrom, G., and Uggla, L. G.: Left auricular pressure measurements in man. Ann. Surg., 138:718, 1953.

Block, P. C., and Palacios, I. F.: Comparison of hemodynamic results of anteriograde versus retrograde percutaneous balloon aortic valvuloplasty. Am. J. Cardiol., 60:659, 1987.

Borow, K., Green, L. H., Mann, T., et al.: End-systolic volume as a predictor of postoperative left ventricular performance in volume overload from valvular regurgitation. Am. J. Med., 68:655, 1980.

Bourassa, M. G., and Noble, J.: Complication rate of coronary arteriography. A review of 5250 cases studied by percutaneous femoral technique. Circulation, 53:106, 1976.

Brannon, E. S., Weens, H. S., and Warren, J. V.: Atrial septal defect: Study of hemodynamics by the technique of right heart catheterization. Am. J. Med. Sci., 210:480, 1948.

Braunwald, E., and Swan, H. J. C.: Cooperative study on cardiac catheterization. Circulation, 37(Suppl. III):1, 1968.

Brock R., Milstein, B. B., and Ross D. N.: Percutaneous left ventricular puncture in the assessment of aortic stenosis. Thorax, 11:163, 1956.

Brockenbrough, E. C., Braunwald, E., and Morrow, A. G.: A hemodynamic technique for the detection of hypertrophic subaortic stenosis. Circulation, 23:189, 1961.

Bush, C. A., Stang, J. M., Wooley, C. F., and Kilman, J. W.: Occult constrictive pericardial disease: Diagnosis by rapid volume expansion and correction by pericardiectomy. Circulation, 56:924, 1977.

Cabin, H. S., and Roberts, W. C.: Left ventricular aneurysm, intraaneurysmal thrombus and systemic embolus in coronary heart disease. Chest, 77:586, 1980.

Cannon, S. E., Richards, K. L., Crawford, M.: Hydraulic estimation of stenotic orifice area: A correction of the Gorlin formula. Circulation, 71:1170, 1985.

Cannon, S. R., Richards, K. L., Crawford, M. H., et al.: Inadequacy of the Gorlin formula for predicting prosthetic valve area. Am. J. Cardiol., 62:113, 1988.

Carabello, B. A.: Advances in the hemodynamic assessment of stenotic cardiac valves. J. Am. Coll. Cardiol., 10:912, 1987.

Carabello, B. A., Barry, W. H., and Grossman, W.: Changes in arterial pressure during left heart pullback in patients with aortic stenosis: A sign of severe aortic stenosis. Am. J. Cardiol., 44:424, 1979.

Carabello, B. A., Nolan, S. P., and McGuire, L. B.: Assessment of preoperative left ventricular function in patients with mitral regurgitation: Value of the end-systolic stress–end-systolic volume ratio. Circulation, 64:1212, 1981.

Carlson, E. B., Mintz, G. S., and Bemis, C. E.: Hemodynamic significance of normal and abnormal fluoroscopic patterns of disc motion in the Beall mitral valve prosthesis. Radiology, 141:335, 1981.

Carpentier, A., Cherard S., and Fahiani, J. N.: Reconstructive surgery of the mitral valve: Ten year appraisal. J. Thorac. Cardiovasc. Surg., 79:338, 1980.

Casale, P. N., Palacios, I. F., Abascal, V. M., et al.: Gorlin valve area varies with cardiac output in aortic stenosis [Abstract]. J. Am. Coll. Cardiol., 11(Suppl. II):63A, 1988.

Cha, S. D., and Gooch, A. S.: Diagnosis of tricuspid regurgitation: Current status. Arch. Intern. Med., 143: 1763, 1983.

Chen, C., Lo, Z., Huang, Z., et al.: Percutaneous transseptal balloon mitral valvuloplasty: The Chinese experience in 30 patients. Am. Heart J., 115:937, 1988.

Choy, M., Beekman, R. H., and Rocchini, A. P.: Percutaneous balloon valvuloplasty for valvular aortic stenosis in infants and children. Am. J. Cardiol., 59:1010, 1987.

Clark, C. E., Henry, W. L., and Epstein, S. E.: Familial prevalence and genetic transmission of idiopathic hypertrophic subaortic stenosis. N. Engl. J. Med., 289:709, 1973.

Cobanoglu, A., and Starr, A.: Tricuspid valve surgery: Indications, methods, and results. In Frankl, W. S., and Berest, A. N. (eds): Cardiovascular Clinics Valvular Heart Disease: Comprehensive Evaluation and Management. Philadelphia, F. A. Davis, 1986, pp. 375–388.

Cohen, M. Y., and Greenberg, M. A.: Constrictive pericarditis: Early and late complication of cardiac surgery. Am. J. Cardiol., 43:657, 1979.

Colle, J. P., Rahal, S., Ohayon, J., et al.: Global left ventricular function and regional wall motion in pure mitral stenosis. Clin. Cardiol., 67:148, 1983.

Come, P. C., and Riley, M. F.: Tricuspid anular dilatation and failure of tricuspid leaflet coaptation in tricuspid regurgitation. Am. J. Cardiol., 55:599, 1985.

Cooke, J. P., Seward, J. B., and Holmes, D. R.: Transluminal balloon valvotomy for pulmonic stenosis in an adult. Mayo Clin. Proc., 62:306, 1987.

Cope, C.: Technique for transseptal catheterization of the left atrium: Preliminary report. J. Thorac. Surg., 37:482, 1959.

Cournand, A.: Cardiac catheterization: Development of the technique, its contribution to experimental medicine, and its initial application in man. Acta Med. Scand., 79(Suppl.):7, 1978.

Cribier, A., Saoudi, N., Berland, J., et al.: Percutaneous transluminal balloon valvuloplasty of acquired aortic stenosis in elderly patients: An alternative to valve replacement? Lancet, 1:63, 1986.

Cribier, A., Savin, T., Berland, J., et al.: Percutaneous transluminal balloon valvuloplasty of adult aortic stenosis: Report of 92 cases. J. Am. Coll. Cardiol., 9:381, 1987.

Curry, T. S., Dowdey, J. E., and Murry, R. C.: Christensen's Introduction to the Physics of Diagnostic Radiology. Philadelphia, Lea & Febiger, 1984.

Davidson, C. J., Harrison, J. K., Leithe, M. E., et al.: Failure of balloon aortic valvuloplasty to result in sustained clinical improvement in patients with depressed left ventricular function. Am. J. Cardiol., 65:72, 1990.

Davidson, C. J., Harrison, J. K., Pieper, K. S., et al: Determinants of 1-year outcome from balloon aortic valvuloplasty. Am. J. Cardiol., 68:75, 1991.

Davidson, C. J., Skelton, T. N., Kisslo, K., et al.: Percutaneous balloon valvuloplasty of calcific aortic stenosis. N. C. Med. J., 48:249, 1987.

Davidson, C. J., Skelton, T. N., Kisslo, K., et al.: A comprehensive evaluation of the risk of systemic embolization associated with percutaneous balloon valvuloplasty in adults. Ann. Intern. Med., 108:557, 1988.

Davis, K., Kennedy, J. W., Kemp, H. G., et al.: Complications of coronary arteriography from the collaborative study of coronary artery surgery (CASS). Circulation, 59:1105, 1979.

DeUbago, J. L. M., DePrada, J. A. V., Bardaji, J. L., et al.: Percutaneous ballon valvotomy for calcific rheumatic mitral stenosis. Am. J. Cardiol., *59*:1007, 1987.

Dexter, L., Haynes, F. W., Burwell, C. S., et al.: Studies of congenital heart disease. II: The pressure and content of blood in the right auricle, right ventricle and pulmonary artery in control patients, with observations on the oxygen saturation and source of pulmonary capillary blood. J. Clin. Invest., *26*:554, 1947.

DiSessa, T. G., Alpert, B. S., Chase, N. A., et al.: Balloon valvuloplasty in children with dysplastic pulmonary valves. Am. J. Cardiol., *60*:405, 1987.

Dodds, G. A., Harrison, J. K., O'Laughlin, M. P., et al.: Relief of superior vena cava syndrome due to fibrosing mediastinitis using the Palmaz stent. Chest, *106*:315, 1994.

Dodge, H. T., Hay, R. E., and Sandler, H.: An angiographic method for determining left ventricular stroke volume in man. Circ. Res., *60*:739, 1962.

Dodge, H. T., and Sheehan, F. H.: Quantitative contrast angiography for assessment of ventricular performance in heart disease. J. Am. Coll. Cardiol., *1*:73, 1983.

Dorros, G., Lewin, R. F., King, J. F., and Janke, L. M.: Percutaneous transluminal valvuloplasty in calcific aortic stenosis: The double balloon technique. Cathet. Cardiovasc. Diagn., *13*:151, 1987.

Driscoll, D. J., Hesslein, P. S., and Mulllins, C. E.: Congenital stenosis of individual pulmonary veins: Clinical spectrum and unsuccessful treatment by transvenous balloon dilation. Am. J. Cardiol., *49*:1767, 1982.

Edmunds, L. H., Stephenson, L. W., Edie, R. N., and Ratcliffe, M. B.: Open-heart surgery in octogenarians. N. Engl. J. Med., *319*:131, 1988.

Emery, R. W., Landes, R. G., Moller, J. H., and Nicoloff, D. M.: Pulmonary valve replacement with a porcine aortic heterograft. Ann. Thorac. Surg., *27*:148, 1979.

Engle, M. A., Gay, W. A., Kaminsky, M. E., et al.: The postpericardiotomy syndrome then and now. Curr. Probl. Cardiol., *3*:1, 1978.

Engle, M. A., Holswade, G. R., Goldberg, H. P., et al.: Regression after pulmonary valvotomy of infundibular stenosis accompanying severe valvular pulmonic stenosis. Circulation, *17*:862, 1958.

Facquet, J. M., Lemoine, J. M., Alhomme, P., and Fefebvre, J.: La measure de la pression auriculaire gauche par voie transbrochique. Arch. Mal. Coeur, *45*:741, 1952.

Fareed, J., Moncada, R., Messmore, H. L., et al.: Molecular markers of contrast-media induced adverse reactors. Semin. Thromb. Hemost., *10*:306, 1984.

Fick, A.: Uber die Messurg des Blutquantums in den Herzventrikeln. Sitz der Physik-Med ges Wurtzberg, 1870, p. 16.

Fischer, H. W., and Thomson, K. R.: Contrast media in coronary arteriography: A review. Invest. Radiol., *13*:450, 1978.

Fisher, M. L.: Coronary angiography: Safety in numbers? Am. J. Cardiol., *52*:898, 1983.

Flamm, M. D., Cohn, K. E., and Hancock, E. W.: Measurement of systemic cardiac output at rest and exercise in patients with atrial septal defect. Am. J. Cardiol., *23*:258, 1969.

Foltz, B. D., Hessel, E. A., and Ivey, T. D.: The early course of pulmonary artery hypertension in patients undergoing mitral valve replacement with cardioplegic arrest. J. Thorac. Cardiovasc. Surg., *88*:238, 1984.

Forssmann, W.: Experiments on myself: Memoirs of a surgeon in Germany. New York, Saint Martin's Press, 1974, pp. 84–85.

Forssmann, W.: Uber kontrastdavstellung der hohler der lebenden vechten erzens und der lungenschlagader. Munch. Med. Wochenschr., *78*:489, 1931.

Fuchs, R. M., Heuser, R. R., Yin, F. C. P., and Brinker, J. A.: Limitations of pulmonary wedge V waves in diagnosing mitral regurgitation. Am. J. Cardiol., *49*:849, 1982.

Gaasch, W. H., Andvias, C. W., and Levine, H. J.: Chronic aortic regurgitation: The effect of aortic valve replacement on left ventricular volume mass and function. Circulation, *58*:825, 1978.

Gaasch, W. H., Blaustein, A. S., and Bing, O. H. L.: Asynchronous (segmental early) relaxation of the left ventricle. J. Am. Coll. Cardiol., *5*:891, 1985.

Gabby, S., and Kresh, J. Y.: Bioengineering of mechanical and biologic heart valve substitutes. *In* Morse D., Steiner, R. M., and

Fernandez, J. (eds): Guide to Prosthetic Cardiac Valves. New York, Springer-Verlag, 1985, pp. 239–256.

Goldstein, J. A., Vlahakes, G. J., Verrier, E. D., et al.: The role of right ventricular systolic dysfunction and elevated intrapericardial pressure in the genesis of low output in experimental right ventricular infarction. Circulation, *65*:513, 1982.

Gorlin, R.: Calculations of cardiac valve stenosis: Restoring an old concept for advanced applications. J. Am. Coll. Cardiol., *19*:920, 1987.

Gorlin, R., and Gorlin, G.: Hydraulic formula for calculation of area of stenotic mitral valve, other cardiac valves and central circulatory shunts. Am. Heart J., *41*:1, 1951.

Graham, T. P., Jr., Jarmakani, J. M., Canent, R. V., Jr., and Morrow, M. N.: Left heart volume estimation in infancy and childhood: Reevaluation of methodology and normal values. Circulation, *43*:895, 1971.

Granger, C. B., Gabriel, D. A., Reece, N. S., et al.: Fibrin modification by ionic and non-ionic contrast media during cardiac catheterization. Am. J. Cardiol., *69*:8217, 1992.

Griffith, B. P., Hardesty, R. L., Siewers, R. D., et al.: Pulmonary valvotomy alone for pulmonic stenosis: Results in children with and without muscular infundibular hypertrophy. J. Thorac. Cardiovasc. Surg., *83*:577, 1982.

Grollman, J. H., Liu, C. K., Astone, R. A., and Lurie, M. D.: Thromboembolic complications in coronary angiography associated with the use of nonionic contrast medium. Cathet. Cardiovasc. Diagn., *14*:159, 1988.

Grondelle, A. van, Ditchey, R. V., Groves, B. M., et al.: Thermodilution method overestimates low cardiac low output in humans. Am. J. Physiol., *245*:H690, 1983.

Grossman, W.: Profiles in constrictive pericarditis, restrictive cardiomyopathy, and cardiac tamponade, Chapter 27. *In* Grossman, W. (ed): Cardiac Catheterization and Angiography. 3rd ed. Philadelphia, Lea & Febiger, 1986, p. 431.

Grossman, W., Jones, W. D., and McLaurin, L. P.: Wall stress and patterns of hypertrophy in the human left ventricle. J. Clin. Invest., *56*:56, 1975.

Gruntzig, A. R., Senning, A., and Siegenthaler, W. F.: Nonoperative dilation of coronary artery stenosis. Percutaneous transluminal coronary angioplasty. N. Engl. J. Med., *301*:61, 1979.

Gunther, S., and Grossman, W.: Determinants of ventricular function in pressure-overload in man. Circulation, *59*:679, 1979.

Hakki, A. H.: A simplified valve formula for the calculation of stenotic cardiac valve areas. Circulation, *63*:1050, 1981.

Halperin, J. L., Brooks, K. M., Rothlauf, E. B., et al.: Effect of nitroglycerin on the pulmonary venous gradient in patients after mitral valve replacement. J. Am. Coll. Cardiol., *5*:34, 1985.

Hamilton, W. F., Moore, J. W., Kinsman, J. M., and Spurling, R. G.: Studies on the circulation. IV: Further analysis of the injection method and of changes in hemodynamics under physiologic and pathologic conditions. Am. J. Physiol., *99*:534, 1932.

Hanrath, P., Mathey, D. G., Siegert, R., and Bleifeld, W.: Left ventricular relaxation and filling pattern in different forms of left ventricular hypertrophy. Am. J. Cardiol., *45*:15, 1980.

Harken, D. E., Black, H., Taylor, W. J., et al.: The surgical correction of calcific aortic stenosis in adults: Results in the first 100 consecutive transaortic valvuloplasties. J. Thorac. Surg., *36*:759, 1958.

Harrison, J. K., Davidson, C. J., Leithe, M. E., et al.: Serial left ventricular performance evaluated by cardiac catheterization before, immediately after and at 6 months after balloon aortic valvuloplasty. J. Am. Coll. Cardiol., *16*:1351, 1990a.

Harrison, J. K., Sheikh, K. H., Davidson, C. J., et al.: Balloon angioplasty of coarctation of the aorta evaluated by intravascular ultrasound. J. Am. Coll. Cardiol., *15*:906, 1990b.

Harrison, J. K., Wilson, J. S., Hearne, S. E., and Bashore, T. M.: Complications related to percutaneous transvenous mitral commissurotomy. Cathet. Cardiovasc. Diagn. *32*:52, 1994.

Haschek, E., and Lindenthol, O.: Ein Beitrag Zur Proktischen Verwerthung Der Photographie Noch Rontgen. Wien. Klin. Wochenschr., *9*:63, 1896.

Hellems, H. K., Haynes, F. W., and Dexter, L.: Pulmonary "capillary" pressure in man. J. Appl. Physiol., *2*:24, 1949.

Herman, M. V., Heinle, R. A., and Klein, M. D.: Localized disorders in myocardial contraction asynergy and its role in congestive heart failure. N. Engl. J. Med., *277*:222, 1967.

Heystraten, F. M. J., and Paalman, H.: Cineradiographic evaluation of the Björk-Shiley mitral and aortic valves. Ann. Radiol., 24:346, 1981.

Higgins, C. B., Sovak, M., Schmidt, W. S., et al.: Direct myocardial effects of intracoronary administration of new contrast agents with low osmolality. Invest. Radiol., 15:39, 1980.

Higgs, L. M., Glancy, D. L., O'Brien, K. P., et al.: Mitral restenosis: An uncommon cause of recurrent symptoms following mitral commissurotomy. Am. J. Cardio., 26:34, 1970.

Hoekenga, D. E., Stevens, G. F., and Ball, W. S.: Percutaneous angioplasty for peripheral pulmonary stenosis in an adult. Am. J. Cardiol., 59:188, 1987.

Hsieh, K. S., Keane, J. F., Nadas, A. S., et al.: Long-term follow-up of valvotomy before 1968 for congenital aortic stenosis. Am. J. Cardiol., 58:338, 1986.

Humes, H. D., Cielinski, D. A., and Messana, J. M.: Effects of radiocontrast agents on renal tubule cell function: Implications regarding the pathogenesis of contrast-induced nephrotoxicity effects of contrast agents on renal function. Cardiology, 5(Suppl.):14, 1988.

Inoue, K., and Feldman, T.: Percutaneous transvenous mitral commissurotomy using the Inoue balloon catheter [Review]. Cathet. Cardiovasc. Diagn., 28:119, 1993.

Inoue, K., Owaki, T., Nakamura, T., et al.: Clinical application of transvenous mitral commissurotomy by a new balloon catheter. J. Thorac. Cardiovasc. Surg., 87:394, 1984.

Isner, J. M., Salem, D. N., Desnoyers, M. R., et al.: Treatment of calcific aortic stenosis by balloon valvuloplasty. Am. J. Cardiol., 59:313, 1987.

Johnson, D. K., and Kostuk, W. J.: Left and right ventricular function during symptom-limited exercise in patients with isolated mitral stenosis. Chest, 89:186, 1986.

Johnson, L. W., Lozner, E. C., Johnson, S., et al.: Registry Committee of Society of Cardiac Angiography. I. Results and complications. Cathet. Cardiovasc. Diagn., 17:5, 1989.

Johnson, R. A., and Palacios, I.: Dilated cardiomyopathy of the adult. Part I, N. Engl. J. Med., 307:1051, 1982; Part II, N. Engl. J. Med., 307:1119, 1982.

Judkins, M. P.: Selective coronary arteriography. I: A percutaneous transfemoral technic. Radiology, 89:815, 1967.

Kan, J., White, R. I., Jr., Mitchell, S. E., et al.: Percutaneous transluminal balloon valvuloplasty for pulmonary valve stenosis. Circulation, 69:554, 1984.

Kan, J., White, R. I., Mitchell, S. E., and Gardner, T. J.: Percutaneous balloon valvuloplasty: A new method for treating congenital pulmonary valve stenosis. N. Engl. J. Med., 307:540, 1982.

Kawanishi, D. T., McKay, C. R., Chandraratna, A. N., et al.: Cardiovascular response to dynamic exercise in patients with chronic symptomatic mild-to-moderate and severe aortic regurgitation. Circulation, 73:62, 1986.

Kazama, S., Nishiguchi, K., Sonoda, K., et al.: Postoperative left ventricular function in patients with mitral stenosis. The effect of commissurotomy and valve replacement on left ventricular systolic function. Jpn. Heart J., 27:35, 1986.

Kennedy, J. W.: Complication associated with cardiac catheterization and angiography. Cathet. Cardiovasc. Diagn., 8:13, 1982.

Kennedy, J. W., Trenholme, S. E., and Kasser, I. S.: Left ventricular volume and mass from single-plane cineangiogram: A comparison of anteroposterior and right anterior oblique methods. Am. Heart J., 80:343, 1970.

Khalilullah, M., Tyagi, S., Lochan, R., et al.: Percutaneous transluminal balloon angioplasty of the aorta in patients with aortitis. Circulation, 76:597, 1987.

King, R. M., Pluth, J. R., Giuliani, E. R., and Piehler, J. M.: Mechanical decalcification of the aortic valve. Ann. Thorac. Surg., 42:269, 1986.

King, T. D., Thompson, S. L., Steiner, C., and Mills, N. L.: Secundum atrial septal defect: Nonoperative closure during cardiac catheterization. J. A. M. A., 235:2506, 1976.

Krevlen, T. H., Gorlin, R., and Herman, M. V.: Ventriculographic patterns and hemodynamics in primary myocardial disease. Circulation, 61:931, 1980.

Kyeselis, D. A., Rocchini, A. P., Beekman, R., et al.: Balloon angioplasty for congenital and rheumatic mitral stenosis. Am. J. Cardiol., 57:348, 1986.

Lababidi, Z., Wu, J. R., and Walls, J. T.: Percutaneous balloon aortic valvuloplasty: Results in 23 patients. Am. J. Cardiol., 53:194, 1984.

Laser, J. A., Fowles, R. E., and Mason, J. W.: Endomyocardial biopsy. In Shroeder, J. S. (ed): Invasive Cardiology (Cardiovascular Clinics, Vol. 14.) Philadelphia, F. A. Davis, 1985, pp. 141–163.

Leithe, M. E., Harrison, J. K., Davidson, C. J., et al.: Surgical aortic valvuloplasty using the cavitron ultrasonic surgical aspiration: An invasive hemodynamic followup study. Cathet. Cardiovasc. Diagn., 24:16, 1991.

Lieberman, E. B., Wilson, E. B., Harrison, J. K., et al.: Aortic valve replacement after balloon aortic valvuloplasty in the elderly. Circulation, 90:II-205, 1994.

Litvack, F., Jakubowski, A. T., Buchbinder, N. A., and Eigler, N.: Lack of sustained clinical improvement in an elderly population after percutaneous aortic valvuloplasty. Am. J. Cardiol., 62:270, 1988.

Lloyd, T. R., Marvin, W. J., Mahoney, L. T., and Laver, R. M.: Balloon dilation valvuloplasty of bioprosthetic valves in extracardiac conduit. Am. Heart J., 114:268, 1987.

Lock, J. E., Bass, J. L., Amplatz, K., et al.: Balloon dilation angioplasty of aortic coarctations in infarcts and children. Circulation, 68:109, 1983a.

Lock, J. E., Bass, J. L., Castaneda-Zuniga, W., et al.: Dilation angioplasty of congenital or operative narrowings of venous channels. Circulation, 70:457, 1984.

Lock, J. E., Block, P. C., McKay, R. G., et al.: Transcatheter closure of ventricular septal defects. Circulation, 78:361, 1988.

Lock, J. E., Castaneda-Zuniga, W. R., Fuhrman, B. P., and Bass, J. L.: Balloon dilation angioplasty of hypoplastic and stenotic pulmonary arteries. Circulation, 67:962, 1983b.

Lock, J. E., Keane, J. F., and Fellows, K. E.: The use of catheter intervention procedrues for cardiac disease. J. Am. Coll. Cardiol., 7:1420, 1986.

Lock, J. E., Khalilullah, M. N., Shrnasta, S., et al.: Percutaneous catheter commissurotomy in rheumatic mitral stenosis. N. Engl. J. Med., 313:1515, 1985.

Lorell, B. H., and Braunwald, E.: Pericardial disease, Chapter 44. In Braunwald, E. (ed): Heart Disease. Philadelphia, W. B. Saunders, 1988, pp. 1484–1534.

Lorell, B. H., Leinbach, R. C., Pohost, G. M., et al.: Right ventricular infarction. Am. J. Cardiol., 43:465, 1979.

Mann, T., Brodie, B. R., Grossman, W., and McLaurin, L.: Effusive-constrictive hemodynamic pattern due to neoplastic involvement of the pericardium. Am. J. Cardiol., 41:781, 1978.

Manske, C. L., Sprafka, J. M., Strony, J. T., Wang, Y.: Contrast nephrotoxicity in a zotemic diabetic patient undergoing coronary angiography. Am. J. Med., 89:615, 1990.

Marantz, P. M., Huhta, J. C., Mullins, et al.: Results of balloon valvuloplasty in typical and dysplastic pulmonary valve stenosis: Doppler echocardiographic followup. J. Am. Coll. Cardiol., 12:476, 1988.

Marcus, M. L., Dot, D. B., Hiratzka, L. F., et al.: Decreased coronary reserve: A mechanism for angina pectoris in patients with aortic stenosis and normal coronary arteries. N. Engl. J. Med., 307:1362, 1982.

Marcus, M. L., Skorton, D. J., Johnson, M. R., et al.: Visual estimates of percent diameter coronary stenosis: "A battered gold standard." J. Am. Coll. Cardiol., 11:882, 1988.

Maron, B. J., Bonow, R. O., Cannon, R. O., III, et al.: Hypertrophic cardiomyopathy. Part I, N. Engl. J. Med., 317:780, 1987; Part II, N. Engl. J. Med., 317:844, 1987.

Maron, B. J., Epstein, S. E., and Roberts, W. C.: Hypertrophic cardiomyopathy and transmural myocardial infarction without significant atherosclerosis of the extramural coronary arteries. Am. J. Cardiol., 43:1089, 1979.

Mason, J. W.: Techniques for right and left ventricular endomyocardial biopsy. Am. J. Cardiol., 41:8874, 1978.

McCristin, J. W., Herman, R. L., Spaccavento, L. J., and Tomlinson, G. C.: Isoproterenol infusion increases Gorlin formula aortic valve area in isolated aortic stenosis [Abstract]. J. Am. Coll. Cardiol., 11(Suppl. II):63A, 1988.

McDonald, D. A., and Taylor, M. G.: The hydrodynamics of the arterial circulation. Prog. Biophys. Biophys. Chem., 9:107, 1959.

McGregor, M., and Sniderman, A.: On pulmonary vascular resistance: The need for a more precise definition. Am. J. Cardiol., 55:217, 1985.

McKay, C. R., Kawanishi, D. T., and Rahimtoola, S. H.: Catheter balloon valvuloplasty of the mitral valve in adults using a double balloon technique. J. A. M. A., 257:1753, 1987.

McKay, R. G.: Balloon valvuloplasty for treating pulmonic, mitral and aortic valve stenosis. Am. J. Cardiol., 61:102G, 1988.

McKay, R. G., Lock, J. E., Keane, J. F., et al.: Percutaneous mitral valvuloplasty in an adult patient with calcific rheumatic stenosis. J. Am. Coll. Cardiol., 7:1410, 1986.

Mehlman, D. J.: A pictorial and radiographic guide for identification of prosthetic heart valves. Prog. Cardiovasc. Dis., 30:441, 1988.

Meier, B., Friedli, B., Oberhaeush, I., et al.: Trefoil balloon for percutaneous valvuloplasty. Cathet. Cardiovasc. Diagn., 12:277, 1986.

Miller, A. J., Pick, R., and Johnson, P. J.: The production of acute pericardial effusion: The effects of various degrees of interference with venous blood and lymph drainage from the heart muscle in the dog. Am. J. Cardiol., 28:463, 1971.

Miller, S. W.: History of angiocardiography. In Miller, S. W. (ed): Cardiac Angiography. Boston, Little Brown, 1984, pp. 3–20.

Morganroth, J., Perloff, J. K., Zeldis, S. M., and Dunkman, W. B.: Acute severe aortic regurgitation. Ann. Intern. Med., 87:225, 1977.

Morrow, W. R., Vick, G. W., Nihill, M. R., et al.: Balloon dilation of unoperated coarctation of the aorta: Short and intermediate-term results. J. Am. Coll. Cardiol., 11:133, 1988.

Morse, D., Steiner, R. M., and Fernandez, J. (eds): A guide to prosthetic valves. New York, Springer-Verlag, 1985.

Mullin, E. M., Jr., Glaucy, D. L., Higgs, L. M., et al.: Current results of operation for mitral stenosis: Clinical and hemodynamic assessment in 124 consecutive patients treated by closed commissurotomy or valve replacement. Circulation, 46:298, 1972.

Murgo, J. P., Alter, B. R., Dorethy, J. F., et al.: Dynamics of left ventricular ejection in obstructive and nonobstructive hypertrophic cardiomyopathy. J. Clin. Invest., 66:105, 1980.

Navetta, F. I., Barber, M. J., Gurbel, P. A., et al.: Myocardial ischemia in constrictive pericarditis. Am. Heart J., 116:1107, 1988.

NHLBI Registry: Percutaneous balloon aortic valvuloplasty. Acute and 30-day follow-up resulting in 674 patients from the NHLBI balloon valvuloplasty registry. Circulation, 84:2383, 1991.

O'Keefe, J. H., Jr., Vliestra, R. E., Hanley, P. C., and Seward, J. C.: Revival of the transseptal approach for catheterization of the left atrium and ventricle. Mayo Clin. Proc., 60:790, 1985.

O'Laughlin, M. P., Slack, M. C., Grifka, R. G., et al.: Implantation and intermediate-term follow-up of stents in congenital heart disease. Circulation, 88:605, 1993.

O'Rourke, M. F.: Pressure and flow waves in systemic arteries and anatomic design of the arterial system. J. Appl. Physiol., 23:139, 1967.

O'Rourke, M. F.: Wave reflections. In O'Rourke, M. F. (ed): Arterial Function in Health and Disease. New York, Churchill Livingstone, 1982, pp. 134, 138.

O'Toole, J. D., Wurtzbacher, J. J., Wearner, N. E., and Jain, A. C.: Pulmonary valve injury and insufficiency during pulmonary artery catheterization. N. Engl. J. Med., 301:1167, 1979.

Otto, C. M., Mickel, M. C., Kennedy, J. W., et al.: Three-year outcome after balloon aortic valvuloplasty. Insights into prognosis of valvular aortic stenosis. Circulation, 89:642, 1994.

Palacios, I. F., Block, P. C., Brandi, S. C., et al.: Percutaneous balloon valvotomy for mitral stenosis [Abstract]. Circulation, 74(Suppl. II):208, 1986a.

Palacios, I. F., Block, P. C., Brandi, S. C., et al.: Percutaneous balloon valvotomy for patients with severe mitral stenosis. Circulation, 75:778, 1987.

Palacios, I. F., Lock, J. E., Keane, J. F., and Block, P. C.: Percutaneous transvenous balloon valvotomy in a patient with severe calcific mitral stenosis. J. Am. Coll. Cardiol., 7:1416, 1986b.

Pelikan, P., French, W. J., Ruiz, C., et al.: Percutaneous double balloon angioplasty of a stenotic modified Fontan aortic homograft conduit. Cathet. Cardiovasc. Diagn., 15:47, 1988.

Pepine, C. J., Gessner, J. H., and Feldman, R. L.: Percutaneous balloon valvuloplasty for pulmonic valve stenosis in the adult. Am. J. Cardiol., 30:1442, 1982.

Pepine, C. J., Gunten, C. V., Hill, J. A., et al.: Percutaneous brachial catheterization using a modified sheath and new catheter system. Cathet. Cardiovasc. Diagn., 10:637, 1984.

Perez, J. A., Hinohara, T., Quigley, P. J., et al.: In-vitro and in-vivo experimental results using a new wire guided concentric atherectomy device [Abstract]. J. Am. Coll. Cardiol., 11(Suppl. II):109A, 1988.

Pichard, A. D., Meller, J., Teichholz, L. E., et al.: Septal perforator compression (narrowing) in idiopathic hypertrophic subaortic stenosis. Am. J. Cardiol., 39:310, 1979.

Portsmann, W., Wierny, L., and Warnke, H.: Closure of persistent ductus arteriosus without thoractomy. Thoraxchirurgie, 15:199, 1967.

Radner, S.: Attempt at roentgenologic visualization of coronary blood vessels in man. Acta Radiol., 26:497, 1945.

Radner, S.: Suprasternal puncture of the left atrium for flow studies. Acta Med. Scand., 148:57, 1954.

Radtke, W., Keane, J. F., Fellows, K. E., et al.: Percutaneous balloon valvotomy of congenital pulmonary stenosis using oversized balloons. J. Am. Coll. Cardiol., 8:909, 1987.

Rahimtoola, S. H.: Catheter balloon valvuloplasty of aortic and mitral stenosis in adults. Circulation, 75:895, 1987.

Rahimtoola, S. H.: The need for cardiac catheterization and angiography in valvular heart disease is not disproven. Ann. Intern. Med., 97:433, 1982.

Rankin, J. S., Gaynor, J. W., Fenely, M. P., et al.: Diastolic myocardial mechanics and the regulation of cardiac performance. In Grossman, W., and Larrell, B. H. (eds): Diastolic Relaxation of the Heart. Boston, Martinus Nijhoff, 1988, pp. 111–124.

Rao, P. S., Fawzy, M. E., Solymar, L., and Mardini, M. K.: Long-term results of balloon pulmonary valvuloplasty for valvular pulmonic stenosis. Am. Heart J., 115:1291, 1988.

Rashkind, W. J.: Transcatheter treatment of congenital heart disease. Circulation, 67:711, 1983.

Rashkind, W. J., and Miller, W. W.: Creation of an atrial septal defect without thoractomy. J. A. M. A., 196:173, 1966.

Rashkind, W. J., and Miller, W. W.: Transposition of the great arteries: Results of palliation by balloon atrioseptostomy in thirty-one infants. Circulation, 38:453, 1968.

Rashkind, W. J., and Tait, M. S.: Interventional cardiac catheterization in congenital heart disease. In Schroeder, J. S. (ed): Invasive cardiology. Cardiovasc. Clin., 15:303, 1985.

Reddy, P. S., Curtiss, E. L., O'Toole, J. D., and Shaver, J. A.: Cardiac tamponade: Hemodynamic observations in man. Circulation, 58:265, 1978.

Reid, C. L., McKay, C. R., Chandraratna, P. A. N., et al.: Mechanisms of increase in mitral valve area and influence of anatomic features in double-balloon, catheter balloon valvuloplasty in adults with rheumatic mitral stenosis: A Doppler and two-dimensional echocardiographic study. Circulation, 76:628, 1987.

Ricci, D. R.: Afterload mismatch and preload reserve in chronic aortic regurgitation. Circulation, 66:826, 1982.

Ricketts, H. J., and Abrams, H. L.: Percutaneous selective coronary cine arteriography. J. A. M. A., 181:140, 1962.

Rigler, L. G., and Watson, J. C.: A combination film changer for rapid or conventional radiography. Radiology, 61:77, 1953.

Ring, J. C., Kulik, T. J., Burke, B. A., and Lock, J. E.: Morphologic changes induced by dilation of the pulmonary valve anulus with overlarge balloons in normal newborn lambs. Am. J. Cardiol., 55:210, 1984.

Roberts, W. C.: Reasons for cardiac catheterization before cardiac valve replacement. N. Engl. J. Med., 306:1291, 1982.

Roberts, W. C., and Spray, T. L.: Pericardial heart disease: A study of its causes, consequences and morphologic features. In Spodick, D. H. (ed): Pericardial Diseases. Vol. 7. Philadelphia, F. A. Davis, 1976, pp. 11–65.

Robicsek, F., and Harbold, N. B., Jr.: Limited value of balloon dilatation in calcified aortic stenosis in adults: Direct observations during open heart surgery. Am. J. Cardiol., 60:857, 1987.

Rocchini, A. P., Kveselis, D. A., Crowley, D., et al.: Percutaneous balloon valvuloplasty for treatment of congenital pulmonary valvular stenosis in children. J. Am. Coll. Cardiol., 3:1005, 1984.

Rosenzweig, A., Watkins, H., Hwang, D. S., et al.: Preclinical diagnosis of familial hypertrophic cardiomyopathy by genetic analysis of blood lymphocytes. N. Engl. J. Med., 325:1753, 1991.

Ross, J., Jr.: Afterload mismatch and preload reserve: A conceptual framework for the analysis of ventricular function. Prog. Cardiovasc. Dis., 18:255, 1976.

Rupprath, G., and Neuhaus, K. L.: Percutaneous balloon valvuloplasty for aortic valve stenosis in infancy. Am. J. Cardiol., 55:1655, 1985.

Safian, R. D., Berman, A. D., Diver, D. J., et al.: Balloon aortic valvuloplasty in 170 consecutive patients. N. Engl. J. Med., 319:125, 1988.

St. John Sutton, M. G., St. John Sutton, M., Oldershaw, P., et al.: Valve replacement without preoperative cardiac catheterization. N. Engl. J. Med., 305:1233, 1981.

Salem, D. N., Findlay, S. R., Isner, J. M., et al.: Comparison of histamine release effects of ionic and nonionic radiographic contrast media. Am. J. Med., 80:382, 1986.

Sanborn, T. A., Haudenschild, C. C., Garber, G. R., et al.: Angiographic and histologic consequences of laser thermal angioplasty: Comparison to balloon angioplasty. Circulation, 75:1281, 1987.

Sandler, H., and Dodge, H. T.: The use of single plane angiocardiograms for the calculation of left ventricular volume in man. Am. Heart J., 75:325, 1968.

Saul, J. P., Keane, J. F., Fellows, K. E., and Lock, J. E.: Balloon dilation angioplasty of postoperative aortic obstructions. Am. J. Cardiol., 59:943, 1987.

Schoenfeld, M. H., Palachios, I. F., Hutter, A. M., et al.: Underestimations of prosthetic mitral valve areas: Role of transseptal catheterization in avoiding unnecessary repeat mitral valve surgery. J. Am. Coll. Cardiol., 5:1387, 1985.

Schoonmaker, F. W., and King, S. B., III: Coronary arteriography by the single catheter percutaneous femoral technique. Circulation, 50:737, 1974.

Schwab, S., Davidson, C. J., Skelton, T. N., et al.: A randomized study of the nephrotoxicity of ionic versus nonionic contrast following cardiac catheterization. N. Engl. J. Med., 320:149, 1989.

Seldinger, S.: Catheter replacement of the needle in percutaneous arteriography, a new technique. Acta Radiol., 39:368, 1953.

Sellers, R. D., Levy, M. J., Amplatz, K., et al.: Left retrograde cardioangiography in acquired cardiac disease: Technique, indications and interpretations in 700 cases. Am. J. Cardiol., 14:437, 1964.

Selzer, A.: Changing aspects of the natural history of valvular aortic stenosis. N. Engl. J. Med., 317:91, 1987.

Sembh, B. K. H., Tjonneland, S., Stake, G., and Aabyholm, G.: Balloon valvotomy of congenital pulmonary valve stenosis with tricuspid insufficiency. Cardiovasc. Radiol., 2:239, 1979.

Sheehan, F. H., Bolson, E. L., Dodge, H. T., et al.: Advantages and applications of the centerline method for characterizing regional ventricular function. Circulation, 74:293, 1986.

Shehadi, W. H.: Contrast media adverse reactions: Occurrence, recurrence and distribution patterns. Radiology, 143:11, 1982.

Sholler, G. F., Keane, J. F., Perry, S. B., et al.: Balloon dilatation of congenital aortic valve stenosis: Results and influence of technical and morphological features in outcome. Circulation, 78:351, 1988.

Sideris, E. B., Baay, J. E., Bradshaw, R. L., and Jones, J. E.: Axillary vein approach for pulmonic valvuloplasty in infants with iliac vein obstruction. Cathet. Cardiovasc. Diagn., 15:61, 1988.

Sigwart, U., Piel, J., Mirkovitch, J., et al.: Intravascular stents to prevent occlusion and restenosis after transluminal angioplasty. N. Engl. J. Med., 316:701, 1987.

Sones, F. M., and Shirey, E. K.: Cine coronary arteriography. Mod. Concepts Cardiovasc. Dis., 31:735, 1962.

Spodick, D. H.: The normal and diseased pericardium: Current concepts of pericardial physiology, diagnosis and treatment. J. Am. Coll. Cardiol., 1:240, 1983.

Stanger, P., Heymann, M. A., Tarnoff, H., et al.: Complications of cardiac catheterization of neonates, infants and children. Circulation, 50:595, 1974.

Stewart, G. N.: Researches on the circulation time and on the influences which affect it. The output of the heart. J. Physiol., (IV) 22:159, 1897.

Stewart, W. H., Hoffman, W. J., and Ghiselin, F. H.: Cinefluorography. Am. J. Roentgenol., 38:465, 1937.

Stott, D. K., Marpole, D. G. F., Bristow, J. D., et al.: The role of left atrial transport in aortic and mitral stenosis. Circulation, 41:1031, 1970.

Sullivan, I. D., Robinson, P. J., and MacArtney, F. J.: Percutaneous balloon valvuloplasty for pulmonary valve stenosis in infants and children. Br. Heart J., 54:285, 1986.

Swan, H. J. C., Ganz, W., Forrester, J. S., et al.: Catheterization of the heart in man with use of a flow-directed balloon-tipped catheter. N. Engl. J. Med., 283:447, 1970.

Terry, P. B., White, R. I., Jr., Barth, K. H., et al.: Pulmonary arteriovenous malformations: Physiologic observations and results of therapeutic balloon embolization. N. Engl. J. Med., 308:1197, 1983.

Tyberg, T. I., Goodyear, A. V. N., Hurst, V. W., et al.: Left ventricular filling in differentiating restrictive amyloid cardiomyopathy and constrictive pericarditis. Am. J. Cardiol., 47:791, 1981.

Ubago, J. L., Figueroa, A., Colman, T., et al.: Right ventriculography as a valid method for the diagnosis of tricuspid regurgitation. Cathet. Cardiovasc. Diagn., 7:433, 1981.

Warren, J. V.: Fifty years of invasive cardiology: Werner Forssmann (1904–1979). Am. J. Med., 69:10, 1980.

White, A. F., Dinsmore, R. E., and Buckley, M. J.: Cineradiographic evaluation of prosthetic cardiac valves. Circulation, 48:882, 1973.

Wigle, E. D., Sasson, Z., Henderson, M. A., et al.: Hypertrophic cardiomyopathy. The importance of the site and the extent of hypertrophy: A review. Prog. Cardiovasc. Dis., 28:1, 1985.

Williams, F. H.: A method for more fully determining the outline of the heart by means of the fluoroscope together with other uses of this instrument. Boston Med. Surg. J., 135:335, 1896.

Worley, S. J., King, R. M., Edwards, W. D., and Holmes, D. R.: Electrohydraulic shock wave decalcification of stenotic aortic valves: Post-mortem and intraoperative studies. J. Am. Coll. Cardiol., 12:458, 1988.

Wynne, J., Green, L. H., Grossman, W., et al.: Estimation of left ventricular volumes in man from biplane cineangiograms filmed in oblique projections. Am. J. Cardiol., 41:726, 1978.

Zimmerman, H. A., Scott, R. W., and Becker, N. O.: Catheterization of the left side of the heart in man. Circulation, 1:357, 1950.

# ■ II Percutaneous Transluminal Coronary Angioplasty

Marino Labinaz, Harry R. Phillips III, and Richard S. Stack

## HISTORICAL ASPECTS

In 1964, Dotter and Judkins inadvertently advanced a diagnostic catheter across a total iliac obstruction and initiated a new era in the treatment of atherosclerotic cardiovascular disease (Dotter, 1980). After this historic event, they observed,

Perhaps it is wishful thinking, but in any event I am convinced that the relief of atheromatous obstruction in small arteries can best be accomplished by catheter technics. A flexible guide introduced percutaneously into an artery proximal to an area of atheromatous narrowing can be manipulated so as to traverse the obstruction. A mechanical attack upon the lesion would then become feasible, perhaps by gradual direct dilatation.

**(Dotter and Judkins, 1964)**

The first intentional angioplasty procedure was done by Dotter on January 16, 1964, in an elderly woman who had gangrene and refused an amputation. An obstruction of the proximal popliteal artery was quickly passed with a guidewire and later dilated by means of several radiolucent, coaxial, polyethylene catheters (Fig. 31–28). The gangrene healed without operation, and the patient became fully ambulatory.

Later in 1964, Dotter and Judkins reported their clinical experience in the first 11 patients treated with percutaneous angioplasty. They advanced a 0.05-inch spring guidewire through an atherosclerotic obstruction, following with a tapered Teflon 0.1-inch dilating catheter over the wire. In appropriately sized vessels, the guidewire was followed by a 0.2-inch Teflon dilating catheter (Fig. 31–29). In the same year, Staple

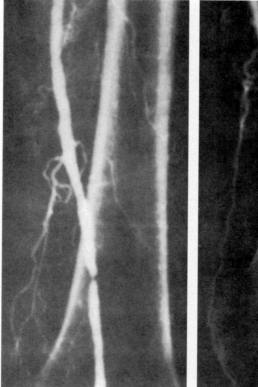
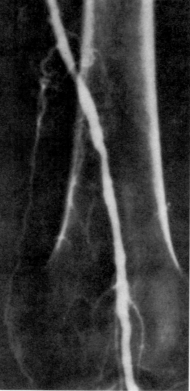
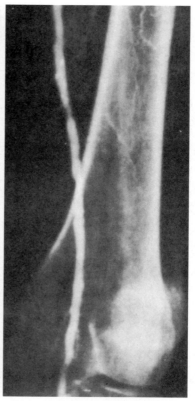

**FIGURE 31–28.** Femoral arteriogram of the first patient to receive percutaneous angioplasty. This 83-year-old woman had refused amputation for advanced gangrene due to a proximal popliteal stenosis and severe distal runoff disease. *Left panel,* Before dilatation; *middle panel,* immediately after dilatation; *right panel,* 2½ years after dilatation. The gangrene healed without operative therapy, and the patient became ambulatory. (From Dotter, C. T.: Transluminal angioplasty: A long view. Radiology, *135*:561, 1980.)

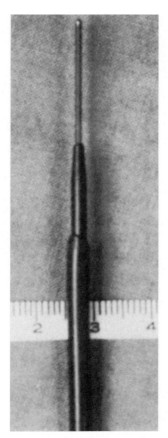

**FIGURE 31–29.** Dotter coaxial dilatation catheter and guidewire. (From Athanasoulis, C. A., Pfister, R. C., Greene, R. E., and Roberson, G. H.: Interventional Radiology. Philadelphia, W. B. Saunders, 1982.)

and co-workers in treating atherosclerotic lesions of the iliac and femoral arteries (Gruentzig et al., 1977). Gruentzig first described the use of percutaneous balloon angioplasty in human coronary arteries in 1977 (Gruentzig, 1978). In 1979, Gruentzig and associates reported a series of 50 patients and initiated the modern era of *percutaneous transluminal coronary angioplasty* (PTCA) in the United States.

A major improvement in balloon catheter system design was Simpson and colleagues' development of a maneuverable inner guidewire system in 1982. Since then, a great expansion of technology and a rapid evolution of coronary angioplasty equipment and methods have occurred. Modern low-profile systems now allow the cardiologist to successfully maneuver the multiple turns and branches of the coronary arterial system with relative ease. An example of a modern low-profile catheter system is shown in Figure 31–33.

## THE ANGIOPLASTY PROCEDURE

### Method of Dilatation

Procedural methods continue to evolve with further improvements in equipment and technique. The fol-

described a system of tapered catheters of increasing size passed sequentially over the guidewire to allow serial dilatations (Staple, 1968). A serial dilatation system was also introduced by van Andel (1976), who used gradually tapering catheters compared with the shorter beveled designs used by Staple (Fig. 31–30). Each of these methods met with reasonable clinical success and became particularly popular in Europe (Waltman et al., 1982).

Initial experience with balloon-tip catheters for peripheral arterial dilatation was less satisfactory. Early balloon catheters used soft, compliant latex balloons that were unable to generate sufficient radial force against the lesion (Waltman et al., 1982). Portsmann (1973) introduced a "corset" type of balloon catheter, which consisted of a latex balloon catheter within a Teflon outer catheter. The outer catheter had longitudinal openings located at the site of the inner balloon, and it allowed adequate force to be applied to the lesion (Fig. 31–31). A problem with this design, however, was the potential for trapping endothelium between the Teflon struts during deflation.

In 1974, Gruentzig introduced an ingenious new double-lumen catheter with a balloon constructed of noncompliant polyvinyl chloride (Fig. 31–32). The use of this balloon catheter system soon became popular in Europe after the successful experience of Gruentzig

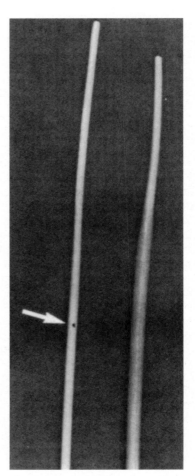

**FIGURE 31–30.** Staple–van Andel dilatation catheters. (From Athanasoulis, C. A., Pfister, R. C., Greene, R. E., and Roberson, G. H.: Interventional Radiology. Philadelphia, W. B. Saunders, 1982.)

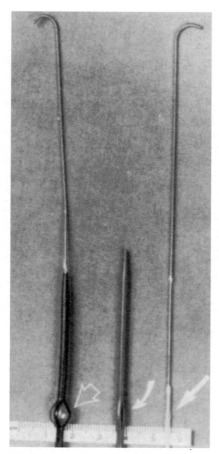

**FIGURE 31–31.** Porstmann corset-type balloon dilatation system. (From Athanasoulis, C. A., Pfister, R. C., Greene, R. E., and Roberson, G. H.: Interventional Radiology. Philadelphia, W. B. Saunders, 1982.)

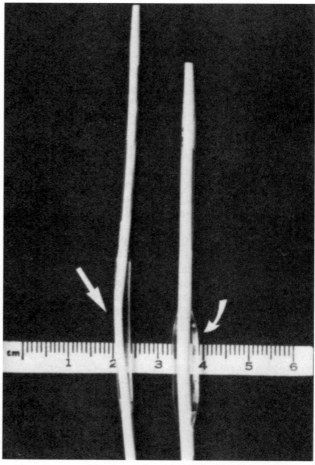

**FIGURE 31–32.** Gruentzig's polyvinyl chloride balloon dilatation catheter. (From Athanasoulis, C. A., Pfister, R. C., Greene, R. E., and Roberson, G. H.: Interventional Radiology. Philadelphia, W. B. Saunders, 1982.)

lowing is a summary of the routine procedures currently used in the Interventional Cardiac Catheterization Laboratory at Duke University Medical Center.

Careful review of each patient's clinical history, functional test data, and cardiac catheterization is performed. These help establish the need for angioplasty and outline a dilatation strategy. Subsequently, the procedure is explained to the patient and her or his family, outlining the risks and benefits of angioplasty, including the potential for emergent bypass surgery, allowing for informed consent to be obtained. The patient prepares for angioplasty by abstaining from any oral intake after midnight on the day of the procedure. The patient is also given at least 48 hours of antiplatelet therapy, either aspirin or ticlopidine in the setting of aspirin allergy, and dipyridamole commencing the day prior to the procedure. All patients are premedicated with diphenhydramine (Benadryl), and if no contraindications exist, they are given 5 mg of diazepam (Valium) on call to the procedure.

Although bypass surgery is available emergently in-hospital, a bypass surgeon is not necessarily notified before every angioplasty procedure. Routinely, however, if the patient is felt to be at high risk or has had previous bypass surgery, a cardiothoracic

surgeon is asked to review the case and state whether back-up surgery is appropriate. Surgical standby is discussed in further detail later in the chapter. In the case of very high-risk patients for whom percutaneous cardiopulmonary support is anticipated, the on-call anesthesiologist and cardiac perfusionist are notified in advance. Each procedure room is equipped with the potential for immediate intra-aortic balloon pumping and percutaneous cardiopulmonary support.

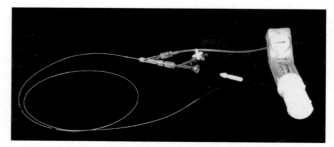

**FIGURE 31–33.** Modern steerable angioplasty system. (Courtesy of Advanced Cardiovascular Systems, Santa Clara, CA.)

The patient is brought to the interventional cardiac catheterization laboratory and is prepped and draped in a sterile manner. Large-screen, high-resolution imaging systems, high-resolution stop-frame recorders, and digital subtraction angiography provide accurate visualization of the coronary tree and allow for immediate decisions during interventional procedures without the need for cine films. The interventional team consists of an interventional cardiac catheterization fellow, an interventional cardiac catheterization senior physician, and an assistant who is scrubbed during the case. An additional assistant who is not sterile is available to administer medications and carefully record procedural details. Furthermore, a technician monitors the hemodynamic status of the patient throughout the procedure.

A No. 6 French introducer sheath is placed in the femoral vein to allow for the rapid administration of fluids or medications, a temporary pacemaker, or a venous catheter for monitoring right-sided heart pressures. An arterial sheath is also placed in the femoral artery. The size of the sheath varies depending on the procedure, but in general a No. 8 French sheath is placed for standard balloon angioplasty, and a larger sheath, such as a No. 10 French, is used during directional coronary atherectomy. Although in most situations the femoral artery and vein are used for central access, the brachial artery is occasionally used.

Following vascular access, intravenous heparin is administered to achieve an activated clotting time (ACT) greater than 300 seconds. The ACT is monitored hourly and additional boluses of heparin are administered as needed. A thin-walled guiding catheter is then advanced to the level of the appropriate coronary ostium. Repeat coronary angiography is performed in orthogonal views to clearly define the lesion and its relationship to important side branches. A coronary guidewire ranging from 0.010 to 0.018 inch in diameter is advanced across the coronary lesion. Once the guidewire is situated across the lesion, with its tip located in the distal artery, the deflated balloon catheter is advanced over the wire (see Fig. 31–33). Subsequently, the balloon is situated across the lesion using fluoroscopic guidance, and its location is confirmed with the aid of markers, which are usually located at the balloon midpoint. The balloon is inflated to several atmospheres of pressure, usually 1 or 2 atmospheres above the pressure at which the waist on the balloon is eliminated. The lesion is dilated for intervals ranging from 60 to 180 seconds or longer. Several inflations may be required to achieve an adequate angiographic result. After adequate dilatation, the balloon is removed while the guidewire is retained across the lesion, and the results of dilatation are assessed angiographically using high-resolution fluoroscopy. If the site appears to be adequately dilated, the guidewire is withdrawn and repeat angiograms are performed immediately and then after 5 to 10 minutes to ensure stability of the dilated segment (Fig. 31–34). In the past, postdilatation pressure gradients were used to assess the adequacy of the dilatation, but owing to several limitations, this technique is no longer used.

The guide catheter is removed from the patient and the patient is returned to the cardiology floor. If there is an acute myocardial infarction (MI) or a potential risk for abrupt closure, the patient is transferred to either the coronary care unit or an intermediate care unit. The femoral sheaths are usually removed 4 to 6 hours after the discontinuation of intravenous heparin. After an additional 6 hours of bedrest, the patient is encouraged to ambulate and is often discharged the following day. The patients are usually sent home with instructions to take an aspirin, a calcium-channel blocker, or long-acting nitrates, or a combination of these. If the patient had sustained a previous MI, the patient also receives a beta blocker for secondary prophylaxis. Furthermore, important clinical risk factors are identified and modification of these factors is instituted. The patient is subsequently followed carefully during the ensuing 6 months to detect restenosis. This can be determined by the recurrence of anginal symptoms, a functional study, or repeat coronary angiography.

## Procedural Outcome

Gruentzig (1978) reported an initial success rate (based on angiographic or clinical evidence of improvement) in 80% of a group of highly selected patients. The original National Institute of Health (NIH) PTCA Registry enrolled 3248 patients from 105 clinical sites in the "early days" of angioplasty between 1979 and 1981. Angiographic success, defined as at least a 20% improvement of luminal diameter, was achieved in 59% of patients (Kent et al., 1982).

In 1988, the results of the second NIH PTCA Registry were reported (Detre et al., 1988). This new registry examined the baseline characteristics, technical outcome, and short-term major complication rate in 1802 consecutive patients who had not had an MI in the 10 days before angioplasty between 1985 and 1986. These results were compared with those of the original registry to document changes in angioplasty technique and outcome.

The new NIH Registry patients were older, and there was a significantly higher proportion of multivessel disease (53% versus 25%; $p < .001$), poor left ventricular function (19% versus 8%; $p < .001$), previous MI (37% versus 21%; $p < .001$), and previous coronary artery bypass graft (CABG) (13% versus 9%; $p < .01$). The new registry cohort also had more complex coronary lesions. Attempts at angioplasty in these patients also involved more multivessel procedures.

Despite these differences, the in-hospital outcome in the new registry was better. Angiographic success rates according to lesion increased from 67 to 88% ($p < .001$), and overall success rates (measured as a reduction of at least 20% in all lesions attempted without mortality, MI, or CABG) increased from 61 to 78% ($p < .001$). In-hospital mortality for the new

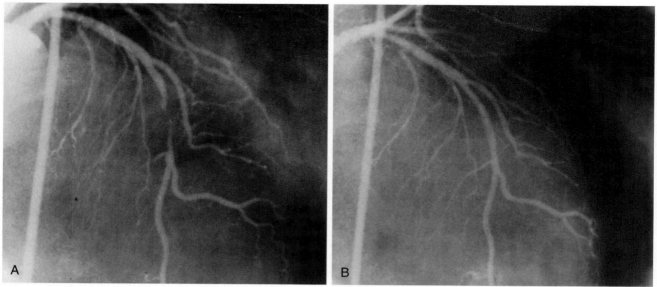

**FIGURE 31–34.** *A,* The patient presented with unstable angina. Angiography revealed a 95% stenosis in the midsection of the left anterior descending coronary artery. *B,* Successful coronary angioplasty reduced the lesion to a minor irregularity.

cohort was 1%, and the nonfatal MI rate was 4.3%. These rates were similar to those of the old registry.

Changes in baseline characteristics between the old and the new registry are shown in Table 31–8. A comparison of the angiographic and clinical success rates between the two registries is shown in Table 31–9. In the original registry, 22% of all lesions could not be crossed with available equipment and techniques. In the new registry, 92% of all lesions were successfully traversed. In the older registry, 68% of patients had one or more lesions reduced by at least 20%, whereas in the new registry, 91% of patients had successful dilatation of at least one lesion. The overall clinical success rate was 61% in the old registry and 78% in the new registry.

Untoward events in patients in the old and new registries are shown in Table 31–10. The incidence of death for patients with single-vessel disease was reduced from 1.3% to 0.2%. The incidence of emergency CABG was reduced from 6.1 to 2.9% in the same group. However, the incidence of death, nonfatal MI, and emergency CABG for all patients combined did not differ between the two registries (Table 31–11).

With continued refinement in technique and newer "bailout" strategies to treat angioplasty complications, further improvements in procedural outcome have occurred. Myler and co-workers (1992) reported on 533 patients treated between July 1990 and February 1991. The procedural success rate was 92%, the incidence of major complications was 4.5%, and emergency bypass surgery was required in 1.3%.

## Surgical Standby

During the developmental phase of angioplasty, immediate surgical backup was essential owing to the relatively high incidence of abrupt and threatened closure. However, with the current improvements in interventional equipment, increased operator experience, and effective interventional strategies for dealing with vessel closure, the need for immediate on-site surgical backup has been questioned.

Angioplasty without on-site surgical backup has been performed for some time in several centers in Europe and Canada. Klinke and Hui (1992) reported a

■ **Table 31–8.** BASELINE CHARACTERISTICS OF OLD–REGISTRY AND NEW–REGISTRY PATIENTS

| Characteristics | Registry | | p Value |
|---|---|---|---|
| | Old (n = 1155) | New (n = 1802) | |
| Mean age (yr) | 53.5 | 57.7 | <.001 |
| Mean duration of chest pain (mo) | 17 | 28 | <.001 |
| | *Number (%)* | | |
| Age ≥65 | 141 (12) | 486 (27) | <.001 |
| Women | 292 (25) | 476 (26) | — |
| Unstable angina | 431 (37) | 890 (49) | <.001 |
| Vessel disease | | | |
| Single | 863 (75) | 839 (47) | <.001 |
| Double | 203 (18) | 568 (32) | |
| Triple | 89 (8) | 395 (22) | |
| Previous infarction | 245 (21) | 662 (37) | <.001 |
| Previous CABG | 108 (9) | 226 (13) | <.01 |
| Ejection fraction <50%* | 76 (8) | 270 (19) | <.001 |
| History of CHF | 37 (3) | 100 (6) | <.01 |
| History of diabetes* | 101 (9) | 244 (14) | <.001 |
| History of hypertension* | 350 (35) | 832 (47) | <.001 |
| Currently smoking* | 398 (37) | 519 (30) | <.001 |

From Detre, K., Holubkov, R., Kelsey, S., et al.: Percutaneous transluminal coronary angioplasty in 1985–1986 and 1977–1981. Reprinted, by permission, from the New England Journal of Medicine, *318:*265, 1988. *Key:* CABG = coronary artery bypass graft; CHF = congestive heart failure.

*Data on these characteristics were missing for some patients. The percentages given are those of patients with known data.

■ **Table 31–9.** ANGIOGRAPHIC AND CLINICAL SUCCESS RATES IN OLD–REGISTRY AND NEW–REGISTRY PATIENTS, ACCORDING TO THE NUMBER OF DISEASED VESSELS*

| Outcome | Single-Vessel (%) | | Double-Vessel (%) | | Triple-Vessel (%) | | Total (%) | |
|---|---|---|---|---|---|---|---|---|
| | Old | New | Old | New | Old | New | Old | New |
| Outcome by Lesion* | (n = 910) | (n = 1060) | (n = 244) | (n = 985) | (n = 109) | (n = 847) | (n = 1263) | (n = 2892) |
| Unable to pass | 21.5 | 6.8 | 23.4 | 9.6 | 20.2 | 7.2 | 21.8 | 7.9 |
| Unable to dilate | 6.3 | 4.2 | 10.7 | 4.0 | 10.1 | 4.8 | 7.4 | 4.3 |
| Not successful, unknown reason | 3.6 | 0.1 | 5.3 | — | 3.7 | — | 4.0 | — |
| Dilated ≥20% | 68.6 | 89.0 | 60.7 | 86.4 | 66.1 | 88.0 | 66.8 | 87.8 |
| Outcome by Patient | (n = 863) | (n = 839) | (n = 203) | (n = 568) | (n = 89) | (n = 395) | (n = 1155) | (n = 1802) |
| One or more lesions reduced ≥20%* | 68.7 | 90.7 | 62.1 | 90.5 | 68.5 | 90.9 | 67.5 | 90.7 |
| All lesions reduced ≥20%† | 67.3 | 86.8 | 55.2 | 78.9 | 60.7 | 77.5 | 64.7 | 82.2 |
| Clinical Success‡ | | | | | | | | |
| All lesions reduced ≥20% and no death, infarction, or CABG | 63.6 | 84.3 | 51.2 | 74.6 | 58.4 | 70.9 | 61.0 | 78.3 |

From Detre, K., Holubkov, R., Kelsey, S., et al.: Percutaneous transluminal coronary angioplasty in 1985–1986 and 1977–1981. Reprinted, by permission, from The New England Journal of Medicine, 318:265, 1988.
*p <.001 for patients in all three groups compared according to registry within each subgroup.
†p <.001 for patients with single- and double-vessel disease, and p < 0.01 for patients with triple-vessel disease.
‡p <.001 for patients with single- and double-vessel disease, and p < 0.05 for patients with triple-vessel disease.

0.9% mortality rate and 1.6% incidence of emergency bypass surgery using a nearby regional surgical hospital in Edmonton, Alberta, Canada. Similar results were obtained by Richardson and associates (1990) at the Belfast City Hospital. In the largest series of patients undergoing interventional procedures with nearby off-site surgical standby, Reifart and colleagues (1993) reported on the outcome of 10,000 patients treated at the Red Cross Hospital in Frankfurt/Main Germany. The procedural success rate was 94%, with a 1.9% incidence of MI, a 0.3% incidence of urgent CABG, and a mortality rate of 0.3%. These results compare favorably with the National Heart, Lung, and Blood Institute (NHLBI) Registry.

Although these results are impressive, several important factors must be considered before the techniques are widely adopted. In the study by Klinke

and Hui (1992), 94.6% of patients underwent only one-vessel PTCA. Also, patients who were deemed high risk and patients requiring nonballoon interventions were referred to PTCA centers with on-site surgical facilities. In the study by Reifart and colleagues (1993), although a number of patients with unfavorable lesion characteristics and multivessel disease were treated, the procedures were performed by experienced interventionists who treated more than 500 cases per year. The importance of operator experience was emphasized in a study by Jollis and colleagues (1993), who examined the United States Medicare database and found an inverse relationship between procedural complication and operator experience.

Although long waiting lists and a paucity of cardiac surgical programs in Europe and Canada were the major incentives for the development of interven-

■ **Table 31–10.** UNTOWARD EVENTS AND ELECTIVE BYPASS GRAFTING IN OLD–REGISTRY AND NEW–REGISTRY PATIENTS, ACCORDING TO THE NUMBER OF DISEASED VESSELS

| Event or CABG | Single-Vessel (%) | | Double-Vessel (%) | | Triple-Vessel (%) | | Total (%) | |
|---|---|---|---|---|---|---|---|---|
| | Old (n = 863) | New (n = 839) | Old (n = 203) | New (n = 568) | Old (n = 89) | New (n = 395) | Old (n = 1155) | New (n = 1802) |
| Death | 1.3* | 0.2* | 0.5 | 0.9 | 2.2 | 2.8 | 1.2 | 1.0 |
| Nonfatal infarction | 5.0 | 3.5 | 3.9 | 5.1 | 6.7 | 5.1 | 4.9 | 4.3 |
| CABG | | | | | | | | |
| Emergency | 6.1† | 2.9† | 5.4 | 3.7 | 3.4 | 4.3 | 5.8 | 3.4 |
| Elective | 19.5‡ | 1.7‡ | 27.6‡ | 2.3‡ | 16.9‡ | 3.3‡ | 20.7 | 2.2 |

From Detre, K., Holubkov, R., Kelsey, S., et al.: Percutaneous transluminal coronary angioplasty in 1985–1986 and 1977–1981. Reprinted, by permission, from The New England Journal of Medicine, 318:265, 1988.
*p <.05.
†p <.01.
‡p <.001.

■ **Table 31–11.** WORST OUTCOMES OF PTCA IN OLD–REGISTRY AND NEW–REGISTRY PATIENTS, ACCORDING TO THE NUMBER OF DISEASED VESSELS

| Outcome | Single-Vessel (%) | | Double-Vessel (%) | | Triple-Vessel (%) | | Total (%) | |
|---|---|---|---|---|---|---|---|---|
| | *Old* (n = 863) | *New* (n = 839) | *Old* (n = 203) | *New* (n = 568) | *Old* (n = 89) | *New* (n = 395) | *Old* (n = 1155) | *New* (n = 1802) |
| Death | 1.3 | 0.2 | 0.5 | 0.9 | 2.2 | 2.8 | 1.2 | 1.0 |
| Myocardial infarction | 5.0 | 3.5 | 3.9 | 5.1 | 6.7 | 5.1 | 4.9 | 4.3 |
| CABG | | | | | | | | |
|   Emergency | 2.3 | 1.8 | 3.9 | 1.8 | 3.4 | 1.8 | 2.7 | 1.8 |
|   Elective | 18.7 | 1.3 | 26.1 | 2.1 | 12.4 | 2.8 | 19.5 | 1.9 |
| Lesions successfully dilated | | | | | | | | |
|   None | 8.2 | 5.8 | 8.9 | 5.5 | 10.1 | 5.6 | 8.5 | 5.7 |
|   Some | 0.9 | 3.1 | 5.4 | 10.0 | 6.7 | 11.1 | 2.2 | 7.0 |
|   All | 63.6 | 84.3 | 51.2 | 74.6 | 58.4 | 70.9 | 61.0 | 78.3 |

From Detre, K., Holubkov, R., Kelsey, S., et al.: Percutaneous transluminal coronary angioplasty in 1985–1986 and 1977–1981. Reprinted, by permission, from *The New England Journal of Medicine, 318*:265, 1988.

tional programs without on-site surgical backup, such is not the case in the United States. Therefore, currently in the United States, it is recommended that angioplasty be performed only in centers with on-site surgical backup. The degree of backup should be determined by the complexity of the procedure and the institution's particular practice pattern. This position is supported by the recently revised American College of Cardiology/American Heart Association (ACC/AHA) guidelines:

The current national standard of accepted medical practice for coronary angioplasty requires that an experienced cardiovascular surgical team be available within the institution to perform emergency coronary bypass surgery should the clinical need arise. Although technical advances, operator experience and alternative reperfusion strategies have somewhat lessened the utilization rates for emergency bypass surgery following failed elective angioplasty, surgical backup has proved life-saving or effectively reduced morbidity such that it is deemed mandatory by this subcommittee for all elective angioplasty procedures.

**(Ryan et al., 1993)**

## INDICATIONS FOR PTCA

### Patient Selection

Selection criteria of patients for coronary angioplasty continue to evolve with improvements in angioplasty equipment and technique. When PTCA was first introduced by Gruentzig, selection of patients was limited to those with the following characteristics:

1. Discrete, concentric lesions
2. Single-vessel involvement
3. Absence of calcification
4. Proximal location distant from major side branches
5. Good left ventricular function

Today, with significant technologic advances, including steerable guidewires, low-profile balloon catheters, increased operator experience, and newer

devices, angioplasty can be performed in multiple lesions, calcified lesions, distal locations, chronic total occlusions, and in patients with significant left ventricular dysfunction. Although there has been a continued trend to expand the clinical indications of angioplasty owing to these advances, careful selection of the patients and attention to their functional data and coronary arteriogram are essential to maximize procedural outcome and minimize morbidity and mortality.

The following are selection criteria commonly used:

1. Patients with significant symptoms of angina pectoris or positive exercise tests in the presence of a significant (>75% luminal diameter narrowing) lesion on the coronary arteriogram
2. Patients with one-, two-, or three-vessel disease without significant left main stenosis
3. Patients with acute MI who may be considered for mechanical balloon dilatation with or without previous thrombolytic therapy

Although multivessel coronary angioplasty is relatively common, some patients—such as those with three-vessel disease accompanied by left ventricular dysfunction—may benefit from bypass surgery. Angioplasty of left main stenosis was previously attempted, but high mortality rates have essentially eliminated this indication for angioplasty. Angioplasty may be attempted for chronic total occlusions, particularly if they are shorter and noncalcified; however, newer devices such as laser angioplasty may prove more effective in this setting.

### PTCA versus CABG versus Medical Therapy

Despite the widespread use of PTCA and CABG, their relative merits compared with each other and with medical therapy have not been extensively studied. Although several randomized clinical trials are currently examining this issue, results will not be available for several years. However, some data are available to help guide therapy. In a large prospective nonrandomized series of patients from the Duke Cardiovascular Disease Databank, Mark and co-workers (1994) described the survival of patients with significant coronary artery disease treated with medicine, PTCA, or CABG between 1984 and 1990. In patients with the least severe form of coronary artery disease, revascularization improved survival, compared with medical therapy, but the difference was not statistically significant. This result is not surprising because, as in most survival studies, differences in mortality in low-risk patients are usually small compared with those noted in high-risk patients. Furthermore, in these low-risk patients with favorable outcome, survival analysis may not be the most relevant endpoint. Symptom relief, quality of life, and patient preference may be more important factors in guiding appropriate therapy. Therefore, in these patients, PTCA or medical therapy should be considered as first-line therapy (Fig. 31–35). Bypass surgery should be reserved for those patients who have symptoms refractory to medical therapy and who are not amenable to PTCA owing to technical factors.

For all other forms of coronary artery disease, revascularization appears to provide a survival advantage compared with medical therapy. For two-vessel disease not including patients with a critical lesion in the proximal left anterior descending artery (LAD), PTCA is superior to CABG. Bypass grafting appears to be the superior mode of revascularization in patients with two-vessel disease in which there is a critical lesion in the proximal LAD and in patients with three-vessel disease (see Fig. 31–35).

Some preliminary information from randomized trials is also available. Parisi and associates (1992) compared angioplasty with medical therapy in the treatment of single-vessel coronary artery disease. PTCA offered earlier and more complete relief of angina than medical therapy, with 64% of the PTCA group free of angina at 6 months compared with only 46% of the medically treated group.

Some of the randomized clinical trials comparing PTCA with CABG include the Randomized Intervention Treatment of Angina (RITA), the Coronary Artery Bypass Revascularisation Investigation (CAPRI), the Emory Angioplasty Surgery Trial (EAST), the German Angioplasty Bypass Investigation (GABI), and the Bypass Angioplasty Revascularization Investigation (BARI) (BARI et al., 1990). Interim results from the RITA trial are now available (RITA Investigators, 1993). This trial compared the long-term effects of PTCA versus CABG in patients with one-, two-, or three-vessel coronary disease in whom revascularization with either procedure appeared possible. The 2½-year follow-up of the 1011 randomized patients revealed no significant difference in the combined primary end-points of death or definite MI. The prevalence of angina was higher in the PTCA group at 6 months (32% vs. 11%), whereas the difference was less at 2 years (31% vs. 22%). In addition, 38% of the PTCA group required revascularization or had had a primary end-point, whereas only 11% of the CABG group required revascularization or had a primary end-point. Although CABG patients at 1 month were

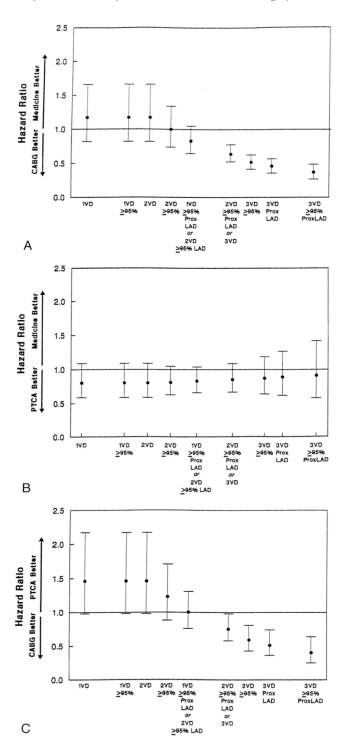

FIGURE 31–35. Hazard ratios for mortality for various forms of therapy for coronary artery disease calculated from the Cox regression model to evaluate relative survival differences. Results are displayed as hazard ratios with 99% confidence intervals. Horizontal line at 1 indicates no difference between the therapies: A, coronary artery bypass grafting (CABG) versus medicine; B, percutaneous transluminal coronary angioplasty (PTCA) versus medicine; C, CABG versus PTCA. (A–C, From Mark, D. B., Nelson, C. L., Califf, R. M., et al.: The continuing evolution of therapy for coronary artery disease: Initial results from the era of coronary angioplasty. Circulation, 89:2015–2025, 1994. Reproduced with permission. Copyright 1994 American Heart Association.)

less physically active and had a lower employment rate, there was no significant difference between the two groups after 1 year. Rodriguez and co-workers reported similar results in a group of 127 patients randomized to either PTCA or CABG (Rodriguez et al., 1993). Interim analysis at 1 year revealed no difference in mortality or in the incidence of MI. Although the bypass patients had fewer cardiac events and less angina during the 1-year follow-up, the cumulative cost at 1 year was greater. Even though these trials suggest that CABG has an advantage over PTCA, early interim analyses emphasize the limitations of angioplasty, since restenosis is known to occur in approximately one-third of patients, but is limited to the initial 6 months following PTCA. In contrast, saphenous vein grafts used during CABG degenerate at a much slower rate and usually produce significant clinical events after approximately 5 years. This important issue should be resolved through long-term follow-up combined with the results from several other randomized trials. Until the results of these studies are known, precise recommendations for either CABG or PTCA in patients with multivessel disease must be individualized to the patient and the experience of the institution.

## PTCA and Acute MI

The ability of thrombolytic agents to recanalize occluded arteries has revolutionized the management of acute MI. Several large clinical trials have demonstrated a significant reduction in mortality (GISSI-2, 1990; ISIS-2, 1988; ISIS-3, 1992). The Global Utilization of Streptokinase Activator for Occluded Coronary Arteries (GUSTO) investigators (1993) demonstrated that accelerated tissue plasminogen activator (TPA), resulting in more rapid reperfusion, correlated with a reduction in mortality compared with other thrombolytic strategies. Despite these benefits, thrombolytic agents fail to restore arterial patency in as many as 20% of patients and are associated with an increased risk of significant hemorrhagic complications and an increased incidence of recurrent ischemia.

In order to overcome some of these limitations, the use of immediate angioplasty in lieu of thrombolytic therapy has been examined by several investigators. Grines and colleagues (1993) reported a significantly lower incidence of nonfatal reinfarction or death (5.1% vs. 12.0%; $p = .02$) and a lower rate of intracranial hemorrhage in patients treated with immediate angioplasty compared with TPA. Similar results were reported by Zijlstra and co-workers (1993), who compared immediate angioplasty with streptokinase. In contrast to Grines and colleagues, they found a significant improvement in left ventricular function with immediate angioplasty.

Although primary angioplasty for MI requires further evaluation before it becomes widely accepted, its use as primary therapy for cardiogenic shock complicating acute MI has been proposed by several researchers. Conservative therapy of this condition is associated with an 80% mortality rate (Hands et al., 1989; Scheidt et al., 1970). In an early report, Stack and associates (1988) found a 41% mortality rate in a group of patients treated with intravenous streptokinase and PTCA. Other investigators examined the use of angioplasty and demonstrated survival rates ranging from 40 to 70% (Brown et al., 1985; O'Neill et al., 1985). Patient selection may account for some of the improved outcomes noted with angioplasty in cardiogenic shock. However, Bengtson and colleagues (1992), in a large consecutive series of patients with cardiogenic shock, reported that patency of the infarct-related artery was the most important predictor of long-term survival. These results emphasize the importance of an aggressive strategy in the management of cardiogenic shock, including rapid restoration of antegrade flow.

Direct angioplasty also appears more beneficial than thrombolytic therapy in patients who have an absolute or relative contraindication to these agents. Some small studies have suggested an increased efficacy in older patients, patients who have had previous bypass surgery, and patients presenting late in the course of an MI (Eckman et al., 1992; Kavanaugh and Topol, 1990). However, these results are preliminary, and further studies are needed to clarify these issues.

Since even the most aggressive thrombolytic strategies achieve patency rates of only 80% (GUSTO Investigators, 1993), the role of angioplasty as a "salvage" procedure has been examined. Several early trials demonstrated relatively low success rates, with high mortality rates when the procedure failed (Ellis et al., 1992). However, in a randomized clinical trial, Califf and co-workers (1991b) demonstrated improved left ventricular function and less recurrent ischemia in patients treated with immediate-rescue PTCA versus delayed coronary angiography and PTCA. Similar favorable results were obtained by Ellis and associates (1994), who demonstrated a significant reduction in the combined end-points of mortality and congestive heart failure in patients treated with rescue PTCA versus patients who did not undergo angioplasty (6.5% vs. 16.4%; $p = .055$).

The role of angioplasty following successful thrombolysis has been carefully studied (Califf et al., 1991a; Thrombolysis in Myocardial Infarction [TIMI] Research Group, 1988; TIMI Study Group, 1989; Topol et al., 1987). Although the two-step approach of thrombolysis followed by angioplasty initially appeared more beneficial than thrombolysis alone, this hypothesis was not borne out by randomized clinical trials. No improvement in left ventricular function was observed with this approach; in fact, routine angioplasty was associated with increased mortality, increased need for repeat emergent revascularization procedures, and increased hemorrhagic complications.

Although routine angioplasty following acute MI is not indicated, these studies should not be misinterpreted to minimize the importance of performing angiography following acute MI. Information obtained from angiography has important prognostic and therapeutic implications, as demonstrated by Topol and colleagues (1991). Patients presenting with left main and severe three-vessel disease can be quickly triaged to surgery. Other forms of multivessel disease may also derive survival benefit from revascularization by either PTCA or CABG. The significant number of patients with single-vessel disease and less than 50% stenosis can be given a favorable prognosis and benefit from early hospital discharge and early return to work. Patients who have greater than 50% residual stenosis and single-vessel disease should undergo functional testing. Predischarge thallium studies revealed that approximately 50% of these patients have a negative test. These patients also have been given a benign prognosis and likely do not require further intervention. However, patients who demonstrate either ischemia on functional study or spontaneous symptomatic ischemia following MI should undergo a revascularization procedure, which in most circumstances of single-vessel disease takes the form of PTCA.

## PATHOPHYSIOLOGY

Although the clinical efficacy of PTCA was established soon after its development by Gruentzig, elucidating the mechanism responsible for luminal enlargement has been much more difficult. In vivo assessment of the effects of angioplasty has been restricted primarily to contrast angiography, which is limited by its inability to provide specific information about intraluminal structures. With the development of intravascular ultrasound and angioscopy, some of these limitations have been overcome but not entirely eliminated. Most of the information that exists on mechanisms has been confined to animal models of arterial disease, which do not completely represent the human condition. Fortunately, some information has been gleaned from human autopsy studies.

In their initial work examining the effects of angioplasty on postmortem peripheral vessels, Dotter and Judkins (1964) concluded that plaque compression causing a "remodeled, compressed, cylindrical remnant of the former core" was the predominant mechanism of the procedure. However, information from necropsy studies performed in humans soon after balloon dilatation suggested that plaque fractures and vessel wall dissections (Fig. 31–36) were responsible for lumen enlargement (Block, 1984; Colavita et al., 1985; Waller, 1987). In contrast, however, studies from patients dying several years after angioplasty failed to reveal fracture sites or areas of dissection. In fact, no unique histopathologic findings were noted in this group.

Besides plaque compression, plaque fracture, and vessel wall dissection, stretching of the arterial wall, particularly the "disease-free wall," was also proposed as an important mechanism of angioplasty (Waller, 1985). This theory proposed that angioplasty initially splits the intima, separating it from the un-

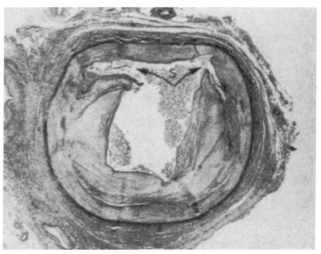

**FIGURE 31–36.** Postmortem cross-section of human atherosclerotic artery after PTCA showing splitting of the plaque. (From Block, P. C.: Mechanism of transluminal angioplasty. Am. J. Cardiol., 53:69C, 1984.)

derlying media and thereby allowing the balloon to further stretch the media and adventitia. By increasing the outer circumference of the artery, the lumen is also enlarged.

Although all three mechanisms—plaque fracture and dissection, plaque compression, and arterial wall stretching—have been observed in autopsy specimens, the relative importance of each has been further clarified with in vivo studies using intravascular ultrasound (IVUS). Losordo and associates (1992) performed IVUS in 40 consecutive patients with iliac stenosis following balloon angioplasty. They found that plaque fracture was responsible for 72% of the increase in luminal cross-sectional area following angioplasty. To a lesser degree, plaque compression was also found to significantly increase the size of the arterial lumen. Although vessel stretching occurred, its overall contribution was minimal. Further research and the application of newer imaging modalities will continue to clarify these important issues.

## LIMITATIONS OF CORONARY ANGIOPLASTY

### Acute Closure

Although it is difficult to determine exactly the success rate for angioplasty in each individual patient, guidelines have been established by the AAC/AHA, based on lesion morphology (Table 31–12). In addition, the presence of significant co-morbid disease also determines the overall success rate of the procedure. Although angioplasty is associated with a relatively high procedural success rate and a low complication rate, abrupt vessel closure may occur in approximately 5% of patients (Detre et al., 1988, 1990; Simpfendorfer et al., 1987).

Abrupt vessel closure may occur through plaque

■ **Table 31–12.** AMERICAN HEART ASSOCIATION/ AMERICAN COLLEGE OF CARDIOLOGY RISK STRATIFICATION (BASED ON LESION–SPECIFIC CHARACTERISTICS)

**Type A (High Success >85%, Low Risk)**

| | |
|---|---|
| Discrete (<10 mm length) | Little or no clarification |
| Concentric | Less than totally occlusive |
| Readily accessible | Not ostial |
| Nonangulated segment (45 degrees) | No major branch involved |
| Smooth contour | Absence of thrombus |

**Type B (Moderate Success 60–85%, Moderate Risk)**

| | |
|---|---|
| Tubular (10–20 mm length) | Moderate to heavy calcium |
| Eccentric | Total occlusion <3 mo |
| Moderate tortuosity | Ostial in location |
| Moderately angulated | Bifurcation lesion (double wire) |
| Irregular contour | Some thrombus present |

**Type C (Low Success 60%, High Risk)**

| | |
|---|---|
| Diffuse (>2 cm length) | Total occlusion >3 mo |
| Excessive tortuosity | Inability to protect brach |
| Extreme angulation | Degenerated vein grafts |

From Guidelines for percutaneous transluminal coronary angioplasty: A report of the American College of Cardiology/American Heart Association Task Force on Assessment of Diagnostic and Therapeutic Cardiovascular Procedures (Subcommittee on Percutaneous Transluminal Coronary Angioplasty). Reprinted with permission from the American College of Cardiology (Journal of the American College of Cardiology, 1993, Vol. 22, pp. 2033–2054).

dissection, thrombus formation, vessel spasm, or any combination of these (Lincoff et al., 1992; Sinclair et al., 1988). A possible schema for treating abrupt closure is outlined in Figure 31–37. Initially, intracoronary nitroglycerin and sublingual nifedipine may be used to eliminate coronary spasm. If this maneuver is not successful, repeat dilatation with the same balloon size or a slightly larger balloon for a longer duration (up to 5 minutes) is attempted. The next commonly employed procedure to treat refractory abrupt closure is prolonged dilatation with an autoperfusion balloon, which allows for antegrade flow to the distal coronary bed during balloon dilatation, permitting dilatations of up to 1 hour with preserved myocardial function. Several studies demonstrated the effectiveness of this strategy (Jackman et al., 1992; Van der Linden et al., 1993). Directional coronary atherectomy can also be used to treat abrupt closure due to dissection. Although atherectomy is successful in many cases, some caution must be exercised in its use in this setting, because there is a risk of arterial perforation. With the development and application of IVUS to guide atherectomy, this form of treatment may become more common. Coronary stenting has become an increasingly popular and successful method for treating arterial dissection. Several clinical studies have demonstrated the clinical utility of these metallic endoluminal prostheses (de Feyter et al., 1990; George et al., 1993). Newer devices, including biodegradable stents, may also prove efficacious in this setting, but will require further development to establish their clinical utility.

Despite these important advances in the management of abrupt closure, emergent coronary bypass surgery is still required in a small number of patients. In most situations, a guidewire or a perfusion balloon catheter is left in place across the lesion to allow for adequate myocardial perfusion while the patient is being prepared for emergent CABG.

## Emergency CABG Following PTCA

With increased operator experience and significant technical advances, the incidence of failed PTCA re-

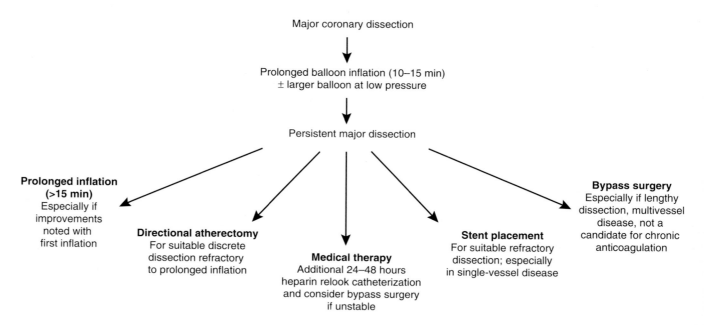

**FIGURE 31–37.** Outline for managing major coronary artery dissection. (Redrawn from Zidar, J. P., et al.: Dissection, abrupt closure, and perforation. *In*, Roubin, G. S., Califf, R. M., O'Neill, W. W., et al. [eds]: Interventional Cardiovascular Medicine: Principles and Practice. Churchill Livingstone, New York, 1993.)

quiring emergency CABG is decreasing. However, with the increasing number of procedures being performed, the prevalence of emergency CABG is increasing. In most high-volume institutions, emergency CABG is required in 2 to 5% of patients (Detre et al., 1988, 1990; Myler et al., 1992).

Several series have examined the in-hospital morbidity and mortality of patients who required emergency CABG following PTCA (Killen et al., 1985; Parsonnet et al., 1988; Pelletier et al., 1985). The operative mortality is approximately 3 to 4% and the incidence of perioperative infarction is 30 to 40%. These patients also appear to experience a more complicated postoperative course, with a higher incidence of postoperative hemorrhage and respiratory failure. Several studies have identified factors that predict poor outcome, including refractory myocardial ischemia, age greater than or equal to 65 years, prior CABG, presence of Class III or IV angina prior to PTCA, cardiogenic shock, and need for cardiopulmonary resuscitation (Buffet et al., 1991; Talley et al., 1990).

Further advances in PTCA with improved treatment strategies for vessel closure, including coronary stenting, will help reduce the need for emergency CABG. Improved methods of myocardial preservation and strategies to reduce reperfusion injury should improve post-CABG outcome.

## Restenosis

Although the clinical utility of PTCA was evident soon after its introduction by Greuntzig, the problem of renarrowing following a successful procedure or restenosis also became quickly apparent. The incidence of restenosis ranges from 20 to 50%, depending on the definition used (Califf et al., 1991a). The most commonly used definition of *angiographic restenosis* is the presence of more than 50% stenosis at the time of follow-up.

Several studies examined the time course of the restenosis process and demonstrated that it appears to be a time-related phenomenon occurring primarily within the first 6 months following angioplasty (Nobuyoshi et al., 1988; Serruys et al., 1988). Within the first 24 hours, there is an initial 10% luminal loss, which is due primarily to elastic recoil and thrombus formation. After this initial loss, there is progressive luminal narrowing, which abates by 6 months.

Clinically, restenosis presents as the recurrence of angina in most patients rather than as unstable rest angina or acute MI (Holmes et al., 1984). Although not proved, this may be due to the fact that restenotic lesions tend to be more fibromuscular and therefore less susceptible to plaque rupture and thrombus formation, as compared with lipid-laden primary atherosclerotic lesions (Mintz et al., 1993). Approximately 25% of patients may have angiographic restenosis in the absence of symptoms—so-called silent restenosis. Although some patients have detectable ischemia on functional testing, most do not, and the long-term clinical course of this group remains undefined (Bengtson et al., 1990).

Even though clinical and angiographic restenosis has been studied extensively, the mechanism of restenosis has not been elucidated. Histologically, the restenotic lesion consists primarily of smooth muscle cells, macrophages, endothelial cells, and extracellular matrix. The dense fibrocellular restenotic lesion appears to be histologically unique compared with the original atherosclerotic plaque, which usually contains greater amounts of lipid, calcium, and necrotic material (Nobuyoshi et al., 1991; Waller et al., 1991).

Several paradigms have been proposed to explain the process of restenosis (Forrester et al., 1991; Ip et al., 1991; Libby et al., 1992). A common hypothesis proposes that injury to the vascular wall produces the secretion of numerous cytokines that promote smooth muscle cell migration and proliferation with subsequent extracellular matrix production leading to luminal narrowing. Other cells, such as endothelial cells, platelets, and macrophages, also play a role by promoting continued smooth muscle proliferation and thrombus formation. This hypothesis has been challenged by O'Brien and associates (1993), who observed that smooth muscle proliferation is a relatively rare occurrence in restenotic tissue obtained by directional coronary atherectomy.

An alternative model proposed by Schwartz and colleagues (1992), based on observations in a pig model of restenosis, suggests that thrombus formation at the site of angioplasty is the initial event inciting subsequent smooth muscle infiltration and proliferation. More recently, using serial IVUS, Mintz and co-workers (1993) suggested that the entire vessel contracts over time, which is termed *chronic remodeling*, and that remodelling rather than neointimal formation is the predominant process in restenosis. Although each model may have a role, the relative importance of each will need to be determined by future studies.

Owing to the significance of restenosis, several studies have sought to identify predictive factors. Some of the more consistent patient-related factors include diabetes mellitus and unstable angina (Hillegass et al., 1994). Other studies examining procedural factors have identified lesion location, length, reference vessel diameter, and baseline and postintervention diameter stenosis as independent predictors (Hillegass et al., 1994). Additional work by Kuntz and Baim (1993) suggests that maximizing luminal enlargement, regardless of the device that is used, is the most important factor in minimizing late restenosis. This hypothesis is the "bigger is better" theory. The authors propose that, although there may be a greater degree of late loss associated with greater acute gains, the initial larger lumen is better able to accommodate the loss, thereby reducing the rate of restenosis. Further studies are required to validate these observations.

To overcome the problem of restenosis, numerous pharmacologic and nonpharmacologic interventions have been attempted. Directional coronary atherectomy was found to produce a marginally lower rate of restenosis in a randomized clinical trial. However, this benefit was achieved at the cost of a higher incidence of procedural complications, including MI (Topol et al., 1993). A multitude of pharmacologic interventions, including antiplatelet, antithrombus, calcium channel blockers, angiotensin converting enzyme (ACE) inhibitors, and fish oil, have been attempted to reduce restenosis (Hillegass et al., 1994). No agent has been shown conclusively to reduce restenosis, but this may be due to a number of factors, including trials insufficiently powered to detect a difference, inadequate duration and concentration of the agents, use of single agents that in themselves may be ineffective but combined with other drugs may have a synergistic response, the "magic bullet" remaining undiscovered, selection of the incorrect target, and the fact that restenosis may simply represent a natural wound-healing response that is unalterable with current technology. The latter hypothesis appears unlikely, since preliminary work from meta-analysis has suggested some benefit with calcium channel blockers and fish oils, whereas newer agents such as ciprostene have also shown some promise (Raizner et al., 1993).

An exciting breakthrough is the demonstration that stenting coronary arteries significantly reduces restenosis (Schatz et al., 1993; Serruys et al., 1993). Although it is tempered somewhat by the increased hospital length of stay and the hemorrhagic complications associated with the obligatory anticoagulant regimes with current designs, this finding represents an important milestone in the field of interventional cardiology.

The future of interventional cardiology rests with the solution to the problem of restenosis. This might best be achieved by a combination of mechanical devices and drugs, such as the development of biodegradable stents loaded with agents able to combat thrombus deposition and neointimal formation and to provide the necessary mechanical support to the vessel wall as it heals.

## NEW DEVICES

Balloon angioplasty is a reliable and effective mode of revascularization in most patients with obstructive coronary artery disease. Limitations of its efficacy have been demonstrated in certain lesion types, including ostial lesions, thrombus-laden lesions, and markedly eccentric and heavily calcified lesions (Ryan et al., 1988). Furthermore, the problems of acute closure and restenosis continue to limit the full potential of balloon angioplasty. New interventional devices have been developed to overcome these important limitations and to expand the role of percutaneous revascularization in coronary artery disease.

### Atherectomy/Ablation

This group of devices includes directional coronary atherectomy (DCA), transluminal extraction endarter-

ectomy (TEC), and rotational ablation (Rotablator). In general, these devices enlarge the arterial lumen by excising or ablating the artheromatous plaque.

### Directional Coronary Atherectomy

The DCA catheter consists of a cutting head housed in a metal cylinder with an open window on one side and a balloon on the other. The entire cutting head is connected to a catheter. The cutting head is a cylindrical cup that is rotated at 2000 rpm by a handheld motor drive unit. To excise plaque, the window is pressed firmly against the arterial lesion by the inflated balloon. The cutter is then slowly advanced while it is spinning, shaving off plaque and storing it in a cylindrical nose cone at the end of the catheter.

DCA has been evaluated in numerous clinical trials (Hinohara et al., 1992; Safian et al., 1990). Its ability to reduce restenosis in comparison with PTCA has been evaluated in two randomized clinical trials. Although the restenosis rate was marginally better with DCA in the Coronary Angioplasty Versus Extraction Atherectomy Trial (CAVEAT), this benefit was modified by a higher incidence of periprocedural MI and bypass surgery (Topol et al., 1993). The Canadian Coronary Atherectomy Trial (CCAT), which compared PTCA and atherectomy in the proximal LAD, found no difference in the restenosis rate or in the complication rate (Adelman et al., 1993). Further analysis of these trials is being conducted to identify certain lesion subsets that may be particularly amenable to atherectomy. The role of atherectomy in saphenous vein grafts is also being evaluated in the ongoing CAVEAT II trial.

### Transluminal Extraction Catheter

The TEC is a forward-cutting atherectomy device that excises atheromatous material using a cylindrical cutting head rotating at 750 rpm. As the plaque is being cut, vacuum suction is applied through the torque tube, thereby removing the material from the patient's body.

Although the TEC catheter has not been evaluated in randomized trials, its use has been examined in several series (O'Neill et al., 1992; Popma et al., 1992; Sketch et al., 1992). The procedural success rate and restenosis rate appear comparable with those of PTCA. Some investigators have suggested a unique role for TEC in thrombus-laden lesions and diffuse lesions, particularly those in saphenous vein grafts (O'Neill et al., 1992; Rosenblum et al., 1991). The utility of TEC in these circumstances and its particular niche in interventional cardiology will be determined by ongoing studies.

### Rotational Ablation

The Rotablator ablates plaque by using a diamond-coated abrasive tip that is connected to a catheter. The tip rotates at 180,000 rpm, thereby pulverizing the atheromatous material into small fragments that pass through the capillary system of the myocardium and are trapped by the reticuloendothelial system (Fourrier et al., 1989). The use of the Rotablator has been described in several series, but its efficacy compared with other interventional devices including PTCA has not been established by randomized clinical trials. Owing to the small burr size, adjunctive PTCA is required in most patients to attain adequate lumen enlargement. The atheromatous particles produced by rotational ablation may pose a more significant problem than anticipated from animal studies as demonstrated by the relatively high incidence of no-reflow and non-Q-wave MI following the procedure. In addition, the major dissection rate with subsequent abrupt closure and the restensosis rate remain high. Although it is unlikely that Rotablator will replace balloon angioplasty, it may have specific niches, including nondilatable plaque, heavily calcified plaque, bifurcation lesions, and possible ostial lesions. Further refinements in the device and increased operator experience may expand its clinical utility.

## Coronary Stents

Although a detailed discussion of all currently available stents is beyond the scope of this chapter, a review of the important principles of this form of coronary intervention is warranted. Stents are endoluminal prosthetic devices that provide a supportive scaffold to the arterial wall. The ability to provide arterial wall support is important for a number of reasons. First, by "tacking" up dissection flaps and ensuring arterial patency, the incidence of acute closure is reduced. Second, by providing a favorable rheologic environment and by maximizing the luminal area at the time of the angioplasty, the effect of late arterial narrowing is minimized, thereby reducing clinical restensois.

The concept of arterial stenting was first introduced in 1968 by Dotter, who implanted stainless-steel coils in the femoral arteries of dogs (Dotter, 1969). The first stents were implanted in humans in 1986 (Sigwart et al., 1987). Despite their relatively recent development, several different stent designs are now available. The initial design was the self-expanding WallStent. This stent was initially used only in Europe and currently is being evaluated in North America (Serruys et al., 1991). The remainder of the stents are balloon expandable and include the Palmaz-Schatz, Gianturco-Roubin, Wiktor, and Strecker stents. These stents are composed of stainless steel except for the Wiktor stent, which consists of tantulum, and the Strecker stent, which is composed of a stainless-steel/tantalum mixture. Two more recent designs, the Advanced Cardiovascular Systems metal stent and the Cordis stents, are now entering initial human studies. The importance of the differences in designs and material has not been established and will require randomized trials to clarify. Currently, the only stents approved for general use by the Food and Drug Administration

in the United States are the Gianturco-Roubin and the Palmaz-Schatz stents.

The successful use of coronary stents depends on several factors, including appropriate patient selection. During the procedure, adequate support from the guiding catheter and coronary guidewire are needed to ensure correct deployment. Meticulous attention to anticoagulation and care of the femoral puncture site are also needed to ensure success. Currently, all patients undergoing stent placement are anticoagulated with aspirin, dipyridamole, dextran, and heparin during the procedure. Patients are also given nitroglycerin and calcium channel blockers to reduce the incidence of coronary artery spasm. Following the procedure, patients are anticoagulated with warfarin sodium (Coumadin) and dipyridamole for 2 months and aspirin indefinitely. However, newer anticoagulation regimes excluding warfarin are currently being evaluated.

As with most new interventional devices, a learning curve was noted with stent deployment. Initial studies reported up to a 20% incidence of subacute closure associated with a 3 to 6% mortality and a 50% incidence of periprocedural MI (Serruys et al., 1991). With increased operator experience and careful attention to anticoagulation, the incidence of subacute closure has dropped significantly. The clinical utility of stents has been demonstrated by several clinical trials. George and associates (1993) reported a 97% success rate with the Gianturco-Roubin stent in 494 patients treated for acute or threatened closure following PTCA. Stents have also had a significant effect on the restenosis rate. Data from randomized trials with the Palmaz-Schatz stents reveal a reduction in restenosis rate of 20 to 29% with stents, compared with 33 to 43% with PTCA (Fischman et al., 1994; Serruys et al., 1994).

Although the initial results with stents are encouraging, current metal stents are limited by several factors. Because metal stents are permanent, there is some concern over potential long-term complications. Despite the improvement in hemorrhagic complications, aggressive systemic anticoagulation is still required, although newer, less aggressive regimes are being evaluated. Metal stents appear to work primarily by mechanically supporting the arterial wall. They do not appear to have any significant effect on the neointimal response. As a result, biodegradable stents with the ability to locally deliver antithrombotic and antiproliferative agents are currently being developed to overcome these important limitations.

## Lasers

Lasers produce pure, coherent, and bright light. Investigation into their ability to ablate atherosclerotic tissue began soon after the discovery of the ruby laser in 1960 (McGuff et al., 1963). Ablation is due predominantly to three mechanisms: thermal vaporization of water and tissue; photodissection, which directly breaks intramolecular bonds; and electrical-mechanical, in which a high density of free electrons (plasma) is created, producing a shock wave that generates tissue dissection (Bittl et al., 1994).

Initial clinical investigation began with continuous wave laser systems in 1984 (Geschwind et al., 1984). These early devices relied predominantly on the application of thermal energy. Unfortunately, owing to the relatively high incidence of restenosis and vessel perforation, these early prototypes were largely abandoned.

More recently, Excimer lasers, which use ultraviolet light, and holmium lasers, which operate in the mid-infrared range, have been used with greater clinical success (Knopf et al., 1991). Both designs ablate atherosclerotic plaque with minimal thermal effect.

Although no direct comparison with other interventional devices has been performed, Excimer lasers appear to be beneficial in the treatment of ostial and aorto-ostial lesions, chronic total occlusions, long lesions, and possibly saphenous vein graft lesions, all of which are not particularly well treated with conventional balloon angioplasty (Bittl et al., 1992; Cook et al., 1991). Lasers appear to produce restenosis rates comparable with those of balloon angioplasty. Current designs remain limited by the inability to selectively ablate atherosclerotic plaque, the risk of vessel perforation and dissection, and difficulty with eccentric and thrombus-laden lesions. With newer innovations and careful patient selection, the utility of the laser is likely to expand, but it will probably remain in the realm of niche devices with specific indications.

## Newer Imaging Devices

Contrast angiography remains the gold standard for assessing the severity and extent of coronary atherosclerosis. Currently, it is the most common imaging modality used for the selection of interventional devices and the assessment of their therapeutic efficacy. However, this technique remains limited by its ability to outline only atherosclerotic lesions, providing relatively little detail about the composition of the arterial wall and intraluminal structures.

In response to these limitations, IVUS and angioscopy have been developed. IVUS was first developed in 1971 by Bom and colleagues for intracardiac imaging, but human coronary arteries were not successfully visualized until 1988 (Bom et al., 1972; Pandian et al., 1988). Currently, there are two basic imaging systems: solid state catheters, which use several transducer elements radially arranged at the catheter tip to produce the ultrasound image, and mechanical catheters, which produce images by rotating the transducer in the tip of the catheter. Each system has unique advantages and disadvantages, but the mechanical systems tend to produce higher-quality images. Newer-generation devices are also being developed that combine IVUS probes with therapeutic devices including DCA, laser, and angioplasty balloons.

IVUS appears to be useful in three conditions: providing further insights into vascular biology; guiding the selection of interventional devices, e.g., lesion-specific therapy; and assessing the results of interventional therapy. IVUS has been particularly helpful in detecting calcium, in intimal dissection, and in characterizing the plaque topography more readily than angiography. Although this information is useful, its impact on selecting and guiding therapy is yet to be determined by prospective trials. Its clinical utility needs to be clearly established before it can be widely accepted, in view of the additional cost and time entailed.

Another promising mode of vascular visualization is coronary angioscopy. These devices involve a high-intensity light source and a fiberoptic imaging bundle. With use of an occlusive balloon and a flushing system, the arterial lumen distal to the catheter is rendered blood-free, allowing for direct visualization of the arterial wall. Early angioscopic studies in patients with acute MI and unstable angina identified plaque rupture with subsequent thrombus formation as the primary event in acute ischemic syndromes (DeWood et al., 1980). This monumental discovery helped to usher in the thrombolytic era. Angioscopy has been used to assess the results of various interventional devices, including conventional balloon angioplasty, coronary stenting, DCA and extraction atherectomy, and lasers (Meaney et al., 1991; Teirstein et al., 1992). Although the angioscope has provided further insight into the mechanisms of luminal enlargement by these various devices, its utility in guiding therapy has not been firmly established. One particularly useful niche appears to be its ability to detect intracoronary thrombus unapparent on contrast angiography. This has been quite common in saphenous vein grafts (White et al., 1993). Since thrombus has been identified as an important risk for periprocedural complications, its identification is important to enable the selection of appropriate forms of therapy. With further refinement of the device and an increase in the number of interventional devices, the concept of lesion-specific therapy may become a reality in the future.

## CONCLUSIONS

PTCA has become well established as an effective method for managing selected patients with coronary artery disease. However, PTCA has at least three major limitations: (1) Many patients are not candidates for PTCA (e.g., patients with diffuse disease or chronic total occlusions). (2) The acute failure rate (>50% residual stenosis after PTCA) remains at 5 to 7%. (3) In approximately one-third of initially successful angioplasties, patients develop restenosis within 6 months.

In an effort to overcome these limitations, investigators have developed new devices to actually remove the plaque by using either laser or mechanical ablation by flexible catheters. Another new approach has been to place short conduits or stents made of stainless steel into dilated segments of arteries to prevent acute occlusion as well as chronic restenosis. Although initial studies with each of these new technologies are encouraging, each must be tested in a prospective randomized manner against the state-of-the-art methods of medical, interventional, and surgical therapy. In the future, it is likely that a number of excellent therapeutic options, both surgical and nonsurgical, will exist and can be tailored to the individual needs of the patient, based on specific clinical and anatomic indications.

## SELECTED BIBLIOGRAPHY

Detre, K., Holubkov, R., Kelsey, S., et al.: Percutaneous transluminal coronary angioplasty in 1985–1986 and 1977–1981. N. Engl. J. Med., 318:265, 1988.

This important study compares the results of the original National Institutes of Health (NIH) Percutaneous Transluminal Angioplasty Registry from 1977 through 1981 with the most recent NIH Registry from 1985 through 1986. The new registry entered 1802 consecutive patients. The angiographic success rates according to lesion increased from 67 to 88% ($p < .001$), and the overall success rate (measured as a reduction of at least 20% in all lesions attempted, without death, myocardial infarction, or coronary bypass grafting) increased from 61 to 78% ($p < .001$) in the registry.

Dotter, C. T.: Transluminal angioplasty: A long view. Radiology, 135:561, 1980.

In this review article, Dotter gives a historical account of the development of percutaneous transluminal coronary angioplasty (PTCA). This is a very interesting perspective from the original developer of percutaneous dilatation techniques.

Dotter, C. T., and Judkins, M. P.: Transluminal treatment of arteriosclerotic obstruction. Circulation, 30:654, 1964.

This is the original study describing the technique and preliminary report of the first group of patients treated with transluminal catheter dilatation for atherosclerotic arteries. The authors describe the methods for dilating plaques with a guidewire and tapered Teflon catheters of increasing diameter. The outcomes of the first 11 patients treated in this manner are described in detail.

Gruentzig, A.: Transluminal dilatation of coronary artery stenosis. Lancet, 1:263, 1978.

In this study, the first five patients to have PTCA are described. The original technique for coronary dilatation with a polyvinyl chloride balloon dilatation catheter is described. Seven dilatations were done in five patients in 1977, with a primary success achieved in six of the seven procedures.

Kent, K. M., Bentivoglio, L. G., Block, P. C., et al.: Percutaneous transluminal coronary angioplasty: Report from the registry of the National Heart, Lung, and Blood Institute. Am. J. Cardiol., 49:2011, 1982.

In this Registry, data were collected from 34 centers in the United States and Europe, where the initial series of angioplasty was performed on 631 patients between 1977 and 1981. Coronary angioplasty was successful (more than 20% decrease of coronary stenosis) in 59% of the stenosed arteries. Emergency coronary bypass operation was required in 40 patients (6%). Myocardial infarction occurred in 29 patients (4%). In-hospital death occurred in 6 patients (1%), 3 with single-vessel disease and 3 with multivessel disease.

Kent, K. M., Mullin, S. M., and Passamani, E. R. (guest eds): Proceedings of the National Heart, Lung, and Blood Institute Workshop on the Outcome of Percutaneous Transluminal Coronary Angioplasty. Am. J. Cardiol., 53:1, 1984.

In this classic journal supplement, 35 articles are compiled from the proceedings of the National Heart, Lung, and Blood Institute Workshop on the outcome of PTCA. Articles in this volume include a report from the NIH Registry, experimental studies, technologic considerations, surgical considerations, acute and chronic outcome of PTCA, and future directions of study.

Roubin, G. S., Califf, R. M., O'Neill, W. W., et al.: Interventional Cardiovascular Medicine: Principles and Practice. New York, Churchill Livingstone, 1993.

A very comprehensive textbook of interventional cardiology with a particular emphasis on the practice of percutaneous interventions.

Stack, R. S., Carlson, E. B., Hinohara, H., and Phillips, H. R.: Interventional cardiac catheterization. Invest. Radiol., 20:333, 1985.

This review article describes historical developments in the field of PTCA, methods of procedure performance, complications, pathology, restenosis, use of PTCA in acute myocardial infarction, and new investigational interventional techniques.

Topol, E. J. (ed): Textbook of Interventional Cardiology. 2nd ed. Philadelphia, W. B. Saunders, 1994.

An excellent authoritative textbook covering all aspects of interventional cardiology. Well illustrated and very up-to-date.

## BIBLIOGRAPHY

Adelman, A. G., Cohen, E. A., Kimball, B. P., et al.: A comparison of directional atherectomy with balloon angioplasty for lesions of the left anterior descending coronary artery. N. Engl. J. Med., 329:228, 1993.

BARI, CABRI, EAST, GABI, and RITA: Coronary angioplasty on trial [Editorial]. Lancet, 335:1315, 1990.

Bengtson, J. R., Kaplan, A. J., Pieper, K. S., et al.: Prognosis in cardiogenic shock after acute myocardial infarction in the interventional era. J. Am. Coll. Cardiol., 20:1482, 1992.

Bengtson, J. R., Mark, D. B., Honan, M. B., et al.: Detection of restenosis after elective coronary angioplasty using the exercise treadmill test. Am. J. Cardiol., 65:28, 1990.

Bittl, J. A., Barbeau, G., and Abela, G. S.: Laser angioplasty: Potential effects and current limitations. In Topol, E. J. (ed): Textbook of Interventional Cardiology. 2nd ed. Philadelphia, W. B. Saunders, 1994, pp. 917–930.

Bittl, J. A., Sanborn, T. A., Tcheng, J. E., et al.: Clinical success, complications and restenosis rates with Excimer laser coronary angioplasty. Am. J. Cardiol., 70:1553, 1992.

Block, P. C.: Mechanism of transluminal coronary angioplasty. Am. J. Cardiol., 53:69C, 1984.

Bom, N., Lancee, C. T., and Egmond, F. C.: An ultrasonic intracardiac scanner. Ultrasonics, 10:72, 1972.

Brown, T. M., Jr., Iannone, L. A., Gordon, D. F., et al.: Percutaneous myocardial perfusion reduces mortality in acute myocardial infarction complicated by cardiogenic shock [Abstract]. Circulation (Suppl.), 72:III-309, 1985.

Buffet, P., Panchin, N., Willemot, J. P., et al.: Early and long-term outcome after emergency coronary artery bypass surgery after failed coronary angioplasty. Circulation, 84:III-254, 1991.

Califf, R. M., Fortin, D. F., Frid, D. J., et al.: Restenosis after coronary angioplasty: An overview. J. Am. Coll. Cardiol., 17:2B, 1991a.

Califf, R. M., Topol, E. J., Stack, R. S., et al.: Evaluation of combination thrombolytic therapy and timing of cardiac catheterization in acute myocardial infarction. Circulation, 83:1543, 1991b.

Colavita, P. G., Ideker, R. E., Reimer, K. A., et al.: The spectrum of pathology associated with percutaneous angioplasty. J. Am. Coll. Cardiol., 5:525, 1985.

Cook, S. L., Eigler, N. L., Shefer, A., et al.: Percutaneous Excimer laser coronary angioplasty of lesions not ideal for balloon angioplasty. Circulation, 84:632, 1991.

de Feyter, P., DeScheerder, I., van den Brand, M., et al.: Emergency stenting for refractory acute coronary occlusion during coronary angioplasty. Am. J. Cardiol., 66:1147, 1990.

Detre, K. M., Holmes, D. R., Holubkov, R., et al.: Incidences and consequences of peri-procedural occlusion. The 1985–1986 National Heart, Lung, and Blood Institute Percutaneous Transluminal Coronary Angioplasty Registry. Circulation, 82:739, 1990.

Detre, K. M., Holubkov, R., Kelsey, S., et al.: Percutaneous transluminal coronary angioplasty in 1985–1986 and 1977–1981. The National Heart, Lung, and Blood Institute Registry. N. Engl. J. Med., 318:265, 1988.

DeWood, M. A., Spores, J., Notske, R., et al.: Prevalance of total coronary occlusion during the early hours of transmural myocardial infarction. N. Engl. J. Med., 303:897, 1980.

Dotter, C. T.: Transluminal angioplasty: A long view. Radiology, 135:561, 1980.

Dotter, C. T.: Transluminally placed coilspring endarterial tube grafts: Long-term patency in canine popliteal artery. Invest. Radiol., 4:329, 1969.

Dotter, C. T., and Judkins, M. P.: Transluminal treatment of atherosclerotic obstructions: Description of a new technic and a preliminary report of its application. Circulation, 30:654, 1964.

Eckman, M. H., Wong, J. B., Salem, O. N., et al.: Direct angioplasty for acute myocardial infarction. Ann. Intern. Med., 117:667, 1992.

Ellis, S. G., Ribeiro-daSilva, E., Heyndrickx, G. R., et al.: Randomized comparison of rescue angioplasty with conservative management of patients with early failure of thrombolysis for acute anterior myocardial infarction. Circulation, 90:2280, 1994.

Ellis, S. G., Van de Werf, F., Ribeiro-daSilva, E., et al.: Present status of rescue coronary angioplasty: Current polarization of opinion and randomized trials [Editorial]. J. Am. Coll. Cardiol., 19:681, 1992.

Fishman, D. L., Leon, M. B., Baim, D. S., et al., for the Stent Restenosis Study Investigators: A randomized comparison of coronary-stent placement and balloon angioplasty in the treatment of coronary artery disease. N. Engl. J. Med., 331:496, 1994.

Forrester, J. S., Fishbein, M., Helfant, R., et al.: A paradigm for restenosis based on cell biology: Clues for the development of new preventive therapies. J. Am. Coll. Cardiol., 17:758, 1991.

Fourrier, J. L., Bertrand, M. E., Auth, D. C., et al.: Percutaneous coronary rational angioplasty in humans: Preliminary report. J. Am. Coll. Cardiol., 14:1278, 1989.

George, B. S., Voorhees, W. D., III, Roubin, G. S., et al.: Multicenter investigation of coronary stenting to treat acute or threatened closure after percutaneous transluminal coronary angioplasty: Clinical and angiographic outcomes. J. Am. Coll. Cardiol., 22:135, 1993.

Geschwind, H., Boussignac, G., and Teissevie, B.: Percutaneous transluminal laser angioplasty in man [Letter]. Lancet, 2:844, 1984.

GISSI-2 (Gruppo Italiano per lo Studio della Sopravvivenza nell' Infarto Miocardio): GISSI-2: A factorial randomised trial of alteplase versus streptokinase and heparin versus no heparin among 12,490 patients with acute myocardial infarction. Lancet, 336:65, 1990.

Grines, C. L., Browne, K. F., Marco, J., et al.: A comparison of immediate angioplasty with thrombolytic therapy for acute myocardial infarction. N. Engl. J. Med., 328:673, 1993.

Gruentzig, A. R.: Transluminal dilatation of coronary artery stenosis. Lancet, 1:263, 1978.

Gruentzig, A. R., Myler, R. K., Hanna, E. S., et al.: Transluminal angioplasty of coronary artery stenosis [Abstract]. Circulation, 56:III-84, 1977.

Gruentzig, A. R., Senning, A., and Siegenthaler, W. E.: Nonoperative dilatation of coronary artery stenosis. N. Engl. J. Med., 301:61, 1979.

GUSTO Investigators: An international randomized trial comparing four thrombolytic strategies for acute myocardial infarction. N. Engl. J. Med., 329:673, 1993.

Hands, M. E., Rutherford, J. D., Muller, J. E., et al.: The in-hospital development of cardiogenic shock after myocardial infarction: Incidence, predictors of occurrence, outcome and prognostic factors. J. Am. Coll. Cardiol., 14:40, 1989.

Hillegass, W. B., Ohman, E. M., and Califf, R. M.: Restenosis: The clinical issues. In Topol E. J. (ed.): Textbook of Interventional Cardiology. 2nd ed. Philadelphia, W. B. Saunders, 1994, pp. 415–435.

Hinohara, T., Safian, R. D., Gihazzal, Z. M. B., et al.: Directional coronary atherectomy: New approaches to coronary interventions experience [Abstract]. Circulation, 86(Suppl.):I-456, 1992.

Holmes, D. R., Vliestra, R. E., Smith, H. C., et al.: Restenosis after percutaneous transluminal coronary angioplasty. A report from the PTCA Registry of the National Heart, Lung, and Blood Institute. Am. J. Cardiol., 53:77C, 1984.

Ip, J. H., Fuster, V., Israel, D., et al.: The role of platelets, thrombin, and hyperplasia in restenosis after coronary angioplasty. J. Am. Coll. Cardiol., 17:77B, 1991.

ISIS-2 (Second International Study of Infarct Survival) Collaborative Group: ISIS-2: Randomised trial of intravenous streptokinase, oral aspirin, both, or neither among 17,187 cases of suspected acute myocardial infarction. Lancet, 2:349, 1988.

ISIS-3 (Third International Study of Infarct Survival) Collaborative Group: ISIS-3: A randomised comparison of streptokinase vs tissue plasminogen activator vs anistreplase and of aspirin plus heparin vs aspirin alone among 41,299 cases of suspected acute myocardial infarction. Lancet, 339:753, 1992.

Jackman, J. D., Zidar, J. P., Tcheng, J. E., et al.: Outcome after prolonged balloon inflations of >20 minutes for initially unsuccessful percutaneous transluminal coronary angioplasty. Am. J. Cardiol., 69:1417, 1992.

Jollis, J. G., DeLong, E. R., Collins, S. R., et al.: The relationship between angioplasty volume and outcome in the elderly in the Medicare database [Abstract]. Circulation, 88(Suppl.):I-480, 1993.

Kavanaugh, K. M., and Topol, E. J.: Acute intervention during myocardial infarction in patients with prior coronary bypass surgery. Am. J. Cardiol., 65:924, 1990.

Kent, K. M., Bentivoglo, L. G., Block, P. C., et al.: Percutaneous transluminal coronary angioplasty: Report from the Registry of the National Heart, Lung, and Blood Institute. Am. J. Cardiol., 9:2011, 1982.

Killen, D. A., Hamaker, W. R, and Reed, W. A.: Coronary artery bypass following percutaneous transluminal coronary angioplasty. Ann. Thorac. Surg., 40:133, 1985.

Klinke, P. W., and Hui, W.: Percutaneous transluminal coronary angioplasty without on-site surgical facilities. Am. J. Cardiol., 70:1520, 1992.

Knopf, W., Fiedotin, A., Cohlmia, G., et al.: Holium laser angioplasty in coronary arteries [Abstract]. J. Am. Coll. Cardiol., 17(Suppl.):279A, 1991.

Kuntz, R. E., and Baim, D. S.: Defining coronary restenosis: Newer clinical and angiographic paradigms. Circulation, 88:1310, 1993.

Libby, P., Schwartz, D., Brogi, E., et al.: A cascade model for restenosis. A special case of atherosclerosis progression. Circulation, 86(Suppl.):III-47, 1992.

Lincoff, A. M., Popma, J. J., Ellis, S. G., et al.: Abrupt vessel closure complicating coronary angioplasty: Clinical, angiographic and therapeutic profile. J. Am. Coll. Cardiol., 19:926, 1992.

Losordo, D. W., Rosenfield, K., Pieczek, A., et al.: How does angioplasty work? Serial analysis of human iliac arteries using intravascular ultrasound. Circulation, 86:1845, 1992.

Mark, D. B., Nelson, C. L., Califf, R. M., et al.: The continuing evolution of therapy for coronary artery disease: Initial results from the era of coronary angioplasty. Circulation, 89:2015, 1994.

McGuff, P. E., Bushnell, D., Soroff, H. S., et al.: Studies of the surgical applications of Laser (light amplification by stimulated emission of radiation. Surg. Forum, 14:143, 1963.

Meaney, T. B., Grines, C. L., Kander, N. H., et al.: Percutaneous coronary angioscopy in the assessment of plaque morphology in conjunction with interventional procedures [Abstract]. J. Am. Coll. Cardiol., 17:125A, 1991.

Mintz, G. S., Douek, P. C., Bonny, R. F., et al.: Intravascular ultrasound comparison of the de novo and restenotic coronary artery lesions [Abstract]. J. Am. Coll. Cardiol., 21:118A, 1993.

Myler, R. K., Shaw, R. E., Stertzer, S. H., et al.: Lesion morphology and coronary angioplasty. Current experience and analysis. J. Am. Coll. Cardiol., 19:1641, 1992.

Nobuyoshi, M., Kimura, T., Nosaka, H., et al.: Restenosis after successful percutaneous transluminal coronary angioplasty. Serial angiographic follow-up of 229 patients. J. Am. Coll. Cardiol., 12:616, 1988.

Nobuyoshi, M., Kimura, T., Ohishi, H., et al.: Restenosis after percutaneous transluminal coronary angioplasty. Pathologic observations in 20 patients. J. Am. Coll. Cardiol., 17:433, 1991.

O'Brien, E. R., Alpers, C. E., Stewart, D. K., et al.: Proliferation in primary and restenotic coronary atherectomy tissue: Implications for antiproliferative therapy. Circ. Res., 73:223, 1993.

O'Neill, W. W., Erbel, R., Laufer, N., et al.: Coronary angioplasty therapy of cardiogenic shock complicating acute myocardial infarction [Abstract]. Circulation, 72(Suppl.):III-309, 1985.

O'Neill, W. W., Kramer, B. L., Sketch, M. H., Jr.: Mechanical extraction atherectomy: Report of the US transluminal extraction catheter investigation [Abstract]. Circulation, 86(Suppl.):I-779, 1992.

Pandian, N. G., Kreis, A., Brockway, B., et al.: Ultrasound angioscopy: Real-time, two-dimensional, intraluminal ultrasound imaging of blood vessels. Am. J. Cardiol., 62:493, 1988.

Parisi, A. F., Folland, E. D., and Hartigan, P.: A comparison of angioplasty with medical therapy in the treatment of single-vessel coronary artery disease. N. Engl. J. Med., 326:10, 1992.

Parsonnet, V., Fisch, D., Gielchinsky, I., et al.: Emergency operation for failed angioplasty. J. Thorac. Cardiovasc. Surg., 96:198, 1988.

Pelletier, L. C., Pardini, A., Renkin, J., et al.: Myocardial revascularization after failure of percutaneous transluminal coronary angioplasty. J. Thorac. Cardiovasc. Surg., 90:265, 1985.

Popma, J. J., Leon, M. B., Mintz, G. S., et al.: Results of coronary angioplasty using the transluminal extraction catheter. Am. J. Cardiol., 70:1526, 1992.

Porstmann, W.: Neuer Korsett-Balloon Katheter zur transluminalen Rekanalisation nach Dotter unter besonderer Berucksichtigung von oblierationen an den Bechenarterien. Radiol. Diagn., 14:239, 1973.

Raizner, A. E., Hollman, J., Abukhalil, J., et al.: Ciprostene for restenosis revisited. Quantitative analysis of angiograms [Abstract]. J. Am. Coll. Cardiol., 21(Suppl.):321A, 1993.

Reifart, N., Preusler, W., Stoger, H., et al.: Outcome of 10,000 coronary interventional procedures without on-site surgical backup [Abstract]. Circulation, 88(Suppl.):I-217, 1993.

Richardson, S. G., Morten, P., Murtagh, J. G., et al.: Management of acute coronary occlusion during percutaneous transluminal coronary angioplasty: Experience of complications in a hospital without on-site facilities for cardiac surgery. Br. Med. J., 300:355, 1990.

RITA Investigators: Coronary angioplasty versus coronary artery bypass surgery: The Randomized Intervention Treatment of Angina (RITA) trial. Lancet, 341:573, 1993.

Rodriguez, A., Boullon, F., Perez-Bolino, N., et al.: Argentine randomized trial of percutaneous transluminal coronary angioplasty versus coronary artery bypass surgery in multivessel disease (ERACI): In-hospital results and 1-year follow-up. J. Am. Coll. Cardiol., 22:1060, 1993.

Rosenblum, J., Pensabene, J. F., and Kramer, B.: The TEC Device: Distal atherectomy and removal of an intracoronary thrombus. J. Invest. Cardiol., 3:41, 1991.

Ryan, T. J., Bauman, W. B., Kennedy, W., et al.: Guidelines for percutaneous transluminal coronary angioplasty: A report of the American College of Cardiology/American Heart Association Task Force on Assessment of Diagnostic and Therapeutic Cardiovascular Procedures (Subcommittee on Percutaneous Transluminal Coronary Angioplasty). J. Am. Coll. Cardiol., 22:2033, 1993.

Ryan, T. J., Faxon, D. P., Gunnar, R. M., et al.: Guidelines for percutaneous transluminal coronary angioplasty: A report of the American College Cardiology/American Heart Association Task Force on Assessment of Diagnostic and Therapeutic Cardiovascular Procedures (Subcommittee on Percutaneous Transluminal Coronary Angioplasty). J. Am. Coll. Cardiol. 12:529, 1988.

Safian, R. D., Gelbfish, J. S., Erny, R. E., et al.: Coronary atherectomy. Clinical, angiographic, and histologic findings and observations regarding potential mechanisms. Circulation, 82:69, 1990.

Schatz, R. A., Penn, I. M., Baim, D. S., et al.: Stent restenosis trial (STRESS): Analysis of in-hospital results [Abstract]. Circulation, 88(Suppl.):I-594, 1993.

Scheidt, S., Ascheim, R., and Killip, T., III: Shock after acute myocardial infarction: A clinical and hemodynamic profile. Am. J. Cardiol., 26:556, 1970.

Schwartz, R. S., Holmes, D. R., Jr., and Topol, E. J.: The restenosis paradigm revisited: An alternative proposal for cellular mechanisms. J. Am. Coll. Cardiol., 20:1284, 1992.

Serruys, P. W., DeJaegere, P., and Kiemeneij, F.: A comparison of balloon-expandable-stent implantation with balloon angioplasty in patients with coronary artery disease. N. Engl. J. Med., 331:489, 1994.

Serruys, P. W., Luijten, H. E., Beatt, K. J., et al.: Incidence of restenosis after successful coronary angioplasty. A time-related phenemenon. A quantitative angiographic study in 342 consecutive patients at 1, 2, 3 and 4 months. Circulation, 77:361, 1988.

Serruys, P. W., Strauss, B. H., Beatt, K. J., et al.: Quantitative follow-up after placement of a self-expanding coronary stent. N. Engl. J. Med., 324:13, 1991.

Sigwart, U., Puel, J., Mirkovitch, V., et al.: Intravascular stents to prevent occlusion and restenosis after transluminal angioplasty. N. Engl. J. Med., 316:701, 1987.

Simpfendorfer, C., Belardi, J., Bellamy, G., et al.: Frequency, management, and follow-up of patients with acute coronary occlusions after percutaneous transluminal coronary angioplasty. Am. J. Cardiol., 59:267, 1987.

Simpson, J. B., Baim, D. S., Robert, E. W., and Harrison, D. C.: A new catheter system for coronary angioplasty. Am. J. Cardiol., 49:1216, 1982.

Sinclair, I. N., McCabe, C. H., Sipperly, M. E., et al.: Predictors, therapeutic options, and long-term outcome of abrupt vessel reclosure. Am. J. Cardiol., 61:61G, 1988.

Sketch, M. H., Jr., O'Neill, W. W., Galichia, J. P., et al.: Restenosis following coronary transluminal extraction-endarterectomy: The final analysis of a multicenter registry. J. Am. Coll. Cardiol., 19:277A, 1992.

Stack, R. S., O'Connor, C. M., Mark, D. B., et al.: Coronary perfusion during acute myocardial infarction with a combined therapy of coronary angioplasty and high-dose intravenous streptokinase. Circulation, 77:151, 1988.

Staple, T. W.: Modified catheter for percutaneous transluminal treatment of atherosclerotic obstructions. Radiology, 91:1041, 1968.

Talley, J. D., Weintraub, W. S., Roubin, G. S., et al.: Failed elective percutaneous transluminal coronary angioplasty requiring coronary artery bypass surgery. In-hospital and late clinical outcome at 5 years. Circulation, 82:1203, 1990.

Teirstein, P. S., Schatz, R. A., Rocha-Singh, K. J., et al.: Coronary stenting with angioscopic guidance [Abstract]. J. Am. Coll. Cardiol., 19:223A, 1992.

TIMI Research Group: Immediate versus delayed catheterization and angioplasty following thrombolytic therapy for acute myocardial infarction. J. A. M. A., 260:2849, 1988.

TIMI Study Group: Comparison of invasive and conservative strategies following intravenous tissue plasminogen activator in acute myocardial infarction: Results of the thrombolysis in myocardial infarction (TIMI) II Trial. N. Engl. J. Med., 320:618, 1989.

Topol, E. J., Callif, R. M., George, B. S., et al.: A randomized trial of immediate versus delayed elective angioplasty after intravenous tissue plasminogen activator in acute myocardial infarction. N. Engl. J. Med., 317:581, 1987.

Topol, E. J., Holmes, D. R., and Rogers, W. J.: Coronary angioplasty after thrombolytic therapy for acute myocardial infarction. Ann. Intern. Med., 144:877, 1991.

Topol, E. J., Leya, F., Pinkerton, C. A., et al.: A comparison of directional atherectomy with balloon angioplasty in patients with coronary artery disease. N. Engl. J. Med., 329:221, 1993.

van Andel, G. J.: Percutaneous Transluminal Angioplasty: The Dotter Procedure. Amsterdam, Excerpta Medica, 1976.

Van der Linden, L. P., Bakx, A. L. M., Sedney, M. I., et al.: Prolonged dilation with an autoperfusion balloon catheter for refractory acute occlusion related to percutaneous transluminal coronary angioplasty. J. Am. Coll. Cardiol., 22:1016, 1993.

Waller, B. F.: Coronary luminal shape and the arc of disease-free wall. Morphologic observations and clinical relevance. J. Am. Coll. Cardiol., 6:1100, 1985.

Waller, B. F.: Pathology of transluminal balloon angioplasty used in the treatment of coronary heart disease. Hum. Pathol., 18:476, 1987.

Waller, B. F., Pinkerton, C. A., Orr, C. M., et al.: Restenosis 1 to 24 months after clinically successful coronary balloon angioplasty: A necropsy study of 20 patients. J. Am. Coll. Cardiol., 17(Suppl.):58B, 1991.

Waltman, A. C., Greenfield, A. J., and Athanasoulis, C. A.: Transluminal angioplasty: General rules and basic considerations. In Athanasoulis, C. A., Pfister, R. C., Greene, R. E., and Roberson, G. H. (eds): Interventional Radiology. Philadelphia, W. B. Saunders, 1982, p. 253.

White, C. J., Ramee, S. R., Collins, T. J., et al.: Percutaneous angioscopy of saphenous vein coronary artery bypass grafts. J. Am. Coll. Cardiol., 21:1181, 1993.

Zijlstra, F., deBoer, M. J., Hoorntje, J. C. A., et al.: A comparison of immediate angioplasty with intravenous streptokinase in acute myocardial infarction. N. Engl. J Med., 328:680, 1993.

# ■ III Fibrinolytic Therapy in the Management of Acute Myocardial Infarction

Robert M. Califf

The evolution of our understanding of the fibrinolytic system, coinciding with safe techniques for evaluating the human coronary circulation during unstable ischemic heart disease syndromes, has dramatically changed the therapy of unstable angina and acute *myocardial infarction* (MI). Both mechanical and pharmacologic techniques to correct the underlying abnormality in coronary blood flow associated with acute MI now form the basis for interventional therapy. Methods of restoring coronary blood flow after acute occlusion will continue to include agents that lyse thrombi, although some centers will prefer mechanical reperfusion with angioplasty. Improved ability to exploit nature and more efficient and elaborate methods of producing human genetic products through recombinant techniques will increase flexibility in altering the structure of these molecules. Thus, the cardiovascular practitioner needs to understand the fibrinolytic system and the consequences of therapeutic manipulation of this system.

## HISTORICAL ASPECTS

Herrick (1912) initially described acute MI as a clinical syndrome representing coronary thrombosis. Subsequent clinicians and researchers continued to describe the problem as one involving a thrombosed coronary artery, until a series of pathologic studies failed to show thrombi in the coronary arteries of patients who died of acute MI. These studies led many prominent cardiologists to doubt the primacy of thrombosis in the pathogenesis of the condition. The issue remained unsettled until the pioneering work of DeWood and colleagues, who reported in 1980 that when acute angiography was done in patients early in acute MI, coronary occlusion was found in more than 80% (DeWood et al., 1980). Moreover, when these patients were referred for *coronary artery bypass grafting* (CABG), thrombus could be removed surgically from the vessel.

Knowledge of the fibrinolytic system was evolving alongside our understanding of the pathophysiology of MI. The instability of blood clots has been recognized since 1838, when Denis described the dissolution of fibrin in human clots (MacFarlane and Biggs, 1948). Nolf and Yudin, from the Soviet Union, began

to use cadaveric blood for transfusion after they noted that clots dissolved several hours after death (Nolf, 1905). Tillett and Garner, at Johns Hopkins, initially described streptokinase in 1933. The possible role of the agent in pharmacologic treatment of thrombotic problems was not generally appreciated until experiments by Tillett and Sherry, reported from 1949 to 1952, showed that streptokinase could successfully lyse clots (Tillett and Sherry, 1949). Most of these early applications were in diseases of the thorax caused by loculation of fluid by blood clots, and the experiments were reported in the surgical literature. In 1949, Johnson and Tillett reported the first model of in vivo fibrinolysis in rabbits (Johnson and Tillett, 1952).

Nydick and colleagues (1961) reported a reduction of infarct size in the animal model with early treatment with streptokinase. The first clinical trial of thrombolytic therapy in acute myocardial infarction was reported by Fletcher and associates in 1958. These initial studies did not evoke tremendous enthusiasm from the clinical community, although a number of large studies of intravenous thrombolytic therapy were initiated in Europe in the 1960s and 1970s. The first large-scale trials of thrombolytic therapy in the United States were initiated by the National Institutes of Health to evaluate this treatment in pulmonary embolism, rather than acute MI, mainly because of skepticism concerning the role of thrombus in the pathogenesis of MI.

Despite the identification of *tissue plasminogen activator* (TPA) in the 1940s, the lack of a suitable method to produce sufficient quantities delayed its evaluation for clinical purposes. In 1979, in Collen's laboratory, a melanoma cell culture was used to isolate sufficient quantities to investigate the structure and biologic properties of TPA (Rijken and Collen, 1981). The first patient was treated with TPA in 1981, and renal vein thrombosis was resolved in two patients after renal transplantation. Through a combination of industry and academic efforts, the TPA gene was cloned and expressed in a mammalian hamster ovary cell line. Large quantities of TPA were thus produced for laboratory and human investigation, beginning in February 1984. Since the early 1980s, a series of large clinical trials have been performed, randomizing over 150,000 patients to either treatment or placebo or to one treatment compared with another. The methodology of the large, simple clinical trial has allowed an excellent understanding of outcomes related to this therapy while providing a paradigm to aid understanding of the impact of other clinical therapies by measuring outcomes in large numbers of patients.

## PATHOPHYSIOLOGY OF UNSTABLE ISCHEMIC HEART DISEASE SYNDROMES

Our understanding of the factors that produce unstable MI is based on demonstration of complete coronary artery occlusion in humans at the time of acute MI and pathologic documentation of abnormal plaque architecture in unstable angina, sudden death, and acute infarction. Atherosclerotic plaques evolve from small yellow fatty streaks to complex lesions, including smooth-muscle cell proliferation, connective tissue proliferation, and collagen and elastin, in addition to pools of cholesterol. Detailed pathoanatomic studies have shown that plaques vary considerably in architecture. Some plaques are predominantly composed of collagen (fibrous plaques), whereas others contain a large lipid pool, which is semifluid at body temperature. These lipid pools are covered by fibrous tissue, which is in turn covered by intact endothelium. Intracellular and extracellular lipid is also found throughout the plaque.

Although the precise mechanism remains to be defined, as "soft" atherosclerotic plaques evolve, sudden disruptions in the endothelium occur and are manifested pathologically as fissures on the surface of the plaques or as more extensive disruption of the undersurface of the plaques, called "plaque rupture." Preliminary evidence has indicated that in some cases, the fibrous plaque is eroded by macrophage digestion, whereas in other cases, a sudden mechanical disruption occurs at stress points where the lipid pool and fibrous portion of the plaque adjoin. Exposure of the contents of the plaque to the bloodstream causes a biochemical sequence that activates the clotting system and precipitates coronary vasospasm. In most cases, the fissure is sealed off, and the lumen of the vessel is not compromised significantly, but in some cases intraluminal thrombus propagates until the artery is totally obstructed. Hemorrhage into the contents of the plaque along planes defined by the geography of the plaque may lead to significant alteration of the degree of lumen compromise without total occlusion (Fig. 31–38). Thus, the process of progressive atherosclerosis is now thought to involve a series of "plaque events" rather than a smooth, steady progression to occlusion of the vessel. Finally, when the clotting system is activated and a thrombus projects into the lumen, the distal vessel may be subject to microemboli of platelets and fibrin.

Platelet activation is mediated by a series of events that are probably initiated through the exposure of platelet receptors to collagen and thrombin (Fig. 31–39). These receptors then activate biochemical pathways that lead to the secretion of vasoactive sub-

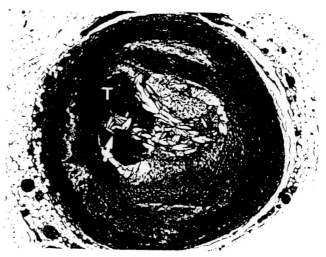

**FIGURE 31–38.** An occluded coronary artery filled with thrombus (T) is depicted. A fissure is present within an intimal pool of lipid, and the thrombus within the lumen contains cholesterol *(arrow)* that has extruded from the plaque. (From Davies, M. J.: Atherogenesis and thrombosis. *In* Califf, R. M., Mark, D. B., and Wagner, G. S. [eds]: Acute Coronary Care in the Thrombolytic Era. Chicago, Year Book Medical, 1988, p. 8. Reprinted with permission.)

stances by the platelets. The initial phase in which platelets become attracted to form a layer on the disrupted endothelial surface is called *platelet adhesion.* Components that have been identified as essential for normal platelet adhesion include the von Willebrand factor, the glycoprotein Ib receptor, and the glycoprotein IIb/IIIa receptor. When platelets adhere to the endothelial surface, a series of events leads to platelet aggregation. The platelets secrete two types of granules: one containing adenine nucleotides, calcium, and serotonin, and the other containing adhesive and coagulation proteins and growth factors. Attention

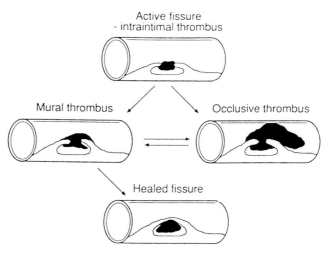

**FIGURE 31–39.** Plaque fissure can lead to mural thrombus that resolves or to an occlusive thrombus leading to myocardial infarction. (From Davies, M. J.: Atherogenesis and thrombosis. *In* Califf, R. M., Mark, D. B., and Wagner, G. S. [eds]: Acute Coronary Care in the Thrombolytic Era. Chicago, Year Book Medical, 1988, p. 9. Reprinted with permission.)

has focused on these growth factors (platelet-derived growth factor and beta growth factor) because of their ability to stimulate smooth-muscle cell proliferation and fibroblast migration. Large amounts of thromboxane $A_2$ are also produced, leading to vasospasm and further platelet aggregation.

As platelets are activated, the blood coagulation system is activated simultaneously (Fig. 31–40). A series of reactions involving coagulation proteins on the surface of the denuded endothelium then produces thrombin. This process is regulated by antithrombin III, which inactivates many components in the coagulation cascade, and proteins C and S, which exert their action predominantly by inactivating Factors Va and VIIIa. The production of thrombin leads to the conversion of fibrinogen to fibrin, thus forming clot; thrombin is also a potent stimulator of platelet activation.

This complex series of events can rapidly convert a "stable" atherosclerotic plaque to a primary initiator of acute ischemic heart disease syndromes (Fig. 31–41). The platelet and fibrin mass causes a progressive narrowing of the arterial lumen. Vasoactive substances are produced, leading to further periodic fluctuations in vascular tone with accompanying unpredictable anginal episodes due to reduced blood supply to the distal myocardium. If the clotting process is not controlled, total occlusion of the vessel ensues, with necrosis downstream within 30 to 45

minutes of occlusion. If the process is controlled before total occlusion, a more high-grade stenosis results, often limiting the lifestyle of the patient.

## FIBRINOLYTIC SYSTEM

Clot formation is actively opposed in nature by a system that acts to restore and maintain vascular patency after thrombus formation. The process of clot formation and dissolution is ubiquitous, and the implications of this complex system for normal biologic processes are now being realized. Just as the conversion of prothrombin to thrombin is the central process in clot formation, the conversion of plasminogen to plasmin is the focal event in clot dissolution (Fig. 31–42). Plasmin degrades both fibrinogen and fibrin to components referred to as fibrin(ogen) degradation products. The action of plasmin to lyse clot is opposed by antiplasmins in the systemic circulation and is activated by a number of activators, just as by the coagulation factors. The predominant antiplasmin in nature is alpha$_2$-antiplasmin, although a number of other antiplasmins have been described.

Plasminogen activators may be divided into three major classifications: exogenous, intrinsic, and extrinsic (Fig. 31–43). The exogenous activators are products from other organisms that can be administered from other biologic systems. The major exogenous activator is streptokinase, a streptococcal protein that forms a complex with plasminogen, causing a shift in the configuration of the plasminogen, thus exposing the active site of the enzyme. The activated enzyme then converts circulating plasminogen to plasmin. The intrinsic pathway includes multiple molecules involved in coagulation and inflammation. The role of this system in nature or pathophysiology is poorly understood. The most clearly understood system is the extrinsic system, which is composed of a series of activators found in the human circulation. TPA is a glycoprotein produced by the vascular endothelium as well as other tissues. The molecular structure and function of this molecule have been defined in a series of eloquent experiments. The molecule contains a serine protease active site and two kringles with a configuration similar to the plasminogen molecule, a "finger" domain resembling the adhesive protein fibronectin, and a portion closely resembling epidermal growth factor. The close affinity of TPA for fibrin is probably conferred by the second kringle and the finger domain. TPA is produced in higher quantity by the vascular endothelium when stimulated by a variety of stressors, including intravascular thrombus formation. In addition, regular exercise, lower body weight, and absence of cigarette smoking have been associated with a more responsive production of TPA by the endothelium. The other known extrinsic native human plasminogen activator is *urokinase plasminogen activator* (UPA). The role of UPA in nature is less well understood, although it is present in the urinary tract in high concentrations and in the circulation in very low concentrations. In its proenzyme or single-chain

## PLATELET ADHESION

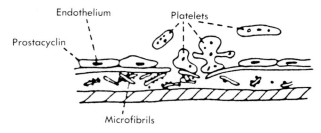

## PLATELET AGGREGATION

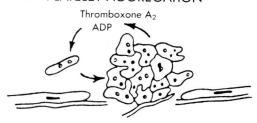

FIGURE 31–40. An overview of the process of primary hemostasis. The initial event is platelet adhesion to the vessel wall, which occurs when the subendothelium is exposed as a result of disruption or injury of endothelial cells. After adhesion, platelets become activated. Under the influence of mediators such as adenosine diphosphate (ADP) and thromboxane $A_2$, circulating platelets are stimulated to the initial monolayer of platelets to form a platelet aggregate. (From Handen, R. I., and Loscalzo, J.: Hemostasis, thrombosis, fibrinolysis, and cardiovascular disease. *In* Braunwald, E. [ed]: Heart Disease. 3rd ed. Philadelphia, W. B. Saunders, 1988, p. 1758.)

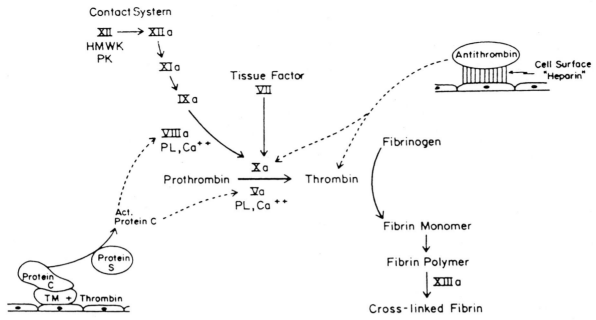

**FIGURE 31–41.** An overview of the coagulation cascade showing the two major pathways of activation. The intrinsic pathway involves Factors XII, XI, IX, and VIII, with the extrinsic or tissue factor system, which involves tissue factor and Factor VII. In both pathways, the conversion of inactive Factor X to its active form, XA, results in the formation of thrombin from prothrombin. Thrombin then converts fibrinogen to fibrin monomers, which are polymerized into cross-links by Factor XIIIA. This illustration also displays the two major anticoagulant systems. The binding of antithrombin to thrombin and Factor XA is accelerated by heparin on endothelial cells. Protein C is activated by thrombin after it is bound to the endothelial cell protein thrombomoduline. Activated protein C and protein S inactivate the two coagulation cofactors VIIIA and VA. (From Handen, R. I.: Bleeding and thrombosis. *In* Braunwald, E., Isselbacher, K. J., and Petersdorf, R. G. [eds]: Harrison's Principles of Internal Medicine. 11th ed. New York, McGraw-Hill, 1987, p. 270.)

form (SCUPA), the molecule has an affinity for fibrin, as TPA does. Each of these activators also has a specific rapid-acting inhibitor that has been isolated. Preliminary information suggests that imbalances between these activators and their inhibitors may be responsible for thrombotic tendencies in many disease states.

The conversion of plasminogen to plasmin and thus

the degradation of fibrin and fibrinogen may occur in one of two compartments: on the surface of a clot (fibrin-specific activation) or in the systemic circulation (nonspecific activation) (Fig. 31–44). Fibrin-spe-

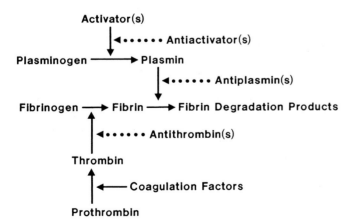

**FIGURE 31–42.** Major pathways of fibrin formation and dissolution. Fibrin is formed, and thrombin is generated by coagulation activation. Fibrin is dissolved when plasma is generated by fibrinolytic activation. (From Stump, D. C., and Collen, D.: Fibrinolytic system: Implications for thrombolytic therapy. *In* Califf, R. M., Mark, D. B., and Wagner, G. S. [eds]: Acute Coronary Care in the Thrombolytic Era. Chicago, Year Book Medical, 1988, p. 59.)

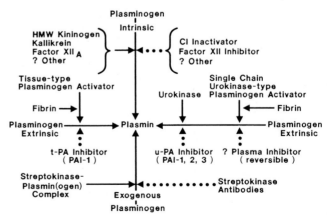

**FIGURE 31–43.** Major pathways of plasminogen activation. Plasma is formed indirectly from the exogenous administration of streptokinase but directly by activation of the intrinsic pathway. Direct plasmin generation also occurs through the action of the extrinsic plasminogen activators t-PA (tissue plasminogen activator) and u-PA (urokinase plasminogen activator). Note the distinction between the pathways of plasminogen activation and what are called *intrinsic* and *extrinsic* pathways of coagulation. (From Stump, D. C., and Collen, D.: Fibrinolytic system: Implications for thrombolytic therapy. *In* Califf, R. M., Mark, D. B., and Wagner, G. S. [eds]: Acute Coronary Care in the Thrombolytic Era. Chicago, Year Book Medical, 1988, p. 62.)

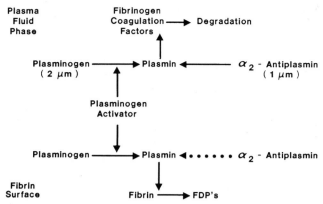

**FIGURE 31–44.** Schematic representation of the fibrin specificity of plasminogen activation. The fact that the activation of plasminogen is targeted to the fibrin surface leads to plasmin and is relatively protected from inhibition by alpha$_2$-antiplasmin. This targeting also avoids the generation of freely circulating plasmin that nonspecifically degrades normal plasma coagulation factors. (From Stump, D. C., and Collen, D.: Fibrinolytic system: Implications for thrombolytic therapy. *In* Califf, R. M., Mark, D. B., and Wagner, G. S. [eds]: Acute Coronary Care in the Thrombolytic Era. Chicago, Year Book Medical, 1988, p. 66.)

cific activation appears to be relatively more efficient, because large quantities of degradation products are not produced, and coagulation factors distant from the site of the thrombus remain relatively intact. TPA is the prototypical fibrin-specific agent, and its affinity for plasminogen increases by 400 times when it is bound directly to fibrin; SCUPA is also relatively fibrin-specific, although the mechanism for this effect is less well understood. However, streptokinase and urokinase have no special affinity for plasminogen in the presence of fibrin. For these agents to produce clot lysis, a sufficient amount is required to convert plasminogen to plasmin throughout the circulation, thus not only destroying the thrombolytic obstruction, but also depleting fibrinogen, Factor V, and Factor VIII in the systemic circulation.

## PATHOPHYSIOLOGY OF MYOCARDIAL NECROSIS

The basic concepts of the impact of coronary occlusion on myocardial necrosis and the pathophysiologic basis for salvage of myocardium have been elucidated by a number of investigators during the last 2 decades after the pioneering work of Reimer and Jennings (1977, 1979). In seminal experiments in the canine model, they showed that irreversible necrosis of the myocardium begins within 30 to 45 minutes of occlusion of an epicardial vessel and that this necrosis advances rapidly from the endocardium toward the epicardium (Fig. 31–45). This process has been called the *wavefront phenomenon of ischemic myocardial necrosis.* The same investigators showed that release of coronary artery occlusion at various times until about 3 hours after occlusion salvaged myocardium that would have become necrotic with continued occlusion. This myocardial salvage tended to occur from the epicardium toward the endocardium, so that an epicardial rim of tissue was spared.

Another important contribution of these investigators was to demonstrate that collateral circulation is important in determining the amount of myocardium that can be salvaged and the time frame for possible salvage (Fig. 31–46). The tremendous variation among species with regard to the time frame of myocardial necrosis and salvage is best explained by differences in collateral supply to the area at risk. Subsequent human studies have corroborated the importance of collateral supply as a mediator of myocardial salvage with reperfusion therapy.

Studies have focused on the process of necrosis in the hope that manipulation of the biochemical substrate could prolong the time frame for myocardial salvage. Many studies in laboratory models of acute occlusion and reocclusion of the coronary arteries have suggested that reperfusion of the acutely ischemic myocardium causes cellular damage that de-

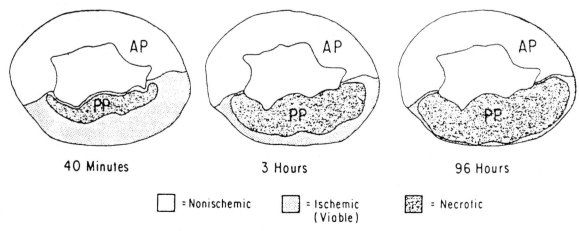

**FIGURE 31–45.** Progression of cell death versus time after left circumflex coronary artery occlusion. Necrosis occurs first in the subendocardial myocardium; with longer occlusions, the cell death moves from the subendocardial zone across the wall. This wavefront of ischemic cell death progressively involves more of the transmural thickness of the ischemic zone. (AP = anterior papillary muscle; PP = posterior papillary muscle.) (From Reimer, K. A.: The relationship between coronary blood flow in reversible and irreversible ischemic injury. *In* Califf, R. M., and Wagner, G. S. [eds]: Acute Coronary Care: Principles and Practice. Dordrecht, Martinus Nijhoff, 1985, p. 10.)

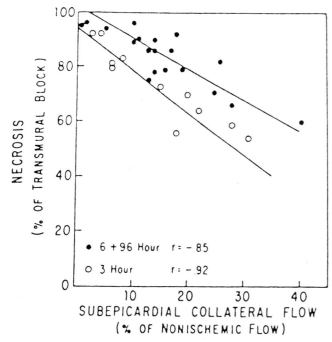

**FIGURE 31–46.** Relationship between transmural necrosis and sub-epicardial blood flow. Regression lines for permanent infarcts (96 hours) and infarcts reperfused at 6 hours were not significantly different and were combined. Infarcts reperfused at 3 hours are indicated by the *open circles.* In both groups, the transmural extent of necrosis was inversely related to subepicardial flow measured at 20 minutes after left circumflex coronary occlusion. However, the 3-hour regression line shifted downward, indicating that reperfusion at 3 hours limited infarct size. (From Reimer, K. A.: The relationship between coronary blood flow in reversible and irreversible ischemic injury. *In* Califf, R. M., and Wagner, G. S. [eds]: Acute Coronary Care: Principles and Practice. Dordrecht, Martinus Nijhoff, 1985, p. 13.)

cell swelling or to platelet and leukocyte accumulation and obstruction of distal vessels. Multiple pharmacologic manipulations of these systems are currently under investigation in animal and human studies, but the first two human clinical trials to limit reperfusion injury (with superoxide dismutase and with fluosol, a perfluorochemical emulsion) have failed.

Finally, demonstration of prolonged survival in patients treated with thrombolytic therapy beyond 6 hours from the onset of symptoms has focused attention on the process of healing of the myocardium. Human and animal studies have shown that during the recovery phase after acute infarction, many ventricles experience progressive dilatation, called *infarct expansion.* This phenomenon at its most extreme creates left ventricular aneurysm and distorts the shape of the left ventricle. In a less extreme form, infarct expansion produces a larger end-diastolic volume and distortion of the shape of the left ventricle, which have been associated with a high risk of death after infarction. Early reperfusion has prevented this process, presumably through greater epicardial sparing of tissue. In some animal models, even when reperfusion occurs after the point at which significant myocardial salvage can be expected, infarct expansion has been prevented. The pathophysiologic basis for this observation is not yet delineated.

## FIBRINOLYTIC AGENTS

Streptokinase is currently the thrombolytic agent most commonly used worldwide. The agent, a streptococcal enzyme with nonfibrin-specific lytic properties, is administered in a dose of 1.5 million units for 30 to 60 minutes and has been associated with a 30 to 70% reperfusion rate in available studies (Kennedy et al., 1985; O'Neill et al., 1986; Stack et al., 1983) (Fig. 31–47). Because of its lack of fibrin specificity, it must be given in sufficient doses to create a systemic lytic state with its prolonged phase of fibrinogen and clotting factor depletion. In addition, because streptokinase is a bacterial enzyme, its use is associated with various systemic effects that are not observed with other thrombolytic agents. Hypotension with an average fall of systolic blood pressure of 30 mm Hg is observed in the average patient. This problem can be treated with volume in most patients, although pressor agents are required in some. Other acute problems range from a rash with fever and chills to bronchospasm to frank anaphylaxis. In addition, a late serum sickness-like reaction has been observed. An *acylated plasminogen-streptokinase activator complex* (APSAC) has been developed. It can be given as a bolus for 5 minutes without hypotension, although the other reactions may occur as the plasminogen deacylates in the circulation (AIMS Trial Study Group, 1988).

Urokinase also has been available for many years. Because of its relative expense and limited quantity, however, it has not yet been approved for routine intravenous use in acute MI. Current studies indicate

tracts from the beneficial overall effects of reperfusion. These deleterious effects appear to be mediated through a series of events that produce myocardial and endothelial cell swelling and rapid accumulation of destructive metabolites and other byproducts of ischemia in the cell. A large overload of calcium occurs shortly after reperfusion, as does explosive cell swelling, which may be caused by an inability of the cells to regulate cell volume. Hemorrhage into the area of infarction caused by loss of endothelial cell integrity also adds to mechanical decompensation. The oxygen free radical system has received much attention as a potential mediator of increased cell death with reperfusion. This system, which usually rids tissues of superoxide anions through a reaction catalyzed by superoxide dismutase, becomes overwhelmed during reperfusion. Consequently, superoxide anions accumulate within the cell, causing rapid tissue destruction and especially loss of structural integrity of the cell membrane. Whether this process of reperfusion injury actually increases infarct size or simply hastens the demise of cells already destined to die remains unsettled. Another possible mechanism of increased damage due to reperfusion is the obstruction of distal arteriolar beds due to endothelial

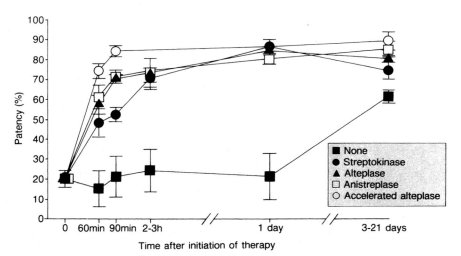

FIGURE 31–47. Pooled analysis of angiographic patency rates over time after various thrombolytic agents: Patency rates are highest following accelerated t-PA, early rates with conventional t-PA and anistreplase are strikingly similar, and the patency rate following streptokinase has "caught up" to conventional t-PA and anistreplase within 2 to 3 hours. Includes 13,728 angiographic observations. (From Granger, C. B., Califf, R. M., and Topol, E. J.: Thrombolytic therapy for acute myocardial infarction: A review. Drugs, 44:293–325, 1992.)

that a dose of 3 million units for 90 minutes will achieve a reperfusion rate of 50 to 70% within 90 minutes of administration. The drug is not associated with hypotension or allergic phenomena because it is a human enzyme. However, it does create a systemic lytic state because it is a nonspecific fibrinolytic agent, like streptokinase.

TPA has now been produced on a large scale through recombinant genetic technology. The enzyme is fibrin-specific at low doses, but as the dose is increased, significant systemic fibrinogenolysis occurs (Collen, 1985). Until recently, the drug was usually administered in a dose of 60 mg in the first hour, with 10 mg as a bolus to produce rapid clot lysis. Patency rates were 60 to 75%. After the first hour, 20 mg/hr was given for 2 hours in an effort to continue clot lysis on the surface of the plaque and to prevent rethrombosis (GISSI-2, 1990. National Heart Foundation, 1988; Rao et al., 1988; Simoons et al., 1988). Recent clinical trials have demonstrated that the initial dosing regimens were suboptimal. Beginning with the pioneering work of Neuhaus, a series of studies indicated that superior rates of infarct artery perfusion could be achieved with "front-loading" or accelerated dosing of TPA. Finally, the large Global Use of Streptokinase and t-PA for Occluded Coronary Arteries (GUSTO, 1993) Trial demonstrated that this regimen is associated with a relative reduction of 14% in mortality rate and improved left ventricular function compared with other currently available thrombolytic regimens.

A comparison of the clinical and hematologic effects of the drugs is shown in Table 31–13. Superior clot lysis rates have been shown with accelerated TPA compared with streptokinase and urokinase (Califf et al., 1989; Topol, 1991; Yusuf et al., 1985). Because TPA has a shorter duration of biologic activity, a maintenance infusion of heparin is often required to prevent reocclusion of the infarct-related artery. Because of their shorter half-life and relative lack of effect on the systemic fibrinolytic system, the fibrin-specific agents were presumed by many to have a lower risk of associated bleeding. With respect to systemic bleeding, this presumption appears to have been validated, although the difference is small. The major reason for bleeding with fibrinolytic therapy appears to be the lysis of hemostatic plugs and not the systemic fibrinolytic state.

The benefit of fibrin-specific drugs in reducing systemic bleeding is overshadowed by the increased risk of intracranial hemorrhage induced by these agents. Streptokinase is associated with a 0.3 to 0.6% rate of intracranial hemorrhage, whereas TPA is associated with a rate in excess of 0.2% (2 per thousand). Intracranial hemorrhage is a devastating complication: The mortality rate is over 50%, with half of the survivors remaining significantly disabled (Gore et al., 1991). All patients treated with fibrinolytic therapy should be carefully observed, although older patients, patients with acute hypertension, light patients, women, and patients with a history of cerebrovascular disease should be watched especially carefully. Immediate reversal of all anticoagulation and consideration of surgical evacuation are necessary when an intracranial bleed is diagnosed. Immediate computed tomographic scanning is recommended for any patient with a few focal neurologic deficits.

## SELECTION OF PATIENTS

The early identification and treatment of candidates for fibrinolytic therapy have become major public

■ Table 31–13. SUMMARY OF AGENTS

| | Streptokinase (%) | TPA (%) |
|---|---|---|
| Speed of lysis | — | + + |
| Coronary patency (90 minutes) | 40–60 | 65–75 |
| Coronary patency (24 hours) | 80 | 80 |
| Left ventricular function | + | + |
| Bleeding risk | + | + |
| Mortality | + | + + |

TPA = tissue plasminogen activator.

health issues. Protocols are needed to rapidly assess and treat patients within 30 minutes of identification, because time is so important in determining the extent of myocardial salvage. Although a physician's supervision is currently required for the use of these agents, several trials of administration in the field by paramedical personnel have yielded promising results. Fibrinolytic therapy is currently reserved for patients with classic signs or symptoms of acute MI and classic ST segment elevation on the electrocardiogram. In general, at least 30 minutes of symptoms without resolution with sublingual nitroglycerin is required. Patients with suspected acute MI who do not meet these electrocardiographic criteria are subjected either to coronary angiography to document the presence of coronary occlusion before treatment or to conservative therapy. Absolute contraindications to thrombolytic therapy include the following situations: known active bleeding sites or disorders, operation within 2 weeks, prolonged (> 5 to 10 minutes) cardiopulmonary resuscitation, previous stroke, recent trauma (within 2 months), and persistent diastolic blood pressure exceeding 100 mm Hg or systolic pressure exceeding 180 mm Hg. Based on an overview of available human studies, a time limit of 12 hours from the onset of symptoms had classically been set for treatment, and the large International Study of Infarct Survival (ISIS)-2 Trial (1987) documented that treatment within 24 hours of the onset of symptoms promoted survival. The mechanism for this late benefit is speculative, but is presumed to include the prevention of infarct expansion and creation of a more electrically stable state.

Physical examination of patients before treatment should focus on excluding other diagnoses that could lead to catastrophe if confused with acute MI. In particular, the cardiovascular examination should carefully assess the probability of aortic dissection or acute pericarditis. The alternative causes of electrocardiographic ST segment elevation should also be excluded if possible (early repolarization normal variant, coronary vasospasm, left ventricular aneurysm, pericarditis, and left ventricular hypertrophy). During infusion of a thrombolytic agent, the patient should be constantly supervised by the nursing staff, with frequent vital sign determination, observation of neurologic status, and clinical and laboratory evaluation of bleeding status.

## IMPACT OF THERAPY ON IMPORTANT CLINICAL OUTCOMES

The beneficial effect of fibrinolytic therapy on mortality has been shown in multiple randomized clinical trials. Although many smaller trials have shown reduced mortality, the Italian GISSI Trial (1986) resolved the issue definitively by randomizing 11,806 patients to receive either 1.5 million units of streptokinase or conservative treatment. The mortality rate was reduced by 47% in patients treated within the first hour of the onset of symptoms and by 25% in patients treated within 12 hours of the onset of symptoms. The longer the treatment was delayed after the onset of symptoms, the less improvement there was in survival compared with conventional treatment. These findings have been replicated with streptokinase in the ISIS-2 Trial, which documented an extension of the benefit to 24 hours from the onset of symptoms, although the benefit was less in patients treated later than with earlier treatment. In addition, this trial clearly documented a benefit in elderly patients and in patients with inferior MI. Despite the wide time allowance for benefit, both trials showed substantially more benefit for patients treated promptly. A large, multicenter trial with APSAC has shown a similar reduction in mortality (AIMS Trial Study Group, 1988). No documentation of reduced mortality exists with regard to urokinase, because no large randomized trials have been done. Pooled data in TPA trials indicate a mortality reduction similar to that observed with streptokinase. A recent overview of over 100,000 patients treated with thrombolysis or conservative therapy in controlled clinical trials found a 27% reduction in the 30-day mortality rate in patients treated with thrombolytic therapy (Fibrinolytic Therapy Trialist [FTT] Collaborative Group, 1994).

An important aspect of fibrinolytic therapy is that it can be initiated safely in the community hospital by a physician who has not had specialized training in cardiology. Thus, the treatment applies to most patients who are identified at an early stage of infarction without a major contraindication. Available information suggests that approximately 30 to 50% of patients who are eventually diagnosed with acute MI reach medical care within 6 hours and do not have a contraindication to this form of treatment, and an additional 15 to 20% of patients come to medical attention within 24 hours. A major public health effort is being devoted to education about the signs and symptoms of MI in an attempt to increase the proportion of patients who might benefit from treatment.

A similar large body of data confirms that all of these agents reduce infarct size and preserve left ventricular function (Fig. 31–48) (Sheehan et al., 1985; Rentrop, 1985; Van de Werf, 1989). Although an entirely satisfactory method of measuring infarct size in patients has not yet been developed, multiple data sources, including enzyme release, left ventricular ejection fraction, and left ventricular volume determinations, emphasize the same result. This outcome translates clinically into a lower incidence of heart failure and related complications and may be responsible for the reduction in sudden death and malignant ventricular arrhythmias in these patients after they have been discharged from the hospital.

All available information indicates an increase in reinfarction rates in patients treated with thrombolytic therapy compared with conservative treatment. The reason relates most probably to the unstable atherosclerotic plaque that remains after fibrinolytic therapy has successfully achieved reperfusion through initial clot lysis. Multiple adjunctive therapies have been used to prevent reocclusion and its often catastrophic

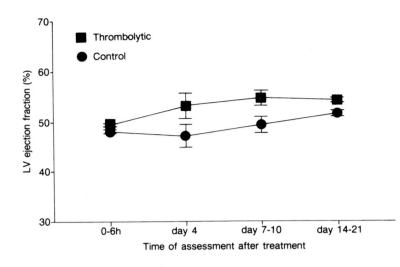

**FIGURE 31–48.** Pooled analysis of left ventricular ejection fraction from randomized trials of thrombolytic therapy versus control: Thrombolytic therapy results in significantly higher ejection fraction ($p \leq .001$ for each time point), and the difference between thrombolytic therapy and control does not increase after day 4. Includes 3066 ventriculographic observations. (From Granger, C. B., Califf, R. M., and Topol, E. J.: Thrombolytic therapy for acute myocardial infarction: A review. Drugs, 44:293–325, 1992.)

outcome (Popma and Topol, 1991). Information from the ISIS group documents that aspirin dramatically improves on survival and essentially doubles the therapeutic benefit of streptokinase alone (ISIS-3, 1993). Heparin, which has now been extensively investigated, has become standard treatment in the first several days after TPA is initiated (Hsai et al., 1990). However, routine anticoagulation with intravenous heparin cannot be recommended when nonspecific agents are used (International Study Group, 1990). Their ability to produce prolonged elevation of the prothrombin time and the activated partial thromboplastin time (aPTT) and to produce an antiplatelet effect between fibrin(ogen) degradation products may obviate the need for heparin. Intravenously administered nitroglycerin has also potentiated the effects of streptokinase on left ventricular function. Future efforts will concentrate on the role of other pharmacologic regimens that alter the coagulation system or platelet function.

Hemorrhagic complications are still the major drawback of this form of therapy. These complications can be divided into three different types: internal, access site, and intracranial. Careful attention to exclusion criteria can significantly reduce the risk of internal bleeding by avoiding thrombolytic therapy for patients with active bleeding sources, particularly the gastrointestinal tract. Nevertheless, a finite rate of such bleeding occurs from previously occult sources or new sources, such as stress ulcers. Vascular intervention of patients immediately before and after thrombolytic therapy should be limited to necessary procedures, because the risk of bleeding is significant with any vascular puncture, particularly in an artery. Depending on the level of vascular invasion, the transfusion requirement after thrombolytic therapy has ranged from 2 to 35% of patients treated.

Intracranial bleeding that cannot be readily reversed is the major complication of this therapy. The event occurs in 0.2 to 0.6% of patients treated with current doses of fibrinolytic therapy despite the exclusion of patients with obvious central nervous system pathology. High-risk patients appear to be the elderly or patients with a long history of poorly controlled hypertension, especially with a wide pulse pressure or acute, severe hypertension with the acute infarction episode. When bleeding occurs, emergency measures for an accurate diagnosis must be taken (cranial tomography or magnetic resonance imaging), and all forms of anticoagulation and antiplatelet therapy must be discontinued. Early consideration of surgical hematoma evacuation may prevent catastrophe.

General measures to reduce bleeding, when it occurs, include discontinuation of anticoagulant and antiplatelet therapy, intravascular volume repletion, and compression of the involved site (Fig. 31–49). Clotting factors may be replaced with fresh frozen plasma and cryoprecipitate. Early surgical intervention should be contemplated to repair sites of loss of vascular integrity if standard measures are unsuccessful. Epsilon aminocaproic acid may be used in life-threatening bleeding, although the risk of rethrombosis of the coronary artery must be considered carefully.

## ROLE OF INVASIVE PROCEDURES

Much research has focused on defining the appropriate use of coronary angiography and coronary angioplasty in patients who have undergone thrombolytic therapy. Routine immediate angiography in acute MI has been shown to be safe and feasible. Between 30 and 50% of patients fail to achieve reperfusion after treatment with fibrinolytic agents. Intermittent monitoring of the electrocardiogram can provide a reasonable assessment 60 to 90 minutes after thrombolytic therapy is begun, and continuous ST segment monitoring is even more accurate. However, coronary angiography is the only definitive method to assess the adequacy of reperfusion. Angiography also identifies patients who have left main or severe three-vessel coronary disease and who might benefit from early surgical intervention. The routine use of angiography is expensive, however, and involves the transfer of many patients in the early phases of in-

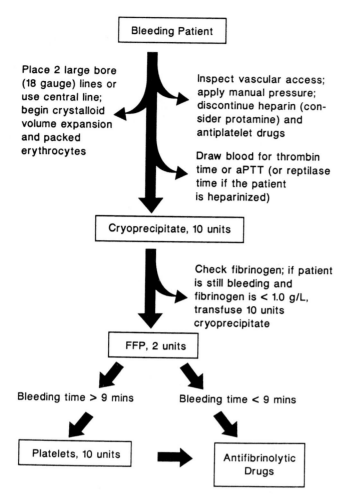

FIGURE 31–49. A typical strategy for the management of major bleeding causing hemodynamic compromise that is not immediately life-threatening. (aPTT = activated partial thromboplastin time; FFP = fresh frozen plasma.) (Reproduced with permission from Sane, D. C., Califf, R. M., Topol, E. J., et al.: Bleeding during thrombolytic therapy for acute myocardial infarction: Mechanisms and management. Ann. Intern. Med., 1989; *111*:1010–1022.)

farction from the community hospital to the interventional center. Our current strategy is to start thrombolytic therapy as expeditiously as possible and then to monitor the ST segment continuously using an online digital electrocardiographic monitor. If the lead with maximal ST segment elevation at baseline has failed to achieve at least 50% resolution within the first 60 to 90 minutes, the artery is assumed to be occluded. Attempts to open the artery with mechanical revascularization are then made if the infarction is deemed substantial or if the patient remains symptomatic or clinically unstable. If the ST segments have resolved by more than 50% during the first 60 to 90 minutes, angiography is deferred and the patient is observed for reocclusion or recurrent ischemia. The strategy of "watchful waiting" with angiography only for recurrent ischemia or heart failure is well supported by clinical trials.

Percutaneous transluminal angioplasty may be used either to replace thrombolytic therapy or as an adjunctive measure after thrombolysis (Stack et al., 1988; SWIFT Trial Study Group, 1991; TIMI Research Group, 1989; TIMI Study Group, 1989; Topol et al., 1987). In patients with a contraindication to fibrinolytic agents, direct angioplasty may be used to achieve vessel patency. In patients who come directly to interventional centers that permit rapid access to the catheterization laboratory, recent studies have suggested that direct angioplasty achieves superior recanalization rates with less bleeding and perhaps with a lower mortality rate.

## SURGICAL ISSUES

The current aggressive strategy of management of acute MI almost certainly leads to earlier and more frequent identification of patients with high-risk anatomy and impaired left ventricular function (Flameng et al., 1987; Hochberg et al., 1984). These findings promote earlier surgical intervention because the convincing data from randomized trials have shown that long-term survival is improved with surgical intervention in patients with multivessel disease and impaired left ventricular function. The multicenter Thrombolysis and Angioplasty in Myocardial Infarction (TAMI) group (Califf et al., 1988) reported an experience with 24 patients undergoing coronary bypass grafting while the TPA infusion was continued. Most of these patients had a failed angioplasty with a perfusion catheter inserted across the infarct lesion to maintain perfusion of the distal myocardial bed. Other patients had early operation for very-high-risk anatomy (left main or combined proximal left anterior descending and circumflex obstruction) with hemodynamic deterioration. Although bleeding complications were more severe than those encountered with elective operation, only three patients required reoperation, and no lethal bleeding complications occurred. Only three in-hospital deaths occurred in the series, all from the eight patients in frank cardiogenic shock at the time of operation. Patients treated surgically had a dramatic improvement in left ventricular function compared with patients not treated with surgery. In a review of the Duke experience, Ferguson and colleagues (1988) found that the complications, mortality, and length of stay were similar in patients who were referred for emergency operation during the acute phase of infarction compared with patients referred because elective angioplasty failed. The major difference was in the need for blood product replacement: The patients with acute infarction required 12.5 units of packed red blood cells, 8.7 units of frozen plasma, 0.9 platelet packs, and 1.2 units of cryoprecipitate. Equivalent figures for the patients with failed elective angioplasty were 8.8, 5.4, 0.48, and 0.48, respectively. Significantly, the internal mammary artery was used in half of the patients in each group, showing that this technique can be used even in emergency cases.

An additional 72 patients in the TAMI I trial (Califf et al., 1988) underwent coronary artery operations before being discharged from the hospital, but not in the acute phase of the infarction. The overall in-hospital mortality rate in all 94 patients who underwent surgery was 6%, despite a risk profile significantly more adverse than that of patients treated without operation. In follow-up to 1 year, only 1 additional patient died, 86% were in functional Class I or II, and 76% rated their health as either excellent or good. This information confirms that coronary surgical procedures can be done safely during the acute phase of infarction or the subsequent hospitalization. Although the exact criteria must still be defined, the results have led me to recommend operation early during hospitalization for patients identified as having multivessel coronary disease and impaired left ventricular function and for patients with ongoing ischemia and anatomy not suitable for angioplasty. Careful attention to repletion of clotting factors and meticulous operative technique produces good results and a shorter stay in the hospital, compared with a more deferred approach to operation.

An issue of growing importance is the proper management of patients with acute infarction after CABG. Thrombolytic therapy is contraindicated for the first several weeks because of the high risk of pericardial hemorrhage and subsequent tamponade. Beyond that point, however, thrombolytic therapy and acute angioplasty are still viable alternatives. Data from the randomized trials indicate that the risk of subsequent nonfatal infarction is not reduced by surgical therapy in patients with chronic angina. Particularly after the first 5 years, graft occlusion becomes a more substantial problem. For many reasons, clinical decision making in these patients is more complex than in patients without previous bypass grafting. The frequent occurrence of conduction disturbances makes the initial diagnosis more difficult than usual. The acute thrombus may be located in a bypass graft rather than in a native vessel. These two possibilities cannot be distinguished except by coronary angiography. A median sternotomy makes acute surgical intervention for failed angioplasty more risky, especially after fibrinolytic therapy. A major practical problem is the frequent occurrence of extensive thrombus throughout the length of the graft. Recent observational studies have demonstrated a 2-fold increase in mortality for patients with acute MI after bypass surgery, compared with patients with acute MI who have undergone no previous surgery. Most of this excess risk is attributable to the fact that patients who have undergone surgery often are older and have preexisting left ventricular dysfunction and multivessel coronary disease. Preliminary studies also suggest a lower rate of successful fibrinolysis in these patients. Data are inadequate to delineate the proper course of action when a patient with previous grafting is identified in the early stages of acute infarction. My current practice is to initiate thrombolytic therapy in the emergency room and then to move quickly to coronary angiography to define the nature of the problem more clearly. Immediate angioplasty in these patients should be approached cautiously, although preliminary results in selected patients have been encouraging.

## SUMMARY

Fibrinolytic therapy for acute ischemic syndromes has become a standard method of treatment. Despite its widespread use, new developments in the biology of thrombosis promise to improve this therapy (see Table 31–13). Modifications of current agents through recombinant genetic engineering may produce more effective therapy with less risk. Even more exciting developments in the production of adjunctive antithrombin and antiplatelet agents are being evaluated in large-scale clinical trials. Improvement in acute survival rates and earlier identification of patients at high risk for recurrent ischemic events will almost certainly increase the frequency of cardiac surgical procedures in this setting.

## SELECTED BIBLIOGRAPHY

Braunwald, E.: Myocardial reperfusion, limitation of infarct size, reduction of left ventricular dysfunction, and improved survival. Should the paradigm be expanded? Circulation, 79:441, 1989.

This article provides an excellent background for the pathophysiologic understanding of the mechanism of benefit of reperfusion. It raises the issue of whether the clinical benefits of reperfusion are simply due to myocardial salvage, or whether prevention of ventricular arrhythmia and maintenance of left ventricular shape are equally important.

Califf, R. M., Fortin, D. F., et al.: Clinical risks of thrombolytic therapy. Am. J. Cardiol., 69:12A, 1992.

This review article outlines the major issues of bleeding risk faced by the clinician using thrombolytic therapy. Methods of identifying high-risk patients and approaches to treating the bleeding patient are covered.

Collen, D.: Human tissue-type plasminogen activator: From the laboratory to the bedside. Circulation, 72:18, 1985.

This editorial reviews the development of tissue plasminogen activator, beginning with its initial isolation and early use in human studies. The use of recombinant DNA technology in the development of this pharmacologic agent is discussed.

Grines, C. L., and DeMaria, A. N.: Optimal utilization of thrombolytic therapy for acute myocardial infarction: Concepts and controversies. J. Am. Coll. Cardiol., 16:223, 1990.

This review article synthesizes information from multiple clinical trials to present a cogent argument for wider use of thrombolytic therapy.

The GUSTO Investigators: An international randomized trial comparing four thrombolytic strategies for acute myocardial infarction. N. Engl. J. Med., 329:673, 1993.

This article presents the initial results of a trial involving over 41,000 patients in which early reperfusion was demonstrated to reduce mortality and other major complications of myocardial infarction. The widespread application of this therapy in multiple countries further establishes thrombolytic therapy as a cornerstone of treatment in myocardial infarction following the groundwork laid by the ISIS and GISSI investigators.

Kereiakes, D. J., Topol, E. J., George, B. S., et al.: Emergency coronary artery bypass surgery preserves global and regional left ventricular function after intravenous tissue plasminogen activator therapy for acute myocardial infarction. J. Am. Coll. Cardiol., 11:899, 1988.

This paper describes an experience with emergency surgical treatment of 27 patients during infusion of TPA for acute myocardial infarction. Although the bleeding complications were greater, the in-hospital and long-term mortality rates were low. Left ventricular function dramatically improved.

Reimer, K. A., Lowe, J. E., Rasmussen, M. M., and Jennings, R. B.:

The wavefront phenomenon of ischemic cell death. I: Myocardial infarct size vs. duration of coronary occlusion in dogs. Circulation, 56:786, 1977.

This important article describes the potential benefits of reperfusion on the salvage of myocardium. The authors used a canine model in which epicardial vessels were occluded, and the occlusion was released at various times. A wavefront of myocardial cell death was described proceeding from the endocardium to the epicardium.

Sane, D. C., Califf, R. M., Topol, E. J., et al.: Bleeding during thrombolytic therapy for acute myocardial infarction: Mechanisms and management. Ann. Intern. Med., 111:1010, 1989.

This article reviews the clinical and pathophysiologic basis of bleeding during thrombolytic therapy. It also provides a detailed rationale for a selection of blood products in the bleeding patient.

Stadius, M. L., Davis, K., Maynard, C., et al.: Risk stratification for 1 year survival based on characteristics identified in the early hours of acute myocardial infarction. Circulation, 74:703, 1986.

This article describes the relationship between baseline characteristics and 1-year survival in a group of patients treated with intracoronary streptokinase. The importance of this work is that it identified an important effect of coronary patency on mortality reduction that was independent of salvage of left ventricular function. The 1-year follow-up of these patients showed a dramatic improvement in survival in patients with a patent coronary artery at the time of initial therapy, compared with patients without a patent coronary artery. This study has raised the issue of the effect of coronary patency during the phase of infarct healing compared with the initial salvage of myocardium.

Topol, E. J., Armstrong, P., Van de Werf, F., et al.: Confronting the issues of patient safety and investigator conflict of interest in an international clinical trial of myocardial reperfusion. J. Am. Coll. Cardiol., 19:1123, 1992.

This article summarizes the thought process behind independent, large clinical trials. It discusses the potential conflicts that can arise in studies funded by industry.

White, H. D., Norris, R. M., Brown, M. A., et al.: Left ventricular end-systolic volume as the major determinant of survival after recovery from myocardial infarction. Circulation, 76:44, 1987.

The authors present definitive evidence that left ventricular volume is a critical determinant of survival in patients treated with reperfusion therapy. Accordingly, the target of reperfusion therapy—aside from opening the vessel—is to provide the best environment for healing of the myocardial infarction.

Yusuf, S., Collins, R., Peto, R., et al.: Intravenous and intracoronary fibrinolytic therapy in acute myocardial infarction: Overview of results on mortality, reinfarction and side-effects from 33 randomized controlled trials. Eur. Heart J., 6:556, 1985.

This review article combines 33 randomized controlled trials of intravenous intracoronary fibrinolytic therapy in a meta-analysis. The finding of this study was that mortality rate was reduced by 22 ± 5%, and that the effects on mortality appeared to be present even in patients treated 12 hours after the onset of symptoms. This important analysis in combination with the GISSI study firmly established the role of thrombolytic therapy as primary treatment for acute myocardial infarction.

## BIBLIOGRAPHY

AIMS Trial Study Group: Effect of intravenous APSAC on mortality after acute myocardial infarction: Preliminary report of a placebo-controlled clinical trial. Lancet, 1:545, 1988.

Califf, R. M., Topol, E. J., George, B. S., et al.: Characteristics and outcome of patients in whom reperfusion with intravenous tissue-type plasminogen activator fails: Results of the thrombolysis and angioplasty in myocardial infarction (TAMI) I trial. Circulation, 77:1090, 1988.

Califf, R. M., Topol, E. J., and Gersh, B. J.: From myocardial salvage to patient salvage in acute myocardial infarction: The role of reperfusion therapy. J. Am. Coll. Cardiol., 14:1382, 1989.

Collen, D.: Human tissue-type plasminogen activator: From the laboratory to the bedside. Circulation, 72:18, 1985.

DeWood, M. A., Spores, J., Notske, R., et al.: Prevalence of total coronary occlusion during the early hours of transmural myocardial infarction. N. Engl. J. Med., 303:897, 1980.

Ferguson, T. B., Muhlbaier, L. H., Salai, D. L., and Wechsler, A. S.: Coronary bypass grafting after failed elective and failed emergent percutaneous angioplasty. Relative risks of emergent surgical intervention. J. Thorac. Cardiovasc. Surg., 95:761, 1988.

Fibrinolytic Therapy Trialists' (FTT) Collaborative Group: Indications for fibrinolytic therapy in suspected acute myocardial infarction: Collaborative overview of early mortality and major morbidity results from all randomised trials of more than 1000 patients. Lancet 343:311, 1994.

Flameng, W., Sargeant, P., Vanhaecke, J., and Suy, R.: Emergency coronary bypass grafting for evolving myocardial infarction. J. Thorac. Cardiovasc. Surg., 94:124, 1987.

Fletcher, A. P., Alkjaersig, N., Smyrniotis, F. G., and Sherry, S.: The treatment of patients suffering from early myocardial infarction with massive and prolonged streptokinase therapy. Trans Assoc. Am. Physicians, 71:287, 1958.

Gore, J. M., Sloan, M., Price, T. R., et al.: Intracerebral hemorrhage, cerebral infarction, and subdural hematoma after acute myocardial infarction and thrombolytic therapy in the thrombolysis in myocardial infarction study. Circulation, 83:448, 1991.

Gruppo Italiano Per Lo Studio Della Sopravvivenza Nell'Infarto Miocardio (GISSI-2): A factorial randomised trial of alteplase versus streptokinase and heparin versus no heparin among 12, 490 patients with acute myocardial infarction. Lancet, 336:65, 1990.

Gruppo Italiano Per Lo Studio Della Streptochinasi Nell'Infarcto Miocardio (GISSI): Effectiveness of intravenous thrombolytic treatment in acute myocardial infarction. Lancet, 1:397, 1986.

Herrick, J. B.: Clinical features of sudden obstruction of the coronary arteries. J. A. M. A., 59:2015, 1912.

Hochberg, M. S., Parsonnet, V., Gielchinsky, I., et al.: Timing of coronary revascularization after acute myocardial infarction. J. Thorac. Cardiovasc. Surg., 88:914, 1984.

Hsai, J., Hamilton, W. P., Kleiman, N., et al.: A comparison between heparin and low-dose aspirin as adjunctive therapy with tissue plasminogen activator for acute myocardial infarction. N. Engl. J. Med., 323:1433, 1990.

The International Study Group: In-hospital mortality and clinical course of 20,891 patients with suspected acute myocardial infarction randomised between alteplase and streptokinase with or without heparin. Lancet, 336:71, 1990.

ISIS Steering Committee: Intravenous streptokinase given within 0–4 hours of onset of myocardial infarction reduced mortality in ISIS-2. Lancet, 1:502, 1987.

ISIS-2: Randomised trial of intravenous streptokinase, oral aspirin, both, or neither among 17,187 cases of suspected acute myocardial infarction: ISIS-2 Lancet, 2:349, 1988.

ISIS-3 (Third International Study of Infarct Survival) Collaborative Group: ISIS-3: A randomised comparison of streptokinase vs tissue plasminogen activator vs anistreplase and of aspirin plus heparin vs aspirin alone among 41, 299 cases of suspected acute myocardial infarction. Lancet, 339:753, 1993.

Johnson, A. J., and Tillett, W. S.: Lysis in rabbits of intravascular blood clots by the streptococcal fibrinolytic system (streptokinase). J. Exp. Med., 95:449, 1952.

Kennedy, J. W., Ritchie, J. L., Davis, K. B., et al.: The western Washington randomized trial of intracoronary streptokinase in acute myocardial infarction. A 12-month follow-up report. N. Engl. J. Med., 312:1073, 1985.

MacFarlane, R. G., Biggs, R.: Fibrinolysis. Its mechanism and significance. Blood, 3:1167, 1948.

National Heart Foundation of Australia Coronary Thrombolysis Group: Coronary thrombolysis and myocardial salvage by tissue plasminogen activator given up to 4 hours after onset of myocardial infarction. Lancet, 1:203, 1988.

Nolf, P. G.: Des modifications de la coagulation due sang chez le chien apres extirpation due foie. Arch. Intern. Physiol., 3:1, 1905.

Nydick, I., Ruegsegger, P., Bouirer, C., et al.: Salvage of heart muscle by fibrinolytic therapy after experimental coronary occlusion. Am. Heart J. 61:93, 1961.

O'Neill, W., Timmis, G., Bourdillon, P., et al.: A prospective randomized clinical trial of intracoronary streptokinase versus coronary angioplasty therapy of acute myocardial infarction. N. Engl. J. Med., 314:812, 1986.

Popma, J. J., and Topol, E. J.: Adjuncts to thrombolysis for myocardial reperfusion. Ann. Intern. Med., 115:34, 1991.

Rao, A. K., Pratt, C., Berke, A., et al.: Thrombolysis in Myocardial Infarction (TIMI) trial. I: Hemorrhagic manifestations and changes in plasma fibrinogen and the fibrinolytic system in patients treated with recombinant tissue plasminogen activator and streptokinase. J. Am. Coll. Cardiol., 11:1, 1988.

Reimer, K. A., and Jennings, R. B.: The "wavefront phenomenon" of myocardial ischemic cell death. II: Transmural progression of necrosis within the framework of ischemic bed size (myocardium at risk) and collateral flow. Lab. Invest., 40:633, 1979.

Rentrop, K. P.: Thrombolytic therapy in patients with acute myocardial infarction. Circulation, 71:627, 1985.

Rijken, D. C., and Collen, D.: Purification and characterization of the plasminogen activator secreted by human melanoma cells in culture. J. Biol. Chem., 256:7035, 1981.

Sheehan, F. H., Mathey, D. G., Schofer, J., et al.: Factors that determine recovery of left ventricular function after thrombolysis in patients with acute myocardial infarction. Circulation, 71:1121, 1985.

Simoons, M. L., Arnold, A. E. R., Betriu, A., et al.: Thrombolysis with rt-PA in acute myocardial infarction: No beneficial effects of immediate PTCA. Lancet, 1:197, 1988.

Stack, R. S., Califf, R. M., Hinohara, T., et al.: Survival and cardiac event rates in the first year following emergency angioplasty for acute myocardial infarction. J. Am. Coll. Cardiol., 6:1141, 1988.

Stack, R. S., Phillips, H. R., Grierson, D. S., et al.: Functional improvement of jeopardized myocardium following intracoronary streptokinase infusion in acute myocardial infarction. J. Clin. Invest., 72:84, 1983.

SWIFT Trial Study Group: SWIFT trial of delayed intervention v. conservative treatment after thrombolysis with anistreplase in acute myocardial infarction. Br. Med. J., 302:555, 1991.

Tillett, W. S., and Garner, R. I.: The fibrinolytic activity of hemolytic streptococci. J. Exp. Med., 58:485, 1933.

Tillett, W. S., and Sherry, S.: The effect in patients of streptococcal fibrinolysin (streptokinase) and streptococcal desoxyribonuclease on fibrinous, purulent, and sanguineous pleural exudations. J. Clin. Invest., 28:173, 1949.

TIMI Research Group: Immediate vs. delayed catheterization and angioplasty following thrombolytic therapy for acute myocardial infarction. TIMI IIA results. J. A. M. A., 260:2849, 1988.

TIMI Study Group: Comparison of invasive and conservative strategies after treatment with intravenous tissue plasminogen activator in acute myocardial infarction. Results of the Thrombolysis in Myocardial Infarction (TIMI) phase II Trial. N. Engl. J. Med., 320:618, 1989.

Topol, E. J.: Which thrombolytic agent should one choose? Prog. Cardiovasc. Dis., 34:165, 1991.

Topol, E. J., Califf, R. M., George, B. S., et al.: A randomized trial of immediate versus delayed elective angioplasty after intravenous tissue plasminogen activator in acute myocardial infarction. N. Engl. J. Med., 317:581, 1987.

Van de Werf, F.: Discrepancies between the effects of coronary reperfusion on survival and left ventricular function. Lancet, 1:1367, 1989.

Yusuf, S., Collins, R., Peto, R., et al.: Intravenous and intracoronary fibrinolytic therapy in acute myocardial infarction: Overview of results on mortality, reinfarction and side-effects from 33 randomized controlled trials. Eur. Heart. J., 6:556, 1985.

# ◼ IV  Role of Computed Tomographic Scans in Cardiovascular Diagnosis

Jessie Chai and Charles E. Spritzer

In 1972, at the Annual Congress of the British Institute of Radiology, G. N. Hounsfield announced the invention of "computerized axial transverse scanning" for imaging the brain. Later known as *computed tomography* (CT), the technique evolved rapidly and has revolutionized the practice of medicine. In 1979, Hounsfield and A. M. Cormack, another investigator, were awarded the Nobel Prize in medicine for their contribution to CT.

The formation of a CT image requires multiple steps (Curry et al., 1990; Sprawls, 1987). The first step is the scanning phase, in which an x-ray beam traverses a section of the body. The radiation that penetrates the slice of tissue is measured by detectors. The x-ray beam is rotated around the body section so that several hundred views are obtained. The data are then stored in computer memory.

The next step is image reconstruction, which converts the scan data for the individual views into a digital image. The image consists of an array of picture elements (pixels). A pixel actually represents a volume element (voxel), because each two-dimensional image represents a slice of the body, ranging from 1 mm to 1 cm. Each pixel is denoted by a CT number that reflects the average attenuation through a thin cross-section of its contained tissues. Spatial resolution is excellent; pixels as small as 0.3 mm are routinely used.

The last step is conversion of the digital image into a video display, where it can be viewed or filmed. This step requires a digital-to-analog converter.

Conventional scan times last approximately 1 to 4 seconds. Images are acquired one at a time, because the cables supplying the x-ray tube in the circular gantry need to be unwound after each image is obtained. The reconstruction step also requires several seconds. Spiral or helical CT, which uses a "slip ring" technology, permits continuous rotation of the x-ray beam and detector and can obtain up to 30 consecutive images in 30 seconds.

*Ultrafast CT* (UFCT) has no moving parts and was developed exclusively for imaging the heart. Moving electrons are bent onto one of four tungsten target rings in the gantry below the patient. The x-rays generated from the tungsten rings then pass through the patient and are sensed by detectors located in the gantry above the patient. Each sweep of the target ring lasts 50 msec, whereas resetting of the beam requires 8 msec. Temporal resolution is 17 frames/sec. The images have a resolution of 0.7 to 2 mm and range in thickness from 3.0 to 10.0 mm. Three scanning modes can be used: Flow mode follows the contrast bolus and is best used for coronary bypass graft visualization; movie mode sequences assess cardiac function; and volume mode, which is similar to images obtained with conventional CT, is used to visualize anatomic abnormalities of the heart, aorta, and pericardium.

Although angiography remains the gold standard for evaluating the heart and great vessels, noninvasive studies are becoming more accurate and more widely used. Echocardiography is a reliable tool for evaluating cardiac diseases, except for coronary artery disease. Radionuclide studies can provide information about ejection fraction and tissue ischemia. CT and *magnetic resonance imaging* (MRI), which are limited by cardiac and respiratory motion, promise to be useful imaging modalites. Conventional CT is excellent for studying diseases of the pericardium and aorta, and UFCT is useful for assessing cardiac function and for evaluating congenital heart disease.

## ANATOMY

Identifying normal cardiovascular anatomy on conventional CT usually does not require intravenous contrast, because mediastinal fat outlines vessels clearly. However, contrast is needed for evaluating the ventricles, intracardiac masses, and coronary artery bypass grafts. Contrast is routinely used with UFCT. The anatomy may be easier to understand if the thorax is arbitrarily divided into the following levels (Sagel and Glazer, 1989): (1) sternoclavicular joints, (2) aortic arch, (3) pulmonary arteries, (4) aortic root and left atrium, and (5) cardiac ventricles.

At the level of the sternoclavicular joints, five vessels are seen anterior to the trachea and esophagus (Fig. 31–50A). The brachiocephalic artery lies just to the right of the trachea. The left common carotid artery lies to the left of the brachiocephalic artery, and the left subclavian artery lies posterolateral to the left common carotid artery. The brachiocephalic veins are posterior to the clavicular heads and anterior to the arteries. The right brachiocephalic vein has a vertical course; the left traverses a more oblique and downward course behind the manubrium.

At the origin of the brachiocephalic arteries lies the aortic arch (Fig. 31–50B), which extends posteriorly and to the left. The superior vena cava abuts the right lateral aspect of the anterior portion of the arch. The trachea lies posterior to the aortic arch, and the esophagus lies posterolateral to the trachea on the left.

The pulmonary arteries (Fig. 31–50C) lie at the base of the heart at a level inferior to the aortic arch and superior to the aortic root. The right pulmonary artery

courses posteriorly and to the right from the main pulmonary artery and passes posterior to the superior vena cava and anterior to the bronchus intermedius and carina. The left pulmonary artery extends posteriorly and to the left from the main pulmonary artery and lies lateral to the carina or left mainstrem bronchus. The ascending aorta lies anteromedial to the superior vena cava.

The aortic root (Fig. 31–50D) is visualized 4 to 5 cm inferior to the carina. To the left of the aortic root lies the main pulmonary artery and ovoid right ventricular outflow tract. Posterior to the aortic root lies the left atrium, which is rectangular. The inferior pulmonary veins drain into the posterolateral aspects of the left atrium bilaterally. To the right of the aortic root lies the right atrium. The right atrial appendage is seen as a triangular structure along the right lateral aspect of the aortic root.

Both ventricles are positioned anterior to their corresponding atria, with the right ventricle positioned anteriorly and to the right of the left ventricle (Fig. 31–50E). Visualization of the interventricular septum requires intravenous administration of contrast. The interventricular septum courses from right posterior to left anterior. Occasionally, the coronary sinus can be seen posterior to the right ventricle. On a more inferior level, the inferior vena cava is visualized as a rounded structure to the right of the spine before its entry into the right atrium.

## CARDIAC APPLICATIONS

Conventional CT evaluation of the heart currently is limited to gross structural information, because scanning times are slow relative to the cardiac cycle. Spatial resolution is consequently degraded. There are a handful of UFCT scanners in the United States that have scanning times of 50 msec and can provide more information, but these machines are not widely available.

UFCT is useful for evaluating coronary artery bypass graft patency. A multicenter study demonstrated UFCT to be 93.4% sensitive for detecting angiographically open grafts and 88.9% specific for detecting angiographically closed grafts (Stanford et al., 1988), with an overall accuracy of 92.1%. The sensitivity, specificity, and accuracy of UFCT between determining patency of internal mammary grafts and determining patency of saphenous venous grafts were not significantly different (Bateman et al., 1987; Stanford et al., 1988). The number of grafts did not influence interpretive accuracy.

Assessment of functional capacity of the grafts has not been totally successful (Stanford et al., 1991). Grafts may be anatomically patent but may function poorly because of nonocclusive thrombus within the graft or vessel bed perfused by the graft. Although preliminary animal studies have shown promise for UFCT assessment of graft flow reserve, UFCT still has not proven to be useful in human patients.

UFCT can accurately assess left and right ventricu-

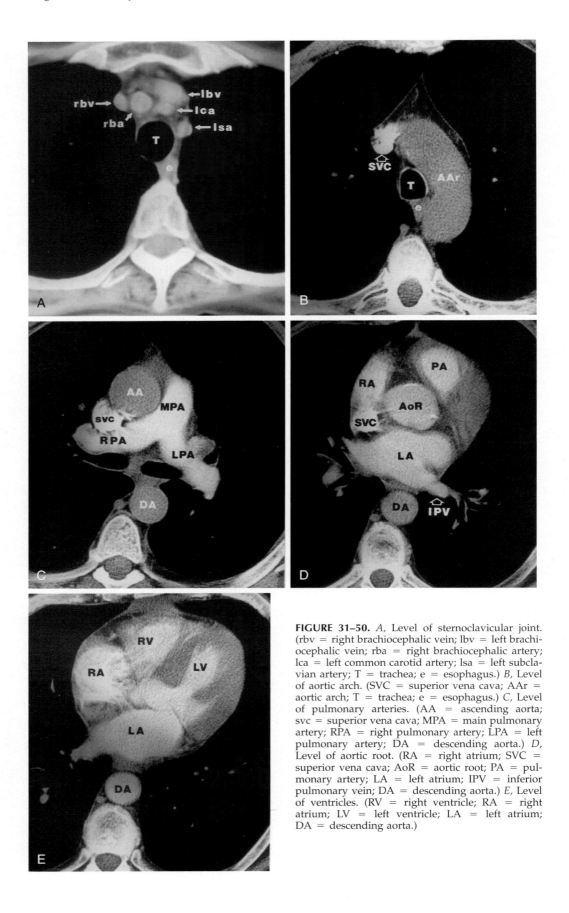

**FIGURE 31–50.** *A*, Level of sternoclavicular joint. (rbv = right brachiocephalic vein; lbv = left brachiocephalic vein; rba = right brachiocephalic artery; lca = left common carotid artery; lsa = left subclavian artery; T = trachea; e = esophagus.) *B*, Level of aortic arch. (SVC = superior vena cava; AAr = aortic arch; T = trachea; e = esophagus.) *C*, Level of pulmonary arteries. (AA = ascending aorta; svc = superior vena cava; MPA = main pulmonary artery; RPA = right pulmonary artery; LPA = left pulmonary artery; DA = descending aorta.) *D*, Level of aortic root. (RA = right atrium; SVC = superior vena cava; AoR = aortic root; PA = pulmonary artery; LA = left atrium; IPV = inferior pulmonary vein; DA = descending aorta.) *E*, Level of ventricles. (RV = right ventricle; RA = right atrium; LV = left ventricle; LA = left atrium; DA = descending aorta.)

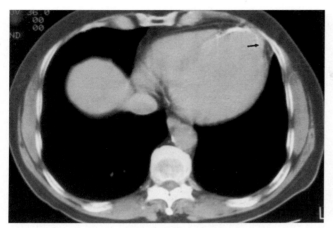

**FIGURE 31–51.** The focal bulge *(arrow)* associated with calcification at the apex of the left ventricle represents an aneurysm. (Courtesy of James T. T. Chen, M.D.)

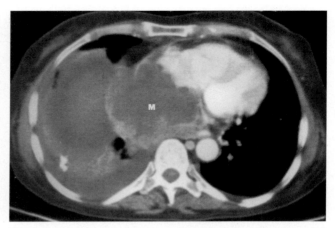

**FIGURE 31–53.** Large lobulated low-density filling defect (M) within the right atrium proved to be a metastatic focus in a patient with malignant melanoma.

lar stroke volumes (Reiter et al., 1986), ventricular mass (Feiring et al., 1985; Hajduczok et al., 1990), and regional and segmental ventricular function (Marcus et al., 1989). Regional myocardial perfusion can be inferred by analysis of left ventricular contrast clearance on UFCT. This technique is currently not clinically established but remains promising (Stanford et al., 1991).

Conventional CT is useful for evaluating complications of myocardial infarctions such as ventricular aneurysm or pseudoaneurysm (Nath et al., 1989). These are visualized as focal thinning of the myocardium, localized dilatation of the wall, and mural thrombus formation. True aneurysms are more commonly located anteriorly or apically (Fig. 31–51), whereas pseudoaneurysms tend to be located posteri-

orly or inferiorly. Both can calcify. The narrow neck of the pseudoaneurysm is rarely seen on CT.

Large intracardiac masses are easily seen on CT, but small ones may be missed because of blurring from cardiac motion. Thrombi may be seen as low-attenuation filling defects within the heart (Fig. 31–52). Myxomas, which typically arise near the left atrial septum, are heterogeneous with lobulated contours. Metastatic tumors of the heart (breast, lung, lymphoma) are more common than primary neoplasms. All appear as irregular low-attenuation masses (Nath et al., 1989) (Figs. 31–53 through 31–55).

Conventional CT can accurately demonstrate congenital anomalies of the aorta, inferior vena cava, superior vena cava (Fig. 31–56) and pulmonary arteries. Vascular rings, including double aortic arch (Fig. 31–57), right aortic arch with aberrant left subclavian artery, left aortic arch with aberrant right subclavian artery, and pulmonary sling, have been accurately demonstrated (Bank and Hernandez, 1988; Schlesinger and Hernandez, 1991). However, echocardiography, UFCT, and MRI are currently the preferred

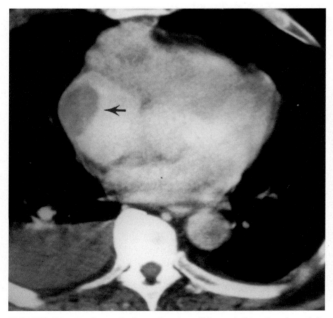

**FIGURE 31–52.** Smooth low-density filling defect in the right atrium *(arrow)* represents a thrombosis.

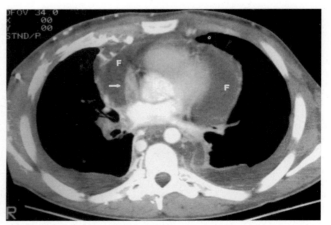

**FIGURE 31–54.** This patient has sarcoma involving a contracted right atrium. The sarcoma is seen as a low-density filling defect *(arrow).* A large amount of pericardial fluid (F) is present.

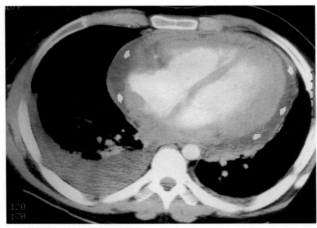

**FIGURE 31–55.** Mass (*arrows*) invading the myocardium proved to be lymphoma.

studies for evaluating congenital heart disease (Caputo and Higgins, 1991; Schlesinger and Hernandez, 1991; Stanford et al., 1991).

## PERICARDIUM

The pericardium is imaged as a thin, dense line measuring no more than 4 mm. It is best seen anterior to the ventricles, where it separates the epicardial fat from the mediastinal fat. It is seen in approximately 95% of adults and less frequently in children. The normal pericardial space between the fibrous parietal pericardium and visceral pericardium normally is not visualized unless the space is increased by effusion.

Echocardiography is the primary diagnostic tool for evaluating pericardial effusions. CT, however, can be used for evaluating patients whose body habitus renders sonography technically difficult and when the

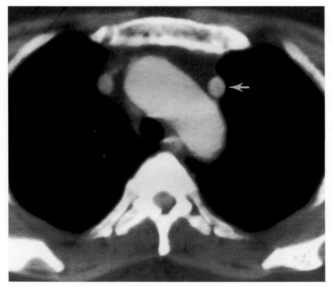

**FIGURE 31–56.** A persistent left superior vena cava (*arrow*). (Courtesy of James T. T. Chen, M.D.)

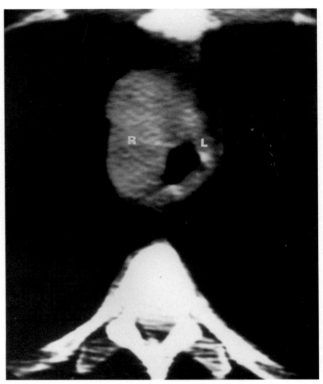

**FIGURE 31–57.** A double aortic arch forms a vascular ring around the trachea. Note that the right arch (R) is larger than the left (L). (Courtesy of James T. T. Chen, M.D.)

clinical findings differ from the echocardiographic interpretations. Moreover, CT is useful for evaluating pericardial thickening, calcific pericarditis, and neoplastic diseases involving the pericardium.

Pericardial effusions are easily visualized on CT because of the different x-ray absorption coefficients between fluid and the fat of the epicardium and mediastinum. Small pericardial effusions tend to layer in a dependent position and are typically seen as curvilinear collections posterior to the left ventricle and left atrium. Moderate-sized effusions extend anterior to the right ventricle. Large effusions form an asymmetric ring around the heart (Fig. 31–58). Hemopericardium and exudates may have higher densities than transudates or chylous effusions (Moncada et al., 1982).

Pericardial calcifications presumably reflect previous inflammatory insults. Etiologies include tuberculosis, trauma, rheumatic fever, bacterial pericarditis, or idiopathic pericarditis. Pathologic determination of the age or etiology of these calcifications is difficult. Encasement of both ventricles by calcified pericardium is needed to produce myocardial constriction (Moncada et al., 1982). About 50% of patients with constrictive pericarditis have pericardial calcifications (Chen, 1992). These calcifications occur primarily over the right heart, atrioventricular grooves, and pulmonary trunk. Involvement over the pulsatile left ventricle is uncommon and is associated with more extensive calcifications in other regions. The left atrium

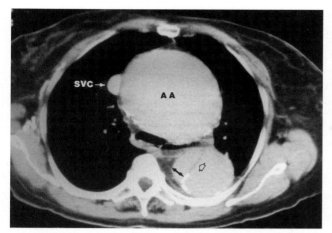

**FIGURE 31–58.** This middle-aged woman with lupus erythematosus has a large pericardial effusion (*arrowheads*).

is almost always spared, presumably because of the relative lack of pericardial coverage.

Conventional CT is useful for distinguishing constrictive pericarditis from restrictive cardiomyopathy (Moncada et al., 1982). In patients with impaired diastolic filling, diffuse pericardial thickening (>5 mm) strongly suggests the diagnosis of constrictive pericarditis, whereas the lack of pericardial abnormality suggests restrictive cardiomyopathy. In a series of seven patients surgically or angiographically proven to have constrictive pericarditis, CT demonstrated diffusely thickened parietal pericardium, measuring 5 mm to 2.0 cm. Two patients with amyloid restrictive cardiomyopathy had normal pericardiums at surgery, although CT raised the question of an area of pericardial thickening anteriorly in one patient. The authors concluded that if CT suggests pericardial thickening in patients with hemodynamic signs of constrictive or restrictive physiology, thoracotomy should be recommended for management.

Metastatic involvement of the pericardium typically presents as an effusion. The pericardium may also become generally or focally thick. Occasionally, one sees nodular masses attached to the pericardium. Primary neoplasms of the pericardium, such as mesothelioma, are rare and can be seen as solid masses within the visceral or parietal pericardium.

Pericardial cysts are congenital fluid-filled structures lined by pericardium that do not communicate with the pericardial cavity. They are typically located in the cardiophrenic angles, more commonly on the right.

## AORTA

Thoracic aortic aneurysms and dissections can be diagnosed on plain radiographs, but definitive diagnosis requires aortography, CT, or MRI. Aortography is considered the gold standard, but drawbacks include radiation exposure, invasiveness of the procedure, and contrast administration. MRI has the ad-

vantage of imaging in multiple planes without radiation exposure or contrast administration. However, scan times can be long, requiring hemodynamically stable patients. CT is more readily available than MRI and produces transaxial images that are less prone to technical artifacts, although intravenous contrast is needed for accurate diagnosis.

The incidence of aortic aneurysms increases with age, and they are estimated to affect 2 to 4% of the population. Most aortic aneurysms are atherosclerotic and tend to affect the distal arch or descending aorta. Aneurysms involving the ascending aorta are associated with disorders of collagen synthesis (such as Marfan's syndrome) and syphilis (Fig. 31–59). CT findings of an aneurysm include localized dilatation, intraluminal thrombus, and wall calcification. The dilatation may be fusiform or saccular. Normal aortic diameters vary with patient age, sex, and size. Absolute numbers, therefore, are not useful for identifying aneurysms. Generally, at a given scan level, the ascending aorta diameter is normally larger than the descending aorta diameter by a ratio of approximately 1:7. With increasing age, the caliber of the descending aorta increases more rapidly than that of the ascending aorta (Aronberg et al., 1984).

The most common complication of aortic aneurysm is rupture. The incidence of rupture of thoracic aortic aneurysms has been reported to be 47%. Saccular aneurysms and aneurysms greater than 6 cm in diameter are more prone to rupture (White et al., 1986). Rupture may be heralded by a rapid increase in size of the aneurysm. CT signs of an aortic rupture or leak include high-density hematoma around the aorta (Kucich et al., 1986), the presence of pleural fluid, and the identification of contrast beyond the aortic wall.

Aortic dissection has been estimated to occur at a rate of 5 to 10 cases per million per year. In most cases, the primary insult is a tear in the intima that allows blood to enter the media and propagate longitudinally. Stanford Type A dissections involve the ascending aorta with or without involvement of the descending aorta. Type B dissections affect only the descending aorta. Type A lesions are generally treated surgically, whereas Type B lesions are generally treated medically. More than 5 mm inward displacement of intimal calcifications from the aortic wall suggests the diagnosis on CT or on plain radiographs and is found in 17% of cases (Vasile et al., 1986). The diagnosis is also suggested on CT by the presence of high-attenuation density material (blood) within the aortic wall, periaortic tissues, or pericardium; these findings are also seen with aortic rupture. The classic finding of contrast filling true and false lumens separated by an intimal flap (Fig. 31–60*A* and *B*) is seen in 70% of cases (Vasile et al., 1986).

CT successfully diagnoses aortic dissections. Thorsen and associates (1983) found no false-negative and one false-positive result in a series of 50 patients with aortography or surgery used as gold standards. Vasile and co-workers (1986) found an accuracy of 94.8% in a series of 137 patients in which angiography or surgery was used as the gold standard for Type A

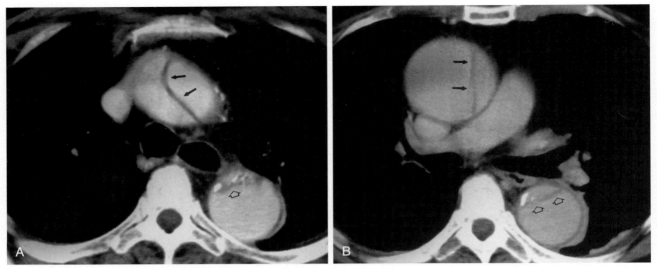

**FIGURE 31–59.** This patient has an aneurysm of the ascending aorta (AA) secondary to syphilis. Type B aortic dissection is also present. Note the displaced intimal calcifications *(double-headed arrow)* and intimal flap *(open arrow)* in the descending aorta. (SVC = superior vena cava.)

dissections, and angiography, follow-up CT, or clinical follow-up for longer than 1 year was used to follow Type B lesions. Oudkerk and associates (1983) found no false-negative or false-positive results in a series of 26 patients when aortography or surgery or both were used as gold standards.

CT is also a convenient method for following patients who have been medically or surgically treated for dissections. Following surgical repair, a dense ring representing the aortic graft is seen in more than 80% of cases (Godwin et al., 1981). The graft should be closely applied to the native aorta if the native aorta

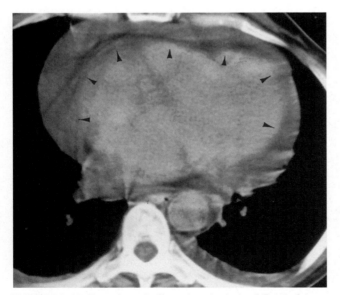

**FIGURE 31–60.** Type A aortic dissection. An intimal flap is demonstrated in the ascending aorta *(solid arrows)* and descending aorta *(open arrow). B,* On a more inferior section, the intimal flap in the descending aorta is more clearly seen *(open arrows).* The intimal flap in the ascending aorta *(solid arrows)* is again demonstrated.

is retained to jacket the graft; when only the dense ring of the graft is identified, the affected segment of aorta is removed and completely replaced by graft.

Post-treatment complications include graft infection, sutural loosening, extension of dissection, aneurysm or pseudoaneurysm formation, or rupture. Gas bubbles may be seen around the graft normally in the early postoperative period; however, the presence of gas weeks or months after surgery implies infection. Contrast entering the space between graft and native aorta indicates sutural dehiscence. Progressive enlargement of the aorta distal to the graft may herald rupture, and progressive dilatation of the native aorta around the graft may necessitate reoperation. Periaortic hematoma suggests a leak (Godwin, 1990).

CT findings of aortic trauma include periaortic hematoma, diffuse mediastinal hemorrhage, and pseudoaneurysm formation. Mediastinal hemorrhage alone is a nonspecific finding; the most common cause in the setting of trauma is venous injury. In the setting of blunt chest trauma, such as a motor vehicle accident, angiography is the first-line modality for excluding aortic transection. The role of CT in the diagnosis of aortic injury is controversial. Some authors (Mirvis et al., 1987) contend that angiography should be the first study performed when chest radiographs clearly demonstrate mediastinal hematoma, and that in the setting of equivocal plain radiographic findings, CT should be used to exclude mediastinal hematoma. CT evidence for mediastinal hematoma can then be used as an indication for angiography. However, at our center, angiography is the study of choice when plain films are equivocal for or demonstrate mediastinal hematoma.

## PULMONARY ARTERIES

CT is a noninvasive method for evaluating the pulmonary arteries. The diameters of the pulmonary ar-

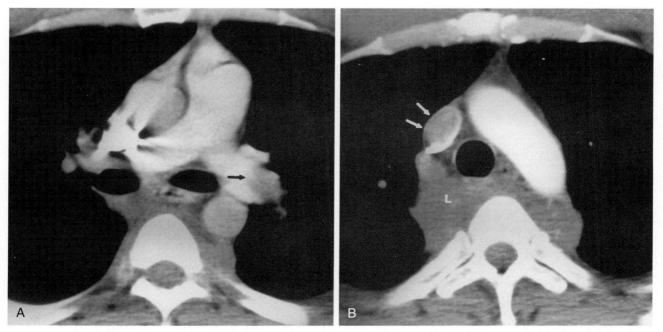

FIGURE 31–61. *A,* A filling defect in the left pulmonary artery *(arrow)* proved to be a pulmonary embolus on angiography. The patient subsequently underwent lytic therapy. *B,* This same patient, who has lymphoma (L), also had thrombus within the superior vena cava *(arrows).*

teries tend to increase with age. The upper limit of normal for the diameter of the main pulmonary artery is 28.6 mm (Kuriyama et al., 1984). The upper limits of normal for the right interlobar pulmonary artery is 16 to 17 mm in men and 15 mm in women (Chang, 1962). The upper limits of normal for the diameter of the left descending pulmonary artery are 16 mm in women and 18 mm in men (Kuriyama et al., 1984). Enlargement of the central pulmonary arteries is associated with pulmonary arterial hypertension. In a series of 27 patients (Kuriyama et al., 1984), the accuracy of the upper limit of normal measurement for the main pulmonary artery diameter was found to be 82% accurate for predicting pulmonary arterial hypertension (> 18 mm Hg.) Sensitivity was found to be 69%, and specificity was found to be 100%.

CT can be used to complement radionuclide scanning for diagnosing pulmonary embolism, particularly with patients suspected of having large central clot who are at high risk for complications with pulmonary angiography. In addition, CT sometimes reveals pulmonary emboli in patients complaining of chest pain who are being scanned to exclude aortic dissection. In a study of 42 patients, the sensitivity of spiral CT in detecting pulmonary emboli in second- to fourth-division pulmonary vessels was demonstrated to be 100% and the specificity 96% with pulmonary angiography as the gold standard (Remy-Jardin et al., 1992).

CT evaluation of pulmonary emboli requires good opacification of the pulmonary arteries. Findings include partial or complete filling defects, mural defects, or "railway track" signs (Godwin et al., 1980; Ovenfors et al., 1981; Remy-Jardin et al., 1992) (Figs.

31–61 and 31–62). Knowledge of intersegmental lymph nodes is essential, because they can be misinterpreted as filling defects (Remy-Jardin et al., 1992).

## FUTURE APPLICATIONS

With the introduction of spiral CT, CT angiography has exciting potential. With spiral CT, scans can be obtained very rapidly with better contrast bolus and lower contrast volume than conventional CT. In addition, fewer artifacts are present, provided that the

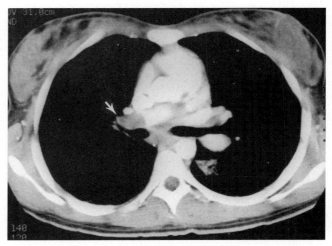

FIGURE 31–62. An elderly woman complained of chest pain and was scanned to exclude an aortic dissection. No dissection was found. Low-density filling defect *(arrow)* within the right pulmonary artery represents a thrombus.

patient can breath-hold. Theoretic advantages over magnetic resonance angiography include less flow artifact, lower cost, and more rapid scanning.

Reconstruction of three-dimensional images is another potential application of spiral CT (Fishman et al., 1991). With future software refinements, high-quality images will routinely facilitate surgical planning.

## SELECTED BIBLIOGRAPHY

Caputo, G. R., and Higgins, C. B.: Advances in cardiac imaging modalities: Fast computed tomography, magnetic resonance imaging, and positron emission tomography. Invest. Radiol., 25(7):838, 1990.

The authors review the applications and strengths of these noninvasive imaging modalities for evaluating cardiac disease.

Godwin, J. D.: Conventional CT of the aorta. J. Thorac. Imaging, 5(4):18, 1990.

This review article discusses the role of CT in evaluating aortic dissections and aneurysms. CT's advantages over MRI include greater compatibility with life-support equipment, fewer artifacts, and detection of calcifications. CT is less invasive than angiography and, unlike angiography, can diagnose dissection when the blood in the false channel is clotted rather than free-flowing.

Schlesinger, A. E., and Hernandez, R. J.: Congenital heart disease: Applications of computed tomography and magnetic resonance imaging. Seminars in Ultrasound, CT, and MR, 12(1):11, 45, 1991.

The article focuses on the practical applications of CT and MRI in patients with congenital heart disease. Conventional CT has a limited role in evaluating congenital heart defects but is useful for evaluating vascular rings, aortic aneurysms, and postoperative grafts and shunts. MRI is increasingly becoming a useful tool for evaluating coarctation of the aorta, vascular rings, vascular aneurysms, postoperative shunts, and abnormalities of the pulmonary arteries.

Stanford, W., Galvin, J. R., Weiss, R. M., et al.: Ultrafast computed tomography in cardiac imaging: A review. Seminars in Ultrasound, CT, and MR, 12(1):45, 1991.

This article reviews the current status of UFCT in cardiac imaging, including assessment of coronary artery bypass graft patency, regional myocardial perfusion, valvular disease, and intracardiac masses. The authors conclude that although UFCT can accurately determine anatomic patency of coronary arterial bypass grafts, assessing functional capacity (nonocclusive obstruction) of the grafts is still problematic. UFCT is currently not clinically useful for evaluating myocardial perfusion but promises to be a useful tool. UFCT excels in assessing valvular calcifications and intracardiac masses. It is reported to be more sensitive than echocardiography for detecting intracardiac thrombi.

## BIBLIOGRAPHY

Aronberg, D. J., Glazer, H. S., Madsen, K., et al.: Normal thoracic diameters by computed tomography. J. Comput. Assist. Tomogr., 8:247, 1984.
Bank, E. R., and Hernandez, R. J.: CT and MR of congenital heart disease. Radiol. Clin. North Am., 26:241, 1988.
Bateman, T. M., Gray, R. J., Whiting, J. S., et al.: Prospective evaluation of ultrafast cardiac computed tomography for determination of coronary bypass graft patency. Circulation, 75:1018, 1987.
Caputo, G. R., and Higgins, C. B.: Advances in cardiac imaging modalities: Fast computed tomography, magnetic resonance imaging, and positron emission tomography. Invest. Radiol., 25:838, 1991.
Chang, C. H. J.: The normal roentgenographic measurement of the right descending pulmonary artery in 1,085 cases. A. J. R., 87:929, 1962.
Chen, J. T. T.: The significance of cardiac calcifications. Appl. Radiol., 21:10, 1992.
Curry, T. S., Dowdey, J. E., Murry, R. C.: Christensen's Physics of Diagnostic Radiology. 4th ed. Philadelphia: Lea & Febiger, 1990, pp. 289–322.
Feiring, A. J., Rumberger, J. A., Reiter, S. K., et al.: Determination of left ventricular mass in dogs with rapid acquisition cardiac CT scanning. Circulation, 72:1355, 1985.
Fishman, E. K., Magid, D., Ney, D. R., et al.: Three-dimensional imaging. Radiology, 181:321, 1991.
Godwin, J. D.: Conventional CT of the aorta. J. Thorac. Imaging, 5:18, 1990.
Godwin, J. D., Turley, K., Herfkens, R. J., et al.: Computed tomography for followup of chronic aortic dissections. Radiology, 139:655, 1981.
Godwin, J. D., Webb, W. R., Gamsu, G., et al.: Computed tomography of pulmonary embolism. A. J. R., 135:691, 1980.
Hajduczok, Z. D., Weiss, R. M., Stanford, W., et al.: Determination of right ventricular mass in humans and dogs with ultrafast cardiac computed tomography. Circulation, 82:202, 1990.
Kucich, V. A., Vogelzang, R. L., Hartz, R. S., et al.: Ruptured thoracic aneurysm: Unusual manifestation and early diagnosis using CT. Radiology, 160:87, 1986.
Kuriyama, K., Gamsu, G., Stern, R. G., et al.: CT-determined pulmonary artery diameters in predicting pulmonary hypertension. Invest. Radiol., 19:16, 1984.
Marcus, M. L., Stanford, W., Rumberger, J. A., et al.: Clinical applications of ultrafast computed tomography. Echocardiography, 6:87, 1989.
Mirvis, S. E., Kostrubiak, I., Whitley, N. O., et al.: Role of CT in excluding major arterial injury after blunt thoracic trauma. A. J. R., 149:601, 1987.
Moncada, R., Baker, M., Salinas, M., et al.: Diagnostic role of computed tomography in pericardial heart disease: Congenital defects, thickening, neoplasms, and effusions. Am. Heart J., 103:263, 1982.
Nath, P. H., Levitt, R. G., and Gutierrez, F.: Heart and pericardium. In Lee, J. T., Sagel, S. S., and Stanley, R. J. (eds): Computed Body Tomography with MRI Correlation. 2nd ed. New York: Raven Press, 1989, pp. 387–413.
Oudkerk, M., Overbosch, E., and Dee, P.: CT recognition of acute aortic dissection. A. J. R., 141:671, 1983.
Ovenfors, C., Godwin, J. D., and Brito, A. C.: Diagnosis of peripheral pulmonary emboli by computed tomography in the living dog. Radiology, 141:519, 1981.
Reiter, S. J., Rumberger, J. A., Feiring, A. F., et al.: Precision of right and left ventricular stroke volume measurements by rapid acquisition cine computed tomography. Circulation, 74:890, 1986.
Remy-Jardin, M., Remy, J., Wattinne, L., et al.: Central pulmonary thromboembolism: Diagnosis with spiral volumetric CT with the single-breath-hold technique—Comparison with pulmonary angiography. Radiology, 185:381, 1992.
Sagel, S. S., and Glazer, H. S.: Thorax: Technique and normal anatomy. In Lee, J. T., Sagel, S. S., and Stanley, R. J. (eds): Computed Body Tomography with MRI Correlation. 2nd ed. New York: Raven Press, 1989, pp. 169–243.
Schlesinger, A. E., and Hernandez, R. J.: Congenital heart disease: Applications of computed tomography and magnetic resonance imaging. Seminars in Ultrasound, CT, and MR, 12:11, 1991.
Sprawls, P.: Physical Principles of Medical Imaging. Rockville, MD, Aspen, 1987, pp. 327–344.
Stanford, W., Brundage, B. H., MacMillan, R., et al.: Sensitivity and specificity of assessing coronary bypass graft patency with ultrafast computed tomography: Results of a multicenter study. J. Am. Coll. Cardiol., 12:1, 1988.
Stanford, W., Galvin, J. R., Weiss, R. M., et al.: Ultrafast computed tomography in cardiac imaging: A review. Seminars in Ultrasound, CT, and MR, 12:45, 1991.
Thorsen, M. K., San Dretto, M. A., Lawson, T. L., et al.: Dissecting aortic aneurysms: Accuracy of computed tomography diagnosis. Radiology, 148:773, 1983.
Vasile, N., Mathieu, D., Keita, K., et al.: Computed tomography of thoracic aortic dissection: Accuracy and pitfalls. J. Comput. Assist. Tomogr., 10:211, 1986.
White, R. D., Lipton, M. J., Higgins, C. B., et al.: Noninvasive evaluation of suspected thoracic aortic disease by contrast-enhanced computed tomography. Am. J. Cardiol., 57:282, 1986.

# ■ V Role of Magnetic Resonance Imaging in Cardiovascular Diagnosis

Charles E. Spritzer

Cardiovascular disease is a primary cause of illness and death in over 60 million people in this country. Coronary heart disease alone is expected to cause the deaths of one-third of the population over the age of 35 years. The significance of the problem has stimulated the development of diagnostic and therapeutic techniques with the goal of improving both the duration and the quality of life in patients with cardiovascular disease (Kannel and Thorn, 1986). Although *magnetic resonance imaging* (MRI) was developed in the late 1970s, it was not until 1981 that R. C. Hawkes and his co-workers reported their initial experience using MRI to study the heart. Three years later, Amparo and associates reported their experience with MRI for visualizing aortic abnormalities (Amparo et al., 1984; Hawkes et al., 1981).

With the advent of electrocardiogram (ECG) gating, various motion control techniques, and higher temporal resolution acquisitions, the use of MRI to evaluate the cardiovascular system has increased dramatically. Given the rapid technologic advances currently taking place, the precise role of MRI in assessing the cardiovascular system continues to be redefined. This chapter explores the current and the potential capabilities of MRI in evaluating the cardiovascular system; more traditional approaches are available and at present may be preferred.

## SAFETY

MRI is generally considered a safe imaging modality (Budinger et al., 1987; Kanal et al., 1990). Except for *radiofrequency* (RF) energy deposition, auditory considerations, and focal heating, no documented lasting harmful effects have been attributed to the MRI experiment. However, there are absolute contraindications to MRI (Kanal et al., 1993). Metallic foreign bodies in the orbit, ferrous intracranial aneurysm clips, cochlear implants, shrapnel in critical locations, and implanted electronic devices, including cardiac pacemakers, all are contraindicated. Potential effects on cardiac pacemakers by MR scanners include triggering of the reed switch, converting the device mode from synchronous to asynchronous (Pavlicek et al., 1983); attraction and torque of the device by the static magnetic field; and "pacing" the heart at the RF pulsing frequency (Pavlicek et al., 1983; Pohost et al.,

1992). Indeed, two deaths have been reported. Both deaths occurred at low field strengths, confirming that all MR scanners are potentially lethal to patients with implanted pacemakers.

In static fields above 0.3 T, reversible ECG changes of no physiologic consequence are routinely noted (Budinger, 1981; Gaffey et al., 1980). The most prominent alteration is superimposition of a voltage potential on the T wave, which is caused by the systolic surge of blood through the aortic arch. Although this alteration of the ECG wave form presents no risk to patients, it presents potential difficulties in monitoring patients who are either acutely ill or undergoing pharmacologic stress.

Soulen and associates (1985) concluded that with the exception of older Starr-Edwards ball-and-cage valve prostheses, artificial heart valves experience no significant RF heating or torque from the static magnetic field (see also Pavlicek et al., 1983). At our institution, we study all but the older Starr-Edwards valves as long as valve loosening is not clinically significant.

At currently used field strengths, an additional risk of MRI is the attraction of ferromagnetic objects by the magnetic field. Pens, scissors, and medical equipment such as otoscopes or stethoscopes all are potentially lethal objects in the scanning room. Meticulous attention to objects on, in, and around the patient is required to avoid a catastrophe.

## IMAGING PRINCIPLES

A detailed description of imaging physics is beyond the purview of this article. The following is provided to acquaint the reader with the somewhat intimidating terminology used in MRI.

Currently, only the $^1$H nucleus (the proton) is routinely used for MRI because of its relative abundance in the body. Such a particle contains a magnetic moment and, when placed in a magnetic field ($B_0$), the nuclei tend to align in the direction of the applied field (also known as the Z axis) because this is the lowest energy state possible. A smaller percentage of nuclei will align against the magnetic field, residing in a slightly higher energy state. The summation of protons aligned with and against the field produces a net magnetic moment that produces the MRI signal.

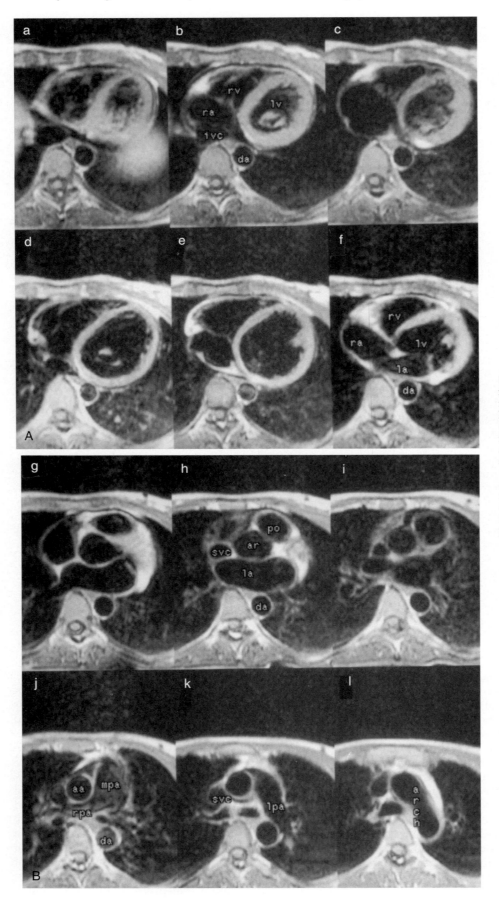

**FIGURE 31–63.** Axial images in a normal volunteer. *A* and *B,* Selected images obtained from the base of the heart *(frame a)* to the aortic arch *(frame l).* Note the absence of signal in the vessels. (aa = ascending aorta; ar = aortic root; da = descending aorta; ivc = inferior vena cava; la = left atrium; lpa = left pulmonary artery; lv = left ventricle; mpa = main pulmonary artery; ra = right atrium; rpa = right pulmonary artery; rv = right ventricle; svc = superior vena cava.)

When energy at the resonant frequency of the protons is applied, the protons move from a low to a higher energy state, and the net magnetic moment vector deviates from its orientation along the applied magnetic field. Typically, enough energy is applied to rotate the net magnetic moment 90 degrees into the X,Y plane. This is known as a 90-degree RF pulse. When the RF pulse is discontinued, the net magnetic moment vector precesses in the X,Y plane. This precession is known as transverse magnetization and creates the MRI signal. Although the nuclei initially precess coherently, with time, energy is transferred from one nucleus to another, resulting in loss of phase coherence. Macroscopically, the net magnetic moment vector decreases, creating a smaller signal. The rate at which this signal decreases depends on intrinsic properties in the tissue, and is described as the tissue's T2 or spin-spin relaxation.

As noted above, the RF energy pulsed into the tissue to be imaged creates a nuclear population existing in a higher energy state. This energy is gradually transferred to the surrounding molecules, commonly called the lattice, allowing the nuclei to return to a lower energy state and realign with the main magnetic field. The rate of transfer of this energy to the lattice is tissue-specific, and is called the T1 or spin lattice relaxation time of the imaged tissue.

MRI is a flexible imaging technique. By adjusting the intensity, number, and timing of the RF pulsations, various image contrasts are produced. Spin echo is currently the most commonly employed MRI sequence. With this sequence, a 90-degree RF excitation pulse is followed by a 180-degree RF pulse. The 180-degree RF pulse reestablishes phase coherence disrupted by imperfections in the main magnetic field. The time from the initial 90-degree RF pulse to the time phase coherence is reestablished and signal is produced is the *echo time* (TE). To produce an image with a resolution of 128 × 128 pixels, this entire excitation and acquisition process is repeated at least 128 times. The timing between the first 90-degree RF pulse and the repetition of the sequence (the second 90-degree RF pulse) is called the *repetition time* (TR). By adjusting both the TR and the TE, image contrast may be altered. Using small values (e.g., TR of 500 msec, TE of 20 msec), contrast is produced by differences in T1 relaxation time creating a "T1-weighted image." By using a longer TR and TE (e.g., 2000 msec TR, 80 msec TE), T2 contrast predominates and a "T2-weighted image" results.

*Gradient recalled echo* (GRE) imaging sequences are increasingly being used to assess the cardiovascular system. Such sequences are known by acronyms such as GRASS, FLASH, and FISP. Unlike spin echo acquisitions, GRE pulse sequences do not employ a 180-degree RF pulse. The 90-degree RF pulse is replaced by an excitation pulse that is typically *not* 90 degrees. Contrast in these sequences depends on the TR, TE, and angle of excitation (amount of RF power used). GRE sequences can produce images quickly, typically in seconds. This is a major advantage over spin echo imaging, which takes minutes to produce an image.

The differences between spin echo and GRE images are most prevalent when viewing the soft tissues. For T1-weighted spin echo images, fat is bright, stationary fluid is dark, and myocardium lies in between. On T2-weighted spin echo images, fluid becomes brighter, myocardium becomes dark, and fat shows signal intermediate between these two. On GRE images, soft tissue contrast is limited to intermediate grays. Fat is brighter than myocardium (Figs. 31–63 and 31–64).

Rapidly flowing blood is dissimilar on spin echo and GRE acquisitions. Using GRE sequences, nonturbulent flowing blood appears bright (Fig. 31–64). The high signal is due to the constant inflow of nuclei that have not been previously excited and are considered unsaturated. On spin echo images, however, rapidly flowing blood is black and is known as a "signal void" (see Fig. 31–63). For a signal to be generated with spin echo imaging, the tissue of interest must experience both the 90- and the 180-degree RF pulses. Blood that is flowing rapidly through the imaging section is not in the plane of imaging long enough to experience both pulses, so it creates a signal void. However, with slow flow, both pulses are experienced, and a signal may be created. Thus, a whole series of flow effects may occur with spin echo imaging, even when schemes such as spatial presaturation are employed to reduce unwanted intraluminal signal. Accordingly, GRE applications are generally considered more robust for assessing flow.

Although spin echo imaging using very short echoes (TE) and repetition times (TR) has produced adequate images of the heart, it was quickly determined that better anatomic visualization could be obtained with gated images (Choyke et al., 1985). Although plethysmography, laser Doppler velocimetry, and optical measurements of capillary blood flow all have been used to gate the MR data acquisition, ECG gating is preferred by most investigators, because it allows precise correlation of the temporal relationship between the obtained image and the QRS complex. Nonetheless, such an approach has limitations, including the inability to handle patients with significant arrhythmias or low QRS voltage potentials.

As a consequence of the relatively long repetition time used in spin echo imaging, data is typically acquired using a gated multislice approach. Following the QRS complex, data are acquired at one section location, and following reception of the first signal, data are then acquired at the second location. This process is continued until the next QRS complex initiates a repetition of the above sequence. As many as 5 to 10 images may be obtained throughout the cardiac cycle. Additionally, multiple echoes may be obtained at each location, providing both T1- and T2-weighted information. However, the disadvantage of this approach is that each image is obtained in a slightly different period of the cardiac cycle. Although strategies have been designed to acquire images through the entire cardiac cycle at each location, they are time-consuming, taking up to 45 minutes. Because GRE techniques work more rapidly, multiple images through the cardiac cycle at multiple locations may

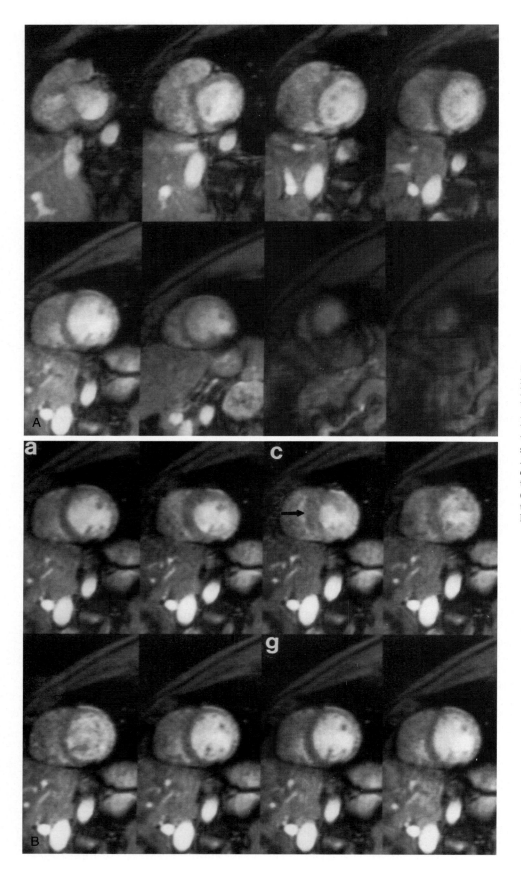

**FIGURE 31–64.** Short-axis cine images in a normal volunteer. *A,* Images obtained form the base of the heart to the apex in diastole. *B,* Images through the mid ventricles showing changes in wall thickness of the intraventricular septum through the cardiac cycle. *Frame a* is in late diastole. *Frame c* is in systole and shows a much thicker intraventricular septum *(arrow). Frame g* shows less contraction of the ventricle in mid to late diastole.

be acquired in reasonable periods. An entire cardiac acquisition may be performed in 10 to 15 minutes. Such techniques are known as "cine MRI" (Fig. 31–64).

Because they differ in speed of acquisition and contrast, both spin echo and GRE sequences are useful in evaluating the cardiovascular system. Often the two techniques are complementary. Because of superior speed, a GRE sequence is selected when images with high temporal resolution are required, such as for evaluating wall motion. However, when high tissue contrast is desired, spin echo sequences are often the first choice. Figure 31–63 is an example of normal anatomy.

## EJECTION FRACTION AND STROKE VOLUME

In patients with cardiomyopathy, congestive heart failure, and coronary artery disease, left ventricular ejection fraction is commonly used as a prognostic indicator. Although early studies reported relatively low correlation with ventriculography, more recent reports using both spin echo and cine techniques quote correlations ranging from 0.85 to 0.95 (Buckwalter et al., 1986; Meese et al., 1990; Stratemeier et al., 1986; Utz et al., 1987). Ejection fractions determined by MRI also agree well with radionuclide studies. Gaudio and associates (1991) obtained a correlation coefficient of 0.98 (see also Pattynama et al., 1993). Equally important, MRI has been demonstrated to be a reproducible technique (Pattynama et al., 1993; Semelka et al., 1990a, 1990b).

Phantom studies also have confirmed the accuracy of MRI. Debatin and co-workers used a biventricular heart model that produced a known ejection fraction. They concluded that cine MRI was more accurate than ventriculography and that the difference was statistically significant (Debatin et al., 1992a, 1992b).

Stroke volumes may also be assessed by MRI (Buser et al., 1989; Kondo et al., 1991; Matsuoka et al., 1993; Sechtem et al., 1987). Cine imaging has been most useful in this regard because of its high temporal resolution and superior contrast between flowing blood and myocardium. Because MRI is a cross-sectional imaging technique, both the left and right ventricles are well visualized, so both left and right ventricular stroke volumes may be obtained. Sechtem and associates (1987) demonstrated that, using cine MRI, the left-to-right ventricular stroke volume ratio was $0.97 \pm 0.006$. This is not statistically different from the expected ratio of 1 (i.e., left and right stroke volumes should be equal). Such measurements allow one to noninvasively quantitate isolated valvular insufficiency and right-to-left and left-to-right shunts. Preliminary studies have in fact demonstrated such capability.

Phase modulation or velocity mapping techniques can determine both velocity and flow volumes (Kondo et al., 1991; Moran, 1982; Mostbeck, 1992; Nayler et al., 1986; Underwood et al., 1987). Flowing blood produces a predictable phase shift compared with the adjacent stationary tissues. Velocity mapping or phase modulation techniques produce images sensitive to such phase shifts. Such techniques can quantitate the degree of flow through a valve and directly measure the amount of regurgitation. These techniques have been combined with cine imaging sequences. Velocity-encoded cine images have been shown to accurately measure right and left ventricular stroke volumes in phantoms and in patients (Kondo et al., 1991; Mostbeck, 1993). Such techniques allow quantitation of blood flow in individual arteries or their branches in addition to global left and right ventricular stroke volumes. Phase-sensitive MRI techniques have been used to evaluate both conduits (Rebergen et al., 1993) and congenital shunts (Sieverding et al., 1992). Additionally, such techniques have been used to characterize as well as quantitate aortic blood flow.

## MYOCARDIAL ISCHEMIA AND INFARCTION

Myocardial infarct size and location are important in both the short- and the long-term prognosis of patients with coronary artery disease (Sobel et al., 1972). A significant body of literature has addressed MRI's ability to detect ischemic or infarcted myocardial tissue. Using gated spin echo techniques, infarcted myocardium has been shown to prolong both T1 and T2 relaxation times. Increases in both T1 and T2 relaxation times correlate with water content, although intracellular versus extracellular compartmentalization of water, hemorrhage, and edema modify the final signal intensity (Higgins et al., 1983; Williams et al., 1980). Transverse (T2) relaxation is generally considered more sensitive in vivo for detecting ischemic myocardium (Fig. 31–65).

Using spin echo techniques, most investigators feel that chronic myocardial infarcts, unlike acute infarctions, show no increase in signal on T2-weighted images (Eichstaedt et al., 1989; Higgins et al., 1984; Thompson et al., 1991). However, Krauss and co-workers in a study of 19 patients, reported that for anterior wall infarctions, the high signal on T2-weighted images could persist for up to 7 months (Krauss et al., 1990).

MRI had been compared with radionuclide angiography, thallium-201 scintigraphy, and cardiac catheterization (Krauss et al., 1989; Matheijssen et al., 1991; Meese et al., 1990; Turnbull et al., 1991). Depending on the reference standard chosen, the reported accuracy of MRI ranges from 82% to 93%. Matheijssen and colleagues (1991) reported that in 20 patients who had suffered infarct 7 to 14 days earlier, MRI correctly identified the territory of infarction in 93% of cases, compared with 79% using thallium-201 scintigraphy and 62% using radionuclide angiography.

Wall thinning is seen with both acute and chronic infarction and can be accurately measured by MRI (Baer et al., 1992; Peshock et al., 1989). In Baer's study

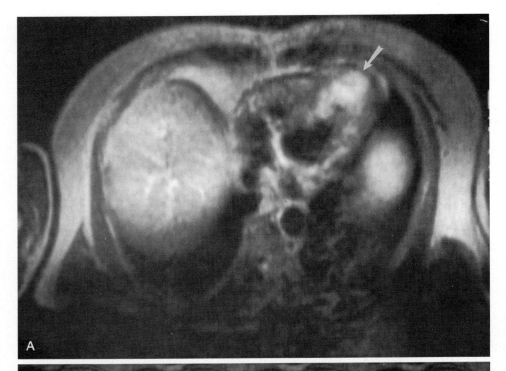

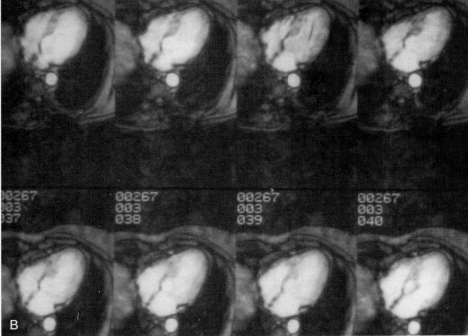

**FIGURE 31–65.** Images from a 64-year-old man with an apical myocardial infarction (MI). *A,* Gated T2-weighted spin-echo image shows increased signal in the area of the infarct *(arrow). B,* Select cine images show no significant myocardial thickening in systole. Apical dyskinesis is evident.

of 20 patients with chronic transmural infarctions, MRI, using a cine technique, agreed with single proton emission computed tomography (SPECT) in 94% of cases.

Meese and co-workers, using cine MRI, studied 24 patients with documented reperfused myocardial infarctions by left ventriculography. Twenty patients had an absolute decrease in myocardial signal and a matched regional wall-motion abnormality (Meese et al., 1990) (see Fig. 31–65). These findings were absent

in normal volunteers. The decrease in signal has been ascribed to hemorrhage (Lotan et al., 1990).

Using techniques analogous to those used in radionuclide imaging, investigators have attempted to induce stress pharmacologically in order to identify tissues at risk for ischemia. In an investigation of 40 patients, cine imaging following dipyridamole administration showed 24 of 36 segments (67%) that had reversible thallium defects (Pennell et al., 1990). Baer and co-workers (1992), also using dipyridamole stress induction, showed 90% sensitivity for detecting two-vessel disease and 69% sensitivity for identifying one-vessel disease using MRI. Specificity in localization ranged from 100% for the left anterior descending artery (LAD) to 87% for the right main coronary artery. Individual vessel sensitivities ranged from 73% to 88%. Pennell and associates (1992), using dobutamine as a pharmacologic stress agent, studied patients with exertional chest pain and abnormal results on exercise ECG. In 21 patients showing reversible ischemia by thallium-201 examination, 20 had corresponding reversible wall-motion abnormalities as detected by MRI. Additionally, compared with baseline, the areas of ischemia also showed reduced myocardial signal.

Gadolinium chelates also have been used to detect and characterize myocardial infarction. On T1-weighted images, acute myocardial infarcts show increased signal due to T1 shortening. No such increase is seen in more chronic infarctions (de Roos et al., 1989b; Nishimura et al., 1989). As with noncontrast spin echo imaging, gadolinium-enhanced images correlated well with radionuclide studies for localizing myocardial infarctions (Nishimura et al., 1989a, 1989b).

Using spin echo techniques, numerous investigators have attempted to use gadolinium chelates to differentiate reperfused from occluded myocardial infarction (de Roos et al., 1989b, 1991; Masui et al., 1991a; Nishimura et al., 1989; van der Wall et al., 1990; van Rossum et al., 1990). The results are somewhat controversial. Van der Wall and co-workers felt that both reperfused and occluded infarction showed enhancement and therefore could not be distinguished. However, others have suggested that the patterns of enhancement are different between the two entities, and that distinction between reperfused and nonreperfused infarction may be possible (de Roos et al., 1991b; Eichenberger et al., 1992; Masui et al., 1991a; van Rossum et al., 1990).

In an attempt to more accurately localize areas of infarction and ischemia as well as differentiate reperfused from nonreperfused infarcted tissue, numerous contrast agents have been tested both in animal models and in humans. A partial list of promising compounds includes Mn DPDP, Ml 25, superparamagnetic iron oxide particles, dextran (gadolinium-DTPA) 15, Dy-DTPA-BMA. In addition, antimyocin-labeled monocrystalline iron oxide nanoparticles have also been studied. Although these are promising, larger studies are necessary to determine which, if any, of these compounds will be clinically useful (Higgins et al., 1993; Pomeroy et al., 1989; Rozenman et al., 1991; Saeed et al., 1989; Weissleder et al., 1992; Wikstrom, 1992).

New pulse sequences such as *echo planar imaging* (EPI) and snap-shot FLASH have become practical with improvements in hardware. These sequences can acquire images in as little as 150 msec. Given such capability, first-pass studies may be performed in real time. Schaefer and associates (1992), using gadopentetate dimeglumine and snap-shot FLASH imaging,

found eight of nine regions of hypoperfusion that had been detected by thallium-201 scintigraphy. Manning and co-workers (1991), using gadolinium DTPA in a first-pass EPI technique, showed that 17 patients with chest pain who had undergone cardiac catheterization had decreased perfusion in the territory of diseased vessels, evidenced by less signal enhancement and a longer interval to maximum enhancement ($p = 0.001$). Of note, four patients underwent revascularization, and each showed increased signal enhancement in the ischemic regions relative to baseline studies (van Rugge et al., 1992; Wendland et al., 1993; Yu et al., 1992).

## CORONARY ARTERIES

To date, most work in assessing coronary artery disease by MRI has explored perfusion abnormalities in a manner analogous to that of thallium-201 studies. Recently, however, visualization of coronary artery disease with *magnetic resonance angiography* (MRA) has become feasible. Manning and colleagues (1993) reported their initial experience in 39 subjects. With segmented k-space GRE acquisitions, breath-held two-dimensional images were obtained that may be displayed as an angiogram is. With the assumption that stenoses greater than or equal to 50% were significant, MRA obtained a sensitivity of 0.90, specificity of 0.92, positive predictive value of 0.85, and a negative predictive value of 0.95 (Figs. 31–66 and 31–67).

However, the variation in sensitivity and specificity from vessel to vessel was significant in the series of Manning and associates. For example, sensitivity and specificity of the left circumflex coronary artery was 71 and 90% respectively, compared with near 100% sensitivity and specificity of the left main coronary artery. The relatively poor accuracy for the left circumflex coronary artery could be ascribed to the chosen pulse sequence, the imaging planes selected, and the need to use surface coils. Although MRA is promising, further refinements in technique will be necessary before it can be used to directly visualize coronary artery abnormalities.

## VALVULAR DISEASE

Although gated spin echo imaging accurately displays most cardiac anatomy, the absence of intravascular signal and the poor temporal resolution preclude assessment of valvular function. On cine images, flowing blood appears white and, assuming nonturbulent flow, the signal emanating from the blood is proportional to its velocity. Utz and associates (1988) reported that with valvular regurgitation or stenosis, turbulence (intravoxel dephasing) eliminates the signal.

In valvular regurgitation, this jet of decreased or absent signal can be seen emanating from the valve plane projecting into the appropriate chamber during

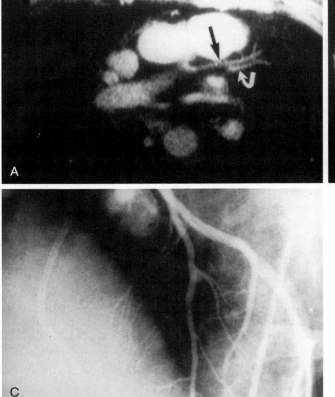

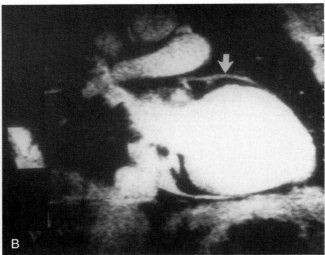

**FIGURE 31–66.** Magnetic resonance coronary angiography in a normal volunteer. *A*, Oblique axial image shows normal main and left anterior descending coronary arteries *(straight arrow).* Several diagonal branches are noted as well as the accompanying vein *(curved arrow).* *B*, Oblique long-axis view shows the normal left anterior descending artery *(arrow).* *C*, Conventional coronary angiogram showing normal left main and anterior descending coronary arteries. (*A–C*, Courtesy of Robert Edelman, M.D., Beth Israel Hospital.)

the appropriate phase of the cardiac cycle on cine images (Utz et al., 1988) (Fig. 31–68). Numerous investigators have reported the ability of cine MRI to detect aortic and mitral regurgitation (Aurigemma et al., 1990, 1991; Nishimura, 1992; Nishimura et al., 1989c; Pflugfelder et al., 1989a, 1989b; Poggessi, 1992; Utz et al., 1988). As the severity of the valvular regurgitation increases, the signal loss in the appropriate chamber increases. Semiquantitative techniques assess the severity of the regurgitation. Such techniques include jet area to chamber area, jet length to chamber area, and maximal valve leaflet separation. In all series, the severity of valvular regurgitation as assessed by MRI correlates well with Doppler ultrasonography, color-flow ultrasonography, or cardiac catheterization. For example, Aurigemma and co-workers (1990, 1991) assessed aortic regurgitation in 35 patients and mitral valve regurgitation in 40 patients. Correlation with ultrasonography was at worst 0.74 (color-flow mitral regurgitation). In terms of detection, MRI had a sensitivity of 94% and a specificity of 95%. In cases of mitral regurgitation, cine MRI has been reported to detect smaller flow disturbances than are detectable by ultrasonography (Aurigemma et al., 1990).

MRI can quantitate regurgitant fractions through both comparison of right-to-left ventricular stroke volumes and velocity phase mapping (Aufferman et al., 1991; Globits et al., 1992; Higgins et al., 1991; Honda et al., 1993; Mohiaddin et al., 1991). Higgins and colleagues (1991) reported an accuracy of 92% in quantitating patients with either mitral regurgitation or aortic regurgitation.

In patients with aortic stenosis, cine images show a jet phenomenon in systole ascending into the aorta. There is associated turbulence within the aorta distal to the jet (see Fig. 31–8). Although not as sensitive as CT, MRI can still identify valvular calcification (de Roos et al., 1989a; Kupari et al., 1992). Mitchell and associates (1989) reported that the length of the signal loss in the aorta correlated with pressure gradients across the valve ($r = 0.86$, $p < .002$).

Using a canine model, Wang and co-workers (1990) showed that left ventricular mass can be quantitated in cases of aortic stenosis. Clinically, Park and associates (1990) have shown that in patients with mitral stenosis, left atrial size decreases following angioplasty. MRI has also been shown to be capable of measuring wall stress in patients with volume overload (Aufferman et al., 1991). Aufferman and his colleagues have demonstrated that wall stress and left ventricular output increase with left ventricular volume overload. Significantly, a disproportionately high

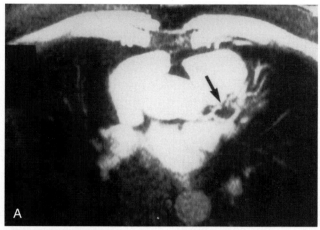

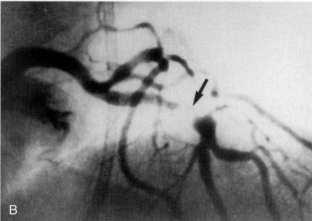

FIGURE 31–67. *A,* Oblique axial imaging showing an area of severe stenosis in the left anterior descending coronary artery *(arrow)* causing focal signal void. *B,* The corresponding conventional coronary angiogram confirms the presence of stenosis *(arrow)*. (*A* and *B,* Courtesy of Robert Edelman M.D., Beth Israel Hospital.)

systolic wall stress relative to regurgitant volume may suggest co-existing myocardial disease. Such information may provide a more objective measure for optimally timing angioplasty or valve replacement (Wang et al., 1990).

MRI has also been used preoperatively to assess the size of the aortic annulus. In 16 patients, MRI was shown to have a higher correlation with surgical assessment than ultrasonography (0.92 vs. 0.69). Additionally, the fact that MRI can identify the coronary arteries is useful in the preoperative assessment of these patients (Kon et al., 1992).

Because it produces poor temporal and spatial resolution compared with echocardiography, MRI has no role to play in assessing valvular vegetations. At present, the published experience of patients suspected of having bacterial endocarditis is small. Akins and colleagues (1991) reported that among 14 patients with complicated bacterial endocarditis, 5 perivalvular pseudoaneurysms were identified by MRI, of which only 3 were seen by ultrasonography. Given such limited data, MRI should be considered only in cases of significant uncertainty (Fig. 31–69).

MRI has little clinical utility in assessing peripros-

thetic leakage or infection due to the susceptibility effect associated with most valve prostheses. Nonetheless, Deutsch and associates (1992) assessed 55 valves in 47 patients. Comparison of MRI with echocardiography and surgery produced agreement in 96% of cases. In only six patients did the origin of leakage differ as assessed by MRI when compared with transesophageal echo.

## CONGENITAL HEART DISEASE

MRI has been used extensively in the noninvasive evaluation of congenital heart disease (Fellows et al., 1992; Kersting-Sommerhoff et al., 1989; Link et al., 1991). Intrinsic contrast between flowing blood combined with the multiplanar capability of MRI allows ready identification of size, position, and course of the great arteries and yield morphologic and quantitative information about the ventricles, shunts, and valvular abnormalities. Experience with transpositions, tetralogy of Fallot, truncus arteriosus, atrial septal defects, ventriculoseptal defects, anomalous venous connections, systemic/pulmonary shunts, and uncommon entities such as double-outlet right ventricle and atrioventricular septal defects have been reported (Baker et al., 1989; Diethelm et al., 1987; Dinsmore et al., 1985; Fisher et al., 1986; Fletcher et al., 1984; Kersting-Sommerhoff et al., 1990a, 1990b; Masui et al., 1991b; Mirowitz et al., 1989; Parsons et al., 1990; Yoo et al., 1991) (Figs. 31–69 through 31–72). Kersting-Sommerhoff and co-workers reported a reader operator curve (ROC) analysis of 51 patients with 110 congenital heart lesions, using only gated spin echo imaging (Kersting-Sommerhoff et al., 1989). At the 90% specificity level, the following sensitivities were reported: (1) great vessel relationships, 100%, (2) thoracic aorta abnormalities, 94%, (3) atrial septal defects, 91%, (4) ventriculoseptal defects, 100%, (5) right ventricular outflow obstructions, 95%, (6) aortic valve abnormalities, 52%, (7) mitral valve abnormalities, 62%, and (8) tricuspid valve abnormalities, 75%. The addition of cine acquisitions to spin echo images should improve valvular assessment.

Diethelm and associates (1987) reported a 97% level of specificity in detecting atrial septal defects when compared with control subjects ($n = 64$). Additionally, the authors felt they were able to separate primum, secundum, and common atrium defects with better than 96% accuracy.

Baker and colleagues (1989) reported their experience with ventricular septal defects and concluded that MRI compares favorably with echocardiography. Mirowitz and co-workers (1989) reported that in patients with tetralogy of Fallot, MRI correctly identified ventricular septal defects in all 17 patients.

In patients with atrial ventricular septal defects, MRI has been equal or superior to both angiography and echocardiography in assessing ventricular size and morphology. However, using spin echo techniques, MRI has not been as accurate in assessing the

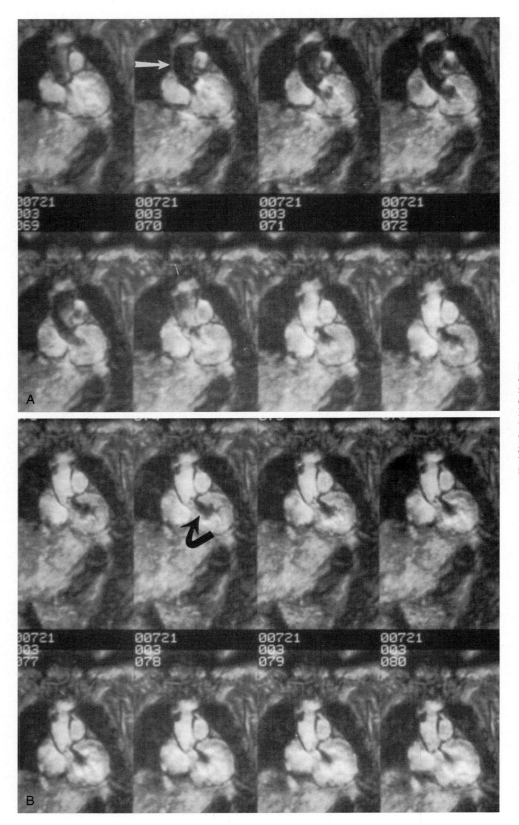

**FIGURE 31–68.** Coronal cine images in a patient with aortic stenosis and insufficiency. *A,* Images obtained in systole show turbulent flow at the aortic jet extending into the ascending aorta *(straight arrow). B,* In diastole, regurgitant flow through the aortic valve into the left ventricle is noted *(curved arrow).*

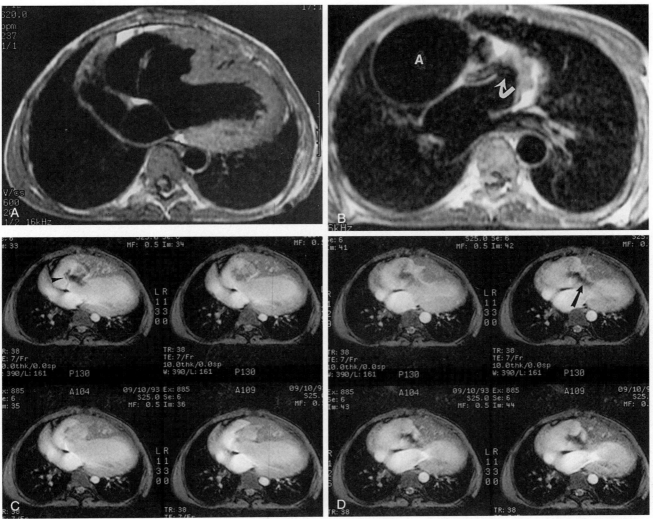

**FIGURE 31–69.** Images from a 13-year-old male with tetralogy of Fallot and subacute bacterial endocarditis. *A,* Axial gated 600/20 spin-echo image shows a large ventriculoseptal defect. Biventricular wall hypertrophy is well identified. *B,* A slightly more cephalad image shows an enlarged overriding aorta (A) and subpulmonic stenosis *(curved arrow). C,* Thickening of cusps *(arrowhead)* around aortic valve raises the question of vegetations confirmed by ultrasonography (not shown). *D,* Breath-held cine images showing small amount of left-to-right flow through the ventricular septal defect (VSD) *(arrow).*

semilunar valves (Kersting-Summerhoff et al., 1990a; Parsons et al., 1990).

MRI may be the imaging modality of choice in the assessment of pulmonary venous connections. The detection rate of MRI for venous abnormalities has been as high as 95%, compared with 69% for angiography and 38% for ultrasonography (Masui et al., 1991b). Similarly, with abnormalities of the pulmonary outflow tract and pulmonary arteries, MRI can identify vessels more peripherally than ultrasonography can, because air keeps sound waves from identifying distal branches. In fact, given a proximal stenotic pulmonary artery, MRI is often required to visualize the peripheral arterial system to determine the feasibility of shunt placement.

MRI has performed comparably to angiography and significantly better than echocardiography in assessing extracardiac shunts (Kastler et al., 1991; Kersting-Summerhoff et al., 1990a; Martinez et al., 1992).

Velocity mapping techniques allow MRI to determine flow rates as well as identify the shunt (Martinez et al., 1992).

Patients with aortic coarctation are readily assessed by MRI (Anderson et al., 1989; Katz et al., 1985; Nymen et al., 1989). Nymen and associates reported that in 11 patients with angiographic confirmation, MRI provided comparable information in terms of the site, severity, and number of collaterals in patients with aortic coarctation. They concluded that MRI is capable of replacing angiography (see Fig. 31–72). Rees and co-workers (1989) reported that in patients having undergone coarctation repair, lumen reduction correlates with an increased pressure gradient, and that greater than 50% stenosis at the isthmus following repair suggests restenosis.

MRI complements or, in specific instances, obviates the need for echocardiography or angiography (Fellows et al., 1992; Mirowitz et al., 1989). Mirowitz and

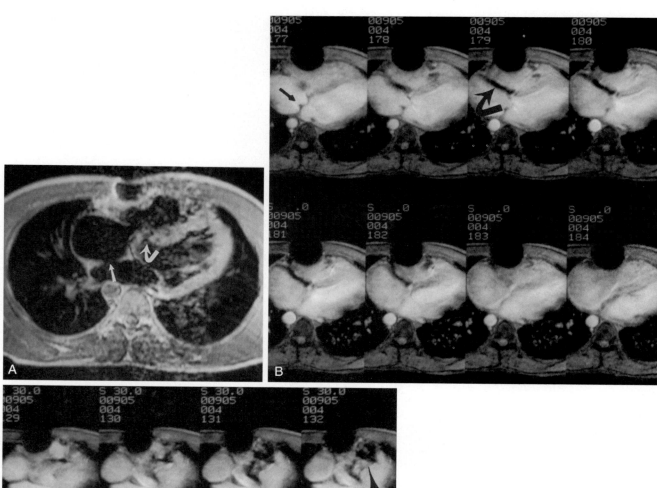

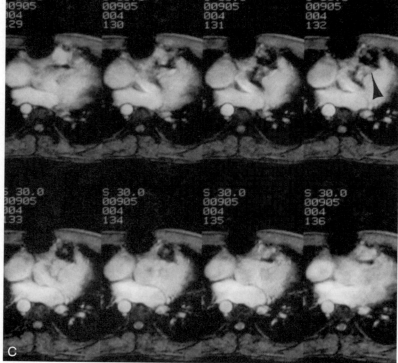

**FIGURE 31–70.** Images from a 20-year-old male with pentalogy of Fallot. *A,* Axial gated spin-echo images show both the atrial septal defect (ASD) and the high-riding VSD *(arrow, curved arrow).* Note the right-sided descending aorta. *B,* Cine image at the same level shows small jet of flow *(curved arrow)* from the left atrium to the right atrium and a larger jet at the level of the VSD. *(Arrow* shows ASD.) *C,* Turbulent flow is identified on the cine image in the pulmonary outflow tract *(arrowhead).*

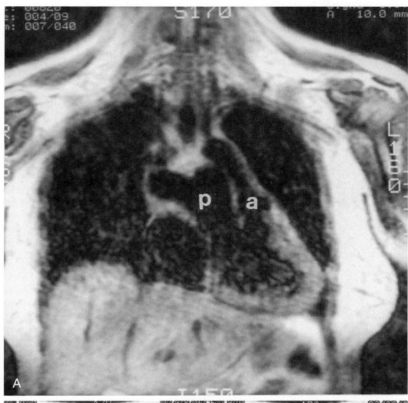

FIGURE 31–71. Images from a 24-year-old woman with a single ventricle and transposition of the great vessels. *A,* Coronal gated spin-echo image showing single ventricle with pulmonary (p) and aortic (a) vessels arising from it. *B,* Four axial gated spin-echo sections show the single ventricle (v), aorta (a), and pulmonary outflow tract (p).

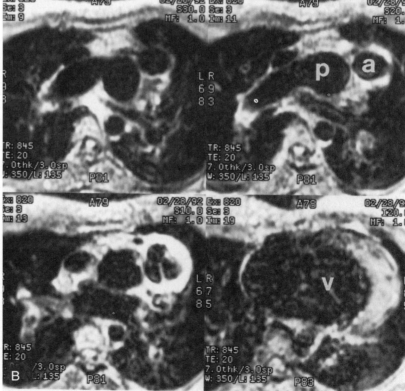

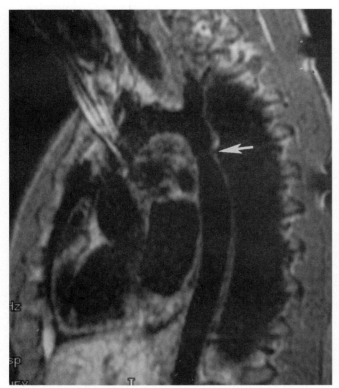

**FIGURE 31–72.** Image from a 16-year-old male with coarctation of the aorta. Oblique sagittal image shows an area of restricturing *(arrow)* consistent with the clinical findings of increased upper extremity blood pressure.

associates report that in patients with tetralogy of Fallot, MRI may replace cardiac catheterization. However, Fellows and co-workers believe that MRI is an ancillary tool despite its superiority in assessing small pulmonary arteries in patients with tetralogy of Fal-

lot, aortic coarctation, and anomalous pulmonary venous connections. At most sites, MRI has remained ancillary because of cost, availability, and the perceived difficulties of attaining diagnostic information in infants and small children. Nonetheless, several series have shown that MRI can effectively obtain images in infants and neonates (Anderson et al., 1989; Kastler et al., 1990b; Parsons et al., 1990). With the series of Anderson and associates and Kastler and co-workers combined, diagnostic studies were reported in 101 of 102 examinations. Relatively limited availability and long study times should be less problematic as faster scanning techniques are implemented clinically.

## HEART TUMORS AND THROMBUS

Primary cardiac neoplasms are rare. Therefore, although the literature is replete with case reports of primary cardiac tumors, large series are scarce. Lund and colleagues (1989) reported their experience in 61 patients suspected of having cardiac tumors. MRI demonstrated neoplasms in 50 (82%), of which 32 were intracardiac, 9 were pericardial, and 9 were in a juxtacardiac location (Fig. 31–73). The authors felt that MRI provided diagnostic information that affected either clinical management or surgical planning in 87% of the patients. This included 11 patients (18%) who by MRI were shown not to have a tumor. However, others have argued that although MRI is better for defining the intra- and extra-cardiac extension of cardiac neoplasms, rhabdomyosarcomas that are intramural are not well visualized with spin echo images (Reinmuller et al., 1989). Therefore, several investigators have suggested using myocardial tagging, gadolinium, or first-pass techniques with high-

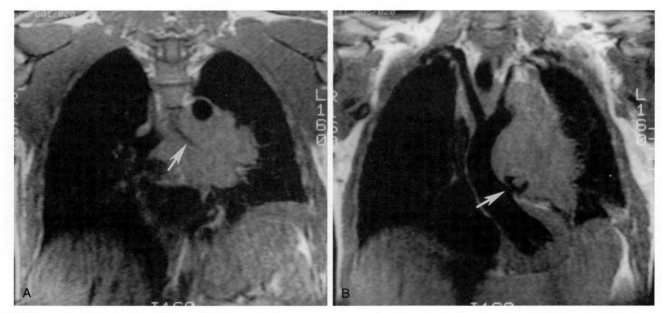

**FIGURE 31–73.** *A,* Image from a 35-year-old man with a large mass encasing the left mainstem bronchus *(arrow). B,* A more anterior image shows invasion into the pulmonary artery *(arrow).*

speed imaging to better identify and demarcate neoplasm from normal contractile myocardium (Bouton et al., 1991; Funari et al., 1991; Semelka et al., 1992).

Except for lipomas, which appear similar to subcutaneous fat on all sequences, the signal characteristics of various tumor types show significant overlap on both T1- and T2-weighted spin echo imaging. However, MRI is capable of distinguishing tumors such as left atrial myxomas from thrombus. With spin echo imaging, thrombus appears bright with more T1 weighting and has variable signal intensity on more T2-weighted images. Conversely, myxomas show decreased signal with T1 weighting and increased signal with more T2 weighting (Figs. 31–74 and 31–75). Also, atrial myxomas are enhanced by gadolinium, whereas thrombi are not (Conces et al., 1985; Dooms and Higgins, 1986; Go et al., 1985; Hananouchi et al., 1990; Kamiya et al., 1990; Kim et al., 1989; Levine et al., 1986; Menegus et al., 1992).

Although echocardiography is used routinely to separate left atrial myxomas from thrombus, the internal architecture of the two lesions is similar by ultrasonography, and separation is usually based on the location of the mass. Left atrial myxomas generally arise from the atrial septum, whereas thrombi arise along the posterior or lateral walls of the atrial ap-

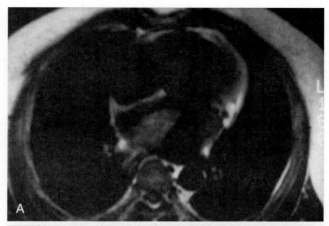
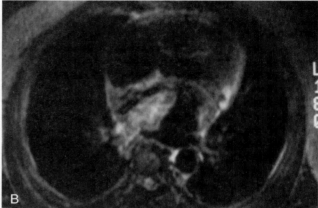

**FIGURE 31–75.** Images from a 52-year-old woman with congestive heart failure. *A,* T1-weighted image and *B,* another T2-weighted spin-echo image show a left atrial mass that increases in signal with T2-weighting, which is consistent with a myxoma.

pendage. When ultrasonography is not definitive, MRI may be helpful.

## PERICARDIAL DISEASE

The normal pericardium is seen as a band of decreased signal surrounding myocardium on spin echo and GRE imaging. The anterior pericardium is better visualized because of the contrast afforded by the adjacent epicardial fat. On gated spin echo acquisitions, the maximum thickness of the pericardium is normally 2.5 mm (Sechtem et al., 1987). Measurements on GRE images are similar. Both animal models and in vivo reports have suggested that MRI may help identify and characterize pericardial effusions (Kastler et al., 1990a; Rokey et al., 1991).

On gated spin echo images, nonhemorrhagic effusions tend to have low signal intensity on T1-weighted images. With increased T2 weighting, the effusion becomes bright. On GRE images, pericardial effusions are bright and are approximately the same intensity as the adjacent fat. No specific criteria have been reported to allow the distinction of transudative from exudative effusions, although Sechtem and associates (1987) have noted that uremic and tuberculous

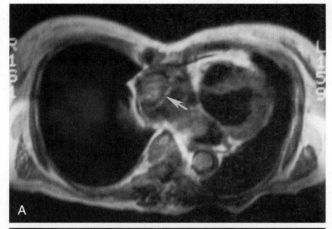
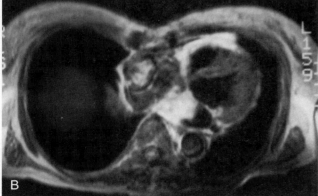

**FIGURE 31–74.** *A,* Gated T1-weighted sequence and *B,* another T2-weighted sequence show a right atrial mass *(arrow in A)* that is bright on all sequences consistent with thrombus. Results from an examination 2 weeks earlier (not shown) were normal.

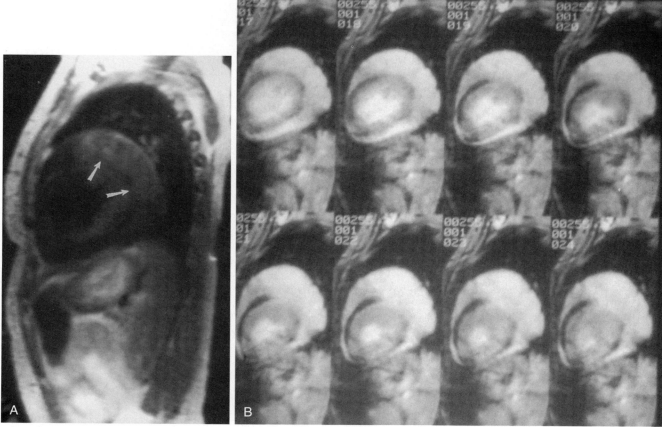

**FIGURE 31–76.** Pericardial effusion. *A,* Sagittal gated T1-weighted spin-echo image shows the effusion *(arrows)* as low signal. *B,* Cine images show the effusion as increased in signal.

effusions tend to have higher signal than simple transudative effusions. Hemorrhagic effusions show high signal on all sequences, including T1-weighted images.

Although fewer reports assess pericardial effusions using GRE images, at our institution cine techniques are preferred because of their superior ability to separate fluid from fibrinous and solid components within the pericardium (Figs. 31–76 and 31–77). MRI is insensitive to calcium (Hammersmith et al., 1991; Olson et al., 1989), a major limitation when using MRI to evaluate pericardial disease.

Although echocardiography remains the primary means of evaluating pericardial effusions because of its availability, portability, low cost, and high accuracy, MRI is an accurate means of assessing pericardial effusions (Mulvagh et al., 1989). A comparison of spin echo MRI and echocardiography revealed that MRI detected several small pericardial effusions not visualized by echocardiography. MRI was especially useful for looking at the superior aortic pericardial reflection, the medial border of the right atrium, and the posterior aspect of the left ventricular apex. Additionally, in 10 patients with both pleural and pericardial effusions, MRI more clearly distinguished the two types of effusions.

Masui and associates (1992) have suggested that MRI may distinguish restrictive cardiomyopathy from constrictive pericarditis. In 29 patients, MRI diagnosed constrictive pericarditis with an 88% sensitivity and 100% specificity, for an overall accuracy of 93%. The diagnosis of constrictive pericarditis is made by

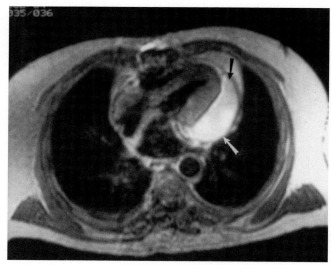

**FIGURE 31–77.** Hemorrhagic pericardial effusion. Axial T1-weighted gated spin-echo image shows high signal in the hemorrhagic pericardial effusion *(arrows)* (500/20 msec).

identifying a thickened pericardium, and pericardial thickening usually surrounds the right ventricle. No pericardial thickening was identified in four patients with restrictive myocarditis (Fig. 31–78). MRI has also helped assess pericardial adhesions after cardiac surgery (Duvernoy et al., 1991).

## AORTIC DISEASE

MRI readily detects dissections of the thoracic aorta. In multiple studies, MRI compares favorably with CT and angiography. The multiplanar capability of MRI facilitates discrimination between type A and type B dissections, facilitating the decision whether to manage the patient surgically or medically (Fig. 31–79).

Several disadvantages have precluded MRI from becoming the primary means of confirming or excluding thoracic aortic dissections: lack of scanner accessibility, the inability to identify intimal flap calcification, and relatively long imaging times. The latter is especially important in patients who are marginally stable. Given the sensitivity of MRI to flowing blood, the

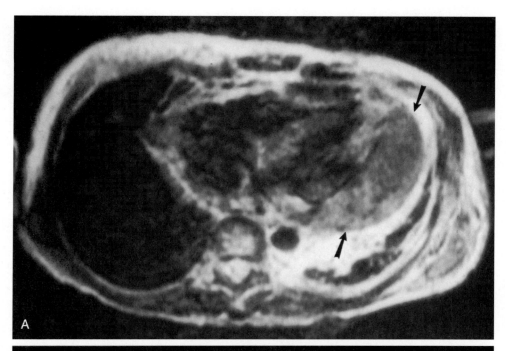

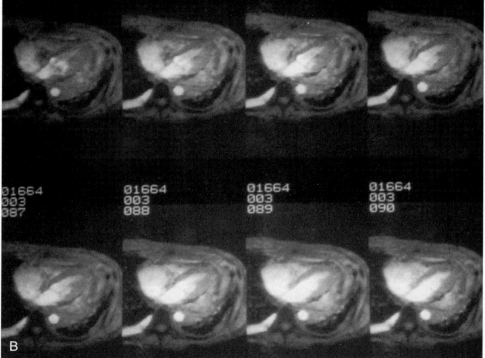

**FIGURE 31–78.** Images from a 37-year-old woman with breast cancer. *A,* Gated T1-weighted image shows a soft tissue mass *(arrows)* in the pericardium. *B,* Cine images show no dilatation of the left ventricle in diastole, confirming constrictive pericarditis.

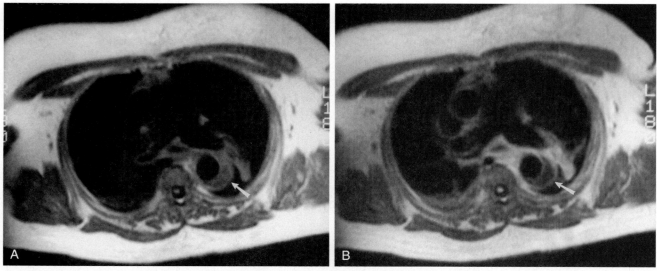

**FIGURE 31–79.** Images from a 66-year-old woman with pain radiating to the back. *A,* Gated T1 (674/20 msec) and *B,* T2 (674/60 msec) images show a Type III dissection *(arrows)* involving the descending aorta. Slow flow causes increased signal in the false lumen on the first echo image that washes out on the second echo image.

inability to see calcium has not been identified as a major problem. Although recent reports have documented the high sensitivity and specificity of MRI in detecting aortic dissections, experience is needed to distinguish flow artifacts and slowly flowing blood from thrombi (Akins et al., 1987; Amparo et al., 1985; Dinsmore et al., 1985; Geisinger et al., 1985; Glazer et al., 1985; Kersting-Summerhof et al., 1988).

The most important advantage of MRI is that an intravenous contrast agent is not required. This is especially crucial for patients who have impaired renal function secondary to atherosclerosis and hypertension and thus are at increased risk for contrast-induced renal failure. Other complications of aortic

dissections, such as pericardial effusions, valvular insufficiency, and hemopericardium, can also be identified by MRI.

Although MRI studies of the aorta traditionally have been lengthy, MRI now takes about as long as state-of-the-art CT does. MRI may become the noninvasive study of choice for assessing the thoracic aorta for intimal dissections (Fig. 31–80).

## CONCLUSION

The potential of MRI to revolutionize the evaluation of the cardiovascular system is enormous. It is

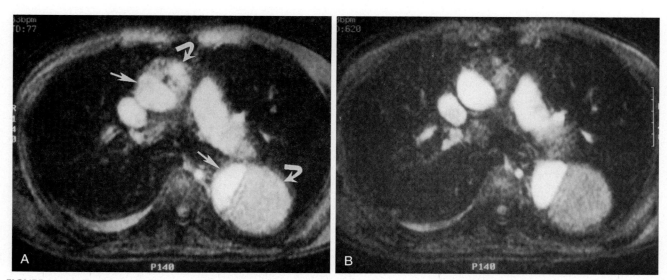

**FIGURE 31–80.** Type I aortic dissection is demonstrated with breath-held cine images. Both images at this slice location were acquired in the same 16-second breath-hold. Image *A* was obtained in systole, image *B* in diastole. Fast bright flow is seen through the true lumen *(straight arrows)* in both the ascending and the descending aorta. Less signal, reflecting slower flow, is present in the false lumen *(curved arrows).*

feasible that MRI will be used to determine ejection fraction, stroke volume, global and regional wall-motion abnormalities, and perfusion abnormalities, as well as for direct visualization of coronary arteries, in a single integrated examination.

The intrinsic sensitivity of MRI to flowing blood suggests that assessment of the great vessels also may be reliable. To date, the limited availability of MR scanners, coupled with long examination times, has precluded MRI from having a significant clinical impact in the cardiovascular arena. With the advent of velocity-sensitive techniques and subsecond imaging, MRI will assume increasing importance in the coming years.

## SELECTED BIBLIOGRAPHY

Auffermann, W., Wagner, S., Holt, W. W., et al.: Noninvasive determination of left ventricular output and wall stress in volume overload and in myocardial disease by cinemagnetic resonance imaging. Am. Heart. J., 121:1750–1758, 1991.

This article recounts a study of patients with myocardial disease and/or valvular regurgitation. The authors demonstrate that regurgitant volumes may be measured and that wall stress may be calculated. The authors conclude that left ventricular output and wall stress rise as left ventricular volume increases, and that a disproportionately high wall stress relative to regurgitant volume suggests myocardial disease. The authors have demonstrated the potential of MRI to objectively determine the timing and feasibility of valve replacement.

Eichenberger, A. C., and von Schulthess, G. K.: Magnetic resonance imaging of the heart and the great vessels: Morphology, function, and perfusion. Curr. Opin. Radiol., 4(1V):41–47, 1992.

This review article discusses the current capabilities of MRI in congenital heart disease, ischemic heart disease, great vessel disease, and wall-motion analysis. Preliminary results using innovative methods are also discussed.

Manning, W. J., Li, W., and Edelman, R. R.: A preliminary report comparing MR coronary angiography with conventional angiography. N. Engl. J. Med., 328(12):828–832, 1993.

This article reports the authors' initial experience with 39 subjects with suspected coronary artery disease. The potential of MRI to accurately detect significant coronary vessel stenosis is documented. Limitations of the MRI technique as performed are addressed. The article heralds the potential of MRI to visualize noninvasively the coronary arteries.

Pennell, D. J., Underwood, R., Manzara, C. C., et al.: Magnetic resonance imaging during Dobutamine stress in coronary artery disease. Am. J. Cardiol., 70:34–40, 1992.

This article describes dobutamine-induced pharmacologic stress as a means of assessing the severity of coronary artery disease by MRI. The study population is 25 patients with exertional chest pain and abnormal results on exercise ECGs. Using thallium tomography as the standard of reference, the authors report that MRI can detect ischemic regions within the heart based on dobutamine-induced wall-motion abnormalities. Such a technique allows assessment of impaired myocardial perfusion by MRI.

## BIBLIOGRAPHY

Akins, E. W., Carmichael, M. J., Hill, J. A., et al.: Preoperative evaluation of the thoracic aorta using MRI and angiography. Ann. Thorac. Surg., 44:499–507, 1987.

Akins, E. W., Slone, R. M., Wiechmann, B. N., et al.: Perivalvular pseudoaneurysm complicating bacterial endocarditis: MR detection in five cases. A. J. R., 156(6):1155–1158, 1991.

Amparo, E. G., Higgins, C. B., Hoddick, W., et al.: Magnetic resonance imaging of aortic disease: Preliminary results. A. J. R., 143:1203–1209, 1984.

Amparo, E. G., Higgins, C. B., Hricak, H., et al.: Aortic dissection: Magnetic resonance imaging. Radiology, 155:399–406, 1985.

Anderson, R. H., Tynan, M., Yates, A. K., et al.: Magnetic resonance imaging of coarctation of the aorta in infants: Use of a high field strength. Br. Heart J., 62(2):97–101, 1989.

Aufferman, W., Wagner, S., Holt, W. W., et al.: Noninvasive determination of left ventricular output and wall stress in volume overload and in myocardial disease by cine magnetic resonance imaging. Am. Heart J., 121(6):1750–1758, 1991.

Aurigemma, G., Reichek, N., Schiebler, M., et al.: Evaluation of aortic regurgitation by cardiac cine magnetic resonance imaging: Planaranalysis and comparison to Doppler echocardiography. Cardiology, 78(4):340–347, 1991.

Aurigemma, G., Reichek, N., Schiebler, M., et al.: Evaluation of mitral regurgitation by cine magnetic resonance imaging. Am. J. Cardiol., 66(5):621–625, 1990.

Baer, F. M., Smolarz, K., Jungehulsing, M., et al.: Chronic myocardial infarction: Assessment of morphology, function, and perfusion by gradient echomagnetic resonance imaging and $^{99m}$Tc-methoxyisobutyl-isonitrile SPECT. Am. Heart. J., 123:636–643, 1992.

Baker, E. J., Ayton, V., Smith, M. A., et al.: MRI at a high field strength of ventricular septal defects in infants. Br. Heart J., 62(4):305–310, 1989.

Bouton, S., Yang, A., McCrindle, B. W., et al.: Differentiation of tumor from viable myocardium using cardiac tagging with MR imaging. J. Comput. Assist. Tomogr., 15(4):676–678, 1991.

Buckwalter, K. A., Aisen, A. M., Dilworth, L. R., et al.: Gated cardiac MRI: Ejection fraction determination using the right anterior oblique view. A. J. R., 147:33, 1986.

Budinger, T. F.: Nuclear magnetic resonance (NMR) in vivo studies: Known thresholds for health effects. J. Comput. Assist. Tomogr., 5:800–811, 1981.

Budinger, T. F.: Potential hazards of nuclear magnetic resonance in in-vivo imaging and spectroscopy. New Concepts in Cardiac Imaging, 3:359–380, 1987.

Buser, P. T., Aufferman, W., Holt, W. W., et al.: Noninvasive evaluation of global left ventricular function with use of cine nuclear magnetic resonance. J. Am. Coll. Cardiol., 13(6):1294–1300, 1989.

Choyke, P. L., Kressel, H. Y., Reichek, N., et al.: Nongated cardiac magnetic resonance imaging: Preliminary experience at 0.12 T. A. J. R., 143:1143–1150, 1985.

Conces, D. J., Vix, V. A., and Klatte, E. C.: Gated MR imaging of left atrial myxomas. Radiology, 156:445–447, 1985.

Debatin, J., Nadel, S. N., Paolini, J., et al.: Cardiac ejection fraction: Phantom study comparing cine MR imaging, radionuclide blood pool imaging and ventriculography. J. M. R. I., 2(2):135–142, 1992a.

Debatin, J., Nadel, S., Sostman, D., et al.: Magnetic resonance imaging—Cardiac ejection fraction measurements: Phantom study comparing four different methods. Invest. Radiol., 27(3):198–204, 1992b.

de Roos, A., Mohanlal, R. W., van Vaals, J. J., et al.: Gadolinium-DTPA-enhanced magnetic resonance imaging of the isolated rat heart after ischemia and reperfusion. Invest. Radiol., 26:1060–1064, 1991.

de Roos, A., Reichek, N., Axel, L., et al.: Cine MR imaging in aortic stenosis. J. C. A. T., 13(3):421–425, 1989a.

de Roos, A., van Rossum, A., C., van der Wall, E., et al.: Reperfused and nonreperfused myocardial infarction: Diagnostic potential of GdDTPA-enhanced MR imaging. Radiology, 172(3):717–720, 1989b.

Deutsch, H. J., Bachmann, R., Sechtem, U., et al.: Regurgitant flow in cardiac valve prostheses: Diagnostic value of gradient echo nuclear magnetic resonance imaging in reference to transesophageal two-dimensional color Doppler echocardiography. J. Am. Coll. Cardiol., 19(7):1500–1507, 1992.

Diethelm, L., Dery, R., Lipton, M. J., et al.: Arterial level shunts: Sensitivity and specificity of MR in diagnosis. Radiology, 162:181–188, 1987.

Dinsmore, R. E., Wismer, G. L., Guyer, D., et al.: MRI of the interatrial septum and atrial septal defects. A. J. R., 145:697–703, 1985.

Dooms, G. C., and Higgins, C. B.: MR imaging of cardiac thrombi. J. Comput. Assist. Tomogr., 10:414–420, 1986.

Duvernoy, O., Malm, T., Thomas, K. A., et al.: CT and MR evaluation of pericardial and retrosternal adhesions after cardiac surgery. J. C. A. T., 15(4):555–560, 1991.

Eichenberger, A. C., and von Schulthess, G. K.: Magnetic resonance imaging of the heart and the great vessels: Morphology, function, and perfusion. Curr. Opin. Radiol., 4:41–47, 1992.

Eichstaedt, H. W., Felix, R., Danne, O., et al.: Imaging of acute myocardial infarction by magnetic resonance tomography (MRT) using the paramagnetic relaxation substance gadolinium-DTPA. Cardiovasc. Drugs Ther., 3(5):779–788, 1989.

Fellows, K. E., Weinberg, P. M., Baffa, J. M., and Hoffman, E. A.: Evaluation of congenital heart disease with MR imaging: Current and coming attractions. A. J. R., 159(5):925–931, 1992.

Fisher, M., and Higgins, C. B.: MRI of congenital heart disease. In Pohost, G. M. (ed): New Concepts in Cardiac Imaging—1986. Chicago, Year Book, 1986, pp. 231–250.

Fletcher, B. D., Jacobstein, M. D., Nelson, A. D., et al.: Gated magnetic resonance imaging of congenital cardiac malformations. Radiology, 150:137–140, 1984.

Fujita, N., Hartiala, J., O'Sullivan, M., et al.: Assessment of left ventricular diastolic function in dilated cardiomyopathy with cine magnetic resonance imaging: Effect of an angiotensin converting enzyme inhibitor, benazepril. Am. Heart J., 125(1):171–178, 1993.

Funari, M., Fujita, N., Peck, W. W., et al.: Cardiac tumors: Assessment with GdDTPA enhanced MR imaging. J. Comput. Assist. Tomogr., 15(6):953–958, 1991.

Gaffey, C. T., Tenforde, T. S., and Dean, E. G.: Alterations in the electrocardiographs of baboons exposed to DC magnetic fields. Bioelectromagnetics, 1:209–215, 1980.

Gaudio, C., Tanzilli, G., Mazzarotto, P., et al.: Comparison of left ventricular ejection fraction by magnetic resonance imaging and radionuclide ventriculography in idiopathic dilated cardiomyopathy. Am. J. Cardiol., 67(5):411–415, 1991.

Geisinger, M. A., Risius, B., O'Donnell, J. A., et al.: Thoracic aortic dissections: Magnetic resonance imaging. Radiology, 155:407–412, 1985.

Glazer, H. S., Gutierrez, F. R., Levitt, R. G., et al.: The thoracic aorta studied by MR imaging. Radiology, 157:149–155, 1985.

Globits, S., Frank, H., Mayr, H., et al.: Quantitative assessment of aortic regurgitation by magnetic resonance imaging. Eur. Heart J., 13(1):78–83, 1992.

Go, R., O'Donnell, J. K., Underwood, D. A., et al.: Comparison of gated cardiac MRI and 2D echocardiography of intracardiac neoplasms. A. J. R., 145:21–25, 1985.

Hammersmith, S. M., Colletti, P. M., Norris, S. L., et al.: Cardiac calcifications: Difficult MRI diagnosis. Magn. Reson. Imag., 9(2):195–200, 1991.

Hananouchi, G. L., and Goff, W. B.: Cardiac lipoma: Six-year follow-up with MRI characteristics, and a review of the literature. Magn. Reson. Imag., 8(6):825–828, 1990.

Hawkes, R. C., Holland, G. N., Moore, W. S., et al.: Nuclear magnetic resonance (NMR) tomography of the normal heart. J. Comput. Assist. Tomogr., 5:605–612, 1981.

Higgins, C. B., Herfkens, R. J., Lipton, M. J., et al.: Nuclear magnetic resonance imaging of acute myocardial infarction in dogs: Alterations in magnetic relaxation times. Am. J. Cardiol., 52:184–188, 1983.

Higgins, C. B., Lanzer, P., Stark, D., et al.: Imaging by nuclear magnetic resonance in patients with chronic ischemic heart disease. Circulation, 69:523–531, 1984.

Higgins, C. B., Saeed, M., Wendland, M., et al.: Contrast media for cardiothoracic MR imaging. J. Magn. Reson. Imag., 3(1):265–276, 1993.

Higgins, C. B., Wagner, S., Kondo, C., et al.: Evaluation of valvular heart disease with cine gradient echo magnetic resonance imaging. Circulation, 84(3):198–207, 1991.

Honda, N., Machida, K., Hashimoto, M., et al.: Aortic regurgitation: Quantitation with MR imaging velocity mapping. Radiology, 186(1):189–194, 1993.

Kamiya, H., Ohno, M., Iwata, H., et al.: Cardiac lipoma in the interventricular septum: Evaluation by computed tomography and MRI. Am. Heart J., 119(5):1215–1217, 1990.

Kanal, E., et al.: Safety considerations in MR imaging. Radiology, 176:593–606, 1990.

Kanal, E., et al.: Survey of reproductive health among female MR workers. Radiology, 187:395–399, 1993.

Kannel, W. B., and Thorn, T. J.: Incidence, prevalence, and mortality of cardiovascular diseases. In Hurst, J. W. (ed): The Heart, Arterial Veins. 5th ed. New York, McGraw-Hill, 1986.

Kastler, B., Germain, P., Dietemann, J. L., et al.: Spin echo MRI in the evaluation of pericardial disease. Comput. Med. Imag. Graphics, 14(4):241–247, 1990a.

Kastler, B., Livolsi, A., Germain, P., et al.: Evaluation of Blalock-Taussig shunts in newborns: Value of oblique MRI planes. Int. J. Card. Imaging, 7:1, 1991.

Kastler, B., Livolsi, A., Germain, P., et al.: MRI in congenital heart disease of newborns: Preliminary results in 23 patients. Eur. J. Radiol., 10(2):109–117, 1990b.

Katz, M. E., Glazer, H. S., Siegel, M. J., et al.: Mediastinal vessels: Postoperative evaluation with MR imaging. Radiology, 161:647–651, 1985.

Kersting-Sommerhoff, B. A., Diethelm, L., Stanger, P., et al.: Evaluation of complex congenital ventricular anomalies with magnetic resonance imaging. Am. Heart J., 120(1):133–142, 1990a.

Kersting-Sommerhoff, B. A., Diethelm, L., Teitel, D. F., et al.: Magnetic resonance imaging of congenital heart disease: Sensitivity and specificity using receiver operating characteristic curve analysis. Am. Heart J., 118(1):155–161, 1989.

Kersting-Sommerhoff, B. A., Higgins, C., White, R., et al.: Aortic dissection: Sensitivity and specificity of MR imaging. Radiology, 166:651–655, 1988.

Kersting-Sommerhoff, B. A., Seelos, K. C., Hardy, C., et al.: Evaluation of surgical procedures for cyanotic congenital heart disease by using MR imaging. A. J. R., 155(2):259–266, 1990b.

Kim, E. E., Wallace, S., Abello, R., et al.: Malignant cardiac fibrous histiocytomas and angiosarcomas: MR features. J. Comput. Assist. Tomogr., 13(4):627–632, 1989.

Kon, N. D., Link, K. M., Buchanan, W. P., et al.: MRI evaluation of recipient for cryopreserved aortic allograph. Ann. Thorac. Surg., 54(1):39–43, 1992.

Kondo, C., Caputo, G., Semelka, R., et al.: Right and left ventricular stroke volume measurements with velocity-encoded cine MR imaging: In vitro and in vivo validation. A. J. R., 157:9–16, 1991.

Krauss, X. H., van der Wall, E. E., Doornbos, J., et al.: Value of magnetic resonance imaging in patients with a recent myocardial infarction: Comparison with planar thallium-201 scintigraphy. Cardiovasc. Intervent. Radiol., 12(3):119–124, 1989.

Krauss, X. H., van der Wall, E. E., van der Laarse, A., et al.: Follow-up of regional myocardial T2 relaxation times in patients with myocardial infarction evaluated with magnetic resonance imaging. Eur. J. Radiol., 11(2):110–119, 1990.

Kupari, M., Hekali, P., Keto, P., et al.: Assessment of aortic valve area in aortic stensis by magnetic resonance imaging. Am. J. Cardiol., 70(9):952–955, 1992.

Levine, R. A., Weyman, A. E., Dinsmore, R. E., et al.: Noninvasive tissue characterization: Diagnosis of lipomatous hypertrophy of the atrial septum by MRI. J. Comput. Assist. Tomogr., 7:688–692, 1986.

Link, K. M., and Lesko, N. M.: Magnetic resonance imaging in the evaluation of congenital heart disease. Magn. Reson. Q., 7(3):173–190, 1991.

Link, K. M., and Lesko, N. M.: The role of MR imaging in the evaluation of acquired diseases of the thoracic aorta. A. J. R., 158(5):1115–1125, 1992.

Lotan, C. S. M., Nukker, S. K., Bouchard, A., et al.: Detection of intramyocardial hemorrhage using high-field proton (1 H) nuclear magnetic resonance imaging. Cathet. Cardiovasc. Diagn., 20:205–211, 1990.

Lund, J. T., Ehman, R. L., Julsrud, P. R., et al.: Cardiac masses: Assessment by MR imaging. A. J. R., 152(3):469–473, 1989.

Manning, W. J., Atkinson, D. J., Grossman, W., et al.: First-pass nuclear magnetic resonance imaging studies using gadolinium-DTPA in patients with coronary artery disease. J. Am. Coll. Cardiol., 18:959–965, 1991.

Manning, W. J., Li, W., Edelman, R. R.: A preliminary report comparing MR coronary angiography with conventional angiography. N. Engl. J. Med., 328(12):828–832, 1993.

Martinez, J. E., Mohiaddin, R. H., Kilner, P. J., et al.: Obstruction in extracardiac ventriculopulmonary conduits: Value of nuclear magnetic resonance imaging with velocity mapping and Doppler echocardiography. J. Am. Coll. Cardiol., 20(2):338–344, 1992.

Masui, T., Finck, S., and Higgins, C.: Constrictive pericarditis and restrictive cardiomyopathy: Evaluation with MR imaging. Radiology, 182(2):369–373, 1992.

Masui, T., Saeed, M., Wendland, M. F., et al.: Occlusive and reperfused myocardial infarcts: MR imaging differentiation with nonionic Gd-DTPA-BMA. Radiology, 181(1):77–83, 1991a.

Masui, T., Seelos, K. C., Kersting-Sommerhoff, B. A., et al.: Abnormalities of the pulmonary veins: Evaluation with MR imaging and comparison with cardiac angiography and echocardiography. Radiology, 181(3):645–649, 1991b.

Matheijssen, N. A., de Roos, A., Blokland, J. A., et al.: Magnetic resonance imaging of myocardial infarction: Correlation with enzymatic, angiographic, and radionuclide findings. Am. Heart. J., 122(5):1274–1283, 1991.

Matsuoka, H., Hamada, M., Honda, T., et al.: Measurement of cardiac chamber volumes by cine magnetic resonance imaging. Angiology, 44(4):321–327, 1993.

Meese, R. B., Spritzer, C. E., Negro-Vilar, R., et al.: Detection, characterization and functional assessment of reperfused Q-wave acute myocardial infarction by cine magnetic resonance imaging. Am. J. Cardiol., 66(1):1–9, 1990.

Menegus, M. A., Greenberg, M. A., Spindola-Franco, H., et al.: MRI of suspected atrial tumors. Am. Heart J., 123(5):1260–1268, 1992.

Mirowitz, S. A., Gutierrez, F. R., Cantaer, C. E., et al.: Tetralogy of Fallot: MR findings. Radiology, 171(1): 207–212, 1989.

Mitchell, L., Jenkins, J. P., Watson, Y., et al.: Diagnosis and assessment of mitral and aortic valve disease by cine-flow magnetic resonance imaging. Magn. Reson. Med., 12(2):181–197, 1989.

Mohiaddin, R. H., Amanuma, M., Kilner, Kilner, P. J., et al.: MR phase shift velocity mapping of mitral and pulmonary venous flow. J. C. A. T., 15(2):237–243, 1991.

Moran, P. R.: A flow zeugmatographic interface for NMR imaging in humans. Magn. Reson. Imag., 1:197–203, 1982.

Mostbeck, G. H., Caputo, G. R., and Higgins, C. B.: MR measurement of blood flow in the cardiovascular system. A. J. R., 159(3):453–461, 1992.

Mostbeck, G. H., Hartiala, J. J., Foster, E., et al.: Right ventricular diastolic filling: Evaluation with velocity-encoded cine MRI. J. Comput. Assist. Tomogr., 17(2):245–252, 1993.

Mulvagh, S. L., Rokey, R., Vick, G. W., et al.: Usefulness of nuclear magnetic resonance imaging for evaluation of pericardia effusions, and comparison with two-dimensional echocardiography. Am. J. Cardiol., 64(16):1002–1009, 1989.

Nayler, G. L., Firmin, D. N., and Longmore, D. B.: Blood flow imaging by cine magnetic resonance. J. Comput. Assist. Tomogr., 10:715–722, 1986.

Nishimura, F.: Oblique cine MRI for the evaluation of aortic regurgitation: Comparison with cineangiography. Clin. Cardiol., 15(2):73–78, 1992.

Nishimura, T., Kobayashi, H., Ohara, Y., et al.: Serial assessment of myocardial infarction by using gated MR imaging and Gd-DTPA. A. J. R., 153:715–720, 1989a.

Nishimura, T., Yamada, Y., Hayashi, M., et al.: Determination of infarct size of acute myocardial infarction in dogs by magnetic resonance imaging and gadolinium-DTPA: Comparison with Indium-111 antimyosin imaging. Am. J. Physiol. Imag., 4:83–88, 1989b.

Nishimura, T., Yamada, N., Itoh, A., et al.: Cine MR imaging in mitral regurgitation: Comparison with color Doppler flow imaging. A. J. R., 153(4):721–724, 1989c.

Nyman, R., Hallberg, M., Sunnegardh, J., et al.: Magnetic resonance imaging and angiography for the assessment of coarctation of the aorta. Acta Radiol., 30(5):481–485, 1989.

Olson, M. C., Posniak, H. V., McDonald, V., et al.: Computed tomography and magnetic resonance imaging of the pericardium. Radiographics, 9(4):633–634, 1989.

Park, J. H., Han, M. C., Im, J. G., et al.: Mitral stenosis: Evaluation with MR imaging after percutaneous balloon valvuloplasty. Radiology, 177(2):533–536, 1990.

Parsons, J. M., Baker, E. J., Anderson, R. H., et al.: Morphological evaluation of arterioventricular septal defects by MRI. Br. Heart J., 64(2):138–145, 1990.

Pattynama, P. M., Lamb, J. H., van der Velde, E. A., et al.: Left ventricular measurements with cine and spin-echo MR imaging: A study of reproducibility with variance component analysis. Radiology, 187(1):261–268, 1993.

Pavlicek, W., et al.: The effects of nuclear magnetic resonance on patients with cardiac pacemakers. Radiology, 147:149–153, 1983.

Pennell, D. J., Underwood, S. R., Ell, P. J., et al.: Dipyridamole magnetic resonance imaging: A comparison with thallium-201 emission tomography. Br. Heart J., 64:362–369, 1990.

Pennell, D. J., Underwood, S. R., Manzara, C. C., et al.: Magnetic resonance imaging during dobutamine stress in coronary artery disease. Am. J. Cardiol., 70:34–40, 1992.

Peshock, R. M., Rokey, R., Malloy, C., et al.: Assessment of myocardial systolic wall thickening using nuclear magnetic resonance imaging. J. Am. Coll. Cardiol., 14:653–659, 1989.

Pflugfelder, P. W., Landzberg, J. S., Cassidy, M. M., et al.: Comparison of cine MR imaging with Doppler echocardiography of the evaluation of aortic regurgitation. A. J. R., 152:4:729–735, 1989a.

Pflugfelder, P. W., Sechtem, U. P., White, R. D., et al.: Noninvasive evaluation of mitral regurgitation by analysis of left atrial signal loss in cinemagnetic resonance. Am. Heart J., 117(5):1112–1119, 1989b.

Poggesi, L.: Evaluation of mitral stenosis by cine magnetic resonance imaging. Am. Heart J., 123(5):1252–1260, 1992.

Pohost, G. M., Blackwell, G., and Shellock, F. G.: Safety of patients with medical devices during application of magnetic resonance methods. Ann. N. Y. Acad. Sci., 649:204–224, 1992.

Pomeroy, O. H., Wendland, M., Wagner, S., et al.: Magnetic resonance imaging of acute myocardial ischemia using a manganese chelate, Mn-DPDP. Invest. Radiol., 24:531–536, 1989.

Rebergen, S. A., Ottenkamp, J., Doornbos, J., et al.: Postoperative pulmonary flow dynamics after Fontan surgery: Assessment with nuclear magnetic resonance velocity mapping. J. Am. Coll. Cardiol., 21(1):123–131, 1993.

Rees, S., Sommerville, J., Ward, C., et al.: Coarctation of the aorta: MR imaging in late postoperative assessment. Radiology, 173(2):499–502, 1989.

Reinmuller, R., Lloret, J. L., Tiling, R., et al.: MRI of pediatric cardiac tumors previously diagnosed by echocardiography. J. Comput. Assist. Tomogr., 13(4):621–626, 1989.

Rokey, R., Vick, G. W., Bolli, R., et al.: Assessment of experimental pericardial effusion using nuclear magnetic resonance imaging techniques. Am. Heart J., 121(4):116–119, 1991.

Rozenman, Y., Zou, X., and Kantor, H. L.: Magnetic resonance imaging with superparamagnetic iron oxide particles for the detection of myocardial reperfusion. Magn. Reson. Imag., 9:933–939, 1991.

Saeed, M., Wendland, M. F., Tomei, E., et al.: Demarcation of myocardial ischemia: Magnetic susceptibility effect of contrast medium in MR imaging. Radiology, 173(3):763–777, 1989.

Schaefer, S., van Tyen, R., and Saloner, D.: Evaluation of myocardial perfusion abnormalities with gadolinium-enhanced snapshot MR imaging in humans. Work in progress. Radiology, 185(3):795–801, 1992.

Sechtem, U., Pflugfelder, P., Gould, R. G., et al.: Measurement of right and left ventricular volumes in healthy individuals with cine MR imaging. Radiology, 163:697–702, 1987.

Semelka, R. C., Shoenut, J. P., Wilson, M. E., et al.: Cardiac masses: Signal intensity features on spin-echo, gradient-echo, gadolinium-enhanced spin-echo, and Turbo FLASH images. J. Magn. Reson. Imag., 2:415–54, 1992.

Semelka, R. C., Tomei, E., Wagner, S., et al.: Interstudy reproducibility of dimensional and functional measurements between cine magnetic resonance studies in the morphologically abnormal left ventricle. Am. Heart J., 119(6):1367–1173, 1990a.

Semelka, R. C., Tomei, E., Wagner, S., et al.: Normal left ventricular dimensions and function: Interstudy reproducibility of measurements with cine MR imaging. Radiology, 174(3 part 1):763–768, 1990b.

Sieverding, L., Jung, W. L., Klose, U., and Apitz, J.: Noninvasive blood flow measurement and quantification of shunt volume by cine magnetic resonance in congenital heart disease. Preliminary results. Pediatr. Radiol., 22(1):48–54, 1992.

Sobel, B. E., Bresnahan, G. F., Shell, W. E., et al.: Estimation of infarct size in man and its relation to prognosis. Circulation, 56:640–648, 1972.

Soulen, R. L., Budinger, T. F., and Higgins, C. B.: Magnetic resonance imaging of prosthetic heart valves. Radiology, 154:704–707, 1985.

Stratemeier, E. J., Thompson, R., Brady, T., et al.: Ejection fraction determination by MR imaging: Comparison with left ventricular angiography. Radiology, 158:775–777, 1986.

Thompson, R. C., Lieu, P., Brady, T. J., et al.: Serial magnetic resonance imaging in patients following acute myocardial infarction. Magn. Reson. Imag., 9(2):155–158, 1991.

Turnbull, L. W., Ridgway, J. P., Nicoll, J. J., et al.: Estimating the size of myocardial infarction by magnetic resonance imaging. Br. Heart J., 66:359–363, 1991.

Underwood, S. R., Firmin, D. N., Kilpstein, R. H., et al.: Magnetic resonance velocity mapping: Clinical application of a new technique. Br. Heart J., 57:404–412, 1987.

Utz, J. A., Herfkens, R. J., Heinsimer, J. A., et al.: Cine MRI determination of left ventricular ejection fraction. A. J. R., 148:839–843, 1987.

Utz, J. A., Herfkens, R. J., Heinsimer, J. A., et al.: Dynamic magnetic resonance imaging in evaluation of cardiac valvular regurgitation. Radiology, 168:91–94, 1988.

van der Wall, E. E., van Dijkman, P. R. M., de Roos, A., et al.: Diagnostic significance of gadolinium-GDTPA enhanced magnetic resonance imaging in thrombolytic treatment for acute myocardial infarction: Its potential in assessing reperfusion. Br. Heart J., 63:12–17, 1990.

van Rossum, A. C., Visser, F. C., van Eenige, M. J., et al.: Value of gadolinium-diethylene-triamine pentaacetic acid dynamics in magnetic resonance imaging of acute myocardial infarction with occluded and reperfused coronary arteries after thrombolysis. Am. J. Cardiol., 65:845–851, 1990.

van Rugge, F. P., van der Wall, E. E., Dijkman, P. R., et al.: Usefulness of ultrafast magnetic resonance imaging in healed myocardial infarction. Am. J. Cardiol., 70(15):1233–1237, 1992.

Wang, J. Z., Mezrich, R. S., Scholz, P., et al.: MRI evaluation of left ventricular hypertrophy in a canine model of aortic stenosis. Invest. Radiol., 25(7):783–788, 1990.

Weissleder, R., Lee, A. S., Khaw, B. A., et al.: Antimyosin-labeled monocrystalline iron oxide allows detection of myocardial infarct: MR antibody imaging. Radiology, 182(2):381–385, 1992.

Wendland, M. F., Saeed, M., Masui, T., et al.: Echo-planar MR imaging of normal and ischemic myocardium with gadodiamide injection. Radiology, 186(2):535–542, 1993.

Wikstrom, M.: MR imaging of experimental myocardial infarction. Acta Radiol., 34(1):64–71, 1992.

Williams, E. S., Raylan, J. L., Thatcher, F., et al.: Prolongation of proton spin lattic relaxation times in regionally ischemic tissue from dog hearts. J. Nucl. Med., 21:449, 1980.

Yoo, S. J. Lim, T. H., Park, T. S., et al.: MR anatomy of ventricular septal defect in double-outlet right ventrical with situs solitus and atrioventricular concordance. Radiology, 181:501, 1991.

Yu, K. K., Saeed, M., Wendland, M. F., et al.: Real-time dynamics of an extravascular magnetic resonance contrast medium in acutely infarcted myocardium using inversion recovery and gradient recalled echo-planar imaging. Invest. Radiol., 27:927–934, 1992.

# ■ VI Radionuclide Imaging in Cardiac Surgery

Robert H. Jones

Radionuclide images provide less spatial resolution of the heart than do ultrasonography, color-flow Doppler, cine computed tomography (CT), and magnetic resonance imaging (MRI), and these images rarely depict sufficient anatomic detail to replace cardiac catheterization before cardiac surgical procedures. However, radionuclide techniques characterize cardiac function in patients more simply and completely than do techniques that excel in anatomic definition. Unique insight into physiologic abnormalities provided by radionuclide tests often aids in the selection and timing of operative therapy in individual patients with cardiac disorders. The simplicity of radionuclide procedures facilitates serial measurements before and after therapy to objectively document the outcome of the operation. Widespread use of these modalities in modern cardiology requires that cardiac surgeons be familiar with the basic aspects of these techniques and their application in common cardiac surgical disorders.

## RADIONUCLIDE TECHNIQUES FOR ASSESSMENT OF CARDIAC FUNCTION

The first use of radioactive tracers to assess any biologic process in humans was for evaluation of blood flow. In 1927, Blumgart and associates injected radon gas into veins of normal subjects and into patients with various cardiac disorders to measure transit times throughout the cardiovascular system. The crude technology then available for detecting radiation and lack of an apparent clinical use for these measurements caused this early insightful work to lapse into obscurity. In 1948, Prinzmetal and associates used newly developed single-probe detectors to quantitate the passage of a tracer bolus of radioactive sodium through the heart, and they called this rediscovered procedure *radiocardiography*. This improvement in technology renewed interest in the use of radionuclide indicator-dilution curves for calculation of cardiac output and measurement of intracardiac shunts in patients (MacIntyre et al., 1951).

In 1963, Bender and Blau first used a gamma camera to image individual cardiac chambers as tracer flowed through the heart. The potential was soon recognized to couple these instruments with computers to obtain data with sufficient anatomic resolution to provide indicator-dilution curves from individual cardiac chambers (Jones et al., 1967, 1972). Initial transit radionuclide angiocardiography evolved primarily as a useful way to measure left ventricular function (Jones et al., 1971; Scholz et al., 1980). This technique

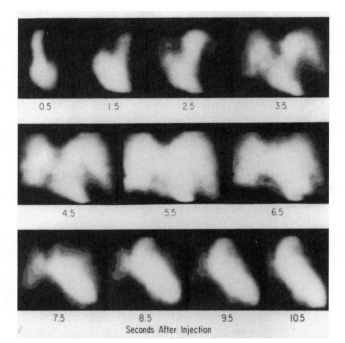

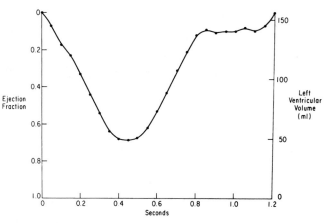

**FIGURE 31–83.** Representative cardiac cycle constructed from radionuclide data obtained during several individual contractions during the initial passage of tracer through the left ventricle. The volume changes are expressed as fractional changes. In addition, planimetry of the end-diastolic image provides an end-diastolic volume in milliliters so that the volume curve can also be calibrated as an absolute change in volume relative to time. The rapid increase in volume during end-diastole reflects left atrial contraction.

**FIGURE 31–81.** Serial 1-second images, each composed of twenty 0.05-second data frames, show the progression of the tracer bolus through the central circulation in the anterior view. The rapid transit through the heart is made apparent by the almost complete clearance of counts from the right ventricle while count rates are maximal in the left ventricle.

requires intravenous injection of a single bolus of radioactive tracer by using a high-sensitivity gamma camera for precordial counting at brief intervals, usually 25 msec. Dynamic counting images blood flow through the right side of the heart, lung, and left side of the heart (Fig. 31–81). To construct left-sided ventriculograms, computerized processing combines phasic-related counts from within the left ventricle during several cardiac cycles into an averaged cardiac beat, which has greater spatial and temporal resolution than the individual beats (Fig. 31–82). After subtraction of background counts arising outside the left ventricle, the remaining left ventricular count changes reflect relative left ventricular volume changes during the cardiac cycle (Fig. 31–83). Geometric assumptions commonly applied to contrast ventriculograms are

applied to the radionuclide image to calculate absolute left ventricular end-diastolic volume. Radionuclide measurements of ejection fraction, cardiac chamber volumes, and volumetric cardiac output compare favorably with contrast ventriculogram measurements. Moreover, the introduction of a high-fidelity micromanometer into the left ventricle to simultaneously record pressure during radionuclide volume measurement permits the construction of pressure-volume loops, which more completely characterize systolic and diastolic left ventricular function than the use of either pressure or volume parameters alone (Purut et al., 1988; Sell et al., 1991) (Fig. 31–84).

The counting sensitivity of standard gamma cameras is insufficient to image the heart from data recorded during the 5 to 10 cardiac beats when an injected tracer bolus first passes through the heart. An alternative approach of gated cardiac imaging acquires data after injected labeled red blood cells reach equilibrium within the blood pool. A simultaneous electrocardiogram synchronizes the acquisition of radionuclide data with the appropriate phase of each of the 100 to 300 heartbeats as counts are added to

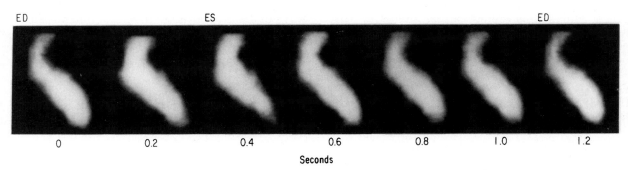

**FIGURE 31–82.** Serial images of the spatial distribution of counts taken from the representative cardiac cycle in Figure 31–83 show normal left ventricular wall motion. (*ED* = end-diastolic; *ES* = end-systolic.)

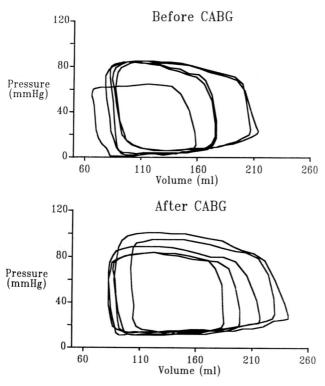

**FIGURE 31–84.** Pressure-volume loops at different levels of filling before and immediately after coronary artery bypass grafting *(CABG)* obtained by David Harpole, M.D., of Duke University Medical Center, show minimal depression of left ventricular function immediately after myocardial revascularization.

form a single averaged cardiac beat that is used to image cardiac motion and calculate ejection fraction. The advantage of gated equilibrium over initial transit cardiac imaging is that it does not require specific instrumentation or a discrete bolus injection. However, the 2 to 3 minutes required to acquire the gated image make the approach less well suited than the initial-transit technique for measuring cardiac function during periods of rapid change in cardiac function, such as during exercise or pharmacologic intervention. Moreover, cardiac volume calculations are less accurate and reproducible with the gated technique because of higher background noise, which results when tracer is at equilibrium in the blood pool. The gated equilibrium technique also requires withdrawal of a blood sample at equilibrium to relate observed counts to absolute cardiac volumes. This step is not required when using the initial-transit approach.

## RADIONUCLIDE TECHNIQUES FOR ASSESSMENT OF MYOCARDIAL PERFUSION AND METABOLISM

Radionuclide methods for noninvasive regional myocardial blood flow measurement are based on the observation of Sapirstein (1958) that the tissue content of any tracer with a high extraction rate during initial capillary transit is determined primarily by blood flow. This principle applies to potassium and the similar cationic tracers cesium, rubidium, and thallium, which accumulate in the myocardium in proportion to blood flow after intravenous injection much as particulate indicators injected directly into the coronary arteries do. Love and Burch (1958) first reported use of [86]Rb in dogs and humans for estimation of myocardial perfusion. The potassium analogue [201]Tl, with a half-life of 73 hours, is a widely used radionuclide for evaluation of regional myocardial perfusion.

After intravenous injection, [201]Tl attains a high initial myocardial concentration as the initial bolus passes through the coronary circulation. The subsequent myocardial distribution changes continually as the intracellular tracer exchanges with that remaining in the blood pool. Therefore, the distribution of [201]Tl during the first few minutes after injection closely reflects regional myocardial blood flow, but several hours after injection, it more closely resembles the amount of potassium in the heart. This characteristic of [201]Tl is used to obtain exercise and delayed redistribution images from a single tracer injection. A large clinical experience with [201]Tl has documented the value and limitations of myocardial scintigraphy in patients with myocardial infarction and ischemia. Sestamibi is a new compound with high myocardial extraction, which can be labeled with [99m]Tc to provide a myocardial perfusion agent with superior physical characteristics for imaging the distribution of coronary blood flow. An added advantage of using this radiopharmaceutical to assess perfusion is that cardiac function can be measured by radionuclide angiocardiography using the same injection (Borges-Neto et al., 1991).

The interaction of specific radiopharmaceuticals with the heart may be used to study regional myocardial metabolism. During myocardial infarction, calcium ions accumulate within injured myocardial cells. The affinity of [99m]Tc pyrophosphate for calcium produces a high accumulation of this tracer in infarcted myocardium (Bonte et al., 1974). Labeled monoclonal antibodies that react with myosin and fibrin have been developed that show promise for detecting myocardial cell breakdown and intravascular thrombosis (Haber, 1986). Cyclotron production of positron-emitting radiopharmaceuticals containing radioisotopes of carbon, oxygen, nitrogen, and fluorine now permit investigation of the full array of biochemical pathways in the myocardium. In addition to measurement of blood flow, regional myocardial accumulation and utilization of glucose, fatty acids, and amino acids can be assessed (Eitzman et al., 1992).

## RADIONUCLIDE IMAGING TECHNIQUES

Images of the distribution of a radioactive tracer in the heart detected by a gamma camera represent two-dimensional projections of counts arising from three dimensions of the cardiac volume. Simultaneous interpretation of several images obtained from different projections offers reasonable approximation of the three-dimensional count distribution in the heart. The most quantitative approach now available for imaging three-dimensional cardiac counts is single photon emission computed tomography (SPECT). During SPECT, the gamma camera detector encircles the patient; data from these multiple projections are later reconstructed into a three-dimensional representation of counts. These count matrices can be quantitated by comparison with normal standards or can be visually interpreted as a series of heart slice images. The accurate regional quantitation of counts provided by SPECT adds objectivity to radionuclide measurements of regional perfusion and metabolism.

Positron emission tomography (PET) is a technique that also uses a number of detectors encircling a patient to image positron-emitting tracers. Positron decay emits high-energy photons in opposite directions simultaneously, and this characteristic is used to accurately position the three-dimensional location of the original event. PET requires more expensive and complicated technology than SPECT does, and present applications are primarily for cardiac metabolism research.

## APPLICATIONS IN PATIENTS WITH CONGENITAL HEART DISORDERS

Surgical treatment of congenital heart disorders has progressed so that most patients with these diseases who previously would have died now survive. Therefore, therapy is no longer evaluated by the survival of the patient alone, and attention has been focused on forms of treatment that minimize myocardial tissue loss and optimally preserve cardiac function. Studies in adults with cardiac disease have documented that many patients with normal resting ventricular function have depressed ejection fractions during exercise. Much of this change appears to be related to exercise-induced myocardial ischemia, but these changes have also been observed in patients with long-standing ventricular volume overload resulting from valvular regurgitation. Therefore, the definition of cardiovascular function should, ideally, describe the performance of the heart both at rest and during the maximal level of activity typical in the daily routine of individual patients. Children studied after undergoing the Fontan and Mustard operations showed increased cardiac output during exercise as much as normal children did (Peterson et al., 1984, 1988). However, cardiac volume changes were abnormal during exercise in both groups of patients, reflecting chronic adaptations to abnormal anatomy of the congenital abnormality altered surgically. These measurements of ventricular function during exercise provide valuable insight into myocardial reserve in children with surgically corrected congenital heart disorders.

## APPLICATIONS IN PATIENTS WITH VALVULAR CARDIAC DISORDERS

Cardiac valvular abnormalities may alter left ventricular function either by the direct effect of the valve disorder on ventricular filling or emptying or by chronic changes within the myocardium in response to the long-standing hemodynamic alteration. Patients with mitral stenosis have restriction of left ventricular filling that becomes more prominent during exercise and limits forward cardiac output. Mitral valvulotomy or replacement eliminates the restriction to filling and returns cardiac function toward normal during rest and exercise (Newman et al., 1979). Aortic stenosis restricts left ventricular emptying, and the decrease in left ventricular ejection fraction that occurs during exercise in these patients may be caused by the large afterload imposed by the stenosis. Also, myocardial ischemia may occur during exercise when myocardial work increases oxygen utilization above that supplied by the coronary blood flow, which is limited by the stenosis. Early in the course of aortic stenosis, left ventricular hypertrophy decreases the end-diastolic volume and causes an abnormally high left ventricular ejection fraction. Late in the natural history of aortic stenosis, the ejection fraction during exercise decreases, and the resting ejection fraction ultimately is also abnormally low. Patients with aortic stenosis who are permitted to progress to resting left ventricular dysfunction have a less favorable prognosis after aortic valve replacement.

Aortic and mitral valve regurgitation increases left ventricular end-diastolic and stroke volumes, and patients with incompetent left-sided valves commonly eject a normal forward cardiac output in addition to the amount of regurgitant blood. An ideal management strategy for patients with aortic and mitral regurgitation would be to withhold valve replacement until such time as further nonoperative therapy would adversely affect the prognosis. Signs or symptoms of cardiac failure in these patients are a frequently used but inconsistent index of cardiac deterioration. The appearance of moderate resting left ventricular dysfunction identifies patients who face greater operative risk if operation is further delayed. Moreover, patients with clinical cardiac failure or left ventricular dysfunction before replacement or repair of an insufficient valve may not regain normal exercise tolerance or cardiac function after valve replacement (Peter et al., 1981). Serial measurements of left ventricular function during rest and exercise by using radionuclide angiocardiography define the time of onset of exercise-induced left ventricular dysfunction that consistently appears before resting dysfunction (Peter and Jones, 1980). Patients with mild exercise-induced left ventricular dysfunction may be safely continued on medical treatment. Patients with more severe dysfunction should be carefully considered for valve replacement.

Simultaneous radionuclide left ventriculography and micromanometry during preload manipulation permit intraoperative assessment of myocardial performance in humans. Despite major alterations in left ventricular systolic loading and ejection fraction after correction of aortic stenosis and mitral regurgitation, intrinsic myocardial contractility showed little change during elective valve replacement (Harpole et al., 1989) (Fig. 31–85).

## APPLICATIONS IN PATIENTS WITH CORONARY ARTERY DISEASE

The major challenge in current management of symptomatic patients with coronary artery disease is risk stratification. The large group of low-risk patients must be separated from the smaller subset of patients with a sufficiently high probability of a cardiac event in the future to require an evaluation for interventional therapy. Previous clinical studies of treatment of coronary artery disease have emphasized that the anatomic severity and extensiveness of coronary atherosclerosis is one of the most important predictors of natural history of the disease in an individual patient. The number, severity, and location of stenoses in coronary arteries dictate the amount of myocardium at jeopardy for ischemic events and identify patients with a higher incidence of myocardial infarction and cardiac death. Patients with the most extensive forms of disease, such as left main coronary artery stenosis, derive the greatest benefit from revascularization procedures. Despite the prognostic importance of coronary angiographic definition of extensiveness of disease, this single parameter does not contain all of the information needed for risk stratification. For example, even in patients who have left main coronary artery stenosis and who are treated medically, 70% survive for at least 5 years; thus, even this strong predictor of risk involves considerable uncertainty when applied to an individual patient.

Radionuclide tests appear particularly well suited for screening large groups of patients. Individuals with the most severe abnormalities can be selected for cardiac catheterization and possible further intervention, whereas those who are defined to be at very low risk would require catheterization in only special circumstances. Myocardial ischemia can be detected clinically by angina pectoris, electrocardiographically by ST segment depression, and functionally by regional perfusion abnormalities and segmental contraction abnormalities with associated hemodynamic alterations. Exercise-induced left ventricular dysfunction is a sensitive marker of ischemia that commonly occurs before an electrocardiographic abnormality as ischemia progressively increases in an individual patient (Upton et al., 1980). Radionuclide techniques measuring ventricular function and myocardial perfusion reflect similar biologic processes because of the close link between myocardial integrity and blood flow. Therefore, perfusion defects on exercise myocardial scintigraphy that disappear after an interval adequate for [201]Tl redistribution are also sensitive markers of ischemia. Myocardial infarction with subsequent fibrosis decreases resting regional and global ventricular function and causes a resting perfusion defect because of loss of myocardial mass and the lower tissue blood flow rate of fibrotic myocardium.

Soon after radionuclide tests were introduced for detecting exercise-induced perfusion defects and functional abnormalities as indicators of myocardial

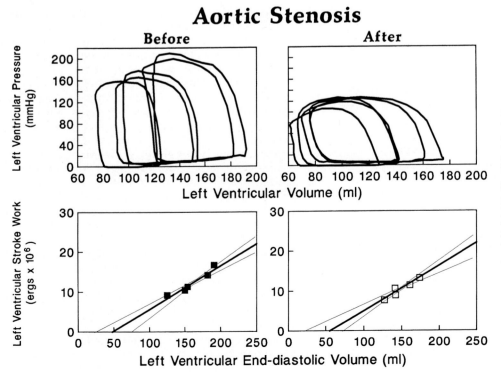

**FIGURE 31–85.** Pressure (mm Hg)-volume (ml) curves *(upper panels)* and stroke work (ergs $\times$ $10^6$)-volume (ml) curves *(lower panels)* for patient with aortic stenosis. Curves before *(left panels)* and after *(right panels)* aortic valve replacement illustrate diminished left ventricular load associated with valvular replacement. Left ventricular ejection fraction increased from 0.38 to 0.51; however, the stroke work/end-diastolic volume relationship ($\pm$2 SD) was unchanged.

ischemia, enthusiastic reports suggested that these procedures were highly accurate for diagnosis of coronary artery disease. Further experience with broader populations of patients shows that resting-exercise perfusion and function tests have an accuracy that ranges between 0.75 and 0.85 for the prediction of coronary disease (Jones et al., 1981). Therefore, the severity of coronary artery disease reflected by the anatomic information from the coronary arteriogram correlates with that suggested by ischemia assessment of radionuclide stress tests in groups of patients. However, a consistent discrepancy occurs between the two approaches in 15 to 25% of patients with coronary artery disease. The early disappointment in the lack of complete agreement between radionuclide tests and coronary angiograms has been interpreted as a benefit, because the two forms of information appear to provide independent prognostic information in patients with coronary artery disease.

[201]Tl imaging more accurately detects coronary artery disease than treadmill electrocardiography does (Brown, 1991; Pollack et al., 1992). The number and location of perfusion defects on [201]Tl scans relate to the extent of coronary artery disease, and the severity of perfusion defects relates to the degree of coronary artery stenosis. Brown and associates (1983) monitored 100 medically treated patients without previous myocardial infarction for a mean of 3.7 years and documented a cardiac event rate of 3% in patients with normal thallium test results and of 33% in patients with three or more defects. In 1689 consecutive patients with suspected coronary artery disease followed for 1 year, Ladenheim and associates (1986) found three variables that provided independent prognostic information: (1) the number of reversible thallium defects—an extent variable, (2) the magnitude of initial reversible defect—a severity variable, and (3) the maximal heart rate achieved during exercise. Combining these variables into a prognostic model categorized risk of a cardiac event from a low cardiac event rate of less than 1% in patients with a normal exercise thallium study to a high event rate of 78% in patients developing severe and extensive reversible defects at a low achieved heart rate.

Reversible left ventricular dysfunction as an indicator of ischemia was first shown in humans by Herman and colleagues (1967), who studied patients with unstable angina during and after periods of spontaneous pain. Sharma and associates (1976) used contrast angiography to show reversible alterations of regional left ventricular function induced by exercise and cardiac pacing. Measurements of ventricular function obtained at rest and during exercise using radionuclide angiocardiography provide a simple approach for assessing the extent of fibrosis and the quantity of potentially ischemic myocardium in individual patients (Rerych et al., 1978).

Pryor and associates (1984) first reported the magnitude of left ventricular dysfunction induced by exercise to relate to later myocardial infarction or cardiovascular death. Lee and associates (1990) compared the prognostic value of exercise radionuclide and cardiac catheterization variables in 571 medically treated patients. The exercise ejection fraction was the most important radionuclide variable that provided prognostic information in patients with coronary artery disease. This simple variable contained more than 70% of the prognostic information provided by combination of other important variables such as the coronary anatomy on arteriogram. The relationship between cardiac event and exercise ejection fraction was not linear, and patients with an exercise ejection fraction above 0.5 had few myocardial infarctions or cardiac deaths (Fig. 31–86). In groups of patients with progressively lower ejection fractions, the number of cardiac events increased dramatically. These observations suggest that measurement of variables such as the exercise ejection fraction, which relates to the magnitude of ischemia, can be used to stratify the risk for individual patients with coronary artery disease. Patients recognized to have a low risk of cardiac events should receive medical treatment. Patients identified to have a high likelihood of myocardial infarction or death benefit most from bypass surgery or other interventional therapy. Although exercise thallium-201 scintigraphy and radionuclide angiocardiography are frequently used for prognosis in patients with coronary artery disease, little is known about the independence, concordance, or relative importance of these two studies. The use of both tests in the same patient has been impractical because of the logistic considerations imposed by two exercise tests on separate days and excessive radiation exposure. New [99m]Tc-labeled radiopharmaceuticals with high myocardial extraction now permit simultaneous assessment of myocardial perfusion and ventricular function during treadmill exercise. Performing all three tests during a single exercise session is an attractive way to risk-stratify patients with coronary artery disease. Moreover, accumulation of more data in patient populations will permit direct comparison of the most useful physiologic variables for identifying

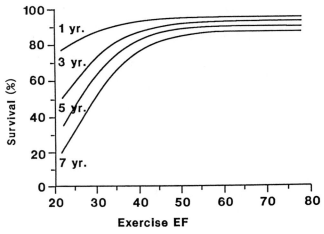

**FIGURE 31–86.** Curve of survival at 1, 3, 5, and 7 years as a function of exercise ejection fraction (EF). Calculated using spline functions with Cox model.

patients likely to benefit from myocardial revascularization.

Perhaps the most important diagnostic use of combined function and perfusion measurements is to add certainty via test redundancy. Test results that are concordantly positive or negative increase the diagnostic weight of the test, which becomes especially important in patients in whom the noninvasive test results appear to contradict other clinical information. In addition, contradictory findings on the function and perfusion study detract from the certainty of diagnosis and raise the need for more careful evaluation for artifacts or spurious results. Discordant test results that appear valid point toward different physiologic mechanisms, because only the distribution of perfusion and not total perfusion is reflected by the procedure in contrast to the function result, which is influenced more by total coronary blood flow than by regional distribution of the flow.

Studies are now being conducted to assess the need for both perfusion and function measurements for risk stratification and prognosis. Some degree of redundancy of information is expected, because a demonstrable correlation has been shown between these two measurements obtained simultaneously in patients with coronary artery disease. However, the relationship between function and perfusion is not identical, and it is likely that both will contribute independent prognostic information.

## RADIONUCLIDE ANGIOCARDIOGRAPHY AFTER CORONARY ARTERY BYPASS GRAFTING

Not every patient who survives coronary artery bypass grafting has an optimal function result. Even the absence of angina after bypass cannot be used as a valid end-point, because either denervation of the heart or perioperative infarction of myocardium that had been ischemic may decrease or obliterate anginal pain.

Patients with good anatomic results documented by angiography after coronary bypass grafting also improve exercise-induced myocardial dysfunction and perfusion deficits after successful bypass. However, coronary blood flow at rest and the potential for flow augmentation during exercise cannot always be predicted from the coronary angiogram. Graft and vessel patency on arteriogram does not always correlate with improvements in regional function and perfusion. Therefore, as before operation, radionuclide tests provide important data that are complementary but that do not always duplicate the information obtained from coronary angiography. Radionuclide procedures objectively document improvement in myocardial perfusion and function, and the end-points are useful to judge effectiveness of operative outcome and predict the future clinical course of individual patients.

Radionuclide measurements of resting left ventricular function before and after bypass operation show

that 10 to 20% of patients have a significant decrease in left ventricular function (Floyd et al., 1983a). This loss in function is permanent and often occurs without clinical symptoms or changes that suggest infarction on the electrocardiogram. A prospective study of 104 patients by Floyd and associates (1983b) showed that QRS change on the electrocardiogram and left ventricular function after coronary artery bypass grafting were unrelated. The loss of left ventricular function did not relate to the duration of hypothermic cardioplegic arrest, and the cause of this functional result probably relates to multiple factors that are now poorly understood. Approximately 10 to 20% of patients show significantly improved resting function after myocardial revascularization, which suggests that reversible resting ischemic dysfunction was present before the operation in the absence of resting pain. Although resting improvement in left ventricular function is modest in most patients, significant abnormal function observed before operation is normalized dramatically after revascularization in some patients.

Physiologic improvement after myocardial revascularization is documented most consistently by radionuclide studies of myocardial function and perfusion during exercise. As early as 8 days after operation, patients have been shown to have greatly improved exercise left ventricular ejection fraction, and this improvement persists in later studies (Austin et al., 1983). This early documentation of reversal of myocardial ischemia provides a useful baseline for patients who later become symptomatic. Subsequent radionuclide studies can quantify the amount of return of ischemia associated with disease progression or graft occlusion and provide a rational basis for the selection of patients who might profit from repeated catheterization and consideration of another revascularization procedure.

### SELECTED BIBLIOGRAPHY

Blumgart, H. L., and Weiss, S.: Clinical studies on the velocity of blood flow. The pulmonary circulation time, the velocity of venous blood flow to the heart, and related aspects of the circulation in patients with cardiovascular disease. J. Clin. Invest., 4:343, 1927.

This series of related articles represents the first use of radioactive tracers in humans and is a model of early insightful clinical investigation.

Jones, R. H., Johnson, S. H., Bigelow, C., et al.: Exercise radionuclide angiocardiography predicts cardiac death in patients with coronary artery disease. Circulation, 84(Suppl. I):52–58, 1991.

This report demonstrated the prognostic information of exercise ejection fraction in 2042 consecutive patients evaluated for coronary artery disease. An exercise ejection fraction of > 0.50 was associated with a good long-term mortality rate, and exercise ejection fractions below this level defined a higher risk of cardiac death.

Zaret, B. L., and Beller, G. A.: Nuclear Cardiology: State of the Art and Future Directions. St. Louis, C. V. Mosby, 1993.

This monograph provides a good review of the state of the art and future directions of nuclear cardiology.

### BIBLIOGRAPHY

Austin, E. H., Oldham, H. N., Jr., Sabiston, D. C., Jr., and Jones, R. H.: Early assessment of rest and exercise left ventricular function following coronary artery surgery. Ann. Thorac. Surg., *35*:159, 1983.

Bender, M. A., and Blau, M.: The autofluoroscope. Nucleonics, *21*:52, 1963.

Bonte, F. J., Parkey, R. W., Graham, K. D., et al.: A new method for radionuclide imaging of myocardial infarcts. Radiology, *110*:473, 1974.

Borges-Neto, S., Coleman, R. E., Potts, J. M., and Jones, R. H.: Combined exercise radionuclide angiocardiography and single photon emission computed tomography perfusion studies for assessment of coronary artery disease. Semin. Nucl. Med., *21*:223, 1991.

Brown, K. A.: Prognostic value of thallium-201 perfusion imaging. A diagnostic tool comes of age. Circulation, *83*:363, 1991.

Brown, K. A., Boucher, C. A., Okada, R. D., et al.: Prognostic value of exercise thallium-201 imaging in patients presenting for evaluation of chest pain. J. Am. Coll. Cardiol., *4*:146, 1983.

Eitzman, D., Al-Aouar, Z., Kanter, H., et al.: Clinical outcome of patients with advanced coronary artery disease after viability studies with positron emission tomography. J. Am. Coll. Cardiol., *29*:559, 1992.

Floyd, R. D., Sabiston, D. C., Jr., Lee, K. L., and Jones, R. H.: The effect of duration of hypothermic cardioplegia on ventricular function. J. Thorac. Cardiovasc. Surg., *85*:606, 1983a.

Floyd, R. D., Wagner, G. S., Austin, E. H., et al.: Relation between QRS changes and left ventricular function after coronary artery bypass grafting. Am. J. Cardiol., *52*:943, 1983b.

Haber, E.: In vivo diagnostic and therapeutic uses of monoclonal antibodies in cardiology. Annu. Rev. Med., *37*:249, 1986.

Harpole, D. H., Rankin, J. S., Wolfe, W. G., et al.: Assessment of left ventricular functional preservation during isolated cardiac valve operations. Circulation, *80*(Suppl. III):1, 1989.

Herman, M. V., Heinle, R. A., Klein, M. D., et al.: Localized disorders in myocardial contraction: Asynergy and its role in congestive heart failure. N. Engl. J. Med., *227*:222, 1967.

Jones, R. H., Goodrich, J. K., Sabiston, D. C., Jr.: Quantitative radionuclide angiocardiography in evaluation of cardiac function. Surg. Forum, *22*:138, 1971.

Jones, R. H., Goodrich, J. K., Sabiston, D. C., Jr.: Radioactive lung scanning in the diagnosis and management of pulmonary disorders. J. Thorac. Cardiovasc. Surg., *54*:520, 1967.

Jones, R. H., McEwan, P., Newman, G. E., et al.: Accuracy of diagnosis of coronary artery disease by radionuclide measurement of left ventricular function during rest and exercise. Circulation, *64*:585, 1981.

Jones, R. H., Sabiston, D. C., Jr., Bates, B. B., et al.: Quantitative radionuclide angiocardiography for determination of chamber-to-chamber cardiac transit times. Am. J. Cardiol., *30*:855, 1972.

Ladenheim, M. L., Pollock, B. H., Rozanski, A., and Berman, D. S.: Extent and severity of myocardial hypoperfusion as predictors of prognosis in patients with suspected coronary artery disease. J. Am. Coll. Cardiol., *7*:464, 1986.

Lee, K. L., Pryor, D. B., and Pieper, K. S.: Prognostic value of radionuclide angiography in medically-treated patients with coronary artery disease. A comparison with clinical and catheterization variables. Circulation, *82*:1705, 1990.

Love, W. D., and Burch, G. E.: Estimation of the rates of uptake of

Rb-86 by the heart, liver and skeletal muscle of man with and without cardiac disease. Int. J. Appl. Radiat. Isot., *3*:207, 1958.

MacIntyre, W. J., Pritchard, W. H., Eckstein, R. W., and Friedell, H. L.: The determination of cardiac output by a continuous recording system utilizing iodinated (I-131) human serum albumin. Circulation, *4*:552, 1951.

Newman, G. E., Rerych, S. K., Bounous, E. P., et al.: Noninvasive assessment of hemodynamic effects of mitral valve commissurotomy during rest and exercise in patients with mitral stenosis. J. Thorac. Cardiovasc. Surg., *78*:750, 1979.

Peter, C. A., Austin, E. H., and Jones, R. H.: Effect of valve replacement for chronic mitral insufficiency on left ventricular function during rest and exercise. J. Thorac. Cardiovasc. Surg., *82*:127, 1981.

Peter, C. A., and Jones, R. H.: Radionuclide measurements of left ventricular function: Their use in patients with aortic insufficiency. Arch. Surg., *115*:1348, 1980.

Peterson, R. J., Franch, R. H., Fajman, W. A., et al.: Noninvasive determination of exercise cardiac function following Fontan operation. J. Thorac. Cardiovasc. Surg., *88*:263, 1984.

Peterson, R. J., Franch, R. H., Fajman, W. A., and Jones, R. H.: Comparison of cardiac function in surgically corrected and congenitally corrected transposition of the great vessels. J. Thorac. Cardiovasc. Surg., *96*:227, 1988.

Pollack, S. G., Abbott, R. D., Boucher, C. A., et al.: Independent and incremental prognostic value of tests performed in hierarchical order to evaluate patients with suspected coronary artery disease and validation of models based on these tests. Circulation, *85*:237, 1992.

Prinzmetal, M., Corday, E., Bergman, H. C., et al.: Radiocardiography: A new method for studying the blood flow through the chambers of the heart in human beings. Science, *108*:340, 1948.

Pryor, D. B., Harrell, F. E., Jr., Lee, K. L., et al.: Prognostic indicators from radionuclide angiography in medically treated patients with coronary artery disease. Am. J. Cardiol., *53*:18, 1984.

Purut, C. M., Sell, T. L., and Jones, R. H.: A new method to determine left ventricular pressure-volume loops in the clinical setting. J. Nucl. Med., *29*:1492, 1988.

Rerych, S. K., Scholz, P. M., Newman, G. E., et al.: Cardiac function at rest and during exercise in normals and in patients with coronary heart disease: Evaluation by radionuclide angiocardiography. Ann. Surg., *187*:449, 1978.

Sapirstein, L. A.: Regional blood flow by fractional distribution of indicators. Am. J. Physiol., *193*:161, 1958.

Scholz, P. M., Rerych, S. K., Moran, J. F., et al.: Quantitative radionuclide angiocardiography. Cathet. Cardiovasc. Diagn., *6*:265, 1980.

Sell, T. L., Purut, C. M., Silva, R., et al.: Recovery of myocardial function during coronary artery bypass grafting. J. Thorac. Cardiovasc. Surg., *101*:681, 1991.

Sharma, B., Goodwin, J. F., Raphael, M. J., et al.: Left ventricular angiography on exercise: A new method of assessing left ventricular function in ischemic heart disease. Br. Heart J., *38*:59, 1976.

Upton, M. T., Rerych, S. K., Newman, G. E., et al.: Detecting abnormalities in left ventricular function during exercise before angina and ST-segment depression. Circulation, *62*:341, 1980.

# ■ VII  Ultrasound Applications in Cardiac Surgery: Echocardiography

Peter K. Smith and Joseph A. Kisslo

In 1954, Edler and Hertz introduced the use of ultrasound to image cardiac structures dynamically. A-mode echocardiography (Fig. 31–87) permitted noninvasive diagnosis of pericardial effusion. The development of M-mode echocardiography provided a spatially limited, time-oriented view of the heart and enabled physicians to assess cardiac valve motion (Fig. 31–88). Obtaining a satisfactory sonogram required a high degree of technical skill, however, and interpretation remained exclusively within the domain of the trained echocardiographer. Despite these limitations, several investigators used this technology to study ventricular function during cardiac procedures in humans (Spotnitz et al., 1979) and in animals (Gaudiani et al., 1978). M-mode echocardiography was also used to assess the efficacy of mitral commissurotomy (Johnson et al., 1972; Mary et al., 1976) and to detect late cardiac tamponade after open heart procedures (Fernando et al., 1977).

Since that time, four technologic developments have significantly broadened the clinical and research applications of ultrasound:

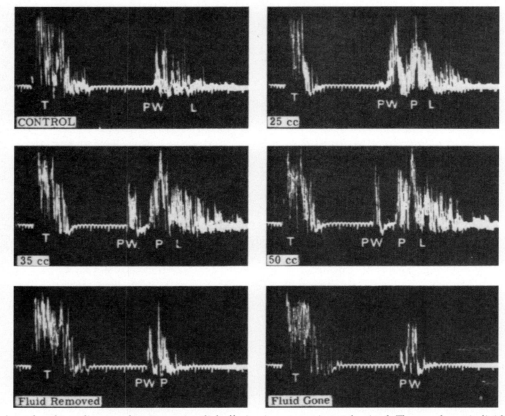

**FIGURE 31–87.** A-mode echocardiogram showing pericardial effusion in an experimental animal. The panels are individually labeled and progress from *top left* to *bottom right*. (T = transducer; PW = posterior wall of ventricle; P = pericardium; L = lung.) The control panel shows no echo-free space between the posterior ventricular wall and the lung. Twenty-five milliliters of saline are infused into the pericardial space, permitting visual separation of the posterior ventricular wall and the pericardium. This space progressively increases as 35 ml and then 50 ml are infused. In the *last two panels,* the fluid is removed, obliterating the pericardial space. (From Feigenbaum, H., Waldhausen, J. A., and Hyde, L. P.: Ultrasound diagnosis of pericardial effusion. J. A. M. A., *191*:711–714. Copyright 1965, American Medical Association.)

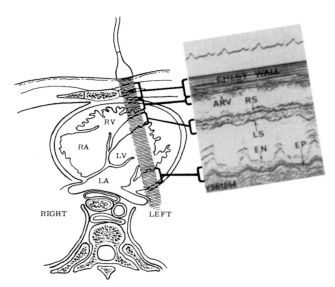

**FIGURE 31–88.** M-mode echocardiogram demonstrating an "ice-pick" view through the heart over time, with the transducer placed parasternally. (ARV = anterior right ventricle; RS = right side of ventricular septum; LS = left side of ventricular septum; EN = endocardium; EP = epicardium.) There is no pericardial effusion. (From Feigenbaum, H.: Echocardiography. 4th ed. Philadelphia, Lea & Febiger, 1986.)

1. Two-dimensional echocardiography
2. Pulsed and continuous-wave Doppler echocardiography
3. Color-flow Doppler echocardiography
4. Transesophageal echocardiography

These developments have made it mandatory that cardiothoracic surgeons understand ultrasound and its applications.

This chapter emphasizes the application of ultrasound techniques in the operating room. Perioperative ultrasound applications that offer *unique* diagnostic and therapeutic options for cardiac surgical patients are also discussed.

## BASIC PRINCIPLES OF ULTRASOUND

Ultrasound is defined as sound with a frequency greater than 20,000 cycles per second (Kossoff, 1966). Sound is composed of a time-oriented series of compressed and rarefied air (Fig. 31–89). Frequencies in the range of 2.5 to 10 million cycles per second (mHz) currently are used for various medical diagnostic applications. Ultrasound is inaudible, is reflected at tissue interfaces, and can be directed into a relatively coherent beam. It is propagated well through a liquid medium and extremely poorly through a gaseous medium. Thus, to visualize cardiac structures, an acoustic pathway or window that is free of air must be found through which the beam and its reflections can be directed appropriately. These features of ultrasound have limited its application in pulmonary medicine but have led to the development of various microbubble echocardiographic contrast agents, which are discussed later.

The acquisition of an ultrasound image begins with the generation of a sound wave from an ultrasound transducer, which changes electrical energy to mechanical (sound) energy. This wave travels through soft tissue and blood at an average speed of 1540 m/sec (Goldman and Jueter, 1956). As it passes through tissue, the sound wave is attenuated and scattered in proportion to the acoustic impedance of each particular tissue (Gregg and Palogallo, 1969). When the sound wave encounters a boundary between two tissues of different acoustic impedance (Fig. 31–90), this mismatch causes reflection and refraction of the sound wave. The amount of reflection is directly proportional to the degree of acoustic impedance mismatch and the angle at which the sound wave inter-

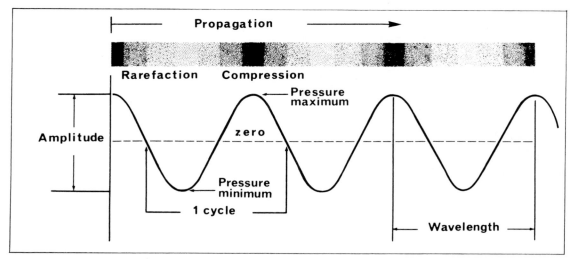

**FIGURE 31–89.** A schematic illustration of a coherent sound wave. A continuous sinusoidal waveform is demonstrated in the direction of propagation showing the amplitude on an arbitrary pressure scale. The cycle length and wave length are shown on an arbitrary time scale. The sound frequency is the reciprocal of wave length. (From Feigenbaum, H.: Echocardiography. 4th ed. Philadelphia, Lea & Febiger, 1986.)

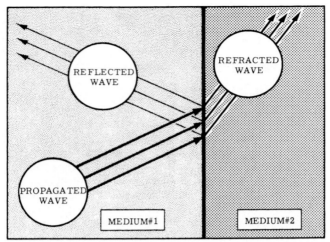

**FIGURE 31–90.** The relative reflection and refraction of a propagated ultrasound wave between two media of differing acoustic impedance. (From Feigenbaum, H.: Echocardiography. 4th ed. Philadelphia, Lea & Febiger, 1986.)

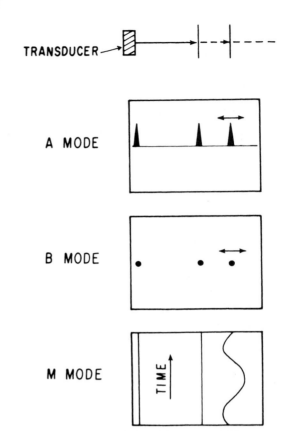

**FIGURE 31–92.** A schematic illustration relating the position of the transducer to two reflecting objects, the second varying in time (*horizontal arrow*). A-, B-, and M-mode echocardiography are illustrated (see text for description). (From DeBruijn, N. P., and Clements, F. M. [eds]: Transesophageal Echocardiography. Boston, Martinus Nijhoff, 1987, p. 22.)

cepts the boundary (Fig. 31–91). Additional factors influencing reflection include the size of the medium traversed and the sound frequency.

Currently available commercial transducers spend approximately 0.1% of the time transmitting ultrasound and the remaining 99.9% of time receiving reflected sound waves. Transducer sensitivity allows the detection of returning sound waves, which are reduced to less than 1% of the transmitted ultrasonic energy. The received signal is related in time to the transmitted signal, and that time is related to the speed of sound in tissue to determine the distance of the reflecting agent. In this way, various "echoes" are arrayed along the line of the ultrasound beam. An oscilloscope can show the relative intensity and timing of the returned signal (A mode, Fig. 31–92). The intensity of returned ultrasound can alternatively be converted into a varying display intensity, whereas the timing is recorded as distance on the oscilloscope screen (B mode, Fig. 31–92). In these modes, positional changes of the ultrasound reflector studied

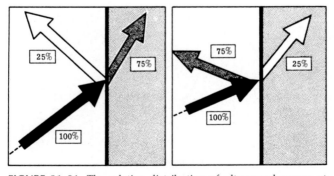

**FIGURE 31–91.** The relative distribution of ultrasound energy at the time of reflection and refraction is shown to be proportionate to the incidence angle when the acoustic impedance mismatch is held constant (propagated wave is shown as the *black arrow*). (From Feigenbaum, H.: Echocardiography. 2nd ed. Philadelphia, Lea & Febiger, 1976.)

(*horizontal arrow* in Fig. 31–92) are shown instantly. By using the second dimension of the display as a time base, these positional changes can be shown continuously (M-mode, Fig. 31–92; see also Fig. 31–88). By sweeping this line throughout an arc, either mechanically or electronically (Fig. 31–93), a tomogram of reflected sound can be obtained (Fig. 31–94). These methods and displays are similar to those used in radar.

The depth and resolution of the tomogram depend highly on the frequency of ultrasound used. With increasing frequency, smaller objects and interfaces cause reflections. At the same time, less ultrasonic energy is available as the acoustic pathway is traversed. Thus, increasing frequency produces better resolution at the expense of penetration. A 2.25-mHz ultrasound wave can effectively penetrate to a depth of approximately 20 cm and yield a range resolution of approximately 1 mm.

## PRINCIPLES OF DOPPLER ECHOCARDIOGRAPHY

The Doppler principle has been applied to ultrasound to quantify regional blood velocity either in

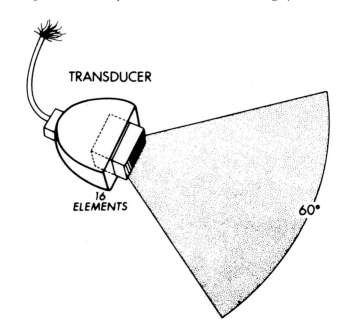

**FIGURE 31–93.** An early phased-array transducer capable of electronically transmitting ultrasound through a 60-degree arc. (From von Ramm, O. T., and Thurstone, F. L.: Cardiac imaging using a phased array ultrasound system. I: System design. Circulation, 53:258, 1976. By permission of the American Heart Association, Inc.)

the heart or great vessels. The physical principle was described originally by Doppler in reference to the effect of motion on the wavelength of light.

The Doppler shift in clinical ultrasound is created by motion of red blood cells (as ultrasound reflectors) either toward or away from the transducer (Fig. 31–95). Motion of red blood cells toward the transducer increases the frequency of the returned signal in proportion to their velocity, which is expressed by the Doppler equation (Fig. 31–96). The angle (the angle between the Doppler beam and the direction of blood flow) also affects the Doppler shift. Similarly, flow away from the transducer reduces the returning frequency. The Doppler equation can be solved for velocity by assuming that the angle is zero (which may

not always be the case). Information about the Doppler shift is also converted into audible sounds, which are broadcast to the equipment operator.

Quantification of this information is accomplished by showing the distribution of velocities detected over time on the echocardiographic monitor (Fig. 31–97). This spectrum can be further analyzed by fast Fourier transformation to display the distribution of the various velocities encompassed by the acoustic pathway over time (Fig. 31–98), and to calculate various indices characterizing portions of the cardiac cycle (Fig. 31–99).

Continuous-wave Doppler echocardiography uses continuous, simultaneous ultrasound generation and reception with a two-crystal transducer (Fig. 31–100).

**FIGURE 31–94.** As the ultrasound beam is swept through a tomographic plane, the returning echo data (depicted as *dots* at the intersection of each discrete ultrasound wave and schematic endocardial and epicardial surfaces) are stored and displayed sequentially as numbered. The time of the return is displayed sequentially as numbered. The time of the return signal is used to determine range, and the time from signal transmission is used to reconstruct the sweep angle. (From DeBruijn, N. P., and Clements, F. M. [eds]: Transesophageal Echocardiography. Boston, Martinus Nijhoff, 1987.)

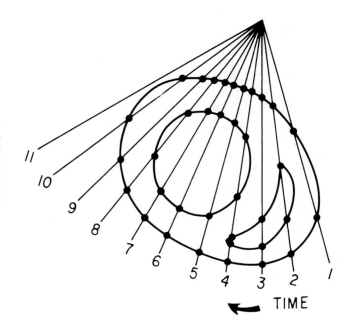

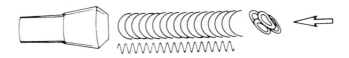

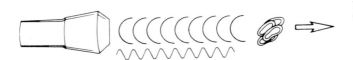

**FIGURE 31–95.** The Doppler shift, showing an increase in the frequency of return sound from red blood cell reflectors moving toward the transducer *(top)* and a corresponding decrease in return frequency from red blood cells moving away from the transducer *(bottom)*. (From Kisslo, J., and Adams, D. B.: An Introduction to Doppler Echocardiography. Vol. 1. New York, Medi Cine Productions, 1987.)

**FIGURE 31–96.** An illustration of the Doppler equation as applied to red blood cells moving toward the transducer within a blood vessel. The angle θ represents the angle of incidence between the ultrasound beam and the direction of flow. As this angle is minimized, cosine θ approaches 1 and the angle effect is removed from the equation. (From Kisslo, J., and Adams, D. B.: An Introduction to Doppler Echocardiography. Vol. 1. New York, Medi Cine Productions, 1987.)

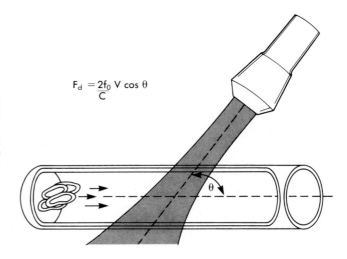

$$F_d = \frac{2f_0 \, V \cos \theta}{C}$$

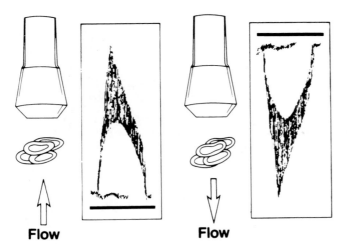

**Flow**      **Flow**

**FIGURE 31–97.** Flowing elements toward the transducer *(left)* are displayed with positive velocities above the baseline. In mid ejection, there is a relatively wide range of velocities within the acoustic pathway, creating a broad band in the velocity spectrum. Similarly, flow away from the transducer *(right)* creates a spectrum of velocities presented below the baseline. (From Kisslo, J., and Adams, D. B.: An Introduction to Doppler Echocardiography. Vol. 1. New York, Medi Cine Productions, 1987.)

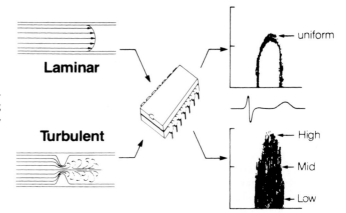

**FIGURE 31–98.** The velocity data detected by the Doppler instruments are processed by fast Fourier transform, and the resulting spectrum of velocities is displayed. Laminar flows are uniform, whereas turbulent flow shows spectral broadening.

**Systolic Velocity Indices**

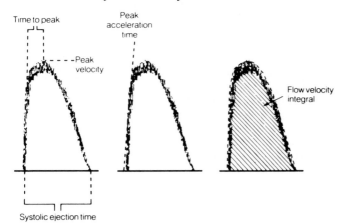

**FIGURE 31–99.** An idealized systolic aortic velocity profile and the derived indices, systolic ejection time, peak velocity, and time to peak velocity are shown on the left side of the panel. Peak acceleration time and the flow velocity integral can also be automatically derived. (From Kisslo, J., and Adams, D. B.: An Introduction to Doppler Echocardiography. Vol. 2. New York, Medi Cine Productions, 1987.)

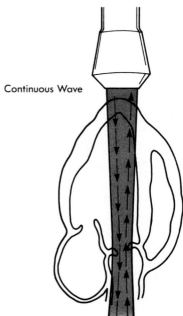

Continuous Wave

**FIGURE 31–100.** Continuous-wave Doppler positioned to interrogate blood velocity along a path from the left ventricular apex through the left ventricular outflow tract and into the aorta. Separate sending and receiving transducers analyze continuous ultrasound, which can be used to determine high velocities occurring along this pathway. As can be seen, these velocities are returned from any position within the acoustic pathway (*outlined in gray*), but the specific location of each discrete velocity subset cannot be determined. (From Kisslo, J., and Adams, D. B.: An Introduction to Doppler Echocardiography. Vol. 1. New York, Medi Cine Productions, 1987.)

Although this can determine high velocities, it cannot discriminate the location of any particular group of velocities shown. With a single transducer that alternates between transmission and reception of ultrasound, it is possible to discriminate the depth at which velocity is determined, again by knowing the average speed of sound through tissues and blood (Fig. 31–101). This range gating, called pulsed-wave Doppler, can be superimposed on a stored *two-dimensional* (2D) echocardiographic image. This combination of geometric and velocity information permits detailed evaluation of valvular regurgitation, stenosis, and intracardiac defects. The main disadvantage of pulsed-wave Doppler is its inability to measure high blood flow velocities (above 1.5 to 2.0 m/sec). This limitation has practical implications because a modification of Bernoulli's equation ($P1 - P2 = 4\ V2$) is used to relate blood flow velocity to the pressure differential across stenotic valvular heart lesions. In practice, these velocities can exceed 6 m/sec and can only be absolutely quantified with the continuous-wave Doppler technique.

## COLOR–FLOW DOPPLER ECHOCARDIOGRAPHY

The returning ultrasound data from a conventional 2D echocardiograph transducer also contains frequency-shift information resulting from encounters with moving structures and blood. The addition of a processor devoted to the analysis of this information, separate from that used to create the 2D echocardiographic image, is used to create color-flow images. Doppler information is obtained from multiple gates along each line and is color-coded according to the direction of flow. By convention, *red hues* indicate flow *toward* the transducer, and *blue hues* indicate flow *away* from the transducer. The brighter the color, the higher the velocity. Additional circuitry compares the spectrum of velocities within each gated sample to

the mean velocity. With great variance, indicating turbulent flow, green is added to the predominant red or blue in proportion to the variance. Thus, the addition of color-flow imaging to 2D echocardiography permits the simultaneous display of cardiac anatomy and physiology.

## DEVELOPMENT AND APPLICATION: GENERAL ASPECTS

The development of real-time 2D echocardiography, initially termed "ultrasound cardiotomography," began in the mid-1960s (Ebina et al., 1967). The provision of spatial orientation and tomographic information greatly enhanced the value of the resulting image. By providing a frame of reference, it became easier to position the M-mode acoustic pathway, the tomogram providing a template of recognizable overall cardiac structure within which to work.

The introduction of 2D and color-flow devices has removed much of the mystery of echocardiographic interpretation and moved the technique into the surgeon's hands. In heart operations, the pathophysiology and anatomy are shown in a format that surgeons intuitively understand. As a result, more and more studies are done in the operating room, and the results are interpreted in real time. The first reported surgical case involved the intraoperative use of 2D echocardiography to localize and successfully remove an intracardiac bullet (Harrison et al., 1981). In early studies, the ultrasound transducer and cable were sterilized with gas before each procedure. More recently, it has been shown to be simple and safe to rinse the transducer in glutaraldehyde (Cidex) and place it in a commercially available, presterilized sheath for intraoperative use.

Transesophageal echocardiography is usually performed and interpreted by the anesthesiologist. The transesophageal approach improves the acoustic window available for cardiac visualization and permits unobtrusive diagnosis. Satisfactory images can be obtained with the chest open or closed and can be useful in the immediate postoperative period.

The importance of echocardiographic information in the cardiac operating room has raised the issue of training in its interpretation. Many cardiac anesthesiology fellowships now incorporate formal experience within the cardiology training program as part of their curriculum.

## TWO–DIMENSIONAL ECHOCARDIOGRAPHY: CLINICAL APPLICATIONS

### Cardiac Function

Although echocardiography has been widely applied in the assessment of cardiac function, credit must be given to Omoto (1982) and to Spotnitz (1982)

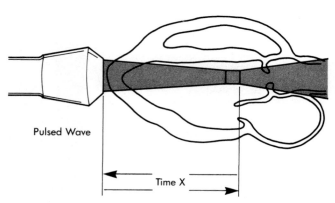

**FIGURE 31–101.** Pulsed-wave Doppler positioned along the same acoustic pathway uses a single transducer alternating between transmission and reception of ultrasound. The information can be range-gated, in this case specifically interrogating the region of the left ventricular outflow tract for velocity information. (From Kisslo, J., and Adams, D. B.: An Introduction to Doppler Echocardiography. Vol. 1. New York, Medi Cine Productions, 1987.)

and associates (Spotnitz et al., 1979) for introducing this application to the operating room.

Global ventricular function has been assessed in many ways. Systolic global ventricular function can be approximated by measuring the ejection fraction. Echocardiography can be used to determine ejection function as a relationship between end-systolic and end-diastolic areas in the short (or minor) axis of the heart, as follows:

$$EF = (EDA - ESA)/EDA$$

where EF = ejection fraction, EDA = end-diastolic area, and ESA = end-systolic area. End-diastolic area is determined by planimetry of the endocardial surface (usually excluding the papillary muscles). The simultaneously recorded electrocardiogram is used to synchronize these determinations over multiple cardiac cycles. End-systolic area is determined similarly at minimal area during ventricular ejection. This process has been automated in newer commercially available systems, which employ automated edge detection algorithms (Sklenar et al., 1992).

There are several potential inaccuracies in this determination. It is important that the ejection fraction be determined in the same plane throughout the cardiac cycle, both before and after any intervention. Intraoperatively, this can be accomplished by referring to external anatomic landmarks or by maintaining constant internal landmarks on the image. Spotnitz (1982) reported the use of the long-axis view of the left ventricle to determine the point at which the short-axis diameter would be maximal as a method to maintain consistency. Accurate determination of the ejection fraction also depends on symmetric global systolic function and minimal cardiac translational motion, neither of which can be assumed in patients undergoing cardiac operations. Additionally, area measurements reflect volume changes only if one of a number of different models of global ventricular geometry is assumed. Nonetheless, use of these methods in humans has shown 0.84 correlation to end-diastolic volume and ejection fraction as determined by radionuclide angiography (Harpole et al., 1989). These methods also have been validated for the estimation of preload recruitable stroke work and end-systolic elastance in animal models (Gorcsan et al., 1994).

The ejection fraction has been shown to improve following aortic valve replacement for aortic stenosis (Spotnitz, 1982), but not for aortic insufficiency (Ren et al., 1985). Similarly, the ejection fraction falls after mitral valve replacement for mitral insufficiency (Ren et al., 1985; Spotnitz, 1982; Wong and Spotnitz, 1981). For unselected patients undergoing coronary artery bypass grafting, the ejection fraction has been reported to change in either direction or to remain the same (Spotnitz, 1982).

Diastolic ventricular function also has been studied before and after cardioplegic arrest in patients. When left ventricular end-diastolic pressure was related to echocardiographically determined end-diastolic di-ameter, left ventricular compliance was unchanged by short periods of ischemia and decreased with longer periods of ischemia (Spotnitz et al., 1979).

The quantitation of regional myocardial wall-motion abnormalities has been a sensitive indicator of regional ischemia (Buda et al., 1986; Meltzer et al., 1979; Wyatt et al., 1981). Changes in regional systolic thickening have been closely correlated with regional blood flow in experimental preparations, although functional deficits tend to slightly overestimate infarct size (Buda et al., 1986). These regions, when identified at coronary operative procedures, have improved immediately after revascularization (Topol et al., 1984). This method may be more applicable in patients having coronary artery procedures, when nonuniform systolic function is expected (Heger et al., 1980; Omoto, 1982; Sheehan et al., 1992).

The sensitivity of echocardiography in detecting regional wall-motion abnormalities has been applied in the development of exercise echocardiography. With exercise, developed regional wall-motion abnormalities have correlated with the number and location of coronary arterial stenosis (Armstrong et al., 1987). This noninvasive method may become a useful screening procedure and may become critical in identifying *physiologically significant* coronary disease. Dobutamine stress echocardiography has been demonstrated to be a cost-effective and reliable screening test for coronary artery disease.

Valvular insufficiency also can be detected using an adjunctive echo-contrast agent and 2D echocardiography. Simple saline solutions, when agitated, produce relatively large microbubbles that are readily imaged. After intracardiac injection, regurgitant lesions are easily identified. This technique has been widely applied, particularly after valve reconstruction. It has been largely replaced by color-flow Doppler echocardiography.

## Cardiac Structure

Two-dimensional echocardiography has been particularly useful in the recognition of abnormalities of intracardiac structure and is the method of choice for evaluation of pericardial effusion (Fig. 31–102) for the intraoperative localization of foreign bodies (Hassett et al., 1986; Sakai et al., 1984) (Figs. 31–103 and 31–104) and for assessing cardiac tumors (Effert and Domanig, 1959).

Mural thrombi associated with myocardial infarction can be studied by using 2D echocardiography (Fig. 31–105). Applied transthoracically, the technique has a sensitivity of 77 to 92% and a specificity of 84 to 94% (Ezekowitz et al., 1982; Stratton et al., 1983; Visser et al., 1983), but an adequate study can be obtained in only 75% of patients (Ezekowitz et al., 1982). The relationship of echocardiographically identified mural thrombi and embolization is by no means certain, however (Ezekowitz, 1985). Further developments in the tissue characterization potential of ultrasound, combined with intraoperative studies during

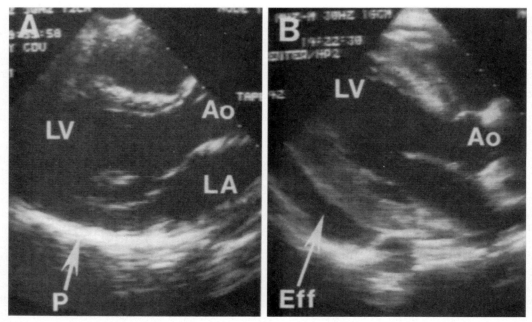

**FIGURE 31–102.** A long-axis parasternal, two-dimensional echocardiogram. *A,* Normal cardiac structure and absence of pericardial effusion are noted. (LV = left ventricle; Ao = aorta; LA = left atrium; P = pericardium.) *B,* Large posterior pericardial effusion (Eff) is shown in a similarly oriented two-dimensional echocardiogram.

coronary bypass grafting for acute myocardial infarction, may clarify this relationship.

Two-dimensional echocardiography has been used extensively in congenital heart operations (Gussenhoven et al., 1987) and was initially applied to evaluate the degree of right ventricular outflow tract obstruction in tetrology of Fallot (Spotnitz et al., 1978). In the pediatric age group, the small size of the subject allows the use of higher-frequency transducers, with consequent better resolution of the intracardiac structures. Direct measurements of pulmonary artery di-

mension have been used for prognostic information (Lappen et al., 1983; Snider et al., 1984), and even structures as small as a patent ductus arteriosus can be directly imaged in 90 to 100% of patients (Huhta et al., 1984; Sahn and Allen, 1978; Vick et al., 1985). When used intraoperatively, the technique often yields additional diagnostic information and permits an accurate assessment of the operative results at the time of weaning from cardiopulmonary bypass (Ungerleider et al., 1990, 1992).

With the injection of intracavitary microbubbles, 2D

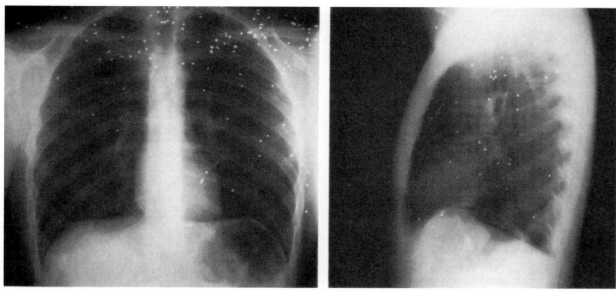

**FIGURE 31–103.** Posteroanterior and lateral chest films of a patient who sustained a shotgun wound to the thorax. Several of the projectiles appear to involve the heart.

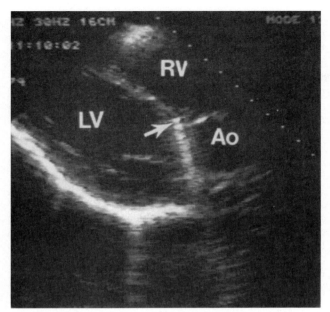

**FIGURE 31–104.** Two-dimensional echocardiography (same patient as seen in Fig. 31–103) confirms the presence of a single pellet *(arrow)* within the ventricular septum near the aortic valve, seen in the parasternal long-axis view. This patient had a newly developed conduction abnormality in association with this injury. (RV = right ventricle; LV = left ventricle; Ao = aorta.)

Two-dimensional echocardiography permits high-resolution evaluation of the intracardiac structures. In endocarditis, echocardiography has been particularly useful in the identification of valvular vegetations and valve destruction and the development of intramyocardial or annular abscesses (Cahalan, 1992). The sensitivity for vegetations in endocarditis is 80 to 85% (Martin et al., 1980), but it does not necessarily follow that the presence of a vegetation is an indication for operative intervention or that the disappearance of vegetation indicative of embolization. Only 32 to 50% of patients with echocardiographically demonstrated vegetations eventually require operation (Martin et al., 1980; Stewart et al., 1980). In complicated cases of endocarditis, it can provide detailed information regarding abscess and fistula formation that is not apparent at cardiac catheterization (Bardy et al., 1982; van Herwerden et al., 1987) (Figs. 31–106 and 31–107).

Two-dimensional echocardiography is sensitive in the detection of intracardiac air bubbles associated with cardiopulmonary bypass or with cardiotomy (Krebber et al., 1982). Air bubbles are identified within the cardiac chambers in 14 to 67% of patients undergoing cardiopulmonary bypass for either coronary artery bypass grafting or valve replacement (Rodigas et al., 1982; Spotnitz, 1982). Although "echo-

echocardiography has been used to detect intracardiac shunts, confirm the preoperative diagnoses, and verify operative repair. In preoperative evaluation, microbubbles can be injected in an arm vein to detect right-to-left shunts or bidirectional shunts at the atrial and ventricular level. In addition, a left arm vein injection provides an easy method to show a persistent left-sided superior vena cava.

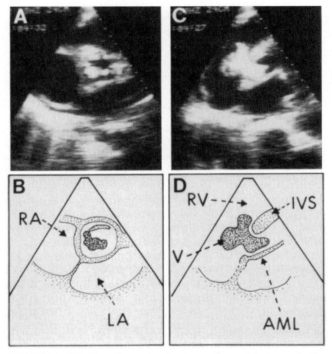

**FIGURE 31–106.** Two-dimensional echocardiographic image in the parasternal short-axis view of the aortic root *(A)* and accompanying schematic diagram *(B)*. The vegetation (V) is heavily stippled and within the aortic root. *C*, A tangential view is obtained through the aortic root and proximal interventricular septum (IVS). As can be seen in the accompanying schematic *(D)*, fistulous tracts surrounding the vegetation are suggested. (AML = anterior mitral leaflet; LA = left atrium; RA = right atrium; RV = right ventricle.) *(A–D* from Bardy, G. H., Valenstein, P., Stack, R. S., et al.: Two-dimensional echocardiographic identification of sinus of Valsalva-right heart fistula due to infective endocarditis. Am. Heart J., *103*:1068, 1982.)

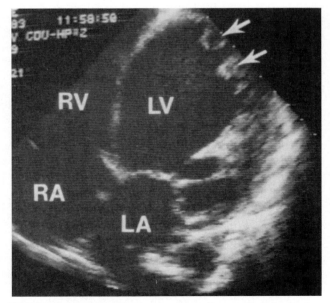

**FIGURE 31–105.** Apical long-axis echocardiogram that clearly demonstrates two large apical thrombi *(arrows).* (LV = left ventricle; RV = right ventricle; RA = right atrium; LA = left atrium)

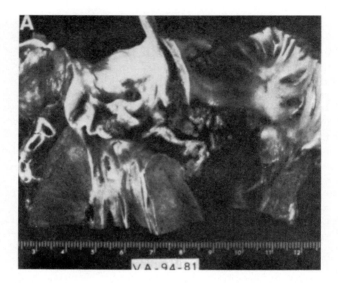

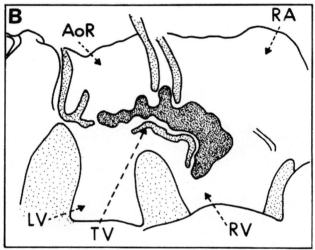

**FIGURE 31–107.** Gross pathologic specimen (A) showing the relationship of the large vegetation to the aortic root (AoR), right atrium (RA), right ventricle (RV), tricuspid valve (TV), and left ventricle (LV) in relation to a schematic drawing in B. The fistulous tracts surround the vegetation and extend through the interventricular system and aortic wall. (A and B, from Bardy, G. H., Valenstein, D., Stack, R. S., et al.: Two-dimensional echocardiographic identification of sinus of Valsalva-right heart fistula due to infective endocarditis. Am. Heart J., *103*:1068, 1982.)

cardiographic bubbles" can cause concern, they have not been correlated with neurologic outcome (Diehl et al., 1987; Topol et al., 1985). Nonetheless, echocardiographic guidance can be used to assist in transcardiac or trans-septal needle aspiration in the operating room (Diehl et al., 1987).

The development of high-frequency epicardial transducers has improved resolution to the extent that human coronary arteries can be directly visualized in the operating room (Hiratzka et al., 1986a, 1986b, 1987; Johnson et al., 1988; Sahn et al., 1982) and even through the chest wall (Douglas et al., 1988; Weyman et al., 1976). A high degree of correlation ($r = 0.91$) between coronary arterial lumen size at echocardiography and at cardiac catheterization has been found

(Sahn et al., 1982). Stenotic lesions are more difficult to characterize when extensive calcification is present. By using a 12-mHz transducer, it is possible to show coronary bypass graft anastomotic defects that might not otherwise be recognized and later to confirm intraoperative correction. Additionally, these probes are able to locate intramyocardial coronary arteries that may otherwise be difficult to identify (Hiratzka et al., 1986a, 1986b, 1987; Johnson et al., 1988). These methods may supplant currently available, highly empiric methods to determine the effectiveness of myocardial revascularization intraoperatively.

Intravascular ultrasound has been introduced as an alternative method to evaluate coronary artery disease (Isner et al., 1991). In vessels with limited calcifications, wall image analysis has correlated well with histologic sections in experimental applications (Siegel et al., 1991). Its use may be further limited by the need to traverse the stenotic lesion to provide adequate images (Coy et al., 1991).

Two-dimensional echocardiography has been advanced as a method to evaluate the operative correction of idiopathic hypertrophic subaortic stenosis (Syracuse et al., 1978), and it has been used to evaluate prosthetic strut encroachment after mitral valve replacement (Spotnitz, 1982). In the latter case, both high- and low-profile prosthetic valves produce severe acoustic artifacts by effectively blocking a large portion of the ultrasound energy. Ventricular pseudoaneurysms secondary to myocardial infarction have been delineated noninvasively and appropriately treated surgically after ultrasound diagnosis (Adamick et al., 1986; Hamilton et al., 1985).

Echocardiography has been used to calculate the overall mass of the left ventricle (Wyatt et al., 1979). Ventricular mass has been monitored in cardiac transplant recipients and has been correlated with transplant rejection (Sagar et al., 1980). Nonetheless, this method has been no more specific than other noninvasive methods, and percutaneous transvenous endomyocardial biopsy has remained the standard method for post-transplant follow-up. Ultrasonography may still have a role in this area because it is highly effective in guiding transvenous manipulation of the bioptome (French et al., 1983). With the use of 2D echocardiography instead of fluoroscopy, both the patient and the surgeon or cardiologist are protected from cumulative radiation hazard. Endomyocardial biopsy can then be accomplished in various locations with portable echocardiography and is not restricted to a specially equipped operating room. Additional attractive features of this method are the simultaneous determination of ventricular function, protection of the tricuspid valve apparatus from injury, and, as described later, noninvasive determination of pulmonary artery pressure and cardiac output. Similarly, echocardiography has been an effective aid in transvenous pacemaker placement (Ren et al., 1987) and in pericardiocentesis (Pandian et al., 1988).

High-frequency direct 2D echocardiography has been used to interrogate the ascending aorta and has been shown to be superior to palpation for detecting severe atherosclerosis (Marshall et al., 1989). This information has been employed to alter the cannulation site, to adjust perfusion techniques, and to direct unanticipated aortic repair (Davila-Roman et al., 1991). Transesophageal echocardiography also has been effective in aortic assessment (Ribakove et al., 1992), but the effectiveness of these adjunctive methods in reducing stroke rate or improving surgical results has yet to be demonstrated.

## PULSED AND CONTINUOUS–WAVE DOPPLER ECHOCARDIOGRAPHY: CLINICAL APPLICATIONS

The combination of pulsed Doppler with 2D echocardiography results in the ability to *quantitate* intracardiac blood velocity in a precisely defined anatomic location. Continuous-wave Doppler can then be used to extend the detectable velocity limit, although there is some ambiguity as to location of velocity along the acoustic pathway. Doppler echocardiography has become most accepted in congenital heart procedures in which it can be used to determine the patency of Blalock-Taussig shunts (Stevenson et al., 1983), and it has been found to be 96% sensitive and 100% specific for the presence of a patent ductus arteriosus (Stevenson et al., 1980).

As described earlier, blood velocity across a regurgitant valve can be used to estimate the transvalvular pressure gradient. The gradient in tricuspid regurgitation has been used to estimate right ventricular systolic pressure (and, in the absence of pulmonic stenosis, systolic pulmonary artery pressure) by calculation with a clinical estimate of the central venous pressure (or right atrial pressure) (Chan et al., 1987; Masuyama et al., 1986).

With the continuity equation, actual valve areas can also be estimated from multiple-gated Doppler velocities along the transvalvular blood path (Rich-

### Continuity Equation

$$Flow_2 = Flow_1$$
$$Area_2 \times V_2 = Area_1 \times V_1$$
$$Area_2 = \frac{Area_1 \times V_1}{V_2}$$

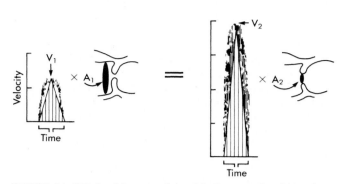

Continuity

**FIGURE 31–109.** In this example, continuity equation is used to calculate valvular stenotic area ($A_2$). $A_1$ is easily determined by two-dimensional echocardiography, and $V_1$ and $V_2$ with pulsed Doppler. In practice, $V_1$ may be obtained with pulsed Doppler, and $V_2$ by continuous-wave Doppler. In this case, a nearly fourfold increase in velocity results from flow through the stenotic area. (From Kisslo, J., and Adams, D. B.: An Introduction to Doppler Echocardiography. Vol. 2. New York, Medi Cine Productions, 1987.)

ards et al., 1986) (Figs. 31–108 and 31–109). These quantitative estimates have been used to evaluate numerous surgical conditions, such as aortic stenosis (Fig. 31–110), mitral stenosis, pulmonary hypertension, idiopathic hypertrophic subaortic stenosis, and congenital heart disease (Williams et al., 1987). Car-

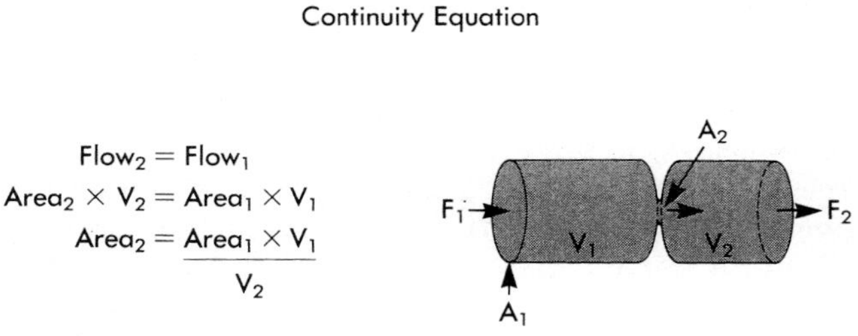

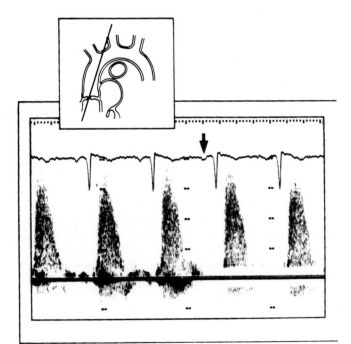

**FIGURE 31–108.** The continuity equation assumes that total volume flow before and after a stenotic lesion are equal ($Flow_2 = Flow_1$). Flow is equal to area × velocity, assuming that the velocity profile is flat. In this example, Area 2 ($A_2$) represents a significant stenosis, and Area 1 ($A_1$) the area just preceding the stenosis. $V_1$ is the velocity just before reaching the stenosis (within Area 1), and $V_2$ represents the velocity within the zone of stenosis ($A_2$). Area 1 can be calculated using two-dimensional echocardiography, and both velocities can be calculated using Doppler echocardiography. Solving the equation for Area 2 yields the effective stenotic orifice area, which may be too geometrically complex to determine by two-dimensional echocardiography. (From Kisslo, J., and Adams, D. B.: An Introduction to Doppler Echocardiography. Vol. 2. New York, Medi Cine Productions, 1987.)

**FIGURE 31–110.** A typical continuous-wave Doppler recording from a patient with aortic stenosis. The ultrasound beam is directed from the suprasternal notch, and the acoustic pathway incorporates the ascending aorta, aortic valve orifice, and left ventricular outflow tract. The velocity profile shows a great degree of variance and high velocity (4 m/sec). A baseline filter *(arrow)* is turned on to remove low-velocity noise. (From Kisslo, J., and Adams, D. B.: An Introduction to Doppler Echocardiography. Vol. 1. New York, Medi Cine Productions, 1987.)

diac tamponade has been associated with a sharp increase in Doppler flow velocity across the pulmonary and tricuspid valves associated with inspiration, combined with a decrease in flow across the aortic and mitral valves. These transvalvular velocities, and the clinical syndrome, have been reversed with therapy (Leeman et al., 1988).

Continuous cardiac output determination also has been made possible by measuring velocity in the ascending aorta and calculating its instantaneous diameter using 2D echocardiography (Mark et al., 1986). Specifically designed Doppler probes have been attached to the ascending aorta during heart procedures and have been safely removed percutaneously. With echocardiographic measure of aortic diameter, the velocity was converted to calculate flow continuously in the postoperative period in 20 patients (Svennevig et al., 1986).

Specific intraoperative applications of Doppler echocardiography include detection of postreparative valve area, determination of residual valvular regurgitation or residual shunts (when high-velocity residua are found, the defects are usually inconsequential), and precise localization of coronary arteriovenous fistulas (Miyatake et al., 1984).

Doppler velocitometry has been useful in the surgical management of coronary artery disease, both clinically and in clinical research. Initially used transthoracically to determine left internal mammary-coronary artery bypass graft patency (Benchimol et al., 1978), this method was introduced in the operating room by Marcus and co-workers (1981). These investigators developed a Doppler probe that can be attached reversibly to the epicardial surface of the heart by suction and that reliably measures coronary velocity in epicardial coronary arteries. In humans, this instrument was used to determine the reactive hyperemic response after occlusion (20 seconds) of both normal and diseased coronary arteries. This measure of physiologic significance was correlated poorly with visual interpretation of the coronary arteriogram (Marcus et al., 1986; White et al., 1984). Even with a computer-assisted definition of the anatomic extent of coronary disease at cardiac catheterization, correlation with reactive hyperemia has been poor (Wilson et al., 1987) unless coronary disease is very limited (Wilson et al., 1987). This method has also been applied to coronary bypass grafting without angiography in a single case of severe adverse dye reaction (Wright et al., 1987). Other physicians have modified the Doppler system to permit measurement of multiple-channel pulsed Doppler velocities in coronary arteries, thus extending its application to lesions that create a nonuniform velocity profile (Kajiya et al., 1986). The major advantage of this technique is the ability to accurately determine the zero velocity level and the fact that it can be done on undissected native coronary arteries. The major disadvantages include difficulty in measuring coronary velocity on posterior coronary arteries and inability to determine actual blood flow. Recent developments have enabled automatic determination of vessel diameter which,

combined with velocity, yields actual blood flow. Thus far, this can only be applied to coronary bypass grafts (Payen et al., 1986).

## COLOR–FLOW DOPPLER ECHOCARDIOGRAPHY: CLINICAL APPLICATIONS

The development of real-time display of tomographic blood velocity, direction, and degree of turbulence has been the most significant recent advance in echocardiography. This information, color-coded and displayed by superimposition on the 2D echocardiograph, is now called color-flow Doppler echocardiography and was introduced by Omoto and others with the development of a new autocorrelator (Bommer et al., 1982; Namekawa et al., 1982; Omoto et al., 1984). Their initial report on 72 patients with acquired valvular heart disease showed that color-flow imaging provides a useful estimate of valve dysfunction, particularly regurgitation (Omoto et al., 1984). Examples of aortic insufficiency (Fig. 31–111) and mitral insufficiency (Fig. 31–112) show the sensitivity of this technique.

This technique has been highly sensitive and specific in the accurate localization of valvular regurgitation and intracardiac shunts. In congenital heart disease, color-flow imaging has been routinely applied in the operating room at several institutions (Hagler et al., 1988; Takamoto et al., 1985), including Duke University Medical Center. The preoperative diagnosis of an atrial septal defect is shown in Figure 31–113.

In the Mayo Clinic series, 21 residual lesions were diagnosed intraoperatively in 30 patients. In Duke's series of 621 consecutive patients, intraoperative color-flow findings were useful in modifying the preoperative diagnosis and in correcting significant residual defects at the time of the original operation (Ungerleider et al., 1992) (Figs. 31–114 and 31–115). Intraoperative echo findings correlated with outcome in 97% of cases.

Surgeons employing reparative techniques for mitral regurgitation have found that color-flow imaging provides an accurate intraoperative evaluation both before and after repair. Analysis of the image by the operating surgeon often clarifies specific portions of the mitral valve apparatus that are defective and adds an important perspective to the direct examination of the mitral valve during cardioplegic arrest (Stewart and Salcedo, 1989). This technique has a sensitivity of 94% and a specificity of 93% for detecting the presence or absence of mitral regurgitation (Czer et al., 1987), and it reliably confirms valve repair (Marwick et al., 1991; Sheikh et al., 1990). In addition, it has great promise for elucidating the mechanisms of mitral regurgitation associated with myocardial infarction and coronary artery disease (Izumi et al., 1987).

Recent specific uses of color-flow echocardiography presage wide application. It has been used in the

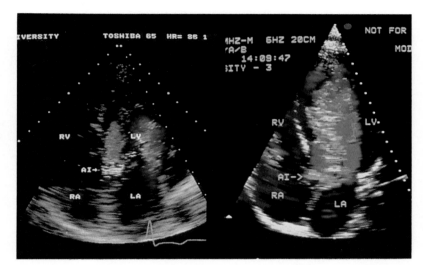

**FIGURE 31–111.** Two patients with aortic insufficiency. One is small in degree *(left)*, and the other is large *(right)*. The mosaic of colors indicates the regurgitant jet.

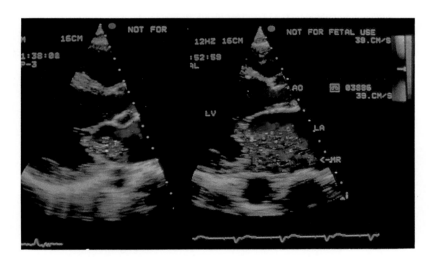

**FIGURE 31–112.** Two patients with mitral regurgitation. One is small in degree *(left)*, and the other is large *(right)*.

**FIGURE 31–113.** Subcostal view of all four cardiac chambers showing a massive interatrial flow communication.

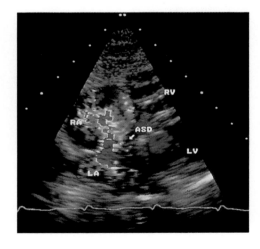

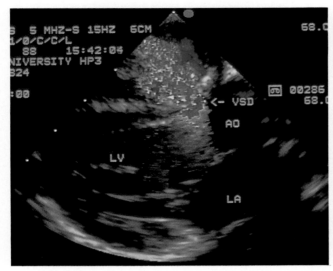

**FIGURE 31–114.** Precardiopulmonary bypass evaluation of a child with a large ventricular septal defect (VSD). The study was done epicardially.

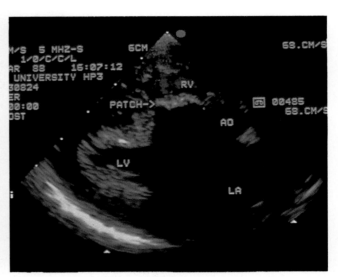

**FIGURE 31–115.** Postcardiopulmonary bypass epicardial scan showing the patch repair and no residual VSD.

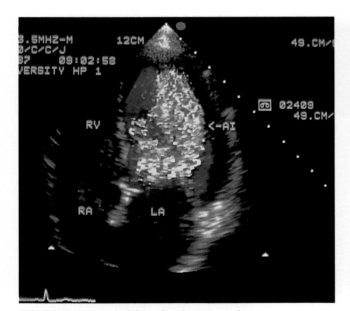

**FIGURE 31–116.** Apical four-chamber image showing massive aortic insufficiency associated with an ascending aortic dissecting aneurysm.

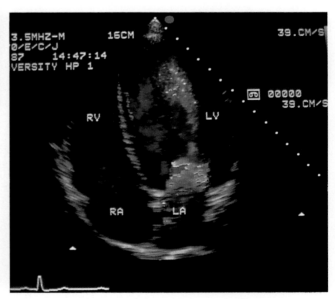

**FIGURE 31–117.** Apical four-chamber image showing no aortic insufficiency after aortic valve resuspension.

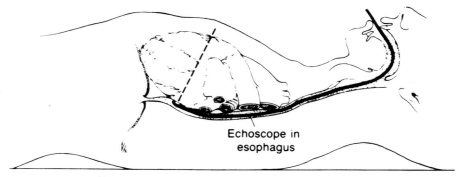

**FIGURE 31–118.** Transducer position for a short-axis view of the left ventricle during transesophageal echocardiography. (From DeBruijn, N. P., and Clements, F. M. [eds]: Transesophageal Echocardiography. Boston, Martinus Nijhoff, 1987, p. 6.)

identification of aortic root abscesses associated with fistulization (Fisher et al., 1987; Khandheria, 1993). Color-flow imaging has been shown to have 99% sensitivity and 98% specificity in the diagnosis of aortic dissection (Iliceto et al., 1987; Omoto et al., 1987; Sheikh et al., 1990). Its value for precisely localizing the intimal flap at the time of operation may alter traditional operative approaches (Ungerleider et al., 1990). Intraoperative confirmation of aortic valve sufficiency (Figs. 31–116 and 31–117) and the identification of anastomotic leaks have also been beneficial. The evolution of color-flow systems for transesophageal echocardiography may have a significant effect on current algorithms for the preoperative diagnosis of this lesion (Simon et al., 1992).

Because of the numerous advantages of color-flow echocardiography, its clinical role is still rapidly evolving. The main drawbacks at this stage are the limitations in frame rate imposed by the sheer volume of data acquired (making examinations at fast heart rates difficult) and the fact that it is so sensitive. The differentiation between color-flow disorders and clinically significant disorders will require reference to pulsed or continuous-wave Doppler findings, as well as further experience.

## TRANSESOPHAGEAL ECHOCARDIOGRAPHY: DEVELOPMENT AND CLINICAL APPLICATIONS

The development of transesophageal echocardiography has greatly increased the use of echocardiographic examinations in the operating room. With the transducer placed in the esophagus, the amount of tissue intervening between the transducer and the heart is greatly reduced, particularly when the patient is in the supine position (Fig. 31–118). In addition, examinations can be done in patients with barrel chests, chronic obstructive pulmonary disease, or obesity, wherein transthoracic acoustic pathways are not available. By placing the ultrasound transducer at the tip of a flexible gastroscope, the image plane can be easily controlled (Fig. 31–119).

Reducing transducer size while maintaining state-of-the-art imaging features has been critical to the

development of transesophageal echocardiography. In 1976, Frazin and co-workers, using a 19 × 13 × 6 mm transducer, obtained M-mode transesophageal echocardiograms (Frazin et al., 1976). Initial real-time transesophageal 2D images were obtained by Hisanaga and associates (1980) with a mechanically rotating transducer. This technique has mainly been replaced by miniature phased-array ultrasound transducers (Schluter et al., 1982). The introduction of multiplane (Decoodt et al., 1992; Flachskampf et al., 1991) and pediatric (Roberson et al., 1990) probes has increased the visuality of the transesophageal approach and removed some of its limitations.

Although the procedure initially was developed by cardiologists for use in awake patients, its predominant application today is in the operating room under the control of the anesthesiologist (DeBruijn and Clements, 1987b). In this setting, it has been safe in patients without manifestations of esophageal disease.

Although transesophageal echocardiography is useful diagnostically; its ability to display various cardiac

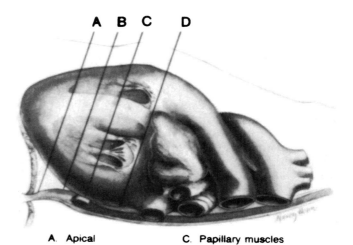

| A. Apical | C. Papillary muscles |
| B. Low left ventricular | D. Mitral valve leaflets |

**FIGURE 31–119.** In transesophageal echocardiography, the gastroscope can be manipulated along the length of the esophagus, and the tip can be flexed to acquire these four typical short-axis views of the heart. (From DeBruijn, N. P., and Clements, F. M. [eds]: Transesophageal Echocardiography. Boston, Martinus Nijhoff, 1987, p. 36.)

dimensions continuously without intruding on the operation has provided a unique monitoring ability. Under the control of anesthesiologists, it has supplied information that was previously unavailable to them despite direct observation of the heart or communication with the surgeon. The addition of color-flow mapping to this equipment has provided physiologic information that was previously unavailable unless the cardiac surgeon was a devoted echocardiographer. These factors have led to a highly cooperative endeavor between operating and nonoperating physicians in the overall management of cardiac surgical patients, and they are certain to have a positive impact greater than the actual technology presently available to each.

Regional wall-motion abnormalities that indicate ischemia can be directly observed by using transesophageal echocardiography (DeBruijn and Clements, 1987b) (Figs. 31–120 and 31–121). This can be particularly helpful for identifying ventricular septal abnormalities (Corya et al., 1981) and appears to be a more effective monitoring technique than continuous electrocardiography (Smith et al., 1985). Although regional systolic thickening can be quantitatively analyzed fairly easily, simple observation by the anesthesiologist has been easily learned and relatively independent of interobserver variability (Clements et al., 1986). Regional wall-motion abnormalities thus detected have responded appropriately both to alterations in anesthetic management and to revascularization (DeBruijn and Clements, 1987a). Transesophageal

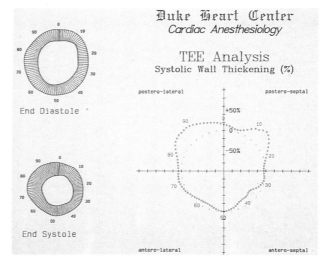

**FIGURE 31–121.** In this example, there is anteroseptal and anterolateral systolic wall thinning, represented by data points *(red boxes)* falling within the circle of unity. Posteriorly, there appears to be a compensatory increase in systolic wall thickening *(green boxes)*. (Courtesy of Dr. Thomas E. Stanley III.)

echocardiography also has been used to optimize ventricular function as it is affected by preload and afterload. These aspects of the overall management of cardiac surgical patients are amenable to quantitation by determining atrial volume (Matsuzaki et al., 1985) and end-diastolic left ventricular area (DeBruijn and Clements, 1987a). In the setting of frequent alterations in left ventricular compliance, these data have provided useful supplemental information in the assessment of intracardiac pressures. The continuous availability of left ventricular global dimensions and wall thickness also permits calculation of wall stress (DeBruijn and Clements, 1987a). Thus, specific manipulations can optimize preload and afterload and monitor efficacy of therapy.

The addition of color-flow capabilities to the transesophageal transducer has made this technique more useful. All applications of transthoracic or epicardial color-flow echocardiography can be similarly made with transesophageal echocardiography, with minimal if any loss of image resolution. Images of the left atrium, mitral valve apparatus, and great vessels may be superior because of their close proximity to the transducer. Many institutions now routinely apply transesophageal echocardiography during cardiac operations to such an extent that equipment availability may become a limiting factor (Beaupre et al., 1984; DeBruijn and Clements, 1987b; Kyo et al., 1987; Smith et al., 1985). Transesophageal echocardiography also has been used to monitor cardiac function during noncardiac procedures, particularly during vascular surgery when the thoracic or abdominal aorta must be occluded. The detection of regional wall-motion abnormalities in response to increased wall stress has been shown to respond to specific modifications of anesthetic technique to the patient's benefit (DeBruijn and Clements, 1987a; Gewertz et al., 1987).

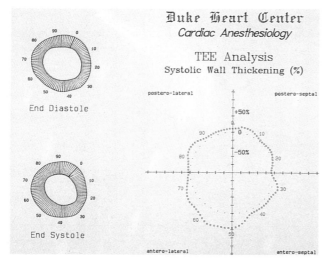

**FIGURE 31–120.** An example of transesophageal analysis of systolic wall thickening. Two hundred transmural chords are defined in end-diastole *(upper left)* and in end-systole *(lower left)*. These results are normalized and graphically displayed for each chord on a polar coordinate system *(right)*. A circle of unity (no change in chord length from diastole to systole) is marked by *small dots,* and actual data points represented by *small squares* arrayed circumferentially as they would appear in a short-axis transesophageal view. In this example, most experimental data reside outside the circle of unity *(green boxes),* indicating systolic wall thickening. Systolic wall thinning *(red boxes)* is seen only in the mid septum. (Courtesy of Dr. Thomas E. Stanley III.)

# FUTURE DIRECTIONS

## Tissue Characterization

Detailed analysis of the myocardial image holds promise for the specific detection and diagnosis of intrinsic structural damage. Early attempts to quantify these changes and associate them with pathologic material (Tanaka and Terasawa, 1979) were complicated by poor resolving capacity and the need to assess transmission rather than reflection of ultrasound (Stefan and Bing, 1972; Tanaka and Terasawa, 1979; von Ramm and Thurstone, 1976; Weiss et al., 1981; Wyatt et al., 1979). Ultrasound was capable of showing only large differences, such as between normal myocardium and myocardium late after infarction. In addition, the images often represent tertiary data that have been log compressed, manipulated in order to enhance boundaries, and in general processed to "please the eye." The resulting data loss, which was beyond the control of clinical investigators, precluded vigorous interpretation. Computer analysis of the average gray level in animal preparations of coronary occlusion has had great difficulty in distinguishing abnormal regions from normal regions under approximated clinical conditions (Skorton et al., 1983).

In the laboratory, the measurement of ultrasonic integrated back scatter, which measures reflected rather than transmitted ultrasound, has been closely correlated with ischemia at 1 and at 6 hours. This is thought to result from an increase in tissue fluid content and contributions of formed elements in the blood (Mimbs et al., 1981).

Methods using analysis of the raw radio frequency signal, such as time-averaged integrated back scatter (Sagar et al., 1987), real-time integrated back scatter (Thomas et al., 1986), and the mean amplitude/standard deviation of the amplitude (Schnittger et al., 1985), have shown promise in the early identification of ischemic areas (Fig. 31–122). Internal calibration and the need for normal reference tissue are obstacles to clinical application (Rasmussen et al., 1984). Cyclic variations in the cardiac cycle ranging from 5 to 10 dB present obstacles to tissue characterization without enhancement (Thomas et al., 1986). The loss of cyclic variation during isometric contraction suggests that the physical arrangement of structures within the tissue may be important (Sagar et al., 1987; Wear et al., 1986). Cyclic back scatter power decreases with ischemia but returns toward normal within 5 hours; it cannot be used alone to distinguish normal from abnormal myocardium, however (Fitzgerald et al., 1987). The Fourier coefficient of the amplitude modulation has been useful in analyzing the cardiac cycle–dependent changes in back scatter (Sagar et al., 1988). In addition to the assessment of myocardial ischemia, back scatter analysis has aided the early recognition of cardiac transplant rejection in an animal model and may have a clinical role (Chandrasekaran et al., 1987).

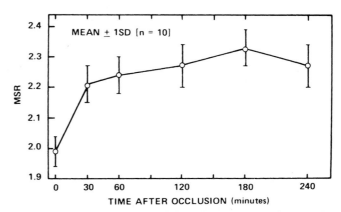

**FIGURE 31–122.** Mean amplitude/standard deviation of the amplitude (MSR) of the unprocessed ultrasound radio frequency signal returned from myocardium supplied by the left anterior descending (LAD) coronary artery, showing a significant increase in this parameter over time after LAD occlusion. (From Schnittger, I., Vieli, A., Heiserman, J. E., et al.: Ultrasonic tissue characterization: Detection of acute myocardial ischemia in dogs. Circulation, 72:193, 1985. By permission of the American Heart Association, Inc.)

## Determination of Regional Perfusion

Advances in tissue characterization depend on similar advances in equipment to distinguish fine changes related to the cardiac cycle and to microscopic characteristics of the tissue. An alternative method is to provide enhancement of the tissue in relationship to its blood supply, which has been accomplished with intravascular microbubbles acting as reflectors specific for regional perfusion. First noted by Gramiak and Shah (1968), contrast enhancement was initially obtained by the forceful injection of indocyanine green. A host of additional contrast agents have been used, such as hydrogen peroxide (Armstrong et al., 1984; Kemper et al., 1983), gelatin-encapsulated microbubbles (Armstrong et al., 1982), and hand-agitated saline or Renografin-76 (Maurer et al., 1984; Taylor et al., 1985). The main disadvantages of these agents has been their relatively short half-lives; large particle size, which causes embolization rather than true perfusion; and large variance in microbubble size. A significant advance in this area has been made by Feinstein and colleagues (1984b), who developed a method to sonicate Renografin-76 to yield a uniform microbubble solution in which the average bubble was smaller than a red blood cell. They showed that these particles traverse the capillary network much as red blood cells do (Feinstein et al., 1984a). They and others have investigated the use of this agent in myocardial perfusion studies in animal models (Lang et al., 1987; Tei et al., 1983) and have shown it to be safe in human application (Feinstein et al., 1986). The more recent development of a stable albumin microbubble with similar size distribution holds great promise for physiologic measurements using 2D echocardiography (Feinstein et al., 1986). This contrast agent is capable of transpulmonary passage and may enable investigators to examine regional myocardial perfusion after arm vein injection Villanueva et al., 1992).

Through the use of intravascular agents, regional brightness changes over time after intravascular administration in relationship to regional perfusion. The enhanced back scatter related to the presence of microbubbles is more easily shown with commercially available equipment. Analysis of these images and the time domain provides a useful estimate of regional perfusion (Ong et al., 1984), although quantitation of that perfusion remains problematic (Klein et al., 1993). Despite this, there is abundant evidence that such contrast enhancement can be a useful method of identifying the area at risk after coronary occlusion in animal preparations. In the operating room, it is a simple matter to inject sonicated Renografin into coronary artery bypass grafts before weaning a patient from cardiopulmonary bypass. Two-dimensional echocardiography then reveals the tomographic region of the heart supplied by each graft, and a qualitative measure of the perfusion rate can be determined by observing the clearance rate of the agent (Fig. 31–123).

## ECHOCARDIOGRAPHY: SURGERY WITHOUT CARDIAC CATHETERIZATION

The advances in echocardiography described earlier, the anticipation of further improvement in resolution, and the development of contrast agents capable of peripheral venous injection raise the question of the degree to which echocardiography can be depended on to replace cardiac catheterization for the preoperative evaluation of surgical patients. The broad institution of such an approach would be less expensive than cardiac catheterization and in some cases may reduce the overall risk of surgical correction to the patient.

This approach was initially undertaken in valvular heart disease (St. John Sutton, 1981) and was applied in approximately 75% of cases without adverse effects on the outcome for patients (Borow et al., 1983; Motro et al., 1980; St. John Sutton et al., 1981).

Even with detailed clinical history and physical examination, as well as routine radiographic and laboratory investigation, approximately 25% of patients with valvular heart disease still require preoperative cardiac catheterization. Thus, it appears to be possible to select a population in which cardiac catheterization can be avoided.

In cases of cardiac trauma, the surgeon is often confronted with a critically ill patient requiring emergency operation. Intraoperative echocardiography has been used successfully to assess intracardiac trauma after life-threatening problems have been solved (Fig. 31–124). Through intraoperative diagnosis, postoperative cardiac catheterization and delayed corrective procedures can be avoided.

In congenital heart disease, the policy of using cardiac catheterization selectively is becoming widespread, probably because of the increased risk of cardiac catheterization in this setting. The low incidence of coronary artery abnormalities in this age group also tends to reduce the necessity of cardiac catheterization (Krabill et al., 1987). A large variety of disorders, as outlined earlier, are suitable for definitive diagnosis by echocardiographic techniques with a high degree of specificity (Freed et al., 1984; Gutgesell et al., 1985; Macartney, 1983; Rice et al., 1983; Stark et al., 1983). In a review of 100 patients undergoing surgery for congenital heart defects without cardiac catheterization, there was a trend toward lower mortality when cardiac catheterization could be avoided (Huhta et al., 1987). In some disorders, particularly left ventricular outflow tract obstruction, avoiding cardiac catheterization has definitely improved results. With the advent of more liberally applied intra-

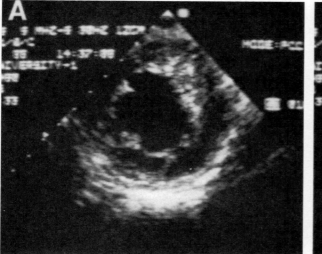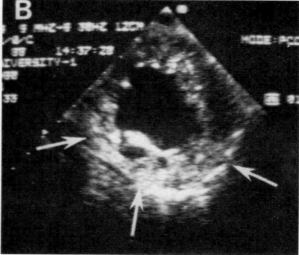

**FIGURE 31–123.** *A,* Intraoperative short-axis two-dimensional echocardiogram done epicardially on cardiopulmonary bypass, after completion of three saphenous vein bypass grafts. *B,* After the injection of 2 ml of sonicated Renografin-76 into the graft supplying the dominant right coronary artery. Note the contrast enhancement of the posterior septum and posterior left ventricle *(arrows),* indicating excellent bypass graft function.

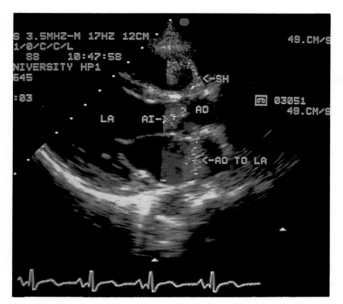

FIGURE 31–124. Parasternal long axis view of a child shot in the chest at close range with an air gun. The child underwent emergency closure of a right ventricular perforation at another institution. No intraoperative or other evaluation was performed. The child was found to have a murmur following discharge. The echocardiogram shows an aorto–right ventricular shunt as well as an aorto–left atrial shunt. Aortic insufficiency from an aortic cusp perforation is also noted.

operative echocardiography, this diagnostic method can be used throughout the procedure to further refine its specificity and to guide the operative procedure in the absence of cardiac catheterization.

## SUMMARY

Recent advances in echocardiography have led to its more general application in the diagnosis and management of cardiac surgical problems. These developments have been technologic and have produced changes in attitude that have made the technique valuable to surgeons.

With rapid advances in computer technology, this trend will likely continue. It is now clear that echocardiography is required for the proper performance of congenital (Ungerleider et al., 1992) and valvular (Stewart and Salcedo, 1989) cardiac surgical procedures. Three-dimensional echocardiography, digital image analysis, and automated data reduction to provide on-line indices of ventricular function and regional myocardial perfusion hold promise in increasing the clinical impact of ultrasound.

### SELECTED BIBLIOGRAPHY

Kisslo, J., and Adams, D. B. (eds): An Introduction to Doppler Echocardiography Vol. 1–4. New York, Medi Cine Productions, 1987.
    Vol. 1: Principles of Doppler Echocardiography and the Doppler Examination
    Vol. 2: Doppler Evaluation of Valvular Regurgitation.
    Vol. 3: Doppler Evaluation of Valvular Stenosis
    Vol. 4: Doppler Color Flow Imaging

This series of monographs describes the principles of Doppler echocardiography and develops physical concepts of the Doppler effect as it is employed in echocardiography in a comprehensive and easy-to-understand manner. There are numerous excellent illustrations (many in color) describing current applications of Doppler echocardiography. These monographs are an excellent resource for the novice, who can rapidly obtain a working knowledge of Doppler echocardiography.

Feigenbaum, H.: Echocardiography. 4th ed. Philadelphia, Lea & Febiger, 1986.

A comprehensive textbook on echocardiography, this is an excellent resource for a full understanding of the physical properties of ultrasonography. It also comprehensively reviews the historical development of all aspects of echocardiography. This book is particularly strong in the area of two-dimensional echocardiography and covers early applications of color flow echocardiography well.

Marshall, W. G., Barzilai, B., Kouchoukos, N. T., et al.: Intraoperative ultrasonic imaging of the ascending aorta. Ann. Thorac. Surg., 48:339, 1989.

This is the seminal article on the use of high-frequency echocardiography to interrogate the ascending aorta during cardiac surgery. It led the authors to pursue large-scale application of this methodology, which they feel results in appropriate modification of cannulation site or perfusion technique, and has led to ascending aortic operations that would not otherwise have been performed.

Ungerleider, R. M., Greeley, W. J., Kanter, R. J., et al.: The learning curve for intraoperative echocardiography during congenital heart surgery. Ann. Thorac. Surg., 54:691, 1992.

In this series of 621 patients undergoing congenital heart surgery, intraoperative echocardiography identified 2 to 3% of patients whose outcome was improved by intraoperative revision that would not have been performed based on standard intraoperative evaluation. The authors demonstrated that a "learning curve" of 200 patients is necessary to gain performance and interpretive skills in intraoperative echocardiography; once these skills are obtained a surgeon can identify 97% of patients intraoperatively who will have a good outcome. They also found echocardiography to be extremely useful in guiding intraoperative revision of incomplete or inadequate congenital repairs.

### BIBLIOGRAPHY

Adamick, R., Sprecher, D., Coleman, R. E., and Kisslo, J.: Pseudoaneurysm of the left ventricle. Echocardiography, 3:237, 1986.
Armstrong, W. F., Mueller, T. M., Kinney, E. L., et al.: Assessment of myocardial perfusion abnormalities with contrast-enhanced two-dimensional echocardiography. Circulation, 66:166, 1982.
Armstrong, W. F., O'Donnell, J., Ryan, T., and Feigenbaum, H.: Effect of prior myocardial infarction and extent and location of coronary disease on accuracy of exercise echocardiography. J. Am. Coll. Cardiol., 10:531, 1987.
Armstrong, W. F., West, S. R., Dillon, J. C., and Feigenbaum, H.: Assessment of location and size of myocardial infarction with contrast-enhanced echocardiography. II. Application of digital imaging techniques. J. Am. Coll. Cardiol., 4:141, 1984.
Bardy, G. H., Valenstein, P., Stack, R. S., et al.: Two-dimensional echocardiographic identification of sinus of Valsalva-right heart fistula due to infective endocarditis. Am. Heart J., 103:1068, 1982.
Beaupre, P. N., Kremer, P. F., Cahalan, M. K., et al.: Intraoperative detection of changes in left ventricular segmental wall motion by transesophageal two-dimensional echocardiography. Am. Heart J., 107:1021, 1984.
Benchimol, A., Reyns, P., Alvarez, S., et al.: Non-invasive assessment of left internal mammary-coronary bypass patency using the external Doppler probe. Am. Heart J., 96:347, 1978.
Bommer, W., and Miller, L.: Real-time two-dimensional color-flow Doppler. Enhanced Doppler flow imaging in the diagnosis of cardiovascular diseases [Abstract]. Am. J. Cardiol., 49:944, 1982.
Borow, K. M., Wynne, J., Sloss, L. J., et al.: Noninvasive assessment of valvular heart disease: Surgery without catheterization. Am. Heart J., 106:443, 1983.
Buda, A. J., Zotz, R. J., and Gallagher, K. P.: Characterization of the functional border zone around regionally ischemic myocar-

dium using circumferential flow-function maps. J. Am. Coll. Cardiol., 8:150, 1986.

Cahalan, M. K.: Intraoperative monitoring. In Dittrich, H. C. (ed): Clinical Transesophageal Echocardiography. St. Louis, Mosby Year Book, 1992, pp. 141–148.

Chan, K., Currie, P. J., Seward, J. B., et al.: Comparison of three Doppler ultrasound methods in the prediction of pulmonary artery pressure. J. Am. Coll. Cardiol., 9:549, 1987.

Chandrasekaran, K., Bansal, R. C., Greenleaf, J. F., et al.: Early recognition of heart transplant rejection by backscatter analysis from serial 2D echos in a herterotopic transplant model. J. Heart Transplant, 6:1, 1987.

Clements, F. M., Hill, R., Kisslo, J., and Orchard, R.: How easily can we learn to recognize regional wall motion abnormalities with 2-D transesophageal echocardiography? Proceedings of the Society of Cardiovascular Anesthesioliology, 7th Annual Meeting, Montreal, May 1986.

Corya, B. C., Phillips, J. F., Black, M. J., et al.: Prevalence of regional left ventricular dysfunction in patients with coronary artery disease. Chest, 79:631, 1981.

Coy, K., Maurer, G., and Siegel, R. J.: Intravascular ultrasound imaging: A current perspective. J. Am. Coll. Cardiol., 18:1811, 1991.

Czer, L. S. C., Maurer, G., Bolger, A. F., et al.: Intraoperative evaluation of mitral regurgitation by Doppler color flow mapping. Circulation, 76(Suppl. 3):108, 1987.

Davila-Roman, V. G., Barzilai, B., Wareing, T. H., et al.: Intraoperative ultrasonographic evaluation of the ascending aorta in 100 consecutive patients undergoing cardiac surgery. Circulation, 84(Suppl 3):47, 1991.

DeBruijn, N. P., and Clements, F. M.: Clinical applications of 2D transesophageal echocardiography. In DeBruijn, N. P., and Clements, F. M. (eds): Transesophageal Echocardiography, Chapter 4. Boston, Martinus Nijhoff, 1987a.

DeBruijn, N. P., and Clements, F. M.: Development of transesophageal echocardiography. In DeBruijn, N. P., and Clements, F. M. (eds): Transesophageal Echocardiography, Chapter 1. Boston, Martinus Nijhoff, 1987b.

Decoodt, P., Kacenelenbogen, R., Bar, J. P., et al.: Clinical usefulness of biplane transesophageal echocardiography. Echocardiography, 9:257, 1992.

Diehl, J. T., Ramos, D., Dougherty, F., et al.: Intraoperative, two-dimensional echocardiography-guided removal of retained intracardiac air. Ann. Thorac. Surg., 43:674, 1987.

Douglas, P. S., Fiolkoski, J., Berko, B., and Reichek, N.: Echocardiographic visualization of coronary artery anatomy in the adult. J. Am. Coll. Cardiol., 11:565, 1988.

Ebina, T., Oka, S., Tanaka, M., et al.: The ultrasono-tomography of the heart and great vessels in living human subjects by means of the ultrasonic reflection technique. Jpn. Heart J., 8:331, 1967.

Edler, I., and Hertz, C. H.: Use of ultrasonic reflectoscope for continuous recording of movement of heart walls. Kung Fysiogr. Sallsk Lund Fordhandle, 24:40, 1954.

Effert, S., and Domanig, E.: The diagnosis of intra-atrial tumor and thrombi by the ultrasonic echo method. German Med. Mth., 4:1, 1959.

Erbel, R., Daniel, W., Visser, C., et al.: Echocardiography in the diagnosis of aortic dissection. Lancet, 46:457, 1989.

Ezekowitz, M. D.: Acute infarction, left ventricular thrombus and systemic embolization: An approach to management. J. Am. Coll. Cardiol., 5:1281, 1985.

Ezekowitz, M. D., Wilson, D. A., Smith, E. O., et al.: Comparison of indium-111 platelet scintigraphy and two-dimensional echocardiography in the diagnosis of left ventricular thrombi. N. Engl. J. Med., 306:1509, 1982.

Feinstein, S. B., Lang, R. M., Dick, C., et al.: Contrast echocardiographic perfusion studies in humans. Am. J. Cardiac Imaging, 1:29, 1986.

Feinstein, S. B., Shah, P. M., Bing, R. J., et al.: Microbubble dynamics visualized in the intact capillary circulation. J. Am. Coll. Cardiol., 4:595, 1984a.

Feinstein, S. B., Ten Cate, F. J., Zwehl, W., et al.: 2D contrast echocardiography. I. In vitro development and quantitative analysis of echo contrast agents. J. Am. Coll. Cardiol., 3:14, 1984b.

Fernando, H. A., Friedman, H. S., Lajam, F., and Sakurai, H.: Late cardiac tamponade following open-heart surgery: Detection by echocardiography. Ann. Thorac. Surg., 24:174, 1977.

Fisher, E. A., Estioko, M. R., Stern, E. H., and Goldman, M. E.: Left ventricular to left atrial communication secondary to a paraaortic abscess: Color flow Doppler documentation. J. Am. Coll. Cardiol., 10:222, 1987.

Fitzgerald, P. J., McDaniel, M. D., Rolett, E. L., et al.: Two-dimensional ultrasonic tissue characterization: Backscatter power, endocardial wall motion, and their phase relationship for normal, ischemic, and infarcted myocardium. Circulation, 76:850, 1987.

Flachskampf, F. A., Hoffman, R., and Hanrath, P.: Experience with a transesophageal echotransducer allowing full rotation of the viewing plane: The omniplane probe [Abstract]. J. Am. Coll. Cardiol., 17:34, 1991.

Frazin, L., Talano, J. V., Stephanides, L., et al.: Esophageal echocardiography. Circulation, 54:102, 1976.

Freed, M. D., Nadas, A. S., Norwood, W. I., and Castaneda, A. R.: Is routine preoperative cardiac catheterization necessary before repair of secundum and sinus venosus atrial septal defects? J. Am. Coll. Cardiol., 4:333, 1984.

French, J. W., Popp, R. L., and Pitlick, P. T.: Cardiac localization of transvascular bioptome using two-dimensional echocardiography. Am. J. Cardiol., 51:219, 1983.

Gaudiani, V. A., Shemin, R. J., Syracuse, D. C., et al.: Continuous epicardial echocardiographic assessment of postoperative left ventricular function. J. Thorac. Cardiovasc. Surg., 76:64, 1978.

Gewertz, B. L., Kremser, P. C., Zarins, C. K., et al.: Transesophageal echocardiographic monitoring of myocardial ischemia during vascular surgery. J. Vasc. Surg., 5:607, 1987.

Goldman, D. E., and Jueter, T. F.: Tabular data of the velocity and absorption of high-frequency sound in a million tissues. J. Acoust. Soc. Am., 28:35, 1956.

Gorcsan, J., Romand, J. A., Mandarino, W. A., et al.: Assessment of left ventricular performance by on-line pressure-area relations using echocardiographic automated border detection. J. Am. Coll. Cardiol., 23:242, 1994.

Gramiak, R., and Shah, P. M.: Echocardiography of the aortic root. Invest. Radiol., 3:356, 1968.

Gregg, E. C., and Palogallo, G. L.: Acoustic impedance of tissue. Invest. Radiol., 4:357, 1969.

Gussenhoven, E. J., van Herwerden, L. A., Roelandt, J., et al.: Intraoperative two-dimensional echocardiography in congenital heart disease. J. Am. Coll. Cardiol., 9:565, 1987.

Gutgesell, H. P., Huhta, J. C., Latson, L. A., et al.: Accuracy of two-dimensional echocardiography in the diagnosis of congenital heart disease. Am. J. Cardiol., 55:514, 1985.

Hagler, D. J., Tajik, J., Seward, J. B., et al.: Intraoperative two-dimensional Doppler echocardiography. A preliminary study for congenital heart disease. J. Thorac. Cardiovasc. Surg., 95:516, 1988.

Hamilton, K., Ellenbogen, K., Lowe, J. E., and Kisslo, J.: Ultrasound diagnosis of pseudoaneurysm and contiguous ventricular septal defect complicating inferior myocardial infarction. J. Am. Coll. Cardiol., 6:1160, 1985.

Harpole, D. H., Clements, F. M., Quill, T., et al.: Right and left ventricular performance during and after abdominal aortic aneurysm repair. Ann. Surg., 209:356, 1989.

Harrison, L. H., Jr., Kisslo, J. A., Jr., and Sabiston, D. C., Jr.: Extraction of intramyocardial foreign body utilizing operative ultrasonography. J. Thorac. Cardiovasc. Surg., 82:345, 1981.

Hassett, A., Moran, J., Sabiston, D. C., and Kisslo, J.: Utility of echocardiography in the management of patients with penetrating missile wounds of the heart. J. Am. Coll. Cardiol., 7:1151, 1986.

Heger, J. J., Weyman, A. E., Wann, L. S., et al.: Cross-sectional echocardiographic analysis of the extent of left ventricular asynergy in acute myocardial infarction. Circulation, 61:1113, 1980.

Hiratzka, L. F., McPherson, D. D., Brandt, B., III, et al.: Intraoperative high-frequency epicardial echocardiography in coronary revascularization: Locating deeply embedded coronary arteries. Ann. Thorac. Surg., 42:S9, 1986a.

Hiratzka, L. F., McPherson, D. D., Brandt, B., III, et al.: The role of intraoperative high-frequency epicardial echocardiography during coronary artery revascularization. Circulation, 76:V-33, 1987.

Hiratzka, L. F., McPherson, D. D., Lamberth, W. C., Jr., et al.: Intraoperative evaluation of coronary artery bypass graft anastomoses with high-frequency epicardial echocardiography: Experimental validation and initial patient studies. Circulation, 73:1199, 1986b.

Hisanaga, K., Hisanaga, A., Hibi, N., et al.: High speed rotating scanner for transesophageal cross-sectional echocardiography. Am. J. Cardiol., 46:837, 1980.

Huhta, J. C., Glascoe, P., Murphy, D. J., Jr., et al.: Surgery without catheterization for congenital heart defects: Management of 100 patients. J. Am. Coll. Cardiol., 9:823, 1987.

Huhta, J. C., Gutgesell, H. P., Latson, L. A., and Huffines, F. D.: Two-dimensional echocardiographic assessment of the aorta in infants and children with congenital heart disease. Circulation, 70:417, 1984.

Iliceto, S., Nanda, N. C., Rizzon, P., et al.: Color Doppler evaluation of aortic dissection. Circulation, 75:748, 1987.

Isner, J., Rosenfield, K., Losordo, D., et al.: Combination balloon-ultrasound imaging catheter for percutaneous transluminal angioplasty. Circulation, 84:739–754, 1991.

Izumi, S., Miyatake, K., Beppu, S., et al.: Mechanism of mitral regurgitation in patients with myocardial infarction: A study using real-time two-dimensional Doppler flow imaging and echocardiography. Circulation, 76:777, 1987.

Johnson, M. L., Holmes, J. H., Spangler, R. D., and Paton, B. C.: Usefulness of echocardiography in patients undergoing mitral valve surgery. J. Thorac. Cardiovasc. Surg., 64:922, 1972.

Johnson, M. R., McPherson, D. D., Fleagle, S. R., et al.: Videodensitometric analysis of human coronary stenoses: Validation in vivo by intraoperative high-frequency epicardial echocardiography. Circulation, 77:328, 1988.

Kajiya, F., Ogasawara, Y., Tsujioka, K., et al.: Evaluation of human coronary blood flow with an 80 channel 20 mHz pulsed Doppler velocimeter and zero-cross and Fourier transform methods during cardiac surgery. Circulation, 74(Suppl. 3):53, 1986.

Kemper, A. J., O'Boyle, J. E., Sharma, S., et al.: Hydrogen peroxide contrast-enhanced two-dimensional echocardiography: Real-time in vivo delineation of regional myocardial perfusion. Circulation, 68:603, 1983.

Khandheria, B. K.: Suspected bacterial endocarditis: To TEE or not to TEE. J. Am. Coll. Cardiol., 21:222, 1993.

Klein, A., L., Bailey, A. S., Moura, A., et al.: Reliability of echocardiographic measurements of myocardial perfusion using commercially produced produced sonicated serum albumin (Albunex). J. Am. Coll. Cardiol., 22:1983, 1993.

Kossoff, G.: Diagnostic applications of ultrasound in cardiology. Aust. Radiol., 10:101, 1966.

Krabill, K. A., Ring, W. S., Foger, J. E., et al.: Echocardiographic versus cardiac catheterization diagnosis of infants with congenital heart disease requiring cardiac surgery. Am. J. Cardiol., 60:351, 1987.

Krebber, H., Hanrath, P., Janzen, R., et al.: Gas emboli during open heart surgery. Thorac. Cardiovasc. Surg., 30:401, 1982.

Kyo, S., Takamoto, S., Matsumura, M., et al.: Immediate and early postoperative evaluation of results of cardiac surgery by transesophageal two-dimensional Doppler echocardiography. Circulation, 76(Suppl. 5):113, 1987.

Lang, R. M., Borow, K. M., Neumann, A., and Feinstein, S. B.: Echocardiographic contrast agents: Effect of microbubbles and carrier solutions on left ventricular contractility. J. Am. Coll. Cardiol., 9:910, 1987.

Lappen, R. S., Riggs, T. W., Lapin, G. D., et al.: Two-dimensional echocardiographic measurement of right pulmonary artery diameter in infants and children. J. Am. Coll. Cardiol., 2:121, 1983.

Leeman, D. E., Levine, M. J., and Come, P. C.: Doppler echocardiography in cardiac tamponade: Exaggerated respiratory variation in transvalvular blood flow velocity integrals. J. Am. Coll. Cardiol., 11:572, 1988.

Macartney, F. J.: Cross-sectional echocardiographic diagnosis of congenital heart disease. Br. Heart J., 50:501, 1983.

Marcus, M., Wright, C., Doty, D., et al.: Measurements of coronary velocity and reactive hyperemia in the coronary circulation of humans. Circ. Res., 49:877, 1981.

Marcus, M. L., Hiratzka, L. F., Doty, D. B., et al.: Coronary obstructive lesions: Assessing their physiological significance in humans. Ann. Thorac. Surg., 42:S5, 1986.

Mark, J. B., Steinbrook, R. A., Gugino, L. D., et al.: Continuous noninvasive monitoring of cardiac output with esophageal Doppler ultrasound during cardiac surgery. Anesth. Analg., 65:1013, 1986.

Marshall, W. G., Barzilai, B., Kouchoukos, N. T., et al.: Intraoperative ultrasonic imaging of the ascending aorta. Ann. Thorac. Surg., 48:339, 1989.

Martin, R. P., Meltzer, R. S., Chia, B. L., et al.: Clinical utility of two-dimensional echocardiography in infective endocarditis. Am. J. Cardiol., 46:379, 1980.

Marwick, T., Currie, P. J., Stewart, W. J., et al.: Mechanisms of failure of mitral valve repair: An echocardiographic study. Am. Heart J., 122:149, 1991.

Mary, D. A. S., Catchpole, L. A., and Ionescu, M. I.: Intraoperative echocardiographic studies of the mitral valve: Assessment of commissurotomy and repair. J. Clin. Ultrasound, 4:349, 1976.

Masuyama, T., Kodama, K., Kitabatake, A., et al.: Continuous-wave Doppler echocardiographic detection of pulmonary regurgitation and its application to noninvasive estimation of pulmonary artery pressure. Circulation, 474:484, 1986.

Matsuzaki, M., Tohma, Y., Anno Y., et al.: Esophageal echocardiographic analysis of atrial dynamics. Am. Heart J., 109:355, 1985.

Maurer, G., Ong, K., Haendchen R., et al.: Myocardial contrast two-dimensional echocardiography: Comparison of contrast disappearance rates in normal and underperfused myocardium. Circulation, 69:418, 1984.

Meltzer, R. S., Woythaler, J. N., Buda, A. J., et al.: Two-dimensional echocardiographic quantification of infarct size alteration by pharmacologic agents. Am. J. Cardiol., 44:257, 1979.

Mimbs, J. W., Bauwens, D., Cohen, R. D., et al.: Effects of myocardial ischemia on quantitative ultrasonic backscatter and identification of responsible determinants. Circ. Res., 49:89, 1981.

Miyatake, K., Okamoto, M., Kinoshita, N., et al.: Doppler echocardiographic features of coronary arteriovenous fistula: Complementary roles of cross-sectional echocardiography and the Doppler technique. Br. Heart J., 51:508, 1984.

Motro, M., and Neufeld, H. N.: Should patients with pure mitral stenosis undergo cardiac catheterization? Am. J. Cardiol., 46:515, 1980.

Namekawa, K., Kasai, C., Tsukamoto, M., and Koyano, A.: Imaging of blood flow using autocorrelation. Ultrasound Med. Biol., 8:138, 1982.

Omoto, R.: Echocardiographic evaluation of left ventricular size, shape and function—Advantages and limitations of this method. Jpn. Circ. J., 46:1121, 1982.

Omoto, R., Takamoto, S., Kyo, S., and Yokote, Y.: The use of two-dimensional color Doppler sonography during the surgical management of aortic dissection. World J. Surg., 11:604, 1987.

Omoto, R., Yokote, Y., Takamoto, S., et al.: The development of real-time two-dimensional Doppler echocardiography and its clinical significance in acquired valvular diseases. With special reference to the evaluation of valvular regurgitation. Jpn. Heart J., 25:325, 1984.

Ong, K., Maurer, G., Feinstein, S., et al.: Computer methods for myocardial contrast two-dimensional echocardiography. J. Am. Coll. Cardiol., 3:1212, 1984.

Pandian, N. G., Brockway, B., Simonetti, J., et al.: Pericardiocentesis under two-dimensional echocardiographic guidance in loculated pericardial effusion. Ann. Thorac. Surg., 45:99, 1988.

Payen, D., Bousseau, D., Laborde, F., et al.: Comparison of perioperative and postoperative phasic blood flow in aortocoronary venous bypass grafts by means of pulsed Doppler echocardiography with implantable microprobes. Circulation, 74(Suppl. 3):61, 1986.

Rasmussen, S., Lovelace D. E., Knoebel, S. B., et al.: Echocardiographic detection of ischemia and infarcted myocardium. J. Am. Coll. Cardiol., 3:733, 1984.

Ren, J., Panidis, I. P., Kotler, M. N., et al.: Effect of coronary bypass surgery and valve replacement on left ventricular function: Assessment by intraoperative two-dimensional echocardiography. Am. Heart J., 109:281, 1985.

Ren, J. Y., Gian, R. H., Huang, W. M., et al.: Two-dimensional echocardiography in the guidance and evaluation of right intraventricular pacemaker implantation. J. Cardiovasc. Ultrason., 6:141, 1987.

Ribakove, G. H., Katz, E. S., Galloway, A. C., et al.: Surgical implications of transesophageal echocardiography to grade atheromatous aortic arch. Ann. Thorac. Surg., 53:758, 1992.

Rice, M. J., Seward, J. B., Hagler, D. J., et al.: Impact of 2-dimensional echocardiography on the management of distressed newborns in whom cardiac disease is suspected. Am. J. Cardiol., 51:288, 1983.

Richards, K. L., Cannon, S. R., Miller, J. F., and Crawford, M. H.: Calculation of aortic valve area by Doppler echocardiography: A direct application of the continuity equation. Circulation, 73:964, 1986.

Roberson, D. A., Muhiudeen, I. A., and Silverman, N. H.: Transesophageal echocardiography in pediatrics: Techniques and limitations. Echocardiography, 7:699, 1990.

Rodigas, P. C., Meyer, F. J., Haasler, G. B., et al.: Intraoperative 2-dimensional echocardiography: Ejection of microbubbles from the left ventricle after cardiac surgery. Am. J. Cardiol., 50:1130, 1982.

Sagar, K. B., Hastillo, A., Wolfgang, T. C., et al.: Echocardiographic left ventricular mass in the detection of acute rejection in cardiac transplantation [Abstract]. Circulation, 62(Suppl. 3):235, 1980.

Sagar, K. B., Pelc, L. E., Rhyne, T. L., et al.: Influence of heart rate, preload, afterload, and inotropic state on myocardial ultrasonic backscatter. Circulation, 77:478, 1988.

Sagar, K. B., Rhyne, T. L., Warltier, D. C., et al.: Intramyocardial variability in integrated backscatter: Effects of coronary occlusion and reperfusion. Circulation, 75:436, 1987.

Sahn, D. J., and Allen, H. D.: Real-time cross-sectional echocardiographic imaging and measurement of the patent ductus arteriosus in infants and children. Circulation, 58:343, 1978.

Sahn, D. J., Barratt-Boyes, B. G., Graham, K., et al.: Ultrasonic imaging of the coronary arteries in open-chest humans: Evaluation of coronary atherosclerotic lesions during cardiac surgery. Circulation, 66:1034, 1982.

Sakai, K., Hoshino, S., and Osawa, M.: Needle in the heart: Two-dimensional echocardiographic findings. Am. J. Cardiol., 53:1482, 1984.

Sheehan, F. H., Feneley, M. P., DeBruijn, M. P., et al.: Quantitative analysis of regional wall thickening by transesophageal echocardiography. J. Thorac. Cardiovasc. Surg., 103:347, 1992.

Sheikh, K. H., de Bruijn, N. P., Rankin, S., et al.: The utility of transesophageal echocardiography and Doppler color flow imaging in patients undergoing cardiac valve surgery. J. Am. Coll. Cardiol., 15:363, 1990.

Siegel, R. J., Ariani, M., Fishbein, M., et al.: Histopathologic validation of angioscopy and intravascular ultrasound. Circulation, 84:109, 1991.

Simon, P., Owen, A. N., Havel, M., et al.: Transesophageal echocardiography in the emergency surgical management of patients with aortic dissection. J. Thorac. Cardiovasc. Surg., 103:1113, 1992.

Sklenar, J., Jayaweera, A. R., and Kaul, S.: A computer-aided approach for the quantitation of regional left ventricular function using two-dimensional echocardiography. J. Am. Soc. Echocardiogr., 5:33, 1992.

Skorton, D. J., Melton, H. E., Jr., Pandian, N. G., et al.: Detection of acute myocardial infarction in closed-chest dogs by analysis of regional two-dimensional echocardiographic gray-level distributions. Circ. Res., 52:36, 1983.

Smith, J. S., Cahalan, M. K., Benefiel, D. J., et al.: Intraoperative detection of myocardial ischemia in high-risk patients: Electrocardiography versus two-dimensional transesophageal echocardiography. Circulation, 72:1015, 1985.

Snider, A. R., Enderlein, M. A., Teitel, D. F., and Juster, R. P.: Two-dimensional echocardiographic determination of aortic and pulmonary artery sizes from infancy to adulthood in normal subjects. Am. J. Cardiol., 53:218, 1984.

Spotnitz, H. M.: Two-dimensional ultrasound and cardiac operations. J. Thorac. Cardiovasc. Surg., 83:43, 1982.

Spotnitz, H. M., Bregman, D., Bowman, F. O., Jr., et al.: Effects of open heart surgery on end-diastolic pressure-diameter relations of the human left ventricle. Circulation, 59:662, 1979.

Spotnitz, H. M., Malm, J. R., King, D. L., et al.: Outflow tract obstruction in tetrology of Fallot: Intraoperative analysis by echocardiography. State J. Med., 6:1100, 1978.

Stark, J., Smallhorn, J., Huhta, J., et al.: Surgery for congenital heart defects diagnosed with cross-sectional echocardiography. Circulation, 68(Suppl. 2):129, 1983.

Stefan, G., and Bing, R. J.: Echocardiographic findings in experimental myocardial infarction of the posterior left ventricular wall. Am. J. Cardiol., 30:629, 1972.

Stevenson, J. G., Kawabori, I., and Bailey, W. W.: Noninvasive evaluation of Blalock-Taussig shunts: Determination of patency and differentiation from patent ductus arteriosus by Doppler echocardiography. Am. Heart J., 106:1121, 1983.

Stevenson, J. G., Kawabori, I., and Guntheroth, W. G.: Pulsed Doppler echocardiographic diagnosis of patent ductus arteriosus: Sensitivity, specificity, limitations, and technical features. Cathet. Cardiovasc. Diagn., 6:255, 1980.

Stewart, W. J., and Salcedo, E. E.: Echocardiography in patients undergoing mitral valve surgery. Semin. Thorac. Cardiovasc. Surg., 1:194, 1989.

Stewart, J. A., Silimperi, D., Harris, P., et al.: Echocardiographic documentation of vegetative lesions in infective endocarditis: Clinical implications. Circulation, 61:374, 1980.

St. John Sutton, M. G.: Routine cardiac catheterization: A prerequistie for valve surgery? Int. J. Cardiol., 1:320, 1981.

St. John Sutton, M. G., St. John Sutton, M. B., Oldershaw, P. J., et al.: Valve replacement without preoperative cardiac catheterization. N. Engl. J. Med., 305:1233, 1981.

Stratton, J. R., Tirchie, J. L., Hamilton, G. W., et al.: Left ventricular thrombi: In vivo detection by indium-111 platelet imaging and two-dimensional echocardiography. Am. J. Cardiol., 47:874, 1983.

Svennevig, J. L., Grip, A., Lindberg, H., et al.: Continuous monitoring of cardiac output postoperatively using an implantable Doppler probe. Scand. J. Thorac. Cardiovasc. Surg., 20:145, 1986.

Syracuse, D. C., Gaudiani, V. A., Kastl, D. G., et al.: Intraoperative intracardiac echocardiography during left ventriculomyotomy and myectomy for hypertrophic subaortic stenosis. Circulation, 58(Suppl. 1):23, 1978.

Takamoto, S., Kyo, S., Adachi, H., et al.: Intraoperative color flow mapping by real-time two-dimensional Doppler echocardiography for evaluation of valvular and congenital heart disease and vascular disease. J. Thorac. Cardiovasc. Surg., 90:802, 1985.

Tanaka, M., and Terasawa, Y.: Echocardiography evaluation of the tissue character in myocardium. Jpn. Circ. J., 43:367, 1979.

Taylor, A. L., Collins, S. M., Skorton, D. J., et al.: Artifactual regional gray level variability in contrast-enhanced two-dimensional echocardiographic images: Effect on measurement of the coronary perfusion bed. J. Am. Coll. Cardiol., 6:831, 1985.

Tei, C., Sakamaki, T., Shah, P. M., et al.: Myocardial contrast echocardiography: A reproducible technique of myocardial opacification for identifying regional perfusion deficits. Circulation, 67:585, 1983.

Thomas, L. J., III, Wickline, S. A., Perea, J. E., et al.: A real-time integrated backscatter measurement system for quantitative cardiac tissue characterization. IEEE Transactions on Ultrasonics, Ferroelectrics, and Frequency Control, UFFC-33, 1:27, 1986.

Topol, E. J., Humphrey, L. S., Borkon, A. M., et al.: Value of intraoperative left ventricular microbubbles detected by transesophageal two-dimensional echocardiography in predicting neurologic outcome after cardiac operations. Am. J. Cardiol., 56:773, 1985.

Topol, E. J., Weiss, J. L., Guzman, P. A., et al.: Immediate improvement of dysfunctional myocardial segments after coronary revascularization: Detection by intraoperative transesophageal echocardiography. J. Am. Coll. Cardiol., 4:1123, 1984.

Ungerleider, R. M., Greeley, W. J., Kanter, R. J., et al.: The learning curve for intraoperative echocardiography during congenital heart surgery. Ann. Thorac. Surg., 54:691, 1992.

Ungerleider, R. M., Greeley, W. J., Sheikh, K. H., et al.: Routine use of intraoperative epicardial echocardiography and Doppler color flow imaging to guide and evaluate repair of congenital heart lesions. J. Thorac. Cardiovasc. Surg., 100:297, 1990.

van Herwerden, L. A., Gussenhoven, E. J., Roelandt, J. R. T. C., et al: Intraoperative two-dimensional echocardiography in complicated infective endocarditis of the aortic valve. J. Thorac. Cardiovasc. Surg., 93:587, 1987.

Vick, G. W., III, Huhta, J. C., and Gutgesell, H. P.: Assessment of the ductus arteriosus in preterm infants utilizing suprasternal two-dimensional/Doppler echocardiography. J. Am. Coll. Cardiol., 5:973, 1985.

Villanueva, F. S., Glasheen, W. P., Sklenar, J., et al.: Successful and reproducible myocardial opacification during two-dimensional echocardiography from right heart injection of contrast. Circulation, 85:1557, 1992.

Visser, C. A., Kan, G., David, G. K., et al.: Two-dimensional echocardiography in the diagnosis of left ventricular thrombus: A prospective study of 67 patients with anatomic validation. Chest, 83:228, 1983.

von Ramm, O. T., and Thurstone, F. L.: Cardiac imaging using a phased array ultrasound system. I. System Design. Circulation, 53:258, 1976.

Wear, K. A., Shoup, T. A., and Popp, R. L.: Ultrasonic characterization of canine myocardium contraction. IEEE Trans. Ultrasonics, Ferroelectrics, and Frequency Control, UFFC-33, 4:347, 1986.

Weiss, J. L., Bulkley, B. H., Hutchins, G. M., and Mason, S. J.: Two-dimensional echocardiographic recognition of myocardial injury in man: Comparison with post-mortem studies. Circulation, 63:401, 1981.

Weyman, A. E., Feigenbaum, H., Dillon, J. C., et al.: Noninvasive visualization of the left main coronary artery by cross-sectional echocardiography. Circulation, 54:169, 1976.

White, C. W., Wright, C. B., Doty, D. B., et al.: Does visual interpretation of the coronary arteriogram predict the physiologic importance of a coronary stenosis? N. Engl. J. Med., 310:819, 1984.

Williams, W. G., Wigle, E. D., Rakowski, H., et al.: Results of surgery for hypertrophic obstructive cardiomyopathy. Circulation, 76(Suppl. 5):104, 1987.

Wilson, R. F., Marcus, M. L., and White, C. W.: Prediction of the physiologic significance of coronary arterial lesions by quantitative lesion geometry in patients with limited coronary artery disease. Circulation, 75:723, 1987.

Wong, C. Y. H., and Spotnitz, H. M.: Systolic and diastolic properties of the human left ventricle during valve replacement of chronic mitral regurgitation. Am. J. Cardiol., 47:40, 1981.

Wright, C. B., Melvin, D. B., Flege, J. B., et al.: Coronary bypass without angiography: An unusual circumstance. J. Thorac. Cardiovasc. Surg., 93:936, 1987.

Wyatt, H. L., Heng, M. K., Meerbaum, S., et al.: Cross-sectional echocardiography. I. Analysis of mathematical models for quantifying mass of the left ventricle in dogs. Circulation, 60:1104, 1979.

Wyatt, H. L., Meerbaum, S., Heng, M. K., et al.: Experimental evaluation of the extent of myocardial dyssynergy and infarct size by two-dimensional echocardiography. Circulation, 63:607, 1981.

# 32 Cardiopulmonary Bypass for Cardiac Surgery

David C. McGiffin and James K. Kirklin

*Cardiopulmonary bypass* (CPB) is a technique by which the pumping action of the heart and the gas exchange functions of the lung are replaced temporarily by a mechanical device—the pump oxygenator—attached to a patient's vascular system. Although some temporary dysfunction of organs and systems is occasionally the sequela of present techniques, CPB has become an indispensable technique for most cardiac surgical procedures.

The temporary provision of arterial blood flow using a pump oxygenator is an abnormal situation in which most if not all of the body's physiologic processes are affected. In total CPB, essentially all systemic venous blood returns to the pump oxygenator instead of to the heart. In partial CPB, some systemic venous blood returns to the heart and is ejected into the aorta.

This chapter outlines the historical development of CPB and discusses the technical aspects, pathophysiology, and damaging effects of CPB.

## HISTORICAL OVERVIEW

CPB and profound hypothermia with circulatory arrest usually are considered mutually exclusive techniques. However, CPB with the addition of hypothermia of some degree, and profound hypothermia with circulatory arrest are, in clinical practice, complementary techniques that may both be required to a greater or lesser extent in a variety of complex procedures for correction of congenital and acquired heart disease. Consequently, the interrelated historical development of these techniques is considered together.

The notion of employing an extracorporeal oxygenator through which the circulation could be diverted can be traced back to at least 1885 (Frey and Gruber, 1985). The next major step was the experimental work of Gibbon, in the late 1930s, who demonstrated support of the circulation by a pump oxygenator system (Gibbon, 1939). Gibbon's work went largely unnoticed for a number of years. During the late 1940s, others, including Dennis at the University of Minnesota, commenced work on pump oxygenators for CPB. This work led to an unsuccessful attempted repair of an atrial septal defect using a pump oxygenator in 1951, allowing Dennis and associates the credit for performing the first cardiac operation using this equipment. An autopsy showed that the lesion was in fact a partial atrioventricular canal, a misinterpretation that contributed to the patient's death. The first successful use of a pump oxygenator, in 1953, was by Gibbon (1954), who closed an atrial septal defect in a young woman. Unfortunately, further success at this time eluded him.

Of important historical interest is the series of operations performed by Lillehei and colleagues at the University of Minnesota beginning in 1954. These operations employed "controlled cross-circulation," with another human (usually a parent of the patient) acting as an oxygenator (Warden et al., 1954). Contemporaneously, other ingenious methods of extracorporeal oxygenation were attempted for intracardiac surgery. Canine lungs (Campbell et al., 1956) and monkey lungs (Mustard et al., 1954; Mustard and Thomason, 1957) were used as extracorporeal oxygenators, but with limited success. Extracorporeal perfusion using a reservoir of oxygenated blood drawn from donors prior to the procedure was used in a number of infants (Warden et al., 1955).

Several other major experimental and clinical contributions to the development of CPB were made by Bjork (1952) and Senning (1952). Of interest is the report of Crafoord and colleagues (1957), who removed an atrial myxoma using CPB. In March 1955, the first intracardiac operations using a pump oxygenator were begun by John Kirklin and colleagues at the Mayo Clinic (1955).

It is interesting to note that one of the early problems with the pump oxygenator was the enormous return of blood to the heart, which made accurate repair impossible (Lillehei, 1993). However, the realization that much lower perfusion flow rates could be used safely, based on the "azygos flow principle," was an important milestone in the development of CPB. The "azygos flow principle" developed from the observation that clamping the inferior and superior venae cavae of dogs allowed sufficient systemic venous return through the azygos vein to support the circulation for 30 minutes (Andreason and Watson, 1952; Cohen et al., 1952).

Hypothermia continues to be an integral part of CPB, with or without low-flow bypass or total circulatory arrest. It was Bigelow and co-workers in Toronto who, in 1950, suggested the advantages of profound hypothermia in intracardiac procedures, a suggestion based on the demonstration that dogs could survive surface cooling to 20° C followed by 15 minutes of total circulatory arrest (Bigelow et al., 1950). Clinical application of this concept can be attributed to Lewis and Taufic, who, in 1953, successfully repaired an atrial septal defect in a 5-year-old girl using surface cooling to achieve profound hypothermia. Swan and colleagues (1953) contemporaneously reported success with the same technique. The combination of hypothermia with CPB was first reported by Sealy and colleagues in 1958. The technique of surface cooling, CPB, profound hypothermia, and total circulatory arrest was reported by a number of surgeons, including Dubost and co-workers (Weiss et al., 1960), Kirklin and colleagues (1961), Horiuchi and associates (1963), Dillard and co-workers (1967), and Barrett-Boyes and colleagues (1970). Core cooling using CPB to achieve profound hypothermia to allow total circulatory arrest was reported by Hamilton and colleagues in 1973.

## ELEMENTS OF CARDIOPULMONARY BYPASS

### Pump Oxygenator

Although the construction of the individual components of the pump oxygenator has changed, the basic components have remained relatively constant. The central component of the system is the *oxygenator,* which allows oxygenation of the blood and elimination of carbon dioxide. Although bubble oxygenators (gas exchange occurring at the blood-gas interface) have the advantages of compactness and economy, they have largely been replaced by membrane oxygenators, in which gas exchange occurs through tiny pores in a membrane. These hollow-fiber membrane oxygenators still have a blood-gas interface, unlike true membrane oxygenators, which incorporate a silicone membrane that eliminates the blood-gas interface. Silicone membrane oxygenators are now used particularly for extracorporeal membrane oxygenation (ECMO) because of their functional stability for long periods. The damaging effects of CPB on the blood appear to be less pronounced with membrane oxygenators than with bubble oxygenators, and membrane oxygenators are therefore preferred (Van Oeveren et al., 1985). The *venous reservoir* stores excess volume and is positioned to allow siphonage of blood by gravity. The *heat exchanger* is required to regulate the temperature of the perfusate.

The *arterial pump* is usually of the roller pump design, which generates a nonpulsatile flow. The centrifugal pump can be used in the CPB circuit. The design of the centrifugal pump incorporates an impeller with vanes within a housing. The impeller is coupled magnetically to an electric motor, and rapid rotation of the impeller produces blood flow. Unlike the roller pump, wherein pump revolution is proportional to flow, the centrifugal pump is totally nonocclusive, and flow (among other variables) depends on downstream resistance. Therefore, flow is not necessarily related to impeller revolutions, and a flow meter is required in the circuit. Centrifugal pumps are used mainly in extracorporeal ventricular assist devices, but they have been used for left-sided heart bypass during thoracic aortic surgery (Diehl et al., 1987; Everts et al., 1991; Olivier et al., 1984; Walls et al., 1989, 1991). Although some benefits have been demonstrated with the centrifugal pump compared with the roller pump (principally less damage to blood cells) (Driessen et al., 1991; Hoerr et al., 1987; Wheeldon et al., 1990), these differences are not sufficient to recommend routine use in CPB.

Blood returning to the operative field is returned to the pump oxygenator by way of *cardiotomy suction lines.* However, this blood usually contains a considerable amount of air, which must be filtered out before being returned to the system. An *arterial line pressure monitor* is required in the system, because line pressures in excess of 300 mm Hg increase the risk of arterial line disruption and cavitation at the arterial cannula. The use of an *arterial line filter* had been considered unnecessary (Walker et al., unpublished data), but more recently it has been demonstrated that gaseous microembolization can be reduced with a 40-μm filter interposed in the arterial line between the pump oxygenator and the patient (Padayachee et al., 1988).

The pump oxygenator should be designed to *minimize priming volume.* This parameter is most critical in infants, in whom the priming volume can greatly exceed blood volume.

### Cannulation

Ascending aortic or, in certain circumstances, femoral arterial cannulation is used. The aortic cannula should be inserted as near to the origin of the innominate artery as is surgically acceptable, and only a short length of cannula is introduced so that its tip cannot actually enter a brachiocephalic vessel or lie near its orifice. The cannula is secured by two concentric purse-string sutures in the aortic adventitia and media. The inner purse-string suture is threaded through a tourniquet to snug down around the cannula (Fig. 32–1).

Venous cannulation in neonates and children involves insertion of right-angle metal-tipped cannulas directly into each vena cava, particularly if one is working through the right atrium or right ventricle. A single venous cannula may be used if the procedure involves working through the left atrium, left ventricle, ascending aorta, and occasionally the right ventricle—for example, when changing a valved external conduit. In infants, a single venous cannula is also used when the repair is to be performed under total circulatory arrest.

In adults, a single large cavoatrial (two-stage) venous cannula may be used for coronary bypass grafting, aortic valve operations, mitral valve operations, and combined procedures. Two venous cannulas are used when working in the right atrium.

The size of arterial (Table 32–1) and venous cannulas (Table 32–2) is determined primarily by the selected total perfusion flow rate. There is an acceptable range of perfusion rates for any given patient size,

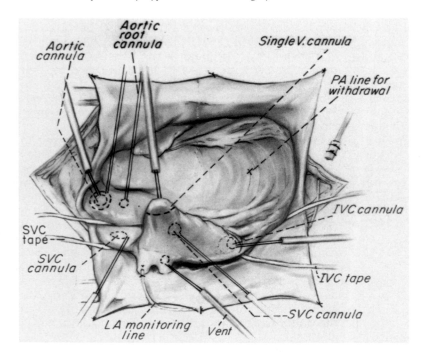

**FIGURE 32–1.** Illustration of the position of possible cannulation sites for cardiopulmonary bypass (CPB). Sites of left atrial (LA) and pulmonary artery (PA) monitoring lines and left atrial vent are also shown. Obviously, not all sites are used in an individual patient. (IVC = inferior vena cava; SVC = superior vena cava; V = venous.) (Modified from Kirklin, J. W., and Barratt-Boyes, B. G.: Hypothermia, circulatory arrest and cardiopulmonary bypass. *In* Kirklin, J. W., and Barratt-Boyes, B. G. [eds]: Cardiac Surgery. Churchill Livingstone, New York, 1993, p. 103.)

which will allow somewhat smaller cannulas to be used if required. The arterial cannula selected should have a pressure gradient of 100 mm Hg or less at the highest flow rate.

## Intracardiac Suction Devices

Suction lines are required to aspirate blood from the opened heart, return it to the pump oxygenator as part of the venous return, and decompress the heart (particularly the left side) when needed. Therefore, just after establishing CPB for some operations, a right-angled catheter vent ($^{2}/_{16}$ or $^{3}/_{16}$ inch internal diameter) is inserted into the left atrium through a small stab wound and protected by a purse-string suture in the right side of the left atrium or in the anterior wall of the superior pulmonary vein near the left atrium. The venting catheter usually is advanced

through the mitral valve into the left ventricle. In most pediatric open heart operations, the left atrium and left ventricle are decompressed by a small metal "infant sump" catheter passed through a patent foramen ovale or a stab wound in the atrial septum. Gentle suction is applied to the vent, ideally by a regulated vacuum system but in practice by a well-controlled occlusive pump.

For aspirating blood from the opened heart, a special sucker that has a guard over the tip is used to minimize the tendency of leaflet and other intracardiac tissue to be drawn up into it. This is used as a sump drain, and therefore functions best when positioned in a pool of blood in a dependent portion of the opened heart. The sucker is attached to one of the intracardiac return lines, again activated by a well-controlled occlusive pump.

## Systemic and Pulmonary Venous Pressure

Systemic venous pressure in the patient during CPB is determined by the following equation:

$$P\overline{v}_{sys} = f \left( \frac{\dot{Q}, \text{Viscosity}}{\text{Cannula size, venous line size, venous line suction}} \right) \quad (1)$$

where $P\overline{v}_{sys}$ = the mean systemic venous pressure and $\dot{Q}$ = systemic blood flow. The cross-sectional area of the single or multiple venous cannulas and their length and, to a lesser extent (because it usually has a large diameter), that of the venous line to the pump oxygenator, are the fixed factors determining venous pressure during total CPB. Thus, the largest venous cannulas that are compatible with the clinical situation are used. When smaller cannulas must be

■ **Table 32–1.** ARTERIAL CANNULA FLOW CHART: PRESSURE GRADIENT IN MILLIMETERS OF MERCURY (mm Hg)

| Cannula Size in French Scale | Flow (l/min) | | | | | | | |
|---|---|---|---|---|---|---|---|---|
| | 0.5 | 1.0 | 1.5 | 2.0 | 2.5 | 3.0 | 3.5 | 4.0 |
| 10 | 60 | 175 | 350 | | | | | |
| 12 | 40 | 100 | 225 | 325 | | | | |
| 14 | 25 | 60 | 140 | 240 | 350 | | | |
| 16 | | 25 | 60 | 90 | 150 | 200 | 260 | |
| 18 | | 20 | 40 | 60 | 80 | 120 | 150 | 200 |
| 20 | | | 25 | 40 | 60 | 80 | 100 | 120 |
| 22 | | | 25 | 40 | 50 | 60 | 75 | 90 |
| 24 | | | | 40 | 50 | 60 | 70 | 80 |

From Kirklin, J. K., and Kirklin, J. W.: Cardiopulmonary bypass for cardiac surgery. *In* Sabiston, D. C., Jr., and Spencer, F. C. [eds]: Surgery of the Chest. 5th ed. Philadelphia, W. B. Saunders, 1990, p. 1109.

■ **Table 32–2.** VENOUS CANNULAS FOR VARIOUS FLOWS

| Total Flow (l/min) | | Cannula Size* | | | | | | |
|---|---|---|---|---|---|---|---|---|
| | | Single Tygon | Single USCI†, ‡ | Two Tygon | Two Ryggs§ | Two USCI† | Pacifico Angled Metal | |
| ≤ | < | | | | | | SVC | IVC |
| | 0.9 | 3⁄16″ (4.75) | 20 Fr (4.7) | | 4 mm | 16 Fr (3.18 mm) | 16 Fr (3.8 mm) | 20 Fr (5.3 mm) |
| 0.9–1.75 | | 4⁄16″ (6.35) | 24 Fr (5.26) | 3⁄16″ (4.75) | 5 mm | | | |
| 0.9–1.2 | | | | | | 20 Fr (4.17) | 20 Fr (5.3 mm) | 24 Fr (5.3 mm) |
| 1.2–1.6 | | | | | | 22 Fr (4.88) | 20 Fr (5.3 mm) | 24 Fr (6.5 mm) |
| 1.6–1.75 | | | | | | 24 Fr (5.26) | 24 Fr (6.5 mm) | 24 Fr (6.5 mm) |
| 1.7–2.2 | | 4⁄16″ (6.35) | 28 Fr (6.60) | 4⁄16″ (6.35) | 6 mm | 28 Fr (6.60) | 24 Fr (6.5 mm) | 28 Fr (7.45 mm) |
| 2.2–2.8 | | 5⁄16″ (7.95) | | 4⁄16″ (6.35) | 6 mm | 30 Fr (7.24) | 28 Fr (7.45 mm) | 29 Fr (7.45 mm) |
| 2.8–3.2 | | 5⁄16″ (7.95) | | 5⁄16″ (7.95) | 6 mm | 32 Fr (8.05) | 28 Fr (7.45 mm) | 28 Fr (7.45 mm) |
| 3.2–3.7 | | 6⁄16″ (9.52) | | 5⁄16″ (7.95) | 7 mm | 34 Fr (9.74) | 28 Fr (7.45 mm) | 32 Fr (8 mm) |
| 3.7 | | 8⁄16″ (12.69) | | 6⁄16″ (9.52) | 7 mm | 36 Fr (9.19) | 32 Fr (8 mm) | 32 Fr (9 mm) |

From Kirklin, J. W., and Barratt-Boyes, B. G. (eds): Cardiac Surgery. Churchill Livingstone, New York, 1993, p. 82.
*Key:* Fr = French; IVC = inferior vena cava; SVC = superior vena cava.
*Outer diameter; internal diameter in mm in parentheses.
†United States Catheter and Instrument, a division of CR Bard, Box 666, Billerica, MA 01821.
‡In adults, at University of Alabama at Birmingham, USCI "two-stage" single cannula is used (46 Fr, 11.84 mm internal diameter, tapering to 34 Fr, 8.74 mm internal diameter).
§Ryggs venous catheters by Polystand (North America), 925 South Curry Pike, Box 1308, Bloomington, IN 47401.

used, the other variables in the equation can be manipulated (e.g., the systemic blood flow may be reduced) to ensure an acceptable venous pressure.

There is no apparent physiologic advantage in having a central venous pressure of more than zero during CPB. Raising the venous pressure requires more intravascular volume and often an additional priming volume.

Pulmonary venous pressure ideally should be at zero during total CPB, and never above 10 mm Hg. Undue rises are dangerous because they tend to produce increased extravascular pulmonary water and eventually pulmonary edema, according to Starling's law of transcapillary fluid exchange:

$$P_c - P_t = \pi_c - \pi_t \tag{2}$$

where $P_c$ = "effective" blood pressure within the capillary; $P_t$ = tissue turgor pressure (interstitial fluid pressure); $\pi_c$ = osmotic pressure of the plasma (colloid) inside the capillary; and $\pi_t$ = osmotic pressure of the extracellular fluid (tissue colloid osmotic pressure). The increase in extracellular pulmonary water is related to the duration of elevation of pulmonary venous or pulmonary capillary pressure, other things being equal.

## Perfusion Flow Rate

The *optimal flow rate* during CPB is still being debated. A few facts are clear. Acidosis with increased lactic acid production, low oxygen consumption, and other features of cardiogenic shock result from normothermic CPB at flows of less than approximately 1.6 l/min/m² (or less than approximately 50 ml/kg/min) (Diesh et al., 1957). Experimental data (Levin et al., 1960; Moffitt et al., 1962) and experience indicate that at normothermia, flows exceeding 1.8 l/min/

m² are acceptable with regard to total body oxygen consumption, but flows of 2.2 to 2.5 l/min/m² are more securely adequate. For large patients (body surface area = 2.0 m²), a flow rate of 1.8 to 2.0 l/min/m² is selected to avoid the potential risks of exceeding the flow capacity of the venous cannulas and increasing the damage to blood elements at the blood-gas interface.

The best criterion of acceptability or adequacy of flow rate at any temperature is the survival of the subject without structural or functional evidence of organ or system damage. We believe that survival without damage is most likely when the entire microcirculation is perfused at flow rates that maintain near-normal tissue oxygen levels. In patients on CPB, this probably pertains to when whole-body oxygen consumption ($\dot{V}O_2$) is near the asymptote of the temperature-specific curve relating flow to $\dot{V}O_2$ (Fig. 32–2).

Low-flow CPB occasionally is required during intracardiac repair to improve visualization. Of all organs, the brain is probably the most sensitive to reductions in oxygen supply. The effects of altered flow rates on brain blood flow and oxygen consumption have been studied in monkeys during CPB at 20° C (Fox et al., 1984). Oxygen consumption of the brain was well maintained as flow was reduced from 1.5 to 0.5 l/min/m² on CPB at 20° C. The resistance to blood flow in the brain remained unchanged, whereas that of the remaining body increased as the flow rate was reduced. Even at the lowest perfusion flow rate (0.25 l/min/m²), all areas of the brain were perfused. It thus appears that the brain, the resistance of which does not change, becomes the passive recipient of proportionally more blood flow during low-flow, hypothermic CPB. In addition to these experimental studies, a large clinical experience indicates that perfusion flow rates can be safely reduced to 0.5 l/min/m² for 30 to 45 minutes at 25° C.

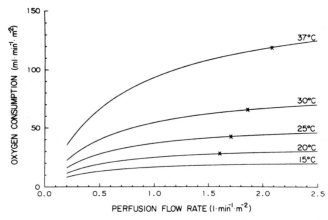

FIGURE 32–2. Nomogram of an equation, expressing the relation of oxygen consumption ($\dot{V}_{O_2}$) to perfusion flow rate ($\dot{Q}$) and temperature (T). The small xs represent the perfusion flow rates that the authors use at these temperatures. The equation is as follows:

$$1 / \dot{V}_{O_2} = 0.168 \times 10^{-0.0387T} + 0.0378 \times \dot{Q}^{-1} \times 10^{-0.0253T}$$

(From Kirklin, J. W., and Barratt-Boyes, B. G.: Hypothermia, circulatory arrest and cardiopulmonary bypass. *In* Kirklin, J. W., and Barrett-Boyes, B. G. [eds]: Cardiac Surgery. Churchill Livingstone, New York, 1993, p. 913.)

## Hematocrit

Hematocrit of the mixed patient and pump oxygenator blood volume is determined by the composition and amounts of blood and fluids infused before and during CPB, the blood loss, and the amount and composition of the initial (priming) volume of the pump oxygenator. The hematocrit is also affected by patient interactions, primarily transcapillary movement of fluid from the intravascular to the interstitial space and into urine volume.

In intact patients at 37° C, the normal hematocrit of 0.4 to 0.5 is optimal for oxygen transport (Chien, 1972). This level provides sufficient oxygen delivery to maintain normal mitochondrial $P_{O_2}$ levels of approximately 0.05 to 1 mm Hg and average intracellular $P_{O_2}$ levels of approximately 5 mm Hg, which are reflected in normal oxygen levels ($P\bar{V}_{O_2}$ of approximately 40 mm Hg, $S\bar{V}_{O_2}$ of approximately 75% in mixed venous blood). The normal hematocrit is also optimal rheologically in intact persons (Chien, 1972). When the hematocrit is abnormally high, oxygen content is high, but the increased viscosity tends to decrease blood flow. Thus, the rate of oxygen transport varies directly with hematocrit (because oxygen content varies directly with hematocrit, assuming normal red blood cell hemoglobin concentrations and adequate oxygenation) and inversely with the blood's (apparent) viscosity (which is also determined primarily by hematocrit). Hypothermia increases the blood's (apparent) viscosity, so that at low temperatures a lower hematocrit is more appropriate than at 37° C. A hematocrit that is less than "normal" appears desirable during hypothermic CPB because of its association with lower apparent blood viscosity and low shear rates, thus presumably producing better

perfusion of the microcirculation. Excessive hemodilution, however, is probably deleterious because of the greater extravascular extravasation of fluid secondary to the decreased intravascular osmotic pressure (Cohn et al., 1971).

Thus, a hematocrit of approximately 0.25 to 0.3 is desirable during hypothermic perfusions. During rewarming, a higher hematocrit ($\geq 0.30$) is desirable because of the increased oxygen demands, and the higher apparent viscosity at these higher hematocrits is appropriate during normothermia. The body's autoregulatory mechanisms, including its capacity to recover from transient abnormalities in oxygen delivery, are so well developed that a considerable range ($\pm 0.05$) of hematocrits around the desirable point is acceptable. This is fortunate; otherwise, the need for homologous blood, with its own economic and medical disadvantages, in the priming volume would be increased. Because at University of Alabama, Birmingham, essentially all CPB procedures are done by using hypothermia (20 to 25° C), an initial hematocrit of 0.25 to 0.3 is accepted. Thus, the authors calculate the mixed patient-machine hematocrit that will result if the pump oxygenator is primed with an asanguineous solution using the following equation, where $Hct_{pm}$ = hematocrit of combined patient-machine blood volume, $Hct_p$ = patient hematocrit, and BV = blood volume. Therefore, when no blood is in the priming volume,

$$Hct_{pm} = \frac{(\text{body weight [kg]} \times f \times 1000) \, Hct_p}{(\text{body weight [kg]} \times f \times 1000) + \text{machine BV}} \quad (3)$$

where f = 0.08 in infants and children (<12 years old) and f = 0.065 in older patients (>12 years old). (These are average values and provide a method of estimating blood volume. More complex regression equations are available for more precise estimates.) If the calculated hematocrit is in the desired range, the clear priming solution is used. Approximately 20% of the priming solution is 5% dextrose and 80% balanced salt solution with sufficient concentrated human albumin added to make it colloidally iso-osmotic. If the calculated hematocrit is too low, an appropriate amount of blood is added by using the following equation to solve for the desired volume of packed red blood cells that will obtain the desired patient-machine hematocrit:

$$Hct_{pm} = \frac{\text{patient RBC volume (ml)} + \text{machine RBC volume (ml)}}{\text{patient BV (ml)} + \text{machine BV (ml)}} \quad (4)$$

Banked blood less than about 48 hours old is used, but older blood for adults is accepted when necessary. The blood has, of course, been rendered $Ca^{2+}$ free by the anticoagulant solution and is acidotic; thus, heparin, calcium, and buffer are added (Table 32–3).

## Temperature of the Perfusate

Virtually all procedures conducted with CPB use some degree of hypothermia of the perfusate and hence of the patient.

**■ Table 32–3.** ADDITIVES TO A UNIT OF CITRATE–PHOSPHATE–DEXTROSE BLOOD FOR THE PUMP OXYGENATOR

| | | |
|---|---|---|
| CPD blood | 500 ml | |
| Heparin | 3 ml | (3000 units—mean 6 units/ml of blood) |
| NaHCO₃ (8.4%) | 10 ml | |
| CaCl₂ (10%) | 5 ml | (added last) |
| | 518 ml | |

From Kirklin, J. K., and Kirklin, J. W.: Cardiopulmonary bypass for cardiac surgery. In Sabiston, D. C., Jr., and Spencer, F. C. (eds): Surgery of the Chest. 5th ed. Philadelphia, W. B. Saunders, 1990, p. 1112.

Considerable experimental information demonstrates that hypothermia reduces oxygen consumption. The relationship between biochemical reaction rates and temperature is described by van't Hoff's law, which states that the logarithm of a chemical reaction is directly related to the temperature. The term $Q_{10}$ is used to describe the multiple by which reaction rates increase for every 10° C increase in temperature.

Several experimental studies of oxygen consumption measured in tissue slices during hypothermia suggest that the $Q_{10}$ is approximately 2.0 (Field et al., 1939; Fuhrman, 1956; Fuhrman et al., 1961). A reanalysis (Kirklin and Barratt-Boyes, 1993) of previously published experimental data (Penrod, 1949; Ross, 1954) suggests a $Q_{10}$ of about 2.7. The use of hypothermia in association with CPB allows lower perfusion flow rates because of the reduced oxygen consumption. A lower perfusion flow rate reduces trauma to the cellular elements of the blood and improves the surgeon's view of the operative field by reducing pulmonary, bronchial, and noncoronary collateral return to the heart. Systemic hypothermia also minimizes warming of the heart that might impair myocardial protection. Systemic hypothermia is also required for cerebral protection if circulatory arrest is to be employed. Finally, systemic hypothermia does afford organ protection during the highly unlikely event of mechanical problems with the pump oxygenator.

An exception to the routine use of hypothermia for CPB is the recent concept of "warm heart surgery." This method is based on the concept that delivery of continuous normothermic cardioplegia causing electromechanical arrest of the myocardium accounts for 90% of the reduction in oxygen requirements, with minimal further reduction due to hypothermia (Lichtenstein et al., 1991). Consequently, with this method, systemic hypothermia to enhance myocardial protection becomes unnecessary. The perfusate is not actively cooled, and the patient's temperature may be allowed to drift to 32 to 34° C or may be held at 37° C according to the preference of the surgeon (Lichtenstein et al., 1991).

## Acid-Base Management

The strategy for managing pH on CPB continues to be controversial, with uncertainty as to the appro-

priate pH and $P_{CO_2}$ values during hypothermia. With hypothermia, the solubility of $CO_2$ increases; hence $P_{CO_2}$ falls and pH rises. This phenomenon can be seen in human tissue—for example, skin on a cold day may have a higher pH than that in exercising muscle, which is at a higher temperature (Davies, 1993). There follow, then, two strategies for managing pH and $P_{CO_2}$ during hypothermic CPB. The pH-stat strategy is based on the assumption that a pH of 7.40 and a $P_{CO_2}$ of 40 mm Hg should be maintained regardless of the temperature. Therefore, during hypothermic CPB, the pH and $P_{CO_2}$ of the patient are measured by a pH electrode at 37° C, and the values obtained are then corrected back to the patient's temperature using a nomogram. To adjust the corrected pH down to 7.40, 5% $CO_2$ is added to the oxygenator gas flow, creating a relative respiratory acidosis and hypercarbia. In the alternative strategy, known as alpha-stat, the pH is allowed to change as temperature changes. (The "alpha" refers to the fraction of unprotonated imidazole groups of histidine, which is the primary determinant of protein charge, and hence buffering; this fraction stays constant as temperature decreases.) Consequently, pH is measured by the pH electrode at 37° C, and no correction is made for the patient's temperature; therefore, at hypothermia, a state of respiratory alkalosis and hypocarbia exists. This system is based on the observations of Rahn and associates (1975), Reeves (1977), and White (1981) concerning acid-base control in poikilothermic animals. Water dissociates less as the temperature falls, but electrochemical neutrality is maintained because the ratio of $H^+$ and $OH^-$ is not disturbed; however, the pH increases because the absolute amount of $H^+$ decreases. Furthermore, the function of a number of enzyme systems depends on electrochemical neutrality being maintained during fluctuations in temperature. Thus, with fluctuations in temperature, the most appropriate pH is linked to neutrality (Fig. 32–3). Williams and Marshall (1982) subsequently suggested the ap-

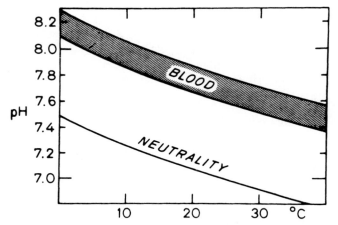

**FIGURE 32–3.** Parallel change in intracellular pH and electrochemical neutrality with changing temperature. (From Ream, A. K., Reitz, B. A., and Silverberg, G.: Temperature correction of $P_{CO_2}$ and pH in estimating acid-base status: An example of the emperor's new clothes? Anesthesiology, 56:41, 1982.)

plication of this approach, which maintains electro-chemical neutrality for acid-base management during hypothermic CPB (alpha-stat).

The disadvantage of the pH-stat method is that autoregulation may be lost, producing excessive cerebral blood flow and increasing the risk of microembolization and cerebral edema (Henriksen, 1986; Lassen, 1966; Murkin et al., 1987). The alpha-stat strategy, however, may reduce cerebral blood flow (Henriksen, 1986; Murkin et al., 1987), and because the milieu is alkalotic, the oxygen/hemoglobin dissociation curve is shifted to the left, and both effects may potentially result in inadequate cerebral oxygen delivery. In clinical practice, no firm recommendation can yet be made as to the optimal pH strategy because of conflicting information. Bashein and co-workers (1990) found no neurobehavioral differences between adults undergoing cardiac surgery with either the alpha-stat or the pH-stat strategy. Baraka and colleagues (1992) found that whole-body oxygen consumption in adult patients undergoing coronary artery bypass surgery was independent of the $CO_2$ management strategy. On the other hand, Tuppurainen and associates (1989), in a study of adult patients, found higher whole-body oxygen consumption during hypothermic CPB using an alpha-stat strategy, compared with a pH-stat strategy, and interpreted these data as reflecting better enzyme function with the alpha-stat strategy. In an animal model (Willford et al., 1990), whole-body oxygen consumption was higher with a pH-stat strategy than with an alpha-stat strategy, but the pH-stat strategy was considered to yield less satisfactory protection of tissues from hypoxic damage during hypothermia. Of some concern is the report by Jonas and associates (1993) that the use of the more alkaline alpha-stat strategy during the cooling phase of CPB prior to circulatory arrest in infants undergoing a Senning repair was associated with developmental impairment suggesting suboptimal cerebral protection.

## Glucose Concentration

The glucose concentration is increased in the priming solution (about 350 mg/100 ml) in order to provide an energy source as well as to promote osmotic diuresis during and for a few hours after CPB.

## Arterial Oxygen

Arterial oxygen levels are usually maintained at a level of 100 to 250 mm Hg with current membrane oxygenators. A higher $Pa_{O_2}$ is unnecessary and exposes the patient to the risk of oxygen toxicity and bubble formation. Shepard (1973) has shown that in dogs undergoing normothermic CPB, arterial oxygen saturation levels less than 65% at normothermia cause decreased $\dot{V}_{O_2}$, indicating hypoxic cell injury. Hypothermic perfusion produces a decrease in $\dot{V}_{O_2}$ and an increase in mixed venous oxygen levels, both of

which cause an increased $Pa_{O_2}$. During rewarming, the increasing $\dot{V}_{O_2}$ produces relatively low mixed venous oxygen levels.

## Perfusion Pressure

No consensus has been reached as to the desirable perfusion pressure during CPB. At least some clinical evidence suggests that cerebral blood flow is reduced with a mean perfusion pressure of less than 50 to 60 mm Hg (Stockard et al., 1973; Treasure et al., 1989; Tufo et al., 1970). Although pharmacologic manipulation of systemic vascular resistance during CPB may not be performed routinely, it does seem a reasonable practice if the perfusion pressure falls below 55 mm Hg, particularly during rewarming. Also, perfusion pressure greater than 100 mm Hg during CPB may be best reduced pharmacologically.

## Anticoagulation for CPB

Heparin is a glycosaminoglycan that produces anticoagulation principally by potentiating the activity of antithrombin III, which then binds with greatly increased avidity to thrombin and to several other factors in the coagulation cascade. During CPB, heparin may be given empirically or monitored either by clotting time, of which *activated clotting time* (ACT) is the mostly widely used method, or by heparin concentration assay. It would appear that a minimum ACT of 300 seconds is adequate (Bull et al., 1975), although lower ACTs may be safe with membrane oxygenators. Although monitored heparin dosing is not clearly superior to unmonitored regimens, it does seem prudent to employ some form of heparin dose monitoring.

Protamine reverses the anticoagulant state by binding ionically to heparin. Several methods are used to calculate the dose of protamine, including a fixed dose based on the amount of heparin administered, ACT/heparin dose response curves, heparin levels, and protamine titration (Moorman et al., 1993). Protamine dose calculation prevents administration of excessive protamine and inadequate heparin reversal, but precision of the dose calculation needs to be balanced against simplicity.

Although we recognize that many other effective anticoagulation and reversal protocols for CPB are in use, the current procedure at the University of Alabama at Birmingham is as follows:

- Baseline ACT
- Heparin administered at a dose of 300 U/kg
- ACT is checked prior to commencing CPB to ensure that it is greater than 480 seconds
- During CPB, ACT is checked every 30 minutes, with additional heparin as required
- Reversal of heparin—1.5 mg of protamine/100 U of initial heparin dose
- For infants, initial dose and heparin dose are added to pump prime

- ACT is checked; if prolonged beyond control, sample is added to an ACT tube containing heparinase to exclude or confirm excess heparin and thus whether more protamine is indicated

An important goal is elimination of the need for systemic heparinization during CPB. A clinical trial of a heparin-coated circuit with a 50% reduction in systemic heparinization significantly decreased postoperative blood loss (Borowiec et al., 1992). Furthermore, the use of a heparin-coated surface with standard heparinization reduced the inflammatory response of CPB (Gu et al., 1993).

## PATHOPHYSIOLOGIC RESPONSE TO CARDIOPULMONARY BYPASS

Understanding of the profound effects of CPB on all tissues continues to evolve. Many responses to CPB have been associated with its damaging effects, but the role of many responses, including the release of numerous autocoids, is not yet understood.

### Catecholamine Response

*Epinephrine* (from the adrenal medulla) and *norepinephrine* (from sympathetic nerve terminals) may reach very high levels during CPB (Hirvonen et al., 1978; Reed et al., 1989; Reves et al., 1982). It appears that plasma epinephrine levels, which decrease following the discontinuation of CPB, remain elevated postoperatively only in those patients with postoperative hypertension (Wallach et al., 1980). Catecholamine release also occurs in neonates and infants undergoing CPB (Anand et al., 1990; Firmin et al., 1985). The marked catecholamine release (especially of norepinephrine) is partly explained by the very much reduced pulmonary blood flow during CPB, the lungs being the site of degradation of norepinephrine (Reves et al., 1982). *Dopamine* does not appear to be released during CPB (Landymore et al., 1979).

### Some Other Hormonal Responses

*Cortisol* secretion in response to CPB appears to be different from the classic stress response to surgery, wherein cortisol levels rise during the procedure, cannot be increased further by adrenocorticotrophic hormone stimulation, and then return to presurgical levels within 24 hours of operation. Although information is conflicting, it is likely that cortisol rises during CPB, but the more marked increase occurs following discontinuation of CPB (Lacoumenta et al., 1987; Uozumi et al., 1972). This response can be significantly modified by anesthetic technique (Raff et al., 1987).

Perturbations to the *renin-angiotensin-aldosterone system* associated with CPB are understandably complex. But despite the role of this system in regulating blood pressure and fluid balance, no consistent relationship is apparent between changes to this hormonal system and postoperative hypertension (Weinstein et al., 1987).

*Triiodothyronine* (T3) is potentially important following cardiac surgery because of its role in the regulation of myocardial beta-adrenergic receptors and hence myocardial contractility and oxygen consumption (Salter et al., 1992). Some information suggests that both total T3 and free T3 levels fall during CPB (Bremner et al., 1978; Holland et al., 1991).

*Atrial natriuretic factor,* under normal circumstances, is released in response to atrial distension, promoting sodium excretion and vascular smooth muscle relaxation. Changes in secretion of this hormone associated with CPB probably depend on the type of cardiac disease. Currello and co-workers (1991) found no alterations in atrial natriuretic factor secretion during CPB in patients undergoing coronary artery bypass grafting, whereas atrial natriuretic factor levels fell during CPB from their elevated preoperative values in patients undergoing mitral valve replacement. Following CPB, atrial natriuretic factor levels rose in both groups of patients.

### Humoral Amplification Systems Response

The *kallikrein-bradykinin cascade* is initiated by Hageman factor, resulting in the production of bradykinin. Bradykinin increases vascular permeability, dilates arterioles, initiates smooth muscle contraction, and elicits pain. Kallikrein activates Hageman factor and activates plasminogen to form plasmin. Several studies have demonstrated elevated levels of bradykinin during CPB (Pang et al., 1979), although the source was thought to be plasma protein solution in the prime (Ellison et al., 1980). Exclusion of the pulmonary circulation during CPB sustains circulating bradykinin levels, because bradykinin is metabolized mainly in the lungs. A study of pulmonary bradykinin inactivation in fetal lambs (Friedli et al., 1973) showed that very young infants may be less able than adults to eliminate bradykinin.

Some evidence suggests that even with heparinization, there is partial activation of the *coagulation cascade* during CPB with the formation of fibrinopeptides (Davies et al., 1980; Gravlee et al., 1990; Tanaka et al., 1989) and thrombin–antithrombin III complexes (Havel et al., 1991). Activation of factor XII occurs at the onset of CPB because of contact of blood with nonendothelial surfaces (Feijen, 1977). At the end of CPB, coagulation factors usually are mildly reduced, (Harker et al., 1980; Kalter et al., 1979), perhaps because of consumption, hemodilution, deposition onto the pump circuit, or denaturation.

The *fibrinolytic cascade* is activated to some extent during CPB. It has been demonstrated that plasmin (converted from the inactive form as plasminogen) can be detected after the commencement of CPB. Evidence suggests that fibrinolysis does play a role in

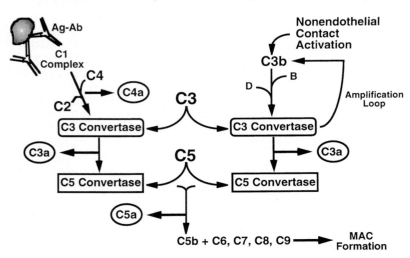

FIGURE 32–4. Schematic representation of the complement pathway. (Ag-Ab = antigen-antibody complex; MAC = membrane attack complex.)

postoperative bleeding after CPB (Blauhut et al., 1991).

The *complement system* involves a group of circulating glycoproteins that is a fundamental component of the body's response to immunologic, traumatic, or foreign body injury. Two pathways exist for activation of the complement sequence (Fig. 32–4). The classic pathway usually is initiated via interaction with antigen-antibody complexes, whereas the alternative pathway is activated by exposure of blood to foreign surfaces. It is this pathway that is primarily activated during CPB (Chenoweth et al., 1981), although some believe that the classic pathway may also be activated (Downing and Edmonds, 1992).

Chenoweth and colleagues (1981) have demonstrated that levels of the complement anaphylatoxin C3a increase shortly after the onset of CPB, with continuing production throughout the duration of bypass (Fig. 32–5). Following CPB, 50% of patients have levels exceeding 1000 ng·ml⁻¹, and 25% have levels above 1600 ng·ml⁻¹. In contrast, patients undergoing cardiac operations without CPB have normal levels of C3a at the end of the operation (Fig. 32–6). An increase in the level of the anaphylatoxin C5a parallels the rise in C3a, but this has been difficult to detect (Chenoweth et al., 1981), perhaps because of the very short half-life of C5a. However, contemporary methods have clearly demonstrated a substantial rise in C5a during CPB (Mollnes et al., 1991). The physiologic effects of C3a and C5a are very similar and include vasoconstriction and increased capillary permeability. Following the administration of protamine, levels of the anaphylatoxin C4a (indicating activation of the classic pathway) become elevated (Cavarocchi et al., 1985; Kirklin et al., 1986).

The *arachidonic acid cascade* is activated during CPB as a result of alterations to the cell membrane (Fig. 32–7). The two major pathways of arachidonic acid metabolism are the cyclo-oxygenase and lipoxygenase pathways, producing prostaglandins and leuko-

trienes, respectively. Faymonville and colleagues (1986) have demonstrated that levels of prostaglandin E₂ and prostacyclin increase at the commencement of CPB and then decline when partial bypass is resumed, allowing blood to pass through the lungs (the primary site of eicosanoid degradation). They also found that thromboxane B₂ (a metabolite of thromboxane A₂) levels rise when partial CPB is commenced following full CPB, presumably because of release of platelet thromboxane in the lungs. Others, however, have found release of prostacyclin and thromboxane during CPB (Davies et al., 1980; Watkins et al., 1982; Ylikorkala et al., 1981). A study by Greeley and colleagues (1988) demonstrated a significant rise

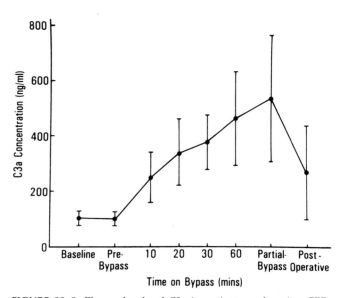

FIGURE 32–5. Plasma levels of C3a in patients undergoing CPB. (From Chenoweth, D. E., Cooper, W. W., Hugli, T. E., et al.: Complement activation during cardiopulmonary bypass. Evidence for generation of C3a and C5a anaphylatoxins. Reprinted, by permission of the New England Journal of Medicine, 304; 497, 1981.)

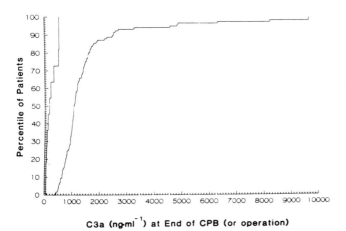

**FIGURE 32–6.** Cumulative percentile plot of C3a levels at the end of operation in patients undergoing closed cardiac surgery (*left*) and patients undergoing cardiopulmonary bypass (CPB) (*right*). Fifty per cent of patients had levels above 1000 ng·ml$^{-1}$ at the end of CPB. (From Kirklin, J. K., Westaby, S., Blackstone, E. H., et al.: Complement and the damaging effects of cardiopulmonary bypass. J. Thorac. Cardiovasc. Surg., *86*:845, 1983.)

in thromboxane $B_2$ in a group of children undergoing CPB; peak levels occurred during full bypass. In the same group of patients, prostacyclin levels rose significantly during CPB; interestingly, a similar rise occurred in a control group of children undergoing a variety of cardiac and vascular procedures without CPB, presumably reflecting surgical manipulation of vascular endothelium. The net physiologic effect of these substances is not clear, because both vasodilatation (prostaglandin $E_2$ and prostacyclin) and vasoconstriction (thromboxane $A_2$) may be produced.

The response of the leukotriene pathway is unclear, but there is some evidence that levels of leukotriene $B_4$, which increases leukocyte chemotaxis and capillary permeability, increase following CPB (Jansen et al., 1991).

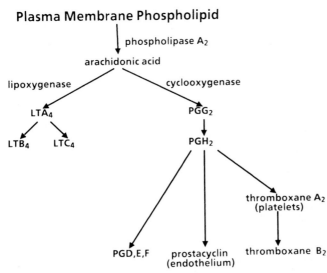

**FIGURE 32–7.** Schematic representation of the arachidonic acid pathway. (LT = leukotriene; PG = prostaglandin.)

## Cytokine Response

Cytokines are polypeptides that are produced endogenously by a number of cell types, and they serve as intercellular messengers during immune and inflammatory responses. Interleukin-1, which mediates many aspects of the inflammatory response, such as fever, acute phase proteins, endothelial permeability, and other cytokine release, has been shown to increase following CPB, the peak production occurring at 24 hours (Haeffner-Cavaillon et al., 1989). Interleukin-6 also has important functions in mediating the inflammatory response, and its level increases following CPB (Butler et al., 1992). Interleukin-8, a neutrophil chemotactic factor, has been detected in the circulation following CPB in children (Finn et al., 1993). These findings should be viewed as preliminary, because at least some information is conflicting and other findings remain to be confirmed.

## Protease Release

Following activation of neutrophils by the complement cascade, proteases (such as elastase) are released, and these substances can injure endothelial and epithelial cells. Evidence of elastase release following CPB is available (Butler et al., 1993; Hashimoto et al., 1992), but there is no evidence to link their release to organ injury.

## Systemic Vascular Resistance

Systemic vascular resistance falls abruptly with the onset of CPB, following which it gradually increases throughout CPB, although there is considerable variation among patients (Cordell et al., 1960; McGoon et al., 1960).

## Body Composition

During and after CPB, extracellular fluid is increased (Breckenridge et al., 1969; Cleland et al., 1966). The major shift of fluid is from the intravascular space to the interstitial space, resulting in increased interstitial fluid pressure (Cleland et al., 1966; Rosenkranz et al., 1980) and decreased plasma volume (Cleland et al., 1966). The amount of exchangeable potassium is decreased, whereas exchangeable sodium is increased (Pacifico et al., 1970).

## DAMAGING EFFECTS OF CARDIOPULMONARY BYPASS

Safe CPB is characterized by the absence of structural or functional damage after the perfusion. Most patients who undergo CPB convalesce without apparently manifesting its damaging effects. However,

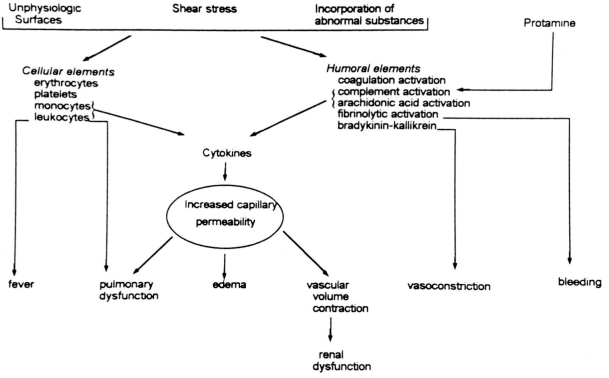

**FIGURE 32–8.** Schematic representation of a current concept of the damaging effects of CPB. (From McGiffin, D. C., and Kirklin, J. K.: Cardiopulmonary bypass, deep hypothermia and total circulatory arrest. *In* Mavroudis, C. and Backer, C. L. [eds]: Pediatric Cardiac Surgery. 2nd ed. St. Louis, Mosby–Year Book, 1994.

probably all patients have some pathophysiologic response to CPB, which in its severest form is identified as "postperfusion syndrome." The clinical manifestations may include pulmonary dysfunction, renal dysfunction, bleeding diathesis, increased interstitial fluid, leukocytosis, fever, vasoconstriction, hemolysis, and increased susceptibility to infection.

There is increasing evidence to support the contention that these damaging effects of CPB are initiated by a whole-body inflammatory response. This inflammatory response involves both cellular and noncellular elements of the blood, and a critical part of the process is the activation of the humoral cascade systems. The initiating factors include exposure of blood to unphysiologic (nonendothelial) surfaces; generation of shear stresses in the pump oxygenator, which causes leukocyte disruption; and incorporation of abnormal substances (microemboli) during CPB, such as fibrin, air bubbles, and tissue debris (Fig. 32–8).

Of particular importance is the association between the clinical manifestations of the damaging effects of CPB and complement activation. A prospective study at the University of Alabama at Birmingham examined the relationship between a number of variables associated with CPB and morbidity after cardiac surgery (Kirklin et al., 1983). For example, cardiac dysfunction during the first 24 hours following operation was significantly related to higher levels of C3a measured 3 hours after CPB, longer duration of CPB, and younger age at operation (Table 32–4). Postoperative pulmonary dysfunction was associated with the same risk factors (Table 32–5). An index of postoperative morbidity was derived, and this was also significantly related to higher levels of C3a, longer duration of CPB, and younger age at operation (Table 32–6 and Fig. 32–9).

Alterations in microvascular permeability are a central physiologic hallmark of the damaging effect of CPB. A number of studies have documented the fluid redistribution with increased extravascular water, but there is little direct evidence for increased capillary permeability. Smith and colleagues (1987), using an experimental model, did provide direct evidence for increased capillary permeability following CPB, however.

■ **Table 32–4.** CARDIAC DYSFUNCTION AFTER OPEN OPERATIONS*

| Incremental Risk Factor | Logistic Coefficient ± SD | p Value |
|---|---|---|
| Higher C3a level | 0.0010 ± 0.0042 | .02 |
| Longer CPB time | 0.014 ± 0.0058 | .02 |
| Younger age | −0.06 ± 0.138 | ≤.0001 |

Modified from Kirklin, J. K., Westaby, S., Blackstone, E. H., et al.: Complement and the damaging effects of cardiopulmonary bypass. J. Thorac. Cardiovasc. Surg., 86:845, 1983.

*Key:* CPB = cardiopulmonary bypass.

*$n$ =116; 27 patients had cardiac events.

■ **Table 32–5.** PULMONARY DYSFUNCTION AFTER OPEN OPERATIONS*

| Incremental Risk Factor | Logistic Coefficient ± SD | p Value |
|---|---|---|
| Higher C3a level | 0.0025 ± 0.00094 | .008 |
| Longer CPB time | 0.025 ± 0.0111 | .02 |
| Younger age | −1.17 ± 0.183 | ≤.0001 |

Modified from Kirklin, J. K., Westaby, S., Blackstone, E. H., et al: Complement and the damaging effects of cardiopulmonary bypass. J. Thorac. Cardiovasc. Surg., 86:845, 1983.
Key: CPB = cardiopulmonary bypass.
*n = 116; 41 patients had cardiac events.

■ **Table 32–6.** IMPORTANT MORBIDITY AFTER OPEN OPERATIONS*

| Incremental Risk Factor | Logistic Coefficient ± SD | p Value |
|---|---|---|
| Higher C3a level | 0.0006 ± 0.00033 | .07 |
| Longer CPB time | 0.017 ± 0.0048 | .0004 |
| Younger age | −0.71 ± 0.131 | <.0001 |

Modified from Kirklin, J. K., Westaby, S., Blackstone, E. H., et al.: Complement and the damaging effects of cardiopulmonary bypass. J. Thorac. Cardiovasc. Surg., 86:845, 1983.
Key: CPB = cardiopulmonary bypass.
*n = 116; 26 patients had cardiac events.

Minimization of the damaging effects of CPB is an important future direction. However, it should be emphasized that robust cardiac performance in the postoperative period significantly reduces the clinical manifestations of the damaging effects of CPB. Blockade of the individual humoral amplification cascades is probably unrealistic, given the complex nature of their interactions, but blockade of the possible final common pathway, the neutrophil, may hold some promise. The finding that the neutrophil adhesion molecule CD-18 can be blocked with an anti–CD-18 monoclonal antibody ameliorating myocardial reperfusion injury suggests that this approach may be useful (Byrne et al., 1992). Furthermore, neutrophil depletion by filtration has been shown to reduce CPB-induced lung injury in an animal model (Bando et al., 1990).

## DEEP HYPOTHERMIC TOTAL CIRCULATORY ARREST

For some operations, particularly in very small neonates, the technique of deep hypothermia and total circulatory arrest provides elegant exposure with a bloodless, uncluttered operative field for the intracardiac repair. The cannulation technique for CPB is simplified by using a single venous cannula in the right atrium for cooling and rewarming. Despite the clinical use of total circulatory arrest for more than 25 years and a number of clinical and experimental studies (Clarkson et al., 1980; Haka-Ikse et al., 1978; Stevenson et al., 1974), controversy continues over the safe duration of total circulatory arrest and the occurrence of neurologic damage associated with its use and duration.

Studies of humans after total circulatory arrest have focused on electroencephalographic change during and after total circulatory arrest, development of postoperative choreoathetosis and seizures, and late studies of motor development. The probability of freedom from a major postoperative neurologic event decreases rapidly when the arrest time exceeds 50 minutes at 18 to 20° C (Fig. 32–10). Most available clinical studies indicate that intellectual and psychomotor development usually are not impaired when circulatory arrest time is less than approximately 60 minutes at 18 to 20° C (Clarkson et al., 1980; Messmer et al., 1976; Wells et al., 1983).

Clinical studies in adult patients undergoing circulatory arrest (Coselli et al., 1988) have suggested that the safe period of total circulatory arrest may be pro-

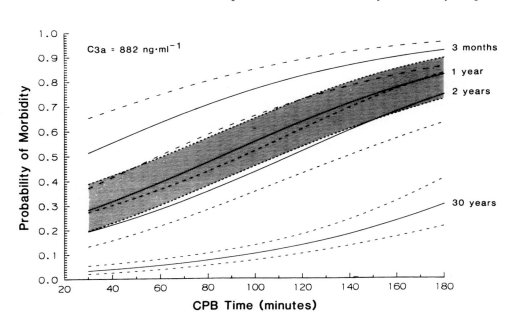

FIGURE 32–9. Nomogram of the probability of morbidity after CPB with increasing duration of CPB (*horizontal axis*) showing relationships for four different ages. The C3a level at the conclusion of CPB was specified as 882 ng·ml⁻¹. (From Kirklin, J. K., Westaby, S., Blackstone, E. H., et al.: Complement and the damaging effects of cardiopulmonary bypass. J. Thorac. Cardiovasc. Surg., 86:845, 1983.)

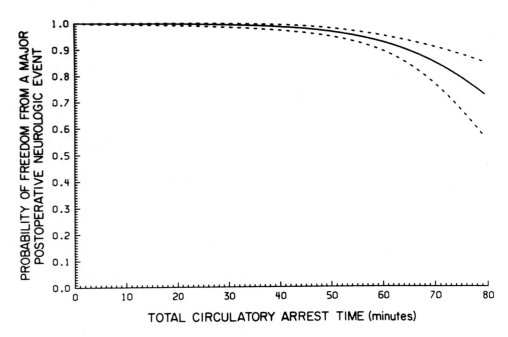

**FIGURE 32–10.** The relation between the probability of a major neurologic event occurring postoperatively and the total circulatory arrest (TCA) time in 219 patients (8 events) undergoing open intracardiac operations at University of Alabama at Birmingham. Among the 211 patients without these events, TCA time was 42 ± 14.0 (SD) minutes versus 59 ± 10.2 for the 8 with such events ($p$ = .0008). The logistic equation for the nomogram is as follows:

$$Z = -7.3 + 0.08 \times TCA$$ where TCA = TCA time in minutes.

(From Kirklin, J. K., Kirklin, J. W., Pacifico, A. D.: Deep hypothermia and total circulatory arrest. *In* Arcinegas, E. [ed]: Pediatric Cardiac Surgery. Chicago, Year Book Medical, 1985.)

longed further by more complete cooling of the brain (as judged by electrocerebral silence on detailed intraoperative electroencephalography) to nasopharyngeal temperatures of 12 to 16° C.

## SELECTED BIBLIOGRAPHY

Chenoweth, D. E., Cooper, S. W., Hugli, T. E., et al.: Complement activation during cardiopulmonary bypass: Evidence for generation of C3a and CSa anaphylatoxins. N. Engl. J. Med., *304*:497, 1981.

CPB is currently a safe support system for most patients who undergo cardiac surgical procedures. An occasional patient, particularly if seriously ill, very young, or very old, suffers additional morbidity related to CPB. Chenoweth and colleagues provided the first direct quantitative evidence for activation of the alternative complement pathway during CPB, resulting from exposure of blood to nonbiologic surfaces. This and other techniques for studying the damaging effects of bypass may ultimately lead to safer support systems for cardiac surgical procedures.

Coselli, J. S., Crawford, E. S., Beall, A. C., Jr., et al.: Determination of brain temperatures for safe circulatory arrest during cardiovascular operation. Ann. Thorac. Surg., *45*:638, 1988.

Profound hypothermia and temporary circulatory arrest have been the basic technique for intracardiac surgical procedures in neonates. A safe period of 45 to 60 minutes of circulatory arrest has generally been accepted, with deep hypothermia to 18 to 20° C. The authors report superb results with the technique of deep hypothermic circulatory arrest in adult patients undergoing aortic procedures. With detailed intraoperative electroencephalography, electrocerebral silence frequently was not achieved until the nasopharyngeal temperature was reduced to 16° C or less. This experience suggests that more complete and profound brain cooling could provide longer periods of safe circulatory arrest than have traditionally been accepted.

Gibbon, J. H.: Application of a mechanical heart and lung apparatus to cardiac surgery. Minn. Med., *37*:171, 1954.

This classic paper describes the first successful use of a heart-lung machine in humans to entirely support the circulation during open heart surgery with closure of an atrial septal defect. The author discusses the physiologic response to CPB, including hemolysis, adequate tissue perfusion, and the problems of cardiac distention and air emboli. Gibbon concluded, "It seems to me that there will always be a place for an extracorporeal blood circuit because it permits a longer safe interval for opening the heart than can ever be obtained by any of the hypothermic methods."

Kirklin, J. W., Dushane, J. W., Patrick, R. T., et al.: Intracardiac surgery with the aid of a mechanical pump oxygenator (Gib-

bon type): Report of eight cases. Proc. Staff Meet. Mayo Clin., *30*:201, 1955.

This is the first report of a series of patients successfully undergoing cardiac procedures with the use of a mechanical pump oxygenator. Four patients had ventricular septal defects, and two survived postoperatively. Two patients had atrioventricular canal defects, and one survived. One patient had tetralogy of Fallot, and he died. One patient underwent closure of an atrial septal defect and survived. At the time of this report, it was widely believed that a totally mechanical support system would not allow successful cardiac surgical procedures.

Kirklin, J. K., Westaby, S., Blackstone, E. H., et al.: Complement and the damaging effects of cardiopulmonary bypass. J. Thorac. Cardiovasc. Surg., *86*:845, 1983.

This prospective clinical study is one of the first rigorous attempts to identify the factors associated with CPB that contribute to organ system dysfunction after cardiac surgical procedures. Complement levels remained normal in patients undergoing cardiac operations without CPB compared with the marked complement activation that occurred during CPB. Cardiac, renal, pulmonary, and hemostatic dysfunction increased with higher levels of the complement anaphylatoxin C3a after bypass, younger age at operation, and longer time on bypass. The authors suggest that a more complete understanding of the biologic response to CPB may eventually lead to the neutralization of these damaging effects.

Lillehei, C. W., Cohen, M., Warden, H. E., and Varco, R. L.: The direct vision intracardiac correction of congenital anomalies by controlled cross circulation. Surgery, *38*:11, 1955.

The authors report the first successful series of intracardiac operations using CPB. The experimental and physiologic bases for the use of another human being as the source of oxygenation and perfusion are discussed. Twenty-two patients underwent repair of a ventricular septal defect (18 survivors), 6 had tetralogy of Fallot (3 survivors), 2 had an atrioventricular canal defect (1 survivor), and 2 had pulmonary stenosis (1 survivor).

Smith, E. E. J., Naftel, D. C., Blackstone, E. H., and Kirklin, J. W.: Microvascular permeability after cardiopulmonary bypass. J. Thorac. Cardiovasc. Surg., *94*:225, 1987.

Since its inception, CPB has been presumed to increase microvascular permeability, but this had not been directly shown. In this controlled experimental study of the small intestinal microvasculature of the dog, the authors provided the first direct evidence that CPB increases microvascular permeability, particularly for large molecules.

## BIBLIOGRAPHY

Anand, K. J., Hansen, D. D., and Hickey, P. R.: Hormonal-metabolic stress responses in neonates undergoing cardiac surgery. Anesthesiology, *73*:661, 1990.

Andreason, A. T., and Watson, F.: Experimental cardiovascular surgery. Br. J. Surg., 39:548, 1952.

Bando, K., Pillai, R., Cammeron, D. E., et al.: Leukocyte depletion ameliorates free radical–mediated lung injury after cardiopulmonary bypass. J. Thorac. Cardiovasc. Surg., 99:873, 1990.

Baraka, A. S., Baroody, M. A., Haroun, S. T., et al.: Effect of alpha-stat versus pH-stat strategy on oxyhemoglobin dissociation and whole-body oxygen consumption during hypothermic cardiopulmonary bypass. Anesth. Analg., 74:32, 1992.

Barratt-Boyes, B. G., Simpson, M. M., and Neutze, J. M.: Intracardiac surgery in neonates and infants using deep hypothermia. Circulation, 61, 62(Suppl. III): III–173, 1970.

Bashein, G., Townes, B. D., Nessly, M. L., et al.: A randomized study of carbon dioxide management during hypothermic cardiopulmonary bypass. Anesthesiology, 72:7, 1990.

Bigelow, W. G., Lindsay, W. K., and Greenwood, W. F.: Hypothermia: Its possible role in cardiac surgery: An investigation of factors governing survival in dogs at low body temperatures. Ann. Surg., 132:849, 1950.

Bjork, V. O.: Brain perfusions in dogs with artificially oxygened blood. Acta Chir. Scand., 96(Suppl.):1, 1952.

Blauhut, B., Gross, C., Necek, S., et al.: Effects of high-dose aprotinin on blood loss, platelet function, fibrinolysis, complement and renal function after cardiopulmonary bypass. J. Thorac. Cardiovasc. Surg., 101:958, 1991.

Borowiec, J., Thelin, S., Bagge, L., et al.: Decreased blood loss after cardiopulmonary bypass using heparin-coated circuit and 50% reduction of heparin dose. Scand. J. Thorac. Cardiovasc. Surg., 26:177, 1992.

Breckenridge, I. M., Digerness, S. B., and Kirklin, J. W.: Validity of concept of increased extracellular fluid after open heart surgery. Surg. Forum, 20:169, 1969.

Bremner, W. F., Taylor, K. M., Baird, S., et al.: Hypothalamo-pituitary-thyroid axis function during cardiopulmonary bypass. J. Thorac. Cardiovasc. Surg., 75:392, 1978.

Bull, B. S., Korpman, R. A., Huse, W. M., and Briggs, B. D.: Heparin therapy during extracorporeal circulation. I. Problems inherent in existing heparin protocols. J. Thorac. Cardiovasc. Surg., 69:674, 1975.

Butler, J., Chong, G. L., Baigrie, R. J., et al.: Cytokine responses to cardiopulmonary bypass with membrane and bubble oxygenation. Ann. Thorac. Surg., 53:833, 1992.

Butler, J., Pillai, R., Rocker, G. M., et al.: Effect of cardiopulmonary bypass on systemic release of neutrophil elastase and tumor necrosis factor. J. Thorac. Cardiovasc. Surg., 105:25, 1993.

Byrne, J. G., Cohn, L., Smith, W., et al.: Complete prevention of myocardial stunning, low reflow and edema after heart transplant by blocking leukocyte adhesion molecule during reperfusion [Abstract]. American Association for Thoracic Association Meeting, Los Angeles, April 26–29, 1992.

Campbell, G. S., Crisp, N. W., Brown, E. B.: Total cardiac bypass in humans utilizing a pump and heterologous lung oxygenator (dog lungs). Surgery, 40:364, 1956.

Cavarocchi, N. C., Schaff, H. V., Orszulak, T. A., et al.: Evidence for complement activation by protamine-heparin interaction after cardiopulmonary bypass. Surgery, 98:525, 1985.

Chenoweth, D. E., Cooper, S. W., Hugli, T. E., et al.: Complement activation during cardiopulmonary bypass: Evidence for generation of C3a and C5a anaphylatoxins. N. Engl. J. Med., 304:497, 1981.

Chien, S.: Present state of blood rheology. In Messemer, K., and Schmid Schonbein, H. (eds): Hemodilution. Theoretical Basis and Clinical Application. New York, Karger, 1972, p. 145.

Clarkson, P. M., MacArthur, B. A., Barratt-Boyes, B., et al.: Developmental progress after cardiac surgery in infancy using hypothermia and circulatory arrest. Circulation, 62:855, 1980.

Cleland, J., Pluth, J. R., Tauxe, W. N., and Kirklin, J. W.: Blood volume and body fluid compartment changes soon after closed and open intracardiac surgery. J. Thorac. Cardiovasc. Surg., 52:698, 1966.

Cohen, M., Hammerstrom, R. N., Spellman, M. W., et al.: The tolerance of the canine heart to temporary complete vena caval occlusion. Surg. Forum, 3:172, 1952.

Cohn, L. H., Angell, W. W., and Shumway, N. E.: Body fluid shifts after cardiopulmonary bypass. I. Effects of congestive heart failure and hemodilution. J. Thorac. Cardiovasc. Surg., 62:423, 1971.

Cordell, A. R., Spencer, M. P., and Meredith, J. H.: Studies of peripheral vascular resistance associated with total cardiopulmonary bypass. I. Peripheral resistance under condition of normothermia and normotension. J. Thorac. Cardiovasc. Surg., 40:421, 1960.

Crafoord, C., Norberg, B., and Senning, A.: Clinical studies in extracorporeal circulation with a heart-lung machine. Acta Chir. Scand., 112:220, 1957.

Curello, S., Ceconi, C., De Giuli, F., et al.: Time course of human atrial natriuretic factor release during cardiopulmonary bypass in mitral valve and coronary artery diseased patients. Eur. J. Cardiothorac. Surg., 5:205, 1991.

Davies, G. C., Sobel, M., and Salzman, E. W.: Elevated plasma fibrinopeptide A and thromboxane B2 levels during cardiopulmonary bypass. Circulation, 61:808, 1980.

Davies, L. K.: Hypothermia: Physiology and clinical use. In Gravlee, G. P., Davis, R. F., and Utley, J. R. (eds): Cardiopulmonary Bypass Principles and Practice. Baltimore, Williams & Wilkins, 1993, p. 140.

Dennis, C., Spreng, D. S., Jr., Nelson, G. E., et al.: Development of a pump oxygenator to replace the heart and lungs: An apparatus applicable to human patients, and application to one case. Ann. Surg., 134:709, 1951.

Diehl, J. T., Payne, D. D., Rastegar, H., and Cleveland, R. J.: Arterial bypass of the descending thoracic aorta with the Bio-Medicus centrifugal pump. Ann. Thorac. Surg., 44:422, 1987.

Diesh, G., Flynn, P. J., Marable, S. A., et al.: Comparison of low (azygous) flow and high flow principles of extracorporeal circulation employing a bubble oxygenator. Surgery, 42:67, 1957.

Dillard, D. H., Mohri, H., Hessel, E. A. II, et al.: Correction of total anomalous pulmonary venous drainage in infancy utilizing deep hypothermia with total circulatory arrest. Circulation, 35, 36(Suppl. 1):105, 1967.

Downing, S. W., and Edmonds, L. H.: Release of vasoactive substances during cardiopulmonary bypass. Ann. Thorac. Surg., 54:1236, 1992.

Driessen, J. J., Fransen, G., Rondelez, L., et al.: Comparison of the standard roller pump and a pulsatile centrifugal pump for extracorporeal circulation during routine coronary artery bypass grafting. Perfusion, 6:303, 1991.

Ellison, N., Behar, M., MacVaugh, H., and Marshall, B. E.: Bradykinin, plasma protein fraction and hypotension. Ann. Thorac. Surg., 29:15, 1980.

Everts, P. A. M., Schonberger, J. P. A. M., Steenbrink, J., and Bredee, J. J.: Partial left heart bypass with centrifugal pump and limited anticoagulation during the resection of coarctation of the aorta. Perfusion, 6:285, 1991.

Faymonville, M.-E., Deby-Dupont, G., Larbuisson, R., et al.: Prostaglandin E2, prostacyclin, and thromboxane changes during nonpulsatile cardiopulmonary bypass in humans. J. Thorac. Cardiovasc. Surg., 91:858, 1986.

Feijen, J.: Thrombogenesis caused by blood foreign surface interaction. In Kenedi, R. M., Courtney, J. M., Gaylor, J. D. S., and Gilchrist, T. (eds): Artificial Organs. Baltimore, University Park Press, 1977, p. 235.

Field, J., II, Belding, H. S., and Martin, A. W.: An analysis of the relation between basal metabolism and summated tissue respiration in the rat: I. The post pubertal albino rat. J. Cell Comp. Physiol., 14:143, 1939.

Finn, A., Naik, S., Klein, N., et al.: Interleukin-8 release and neutrophil degranulation after pediatric cardiopulmonary bypass. J. Thorac. Cardiovasc. Surg., 105:234, 1993.

Firmin, R. K., Bouloux, P., Allen, P., et al.: Sympathoadrenal function during cardiac operations in infants with the technique of surface cooling, limited cardiopulmonary bypass, and circulatory arrest. J. Thorac. Cardiovasc. Surg., 90:729, 1985.

Fox, L. S., Blackstone, E. H., Kirklin, J. W., et al.: Relationship of brain blood flow and oxygen consumption to perfusion flow rate during hypothermic cardiopulmonary bypass. J. Thorac. Cardiovasc. Surg., 87:658, 1984.

Friedli, B., Kent, G., and Olley, P. M.: Inactivation of bradykinin in the pulmonary vascular bed of newborn and fetal lambs. Circ. Res., 33:421, 1973.

Frey, M. V., and Gruber, M.: Untersuchungen über den Stoffwechsel isolierter Organe: Ein Respirationsapparat für isolierte Organe. Arch. Fr. Physiol., 9:519, 1885.

Fuhrman, F. A.: Oxygen consumption of mammalian tissues at reduced temperatures. In Dripps, R. D. (ed): The Physiology of Induced Hypothermia. Washington, DC, National Academy of Sciences–National Research Council, 1956, pp. 50–51.

Fuhrman, F. A., Fuhrman, G. J., Farr, D. A., and Fail, J. H.: Relationship between tissue respiration and total metabolic rate in hypo- and normothermic rats. Am. J. Physiol., 201:231, 1961.

Gibbon, J. H., Jr.: Application of a mechanical heart and lung apparatus to cardiac surgery. Minn. Med., 37:171, 1954.

Gibbon, J. H., Jr.: The maintenance of life during experimental occlusion of the pulmonary artery followed by survival. Surg. Gynecol. Obstet., 69:602, 1939.

Gravlee, G. P., Haddon, W. S., Rothberger, H. K., et al.: Heparin dosing and monitoring for cardiopulmonary bypass. J. Thorac. Cardiovasc. Surg., 99:518, 1990.

Greeley, W. J., Bushman, G. A., Kong, D. L., et al.: Effects of cardiopulmonary bypass on eicosanoid metabolism during pediatric cardiovascular surgery. J. Thorac. Cardiovasc. Surg., 95:842, 1988.

Gu, Y. J., van Oeveren, W., Akkerman, C., et al.: Heparin-coated circuits reduce the inflammatory response to cardiopulmonary bypass. Ann. Thorac. Surg., 55:917, 1993.

Haeffner-Cavaillon, N., Roussellier, N., Ponzio, O., et al.: Induction of interleukin-1 production in patients undergoing cardiopulmonary bypass. J. Thorac. Cardiovasc. Surg., 98:1100, 1989.

Haka-Ikse, K., Blackwood, M. J. A., and Steward, D. J.: Psychomotor development of infants and children after profound hypothermia during surgery for congenital heart disease. Dev. Med. Child Neurol., 29:62–70, 1978.

Hamilton, D. I., Shackleton, J., Rees, G. J., and Abbot, T.: Experience with deep hypothermia in infancy using core cooling. In Barratt-Boyes, B. G., Houtze, J. M., and Harris, E. A. (eds): Heart Disease in Infancy. Baltimore, Williams & Wilkins, 1973, p. 52.

Harker, L. A., Malpass, T. W., Branson, H. E., et al.: Mechanism of abnormal bleeding in patients undergoing cardiopulmonary bypass: Acquired transient platelet dysfunction associated with selective alpha-granule release. Blood, 56:824, 1980.

Hashimoto, K., Miyamoto, H., Suzuki, K., et al.: Evidence of organ damage after cardiopulmonary bypass. J. Thorac. Cardiovasc. Surg., 104:666, 1992.

Havel, M., Teufelsbauer, H., Knobl, P., et al.: Effect of intraoperative aprotinin administration on postoperative bleeding in patients undergoing cardiopulmonary bypass operation. J. Thorac. Cardiovasc. Surg., 101:968–972, 1991.

Henriksen, L.: Brain luxury perfusion during cardiopulmonary bypass in humans. A study of the cerebral blood flow response to changes in $CO_2$, $O_2$ and blood pressure. J. Cereb. Blood Flow Metab., 6:366, 1986.

Hirvonen, J., Huttunen, P., Nuutinen, L., and Pekkarinen, A.: Catecholamines and free fatty acids in plasma of patients undergoing cardiac operations with hypothermia and bypass. J. Clin. Pathol., 31:949, 1978.

Hoerr, H. R., Kraemer, M. F., Williams, J. L., et al.: In vitro comparison of the blood handling by the constrained vortex and twin roller blood pumps. J. Extracorpor. Technol., 19:316, 1987.

Holland, F. W., II, Brown, P. S., Jr., Weintraub, B. D., and Clark, R. E.: Cardiopulmonary bypass and thyroid function: A "euthyroid sick syndrome." Ann. Thorac. Surg., 52:46, 1991.

Horiuchi, T., Koyamada, K., Matano, I., et al.: Radical operation for ventricular septal defect in infancy. J. Thorac. Cardiovasc. Surg., 46:180, 1963.

Jansen, N. J. G., van Oeveren, W., Broek, L. V. D., et al.: Inhibition by dexamethasone of the reperfusion phenomena in cardiopulmonary bypass. J. Thorac. Cardiovasc. Surg., 102:515, 1991.

Jonas, R. A., Bellinger, D. C., Rappaport, L. A., et al.: Relation of pH strategy and developmental outcome after hypothermic circulatory arrest. J. Thorac. Cardiovasc. Surg., 106:362, 1993.

Kalter, R. D., Saul, C. M., Wetstein, L., et al.: Cardiopulmonary bypass. Associated hemostatic abnormalities. J. Thorac. Cardiovasc. Surg., 77:427, 1979.

Kirklin, J. K., Chenoweth, D. E., Naftel, D. C., et al.: Effects of protamine administration after cardiopulmonary bypass on complement, blood elements and the hemodynamic state. Ann. Thorac. Surg., 41:193, 1986.

Kirklin, J. K., Westaby, S., Blackstone, E. H., et al.: Complement and the damaging effects of cardiopulmonary bypass. J. Thorac. Cardiovasc. Surg., 86:845, 1983.

Kirklin, J. W., Dawson, B., Devloo, R. A., and Theye, R. A.: Open intracardiac operations: Use of circulatory arrest during hypothermia induced by blood cooling. Ann. Surg., 154:769, 1961.

Kirklin, J. W., DuShane, J. W., Patrick, R. T., et al.: Intracardiac surgery with the aid of a mechanical pump-oxygenater system (Gibbon type): Report of eight cases. Proc. Staff Meet. Mayo Clin., 30:201, 1955.

Lacoumenta, S., Yeo, T. H., Paterson, J. L., et al.: Hormonal and metabolic responses to cardiac surgery with sufentanil-oxygen anaesthesia. Acta Anesthesiol. Scand., 31:258, 1987.

Landymore, R. W., Murphy, D. A., Kinley, C. E., et al.: Does pulsatile flow influence the incidence of postoperative hypertension? Ann. Thorac. Surg., 28:261, 1979.

Lassen, N. A.: The luxury-perfusion syndrome and its possible relation to acute metabolic acidosis localized within the brain. Lancet, 2:1113, 1966.

Levin, M. B., Theye, R. A., Fowler, W. S., and Kirklin, J. W.: Performance of the stationary vertical-screen oxygenator (Mayo-Gibbon). J. Thorac. Cardiovasc. Surg., 39:417, 1960.

Lewis, F. J., and Taufic, M.: Closure of atrial septal defects with the aid of hypothermia: Experimental accomplishments and the report of one successful case. Surgery, 33:52, 1953.

Lichtenstein, S. V., Fremes, S. E., Abel, J. G., et al.: Technical aspects of warm heart surgery. J. Cardiovasc. Surg., 6:278, 1991.

Lillehei, C. W.: Historical development of cardiopulmonary bypass. In Gravlee, G. P., Davis, R. F., Utley, J. R. (eds): Cardiopulmonary Bypass Principles and Practice. Baltimore, Williams & Wilkins, 1993, p. 1.

McGoon, D. C., Moffitt, E. A., Theye, R. A., and Kirklin, J. W.: Physiologic studies during high flow, normothermic, whole body perfusion. J. Thorac. Cardiovasc. Surg., 39:275, 1960.

Messmer, B. J., Schallberger, U., Gattiker, R., and Senning, A.: Psychomotor and intellectual development after deep hypothermia and circulatory arrest in early infancy. J. Thorac. Cardiovasc. Surg., 72:495, 1976.

Moffitt, E. A., Kirklin, J. W., and Theye, R. A.: Physiologic studies during whole-body perfusion in tetralogy of Fallot. J. Thorac. Cardiovasc. Surg., 44:180, 1962.

Mollnes, T. E., Videm, V., Gotze, O., et al.: Formation of C5a during cardiopulmonary bypass: Inhibition by precoating with heparin. Ann. Thorac. Surg., 52:92, 1991.

Moorman, R. M., Zapol, W. M., and Lowenstein, E.: Neutralization of heparin anticoagulation. In Gravlee, G. P., Davis, R. F., and Utley, J. R. (eds): Cardiopulmonary Bypass Principles and Practice. Baltimore, Williams & Wilkins, 1993, p. 140.

Murkin, J. M., Farrar, J. K., Tweed, W. A., et al.: Cerebral autoregulation and flow/metabolism coupling during cardiopulmonary bypass: The influence of $PA_{CO_2}$. Anesth. Analg., 66:825, 1987.

Mustard, W. T., Chute, A. L., Keith, J. D., et al.: A surgical approach to transposition of the great vessels with extracorporeal circuit. Surgery, 36:39, 1954.

Mustard, W. T., and Thomason, J. A.: Clinical experience with the artificial heart lung preparation. J. Can. Med. Assoc., 76:265, 1957.

Olivier, H. F., Jr., Maher, T. D., Liebler, G. A., et al.: Use of the BioMedicus centrifugal pump in traumatic tears of the thoracic aorta. Ann. Thorac. Surg., 38:586, 1984.

Pacifico, A. D., Digerness, S., and Kirklin, J. W.: Acute alterations of body composition after open intracardiac operations. Circulation, 41:331, 1970.

Padayachee, T. S., Parsons, S., Theobold, R. G., et al.: The effect of arterial filtration on reduction of gaseous microemboli in the middle cerebral artery during cardiopulmonary bypass. Ann. Thorac. Surg., 45:647, 1988.

Pang, L. M., Stalcup, S. A., Lipset, J. S., et al.: Increased circulating bradykinin during hypothermia and cardiopulmonary bypass in children. Circulation, 60:1503, 1979.

Penrod, K. E.: Oxygen consumption and cooling rates in immersion hypothermia in the dog. Am. J. Physiol., 157:436, 1949.

Raff, H., Norton, A. J., Flemma, R. J., and Findling, J. W.: Inhibition of the adrenocorticotropin response to surgery in humans: Interaction between dexamethasone and fentanyl. J. Clin. Endocrinol. Metab., 65:295, 1987.

Rahn, H., Reeves, R. B., and Howell, B. J.: Hydrogen ion regulation, temperature, and evolution. Am. Rev. Respir. Dis., 112:165, 1975.

Reed, H. L., Chernow, B., Lake, C. R., et al.: Alterations in sympathetic nervous system activity with intraoperative hypothermia during coronary artery bypass surgery. Chest, 95:616, 1989.

Reeves, R. B.: The interaction of body temperature and acid-base balance in ectothermic vertebrates. Ann. Rev. Physiol., 39:559, 1977.

Reves, J. G., Karp, R. B., Buttner, E. E., et al.: Neuronal and adrenomedullary catecholamine release in response to cardiopulmonary bypass in man. Circulation, 66:49, 1982.

Rosenkranz, E. R., Utley, J. R., Menninger, F. J., III, et al.: Interstitial fluid pressure changes during cardiopulmonary bypass. Ann. Thorac. Surg., 30:536, 1980.

Ross, D. N.: Hypothermia: Part 2. Physiological observations during hypothermia. Guys Hosp. Rep., 103:116, 1954.

Salter, D. R., Dyke, C. M., and Wechsler, A. S.: Triiodothyronine (T3) and cardiovascular therapeutics: A review. J. Cardiac Surg., 7:363, 1992.

Sealy, W. C., Brown, I. W., and Young, W. G.: A report on the use of both extracorporeal circulation and hypothermia for open heart surgery. Ann. Surg., 147:603, 1958.

Senning, A.: Ventricular fibrillation during extracorporeal circulation: Used as a method to prevent air embolisms and to facilitate intracardiac operations. Acta Chir. Scand., 171 (Suppl.):1, 1952.

Shepard, R. B.: Whole body oxygen consumption during hypoxic hypoxemia and cardiopulmonary bypass circulation. Proceedings Tenth International Symposium on Space Technology and Science, Tokyo, 1973, p. 1307.

Smith, E. E. J., Naftel, D. C., Blackstone, E. H., and Kirklin, J. W.: Microvascular permeability after cardiopulmonary bypass. J. Thorac. Cardiovasc. Surg., 94:225, 1987.

Stevenson, J. G., Stone, E. F., Dillard, D. H., and Morgan, B. C.: Intellectual development of children subjected to prolonged circulatory arrest during hypothermic open heart surgery in infancy. Circulation, 49/50(Suppl. 2):54, 1974.

Stockard, J. J., Bickford, R. G., and Schauble, J. F.: Pressure dependent cerebral ischemia during cardiopulmonary bypass. Neurology, 23:521, 1973.

Swan, H., Zeavin, I., Blount, S. G., Jr., and Virtue R. W.: Surgery by direct vision in the open heart during hypothermia. J. A. M. A., 153:1081, 1953.

Tanaka, K., Takao, M., Yada, I., et al.: Alterations in coagulation and fibrinolysis associated with cardiopulmonary bypass during open heart surgery. J. Cardiothorac. Vasc. Anesth., 3:181, 1989.

Treasure, T., Smith, P. L. C., Newman, S., et al.: Impairment of cerebral function following cardiac and other major surgery. Eur. J. Cardiothorac. Surg., 3:216, 1989.

Tufo, H. M., Ostfeld, A. M., and Shekelle, R.: Central nervous system dysfunction following open heart surgery. J. A. M. A., 212:1333, 1970.

Tuppurainen, T., Settergren, G., and Stensved, P.: The effect of arterial pH on whole body oxygen uptake during hypothermic cardiopulmonary bypass in man. J. Thorac. Cardiovasc. Surg., 98:769, 1989.

Uozumi, T., Manabe, H., Kawashima, Y., et al.: Plasma cortisol, corticosterone, and non–protein-bound cortisol in extra-corporeal circulation. Acta Endocrinol., 69:517, 1972.

Van Oeveren, W., Kazatchkine, M. D., Descamps-Latscha, B., et al.: Deleterious effects of cardiopulmonary bypass. A prospective study of bubble versus membrane oxygenation. J. Thorac. Cardiovasc. Surg., 89:888, 1985.

Walker, D. R., Blackstone, E. H., Kirklin, J. W., et al.: The effect of micropore filtration of the arterial return during cardiopulmonary bypass: A randomized clinical study (unpublished data).

Wallach, R., Karp, R. B., Reves, J. G., et al.: Pathogenesis of paroxysmal hypertension developing during and after coronary bypass surgery: A study of hemodynamic and humoral factors. Am. J. Cardiol., 46:559, 1980.

Walls, J. T., Boley, T., Curtis, J., et al.: Centrifugal pump support for repair of thoracic aortic injury. Mo. Med., 88:811, 1991.

Walls, J. T., Curtis, J. J., and Boley, T. M.: Sarns centrifugal pump for repair of thoracic aortic injury: Case reports. J. Trauma, 29:1283, 1989.

Warden, H. E., Cohen, M., Read, R. C., and Lillehei, C. W.: Controlled cross circulation for open intracardiac surgery. J. Thorac. Surg., 28:331, 1954.

Warden, H. E., DeWall, R. A., Read, R. C., et al.: Total cardiac bypass utilizing continuous perfusion from a reservoir of oxygenated blood. Proc. Soc. Exp. Biol. Med., 90:246, 1955.

Watkins, W. D., Peterson, M. B., Kong, D. L., et al.: Thromboxane and prostacyclin changes during cardiopulmonary bypass with and without pulsatile flow. J. Thorac. Cardiovasc. Surg., 84:250, 1982.

Weinstein, G. S., Zabetakis, P. M., Clavel, A., et al.: The renin-angiotensin system is not responsible for hypertension following coronary artery bypass grafting. Ann. Thorac. Surg., 43:74, 1987.

Weiss, M., Piwnica, A., Lenfant, C., et al.: Deep hypothermia with total circulatory arrest. Trans. Am. Soc. Artif. Intern. Organs, 6:227, 1960.

Wells, F. C., Coghill, S., Caplan, H. L., and Lincoln, C.: Duration of circulatory arrest does influence the psychological development of children after cardiac operations in early life. J. Thorac. Cardiovasc. Surg., 86:823, 1983.

Wheeldon, D. R., Bethune, D. W., and Gill, R. D.: Vortex pumping for routine cardiac surgery: A comparative study. Perfusion, 5:135, 1990.

White, F. N.: A comparative physiological approach to hypothermia. J. Thorac. Cardiovasc. Surg., 82:821, 1981.

Willford, D. C., Moores, W. Y., Ji, S., et al.: Importance of acid-base strategy in reducing myocardial and whole body oxygen consumption during perfusion hypothermia. J. Thorac. Cardiovasc. Surg., 100:699, 1990.

Williams, J. J., and Marshall, B. E.: A fresh look at an old question [Editorial]. Anesthesiology, 56:1, 1982.

Ylikorkala, O., Saarela, E., and Viinikka, L.: Increased prostacyclin and thromboxane production in man during cardiopulmonary bypass. J. Thorac. Cardiovasc. Surg., 82:245, 1981.

# 33 The Aorta

## ■ I Aortic Grafts and Prostheses

Robert B. Peyton and O. Wayne Isom

Aortic grafts and prostheses were developed to replace or bypass diseased segments of the aorta. Early experimental attempts by Jaboulay, Exner, Ward, and Breer met with failure. In 1949, Gross and associates reported the first use of human arterial homografts for the correction of aortic defects. These grafts were removed from trauma victims and stored in a balanced salt solution of 10% human serum at 4° C. The increased demands for homografts led to the development of blood vessel banks and a variety of techniques for collecting, sterilizing, preserving, and storing homografts. In 1952, Dubost and co-workers described the first successful resection of an abdominal aneurysm and insertion of a homograft; in 1953, DeBakey and Cooley successfully resected an aneurysm of the thoracic aorta and restored continuity with an aortic homograft. Improved preservation techniques, including antibiotic preservation, have produced acceptable durability (Matsuki et al., 1988). However, the limited supply and difficulties associated with the harvest, sterilization, and preservation of homograft material provided the impetus to find suitable arterial synthetic substitutes (Wesolowski et al., 1963).

Experimentation with arterial synthetic substitutes included cylinders of glass, aluminum, plated gold, paraffin-lined silver, methyl methacrylate, and polyethylene plastics (Carrel, 1912; Hufnagel, 1947; McGee et al., 1987; Sawyer, 1987). These materials were associated with thrombus formation that caused distal embolization. Voorhees noted that silk within the right ventricle of the dog became coated with an endothelial surface, and reasoned that cylindrical prostheses of fine-mesh synthetic fibers might be useful to restore arterial defects (Sawyer, 1987). In 1952, Voorhees and colleagues reported their successful experimental use of Vinyon "N" cloth tube as an aortic substitute and are credited with stimulating the present era of reconstructive arterial surgery with synthetic fiber conduits.

Numerous substances, including Vinyon "N," nylon, Teflon, Orlon, and Dacron, have been used to construct vascular grafts in a knitted (highly porous) or woven (tight) weave, with or without velour (Mathisen et al., 1986). Velour is a warp-knitted cloth with a surface resembling velvet, and small loops of yarn extend perpendicularly from the fabric surface. The addition of a double velour surface is reported to provide a superior matrix for improved luminal healing and a decreased incidence of thromboembolic episodes (Lindenauer et al., 1984; Mitchell et al., 1980; Muto et al., 1988; Scott et al., 1985; Zammit et al., 1986). Based on experimentation with numerous synthetics, Wesolowski and associates (1961) defined the characteristics of an "ideal" vascular graft: durability, nontoxicity, minimal implantation porosity, maximal tissue permeability, and ease of mechanical handling.

The healing of implanted synthetic grafts has been well described (Berger et al., 1972; Burkel et al., 1981; Goldman et al., 1982b; Graham et al., 1980; Noishiki, 1978; Scott et al., 1985; Sawyer, 1987). The lumen becomes coated with fibrinogen, albumin, and other plasma proteins. If the patient is heparinized, a white thrombus of platelets and leukocytes forms on the graft surface and the prosthesis is gradually converted to a fibrin-coated tube. Healing is characterized by slow cellular infiltration (fibroblasts) and capillary formation. For optimal healing, the neointima should be thin, with an excellent blood supply. Endothelial cells gradually cover the luminal surface, although in humans the process may remain incomplete.

It was recognized early on that the degree of porosity of the prosthesis was an important determinant of luminal surface thrombogenicity (Goldman et al., 1982a; Harrison and Davalos, 1961; Weslowski et al., 1961). The larger interstices of the more porous knitted grafts provide less resistance to the ingrowth of fibrous tissues and neointima from the surrounding tissue and provide more complete healing. The more porous knitted grafts are reported to be less thrombogenic, more durable, and more resistant to ulceration and degeneration (Haverich et al., 1984). In general, porosity corresponds directly to endothelial regeneration, which corresponds inversely with platelet deposition and thrombogenicity. More recently, investigators have explored the effectiveness of endothelial seeding of grafts to improve patency and decrease thrombogenicity, although this may be more significant for small-diameter grafts than for aortic grafts (Clagett et al., 1987; Kadletz et al., 1992).

Complex proximal aortic reconstruction requires full heparinization and cardiopulmonary bypass. Tightly woven low-porosity Dacron grafts, preclotted with standard techniques, can frequently *declot* and operative blood loss can be excessive. Additional preclotting techniques have been proposed, consisting of autoclaving the graft previously soaked in heparinized blood (Bethea and Reemtsma, 1979), autogenous platelet-rich plasma (Cooley et al., 1981), or albumin (Gloviczki et al., 1984; Glynn and Williams, 1980; McGee et al., 1987; Rumisek et al., 1986; Thurer et al., 1982). Preclotted tightly woven Dacron prostheses continue to be the most common graft used (Cabrol et al., 1986; Crawford et al., 1981, 1984; Kouchoukos et al., 1980). Dacron has excellent durability, is relatively inert in the body, and is well incorporated into the tissues. Tightly woven Dacron prostheses nevertheless have been associated with early and late thromboembolic complications (Agarwal et al., 1982; Makin, 1988; Stratton and Hall, 1979).

With the advent of *biologic sealants,* knitted Dacron grafts are being implanted in the thoracic aorta. Dacron knitted grafts are reported to have superior tissue ingrowth, minimal intimal dissection, and minimal luminal thrombogenicity, as described previously. The Dacron knitted grafts are made leak-proof by albumin impregnation (Guidoin et al., 1984; McGee et al., 1987), collagen coating (Quinones-Baldrich et al., 1986), or fibrin gluing (Borst et al., 1982; Haverich et al., 1981, 1984; Zammit and Wu, 1986).

The sutureless intraluminal prosthesis (Fig. 33–1) is a further innovation currently available; it offers the advantage of being placed without a suture line, which is especially useful in conditions of poor tissue quality, such as with aortic dissection. The graft ends

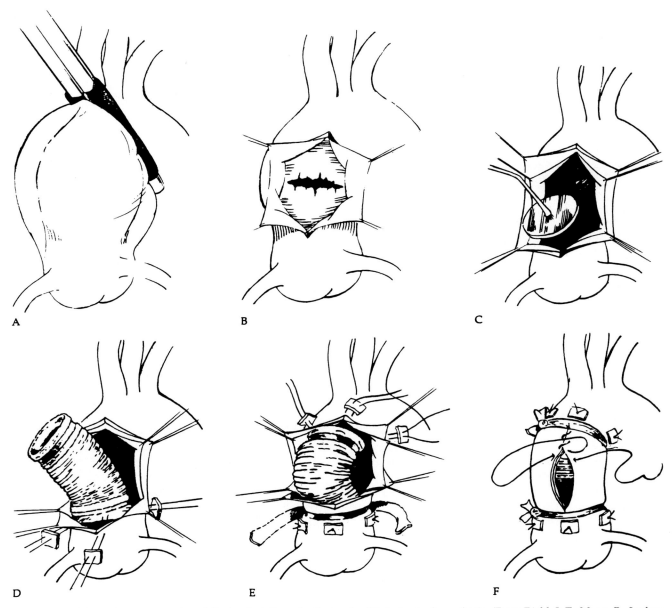

**FIGURE 33–1.** Schematic representation of the implantation of a "sutureless" intraluminal prosthesis. (From Diehl, J. T., Moon, B., Leclerc, Y., and Weisel, R. D.: Acute type A dissections of the aorta: Surgical management with the sutureless intraluminal prosthesis. Reprinted with permission from the Society of Thoracic Surgeons [The Annals of Thoracic Surgery, 1987, Vol. 43, pp. 502–507].)

are attached to a plastic spool, which is placed intra-luminally and secured in place with tapes tied around the aorta over the spools. The intraluminal graft can be applied for most aortic operations (Diehl et al., 1987).

## BIBLIOGRAPHY

Agarwal, K. C., Edwards, W. D., and Feldt, R. H.: Pathogenesis of nonobstructive fibrous peels in right-sided porcine-valved extracardiac conduits. J. Thorac. Cardiovasc. Surg., 83:584, 1982.

Berger, K., Sauvage, L. R., Rao, A. M., and Wood, S. J.: Healing of arterial prostheses in man: Its incompleteness. Ann. Surg., 175:118, 1972.

Bethea, M. C., and Reemtsma, K.: Graft hemostasis: An alternative to preclotting. Ann. Thorac. Surg., 27:374, 1979.

Borst, H. G., Haverich, A., Walterbusch, G., and Maatz, W.: Fibrin adhesive: An important hemostatic adjunct in cardiovascular operations. J. Thorac. Cardiovasc. Surg., 84:549, 1982.

Burkel, W. E., Vinter, D. W., Ford, J. W., et al.: Sequential studies of healing endothelial seeded vascular prostheses: Histologic and ultrastructure characteristics of graft incorporation. J. Surg. Res., 30:305, 1981.

Cabrol, C., Pavie, A., Mesnildrey, P., et al.: Long-term results with total replacement of the ascending aorta and reimplantation of the coronary arteries. J. Thorac. Cardiovasc. Surg., 91:17, 1986.

Carrel, A.: Permanent intubation of the thoracic aorta. J. Exp. Med., 16:17, 1912.

Clagett, C. P., Burke, W. E., and Sharcfkin, J. B.: Platelet reactivity in vivo in dogs with arterial prostheses seeded with endothelial cells. Circulation, 69:632, 1987.

Cooley, D. A., Romagnoli, A., Milam, J. D., and Bossart, M. I.: A method of preparing woven Dacron aortic grafts to prevent interstitial hemorrhage. Cardiovasc. Dis. Bull. Tex. Heart Inst., 8:48, 1981.

Crawford, E. S., Stowe, C. L., Crawford, J. L., et al.: Aortic arch aneurysm: A sentinel of extensive aortic disease requiring sub-total and total aortic replacement. Ann. Surg., 199:742, 1984.

Crawford, E. S., Walker, H. S. J., Saleh, S. A., and Normann, N. A.: Graft replacement of aneurysm in descending thoracic aorta: Results without bypass or shunting. Surgery, 89:73, 1981.

DeBakey, M. E., and Cooley, D. A.: Successful resection of aneurysm of the thoracic aorta and replacement by graft. J. A. M. A., 152:673, 1953.

Diehl, J. T., Moon, B., Leclerc, Y., and Weisel, R. D.: Acute type A dissections of the aorta: Surgical management with the su-tureless intraluminal prosthesis. Ann. Thorac. Surg., 43:502, 1987.

Dubost, C., Allary, M., and Oeconomos, N.: Resection of an aneurysm of the abdominal aorta. Arch. Surg., 64:405, 1952.

Gloviczki, P., Hollier, L. H., Hoffman, E. A., et al.: The effect of preclotting on surface thrombogenicity and thromboembolic complications of Dacron grafts in the canine aorta. J. Thorac. Cardiovasc. Surg., 88:253, 1984.

Glynn, M. F. X., and Williams, W. G.: A technique for preclotting vascular grafts. Ann. Thorac. Surg., 29:182, 1980.

Goldman, M., McCollum, C. N., Hawker, R. J., et al.: Dacron arterial grafts: The influence of porosity, velour, and maturity on thrombogenicity. Surgery, 92:947, 1982a.

Goldman, M., Norcott, H. C., Hawker, R. J., et al.: Platelet accumulation on mature Dacron grafts in man. Br. J. Surg., 69(Suppl.):38, 1982b.

Graham, L. M., Vinter, D. W., Ford, J. W., et al.: Endothelial cell seeding of prosthetic vascular grafts: Early experimental studies with cultured autologous canine endothelium. Arch. Surg., 115:929, 1980.

Gross, R. E., Bill, A. H., and Pierce, E. C.: Methods for preservation and transplantation of arterial grafts: Observations on arterial grafts in dogs: Report of transplantation of preserved arterial grafts in 9 human cases. Surg. Gynecol. Obstet., 88:689, 1949.

Guidoin, R., Synder, R., Martin, L., et al.: Albumin coating of a knitted polyester arterial prosthesis: An alternative to preclotting. Ann. Thorac. Surg., 37:457, 1984.

Harrison, J. H., and Davalos, P. A.: Influence of porosity on synthetic grafts: Fate in animals. Arch. Surg., 82:28, 1961.

Haverich, A., Oelert, H., Maatz, W., and Borst, H. G.: Histopathological evaluation of woven and knitted Dacron grafts for right ventricular conduits: A comparative experimental study. Ann. Thorac. Surg., 37:404, 1984.

Haverich, A., Waterbusch, G., and Borst, H. G.: The use of fibrin glue for sealing vascular prosthesis of high porosity. Thorac. Cardiovasc. Surg., 29:252, 1981.

Hufnagel, C. A.: Permanent intubation of the thoracic aorta. Arch. Surg., 54:382, 1947.

Kadletz, M., Magometschnigg, M., Minar, E., et al.: Implantation of in vitro endothelialized polytetrafluoroethylene grafts in human beings: A preliminary report. J. Thorac. Cardiovasc. Surg., 104:736, 1992.

Kouchoukos, N. T., Karp, R. B., Blackstone, E. H., et al.: Replacement of the ascending aorta and aortic valve with a composite graft. Results in 86 patients. Ann. Surg., 3:403, 1980.

Lindenauer, S. M., Stanley, J. C., Zelenock, G. B., et al.: Aorto-iliac reconstruction with Dacron double velour. J. Cardiovasc. Surg., 25:36, 1984.

Makin, G. S.: Peripheral emboli following aortic grafting. Br. J. Surg., 54:650, 1988.

Mathisen, S. R., Wu, H. D., Sauvage, L. R., et al.: An experimental study of eight current arterial prostheses. J. Vasc. Surg., 4:33, 1986.

Matsuki, O., Robles, A., Gibbs, S., et al.: Long-term performance of aortic homografts in the aortic position. Ann. Thorac. Surg., 46:187, 1988.

McGee, G. S., Shuman, T. A., Atkinson, J. B., et al.: Experimental evaluation of a new albumin-impregnated knitted Dacron prosthesis. Am. Surg., 53:695, 1987.

Mitchell, R. S., Miller, D. C., Billingham, M. E., et al.: Comprehensive assessment of the safety, durability, clinical performance, and healing characteristics of a double velour knitted Dacron arterial prosthesis. Vasc. Surg., 14:197, 1980.

Muto, Y., Miyazaki, T., Eguchi, H., et al.: Aneurysm in a double velour knitted Dacron graft. J. Cardiovasc. Surg., 28:723, 1988.

Noishiki, Y.: Pattern of arrangement of smooth muscle cells in neointimae of synthetic vascular prostheses. J. Thorac. Cardiovasc. Surg., 75:894, 1978.

Quinones-Baldrich, W. J., Moore, W. S., Ziomek, S., and Chvapil, M.: Development of a "leak-proof," knitted Dacron vascular prosthesis. Vasc. Surg., 3:895, 1986.

Rumisek, J. D., Wade, C. E., Brooks, D. E., et al.: Heat-denatured albumin-coated Dacron vascular grafts: Physical characteristics and in vivo performance. J. Vasc. Surg., 4:136, 1986.

Sawyer, P. N.: Patency of small-diameter negatively charged glutaraldehyde-tanned (St. Jude Medical Biopolymeric) grafts. In Sawyer, P. N. (ed): Modern Vascular Grafts. New York, McGraw-Hill, 1987.

Scott, S. M., Hoffman, H., Gaddy, L. R., et al.: A new woven double velour vascular prosthesis. J. Cardiovasc. Surg., 26:175, 1985.

Stratton, J. W., and Hall, R. V.: Pseudointimal embolism from a woven Dacron graft. Surgery, 86:772, 1979.

Thurer, R. L., Hauer, J. M., and Weintraub, R. M.: A comparison of preclotting techniques for prosthetic aortic replacement. Circulation, 66(Suppl.):I-143, 1982.

Voorhees, A. B., Jr., Jaretzki, A., III, and Blakemore, A. H.: The use of tubes constructed from Vinyon "N" cloth in bridging arterial defects: Preliminary report. Ann. Surg., 135:332, 1952.

Wesolowski, S. A., Fries, C. C., Domingo, R. T., et al.: The compound prosthetic vascular graft: A pathologic survey. Surgery, 53:19, 1963.

Wesolowski, S. A., Fries, C. C., Karlson, K. E., et al.: Porosity: Primary determinant of ultimate fate of synthetic vascular grafts. Surgery, 50:91, 1961.

Zammit, M., and Wu, H. D.: A comparison of external velour and double velour Dacron grafts in the canine thoracic aorta. Am. Surg., 51:637, 1985.

Zammit, M., Wu, H. D., Mathisen, S. R., and Sauvage, L. R.: Influence on healing in the canine thoracic aorta of three substances used to close the interstices of macroporous Dacron grafts. Am. Surg., 52:667, 1986.

# ■ II Patent Ductus Arteriosus, Coarctation of the Aorta, Aortopulmonary Window, and Anomalies of the Aortic Arch

J. William Gaynor and David C. Sabiston, Jr.

## PATENT DUCTUS ARTERIOSUS

The ductus arteriosus was first described by Galen, and its role in the fetal circulation was first demonstrated by Harvey in 1628 (Boyer, 1967). During the 19th century, the morbidity associated with *patent ductus arteriosus* (PDA) was recognized, and Gibson (1900) described the characteristic murmur. Surgical correction by ligating or crushing the ductus was proposed by Munro in 1907. The first attempt at surgical intervention was by Strieder and colleagues in 1937 in a patient with bacterial endocarditis (Graybiel et al., 1938). Because of the friable tissues, the ductus could not be ligated and an attempt was made to obliterate it with plicating sutures. The patient survived the operation with a persistent murmur, and died of aspiration 4 days postoperatively. In 1938, Gross successfully ligated a PDA in a 7-year-old girl, initiating the modern era (Gross and Hubbard, 1939). The first successful treatment of an infected PDA was done in 1939 by Tubbs, who successfully performed ligation (Bourne et al., 1941; Hurt, 1992). Touroff and Vesell (1940) subsequently performed the first successful ductal division in a patient with bacterial endocarditis, curing the infection. An increased incidence of PDA in premature infants was reported by Burnard (1959). Powell (1963) and Decancq (1963) independently reported ligation of a PDA in premature infants. In 1966, Porstmann and co-workers first described catheter closure of a PDA using an Ivalon plug (Porstmann et al., 1971). Successful closure of PDA in premature infants by pharmacologic methods was reported independently in 1976 by Friedman and colleagues and by Heymann and associates. Rashkind and Cuaso (1979) reported the use of a transcatheter device to close a PDA in an infant. Wessel and co-workers (1988) reported the use of this device for closure of PDA as an outpatient procedure. Video-assisted thoracoscopic interruption of PDA was reported by Laborde and colleagues in 1993.

### Embryology and Pathologic Anatomy

The ductus arteriosus is derived from the sixth aortic arch and normally extends from the main or left pulmonary artery to the descending aorta just distal to the origin of the subclavian artery. Rarely, the ductus may be right-sided, bilateral, or absent. The ductus is usually 5 to 10 mm long and varies from a few millimeters to 1 to 2 cm in diameter. The aortic orifice is usually larger than the pulmonary orifice. In utero, blood ejected by the right ventricle flows almost exclusively through the ductus to the lower extremities and placenta, bypassing the high-resistance pulmonary circulation. The anatomic relationship of the ductus to the aorta is determined primarily by the hemodynamics of any associated anomalies. In pulmonary atresia, pulmonary blood flow is ductal-dependent with flow from the aorta to the pulmonary artery; thus, the ductus may appear to be a downward-directed branch of the aorta. In coarctation of the aorta or interruption of the aortic arch with ductal-dependent systemic blood flow, the descending aorta often appears to be a continuation of the large ductus.

Closure of the ductus occurs following birth during the transition from the fetal to the adult circulation. The lungs expand with the first breath, and pulmonary vascular resistance (PVR) decreases, increasing pulmonary blood flow and arterial oxygen concentration. Closure occurs secondary to constriction of smooth muscle in the ductal wall, causing apposition of intimal cushions, and is mediated by various substances that constrict or dilate ductal smooth muscle. Proliferation of the intima and media produces mounds, mucoid-filled spaces, and disruption of the internal elastic membrane (Ho and Anderson, 1979a). Doppler echocardiography reveals intraluminal protrusions in the ductus in 30% of normal full-term infants within 1 hour of birth and in 96% by 8 hours of age (Hiraishi et al., 1987). Closure by Doppler echocardiography is complete in 82 to 96% of full-term infants by 48 hours of age, although intermittent patency may occur even in healthy newborn infants (Gentile et al., 1981; Lim et al., 1992). The sensitivity of ductal smooth muscle depends on gestational age. In full-term infants, rising arterial oxygen tension constricts muscle fibers in the wall of the ductus. Prostaglandins of the E series dilate the ductus, so lower concentrations after birth effect closure. Ductal smooth muscle in premature infants is less sensitive to oxygen-induced constriction and more sensitive to the vasodilatory effects of certain prostaglandins. Anatomic closure by fibrosis usually is complete by 2 to 3 weeks postnatally, producing the ligamentum arteriosum connecting the pulmonary artery and the aorta.

Failure of the ductus to close causes persistent patency. Final closure may occur at any age, but is uncommon after 6 months. Persistent patency of the ductus may occur as an isolated lesion or may be associated with a variety of other congenital defects. Histologic examination of a persistently patent ductus reveals significant differences in the subendothelial elastic lamina when compared with a ductus that closes normally, suggesting that a primary defect in the composition of the ductal wall may be responsible for failure of closure (Gittenberger-deGroot, 1977). In infants with complex congenital heart disease, pulmonary or systemic blood flow often depends on patency of the ductus, and sudden decompensation may occur if the ductus closes. Infusion of prostaglandins to dilate the ductus often produces dramatic improvement, allowing stabilization and resuscitation before surgical intervention.

Prolonged patency of the ductus causes a left-to-right shunt of blood with pulmonary congestion and left ventricular volume overload. The magnitude of this shunt depends on the size of the ductus. With a large nonrestrictive ductus, the relative levels of PVR and systemic vascular resistance (SVR) are important in determining the severity of shunting. Shunting occurs throughout systole and diastole, and may cause hypotension with impaired perfusion of the brain, lower extremities, and abdominal organs. Myocardial dysfunction may result and lead to increasing left ventricular failure.

## Incidence, Mortality, and Morbidity

Isolated PDA occurs approximately once in 2500 to 5000 live births. The incidence increases with prematurity and with decreasing birth weight, and may be more than 80% in infants weighing less than 1000 g. The increased incidence is related to several factors, including decreased smooth muscle in the ductal wall, diminished responsiveness of ductal smooth muscle to oxygen, and possibly elevated levels of circulating vasodilatory prostaglandins. Genetic factors may be involved in PDA and persistent patency of the ductus occurs more commonly in females than males, with a 2:1 ratio.

PDA is not a benign entity, although prolonged survival is possible. The mortality in infants with untreated PDA may be as high as 30%. In a classic series, Abbott (1936) reported an average age at death of 24 years (Campbell, 1968). In a study of the natural history of untreated PDA, Shapiro and Keys (1943) found that 80% of the patients with PDA would eventually die of their cardiac disease. In this series, the life expectancy of patients alive at 17 years was a mean of 18 years. Before antibiotics, 40% of patients with PDA died of bacterial endocarditis, and most of

the remainder died of congestive heart failure (CHF). Campbell (1968) calculated that 42% of patients with untreated PDA will die by 45 years of age. Patients surviving to adulthood may develop CHF or pulmonary hypertension with reversed shunting through the ductus. Premature infants with PDA often have problems associated with prematurity, including respiratory distress syndrome, necrotizing enterocolitis, and intraventricular hemorrhage, which may be aggravated by the abnormal hemodynamics. CHF often results and may respond poorly to medical management. The incidence of long-term sequelae or prematurity, such as bronchopulmonary dysplasia, may be increased by the presence of a PDA. Infants with a large PDA can develop severe pulmonary hypertension at an early age. Young children with persistent patency of the ductus may show growth retardation.

## Clinical Manifestations and Diagnosis

The signs and symptoms of PDA depend on the size of the ductus, the PVR, the age at presentation, and associated anomalies. Full-term infants usually do not become symptomatic until the PVR decreases at 6 to 8 weeks of age, producing a significant left-to-right shunt. Because premature infants have less smooth muscle in the pulmonary arterioles, PVR decreases earlier and symptoms may develop during the first week of life. Up to 60% of very low birth weight infants (<1000 g) may show ductal shunting echocardiographically at 2 to 3 days of life without evidence of a murmur or other clinical signs of PDA (Dudell and Gersony, 1984; Hammerman et al., 1986). Approximately 40% of these infants eventually develop a hemodynamically significant left-to-right shunt. Infants with a birth weight greater than 1000 g have a much lower risk of developing a clinically significant shunt even if a murmur is present (Clyman and Campbell, 1987).

A large hemodynamically significant PDA usually presents in infancy with CHF. Afflicted infants are irritable, tachycardic, and tachypneic and tolerate feeding poorly. Physical examination often reveals a hyperdynamic precordium and bounding peripheral pulses. The systolic blood pressure is usually normal but diastolic hypotension may be present. Auscultation reveals a systolic or continuous murmur, often called a *machinery murmur*, which is heard best in the pulmonic area and radiates toward the middle third of the clavicle. A mid-diastolic apical murmur may be present secondary to increased flow across the mitral valve. If cardiac failure is present, a gallop may also be heard. Hepatomegaly is frequently present. Cyanosis is not present in uncomplicated, isolated PDA. Absence of these findings, however, does not exclude the presence of a significant PDA, especially in premature infants (Evans, 1993). A study of infants with symptomatic PDA found that the most sensitive clinical sign was a hyperdynamic precordium, which was present in 95% of patients. Bounding pulses and a murmur were absent in 15% and 20% of the patients, respectively (Kupferschmid et al., 1988).

The diagnosis of PDA can often be made noninvasively and the physical examination may be almost diagnostic. The chest film often demonstrates cardiomegaly and pulmonary congestion. However, 22% of infants with a symptomatic PDA show no increase in radiologic heart size (Higgins et al., 1977). In older children and adults, the electrocardiogram (ECG) may show left ventricular hypertrophy. Two-dimensional echocardiography may demonstrate the ductus and associated anomalies. The left atrial and aortic root diameters may be measured with M-mode echocardiography and, if the ratio is greater than 1.4 to 1.5, a significant left-to-right shunt is likely. This ratio may be normal, however, in infants with a significant PDA whose fluids have been restricted and who have been treated with diuretics. Continuous-wave and pulsed Doppler echocardiography may be used to demonstrate abnormal pulmonary artery flow patterns and estimate the magnitude of ductal flow. Color Doppler flow imaging may be used to demonstrate flow in a PDA and reveal the direction of shunting (see Fig. 33–2, color plate). Echocardiography may show a significant left-to-right shunt before the onset of clinical symptoms. The sensitivity of these techniques has made it possible to recognize a subgroup of patients who have a small PDA with normal pulmonary pressures who cannot be identified clinically (Houston et al., 1991). Tiny residual leaks may also be detected after either surgical or catheter closure of PDA (Sorenson et al., 1991; Zucker et al., 1993). The significance and possible morbidity of a "silent" PDA is unknown, as are the implications for further therapy. Formal cardiac catheterization is not required in children or young adults with classic findings of PDA, and this should be reserved for older patients as well as those with atypical findings, suspicion of associated anomalies, or pulmonary hypertension.

Patients with a moderate-sized PDA may remain asymptomatic until the second or third decade of life, when left ventricular failure or pulmonary hypertension occur. The earliest symptom is usually dyspnea on exertion followed by increasing CHF. Auscultation may reveal the typical murmur. The ECG and chest film may show left ventricular enlargement and hypertrophy. A small PDA usually causes no symptoms or growth retardation. A systolic or continuous murmur is present. The ECG and chest film usually appear normal. Some patients with PDA present with bacterial endocarditis as the first clinical manifestation. Bacterial endocarditis usually develops at the pulmonary orifice of the ductus.

Aneurysmal dilatation and rupture of the ductus arteriosus, although rare, may occur in infants and adults (Lund et al., 1992). Ductal aneurysm was first described by Martin in 1927 (Falcone et al., 1972). Closure of the pulmonary orifice with patency of the aortic orifice of the ductus, exposing the ductal tissue to systemic blood pressure, may be caused by progressive dilatation. Aneurysmal dilatation of a PDA has also been described and is usually associated with pulmonary hypertension (Green and Rollason, 1992). Neonatal aneurysm of the ductus must be differentiated from the ductus bump, a transient dilatation of the ductus seen on chest film. This is a benign finding that usually resolves by 48 hours of age. The ductus bump may persist into adulthood, however. Ductal aneurysm may present as an asymptomatic mediastinal mass on the chest film, or if significant enlarge-

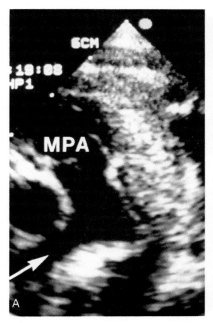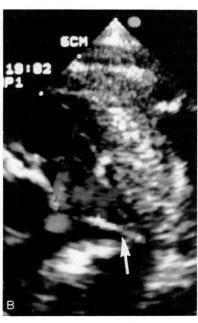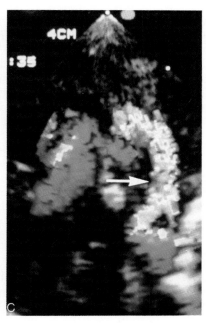

FIGURE 33–2. *A,* Two-dimensional echocardiogram in an infant with a small patent ductus arteriosus (PDA) showing main pulmonary artery (MPA), right pulmonary artery *(arrow),* and left pulmonary artery. *B,* Same patient with color Doppler image *(arrow)* of turbulent flow in pulmonary artery secondary to the PDA. *C,* Infant with large PDA. Color Doppler image shows large left-to-right shunt with turbulent flow in the main pulmonary artery *(arrow). (A–C,* Courtesy of Dr. Joseph Kisslo.)

ment has occurred, respiratory distress may occur secondary to bronchial compression and hoarseness may be present secondary to recurrent nerve involvement. Calcification of the wall and thrombus within the aneurysm are frequently seen. Because of a risk of progressive enlargement and rupture, surgical therapy should be undertaken at the time of diagnosis. Frequently, a discrete neck is present and aneurysmorrhaphy is indicated, rather than resection and grafting of the aorta.

The development of pulmonary hypertension in a patient with PDA is a serious prognostic sign. Pulmonary hypertension may be occasionally encountered in children who are under 2 years of age and who have nonrestrictive ductus and greatly increased pulmonary blood flow, but significant pulmonary hypertension is usually noted in older patients with PDA. The elevated pulmonary pressures may be secondary to the increased blood flow and may normalize after surgical closure of the PDA. In some patients, irreversible pulmonary vascular changes occur and pulmonary hypertension persists despite closure of the PDA. These patients usually have systemic pulmonary artery pressures and show evidence of Eisenmenger's physiology, with a bidirectional or right-to-left shunt causing cyanosis. Closure of the PDA in these patients is hazardous and may not lower pulmonary artery pressure.

## Management

The presence of a persistent PDA in a child or adult is a sufficient indication for surgical closure because of the increased mortality and risk of endocarditis. In symptomatic patients, closure should be performed when the diagnosis is made. In asymptomatic children, intervention can be postponed, if desired, but it should be done in the preschool years. Older patients should have the ductus closed when the diagnosis is made. If severe pulmonary hypertension has occurred with reversal of the ductal shunt, closure is associated with a higher mortality and may not improve symptoms. The increasing use of echocardiography has revealed a group of patients with a clinically silent PDA in which a very small amount of flow can be identified. The risk of endocarditis in these patients is unknown and indications for intervention have not been defined (Glickstein et al., 1993; Houston et al., 1991; Sorenson et al., 1991; Zucker et al., 1993). The appropriate management of a PDA in premature infants remains controversial.

### Surgical Procedures

Gross and Hubbard (1939) initially used simple ligation to interrupt the PDA. Because of difficulties with recannulization, they attempted ligation and wrapping with cellophane to induce fibrosis. However, recannulization still occurred. Touroff and Vesell (1940) were the first to report successful division of a PDA. During an attempt to ligate a PDA in a patient

with bacterial endocarditis, significant hemorrhage occurred and the ductus was successfully divided to control the bleeding. Gross (1944) pioneered division of PDA as the therapy of choice because of difficulties with recannulization. Blalock (1946) suggested ligation with multiple transfixion sutures as a preferred method because of concern over the safety of ductal division. In children and adults, either division or multiple suture ligation in the ductus is appropriate. Simple ligation is usually performed in neonates. In adults with a large ductus (10 mm or more) or patients with pulmonary hypertension, division is indicated.

The operation may be performed through either a left anterior or a left posterior thoracotomy. The lung is retracted and an incision is made in the pleura overlying the aorta. The pleura is reflected medially, exposing the ductus, with care taken to avoid damage to the phrenic and recurrent laryngeal nerves. The anatomy must be carefully defined to avoid inadvertent ligation of the left pulmonary artery. After the ductus has been mobilized, it may be obliterated with multiple suture ligatures (Fig. 33–3) or divided (Fig. 33–4). If division is planned, vascular clamps are placed across the ductus, which is then divided. Closure of each end is accomplished with two rows of nonabsorbable suture. If the ductus is particularly short and wide, it may be necessary to cross-clamp the aorta above and below the ductus, as in a coarctation repair. The pulmonary end of the ductus is clamped and the ductus is divided at the aorta, leaving a sufficient margin for closure. The open end of the aorta is closed and the cross-clamps removed. The pulmonary end of the ductus is then closed. In patients with a noncalcified ductus arteriosus and associated cardiac anomalies that require correction, the ductus arteriosus may be ligated via a median sternotomy before cardiopulmonary bypass is instituted.

In neonates, single or double ligation of PDA is usually the procedure of choice. Closure of the ductus in neonates by applying surgical clips has been described (Adzick et al., 1986; Kron et al., 1984). Several authors have advocated closing a PDA in the neonatal intensive care unit rather than transporting critically ill neonates to the operating room (Pate et al., 1981). There has been interest in video-assisted thoracoscopic interruption of PDA. Between 1991 and 1992, Laborde and colleagues (1993) performed thoracoscopic PDA closure using surgical clips in 38 patients with a mean age of 23.3 months and a mean weight of 9.5 kg. The procedure was initially successful in 36 patients, although 2 patients required a second procedure because of incomplete closure. No patient required open ligation and there were no operative deaths.

A calcified PDA is a difficult surgical problem. Simple ligation or division is not possible if diffuse circumferential calcification is present. Several techniques using cardiopulmonary bypass and closure from within the aorta or pulmonary artery have been described (Goncalves-Estella et al., 1975). A median

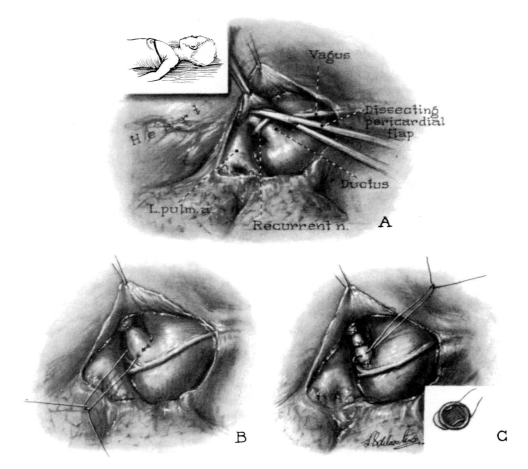

**FIGURE 33–3.** Operative treatment of PDA by ligation. Incision is anterolateral in the third interspace. In females, the incision circles beneath the breast. Elevation of pericardial lappet exposes the ductus. A purse-string suture, which does not enter the lumen, is placed at each end, and perforating mattress sutures are placed in between. The ductus should be obliterated over an 8- to 10-mm distance.

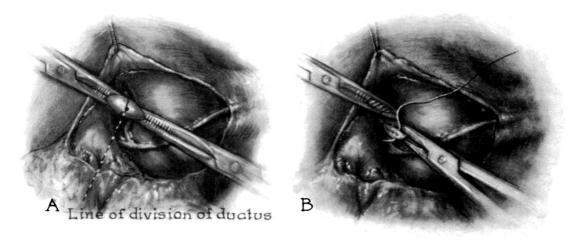

**FIGURE 33–4.** Treatment of PDA by division. Anterolateral third interspace incision is used with exposure, as for ligation. *A,* A thin occluding clamp is placed at each end, and the ductus is divided. Pressing the clamp against the pulmonary artery or aorta after division reduces the likelihood of slipping. *B,* Suture of the ductus is by a continuous mattress suture adjacent to clamp, followed by whipstitch backup over the free edge. Suture of the pulmonary artery is easier when performed from the patient's right side.

sternotomy is performed and cardiopulmonary by-pass instituted. As the patient is cooled, the PDA is occluded by compression of the left pulmonary artery to prevent overdistension of the pulmonary vasculature. The aorta is cross-clamped, cardioplegia is infused, and the pump flow is reduced. A pulmonary arteriotomy is performed and the pulmonary orifice of the ductus closed using direct suture of a patch. Patch closure of the aortic orifice of a PDA has also been described and may be performed using either cardiopulmonary bypass or a heparin-bonded shunt. The aorta is cross-clamped above and below the ductus arteriosus and an aortotomy performed. The ductus is occluded with a balloon catheter and a Dacron patch is used to close the aortic orifice (Wernly and Ameriso, 1980). A similar technique has been reported without the use of shunts or bypass (Johnson and Kron, 1988).

Treatment of an infected PDA can be hazardous. Infected PDA has been successfully treated by ligation or division with antibiotic therapy. Complete resection of the ductus and infected pulmonary artery wall using cardiopulmonary bypass has also been reported (Stejskal and Stark, 1992).

Closure of a PDA in patients with pulmonary hypertension presents special difficulties. In patients with irreversible pulmonary vascular changes, closure may further elevate the pulmonary pressures, producing right ventricular failure. Ellis and associates (1956) reported closure of a PDA in 72 patients with pulmonary hypertension. The overall mortality was 18% and was 56% in patients with right-to-left shunting. John and co-workers (1981) reported 5 deaths after PDA closures in 22 patients with pulmonary artery pressures greater than 70 mm Hg. Patients who have marked pulmonary hypertension and right-to-left shunting who survive closure may not improve and may develop progressive cor pulmonale.

Surgical closure of PDA may be complicated by hemorrhage, pneumothorax, chylothorax, left recurrent laryngeal nerve damage (Davis et al., 1988), and infection. Phrenic nerve paralysis has also been reported after closure of PDA. Great care must be exercised when dissecting or placing clamps on the ductus because the ductal tissue may be friable and a tear may cause hemorrhage that is difficult to control. Ligation or division of the left pulmonary artery has been reported following attempts at ductal ligation (Pontius et al., 1981). Inadvertent ligation of the pulmonary artery should be considered if the patient fails to improve postoperatively, if the chest film shows decreased pulmonary vascular markings of the left lung, or if there is continued evidence of a PDA. The diagnosis can be confirmed by perfusion scan (Orzel and Monaco, 1986) or pulmonary arteriography. Removal of the ligature or reanastomosis usually results in reperfusion of the lung (Fleming et al., 1983).

In the early days of surgical closure of PDA, recannulization presented a major problem. However, the instance of clinically significant recurrent ductal patency should approach zero after division or multiple-suture ligation. With color-flow Doppler echocardiography, a highly sensitive method for identification of PDA flow, evaluation of patients following surgical closure of a PDA shows an incidence of residual patency of 6 to 23%. Most of these patients are asymptomatic, with no clinical evidence of a residual shunt (Musewe et al., 1989; Sorensen et al., 1991; Zucker et al., 1993). The risk of endocarditis is unknown and the indications for reintervention in asymptomatic patients with minimal flow have not been defined.

### Transcatheter Closure

There has been increased interest in catheter closure of PDA. In 1966, Porstmann and co-workers successfully used a transcatheter technique to occlude a PDA with an Ivalon plug (Porstmann et al., 1971). Rashkind and Cuaso (1979) developed a double-umbrella device inserted via a right-sided catheter for ductal closure. Long-term follow-up on 208 patients who had closure of PDA with an Ivalon plug was reported in 1986 (Wierny et al., 1986). Ductal closure was successful in 94.7% of the patients. There were no deaths, and no patients required thoracotomy to retrieve the plug after dislodgement. Arterial complications occurred in 16 patients, 9 of whom required surgical intervention. Rashkind and colleagues (1987) reported attempted ductal closure by using the double-umbrella device in 146 patients. Closure was successful in 94 patients. Embolization occurred after release in 19 patients, 1 of whom required emergency operation.

Wessel and co-workers (1988) reported transcatheter closure using Rashkind's device in 22 children, 19 of whom were discharged on the same day. Khan and associates (1992) reported attempted transcatheter closure of PDA in 182 patients. Initial implantation was achieved in 174 patients (96%) with no deaths. At the 6-month follow-up, 37 of 167 patients (22%) had residual ductal flow. Twenty-one patients underwent implantation of a second device. The collective European experience was reported by the European Registry for Transcatheter Occlusion of Persistent Arterial Duct in 1992 (Tynan, 1992). The study enrolled 686 patients and the device was successfully implanted in 642 patients. The actuarial complete occlusion rate was 82.5% at 1 year. Forty-one patients have required a second device for persistent flow. Mechanical hemolysis occurred in 4 patients (0.5%), and there were 2 early deaths (0.3% mortality). Transcatheter occlusion of PDA has also been accomplished using Gianturco coils (Lloyd et al., 1993). Complications of transcatheter closure include failure of occlusion, embolization, vascular complications, mechanical hemolysis, protrusion of the device into the aorta, and left pulmonary artery stenosis (Fadley et al., 1993; Hayes et al., 1992; Ottenkamp et al., 1992).

### Management of PDA in Premature Infants

Premature infants often require mechanical ventilation and prolonged oxygen therapy. An increased instance of PDA in these neonates correlates with increasing prematurity and decreasing birth weight. A review of 21 randomized trials of treatment of PDA in premature infants found that the incidence of PDA at 3 days of life in very low birth weight infants did not correlate with birth weight or gestational age, but rather correlated with indices of clinical condition (ventilation indices, blood product administration) (Knight, 1992). The additional hemodynamic burden of a PDA may be poorly tolerated in these infants. The increased pulmonary blood flow causes pulmonary hypertension, diminished lung compliance, hypercarbia, and hypoxia. Differentiation of the effects of PDA from underlying pulmonary disease can be difficult. If the pulmonary disease is severe, ligation of the PDA may produce little or no improvement. A hemodynamically significant PDA is suggested by the presence of a hyperdynamic precordium, a continuous murmur, and bounding pulses. The chest x-ray usually shows cardiomegaly, pulmonary congestion, or the changes of hyaline membrane disease. Echocardiography is very useful in determining the presence of a left-to-right shunt in these patients.

Management of the PDA in premature infants is controversial because the ductus may close as the child matures. Some children may be managed conservatively with fluid restriction and diuretics. Treatment with digoxin is of no benefit. However, if there is persistent left-to-right shunting, CHF, need for mechanical ventilation, or an inability to receive adequate nutrition secondary to fluid restriction, further intervention is indicated. Two therapeutic options exist at this point. Pharmacologic closure can be attempted with prostaglandin inhibitors such as indomethacin (Friedman et al., 1976; Heymann et al., 1976). Final closure may be achieved in more than 70% of infants, but the ductus may reopen. Reopening occurs most frequently in the most premature infants and may be treated with a second course of indomethacin, although the success rate is lower. The success of therapy with indomethacin is related to the birth weight and postnatal age of the infant (Achanti et al., 1986). Adverse effects of indomethacin include renal dysfunction, hypernatremia, impaired platelet function, altered cerebral blood flow, and gastrointestinal hemorrhage. No adverse long-term sequelae of successful indomethacin therapy has been identified. Surgical closure can be used if there is a contraindication to indomethacin or if the duct fails to close. In some centers, surgical intervention is the primary therapy after conservative medical therapy fails.

Early closure of PDA in premature infants has been shown to decrease the need for mechanical ventilation and to decrease complications such as bronchopulmonary dysplasia, necrotizing endocarditis, and intolerance of enteral feeding. Closure with indomethacin is as effective as surgical ligation in preventing these complications. There has been a trend toward early intervention in premature infants, and the prophylactic use of indomethacin before development of hemodynamically significant shunt has been suggested. Studies suggest that indomethacin is indicated in very low birth weight infants (<1000 g) when clinical signs of a PDA first appear, because most of these infants develop significant shunting. In infants with a birth weight of more than 1000 g, however, there is no benefit in initiating therapy before the development of significant shunting (Clyman and Campbell, 1987). If indomethacin fails to close the ductus or if the ductus closes and reopens, surgical ligation is indicated. One study has reported a 42% failure rate with indomethacin in infants of very low birth weight and has suggested that primary surgical closure is more predictable with minimal morbidity (Palder et al., 1987). A review of 21 randomized trials of either surgical closure of the ductus or indomethacin therapy in preterm infants showed no significant effect of either method on mortality or chronic lung disease. All of the trials included backup treatment if the PDA persisted, so the effect of closure versus nonclosure was not tested. However, treatment before the development of symptoms tended to reduce the incidence of chronic lung disease (Knight, 1992).

### Results

Surgical closure of an isolated PDA has become a very safe procedure. Operative mortality approaches zero even in critically ill neonates. In premature infants, hospital mortality and long-term results depend primarily on associated pulmonary disease, coexistent anomalies, and the degree of prematurity. Mortality is increased and the long-term results are poor in older patients with a calcified ductus, and are poorest in those patients with severe pulmonary hypertension and reversed shunting. Most patients with PDA become functionally normal and have a normal life expectancy after closure.

## COARCTATION OF THE AORTA

The term *coarctation* is derived from the Latin *coarctatio* (a drawing or pressing together). *Coarctation of the aorta* is defined as a narrowing that diminishes the lumen and produces an obstruction to the flow of blood. The lesion may be a definite localized obstruction or may be a diffusely narrowed segment, called *tubular hypoplasia*. Localized coarctation of the aorta and tubular hypoplasia may occur separately or may coexist. Isolated coarctation may occur at any site within the aorta, but the most common location is at the insertion of the ductus (or ligamentum arteriosus). Externally, the aorta appears to be sharply indented or constricted. Internally, an obstructing diaphragm or shell on the posterior wall is usually more marked than is apparent by external appearance. The shelf consists of an infolding of the aortic media with a ridge of intimal hypoplasia, and may include tissue extending from the ductus arteriosus (Fig. 33–5). Tubular hypoplasia most often occurs in the aortic isthmus (the segment of aorta between the left subclavian artery and the insertion of the ductus arteriosus), but in some patients with coarctation, a hypoplastic transverse arch is also present. Localized coarctation

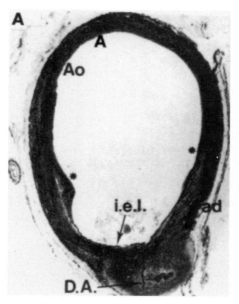
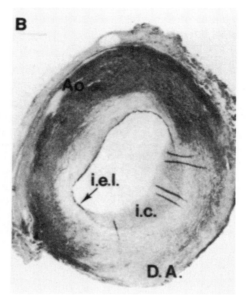

**FIGURE 33–5.** *A,* Transverse section of a normal aorta of a newborn at the level of the ductus arteriosus (D.A.). Ductal tissue stains lighter than aortic tissue because it is relatively poor in elastin. The inner third of the elastic lamellae of the aorta (Ao) merges into the internal elastic lamina (i.e.l.) of the ductus whereas the outer two-thirds merge into the adventitia (ad), resulting in a fish tail–like *(asterisk)* connection of the walls of the two vessels (more clearly visible on the right side of the figure than on the left). Ductal tissue does not extend beyond one-third of the total circumference of the aorta. (Elastic tissue stain; original magnification × 10). *B,* Transverse section of the aorta of a young infant with preductal coarctation (1) at the level of the ductus arteriosus. The lightly stained tissue of the ductus is clearly seen to encircle the lumen of the aorta. A small intimal cushion (i.c.) is present in this specimen. (Elastic tissue stain; original magnification × 10.) (*A* and *B,* From Elzenga, N. J., and Gittenberger-deGroot, A. C.: Localized coarctation of the aorta: An age-dependent spectrum. Br. Heart J., *49:*317, 1983.)

and tubular hypoplasia are part of the spectrum of disorders ranging from pseudocoarctation (a kinking or buckling of the aorta without producing obstruction of flow) to complete interruption of the aorta.

## Historical Aspects

Paris provided the first accurate description of co-arctation of the aorta in 1791, although Meckel in 1750 and Morgagni in 1760 had reported finding aortic narrowing at autopsy (Jarcho, 1961). Throughout the 19th century, coarctation of the aorta was considered a rare disorder. Legrand, in 1835, made the first pre-mortem diagnosis of obstruction of the thoracic aorta (Jarcho, 1962b). In 1903, Bonnet published an extensive review and distinguished between preductal co-arctation (infantile) and postductal coarctation (adult). In 1928, Abbott documented 200 cases of coarctation in patients over 2 years of age. This historical report stimulated much interest in the disorder, and in 1944, Blalock and Park proposed anastomosis of the left subclavian artery to the descending aorta to bypass the obstruction. In 1945, Craford and Nylin performed the first surgical correction with resection of the coarctation and end-to-end anastomosis. Gross and Hufnagel independently performed a similar procedure in 1945 (Gross, 1945a; Gross and Hufnagel, 1945). Subsequently, Gross (1951) was the first to use aortic homografts to replace a narrow segment of the aorta. Lynxwiler and co-workers (1951) reported the first successful repair of coarctation in an infant. The use of prosthetic onlay grafts was reported in 1957 by Vossschulte (1961), and in 1966, Waldhausen and Nahrwold described the subclavian flap aortoplasty. Recent years have seen increasing interest in the use

of percutaneous transluminal angioplasty for native and recurrent coarctation.

## Embryology and Pathologic Anatomy

The cause of the coarctation of the aorta and hypo-plasia of the aortic arch is still controversial. Two major theories have been proposed to explain the embryologic development of aortic narrowing. In some patients with coarctation, tissue from the ductus arteriosus (a muscular artery) extends circumferentially into the aortic wall (an elastic artery). Contraction and fibrosis of this ductal tissue at the time of ductal closure could lead to a localized narrowing (see Fig. 33–5). Extension of ductal tissue into the aortic wall has been shown histologically by Wielenga and Dankmeijer (1968), Ho and Anderson (1979b), and Elzenga and Gittenberger-deGroot (1983). Russell and colleagues (1991) performed pathologic examination of tissue resected during coarctation repair in patients less than 3 months of age and found a circumferential sling of ductal tissue extending from the ductus arteriosus into the aorta at the level of the coarctation shelf in 22 of 23 specimens. Fifteen of the patients had one or two tongue-like protrusions of ductal tissue that arose from the circumferential sling (opposite the ductal insertion) extended into the descending aorta below the insertion of the ductus. Van Son and associates (1993) reported proximal extension of similar tongues of ductal tissue into the isthmus. Other investigators have not found this abnormal tissue and have hypothesized that coarctation results from abnormal fetal blood flow patterns (Rudolph et al., 1972; Shinebourne and Elseed, 1974). In the normal fetus, blood flow across the isthmus is less than flow in either the ascending or the descending aorta (which receives the ductal flow), and thus the diameter of the isthmus is smaller than that of either the ascending or the descending aorta.

An increased incidence of coarctation is seen with lesions that produce left ventricular outflow tract obstruction (ventricular septal defects [VSDs], aortic stenosis, mitral valve anomalies) and diminishing ascending aortic flow, which might cause abnormal narrowing of the isthmus. Coarctation is rarely associated with anomalies that decrease ductal flow and increase ascending aortic flow (e.g., tetralogy of Fallot). Van Son and associates (1993) hypothesize that both abnormal extension of ductal tissue and hemodynamic factors play a role in the pathogenesis of coarctation. Preductal coarctation is frequently found in children with augmented flow through the ductus arteriosus and decreased flow through the aortic arch. A well-developed ductus arteriosus secondary to increased flow may have disproportionate growth, facilitating proliferation of the ductal tissue into the aorta. The presence and extent of abnormal ductal tissue is important in determining appropriate surgical therapy. If abnormal ductal tissue is present, failure to completely excise this abnormal tissue may allow further contraction and recurrent coarctation. There is also evidence of an increased incidence of cystic medial necrosis in patients with coarctation (Lindsay, 1988). It is uncertain whether this is a primary weakness of the aortic wall or secondary disease produced by the coarctation. Increased fragility of the wall may lead to aneurysmal dilatation, aortic dissection, and rupture of the aorta.

## Incidence and Associated Anomalies

Coarctation of the aorta represents 5 to 10% of congenital heart disease and the autopsy incidence is 1 in 3000 to 4000 autopsies. Isolated coarctation occurs more commonly in males, but there is no sex predisposition among patients with more complex lesions. Several anomalies are found commonly in patients with coarctation of the aorta, including bicuspid aortic valve, VSDs, PDA, and various mitral valve disorders (Becker et al., 1970). Congenital aortic stenosis, aortic atresia, and hypoplastic left-sided heart syndrome may also occur. VSDs that occur with coarctation are often associated with posterior septal malalignment, which compromises the left ventricular outflow tract and decreases ascending aortic flow, possibly causing coarctation. Moene and co-workers (1987) found that up to 70% of VSDs that occur in association with coarctation of the aorta are of types characterized by frequent spontaneous closure. This has also been confirmed in recent surgical series where many infants did not require closure of VSD after initial repair of coarctation (Park et al., 1992). Mitral valve anomalies with stenosis or regurgitation secondary to the abnormalities of the chordae tendinae and papillary muscles are frequently seen in patients with coarctation (Celano et al., 1984; Freed et al., 1974; Rosenquist, 1974). Shone's syndrome is a complex of parachute mitral valve, cor triatriatum, subaortic stenosis, and coarctation (Shone et al., 1963). Coarctation of the aorta is occasionally found in patients with transposition of the great arteries, and usually occurs in patients with associated right ventricular outflow tract obstruction (Moene et al., 1985; Vogel et al., 1984). Coarctation may be encountered in up to 50% of patients with the Taussig-Bing anomaly (Parr et al., 1983; Sadow et al., 1985). Genetic factors may have a role: There are reports of familial occurrences, and 15 to 36% of patients with Turner's syndrome are found to have a coarctation (Ravelo et al., 1980). Patients with severe associated defects tend to have associated tubular hypoplasia or a hypoplastic transverse aortic arch rather than isolated coarctation.

## Clinical Manifestations

The age and symptoms at presentation depend on the location and severity of the coarctation and the associated anomalies. A preductal coarctation entails an increased incidence of cardiac defects, and patients frequently present in infancy with CHF. Preductal coarctation frequently consists of hypoplasia of the transverse arch and isthmus terminating in an obstructive shelf. Paraductal and postductal coarctation are usually isolated obstructions and have a low incidence of associated defects. Bonnet considered preductal coarctation to be the infantile form because of its usual presentation in infancy. However, the terms *infantile* and *adult* are inappropriate, because patients with the so-called infantile form can survive to adulthood and some patients with the so-called adult type develop clinical manifestations in infancy.

Preductal coarctation may not seriously alter the normal fetal circulation and therefore does not stimulate development of a collateral circulation in utero. Infants with severe narrowing may appear normal at birth and have palpable femoral pulses if a PDA allows blood flow past the obstructive shelf. Symptoms develop as the ductus closes, causing significant aortic obstruction. The infants become irritable, tachypneic, and disinterested in feeding. A systolic murmur may be present over the left precordium and posteriorly between the scapulae. Although blood pressure is difficult to record accurately in neonates, moderate upper extremity hypertension and an arm/leg systolic pressure gradient are usually present. These findings may be absent in critically ill infants with a low cardiac output. Hypotension, oliguria, and severe metabolic acidosis are frequently present in critically ill infants. The diagnosis may be obscured in patients with severe obstruction or complete aortic interruption whose pulmonary artery pulse may be felt in the femoral arteries when the ductus is open. Differential cyanosis may be present between the upper and the lower extremities. Left-to-right shunting may occur through a patent foramen ovale. In neonates, signs of a collateral circulation are not present.

Older children and adults often present with unexplained hypertension or complications of hypertension, and some may be asymptomatic for many years and lead an active life. Presenting complaints include headache, epistaxis, visual disturbances, and exertional dyspnea. Some patients present with a cerebrovascular accident (secondary to an aneurysm of the circle of Willis, aortic rupture, dissecting aneurysm, or bacterial endocarditis) (Shearer et al., 1970). Many patients are discovered through evaluation of hypertension or of a murmur heard on routine examination.

## Diagnosis

The diagnosis of a coarctation of the aorta usually can be made clinically and it depends on evidence of obstruction to blood flow in the thoracic aorta. The findings include hypertension, a systolic pressure gradient between the arms and the legs, a systolic murmur heard over the left precordium and posteriorly between the scapulae, and diminished or absent femoral pulses with a delayed upstroke. The presence of an anterior diastolic murmur may indicate aortic regurgitation secondary to a bicuspid aortic valve. Because anomalous origin of the right subclavian artery can occur distal to the coarctation, the blood pressure must be obtained in *both* arms, as the orifice of either subclavian artery may be involved in the coarctation. In older children and adults, evidence of a collateral circulation may be found involving branches of the subclavian arteries proximal to the obstruction (the internal mammary, vertebral, thyrocervical, and costocervical arteries) that anastomose with intercostal arteries and other arteries below the obstruction. Enlarged collateral vessels may be seen or occasionally palpated between the scapulae, and a bruit may be audible as well. Aneurysmal dilatation of the intercostal arteries can occur and may complicate surgical reconstruction. Poststenotic dilatation of

the descending aorta is common, but an aneurysm of the ascending or descending aorta may be present only rarely.

The ECG in infancy may show right ventricular, left ventricular, or biventricular hypertrophy. In older children and adults, the ECG may be normal or show evidence of left ventricular hypertrophy, often with a strain pattern. The chest film may reveal cardiomegaly with left ventricular hypertrophy. Infants with heart failure may demonstrate extreme cardiomegaly and pulmonary congestion. Rib notching secondary to the enlarged tortuous intercostal vessels is almost pathognomonic and was first described by Meckel in 1827 (Jarcho, 1962a). In 1929, Rosler (Christiansen, 1948) and Railsback and Dock (1929) emphasized the radiologic appearance of rib notching, erosions that occur on the underside of the rib. These may be unilateral if the orifice of the left subclavian artery is narrowed by the coarctation or if there is anomalous origin of the right subclavian artery distal to the coarctation. Absence of rib notching in older patients may indicate a poor collateral circulation. The "3" sign—consisting of proximal dilatation of the aorta, aortic constriction, and poststenotic dilatation—may be present (Fig. 33–6).

Angiocardiography is still the most objective method of visualizing the coarctation. It shows the location and extent of narrowing, the involvement of the great vessels, and the extent of the collateral circulation. The pressure gradient can be measured, and associated cardiac defects can be evaluated by cardiac catheterization. Two-dimensional echocardiography with color-flow Doppler echocardiography helps show the site of the obstruction, suggest or exclude associated anomalies, and estimate the arterial pressure gradient (see Fig. 33–7, color plate). Echocardiography is the diagnostic method of choice in critically ill neonates with suspected coarctation. Cardiac catheterization is usually not necessary in

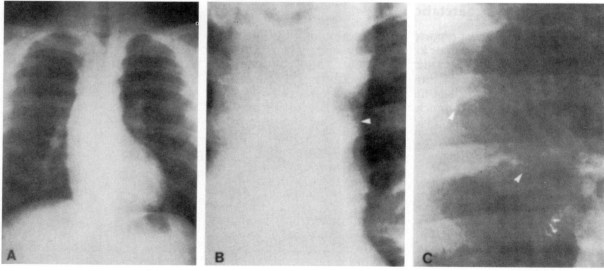

**FIGURE 33–6.** Patient with coarctation of the aorta. *A,* Chest roentgenogram. *B,* Detail showing "3" sign formed by proximal dilated aorta, area of constriction *(arrow),* and distal dilated aorta. *C,* Detail showing rib notching *(arrows)* secondary to dilated intercostal vessels. *(A–C,* Courtesy of Dr. James Chen.)

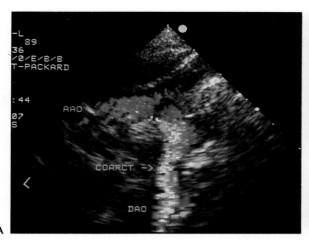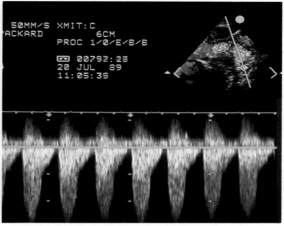

**FIGURE 33–7.** *A,* Freeze frame two-dimensional color Doppler echocardiogram of the aortic arch in a child with coarctation of the aorta. This is a suprasternal view showing the ascending aorta (AAO) at the left and the descending aorta (DAO) at the bottom. Note the coarctation (coarct) with narrowing of the aorta and turbulent flow. *B,* Steerable continuous-wave spectral velocity recording from the child shown in *A.* The two-dimensional image in the upper right-hand corner shows the location and the direction of the continuous wave Doppler beam. The flow is away from the transducer and therefore is represented below the baseline. The velocity is proportional to the degree of stenosis in most cases. Peak velocity in this patient is 3 m/sec. (*A* and *B,* Courtesy of Dr. Joseph Kisslo.)

these patients before surgical correction. Echocardiography is also useful in postoperative patients to evaluate the surgical result. However, it is important to realize that Doppler echocardiography may not accurately estimate the magnitude of the pressure gradient either preoperatively or postoperatively (Chan et al., 1992). Computed tomography (CT), digital subtraction angiography (DSA), and magnetic resonance imaging (MRI) are also helpful in difficult cases (Fig. 33–8).

## Natural History

The natural history of untreated coarctation of the aorta depends on the age at presentation and associated anomalies. Symptomatic infants have a very high mortality depending on the severity of the coarctation and the presence of associated defects. Patients surviving until adulthood have a greatly decreased life expectancy. In 1928, before the development of antibiotics and surgical methods of correction of coarctation, Abbott reviewed 200 cases of coarctation confirmed at autopsy in patients older than 2 years. Death occurred in 34% of the patients by 40 years of age, and the average age at death was 42 years. The most common causes of death were spontaneous rupture of the aorta, bacterial endocarditis, and cerebral hemorrhage. Reifenstein and colleagues reported 104 cases of coarctation in 1947. The average age at death was 35 years, with 23% of the patients dying of aortic rupture, 22% of bacterial endocarditis or aortitis, 18% of CHF, and 11% of cerebrovascular accident. Rupture of the aorta or an intracranial aneurysm occurred usually in the second or third decade of life. Endocarditis was most commonly associated with a bicuspid aortic valve. Campbell (1970) calculated that of patients with coarctation surviving the first 2 years of life, 25% would die by 20 years of age, 50% by 32

years of age, 75% by 46 years of age, and 90% by 58 years of age. However, the presence of a coarctation does not preclude prolonged survival; 1 patient is known to have lived to the age of 92 years. The coronary arteries in patients with untreated coarctation show striking intimal degeneration, medial thickening, and increase in mineralization. These changes can occur even in young children and may predispose patients to early atherosclerosis. Hypertension secondary to the coarctation has been the most important factor in the pathogenesis of these changes. Surgical therapy has significantly increased the life expectancy of patients with coarctation, although they do not become fully normal.

## Pseudocoarctation

Pseudocoarctation was first reported by Souders and associates (1951). This is a buckling or kinking of the aorta that does not produce an obstruction to flow. The chest film usually reveals an abnormal aortic contour that mimics a left superior mediastinal mass. There is no evidence of collateral circulation and the diagnosis is confirmed by aortography showing a tortuous kinked aorta with no measurable pressure gradient. Although pseudocoarctation was thought to be a benign entity, aneurysmal dilatation can occur in the segment distal to the buckle area. Gay and Young (1969) reported a patient who had pseudocoarctation and died secondary to aortic rupture. They recommended careful evaluation of patients with pseudocoarctation for aneurysm formation. Surgical intervention should be undertaken in patients developing progressive aortic dilatation.

## Physiology of Hypertension

The pathogenesis of hypertension in coarctation is multifactorial. The most prominent causes appear to

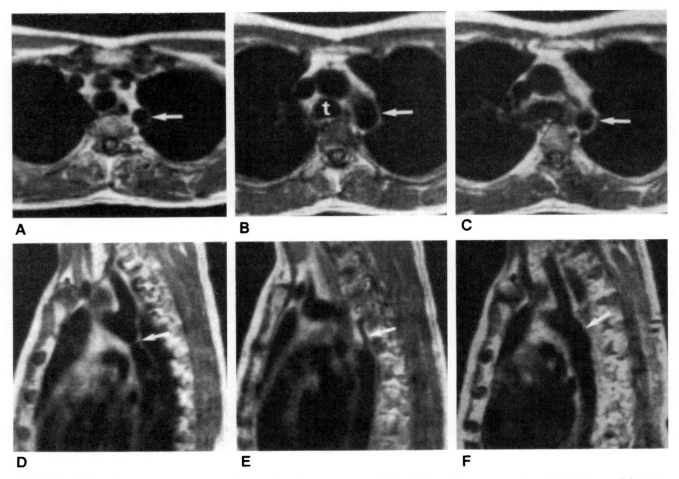

A

B

C

D

E

F

**FIGURE 33–8.** Magnetic resonance images. *A,* Transaxial section above arch. Dilated left subclavian artery *(arrow). B,* More caudal section. Posterior aortic arch immediately proximal to coarctation *(arrow).* (t = trachea). *C,* Section taken 1 cm below *B.* Reduction in caliber of descending aorta *(arrow). D,* Parasagittal section. Coarctation distal to dilated left subclavian artery *(arrow).* Diaphragm-like stricture is better appreciated than on transaxial sections. *E,* Parasagittal section through the distal descending aorta. Dilated collateral artery *(arrow).* *F,* Postoperative parasagittal section through distal descending aorta. Dilated collateral artery *(arrow).* Widely patent lumen at the previous site of coarctation. (A–F, From Amparo, E. G. Higgins, C. B., and Shafton, E. P.: Demonstration of coarctation of the aorta by magnetic resonance imaging. Am. J. Roentgenol., *143:*1192–1194. Copyright 1984 by Williams & Wilkins Company.)

be mechanical and renal, although recent investigations suggest that abnormal endothelial function may also be a factor. Abbott (1928) and Lewis (1933) emphasized the importance of hypertension in the natural history of coarctation of the aorta. Rytand (1938) and others noted an increase in vascular resistance proximal and distal to the narrow segment, causing in diastolic hypotension. Gupta and Wiggers (1951) showed that it was necessary to diminish the aortic lumen by 40 to 45% to cause an elevation in the blood pressure, and they suggested that mechanical factors alone were responsible for the hypertension. Scott and Bahnson (1951) were the first to definitively demonstrate the role of the kidneys in the pathogenesis of the hypertension of coarctation and experimental coarctation. In experimental coarctation, hypertension could be eliminated by transplanting one kidney to the neck (proximal to the obstruction) with contralateral nephrectomy. Young and colleagues (1950) later found normal renal blood flow in experimental coarctation. Renal blood flow is usually normal in patients

with coarctation and studies of the renin-angiotensin system have yielded conflicting results. Renin and angiotensin levels have been reported to be normal in both experimental animals and patients with coarctation. However, with a canine model, Bagby and associates (1975, 1980) showed greater than expected elevation of plasma renin activity during sodium restriction. During low-, normal-, and high-sodium intake, plasma volume, extracellular volume, and plasma renin activity were higher in animals with coarctation than in control animals. Alpert and co-workers (1979) showed significant increases in plasma renin activity during volume depletion in coarctation patients compared with normal controls. These findings suggest that the hypertension of coarctation is similar to a one-kidney one-clip Goldblatt model of hypertension. Plasma renin activity is initially elevated, increasing plasma volume and restoring renal perfusion to normal levels. The stimulus for increased renin secretion is diminished and plasma renin activity returns to normal levels with the hypertension maintained by volume expansion (Parker et al., 1980). Angiotensin blockade has not been consistently useful in treating the hypertension of coarctation. Ferguson and colleagues (1977), using a model of coarctation similar to that of Scott and Bahnson, showed that animals with coarctation developed generalized hypertension; but when a graft was used to reestablish renal blood flow, hypertension developed only proximal to the stenosis. Other investigators have shown abnormal stiffness of the prestenotic aortic wall (Sehested et al., 1982) and abnormal baroreceptor function (Beekman et al., 1983). Gardiner and associates (1993) showed abnormal endothelium-mediated vasodilatation in normotensive adults following coarctation repair, suggesting that abnormal endothelial function may contribute to the pathogenesis of hypertension.

## Management

Medical therapy plays only a small role in patients with coarctation. The presence of coarctation is usually sufficient indication for surgical intervention; the major questions are the timing and method of repair. Symptomatic infants usually require intervention, although a few improve with conservative medical treatment of CHF and can then undergo elective surgical correction. A major advance in the treatment of critically ill neonates with coarctation and interrupted aortic arch has been the introduction of prostaglandin E$_1$ (PGE$_1$) therapy (Leoni et al., 1984). Infusion of PGE$_1$ can reopen and maintain patency of the ductus arteriosus in many neonates, allowing perfusion in the lower body and correction of the severe metabolic acidosis and oliguria that are often present (Heymann et al., 1979). Stabilization of these severely ill infants allows surgical correction to be accomplished in more optimal conditions with decreased mortality.

The timing of elective repair of the coarctation of the aorta is perhaps the most important determinant of long-term outcome. Although it provides relief of some symptoms, repair in late childhood or adulthood has an increased incidence of persistent hypertension with its associated morbidity. Repair in infants using resection and end-to-end anastomosis was reported to cause a high incidence (up to 60%) of recurrent coarctation, although recent series have shown a much lower rate of recurrence. Alternative techniques of repair were developed to allow repair at an early age with fewer recoarctations. The current trend is for elective repair at an early age, and some authors believe that repair should be undertaken at the time of diagnosis in symptomatic and asymptomatic infants to prevent complications (Waldhausen et al., 1981). In recent years, percutaneous transluminal balloon angioplasty has been an alternative therapy for coarctation. The long-term possibility of recoarctation after balloon angioplasty for a native coarctation of the aorta are unknown.

### Surgical Correction

The classic method of repair of coarctation developed by Crafoord and by Gross is resection of the obstruction with a primary end-to-end anastomosis. Because recoarctation often occurred, particularly in infants, other techniques were developed. In 1957, Vossschulte introduced the prosthetic patch onlay graft technique, which uses a prosthetic patch to enlarge the area of constriction (Vossschulte, 1961). Subclavian flap aortoplasty was introduced by Waldhausen and Nahrwold in 1966. In this repair, a flap of the left subclavian artery is turned down onto the aorta to enlarge the area of constriction. More extensive forms of the classic repair have been developed. Amato and co-workers (1977) proposed anastomosis of the distal aorta to the inferior aspect of the arch, with anastomosis of the contiguous walls of the left carotid and subclavian arteries, if necessary, to alleviate the obstruction. Lansman and colleagues (1986) proposed an extended resection with primary anastomosis. The coarcted segment is excised and the anastomosis enlarged by an incision proximally on the inferior aspect of the arch. Elliott (1987) has described a more extensive procedure in which the arch is completely dissected, the descending aorta is mobilized to the diaphragm, an incision is made on the inferior aspect of the arch as proximal as possible, the descending aorta is spatulated posteriorly, and the anastomosis is completed. Various modifications of these repairs have also been described.

#### METHOD OF REPAIR

**Resection and End-to-End Anastomosis.** The patient is positioned in the right lateral decubitus position, and a left posterolateral thoracotomy is performed. The lung is retracted inferiorly and anteriorly and the pleura overlying the descending aorta is incised. The proximal aorta and left subclavian artery, area of coarctation, and ligamentum (or ductus arteriosum) are carefully dissected, avoiding damage to the recurrent laryngeal nerve (Fig. 33–9). Abbott's artery, an anomalous aortic branch that may be a remnant of the fifth aortic arch, sometimes originates from the isthmus and may be divided. Care is taken not to injure any enlarged intercostal arteries during the dissection. Division of these arteries may be necessary, especially if aneurysm dilatation has occurred, but it is preferable to preserve all collaterals. To obtain an optimal result with this technique, it is necessary to resect the entire constricting segment and construct the anastomosis without tension (Fig. 33–10). The extent of the dissection needed depends on the extent of the resection planned. If an extended resection and anastomosis to the inferior aspect of the arch is planned, it is necessary to completely dissect and mobilize the aortic arch to the innominate artery. The descending aorta must be fully mobilized in order to construct an anastomosis without tension. When the repair is performed in infants, heparin is not administered and the aorta is cross-clamped proximally and distally. If an extended resection is planned, it may be necessary to place the proximal clamp so that the left carotid artery is occluded and the clamp extends on to the ascending aorta (Fig. 33–11). The ductus is

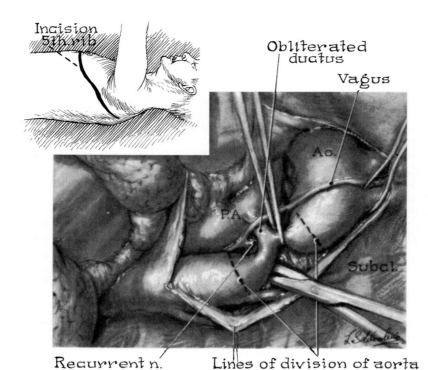

Incision 5th rib

Obliterated ductus

Vagus

Ao.

PA

Subcl.

Recurrent n.          Lines of division of aorta

**FIGURE 33–9.** Operative exposure for resection of coarctation of the aorta is through the bed of the fifth rib. The entire rib is removed from neck to cartilage. The constricted segment is usually held medially by an obliterated ductus, division of which allows considerable mobility. The coarctation is held forward to facilitate dissection posteriorly. Large intercostal arteries must be carefully avoided. Division of the aorta should be through a point of normal diameter.

ligated and divided and the coarcted segment completely excised. Complete excision of all tissue that appears to be ductal in origin is very important. Care should be taken to preserve as much of the lateral isthmus as possible. The undersized aortic arch is incised to a point more proximal than the area of hypoplasia, and the incision can be continued to the medial aspect of the ascending aorta, if necessary. An incision is then made on the posterolateral aspect of the descending aorta. This incision is important because it will divide any constricting ring of ductal tissue that may be present. The anastomosis is then performed using a continuous polypropylene suture, and the aortic clamps are removed. Following completion of the repair, the pressure should be measured in the descending aorta and compared with the right arm pressure to determine whether any obstruction remains. Advantages of this technique include complete relief of left ventricular obstruction, wide resection of ductal tissue, absence of prosthetic material, and preservation of the left subclavian artery.

**Subclavian Flap Aortoplasty.** Subclavian flap aortoplasty is performed through a left thoracotomy (Fig. 33–12). The initial dissection and exposure are similar to that for resection and anastomosis, although less dissection is required. The left subclavian artery is fully mobilized and ligated at its first branch. The vertebral artery should be ligated to prevent a subclavian steal phenomenon. A longitudinal incision is then made through the region of the coarctation and continued on to the subclavian artery to create a flap. The posterior obstructing shelf is resected and the flap of the subclavian artery is turned down to enlarge the area of constriction. The flap must be of sufficient length to bridge the obstruction. Advantages of this

technique include avoidance of prosthetic material, decreased dissection, decreased aortic cross-clamp period, and a possible increase in anastomotic growth because there is no circumferential suture line. If the area of narrowing occurs proximal to the left subclavian artery, the flap may be directed proximally and a reversed subclavian flap aortoplasty performed to enlarge the aortic arch.

**Prosthetic Patch Onlay Graft.** The use of prosthetic patches to enlarge the area of constriction was introduced in 1957. A left thoracotomy is performed (Fig. 33–13). The area of constriction is incised longitudinally, although the obstructing shelf is not excised (previous reports suggest an increased risk of aneurysm if the shelf is resected), and a prosthetic patch is used to enlarge the lumen. Yee and associates (1984) used Gore-Tex patches. They found that the advantages of the technique include decreased operative time, decreased dissection, maximal augmented area of stenosis preservation of collateral vessels, and no sacrifice of normal vascular structures. Ungerleider and Ebert (1987) demonstrated the applicability of patch aortoplasty via a median sternotomy in selected infants who required simultaneous correction of coarctation and intracardiac defects. There have been increasingly frequent reports of the formation of aneurysms and pseudoaneurysms (Aebert et al., 1993; Bergdahl and Ljungqvist, 1980; Mendelsohn et al., 1992) following prosthetic patch repairs of coarctation.

**Interposition Grafts.** In some older patients with tubular hypoplasia and inelastic aortas, it may not be possible to resect the narrow segment completely and restore aortic continuity by primary anastomosis. Gross (1951) pioneered the use of aortic homografts as

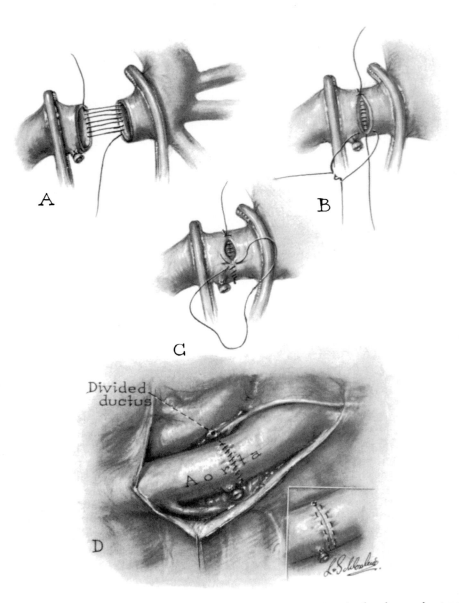

**FIGURE 33–10.** Anastomosis after excision of coarctation. *A*, An everting mattress suture is placed over about one-third of the posterior row before the vessels are approximated and the suture is pulled up *(B)*. *C*, The anastomosis is completed with continuous over-and-over suture. *Inset* in *D* shows the everting mattress suture sometimes used. In children, interrupted mattress sutures can be used for the entire anterior row.

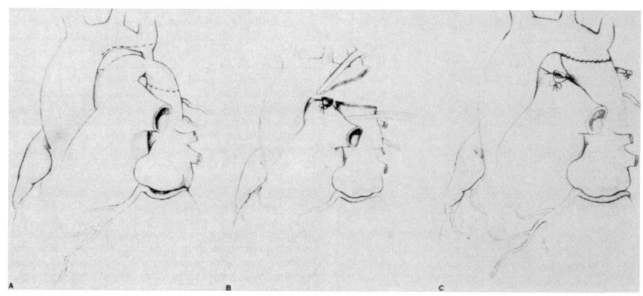

**FIGURE 33–11.** The operative technique for extended aortic arch anastomosis for repair of coarctation. *A,* Region of coarctation to be excised. *B,* The aortic arch and descending aorta have been mobilized and the PDA ligated. The entire segment of abnormal aorta has been resected with extension of the incision onto the inferior aspect of the arch. *C,* Completed repair. (*A–C,* From Lansman, S., Shapiro, A. J., Schiller, M. S., et al.: Extended aortic arch anastomosis for repair of coarctation in infancy. Circulation, *74*[Suppl. I]:I-37, 1986.)

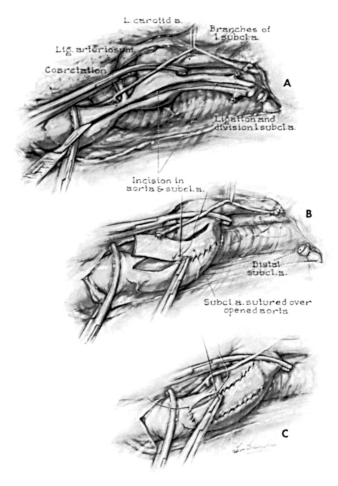

**FIGURE 33–12.** Subclavian flap aortoplasty. *A,* Through a left posterolateral thoracotomy, the proximal and distal aorta is mobilized and the aorta is cross-clamped between the left subclavian and the left carotid arteries. The aorta is also clamped distally. The subclavian artery is divided, and a longitudinal incision is made through the entire length of the subclavian artery and the coarctation segment. *B,* the subclavian artery is rolled down over the coarctation to enlarge the segment. *C,* The suture line is completed. Care must be taken to ensure that the length of the subclavian artery is adequate to cover the entire coarctation segment. (*A–C,* From Elbert, P. A.: Atlas of Congenital Cardiac Surgery. New York, Churchill Livingstone, 1989.)

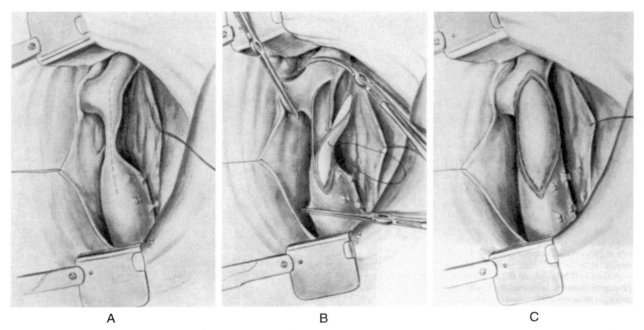

A          B          C

**FIGURE 33–13.** Operative technique for repair of coarctation of the aorta with a synthetic patch aortoplasty. *A,* Operative view showing the line of incision across coarctation. *B,* Placement of patch to enlarge area of constriction. *C,* Completed repair. (*A–C,* From Vossschulte, K.: Surgical correction of coarctation of the aorta by an "isthmusplastic" operation. Thorax, *16*:338, 1961.)

an interposition graft in these patients, and reported follow-up of 70 patients who had undergone homograft insertion (Schuster and Gross, 1962). No complications other than calcification of the graft (which was present in less than 50% of the patients) were reported. No aneurysms formed. Prosthetic interposition grafts are rarely indicated but may be useful in patients with complex coarctation, recurrent coarctation, or aneurysm formation.

**Alternative Repairs.** Numerous alternative procedures have been proposed for correction of coarctation. The Blalock-Park anastomosis divides the left subclavian artery with anastomosis to the descending aorta to bypass the obstruction (Blalock and Park, 1944). Modifications of the subclavian flap aortoplasty include subclavian artery reimplantation, end-to-end anastomosis with use of a subclavian flap to enlarge the anastomosis, and end-to-end anastomosis with reimplantation of the subclavian artery. Ascending aorta to descending aorta bypass grafts have been used and may also be useful at reoperation.

### Management of Associated Anomalies

Outcome after surgical correction depends on the patient's age at the time of operation, the method of repair chosen, and especially the presence of associated anomalies. The optimal management of infants with associated anomalies is still controversial. A PDA is frequently present and should be divided and ligated. A bicuspid aortic valve may be present but often requires no intervention at the time the coarctation is corrected. Appropriate management of associated VSDs is less clear. Several therapeutic options are available. In the past, the pulmonary artery was

often banded at the time of coarctation repair in infants with an unrestrictive VSD. However, VSDs associated with coarctation have a high incidence of spontaneous closure. In infants with coarctation and a VSD and no other associated anomalies, some experts advocate repair of the coarctation alone. If the CHF does not resolve, the VSD is closed at a second operation. Hammon and co-workers (1985) reported improved survival when pulmonary banding was performed at the time of coarctation repair and the VSD was closed later. Leanage and colleagues (1981) suggested that banding should be performed only in infants with an associated large VSD. Goldman and colleagues (1986) found no survival benefit with pulmonary artery banding even in infants with a large VSD. They did, however, report decreased mortality with the use of pulmonary banding in patients with coarctation, VSD, and associated intracardiac anomalies. Park and associates (1992) reported 23 infants under the age of 3 months with VSD and coarctation managed with coarctation repair alone. Nine needed no further surgical treatment, 6 required early closure of the VSD, and 8 required late repair of the VSD. Eight patients were treated after 3 months of age. Seven of these patients underwent coarctation repair alone and none required a second operation for VSD closure. If pulmonary artery banding is to be performed, some experts advocate banding before clamping the aorta to prevent increased shunting due to the increased left ventricular afterload; others contend that the timing of banding is not critical. Children with associated complex anomalies may improve sufficiently after coarctation repair to allow elective repair of the associated defects at a later date. One-stage repair of coarctation and associated anomalies via a median sternotomy may be the optimal procedure for patients with coarctation and associated complex anomalies.

COMPLICATIONS

Correction of coarctation may be complicated by hemorrhage, chylothorax, recurrent nerve paralysis, infection, and suture line thrombosis. It has been suggested that the patients with Turner's syndrome may be at increased risk for hemorrhage because of friable tissues (Brandt et al., 1984; Ravelo et al., 1980). Several unique problems may develop postoperatively. Paradoxical elevation of the blood pressure to greater than preoperative levels may occur. This two-phased phenomenon is characterized by a rise of a systolic blood pressure during the first 24 to 36 hours after operation and a later increase in the diastolic pressure. The first phase is characterized by activation of the sympathetic nervous system with elevation of serum catecholamines (Benedict et al., 1978). The late phase is characterized by elevation of plasma renin and angiotensin levels (Fox et al., 1980). Postoperative elevation of blood pressure has not been described in children having thoracotomy for repair of other cardiac lesions. Paradoxical hypertension may be associated with the post-coarctectomy syndrome of abdominal pain and distention first reported by Sealy in 1953 (Sealy et al., 1957). Up to 20% of patients having repair of coarctation of the aorta experience abdominal pain and distention postoperatively. Laparotomy is occasionally indicated and may reveal evidence of mesenteric ischemia. Bowel resection may be necessary in some cases (Downing et al., 1958). Arteriography shows changes in mesenteric vessels and pathologic examination reveals necrotizing mesenteric arteritis (Kawauchi et al., 1985). The syndrome is possibly related to elevated renin levels. Aggressive therapy of hypertension appears to prevent the full manifestation of the post-coarctectomy syndrome. Many drugs have controlled postoperative hypertension, and vasodilators such as sodium nitroprusside with beta blockade have also been useful (Will et al., 1978). Interestingly, a small series suggests that paradoxical hypertension may not occur after balloon angioplasty of the constructing lesion (Choy et al., 1987). This result may be related to less effective relief of the stenosis or lack of surgical manipulation of the aorta and periaortic neural fibers.

The most dreaded complication of coarctation repair is paraplegia, which occurs in 0.1 to 1% of patients. Poor collaterals, anomalous origin of the right subclavian artery, distal hypertension during aortic cross-clamping, reoperation, or hyperthermia may predispose to paraplegia during the procedure. Brewer and co-workers (1972) reviewed 66 cases of paraplegia after 12,532 procedures for repair of coarctation, an incidence of 0.41%. In this study, neither sacrifice of intercostals nor duration of aortic cross-clamping could be related to the occurrence of paraplegia. Brewer emphasized the marked variation in spinal cord blood supply and suggested that measurement of distal pressure after cross-clamping of the aorta be done to assess the adequacy of the collateral circulation. A survey of surgeons in the United Kingdom and Ireland revealed that paraplegia occurred in 16 patients out of 5492 operations (an incidence of 0.3%) (Keen, 1987). Hughes and Reemtsma (1971), based on results in two patients, suggested monitoring distal perfusion pressure with bypass if the pressure fell below 60 mm Hg. Others have recommended monitoring of the cerebrospinal fluid pressure with bypass and drainage of spinal fluid if necessary to maintain an adequate perfusion pressure of the spinal cord. The use of somatosensory evolved potentials to assess the adequacy of spinal cord perfusion has been extensively investigated (Krieger and Spencer, 1985; Laschinger et al., 1987a, 1987b; Pollock et al., 1986). Loss of somatosensory evoked potentials is a sensitive indicator of spinal cord ischemia. Maintenance of the distal aortic pressure during aortic cross-clamping above 60 mm Hg correlated with preservation of the somatosensory evoked potentials. Distal hypertension with the loss of somatosensory evoked potentials for more than 30 minutes was associated with a greater than 70% incidence of paraplegia (Cunningham et al., 1987). In patients other than neonates and small infants undergoing repair of coarctation, the distal aortic pressure should be measured and distal perfusion pressure maintained above 60 mm Hg with a shunt or bypass techniques as necessary.

### Nonsurgical Therapy

Percutaneous transluminal balloon angioplasty has been introduced as an alternative therapy for coarctation. Although initial results were encouraging, later reports described aneurysmal dilatation following balloon angioplasty of previously unoperated coarctations. Dilatation of recurrent stenosis had been more successful and there had been fewer reports of aneurysm formation, presumably secondary to surrounding scar tissue (Fig. 33–14). Morrow and colleagues (1988) reported successful angioplasty in 31 of 33 patients with native coarctation. Follow-up angiography in 10 patients showed no restenosis. However, aneurysmal dilatation was present in 2 patients. Rao and Chopra (1991) reported balloon angioplasty of native coarctation in 20 neonates and infants under the age of 1 year. The peak systolic gradient was reduced from 40 mm Hg to 11 mm Hg, and no patient required immediate surgical intervention. The residual gradient at a mean follow-up of 12 months was 18 ± 15 mm Hg. No patient developed an aneurysm. Recoarctation developed in 5 infants and was successfully treated by surgical resection in 2 and by repeat angioplasty in 3. Cystic medial necrosis has been described as a consistent histologic finding in patients with coarctation, suggesting that balloon-induced tears into an abnormal media may provide the substrate for aneurysm formation (Isner et al., 1987; Lindsay, 1988). The long-term results of balloon angioplasty for native coarctation in terms of recoarctation and especially aneurysm formation are unknown.

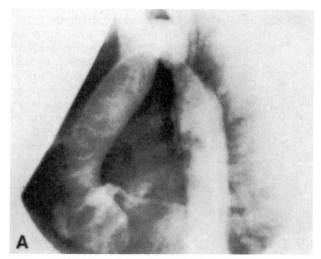

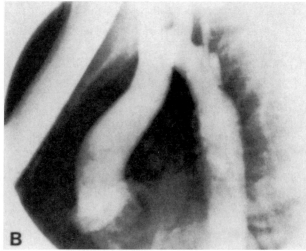

**FIGURE 33–14.** *A,* Aortogram showing recurrent stenosis after surgical correction of coarctation of the aorta. *B,* Aortogram after balloon angioplasty of the recoarctation. (*A* and *B,* Courtesy of Dr. Bennett Pearce.)

Rupture of the aorta has been reported during balloon dilatation of coarctation (Balaji, 1991b). The indications for balloon angioplasty for native coarctation are uncertain, and many centers still employ surgical therapy as the primary therapy. Angioplasty of postoperative recoarctation produces good results and may be associated with less mortality and morbidity than is reoperation. However, long-term follow-up is necessary (Saul et al., 1987).

## Results

The results of surgical correction depend on the anatomy of the defect, including the presence or absence of hypoplasia of the aortic arch, the age at repair, the type of repair used, and the presence of associated anomalies. Operative mortality in neonates with isolated coarctation has decreased to 5 to 10% and is lower in older children. Mortality is very low

in patients with isolated coarctations. The rate of recoarctation for resection with end-to-end anastomosis in infancy has been reported to be as high as 60%. A decreased incidence of recurrent coarctation has been reported with subclavian patch aortoplasty and the prosthetic patch graft repair, compared with historical series. However, the most recent series using resection and end-to-end anastomosis shows results even in neonates that compare favorably with other methods in terms of mortality and recoarctation.

Any comparison of techniques for repair of coarctation must consider the historical time frame (Ziemer et al., 1986). Advances in the care of critically ill infants, including the introduction of neonatal intensive care units and the use of prostaglandin infusions, have dramatically improved the preoperative condition of patients with coarctation, and these changes may affect mortality as much as the choice of repair. Advances in suture materials and vascular surgical technique also make it difficult to compare results from different time periods. Circumferential arterial suture lines have been effective in the arterial switch operation for transposition of the great vessels and other congenital cardiac anomalies, and therefore should be successful in coarctation repair. Since a prospective randomized trial of the various repair techniques has not been performed, long-term results with different techniques cannot be accurately compared.

Recent series of resection and primary anastomosis have shown excellent results, even in neonates. Cobanoglu and associates (1985) reported a 5-year reoperation-free rate of 92% in neonates with coarctation after resection and primary anastomosis. Korfer and coworkers (1985) reported 55 infants under 3 years of age who had resection with end-to-end anastomosis with a hospital mortality of 3.6%. At a mean follow-up of 5 years, only 3 showed evidence of significant restenosis. Lacour-Gayet and colleagues (1990) reported results in 66 consecutive neonates treated with extended resection and anastomosis with reconstruction of the aortic arch. The overall early mortality rate was 14% and freedom from reoperation was 89.5% at 5 years. Van Heurn and associates (1994), from the Hospital for Sick Children in London, reported 151 infants under the age of 3 months who underwent repair of coarctation between 1985 and 1990. Over 50% of these children had hypoplasia of a portion of the aortic arch. The subclavian flap angioplasty was used in 15 patients, resection with a traditional end-to-end anastomosis in 43, and an extended end-to-end anastomosis in 77. The actuarial freedom from recoarctation at 4 years was 57% after subclavian flap angioplasty, 83% after extended end-to-end anastomosis, and 96% after radically extended end-to-end anastomosis (proximal to the origin of the left carotid artery). These authors felt that extended end-to-end anastomosis could be successfully applied to almost all types of arch anomalies and that it produced the lowest incidence of recoarctation. There is evidence, however, that a hypoplastic arch can grow if the localized obstruction is relieved by either a simple resection and end-to-end anastomosis or a subclavian flap aortoplasty, so that an extended repair may not be necessary (Brouwer et al., 1992; Myers et al., 1992).

Equally good results have been reported for the subclavian flap angioplasty. Campbell and associates (1984) reported use of the subclavian flap repair in 53 patients under 1 year of age. The operative mortality was 4%, and follow-up revealed no pressure gradient greater than 20 mm Hg. Hamilton and co-workers (1978) reported 45 infants who underwent subclavian flap aortoplasty with an overall mortality of 24%. All deaths occurred in children who had associated anomalies and who underwent operation before 2 months of age. There was no evidence of residual or recurrent coarctation in the survivors. Sciolaro and colleagues (1991) reviewed 56 children under 4 years of age. Thirty-four had a subclavian flap angioplasty and 22 had resection with end-to-end anastomosis. Among the 23 infants under 3 months of age, the 6-year actuarial freedom from recoarctation was 93% in the subclavian flap group compared with 53% in the end-to-end group. These investigators therefore recommended the subclavian flap angioplasty in patients under 3 months of age.

However, there has been concern that the subclavian flap aortoplasty may not be the best method for repairing coarctation in very young infants. Cobanoglu and associates (1985) reported an increased incidence of early recoarctation in infants under 3 months of age after subclavian flap aortoplasty when compared with the resection of primary anastomosis. They propose that the cause of restenosis was inadequate resection of ductal tissue in the aortic wall with continued constriction and fibrosis. Sanchez and associates (1986) reported a 22% incidence of early recoarctation following subclavian flap angioplasty secondary to a posterior shelf in infants under 3 months of age. Restenosis was strongly correlated with younger age at the time of surgical correction and was thought to be secondary to persistent ductal tissue in the aortic wall. Trinquet and co-workers (1988) reported follow-up on 178 infants undergoing coarctation repair at less than 3 months of age; 63 infants had an isolated coarctation, 47 had associated VSDs, and 68 had other associated anomalies. Actuarial survival at 5 years was 90% for infants with isolated coarctation, 84% for those with associated VSDs, and 40% for those with complex anomalies. The rate of restenosis was the same for subclavian flap angioplasty, resection with primary anastomosis, and extended resection and anastomosis.

Further, there is concern about sacrifice of the major vascular supply to the left upper extremity. The subclavian artery is frequently divided to create systemic-to-pulmonary shunts, and adverse sequelae have been rare. There is evidence of decreased growth in the length and mass of the extremity, and rare reports have shown vascular insufficiency with gangrene of the arm (Geiss et al., 1980; Mellgren et al., 1987; Todd et al., 1983; Webb and Burford, 1952), especially if branches of the subclavian artery distal to the vertebral artery are ligated.

The prosthetic patch onlay graft technique has been used in patients of all ages for correction of coarctation of the aorta. Yee and associates (1984) reported the use of Gore-Tex patches, and emphasized the advantages of decreased operative time, decreased dissection, maximal augmentation of the area of stenosis, preservation of the collateral vessels, and no sacrifice of normal vascular structures. A thoracotomy incision has commonly been used for synthetic patch aortoplasty. Ungerleider and Ebert (1987) demonstrated the applicability of patch aortoplasty via a median sternotomy in selected infants who require simultaneous correction of coarctation and intracardiac defects. Sade and colleagues (1984) documented growth of the posterior wall of the aorta after patch aortoplasty. Patch aortoplasty is highly effective in relieving the aortic obstruction (Sade et al., 1979) and has a low incidence of restenosis and persistent hypertension (at rest and following exercise) (Smith et al., 1984). However, the use of prosthetic material may predispose to infection and there are increasingly frequent reports of formation of aneurysms and pseudoaneurysms (Aebert et al., 1993; Bergdahl and Ljungqvist, 1980; Mendelsohn et al., 1992). Aneurysmal dilatation of the posterior aortic wall opposite the prosthetic patch has been reported in up to 38% of patients (Clarkson et al., 1985), but the true incidence is unknown. An experimental study suggested that damage to the posterior wall during excision of the obstructing shelf may form an aneurysm (DeSanto et al., 1987). Microscopic examination of the aneurysm wall in patients with aneurysmal dilatation following patch aortoplasty demonstrated degeneration of the media (Hehrlein et al., 1986). Differences in the tensile strength between the prosthetic patch and the native aortic wall may also be a factor in the formation of true and false aneurysms. Aebert and associates (1993) reported significant dilatation of the operative site in 35% of patients following patch graft repair for coarctation of the aorta; reoperation was required in 19.5%. Mendelsohn and co-workers (1992) examined the ratio of the aortic diameter at the repair site to the aortic diameter at the diaphragm in 29 patients following patch repair of coarctation of the aorta. Patients with a ratio of greater than 1.5% progressed to aneurysmal dilatation within 3 to 5 years. All patients who have undergone synthetic patch aortoplasty must be carefully monitored to evaluate possible aneurysm formation (del Nido et al., 1986). Aortic aneurysms have also been reported following the subclavian aortoplasty repair for coarctation of the aorta (Berri et al., 1993; Martin et al., 1988).

Recoarctation usually manifests as persistent hypertension or an arm/leg pressure gradient. The arm/leg gradient should be measured in the immediate postoperative period to distinguish residual stenosis secondary to inadequate repair from true recoarctation. Causes of recoarctation include failure of growth of the anastomosis, inadequate resection of the narrowed segment, residual abnormal ductal tissue, and suture line thrombosis. Exercise testing with measurement of the arm/leg gradient can be performed to evaluate postoperative repair in patients (Connors, 1979). Some patients who are normotensive at rest without an arm/leg gradient develop severe hypertension with a measured gradient after exercise and may have a significant restenosis. It is important to measure the arm and leg pressure simultaneously to assess the gradient accurately. This can be done easily using Doppler pressure measurements at rest and immediately after exercise. In infants, the arm/leg gradient can be assessed before and after a noxious stimulus. The long-term consequences of exercise-induced hypertension after correction of coarctation are unknown, but this finding may adversely affect the prognosis (Freed et al., 1979; Leandro et al., 1992; Markel et al., 1986).

Reoperation is indicated if significant hypertension or other symptoms occur and a pressure gradient can be demonstrated (Foster, 1984). Reoperation is more difficult because of scarring and there is an increased morbidity and mortality. Lack of a collateral circulation may increase the incidence of paraplegia. In patients who have had previous resection and end-to-end anastomosis or subclavian flap aortoplasty, a prosthetic patch onlay graft is an appropriate method to repair recoarctation (Pollack et al., 1983). Sweeney and colleagues (1985) reported follow-up of 53 patients who required reoperation. Patch aortoplasty was used in 26 patients, bypass grafting was used in 16 patients, and interposition grafts were required in 8 patients; 3 patients underwent resection with end-to-end anastomosis. Temporary shunts and bypass techniques were not used. No operative deaths or neurologic complications occurred. Jacob and associates (1988) reported the use of ascending aorta-to-descending aorta bypass in 10 patients with recoarctation without mortality, paraplegia, or hypertension. They used a two-incision approach via a left thoracotomy and median sternotomy without cardiopulmonary bypass. Balloon angioplasty has become frequently used in patients with recoarctation and may be the optimal initial therapy for recoarctation (Kan et al., 1983).

Follow-up of surgical patients indicates that they are not rendered entirely normal (Simon and Zloto, 1974). Some patients who have had a technically excellent repair may not have complete resolution of hypertension (Nanton and Olley, 1976). The cause of persistent hypertension following repair is unclear but is related to the age at repair and the duration of preoperative hypertension. Maron and associates (1973), reporting long-term follow-up of 248 patients who had correction of aortic coarctation, found an increased incidence of premature death, usually secondary to cardiovascular disease, and related this to the duration of preoperative hypertension. Evidence shows increased coronary atherosclerosis in patients with coarctation (Cokkinos et al., 1979). Koller and co-workers (1987) found that patients operated on between the ages of 2 and 4 years had a lower risk of persistent hypertension. Cohen and colleagues (1989) at the Mayo Clinic reported long-term follow-up on 571 patients following repair of coarctation. Age at

the time of surgery was the most important predictor of survival. If the repair was performed before 14 years of age, survival to 20 years was 91%, but if the repair was performed after 14 years of age, 20-year survival was 79%. The best survivorship was for patients repaired before the age of 9 years. Age at the time of repair was also the most important predictor of persistent hypertension. Coronary artery disease was the most common cause of late death.

There is evidence of abnormal left ventricular function despite relief of the obstruction (Carpenter et al., 1985). Kimball and associates (1986a) showed a persistent increase in ventricular contractility after successful coarctation repair. This may result from cardiac ultrastructural changes due to congenital pressure overload. These authors have also documented abnormal thallium scans after successful coarctation repair, suggesting persistent changes in the coronary arteries (Kimball et al., 1986b). Gardiner and associates (1993) have documented abnormal endothelial response to nitroglycerin in normotensive patients following successful coarctation repair, suggesting that damage occurs early in vessels proximal to the coarctation and may persist even after successful repair in the neonatal period. The relationship of abnormal endothelial function to persistent hypertension and coronary artery disease is unknown. Aortic stenosis and regurgitation secondary to a bicuspid aortic valve may develop and require valve replacement. As has been emphasized, the long-term prognosis of many patients is determined primarily by the associated anomalies.

## INTERRUPTION OF THE AORTIC ARCH

Complete absence of a segment of the aortic arch without any anatomic connection between the proximal and the distal segments is termed *interruption of the aortic arch* (IAA). IAA at the aortic isthmus was first described by Steidele (1778). Seidel (1818) reported absence of the segment between the left subclavian and the left common carotids. IAA between the left common carotid and the innominate arteries was first reported by Weisman and Kesten (1948). Samson and co-workers reported the first successful correction of IAA in 1955 (Merrill et al., 1957). Sirak and colleagues (1968) were the first to successfully correct an IAA in a neonate. Barratt-Boyes and associates (1972) reported the first simultaneous correction of IAA and all associated anomalies. In 1976, the introduction of prostaglandin therapy to maintain ductal patency allowed preoperative stabilization of infants with IAA, and greatly improved surgical results.

### Incidence, Pathologic Anatomy, and Natural History

IAA is a rare anomaly constituting less than 1.5% of congenital heart disease. IAA may be an isolated

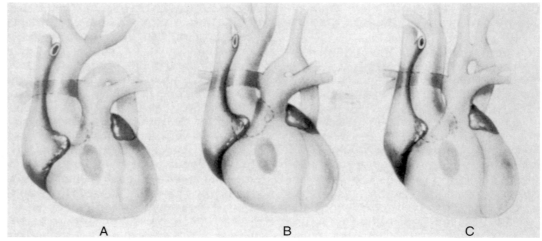

**FIGURE 33–15.** Three types of interrupted arch. *Type A* is between the left subclavian artery and the descending aorta; *Type B* is between the left carotid and the left subclavian arteries; and *Type C* is between the innominate and the left carotid arteries. Incidence is 43% for Type A; 53% for Type B; and 4% for Type C. (*A–C*, From Turley, K., Yee, E. S., and Ebert, P. A.: The total repair of interrupted arch complex in infants: The anterior approach. Circulation, *70*[Suppl. I]:I-16, 1984.)

defect but is usually associated with other anomalies. Celoria and Patton (1959) classified IAA based on the absent segment (Fig. 33–15). In IAA Type A, the interruption occurs only to the left subclavian artery. In IAA Type B, the interruption occurs between the left subclavian and the left common carotid arteries. With IAA Type C, the interruption occurs between the left common carotid artery and the innominate artery. These classifications may be further subdivided by the presence or absence of anomalous origin of the right subclavian artery from the distal aorta, and are designated A1, B1, and C1 if an anomalous origin is present. In a review of 165 cases of IAA, Van Praagh and co-workers (1971) found that 43% were Type A, 53% were Type B, and 4% were Type C.

The cause of IAA is unclear. As with coarctation, there is an association with defects that decrease ascending aortic flow and increase ductal flow, which suggests that abnormal fetal blood patterns are a causative factor. IAA Type B is frequently found in association with DiGeorge's syndrome (absence of the third and fourth pharyngeal pouches) (Van Mierop and Kutsche, 1986). In DiGeorge's syndrome, the thymus and parathyroid glands are absent and the patients are hypocalcemic and suffer from defects in cellular immunity. Defects in the development of the neural crest may be responsible for DiGeorge's syndrome and IAA Type B. Genetic factors may also be important and familial occurrence of IAA has been reported (Gobel et al., 1993). Everts-Suarez and Carson (1959) noted the frequent association of IAA, PDA, and VSD. IAA may be associated with a wide variety of cardiac anomalies and is often found coexistent with truncus arteriosus or aortopulmonary window.

The prognosis of uncorrected IAA is poor. The mean age at death has been reported to be 4 to 10 days (Moulton and Bowman, 1981). Ninety per cent of infants with IAA die in the first year of life without operation.

## Diagnosis

Most infants with IAA present with CHF secondary to left-to-right shunting through a VSD and increased left ventricular afterload. Lower body perfusion is maintained by right-to-left shunting through a PDA. When the ductus closes, perfusion of the lower body essentially ceases and the infants become anuric and severely acidotic and the femoral pulses become nonpalpable. The CHF and acidosis resist medical therapy, and death occurs within a few days. PGE$_1$ therapy, however, has made it possible to maintain ductal patency and improve lower body perfusion, reverse the acidosis, and increase urinary output (Zahka et al., 1980). The physical examination is not specific for IAA and there are no characteristic murmurs. The ECG is not useful, although the chest film reveals an enlarged heart with pulmonary congestion. Cardiac catheterization with angiography has been the gold standard for diagnosis. Contrast injection was performed in both the proximal and the distal segments to define the anatomy. However, in critically ill neonates, echocardiography can be used to make the diagnosis, so that catheterization is not required. In infants with IAA Type B, there is a high incidence of DiGeorge's syndrome and great care must be taken to avoid hypocalcemia. Because of possible immunologic defects, these patients should receive irradiated blood products to prevent the development of graft versus host disease.

## Management and Results

Various procedures have been used to either palliate or correct IAA. The ultimate goal is to restore aortic continuity and correct associated anomalies. Aortic continuity may be restored by direct anastomosis of the aortic segments or by end-to-side anastomosis of an arch vessel to either the proximal or the distal segment, or through use of an interposition graft.

Palliative procedures are usually performed using a left thoracotomy, and aortic continuity is restored by using one of the arch vessels as a conduit. In IAA Type A, a Blalock-Park anastomosis can be used. In IAA Type B, the left common carotid is anastomosed to the distal segment, or a reversed Blalock-Park anastomosis may be created. In IAA Type C, the left common carotid may be anastomosed to the ascending aorta. Use of ductal tissue in the anastomosis should be avoided because obstruction may occur if the tissue contracts and fibroses. Alternatively, a prosthetic graft may be interposed to restore continuity. Simultaneous correction of intracardiac anomalies is not possible through a left thoracotomy. However, pulmonary artery banding can be performed if indicated. Repair of a VSD and other anomalies may be performed at a later date through a median sternotomy.

Norwood and colleagues (1983) reported improved survival after primary correction of IAA. A prosthetic graft is used to restore aortic continuity and the distal anastomosis is performed via a left thoracotomy after ductal division. A median sternotomy is then performed and the proximal anastomosis completed. Cardiopulmonary bypass is instituted for closure of VSD. Ten of 13 patients survived repair with good results despite the eventual development of subaortic stenosis in several patients. Turley and associates (1984) reported total correction via an anterior approach (Fig. 33–16). Cardiopulmonary bypass with cannulation of the ascending aorta and of the descending aorta through the ductus was instituted with profound hypothermia and circulatory arrest during the arch repair. The ductus is divided, the aorta is mobilized to the diaphragm, and aortic continuity is restored by direct anastomosis of the proximal and distal aortic segments. The VSD is repaired through a right ventriculotomy. Early mortality was 20%, com-

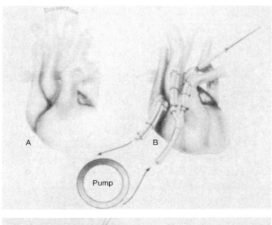
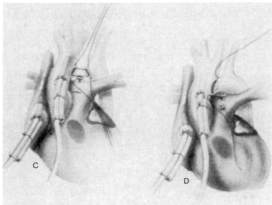
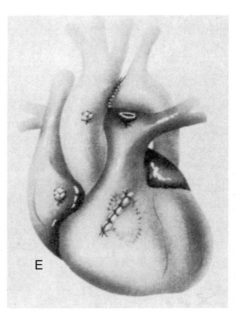

FIGURE 33–16. *A,* Dissection. The arch vessels are dissected to the thoracic outlet laterally, the carotid bifurcations superiorly, and the descending aorta inferiorly with the use of electrocautery to the diaphragm. This dissection maximizes anteroposterior displacement of both vessels, minimizing anastomotic tension not possible when mobilization of the descending aorta alone from the lateral approach is used. *B,* Single atrial-to-biaortic cannulation. Ascending aortic and transductal descending aortic cannulation is used, and a tourniquet is used to isolate the pulmonary circulation, preventing flooding of the lungs during bypass and affording continued total perfusion of the entire body until deep hypothermia is achieved. *C* and *D,* Removal of the descending aortic cannula after total circulatory arrest affords a bloodless field for precise repair and maximal anastomotic size when the descending aorta is anastomosed to the posterior aspect of the ascending aorta. The pulmonary arteriotomy and ductus are simultaneously repaired. *E,* During rewarming with single atrial-to-ascending aortic cannulation the aortic anastomosis can be assessed, and through a right ventriculotomy (outflow tract), the ventricular septal defect is repaired. (*A–E,* From Turley, K., Yee, E. S., and Ebert, P. A.: The total repair of interrupted arch complex in infants: The anterior approach. Circulation, *70*[Suppl. I]:I-16, 1984.)

pared with 33 to 44% for a staged procedure at the same institution.

Sell and co-workers (1988) reported 71 patients seen with IAA between 1974 and 1987. In the early years, an interposition graft repair was performed, but more recently, direct anastomosis with closure of the VSD has been performed. Actuarial survival at 10 years was 47% and mortality declined with increasing experience. Recurrent arch obstruction was managed with reoperation or balloon angioplasty. Karl and colleagues (1992) reported repair of IAA or coarctation plus hypoplastic arch in 55 infants via a median sternotomy. The operative mortality for arch repair plus biventricular intracardiac repair was 9%. Mortality for arch repair plus palliative repair was 40%, suggesting that primary repair of IAA and associated anomalies should be undertaken even when complex intracardiac anomalies are present. Improved results with primary complete repair have also been reported by others (Menahem et al., 1992; Scott et al., 1988; Vouhe et al., 1990).

Subaortic stenosis has been reported after successful repair of IAA and may necessitate further surgical intervention. Bove and colleagues (1993) reported correction of severe subaortic stenosis, VSDs, and aortic arch obstruction in seven neonates. Patients underwent direct anastomosis for repair of the arch obstruction, and the subaortic stenosis was relieved via a transatrial resection of the infundibular septum with closure of the VSD. All patients survived the operation, one late death occurred, and no patient had significant residual subaortic stenosis.

Some authors, however, continue to advocate a staged repair for IAA and VSD. Irwin and associates (1991) reported correction of staged repair of IAA and VSD in 20 infants. Initially, a left thoracotomy was performed to restore arch continuity using a Gore-Tex graft, and a pulmonary artery banding was performed. Within 2 to 3 months, the pulmonary artery band was removed and the VSD closed. Only 1 infant subsequently developed aortic arch obstruction and required replacement of the conduit.

IAA remains a difficult surgical problem. Advances in surgical techniques in neonatal intensive care and in the use of $PGE_1$ therapy have greatly improved survival. After stabilization, these critically ill infants should undergo total correction of the IAA and associated anomalies via a median sternotomy.

## AORTOPULMONARY WINDOW

*Aortopulmonary window* (APW) is a rare congenital defect resulting from abnormal septation of the truncus arteriosus into the aorta and the pulmonary artery. An APW is found in 0.2% of patients with congenital heart disease. Various terms have been applied to this defect, including aorticopulmonary fistula, aortic septal defect, aorticopulmonary septal defect, and aorticopulmonary fenestration. APW was first described by Elliotson in 1830, and Cotton reported the

first case in the United States in 1899. Abbott's classic review (1936) of 1000 cases of congenital heart disease included only 10 cases of APW. In 1948, Gross successfully ligated an APW in a patient undergoing thoracotomy for the mistaken diagnosis of PDA (Gross, 1952). Gasul and co-workers (1951) diagnosed APW using retrograde aortography. Scott and Sabiston (1953) described a closed method for division of an APW in 1953. In 1957, Cooley and colleagues reported the first successful division of an APW using cardiopulmonary bypass. Putnam and Gross (1966) suggested a transpulmonary approach for closure of APW. In 1967 and 1968, Negre in France, Burks in Germany, and Aberg in Sweden and their colleagues independently repaired APW using an anterior sandwich patch closure (Johansson et al., 1978; Negre, 1979; Negre et al., 1968; Preusse, 1988; Ravikumar et al., 1988). Wright and associates (1968) reported direct suture closure of an APW via a transaortic approach, and in 1969, Deverall and associates recommended patch closure of the defect using this approach.

A closely related defect is anomalous origin of either pulmonary artery from the aorta (Fong et al., 1989). Aortic origin of the right pulmonary artery was first reported by Fraentzel in 1868 (Fontana et al., 1987). Caro and co-workers (1957) first attempted surgical correction using an interposition graft, but the patient died shortly after the operation. Armer and colleagues (1961) reported the first successful correction using an interposition graft. Kirkpatrick and associates (1967) reported successful direct anastomosis of the right pulmonary artery to the main pulmonary artery. Aortic origin of the left pulmonary artery from the aorta occurs less commonly. Herbert and co-workers (1973) reported the first successful correction of this anomaly.

## Embryology and Pathologic Anatomy

In the truncus arteriosus, two opposing truncal cushions form on the right superior and left inferior walls and fuse to create the proximal portion of the septum between the aortic and the pulmonary chambers (Van Mierop and Kutsche, 1990). Distally, the fourth aortic arch is aligned with the aortic channel and the sixth aortic arch is aligned with the pulmonary channel. The distal aortopulmonary septum that fuses with the proximal truncal cushions is formed by the wall between the origins of the fourth and sixth aortic arches (Van Mierop and Kustche, 1990). Failure to fuse or malalignment of the truncal divisions may produce a proximal defect in the aortopulmonary septum. Abnormal migration of the sixth aortic arches may create a distal defect. The aortic and pulmonary valves are normally formed, unlike those in persistent truncus arteriosus. Unlike persistent truncus arteriosus and Type B IAA, APW is not associated with DiGeorge's syndrome.

An APW is usually a single large defect beginning a few millimeters above the aortic valve on the left lateral wall of the aorta (Fig. 33–17). Multiple defects have rarely been reported. Defects may occasionally be found more distally overlying the origin of the right pulmonary artery, and rarely, absence of the entire aortopulmonary septum may be encountered. As the term *window* implies, there is usually minimal length to the defect, but occasionally, a structure similar to a ductus is present. Origin of the right coronary artery (Luisi et al., 1980) and, rarely, the left coronary artery (Agius et al., 1970) from the pulmonary artery can complicate surgical correction. APW is usually an isolated lesion, although associated anomalies, including PDA, Type A IAA, VSD, and tetralogy of Fallot, may be found in up to 50% of patients. Aortic origin of a pulmonary artery may be seen in association with tetralogy of Fallot.

An APW allows a large left-to-right shunt that causes pulmonary hypertension and CHF. As with a nonrestrictive VSD, irreversible pulmonary vascular disease may occur at an early age. In patients with aortic origin of the right pulmonary artery, pulmonary hypertension is also present in the left pulmonary artery. The cause of this contralateral pulmonary hypertension is uncertain, and a reflex mechanism has been postulated.

Because APW and aortic origin of a pulmonary artery are rare defects, the natural history is not well defined. Patients with a large APW usually do not survive infancy. Irreversible pulmonary vascular disease may occur at an early age. Children or young adults with an APW are encountered occasionally and have usually developed significant pulmonary vascular disease. The clinical course is likely to be similar to that of untreated patients with a large VSD.

## Diagnosis

Infants with APW usually present with CHF, growth retardation, and recurrent pulmonary infections early in life (Blieden and Moller, 1974). Physical examination reveals a systolic murmur and occasionally a continuous murmur, which suggests the presence of a PDA. The chest film shows cardiomegaly with pulmonary vascular engorgement or CHF. APW must be distinguished from PDA, persistent truncus arteriosus, VSD with aortic regurgitation, and ruptured aneurysm of the sinus of Valsalva. Two-dimensional echocardiography can be used to show the defect. Cardiac catheterization reveals an oxygen saturation step-up at the level of the pulmonary artery and the course of the catheter may suggest the diagnosis. Retrograde aortography provides accurate visualization of the defect. It is necessary to document the presence of normal aortic and pulmonic valves to confirm the diagnosis. The location of the coronary ostium must be carefully demonstrated before surgical intervention. In general, cardiac catheterization and angiography are the optimal methods for diagnosing APW. However, two-dimensional echocardiography has become even more important in diagnosing this defect (Balaji et al., 1991a; Rice et al., 1982). Echocardiography can provide excellent visualization of an APW, although a high index of suspicion is required especially in patients with associated anomalies. In a recent series, five of six patients with an isolated APW were correctly diagnosed (Balaji et al., 1991a), but the correct diagnosis was established at the first examination in only three of eight patients with associated anomalies. A retrospective review,

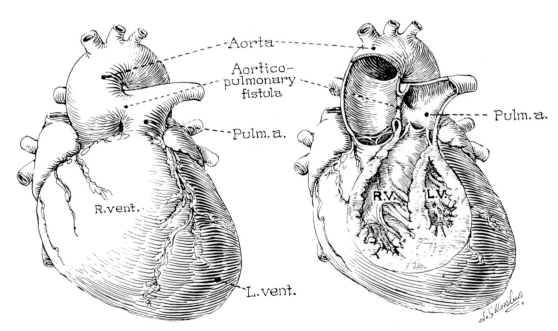

**FIGURE 33–17.** Aortopulmonary window. The size of the fistula and its relation to the semilunar valves vary. (From Scott, H. W., Jr., and Sabiston, D. C., Jr.: Surgical treatment for congenital aorticopulmonary fistula. J Thorac Surg, 25:26, 1953.)

however, revealed that the APW actually had been imaged in five of the six patients but had been incorrectly diagnosed.

## Method of Surgical Correction

The presence of an APW is sufficient indication for repair unless severe pulmonary vascular disease has occurred. In general, repair is undertaken at the time of diagnosis. However, in asymptomatic patients with small defects, elective operation may be performed after infancy. Various techniques have been suggested. Simple ligation should not be performed because of the risk of hemorrhage from the friable tissues. Division with primary closure may cause narrowing of the aorta or pulmonary artery. Transpulmonary patch closure of the defect is not recommended because it is difficult to visualize the coronary ostia. The preferred method for repair is either transaortic closure by direct suture or patch closure or division of the APW, with patch closure of both the aorta and the pulmonary artery to prevent narrowing. The operation is performed via a median sternotomy using either cardiopulmonary bypass or hypothermic circulatory arrest. If transaortic closure is planned, a longitudinal aortotomy at the level of the window is performed and the anatomy is carefully defined. Particular attention must be given to the location of the coronary ostia and the origin of the right pulmonary artery. Small defects may be closed by direct suture. Larger defects should be closed with a prosthetic patch. Care must be taken to place the patch so the coronary ostia are on the aortic side. If the defect involves the origin of the right pulmonary artery, a teardrop-shaped patch extending along the right pulmonary artery may be used to repair the defect. Several authors have described repair by opening the anterior aspect of the APW, suturing a patch to the posterior wall, and continuing the suture to close the incision, incorporating the patch with suture line.

Repair may also be undertaken by division of the APW with patch closure of the aorta and pulmonary artery with either prosthetic material or a homograft. After aortic cross-clamping, the APW is opened anteriorly and the coronary ostia and right pulmonary artery are visualized. The APW is then divided posteriorly, including the coronary ostia with the aorta and the right pulmonary artery with the main pulmonary artery. The aorta and pulmonary artery defects are then closed with patches to prevent the stenosis. Aortic origin of the right pulmonary artery is best repaired by division of the right pulmonary artery and direct anastomosis to the main pulmonary artery. The optimal management of associated anomalies is uncertain and must be individualized, although usually total correction is undertaken (Fong et al., 1989). The postoperative course is generally routine following closure of an APW, although severe pulmonary hypertension may develop. These episodes are characterized by increased pulmonary arterial pressure, hypoxia, hypotension, and worsening peripheral perfusion (Ravikumar et al., 1988) and can be managed by sedation, paralysis, and hyperventilation with 100% oxygen.

## Mortality

The operative mortality is low for repair of isolated APW or aortic origin of a pulmonary artery in infancy. The long-term results are good if there are no associated anomalies. In older infants and children, the results depend on the severity and reversibility of the pulmonary vascular disease.

## ANOMALIES OF THE AORTIC ARCH

At length, by mere accident I discovered an extraordinary lusus naturae in the disposition of the right subclavian artery.
**David Bayford**

Vascular rings are developmental anomalies of the aorta and great vessels that form a circle and may constrict the esophagus and trachea. In 1735, Hunauld reported the necropsy finding of anomalous origin of the right subclavian artery for the descending aorta (Shannon, 1961). Persistent double aortic arch was described in 1737 by Hommel (Blake and Manion, 1962). In a case report read before the Medical Society of London in 1787 and published in 1794, Bayford presented the case history and autopsy findings of a 62-year-old woman who died of starvation secondary to severe dysphagia. Anomalous origin of the right subclavian artery from the descending aorta was present, and Bayford attributed the dysphasia to this anomaly even though the artery coursed between the trachea and the esophagus rather than posterior to the esophagus. He called the finding a *lusus naturae* or "prank of nature," and coined the term *dysphasia lusoria*. Throughout the 19th century, aortic arch anomalies remained anatomic curiosities. Congdon (1922) greatly clarified the embryology of the aortic arches. In 1936, Kommerell described the origin of the right subclavian artery from a diverticulum of the descending aorta (Shannon, 1961). The clinical syndrome of stridor and dysphagia in early infancy secondary to persistent double aortic arch was clearly delineated by Wolman (1939). Surgical correction of constricting vascular rings was not performed until 1945, when Gross successfully divided a double aortic arch and aberrant right subclavian artery (Gross, 1945b, 1946). Neuhauser (1946) later pioneered the use of the barium esophagogram for diagnosis of vascular rings (Gross and Neuhauser, 1951). Edwards (1948) presented the concept of a hypothetical double arch to allow classification of the multiple possible arch anomalies (Figs. 33–18 and 33–19).

## Embryology and Pathologic Anatomy

In the embryo, six pairs of aortic arches arise sequentially from the truncus arteriosus and join paired proximal right and left sixth aortic arches. The distal left sixth arch develops into the ductus arteriosus, whereas the distal right sixth arch regresses. Failure of a segment to regress normally may cause a constricting ring.

Various anomalies occur and may be easily visualized using the hypothetical scheme of Edwards, which consists of an ascending aorta, right and left aortic arches, a descending aorta on either the right

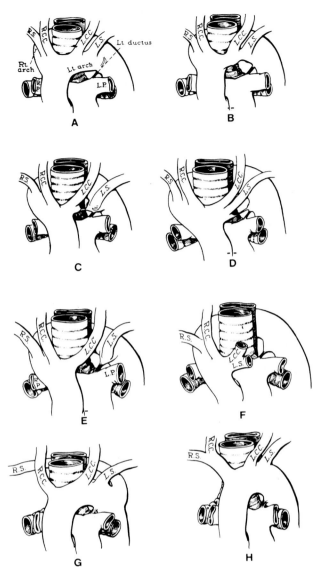

**FIGURE 33–18.** Aortic arch anomalies (left descending aorta and ligamentum arteriosum). *A,* Double aortic arch with equal anterior and posterior arches. *B,* Double aortic arch with smaller anterior (left) arch. *C,* Double aortic arch with atresia of anterior arch between the carotid and the subclavian arteries. *D,* Double aortic arch with atresia of anterior arch distal to subclavian artery. *E,* Right aortic arch with retroesophageal segment and anomalous origin of the left subclavian artery from Kommerell's diverticulum. *F,* Right aortic arch with retroesophageal segment and mirror image branching. (Note the ligamentum arteriosum inserting onto diverticulum of the descending aorta.) *G,* Left aortic arch with anomalous origin of the right subclavian artery. *H,* Normal pattern. (*A–H,* From Edwards, J. E.: Anomalies of the derivatives of the aortic arch system. Med. Clin. North Am., July 1948, p. 925.)

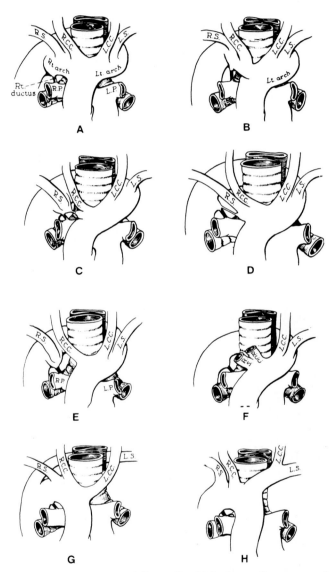

**FIGURE 33–19.** Aortic arch anomalies (right descending aorta and ligamentum arteriosum). *A,* Double aortic arch with equal anterior and posterior arches. *B,* Double aortic arch with smaller anterior (right) arch. *C,* Double aortic arch with atresia of anterior arch between carotid and subclavian arteries. *D,* Double aortic arch with atresia of anterior arch distal to subclavian artery. *E,* Left aortic arch with retroesophageal segment and anomalous origin of right subclavian artery from Kommerell's diverticulum. *F,* Left aortic arch with retroesophageal segment. (Note the insertion of the ligamentum arteriosum onto the diverticulum of the descending aorta.) *G,* Right aortic arch with mirror image branching. *H,* Normal pattern. (*A–H,* From Edwards, J. E.: Anomalies of the derivatives of the aortic arch system. Med. Clin. North Am., July 1948, p. 925.)

dorsal aortas. Persistence or regression of various segments of these arches creates the normal pattern of the aorta and pulmonary artery and great vessels. In normal development, the third pair of arches form parts of the common carotid arteries. The left fourth arch forms the adult aortic arch and the proximal portion of the right fourth arch persists as the innominate artery. The pulmonary arteries develop from the or the left, and bilateral ductus arteriosi. Theoretically, involution of the ring at any one point allows 36 possible configurations, although not all have been reported in humans (Blake and Manion, 1962). Involution at two or more points would produce even more possibilities. Some of the possible configurations are shown in Figures 33–18 and 33–19. Associated cardiac defects, frequently the tetralogy of Fallot, may occur especially in patients with a persistent right aortic arch.

## Clinical Manifestations and Natural History

The natural history of vascular rings is obscured by the wide spectrum of anomalies and the range of symptoms. Vascular rings should be suspected in any infant with stridor, dysphagia, recurrent respiratory tract infections, difficulty in feeding, or failure to thrive. Vascular rings are not necessarily inconsistent with prolonged survival, and many patients are totally asymptomatic. Anomalies that become symptomatic are usually diagnosed by 6 months of age, although some adults present when atherosclerosis causes dilatation of the aorta and increasing constriction. Children with mild symptoms may show marked improvement as they grow (Godtfredsen et al., 1977). Afflicted infants most commonly present with respiratory difficulties; the breathing is stridorous and may be exacerbated by feeding. Hyperexten-

sion of the neck reduces the constriction, and marked respiratory difficulties may occur if the neck is flexed. The physical examination is usually nonrevealing, although signs of associated cardiovascular anomalies may be found.

The plain chest film may be normal, may show pneumonia, or may occasionally show compression of the air-filled trachea. A right aortic arch is seen in some anomalies. The barium esophagogram is a particularly valuable study and is the most useful screening test (Lillehei and Colan, 1992). The combination of posterior compression of the esophagus on barium swallow and anterior tracheal compression is almost pathognomonic for a vascular ring. Angiocardiography accurately delineates the anatomy of vascular rings and allows evaluation of associated anomalies; however, some atretic segments may not be visualized with angiocardiography. Although most rings can be divided without preoperative catheterization, some centers routinely perform catheterization to avoid misdiagnosis. Other diagnostic modalities have become increasingly useful, especially echocardiography and MRI (Azarow et al., 1992; Lillehei and Colan, 1992). Bronchoscopy is indicated in some patients, especially those with suspected anomalous origin of the innominate artery.

## Management

Although a few patients with constricting vascular rings improve with growth, the long-term prognosis

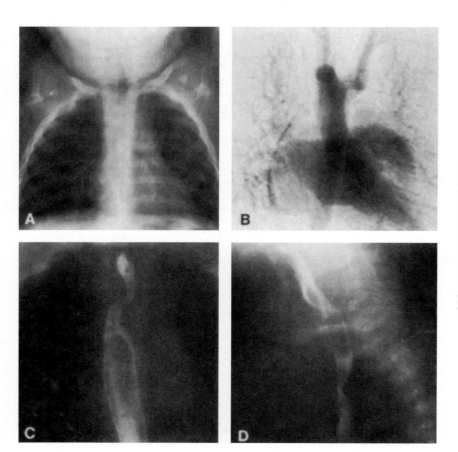

FIGURE 33–20. Infant with double aortic arch. *A,* Plain chest film. (Note the increased width of mediastinal soft tissue to the right of the trachea.) *B,* Digital subtraction angiogram showing double aortic arch. (Note the larger right arch to the right and posterior to trachea.) *C,* Barium esophagogram (AP) showing double indentation characteristic of double aortic arch. (Note the higher, deeper indentation on the right caused by the larger right posterior arch.) *D,* Barium esophagogram (lateral) showing posterior indentation of the esophagus. (*A–D,* Courtesy of Dr. Eric Effman.)

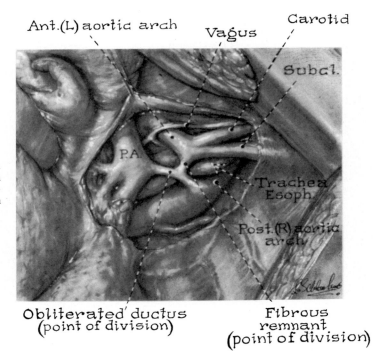

Ant.(L) aortic arch    Vagus    Carotid
Subcl.
P.A.
Trachea
Esoph
Post.(R) aortic arch
Obliterated ductus (point of division)    Fibrous remnant (point of division)

**FIGURE 33–21.** Operative view of tracheal ring completed by obliterated remnant of distal left arch and ligamentum arteriosum. After complete exposure of the vascular components, the proper point of division of the ligaments can easily be determined.

of medical therapy is poor in most symptomatic patients. Despite the wide spectrum of anomalies, the principles of surgical therapy are simple (Arciniegas et al., 1979; Backer et al., 1989; Binet and Langlois, 1977). Surgical intervention should be undertaken at the time of diagnosis and is designed to divide the vascular ring, relieve the constriction, and preserve circulation to the aortic arches. Adequate exposure is absolutely necessary. Gross and Neuhauser (1951) stated that all vascular rings could safely be divided through a left thoracotomy; however, a few anomalies require approach via a right-sided thoracotomy (McFaul et al., 1981).

## Double Aortic Arch

The most common anomaly that causes a true vascular ring is a persistence of the right and left fourth aortic arches, forming a double aortic arch. The right posterior arch is usually larger and there is a left ascending aorta and a left ductus arteriosus (see Fig. 33–18B). But, occasionally, the arches are of equal size or the anterior left arch is larger (see Fig. 33–18A). Rarely, a right descending aorta is encountered, in which case, the right arch is anterior (see Fig. 33–19A). Partial atresia of an arch may be noted usually in the smaller anterior arch (see Fig. 33–18C and D). The right carotid and right subclavian arteries arise from the right arch, and the left carotid and subclavian arteries arise from the left arch. Patients with double aortic arch usually present early in infancy and are severely symptomatic. The diagnosis of a double aortic arch can be easily made from the barium esophagogram (Fig. 33–20). In the common situation, the

anteroposterior projection shows right- and left-sided indentation of the barium-filled esophagus, with the right indentation being higher and larger. The lateral projection shows posterior esophageal compression from the retroesophageal posterior arch. Arteriography may also help diagnose the condition, although it will not show atretic segments (Fig. 33–20). Surgical division is indicated at the time of diagnosis.

Commonly, a left thoracotomy is performed and the small anterior arch divided and oversewn at its junction with the descending aorta so that the left carotid and subclavian arteries arise from the ascending aorta (Fig. 33–21). If an atretic segment is present, the double aortic arch is divided at that point. The ligamentum arteriosum is also divided and the constricting vessels are dissected away from the trachea and esophagus. If necessary, the divided left arch may be suspended from the posterior surface of the sternum to further relieve the constriction (Fig. 33–22). If atresia of the posterior (right) arch is present, a right-sided thoracotomy will provide optimal exposure.

## Left Aortic Arch with Anomalous Right Subclavian Artery

Aberrant origin of the right subclavian artery is a common anomaly, but it rarely causes symptoms (see Fig. 33–18G). This defect results from regression of the right fourth aortic arch between the carotid and the subclavian arteries rather than distal to the subclavian. The artery may appear to arise from a diverticulum of the descending aorta (Kommerell's diverticulum) that is actually a remnant of the distal right

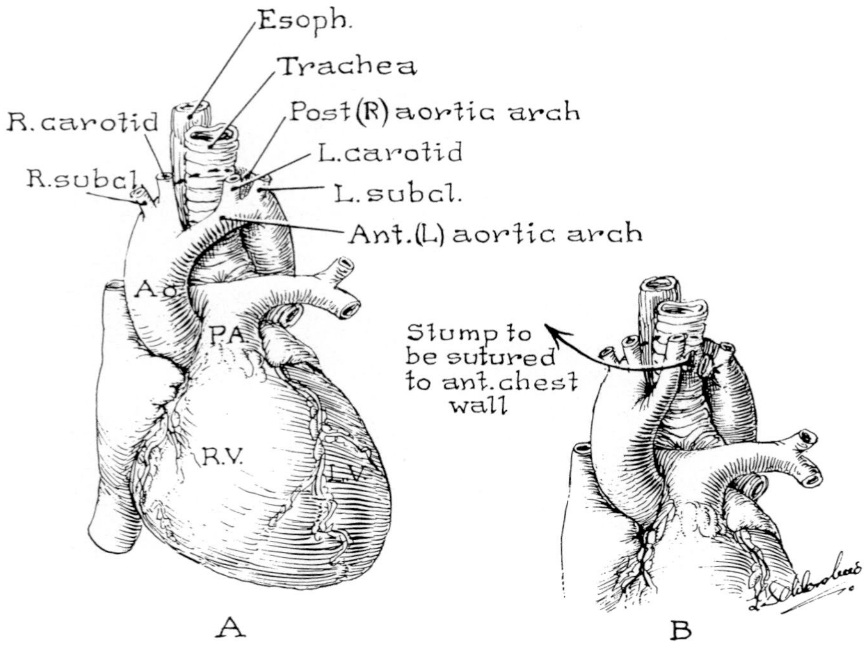


**FIGURE 33–22.** Double aortic arch. *A,* The larger channel is usually posterior and on the right. Branches of the arch arise independently. In almost all cases, the descending thoracic aortic arch is on the left as shown. *B,* Point of division of the smaller arch is selected to preserve circulation to the branches. The left common carotid artery is then tacked to the anterior chest wall to further relieve tracheal compression.

fourth arch (Shannon, 1961). The anomalous artery most often courses posterior to the esophagus, but may pass between the trachea and the esophagus or anterior to the trachea. Anomalous origin of the right subclavian artery is not a true vascular ring encircling the trachea and esophagus. However, the aberrant artery or occasionally the diverticulum may compress the esophagus, causing dysphagia lusoria. If a right ligamentum arteriosum is present connecting the right subclavian to the right pulmonary artery, a true vascular ring is formed. Aneurysmal dilatation of Kommerell's diverticulum was first reported by McCallen and Schaff in 1956. The diagnosis of aberrant origin of the right subclavian artery can be made by barium swallow. The lateral esophagogram shows an oblique posterior impression coursing upward from left to right, as well as arterial pulsations. This anomaly may be an incidental finding for other indications at the time of barium swallow.

Gross (1946) pioneered surgical therapy for anomalous origin of the right subclavian artery. In children, the artery may simply be ligated and divided without sequelae. A subclavian steal syndrome may result after simple division in adults, so reanastomosis to the aorta may be necessary. An aneurysmal aortic diverticulum may require excision with grafting of the subclavian artery (Austin and Wolfe, 1985; Esposito et al., 1988).

## Left Aortic Arch with Right Descending Aorta

Left aortic arch with a retroesophageal segment and a right descending aorta is a rare arch anomaly first reported by Paul (1948) (see Fig. 33–19*E*). The right subclavian artery arises from the descending aorta and the ring is completed by a right ligamentum arteriosum. Most of the patients reported with this anomaly have had few symptoms (de Balsac, 1960). However, a short ligamentum may create a symptomatic constricting ring. The diagnosis is suggested by plain chest film and confirmed by barium swallow or aortography. Surgical therapy divides the right-sided ligamentum arteriosus through a right-sided thoracotomy.

## Anomalous Origin of the Innominate Artery

Compression of the anterior trachea by an innominate artery that originates farther to the left on the aortic arch was first described by Gross and Neuhauser (1948) (Fig. 33–23). Fearon and Shortreed (1963) described 69 patients with compression of the aorta by an anomalous innominate artery. They emphasized the importance of endoscopy as a diagnostic modality and described reflex apnea with respiratory arrest followed by stimulation of the compressed area of the trachea. Mustard and colleagues (1969) reported 285 cases of innominate artery compression. Less than 14% of the patients required surgical intervention, and reflex apnea was a major indication for surgery.

Children with anomalous origin of the innominate artery present with respiratory distress, stridor, and occasionally respiratory arrest. Dysphagia does not occur because the esophagus is not obstructed. Reflex apnea may result from irritation of the trachea by accumulation of secretions or from further compression of the trachea by a bolus of food in the esophagus (see Fig. 33–23). Recurrent pneumonia and atelectasis may also occur. The physical examination is not helpful in the diagnosis, although the chest film may show pneumonia or atelectasis. The barium esophagogram is normal. Aortography may show an abnormal position of the innominate artery, but this finding does not indicate tracheal compression. Bronchoscopy is the optimal method for confirming tracheal compression, and will show buckling of the tracheal cartilages in affected infants (Filston et al., 1987). Many infants with innominate artery compression have mild symptoms and improve as they grow. The primary indication for surgical intervention is reflex apnea.

Aortopexy may be performed via a median sternotomy or right-sided anterior thoracotomy. Using multiple adventitial sutures, the aorta and innominate artery are suspended from the posterior aspect of the sternum (see Fig. 33–23). The innominate artery should not be dissected free from the trachea but suspended from the aorta in order to exert traction on the buckled tracheal cartilages.

Division and reimplantation of the innominate artery may also be used to relieve tracheal compression. Hawkins and associates (1992) reported reimplanta-

tion of the innominate artery in 29 infants and children. Using a median sternotomy, the innominate artery is reimplanted more proximally on the ascending aorta so that the artery lies to the right of the trachea. There were no early or later deaths, and 27 patients had complete resolution of symptoms.

## Right Aortic Arch

Fiorratti and Aglietta reported a right aortic arch in 1763 (Hastreiter et al., 1966). Corvisart described a right aortic arch in a patient with tetralogy of Fallot in 1818 (Hastreiter et al., 1966). Persistence of the right aortic arch occurs commonly, but a vascular ring cannot result unless there is a retroesophageal segment or aberrant vessel (Knight and Edwards, 1974). A right aortic arch with mirror-image origin of the branches frequently accompanies tetralogy of Fallot (see Fig. 33–19G). In some patients, the left subclavian artery arises aberrantly from the descending

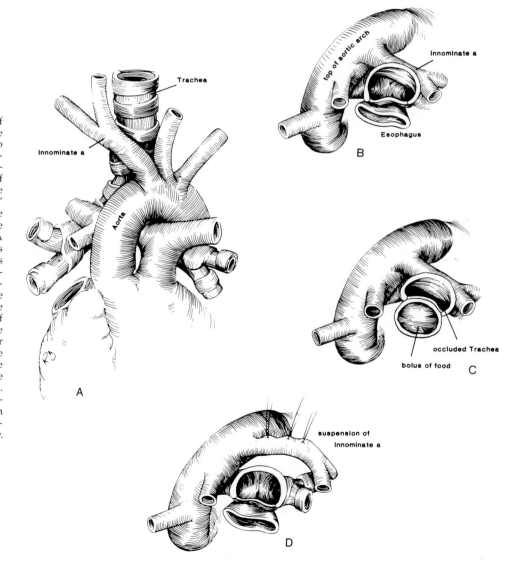

FIGURE 33–23. A, Depiction of the normal relationships of the aorta and its major branches to the trachea showing the innominate artery crossing the lower trachea, producing compression of the trachea and buckling of the cartilages. B, "Endoscopic view" of these relationships shows the buckled arch impinging on the lumen of the distal trachea. C, A bolus of food in the esophagus forces the posterior membranous portion of the trachea into the tracheal lumen, causing almost complete airway obliteration by the anterior compression and the posterior bulge. D, Suspension of the aorta and the innominate artery eliminates the anterior compression and buckling of the tracheal rings, increasing the cross-sectional diameter of the trachea. (A–D, From Filston, H. C., Ferguson, T. B., Jr., and Oldham, H. N.: Airway obstruction by vascular anomalies: Importance of telescopic bronchoscopy. Ann. Surg., 205:541, 1987.)

aorta and courses posterior to the esophagus. A Kommerell diverticulum may be present representing the distal left arch. This anomaly may cause dysphagia, and a true vascular ring is formed if a left ligamentum arteriosum connects to the aberrant subclavian artery. In some patients, a right aortic arch is found with a retroesophageal segment and a left descending aorta, the branches may arise in mirror image (see Fig. 33–18F), or the left subclavian may arise from a diverticulum of the descending aorta (see Fig. 33–18E). In any case, the presence of a left ligamentum that attaches to the descending aorta constitutes a true vascular ring. There have been rare reports of right aortic arches with a retroesophageal left innominate artery and of right aortic arch with isolation of the left subclavian artery. The latter defect requires involution of the left arch at two sites. The subclavian artery arises from the ductus or ligamentum arteriosum, and a subclavian steal syndrome may occur.

In symptomatic patients with a right aortic arch, retroesophageal segment and left descending aorta, or an aberrant left subclavian artery, a left ligamentum arteriosum usually must be present for significant tracheal and esophageal compression to occur. The surgical procedure divides the ligamentum arteriosum through a left thoracotomy. Patients occasionally may develop dysphagia secondary to an anomalous left subclavian artery or enlarged Kommerell's diverticulum. In these patients, the aberrant artery may be divided via a left thoracotomy, or right-sided thoracotomy may be necessary to excise the diverticulum.

### Cervical Aortic Arch

The cervical aortic arch is a rare anomaly in which the aorta arises to a point above the clavicle. Beaven and Fatti (1947) reported the first case in a 9-year-old girl who rapidly expired after ligation of a presumed carotid artery aneurysm. The cervical aortic arch is thought to represent persistence of the third rather than the fourth aortic arch. The cervical aortic arch may be an isolated finding or may occur in association with other arch anomalies. The presence of a cervical aortic arch can be confirmed with compression of a pulsatile neck mass, which extinguishes the femoral pulses. No intervention is necessary unless another symptomatic anomaly is present (Mullins et al., 1973).

### Results

Survival and relief of symptoms through surgical therapy are good in infants with isolated vascular rings. Operative mortality is low but not zero. Postoperative morbidity is often related to tracheomalacia secondary to vascular compression (Roesler et al., 1983). Chun and co-workers (1992) reported 39 patients treated for vascular rings at the Johns Hopkins Hospital between 1968 and 1990. There were 2 hospi-

tal deaths and 1 child had persistence of severe symptoms. At a median follow-up of 1 year, 97% of survivors were completely or nearly completely free from symptoms. Some infants may continue to have residual obstruction following repair, leading to recurrent respiratory distress and infection. These problems usually diminish as the child grows. In children with associated cardiac anomalies, the long-term outcome is related to the severity of the cardiac defect.

## PULMONARY ARTERY SLING

Pulmonary artery sling is a rare cardiac anomaly that occurs when the left pulmonary artery arises aberrantly from the right pulmonary artery and courses between the trachea and the esophagus. A true vascular ring is not present. However, compression of the distal trachea and mainstem bronchi usually occurs. Glaevecke and Doehle (1897) first described pulmonary artery sling. Scheid (1938) reported a pulmonary artery sling with associated tracheal stenosis and complete cartilaginous rings. Welsh and Munro (1954) reported a patient with an aberrant left pulmonary artery and suggested that this anomaly would produce an anterior defect in the barium esophagogram, a finding that was later described by Wittenborg and colleagues (1956).

Potts and associates (1954) performed a thoracotomy on a child with a suspected vascular ring and discovered a pulmonary artery sling. They divided the anomalous left subclavian artery and reanastomosed the artery to the proximal portion of the pulmonary artery anterior to the trachea. A similar procedure was reported by Hiller and MacLean (1957), although they anastomosed the left pulmonary artery to the main pulmonary artery rather than to the proximal left pulmonary artery.

### Embryology and Pathologic Anatomy

The aberrant left pulmonary artery arises from the posterior aspect of the right pulmonary artery and courses posteriorly over the right mainstem bronchus between the trachea and the esophagus. The hilum of the left lung is lower than normal. Tracheal stenosis with complete cartilaginous rings and absence of the membranous portion of the trachea occurs frequently. Tracheal stenosis may extend proximally, may include the left mainstem bronchus, and may also be present in segments not actually compressed by the anomalous vessel. Tracheomalacia and origin of the right mainstem bronchus from the trachea (bronchus suis) are also commonly associated with pulmonary artery sling.

The proximal pulmonary arteries normally develop from the proximal portion of the right and left sixth aortic arches (Bamman et al., 1977). The distal portions of the pulmonary arteries develop from the vascular plexus of the lung buds. If the sixth aortic arch develops abnormally, the lung bud may establish a vascular connection with any nearby artery. If a connection is established with the systemic artery, complete absence of a pulmonary artery occurs. If a connection is established across the midline to the right sixth aortic arch and posterior to the trachea, a pulmonary artery sling results. The ductus arteriosus arises from the main pulmonary artery and passes anterior to the trachea to connect with the aorta in the usual manner. The cause of the tracheobronchial anomalies is unclear but may be related to compression by the aberrant vessel. Various associated cardiac anomalies have been reported, including PDA, persistent left superior vena cava, atrial septal defect, VSD, and aortic arch anomalies.

## Clinical Findings and Diagnosis

Infants with pulmonary artery sling often present with respiratory symptoms at birth and most are symptomatic by 1 month of age. It is impossible, however, to estimate the number of asymptomatic patients with pulmonary artery sling (Dupuis et al., 1988). The most common findings are respiratory distress, wheezing, and expiratory stridor. Acute respiratory failure secondary to obstruction may occur and require intubation. Signs and symptoms of esophageal obstruction are rare. Repeated respiratory tract infections may occur.

The physical examination does not help diagnose pulmonary artery sling. The chest film may be normal and may show a number of findings suggestive of pulmonary artery sling, including hyperinflation of one lung (most commonly the right but occasionally the left), anterior bowing of the tracheal air column, and a low hilum of the left lung (Fig. 33–24). Infants may present at birth with opacification of one lung secondary to retention of fetal fluid (Zumbro et al., 1974). Pulmonary artery sling may be present in adults as a mediastinal or paratracheal mass. The barium esophagogram is particularly useful and shows anterior pulsatile compression of the esophagus (Fig. 33–24). This finding strongly suggests a pulmonary artery sling, but can be seen if an anomalous subclavian artery courses between the trachea and the esophagus. Mediastinal tumors, cysts, or lymph nodes may occasionally cause anterior esophageal compression, but these lesions are nonpulsatile. Angiocardiography shows the aberrant vessel and evaluate associated anomalies (Fig. 33–24). Alternative diagnostic techniques that help diagnose pulmonary artery sling include DSA, two-dimensional echocardiography, CT scans, and MRI. Bronchoscopy is particularly useful in these patients for evaluation of associated tracheobronchial anomalies. Bronchography is now rarely used.

## Natural History

The exact incidence of pulmonary artery sling is unknown. Patients may present with symptoms in

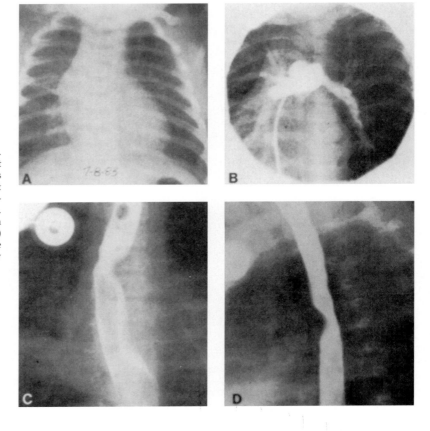

FIGURE 33–24. Infant with pulmonary artery sling. *A,* Plain chest film shows hyperaeration of the left lung. *B,* Pulmonary arteriogram shows anomalous origin of the left pulmonary artery from the right pulmonary artery. (Note the course of the left pulmonary artery around the tracheal air column.) *C,* Barium esophagogram (AP) showing compression of the esophagus. *D,* Barium esophagogram (lateral) showing characteristic anterior indentation of the esophagus behind the distal trachea. (*A–D,* Courtesy of Dr. Eric Effman and Dr. Bennett Pearce.)

infancy but may survive to an advanced age. The oldest reported patient was 78 years old and he was asymptomatic until a few months before his death. Increasing reports show children and adults who have pulmonary artery sling with minimal or no symptoms, in whom the anomaly is discovered during evaluation for unrelated complaints (Dupuis et al., 1988).

The natural history of patients with pulmonary artery sling depends on the degree of respiratory obstruction and associated tracheobronchial and cardiac anomalies (Sade et al., 1975). Infants who present with respiratory obstruction may succumb to the acute event. If they survive, their prognosis is poor without surgical intervention. Phelan and Venables (1978), however, reported nonsurgical management in five patients (one patient had division of a ligamentum arteriosum) with resolution or marked diminution in symptoms in all other patients. Three of these patients had associated tracheobronchial stenosis, which was thought to contribute to the residual symptoms.

## Surgical Intervention

Surgical intervention is indicated in any patient with pulmonary artery sling and symptoms of significant respiratory obstruction. Nonsurgical management may be possible in patients with minor symptoms. The recommended procedure is division of the anomalous artery with anastomosis to the main pulmonary artery rather than to the proximal left pulmonary artery, to avoid kinking. This may be performed using either a left thoracotomy or a median sternotomy with cardiopulmonary bypass. Although a right-sided thoracotomy was occasionally used in the past, it should be avoided because patients usually do not tolerate collapse of the right lung with simultaneous interruption of the vascular supply to the left lung.

A left thoracotomy is performed through the fourth interspace and the ligamentum arteriosum is divided (Fig. 33–25). The anomalous pulmonary artery is dissected free from the trachea and surrounding mediastinal structures. Heparin is administered and the left pulmonary artery is divided between clamps. The proximal portion is doubly oversewn with a continuous nonabsorbable suture. The pericardium is opened and the left pulmonary artery is passed through a second pericardial incision posterior to the phrenic nerve. The artery is positioned so the anastomosis may be constructed without kinking or tension. A partial occlusion clamp is placed on the main pulmonary artery and an ellipse of arterial wall is excised. An end-to-side anastomosis is performed using a continuous monofilament suture. Alternatively, the posterior wall may be performed with a continuous suture and the anterior wall may be done with interrupted sutures.

A median sternotomy with or without cardiopulmonary bypass may also be used for repair of pulmonary artery sling. After cannulation and initiation of cardiopulmonary bypass, the left pulmonary artery is dissected free and divided at the right pulmonary

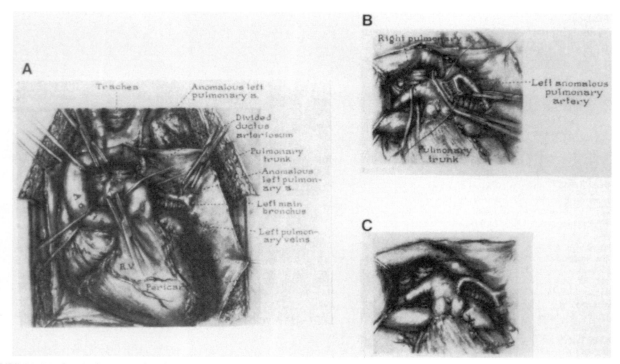

**FIGURE 33–25.** Surgical repair of pulmonary artery sling. *A,* The ligamentum is divided, and the anomalous vessel is transected and transferred anterior to the trachea. *B,* The left pulmonary artery is anastomosed in an end-to-side manner to the main pulmonary artery. *C,* Completed repair. (*A–C,* From Campbell, C. D., Wernly, J. A., Koltip, P. C., et al.: Aberrant left pulmonary artery [pulmonary artery sling]: Successful repair and 24-year follow-up report. Am. J. Cardiol., *45*:316, 1980.)

artery. The proximal defect is closed and the left pulmonary artery is passed anterior to the trachea and through the pericardium posterior to the phrenic nerve. An ellipse of the main pulmonary artery is excised and the anastomosis is performed so that the left pulmonary artery lies without kinking or tension.

The management of associated tracheobronchial anomalies continues to be a difficult problem. If significant obstruction remains after correction of the pulmonary artery sling, resection of the stenotic segment of the trachea or bronchus may be necessary (Pawade et al., 1992). If complete tracheal rings are present, either resection of the stenotic segment or an anterior tracheoplasty with autologous pericardium may be used to relieve the stenosis (Backer et al., 1992; Idriss et al., 1984; Pawade et al., 1992). Hickey and Wood (1987) reported single-stage correction of the pulmonary artery sling by reimplantation of the left pulmonary artery and tracheal resection using cardiopulmonary bypass. Jonas and co-workers (1989) reported single-stage correction without a vascular anastomosis by resecting the stenotic area, mobilizing the left pulmonary artery anteriorly, and reanastomosing the trachea posterior to the artery.

## Results

The results of surgical therapy for pulmonary artery sling have been somewhat disappointing but have improved significantly in recent series. Potts and associates' first patient in 1953 fared very well and was discharged on the 11th postoperative day. Follow-up 24 years later showed that the child had developed normally and had normal exercise tolerance; however, a ventilation-perfusion scan showed minimal perfusion of the left lung (Campbell et al., 1980). Sade and colleagues (1975) reviewed 40 cases of pulmonary artery sling treated surgically with a 50% mortality. The survivors were generally asymptomatic; however, 9 of 10 patients studied had occluded left pulmonary arteries. Dunn and associates (1979) reported 4 patients who had repair of pulmonary artery sling, with patency of the left pulmonary artery documented in all patients. Pawade and co-workers (1992) from the Hospital for Sick Children in London reported 18 patients treated for pulmonary artery sling. Patients with isolated pulmonary artery sling underwent reimplantation of the left pulmonary artery via a left thoracotomy. Four patients with stovepipe trachea and complete cartilaginous rings underwent tracheal resection and cardiopulmonary bypass and reanastomosis of the left pulmonary artery to the main pulmonary artery. There were no early deaths. There was 1 late death, and the pulmonary artery anastomosis was patent in 14 patients investigated postoperatively. Backer and colleagues (1992) reported 12 infants who underwent surgical repair of pulmonary artery sling at a mean age of 5 months. Three patients had simultaneous pericardial patch tracheoplasty for complete tracheal rings. There were no operative deaths and 2 late deaths. The pulmonary

artery anastomosis was patent in 7 of 9 patients studied postoperatively.

Morbidity and mortality following repair of pulmonary artery sling are usually related to the severity of the tracheal stenosis and associated defects. Survivors generally have a benign course if the tracheal stenosis has been adequately relieved, even if occlusion of the left pulmonary artery occurs. Although there has been concern that patients with an occluded left pulmonary artery might develop pulmonary hypertension in the right lung or hemoptysis secondary to bronchial collaterals, neither has been encountered. Attempts to restore patency to occluded left pulmonary arteries have not met with success and are generally not recommended.

## SELECTED BIBLIOGRAPHY

Lacour-Gayet, F., Bruniaux, J., Serraf, A., et al.: Hypoplastic transverse arch and coarctation in neonates: Surgical reconstruction of the aortic arch: A study of sixty-six patients. J. Thorac. Cardiovasc. Surg., 100:808, 1990.
Sciolaro, C., Copeland, J., Cork, R., et al.: Long-term follow-up comparing subclavian flap angioplasty to resection with modified oblique end-to-end anastomosis. J. Thorac. Cardiovasc. Surg., 101:1, 1991.
Van Heurn, L. W. E., Wong, C. M., Spiegelhalter, D. J., et al.: Surgical treatment of aortic coarctation in infants age less than three months, 1985–1991. J. Thorac. Cardiovasc. Surg., 107:74, 1994.

These three articles report the experience with neonatal coarctation of the aorta at three centers, comparing the advantages and disadvantages of subclavian flap angioplasty with repair by resection and end-to-end anastomosis. The conflicting results with these techniques obtained at different centers illustrate the difficulties in recommending one type of repair for coarctation of the aorta over another.

Brewer, L. A., III, Fosburg, R. G., Mulder, G. A., and Verska, J. J.: Spinal cord complications following surgery for coarctation of the aorta: A study of 66 cases. J. Thorac. Cardiovasc. Surg., 64:368, 1972.
Keen, G.: Spinal cord damage and operations for coarctation of the aorta: Aetiology, practice, and prospects. Thorax, 42:11, 1987.

These two articles are extensive retrospective reviews of spinal cord complications after repair of coarctation of the aorta. The first encompasses 12,532 cases and the second 5492 cases. These reviews delineate the incidence of spinal cord complications following repair of coarctation of the aorta and possible contributing factors.

Karl, T. R., Sano, S., Brawn, W., and Mee, R. B. B.: Repair of hypoplastic or interrupted aortic arch via sternotomy. J. Thorac. Cardiovasc. Surg., 104:688, 1992.

This study reports a large series from a single institution of infants with aortic arch obstruction and hypoplastic aortic arch who underwent a primary complete intracardiac repair with excellent results.

Chun, K., Colombani, P. M., Dudgeon, D. L., and Haller, J. A.: Diagnosis and management of congenital vascular rings: A 22-year experience. Ann. Thorac. Surg., 53:597, 1992.

This large series of congenital aortic arch anomalies treated at a single institution outlines the management principles for successful treatment of vascular rings.

Pawade, A., de Leval, M. R., Elliott, M. J., and Stark, J.: Pulmonary artery sling. Ann. Thorac. Surg., 54:967, 1992.

This series of 18 patients with pulmonary artery sling was treated at the Hospital for Sick Children in London. Patients with isolated pulmonary artery sling were treated by division and reimplantation of the left pulmonary artery. Patients with tracheal stenosis were treated by tracheal resection as well as reimplantation of the left pulmonary artery. Methods for diagnosis and treatment of patients with pulmonary artery sling with and without complete cartilaginous tracheal rings are reviewed.

# BIBLIOGRAPHY

Abbott, M. E.: Atlas of Congenital Heart Disease. New York, American Heart Association, 1936.

Abbott, M. E.: Coarctation of the aorta of the adult type. Am. Heart J., 3:574, 1928.

Achanti, B., Yeh, T. F., and Pildes, R. S.: Indomethacin therapy in infants with advanced postnatal age and patent ductus arteriosus. Clin. Invest. Med., 9:250, 1986.

Adzick, W. S., Harrison, M. R., and Delorimier, A. A.: Surgical clip ligation of patent ductus arteriosus in premature infants. J. Pediatr. Surg., 21:158, 1986.

Aebert, H., Laas, J., Bednarski, P., et al.: High incidence of aneurysm formation following patch plasty repair of coarctation. Eur. J. Cardiothorac. Surg., 7:200, 1993.

Agius, P. V., Rushworth, A., and Connolly, N.: Anomalous origin of left coronary artery from pulmonary artery associated with an aortopulmonary septal defect. Br. Heart J., 32:708, 1970.

Alpert, B. S., Bain, H. H., Balfe, J. W., et al.: Role of the renin-angiotensin-aldosterone system in hypertensive children with coarctation of the aorta. Am. J. Cardiol., 43:828, 1979.

Amato, J. J., Rheinlander, H. F., and Cleveland, R. J.: A method of enlarging the distal transverse arch in infants with hypoplasia and coarctation of the aorta. Ann. Thorac. Surg., 23:261, 1977.

Arciniegas, E., Hakimi, M., Hertzler, J. H., et al.: Surgical management of congenital vascular rings. J. Thorac. Cardiovasc. Surg., 77:721, 1979.

Armer, R. M., Shumacker, H. B., and Klatte, E. C.: Origin of the right pulmonary artery from the ascending aorta: Report of a surgically correlated case. Circulation, 24:662, 1961.

Austin, E. H., and Wolfe, W. G.: Aneurysm of aberrant subclavian artery with a review of the literature. J. Vasc. Surg., 2:511, 1985.

Azarow, K. S., Pearl, R. H., Hoffman, M. A., et al.: Vascular ring: Does magnetic resonance imaging replace angiography? Ann. Thorac. Surg., 53:882, 1992.

Backer, C. I., Idriss, F. S., Holinger, L. D., and Mavroudis, C.: Pulmonary artery sling: Results of surgical repair in infancy. J. Thorac. Cardiovasc. Surg., 103:683, 1992.

Backer, C. I., Ilbawi, M. N., Idriss, P. S., and DeLeon, S. Y.: Vascular anomalies causing tracheoesophageal compression. J. Thorac. Cardiovasc. Surg., 97:725, 1989.

Bagby, S. P., and Mass, R. D.: Abnormality of the renin/body-fluid-volume relationship in serially studied inbred dogs with neonatally induced coarctation hypertension. Hypertension, 2:631, 1980.

Bagby, S. P., McDonald, W. J., Strong, D. W., et al.: Abnormalities of renal perfusion and the renal pressor system in dogs with chronic aortic coarctation. Circ. Res., 37:615, 1975.

Balaji, S., Burch, M., and Sullivan, I. D.: Accuracy of cross-sectional echocardiography in diagnosis of aortopulmonary window. Am. J. Cardiol., 67:650, 1991a.

Balaji, S., Oommen, R., and Rees, P. G.: Fatal aortic rupture during balloon dilatation of recoarctation. Br. Heart J., 65:100, 1991b.

Bamman, J. L., Ward, B. H., and Woodrum, D. W.: Aberrant left pulmonary artery: Clinical and embryologic factors. Chest, 72:67, 1977.

Barratt-Boyes, B. G., Nicholls, T. T., Brandt, P. W. T., and Neutze, J. M.: Aortic arch interruption associated with patent ductus arteriosus, ventricular septal defect, and total anomalous pulmonary venous connection. Total correction in an 8-day-old infant by means of profound hypothermia and limited cardiopulmonary bypass. J. Thorac. Cardiovasc. Surg., 63:367, 1972.

Bayford, D.: An account of a singular case of obstructed deglutition. Memoirs Med. Soc. Lond., 2:275, 1794.

Beaven, T. E. D., and Fatti, L.: Ligature of aortic arch in the neck. Br. J. Surg., 34:414, 1947.

Becker, A. E., Becker, M. J., and Edwards, J. E.: Anomalies associated with coarctation of aorta: Particular reference to infancy. Circulation, 41:1067, 1970.

Beekman, R. H., Katz, B. P., Moorehead-Steffens, C., and Rocchini, A. P.: Altered baroreceptor function in children with systolic hypertension after coarctation repair. Am. J. Cardiol., 52:112, 1983.

Benedict, C. R., Phil, D., Grahame-Smith, D. G., and Fisher, A.: Changes in plasma catecholamines and dopamine beta-hydroxylase after corrective surgery for coarctation of the aorta. Circulation, 57:598, 1978.

Bergdahl, L., and Ljungqvist, A.: Long-term results after repair of coarctation of the aorta by patch grafting. J. Thorac. Cardiovasc. Surg., 80:177, 1980.

Berri, G., Welsh, P., and Capelli, H.: Aortic aneurysm after subclavian arterial flap angioplasty for coarctation of the aorta. J. Thorac. Cardiovasc. Surg., 105:951, 1993.

Binet, J. P., and Langlois, J.: Aortic arch anomalies in children and infants. J. Thorac. Cardiovasc. Surg., 73:248, 1977.

Blake, H. A., and Manion, W. C.: Thoracic arterial arch anomalies. Circulation, 26:251, 1962.

Blalock, A.: Operative closure of the patent ductus arteriosus. Surg. Gynecol. Obstet., 82:113, 1946.

Blalock, A., and Park, E. A.: The surgical treatment of experimental coarctation (atresia) of the aorta. Ann. Surg., 119:445, 1944.

Blieden, L. C., and Moller, J. H.: Aorticopulmonary septal defect: An experience with 17 patients. Br. Heart J., 36:630, 1974.

Bonnet, L. M.: Stenose congenitale de l'aorte. Rev. Med. Paris, 23:108, 1903.

Bourne, G., Keele, K. D., and Tubbs, O. S.: Ligation and chemotherapy for infection of patent ductus arteriosus. Lancet, 2:444, 1941.

Bove, E. L., Minich, L. L., Pridjian, A. K., et al.: The management of severe subaortic stenosis, ventricular septal defect, and aortic arch obstruction in the neonate. J. Thorac. Cardiovasc. Surg., 105:289, 1993.

Boyer, N. H.: Patent ductus arteriosus: Some historical highlights. Ann. Thorac. Surg., 4:570, 1967.

Brandt, B., III, Heintz, S. E., Rose, E. F., et al.: Repair of coarctation of the aorta in children with Turner's syndrome. Pediatr. Cardiol., 5:175, 1984.

Brewer, L. A., III, Fosburg, R. G., Mulder, G. A., and Verska, J. J.: Spinal cord complications following surgery for coarctation of the aorta: A study of 66 cases. J. Thorac. Cardiovasc. Surg., 64:368, 1972.

Brouwer, M. H. J., Cromme-Dijkhuis, A. H., Ebels, T., and Eijgelaar, A.: Growth of the hypoplastic aortic arch after simple coarctation resection and end-to-end anastomosis. J. Thorac. Cardiovasc. Surg., 104:426, 1992.

Burnard, E. D.: Discussion on the significance of continuous murmurs in the first days of life. Proc. R. Soc. Med., 52:77, 1959.

Campbell, C. D., Wernly, J. A., Koltip, P. C., et al.: Aberrant left pulmonary artery (pulmonary artery sling): Successful repair and 24-year follow-up report. Am. J. Cardiol., 45:316, 1980.

Campbell, D. B., Waldhausen, J. A., Pierce, W. S., et al.: Should elective repair of coarctation of the aorta be done in infancy? J. Thorac. Cardiovasc. Surg., 88:979, 1984.

Campbell, M.: Natural history of coarctation of the aorta. Br. Heart J., 32:633, 1970.

Campbell, M.: Natural history of persistent ductus arteriosus. Br. Heart J., 30:4, 1968.

Caro, C., Lermanda, V. C., and Lyons, H. A.: Aortic origin of the right pulmonary artery. Br. Heart J., 19:345, 1957.

Carpenter, M. A., Dammann, J. F., Watson, D. D., et al.: Left ventricular hyperkinesia at rest and during exercise in normotensive patients 2 to 27 years after coarctation repair. J. Am. Coll. Cardiol., 6:879, 1985.

Celano, V., Pieroni, D. R., Morera, J. A., et al.: Two-dimensional echocardiographic examination of mitral valve abnormalities associated with coarctation of the aorta. Circulation, 69:924, 1984.

Celoria, G. C., and Patton, R. B.: Congenital absence of the aortic arch. Am. Heart J., 58:408, 1959.

Chan, K. C., Dickinson, D. F., Wharton, G. A., and Gibbs, J. L.: Continuous wave Doppler echocardiography after surgical repair of coarctation of the aorta. Br. Heart J., 68:192, 1992.

Choy, M., Rocchini, A. P., Beekman, R. H., et al.: Paradoxical hypertension after repair of coarctation of the aorta in children: Balloon angioplasty versus surgical repair. Circulation, 75:1186, 1987.

Christiansen, N. A.: Coarctation of the aorta: Historical review. Proc. Staff Meet. Mayo Clin., 23:322, 1948.

Chun, K., Colombani, P. M., Dudgeon, D. L., and Haller, J. A.: Diagnosis and management of congenital vascular rings: A 22-year experience. Ann. Thorac. Surg., 53:597, 1992.

Clarkson, P. M., Brandt, P. W. T., Barratt-Boyes, B. G., et al.: Prosthetic repair of coarctation of the aorta with particular reference to Dacron onlay patch grafts and late aneurysm formation. Am. J. Cardiol., 56:342, 1985.

Clyman, R. I., and Campbell, D.: Indomethacin therapy for patent ductus arteriosus: When is prophylaxis not prophylactic? J. Pediatr., 111:718, 1987.

Cobanoglu, A., Teply, J. F., Grunkemeier, G. L., et al.: Coarctation of the aorta in patients younger than three months. J. Thorac. Cardiovasc. Surg., 89:128, 1985.

Cohen, M., Fuster, V., Steele, M. P., et al.: Coarctation of the aorta: Long-term follow-up and prediction of outcome after surgical correction. Circulation, 80:840, 1989.

Cokkinos, D. V., Leachman, R. D., and Cooley, D. A.: Increased mortality rate from coronary artery disease following operation for coarctation of the aorta at a late age. J. Thorac. Cardiovasc. Surg., 77:315, 1979.

Congdon, E. D.: Transformation of the aortic-arch system during the development of the human embryo. Contrib. Embryol., 68:47, 1922.

Connors, T. M.: Evaluation of persistent coarctation of aorta after surgery with blood pressure measurement and exercise testing. Am. J. Cardiol., 43:75, 1979.

Cooley, D. A., McNamara, D. G., and Latson, J. R.: Aorticopulmonary septal defect: Diagnosis and surgical treatment. Surgery, 42:101, 1957.

Cotton, A. C.: Report of a case of anuria. Arch. Pediatr., 16:774, 1899.

Crafoord, C., and Nylin, G.: Congenital coarctation of the aorta and its surgical treatment. J. Thorac. Cardiovasc. Surg., 14:347, 1945.

Cunningham, H. N., Jr., Laschinger, J. C., and Spencer, F. C.: Monitoring of somatosensory evoked potentials during surgical procedures on the thoracoabdominal aorta. IV: Clinical observations and results. J. Thorac. Cardiovasc. Surg., 94:275, 1987.

Davis, J. T., Baciewicz, F. A., Suriyapa, S., et al.: Vocal cord paralysis in premature infants undergoing ductal closure. Ann. Thorac. Surg., 46:214, 1988.

de Balsac, R. H.: Left aortic arch (posterior or circumflex type) with right descending aorta. Am. J. Cardiol., 5:546, 1960.

Decancq, H. G., Jr.: Repair of patent ductus arteriosus in a 1417-gram infant. Am. J. Dis. Child., 106:402, 1963.

del Nido, P. J., Williams, W. G., Wilson, G. J., et al.: Synthetic patch angioplasty for repair of coarctation of the aorta: Experience with aneurysm formation. Circulation, 74(Suppl. I):32, 1986.

DeSanto, A., Bills, R. G., King, H., et al.: Pathogenesis of aneurysm formation opposite prosthetic patches used for coarctation repair: An experimental study. J. Thorac. Cardiovasc. Surg., 94:720, 1987.

Deverall, P. B., Lincoln, J. C. R., Aberdeen, E., et al.: Aortopulmonary window. J. Thorac. Cardiovasc. Surg., 57:479, 1969.

Downing, D. F., Grotzinger, P. J., and Weller, R. W.: Coarctation of the aorta: The syndrome of necrotizing arteritis of the small intestine following surgical therapy. Am. J. Dis. Child., 96:711, 1958.

Dudell, G. G., and Gersony, W. M.: Patent ductus arteriosus in neonates with severe respiratory disease. J. Pediatr., 104:915, 1984.

Dunn, J. M., Gordon, I., Chrispin, A. R., et al.: Early and late results of surgical correction of pulmonary artery sling. Ann. Thorac. Surg., 28:230, 1979.

Dupuis, C., Vaksmann, G., Pernot, C., et al.: Asymptomatic form of left pulmonary artery sling. Am. J. Cardiol., 61:177, 1988.

Edwards, J. E.: Anomalies of the derivatives of the aortic arch system. Med. Clin. North Am., 32:925, 1948.

Elliotson, J.: Case of malformations of the pulmonary artery and aorta. Lancet, 1:247, 1830.

Elliott, M. J.: Coarctation of the aorta with arch hypoplasia: Improvements on a new technique. Ann. Thorac. Surg., 44:321, 1987.

Ellis, F. H., Jr., Kirklin, J. W., Callahan, J. A., and Wood, E. H.: Patent ductus arteriosus with pulmonary hypertension. J. Thorac. Surg., 31:268, 1956.

Elzenga, N. J., and Gittenberger-deGroot, A. C.: Localized coarctation of the aorta: An age-dependent spectrum. Br. Heart J., 49:317, 1983.

Esposito, R. A., Khalil, F., Galloway, A. C., and Spencer, F. C.: Surgical treatment for aneurysm of aberrant subclavian artery based on a case report and a review of the literature. J. Thorac. Cardiovasc. Surg., 95:888, 1988.

Evans, N.: Diagnosis of patent ductus arteriosus in the preterm newborn. Arch. Dis. Child., 68:58, 1993.

Everts-Suarez, E. A., and Carson, C. P.: The triad of congenital absence of aortic arch (isthmus aortae), patent ductus arteriosus, and interventricular septal defect—A trilogy. Ann. Surg., 150:153, 1959.

Fadley, F., Al-Halees, Z., Galal, O., et al.: Left pulmonary artery stenosis after transcatheter occlusion of persistent arterial duct. Lancet, 341:559, 1993.

Falcone, M. W., Perloff, J. K., and Roberts, W. C.: Aneurysm of the nonpatent ductus arteriosus. Am. J. Cardiol., 29:422, 1972.

Fearon, B., and Shortreed, R.: Tracheobronchial compression by congenital cardiovascular anomalies in children: Syndrome of apnea. Ann. Otol. Rhinol. Laryngol., 72:949, 1963.

Ferguson, J. C., Barrie, W. W., and Schenk, W. G., Jr.: Hypertension of aortic coarctation: The role of renal and other factors. Ann. Surg., 185:423, 1977.

Filston, H. C., Ferguson, T. B., Jr., and Oldham, H. N.: Airway obstruction by vascular anomalies: Importance of telescopic bronchoscopy. Ann. Surg., 205:541, 1987.

Fleming, W. H., Sarafian, L. B., Kugler, J. D., and Nelson, R. M., Jr.: Ligation of patent ductus arteriosus in premature infants: Importance of accurate anatomic definition. Pediatrics, 71:373, 1983.

Fong, L. V., Anderson, R. H., Siewers, R. D., et al.: Anomalous origin of one pulmonary artery from the ascending aorta: A review of echocardiographic, catheter, and morphological features. Br. Heart J., 62:389, 1989.

Fontana, G. P., Spach, M. S., Effmann, E. L., and Sabiston, D. C., Jr.: Origin of the right pulmonary artery from the ascending aorta. Ann. Surg., 206:102, 1987.

Foster, E. D.: Reoperation for aortic coarctation. Ann. Thorac. Surg., 38:81, 1984.

Fox, S., Pierce, W. S., and Waldhausen, J. A.: Pathogenesis of paradoxical hypertension after coarctation repair. Ann. Thorac. Surg., 29:135, 1980.

Freed, M. D., Keane, J. F., Van Praagh, R., et al.: Coarctation of the aorta with congenital mitral regurgitation. Circulation, 49:1175, 1974.

Freed, M. D., Rocchini, A., Rosenthal, A.., et al: Exercise-induced hypertension after surgical repair of coarctation of the aorta. Am. J. Cardiol., 43:253, 1979.

Friedman, W. F., Hirschklau, M. J., Printz, M. P., et al.: Pharmacologic closure of patent ductus arteriosus in the premature infant. N. Engl. J. Med., 295:526, 1976.

Gardiner, H. M., Celermajer, D. S., Sorenson, K. E., and Deanfield, J. E.: Abnormal endothelial response in the precoarctation vascular bed of young normotensive adults after successful coarctation repair. Br. Heart J., 69:18, 1993.

Gasul, B. M., Fell, E. H., and Casas, R.: The diagnosis of aortic septal defect by retrograde aortography: Report of a case. Circulation, 4:251, 1951.

Gay, W. A., Jr., and Young, W. G., Jr.: Pseudocoarctation of the aorta: A reappraisal. J. Thorac. Cardiovasc. Surg., 58:739, 1969.

Geiss, D., Williams, W. G., Lindsay, W. K., and Rowe, R. D.: Upper extremity gangrene: A complication of subclavian artery division. Ann. Thorac. Surg., 30:487, 1980.

Gentile, R., Stevenson, G., Dooley, J., et al.: Pulsed Doppler echocardiographic determination of time of ductal closure in normal newborn infants. J. Pediatr., 98:443, 1981.

Gibson, G. A.: Clinical lectures on circulatory affections. Lecture 1. Persistence of the arterial duct and its diagnosis. Edinb. Med. J., 8:1, 1900.

Gittenberger-deGroot, A. C.: Persistent ductus arteriosus: Most probably a primary congenital malformation. Br. Heart J., 39:610, 1977.

Glaevecke, H., and Doehle, H.: Ueber eine saltene angeborne anomolie des pulmonalarterie. Munchen Med. Wschr., 44:950, 1897.

Glickstein, J., Friedman, D., Langsner, A., and Rutkowski, M.: Doppler ultrasound and the silent ductus arteriosus. Br. Heart J., 69:193, 1993.

Gobel, J. W., Pierpont, M. E. M.., Moller, J. H., et al.: Familial interruption of the aortic arch. Pediatr. Cardiol., 14:110, 1993.

Godtfredsen, J., Wennenvold, A., Efsen, F., and Lauridsen, P. B.: Natural history of vascular ring with clinical manifestations: A follow-up study of eleven unoperated cases. Scand. J. Thorac. Cardiovasc. Surg., 11:75, 1977.

Goldman, S., Hernandez, J., and Pappas, G.: Results of surgical treatment of coarctation of the aorta in the critically ill neonate, including the influence of pulmonary artery banding. J. Thorac. Cardiovasc. Surg., 92:732, 1986.

Goncalves-Estella, A., Perez-Villoria, J., Gonzalez-Reoyo, F., et al.: Closure of a complicated ductus arteriosus through the transpulmonary route using hypothermia: Surgical considerations in one case. J. Thorac. Cardiovasc. Surg., 69:698, 1975.

Graybiel, A., Strieder, J. W., and Boyer, N.: An attempt to obliterate the patent ductus arteriosus in a patient with subacute bacterial endarteritis. Am. Heart J., 15:621, 1938.

Green, N. J., and Rollason, T. P.: Pulmonary artery rupture in pregnancy complicating patent ductus arteriosus. Br. Heart J., 68:616, 1992.

Gross, R. E.: Complete surgical division of the patent ductus arteriosus: A report of fourteen successful cases. Surg. Obstet. Gynecol., 78:36, 1944.

Gross, R. E.: Surgical closure of an aortic septal defect. Circulation, 5:858, 1952.

Gross, R. E.: Surgical correction for coarctations of the aorta. Surgery, 18:673, 1945a.

Gross, R. E.: Surgical relief for tracheal obstruction from a vascular ring. N. Engl. J. Med., 233:586, 1945b.

Gross, R. E.: Surgical treatment for dysphagia lusoria. Ann. Surg., 124:532, 1946.

Gross, R. E.: Treatment of certain aortic coarctations by homologous grafts. Ann. Surg., 134:753, 1951.

Gross, R. E., and Hubbard, J. P.: Surgical ligation of a patent ductus arteriosus: Report of first successful case. J. A. M. A., 112:729, 1939.

Gross, R. E., and Hufnagel, C. A.: Coarctation of the aorta: Experimental studies regarding its surgical corrections. N. Engl. J. Med., 233:287, 1945.

Gross, R. E., and Neuhauser, E. B. D.: Compression of the trachea by an anomalous innominate artery: An operation for its relief. Am. J. Dis. Child., 75:570, 1948.

Gross, R. E., and Neuhauser, E. B. D.: Compression of the trachea or esophagus by vascular anomalies. J. Pediatr., 7:69, 1951.

Gupta, T. C., and Wiggers, C. J.: Basic hemodynamic changes produced by aortic coarctation and different degrees. Circulation, 3:17, 1951.

Hamilton, D. I., Di Eusanio, G., Sandrasagra, F. A., and Donnelly, R. J.: Early and late results of aortoplasty with a left subclavian flap for coarctation of the aorta in infancy. J. Thorac. Cardiovasc. Surg., 75:699, 1978.

Hammerman, C., Strates, E., and Valaitis, S.: The silent ductus: Its precursors and its aftermath. Pediatr. Cardiol., 7:121, 1986.

Hammon, J. W., Jr., Graham, T. P., Jr., Boucek, R. J., Jr., and Bender, H. W., Jr.: Operative repair of coarctation of the aorta in infancy: Results with and without ventricular septal defect. Am. J. Cardiol., 55:1555, 1985.

Hastreiter, A. R., D'Cruz, I. A., and Cantez, T.: Right-sided aorta: Occurrence of right aortic arch in various types of congenital heart disease. Br. Heart J., 28:722, 1966.

Hawkins, J. A., Bailey, W. W., and Clark, S. M.: Innominate artery compression of the trachea. J. Thorac. Cardiovasc. Surg., 103:678, 1992.

Hayes, A. M., Redington, A. N., and Rigby, M. L.: Severe haemolysis after transcatheter duct occlusion: A non-surgical remedy. Br. Heart J., 67:321, 1992.

Hehrlein, F. W., Mulch, J., Rautenburg, H. W., et al.: Incidence and pathogenesis of late aneurysms after patch graft aortoplasty for coarctation. J. Thorac. Cardiovasc. Surg., 92:226, 1986.

Herbert, W. H., Rohman, M., Farnsworth, P., and Saraswathi, S.: Anomalous origin of left pulmonary artery from ascending aorta, right aortic arch and right patent ductus arteriosus. Chest, 63:459, 1973.

Heymann, M. A., Berman, W., Jr., Rudolph, A. M., and Whitman, V.: Dilatation of the ductus arteriosus by prostaglandin $E_1$ in aortic arch abnormalities. Circulation, 59:169, 1979.

Heymann, M. A., Rudolph, A. M., and Silberman, N. H.: Closure of the ductus arteriosus in premature infants by inhibition of prostaglandin synthesis. N. Engl. J. Med., 295:530, 1976.

Hickey, M. St. J., and Wood, A. E.: Pulmonary artery sling with tracheal stenosis. Ann. Thorac. Surg., 44:416, 1987.

Higgins, C. B., Rausch, J., Friedman, W. F., et al.: Patent ductus arteriosus in preterm infants with idiopathic respiratory distress syndrome. Radiology, 124:189, 1977.

Hiller, H. G., and MacLean, A. D.: Pulmonary artery ring. Acta Radiol., 48:434, 1957.

Hiraishi, S., Misawa, H., Oyuchi, K., et al.: Two-dimensional Doppler echocardiographic assessment of closure of the ductus arteriosus in normal newborn infants. J. Pediatr., 111:755, 1987.

Ho, S. Y., and Anderson, R. H.: Anatomical closure of the ductus arteriosus: A study in 35 specimens. J. Anat., 128:829, 1979a.

Ho, S. Y., and Anderson, R. H.: Coarctation, tubular hypoplasia, and the ductus arteriosus: Histological study of 35 specimens. Br. Heart J., 41:268, 1979b.

Houston, A. B., Gnanapragasam, J. P., Lim, M. K., et al.: Doppler ultrasound and the silent ductus arteriosus. Br. Heart J., 65:97, 1991.

Hughes, R. K., and Reemtsma, K.: Correction of coarctation of the aorta. Manometric determination of safety during test occlusion. J. Thorac. Cardiovasc. Surg., 62:31, 1971.

Hurt, R.: Surgical treatment of infected persistent ductus arteriosus. Eur. J. Cardiothorac. Surg., 6:677, 1992.

Idriss, F. S., DeLeon, S. Y., Ilbawi, M. N.., et al: Tracheoplasty with pericardial patch for extensive tracheal stenosis in infants and children. J. Thorac. Cardiovasc. Surg., 88:527, 1984.

Irwin, E. D., Braunlin, E. A., and Foker, J. E.: Staged repair of interrupted aortic arch and ventricular septal defect in infancy. Ann. Thorac. Surg., 52:632, 1991.

Isner, J. M., Donaldson, R. F., Fulton, D., et al.: Cystic medial necrosis in coarctation of the aorta: A potential factor contributing to adverse consequences observed after percutaneous balloon angioplasty of coarctation sites. Circulation, 75:689, 1987.

Jacob, T., Cobanoglu, A., and Starr, A: Late results of ascending aorta–descending aorta bypass grafts for recurrent coarctation of the aorta. J. Thorac. Cardiovasc. Surg., 95:782, 1988.

Jarcho, S.: Coarctation of the aorta (Albrecht Meckel, 1827). Am. J. Cardiol., 9:307, 1962a.

Jarcho, S.: Coarctation of the aorta (Legrand, 1833). Am. J. Cardiol., 10:266, 1962b.

Jarcho, S.: Coarctation of the aorta (Meckel, 1750; Paris, 1791). Am. J. Cardiol., 7:844, 1961.

Johansson, L., Michaelsson, M., Westerholm, C. J., and Aberg, T.: Aortopulmonary window: A new operative approach. Ann. Thorac. Surg., 25:564, 1978.

John, S., Muralidharan, S., Jairaj, P. S., et al.: The adult ductus: Review of surgical experience with 131 patients. J. Thorac. Cardiovasc. Surg., 82:314, 1981.

Johnson, A. M., and Kron, I. L.: Closure of the calcified patent ductus in the elderly: Avoidance of ductal clamps and shunts. Ann. Thorac. Surg., 45:572, 1988.

Jonas, R. A., Spevak, P. T., McGill, T., and Castenada, A. R.: Pulmonary artery sling: Primary repair by tracheal resection in infancy. J. Thorac. Cardiovasc. Surg., 97:548, 1989.

Kan, J. S., White, R. I., Jr., Mitchell, S. E., et al.: Treatment of restenosis of coarctation by percutaneous transluminal angioplasty. Circulation, 68:1087, 1983.

Karl, T. R., Sano, S., Brawn, W., and Mee, R. B. B.: Repair of hypoplastic or interrupted aortic arch via sternotomy. J. Thorac. Cardiovasc. Surg., 104:688, 1992.

Kawauchi, M., Tada, Y., Asano, K., and Sudo, K.: Angiographic demonstration of mesenteric arterial changes in postcoarctectomy syndrome. Surgery, 98:602, 1985.

Keen, G.: Spinal cord damage and operations for coarctation of the aorta: Aetiology, practice, and prospects. Thorax, 42:11, 1987.

Khan, M. A. A., Yousef, S. A., Mullins, C. E., and Sawyer, W.: Experience with 205 procedures of transcatheter closure of ductus arteriosus in 182 patients, with special reference to residual shunts and long-term follow-up. J. Thorac. Cardiovasc. Surg., 104:1721, 1992.

Kimball, B. P., Shurvell, B. L., Houle, S., et al.: Persistent ventricular adaptations in postoperative coarctation of the aorta. J. Am. Coll. Cardiol., 8:172, 1986a.

Kimball, B. P., Shurvell, B. L., Mildenberger, R. R., et al.: Abnormal thalium kinetics in postoperative coarctation of the aorta: Evidence for diffuse hypertension-induced vascular pathology. J. Am. Coll. Cardiol., 7:538, 1986b.

Kirkpatrick, S. E., Girod, D. A., and King, H.: Aortic origin of the right pulmonary artery. Circulation, 36:771, 1967.

Knight, D. B.: Patent ductus arteriosus: How important to which babies? Early Hum. Dev., 29:287, 1992.

Knight, L., and Edwards, J. E.: Right aortic arch: Types and associated cardiac anomalies. Circulation, 50:1047, 1974.

Koller, M., Rothlin, M., and Sinning, A.: Coarctation of the aorta: Review of 362 operated patients. Long-term follow-up and assessment of prognostic variables. Eur. Heart J., 8:670, 1987.

Korfer, R., Meyer, H., Kleikamp, G., and Bircks, W.: Early and late results after resection and end-to-end anastomosis of coarctation of the thoracic aorta in early infancy. J. Thorac. Cardiovasc. Surg., 89:616, 1985.

Krieger, K. H., and Spencer, F. C.: Is paraplegia after repair of coarctation of the aorta due principally to distal hypotension during aortic cross-clamping? Surgery, 2:97, 1985.

Kron, I. L., Mentzer, R. M., Jr., Rheuban, K. S., and Nolan, S. P.: A simple, rapid technique for operative closure of patent ductus arteriosus in the premature infant. Ann. Thorac. Surg., 37:422, 1984.

Kupferschmid, C. H., Lang, D., and Pohlandt, F.: Sensitivity, specificity and predictive value of clinical findings, M-mode echocardiography and continuous wave Doppler sonography in the diagnosis of symptomatic patent ductus arteriosus in preterm infants. Eur. J. Pediatr., 147:279, 1988.

Laborde, F., Noirhomme, P., Karam, J., et al.: A new video-assisted thoracoscopic surgical technique for interruption of patent ductus arteriosus in infants and children. J. Thorac. Cardiovasc. Surg., 105:278, 1993.

Lacour-Gayet, F., Bruniaux, J., Serraf, A., et al.: Hypoplastic transverse arch and coarctation in neonates. Surgical reconstruction of the aortic arch: A study of sixty-six patients. J. Thorac. Cardiovasc. Surg., 100:808, 1990.

Lansman, S. Shapiro, A. J., Schiller, M. S., et al.: Extended aortic arch anastomosis for repair of coarctation in infancy. Circulation, 74(Suppl. I):37, 1986.

Laschinger, J. C., Cunningham, J. N., Baumann, F. G., et al.: Monitoring of somatosensory evoked potentials during surgical procedures on the thoracoabdominal aorta. II: Use of somatosensory evoked potentials to assess adequacy of distal aortic bypass and perfusion after thoracic aortic cross-clamping. J. Thorac. Cardiovasc. Surg., 94:266, 1987a.

Laschinger, J. C., Cunningham, J. N., Baumann, F. G., et al.: Monitoring of somatosensory evoked potentials during surgical procedures on the thoracoabdominal aorta. III: Intraoperative identification of vessels critical to spinal cord blood supply. J. Thorac. Cardiovasc. Surg., 94:271, 1987b.

Leanage, R., Taylor, J. F. N., DeLeval, M., et al.: Surgical management of coarctation of aorta with ventricular septal defect. Br. Heart J., 46:269, 1981.

Leandro, J., Smallhorn, J. F., Benson, L., et al.: Ambulatory blood pressure monitoring and left ventricular mass and function after successful surgical repair of coarctation of the aorta. J. Am. Coll. Cardiol., 20:197, 1992.

Leoni, F., Huhta, J. C., Douglas, J., et al.: Effect of prostaglandin on early surgical mortality in obstructive lesions of the systemic circulation. Br. Heart J., 52:654, 1984.

Lewis, T.: Material relating to coarctation of the aorta of the adult type. Heart, 16:205, 1933.

Lillehei, C. W., and Colan, S.: Echocardiography in the preoperative evaluation of vascular rings. J. Pediatr. Surg., 27:1118, 1992.

Lim, M. K., Hanretty, K., Houston, A. B., et al.: Intermittent ductal patency in healthy newborn infants: Demonstration by colour Doppler flow mapping. Arch. Dis. Child., 67:1217, 1992.

Lindsay, J., Jr.: Coarctation of the aorta, bicuspid aortic valve and abnormal ascending aortic wall. Am. J. Cardiol., 61:182, 1988.

Lloyd, T. R., Fedderly, R., Mendelsohn, A. M., et al.: Transcatheter occlusion of patent ductus arteriosus with Gianturco coils. Circulation, 88(Part 1):1412, 1993.

Luisi, S. V., Ashraf, M. H., Gula, G., et al.: Anomalous origin of the right coronary artery with aortopulmonary window: Functional and surgical considerations. Thorax, 35:446, 1980.

Lund, J. T., Hansen, D., Brocks, V., et al.: Aneurysm of the ductus arteriosus in the neonate: Three case reports with a review of the literature. Pediatr. Cardiol., 13:222, 1992.

Lynxwiler, C. P., Smith, S., and Babich, J.: Coarctation of the aorta. Arch. Pediatr., 68:203, 1951.

Markel, H., Rocchini, A. P., Beekman, R. H., et al.: Exercise-induced hypertension after repair of coarctation of the aorta: Arm versus leg exercise. J. Am. Coll. Cardiol., 8:165, 1986.

Maron, B. J., Humphries, J. O., Rowe, R. D., and Mellits, E. D.: Prognosis of surgically corrected coarctation of the aorta: A 20-year postoperative appraisal. Circulation, 47:119, 1973.

Martin, M. M., Beekman, R. H., Rocchini, A. P., et al.: Aortic aneurysms after subclavian angioplasty repair of coarctation of the aorta. Am. J. Cardiol., 61:951, 1988.

McCallen, A. M., and Schaff, B.: Aneurysm of an anomalous right subclavian artery. Radiology, 66:561, 1956.

McFaul, R., Millard, P., and Nowicki, E.: Vascular rings necessitating right thoracotomy. J. Thorac. Cardiovasc. Surg., 82:306, 1981.

Mellgren, G., Friberg, L. G., Eriksson, B. O., et al.: Neonatal surgery for coarctation of the aorta. Scand. J. Thorac. Cardiovasc. Surg., 21:193, 1987.

Menahem, S., Rahayoe, A. U., Brawn, W. J., and Mee, R. B. B.: Interrupted aortic arch in infancy: A 10-year experience. Pediatr. Cardiol., 13:214, 1992.

Mendelsohn, A. M., Crowley, D. C., Lindauer, A., and Beekman, R. H.: Rapid progression of aortic aneurysms after patch aortoplasty repair of coarctation of the aorta. J. Am. Coll. Cardiol., 20:381, 1992.

Merrill, D. L., Webster, C. A., and Samson, P. C.: Congenital absence of the aortic isthmus. J. Thorac. Surg., 33:311, 1957.

Moene, R. J., Gittenberger-DeGroot, A. C., Oppenheimer-Dekker, A., and Bartelings, M. M.: Anatomic characteristics of ventricular septal defect associated with coarctation of the aorta. Am. J. Cardiol., 59:952, 1987.

Moene, R. J., Ottenkamp, J., Oppenheimer-Dekker, A., and Bartelings, M. M.: Transposition of the great arteries and narrowing of the aortic arch: Emphasis on right ventricular characteristics. Br. Heart J., 53:58, 1985.

Morrow, W. R., Vick, G. W., Nihill, M. R., et al.: Balloon dilatation of unopened coarctation of the aorta: Short- and intermediate-term results. J. Am. Coll. Cardiol., 11:113, 1988.

Moulton, A. L., and Bowman, F. O., Jr.: Primary definitive repair of type B interrupted aortic arch, ventricular septal defect, and patent ductus arteriosus. J. Thorac. Cardiovasc. Surg., 82:501, 1981.

Mullins, C. E., Gillette, P. C., and McNamara, D. G.: The complex of cervical aortic arch. Pediatrics, 51:210, 1973.

Munro, J. C.: Surgery of the vascular system. I: Ligation of the ductus arteriosus. Ann. Surg., 46:335, 1907.

Musewe, N. N., Benson, L. N., Smallhorn, J. F., and Freedom, R. M.: Two-dimensional echocardiographic and color-flow Doppler evaluation of ductal occlusion with the Rashkind prosthesis. Circulation, 80:1706, 1989.

Mustard, W. T., Bayliss, C. E., Fearon, B., et al.: Tracheal compression by the innominate artery in children. Ann. Thorac. Surg., 8:312, 1969.

Myers, J. L., McConnell, B. A., and Waldhausen, J. A.: Coarctation of the aorta in infants: Does the aortic arch grow after repair? Ann. Thorac. Surg., 54:869, 1992.

Nanton, M. A., and Olley, P. M.: Residual hypertension after coarctectomy in children. Am. J. Cardiol., 37:769, 1976.

Negre, E.: Aortopulmonary window. Ann. Thorac. Surg., 28:493, 1979.

Negre, E., Chaptal, P. A., Mary, H.: Fistules aortopulmonaires: Details techniques de leur fermelure. Ann. Chir. Thorac. Cardiovasc., 65:7, 1968.

Neuhauser, E. B. D.: The roentgen diagnosis of double aortic arch and other anomalies of the great vessels. Am. J. Roentgenol. Rad. Ther., 56:1, 1946.

Norwood, W. I., Lang, P., Castaneda, A. R., and Hougen, T. J.: Reparative operations for interrupted aortic arch with ventricular septal defect. J. Thorac. Cardiovasc. Surg., 86:832, 1983.

Orzel, J. A., and Monaco, M. P.: Inadvertent ligation of the left pulmonary artery instead of patent ductus arteriosus: Noninvasive diagnosis by pulmonary perfusion imaging. Clin. Nucl. Med., 11:629, 1986.

Ottenkamp, J., Hess, J., Talsma, M. D., and Buis-Liem, T. N.: Protrusion of the device: A complication of catheter closure of patent ductus arteriosus. Br. Heart J., 68:301, 1992.

Palder, S. B., Schwartz, M. Z., Tyson, K. R. T., and Marr, C. C.: Management of patent ductus arteriosus: A comparison of operative vs. pharmacologic treatment. J. Pediatr. Surg., 22:1171, 1987.

Park, J. K., Dell, R. B., Ellis, K., and Gersony, W. M.: Surgical management of the infant with coarctation of the aorta and ventricular septal defect. J. Am. Coll. Cardiol., 20:176, 1992.

Parker, F. B., Farrell, B., Streeten, D. H. P., et al.: Hypertensive mechanisms in coarctation of the aorta: Further studies of the renin-angiotensin system. J. Thorac. Cardiovasc. Surg., 80:568, 1980.

Parr, G. V. S., Waldhausen, J. A., Bharati, S., et al.: Coarctation of Taussig-Bing malformation of the heart. J. Thorac. Cardiovasc. Surg., 86:280, 1983.

Pate, J. W., Korones, S., and Sarasohn, C.: Surgical closure of patent ductus arteriosus outside the operating theater. World J. Surg., 5:873, 1981.

Paul, R. N.: A new anomaly of the aorta: Left aortic arch with right descending aorta. J. Pediatr., 32:19, 1948.

Pawade, A., de Leval, M. R., Elliott, M. J., and Stark, J.: Pulmonary artery sling. Ann. Thorac. Surg., 54:967, 1992.

Phelan, P. D., and Venables, A. W.: Management of pulmonary artery sling (anomalous left pulmonary artery arising from right pulmonary artery): A conservative approach. Thorax, 33:67, 1978.

Pollack, P., Freed, M. D., Castaneda, A. R., and Norwood, W. I.: Reoperation for isthmic coarctation of the aorta: Follow-up of 26 patients. Am. J. Cardiol., 51:1690, 1983.

Pollock, J. C., Jamieson, M. P., and McWilliam, R.: Somatosensory evoked potentials in the detection of spinal cord ischemia in aortic coarctation repair. Ann. Thorac. Surg., 41:251, 1986.

Pontius, R. G., Danielson, G. K., Noonan, J. A., and Judson, J. P.: Illusions leading to surgical closure of the distal left pulmonary artery instead of the ductus arteriosus. J. Thorac. Cardiovasc. Surg., 82:107, 1981.

Porstmann, W., Wierny, L., Warnke, H., et al.: Catheter closure of patent ductus arteriosus: 62 cases treated without thoracotomy. Radiol. Clin. North Am., 9:203, 1971.

Potts, W. J., Holinger, P. H., and Rosenblum, A. H.: Anomalous left pulmonary artery causing obstruction to right main bronchus: Report of a case. J. A. M. A., 155:1409, 1954.

Powell, M. L.: Patent ductus arteriosus in premature infants. Med. J. Aust., 2:58, 1963.

Preusse, C. J.: The surgical management of aortopulmonary window using the anterior sandwich patch closure technique. J. Cardiovasc. Surg., 29:629, 1988.

Putnam, T. C., and Gross, R. E.: Surgical management of aortopulmonary fenestration. Surgery, 59:727, 1966.

Railsback, O. C., and Dock, W.: Erosion of the ribs due to stenosis of the isthmus (coarctation) of the aorta. Radiology, 12:58, 1929.

Rao, P. S., and Chopra, P. S.: Role of balloon angioplasty in the treatment of aortic coarctation. Ann. Thorac. Surg., 52:621, 1991.

Rashkind, W. J., and Cuaso, C. C.: Transcatheter closure of patent ductus arteriosus: Successful use in a 3.5-kilogram infant. Pediatr. Cardiol., 1:3, 1979.

Rashkind, W. J., Mullins, C. E., Hellenbrand, W. E., and Tait, M. A.: Nonsurgical closure of patent ductus arteriosus: Clinical application of the Rashkind PDA occluder system. Circulation, 75:583, 1987.

Ravelo, H. R., Stephenson, L. W., Friedman, S., et al.: Coarctation resection in children with Turner's syndrome: A note of caution. J. Thorac. Cardiovasc. Surg., 80:427, 1980.

Ravikumar, F., Whight, C. M., Hawker, R. E., et al.: The surgical management of aortopulmonary window using the anterior sandwich patch closure technique. J. Cardiovasc. Surg., 29:629, 1988.

Reifenstein, G. H., Levine, S. A., and Gross, R. E.: Coarctation of the aorta: A review of 104 autopsied cases of the "adult type" 2 years of age or older. Am. Heart J., 33:146, 1947.

Rice, M. J., Seward, J. B., Hagler, D. J., et al.: Visualization of aortopulmonary window by two-dimensional echocardiography. Mayo Clin. Proc., 57:482, 1982.

Roesler, M., deLeval, M., Chrispin, A., and Stark, J.: Surgical management of vascular ring. Ann. Surg., 197:129, 1983.

Rosenquist, G. C.: Congenital mitral valve disease associated with coarctation of the aorta. Circulation, 49:985, 1974.

Rudolph, A. M., Heymann, M. A., and Spitznas, U.: Hemodynamic considerations in the development of narrowing of the aorta. Am. J. Cardiol., 30:514, 1972.

Russell, G. A., Berry, P. J., Watterson, K., et al.: Patterns of ductal tissue in coarctation of the aorta in the first three months of life. J. Thorac. Cardiovasc. Surg., 102:596, 1991.

Rytand, D. A.: The renal factor in arterial hypertension with coarctation of the aorta. J. Clin. Invest., 17:391, 1938.

Sade, R. M., Crawford, F. A., Hohn, A. R., et al.: Growth of the aorta after prosthetic patch aortoplasty for coarctation in infants. Ann. Thorac. Surg., 38:21, 1984.

Sade, R. M., Rosenthal, A., Fellows, K., and Castaneda, R.: Pulmonary artery sling. J. Thorac. Cardiovasc. Surg., 69:333, 1975.

Sade, R. M., Taylor, A. B., and Chariker, E. P.: Aortoplasty compared with resection for coarctation of the aorta in young children. Ann. Thorac. Surg., 28:346, 1979.

Sadow, S. H., Synhorst, D. P., and Pappas, G.: Taussig-Bing anomaly and coarctation of the aorta in infancy. Surgical options. Pediatr. Cardiol., 6:83, 1985.

Sanchez, G. R., Balsara, R. K., Dunn, J. M., et al.: Recurrent obstruction after subclavian flap repair of coarctation of the aorta in infants. J. Thorac.. Cardiovasc Surg., 91:738, 1986.

Saul, J. P., Keane, J. F., Fellows, K. E., and Lock, J. E.: Balloon dilatation angioplasty of postoperative aortic obstructions. Am. J. Cardiol., 59:943, 1987.

Scheid, P.: Missbilclung des tracheal skelettes un der linken arteria pulmonalis mit erstickangstad bei 2 monate alten. Kind. Z. Path., 52:114, 1938.

Schuster, S. R., and Gross, R. E.: Surgery for coarctation of the aorta: A review of 500 cases. J. Thorac. Cardiovasc. Surg., 43:54, 1962.

Sciolaro, C., Copeland, J., Cork, R., et al.: Long-term follow-up comparing subclavian flap angioplasty to resection with modified oblique end-to-end anastomosis. J. Thorac. Cardiovasc. Surg., 101:1, 1991.

Scott, H. W., Jr., and Bahnson, H. T.: Evidence for a renal factor in the hypertension of experimental coarctation of the aorta. Surgery, 30:206, 1951.

Scott, H. W., Jr., and Sabiston, D. C., Jr.: Surgical treatment for congenital aorticopulmonary fistula. J. Thorac. Surg., 25:26, 1953.

Scott, W. A., Rocchini, A. P., Bove, E. L., et al.: Repair of interrupted aortic arch in infancy. J. Thorac. Cardiovasc. Surg., 96:564, 1988.

Sealy, W. C., Harris, J. S., Young, W. G., Jr., and Callaway, H. A.: Paradoxical hypertension following resection of coarctation of aorta. Surgery, 42:135, 1957.

Sehested, J., Baandrup, U., and Mikkelsen, E.: Different reactivity and structure of the prestenotic and poststenotic aorta in human coarctation. Circulation, 65:1060, 1982.

Seidel, J. F.: Index Musei Anatomici Killiensis. C. F. Mohr, 1818, p. 61.

Sell, J. E., Jonas, R. A., Mayer, J. E.., et al: The results of a surgical program for interrupted aortic arch. J. Thorac. Cardiovasc. Surg., 96:864, 1988.

Shannon, J. M.: Aberrant right subclavian artery with Kommerell's diverticulum: Report of a case. J. Thorac. Cardiovasc. Surg., 41:408, 1961.

Shapiro, M. J., and Keys, A.: The prognosis of untreated patent ductus arteriosus and the results of surgical intervention. Am. J. Med. Sci., 206:174, 1943.

Shearer, W. T., Rutman, J. Y., Weinberg, W. A., and Goldring, D.: Coarctation of the aorta and cerebrovascular accident: A proposal for early corrective surgery. J. Pediatr., 77:1004, 1970.

Shinebourne, E. A., and Elseed, A. M.: Relation between fetal flow patterns, coarctation of the aorta, and pulmonary blood flow. Br. Heart J., 36:492, 1974.

Shone, J. D., Sellers, R. D., Anderson, R. C., et al.: The developmental complex of "parachute mitral valve," supravalvular ring of left atrium, subaortic stenosis, and coarctation of aorta. Am. J. Cardiol., 11:714, 1963.

Simon, A. B., and Zloto, A. E.: Coarctation of the aorta: Longitudinal assessment of operated patients. Circulation, 50:456, 1974.

Sirak, H. D., Ressahat, M., Hosier, D. M., and Delorimer, A. A.: A new operation for repairing aortic arch atresia in infancy: Report of 3 cases. Circulation, 37:II43, 1968.

Smith, R. T., Jr., Sade, R. M., Riopel, D. A., et al.: Stress testing for comparison of synthetic patch aortoplasty with resection and end-to-end anastomosis for repair of coarctation in childhood. J. Am. Coll. Cardiol., 4:765, 1984.

Sorensen, K. E., Kristensen, B. O., and Hansen, O. K.: Frequency of occurrence of residual ductal flow after surgical ligation by color-flow mapping. Am. J. Cardiol., 67:653, 1991.

Souders, C. R., Pearson, C. M., and Adams, H.D.: An aortic deformity stimulating mediastinal tumor. A subclinical form of coarctation. Dis. Chest, 20:35, 1951.

Steidele, R. V.: Chir. Med. Beob. Vienna, 2:114, 1778.

Stejskal, L., and Stark, J.: Surgical treatment of persistent ductus arteriosus complicated by bacterial endocarditis. Eur. J. Cardiothorac. Surg., 6:272, 1992.

Sweeney, M. S., Walker, W. E., Duncan, J. M., et al.: Reoperation for aortic coarctation: Techniques, results, and indications for various approaches. Ann. Thorac. Surg., 40:48, 1985.

Todd, P. J., Dangerfield, P. H., Hamilton, D. I., and Wilkinson, J. L.: Late effects on the left upper limb of subclavian flap aortoplasty. J. Thorac. Cardiovasc. Surg., 85:678, 1983.

Touroff, A. S. W., and Vesell, H.: Subacute *Streptococcus viridans* endarteritis complicating patent ductus arteriosus. J. A. M. A., 115:1270, 1940.

Trinquet, F., Vouhe, P. R., Vernant, F., et al.: Coarctation of the aorta in infants: Which operation? Ann. Thorac. Surg., 45:186, 1988.

Turley, K., Yee, E. S., and Ebert, P. A.: The total repair of interrupted arch complex in infants: The anterior approach. Circulation, 70:16, 1984.

Tynan, M.: Transcatheter occlusion of persistent arterial duct. Lancet, 340:1062, 1992.

Ungerleider, R. M., and Ebert, P. E.: Indications and techniques for midline approach to aortic coarctation in infants and children. Ann. Thorac. Surg., 44:517, 1987.

Van Heurn, L. W. E., Wong, C. M., Spiegelhalter, D. J., et al.: Surgical treatment of aortic coarctation in infants age less than three months, 1985–1991. J. Thorac. Cardiovasc. Surg., 107:74, 1994.

Van Mierop, L. H. S., and Kutsche, L. M.: Cardiovascular anomalies in DiGeorge syndrome and importance of neural crest as a possible pathogenetic factor. Am. J. Cardiol., 58:133, 1986.

Van Mierop, L. H. S., and Kutsche, L. M.: Embryology of the Heart. *In* Hurst, J. W. (ed-in-chief): The Heart, Arteries and Veins. 7th ed. New York, McGraw-Hill Information Services, 1990.

Van Praagh, R., Bernard, W. F., Rosenthal, A., et al.: Interrupted aortic arch: Surgical treatment. Am. J. Cardiol., 27:200, 1971.

Van Son, J. A. M., Lacquet, L. K., and Smedts, F.: Patterns of ductal tissue in coarctation of the aorta in early infancy. J. Thorac. Cardiovasc. Surg., 105:368, 1993.

Vogel, M., Freedom, R. M., Smallhorn, J. F., et al.: Complete transposition of the great arteries of coarctation of the aorta. Am. J. Cardiol., 53:1627, 1984.

Vossschulte, K.: Surgical correction of coarctation of the aorta by an "isthmusplastic" operation. Thorax, 16:338, 1961.

Vouhe, P. R., Mace, L., Vernant, F., et al.: Primary definitive repair of interrupted aortic arch with ventricular septal defect. Eur. J. Cardiothorac. Surg., 4:365, 1990.

Waldhausen, J. A., and Nahrwold, D. L.: Repair of coarctation of the aorta with a subclavian flap. J. Thorac. Cardiovasc. Surg., 51:532, 1966.

Waldhausen, J. A., Whitman, V., Werner, J. C., and Pierce, W. S.: Surgical intervention in infants with coarctation of the aorta. J. Thorac. Cardiovasc. Surg., 81:323, 1981.

Webb, W. R., and Burford, T. H.: Gangrene of the arm following use of the subclavian artery in a pulmonosystemic (Blalock) anastomosis. J. Thorac. Surg., 23:199, 1952.

Weisman, D., and Kesten, H. D.: Absence of the transverse aortic arch with defects of cardiac septums: Report of a case simulating acute abdominal disease in a newborn infant. Am. J. Dis. Child., 76:326, 1948.

Welsh, T. M., and Munro, I. B.: Congenital stridor caused by an aberrant pulmonary artery. Arch. Dis. Child., 29:101, 1954.

Wernly, J. A., and Ameriso, J. L.: Intra-aortic closure of the calcified patent ductus. J. Thorac. Cardiovasc. Surg., 80:206, 1980.

Wessel, D. L., Keane, J. F., Parness, I., and Lock, J. E.: Outpatient closure of the patent ductus arteriosus. Circulation, 77:1068, 1988.

Wielenga, G., and Dankmeijer, J.: Coarctation of the aorta. J. Pathol. Bacteriol., 95:265, 1968.

Wierny, L., Plass, R., and Porstmann, W.: Transluminal closure of patent ductus arteriosus: Long-term results of 208 cases treated without thoracotomy. Cardiovasc. Intervent. Radiol., 9:279, 1986.

Will, R. J., Walker, O. M., Traugott, R. C., and Treasure, R. L.: Sodium nitroprusside and propranolol therapy for management of postcoarctectomy hypertension. J. Thorac. Cardiovasc. Surg., 75:722, 1978.

Wittenborg, M. H., Tantiwongse, T., and Rosenberg, B. F.: Anomalous course of left pulmonary artery with respiratory obstruction. Radiology, 67:339, 1956.

Wolman, I. J.: Syndrome of constricting double aortic arch in infancy. J. Pediatr., 14:527, 1939.

Wright, J. S., Freeman, R. R., and Johnston, J. B.: Aortopulmonary fenestration: A technique of surgical management. J. Thorac. Cardiovasc. Surg., 55:280, 1968.

Yee, E. S., Turley, K., Soifer, S., and Ebert, P. A.: Synthetic patch aortoplasty. Am. J. Surg., 148:240, 1984.

Young, W. G., Sealy, W. C., and Harris, J. S.: Effects of chronic constriction of the thoracic aorta upon renal dynamics. Surg. Forum, 1:200, 1950.

Zahka, K. G., Roland, J. M., Cutilletta, A. F., et al.: Management of aortic arch interruption with prostaglandin E$_1$ infusion and microporous expanded polytetrafluoroethylene grafts. Am. J. Cardiol., 46:1001, 1980.

Ziemer, G., Jonas, R. A., Perry, S. B., et al.: Surgery for coarctation of the aorta in the neonate. Circulation, 74(Suppl. I):25, 1986.

Zucker, N., Qureshi, S. A., Baker, E. J., et al.: Residual patency of the arterial duct after surgical ligation. J. Am. Coll. Cardiol., 21:323A, 1993.

Zumbro, G. L., Treasure, R. L., and Geiger, J. P.: Respiratory obstruction in the newborn associated with increased volume and opacification of the hemithorax. Ann. Thorac. Surg., 18:622, 1974.

# 33

■ **III** Aneurysms of the Sinuses of Valsalva

William L. Holman

The three sinuses of Valsalva are outpouchings in the aortic root that arise immediately distal to the aortic valve and are named either by their anatomic position (anterior, left posterior, and right posterior) or, more commonly, according to the coronary artery ostia that arise from the sinuses of Valsalva (right, left, and noncoronary). The first description of aneurysmal enlargement of one of these sinuses with intracardiac rupture is attributed to Hope (1839). Subsequently, Thurnam (1840) published a series of six cases, including the one described by Hope, and noted the importance of the anatomic relationship of these aneurysms to the chambers of the heart. The syphilitic etiology of sinus of Valsalva aneurysms was initially emphasized by Smith (1914). However, the work of Abbott (1919) clearly established a congenital etiology for sinus of Valsalva aneurysms. Dr. Abbott's concept of the congenital etiology for sinus of Valsalva aneurysms was subsequently furthered by Edwards and Burchell (1957), who histologically demonstrated the deficiency of elastic and muscular tissue at the site of congenital sinus of Valsalva aneurysms, and by Sakakibara and Konno (1962), who developed a classification system for congenital sinus of Valsalva aneurysms.

The advent of invasive cardiac diagnostic procedures and the development of cardiac surgery in the first half of the 20th century eventually led to the successful surgical treatment of sinus of Valsalva aneurysms. Ingenious methods were devised for the direct closure of ruptured sinus of Valsalva aneurysms, utilizing hypothermia with inflow occlusion (Bigelow and Barnes, 1959; Morrow et al., 1957). However, the open approach supported by extracorporeal circulation, as first described by McGoon and colleagues (1958) and Lillehei and associates (1957), eventually became the accepted method of treatment. Interestingly, the 1957 report by Lillehei and associates also included descriptions of an early bubble oxygenator and novel methods (e.g., cardioplegic arrest and continuous retrograde myocardial perfusion) to permit open surgical repair of ruptured sinus of Valsalva aneurysms (Holman, 1993).

## ANATOMY, PATHOPHYSIOLOGY, AND NATURAL HISTORY

An aneurysm of the sinus of Valsalva represents the pathologic enlargement of the sinus into a thin-walled sac. The aneurysm may be entirely asymptomatic, or it can produce symptoms by becoming infected, impinging on adjacent structures, or rupturing. The sinuses of Valsalva lie immediately distal to the aortic valve and its annulus within the aortic root (Sud et al., 1984). The right and left coronary arteries each arise from the corresponding sinus of Valsalva before the sinuses narrow distally to form the ascending aorta. An accurate conceptualization of the anatomic relations of the aortic root is crucial to understanding the pathophysiology associated with sinus of Valsalva aneurysms as well as their surgical treatment (Figs. 33–26 and 33–27).

Sinus of Valsalva aneurysms are uncommon, being noted in 7 of 8138 autopsies (Smith, 1914) and in 0.43%, 0.14%, and 0.96% of open heart cases performed at three cardiac surgical centers (Chu et al., 1990; Henze et al., 1983; Mayer et al., 1975). The differences between the anatomy of congenital and acquired sinus of Valsalva aneurysms stem from their different etiologies. Congenital aneurysms stem from a deficiency or absence of muscular and elastic tissue at the base of the aorta, as illustrated by Edwards and Burchell (1957) (Fig. 33–28). This structural deficiency may be related to an abnormality in the development of the distal bulbar septum (Abbott, 1919), a concept that is strengthened by the frequent (30 to 60%) association of ventricular septal defects (VSDs) and congenital sinus of Valsalva aneurysms (Bonfils-Roberts et al., 1971; Chih et al., 1981; Nowicki et al., 1977). The frequency of congenital sinus of Valsalva aneurysms is, therefore, highest in the right coronary cusp because this cusp abuts the largest portion of the septum. Sinus of Valsalva aneurysms occur less frequently in the noncoronary cusp, and rarely have congenital aneurysms been reported from the left coronary cusp (Jones and Langley, 1949; Mayer et al., 1975; Nowicki et al., 1977) (Table 33–1). The incidence of congenital sinus of Valsalva aneurysms appears to be higher in Asian populations, but the reason for this is not clear (Chu et al., 1990).

The anatomic classification system of Sakakibara and Konno defines congenital sinus of Valsalva aneurysms according to the their exact position relative to each aortic valve cusp (Sakakibara and Konno, 1962). Direct extension of aneurysms from the left or midportion of the right coronary sinus (Types I and II) directs the aneurysm into the right ventricle, whereas an aneurysm originating in the right portion of the right coronary sinus may penetrate either the right

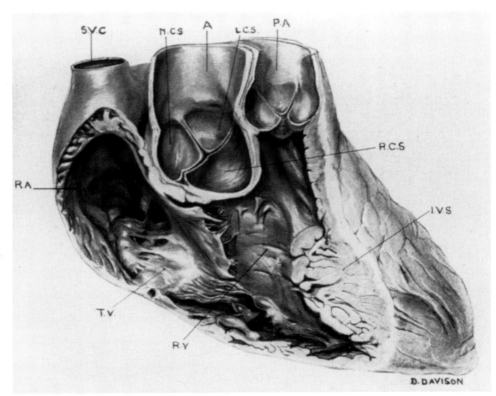

**FIGURE 33–26.** The relationship of the sinuses of Valsalva with the aortic root to the structures of the right heart. The anatomic distribution of fistulas resulting from the intracardiac rupture of aneurysms of the sinus of Valsalva can be understood by studying the anatomic relationships. (SVC = superior vena cava; RA = right atrium; TV = tricuspid valve; RV = right ventricle; NCS = noncoronary sinus; RCS = right coronary sinus; LCS = left coronary sinus; A = aorta; PA = pulmonary artery; IVS = intraventricular septum.) (From Jones, A. M., and Langley, F. A.: Aortic sinus aneurysms. Br. Heart. J., *11*:325, 1949.)

atrium or the right ventricle (Types III–V and IIIA). Aneurysms from the noncoronary sinus (Type IV) extend into the right atrium immediately above the septal leaflet of the tricuspid valve. The rare left coronary sinus aneurysms were not classified by Sakakibara and Konno (1962) but have been reported to pass into the right atrium, right ventricle, left atrium, left ventricle, and pericardial space. Besides VSDs, other congenital cardiac lesions associated with sinus of Valsalva aneurysms include aortic valve abnormalities (prolapsing cusp, bicuspid valve, or other valve deformity) in roughly 10% of patients and, rarely, pulmonary stenosis or regurgitation, atrial septal defects, or a patent ductus arteriosus (Bonfils-Roberts et al., 1971; Chih et al., 1981; Nowicki et al., 1977).

Acquired sinus of Valsalva aneurysms can be the result of several pathologic processes, including luetic degeneration (Smith, 1914), bacterial endocarditis (Bardy et al., 1982; Qizilbash, 1974; Shumacker, 1972), trauma (Morris et al., 1958; Murray et al., 1993), cystic medial necrosis (DeBakey et al., 1967), and atherosclerosis (DeBakey and Lawrie, 1979). The acquired aneurysms are more evenly distributed among the three sinuses, with 44% of reported cases arising from the right coronary sinus, 23% arising from the left coronary sinus, and 10% arising from multiple sinuses. As compared with congenital aneurysms, acquired aneurysms tend to occupy larger regions of the aortic root and may involve multiple sinuses of Valsalva and even the ascending aorta. In contradistinction to congenital aneurysms, the site of the acquired aneurysmal rupture is less frequently intracardiac (25%) and is more often a catastrophic hemorrhage into the pericardium or pleural space or externally (13%)

■ **Table 33–1.** THE ANATOMY OF RUPTURED AND NONRUPTURED CONGENITAL SINUS OF VALSALVA ANEURYSMS

| Site of Origin | Total | | Nonruptured | RA | RV | RA + RV | Site of Rupture | | | |
| | N | % | | | | | LA | LV | PA | Pericardium |
|---|---|---|---|---|---|---|---|---|---|---|
| RCS | 128 | 65% | 13 (10%) | 19 (14%) | 86 (67%) | 2 (2%) | 0 (0%) | 5 (4%) | 2 (2%) | 1 (1%) |
| NCS | 54 | 28% | 15 (28%) | 28 (51%) | 7 (13%) | 0 (0%) | 2 (4%) | 1 (2%) | 0 (0%) | 1 (2%) |
| LCS | 14 | 7% | 5 (36%) | 4 (29%) | 3 (21%) | 0 (0%) | 1 (7%) | 1 (7%) | 0 (0%) | 0 (0%) |

Data from Jones and Langley, 1949; Nowicki et al., 1977; and Mayer et al., 1986.
*Key*: RCS = right coronary sinus; NCS = noncoronary sinus; LCS = left coronary sinus; RA = right atrium; RV = right ventricle; LA = left atrium; LV = left ventricle; PA = pulmonary artery.

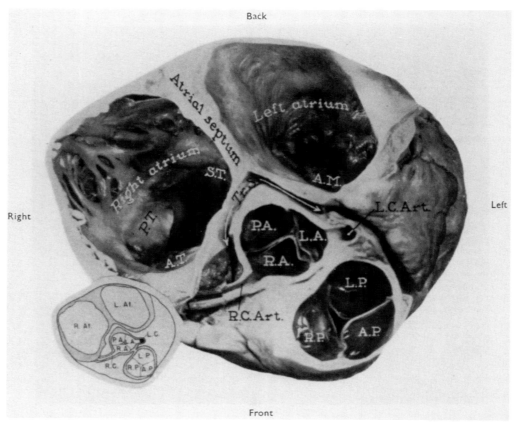

**FIGURE 33–27.** On coronal section, the aortic root is seen nestled within the central portion of the heart. The relationship of the sinuses of Valsalva to the right and left main coronary arteries is also emphasized. (PT, ST, AT = posterior, septal, and anterior tricuspid leaflets; AM = anterior mitral leaflet; TrS = transverse sinus; RA, PA, LA = right, posterior, and left aortic valve leaflets; LCArt = left main coronary artery; RCArt = right coronary artery; AP, RP, LP = anterior, right, and left pulmonary valve leaflets.) (From Edwards, J. E., and Burchell, H. R.: The pathologic anatomy of deficiencies between the aortic root and the heart, including aortic sinus aneurysms. Thorax, *12*:125, 1957.)

(DeBakey et al., 1979; Jones and Langley, 1949; Qizilbash, 1974).

Most patients with unruptured sinus of Valsalva aneurysms are asymptomatic, with a diagnosis made incidentally from cardiac diagnostic tests performed to examine other cardiac pathology. However, unruptured aneurysms may produce symptoms when they become infected or impinge on other structures. Aneurysmal extension into the right ventricular outflow tract may produce obstruction (Desai et al., 1985; Warnes et al., 1984), and extension into the ventricular septum can cause medically refractory ventricular tachycardia (Raizes et al., 1979) or other conduction abnormalities (Heydorn et al., 1976; Mayer et al., 1986). Enlargement of the sinus and intramural thrombus formation can cause deformation or obstruction of the left or right coronary arteries at their ostia, which then causes myocardial ischemia (Hiyamuta et al., 1983) or infarction (Brandt et al., 1985; Faillace et al., 1985). Embolic stroke associated with a large, thrombus-filled sinus of Valsalva aneurysm has been reported (Wortham et al., 1993).

Expansion of a sinus of Valsalva aneurysm into an adjacent cardiac chamber may be followed by rupture of the aneurysm. On gross inspection, this communication may appear either as a simple fistula tract or as a thin-walled windsock protrusion into a cardiac chamber, with distal perforation of the windsock (Fig. 33–29). The fistula tract formed after aneurysmal rupture allows blood to flow from the aorta into the affected cardiac chamber, and if the recipient chamber is the right atrium, right ventricle, or pulmonary artery, a net left-to-right shunting of blood occurs. As well described by Morch and Greenwood (1966), the murmur associated with the most commonly ruptured sinus of Valsalva aneurysms (aorta to right ventricle or right atrium) is a harsh continuous murmur that for diagnostic purposes must be distinguished from the murmur of a patent ductus arteriosus, VSD associated with aortic insufficiency, aortopulmonary window, coronary arteriovenous malformation, or pulmonary arteriovenous malformation.

In one-third of patients, left-to-right shunting immediately following the rupture of a sinus of Valsalva aneurysm into the right side of the heart produces acute dyspnea and substernal chest pain that is often associated with epigastric or right upper quadrant abdominal pain. However, one-half of patients note the *gradual* onset of dyspnea, fatigue, chest pain, and peripheral edema over several months or even years

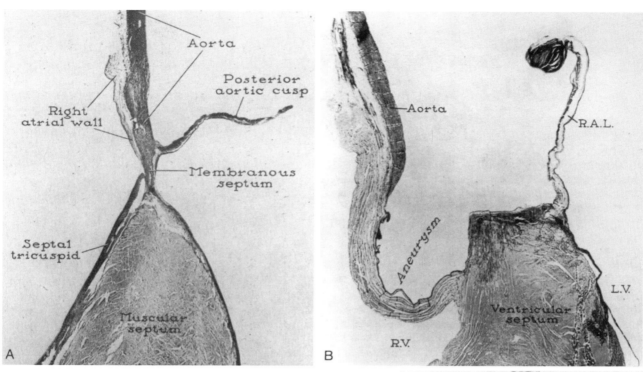

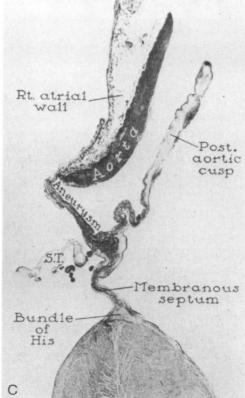

**FIGURE 33–28.** *A,* Longitudinal section of normal heart taken through noncoronary sinus of Valsalva. *B,* Longitudinal section of heart taken through aneurysm of the right sinus of Valsalva. Note the attenuated wall of the aneurysm descending along the right side of the ventricular septum toward the right ventricle. (RV = right ventricle; LV = left ventricle; RAL = right aortic valve leaflet.) *C,* Longitudinal section of aorta taken through the noncoronary cusp. A thin-walled sinus of Valsalva aneurysm is protruding into the right atrium immediately above the septal leaflet of the tricuspid valve. (ST = septal leaflet of tricuspid valve; post. aortic cusp = posterior [noncoronary] aortic valve cusp.) (*A–C,* From Edwards, J. E., and Burchell, H. B.: The pathologic anatomy of deficiencies between the aortic root and the heart, including aortic sinus aneurysms. Thorax, *12*:125, 1957.)

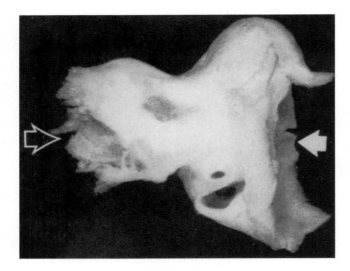

**FIGURE 33–29.** Gross appearance of ruptured aneurysm of the sinus of Valsalva. The *white arrow* designates the aortic side of the aneurysm and the *black arrow* designates the point of rupture. (From McKenney, P. A., Shemin, R. J., and Wiegers, S. E.: Role of transesophageal echocardiography in sinus of Valsalva aneurysm. Am. Heart J., *123*:229, 1992.)

following rupture of a sinus of Valsalva aneurysm, and the remainder of patients remain asymptomatic at the time of diagnosis (Bonfils-Roberts et al., 1971; Mayer et al., 1986; Nowicki et al., 1977). Patients with ruptured sinus of Valsalva aneurysms are most commonly men (two-thirds of patients) in the third or fourth decade of life (50 to 60% of patients), although neonates (Perry et al., 1991) and elderly patients have been reported. A continuous murmur at the left sternal border is almost always audible (90 to 95% of patients), and in roughly one-half of patients, physical signs of congestive heart failure, including rales, peripheral edema, ascites, and hepatomegaly, are present at the time of presentation (Mayer et al., 1986; Nowicki et al., 1977). The natural history of unruptured sinus of Valsalva aneurysms is impossible to

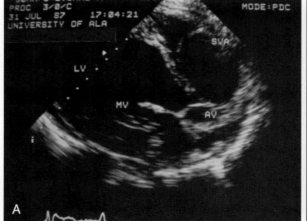

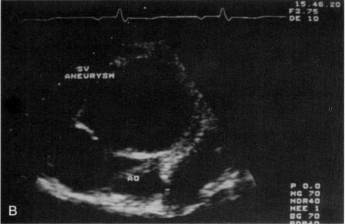

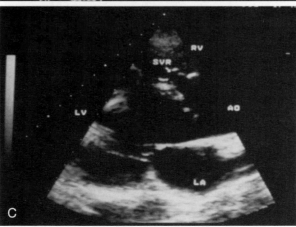

**FIGURE 33–30.** *A,* This echocardiographic image is a modified parasternal long-axis view that demonstrates a large sinus of Valsalva aneurysm (SVA) bulging into the right ventricle. (LV = left ventricle; MV = mitral valve; AV = aortic valve.) *B,* This short-axis view demonstrates enlargement of single sinus as well as central noncoaptation of the aortic valve leaflets. (SV aneurysm = sinus of Valsalva aneurysm; AO = aorta.) *C,* This patient had discontinuity of the sinus of Valsalva aneurysm at the point where the aneurysm ruptured into the right ventricle. Flow through the ruptured sinus of Valsalva aneurysm as well as through a ventricular septal defect was noted on color Doppler examination (not shown). (SVR = sinus of Valsalva rupture; RV = right ventricle; LV = left ventricle; AO = aorta; LA = left atrium.) (*A–C,* From Nanda, N. C.: Atlas of Color Doppler Echocardiography. Philadelphia, Lea & Febiger, 1989, pp. 524–525.)

define accurately, because most unruptured aneurysms are asymptomatic and probably remain undiagnosed. Although there is at least one report of an asymptomatic congenital sinus of Valsalva aneurysm that was followed without surgical intervention for 19 years (Martin et al., 1986), the excellent surgical results reported for nonruptured sinus of Valsalva aneurysms support surgical intervention (Jebara et al., 1992).

Rupture of a sinus of Valsalva aneurysm usually produces serious pathologic changes. Extracardiac rupture is generally fatal (Brabham and Roberts, 1990), although there is one reported survivor of an intrapericardial rupture (Killen et al., 1987). Intracardiac rupture of a sinus of Valsalva aneurysm may produce symptoms that improve spontaneously following the event. However, over time, cardiac decompensation occurs with cardiac failure that is eventually fatal if the aneurysm is not surgically treated. In addition, the associated problems of bacterial endocarditis and aortic insufficiency due to weakening of the annulus with cusp prolapse may occur and cause significant additional morbidity and mortality. In patients not surgically treated, the mean survival time after diagnosis of a ruptured sinus of Valsalva aneurysm has been reported to be 3.9 years, although if 2 unusual patients who survived for 10 and 15 years are excluded from this series of 45 cases, the mean survival time would be roughly 1 year (Sawyers et al., 1957).

The diagnosis of ruptured sinus of Valsalva aneurysm is generally made by history and physical examination in connection with echocardiography and angiography (Figs. 33–30 and 33-31) to define the precise anatomy of the aneurysm. Magnetic resonance imaging has also been used (Ogawa et al., 1991). Several points should be considered and clearly defined prior to surgery. VSDs associated with sinus of Valsalva aneurysms generally lie immediately below the aneurysm. Without careful attention, these VSDs may remain undiagnosed, particularly if the wall of the aneurysm descends to particularly occlude the flow through the VSD (Sakakibara and Konno, 1963). Aortic valve abnormalities, primarily abnormalities that lead to aortic insufficiency, are common. The degree of aortic insufficiency and an assessment of its effect on left ventricular function are therefore important. The position and patency of the coronary arteries should also be confirmed, particularly in larger aneurysms.

Over the past several years, echocardiography with color-flow Doppler mapping has had an increasingly important role in the diagnosis of sinus of Valsalva aneurysms. In one series, patients underwent surgery after echocardiography without additional diagnostic evaluation (Sahasakul et al., 1990).

## SURGICAL TREATMENT AND RESULTS

The repair of congenital sinus of Valsalva aneurysms may be accomplished by approaching the lesion from either the chamber of origin (e.g., the aorta) or the chamber of termination. The exact approach

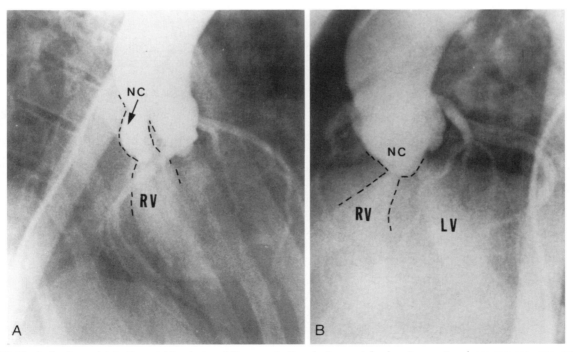

FIGURE 33–31. *A*, Aortic root injection, right anterior oblique projection during systole showing ruptured noncoronary aneurysm of the sinus of Valsalva terminating in the right ventricle. *B*, Left anterior oblique projection, aortic root injection during diastole in the same patient demonstrating regurgitation of aortic blood into the right ventricle via the aneurysm of the sinus of Valsalva, and regurgitation into the left ventricle related to mild aortic insufficiency. (NC = noncoronary cusp; RV = right ventricle; LV = left ventricle.) (*A* and *B*, Courtesy of Dr. Benigno Soto, University of Alabama at Birmingham.)

chosen depends on several factors, including whether the aneurysm has ruptured and whether there is associated aortic valvular insufficiency or a VSD. The goal is to close the aneurysm securely and obliterate or excise the aneurysmal sac, while avoiding the creation of aortic valve dysfunction or heart block. Standard dual venous cannulation and aortic cannulation are performed, and the left ventricle may be vented.

Prior to ventricular fibrillation, the aorta is cross-clamped and cardioplegia solution is infused. If aortic insufficiency is not present and rupture of the aneurysm has not occurred, or if the fistula is digitally occluded, the cardioplegic solution may be infused directly into the aortic root. Otherwise, ostial cardioplegia infusion or retrograde cardioplegia infusion is used.

The aortic root is inspected to assess valvular competence and the severity of pathologic changes in the structure of the aortic root. The ventricular septum is examined carefully for defects, and the position and patency of the coronary artery ostia are checked. If the aneurysm is reasonably small and has not ruptured, closure of the aneurysm via a transaortic exposure of the sinus of Valsalva is sufficient (Henze et al., 1983; Mayer et al., 1975; Shumacker et al., 1965) (Fig. 33–32). The closure of the aortic aspect of the aneurysm can occasionally be accomplished with interrupted sutures with or without Teflon felt buttressing. However, this closure is best accomplished using a Dacron patch, possibly with an added layer of pericardium, to avoid deforming the normal coaptation of the aortic valve and to diminish stress on the suture line. If the aneurysm has ruptured, the chamber of termination (usually the right atrium, right ventricle, or pulmonary artery) should also be opened to expose the fistula tract (Bonfils-Roberts et al., 1971; Chih et al., 1981; DeBakey et al., 1967; Lillehei et al., 1957; Mayer et al., 1986; McGoon et al., 1958). If a windsock deformity is present, it is excised, and the terminal orifice of the fistula is occluded with sutures or a patch. The ventricular surface is also closely examined for a VSD. If one is found, both the sinus of Valsalva aneurysm and the VSD orifices may be occluded with a single patch (Fig. 33–33). Transaortic repair of the VSD has been reported; however, because of the risk of injury to the His bundle and complete heart block, the right-sided approach is usually preferable.

If there is aortic valve insufficiency due to cusp prolapse, the native valve may be salvaged using the technique of aortic valvuloplasty described by Trusler and co-workers (1973). If there is other valvular pathology that does not lend itself to correction via this technique, then valve replacement is performed using the standard criteria for aortic valve replacement. All valve procedures should be performed after the sinus of Valsalva aneurysm repair has been completed.

Compared with congenital sinus of Valsalva aneurysms, acquired aneurysms are a more heterogeneous

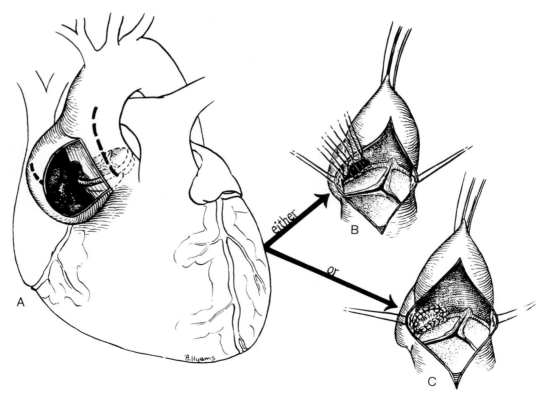

**FIGURE 33–32.** Transaortic repair of aneurysm of the sinus of Valsalva may be accomplished either by direct closure of the mouth of the aneurysm with interrupted sutures or by patching of the orifice of the aneurysm. (From Meyer, J., Wukash, D. C., Hallman, G. L., and Cooley, D. A.: Aneurysm and fistula of the sinus of Valsalva. Reprinted with permission from the Society of Thoracic Surgeons [The Annals of Thoracic Surgery, Vol. 19, 1975, pp. 170–179].)

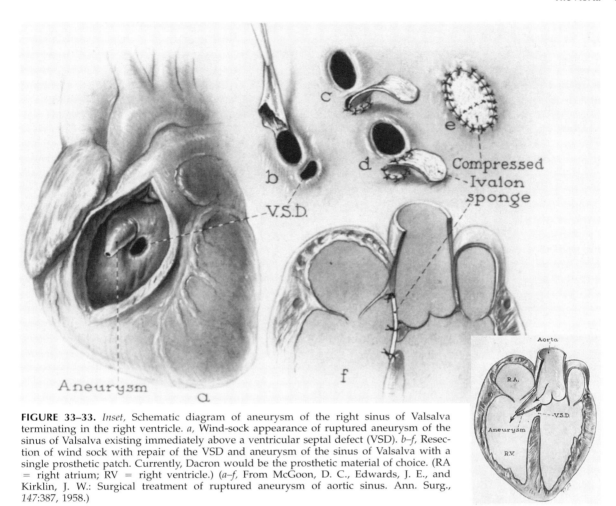

**FIGURE 33–33.** *Inset,* Schematic diagram of aneurysm of the right sinus of Valsalva terminating in the right ventricle. *a,* Wind-sock appearance of ruptured aneurysm of the sinus of Valsalva existing immediately above a ventricular septal defect (VSD). *b–f,* Resection of wind sock with repair of the VSD and aneurysm of the sinus of Valsalva with a single prosthetic patch. Currently, Dacron would be the prosthetic material of choice. (RA = right atrium; RV = right ventricle.) (*a–f,* From McGoon, D. C., Edwards, J. E., and Kirklin, J. W.: Surgical treatment of ruptured aneurysm of aortic sinus. Ann. Surg., *147*:387, 1958.)

group in terms of etiology and anatomic extent of disease. Sinus of Valsalva aneurysms due to luetic degeneration or cystic medical necrosis may be confined to a single sinus, but often the entire aortic root is affected with aneurysmal enlargement of the ascending aorta distally and severe aortic valvular insufficiency proximally. As described by DeBakey and colleagues (1967), some of these lesions can be managed occasionally by excision of the aneurysmal region and primary closure or Dacron patching with reimplantation of coronary arteries as necessary (Fig. 33–34). More often, acquired sinus of Valsalva aneurysms require complete replacement of the aortic root.

Sinus of Valsalva aneurysms due to advanced bacterial endocarditis are often associated with extensive burrowing abscesses and destruction of tissue in the region of the aortic annulus. Débridement and reconstruction of the aortic root are usually the only therapeutic options, and these are attempted despite the attendant risks of reinfection and high operative mortality (Bardy et al., 1982; Qizilbash, 1974; Shumacker, 1972). Aortic root replacement with a homograft minimizes the risk of reinfection in this setting.

Sinus of Valsalva aneurysms have been associated with both atherosclerotic coronary artery disease and atherosclerotic degeneration of the aorta (DeBakey and Lawrie, 1979), and they have been managed successfully by excision and patching of the aneurysmal region and coronary artery bypass grafting in lieu of coronary reimplantation.

Management of unruptured asymptomatic sinus of Valsalva aneurysms remains an unresolved controversy. The importance of this controversy is increasing as noninvasive cardiac diagnostic procedures become more accurate and widely available. Some authorities feel that this subgroup of aneurysms can be followed by serial observations and argue that if the aneurysm enlarges, ruptures, or begins to cause symptoms related to impingement on adjacent structures, surgical therapy can be initiated with no additional risk (Martin et al., 1986; Mayer et al., 1975). The one report of a patient followed successfully for 19 years would support this contention. However, most surgeons reporting on sinus of Valsalva aneurysms feel that the risks of surgical correction are acceptable in light of the many serious potential complications of unruptured sinus of Valsalva aneurysms, including right ventricular outflow tract obstruction, infection, malignant arrhythmias, or acute ostial coronary artery obstruction (Faillace et al., 1985; Heydorn et al., 1976;

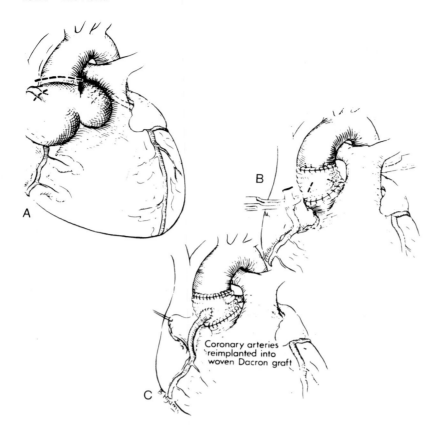

Coronary arteries
reimplanted into
woven Dacron graft

**FIGURE 33–34.** *A,* Acquired aneurysm of the sinus of Valsalva involving multiple sinuses. *B,* Resection of aneurysm of the sinus of Valsalva with prosthetic tube graft. *C,* Coronary reimplantation to restore coronary arterial flow. (*A–C,* From Meyer, J., Wukash, D. C., Hallman, G. L., and Cooley, D. A.: Aneurysm and fistula of the sinus of Valsalva. Reprinted with permission from the Society of Thoracic Surgeons [The Annals of Thoracic Surgery, Vol. 19, 1975, pp. 170–179].)

Jebara et al., 1992; Mayer et al., 1975). Once symptoms related to a sinus of Valsalva aneurysm are identified or once rupture of the aneurysm has occurred, operative repair should be advised. Sinus of Valsalva aneurysms that are discovered incidentally at the time of surgery for other cardiac pathology also should be repaired unless specific contraindications exist.

The results of repair reported for a small number of asymptomatic patients with unruptured aneurysms is excellent (Jebara et al., 1992). In contrast, the short- and long-term results of surgical therapy for sinus of Valsalva aneurysms associated with bacterial endocarditis has been poor (Bardy et al., 1982; Qizilbash, 1974; Shumacker, 1972). The early postoperative mortality following repair in patients with noninfected congenital sinus of Valsalva aneurysms has ranged from 0% (Bonfils-Roberts et al., 1971; Mayer et al., 1986; Pasic et al., 1992) to 10 to 12% (Chih et al., 1981; Nowicki et al., 1977). The perioperative deaths were primarily related to low postoperative cardiac output, and often occurred in patients undergoing simultaneous correction of coexisting cardiac anomalies. Longer-term surgical follow-up has been reported by several groups (Bonfils-Roberts et al., 1971; Chih et al., 1981; Chu et al., 1990; DeBakey et al., 1967; Mayer et al., 1975; Nowicki et al., 1977) and ranges up to 20 years in one series. Postrepair recurrence of the aneurysm is rare, and has led to a fatality in only one reported case. Persistent improvement in symptoms as determined by assessment of New York Heart Association functional class after closure of a ruptured sinus of Valsalva aneurysm has been shown to occur

in 80 to 90% of patients. Late cardiovascular morbidity and mortality are uncommon in these series, but include native valve endocarditis, recurrence of previously repaired VSDs, and problems associated with prosthetic aortic valve replacement (e.g., thrombosis, dehiscence, infection, degeneration, and embolization). If there is mild to moderate postrepair aortic insufficiency, it tends to increase slowly over time and ultimately may lead to a second operation for valve replacement. In general, the prognosis for patients undergoing surgical repair of sinus of Valsalva aneurysms is excellent unless their condition is complicated by extensive involvement of the aortic root and ascending aorta, infection, aortic valve dysfunction requiring valve replacement, or impaired ventricular function related to chronic aortic insufficiency or other coexisting cardiac disorders.

## SELECTED BIBLIOGRAPHY

Chu, S. H., Hung, C. R., How, S. S., et al.: Ruptured aneurysms of the sinus of Valsalva aneurysms in Oriental patients. J. Thorac. Cardiovasc. Surg., *99*:288, 1990.

Fifty-seven cases of ruptured sinus of Valsalva aneurysms treated by the authors were combined with 361 additional cases collected from previous publications. Asian patients had a higher incidence of sinus of Valsalva aneurysms arising from the right coronary sinus and a higher incidence of associated ventricular septal defects. However, there were fewer other congenital cardiac abnormalities in the Asian group compared with the non-Asian group.

Jebara, B. A., Chauvaud, S., Portoghese, M., et al.: Isolated extracardiac unruptured sinus of Valsalva aneurysms. Ann. Thorac. Surg., *54*:323, 1992.

This report describes four cases of isolated unruptured sinus of Valsalva aneurysms that underwent elective repair. Repair was achieved by patch reconstruction of the involved sinus and did not require aortic valve replacement in any of the patients. Subsequent examinations showed excellent surgical results. This report supports surgical intervention in patients with large sinus of Valsalva aneurysms even though they are asymptomatic at initial presentation.

Jones, A. M., and Langley, F. A.: Aortic sinus aneurysms. Br. Heart J., 11:325, 1949.

In this beautifully written and illustrated article, the authors define the anatomy of the aortic root as it relates to sinus of Valsalva aneurysms, then carefully define the clinical features and pathophysiology of this condition. The distinction between congenital and acquired sinus of Valsalva aneurysms is emphasized, and a collected review of patients is included which illustrates the natural history of this condition.

Mayer, E. D., Ruffman, K., Saggau W., et al.: Ruptured aneurysms of the sinus of Valsalva. Ann. Thorac. Surg., 42:81, 1986.

This review of 15 patients treated for both congenital and acquired sinus of Valsalva aneurysms includes a summary of the incidence and clinical features of this disorder. All of the patients underwent surgery, and there were no early or late postoperative deaths. The clinical condition of the patients is described for a follow-up period that averaged 7.9 years, with a range of 10 months to 20 years.

Nowicki, E. R., Aberdeen, E., Friedman, S., and Rashkind, W. J.: Congenital left aortic sinus–left ventricle fistula and review of aortocardiac fistulas. Ann. Thorac. Surg., 23:378, 1977.

This review article summarizes the findings previously published for 175 cases of aortocardiac fistulas published in the English literature from 1839 through 1972. There is an excellent summary of the clinical syndrome resulting from the formation of an aortocardiac fistula, and the principles of operative treatment are well reviewed.

Sakakibara, S., and Konno, S.: Congenital aneurysm of the sinus of Valsalva. Anatomy and classification. Am. Heart J., 63:405, 1962.

The authors draw on their own extensive personal experience, as well as an excellent review of previous literature, to summarize the anatomy of congenital sinus of Valsalva aneurysms and to organize these aneurysms into a classification system that defines four basic groups. The etiology and development of sinus of Valsalva aneurysms and the relationship of these aneurysms to ventricular septal defects are discussed.

## BIBLIOGRAPHY

Abbott, M. E.: Clinical and developmental study of a case of ruptured aneurysm of the right anterior aortic sinus of Valsalva, leading to communication between the aorta and base of the right ventricle, diagnosed during life, opening in anterior interventricular septum (probably bulbar septal defect) malignant endocarditis. In Contributions to Medical and Biological Research. New York, Paul B. Hoeber, 1919, p. 899.

Bardy, G. H., Valenstein, P., Stack, R. S., et al.: Two-dimensional echocardiographic identification of sinus of Valsalva–right heart fistula due to infective endocarditis. Am. Heart J., 103:1068, 1982.

Bigelow, W. G., and Barnes, W. T.: Ruptured aneurysm of aortic sinus. Ann. Surg., 150:117, 1959.

Bonfils-Roberts, E. A., Dushane, J. W., McGoon, D. C., et al.: Aortic sinus fistula: Surgical considerations and results of operation. Ann. Thorac. Surg., 12:492, 1971.

Brabham, K. R., and Roberts, W. C.: Fatal intrapericardial rupture of sinus of Valsalva aneurysm. Am. Heart J., 120:1455, 1990.

Brandt, J., Jogi, P., and Luhrs, C.: Sinus of Valsalva aneurysm obstructing coronary arterial flow: Case report and collective review of the literature. Eur. Heart J., 6:1069, 1985.

Chih, P., Heng, T. C., Chun, C., et al.: Surgical treatment of the ruptured aneurysm of the aortic sinuses. Ann. Thorac. Surg., 32:162, 1981.

Chu, S. H., Hung, C. R., How, S. S., et al.: Ruptured aneurysms of the sinus of Valsalva in Oriental patients. J. Thorac. Cardiovasc. Surg., 99:288, 1990.

DeBakey, M. E., Diethrich, E. B., Liddicoat, J. E., et al.: Abnormalities of the sinuses of Valsalva: Experience with 35 patients. J. Thorac. Cardiovasc. Surg., 54:312, 1967.

DeBakey, M. E., and Lawrie, G. M.: Aneurysm of sinus of Valsalva with coronary atherosclerosis: Successful surgical correction. Ann. Surg., 189:303, 1979.

Desai, A. G., Sharma, S., Kumar, A., et al.: Echocardiographic diagnosis of unruptured aneurysm of right sinus of Valsalva: An unusual cause of right ventricular outflow obstruction. Am. Heart J., 109:363, 1985.

Edwards, J. E., and Burchell, H. B.: The pathological anatomy of deficiencies between the aortic root and the heart, including aortic sinus aneurysms. Thorax, 12:125, 1957.

Faillace, R. T., Greenland, P., and Nanda, N. C.: Rapid expansion of a saccular aneurysm on the left coronary sinus of Valsalva: A role for early surgical repair? Br. Heart J., 54:442, 1985.

Henze, A., Huttunen, H., and Bjork, V. O.: Ruptured sinus of Valsalva aneurysms. Scand. J. Thorac. Cardiovasc. Surg., 17: 249, 1983.

Heydorn, W. H., Nelson, W. P., Fitterer, J. D., et al.: Congenital aneurysm of the sinus of Valsalva protruding into the left ventricle: Review of diagnosis and treatment of the unruptured aneurysm. J. Thorac. Cardiovasc. Surg., 71:839, 1976.

Hiyamuta, K., Ohtsuki, T., Shimamatsu, M., et al.: Aneurysm of the left aortic sinus causing acute myocardial infarction. Circulation, 67:1151, 1983.

Holman, W. L.: Sinus of Valsalva aneurysms and application of surgical science to their repair. Ann. Thorac. Surg., 55:545, 1993.

Hope, J. (ed): A Treatise on the Diseases of the Heart and Great Vessels. 3rd ed. Philadelphia, Lea & Blanchard, 1839, pp. 466–471.

Jebara, V. A., Chauvaud, S., Portoghese, M., et al.: Isolated extracardiac unruptured sinus of Valsalva aneurysms. Ann. Thorac. Surg., 54:323, 1992.

Jones, A. M., and Langley, F. A.: Aortic sinus aneurysms. Br. Heart J., 11:325, 1949.

Killen, D. A., Wathanacharoen, S., and Pogson, G. W., Jr.: Repair of intrapericardial rupture of left sinus of Valsalva aneurysm. Ann. Thorac. Surg., 44:310, 1987.

Lillehei, C. W., Stanley, P., and Varco, R. L.: Surgical treatment of ruptured aneurysms of the sinus of Valsalva. Ann. Surg., 146:459, 1957.

Martin, L. W., Hsu, I., Schwartz, H., et al.: Congenital aneurysm of the left sinus of Valsalva: Report of a patient with 19-year survival without surgery. Chest, 90:143, 1986.

Mayer, E. D., Ruffman, K., Saggau, W., et al.: Ruptured aneurysms of the sinus of Valsalva. Ann. Thorac. Surg., 42:81, 1986.

Mayer, J. H., III, Holder, T. M., and Canent, R. V.: Isolated, unruptured sinus of Valsalva aneurysm: Serendipitous detection and correction. J. Thorac. Cardiovasc. Surg., 69:429, 1975.

McGoon, D. C., Edwards, J. E., and Kirklin, J. W.: Surgical treatment of ruptured aneurysm of aortic sinus. Ann. Surg., 147:387, 1958.

McKenney, P. A., Shemin, R. J., Wiegers, S. E.: Role of transesophageal echocardiography in sinus of Valsalva aneurysm. Am. Heart J., 123:228, 1992.

Morch, J. E., and Greenwood, W. F.: Rupture of the sinus of Valsalva: A study of eight cases with discussion on the differential diagnosis of continuous murmurs. Am. J. Cardiol., 18:827, 1966.

Morris, G. C., Jr., Foster, R. P., Dunn, J. R., et al.: Traumatic aortico-ventricular fistula: Report of two cases successfully repaired. Am. Surg., 24:883, 1958.

Morrow, A. G., Baker, R. R., Hanson, H. E., et al.: Successful surgical repair of a ruptured aneurysm of the sinus of Valsalva. Circulation, 16:533, 1957.

Murray, E. G., Minami, K., Kortke, H., et al.: Traumatic sinus of Valsalva fistula and aortic valve rupture. Ann. Thorac. Surg., 55:760, 1993.

Nowicki, E. R., Aberdeen, E., Friedman, S., et al.: Congenital left aortic sinus–left ventricle fistula and review of aortocardiac fistulas. Ann. Thorac. Surg., 23:378, 1977.

Ogawa, T., Iwama, Y., and Hashimoto, H.: Noninvasive methods in the diagnosis of ruptured aneurysm of Valsalva. Chest, 100:579, 1991.

Pasic, M., von Segesser, L., Carrel, T. H., et al.: Ruptured congenital aneurysm of the sinus of Valsalva: Surgical technique and long-term follow-up. Eur. J. Cardiothorac. Surg., 6:542, 1992.

Perry, L. W., Martin, G. R., Galioto, F. M., et al.: Rupture of congenital sinus of Valsalva aneurysm in a newborn. Am. J. Cardiol., 68:1255, 1991.

Qizilbash, A. H.: Myotic aneurysm of the aortic sinus of Valsalva with rupture. Arch. Pathol., 98:414, 1974.

Raizes, G. S., Smith, H. C., Vlietstra, R. E., et al.: Ventricular tachycardia secondary to aneurysm of sinus of Valsalva. J. Thorac. Cardiovasc. Surg., 78:110, 1979.

Sahasakul, Y., Panchavinnin, P., Chaithiraphan, S., et al.: Echocardiographic diagnosis of a ruptured aneurysm of the sinus of Valsalva: Operation without catheterization in seven patients. Br. Heart J., 54:195, 1990.

Sakakibara, S., and Konno, S.: Congenital aneurysm of the sinus of Valsalva: Anatomy and classification. Am. Heart J., 63:405, 1962.

Sakakibara, S., and Konno, S.: Congenital aneurysm of the sinus of Valsalva: Criteria for recommending surgery. Am. J. Cardiol., 12:100, 1963.

Sawyers, J. L., Adams, J. E., and Scott, H. W., Jr.: Surgical treatment for aneurysms of the aortic sinuses with aorticoatrial fistula: Experimental and clinical study. Surgery, 41:26, 1957.

Shumacker, H. B., Jr.: Aneurysms of the aortic sinuses of Valsalva due to bacterial endocarditis, with special reference to their operative management. J. Thorac. Cardiovasc. Surg., 63:896, 1972.

Shumacker, H. B., Jr., King, H., and Waldhausen, J. A.: Transaortic approach for the repair of ruptured aneurysms of the sinuses of Valsalva. Ann. Surg., 161:946, 1965.

Smith, W. A.: Aneurysm of the sinus of Valsalva, with report of two cases. J. A. M. A., 62:1878, 1914.

Sud, A. Parker, F., and Magilligan, D. J., Jr.: Anatomy of the aortic root. Ann. Thorac. Surg., 38:76, 1984.

Thurnam, J.: On aneurysms, and especially spontaneous varicose aneurysms of ascending aorta and sinus of Valsalva, with cases. Medicochir. Trans., 23:323, 1840.

Trusler, G. A., Moes, C. A. F., and Kidd, B. S. L.: Repair of ventricular septal defect with aortic insufficiency. J. Thorac. Cardiovasc. Surg., 66:394, 1973.

Warnes, C. A., Maron, B. J., Jones, M., et al.: Asymptomatic sinus of Valsalva aneurysm causing right ventricular outflow obstruction before and after rupture. Am. J. Cardiol., 54:1383, 1984.

Wortham, D. C., Gorman, P. D., Hull, R. W., et al.: Unruptured sinus of Valsalva aneurysm presenting with embolization. Am. Heart J., 125:896, 1993.

# ■ IV  Thoracic Aortic Aneurysms and Aortic Dissection

Lawrence H. Cohn

## THORACIC AORTIC ANEURYSMS

A true aneurysm of the aorta is a localized enlargement of the aorta contained by all layers of the normal aortic wall, whereas a false aneurysm of the aorta consists only of aortic adventitia and periaortic fibrous tissue. The intrathoracic aorta may be aneurysmal from the ascending aorta above the aortic valve to the diaphragm and into the abdomen, forming a thoracoabdominal aneurysm. Approximately one-fourth of all arteriosclerotic aneurysms involve the thoracic aorta (Crisler and Bahnson, 1972; Joyce et al., 1964; Lindsay, 1979a). The degenerative pathologic process that causes an aneurysm to form includes medial degeneration and increased local dilatation. Other causes of aneurysms of the thoracic aorta include syphilis (ascending only), bacterial infections (mycotic), congenital abnormalities, trauma, and annuloaortic ectasia usually associated with Marfan's syndrome. Although the pathologic processes may differ microscopically and etiologically, the fundamental process of dilatation, continued expansion with local pressure-related symptoms, and eventual rupture is the same for all aneurysms.

The ultimate therapy for aneurysmal disease of the thoracic aorta is excision and prosthetic grafting. Within that context there are a wide variety of surgical approaches to the different anatomic segments of the aorta: (1) the ascending aorta, (2) the arch of the aorta, (3) the descending thoracic aorta, and (4) the thoracoabdominal aorta.

Surgical treatment of thoracic aneurysms began in the early 1950s by Lam and Aram (1951), who introduced homografts for descending thoracic aneurysms; DeBakey and Cooley (1953), who pioneered the use of artificial grafts; and Bahnson (1953), who introduced aneurysmorrhaphy. After these initial operations, the surgical treatment of thoracic aneurysms expanded to many centers and artificial grafts became generally available.

The ascending aorta and arch of the aorta were first successfully approached using modern *cardiopulmonary bypass* (CPB) techniques (Cooley and DeBakey, 1956; DeBakey et al., 1957). Continuing technical modifications have improved the surgical treatment of ascending, arch, and descending aortic aneurysms through development of new graft prostheses and conceptual advances in protection of the spinal cord and perfusion techniques. The one-piece valve graft conduit first proposed by Bentall and deBono (1968) and by Edwards and Kerr (1970) was an important advance in the treatment of Marfan's syndrome and annuloaortic ectasia. Considerable improvement in survival after arch aneurysms has followed the technical advances of using a single anastomosis for the cerebral vessel button (Bloodwell et al., 1968), profound hypothermia, and circulatory arrest with new support techniques (Griepp et al., 1975) and graft technology (Crawford and Crawford, 1984).

## Natural History

The natural history of thoracic aortic aneurysms is not as well documented as that for abdominal aneurysms, but it appears similar to that of any arterial aneurysms—that is, the signs, symptoms, and prognosis in a patient with an aneurysm are related to the size of the aneurysm. The law of Laplace states that as a sphere increases in size, the wall tension of that sphere increases. Thus, thoracic aneurysms larger than 6 cm are more prone to rupture than are smaller ones (Lindsay, 1979b). The natural history of thoracic aneurysms has been difficult to document because so many patients have generalized arteriosclerosis that more than half with a diagnosed thoracic aneurysm will not be alive in 5 years. In a classic study by Joyce and colleagues (1964), the 5-year survival rate was 27% for symptomatic aneurysms, whereas 58% of patients survived for 5 years with an asymptomatic aneurysm. One-third of the deaths were attributed to aneurysm rupture, and more than half of the mortality was due to the effects of generalized arteriosclerosis in other vascular beds. Bickerstaff and co-workers (1982) reported a 5-year survival rate of only 19% after diagnosis of a thoracic aneurysm. In this study,

aneurysm rupture occurred in 74% of patients. A large study by Pressler and McNamara (1985) revealed that rupture was also the most common cause of death. In this series, rupture accounted for 44% of the deaths, whereas the surgical mortality for aneurysm resection was significantly lower than the risk of late death in untreated patients.

## Pathophysiologic Anatomic Correlations

### Arteriosclerotic Aneurysms

Arteriosclerosis, the most common cause of thoracic aortic aneurysms, produces a nonspecific degenerative process in the aortic wall. Approximately half of the aneurysms that require surgical therapy are related to this diagnosis (Crawford and Crawford, 1984). These aneurysms are usually fusiform but may be saccular. They are more common in the ascending than the descending thoracic aorta, and least common in the aortic arch (Bickerstaff et al., 1982).

### Annuloaortic Ectasia

Annuloaortic ectasia in the ascending aorta is commonly associated with cystic medial necrosis (Lemon and White, 1978; Lindsay, 1979a; Pyeritz and McKusick, 1979). These changes include necrosis and absence of muscle cells in the elastic laminar and cystic spaces filled with the mucoid material (Fig. 33–35).

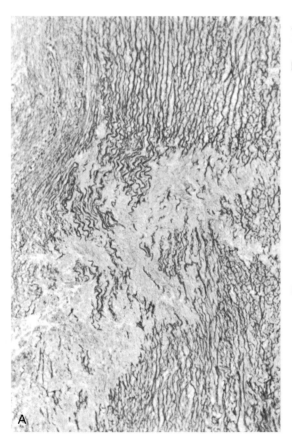

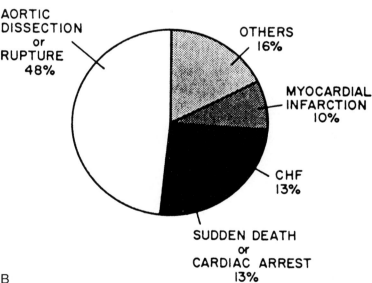

FIGURE 33–35. *A,* Medial degeneration of aorta. Focal disintegration and disruption of elastic lamina characterizes the elastic-tissue type of medial degeneration. *B,* Causes of death for 81 of 84 patients with Marfan's syndrome. Of the known causes of death, 84% were from involvement of the cardiovascular system. (CHF = congestive heart failure.) (*A,* From Gore, I.: Lesions of the aorta. *In* Gould, S. E. [ed]: Pathology of the Heart. 2nd ed. Springfield, IL, Charles C. Thomas, 1960; *B,* From Marselese, D. L., Moodie, D. S., Vacante, M., et al.: Marfan's syndrome: Natural history and long-term follow-up of cardiovascular involvement. Reprinted with permission from the American College of Cardiology [Journal of the American College of Cardiology, 1989, Vol. 14, pp. 422–428].)

The resultant aneurysm is fusiform and has an equal circumference on all sides. As the media degenerates, the aorta widens, the root is involved, and the annulus dilates. The aortic leaflets are separated and do not coapt, and aortic regurgitation results. Dissection of the aorta is the most common cause of death in these individuals (Marsalese et al., 1989) (Fig. 33–35B). Marfan's syndrome is commonly associated with severe aortic valvular incompetence from annuloaortic ectasia. In some series of aortic aneurysms, patients without classic Marfan's syndrome have annuloaortic ectasia as the most common lesion (Lewis et al., 1992).

### Traumatic Aneurysm

Severe deceleration injuries may cause disruption of the ascending aorta, but patients with such injuries rarely live to obtain surgical treatment. Trauma most commonly causes treatable injuries of the descending thoracic aorta at the level of the ligamentum arteriosum because of the hinge point of the ligamentum. A partial tear through the intima results. In the most serious situation, a traumatic transection of the descending aorta may occur. In this case, blood remains in communication with the descending aorta only because of the integrity of the adventitia and periadventitial hematoma, which forms a false aneurysm. A false aneurysm, if diagnosed late, may enlarge and form a typical thoracic aneurysm. Repair is required when the manifestations of the thoracic aneurysm become apparent either by diagnostic techniques or by symptoms of pressure. Kirklin and Barratt-Boyes (1993) have estimated that approximately 10% of descending thoracic aneurysms follow trauma. Traumatic tears may occur throughout the entire thoracic aorta, with those in the descending aorta being more common than those in the ascending aorta, which are more common than those in the arch.

### Infection

The term *mycotic aneurysm* was first used by Osler to define any localized dilatation caused by sepsis in the aortic wall. Mycotic aneurysms may result from various bacterial infections and are often localized saccular lesions with culture-positive organisms in the aortic wall. The pathogenesis is septic embolism from bacterial endocarditis to the normal or atherosclerotic aorta; contiguous spread from recent abscesses, infected lymph nodes, or empyema; or sepsis as a result of trauma, intravenous injections, or a previous surgical procedure (Bakker-de Wekker et al., 1984; Crawford and Crawford, 1984; Jarrett et al., 1975). Any organism may invade the arterial wall, but *Salmonella* particularly appears to infect arteriosclerotic aneurysms. Granulomatous aortitis, tuberculosis, and syphilis may occasionally be encountered in mycotic aneurysms of the ascending aorta.

### Chronic Aortic Dissection

Dilatation of the persistent false lumen after an aortic dissection may also produce a localized aneurysm as a result of the law of Laplace.

## Clinical Signs and Symptoms

Most patients with aneurysms are males, and most have a history of hypertension. The symptoms of thoracic aneurysm are usually caused by local pressure or obstruction of adjacent thoracic structures. Acute symptoms follow rapid expansion or rupture with signs of cardiopulmonary collapse. In the ascending aorta, until the aneurysm increases to large dimensions, it may be asymptomatic and may be found only by chest x-ray. Without annuloaortic ectasia and aortic regurgitation, a large aneurysm of the ascending aorta may obstruct the superior vena cava (SVC), producing the superior vena caval syndrome, or may exert pressure on the posterior table of the sternum, causing, in the extreme case, compression necroses of parts of the sternum and erosion of ribs.

In the arch of the aorta, the only symptom or sign noted may be compression of adjacent structures, including the trachea (tracheal tug), as well as protrusion above the suprasternal notch. Enlarging size may compress one of the cerebral arch vessels, producing cerebral ischemia.

The descending thoracic aorta may show a number of signs and symptoms related to enlarging size and stretching of various nerves. A common complaint is hoarseness due to compression and stretching of the left vagus and the recurrent laryngeal nerves as they course over and under the enlarged descending thoracic aorta. Phrenic paralysis may produce an elevated, nonfunctional left hemidiaphragm. Pressure on the esophagus, causing dysphagia, or on the bronchial tree, causing wheezing, may also occur. An aneurysm that is expanding or rupturing may leak into the pulmonary parenchyma, causing hemoptysis (St. Cyr et al., 1987). Erosion of the aortic aneurysm posteriorly into the rib cage or vertebrae can produce severe chronic back pain.

## Diagnosis

Most thoracic aortic aneurysms are readily visible on radiograph, and fluoroscopy may differentiate an aneurysm from other types of masses, such as solid tumors in the mediastinum or lung. The chest films, as shown in Figure 33–36, may show a convex shadow to the right of the cardiac shadow for ascending aneurysms (Fig. 33–36A), left-sided shadow in aneurysms of the transverse arch (Fig. 33–36B), and a shadow to the left and posterior in aneurysms of the descending thoracic aorta (Fig. 33–36C). The main differential diagnosis of the mass, particularly in the descending thoracic aorta, is a tortuous aorta.

The previous gold standard of radiologic diagnosis was the contrast thoracic aortogram (Fig. 33–37), which is now used much less frequently because it is costly and can produce certain complications, particularly in the elderly patient, such as stroke from emboli of the aneurysm. Thus, the use of thoracic aortograms has decreased as the incidence of noninvasive imaging techniques has increased. Despite reduced us-

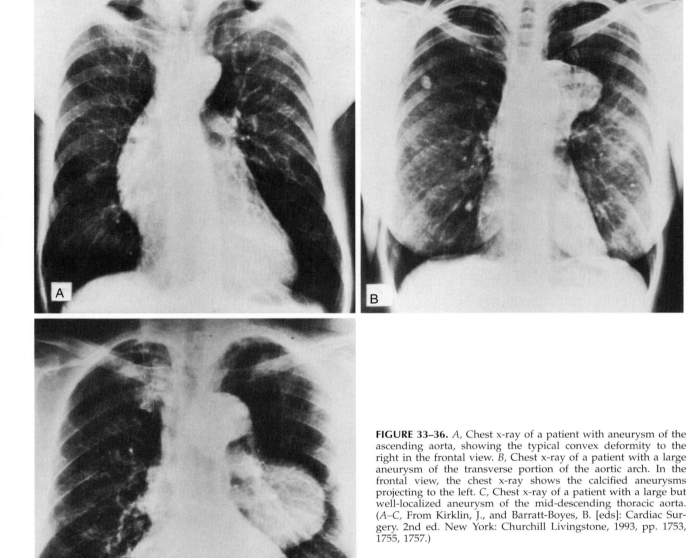

**FIGURE 33–36.** *A,* Chest x-ray of a patient with aneurysm of the ascending aorta, showing the typical convex deformity to the right in the frontal view. *B,* Chest x-ray of a patient with a large aneurysm of the transverse portion of the aortic arch. In the frontal view, the chest x-ray shows the calcified aneurysms projecting to the left. *C,* Chest x-ray of a patient with a large but well-localized aneurysm of the mid-descending thoracic aorta. (*A–C,* From Kirklin, J., and Barratt-Boyes, B. [eds]: Cardiac Surgery. 2nd ed. New York: Churchill Livingstone, 1993, pp. 1753, 1755, 1757.)

age, aortography continues to be very useful in certain situations. It can precisely denote the origin of various important arterial vessels, particularly in the arch where this differentiation may be difficult to detect with the computed tomography (CT) scan, and it can substantiate a difficult diagnosis of aneurysm not diagnostic on CT scan, echocardiogram, or magnetic resonance imaging (MRI).

The *standard* of radiologic diagnosis at the present time is the CT scan, the screening test of choice for all patients with aneurysms (Kubicka and Smith, 1992) (Fig. 33–38). The CT scan can portray aneu-

rysms at any level in the thoracic aorta and in all of the ascending arch and descending thoracic aorta. Intraluminal thrombus, dissected intima, and the like can be seen with this technique. Further and most important, the CT scan is the one examination that can be used not only as a screening device but also as a method to assess a patient's condition after surgical treatment. In conjunction with the CT scan, particularly in ascending aneurysms, the Doppler echocardiogram can demonstrate the amount of aortic regurgitation. Together with the CT scan, this method can make a complete noninvasive diagnosis, estimating

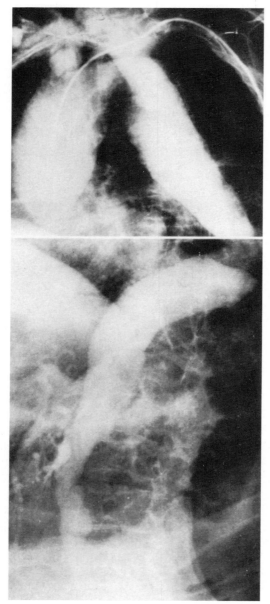

**FIGURE 33–37.** Aneurysm of the ascending aorta and aortic arch, the descending thoracic aorta, and dilatation of entire distal aorta in a 69-year-old-woman. (From Crawford, E. S., and Crawford, J. L. [eds]: Diseases of the Aorta, Including an Atlas of Angiographic Pathology and Surgical Technique. Baltimore, Williams & Wilkins, 1984, p. 50.)

the size and location of the aneurysm and the degree of aortic regurgitation.

More recently, the use of MRI has been even more useful in diagnosing noninvasively the nature and extent of thoracic aneurysms (Fig. 33–39). This technique, which actually shows the extent of aneurysm, is growing in popularity, but its use is limited by its expense and its unavailability for acutely ill patients.

## Surgical Treatment

Excision with graft replacement of enlarged thoracic aneurysms is the standard therapy and treat-

ment of choice. Excision of aneurysms depends on their location and whether they are saccular or fusiform. However, before operative therapy, the necessary preparations must be accomplished to ensure maximal safety for the patient during operation. Careful evaluation of all organ subsystems, especially renal and pulmonary, should be done preoperatively, particularly on individuals with aneurysms of the descending thoracic aorta. In the operating room, arterial pressure monitoring, multiple intravenous lines for volume replacement, urinary catheters, right atrial pressure lines, and a pulmonary artery catheter for the measurement of left atrial wedge pressure are important. For left-sided thoracotomy incisions for descending thoracoabdominal aneurysms, using a double-lumen endotracheal tube to produce anesthesia using one lung is helpful: The left lung is deflated and out of the field during operation. Blood salvage systems are essential for all thoracic aortic operations. Appropriate shunts around the aneurysm or CPB, or both, may be needed depending on the location of the aneurysms, and these are discussed later in the section on repair of aneurysms.

Sutures used for repair of aneurysms are monofil-

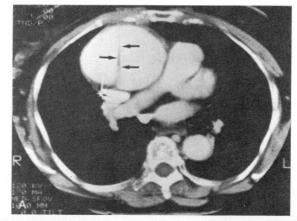

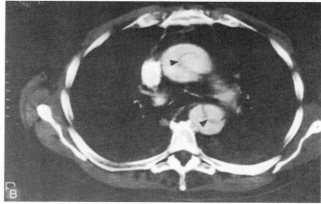

**FIGURE 33–38.** *A* and *B,* This contrast-enhanced computed tomography (CT) scan shows an aneurysmally dilated ascending aorta and intimal flap dividing the aorta into true and false channels (*arrowheads* in *B*). (*Arrows* in *A* show the dissected intima of the aorta.) (*A* and *B,* From Kubicka, R. A., and Smith, C.: Diagnostic considerations for thoracic aortic aneurysms or dissection. Chest Surg. North Am., 2:225, 1992.)

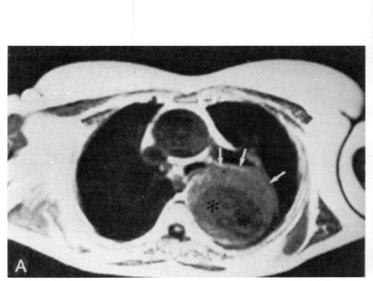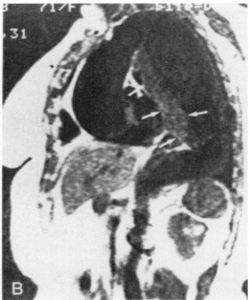

**FIGURE 33–39.** Thoracic aortic aneurysm diagnosed by a transaxial magnetic resonance imaging (MRI) scan. *A,* The left transaxial MRI is centered below the carina. *B,* A left interior black MRI of the midportion of the chest shows annulodilatation of the ascending aorta. (*Asterisk* in *A* and *arrows* in *A* and *B* show dissected intima of the aorta.) (*A* and *B,* From Kubicka, R. A., and Smith, C.: Diagnostic considerations for thoracic aortic aneurysms or dissection. Chest Surg. North Am., 2:225, 1992.)

ament polypropylene, to minimize tissue resistance and infection. Preclotting of grafts is appropriate, but increasingly popular is the technique of soaking synthetic grafts in albumin and autoclaving them to decrease blood leakage through the graft pores after anastomosis (Cooley et al., 1981). A commercially available albumin-soaked graft has been developed for usage with thoracic aneurysms (Meadox Corporation). Complete heparinization is necessary for patients on CPB, whereas only limited heparin is needed for patients in whom left atrium– or left ventricle–to-femoral artery bypass is used for treatment of descending thoracic aortic aneurysms.

### Resection and Repair of Ascending Aortic Aneurysm

Right atrial and femoral arterial cannulation is the preferred CPB technique for ascending aneurysm. The femoral artery is preferred to maximize the working area at the ascending distal aorta. It has become evident, however, that embolization from retrograde cannulation and perfusion can occur in patients who have descending thoracic aortic atherosclerosis with debris, blood clot, and the like. In fact, atherosclerotic material in the entire aorta is now recognized as a major risk factor for stroke, and Doppler scan of the aorta in all situations is increasingly important (Blauth et al., 1992; Ribakove et al., 1992). It is now recommended that transesophageal echocardiography also be used to scan the *descending* thoracic aorta before implementing retrograde CPB via the femoral route. If severe atherogenic material or thrombus, or both, is found, it is recommended that antegrade perfusion be done through the proximal aortic arch,

through the right subclavian artery, or in extreme cases, through the aneurysm itself, with removal of the perfusion cannula during hypothermic arrest and placement into the graft after completion on the ascending aorta. Systemic and local hypothermia is used to cool the heart. During the interruption of the circulation to the heart by the ascending aortic cross-clamp, intracoronary crystalloid or blood cardioplegia is administered. Because of aortic regurgitation, retrograde cardioplegia via the coronary sinus has become standard procedure as well. A left ventricular vent is placed in the right superior pulmonary vein with or without aortic valve replacement.

To assess the extent of the aneurysm resection needed requires considerable judgment. Patients with a large aneurysm extending into the aortic arch pose a more complex problem with a higher operative mortality. Therefore, the surgeon must be prudent in extending into the arch when the primary pathology is in the ascending aorta. The type of ascending aortic operation depends on the pathology in the lower aspect of the ascending aorta—specifically, whether the sinuses of Valsalva are involved and whether the patient has severe aortic regurgitation requiring valve replacement. If the aneurysm is confined to the ridge of the aorta above the coronary arteries, which is the case with most arteriosclerotic aneurysms, simple excision and grafting of the aneurysm is satisfactory (Fig. 33–40). The inclusion technique for anastomosis of the graft into the ascending aorta is adapted from the abdominal aneurysm technique first reported by Creech (1966), in which the back wall of the aorta distally and proximally is left completely intact (Fig. 33–41). This technique is the subject of controversy because of its higher incidence of false aneurysms

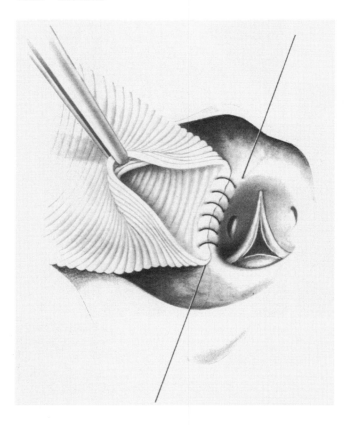

FIGURE 33–40. Replacement of the suprabulbar aorta. The graft is anastomosed to the aorta above the level of the aortic commissures, suturing entirely within the lumen. (From Borst, H. G.: Ascending aortic aneurysms. *In* Cohn, L. H. [ed]: Modern Techniques in Surgery/Cardiac Thoracic Surgery. Mt. Kisco, NY, Futura Publishing, 1984.)

(Crawford, 1983), and most surgeons now use the exclusion technique for the distal anastomosis (Fig. 33–42). If the aneurysm is produced by a chronic dissection, it may be managed in a different manner, as discussed in the next section.

If the aortic sinuses are dilated and there is concomitant aortic regurgitation from annuloaortic ectasia, a composite one-piece valve-graft conduit technique may be required. The applications for this operation vary, depending on the type of pathology. Annuloaortic ectasia secondary to Marfan's syndrome (Fig. 33–43) is an absolute indication for the use of this technique, and replacement of the Marfan ascending aorta is indicated when the echocardiographic dimensions of the ascending aorta exceed 5 to 6 cm (Gott et al., 1991). In other pathologic states, there are relative indications for this operation, depending on coronary displacement from the aortic annulus. The classic Bentall procedure (Bentall and deBono, 1968) for replacing the ascending aorta with a valve conduit in patients with annuloaortic ectasia, with or without aortic regurgitation, is shown in Figure 33–44. The operation consists of placing the proximal end first, with a series of interrupted mattress sutures around the annulus. These sutures should include a Teflon pledget, because the strength of the tissue in the Marfan aortic annulus is relatively poor. After completion of the proximal anastomosis, the graft should be

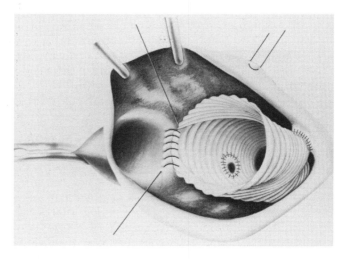

FIGURE 33–41. Distal graft-to-aorta inclusion anastomosis. The over-and-over suture begins posteriorly and proceeds anteriorly on both sides, stitching entirely from within the aortic lumen. (From Borst, H. G.: Ascending aortic aneurysms. *In* Cohn, L. H. [ed]: Modern Techniques in Surgery/Cardiac Thoracic Surgery. Mt. Kisco, NY, Futura Publishing, 1984.)

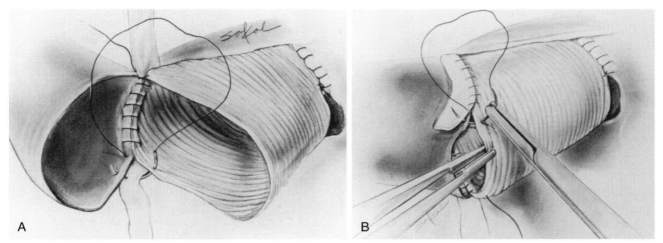

**FIGURE 33–42.** *A,* The aorta is completely transected and the posterior half is anastomosed by exclusion technique to graft with 3-0 polypropylene suture. The suture line is reinforced with a strip of Teflon felt. *B,* The anterior half of the anastomosis is then completed. (*A* and *B,* From Kouchoukos, N. T., and Marshall, W. G.: Treatment of ascending aortic dissection in Marfan's syndrome. J. Cardiac Surg., *1:*341, 1986.)

stretched to the appropriate length and the coronary anastomosis should be performed. The orifices in the prosthetic graft for the coronary arteries are created with a cautery. In annuloaortic ectasia, the coronary arteries are usually displaced a considerable distance from the annulus. The graft orifices for coronary implantation are made so that they are larger than the actual coronary orifices, leaving some pericoronary tissue for the 4-0 polypropylene sutures used in the running anastomoses.

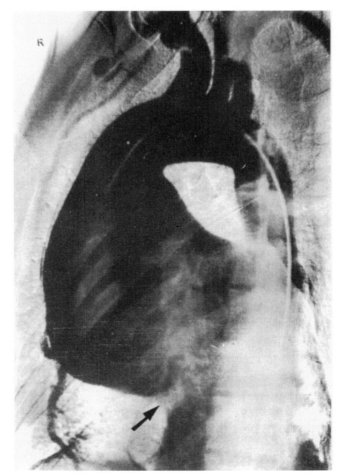

**FIGURE 33–43.** Aortogram of massive annuloaortic ectasia secondary to Marfan's syndrome in a 21-year-old woman. *Arrow* indicates level of aortic valve. (From Cohn, L. H.: The long-term results of aortic valve replacement. Chest, *85:*389, 1984.)

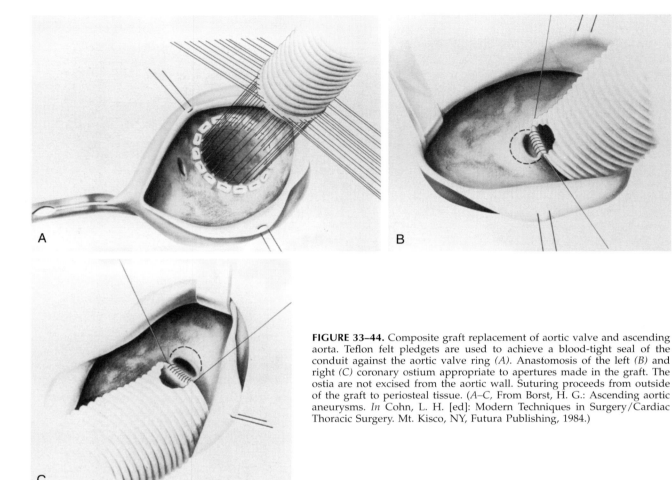

**FIGURE 33–44.** Composite graft replacement of aortic valve and ascending aorta. Teflon felt pledgets are used to achieve a blood-tight seal of the conduit against the aortic valve ring *(A)*. Anastomosis of the left *(B)* and right *(C)* coronary ostium appropriate to apertures made in the graft. The ostia are not excised from the aortic wall. Suturing proceeds from outside of the graft to periosteal tissue. *(A–C, From Borst, H. G.: Ascending aortic aneurysms. In Cohn, L. H. [ed]: Modern Techniques in Surgery/Cardiac Thoracic Surgery. Mt. Kisco, NY, Futura Publishing, 1984.)*

Coronary implantation from hemorrhage or false aneurysm is the major risk factor of this operation, and if coronary displacement is not great (<5 mm), other techniques may be necessary. In Cabrol and associates' technique (Cabrol et al., 1986), the 8-mm graft is sewn to both coronary orifices and then side-to-side to the ascending aorta graft (Fig. 33–45). Direct extension of a saphenous vein or Gore-Tex graft from the coronary orifice directly to the graft itself can also be used (Piehler and Pluth, 1982). Increasingly popular is reimplantation of the coronary arteries by excising a button of pericoronary aortic wall and suturing this button to the graft (Fig. 33–46). The posteriorly placed left coronary artery is reimplanted first, followed by the anterior right coronary artery. The distal aortic anastomosis is then performed in the usual manner, using the exclusion technique. As the last anastomotic suture line is begun, systemic rewarming is started and air is aspirated from the ascending aortic graft and left ventricle.

Some controversy exists about the use of the valve-graft conduit, even in Marfan's syndrome. Frist and Miller (1986) suggested that careful scalloping of the aorta and meticulous suturing around the coronary orifices may be as successful as the combined valve-graft conduit concept (Fig. 33–47). Leaving even a

centimeter of sinus tissue in a patient with Marfan's syndrome may cause recurrence of a false aneurysm, which is a difficult entity to treat. If the inclusion technique is used, the aortic wall is wrapped around the aneurysm and sutured closed to promote hemostasis. The common association of mitral valve prolapse and insufficiency may also allow mitral valve replacement via the aortic root in this syndrome (Crawford and Coselli, 1988).

David and Feindel (1992) advocated a new operation to spare the aortic valve for patients with aortic incompetence and aneurysm of the ascending aorta even with Marfan's syndrome. In this technique (Fig. 33–48), the entire diseased ascending aorta is excised down to a small portion of aortic wall and left ventricular outflow tract. The coronary arteries are dissected and removed with a button of periaortic tissue. A series of sutures is placed to solidify the aortic annulus, and a scalloped vascular graft prosthesis is dropped over the valve, which is anchored by the annular sutures, reinforcing the valve annulus. The native, normal aortic valve is reattached to the Dacron graft and the coronary buttons are reimplanted. This method has been used in patients with Marfan's syndrome, who have totally normal valves and have aortic regurgitation due to annuloaortic ectasia. Al-

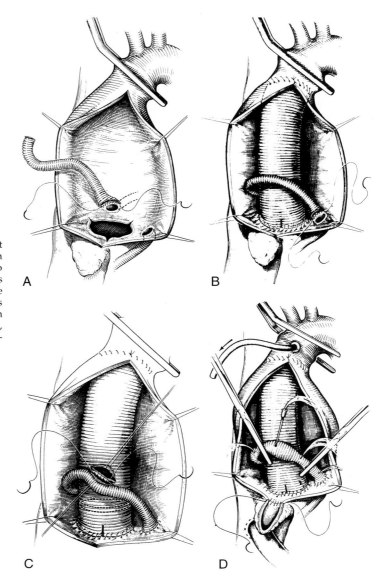

A

B

C

D

**FIGURE 33–45.** *A,* After excision of the aortic valve, the left coronary artery ostia is anastomosed to the 8-mm Dacron graft. *B,* The right coronary artery ostia is anastomosed to the 8-mm Dacron graft. *C,* The Dacron coronary graft is anastomosed side-to-side to the valved conduit above the aortic valvular prosthesis. *D,* The aorta is unclamped; air is carefully evacuated from the aortic graft and from both segments of the coronary graft. (*A–D,* From Cabrol, C., Gandjbakhch, I., and Pavie, A.: Surgical treatment of ascending aortic pathology. J. Cardiac Surg., *3:*167, 1988.)

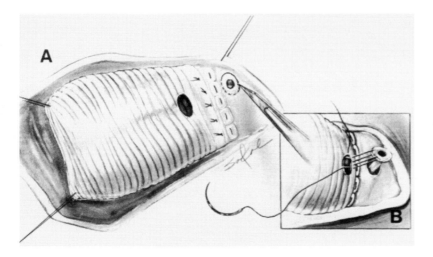

**FIGURE 33–46.** *A,* Technique for excision of a full-thickness button of aortic wall adjacent to coronary ostium. *B,* Mobilization and direct anastomosis to aortic graft. (*A* and *B,* From Kouchoukos, N. T., and Marshall, W. G.: Treatment of ascending aortic dissection in Marfan's syndrome. J. Cardiac Surg., *1:*340, 1986.)

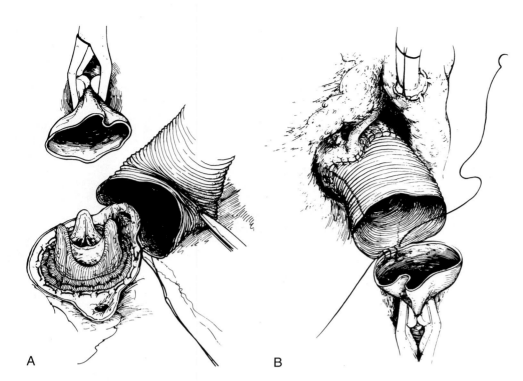

A

B

FIGURE 33–47. *A*, Using the scalloping technique (which entails insertion of the aortic valve prosthesis and the tubular synthetic graft separately), essentially the entire aortic root is either excised or obliterated. If aortic valve replacement is not necessary, the sinuses of Valsalva are not resected. *B*, Completion of the anterior aspect of the proximal anastomosis; care is necessary to ensure that the right coronary artery (lying in the proximal right atrial-ventricular groove, not at the ostium) is not inadvertently compromised. (*A* and *B*, From Frist, W. H., and Miller, D. C.: Repair of ascending aortic aneurysms and dissections. J. Cardiac Surg., *1*:33, 40, 1986.)

FIGURE 33–48. Aortic valve reimplantation into Dacron graft, secured at two levels: below the leaflets by horizontal mattress sutures and above the leaflets by suturing the remnants of arterial wall to the Dacron graft. The coronary arteries are reimplanted. (From David, T. E., and Feindel, C. M.: Aortic valve-sparing operation for patients with aortic incompetence and aneurysms of ascending aorta. J. Thorac. Cardiovasc. Surg., *103*:617, 1992.)

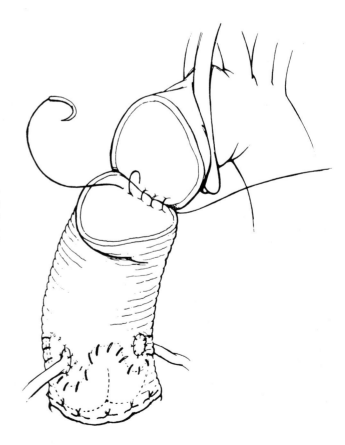

though follow-up is relatively short, the results thus far appear encouraging and may preclude the use of aortic valves in patients who have normal valves despite aortic regurgitation.

Another technique for ascending aortic aneurysms, particularly in elderly patients who are critically ill, is aortoplasty for the greatly dilated ascending aorta. This procedure involves tailoring the aortic size to prevent rupture by reducing wall stress in the relatively normal aorta, and external graft wrapping (Robicsek, 1982). However, in this author's experience, recurrence is not uncommon. The operative mortality rate ranges from 5 to 10% (Cohn, 1988–1993; Crawford and Crawford, 1984; Kouchoukos et al., 1986; Lewis et al., 1992). Rates of late survival and freedom from reoperation are shown in Figure 33–49.

### Resection of Aneurysms of the Transverse Arch of the Aorta

Aneurysms of the transverse arch aorta are more complex clinically because resection involves preserv-

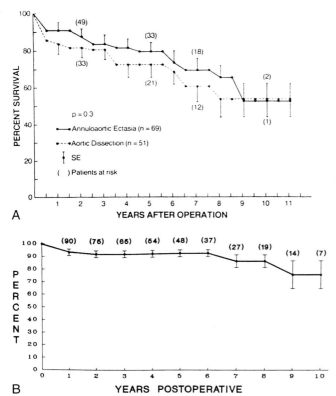

FIGURE 33–49. *A*, Actuarial survival of 69 patients with annuloaortic ectasia and 51 patients with aortic dissection. *B*, Actuarial survival of 99 patients discharged from the hospital after composite graft repair from Marfan's syndrome ascending aortic aneurysm. Number of patients at risk is shown in parenthesis. *Horizontal bars* show 70% confidence limit. (*A*, From Kouchoukos, N. T., Marshall, W. G., Jr., and Wedige-Stecher, T. A.: Eleven-year experience with composite graft replacement of the ascending aorta and aortic valve. J. Thorac. Cardiovasc. Surg., *92*:696, 1986; *B*, From Gott, V. L., Pyeritz, R. E., Cameron, D. E., et al.: Composite graft repair of Marfan aneurysm of the ascending aorta: Results in 100 patients. Reprinted with permission from the Society of Thoracic Surgeons [The Annals of Thoracic Surgery, 1991, Vol. 52, p. 38].)

ing the integrity of the blood supply to the central nervous system and protecting cerebral function while cerebral blood flow is necessarily interrupted by deep hypothermic circulatory arrest. Early techniques involved separate cannulation of the individual cerebral vessels. More recent procedures, however, have emphasized simplicity of repair and have used deep hypothermic circulatory arrest or very low CPB flow rates, or both (Cooley, 1992; Crawford and Crawford, 1984; Ergin et al., 1982; Kay et al., 1986). The basic principles of resection of the arch are shown in Figure 33–50. The brachiocephalic vessels are occluded, and flow from the CPB machine is totally interrupted. At body temperatures of 15 to 20° C, it is usually safe to arrest circulation in an adult for as long as 60 minutes following removal of the aneurysm, and to reimplant the cerebral vessel aortic button. When the aneurysm is opened, various repair techniques may be used. If the entire aorta is aneurysmal and the cerebral vessels require implantation, a graft is sutured to the descending aorta and then the cerebral button is sewn in as a patch graft. For an inferior aneurysm, however, a graft may be placed excluding an anastomosis into the descending aorta, but basically into the underside of the arch as a funnel-shaped graft (Fig. 33–51). If there is simply an opening into a saccular aneurysm, it may be repaired by Dacron patch (Fig. 33–52).

For the patient who has not only an ascending and an arch aneurysm but also a descending thoracic component that cannot be resected by the operation via median sternotomy but will have to be resected at a subsequent operation, an additional technique is the "elephant trunk" procedure developed by Borst and colleagues (1988). This technique (Fig. 33–53) uses the same principles as that of repair of such aneurysms, but extends a graft that is sutured at the origin of the descending thoracic aorta into the distal thoracic aorta and is allowed to float free in the descending aorta. This allows for later, easy retrieval of the prosthetic graft when the aneurysm is exposed and opened and the graft cross-clamped. The remaining lower part of the descending thoracic aneurysm procedure is carried out with an approach similar to that for a patient with a total thoracic aortic aneurysm. Results have been quite satisfactory and the descending aorta resection has been uncomplicated in most cases.

Failure to remove air from the circulation when circulatory arrest occurs is, of course, one of the major risks. Retrograde SVC perfusion during hypothermic arrest or simply clamping of the SVC to produce cerebral venous hypertension to help force air out the orifices of the cerebral arch vessels is a new concept. After completion of the anastomosis, the patient is placed in the Trendelenburg position, CPB is slowly begun, and air is removed from the ascending aorta and the cerebral vessels. When the cerebral vessel button is in position, the aortic graft is clamped proximally and distal perfusion is restarted. Completion of the ascending graft portion is accomplished, air is evacuated from this segment of aorta, and the patient

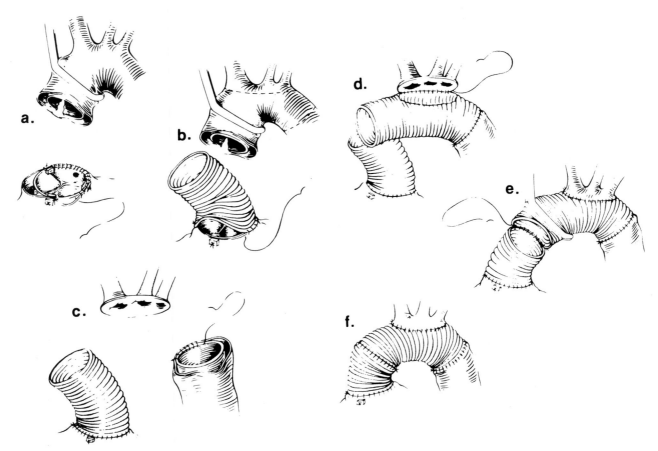

**FIGURE 33–50.** Techniques for replacement of arch of the aorta utilizing a cerebrovascular button. The anastomosis is first made to the graft in the ascending aorta (*a* and *b*) and then a graft is placed in the descending aorta *(c)*. The cerebral button, which has the orifices of all three cerebral vessels, is then anastomosed to the apex of the transverse aortic arch graft *(d)*. The final step is anastomosis of the transverse arch graft to the ascending aortic graft *(e)*. *f*, The completed graft. (*a–f*, From Ergin, M. A., and Griepp, R. B.: Progress in treatment of aneurysms of the aortic arch. World J. Surg., *4*:535, 1980.)

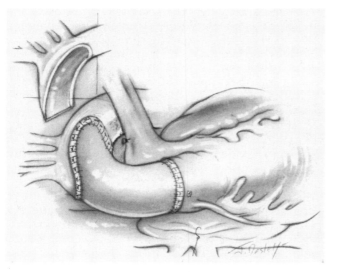

**FIGURE 33–51.** Funnel-shaped prosthestic graft to the underside of the arch of the aorta for segmental replacement of the aneurysm of the arch of the aorta with button replacement of the cerebral vessels. (From Kirklin, J. W., and Barratt-Boyes, B. G. [eds]: Cardiac Surgery. 2nd ed. New York, Churchill Livingstone, 1993.)

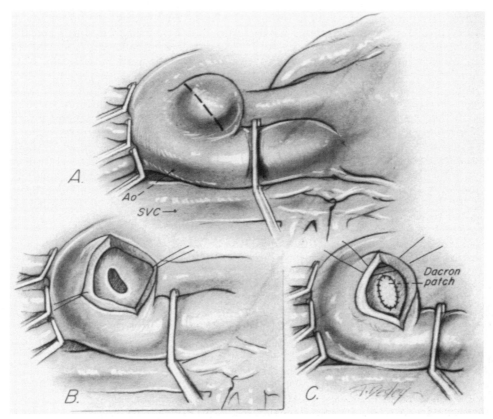

**FIGURE 33–52.** Repair of a saccular aneurysm arising from the undersurface of the portion of the aortic arch *(A)*. The innominate left common carotid and subclavian arteries have been dissected out, as has the proximal aspect of the transverse portion of the arch. Clamps have been placed on the aortic origin of the three brachiocephalic vessels and on the midportion of the ascending aorta *(B)*. After the aneurysm has been opened and the thrombotic material removed, a discrete opening between the transverse arch and the aneurysm is identified *(C)*. This opening is closed with a preclotted woven Dacron patch. *(A–C, From Kirklin, J. W., and Barratt-Boyes, B. [eds]: Cardiac Surgery. 2nd ed. Churchill Livingstone, New York, 1993, p. 1761.)*

**FIGURE 33–53.** *A–F,* The "elephant trunk" technique used to repair aneurysms of the distal transverse arch facilitates subsequent repair of an extension of the aneurysm into the descending aorta, which must be done through a lateral thoracotomy. At the lateral thoracotomy *(F)*, the freely hanging graft in the descending thoracic aorta is grasp-clamped and the rest of the aneurysm is excised in a much simplified fashion. *(A–F, From Cooley, D. A.: Aneurysms involving the transverse aortic arch. Chest Surg. Clin. North Am., 2:279, 1992.)*

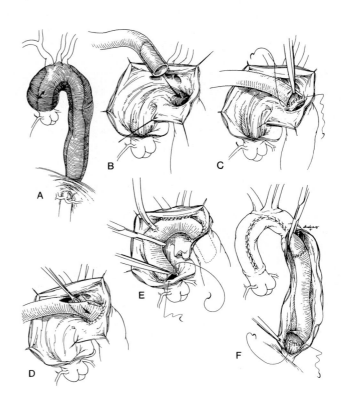

is resuscitated and taken off CPB. Perioperative complications may include embolic air or particulate material in the cerebral circulation, coagulation problems, and respiratory problems. Some surgeons have reported that aneurysms of the left common carotid and the subclavian arteries may be repaired only with perfusion of the innominate artery with excellent results (Kay et al., 1986). Although the median approach is the standard incision with CPB, some of these procedures can be performed by a posterolateral incision with partial CPB (Crawford et al., 1985; Szentpetery et al., 1993). It is necessary to screen the descending thoracic aorta with a transesophageal echocardiogram of the descending aorta before femoral cannulation. If atherogenic material appears, then retrograde cannulation through the femoral artery might produce embolization into the cerebral circulation. Therefore, the cannula for arterial perfusion may be placed in the right subclavian artery or actually in the aneurysm itself. The cannula is removed after the patient has achieved deep hypothermic levels, the prosthetic graft is then placed, and the cannula is reinserted into the ascending aortic graft to rewarm and resuscitate.

With the advent of the technique using hypothermic arrest and one-step attachment of the cerebral button, the mortality rate has declined from prohibitive levels to approximately 10 to 20%. The age of the patient and concomitant subsystem organ failure are important preoperative risk factors, and surgical treatment must be tailored to each patient.

### Resection of Descending Thoracic Aortic Aneurysms

Aneurysms distal to the left subclavian artery are the most commonly encountered thoracic aortic aneurysms. Operation is indicated for aneurysms greater than 5 cm with documented enlargement or chest or back pain indicating expansion. Aneurysms in this area of the aorta are second in incidence only to infrarenal abdominal aortic aneurysms. Traumatic aneurysms are invariably found at this location because the ligamentum arteriosum offers an anchoring point of the thoracic aorta, and shear forces create a tear, producing the traumatic aneurysm, which may be evident many years after its production. Chronic dissections from aortic degeneration may occur and produce aneurysmal dilatation. Patients with aneurysms of the descending aorta are older and often have complicated multisystem disease, including pulmonary and renal disease and especially coronary artery disease. All of these organ systems should be evaluated carefully before elective operative intervention is undertaken. For patients, the highest risk factor in repair of descending thoracic aneurysms is the presence of coronary artery disease. It is now suggested that all patients with descending thoracic aneurysms planned for resection undergo careful evaluation of *coronary artery disease*, including, in most instances, a coronary arteriogram. In some cases, the presence of severe coronary disease may preclude a direct intervention of the thoracic aneurysm, and the patient may

first undergo a coronary bypass operation, followed several weeks later by the aneurysm resection.

These aneurysms are approached through a left thoracotomy, using one-lung anesthesia. The fourth interspace generally provides the best exposure of upper thoracic aortic aneurysms, but if the aneurysm is located in the lower part of the thoracic aorta, which is not uncommon, or is a very long aneurysm extending from left subclavian artery to diaphragm, an appropriately placed second lower intercostal incision may also be necessary. The parasympathetic nerves in this region—the left phrenic, vagus, and recurrent laryngeal nerves—complicate aneurysm repair. Identification and avoidance of these structures during the course of the operation are mandatory. The lung often adheres to the aneurysm, and resection

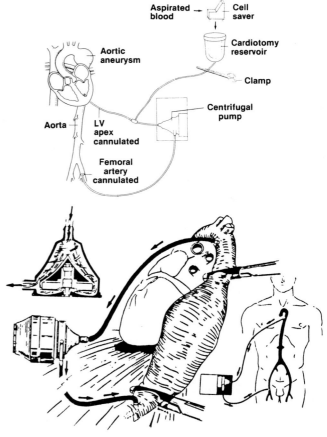

**FIGURE 33–54.** *A,* An example of left ventricular-femoral artery bypass graft for the protection of the lower half of the body during resection of a descending thoracic aortic aneurysm. *B,* Cannula placement for arterial bypass of the descending thoracic aorta. Aortoaortic bypass or aortofemoral bypass may be used in conjunction with the Bio-Medicus pump. *Inset* of pump head demonstrates the vortex, which is the basis of the kinetic pump. *Arrows* indicate direction of flow. (*A,* From Griepp, R. B., Stinson, E. B., Hollingsworth, J. F., and Buehler, D.: Prosthetic replacement of the aortic arch. J. Thorac. Cardiovasc. Surg., 70:1051, 1975; *B,* From Diehl, J. T., Payne, D. D., Rastegar, H., and Cleveland, R. J.: Arterial bypass of the descending aorta with the Bio-Medicus centrifugal pump. Reprinted with permission from the Society of Thoracic Surgeons [The Annals of Thoracic Surgery, 1987, Vol. 44, p. 423].)

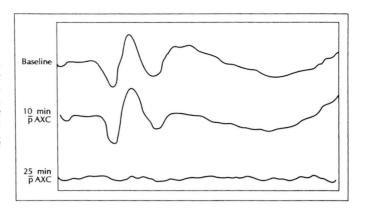

FIGURE 33–55. Somatosensory evoked potential changes produced by prolonged distal hypotension despite the use of a shunt or bypass. Potential is lost within 25 minutes of aortic cross-clamping (AXC). (From Laschinger, J. C., Cunningham, J. N., Jr., Nathan, I. M., et al.: Experimental and clinical assessment of the adequacy of partial bypass in maintenance of spinal cord blood flow during operations on the thoracic aorta. Reprinted with permission from the Society of Thoracic Surgeons [The Annals of Thoracic Surgery, 1983, Vol. 36, pp. 417–426].)

of the lung may occasionally be necessary before the aneurysm can be exposed and resected.

The major risk factor of descending aortic aneurysm resection is paraplegia due to spinal cord ischemia. Debate continues concerning the preferred procedure to protect the lower half of the body when the thoracic aorta is clamped, although most experts suggest a mechanized shunt around the aneurysm to the lower half of the body. Protective methods vary from complete heparinization and femorofemoral bypass with a pump oxygenator to simple cross-clamping of the aorta and manipulation of the upper circulatory afterload increase by vasodilators, with rapid restoration of the blood volume after removal of the aortic cross-clamp. In addition to organ perfusion below the aneurysm, bleeding from the inserted grafts is a serious risk, sometimes prohibiting complete heparinization in patients with a descending thoracic aortic graft. Crawford and co-workers (1981) originally suggested that bypass shunts were not necessary but that simple clamping with performance of the aortic anastomosis with the patient under pharmacologic control was satisfactory. This technique places pressure on the surgeon to accomplish this within a relatively short time (less than 30 minutes) and does not take into account extra time that may be needed for the more anatomically complicated aneurysms. In addition, postclamp hypotension is a major risk factor with the large amounts of blood used. Most surgeons now use some form of descending aortic bypass (Carlson et al., 1983; Culliford et al., 1983; Diehl et al., 1987) (Fig. 33–54).

It is now commonplace to use a left atrial–to-femoral bypass with limited heparinization (approximately 5000 units). This left-sided aortic shunt utilizes heparin-bonded right perfusion equipment and low-dose heparin to minimize blood loss. With radial and femoral arterial pressure monitorings, perfusion to the lower half of the body is exquisitely monitored. Especially important is that postclamp shock does not occur because the perfusion cycle restores blood volume accurately.

Monitoring of spinal cord ischemia is now possible with measurement of somatosensory evoked potentials, a technique popularized by Laschinger and associates (1982) (Fig. 33–55). In this technique, ischemia

of the cord can be recognized by the decrease in the somatosensory evoked potential of the lower extremities, and techniques to provide more blood to the lower aorta must be used. No technique guarantees that paraplegia will not occur, but it now appears that the shunt techniques described previously lead to a lower incidence of paraplegia, which occurs in approximately 5% of patients with aneurysmectomy of the descending thoracic aorta. The probability of paraplegia with and without shunts is shown in Figure 33–56. If large lateral intercostal arteries are identified within the aneurysm, these may be preserved and inserted into the graft by the patch angioplasty technique (Fig. 33–57). The basic technique for graft replacement using graft inclusion is shown in Figure 33–58. In unusual circumstances, particularly with various forms of traumatic aneurysms and chronic dissection, small entry points from the lumen to the exterior may appear; these may be closed with a patch and the false lumen may be obliterated.

The operative mortality rate after resection of a descending aneurysm varies from 5 to 15%, depending on the acuity and the demography of the

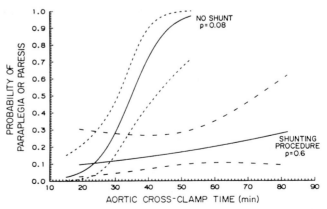

FIGURE 33–56. Nomogram of the logistic equations relating the probability of evidence for spinal cord injury (paraplegia or paresis) to aortic cross-clamp time (minutes) for patients in whom no shunting procedure was used and for those in whom it was used. The *dashed lines* are the 70% confidence limits. (From Katz, N. M., Blackstone, E. H., Kirklin, J. W., and Karp, R. B.: Incremental risk factors for spinal cord injury following operation for acute traumatic aortic transection. J. Thorac. Cardiovasc. Surg., 81:672, 1981.)

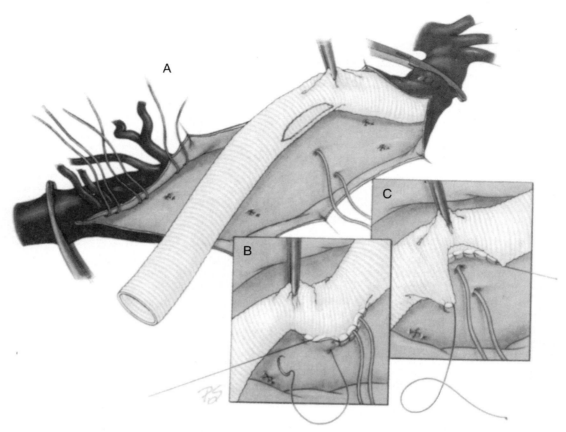

**FIGURE 33–57.** Steps in descending thoracic aortic aneurysm resection incorporating intercostal arteries. The graft is placed under tension and an oval opening is made in it opposite the intercostal arteries to be reattached *(A)*. This opening is sutured around the origin of these arteries. The inside or medial part of the anastomosis is performed first for convenience *(B)*. *C*, The other side is then performed, completing the anastomosis over the balloon. (*A–C*, From Crawford, E. S., and Crawford, J. L. [eds]: Diseases of the Aorta, Including an Atlas of Angiographic Pathology and Surgical Technique. Baltimore, Williams & Wilkins, 1984, p. 86.)

groups of patients. Small midthoracic aortic aneurysms of an arteriosclerotic nature should be operated electively with a risk of no more than 5%, whereas large proximal descending aneurysms in elderly patients with multiple subsystem organ failure have a strikingly high risk. Long-term survival after resection, with comparison of ascending to descending aneurysms, is shown in Figure 33–59.

### *Resection of Thoracoabdominal Aortic Aneurysms*

Thoracoabdominal aortic aneurysms are perhaps the most complex to repair because they require reimplantation of all the abdominal visceral arterial supply and may produce serious injury to subsystem organ function, particularly the kidneys. DeBakey and colleagues (1956) were the first to treat this problem in large numbers of patients. These aneurysms are approached through a posterior thoracoabdominal incision, retroperitoneally, beginning in the seventh intercostal space and extending to the pubis. The aorta is approached retroperitoneally and the diaphragm is incised (Fig. 33–60). The thoracic portion is removed, and the proximal aortic graft is anastomosed. If intercostal arteries are encountered, they may be reim-

planted into the thoracic aortic graft as a patch graft. This graft may include a significant spinal accessory artery to provide the best possible blood supply to the spinal cord. The entire arterial supply to the abdominal viscera is anastomosed as a large patch graft to the aorta. One-lung anesthesia with meticulous hemodynamic monitoring is critical, and afterload manipulation by nitroprusside is necessary. As with other thoracic aortic aneurysms, the aneurysmal sac is usually placed over the aortic graft and oversewn. The inclusion technique for graft replacement is generally used.

The operative techniques in this most complicated of aneurysms are directed toward reducing the time of ischemia, including in the spinal chord. The technique involves sequential clamping and reanastomosis and reperfusion of various organ beds. Techniques for the use of left atrial–to-femoral bypass have been used in some patients who have extensive aneurysmal disease from the arch to the aortic bifurcation.

The largest series and best results are attributed to Crawford and co-workers (1988), Cambria and associates (1989), and Golden and colleagues (1991). Current operative mortality ranges from 5 to 10%. Paraplegia is a major risk factor following repair of these aneurysms, and is higher than with thoracic aneu-

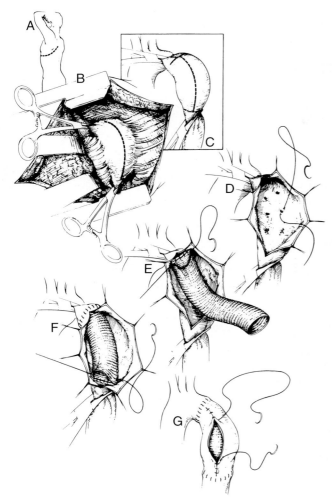

**FIGURE 33–58.** Illustrations of method for graft replacement of fusiform aneurysm of descending thoracic aorta employing graft inclusion technique. (*A–G,* From Crawford, E. S., Snyder, D. M., and Graham, J. M.: Aneurysm of the descending thoracic aorta. *In* Cohn, L. H. [ed]: Modern Techniques in Surgery/Cardiac Thoracic Surgery. Mt. Kisco, NY, Futura Publishing, 1984.)

rysms (10%) (Crawford and Crawford, 1984). Actuarial survival of patients after chronic thoracoabdominal aneurysm surgery is approximately 60% at 5 years (Crawford et al., 1985).

## Special Technical Features

### Surgical Glue

Fibrin glue (Walterbusch et al., 1982) is used in the suture lines of a friable aorta in aneurysm repair to minimize hemorrhage and promote tissue ingrowth in porous grafts by producing a neointima. Use of this material is increasing, and the United States Food and Drug Administration (FDA) is considering its approval.

The use of gelatin-resorcinol-formalin (GFR) glue technique has been increasing in major cardiovascular centers outside the United States by Fabiani and co-

workers (1990) and Bachet and associates (1990). This material, which is not approved by the FDA in the United States, allows for a "leathering" of the aorta, and has been very helpful in extremely fragile aortas, even occasionally allowing direct anastomosis without graft insertion.

### Sutureless Intraluminal Grafts

Sutureless intramural grafts were first adopted by Ablaza and colleagues (1978) and were popularized by Spagna and co-workers (1985) and Lemole (1990). They have been used increasingly for complex ascending and descending aneurysms and aortic dissections when rapid operating time is desirable. The sutureless intraluminal graft is anchored with two sutures, and a very strong circumferential umbilical tape is placed around the aneurysm and tied down on the ring of the intraluminal graft. In some cases, one end of the ring may be used while the other end is sutured to the aorta, especially in the ascending aorta. The long-term results of these grafts are unknown, and false aneurysms occasionally occur when the umbilical tapes slip or loosen and blood permeates the ring inside the aorta. This important graft adjunct will be used more in future years for more complex operations, especially in elderly, seriously ill patients needing urgent, efficient operations.

### Stapling

To exclude large thoracic aneurysms and placement of bypass, shunts may be necessary in some debilitated patients who cannot have conventional procedures. Ergin and associates (1983) have used stapling in seven patients, reporting long-term success and no recurrence. In these patients, the aneurysm was excluded and Dacron/Teflon grafts were placed around the aneurysm site without disturbing the aneurysms. Carpentier and colleagues (1981) have also used a stapling technique for thrombus exclusion for large aneurysms in high-risk patients.

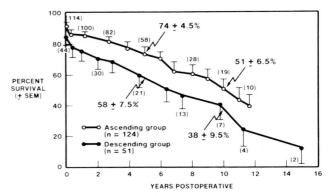

**FIGURE 33–59.** Actuarial survival rates for patients with thoracic aortic aneurysms, excluding dissection. (SEM = standard error of the mean.) (From Moreno-Cabral, E. C., Miller, D. C., Mitchell, R. S., et al.: Degenerative and atherosclerotic aneurysms of the thoracic aorta. J. Thorac. Cardiovasc. Surg., *88*:1025, 1984.)

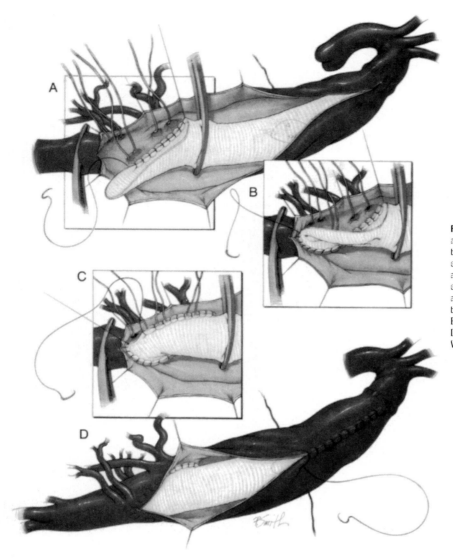

**FIGURE 33–60.** Steps in thoracoabdominal aneurysm resection and visceral artery reattachment. The distal end of the graft is beveled and attached to restore aortic continuity and to replace the involved aortic circumference behind the visceral artery openings (*A* and *B*). The anastomosis is completed by suturing the lateral margin (*C* and *D*). (*A–D*, From Crawford, E. S., and Crawford, J. L.: Diseases of the Aorta. Baltimore, Williams & Wilkins, 1984, p. 87.)

## AORTIC DISSECTION AND DISSECTING AORTIC ANEURYSMS

Acute aortic dissection is a sudden catastrophic event in which a tear in the intima allows blood to escape from the true lumen of the aorta, rapidly separating the inner from the outer layer of the media. This column of blood is driven by the force of the left ventricular systolic pressure, which strips the intima from the adventitia for various distances along the length of the aorta. The process is considered to be acute when less than 14 days old. It is actually unclear whether the rupture of the intima is caused primarily by hemorrhage occurring within a diseased media, followed by disruption of the intima, or whether it is a dissecting hematoma into the intimal tear. The clinical and pathologic manifestations of the aortic dissection are determined by the path that is taken by the dissecting hematoma as it progresses between the layers of aorta around its entire length. The circulation in any major artery that arises from the aorta may be compromised, and disruption of the aortic root and actual rupture through the adventitia anywhere along the aorta may produce a fatal hemorrhage.

Aortic dissection has been recognized for centuries. The term *dissecting aneurysm* was introduced by Laënnec (1826), but until the classic studies by Shennan (1934) and by Hurst and co-workers (1958), there was little evidence that the entity was as common as is now recognized and that it predisposes the patient to acute catastrophic cardiovascular events. Early operations for aortic dissection were designed to produce distal internal fenestration to cause downstream decompression in the aorta such as that proposed by Shaw (1955). DeBakey and associates (1955) first successfully repaired an acute dissection of the descending thoracic aorta with resection of both dissected ends and placement of an interposition graft. Spencer and Blake (1962) first repaired a chronic ascending aortic dissection, and Morris and colleagues (1963) first successfully repaired an acute ascending dissection. Wheat and co-workers (1965) advocated a major advance in the general management of acute aortic dissection by integrating surgical therapy with anti-hypertensive and beta-blockade therapy before surgical treatment.

## Etiology and Pathogenesis

The most common cause of dissection was once believed to be degeneration of the aortic media associated with cystic changes—the source of the term *cystic medial necrosis,* which was encountered in patients with Marfan's syndrome and other inherited connective tissue disorders. Only a few patients with dissection show these classic changes (Larson and Edwards, 1984), but all patients probably have some inherent anatomic weakness of the aortic wall. A number of predisposing conditions are associated with aortic dissection. Hypertension most commonly contributes to aortic dissection and is found in approximately 70 to 90% of all dissections, more often in distal than in proximal dissections. Although many patients do have cystic medial necrosis and Marfan's syndrome, many have a normal aorta and may not have chronic hypertension. Pregnancy has been associated with acute aortic dissection, but the number of patients reported is small and may reflect the hypertension of pregnancy (Pumphrey et al., 1986). Iatrogenic aortic dissection has become increasingly frequent as more patients have had cardiac operations; it may occur at the aortic cannulation site, from aorta–saphenous vein bypass, during the course of aortic valve replacement, or from retrograde femoral artery perfusion (Dabir and Serry, 1988; Murphy et al., 1983) and also as a late consequence of aortic valve replacement (Derkac et al., 1974; Muna et al., 1977; Orszulak et al., 1982). Bicuspid aortic valves and coarctation of the aorta are more frequently associated with aortic dissection (Roberts, 1981). Closed chest trauma may also be a cause of dissection, especially in the descending thoracic aorta (Wilson and Hutchins, 1982).

## Pathoanatomy

In approximately 95% of patients, dissections of the thoracic aorta arise in one of two locations: in the ascending aorta within several centimeters of the aortic valve (approximately 66%), and in the descending thoracic aorta just beyond the origin of the left subclavian artery at the site of the ligamentum arteriosum. In a small percentage of patients, the intimal laceration begins in the aortic arch or in the distal descending thoracic aorta. The tear is usually transverse and separates the aortic media for various lengths. Ascending dissection may extend into the descending aorta, but retrograde extension is relatively uncommon. Most experts now believe that in the immediate period after dissection occurs in the media, blood rushes into the dissected area between the two layers of the aorta and the pathology is established. Ac-

cording to Najafi (1983), evidence for this theory is confirmed by the events after retrograde aortic dissections during CPB, when the dissection of the entire aorta occurs almost instantaneously. Blood in the false lumen in dissections is separated from the exterior by the thin outer media and adventitia, and unless pressure is controlled, rupture may ensue. Several days after the onset of dissection, necrosis of the aortic wall may develop, causing the aorta to rupture. Necrosis of the aortic wall was observed in 62% of dissections (Barsky and Rosen, 1978). Clinical complications of dissection include aortic rupture through the false lumen and obstruction and occlusion of aortic branches, producing major clinical sequelae.

## Clinical Classification of Aortic Dissections

There are two basic clinical classifications of aortic dissections. In the DeBakey classification (Debakey et al., 1965) (Fig. 33–61), Type I involves the ascending aorta, the transverse arch, and the descending aorta. The intimal tear occurs in the anterior wall of the ascending aorta; but in some patients with intimal tears in the left subclavian artery, the dissection may evolve into the ascending aorta, thus becoming an anatomic DeBakey's Type I. In DeBakey's Type II, only the ascending aorta is involved and the dissection stops proximal to the innominate artery. In DeBakey's Type III, the aortic dissection involves the descending thoracic aorta from a tear at the left subclavian and commonly extends into the abdominal aorta.

The other commonly used clinical classification is that proposed by Daily and associates (1970) from Stanford (Fig. 33–62), which categorizes the dissections as beginning in the ascending aorta (Type A) or the descending aorta (Type B). This simplified classi-

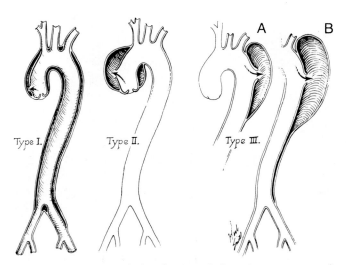

**FIGURE 33–61.** Surgical classification of dissecting aneurysm of aorta into three basic types in accordance with origin and extent of dissecting process. (From DeBakey, M. E., Henly, W. S., Cooley, D. A., et al.: Surgical management of dissecting aneurysms of the aorta. J. Thorac. Cardiovasc. Surg., *49*:131, 1965.)

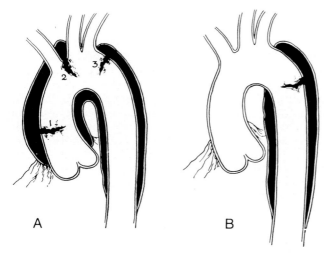

**FIGURE 33–62.** Classification of aortic dissections (Stanford). In type *A*, the ascending aorta is dissected. The intimal tear has always been at position 1, but it can occur at position 2 or 3. In Type *B* dissection, the dissection is limited to the descending aorta, and the intimal tear is usually within 2 to 5 cm of the left subclavian artery. (*A* and *B*, From Daily, P. O., Trueblood, H. W., Stinson, E. B., et al.: Management of acute aortic dissections. Reprinted with permission from the Society of Thoracic Surgeons [The Annals of Thoracic Surgery, 1970, Vol. 10, p. 244].)

fication does not provide as much detail about the pathologic involvement as does that of DeBakey, but it is more usable clinically.

## Clinical Signs and Symptoms

Acute aortic dissection affects more males than females, by a ratio of 3:1 (although it is as high as 7:1 in some series [Wolfe et al., 1983]), and the most common age of presentation is in the sixth or seventh decade of life (Doroghazi et al., 1984). Patients presenting with dissection of the ascending aorta are about 10 years younger than the average age of patients presenting with a dissection of the descending aorta. The most common manifestation is sudden severe chest pain, which signifies the onset of the dissection and the formation of the false channel. The chest pain is usually described as a tearing sensation felt in the anterior chest with ascending thoracic aortic dissections and in the back between the scapulae with descending thoracic aortic dissections. The absence of posterior scapular pain is a strong indication that a posterior dissection is not present. The pain may often be in the jaw or neck, or it may simulate upper esophageal pain. Pain occurs in almost every patient (DeSanctis et al., 1987), although painless dissections have been reported (Greenwood and Robinson, 1986). With the onset of pain, hypovolemic shock of various degrees may follow loss of blood into the false channel. This may be caused by acute aortic valve regurgitation secondary to cardiac tamponade when the dissected aorta tears into the pericardial space below the pericardial reflection. Sudden death may follow dissection of the right or left coronary artery.

Rarely, a patient with dissection may present with severe neurologic complications because the dissection immediately obstructs one of the major arch cerebral arteries, such as the innominate or the left common carotid, producing a stroke. Paraplegia may develop as the intercostal arteries are separated from the aortic lumen, or ischemic neuropathy may result from limb ischemia. Similarly, occlusion of the arteries in the lower leg may indicate acute obstruction of the arterial supply of the lower leg, stimulating embolism or thrombotic occlusion. Occlusion of the renal arteries may be associated with acute hypertension or renal shutdown. Thus, the clinical manifestations of acute aortic dissection depend on the variation in

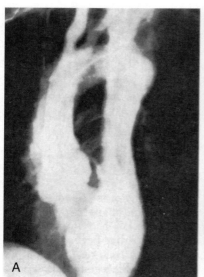

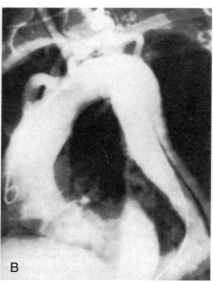

**FIGURE 33–63.** *A,* Thoracic aortogram in the left anterior oblique projection showing a dissection beginning in the ascending aorta and spiraling through the aortic arch into the descending aorta. The false lumen can be faintly visualized. *B,* Left oblique anterior view of the aorta outlined angiographically showing a distal aortic dissection in a 63-year-old man. The true and false channels are clearly seen. The false channel is heavily opacified. (*A* and *B,* From Braunwald, E. [ed.]: Heart Disease: A Textbook of Cardiovascular Medicine. Philadelphia, W. B. Saunders, 1984, p. 1553.)

flow of blood in the false channel and the extent to which peripheral or central arterial occlusions occur.

## Diagnostic Tests

### Plain Thoracic X-ray

Patients with acute aortic dissection usually have a widened mediastinum, particularly in the upper mediastinum and toward the left thorax. In ascending aortic dissection, concomitant cardiomegaly may be secondary to pericardial effusion. There may be successive changes in the configuration of the aorta, such as displacement of intimal calcification, a localized hump in the aortic arch, disparity of size in the ascending versus the descending aorta, and often a left pleural effusion (Smith and Jang, 1983).

### Electrocardiogram

Electrocardiography helps to exclude the most common differential diagnostic problem, acute myocardial infarction. Absence of an acute injury pattern in the electrocardiogram (ECG), together with negative serum cardiac enzymes, supports the diagnosis of dissection. If an ascending dissection occludes a coronary artery, the distinction may be impossible to make because the patient may manifest an acute myocardial injury pattern.

### Diagnostic Radiographic Techniques

The aortic angiogram has been a standard method for identifying patients suspected of having an acute aortic dissection and has been frequently performed before operation (Kirklin and Barratt-Boyes, 1993) (Fig. 33–63). The accuracy of this test is approximately 90%. The angiogram can establish the diagnosis of the dissection, determine the site of the tear, and delineate the extent of dissection distally. It has become clear, however, that this test is more lengthy than newer imaging techniques, and it prolongs the time from onset of intimal tear to time of operation and increases morbidity and mortality. Thus, an imaging technique that can accurately establish the origin of the intimal tear and the extent of dissection in the fastest possible time is preferable. A change in management has occurred since 1990 to decrease the time from diagnosis to the time of operation. It has been shown that the CT scan, echocardiography, or MRI can be very reliable in documenting the origin of the dissection (Barbant et al., 1992; Nienaber et al., 1992; Wilbers et al., 1990). Double aortic channels, location of the tear, presence or absence of hematoma, presence or absence of false channel communication, presence of aortic regurgitation, and the like can each be determined by Doppler echocardiography. In fact, the new algorithmic approach to diagnosis and treatment (Fig. 33–64) indicates that echocardiography (Erbel et al., 1993) and CT scan (Adachi et al., 1991; Ballal et al., 1991; Singh et al., 1986; White et al., 1986)

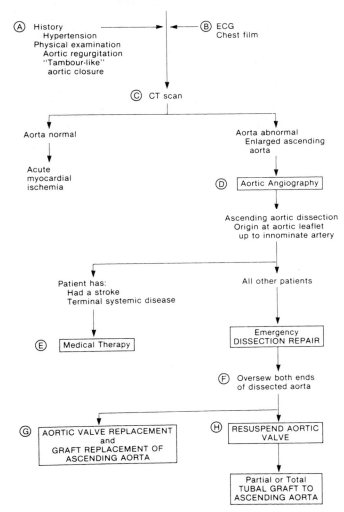

FIGURE 33–64. Algorithm for decision making in acute aortic dissection. (From Cohn, L. H., Doty, D. B., McElvein, R. B.: Decision Making in Cardiothoracic Surgery. St. Louis, Mosby-Year Book, 1987, p. 63.)

should be the emergency diagnostic techniques of choice (Fig. 33–65).

MRI is extremely accurate in dissection diagnosis (Amparo et al., 1985; Goldman et al., 1986; Sax, 1990) but placing an extremely sick patient in an MRI scanner may be impractical or unsafe. Thus, imaging techniques for diagnosis have become the routine, leading to faster operative therapy.

Many surgeons have expressed concern about the inability of imaging techniques to diagnose the presence of concomitant coronary arterial obstruction. In fact, the incidence of coronary artery disease appears to be relatively low in ascending dissections but moderately high in acute descending thoracic dissections. In addition, in the ascending dissection when there is a torn proximal intima where the valve may be deformed, it is often difficult to selectively cannulate

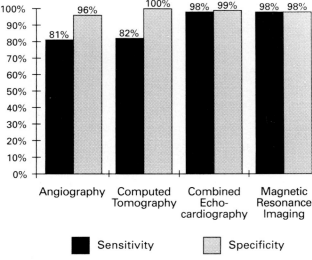

FIGURE 33–65. Comparative sensitivity and specificity of various imaging techniques in diagnosing aortic dissection. (From Wilbers, C. R. H., Carrol, C. L., Hnilica, M. A.: Optimal diagnostic imaging or aortic dissection. Tex. Heart Inst. J., *17*:271, 1990.)

coronary arteries, thus prolonging the procedure. Rizzo and co-workers (1994) discussed the incidence of coronary artery disease and the rapidity and accuracy of the various imaging techniques for acute ascending dissection. The diagnostic imaging technique of choice would first be transthoracic echocardiography, followed by transesophageal echocardiography, and then CT scan. If none of these imaging techniques can reliably diagnose the resection, then standard aortography should be performed to define the intimal lesion.

## Therapy

### Natural History

The overall survival of patients with acute aortic dissection is difficult to predict because many patients die acutely, particularly with ascending dissection by aortic rupture into the pericardial cavity (Joyce et al., 1964) or by dissecting a main coronary artery. Without treatment, approximately 8% of patients with ascending dissection survive for more than 1 month, whereas more than 75% may survive after dissection of the descending aorta (Kay et al., 1986). The accompanying data (Fig. 33–66) show the estimates of 1-year survival without surgical treatment of acute dissection: for the ascending aorta, 5%; for the descending aorta, about 70%.

### Medical Therapy

Patients suspected of having aortic dissection should be admitted immediately to the intensive care unit for monitoring of arterial, central venous, and pulmonary artery pressures, as well as urinary volume and electrocardiographic changes. The arterial

blood pressure is immediately lowered with vasodilators such as sodium nitroprusside, trimethaphan, or reserpine (Wheat et al., 1965).

The drug most commonly used is sodium nitroprusside, 50 to 100 mg in 500 ml of saline infused at 25 to 50 μg/min, to reduce the systolic blood pressure to the lowest level that still allows normal function of the cerebral, cardiac, and renal organs. The side effects of prolonged use of nitroprusside may include cyanide toxicity developing after 48 hours of intensive use. If nitroprusside is insufficient or contraindicated, trimethaphan, 1 to 2 mg/min, can be used. Routine simultaneous beta-blockade is particularly important when sodium nitroprusside is used, because the latter may cause an increase in dV/dT (DeSanctis et al., 1987). To reduce dV/dT, beta-blockade is used. Propranolol (1 mg every 5 minutes) has been commonly used, but esmolol, a faster-acting beta-blocker, is increasingly utilized and is administered until there is evidence of beta-blockade indicated by a slowing pulse rate. Esmolol may be more effective because of its more rapid action (Gray, 1988). When the patient is monitored and stabilized, preparations are made for immediate diagnostic testing (see Fig. 33–64).

For descending thoracic aortic dissections, primary treatment is usually considered to be medical therapy consisting of beta-blockade, antihypertensive therapy, and general supportive measures. Such treatment involves less chance of catastrophic compromise of an artery to the vital organs. Further, the average patient is considerably older and has other cardiovascular disease, factors that may compromise operative results. Surgical repair is the treatment of choice for all ascending aortic dissections, and medical care is appropriate only as preparation for operation. Medical therapy may be used in patients with an ascending dissection if there are serious associated medical problems that make the patient a prohibitive risk or if the aneurysm dissection occurs in the setting of other

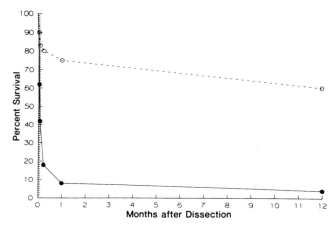

FIGURE 33–66. Estimate of survival without surgical treatment after acute aortic dissection. (*Solid circles* = patients with ascending aortic involvement; *open circles* = patients with only descending aortic involvement with or without abdominal aortic extension.) The estimate is based on data from the literature. (From Kirklin, J. W., and Barratt-Boyes, B. [eds]: Cardiac Surgery. 2nd ed. Churchill Livingstone, New York, 1993.)

systemic incurable disease, such as terminal cancer or severe organic brain syndrome. Aortic arch dissection is relatively rare. It should be treated successfully by operative intervention after preparatory medical therapy including antihypertensive beta-blockade, diuretics, and the like. Operative therapy must be carefully considered, especially in the elderly, because of the necessary hypothermic arrest and common comorbidities.

### Surgical Therapy

DISSECTION OF THE ASCENDING AORTA

The optimal therapy for acute ascending dissections is emergency surgical repair. The purpose of surgical treatment is to prevent exsanguination due to rupture and to reestablish blood flow to areas that may be occluded by the development of the intimal flap and false lumen. Operation is indicated even with serious complications related to the dissection, such as an acute stroke related to obstruction of a cerebral vessel. Obviously, considerable judgment regarding surgical intervention is required for patients with evolving stroke. Emergency repair of ascending dissections has become the treatment of choice, evolving from retrospective analyses of a number of medical and surgically treated cases in the 1960s and 1970s (Appelbaum et al, 1976; Daily et al., 1970; Dalen et al., 1974). In the very early attempts to repair ascending dissections in the 1950s, the high mortality and morbidity were prohibitive. However, in the 1960s and 1970s, when the number of surgical operations increased as perfusion techniques and graft material improved, repair of ascending aortic dissection proved to be more successful than medical therapy. These data have been duplicated by several other investigators and apply to any patient with acute dissection of the ascending aorta (Crawford et al, 1988; DeBakey et al., 1982; DeSanctis et al., 1987; Galloway et al., 1993; Rizzo et al., 1994), provided there are no other severe comorbidities.

The objectives of repair of the dissected ascending aorta are obliteration of the site of the intimal tear and the false lumen, proximally and distally, and reapproximation of the dissected aorta proximally and distally by a prosthetic interposition graft (Fig. 33–67). Valvar aortic regurgitation often accompanies acute ascending dissection, caused by intimal distortion producing prolapse of a leaflet. Controversy continues concerning treatment of the regurgitant aortic valve in acute proximal dissections. Many surgeons have suggested routine aortic valve replacement with proximal dissection, using a valve-graft conduit for

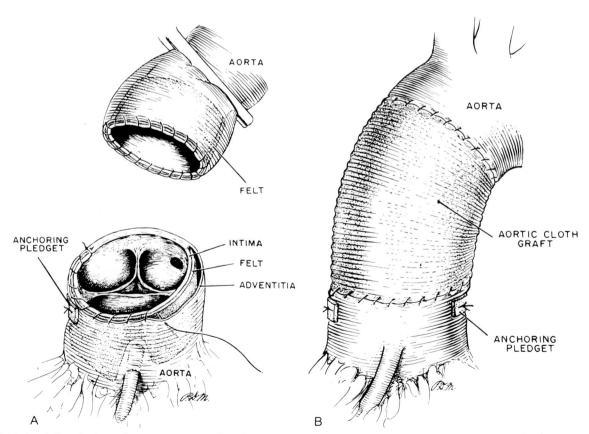

**FIGURE 33–67.** *A,* Prosthetic media reconstruction when the ascending aorta has been transected. *B,* Circumferential woven cloth graft to replace excised ascending aorta. (*A* and *B,* From Koster, J. K., Jr., Cohn, L. H., Mee, R. B. B., and Collins, J. J., Jr.: Late results of operation for acute aortic dissection producing aortic insufficiency. Reprinted with permission of the Society of Thoracic Surgeons [The Annals of Thoracic Surgery, 1978, Vol. 26, p. 463].)

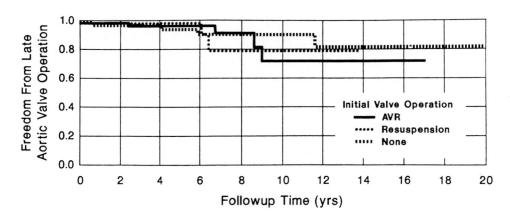

**FIGURE 33–68.** Actuarial estimates of freedom from late aortic valve replacement (AVR) according to type of initial concomitant aortic valve procedure performed. There is no difference in the prevalence of late aortic valve replacement among the three subgroups. (From Fann, J. I., Glower, D. D., Miller, D. C., et al.: Preservation of aortic valve in type A aortic dissection complicated by aortic regurgitation. J. Thorac. Cardiovasc. Surg., *102*:62, 1991.)

acute and chronic dissections (Cabrol et al., 1986; Crawford, 1983; Gott et al., 1991; Kouchoukos et al., 1986). Others prefer reconstructive procedures when possible, preserving the native aortic valve by tacking the commissure with pledgeted sutures to preserve the valve, yet obliterating the aortic dissection (Kirklin and Barratt-Boyes, 1993; Koster et al., 1978; Meng et al., 1981). The actuarial probability of freedom of late aortic valve replacement comparing resuspension with valve replacement is shown in Figure 33–68.

In chronic dissection (greater than 14 days), a more studied diagnostic approach may be taken because these patients have survived the acute episode. In chronic dissection, patients are operated on for expanding aortic aneurysm associated with the false aneurysm or, more commonly, severe aortic regurgita-

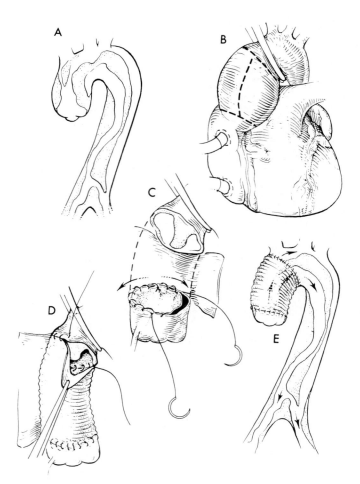

**FIGURE 33–69.** *A*, Chronic dissection of the entire aorta with a fragmented intima-medial flap. *B*, Limited transverse aortic root incision followed by H extension to facilitate graft replacement of the ascending aorta. *C*, Whipstitch used to obliterate the proximal false lumen and resuspend the aortic valve. The chronic false lumen is visible at the distal cut margin. *D*, A woven Dacron graft is interposed between the oversewn ends of the aorta and sewn into place with a continuous suture. *E*, Completed repair demonstrates perforation of both the true lumen and the false lumen distally, thereby reconstituting aortic blood flow. (*A–E*, From Gold, J. P., and Cohn, L. H.: Repair of chronic aortic dissection. *In* Cohn, L. H. [ed]: Modern Techniques in Surgery/Cardiac Thoracic Surgery. Mt. Kisco, NY, Futura Publishing, 1984.)

tion (Fig. 33–69). In some patients, primary repair without an interposition graft has been reported (Olinger et al., 1987). However, these cases are unusual owing to tissue disparity after the aortic transection and concern about suture line tension. Another technique for repairing ascending aortic dissections that has received some attention is use of the intraluminal graft, developed because of the hemorrhagic complications secondary to the friable aortic suture lines. Reports by Spagna and co-workers (1985) and Berger and associates (1983) indicate favorable results and a decrease in the incidence of hemorrhagic complications, but the use of this technique is limited in the ascending aorta.

Another important problem that has undergone revision is the management of the ascending aorta when the dissection is exposed. There has been an increasing trend toward deep hypothermic circulatory arrest and not cross-clamping the ascending aorta because of concern about clamp trauma, even if the clamp is placed well above the intimal tear (Galloway et al., 1993). Similarly, if the tear is seen to go into the aortic arch, it is considered mandatory to go into the arch to completely obliterate the intimal tear to prevent recurrent dissection (Bachet et al., 1988). Newer techniques of hypothermic arrest, better protection of the cerebral vasculature, and better use of perfusion techniques to prevent air in the cerebral circulation have become relatively standard. The incidence of redissection and false aneurysm, therefore, appear to be considerably lessened when the entire aortic intimal lesion is resected (Crawford and Coselli, 1988; Yun et al., 1991) (Fig. 33–70). However, arch repair does lead to decreased survival (Crawford and Coselli, 1988).

Bachet and colleagues (1982) reported the use of gelatin-resorcinol-formalin (GRF) adhesive to literally "glue" the edges of the dissected aorta together and also to toughen and tan the aorta at the point of dissection. This glue has been used extensively in Western Europe and South America, and the experience indicates considerable improvement in results because proximal and distal suture lines are much stronger and less friable. Many others (Weinschelbaum et al., 1992) have reported excellent results with this technique. It is not FDA-approved in the United States at this time.

DISSECTION OF THE DESCENDING AORTA

Controversy still exists about the best timing of surgical intervention for dissection of the descending thoracic aorta. In some series, medically treated patients do better than surgically treated patients because of co-morbidities. Repair of dissecting descending aortic aneurysms in most clinics is reserved for patients who have had (1) distal dissection with leakage of blood from the aorta, (2) compromise of arterial supply to a specific organ or limb, (3) continued thoracic pain, or (4) extension of the dissection while receiving satisfactory medical treatment. Inability to treat hypertension by maximal medical therapy is also an indication for repair. Some centers have excellent results with operative intervention, however, and believe that most patients at some time during the first year after the acute event require operation for acute dissection of the thoracic descending aorta (Elefteriades et al., 1992; Jex et al., 1986; Miller et al., 1984) unless the false lumen is clotted. Acute dissection of the descending thoracic aorta should be aggressively treated medially if no complications exist. The patient is stabilized for approximately 4 to 6 weeks after treatment of the acute event in preparation for definitive resection. At this time, edema of the aortic wall has resolved and the technical repair is easier and more secure.

The technical aspects of surgical intervention for descending thoracic aortic dissection are similar to those for the ascending aorta. Grafts are sewn in with the inclusion technique or intraluminal graft techniques (Fig. 33–71) by using one-lung anesthesia and intensive monitoring. For repair of the descending thoracic aortic dissection, various techniques may be used to protect the spinal cord, as for descending aortic aneurysm: femorofemoral bypass, left atrial–femoral bypass, or left ventricular–femoral bypass. In

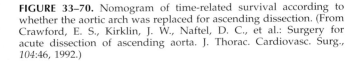

FIGURE 33–70. Nomogram of time-related survival according to whether the aortic arch was replaced for ascending dissection. (From Crawford, E. S., Kirklin, J. W., Naftel, D. C., et al.: Surgery for acute dissection of ascending aorta. J. Thorac. Cardiovasc. Surg., 104:46, 1992.)

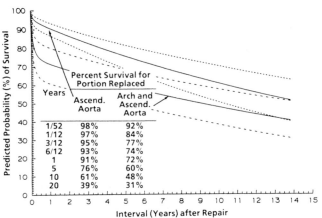

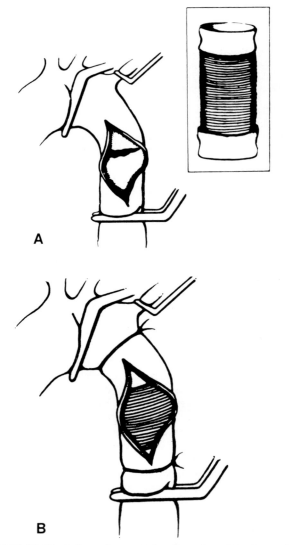

**FIGURE 33–71.** *A,* Sutureless graft for dissection of the descending aorta—the tear and graft. *B,* The graft in place, secured by heavy ties. (*A* and *B,* From Ergin, M. A., Lansman, S. L., and Griepp, R. B.: Acute dissections of the aorta. Cardiac Surg., *1:*377, 1987.)

acute dissections, the aorta is very friable and insertion of bypass shunts or cannulas into the thoracic aorta is contraindicated. One other technique of choice is left atrial–femoral bypass with reduced heparinization. The incidence of paraplegia is approximately 5 to 10% (Jex et al., 1986), although bypass shunts reduce this complication to less than 5%.

DISSECTION OF THE AORTIC ARCH

Dissection of the arch of the aorta presents a formidable problem that, until recently, has been treated medically unless rupture has occurred. Some investigators have reported reasonable success with profound hypothermia and circulatory arrest (Cooley, 1992; Ergin et al., 1982) or low flow and moderate hypothermia with cerebral perfusion (Frist et al., 1986). With emergency operation, the risk is still 20 to 40% (Lansman et al., 1993). A simplified technique to reimplant cerebral vessels and obliterate arch dissection is shown in Figure 33–72*A–E.*

Dissections that begin distally and extend proximally with the development of late false aneurysms requiring reoperation represent another problem. Although surgical attempts are used to obliterate the false channel, an intimal tear may extend beyond the cross-clamp of the aorta or may not be detected at the time of the exploration. Haverich and colleagues (1985), Ergin and co-workers (1987), and Yun and associates (1991) believe that the total extent of the intimal tear should be identified and repair of the arch of the aorta carried out.

### Results of Surgical Therapy for Dissection

Operative mortality for ascending aorta dissection is 5 to 20%, depending on the time between onset of the dissection and surgery; chronic dissections have a much lower mortality rate (5 to 10%). In the descending thoracic aorta, acute operations for dissection have an operative mortality of approximately 10 to 20%, primarily because most operations are not performed unless there is a complication. Chronic dissection aneurysms, in comparison, have much lower mortality, approximately 5 to 10%. Miller and colleagues (1984) analyzed 175 patients with aortic dissection by logistic descriptive analysis to identify high operative risk factors. After univariant screening, most predictive factors of operative mortality for Type A patients were renal dysfunction, tamponade, ischemia, and the time of operation. In Type B (descending) rupture, renal or visceral ischemia and age were the significant risk factors. Hemorrhage due to bleeding through and around the grafts from suture lines in the friable aorta has been the most common cause of operative mortality. The largest series in the literature of surgically treated patients with dissection is that of Crawford and co-workers (1988) with 546 patients. The most common causes of late death in this series were vascular myocardial *infarction* and *stroke.* Actuarial survival curves from the large series are shown in Figure 33–73.

Redissection is an important consideration in the therapy of aortic dissection. Patients with chronic untreated dissections and those who are postoperative must have continual long-term follow-up with chest films and noninvasive imaging to detect redissection. Reoperations pose an additional risk, and are approached for expansion or leakage or recurrent aortic insufficiency in patients treated by valve resuspension. In Crawford and co-workers' experience (1988), the interval between operations varied from 2 months to 11 years in acute dissection in 12 patients treated initially for Type I aortic dissection. Recurrent false aneurysms have been prevented in many patients by new suturing techniques with the use of more reinforced Teflon strips and GRF glue and the exclusion technique. In reoperations, CPB reduction of body temperature to deep hypothermic levels of 15 to 18° C is standard therapy. The circulation is ar-

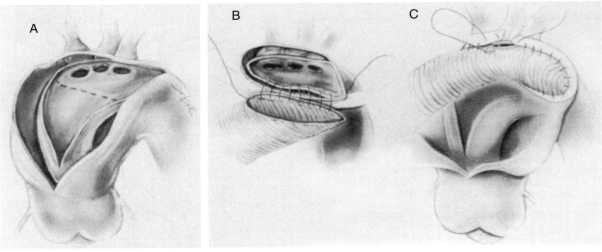

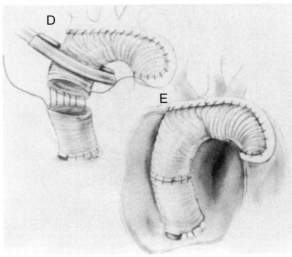

**FIGURE 33–72.** Repair of dissection of the aortic arch. *A,* The line of incision for distal aortic anastomosis when dissection extends into the aortic arch. *B* and *C,* The aorta is completely transected and anastomosed to tube graft using an outer strip of Teflon felt. *D,* The tube graft is clamped proximal to the innominate artery after reestablishing bypass and evacuating air. *E,* The tube graft is sutured to the composite graft with 3-0 polypropylene. (*A–E,* From Kouchoukos, N. T., and Marshall, W. G.: Treatment of ascending aortic dissection in Marfan's syndrome. J. Cardiac Surg., *1:*342, 343, 1986.)

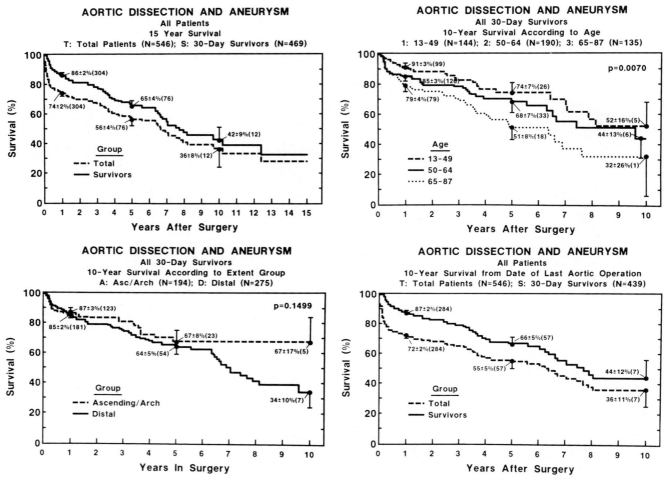

**FIGURE 33–73.** Results of aortic dissection. *A,* Fifteen-year survival of all patients and all survivors of first operation. *B,* Ten-year survival of first operative survivors according to age. *C,* Ten-year survival of first operation survivors according to extent of resection. *D,* Ten-year survival from date of last aortic operation of all patients and those who survived for 30 days. (*A–D,* From Crawford, E. E., Svensson, L. G., Coselli, J. S., et al.: Aortic dissection and dissection aortic aneurysms. Ann. Surg., *208*:254, 1988.)

rested and the patient's pseudoaneurysm is repaired during the period of hypothermic arrest (Crawford et al., 1988).

## SELECTED BIBLIOGRAPHY

Crawford, E. S., and Crawford, J. L.: Diseases of the Aorta Including an Atlas of Angiographic Pathology and Surgical Technique. Baltimore, Williams & Wilkins, 1984.

This is a comprehensive atlas and treatise on surgical technique and summary of results of one of the leading aortic surgeons in the world. The illustrations are magnificent and the philosophy of the surgeon permeates the entire volume, which includes sections on all forms of aortic pathology, including arteriosclerosis, Marfan's syndrome, inflammatory diseases, and dissections. There is also a concomitant wealth of angiographic anatomy.

Crawford, E. S., Svensson, L. G., Coselli, J. S., et al.: Aortic dissection and aortic aneurysms. Ann. Surg., 208:254, 1988.

This is the largest series of acute aortic dissections in the world's literature treated over a 32-year period, 1956–1988. Current concepts and operative techniques are shown to evolve and the wealth of data here provided by the late master aortic surgeon is simply unparalleled.

DeSanctis, R. W., Doroghazi, R. M., Austen, W. G., and Buckley, M.J.: Aortic dissection. N. Engl. J. Med., 317:1060, 1987.

A classic overview of current diagnostic and therapeutic advances in the treatment of aortic dissection. The comprehensive article, written by one of the leading cardiologists in the United States, discusses the current diagnostic techniques including magnetic resonance imaging.

Fann, J. I., Glower, D. D., Miller, D. C., et al.: Presevation of aortic valve in type A aortic dissection complicated by aortic regurgitation. J. Thorac. Cardiovasc. Surg., 102:62, 1991.

A large retrospective two-center study (Stanford and Duke) over a 30-year period discusses the acute Type A dissections and the attempts to preserve the aortic valve. The series is impressive, not only for the surgical attempts at valve preservation but also for the comprehensive statistical methods that serve as a model for reporting of surgical results.

Gott, V. L., Pyeritz, R. E., Cameron, D. E., et al.: Composite graft repair of Marfan aneurysm of the ascending aorta: Results in 100 patients. Ann. Thorac. Surg., 52:38, 1991.

This superb series integrates pathophysiology, surgical techniques, and long-term results in patients with Marfan's syndrome from one of the largest medical genetics clinics in the world. An excellent article on guidelines for surgical interventions provides superb long-term follow-up, giving a rather optimistic look for these patients who have undergone valve-graft conduit replacement of the ascending aorta and aortic valve.

Najafi, H.: Aneurysms of the thoracic aorta. In Najafi, H. (ed): Chest Surgery Clinics of North America. Philadelphia, W. B. Saunders, May, 1992.

A comprehensive small monograph that has the current individual articles by the leading thoracic aortic surgeons of the world, each on a topic with quite concise and authoritative analysis of the entire spectrum of thoracic aortic disease.

Rizzo, R. J., Aranki, S., Aklog, L., et al.: Rapid noninvasive diagnosis and surgical repair of acute ascending aortic dissection and improved survival with less angiography. J. Thorac. Cardiovasc. Surg., 108:567, 1994; Discussion, 574.

A hallmark paper that presents the first report by an American surgical group on dissections of the aorta with reliance on noninvasive testing rather than aortography, proving that results were improved and the threat of coronary disease appeared to be nonexistent.

## BIBLIOGRAPHY

Ablaza, S. G., Ghosh, S. C., and Grana, V. P.: Use of a ringed intraluminal graft in the surgical treatment of dissecting aneurysms of the thoracic aorta. J. Thorac. Cardiovasc. Surg., 76:390, 1978.

Adachi, H., Omoto, R., Kyo, S., et al.: Emergency surgical intervention of acute aortic dissection with the rapid diagnosis by transesophageal echocardiography. Circulation, (Suppl.)84:III-14, 1991.

Amparo, E. G., Higgins, C. B., Hricak, H., and Solitto, R.: Aortic dissection: Magnetic resonance imaging. Radiology, 155:399, 1985.

Appelbaum, A., Karp, R. B., and Kirklin, J. W.: Ascending vs. descending aortic dissections. Ann. Surg., 183:296, 1976.

Bachet, J., Goudot, B., Teodori, G., et al.: Surgery of type A acute aortic dissection with Gelatine-Resorcine-Formol biological glue: A twelve-year experience. J. Cardiovasc. Surg., 31:263, 1990.

Bachet, J., Laurian, C., Goudot, B., and Guilmet, D.: Four-year clinical experience with the Gelatine-Resorcine-Formol biological glue in acute aortic dissection. J. Thorac. Cardiovasc. Surg., 83:212, 1982.

Bachet, J., Teodori, G., Goudot, B., et al: Replacement of the transverse aortic arch during emergency operations for type A acute aortic dissection. J. Thorac. Cardiovasc. Surg. 96:878, 1988.

Bahnson, H. T.: Definitive treatment of saccular aneurysms of the aorta with excision and suture. Surg. Gynecol. Obstet., 96:383, 1953.

Bakker-de Wekker, P., Alfuri, O., Vermeulen, F., et al.: Surgical treatment of infected pseudoaneurysm. J. Thorac. Cardiovasc. Surg., 88:447, 1984.

Ballal, R., Nanda, N., Gatewood, R., et al.: Usefulness of transesophageal echocardiography in assessment of aortic dissection. Circulation, 84:1903, 1991.

Barbant, S., Eisenberg, M., and Schiller, N.: The diagnostic value of imaging techniques for aortic dissection. Am. Heart J., 124:541, 1992.

Barsky, S. H., and Rosen, S.: Aortic infarction following dissecting aortic aneurysm. Circulation, 58:876, 1978.

Bentall, H., and deBono, A.: A technique for complete replacement of the ascending aorta. Thorax, 23:338, 1968.

Berger, R. L., Romero, L., Chaudry, A. G., and Dobnik, D. B.: Graft replacement of the thoracic aorta with a sutureless technique. Ann. Thorac. Surg., 35:231, 1983.

Bickerstaff, L. K., Pairolero, P. C., Hollier, L H., et al.: Thoracic aortic aneurysms: A population-based study. Surgery, 92:1103, 1982.

Blauth, C. I., Cosgrove, D. M., Webb, B. W., et al.: Atheroembolism from the ascending aorta. An emerging problem in cardiac surgery. J. Thorac. Cardiovasc. Surg., 103:1104, 1992.

Bloodwell, R. D., Hallman, G. L., and Cooley, D. A.: Total replacement of the aortic arch and the "subclavian steal" phenomenon. Ann. Thorac. Surg., 5:236, 1968.

Borst, H. G., Frank, G., and Schaps, D.: Treatment of extensive aortic aneurysms by a new multiple-stage approach. J. Thorac. Cardiovasc. Surg., 95:11, 1988.

Cabrol, C., Pavie, A., Mesnildrey, P., et al.: Long-term results with total replacement of the ascending aorta and reimplantation of the coronary arteries. J. Thorac. Cardiovasc. Surg., 91:17, 1986.

Carlson, D. E., Karp, R. B., and Kouchoukos, N. T.: Surgical treatment of aneurysms of the descending thoracic aorta: An analysis of 85 patients. Ann. Thorac. Surg., 35:58, 1983.

Cambria, R. P., Brewster, D. C., and Moncure, A. C.: Recent experience with thoracoabdominal aneurysm repair. Arch. Surg., 124:620, 1989.

Carpentier, A., Deloche, A., Fabiani, J. N., et al.: New surgical approach to aortic dissection: Flow reversal and thromboexclusion. J. Thorac. Cardiovasc. Surg., 81:659, 1981.

Cohn, L. H.: Unpublished data. Brigham Cardiac Surgery Data Bank, 1988–1993.

Cooley, D. A.: Aneurysms involving the transverse aortic arch. Chest Surg. Clin. North Am., 2:279, 1992.

Cooley, D. A., and DeBakey, M. E.: Resection of entire ascending aorta in fusiform aneurysms using cardiac bypass. J. A. M. A., 162:1158, 1956.

Cooley, D. A., Romagnoli, A., and Milani, J. D.: A method of preparing woven Dacron grafts to prevent interstitial hemorrhage. Bull. Tex. Heart Inst., 8:48, 1981.

Crawford, E. S.: Marfan's syndrome: Broad-spectrum surgical treatment of cardiovascular manifestations. Ann. Surg., 198:487, 1983.

Crawford, E. S., and Coselli, J. S.: Marfan's syndrome: Combined composite valve graft replacement of the aortic root and transaortic mitral valve replacement. Ann. Thorac. Surg., 45:296, 1988.

Crawford, E. S., and Crawford, J. L.: Diseases of the Aorta Including an Atlas of Angiographic Pathology and Surgical Technique. Baltimore, Williams & Wilkins, 1984.

Crawford, E. S., Crawford, J. L., Safi, H. J., and Coselli, J. S.: Redo operations for recurrent aneurysmal disease of the ascending aorta and transverse aortic arch. Ann. Thorac. Surg., 40:439, 1985.

Crawford, E. S., Crawford, J. L., Safi, H. J., et al.: Thoracoabdominal aortic aneurysms: Preoperative and intraoperative factors determining immediate and long-term results of operations in 605 patients. J. Vasc. Surg., 3:389, 1986.

Crawford, E. S., Walker, H. S. J., Saleh, S. A., and Normann, N. A.: Graft replacement of aneurysm in descending thoracic aorta: Results without bypass or shunting. Surgery, 89:73, 1981.

Crawford, E. S., Svensson, L. G., Coselli, J. S., et al.: Aortic dissection and dissecting aortic aneurysms. Ann. Surg., 208:254, 1988.

Creech, O., Jr.: Endoaneurysmorrhaphy and treatment of aortic aneurysm. Ann. Surg., 164:935, 1966.

Crisler, C., and Bahnson, H. T.: Aneurysm of the aorta. Curr. Probl. Surg., 1:64, 1972.

Culliford, A. T., Ayvaliotis, B., Shemin, R., et al.: Aneurysms of the descending aorta. J. Thorac. Cardiovasc. Surg., 85:98, 1983.

Dabir, R., and Serry, C.: Mycotic disruption of aortic cannulation site. J. Card. Surg., 3:77, 1988.

Daily, P. O., Trueblood, W., Stinson, E. B., et al.: Management of acute aortic dissections. Ann. Thorac. Surg., 10:237, 1970.

Dalen, J. E., Alpert, J. S., Cohn, L. H., et al.: Dissection of the thoracic aorta: Medical or surgical therapy? Am. J. Cardiol., 34:803, 1974.

David, T. E., and Feindel, C. M.: An aortic valve–sparing operation for patients with aortic incompetence and aneurysm of the ascending aorta. J. Thorac. Cardiovasc. Surg., 103:617, 1992.

DeBakey, M. E., and Cooley, D. A.: Successful resection of aneurysm of thoracic aorta and replacement by graft. J. A. M. A., 152:673, 1953.

DeBakey, M. E., Cooley, D. A., and Creech, O., Jr.: Surgical considerations of dissecting aneurysms of the aorta. Ann. Surg., 142:586, 1955.

DeBakey, M. E., Crawford, E. S., Cooley, D. A., and Morris, G. C., Jr.: Successful resection of fusiform aneurysm of aortic arch with replacement by homograft. Surg. Gynecol. Obstet., 105:657, 1957.

DeBakey, M. E., Creech, O., Jr., and Morris, G. C., Jr.: Aneurysm of thoracoabdominal aorta involving the celiac, superior mesenteric, and renal arteries: Report of four cases treated by resection and homograft replacement. Ann. Surg., 144:549, 1956.

DeBakey, M. E., Henly, W. S., Cooley, D. A., et al.: Surgical management of dissecting aneurysms of the aorta. J. Thorac. Cardiovasc. Surg., 49:130, 1965.

DeBakey, M. E., McCollum, C. H., Crawford, E. S., et al.: Dissection and dissecting aneurysms of the aorta: Twenty-year follow-up of 527 patients treated surgically. Surgery, 92:1118, 1982.

Derkac, W., Laks, H., Cohn, L. H., and Collins, J. J., Jr.: Dissecting aneurysm after aortic valve replacement. Arch. Surg., 109:388, 1974.

DeSanctis, R. W., Doroghazi, R. M., Austen, W. G., and Buckley, M. J.: Aortic dissection. N. Engl. J. Med., 317:1060, 1987.

Diehl, J. T., Payne, D. D., Rastegar, H., and Cleveland, R. J.: Arterial bypass of the descending thoracic aorta with the Bio-Medicus centrifugal pump. Ann. Thorac. Surg., 44:422, 1987.

Doroghazi, R. M., Slater, E. E., DeSanctis, R. W., et al.: Long-term survival of patients with treated aortic dissection. J. Am. Coll. Cardiol., 3:1026, 1984.

Edwards, W. S., and Kerr, A. R.: A safer technique for replacement of the entire ascending aorta and aortic valve. J. Thorac. Cardiovasc. Surg., 59:837, 1970.

Elefteriades, J. A., Hartleroad, B. S., and Gusberg, R. J., et al.: Long-term experience with descending aortic dissection: The complication-specific approach. Ann. Thorac. Surg., 53:11, 1992.

Erbel, R., Oelert, H., Meyer, J., et al.: Effect of medical and surgical therapy on aortic dissection evaluated by transesophageal echocardiography. Implications for prognosis and therapy. Circulation, 87:1604, 1993.

Ergin, M. A., Lansman, S. L., and Griepp, R. B.: Acute dissections of the aorta. Cardiac Surgery: State of the Art Reviews, 1:721, 1987.

Ergin, M. A., O'Connor, J. V., Blanche, C., and Griepp, R. B.: Use of stapling instruments in surgery for aneurysms of the aorta. Ann. Thorac. Surg., 36:161, 1983.

Ergin, M. A., O'Connor, J., Guinto, R., and Griepp, R. B.: Experience with profound hypothermia and circulatory arrest in the treatment of aneurysms of the aortic arch: Aortic arch replacement for acute arch dissections. J. Thorac. Cardiovasc. Surg., 84:649, 1982.

Fabiani, J. N., Jebara, V. A., DeLoche, A., and Carpentier, A.: Use of glue without graft replacement for type A dissections: A new surgical technique. Ann. Thorac. Surg., 50:143, 1990.

Frist, W. H., Baldwin, J. C., Starnes, V. A., et al.: Reconsideration of cerebral perfusion in aortic arch replacement. Ann. Thorac. Surg., 42:273, 1986.

Frist, W. H., and Miller, D. C.: Repair of ascending aortic aneurysms and dissections. J. Card. Surg., 1:33, 1986.

Galloway, A. C., Colvin, S. B., Grossi, E. A., et al.: Surgical repair of type A aortic dissection by the circulatory arrest–graft inclusion technique in 66 patients. J. Thorac. Cardiovasc. Surg., 105:781, 1993.

Golden, M. A., Donaldson, M. C., and Whittemore, A. D.: Evolving experience with thoracoabdominal aortic aneurysms repair at a single institution. J. Vasc. Surg., 13:792, 1991.

Goldman, A. P., Kotler, M. N., Scanlon, M. H., et al.: The complementary role of magnetic resonance imaging, Doppler echocardiography, and computed tomography in the diagnosis of dissecting thoracic aneurysm. Am. Heart J., 111:970, 1986.

Gott, V., Pyeritz, R.E., Cameron, D.E., et al: Composite graft repair of Marfan aneurysm of the ascending aorta: Results in 100 patients. Ann. Thorac. Surg., 52:38, 1991.

Gray, R. J.: Managing critically ill patients with esmolol, an ultra short-acting adrenergic blocker. Chest, 93:398, 1988.

Greenwood, W. R., and Robinson, M. D.: Painless dissection of the thoracic aorta. Am. J. Emerg. Med., 4:330, 1986.

Griepp, R. B., Stinson, E. B., Hollingsworth, J. F., and Buehler, D.: Prosthetic replacement of the aortic arch. J. Thorac. Cardiovasc. Surg., 70:1051, 1975.

Haverich, A., Miller, D. C., Scott, W. C., et al.: Acute and chronic aortic dissections: Determinants of long-term outcome for operative survivors. Circulation, 72(Suppl. II):II-22, 1985.

Hurst, A. E., Jr., Johns, V. J., Jr., and Kime, S. W., Jr.: Dissecting aneurysm of the aorta: A review of 505 cases. Medicine, 37:217, 1958.

Jarrett, F., Darling, R. C., Mundth, E. D., and Austen, W. G.: Experience with infected aneurysms of the abdominal aorta. Arch. Surg., 110:1281, 1975.

Jex, R. K., Schaff, H. V., Piehler, J. M., et al.: Early and late results following repair of dissections of the descending thoracic aorta. J. Vasc. Surg., 3:226, 1986.

Joyce, J. W., Fairbairn, J. F., Kincaid, O. W., and Juergens, J. L.: Aneurysms of the thoracic aorta—A clinical study with special reference to prognosis. Circulation, 29:176, 1964.

Kay, G. L., Cooley, D. A., Livesay, J. J., et al.: Surgical repair of aneurysms involving the distal aortic arch. J. Thorac. Cardiovasc. Surg., 91:397, 1986.

Kirklin, J., and Barratt-Boyes, B.: Cardiac Surgery. 2nd ed. New York, Churchill-Livingstone, 1993, p. 1779.

Koster, J. K., Jr., Cohn, L. H., Mee, R. B. B., and Collins, J. J., Jr.: Late results of operation for acute aortic dissection producing aortic insufficiency. Ann. Thorac. Surg., 26:461, 1978.

Kouchoukos, N. T., Marshall, W. G., and Wedige-Stecher, T. A.: Eleven-year experience with composite graft replacement of the ascending aorta and aortic valve. J. Thorac. Cardiovasc. Surg., 92:691, 1986.

Kubicka, R. A., and Smith, C.: Diagnostic considerations for thoracic aortic aneurysms or dissection. Chest Surg. Clin. North Am., 2:225, 1992.

Laënnec, R. T. H.: Traite de l'auscultation mediate et des maladies des poumons et du coeur. 2nd ed. Vol. 2. Paris, J. J. Chand, 1826, p. 696.

Lam, C. R., and Aram, H. H.: Resection of the descending thoracic aorta for aneurysm: A report of the use of a homograft in a case and an experimental study. Ann. Surg., 134:743, 1951.

Lansman, S. L., Ergin, M. A., and Griepp, R. B.: Treatment of acute aortic arch dissection. Ann. Thorac. Surg., 55:816, 1993.

Larson, E. W., and Edwards, W. D.: Risk factors for aortic dissection: A necropsy study of 161 cases. Am. J. Cardiol., 53:849, 1984.

Laschinger, J. C., Cunningham, J. N., Jr., Catinella, F. P., et al.: Detection and prevention of intraoperative spinal cord ischemia after cross-clamping of the thoracic aorta: Use of somatosensory evoked potentials. Surgery, 92:1109, 1982.

Lemole, G. M.: Aortic replacement with sutureless intraluminal grafts. Tex. Heart Inst. J., 17:302, 1990.

Lemon, D. K., and White, C. W.: Annuloaortic ectasia: Angiographic, hemodynamic, and clinical comparison with aortic valve insufficiency. Am. J. Cardiol., 41:482, 1978.

Lewis, C. T. P., Cooley, D. A., Murphy, M. C., et al.: Surgical repair of aortic root aneurysms in 280 patients. Ann. Thorac. Surg., 53:38, 1992.

Lindsay, J., Jr.: The Marfan syndrome and idiopathic cystic medial degeneration. In Lindsay, J., Jr., and Hurst, J. W. (eds): The Aorta. New York, Grune & Stratton, 1979a, p. 263.

Lindsay, J., Jr.: Thoracic aneurysms. In Lindsay, J., Jr., and Hurst, J. W. (eds): The Aorta. New York, Grune & Stratton, 1979b, p. 121.

Marsalese, D. L., Moodie, D. S., Vacante, M., et al.: Marfan's syndrome: Natural history and long-term follow-up of cardiovascular involvement. J. Am. Coll. Cardiol., 14:422, 1989.

Meng, R. L., Najafi, H., Javid, H., et al.: Acute ascending aortic dissection: Surgical management. Circulation, 64(Suppl. II):II-231, 1981.

Miller, D. C., Mitchell, R. S., Oyer, P. E., et al.: Independent determinants of operative mortality for patients with aortic dissections. Circulation, 70(Suppl. I):I-153, 1984.

Morris, G. C., Jr., Henly, W. S., and DeBakey, M. E.: Correction of acute dissecting aneurysm of aorta with valvular insufficiency. J. A. M. A., 184:63, 1963.

Muna, W. F., Spray, T. L., Morrow, A. G., and Roberts, W. C.: Aortic dissection after aortic valve replacement in patients with valvular aortic stenosis. J. Thorac. Cardiovasc. Surg., 74:65, 1977.

Murphy, D. A., Craver, J. M., Jones, E. L., et al.: Recognition and management of ascending aortic dissection complicating cardiac surgical operations. J. Thorac. Cardiovasc. Surg., 85:247, 1983.

Najafi, H.: Aortic dissection. In Sabiston, D. C., Jr., and Spencer, F. C. (eds): Gibbon's Surgery of the Chest. 4th ed. Philadelphia, W. B. Saunders, 1983, pp. 956–957.

Nienaber, C. A., Spielmann, R. P., von Kodolitsch, Y., et al.: Diagnosis of thoracic aortic dissection. Magnetic resonance imaging versus transesophageal echocardiography. Circulation, 85:434, 1992.

Olinger, G. N., Schweiger, J. A., and Galbraith, T. A.: Primary repair of acute ascending aortic dissection. Ann. Thorac. Surg., 44:389, 1987.

Orszulak, T. A., Pluth, J. R., Schaff, H. V., et al.: Results of surgical treatment of ascending aortic dissections occurring late after cardiac operation. J. Thorac. Cardiovasc. Surg., 83:538, 1982.

Piehler, J. M., and Pluth, J. R.: Replacement of the ascending aorta and aortic valve with a composite graft in patients with nondisplaced coronary ostia. Ann. Thorac. Surg., 33:406, 1982.

Pressler, V., and McNamara, J. J.: Aneurysm of the thoracic aorta. Review of 260 cases. J. Thorac. Cardiovasc. Surg., 89:50, 1985.

Pumphrey, C. W., Fay, T., and Weir, I.: Aortic dissection during pregnancy. Br. Heart J., 55:106, 1986.

Pyeritz, R. E., and McKusick, V. A.: The Marfan syndrome: Diagnosis and management. N. Engl. J. Med., 300:772, 1979.

Ribakove, G. H., Katz, E. S., Galloway, A. C., et al.: Surgical implications of transesophageal echocardiography to grade the atheromatous aortic arch. Ann. Thorac. Surg., 53:758, 1992.

Rizzo, R. J., Aranki, S. F., Aklog, L., et al.: Rapid noninvasive diagnosis and surgical repair of acute ascending aortic dissection: Improved survival with less angiography. J. Thorac. Cardiovasc. Surg., 108:567, 1994; Discussion, 574.

Roberts, W. C.: Aortic dissection: Anatomy, consequences, and causes. Am. Heart J., 101:195, 1981.

Robicsek, F.: A new method to treat fusiform aneurysms of the ascending aorta associated with aortic valve disease: An alternative to radical resection. Ann. Thorac. Surg., 34:92, 1982.

Sax, S. L.: Magnetic resonance imaging of thoracic aortic dissections. Tex. Heart Inst. J., 17:262, 1990.

Shaw, R. S.: Acute dissecting aortic aneurysm: Treatment by fenestration of the internal wall of the aneurysm. N. Engl. J. Med., 253:331, 1955.

Shennan, T.: Dissecting aneurysms. Medical Research Clinical Special Report Series No. 193. London: His Majesty's Stationery Office, 1934.

Singh, H., Fitzgerald, E., and Ruttley, M. S.: Computed tomography: The investigation of choice for aortic dissection? Br. Heart J., 56:171, 1986.

Smith, D. C., and Jang, G. C.: Radiological diagnosis of aortic dissection. In Doroghazi, R. M., and Slater, E. E. (eds): Aortic Dissection. New York, McGraw-Hill, 1983, pp. 71–132.

Spagna, P. M., Lemole, G. M., Strong, M. D., and Karmilowicz, N. P.: Rigid intraluminal prostheses for replacement of thoracic or abdominal aorta. Ann. Thorac. Surg., 39:47, 1985.

Spencer, F. C., and Blake, H.: A report of the successful surgical treatment of aortic regurgitation from a dissecting aortic aneurysms in a patient with the Marfan syndrome. J. Thorac. Cardiovasc. Surg., 44:238, 1962.

St. Cyr, J. A., Ward, H. B., and Molena, J. E.: Correction of thoracic aortic aneurysm bronchial fistula. J. Card. Surg., 2:109, 1987.

Szentpetery, S., Crisler, C., and Grinnan, G. L. B.: Deep hypothermic arrest and left thoracotomy for repair of difficult thoracic aneurysms. Ann. Thorac. Surg., 55:830, 1993.

Walterbusch, G., Haverich, A., and Borst, H. G.: Clinical experience with fibrin glue for local bleeding control and sealing of vascular prostheses. Thorac. Cardiovasc. Surg., 30:234, 1982.

Weinschelbaum, E. E., Schamun, C., and Caramutti, V.: Surgical treatment of acute type A dissecting aneurysms, with preservation of the native aortic valve and use of biologic glue. J. Thorac. Cardiovasc. Surg., 103:369, 1992.

Wheat, M. W., Jr., Palmer, R. F., Bartley, T. D., and Seelman, R. C.: Treatment of dissecting aneurysms of the aorta without surgery. J. Thorac. Cardiovasc. Surg., 50:364, 1965.

White, R. D., Lipton, M. J., and Higgins, C. B., et al.: Noninvasive evaluation of suspected thoracic aortic disease by contrast-enhanced computed tomography. Am. J. Cardiol., 57:282, 1986.

Wilbers, C. R. H., Carrol, C. L, and Hnilica, M. A.: Optimal diagnostic imaging of aortic dissection. Tex. Heart Inst. J., 17:271, 1990.

Wilson, S. K., and Hutchins, G. M.: Aortic dissecting aneurysms: Causative factors in 204 subjects. Arch. Pathol. Lab. Med., 206:175, 1982.

Wolfe, W. G., Oldham, H. N., Rankin, J. S., and Moran, J. F.: Surgical treatment of acute ascending aortic dissection. Ann. Surg., 197:738, 1983.

Yun, K. L., Glower, D. D., Miller, D. C., et al.: Aortic dissection resulting from tear of transverse arch: Is concomitant arch repair warranted? J. Thorac. Cardiovasc. Surg., 102:355, 1991.

# ■ V Occlusive Disease of Branches of the Aorta

Robert B. Peyton and O. Wayne Isom

Occlusive disease of the arch vessels presents as ischemic disturbances of the head, neck, or upper extremities associated with absent or decreased pulses in the corresponding arteries. Savory first described this condition in 1856 in a young woman in whom both subclavian arteries and the left carotid artery were completely occluded. Since that time, aortic arch syndrome (Ross and McKusick, 1953), Takayasu's disease (Takayasu, 1908), pulseless disease (Davis et al., 1956), reverse coarctation (Crawford et al., 1962), Martorell's syndrome (Davis et al., 1956), thrombotic obliteration of the branches of the aortic arch (Crawford et al., 1962), and aortic dome syndrome (Thevenet, 1979) are terms that have been applied to this condition (Crawford et al., 1983).

In early reports, most patients demonstrated advanced clinical manifestations with extensive arterial occlusion. These lesions were considered rare and incurable. With the advent of cerebral angiography, this disease has been recognized with increasing frequency. Early, well-localized occlusive pathology, with relatively normal proximal and distal arterial segments, is now more readily appreciated. This form of the disease has led to the development of numerous successful operative techniques since the mid-1960s.

## PATHOLOGY

Occlusive lesions in the branches of the aortic arch have been reported to account for only 5 to 15% of extracranial lesions producing cerebral symptoms (Fields and Lemak, 1972; Hass et al., 1968; Zelenock et al., 1985). The left subclavian artery is the most common arch vessel involved (Thompson et al., 1980), with most of these obstructive lesions due to atherosclerosis. Atherosclerosis of the aortic arch branches is usually a multifocal disease, with some degree of pathology at the origins of all three of the aortic arch branches—the innominate, common carotid, and left subclavian arteries. However, the most common cause of common carotid artery occlusion is retrograde thrombosis following progression of atheromatous plaque of the common carotid bifurcation (Moore et al., 1976). Proximal carotid lesions causing prograde thrombosis are rare, and midcarotid occlusions are usually due to previous neck irradiation (Ehrenfeld

and Rapp, 1985; Rapp et al., 1986). Atherosclerotic lesions of the innominate artery most commonly occur in the proximal one-third of the vessel and usually involve the full circumference of the vessel origin, tapering into a posterior plaque extending into the subclavian artery, sparing the common carotid artery.

Occlusive lesions of the aortic arch are more common in males and are found predominantly in patients over 50 years of age. Uncommon in younger patients, occlusive lesions at the origins of the arch vessels are relatively common in patients over 65 years of age, who have associated risk factors of smoking, hypertension, hyperlipidemia, cardiovascular disease, and diabetes (Brewster et al., 1985). In young women, especially Asian women, the syndrome of multiple occlusions rather than stenoses of the aortic arch vessels is due to a nonspecific arteritis first described by Takayasu in 1908 (Fig. 33–74). Takayasu's disease represents a specific entity that is distinct from atherosclerotic lesions of the arch vessels. The arteritis involves all layers of the aortic wall, with degeneration of the elastic fibers and proliferation of connective tissue, with granulomatous inflammation and mononuclear and multinucleated giant cell formation. Alternating stenosis and aneurysmal dilatation of involved vessels may yield a "beading" pattern on angiography. Involvement of the pulmonary arteries is one distinguishing feature of this syndrome. In a series of patients studied angiographically, the left subclavian artery was the most frequent site of involvement (Ishikawa, 1978; Park et al., 1989).

Other causes of occlusive disease of the branches of the aorta include syphilis, tuberculosis, periarteritis nodosa, collagen vascular disease, rheumatic fever, trauma, congenital malformations, radiation injury, fibromuscular dysplasia (Manns et al., 1987; McCready et al., 1982), aneurysmal disease, aortic dissection, and tumor/scar (Brewster et al., 1985; Harris et al., 1984; Najafi et al., 1979).

## CLINICAL MANIFESTATIONS— PATHOPHYSIOLOGY

Most atherosclerotic disease at the origin of the arch vessels is clinically silent, either because the obstructing lesion is not hemodynamically significant or be-

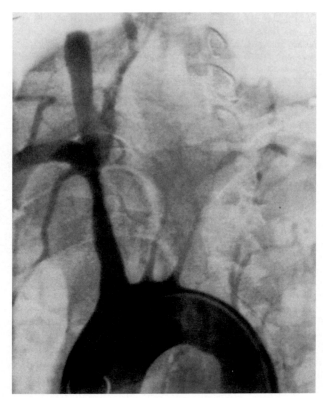

**FIGURE 33-74.** Arch arteriogram of a 32-year-old woman with Takayasu's disease.

cause the obstruction is compensated for by the extensive collateral circulation across the thoracic outlet, neck, and face. Because of this "watershed" effect, occlusions of one or more vessels may produce symptoms from reduction of total cerebral perfusion rather than irreversible neurologic changes confined to one area of the brain (Wylie et al., 1980). Subclavian occlusive disease is unlikely to be symptomatic without concomitant carotid disease.

Patients with symptoms tend to have ulcerative lesions, multiple proximal arch vessel obstructions, or sequential obstructions in one or more distal vessels, including the internal carotid or vertebral arteries (Crawford et al., 1983) (Tables 33-2 and 33-3). Three pathophysiologic mechanisms are responsible for the development of the wide range of clinical features found with these lesions: the diminished forward flow through the involved vessel; embolization from ulcerative lesions; and the reversal of cerebral blood flow away from the brain—the "steal" phenomenon, which is usually associated with atherosclerotic stenosis or occlusion of the subclavian artery proximal to the vertebral artery origin. Decreased distal pressure produces a gradient away from the brain. Retrograde flow in the ipsilateral vertebral artery can be demonstrated, but does not always correspond to symptoms.

Specific sequelae of inadequate cerebral circulation include unilateral impairment of motor or sensory functions, syncope, headaches, confusion, speech disorders, tinnitus, impairment of vision, and sometimes convulsions and paralysis, all of which tend to be intermittent and transient in nature (Campbell and Simons, 1987; Carlson et al., 1977). Cerebellar transient ischemic attacks or basal artery hypoperfusion is caused by diminished or reversed vertebral artery blood flow and may be manifested by episodic vision loss, vertigo, ataxia, dizziness, syncope, visual hallucinations, and "drop" attacks (Edwards and Muhlerin, 1983).

Upper extremity ischemic symptoms are usually mild because of the abundance of collateral to the arms and the small muscle mass affected. The patient may complain of weakness, easy fatigability, or intermittent claudication of the involved extremity. Ischemic changes in the fingers may be produced by microemboli. Advanced disease may cause rest pain or gangrene of the extremity (Gross et al., 1978; Harris et al., 1984; Rapp et al., 1986). Other clinical manifestations of aortic occlusive disease include facial atrophy, inequality of pulses of the cervical and brachial arteries, optic atrophy without papilledema, and presenile cataracts (Davis et al., 1956; Najafi et al., 1979).

## DIAGNOSIS

The symptoms described previously, together with bruits, pulse deficits, or upper extremity pressure gradients on physical examination, help establish the appropriate diagnosis in most cases. Digital arch arteriography is the diagnostic roentgenographic technique most frequently used today to visualize stenotic arch and cerebral vascular lesions, and it remains the diagnostic standard. The addition of selected cerebral

■ **Table 33-2.** LOCATION OF GREAT VESSEL LESION AND PREOPERATIVE SYMPTOMS

| Location | No. of Patients | No. of Symptoms | | | | |
|---|---|---|---|---|---|---|
| | | Carotid | Vertebrobasilar | Extremity Ischemia | Multiple | None |
| Subclavian | 80 | 6 | 22 | 24 | 24 | 4 |
| Innominate | 18 | 2 | 8 | 4 | 4 | 0 |
| Common carotid | 8 | 2 | 3 | 0 | 3 | 0 |
| Multiple proximal lesions | 36 | 5 | 17 | 2 | 11 | 1 |
| Total | 142 | 15 | 50 | 30 | 42 | 5 |

From Crawford, E. S., Stowe, C. L., and Powers, R. W., Jr.: Occlusion of the innominate, common carotid, and subclavian arteries: Long-term results of surgical treatment. Surgery, 94:781, 1983.

■ **Table 33–3.** INCIDENCE AND LOCATION OF DISTAL DISEASE ACCORDING TO LOCATION OF PROXIMAL LESION

| Proximal Lesion | Total No. of Patients | No. (%) with Distal Disease | No. with Distal Disease at | | | |
| --- | --- | --- | --- | --- | --- | --- |
| | | | *Internal Carotid* | *Vertebral* | *Intracranial* | *Mixed* |
| Subclavian | 80 | 28 (35) | 12 | 8 | 0 | 8 |
| Innominate | 18 | 3 (17) | 1 | 1 | 0 | 1 |
| Common carotid | 8 | 4 (50) | 2 | 2 | 0 | 0 |
| Multiple lesions | 36 | 23 (64) | 11 | 4 | 0 | 8 |
| Total | 142 | 58 (41) | 26 | 15 | 0 | 17 |

From Crawford, E. S., Stowe, C. L., and Powers, R. W., Jr.: Occlusion of the innominate, common carotid, and subclavian arteries: Long-term results of surgical treatment. Surgery, 94:781, 1983.

angiography further delineates the cerebral arteriographic anatomy and is needed to further define ulcerative or stenotic lesions and distal disease. Computed tomography and magnetic resonance imaging may serve as an adjunct to aortography in patients with complex aortic problems. Ultrasonic duplex scanning with hemodynamic arm exercise may also prove useful in delineating and noninvasively screening for hemodynamically significant obstruction.

## THERAPY

Brachiocephalic disease severe enough to warrant surgical correction is relatively uncommon when compared with atherosclerosis of the carotid bifurcation. This is exemplified by a report from the Cleveland Clinic that reviewed a series of patients from 1965 to 1980, in whom 1500 carotid endarterectomies were performed, compared with only 100 reconstructive brachiocephalic procedures (Vogt et al., 1982; Zelenock et al., 1985).

Intervention for brachiocephalic occlusive disease may be indicated for symptomatic obstruction or severe anatomic lesions (80% stenosis) or severely ulcerated plaques with greater than 50% stenosis (Reul et al., 1991). Takayasu's disease is approached as a distinct entity, with surgical therapy usually held in reserve because of the recurring nature of this disease.

■ **Table 33–4.** MULTIPLE SURGICAL APPROACHES TO VASCULAR LESIONS

| Arterial Lesion | Surgical Therapy | Figure | Study |
| --- | --- | --- | --- |
| *Single Vessel* | | | |
| Innominate | Aorta-distal artery bypass | Figure 33–76 | Brewster et al., 1985; Crawford et al., 1983; Deriu and Ballotta, 1981; Thevenet, 1979; Vogt et al., 1982; Zelenock et al., 1985 |
| | Endarterectomy | Figure 33–75 | Brewster et al., 1985; Carlson et al., 1977; Crawford et al., 1983; Ehrenfeld and Rapp, 1985; Ekestrom et al., 1983; Thevenet and Ruotolo, 1984; Vogt et al., 1982; Zelenock et al., 1985 |
| | Axilloaxillary bypass | | Brewster et al., 1985; Moore, 1988 |
| | Subclavian-subclavian bypass | | Brewster et al., 1985 |
| | Carotid-carotid bypass | | Brewster et al., 1985; Moore, 1988 |
| Carotid | | | |
| Right | Carotid-subclavian bypass | | Brown et al., 1983; Crawford et al., 1983; Maggisano and Provan, 1981; Thompson et al., 1980 |
| | Endarterectomy (patch) | | Najafi et al., 1979 |
| Left | Carotid-subclavian bypass | Figure 33–77 | Brown et al., 1983; Crawford et al., 1983; Gerety et al., 1981; Moore, 1988; Vogt et al., 1982 |
| | Endarterectomy | | Moore, 1988; Najafi et al., 1979; Thevenet and Ruotolo, 1984; Vogt et al., 1982; Zelenock et al., 1985 |
| | Carotid-subclavian implantation | | Vogt et al., 1982 |
| | Carotid-innominate implantation | | Ehrenfeld and Rapp, 1985 |
| Subclavian | | | |
| Right | Carotid-subclavian bypass | | Crawford et al., 1983; Raithel, 1980; Vogt et al., 1982 |
| | Carotid-subclavian implantation | | Edwards and Mulherin, 1983; Moore, 1988; Vogt et al., 1982 |
| Left | Carotid-subclavian bypass | | Posner et al., 1983; Vogt et al., 1982 |
| | Axilloaxillary bypass | | Posner et al., 1983; Schanzer et al., 1987; Vogt et al., 1982 |
| | Endarterectomy | | Ehrenfeld and Rapp, 1985; Thevenet and Ruotolo, 1984; Vogt et al., 1982 |
| Vertebral | Endarterectomy | | Edwards and Mulherin, 1983; Ehrenfeld and Ruotolo, 1985 |
| | Vertebral-carotid implantation | | Imparato, 1985; Thevenet and Ruotolo, 1984; Vogt et al., 1982 |
| | Internal mammary-vertebral artery bypass | | Baker et al., 1986 |
| *Multivessel* | | | |
| | Aorta–distal artery bypass | | Crawford et al., 1983 |

Corticosteroids are generally the mainstay of treatment for Takayasu's disease. On the other hand, the efficacy of medical treatment for significant atherosclerotic occlusive disease is limited. Arterial reconstruction of branches of the aortic arch has undergone considerable advancement since its first description (Cate and Scott, 1959; DeBakey et al., 1959). Table 33–4 summarizes the variety of surgical approaches applied to these lesions. Most recently, percutaneous transluminal angioplasty has been offered as an alternative to surgical intervention and for occlusive atherosclerotic occlusion of the subclavian artery to treat Takayasu's disease, where reocclusion frequently complicates surgical endarterectomy. Encouraging initial results have been reported (Hebrang et al., 1991; Park et al., 1989; Shapira et al., 1991).

Most aortic arch lesions can readily be remedied by one of three surgical techniques: extrathoracic or intrathoracic endarterectomy (see Fig. 33–75); intrathoracic aorta-distal artery bypass (see Fig. 33–76);

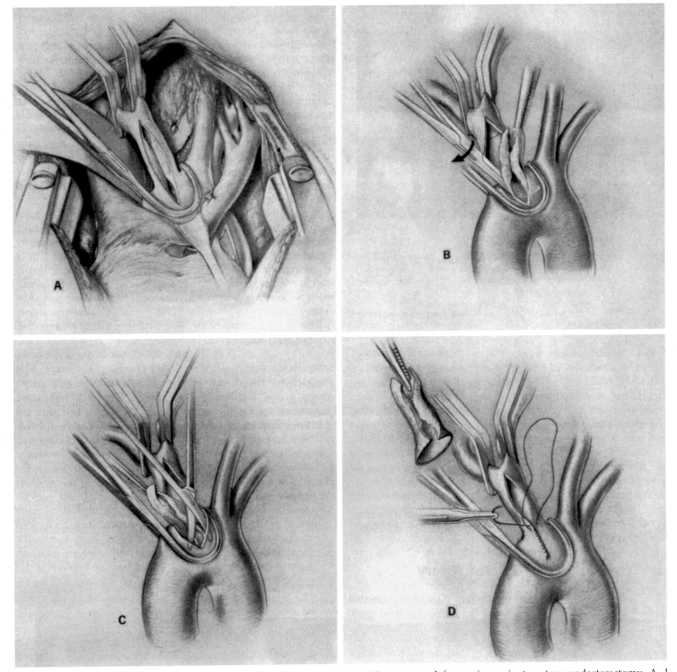

**FIGURE 33–75.** *A–D*, A full-length sternotomy and upper cutaneous incision are used for an innominate artery endarterectomy. A J-shaped clamp is used to occlude the side of the aorta adjacent to the innominate orifice, and the endarterectomy is completed. (*A–D*, From Carlson, R. E., Ehrenfeld, W. K., Stoney, R. J., and Wylie, E. J.: Innominate artery endarterectomy. Arch. Surg., *112*:1389–1393. Copyright 1977, American Medical Association.)

or extrathoracic carotid-subclavian bypass (see Fig. 33–77). Of these, the most commonly employed approach is the implantation of a synthetic bypass graft, either Dacron or expanded polytetrafluoroethylene (ePTFE), or the use of autogenous saphenous vein. Most lesions can be bypassed successfully with a graft from the carotid to the unilateral distal subclavian artery (Otis et al., 1984), and most authors try to implant unilateral short grafts that avoid crossing the midline owing to the possibility of tracheal compression-erosion or future interference with a tracheostomy or median sternotomy. Much debate has existed over the use of *extrathoracic* versus *intrathoracic* procedures. In early reports, intrathoracic procedures were associated with a 20 to 40% mortality. However, contemporary experience using better patient selection and improved surgical and anesthetic techniques has lowered the mortality rate to less than 5% (Brewster et al., 1985).

## Innominate Artery

Multiple surgical approaches to occlusive innominate artery disease are well described (see Table 33–4). The transsternal approach is now favored over the variety of extrathoracic procedures for several reasons: Median sternotomy is well tolerated with minimal postoperative pain or respiratory difficulties; anatomic transsternal repair provides superior long-term patency and relief of symptoms; either endarterectomy or anatomic graft reconstruction eliminates the embolic potential of innominate lesions; and the most reliable extrathoracic graft, ipsilateral carotid subclavian bypass, is not applicable for innominate lesions (Brewster et al., 1985). Transsternal innominate endarterectomy has been well described as the simplest and most satisfactory operation when dealing with innominate occlusive disease (Fig. 33–75). Aorta-distal artery bypass is also accepted as a technically easy, well-tolerated procedure with excellent relief of symptoms and long-term patency (Fig. 33–76). Extrathoracic grafts are used selectively when anticipating technical problems. Patients with prior mediastinal operations, aortic dissection, mediastinal infections, or complex anatomic problems or truly high-risk patients may be treated with one of the available extrathoracic graft procedures (Brewster et al., 1985).

## Common Carotid Artery

Treatment of left common carotid occlusions involves a variety of approaches, including a carotid bifurcation endarterectomy followed by a retrograde thrombectomy (Moore et al., 1976); common carotid transection caudal to the clavicle followed by thrombectomy and end-to-side anastomosis to the left subclavian; median sternotomy with common carotid thrombectomy; median sternotomy with proximal common carotid transection anastomosed into the innominate artery (Ehrenfeld and Rapp, 1985; Rapp et

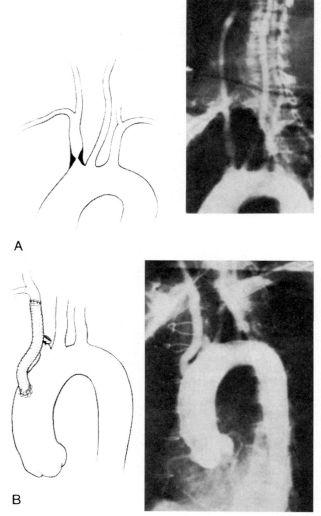

**FIGURE 33–76.** Illustration of proximal occlusion of the innominate artery causing amaurosis fugax, which is treated by bypass grafting of the ascending aorta to the distal end of the innominate artery. *A,* Drawing and aortogram made before operation show the location and the extent of occlusion. *B,* Drawing and aortogram made after operation show the location and method of operation. (*A* and *B,* From Crawford, E. S., Stowe, C. L., and Powers, R. W.: Occlusion of the innominate, common carotid, and subclavian arteries: Long-term results of surgical treatment. Surgery, *94*:781, 1983.)

al., 1986); and carotid subclavian bypass (Brown et al., 1983; Crawford et al., 1983; Vogt et al., 1982).

## Subclavian Artery

The relief of vertebral basal insufficiency is the most common indication for subclavian-vertebral operations. Four principal extrathoracic construction options are available: a bypass graft placed between the ipsilateral carotid artery and the subclavian artery distal to its obstruction (Fig. 33–77); detachment of the subclavian artery proximal to the origin of the vertebral artery with reconstruction to the ipsilateral carotid in an end-to-side manner; a bypass graft from

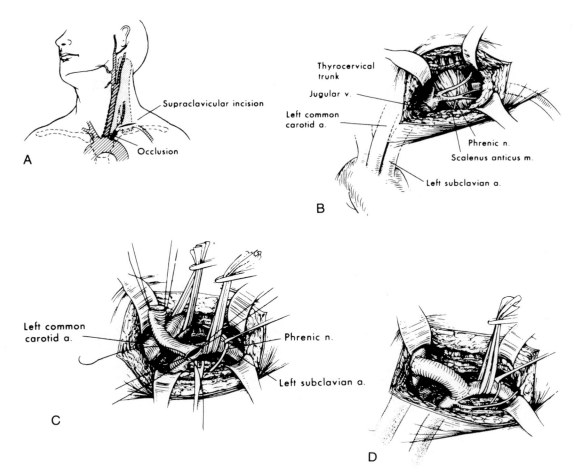

**FIGURE 33–77.** *A,* Demonstration of the placement of the supraclavicular incision. It is centered over the clavicular head of the sternomastoid muscle. *B,* After division of the clavicular head of the sternomastoid muscle, the relationships of the phrenic nerve, scalenus anticus, and subclavian artery are shown. *C,* After mobilization of the carotid and subclavian arteries, preparation is made for a graft connection. *D,* Completion of the subclavian-carotid artery bypass is shown and denotes the proximity of the two arteries and the short length of graft that is required. (*A–D,* From Moore, W. S., Malone, J. M., and Goldstone, J.: Extrathoracic repair of branch occlusions of the aortic arch. Am. J. Surg., *132*:249, 1976.)

the contralateral axillary artery passed subcutaneously across the sternum and anastomosed in an end-to-side manner into ipsilateral artery providing bidirectional flow (Moore et al., 1976; Posner et al., 1983; Schanzer et al., 1987); and transposition of the left vertebral artery to the side of the left common carotid artery (Ehrenfeld and Rapp, 1985; Moore et al., 1976). Intrathoracic procedures preferred by other authors consist of subclavian and vertebral endarterectomies (Ehrenfeld and Rapp, 1985).

## RESULTS OF SURGICAL THERAPY

The results with surgical therapy are excellent, with most large series reporting an operative mortality rate of 2 to 5% and a postoperative stroke rate of 2 to 5%. Approximately 95% of patients have early relief of symptoms, and 85% remain asymptomatic on long-term follow-up. Graft patency at 7 years is reported to be approximately 85% for carotid-subclavian bypass, with a 3% synthetic graft failure rate versus 25% for

vein grafts (Ziomek et al., 1986). Actuarial survival curves show an 85% or better 5-year survival and a 50 to 80% 10-year survival (Brewster et al., 1985; Crawford et al., 1983; Deriu and Ballotta, 1981; Edwards and Muhlerin, 1980; Maggisano and Provan, 1981; Reul et al., 1991; Schroeder and Hansen, 1980; Vogt et al., 1982).

## BIBLIOGRAPHY

Baker, N. H., Ewy, H. G., Moore, P. J., et al.: Direct internal mammary–vertebral artery anastomosis: An eighteen-year follow-up. J. Thorac. Cardiovasc. Surg., *92*:1103, 1986.

Brewster, D. C., Moncure, A. C., Darling, C., et al.: Innominate artery lesions: Problems encountered and lessons learned. J. Vasc. Surg., *2*:99, 1985.

Brown, O. W., Hollier, L. H., and Pairolero, P. C.: Amaurosis fugax and transient ischemic attacks secondary to proximal carotid artery lesions. Am. Surg., *49*:18, 1983.

Campbell, J. B., and Simons, R. M.: Brachiocephalic artery stenosis presenting with objective tinnitus. J. Laryngol. Otol., *101*:718, 1987.

Carlson, R. E., Ehrenfeld, W. K., Stoney, R. J., and Wylie, E. J.: Innominate artery endarterectomy. Arch. Surg., *112*:1389, 1977.

Cate, W. R., and Scott, H. W., Jr.: Cerebral ischemia of central origin: Relief by subclavian-vertebral artery thromboendarterectomy. Surgery, 45:19, 1959.

Crawford, E. S., DeBakey, M. E., Morris, G. C., and Cooley, D. A.: Thrombo-obliterative disease of the great vessels arising from the aortic arch. J. Thorac. Cardiovasc. Surg., 43:38, 1962.

Crawford, E. S., Stowe, C. L., and Powers, R. W.: Occlusion of the innominate, common carotid, and subclavian arteries: Long-term results of surgical treatment. Surgery, 94:781, 1983.

Davis, J. B., Grove, W. J., and Julian, O. C.: Thrombic occlusion of the branches of the aortic arch, Martorell's syndrome: Report of a case treated surgically. Ann. Surg., 144:124, 1956.

DeBakey, M. E., Crawford, E. S., and Cooley, D. A.: Surgical considerations of occlusive disease of innominate, carotid, subclavian, and vertebral arteries. Ann. Surg., 149:690, 1959.

Deriu, G. P., and Ballotta, E.: The surgical treatment of atherosclerotic occlusion of the innominate and subclavian arteries. J. Cardiovasc. Surg., 22:532, 1981.

Edwards, W. H., and Muhlerin, J. L., Jr.: The management of brachiocephalic occlusive disease. Am. Surg., 49:465, 1983.

Edwards, W. H., and Muhlerin, J. L., Jr.: The surgical approach to significant stenosis of vertebral and subclavian arteries. Surgery, 87:20, 1980.

Ehrenfeld, W. K., and Rapp, J. H.: Direct revascularization for occlusion of the trunks of the aortic arch. J. Vasc. Surg., 2:228, 1985.

Ekestrom, S., Liljeqvist, L., and Nordhus, O.: Surgical management of obliterative disease of the brachiocephalic trunk: Experience from 24 cases. Scand. J. Thorac. Cardiovasc. Surg., 17:305, 309, 1983.

Fields, W. S., and Lemak, N. A.: Joint study of extracranial arterial occlusion. VII: Subclavian steal—A review of 168 cases. J. A. M. A., 222:1130, 1972.

Gross, W. S., Flanigan, P., Kraft, R. O., and Stanley, J. C.: Chronic upper extremity arterial insufficiency: Etiology, manifestations, and operative management. Arch. Surg., 113:419, 1978.

Harris, R. W., Andros, G., Dulawa, L. B., et al.: Large vessel arterial occlusive disease in symptomatic upper extremity. Arch. Surg., 119:1277, 1984.

Hass, W. K., Field, W. S., North, R. R., et al.: Joint study of extracranial arterial occlusion: II. Arteriography, techniques, sites, and complications.

Hebrang, A., Maskovic, J., and Tomac, B.: Percutaneous transluminal angioplasty of the subclavian arteries: Long-term results in 52 patients. A. J. R., 156:1091, 1991.

Imparato, A. M.: Vertebral arterial reconstruction: A nineteen-year experience. J. Vasc. Surg., 2:626, 1985.

Ishikawa, K.: Natural history and classification of occlusive thromboaortopathy (Takayasu's disease). Circulation, 57:27, 1978.

Maggisano, R., and Provan, J. L.: Surgical management of chronic occlusive disease of the aortic arch vessels and vertebral arteries. Can. Med. Assoc. J., 124:972, 1981.

Manns, R. A., Nanda, K. K., and Mackie, G.: Case report: Fibromuscular dysplasia of the cephalic and renal arteries. Clin. Radiol., 38:427, 1987.

McCready, R. A., Pairolero, P. C., Hollier, L. H., et al.: Fibromuscular dysplasia of the right subclavian artery. Arch. Surg., 117:1243, 1982.

Moore, W. S.: Extra-anatomic bypass for revascularization of occlusive lesions involving the branches of the aortic arch. J. Vasc. Surg., 2:230, 1988.

Moore, W. S., Malone, J. M., and Goldstone, J.: Extrathoracic repair of branch occlusions of the aortic arch. Am. J. Surg., 132:249, 1976.

Najafi, H., Javid, H., Hunter, J. A., et al.: Occlusive disease of the branches of the aortic arch. In Bergan, J. J., and Yao, J. S. T. (eds): Surgery of the Aorta and Its Body Branches. New York, Grune & Stratton, 1979.

Otis, S., Rush, M., Thomas, M., and Dilley, R.: Carotid steal syndrome following carotid subclavian bypass. J. Vasc. Surg., 1:649, 1984.

Park, J. H., Han, M. C., Kim, S. H., et al.: Takayasu arteritis: Angiographic findings and results of angioplasty. A. J. R., 153:1069, 1989.

Posner, M. P., Riles, T. S., Ramirez, A. A., et al.: Axillo-axillary bypass for symptomatic stenosis of the subclavian artery. Am. J. Surg., 145:644, 1983.

Raithel, D.: Our experience of surgery for innominate and subclavian lesions. J. Cardiovasc. Surg., 21:423, 1980.

Rapp, J. H., Reilly, L. M., Goldstone, J., et al.: Ischemia of the upper extremity: Significance of proximal arterial disease. Am. J. Surg., 152:122, 1986.

Reul, G. J., Jacobs, M. J., Gregoric, I. D., et al.: Innominate artery occlusive disease: Surgical approach and long-term results. J. Vasc. Surg., 14:405, 1991.

Ross, R. S., and McKusick, V. A.: Aortic arch syndromes. Arch. Intern. Med., 92:701, 1953.

Savory, W. S.: Case of a young woman in whom the main arteries of both upper extremities and of the left side of the neck were throughout completely obliterated. Trans. Med. Chir. Soc., 39:205, 1856.

Schanzer, H., Chung-Loy, H., Kotok, M., et al.: Evaluation of axillo-axillary artery bypass for the treatment of subclavian or innominate artery occlusive disease. J. Cardiovasc. Surg., 28:258, 1987.

Schroeder, T., and Hansen, H. J. B.: Arterial reconstruction of the brachiocephalic trunk and the subclavian arteries. Ten years' experience with a follow-up study. Acta Chir. Scand., 502:122, 1980.

Shapira, S., Braun, S. D., Puram, B., et al.: Percutaneous transluminal angioplasty of proximal subclavian artery stenosis after left internal mammary to the left anterior descending artery bypass surgery. J. Am. Coll. Cardiol., 18:1120, 1991.

Takayasu, M.: Case of queer changes in central blood vessels of retina. Acta Soc. Ophthal. Jap., 12:2554, 1908.

Thevenet, A.: Surgical management of the aortic dome and origin of supra-aortic trunks. World J. Surg., 3:187, 1979.

Thevenet, A., and Ruotolo, C.: Surgical repair of vertebral artery stenosis. J. Cardiovasc. Surg., 25:101, 1984.

Thompson, B. W., Read, R. C., and Campbell, G. S.: Operative correction of proximal blocks of the subclavian or innominate arteries. J. Cardiovasc. Surg., 21:125, 1980.

Vogt, D. P., Hertzer, N. R., O'Hara, P. J., and Beven, E. G.: Brachiocephalic arterial reconstruction. Ann. Surg., 196:541, 1982.

Wylie, E. J., Stoney, R. J., and Ehrenfeld, W. K.: Manual of Vascular Surgery. New York, Heidelberg, Berlin, Springer-Verlag, 1980, pp. 85–106.

Zelenock, G. B., Cronenwett, J. L., Graham, L. M., et al.: Brachiocephalic arterial occlusions and stenoses: Manifestations and management of complex lesions. Arch. Surg., 120:370, 1985.

Ziomek, S., Quinones-Baldrich, W. J., Busuttil, R. W., et al.: The superiority of synthetic arterial grafts over autologous veins in carotid-subclavian bypass. J. Vasc. Surg., 3:140, 1986.

# 34 The Pericardium

James M. Douglas, Jr.

## HISTORICAL PERSPECTIVES

Medical writings concerning the pericardium began with the descriptions of the normal pericardium by Hippocrates. The early Greeks noted the characteristics of the heart in certain battlefield heroes, describing it as "hairy." Extrapolation has led some authors to suggest that these descriptions refer to inflammatory diseases of the pericardium (Spodick, 1970). Galen recognized the protective function of the pericardium surrounding the heart. His animal dissections provided one of the earliest descriptions of pericardial effusion. Further, Galen may have performed the first pericardial resection: A young man with septic anterior mediastinitis underwent trephination of the sternum and probable removal of a portion of the pericardium.

The pericardium was increasingly recognized as an entity during the Renaissance. Vesalius carefully described the gross anatomy of the pericardium, and Ambroise Paré recognized that wounds to the heart were not always immediately fatal. This led to acknowledgment of the association between hemopericardium and delayed death (Ballance, 1920).

In the early 17th century, Rondelet described pericarditis and pleuritis. Jean Riolan (1649) suggested trephining the sternum to perform pericardiotomy as treatment for pericarditis. William Harvey (1649) described a case of hemopericardium and determined that the surface of the heart was insensitive to touch. Richard Lower (1669) accurately described the concepts of cardiac tamponade and constrictive pericarditis. His descriptions are poetic in structure yet accurate in content. In 1674, John Mayow described constrictive pericarditis and its physiologic consequences, 200 years before its recognition as the so-called Pick's syndrome. Vieussens was able to diagnose cardiac tamponade in living persons by the close of the 17th century.

Advances in knowledge of the pericardium and its diseases were dominated in the 18th century by Morgagni, who described constrictive pericarditis and its association with pleuritis and offered 45 pathologic cases to exemplify his findings (Morgagni, 1756). Additionally, Morgagni reluctantly advocated pericardiocentesis and recognized its attendant danger. The physical diagnosis of pericardial effusion was refined by Leopold Auenbrugger (1761), who not only popularized precordial percussion as a diagnostic modality but also recorded his observations of other clinical signs of cardiac tamponade.

During the 19th century, enthusiasm grew for direct intervention into the pericardium. Although Corvisart (1818) and his student, Laënnec (1819), were quite hesitant to use either incision or blind puncture of the pericardium, their clinical observations formed a sound basis for future interventions. In 1819, Romero performed the first successful pericardiotomy (Baizeau, 1868). In 1840, Franz Schuh performed the first blind pericardiocentesis (Dumreicher, 1866). The 19th century also saw increasing understanding of the pathophysiology of constrictive pericarditis. In 1842, Cheevers pointed out that the contraction of fibrous tissue around the heart interfered with cardiac function and produced the symptoms associated with constrictive pericarditis. In 1873, Kussmaul identified the association of paradoxic pulse with constrictive pericarditis. The term *pulsus paradoxus* arose as a result of his observation that the peripheral pulse seemed to disappear when the cardiac impulse was known to be present. Kussmaul also described the rise in venous pressure occurring during inspiration in patients with pericardial constriction. In 1896, Pick described three patients with hepatic congestion and fibrosis attributed to cirrhosis of the liver, which later proved pathologically to be due to chronic constrictive pericarditis (Pick, 1896). Surgical attack on pericardial constriction was proposed by Weill in 1895 and Délorme in 1898.

The early 20th century marked a time of widespread surgical attack on diseases of the pericardium, particularly constrictive pericarditis. Rehn (1913) and Sauerbruch (1925) each described pericardial resection for constrictive pericarditis. Schmieden and Fischer (1926) offered their experience with seven cases of pericardial resection in the German literature. Landmark experiences with the surgical treatment of constrictive pericarditis in America were published by Churchill (1936), Beck and Griswold (1930), and Blalock and Levy (1937). Beck's experiment with the induction of constrictive pericarditis following injection of Dakin's solution into the pericardial cavity of dogs proved that the development of the symptoms of pericardial constriction required mechanical constriction of the myocardium by the encompassing scar, not simply the obliteration of the pericardial cavity. He further showed that pericardiectomy would relieve the syndrome. Parsons and Holman (1951) performed similar experiments on right-sided constrictive pericarditis, following which Isaacs (Isaacs et al., 1952) performed exceedingly detailed experimental studies of localized and generalized pericarditis and the associated hemodynamic findings. Holman, in his chairman's address to the Surgical Session of the American Medical Association, expounded on the advantages of radical pericardiectomy, including excision of thickened epicardium when necessary (Holman and Willett, 1955).

Much of our current understanding of the pericardium and its associated diseases has been elucidated by the works of Spodick and Shabetai. These authors, as well as many others, continue to teach us about the surprising complexity that is discovered through dedicated study of seemingly simple phenomena.

## ANATOMY AND PHYSIOLOGY OF THE PERICARDIUM

What is called the *pericardium* is actually the *parietal pericardium,* which is, not simply, a fibrous sac surrounding the heart. This sac is composed of an outer serosa and an inner fibrosa. The visceral pericardium is a monocellular serosal layer comprising the epicardium of the cardiac surface (Holt, 1970). The visceral and parietal pericardium fuse over the great vessels and pulmonary veins. The fibrosa of the parietal pericardium continues up over the arch of the aorta, where it blends with the deep cervical fascia. Two major developmental recesses may be identified within the pericardial sac (Fig. 34–1). The *transverse sinus* is located behind the proximal ascending aorta and the pulmonary artery, and in front of the atria and superior vena cava. The *oblique sinus* lies inferior to the transverse sinus, between the right and the left pulmonary veins, and medial to the inferior vena cava (Spodick, 1992).

The pericardium is innervated by the phrenic and vagal nerves. The arterial supply originates from small aortic branches dorsally and from the pericardiacophrenic vessels branching from the internal thoracic artery. Venous drainage occurs from corresponding veins. A superficial plexus of cardiac lymphatics drains the visceral pericardium into the tracheal and bronchial mediastinal lymph nodes. The lymphatic drainage of the anterior and posterior parietal pericardium is directed into corresponding mediastinal lymph nodes. One or two identifiable lymph nodes may be found within the fibrosa near the junction of the inferior vena cava with the heart (Spodick, 1992).

The fibrosa of the parietal pericardium is loosely anchored by ligamentous structures to the sternal manubrium and xiphoid process. However, it is firmly attached to the central tendon of the diaphragm.

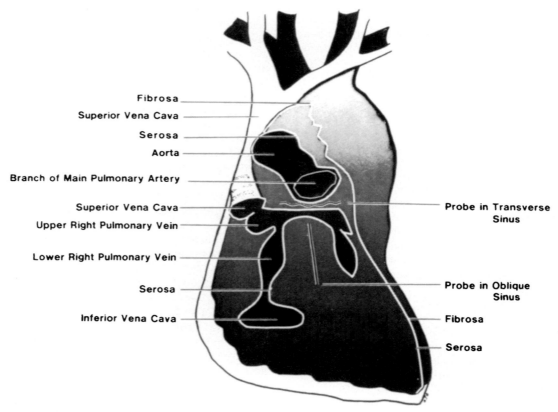

**FIGURE 34–1.** Anatomy of the posterior cardiac bed of the pericardium. Major pericardial sinuses are shown with probes lying in them. The upper recess, the *transverse sinus*, is a small tube. In the *oblique sinus* is a relatively large pericardial outpouching where the pericardium splits to permit passage of the four pulmonary veins and the venae cavae. (From Spodick, D. H.: Macrophysiology, microphysiology, and anatomy of the pericardium: A synopsis. Am. Heart J., *124*:1046, 1992.)

## Microscopic Anatomy

The serosa is composed of interdigitating mesothelial cells. These cells contain microvilli and a cytoskeletal filament structural support system. The basal lamina beneath the serosal cells provides little resistance to exfoliation.

The fibrosa is composed of fibrocollagenous tissue containing elastic fibers that decrease in density with age. The fibrous tissue is thickest over the thinner parts of the myocardium. They are oriented according to mechanical stress (Spodick, 1992).

## Pericardial Fluid

There is normally about 15 to 50 ml of serous fluid between the visceral and the parietal pericardia. This fluid is an ultrafiltrate of plasma containing an overall protein concentration lower than plasma but a higher albumin content. The electrolyte concentrations are those of any plasma ultrafiltrate. Consequently, the osmolarity is less than plasma osmolarity (Spodick, 1992).

## PHYSIOLOGIC FUNCTIONS OF THE PERICARDIUM

Because of its location and the presence of pericardial fluid, the pericardium mechanically protects the heart from external friction and provides a barrier to inflammation from contiguous structures. Thinner portions of the myocardium, including the atria and right ventricle, may be protected and supported by its relatively tough composition. Through its attachments to the diaphragm and sternum, it also maintains cardiac position against gravitational forces and other sources of acceleration (Holt, 1970).

Detailed research studies have identified other regulatory and serologic functions of the pericardium. Mechanoreceptors are present, and they can contract the spleen and lower blood pressure. These mechanoreceptors, with their associated phrenic nerve afferents, have been identified in dogs (Kostreva and Pontus, 1993). Additionally, neuroreceptors operating through feedback mechanisms can cause vagally generated lowering of the blood pressure and heart rate. The pericardial fluid contains immunologic constituents, including complement, as well as prostacyclin and prostacyclin synthetase, which can affect coronary artery vasomotor tone. Furthermore, the fibrinolytic activity of the pericardial fluid has long been observed to oppose intrapericardial blood clotting following intrapericardial hemorrhage.

## NORMAL AND PATHOLOGIC HEMODYNAMIC EFFECTS OF THE PERICARDIUM

Although it has been amply demonstrated that the normal animal or human can function satisfactorily without a pericardium, whether surgically removed or congenitally absent, it is also clear that the presence of the pericardium has definite hemodynamic and physiologic consequences (Tyson et al., 1984; Watkins and LeWinter, 1993). Under conditions of left ventricular stress, the resulting pericardial tension may limit right ventricular diastolic filling. Similarly, ventriculoatrial regurgitation may be limited by the presence of the pericardium (Berglund et al., 1955). Following cardiac surgery, closure of the pericardium has been shown to significantly constrain diastolic filling of the left ventricle (Daughters et al., 1992). In pathologic conditions of the pericardium or the encompassed cardiac structures, the pericardium can have dramatic effects.

To understand the hemodynamic effects of the pericardium and how the measurement of these effects aids diagnosis of pathologic conditions, one must firmly understand basic cardiac mechanics and cardiac chamber pressure fluctuations over the cardiac cycle. The combination of these intracardiac processes and the pressure gradients within and outside the pericardium determines the ultimate hemodynamic changes that may be identified. Despite decades of study, certain long-standing physiologic observations continue to generate controversy.

### Hemodynamic Effects of Respiration in Normal Subjects

Normally, the measured intrapericardial pressure is approximately 2 mm Hg in the absence of active inspiration or expiration. This measured pressure approximates and varies with intrapleural pressure measured at the same hydrostatic level. Consequently, transmural pericardial pressure, defined as intrapericardial pressure minus intrapleural pressure, approximates zero as long as cardiac cavitary pressures are normal. On the other hand, myocardial transmural pressure, defined as intracavitary chamber pressure minus adjacent intrapericardial pressure, is positive during diastole, ensuring that the distending cardiac pressures are greater than the cavitary pressure. For example, a diastolic pressure of 5 mm Hg relative to atmospheric pressure would translate into a transmural pressure of 7 mm Hg (i.e., $5-(-2) = 7$) when referenced to the intrapericardial pressure. The transmural pressure then becomes the actual chamber pressure-distending pressure, or filling pressure, in contrast to the cavitary pressure measured with reference to atmospheric pressure (Spodick, 1992). During inspiration, pleural, pericardial, right atrial, right ventricular, pulmonary wedge, and systemic arterial pressures all decrease slightly. However, pericardial pressure decreases more than atrial pressure, such that the right atrial and other central transmural pressures increase, thereby augmenting right-sided heart filling and, consequently, right ventricular preload. Pulmonary arterial flow velocity increases while aortic flow and aortic transmural pressure decrease. This activity occurs as systemic venous return is increasing. Pulmonary vascular capacity increases as the right ventricular output tends to pool in the lungs during inspiration. This reduces pulmonary venous return to the left atrium during inspiration.

It has long been noted that the left ventricular stroke volume, aortic blood flow, and aortic blood pressure all decrease during inspiration. The decrease in blood pressure is less than 10 mm Hg in normal subjects. Despite the long-standing recognition of this phenomenon, its function has not been easy to explain, and it has been the source of extensive experimental investigations. It now seems evident that the decrease in left ventricular output and subsequent aortic blood pressure results from several factors. The relative importance of each factor probably varies with physiologic conditions. Several explanations have been offered: (1) Increased pooling of blood in the lungs during inspiration causes a decrease in left ventricular end diastolic volume and the subsequent fall in left ventricular stroke shortening and peak aortic blood flow (Franklin et al., 1962; Macklin, 1946). (2) Increased filling of the right ventricle during inspiration causes a leftward shift of the intraventricular septum with resultant decrease in left ventricular filling and subsequent stroke volumes (Brinker et al., 1980; Santamore et al., 1976). (3) Leftward shifting of the intraventricular septum as a result of increased right-sided heart filling during inspiration alters the left ventricular geometry such that the flattened intraventricular septum develops a greater septal radius of curvature. This increased radius of curvature would be associated with an increased wall tension, according to La Place's law, and thereby cause an increased left ventricular afterload, with associated decrease in the left ventricular stroke volume during ejection (Hoffman et al., 1965). (4) Left ventricular transmural pressure (left ventricular intracavitary pressure minus pleural pressure) increases during inspiration and causes a fall in left ventricular stroke volume (Charlier et al., 1974; Schrijen et al., 1975; Summer et al., 1979). (5) During inspiration, the intracavitary left ventricular pressure is decreased relative to atmospheric pressure. The effective ejection pressure during systole becomes the intracavitary left ventricular pressure relative to atmospheric pressure, because the peripheral vasculature is subjected to atmospheric pressure as the appropriate external pressure force. This has been called the reverse thoracic pump mechanism of decreased left ventricular stroke volume during inspiration (Olsen et al., 1985).

The authors of the last hypothesis have questioned each of the first four explanations following very elegant experimental observations.

## Normal Venous Pulse

The jugular venous pulse as examined externally directly reflects the central venous pressure waves and, in turn, the right atrial pressure fluctuations occurring during the cardiac cycle. These pressure waves have a characteristic configuration that varies with respiration and with each component of the cardiac contraction (Hurst, 1978; Shabetai et al., 1970) (Fig. 34–2). The pulse contour consists of three positive pulse waves, called a, c, and v waves, and two negative pulse waves, called x and y. The a wave occurs as a result of normal atrial contraction. If an S4 atrial gallop sound is heard, it occurs at the peak of the a wave. As the atrium relaxes, the venous pressure decreases slightly until the onset of ventricular contraction. Right ventricular systole causes bulging of the tricuspid valve into the right atrium and a consequent pressure elevation, inscribed as the c wave. The c wave begins at the end of the first heart sound and peaks shortly after the first heart sound. Soon after the summit of the c wave, the venous pulse contour rapidly declines ("x descent") from the fall in pressure produced by downward displacement of the base of the ventricles, including the tricuspid valve, during ventricular systole. Atrial relaxation also contributes to this fall in pressure. If pressure is measured in the right atrium, the lowest point of the x wave occurs in early or mid-ventricular systole, whereas in the jugular vein it usually occurs in late systole, shortly before the second heart sound.

While ventricular systole is nearing its completion, blood continues to fill the venae cavae and the right atrium, thereby increasing volume and pressure within those chambers. This is reflected in a rising venous pulse pressure known as the v wave. The peak of the v wave occurs just after the second heart sound. The right atrial pressure rapidly decreases following opening of the tricuspid valve, thereby inscribing the descending limb of the y wave, or *y descent*, also called the jugular venous *diastolic collapse*. The initial portion of the y descent corresponds to rapid right ventricular filling. If the patient has a right-sided S3 gallop, it usually occurs at the nadir of the recorded y wave. A left-sided S3 gallop would

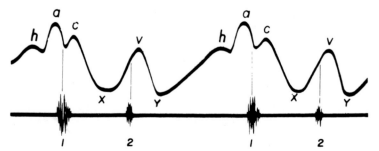

**FIGURE 34–2.** Tracing of venous pulse waves overlying phonocardiogram recording of first and second heart sounds. See text for details. (From Hurst, J. W.: The Heart. 4th ed. New York, McGraw-Hill, 1978. Reproduced with permission of McGraw-Hill, Inc.)

occur shortly before the nadir. The subsequent rise in pressure occurs as diastole continues and the heart fills with blood prior to atrial systole. The rate of rise of the ascending limb of the y wave depends on the rate of venous return and the distensibility of the cardiac chambers and venae cavae. A small, brief, positive wave known as the h wave may be noted following recording of the ascending limb of the y wave if diastole is particularly long. This marks the end of slow filling of the right ventricle and occurs just prior to atrial contraction and the accompanying a wave. As the heart rate increases, the h wave disappears, and the y descent and ascent are followed immediately by the positive a wave. With extremely fast heart rates, the entire y wave may be eliminated as the v wave fuses with the following a wave.

To further understand the use of these pressure waves in the diagnosis of pericardial diseases, it is important to highlight the characteristics of the x and y descents. The x descent occurs during the so-called systolic collapse of the venous pulse, and the y descent occurs during the diastolic collapse of the venous pulse. Furthermore, during inspiration, the x wave is usually lower than the y wave at a time when intrathoracic pressure is decreasing and pulmonary vascular capacity is increasing. During expiration, the y wave may be as low as the x wave or lower when intrathoracic pressure is more positive and venous return is reduced.

## HEMODYNAMIC CONSEQUENCES OF PERICARDIAL DISEASE

Although the normal heart can function quite satisfactorily in the absence of the parietal pericardium, disease states can profoundly influence normal hemodynamics. Of particular interest in this regard are the two conditions known as *cardiac tamponade* and *constrictive pericarditis*. Each may be caused by a variety of diseases and abnormal circumstances. However, the common end-point of impairment in cardiac function is characterized by distinctive clinical findings. This section addresses these two entities in terms of their physiologic effects, with little regard to the inciting disease state. Additionally, it compares the physiology of these conditions with that of restrictive cardiomyopathy, which may be confused with either of these conditions when hemodynamic data alone are available. Subsequent sections discuss specific diseases that may cause these syndromes.

### Cardiac Tamponade

Cardiac tamponade has been eloquently defined by Spodick as hemodynamically significant cardiac compression due to accumulating pericardial contents that evoke and defeat compensatory mechanisms (Spodick, 1983). The offending pericardial contents may be effusion, pus, blood, gas, or tumor. Because the pericardium can accommodate increasing pericar-

dial contents over time, the development of hemodynamic compromise depends on both the volume of pericardial contents and the rate at which these contents accumulate. Even pericardial effusions as large as a liter in volume may be unaccompanied by hemodynamic embarrassment if this fluid accumulates over a long period. On the other hand, the acute accumulation of 200 ml of fluid may cause profound impairment in cardiac function in otherwise normal individuals.

The pathophysiology of cardiac tamponade is primarily based on impaired diastolic filling of the heart by other intrapericardial contents. The greatest initial effect is on the right side of the heart, and this is reflected in most cases by high central venous, mean atrial, and ventricular diastolic pressures. Central venous pressures in the 12 to 25 mm Hg range are common and may exceed 30 mm Hg in exceptional circumstances. The ventricular diastolic and mean right atrial pressures usually equilibrate within 4 mm Hg of these levels. These central venous pressures are rarely less than 10 mm Hg. This so-called "low pressure tamponade" occurs in patients in whom volume depletion is extreme (Kern and Aguirre, 1992a). As the intrapericardial pressure rises, the transmural pressure (intracavitary pressure minus intrapericardial pressure) is progressively reduced. In fact, during extreme cardiac tamponade, the transmural pressure may actually become negative, so that the ventricles fill partly by diastolic suction. This impairment in ventricular filling decreases stroke volume even in the presence of a normal ejection fraction and increased heart rate.

Although the compressive effects of cardiac tamponade on the low-pressure, thin-walled chambers of the right side of the heart occur early and are easy to identify, left ventricular function also is impaired. This seems to stem not only from external compression of the left ventricular and left atrial walls by the other intrapericardial contents, but also from the leftward shifting of the intraventricular septum exaggerated by the increased filling pressures in the right side of the heart.

The dynamic pressure changes occurring within the cardiac chambers during cardiac tamponade are reflected in the venous wave forms. During cardiac tamponade, the increased pericardial pressure surrounds the heart throughout the cardiac cycle, and its effect on cardiac filling increases as diastole progresses. Because the "systolic collapse" of the venous pressure persists during ventricular systole, the x descent remains on the venous pressure wave tracing. However, the normal y descent reflecting the "diastolic collapse" of the venous pressure wave is amputated because of impairment of atrial filling and emptying by the increasing intrapericardial pressure as the heart attempts to fill.

Cardiac tamponade exaggerates the normal inspiratory fall in left ventricular stroke volume and systolic blood pressure. This is called *pulsus paradoxus*, and is said to be present when the fall in systolic blood pressure is greater than or equal to 10 mm Hg (Kussmaul, 1873). The factors considered responsible for the normal decrease in systolic blood pressure during inspiration were described earlier. These factors undoubtedly come to play in the production of pulsus paradoxus during cardiac tamponade. However, the exaggeration of this effect is most likely due to further shifting of the left ventricular septum, which results from increased right-sided heart pressures caused by impairment of right-sided heart filling secondary to external compression. Left ventricular filling is further impaired by external compression. This reduced left ventricular filling is reflected in a reduced stroke volume.

Pulsus paradoxus is a characteristic finding in cardiac tamponade, but it may also be detected in other clinical states, including chronic obstructive pulmonary disease, pulmonary embolism, obesity, right-sided heart failure, and tense ascites, among other conditions. The mechanism that produces pulsus paradoxus is multifactorial in each of these conditions, but ultimately seems to be related to an exaggeration of one or more factors responsible for the reduction in stroke volume seen during normal inspiration. On the other hand, pulsus paradoxus may be absent in some patients with tamponade in the setting of left ventricular dysfunction, atrial septal defect, regional tamponade, or positive-pressure breathing (Fowler, 1993).

## Constrictive Pericarditis

Pericardial constriction may be a consequence of pericardial inflammation following most causes of pericarditis. The accompanying scarring may affect the parietal and visceral pericardium, obliterating the pericardial space and restricting cardiac filling. In contrast to cardiac tamponade, constrictive pericarditis does not impair cardiac filling in the very early phases of diastole. This delayed effect is responsible for the characteristic diastolic pressure tracings and is the basis for diagnosing the condition and differentiating it from cardiac tamponade.

With pericardial constriction, the ventricles relax without impediment during the early phases of diastole until they are suddenly limited by the encompassing scar. This is reflected in the characteristic "square root" configuration of the diastolic pressure tracings. The venous pulse tracing will show prominent y as well as x descents. The y descent, or diastolic collapse, tends to be deeper and very rapid compared with those of the cardiac tamponade. Figure 34–3 illustrates the distinguishing characteristics of pericardial constriction versus cardiac tamponade.

Restrictive cardiomyopathies such as amyloidosis and other myocardial infiltrative diseases may produce hemodynamic findings that have characteristics of both cardiac tamponade and pericardial constriction (Schoenfeld, 1990). In fact, restrictive cardiomyopathies may occur in concert with elements of pericardial constriction and compression. The differentiation of restrictive cardiomyopathies from cardiac tamponade or restrictive cardiomyopathies may be exceedingly difficult. Ultimately, myocardial biopsy may be required to make the definitive diagnosis. However, certain characteristics, including impair-

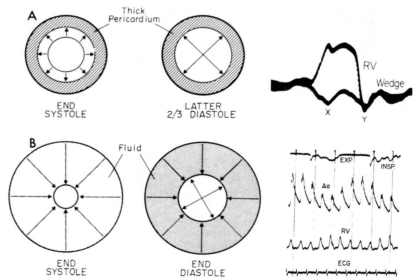

**FIGURE 34–3.** Diagram highlighting the differences between constrictive pericarditis and cardiac tamponade. *A*, Constrictive pericarditis. At end-systole and during early diastole, compression is absent or minimal. During this period, ventricular volume expands rapidly and ventricular filling is rapid. This is reflected in the early diastolic dip of right ventricular pressure and the corresponding Y descent of right atrial and wedge pressure. At the end of the first third of diastole, ventricular volume reaches the volume of the pericardium and cannot increase further; therefore, ventricular diastolic pressure plateaus. Note that in the latter part of diastole, right ventricular and pulmonary wedge pressures are equal. Normal systolic filling of the right ventricle occurs, reflected by the X descent of right atrial and wedge pressures. *B*, Cardiac tamponade. Severe compression is present throughout the cardiac cycle, but at end-diastole, the heart is at its largest volume, and therefore pericardial pressure is at its highest. For this reason, there is no filling of the heart during diastole. This is shown in the right ventricular pressure tracing, from which an early diastolic dip is absent. Note severe pulsus paradoxus in the aortic tracing. (RV = right ventricle; EXP. = expiration; INSP. = inspiration; Ao = aorta; ECG = electrocardiogram.) (From Shabetai, R.: The Pericardium. New York, Grune & Stratton, 1981, p. 241.)

ment in cardiac systolic function, left-sided cardiac pressures exceeding right-sided pressures, and slower early to mid-diastolic cardiac filling, are suggestive of restrictive cardiomyopathy. Echocardiography may help but may not be diagnostic. A thorough discussion of the problems in differentiating these diseases is beyond the scope of this chapter. The reader is referred to the works of Brockington and colleagues (1990) and Schoenfeld (1990).

## DIAGNOSTIC TESTS FOR PERICARDIAL DISEASES

Pericardial disease may be suggested by the inflammatory response or hemodynamic consequences of the disease. Pericardial inflammation may be indicated by the presence of chest pain, fever, or systemic symptoms. The presence of myocardial compression or constriction may be reflected in hemodynamic deterioration, abdominal pain, ascites, or peripheral edema. Occasionally, pericardial disease is asymptomatic. A variety of diagnostic tests may indicate the presence of pericardial disease.

The electrocardiogram is a fairly nonspecific modality for the diagnosis of pericardial disease, but in the presence of large pericardial effusions, the QRS voltage may be diminished. Pericarditis may be reflected in more characteristic changes. Pericarditis typically goes through four stages that can be recognized by the electrocardiogram (Spodick, 1983). Stage I is characterized by diffuse ST segment elevation in all leads except for AVR and $V_1$. In Stage II, which develops several days following Stage I, the ST segments are normal, and the T waves are flattened. In Stage III, the T-wave inversion returns but is not associated with the loss of R-wave voltage and the appearance of Q waves as seen during the evolution of myocardial infarction. Finally, in Stage IV, which occurs weeks or months later, the T waves revert to normal.

The chest film may indicate the presence of pericardial disease by revealing pericardial calcifications, as seen in chronic constrictive pericarditis, or enlargement of the cardiac silhouette, seen when pericardial effusion, hemopericardium, or intrapericardial tumor is present. Additionally, pneumopericardium may be visualized on chest film. Occasionally, pericardial cysts may be identified by chest radiographs.

Echocardiography, particularly in the two-dimensional mode, currently provides the greatest amount of information with the least invasiveness required to diagnose pericardial diseases. Echocardiography can define the presence of intrapericardial fluid or masses, pericardial cysts, pericardial calcification, and accompanying cardiac or intracardiac pathology. Additionally, echocardiography can help evaluate the hemodynamic consequences of pericardial disease. It may be used to diagnose cardiac tamponade and is useful in distinguishing pericardial constriction. It may also monitor the course of therapy. Echocardiography

markedly increases the accuracy and safety of pericardiocentesis.

Computed tomography (CT) and electrocardiographically gated magnetic resonance imaging (MRI) have been used to evaluate diseases of the pericardium (Brown et al., 1989). Each study has particular advantages under certain circumstances, but the two overlap considerably in their generation of useful information. MRI has the advantage of not requiring injection of contrast medium into the circulation. Additionally, it can enhance the contrast of soft tissue. On the other hand, CT has better spatial resolution and greater sensitivity to calcification. Intracardiac masses are better delineated by MRI (Pennell and Underwood, 1993). Of particular interest are the data suggesting that CT and MRI may be useful in identifying myocardial atrophy and restrictive cardiomyopathy in association with pericardial constriction (Reinmuller et al., 1993; Suchet and Horwitz, 1992).

Angiocardiography is useful primarily in detecting the hemodynamic consequences of pericardial disease. The pressure tracings obtained during this study may be used to diagnose cardiac tamponade and pericardial constriction (described earlier). Furthermore, with the exchange of catheters for biotomes, intramyocardial biopsies may be obtained for the diagnosis of associated myocardial disease. These biopsies are frequently required to distinguish restrictive cardiomyopathies from pericardial constriction.

## CLINICAL PRESENTATION AND MANAGEMENT OF CARDIAC TAMPONADE AND PERICARDIAL CONSTRICTION

Cardiac tamponade may derive from the accumulation of any intrapericardial contents to a degree sufficient to compress the heart and interfere with cardiac filling. Acute cardiac tamponade occurs most often as a result of hemopericardium. This may follow trauma, such as that produced by knife or bullet wounds, iatrogenic injury from pericardiocentesis, or aortic rupture (Fig. 34–4). These patients can present with cardiovascular collapse and shock. Jugular venous distention, a hallmark of cardiac tamponade, may not be present if the intravascular volume is diminished. More chronic cardiac tamponade may derive from the accumulation of pericardial effusion following pericarditis, malignancy, or connective tissue disorders. Symptoms may include the insidious onset of malaise and accompanying signs of tachypnea, tachycardia, pallor, cyanosis, diaphoresis, cool periphery, and impairment of cerebral and renal function. These findings reflect the body's attempt to compensate for the diminished cardiac output by increasing adrenergic stimulation to preserve blood pressure and maintain blood volume.

The therapeutic interventions required for the treatment of cardiac tamponade depend on the acuity of onset, the degree of hemodynamic compromise, and the disease process responsible for the syndrome.

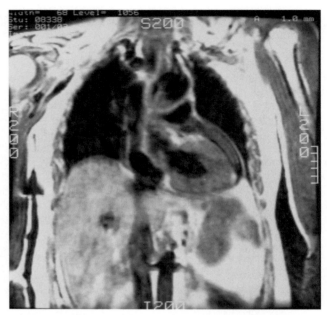

**FIGURE 34–4.** Magnetic resonance imaging scan demonstrating an ascending aortic dissection with associated hemopericardium.

Medical therapy alone is rarely indicated. However, in cases of chronic cardiac tamponade, patients may be prepared for more definitive therapy by blood volume expansion, inotropic support, or afterload-reducing agents, or a combination of these. Regardless of the cause, definitive treatment of cardiac tamponade requires removal of the agent responsible for the cardiac compression. In the setting of acute cardiac decompensation following intrapericardial hemorrhage, for example, the evacuation of as little as 50 ml of blood can produce marked clinical improvement. This may be accomplished quickly by percutaneous pericardiocentesis. The safety of this procedure, which may have a complication rate ranging from 7 to 20%, may be significantly improved by the use of electrocardiographic monitoring or echocardiographically directed pericardial aspiration (Kirkland and Taylor, 1992; Susini et al., 1993; Wang et al., 1992). Following initial stabilization with pericardiocentesis, a definitive approach to the inciting process is frequently necessary. In the event of hemopericardium, adequate exposure to allow repair of the compromising process and evacuation of blood may require full median sternotomy. Alternatively, left-sided anterior thoracotomy provides quick, but more limited, access to the heart.

In the setting of more chronic effusion, a subxiphoid approach may be used to evacuate the effusion and resect pericardial tissue for pathologic examination. With loculated effusions or recurrent effusions, or when recurrence of effusion is likely, the thoracotomy approach may be preferable to a subxiphoid pericardial window. A thoracoscopic approach through the left side of the chest has been shown to be effective for wide pericardial resection (Mack et al., 1992).

## CARDIAC TAMPONADE FOLLOWING CARDIAC OPERATIONS

In the early postoperative period following cardiac surgery, cardiac tamponade may begin with clinical findings that differ from those more typical of nonsurgical patients. Although sudden cardiac hemorrhage may be accompanied by classic signs of shock with high venous pressures, the slow accumulation of pericardial clot may present quite differently. The diagnosis of cardiac tamponade following surgery requires a great deal of clinical judgment. Because the patient may have cardiac deterioration from ventricular failure as well as compressive disorders, the surgeon must determine which factors are responsible.

The development of increasing right-sided pressures accompanied by deteriorating cardiac output and diminished urine output should alert the surgeon to the possibility of ongoing cardiac tamponade. Its likelihood is increased when excessive bleeding has been recognized. Classic right-sided pressure tracings may not be present. In fact, the tracings may be more like those seen in constrictive pericarditis, in that the y descent is frequently prominent (Beppu et al., 1993). This appears to reflect the fact that pericardial clot and its accompanying compression causes a more localized cardiac impairment, becoming most evident after the onset of diastole. Although the clot may be rather localized, intrapericardial pressures will be elevated in general.

Echocardiography may help to determine the presence of cardiac tamponade postoperatively. However, its value lies more in its ability to document adequate ventricular function than in its identification of pericardial clot. Because blood and clot may occur in the absence of cardiac tamponade, the identification of either of these does not necessarily confirm its presence. Transesophageal echocardiography is more accurate than surface echocardiography in identifying the presence of clot anteriorly or inferiorly.

A high degree of clinical suspicion is necessary to avoid catastrophic results from missing the diagnosis of cardiac tamponade. None of the previously mentioned findings are diagnostic when taken alone. However, when they are considered in the overall clinical setting, suspicion of cardiac tamponade is reasonable. In some cases, it is much better to explore the patient for possible cardiac tamponade and risk negative results than to allow the condition to persist and cause serious morbidity.

## PERICARDITIS

Pericarditis refers to many inflammatory and infectious diseases that affect the pericardium. The diseases may be primary processes involving the pericardium, contiguous disease processes from the lungs or myocardium, or secondary manifestations of systemic diseases. The conditions may be characterized as either acute or chronic according to the rapidity of onset and course of progression. Furthermore, pericarditis may be characterized according to the morphologic and pathologic nature of the reaction: it may be called dry, transudative, effusive, hemorrhagic, fibrinous, effusive, exudative, purulent, constrictive, or effusive-constrictive. Although these terms do not apply exclusively to individual disease processes, characteristic pathologic appearances do accompany specific disease states.

In its acute, inflammatory stages, pericarditis is frequently accompanied by chest pain. This pain may be pleuritic and may radiate to the trapezius muscle regions. Accompanying cardiac, bronchopulmonary, or pleural disease may produce dyspnea. Low-grade fever is not unusual, and anorexia is common. Physical examination may reveal a pericardial friction rub. Hematologic parameters vary with the disease process responsible for the pericarditis. Electrocardiographic changes (described earlier) are nonspecific but progress characteristically. Echocardiography may reveal increased pericardial fluid (Spodick, 1992).

Chronic pericarditis is more likely to be symptomatic because it is accompanied by accumulation of pericardial fluid or the development of pericardial constriction. The signs and symptoms of cardiac tamponade and pericardial constriction then accompany this development. The following sections explore the clinical and pathologic features of some specific pericardial diseases.

## Idiopathic and Viral Pericarditis

So-called benign or idiopathic pericarditis is a syndrome characterized by pericardial inflammation, usually accompanied by increased pericardial fluid, without clearly definable cause. Patients become symptomatic either from the inflammatory response or the compressive effects of the fluid. Some cases are identified incidentally. The findings are identical to those accompanying documented viral pericarditis from viruses such as Coxsackie A and B and influenza A and B. The difference lies only in the ability to culture these organisms from pericardial tissue and fluid (Waller et al., 1992).

Treatment of these forms of pericarditis is primarily medical. Nonsteroidal anti-inflammatory agents such as ibuprofen and indomethacin are the first lines of therapy. Aspirin also may be used. Because experimental work has suggested that indomethacin can reduce coronary artery blood flow and increase blood pressure, it is prudent to avoid this medication in patients with known coronary artery disease and hypertension. When patients do not respond to either of these medications, corticosteroid therapy may be necessary. Because of the known side effects of chronic steroid therapy, chronic administration is avoided; usually it is applied only after other anti-inflammatory agents have been unsuccessful.

Surgery may be required if accompanying pericardial effusion or subsequent constriction impairs cardiac function. In rare cases when medical treatment of inflammatory symptoms has been unsuccessful, pericardiectomy may be tried.

## Uremic Pericarditis

Uremic pericarditis occurs in approximately 50% of patients with untreated renal disease and approximately 20% of patients on hemodialysis (Frame et al., 1983). It is less often seen in patients on peritoneal dialysis. Uremic pericarditis appears to be unrelated to the absolute level of the blood urea nitrogen and the serum creatinine. The pathogenesis of the disease process is unclear (Fig. 34–5).

Individuals with the disorder may present with signs and symptoms of typical acute pericarditis. They most often come to the attention of the surgical service as a result of accompanying effusions. Additionally, the disease may develop into constrictive pericarditis and thus require surgical intervention.

Initially, symptomatic patients should be treated

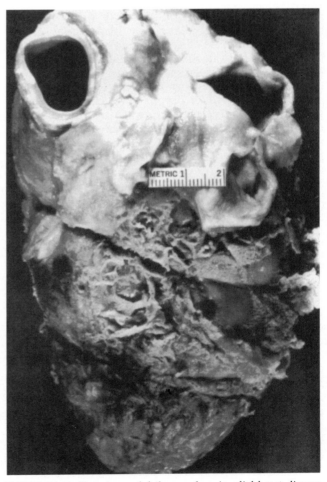

**FIGURE 34–5.** Chronic renal failure and pericardial heart disease. Diffuse fibrinous deposits over the visceral pericardial surface. (From Waller B. F., Taliercio, C. P., Howard, J., et al.: Morphologic aspects of pericardial heart disease: Part II. Clin. Cardiol., 15:291, 1992. Copyrighted and reprinted with the permission of Clinical Cardiology Publishing Company, Inc., and/or Foundation for Advances in Medicine and Sciences, Inc.)

with daily dialysis. This allows recovery in approximately half of these individuals. Short courses of steroids or nonsteroidal inflammatory agents may be added, particularly for the treatment of chest pain and fever. Pericardiocentesis should be performed for the treatment of hemodynamic compromise. In patients with significant hemodynamic instability, a pericardial window for drainage is mandatory. Additionally, patients who develop an enlarging effusion or an effusion unresponsive to 10 days of medical therapy should be considered for pericardial window (Frame et al., 1983). A subxiphoid approach is commonly used. However, complex, loculated effusions and recurrent effusions are best treated by a left-sided anterior thoracotomy or perhaps a thoracoscopic approach.

## Tuberculous Pericarditis

Tuberculous pericarditis occurs in approximately 1 to 2% of cases of tuberculosis. It most likely rises from blood-borne infection, though some cases may come from retrograde lymphatic spread or direct invasion from infected lung, pleura, or mediastinal lymph nodes. The four stages of tuberculous involvement of the pericardium have been described by Peel (Waller et al., 1992). The disease begins with an early stage of fibrinous pericarditis and slowly progresses to effusive (nonconstrictive), fibrous (nonconstrictive), and fibrous (constrictive). Patients may present with typical signs of tuberculosis, including malaise, fever, sweats, and a cough. The presence of chest pain, pleural pain, and a pericardial friction rub would easily lead one to diagnose tuberculous pericarditis. However, many patients have very nonspecific and insidious symptoms that may not be identified as being secondary to tuberculosis until the disease has progressed.

The effusion associated with tuberculous pericarditis may be clear, straw-colored, or sanguineous. As the fluid is absorbed, it becomes viscous and is associated with the deposition of fibrous tissue. With chronic disease, this fibrosis may calcify; in fact, tuberculosis is one of the most common causes of calcific pericardial heart disease. Chronic constriction is a consequence of late intervention.

Tuberculous pericarditis may be diagnosed from culture of pericardial fluid or tissue containing acid-fast bacilli. Skin test results for tuberculosis may be negative because of anergy resulting from diffuse disease. In some cases, treatment for tuberculosis is indicated in patients who have the clinical characteristics of the disease even when culture studies cannot confirm its presence.

Treatment of tuberculous pericarditis requires intensive multiple antituberculosis drug therapy. Aspiration of pericardial fluid may be required to diagnose or treat compressive symptoms. Chronic, open drainage is to be avoided. Following the initiation of therapy, clinical signs of improvement usually appear in 2 to 3 weeks.

Tuberculous pericarditis that goes untreated predictably causes progressive pericardial effusion and subsequent pericardial constriction. Constrictive pericarditis following tuberculosis may cause calcified pericardial disease, which is difficult to treat. Because of these recognized complications, early treatment of tuberculous pericarditis is recommended. Aspiration and drainage of a tuberculous effusion early in the course of the disease may avert the subsequent development of constrictive pericarditis. Once constrictive pericarditis is diagnosed, pericardiectomy via a median sternotomy or left-sided anterior thoracotomy should be performed.

## Purulent Pericarditis

Bacterial infection of the pericardium is most commonly caused by *Staphylococcus* or gram-negative organisms in adults, and *Hemophilus influenzae* or *Staphylococcus* in children (Fig. 34–6). It may follow direct contamination from an injury or spread from a contiguous pneumonic or subdiaphragmatic infection. Blood-borne infection also may cause purulent pericarditis.

Most commonly, purulent pericarditis produces

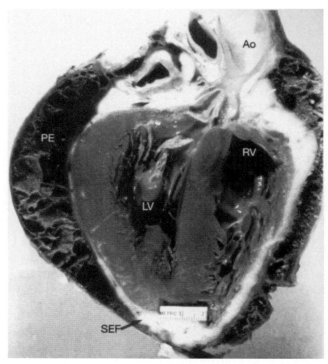

**FIGURE 34–6.** Bacterial pericarditis. Tomographic view of the heart showing large, bloody, purulent pericardial effusion (PE). The patient had repeated episodes of *Staphylococcus* septicemia. Various pericardial responses are present: fibrin *(arrow)*, blood, pus, neutrophils, necrotic debris, and pericardial thickening. (Ao = aorta; LV = left ventricle; RV = right ventricle; SEF = subepicardial fat.) (From Waller, B. F., Taliercio, C. P., Howard, J., et al.: Morphologic aspects of pericardial heart disease: Part II. Clin. Cardiol., 15:291, 1992. Copyrighted and reprinted with the permission of Clinical Cardiology Publishing Company, Inc., and/or Foundation for Advances in Medicine and Sciences, Inc.)

symptoms of chest pain and fever. The sudden accumulation of intrapericardial fluid may cause cardiac tamponade. Additionally, children may present with respiratory distress, anorexia, or abdominal discomfort.

Purulent pericarditis is diagnosed with pericardiocentesis. Initial therapy usually consists of appropriate antibiotics and aspiration of the purulent fluid. Early aggressive tube drainage by means of a subxiphoid pericardial window has been advocated by some authors. Because of the thick purulent drainage associated with *Hemophilus influenzae* pericarditis, some authors have recommended early pericardiectomy (Morgan et al., 1983). Pericardiectomy is also indicated as treatment for cardiac tamponade or persistent fever.

## Other Forms of Infectious Pericarditis

Amebic abscesses originating in the liver may rupture into the neighboring pericardium as a direct extension of the process from the left lobe of the liver. Sudden rupture may be accompanied by severe pain, dyspnea, and cardiovascular collapse. Immediate pericardial aspiration is indicated (Waller et al., 1992).

Echinococcal cysts may originate in the myocardium and rupture into the pericardium. The resultant reaction may be mild or, following multiplication of the organisms, the entire pericardial sac may become involved.

## Neoplastic Pericarditis

Cardiac involvement occurs in approximately 10% of patients with noncardiac neoplasms. Tumors affect the pericardium in 85% of those patients (Hawkins and Vacek, 1989). Most cases of pericardial involvement with metastatic disease occur from carcinomas of the lung and breast, in addition to leukemias and lymphomas. The primary tumors most likely to spread to the pericardium are melanoma, leukemia, and lymphoma. Primary neoplasms of the pericardium are rare. Sarcomas and malignant teratomas have been reported. Additionally, some cases of primary mesothelioma have been described. Benign tumors, including lipomas, hemangiomas, and fibromas, have been reported.

Neoplastic diseases of the pericardium usually present clinically as a result of the associated pericardial effusion (Fig. 34–7). Signs and symptoms of cardiac tamponade are common modes of presentation. Rarely, lymphomas present with pericardial constriction (Lawrence and Rochmis, 1967; Scully et al., 1987). In the setting of known malignant disease, other processes in the differential diagnosis include superior vena caval obstruction, pulmonary hypertension related to tumor embolization in the pulmonary arterial tree, or thrombosis and pericardial constriction.

Malignant pericardial effusion is most easily diagnosed by echocardiography. Cardiac catheterization

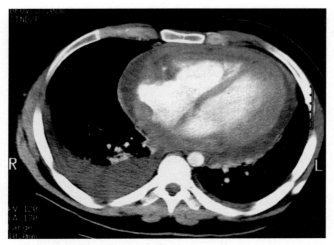

**FIGURE 34–7.** Computed tomographic scan of patient with neoplastic pericarditis. Note the thickened pericardium and circumferential effusion.

provides hemodynamic data and may be useful in discriminating other processes in the differential diagnosis. Aspiration of the pericardial fluid reveals a cytologically positive diagnosis of malignancy in approximately 75% of patients (Hawkins and Vacek, 1989). Firm diagnosis may require pericardial biopsy. CT or MRI can aid in visualizing tumor masses (Moncada et al., 1986).

Because neoplastic pericardial disease most commonly results from accompanying pericardial effusion, the first step in diagnosis and/or treatment is typically echocardiography followed by pericardiocentesis. Bedside echo-directed pericardiocentesis is frequently performed. Pericardiocentesis done with Swan-Ganz catheter monitoring allows documentation of the hemodynamic effects of the fluid aspiration. The insertion of a drainage catheter within the pericardium allows for several days of drainage and multiple aspirations. Recurrent or large effusions are treated best with a pericardial window, most often using the subxiphoid approach. Though the recurrence rate is probably lower when pericardiectomy is performed through a left-sided anterior thoracotomy, the generally poor prognosis in patients with malignancy and the less invasive nature of the subxiphoid approach make it preferable in most cases. Of 25 patients at Duke University with malignancy and pericardial effusion, 91% died in less than 1 year (Campbell et al., 1992). Experience is growing with a thoracoscopic approach to pericardial window, with drainage of the fluid into the left chest (Mack, 1992). This technique avoids a larger thoracotomy incision and allows for essentially the same operation to be performed. However, it may be more time-consuming and more challenging in inexperienced hands.

Some authors have recommended the intrapericardial administration of tetracycline as a sclerosing agent to prevent recurrence of malignant pericardial effusion. However, because tetracycline is no longer available for such use, the use of doxycycline has been described (Robinson et al., 1993). Antineoplastic agents have also been used. The appropriate use of these agents has yet to be elucidated fully. Some physicians have been wary of these treatments because of the risks for producing constrictive pericarditis. It seems prudent to reserve this form of therapy for patients who are particularly resistant to more standard treatment or those who are very poor surgical candidates.

## POSTPERICARDIOTOMY SYNDROME

The postpericardiotomy syndrome typically occurs between 2 and 4 weeks following surgical intervention within the pericardium. The development of the syndrome does not depend on the operation performed or even the degree of incision into the pericardium. It is characterized by the development of pericardial and/or pleural effusions. Patients suffering from the disorder may present with symptoms of fever, chest pain, or cardiac compression. Other symptoms include dyspnea, nonproductive cough, fatigue, and myalgias. The severity varies from a very mild complex to severe, incapacitating malaise. This syndrome occurs to some degree in approximately 10 to 40% of patients following cardiac surgery. The etiology of postpericardiotomy syndrome is unknown, but it is thought to be due to an autoimmune reaction directed against the epicardium. An association between elevated antiheart antibody titers and elevated antiviral titers suggests that a viral infection may somehow trigger these symptom complexes (Engle et al., 1974).

Mild to moderate cases of postpericardiotomy syndrome are treated with anti-inflammatory agents. Steroid therapy may be required in severe cases. If symptomatic pleural or pericardial fluid accumulation occurs, thoracentesis or pericardiocentesis may be necessary. Constrictive pericarditis has been known to occur following cardiac surgery, and it may or may not be associated with a previous postpericardiotomy syndrome (Bonchek et al., 1988; Kendall et al., 1972). Pericardiectomy is required for recurrent symptomatic effusions or constrictive pericarditis.

## CONSTRICTIVE PERICARDITIS

Chronic fibrosis and thickening of the pericardium, impairing diastolic filling of the heart, may occasionally follow almost any of the identified causes of pericarditis. Encasement of the heart by constrictive pericarditis is frequently a result of both parietal and visceral pericardial involvement. There may also be myocardial atrophy in some cases (Bashi et al., 1988; Vogel et al., 1971). Pericardial constriction may occur in association with pericardial effusion, producing *effusive constrictive pericarditis.* Tuberculosis was once the most frequent cause of constrictive pericarditis in the United States, before effective antituberculous therapy became available (Cameron et al., 1987). Furthermore, in countries in which tuberculosis remains

endemic, it continues to be a leading cause of constrictive pericarditis. However, most cases in the United States develop from cardiac surgery, radiation therapy, and viral and undiagnosed causes of pericarditis.

Patients with constrictive pericarditis present with progressive dyspnea and fatigue. Physical findings may include peripheral edema, ascites, and hepatosplenomegaly (Sellors, 1944). There is usually jugular venous distention, which increases with inspiration (Kussmaul's sign) (Meyer et al., 1989). Cardiac examination reveals wide inspiratory splitting of the first heart sound. A third heart sound or pericardial knock may be heard as a result of rapid ventricular filling. Pulsus paradoxus is unusual in pure constriction, but may be seen when pericardial fluid is present and sinus rhythm persists.

The electrocardiogram may show atrial fibrillation. The T waves can be flat or inverted, and the QRS voltage is low. Chest radiographs may reveal pericardial calcifications and pleural effusions. The cardiac silhouette usually is not enlarged. Echocardiography is nondiagnostic by itself but may be useful in demonstrating pericardial thickening, the presence or absence of pericardial effusion, and myocardial function. CT or MRI may show thickening of the pericardium.

Cardiac catheterization is most useful for revealing the dip and plateau of the right ventricular pressure tracing ("square root sign"), as described earlier. Cardiac catheterization may also be used to evaluate ventricular function and define the presence or absence of associated coronary artery disease. Myocardial biopsies may be required to differentiate restrictive cardiomyopathies.

The management of constrictive pericarditis is primarily surgical (Bigelow et al., 1956; Churchill, 1936; Somerville, 1968). However, preoperative medical treatment consists primarily of the administration of diuretics for symptomatic relief. Digitalis or other antiarrhythmic drugs may be required to control ventricular response in the presence of atrial fibrillation or other arrhythmias (Brockington et al., 1990). Surgical intervention is then indicated in all symptomatic patients who can tolerate an operation. Ideally, total pericardiectomy with pedicles of pericardium left along the phrenic nerves should be performed. Delayed recovery or failure to recover postoperatively has been attributed by some authors to inadequate pericardial resection (Fitzpatrick et al., 1962). This has led to the recommendation that the pericardium be removed over the cavae, atria, ventricles, and great vessels. Furthermore, constrictive epicardial disease should also be resected. However, experience has shown that the degree of required pericardial resection varies with the distribution of the disease in individual patients and that surgical technique must be modified to make pericardial resection complete and safe. Furthermore, some patients have an accompanying myocardial atrophy that accounts for low cardiac output syndrome following adequate pericardial resection (McCaughan et al., 1985; Vogel et al., 1971). The development of low cardiac output syndrome following pericardiectomy is the leading cause of death in these patients. Sophisticated preoperative studies may be able to predict those patients at risk. Reinmuller and associates performed MRI and CT on 79 patients with constrictive pericarditis, identifying 17 who had myocardial atrophy. Seven of these patients underwent pericardiectomy, and all of them died of low cardiac output syndrome in the postoperative period (Reinmuller et al., 1993).

The results following surgical treatment of constrictive pericarditis vary with the preoperative characteristics of the patients. Advanced degrees of preoperative disability, as seen in patients with Class III to IV New York Heart Association symptoms, accompanied by severe ascites or peripheral edema and high right ventricular end-diastolic pressures are associated with a worse prognosis. A large study from Stanford University revealed an operative mortality rate of 5% in patients with a right ventricular end-diastolic pressure of 16 mm Hg or less, 10% with 20 mm Hg, and 30% with a right ventricular end-diastolic pressure of 30 mm Hg. These and other authors have noted that patients with radiation-induced constriction have a generally worse outcome, probably because of associated radiation-induced myocardial injury (DeValeria et al., 1991; Seifert et al., 1985). Other poor prognostic signs include renal failure, pericardiectomy for malignant disease, and repeat pericardiectomy following a failed pericardial procedure. Patients who are not in the previously mentioned high-risk groups tend to have excellent outcomes and return to New York Heart Association Class I or II symptoms.

Pericardiectomy for pericardial constriction is most often approached by either a left-sided anterior thoracotomy or a median sternotomy. Each of these approaches has its relative advantages and disadvantages. The left-sided anterior thoracotomy approach provides easy access to the left ventricle, including the area posterior to the left phrenic nerve (Astudillo and Ivert, 1989; McCaughan et al., 1985). Exposure of the right ventricle is also adequate, although complete exposure and extension to the right atrium and venae cavae are difficult. A more radical extension of the thoracotomy across the sternum occasionally has been used to allow better access to these areas. If cardiopulmonary bypass is required, femoral artery and vein cannulation would be required. The median sternotomy has been the most frequently used approach at our institution. This allows excellent access to the anterior surface of the heart, including all of the right ventricle, atria, and venae cavae. Complete exposure of the left ventricle requires careful manipulation of the heart. The pericardium may be resected from phrenic nerve to phrenic nerve (DeValeria et al., 1991). However, excision of pericardium posterior to the left phrenic nerve is hazardous. Cardiopulmonary bypass can be instituted easily through this approach.

## CONGENITAL DEFECTS OF THE PERICARDIUM

Congenital defects of the pericardium are rare anomalies, ranging from complete absence to the more common localized defects of the pericardial sac. The incidence is said to be approximately 1 in 10,000 postmortem examinations (Southworth and Stevenson, 1938). Left-sided pericardial defects predominate, though occasionally right-sided defects have been described. The male/female ratio is approximately 3:1 (Nasser, 1976). The pathogenesis of left-sided defects is thought to be secondary to premature atrophy of the left duct of Cuvier, compromising the blood supply to the left pleuropericardial membrane, normally formed from the left pericardium. Other explanations include herniation of an abnormal lung bud through the pleuropericardial foramen. Approximately 30% of patients with pericardial defects have other associated cardiac or pulmonary anomalies (Nasser, 1976).

Although complete absence of the pericardium normally has no significant hemodynamic effects, partial pericardial defects can be associated with significant clinical problems. These problems can result from herniation of the left atrial appendage or ventricles through the defect, producing torsion or strain of the great vessels and compromise of venous return. Pleuromyocardial adhesions or compression of the coronary vessels by a thickened pericardial edge can occur (Wallace et al., 1971). Patients may present with chest pain, dyspnea, dizziness, syncope, or sudden death.

It is quite unusual to base suspicion of congenital defect of the pericardium on physical examination, although patients may have an associated systolic ejection murmur heard best along the left sternal border or a prominent second heart sound. Typically, the diagnosis is based on chest radiographic findings. Characteristic plain radiographic findings in complete absence of the left pericardium include rotation of the heart with leftward displacement. The right cardiac border often overlies the spine and is therefore not visible. The pulmonary artery may be prominent and appear as a convexity between aortic knob and ventricle (Taysi et al., 1985). Both CT and nuclear MRI can be extremely helpful in demonstrating pericardial defects (Moncada et al., 1986).

Because of the risk for cardiac herniation and sudden death in patients with partial defects of the pericardium, surgical therapy is indicated for all patients in whom the diagnosis is made. Surgical options include pericardiectomy, primary closure, or patching of the defect with Teflon, fascia lata, Dacron, bovine pericardial substitutes, or PTFE (Gore-Tex) (Chapman et al., 1988). Complete absence of the pericardium requires no specific treatment.

## Pericardial Cysts and Diverticula

Pericardial cysts are typically asymptomatic masses found on chest film in middle-aged adults (Fig. 34–8). The incidence is slightly greater for men than for women, by a 3:2 ratio. The classic pericardial cyst is located in the costophrenic angle, typically on the right side. Such cysts may be round or elliptical and are usually unilocular. Unlike pericardial cysts, peri-

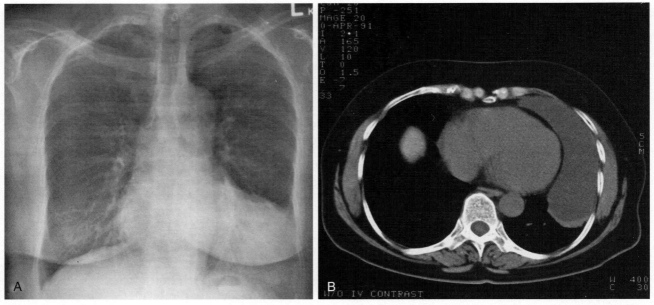

**FIGURE 34–8.** *A*, Frontal radiograph of patient with large pericardial cyst. *B*, Computed tomographic scan of same patient showing pericardial cyst extending into left hemithorax.

cardial diverticula openly communicate with the pericardial sac (Moncada et al., 1986).

The pericardial cyst contains fluid that is a clear transudate of plasma. Specific diagnosis of the entity may be possible through CT. When computed tomographic density readings reveal fluid of water density in a cystic mass adjacent to the pericardium, pericardial cyst can be confidently diagnosed. However, higher-density fluids or uneven density makes the diagnosis less certain (Moncada et al., 1986).

In asymptomatic patients with characteristic computed tomographic findings of pericardial cysts or diverticula containing water-density fluid, surgical intervention is not necessary (Moncada et al., 1986). However, when high-density fluid is present, aspiration or surgical resection may be required for diagnosis. Also, in the unusual patient in whom the cyst or diverticulum causes a mass effect with impingement on surrounding structures, resection may be necessary.

## PNEUMOPERICARDIUM

Air within the pericardial sac is an unusual finding but has been recognized since 1844, when Bricheteau reported on a case in the French literature (Bricheteau, 1844). The spontaneous development of pneumopericardium is extremely rare (Taupin et al., 1992). In this form, alveolar rupture releases air that courses along the bronchi into the tissue planes leading into the pericardium. More commonly, pneumopericardium results from severe chest trauma with associated alveolar rupture (Fig. 34–9). Frequently, an associated pneumothorax is identified. Pneumopericardium has become a more commonly observed phenomenon

since the introduction of mechanical ventilatory support. Particularly in young infants receiving high-pressure ventilation, pneumopericardium resulting from barotrauma to the stiffened lungs has produced a more frequent diagnosis of the disease (Finer et al., 1993; Fiser and Walker, 1992). High-frequency, low-pressure ventilation lessens the risk of this complication.

In general, pneumopericardium causes few clinical effects. However, cardiac tamponade may result from the progressive accumulation of air around the heart. Additionally, the presence of bacterial organisms may signal infection.

Treatment of pneumopericardium is directed primarily toward its complications, most specifically the development of cardiac decompensation. Needle aspi-

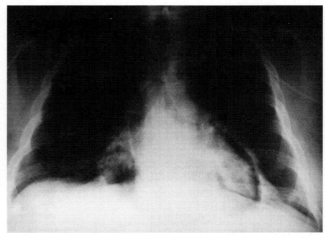

**FIGURE 34–9.** Frontal chest radiograph revealing post-traumatic pneumopericardium.

ration of the pericardium can produce prompt hemodynamic improvement. This is typically followed by either percutaneous passage of an inlying catheter or direct surgical drainage of the pericardial space (Fiser and Walker, 1992). If infection is present, appropriate systemic antibiotics should be administered in concert with pericardial drainage.

## TECHNICAL APPROACHES TO DRAINAGE AND RESECTION OF THE PERICARDIUM

### Pericardial Aspiration

Pericardiocentesis is most effectively employed as an emergency drainage procedure for the treatment of severe cardiac tamponade (Kirkland and Taylor, 1992). It is also used diagnostically in the presence of undefined pericardial effusions. Because of the risk of cardiac penetration and/or laceration of coronary vessels, various adjunctive measures have been em-

ployed to increase safety. The risk of cardiac injury clearly is lessened with larger effusions.

The procedure is most often performed with the patient in the supine position. Following sterile skin preparation and administration of cutaneous local anesthesia, the pericardiocentesis needle is passed just to the left of the patient's xiphoid process and aimed toward the midscapular region (Fig. 34–10). Classically, electrocardiographic monitoring has allowed early recognition of myocardial contact (Bishop et al., 1956). A negative deflection of the QRS complex reveals myocardial contact and mandates slow withdrawal of the needle until the electrocardiogram returns to normal. More recently, bedside monitoring of the pericardiocentesis by means of echocardiography has been used (Kirkland and Taylor, 1992; Susini et al., 1993; Wang et al., 1992). Contrast enhancement techniques also have been added to echocardiography. Transesophageal echocardiography can also be employed. In elective circumstances, continuous hemodynamic measurements during pericardial aspira-

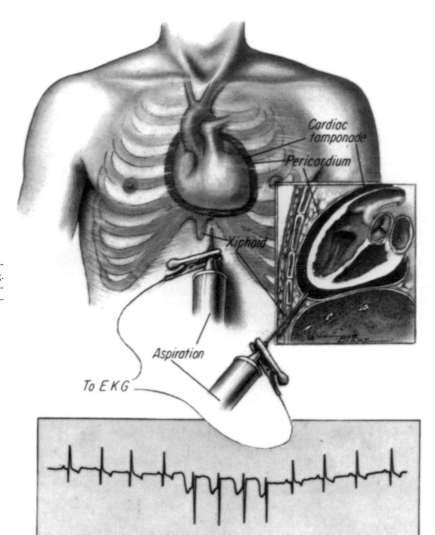

**FIGURE 34–10.** Illustration of subxiphoid pericardiocentesis with electrocardiographic monitoring. Note negative QRS deflection indicating myocardial contact. See text for details. (EKG = electrocardiogram.)

tion may also be used to confirm or disprove a diagnosis of cardiac tamponade (Kern and Aguirre, 1992b).

## Pericardial Biopsy

It is not uncommon for pericardial aspiration to be nondiagnostic for specific pericardial diseases. For example, in malignant pericarditis, cytologic examination of the pericardial fluid may yield positive results in only 50 to 80% of patients. Additionally, culture results of *Mycobacterium tuberculosis* may be negative from pericardial fluid, even in the presence of active tuberculous pericarditis. To avoid these problems, pericardial biopsy in addition to pericardial drainage has been recommended.

Several techniques have been used to obtain pericardial biopsies through less invasive modalities than open surgery. These include placement of a subxiphoid No. 7 French catheter with passage of a transluminal endomyocardial bioptome, use of the flexible fiberoptic bronchoscope with bronchoscopic forceps, and percutaneous subxiphoid transluminal biopsy using bronchoscopic forceps under echocardiographic guidance (Inderbitzi et al., 1993; Urschel and Horan, 1993). The safety and efficacy of these procedures is currently under investigation.

## Catheter Drainage

Because pericardiocentesis alone is commonly followed by reaccumulation of the pericardial fluid, a more chronic form of drainage has been required. Several days of drainage may be accomplished by percutaneous insertion of a guidewire into the pericardium followed by passage of a multiple-hole No. 6 French, 30-cm catheter over the wire into the pericardium and removal of the wire (Susini et al., 1993). This procedure is useful for draining thin, uncomplicated pericardial effusions, but it is unsuccessful when clot or fibrous exudate is prominent. This method has been used in adults and children, but may be more complicated in children under 2 years of age (Zahn et al., 1992). Overall morbidity and mortality has been low (Duvernoy et al., 1992).

## Pericardioplasty

Because pericardial effusions tend to reaccumulate following drainage, various techniques can be employed to minimize this occurrence (Selig, 1993). Most open procedures have developed in response to this need. However, procedures designed to minimize the need for open operation remain unproved. A small experience with the use of a catheter-based technique employing a valvuloplasty balloon under fluoroscopic guidance has been reported by Palacios and colleagues (1991). This procedure involves puncture of the pericardium and dilatation of the hole to allow

drainage into the left side of the chest. An echocardiographically guided modification of this technique has been reported by Vora and co-workers (1992). Ziskind and associates (1993) reported a multicenter registry experience using balloon catheter techniques in 50 patients, with good results. They recommended this procedure for patients with malignant pericardial effusions. The ultimate utility of these procedures is under continued investigation.

## Subxiphoid Pericardial Window

The subxiphoid pericardial window is the most common open surgical procedure used for the treatment of pericardial disease. This approach allows good drainage of the pericardium and the placement of mediastinal tubes for prolonged evacuation. The approach yields access for digital break-up of loculations and removal of pericardial tissue for pathologic examination. When used as treatment for pericardial effusion, it has produced a low incidence of recurrence, approximately 5% (Campbell et al., 1992; Naunheim et al., 1991). It is particularly useful for the treatment of chronic effusions secondary to malignant diseases. Many of these very ill patients will succumb to other causes before pericardial fluid reaccumulates.

The procedure may be performed with local or general anesthesia (Fig. 34–11). A skin incision placed in the midline over the xiphoid process and extending for several centimeters below the process is the preferred route. Rarely is more than 10 cm of skin incision necessary to accomplish the procedure. Dissection then continues through subcutaneous tissues through the linea alba. The linea alba is divided, and the underlying peritoneum is left intact. The xiphoid process usually is removed, but occasionally it is retracted. However, if it is retracted, care must be taken to identify any breakage or loosening; patients occasionally develop a chronic, painful costochondritis-type syndrome when the xiphoid process is dislocated and healing is impaired. Blunt dissection is then performed superiorly and toward the left shoulder. Care is taken to avoid entry into the right pleural cavity by keeping dissection toward the left. Pericardial fat is identified and swept away from the underlying pericardium, with care taken to control any bleeding. The underlying pericardium frequently is very tense, so grasping of the tissue may be difficult. Occasionally, superficial placement of a suture allows a handle to raise the pericardium. Direct pericardiocentesis is advisable before opening the pericardium in order to confirm the presence of free pericardial fluid. If bloody fluid is obtained, it should be nonclotting if it has been within the pericardial space for some time. A window of pericardial tissue is then excised. A large sample measuring approximately 4 × 4 cm is considered optimal, although smaller excisions have been effective both diagnostically and therapeutically.

## Left-Sided Anterior Thoracotomy

Because a wider excision of pericardium can be obtained, the left-sided anterior thoracotomy ap-

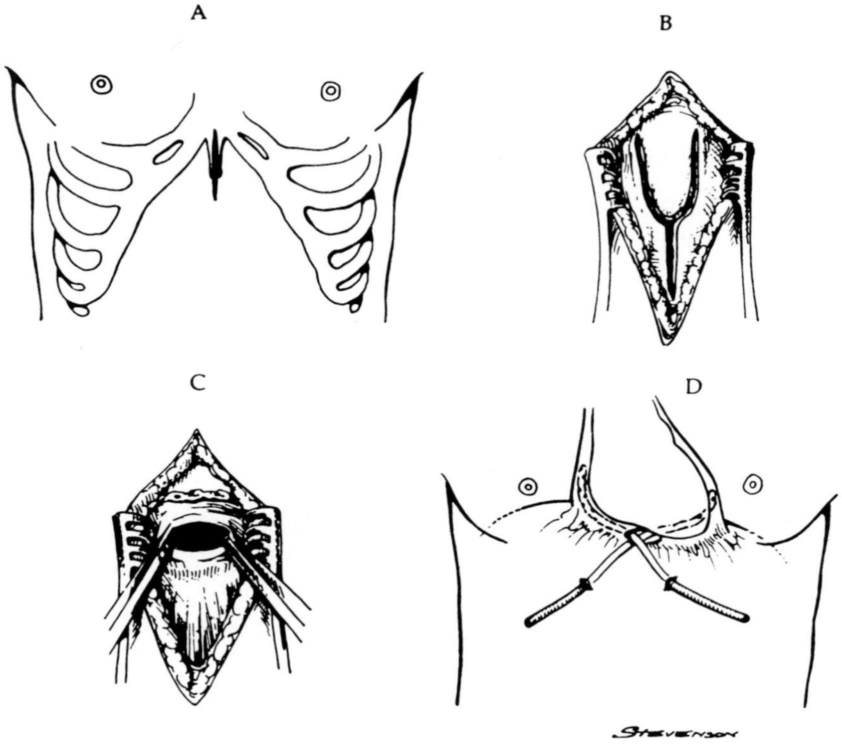

**FIGURE 34–11.** Subxiphoid pericardial window. *A,* A 6- to 10-cm incision is made centered over the xiphoid process. *B,* The linea alba is divided superficial to the peritoneum, and the xiphoid process is dissected free of surrounding tissues. *C,* Blunt dissection beneath the sternum reveals the pericardium. *D,* A 4 × 4 section of pericardium is excised, and drainage catheters are placed. (See text for details.) (*A–D,* From Hankins, J. R., Satterfield, J. R., Aisner, J., et al.: Pericardial window for malignant pericardial effusion. Reprinted with permission from the Society of Thoracic Surgeons [The Annals of Thoracic Surgery, 1980, Vol. 30, pp. 465–471].)

proach is preferable for treatment of pericardial effusions that are recurrent or likely to recur. It is rarely used in patients with malignant pericardial effusions because of their generally poor prognosis. However, in benign disease and when loculations are present, the left-sided anterior thoracotomy approach provides excellent access. It may be used for pericardiectomy in patients with pericardial constriction (Astudillo and Ivert, 1989). In this instance, it provides excellent access to the pericardium, encompassing the entire left ventricle and most of the right ventricle. More extensive right-sided dissection is difficult. Likewise, access for cardiopulmonary bypass requires femoral cannulation techniques.

The patient is placed in the supine position with the left side of the chest elevated approximately 30 degrees. General anesthesia is required. A submammary skin incision is performed, and entrance is gained through the fifth intercostal space. Typically, the internal mammary artery is avoided, although this may be ligated and divided if desired. If a pericardial window is performed, aspiration, as described for the subxiphoid approach, before opening the pericardium may help prevent cardiac entry. Care is taken during the incision of the pericardium to obtain meticulous hemostasis. However, overzealous electrocautery may be associated with ventricular arrhythmias and possible fibrillation.

If pericardiectomy is being performed for constrictive pericarditis, the initial incision into the pericardium usually is made parallel and anterior to the phrenic nerve. This incision should be made over more bare pericardium, not through pericardial fat.

The incision is made carefully until the underlying myocardium begins to bulge through the opening. This allows definition of the plane of dissection, which then proceeds anteriorly and to the patient's right. Following removal of the pericardium over the anterior and lateral left ventricle, dissection is continued over the right ventricle as far as possible. The left ventricle is then dissected away from the posterior pericardium. A pedicle of pericardium containing phrenic nerve is preserved. The posterior pericardium is then resected. If the epicardium also constricts the myocardium, epicardial stripping is performed very gingerly. Areas of calcification extending into the myocardium are not removed. When epicardial stripping is difficult, carefully placed criss-crossing incisions will break-up the scar and allow some bulging of the underlying myocardium (Bonchek et al., 1991; Faggian et al., 1990).

## Thoracoscopic Pericardiectomy

Pericardial resection may also be accomplished thoracoscopically (Mack et al., 1992; Rees et al., 1993). This technique is particularly useful in patients who otherwise might undergo a left-sided anterior thoracotomy approach for pericardial drainage. The tedious nature of the dissection and dangers associated with pericardiectomy for pericardial constriction make the thoracoscopic approach for treatment of this disease unsatisfactory. Furthermore, in patients who might otherwise be treated by means of a subxiphoid pericardial window, more selective use of the thoracoscopic procedure is probably indicated.

The patient is placed on the operating table in the right lateral decubitus position (Fig. 34–12). This allows maximum access for trocar placements. Additionally, the heart may shift somewhat away from the left chest wall, thereby making the procedure technically easier. When the thoracoscopic approach is used, crowding of the chest by a distended pericardium must be taken into consideration. Accordingly, the initial trocar placement for the video camera should be high around the third intercostal space. Working ports are then placed in lower intercostal spaces anterior and posterior to the pericardial sac to allow for a triangulated pattern of access. This provides maximal mobility and prevents dueling of the instrumentation during the procedure.

Following positioning of the instrumentation, the approach to the pericardial resection is generally the same as described for the open techniques. Some surgeons have made certain modifications. For example, the endoscopic cutting stapler has occasionally been employed to divide the pericardium, particularly in areas with thick overlying pericardial fat. A laparoscopic transabdominal approach has also been described (Sastic et al., 1992).

## Bilateral Anterior Thoracotomy

Some authors have employed bilateral anterior thoracotomy through the fifth intercostal space with transection of the body of the sternum to provide wide exposure of the pericardium. This has been used particularly to treat constrictive pericarditis. Although the procedure provides excellent access to all areas of the pericardium, morbidity associated with this incision seems to be greater than that accompanying either median sternotomy or left-sided anterior thoracotomy. Consequently, in our institution, we have avoided this particular incision. This approach may be helpful in the emergency room, where emergency anterior thoracotomy may be inadequate for exposure. Extending the incision across the sternum into the opposite side of the chest will allow rapid exposure of the cardiac structures and vasculature.

## Median Sternotomy

The median sternotomy is the most versatile incision employed for access to all anterior and middle mediastinal structures (Hehrlein et al., 1991). Most major pericardial or cardiac operations may be approached through this incision. For the treatment of constrictive pericarditis, this provides excellent exposure of the anterior and right lateral pericardium (De-Valeria et al., 1991). Access to the left lateral and posterior pericardium requires significant manipulation of the heart. Cardiopulmonary bypass may be instituted quite readily from a median sternotomy approach (Copeland et al., 1975). Although resection of the posterior pericardium is quite difficult from this approach, particularly off cardiopulmonary bypass, sufficient pericardial resection usually is possible.

A midline incision is performed extending from 2

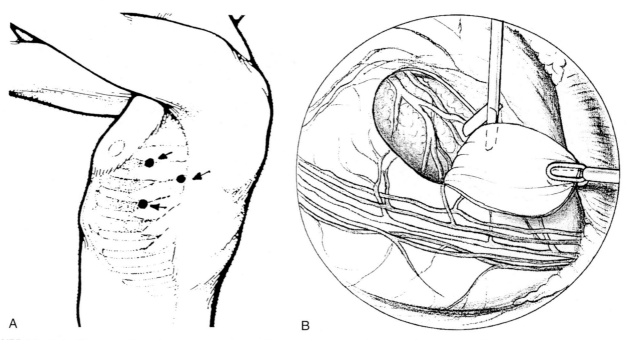

**FIGURE 34–12.** *A,* Trocar positions for patient in preparation for thoracoscopic pericardial window. The patient is placed in the right lateral decubitus position. The camera trocar site lies most posteriorly. The remaining two sites are used for manipulating instruments. *B,* Thoracoscopic view of pericardial resection. (*A* and *B,* From Inderbitzi, R., Furrer, M., and Leupi, F.: Pericardial biopsy and fenestration. Eur. Heart J., *14:*135–137, 1993.)

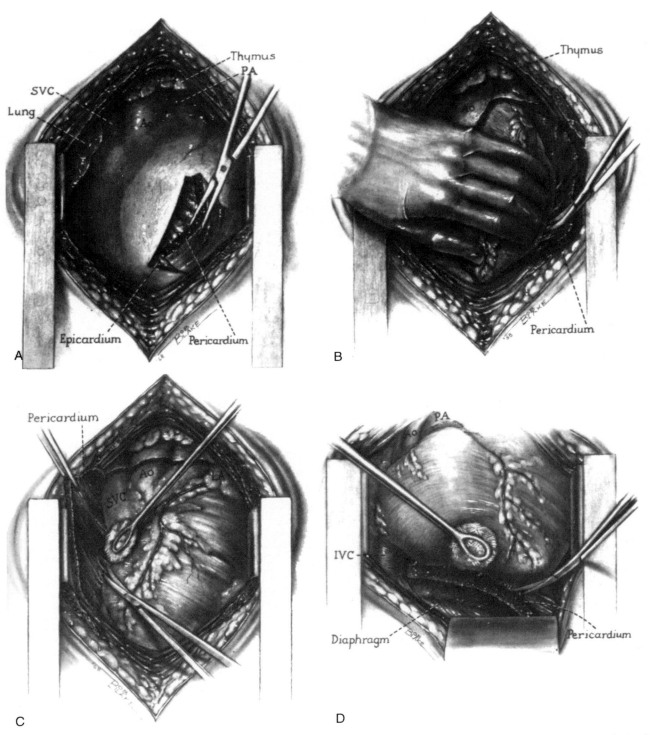

**FIGURE 34–13.** *A,* The pericardium is exposed through a midline sternal splitting incision. A longitudinal incision is made in the pericardium, and a plane of dissection is established so that the thickened pericardium can be removed from the left ventricle. (Ao = aorta; PA = pulmonary artery; SVC = superior vena cava.) *B,* The heart is held to the right so that the posterior left ventricle can be freed. The phrenic nerve must be isolated to avoid injuring this structure. The large pericardial flap will be excised. *C,* The pericardium is freed from the right atrium and the venae cavae. These thin-walled structures are easily torn, and adequate exposure is mandatory for this part of the dissection. *D,* The thick pericardium attached between the apex of the heart and the diaphragm must be excised to prevent recurrent adherent bands and inferior vena cava (IVC) obstruction.

cm below the sternal notch to approximately 2 to 3 cm beyond the tip of the xiphoid process. Dissection is carried down through subcutaneous tissues to the midline of the sternum. Careful identification of the midline of the sternum is important and can be assured by placing the incision equidistant from the sternal attachments of the pectoralis muscles. The suprasternal ligament should be defined by blunt finger dissection, and a plane should be established beneath the ligament posterior to the upper portion of the manubrium. The sternal saw is then employed to divide the sternum in the midline. A sternal retractor is then placed and carefully opened. Placement of the retractor should be as inferior as possible to minimize stretch on the brachial plexi. Additionally, opening should be stepwise to allow muscle relaxation and as much protection of the brachial plexus as possible. If pericardial resection is to be performed for constriction, the technique is as described in Figure 34–13.

## SELECTED BIBLIOGRAPHY

McCaughan, C., Schaff, H. V., Piehler, J. M., et al.: Early and late results of pericardiectomy for constrictive pericarditis. J. Thorac. Cardiovasc. Surg., 89:340, 1985.

This study reported from the experience at the Mayo Clinic represents one of the largest groups of patients treated with pericardiectomy for constrictive pericarditis. Drawing on an experience with 231 patients being treated for constrictive pericarditis, the authors describe the risk factors, survival statistics, and relative merits of various surgical approaches. Operative risk was found to be directly related to preoperative disability, with a mortality rate of 46% in patients with Class IV symptoms. In contrast, patients discharged alive from the hospital had a 5-year survival rate of 84%. The relative merits of left-sided anterior lateral thoracotomy, median sternotomy, Harrington incision, or bilateral anterior thoracotomy are discussed.

Moncada, R., Kotler, M. N., Churchill, R. J., et al.: Multimodality approach to pericardial imaging. Cardiovasc. Clin., 17:409, 1986.

This is an excellent review of the radiologic studies currently used to evaluate diseases of the pericardium. The authors broadly discuss computed tomography and magnetic resonance imaging, as well as echocardiography, in the diagnosis of pericardial diseases. The illustrations and photographs are clear and helpful.

Seifert, F. C., Miller, D. C., Oesterle, S. N., et al.: Surgical treatment of constrictive pericarditis: Analysis of outcome and diagnostic error. Circulation, 72(Suppl. II):II-264, 1985.

In this study from Stanford University, the authors report on their experience with 61 patients treated for constrictive pericarditis. This study is frequently quoted because of its excellent statistical analyses of the risk factors and postoperative results in patients with these diseases. The authors clearly demonstrate the effect of preoperative functional status on postoperative outcome. The strongly negative impact of radiation-induced pericardial constriction on survival also is clearly demonstrated.

Shabetai, R., Fowler, N. O., and Guntheroth, W. G.: The hemodynamics of cardiac tamponade and constrictive pericarditis. Am. J. Cardiol., 26:480, 1970.

This article is written by a noted expert in the physiology of the pericardium and his colleagues. The hemodynamic characteristics of cardiac tamponade and constrictive pericarditis are thoroughly discussed, and the article is readable and informative.

Spodick, D. H.: Macrophysiology, microphysiology, and anatomy of the pericardium: A synopsis. Am. Heart J., 124:1046, 1992.

This review article reflects years of accumulated knowledge on the physiology of the pericardium. It encompasses all areas of interest relative to the pericardium and its effects on cardiovascular hemodynamics.

## BIBLIOGRAPHY

Astudillo, R., and Ivert, T.: Late results after pericardectomy for constrictive pericarditis via left thoracotomy. Scand. J. Thorac. Cardiovasc. Surg., 23:115, 1989.

Baizeau, J.: Mémoire sur le ponction du péricarde au point de vue chirurgical. Gaz. Med. Chir., 1:565, 1868.

Ballance, C. S.: The surgery of the heart. Lancet, 1:1, 1920.

Bashi, V., John, S., Ravikumar, E., et al.: Early and late results of pericardiectomy in 118 cases of constrictive pericarditis. Thorax, 43:637, 1988.

Beck, C. S., and Griswold, R. A.: Pericardiectomy in the treatment of the Pick syndrome: Experimental and clinical observations. Arch. Surg., 21:1064, 1930.

Beppu, S., Tanaka, N., Nakatani, S., et al.: Pericardial clot after open heart surgery: Its specific localization and haemodynamics. Eur. Heart J., 14:230, 1993.

Berglund, E., Sarnoff, S. J., and Isaacs, J. P.: Ventricular function role of the pericardium in regulation of cardiovascular hemodynamics. Circ. Res., 3:133, 1955.

Bigelow, W. G., Dolan, F. G., Wilson, D. R., and Gunton, R. W.: The surgical treatment of chronic constrictive pericarditis. Can. Med. Assoc. J., 75:814, 1956.

Bishop, L. H., Estes, E. H., and MacIntosh, H. D.: The electrocardiogram as a safeguard in pericardiocentesis. J. A. M. A., 62:264, 1956.

Blalock, A., and Levy, S. E.: Tuberculous pericarditis. J. Thorac. Surg., 7:132, 1937.

Bonchek, L. I., Burlingame, M. W., and Vazales, B. E.: Constrictive epicarditis after open heart surgery: The turtle cage operation [letter; comment]. J. Cardiovasc. Surg., 6:355, 1991.

Bonchek, L. I., Burlingame, M. W., and Vazales, B. E.: Postoperative fibrous cardiac constriction. Ann. Thorac. Surg., 45:311, 1988.

Bricheteau, I.: Observations d' hydropneumopericarde. Arch. Gén. Méd., 4:334, 1844.

Brinker, J. A., Weiss, J. L., Lappé, D. L., et al.: Leftward septal displacement during right ventricular loading in man. Circulation, 61:626, 1980.

Brockington, G. M., Zebede, J., and Pandian, N. G.: Constrictive pericarditis. Card. Clin., 8:645, 1990.

Brown, J., Barakos, J., and Higgins, C. B.: Magnetic resonance imaging of cardiac and paracardiac masses. J. Thorac. Imag., 4(2):58, 1989.

Cameron, J., Oesterle, S. N., Baldwin, J. C., and Hancock, E. W.: The etiologic spectrum of constrictive pericarditis. Am. Heart J., 113:354, 1987.

Campbell, P. T., Van, T. P., Wall, T. C., et al.: Subxiphoid pericardiotomy in the diagnosis and management of large pericardial effusions associated with malignancy. Chest, 101:938, 1992.

Chapman, J. E. J., Rubin, J. W., Gross, C. M., and Janssen, M. E.: Congenital absence of pericardium: An unusual cause of atypical angina. Ann. Thorac. Surg., 45:91, 1988.

Charlier, A. A., Jaumin, P. M., and Pouleur, H.: Circulatory effects of deep inspirations, blocked expirations and positive pressure inflations at equal transpulmonary pressures in conscious dogs. J. Physiol., 241:589, 1974.

Cheevers, N.: Observations on diseases of the orifice and valves of the aorta. Guy's Hosp. Rep., 7:387, 1842.

Churchill, E. D.: Pericardial resection in chronic constrictive pericarditis. Ann. Surg., 104:516, 1936.

Copeland, J. G., Stinson, E. B., Griepp, R. B., and Shumway, N. E.: Surgical treatment of chronic constrictive pericarditis using cardiopulmonary bypass. J. Thorac. Cardiovasc. Surg., 69:236, 1975.

Daughters, G. T., Frist, W. H., Alderman, E. L., et al.: Effects of the pericardium on left ventricular diastolic filling and systolic performance early after cardiac operations [see comments]. J. Thorac. Cardiovasc. Surg., 104:1084, 1992.

Délorme, E.: Sur un traitement chirurgical de la symphyse cardopericardique. Gaz. Hop., 71:1150, 1898.

DeValeria, P. A., Baumgartner, W. A., Casale, A. S., et al.: Current indications, risks, and outcome after pericardiectomy. Ann. Thorac. Surg., 52:219, 1991.

Dumreicher, J. V.: Zur Erinnerung an weil. Wien Med. Wschr., 16:409, 1866.

Duvernoy, O., Borowiec, J., Helmius, G., and Erikson, U.: Complications of percutaneous pericardiocentesis under fluoroscopic guidance. Acta Radiol., 33:309, 1992.

Ebert, P.A., and Najafi, H.: The pericardium. In Sabiston, D. C., Jr., and Spencer, F. C., (eds.): Surgery of the Chest. 5th ed. Philadelphia, W. B. Saunders, 1990.

Engle, M. A., McCabe, J. C., Ebert, P. A., and Zabriskie, J.: The postpericardiotomy syndrome and antiheart antibodies. Circulation, 49:401, 1974.

Faggian, G., Mazzucco, A., Tursi, V., et al.: Constrictive epicarditis after open heart surgery: The turtle cage operation [see comments]. J. Cardiovasc. Surg., 5:318, 1990.

Finer, N. N., Peliowski, A., and Hayashi, A.: Tension hemopericardium complicating neonatal pneumopericardium. Am. J. Perinatol., 10:50, 1993.

Fiser, D. H., and Walker, W. M.: Tension pneumopericardium in an infant. Chest, 102:1888, 1992.

Fitzpatrick, D. P., Wyso, E. M., Bosher, L. H., and Richardson, D. W.: Restoration of normal intracardiac pressures after extensive pericardiectomy for constrictive pericarditis. Circulation, 25:484, 1962.

Fowler, N. O.: Cardiac tamponade. A clinical or an echocardiographic diagnosis? Circulation, 87:1738, 1993.

Frame, J. R., Lucas, S. K., Pederson, J. A., and Elkins, R. C.: Surgical treatment of pericarditis in the dialysis patient. Am. J. Surg., 146:800, 1983.

Franklin, D. L., Van Critters, R. L., and Rushmer, R. F.: Balance between right and left ventricular output. Circ. Res., 10:17, 1962.

Hawkins, J. W., and Vacek, J. L.: What constitutes definitive therapy of malignant pericardial effusion? "Medical" versus surgical treatment. Am. Heart J., 118:428, 1989.

Hehrlein, F. W., Moosdorf, R., Pitton, M., and Dapper, F.: The role of pericardiectomy in pericardial disorders. Eur. Heart J., 12(Suppl. D):7, 1991.

Hoffman, J. I. E., Guz, A., Charlier, A. A., and Wicken, D. E. L.: Stroke volume in conscious dogs: Effects of respiration, posture, and vascular occlusion. J. Appl. Physiol., 20:865, 1965.

Holman, E., and Willett, F. W.: Results of radical pericardiectomy for constrictive pericarditis. J. A. M. A., 157:789, 1955.

Holt, J. P.: The normal pericardium. Am. J. Cardiol., 26:455, 1970.

Inderbitzi, R., Furrer, M., and Leupi, F.: Pericardial biopsy and fenestration. Eur. Heart J., 14:135, 1993.

Isaacs, J. P., Carter, B. N., II, and Haller, J. A., Jr.: Experimental pericarditis: The pathologic physiology of constrictive pericarditis. Bull. Johns Hopkins Hosp., 90:259, 1952.

Kendall, M. E., Rhodes, G. R., and Wolfe, W.: Cardiac constriction following aorta-to-coronary bypass surgery. J. Thorac. Cardiovasc. Surg., 64:142, 1972.

Kern, M. J., and Aguirre, F.: Interpretation of cardiac pathophysiology from pressure waveform analysis: Pericardial compressive hemodynamics, Part II. Cathet. Cardiovasc. Diagn., 26:34, 1992a.

Kern, M. J., and Aguirre, F. V.: Interpretation of cardiac pathophysiology from pressure waveform analysis: Pericardial compressive hemodynamics, Part III. Cathet. Cardiovasc. Diagn., 26:152, 1992b.

Kirkland, L. L., and Taylor, R. W.: Pericardiocentesis. Crit. Care Clin., 8:699, 1992.

Kostreva, D. R., and Pontus, S. P.: Pericardial mechanoreceptors with phrenic afferents. Am. J. Physiol., 1993.

Kussmaul, A.: Ueber schwielige mediastino-pericarditis und den paradoxen puls. Berl. Klin. Wochenschr., 10:433, 445, 461, 1873.

Lawrence, L. T., and Rochmis, P. G.: Chronic constrictive pericarditis with unexpected remission. J. A. M. A., 202:66, 1967.

Mack, M. J., Aronoff, R. J., Acuff, T. E., et al.: Present role of thoracoscopy in the diagnosis and treatment of diseases of the chest. Ann. Thorac. Surg., 54:403, 1992.

Macklin, C. C.: Evidences of increases in the capacity of the pulmonary arteries and veins of dogs, cats, and rabbits during inflation of the freshly excised lung. Rev. Can. Biol., 5:199, 1946.

McCaughan, C., Schaff, H. V., Piehler, J. M., et al.: Early and late results of pericardiectomy for constrictive pericarditis. J. Thorac. Cardiovasc. Surg., 89:340, 1985.

Meyer, T. E., Sareli, P., Marcus, R. H., et al.: Mechanism underlying Kussmaul's sign in chronic constrictive pericarditis. Am. J. Cardiol., 64:1069, 1989.

Moncada, R., Kotler, M. N., Churchill, R. J., et al.: Multimodality approach to pericardial imaging. Cardiovasc. Clin., 17:409, 1986.

Morgan, R. J., Stephenson, L. W., Woolf, P. K., et al.: Surgical treatment of pericarditis in children. J. Thorac. Cardiovasc. Surg., 85:527, 1983.

Nasser, W. K.: Congenital diseases of pericardium. Cardiovasc. Clin., 7:271, 1976.

Naunheim, K. S., Kesler, K. A., Fiore, A. C., et al.: Pericardial drainage: Subxiphoid vs. transthoracic approach. Eur. J. Cardiothorac. Surg., 5:99, 1991.

Olsen, C. O., Tyson, G. S., Maier, G. W., et al.: Diminished stroke volume during inspiration: A reverse thoracic pump. Circulation, 72:668, 1985.

Palacios, I. F., Tuzcu, M., Ziskind, A., et al.: Percutaneous balloon pericardial window for patients with maligant pericardial effusion and tamponade. Cathet. Cardiovasc. Diagn., 22:244–249, 1991.

Parsons, H. G., and Holman, E.: Experimental Ascites. Philadelphia, W. B. Saunders, 1951.

Pennell, D. J., and Underwood, R.: Magnetic resonance imaging of the heart. Br. J. Hosp. Med., 49:90, 1993.

Pick, F.: Ueber chronische, unter dem Bilde der Lebercirrhose verlaufende Pericarditis (pericarditische Pseudolebercirrhose) nebst Bemerkungen ueber Zuckergussleber (Curshmann). Z. Klin. Med., 29:385, 1896.

Rees, A. P., Risher, W., McFadden, P. M., et al.: Partial congenital defect of the left pericardium: Angiographic diagnosis and treatment by thoracoscopic pericardiectomy: Case report. Cathet. Cardiovasc. Diagn., 28:231, 1993.

Rehn, I.: Zur experimentellen Pathologie des Herzbeutels. Verh. Dtsch. Ges. Chir., 42:339, 1913.

Reinmuller, R., Gurgan, M., Erdmann, E., et al.: CT and MR evaluation of pericardial constriction: A new diagnostic and therapeutic concept. J. Thorac. Imaging, 8:108, 1993.

Riolan, J.: Encheridium Anatomicum et Pathologicum. Lugdu, Batavorum, Ex Officini Adriani, Wyngaarden, 1649, p. 206.

Robinson, L. A., Fleming, W. H., and Galbraith, T. A.: Original articles: Intrapleural doxycycline control of malignant pleural effusions. Ann. Thorac. Surg., 55:1115, 1993.

Santamore, W. P., Lynch, P. R., Meier, G., et al.: Myocardial interaction between the ventricles. J. Appl. Physiol., 41:362, 1976.

Sastic, J. W., Stalter, K. D., and Goddard, R. L.: Laparoscopic pericardial window. J. Laparoendosc. Surg., 2:263, 1992.

Sauerbruch, F.: Die Chirurgie der Brustorgane. Vol. 2. Berlin, 1925.

Schmieden, V., and Fischer, H.: Die Herzbeutelentzundung und ihre Folgezustande. Ergeb. Chir. Orthop., 19:98, 1926.

Schoenfeld, M. H.: The differentiation of restrictive cardiomyopathy from constrictive pericarditis. Cardiol. Clin., 8:663, 1990.

Schrijen, F., Ehrlich, W., and Permutt, S.: Cardiovascular changes in conscious dogs during spontaneous deep breaths. Pfluegers Arch., 355:205, 1975.

Scully, R. E., Mark, E. J., McNeely, W. F., and McNeely, B. U.: Case records of the Massachusetts General Hospital. N. Engl. J. Med., 316:1394, 1987.

Seifert, F. C., Miller, D. C., Oesterle, S. N., et al.: Surgical treatment of constrictive pericarditis: Analysis of outcome and diagnostic error. Circulation, 72(Suppl. II):264, 1985.

Selig, M. B.: Percutaneous transcatheter pericardial interventions: Aspiration, biopsy, and pericardioplasty [editorial]. Am. Heart J., 125:269, 1993.

Sellors, T. H.: Constrictive pericarditis. Br. J. Surg., 33:215, 1944.

Shabetai, R., Fowler, N. O., and Guntheroth, W. G.: The hemodynamics of cardiac tamponade and constrictive pericarditis. Am. J. Cardiol., 26:480, 1970.

Somerville, W.: Constrictive pericarditis with special reference to the change in natural history brought about by surgical intervention. Circulation, 37, 38(Suppl. 5):102, 1968.

Southworth, H., and Stevenson, C. S.: Congenital defects of pericardium. Arch. Intern. Med., 61:223, 1938.

Spodick, D. H.: Macrophysiology, microphysiology, and anatomy of the pericardium: A synopsis. Am. Heart J., 124:1046, 1992.

Spodick, D. H.: Medical history of the pericardium: The hairy hearts of hoary heroes. Am. J. Cardiol., 26:447, 1970.

Spodick, D. H.: The normal and diseased pericardium: Current concepts of pericardial physiology, diagnosis and treatment. J. Am. Coll. Cardiol., 1:240, 1983.

Suchet, I. B., and Horwitz, T. A.: CT in tuberculous constrictive pericarditis. J. Comput. Assist. Tomogr., 16:391, 1992.

Summer, W. R., Permutt, S., Sagawa, K., et al.: Effects of spontaneous respiration on canine left ventricular function. Circ. Res., 45:719, 1979.

Susini, G., Pepi, M., Sisillo, E., et al.: Percutaneous pericardiocentesis versus subxiphoid pericardiotomy in cardiac tamponade due to postoperative pericardial effusion. J. Cardiothorac. Vasc. Anesth., 7:178, 1993.

Taupin, J. M., Laudinat, J. M., Fellinger, F., et al.: [Spontaneous idiopathic pneumopericardium in young patients. Review of the literature. Apropos of a new case]. Ann. Cardiol. Angeiol. (Paris), 41:485, 1992.

Taysi, K., Hartmann, A. F., Shackelford, G. D., and Sundaram, V.: Congenital absence of left pericardium in a family. Am. J. Med. Genet., 21:77, 1985.

Tyson, G. S., Maier, G. W., Olsen, C. O., et al.: Pericardial influences on ventricular filing in the conscious dog: An analysis based on pericardial pressure. Circ. Res., 54:173, 1984.

Urschel, J. D., and Horan, T. A.: Pericardioscopy and biopsy. Surg. Endosc., 7:100, 1993.

Vogel, J. H. K., Horgan, J. A., and Strahl, C. L.: Left ventricular dysfunction in chronic constrictive pericarditis. Chest, 59:484, 1971.

Vora, A. M., Lokhandwala, Y. Y., and Kale, P. A.: Echocardiography guided creation of balloon pericardial window [letter; comment]. Cathet. Cardiovasc. Diagn., 25:164, 1992.

Wallace, H. W., Shen, D., Baum, S., Blakemore, W. S., and Zinsser, H. F.: Angina pectoris associated with a pericardial defect. 61:461, 1971.

Waller, B. F., Taliercio, C. P., Howard, J., et al.: Morphologic aspects of pericardial heart disease: Part II. Clin. Cardiol., 15:291, 1992.

Wang, K. Y., Hwang, C. L., Lee, D. Y., et al.: Pericardiocentesis: A 20 patients study. Chung Hua I Hsueh Tsa Chih, 50:208, 1992.

Watkins, M. W., and LeWinter, M. M.: Physiologic role of the normal pericardium. Ann. Rev. Med., 44:171, 1993.

Zahn, E. M., Houde, C., Benson, L., and Freedom, R. M.: Percutaneous pericardial catheter drainage in childhood. Am. J. Cardiol., 70:678, 1992.

Ziskind, A. A., Pearce, A. C., Lemmon, C. C., et al.: Percutaneous balloon pericardiotomy for the treatment of cardiac tamponade and large pericardial effusions: Description of technique and report of the first 50 cases. J. Am. Coll. Cardiol., 21:1, 1993.

# 35 Atrial Septal Defects, Atrioventricular Canal Defects, and Total Anomalous Pulmonary Venous Return

Aubrey C. Galloway, Stephen B. Colvin, and Frank C. Spencer

Defects in the atrial septum range from the simple, uncomplicated ostium secundum defect to the more complex ostium primum defect. Partial anomalous drainage of the pulmonary veins is possible in a small number of secundum defects but almost always present with the high sinus venosus defect. Because the physiologic burden with a secundum defect is identical to that of partial anomalous drainage of pulmonary veins with sinus venosus defect, consisting of a left-to-right shunt, these two abnormalities are considered together in the following section. Later sections discuss the more severe abnormalities—incomplete atrioventricular (AV) canal or ostium primum defect, complete AV canal, and total anomalous pulmonary venous return (TAPVR).

## SECUNDUM DEFECT AND SINUS VENOSUS DEFECT WITH PARTIAL ANOMALOUS PULMONARY VENOUS RETURN

### Historical Considerations

The modern era of extracorporeal circulation (ECC) began in 1953, when the first successful intracardiac operation in humans was done by Gibbon to close an atrial septal defect (Gibbon, 1954). Also in 1953, Lewis successfully closed a defect under direct vision by using hypothermia and inflow occlusion (Lewis and Taufic, 1953). These two pioneering achievements soon launched the modern era of ECC. Several ingenious techniques that did not require ECC were developed in earlier years but quickly became of historical interest only. The technique of hypothermia and inflow occlusion was effective and safe, because temporary occlusion of the vena cava for 10 to 12 minutes at 28 to 30° C was well tolerated. This technique was used for several years until ECC became safer (Spencer and Bahnson, 1959). By 1960, ECC had developed to such an extent that other techniques were abandoned.

## Pathologic Features

Secundum-type atrial defects are among the most common cardiac malformations, occuring in 10 to 15% of all patients with congenital heart disease. Women are affected about twice as often as are men. No etiologic factors are known.

Atrial defects vary widely in size and location (Fig. 35–1). Most are 2 to 3 cm in diameter and range from as small as 1 cm to virtual absence of the atrial septum. Occasionally, the atrial septum is fenestrated with multiple defects. A foramen ovale is a normal opening, not an abnormality, because it occurs in 10 to 25% of adult hearts. With its slit-like construction, it is normally sealed, unless there is a sharp rise in right atrial pressure.

Most secundum defects are in the midportion of the septum. *Low* defects may involve the orifice of the inferior vena cava; caution is required at operation to avoid constriction of the caval orifice. In 5 to 10% of patients, a *high* defect occurs at the junction of the superior vena cava and the right atrium; this is called a sinus venosus defect because of its embryologic origin. Anomalous drainage of the pulmonary veins from the right upper and middle lobes into the superior vena cava occurs in almost all of these patients. Rarely, anomalous pulmonary veins enter the superior cava, but the atrial septal defect is small or absent. This requires the creation of an atrial septal defect at the time of operative correction. The "high" sinus venosus defect is the most common variety of atrial septal defect associated with anomalous pulmonary veins.

Less frequently, anomalous pulmonary veins enter directly into the posterior wall of the right atrium, anterior to the margin of a posterior atrial septal defect. The rarest abnormality is entry of the pulmonary veins into the inferior vena cava. A variation of this unusual anomaly, associated with other malformations, has been called the "scimitar" syndrome, because of the radiologic appearance produced by the shadow of the anomalous pulmonary vein parallel to the right border of the heart. Usually there is an associated hypoplasia of the right lung and anomalous origin of the pulmonary arteries from the aorta.

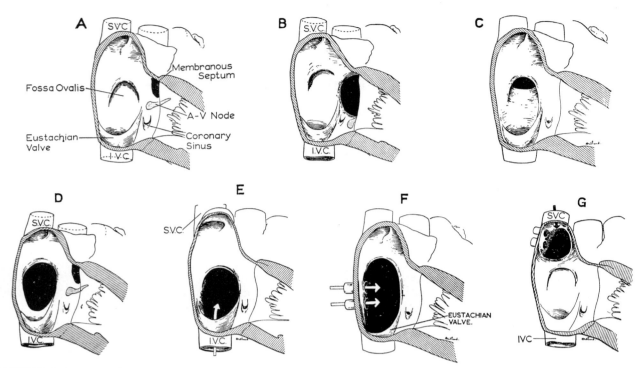

**FIGURE 35–1.** Anatomy of atrial septal defects, seen from the right atrium, as accurately shown and described in 1957 by Bedford and associates. The terminology is theirs. (SVC = superior vena cava; IVC = inferior vena cava; A-V = atrioventricular.) *A,* Normal atrial septum. *B,* AV (Now called ostium primum or incomplete AV canal) type of defect. *C,* Widely patent foramen ovale. *D,* Fossa ovalis (secundum) defect with complete septal rim. *E,* Low (secundum) fossa ovalis defect astride inferior caval orifice with large eustachian valve. *F,* Large (secundum) fossa ovalis defect without any posterior septal rim; pseudoanomalous right pulmonary veins. *G,* Superior caval (Now called sinus venosus) type of defect, showing entrance of right upper pulmonary veins. (*A–G,* From Bedford, D. E., Sellors, T. H., Somerville, W., et al: Atrial septal defect and its surgical treatment. Lancet, 272:1255, 1957.)

Because little blood is shunted through the hypoplastic lung, the physiologic left-to-right shunt is not severe.

Partial anomalous drainage of pulmonary veins usually involves the veins of only one lung, but a few examples of partial drainage of pulmonary veins from both lungs have been reported. One of the most detailed reports of the variety of pathologic patterns that occurs with anomalous pulmonary veins, published by Blake and associates (1965), analyzed 113 patients from the Armed Forces Institute of Pathology. Twenty-seven patterns were found. This fact emphasizes the importance of routinely identifying the location of all pulmonary veins at the time of operation.

In a small percentage of patients with a secundum defect, mitral stenosis is also present, a combination called Lutembacher's syndrome. With restriction of flow of blood into the left ventricle because of the mitral stenosis, an enormous left-to-right shunt develops, with massive dilatation of the pulmonary arteries. Craig and Selzer (1968) emphasized that the combination of lesions represented a true susceptibility of patients with secundum defects to rheumatic fever, because the frequency of the syndrome was greater than would occur from random association. Mitral prolapse occurs in 10 to 20% of patients in association with a secundum defect. It may be overlooked, unless specifically excluded by echocardiography or angiocardiography. In most of these patients, mild mitral

insufficiency improves simply through closure of the septal defect, probably by increasing the left ventricular end-diastolic volume, which changes the closing plane of the valve. Less than 5% of cases require mitral valve correction; when necessary, valve repair using Carpentier's techniques or suture annuloplasty is usually possible. Moderate to severe mitral insufficiency should be corrected to avoid serious pulmonary congestion.

## Pathophysiology

An atrial septal defect produces a shunt of oxygenated blood from the left atrium to the right atrium because the left ventricle is a thicker muscle than the right ventricle. The difference in thickness (10 to 12 mm vs. 4 to 5 mm) is reflected by a difference in distensibility, or compliance, of the two ventricles. As a result, with an intact atrial septum, normal mean left atrial pressure is almost 8 to 10 mm Hg, whereas normal mean right atrial pressure is seldom more than 4 to 5 mm Hg. During the first 2 years of life, the right ventricle is similar to the left. Thus, only a small shunt may exist across an atrial septal defect early in life, but the shunt may increase in magnitude with growth of the child. Often, an atrial septal defect is not clinically evident in the first 2 years of life.

Rudolph (1974) offered an alternative explanation

for infants in whom catheterization a few hours after birth detects a large shunt at the atrial level. Rudolph suggested that differences in the vascular resistance in the pulmonary and systemic circulations may be as important as the difference in distensibility of the two ventricles. Because the pulmonary vascular resistance is increased during the first year of life, the shunt would be small but would increase thereafter as the pulmonary resistance drops.

Both compliance and pulmonary vascular resistance probably are important in determining the degree of shunting. Depending on the size of the defect, the compliance of the ventricles, and the relative vascular resistances, the size of the shunt varies from as little as 1 l/min to as much as 20 l/min. Usually, the pulmonary blood flow is 2 to 3 times greater than the systemic blood flow. There is a reciprocal decrease in pulmonary vascular resistance with the increased pulmonary blood flow, so pulmonary hypertension is rare. In adults, pulmonary hypertension eventually develops in 15 to 20% of patients. An enigma of the pathophysiology of congenital heart disease is the frequency of a progressive increase in pulmonary vascular resistance, ultimately to a lethal degree, with an untreated ventricular septal defect or aortopulmonary window. Conversely, with an atrial septal defect, even with a large shunt, such an increase in pulmonary vascular resistance almost never develops in the first several years of life.

Because the intracardiac shunt reduces systemic blood flow, growth and development may be retarded, producing a gracile habitus. In adults, the cardiac index is usually near the lower limits of normal (2.5 l/m$^2$/min). In a group of 128 adult patients studied by Craig and Selzer (1968), only 9 had a cardiac index of less than 2.0. A slight decrease in arterial oxygen saturation is frequent and probably results from mixing of oxygenated and unoxygenated blood in the atria. In the group studied by Craig and Selzer, 51 had an arterial oxygen saturation of 90 to 94%, and 17 had saturations of less than 90%. Severe hypoxia appears only when there is a marked increase in pulmonary vascular resistance.

The handicap from a pulmonary blood flow 2 to 3 times greater than normal is surprisingly well tolerated in most children. Most are asymptomatic; a few have dyspnea on extreme exertion. With modern cardiorespiratory exercise testing, performance capacity may be decreased, however. In a 1991 study by Reybrouck and associates, children with atrial septal defect who were over 5 years of age at the time of repair had a decreased ventilatory threshold during exercise (85% predicted), compared with normal exercise capacity in patients undergoing repair earlier in life. Susceptibility to pneumonia may increase, as may susceptibility to rheumatic fever. Bacterial endocarditis is almost unknown. In the 1968 report by Craig and Selzer (128 patients over 18 years of age), most patients were limited only by dyspnea on exertion. Cardiac failure, with or without atrial fibrillation, was unusual before 40 years of age. Arrhythmias become much more common in the third and forth decades of

life, however, as does heart failure. The most alarming finding was an increase in pulmonary vascular resistance above the upper limits of normal (400 dyn-sec/cm$^5$) in 13% of patients. This finding represented a catastrophe, because the development of a major increase in pulmonary vascular resistance changed an atrial septal defect from an easily curable lesion to an inevitably lethal one. The pattern of development of the increase in pulmonary vascular resistance was studied in some detail in the 18 patients in whom it occurred and could not be correlated with age or with the degree of increase in pulmonary blood flow. Thus, it was not a "wear and tear" phenomenon. Apparently, an unknown individual susceptibility was the basic factor. The increased resistance occurred in approximately one-third of patients before 20 years of age, in another one-third in the third and fourth decades of life, and in the remainder after 40 years of age. In a few patients studied with serial catheterizations, the rise in pulmonary vascular resistance, once it began, continued rapidly. In two patients, it continued despite surgical closure of the defect.

The unpredictability of the development of an increase in pulmonary vascular resistance, although it never occurs in most patients, is sufficient reason in itself to close atrial septal defects routinely in all patients whenever they are diagnosed, even though most are asymptomatic. The previously cited exercise testing results reported by Reybrouck and co-workers suggest that closure prior to 5 years of age is important if subtle changes in exercise performance are to be prevented.

Also in 1968, Gault and associates reported studies of 62 patients over 40 years of age. Compared with the younger group reported by Craig and Selzer, most patients were symptomatic, with 45% classified as Class III or Class IV cardiac patients. An increase in pulmonary vascular resistance was seen in 70%, a frequency identical to that found by Craig and Selzer.

Craig and Selzer commented on the rarity of a patient over 50 years of age with an atrial septal defect. Statistical analyses indicated that this low frequency was less than would occur in the normal population, suggesting that most patients succumbed to cardiac failure or pulmonary hypertension before the sixth decade of life. The average life expectancy of all patients with atrial septal defects has been estimated to be near 40 years, with 75% of patients dying by age 50, and 90% by age 60 (Fig. 35–2). Fifteen to 20% of patients die of pulmonary hypertension. The others die of cardiac failure 15 to 20 years earlier than the normal population.

## Clinical Features

When they are present, the most common symptoms are exertional dyspnea, fatigue, and palpitations. In a 1966 study of 275 patients undergoing surgery, Sellers and colleagues found that 113 were asymptomatic. As mentioned earlier, dyspnea is more frequent in adults and results from either pulmonary

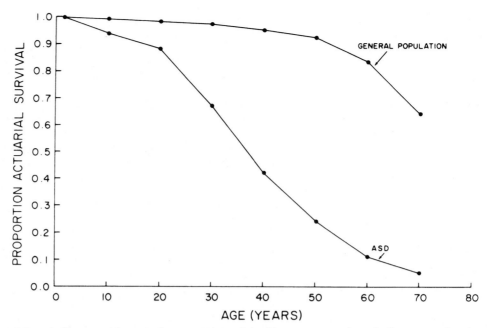

**FIGURE 35–2.** Plot of Campbell's actuarial survival computations of the life expectancy of surgically untreated patients with atrial septal defects who reach the age of 1 year (Campbell, 1970). The plot is based on three sets of collected data. There is some spread between the three sets of data, which indicates confidence limits of modest width around the point estimates (they cannot be calculated from the data). The life expectancy of the general population of 1-year-olds is also from Campbell and is very close to that computed from United States life tables (UAB). The data (see "Natural History") suggest that 99.9% of patients born with atrial septal defects reach the first year of life unless unrelated conditions cause death. (From Kirklin, J. W., and Barratt-Boyes, B. G.: Cardiac Surgery. Churchill Livingstone, New York, 1993.)

hypertension or cardiac failure. Atrial arrhythmias become more frequent in the fourth decade of life, probably from hypertrophy of the right atrium, and may precipitate or intensify symptoms of congestive failure. As with the atrial fibrillation that develops with chronic mitral stenosis, these arrhythmias may be permanent and may remain even after closure of the septal defect. Cyanosis is rare except in the small percentage of patients in whom pulmonary vascular resistance has increased sufficiently to produce a large right-to-left shunt.

On physical examination, the most common finding is a soft, systolic murmur in the left second or third intercostal space near the sternum. The murmur arises from the increased flow of blood through the pulmonic valve. Wide, fixed splitting of the second sound is another important auscultatory finding.

The chest film may show slight to moderate cardiac enlargement from dilatation of the right ventricle. Enlargement of the pulmonary artery is frequent. The electrocardiogram usually shows typical abnormalities that include right ventricular hypertrophy with a right axis deviation and conduction abnormalities. Two-dimensional echocardiography usually can confirm the diagnosis; thus, most cardiac centers no longer routinely catheterize children or young adults.

The diagnosis obviously can be made by cardiac catheterization when necessary, and the procedure shows an oxygen step-up in the right atrium compared with the venae cavae. The presence of anomalous pulmonary veins can be recognized if the cardiac catheter enters a pulmonary vein directly from the superior vena cava. If the pulmonary vein is entered from the right atrium, the diagnosis is uncertain, because the catheter may have traversed an atrial septal defect. Precise delineation of the pulmonary veins is possible with selective angiography. In most patients, the systolic right ventricular pressure is between 30 and 40 mm Hg. With large shunts, a gradient of 20 to 40 mm Hg may be found across a normal pulmonic valve because of the increased flow of blood. Cardiac catheterization is now primarily performed in the older population to assess the pulmonary resistance and to evaluate associated cardiac defects.

## Surgical Treatment

### Indications and Contraindications

Operation is recommended for most patients with defects 1 to 2 cm or larger, particularly when pulmonary blood flow is increased, with a pulmonary blood flow/systemic blood flow ($\dot{Q}_P/\dot{Q}_S$) ratio greater than 1.5:1. Because most children are asymptomatic, the decision for operation is usually based on clinical findings and the chest film, electrocardiogram, and echocardiographic studies. The ideal time for operation is between 2 and 5 years of age, before the child develops physiologic changes in exercise capacity and before beginning school. A study by Murphy and associates reported in 1990 demonstrated that in patients undergoing repair of atrial septal defect prior to 24 years of age, long-term survival was equal to that of the age- and sex-matched control population. Thus, survival is not adversely affected by this lesion when surgical correction is performed early in life. When repair was postponed to later in life, survival was significantly worse. Repair of atrial septal defect should be performed in childhood for optimal long-term results.

The only contraindication to operation is irreversible pulmonary hypertension, with a pulmonary vascular resistance of 8 to 12 units/m$^2$ and a $\dot{Q}_P/\dot{Q}_S$ ratio of less than 1.2:1. When irreversible pulmonary vascular disease is present, the patient may present with cyanosis secondary to right-to-left shunting, the Eisenmenger syndrome. Although this rarely occurs before the fifth to sixth decades of life, sporadic and unpredictable cases of irreversible pulmonary hypertension have been reported much earlier in life in patients with atrial septal defect. Because operation in patients with a pulmonary vascular resistance near systemic levels is dangerous and may produce little benefit, oxygen studies at the time of catheterization sometimes may help to determine if the pulmonary resistance is fixed or reactive. A more modest increase in pulmonary vascular resistance does not contraindicate operative repair as long as the shunt is still left-to-right, with a $\dot{Q}_P/\dot{Q}_S$ ratio of at least 1.3 to 1.5:1.

Age, per se, and heart failure do not contraindicate operation. In 1988, Fiore and associates reported no operative deaths in 51 patients over 50 years of age, with a 10-year survival rate of 86%. All patients improved by at least one New York Heart Association (NYHA) functional category, demonstrating the excellent results achievable in the older population. Nevertheless, the previously cited report by Murphy and associates noted decreased late survival in patients over 24 years of age undergoing operative closure of atrial septal defect; the 27-year survival rate was only 40% in patients repaired after 40 years of age. Despite this, repair is still clearly indicated in older patients, because operation is their only chance for long-term survival.

**Operative Technique.** All patients undergo surgery with ECC. At New York University, both sternotomy and right-sided anterolateral thoracotomy incisions have been used, with equal success. The anterolateral incision is used primarily for cosmetic purposes in young females, and it requires positioning of the patient with a padded roll to elevate the right side of the body 30 to 40 degrees from the horizontal plane. A submammary incision is made, extending to but not dividing the latissimus dorsi muscle, and elevating a small flap so that the fourth intercostal space is entered. A median sternotomy incision usually is used, particularly if cosmetics are not an issue or if the diagnosis may be uncertain.

Once the pericardium is entered, the superior vena cava and innominate vein are inspected. A large superior vena cava suggests partial anomalous pulmonary venous drainage with a sinus venosus type of septal defect. A small superior vena cava or absent innominate vein suggests a persistent left superior vena cava, which is also detected by noting an enlarged coronary sinus. The persistent left vena cava is confirmed by lifting the heart and noting its entry into the coronary sinus above the left atrial appendage. Another helpful maneuver is palpation of the internal aspects of the atrium, where several anatomic features can be identified, including the size and location of the atrial defect, the location of the pulmonary veins, and the presence of mitral or tricuspid valvular insufficiency. This maneuver is particularly useful in adult patients or larger children if the diagnosis is uncertain, and has been used by the senior author for many years.

Once cardiopulmonary bypass has been established, the patient is cooled to 30 to 32° degrees C, the aortic cross-clamp is applied, and the heart is arrested with potassium cardioplegia. Other groups have used electrical fibrillation for repair with similar success. A vertical incision is made in the right atrium, slightly anterior to the sulcus terminalis, in the body of the atrium, after which the intracardiac structures are identified. To minimize the risk of air embolism, care is taken not to aspirate excessive intracardiac blood from the left atrium.

The usual secundum defect can be identified as a 1- to 4-cm opening in the midportion of the atrial septum. Variations are numerous and range from a common atrium with no appreciable posterior septum to a "low" defect that extends close to the inferior vena cava. The location of the coronary sinus and tricuspid valve in relation to the defect should be confirmed. When a persistent left superior vena cava is present, a large amount of blue blood returns from the enlarged coronary sinus. This is easily controlled by placing the coronary suction into the coronary sinus to collect venous return while repair is completed.

Most secundum defects in children or young adults can be closed primarily with a simple continuous suture, usually with 4-0 or 5-0 polypropylene. Attenuated or fenestrated tissue should be removed. The septum must be appropriately flexible if direct closure is to be used. Patch closure with autogenous pericardium is often done in older adults and in some children with large defects when the atrial septum is less pliable. The pericardial patch is cleared of fat and tailored to avoid distortion of the atrium; a continuous suture is used. Similarly, a large secundum defect, such as a common atrium with partial anomalous venous drainage into the right atrium, is corrected by recreating the septum with pericardium, simultaneously redirecting the pulmonary venous drainage into the left atrium. After the septal defect is repaired, but before the septal suture line is tied, the lungs are held in the inflated position to de-air the left atrium, after which sutures are tied under blood.

Patients with sinus venosus defect and partial anomalous pulmonary venous drainage require a more complex correction to avoid obstructing the pulmonary veins or the superior vena cava. The first principle is to dissect the extrapericardial superior vena cava superiorly to above the entry point of the azygous vein. The anomalous veins almost always enter the vena cava below the level of the azygous vein; cannulation above this point with a metal right-angle cannula often simplifies exposure. The atrial incision is extended either well laterally or medially up the superior vena cava; care must be taken to avoid the sinus node, which is usually at the junction of the sulcus terminalis and the superior vena cava. A pericardial patch is used in all cases, starting the patch at the upper border of the most superior anomalous pulmonary vein in the vena cava and redirecting flow from the anomalous veins across the sinus venosus defect, simultaneously correcting the pulmonary venous return and the atrial septal defect. In rare cases when the septal defect is absent, a defect must be created, after which the repair proceeds as usual. The junction of the superior vena cava and right atrium is often enlarged to avoid vena caval obstruction, especially in children. This may be done with an inverted Y to V advancement flap, or else a pericardial patch may be used.

After repair is completed and the right atriotomy incision is closed, electrical fibrillation of the ventricle is induced, the aorta is vented, and the cross-clamp is removed. Care is taken to de-air each chamber of the heart, usually by aspiration with a large needle. After all apparent air is removed, the aortic root is placed on gentle suction as a final precaution, after which the heart is defibrillated.

In adult patients with chronic left-to-right shunting, the left side of the heart may be small and noncompliant; in such patients, left atrial pressure monitoring may be helpful after discontinuing cardiopulmonary bypass. Similarly, transesophageal echocardiography may be helpful in patients with associated mitral insufficiency. Following bypass, blood samples for oxygen saturation routinely are obtained from the superior vena cava and pulmonary artery to confirm the absence of a residual shunt.

**Operative Results.** Operative risk is less than 1%, approaching 0%. At New York University, no deaths have occurred in children with uncomplicated secundum defect for the last 15 years, which supports the policy of routine closure of significant secundum defects. Long-term survival is related primarily to age and pulmonary artery systolic pressure before operation, according to the report by Murphy and associates (1990), which included 123 patients followed for 30 years. Survival was equal to that of the normal population in patients undergoing surgery early in life, before the development of atrial fibrillation, heart failure, and pulmonary hypertension. The 27-year survival rate was 97% in patients repaired before age 12 and 40% in those repaired after age 40.

Current data support a policy of routine closure of atrial septal defects regardless of age, as long as a significant left-to-right shunt is still present. The life expectancy of surgically untreated patients, as described by Campbell in 1970, is shown in an actuarial curve in Figure 35–2. The results reported by Fiore and associates (1988) for surgical repair in older pa-tients described survival that was superior to the natural history of nonsurgically treated patients.

If the pulmonary vascular resistance is elevated, the risk of operation is increased and long-term benefit is decreased. The question as to when operation should not be done because of increased vascular resistance remains uncertain. We prefer to see a decrease in pulmonary vascular resistance in response to oxygen and a $\dot{Q}_P/\dot{Q}_S$ ratio of greater than 1.2:1, suggesting some reactivity in the pulmonary vascular bed. A 1987 report from the Mayo Clinic by Steele and associates contains excellent data. During a period of 25 years, 40 patients with significant elevation of pulmonary vascular resistance (total resistance greater than 7 units/m$^2$) were treated, 26 surgically. Excellent results after operation were obtained in those with pulmonary vascular resistance less than 15 units/m$^2$; 19 of the 22 were in good condition with follow-up of over 10 years. In patients with a pulmonary resistance above 15 units/m$^2$, the mortality rate was 75%. With medical treatment, the mortality rate was 80% when resistance was less than 15 units/m$^2$ and 66% when the resistance was higher than this. Thus, in this series, a pulmonary vascular resistance over 15 units/m$^2$ defined a level at which surgical therapy was no longer beneficial.

**Postoperative Course and Complications.** Postoperative convalescence and recovery are prompt and uncomplicated in most patients. The average hospital stay is less than a week. Heart block is extremely rare, but sinus node dysfunction may occur after repair of patients with sinus venosus defect. The most frequent late complications are atrial fibrillation and embolism.

Atrial fibrillation is transient unless chronic preoperatively; the condition in most patients can be converted into a sinus mechanism with medications. According to Hawe and associates (1969), atrial fibrillation is present in 30 to 40% of the patients with atrial septal defect over 40 years of age. Embolism is a bigger hazard in this group; chronic anticoagulation with warfarin is recommended when chronic atrial fibrillation persists postoperatively. Antiplatelet therapy for 2 to 3 months postoperatively may be appropriate when a patch is used, although the report by Fiore and associates (1988) suggests that long-term anticoagulation is unnecessary. Continuous antiplatelet therapy or anticoagulation with warfarin is not recommended for patients in sinus rhythm.

## PARTIAL ATRIOVENTRICULAR CANAL DEFECT (OSTIUM PRIMUM)

The term *AV canal defect*, partial or complete, best describes this spectrum of malformations, which vary in severity with the extent of the deficiency in the AV septum. This concept of defective development of the endocardial cushions is discussed well by Kirklin and Barratt-Boyes (1993). The defects range from an atrial septal defect (ostium primum) to a severe defect with a common AV valve orifice and septal defect at both the lower atrial and ventricular levels (old term: *atrio-*

*ventricularis communis*). The current terminology is based on the pathologic anatomy rather than on the embryologic concepts, on which the previous terminology was based. These defects account for approximately 5% of all atrial septal defects and are found in 20 to 30% of children with Down syndrome; other than this association, no etiologic factors are known. Complete AV canal defects with a common AV orifice are discussed in a later section.

Anatomic studies over the past 2 decades have clarified the pathologic abnormality in these malformations. After the initial observations by Rastelli and colleagues in 1966, further important observations were made by Piccoli, Carpentier, and Anderson. The 1985 paper by Penkoske and co-workers described observations of 130 AV canal defects from specimens in the pathologic collection of the Children's Hospital in Pittsburgh and summarized several important anatomic characteristics. First, the cardiac anatomy is similar in both partial and complete AV canal defects, varying only with the presence of the defect in the ventricular septum and the degree of malformation in the valve leaflets. Both the valve leaflets and the ventricular cavities are different from those found in normal hearts or other malformations. The left ventricular "mitral" valve is a trileaflet structure that comprises the left lateral, left superior, and left inferior leaflets. The "cleft" (Fig. 35–3) dividing the left superior and left inferior leaflets (which is the anterior leaflet of the mitral valve in standard anatomy) is actually a normal commissure. The extent of the cleft, which ranges from a small vertical opening to a triangular defect, is the principal determinant of the degree of mitral insufficiency. This subject is discussed well in the 1985 paper by Anderson and colleagues. The conduction bundle is displaced posteriorly and inferiorly to lie between the inferior margin of the primum defect and the annulus of the tricuspid orifice.

The atrial septal defect is recognized readily at op-
eration through palpation or inspection. The superior border of the defect is a low, crescent-shaped defect in the atrial septum, with the inferior border adjacent to the top of the ventricular septum, bridging the leaflet tissue or annulus between the mitral and tricuspid valves.

If the trileaflet mitral valve functions normally, there is no insufficiency. At least 30 to 40% of patients experience moderate or severe insufficiency, either from the presence of the defect between the left superior and left inferior leaflets (the cleft) or from the absence of a varying extent of leaflet tissue that results in a triangular-shaped defect rather than in a simple cleft. Complete repair of incompetence may not be achieved in a few patients because of significant absence of leaflet tissue.

The chordae tendineae are usually normally attached along the margins of the two halves of the cleft leaflet (the commissure between the left superior and the left inferior leaflets) and are valuable guidelines during repair. Anomalous chordae may attach directly to the ventricular septum because of the bridging of the leaflet tissue; these may partly constrict the left ventricular outflow tract.

The anatomy of the different leaflets of the tricuspid valve varies. The septal leaflet is deficient or absent in almost 80% of patients, but significant tricuspid insufficiency is rare and does not require surgical treatment. Associated abnormalities are found in 10 to 15% of patients (40 of 232 patients described by McMullan and associates in 1973); the most common abnormalities were secundum defect, pulmonary stenosis, and anomalous vena cava.

## Pathophysiology

The two physiologic abnormalities are a left-to-right shunt at the atrial level and mitral insufficiency. When mitral insufficiency is small, the disability is

FIGURE 35–3. Operative photograph of incomplete atrioventricular canal–ostium primum atrial septal defect. Note the cleft in the anterior leaflet of the mitral valve (MV).

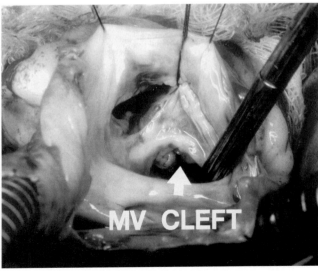

identical to that of a secundum atrial septal defect. When mitral insufficiency is severe, cardiac failure and pulmonary hypertension often develop in the first 1 to 3 years of life. The series by McMullan and associates (1973) described catheterization data for 74 patients. The ratio of pulmonary flow to systemic flow was 2.7:1 and ranged from 1.3:1 to 5.6:1. Pulmonary resistance averaged 2.7 units/$m^2$ and ranged from 0.5 to 7.5 units/$m^2$. Systolic pulmonary artery pressure greater than 30 mm Hg was found in 36 patients. Pulmonary hypertension with increased pulmonary vascular resistance occurs more frequently than in patients with secundum atrial septal defects but is less frequent than with complete AV canal defects.

With the varying degrees of mitral insufficiency is a corresponding wide range in symptoms. With severe mitral insufficiency, exertional dyspnea, pulmonary congestion, and cardiac failure are common. In 30 patients described by Braunwald and Morrow (1966), only 30 to 50% were asymptomatic. On physical examination, the dominant finding is a loud systolic murmur along the left sternal border as well as at the cardiac apex, which indicates an abnormality other than a simple secundum defect. The pulmonic second sound is more intense and widely split. If cardiac failure is present, there may be signs of pulmonary and hepatic congestion. Findings on the chest film vary. Enlargement of the pulmonary artery is the most frequent abnormality. With severe abnormalities, there is corresponding enlargement of the right ventricle. If mitral insufficiency is dominant, there is preponderant enlargement of the left ventricle.

The electrocardiogram almost always shows a left axis deviation, and may provide the first clue to the correct diagnosis. Right and left ventricular hypertrophy can occur to various degrees. Conduction defects, with prolongation of the P-R interval, are frequent. The electrocardiographic abnormalities stem primarily from the conduction defect resulting from inferior displacement of the conduction bundle.

A characteristic abnormality is usually present on the vector cardiogram; the frontal plane is inscribed in a counterclockwise loop, almost diagnostic of an endocardial cushion defect. The two-dimensional echocardiogram is virtually diagnostic; some physicians consider cardiac catheterization superfluous for uncomplicated defects. Cardiac catheterization and angiography are done occasionally, however, to determine the degree of mitral insufficiency and the level of pulmonary hypertension and to identify associated cardiac anomalies.

## Surgical Treatment

Most patients with significant mitral insufficiency, cardiac failure, or pulmonary hypertension should undergo surgery before 6 to 8 months of age. When mitral insufficiency is not present, the physiologic defect is the same as with a simple secundum defect. In uncomplicated cases, there is little urgency in oper-

ation, but correction before age 3 to 4 years is preferred. An adult occasionally is seen in the third or fourth decade of life with little disability from an incomplete AV canal defect. These patients are without mitral insufficiency and without a predisposition to pulmonary hypertension. More commonly, the large left-to-right shunt combined with mild-to-moderate mitral insufficiency causes congestive heart failure, cardiomegaly, and moderate pulmonary hypertension during childhood.

The risk of operation is related to the degree of mitral insufficiency and pulmonary hypertension. The operative mortality rate averages 2 to 5%. Without these abnormalities, the operative mortality rate is less than 1%.

**Technique of Operation.** The principal objectives are repair of the mitral insufficiency, avoidance of heart block, and closure of the atrial septal defect. A median sternotomy is preferable. A right-sided anterior thoracotomy in the fourth intercostal space is less satisfactory. Palpation of the intracardiac chambers through the right atrial appendage readily confirms the diagnosis, noting the characteristic upper curved margin of the septal defect, as described earlier. The degree of mitral insufficiency can be estimated from the vigor of the regurgitant jet. Intraoperative transesophageal echocardiography is also helpful in assessing mitral insufficiency.

The heart is arrested with the cold blood potassium cardioplegia technique. The right atrium is then opened widely, and appropriate retractors are inserted. The intracardiac anatomy is carefully examined, noting the size of the atrial septal defect, the extent and dimensions of the "cleft" in the mitral valve, the presence of abnormal chordae that might obstruct the aortic outflow tract, any abnormalities in the tricuspid valve, and the presence of any ventricular septal defect.

The site and severity of the mitral insufficiency can be evaluated by injection of saline with a bulb syringe into the ventricular cavity to distend the valve leaflets.

The cleft in the mitral valve is repaired first, with figure-of-eight 4-0 or 5-0 polypropylene sutures. Two or three sutures are usually necessary, but the cleft is not totally closed to the free margin, so that the leaflet is not restricted. The insertion points of the chordae tendineae are carefully noted. Care is taken with the sutures to avoid stretching the valve leaflets or tethering the chordae, which might create rather than correct insufficiency.

There has been a great deal of discussion about whether or not the cleft should be sutured, because it is recognized anatomically as a commissure, not as a cleft. The surgical significance of this debate seems to be minimal. We have not recognized injury from routine suturing of the cleft and consider partial closure important. The extensive 1986 report from the Mayo Clinic by King and associates describes experiences with 199 patients during the previous 22 years. The cleft was routinely closed, regardless of the degree of preoperative valvular insufficiency. In two patients who had developed mitral insufficiency years after closure of the ostium primum defect in childhood without suture of the cleft, closure of the cleft at a second operation successfully eliminated regurgitation. In the 1987 report by Stewart and associates, which described experiences with 35 patients, the cleft was routinely closed. In the 1986 report by Pillai and associates, which described experiences with 84 patients at the Brompton Hospital in London during the previous 10 years, the cleft was sutured completely or partly in 72 members of the group and was left alone in 11 patients.

Competency of the reconstructed leaflets is evaluated by injection of saline through a bulb syringe. In a few patients, a diffuse, central insufficiency can be seen through annular dilation. This is not amenable to simple suturing of the cleft. Annuloplasty sutures at the commissure to narrow the mitral orifice have been used in these patients with good results.

After repair of the cleft in the mitral valve, the atrial defect is closed with a pericardial patch. It is crucial to avoid heart block caused by the sutures injuring the conduction bundle. The AV conduction bundle is at the inferior border of the defect adjacent to the apex of the triangle of Koch and courses along the crest of the muscular ventricular septum below. This bundle is displaced inferiorly from its usual course because the AV septum is absent. With proper technique, heart block can be avoided in most patients, but the importance of technique is indicated by the variation in the frequency of heart block after operation, which ranges from 20% in operations done over 20 years ago to 1 to 2% in current reports.

Either a series of interrupted sutures or a continuous polypropylene suture is placed superficially to the left of the rim of the defect, directly in the annulus of the mitral valve. This is done carefully, with traction on the mitral valve leaflet to stretch the tissue and define the annulus precisely. Excellent visualization is required; the sutures must be placed very superficially when near the apex of the triangle of Koch. Kirklin and Barratt-Boyes (1993) noted that McGoon used this method for many years with excellent results. This method also was used in the 199 patients described in King's report in 1986 and in the report of Stewart and associates (1987).

When the crucial sutures have been inserted through the patch and tied, the patch can be attached to the remaining margins of the defect with a continuous suture of 4-0 Prolene.

An alternative method places the sutures to the *right* of the conduction bundle and the coronary sinus, which diverts the coronary sinus blood into the left atrium. This is described well by Kirklin and Barratt-Boyes (1993) and by Pillai and colleagues (1986). Heart block is rare with this technique; either method appears to give excellent results.

After the different cardiac incisions are sutured, air is carefully removed from the heart; air embolism was a frequent complication years ago but now is rare when appropriate techniques are used. After bypass, left atrial pressure should be measured as an index of residual mitral insufficiency. Intracardiac left atrial and right atrial catheters are left in place for postoperative monitoring. Pacemaker wires also are routinely left on the atrium and ventricle for a few days after operation, because transitory conduction defects are common, probably from edema near the conduction bundle.

## Results

Postoperative recovery usually is uneventful if the hazards described earlier are avoided. Complete heart block is now uncommon with proper technique, occurring in less than 1% of cases. If complete heart block is present in the operating room, one should consider redoing the patch and aligning it to the right of the coronary sinuses, if this was not done initially. If permanent heart block occurs, it should be treated by implanting a pacemaker before the patient is discharged from the hospital.

Some residual mitral insufficiency occurs in less than 10% of patients. Occasionally, patients have a mild residual systolic murmur, usually of no hemodynamic significance. A loud systolic murmur warns of significant mitral insufficiency that may remain; this should be evaluated using echocardiography and possibly ventriculography.

The risk inherent in operation is small, now in the range of 1 to 3%. The mortality rate was 5.5% in the 199 patients in King's report and has decreased to 3% since 1980. The mortality rate was 1.8% in Ceithaml's report, 2% in Pillai's report, and 5% in Stewart's report. The principal factors that influence mortality are the degree of mitral insufficiency, the presence of pulmonary vascular disease, and the age of the patient. Several reports describe early and late results (Castaneda et al., 1985; Ceithaml et al., 1989; King et al., 1986; Pillai et al., 1986; Portman et al., 1985; Stewart et al., 1987). Residual mitral insufficiency may be found after operation in 5 to 10% of patients. With severe insufficiency, patients often require another operation within a few years. Except for this group, long-term prognosis is excellent. In the Mayo Clinic series, 20 years after operation, the survival rate was 96% and freedom from reoperation was 86%. Ceithaml reported that 89% of the survivors were in NYHA Functional Class I or II late postoperatively.

We have not seen the unusual syndrome of severe hemolytic anemia after operation, described by Neill in 1964, for more than 20 years. This syndrome has been avoided by using pericardium as the patch material and by using an operative technique that prevents the development of localized mitral insufficiency.

## COMPLETE ATRIOVENTRICULAR CANAL DEFECT

As described earlier, this defect results from a more severe arrest in the development of the endocardial cushions than that which produces an ostium primum defect (partial AV canal). The basic defect is absence of the common AV septum from failure of development of the endocardial cushions. Both the left-sided and right-sided AV valves are malformed into a single six-leaflet structure and a large septal defect that consists of a continuous atrial and a ventricular septal defect. The atrial septal defect is low, identical to that with the ostium primum defect. The ventricular septal defect ranges from a small opening to a large posterior defect.

The classic pathologic studies by Rastelli and associates (1965, 1966, 1968) identified distinct anatomic types, called Types A, B, and C. These categories were based on the degree of bridging of the left superior leaflet of the mitral valve. In Type A, the left superior leaflet does not bridge the septum, and the chordae extend to the rim of the ventricular septal defect. Types B and C show more extensive bridging of the left superior leaflet, with attachment of the chordae of the left superior leaflet to papillary muscles in the right ventricle. These concepts are illustrated well in

Figure 35–4. The 1985 publication by Penkoske and associates, based on a study of 130 specimens, clarified and redefined the different Rastelli types. Currently, this classification is less useful, because a more practical approach is to visualize the common AV canal as a five- or six-leaflet structure that provides a common inlet to the ventricles, overlaying a large ventricular septal defect, and contiguous with an ostium primum atrial septal defect. Common AV valvular leaflets include left superior, left lateral, left inferior, right superior, right lateral, and right inferior leaflets. The degree of fusion and overriding in the superior and inferior leaflets varies highly.

The physiologic handicap with complete AV canal defect is far more severe than with an ostium primum defect. Cardiac failure occurs at an early age to the extent that 80% of untreated infants die within 2 years, and pulmonary hypertension develops in almost all infants by 3 to 5 years of age. Diagnostic evaluation is identical to that described for the partial AV defect. The echocardiogram is normally diagnostic. The cardiac catheterization shows a typical "goose

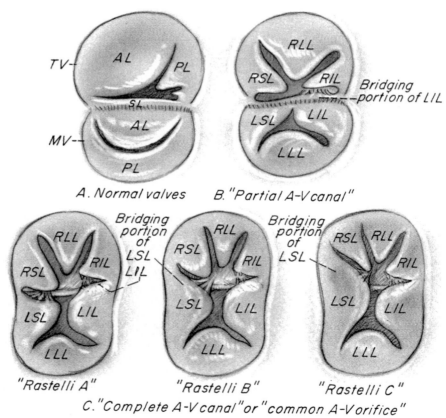

**FIGURE 35–4.** Diagrammatic representation of the AV valves seen from the atrial side (surgical orientation). *A*, Normal, with anterior and posterior mitral valve (MV) leaflets and septal, anterior, and posterior tricuspid valve (TV) leaflets. *B*, The leaflets in partial AV canal defects. The left superior, left inferior, and left lateral leaflets form the left AV valve; the right superior, right inferior, and right lateral leaflets form the right AV valve. *C*, The leaflets in complete AV canal defects are similar to those in *B*. However, the left superior and left inferior leaflets are not connected. The left inferior leaflet usually bridges a little (grade 1 or 2, on the basis of 1 to 5) across the crest of the ventricular septum. The left superior leaflet may bridge little or not at all (grade 0 or 1, Rastelli Type A) or moderately (grade 2 or 3, Rastelli Type B), or markedly (grade 4 or 5, Rastelli Type C). (AL = anterior leaflet; LIL = left inferior leaflet; LLL = left lateral leaflet; LSL = left superior leaflet; PL = posterior leaflet; RIL = right inferior leaflet; RLL = right lateral leaflet; RSL = right superior leaflet; SL = septal leaflet.) (*A–C*, From Kirklin, J. W., Pacifico, A. D., and Kirklin, J. K.: The surgical treatment of atrioventricular canal defects. *In* Arciniegas, E. [ed]: Pediatric Cardiac Surgery. Chicago, Year Book Medical, 1985.)

neck" deformity. Catheterization is done primarily to evaluate associated cardiac defects. Down syndrome is present in over 50% of the patients with complete AV canal defects.

## Surgical Treatment

The concepts of modern surgical treatment originated with Rastelli and associates at the Mayo Clinic, who developed an operative technique based on their anatomic studies (1968). This procedure was described in detail in the 1972 report by McMullan and associates.

Most infants should undergo primary operative repair in the first 6 months of life—earlier if severe symptoms are present. Palliative pulmonary artery banding now is seldom used except in extremely "unbalanced" AV canals, when the left ventricle is underdeveloped. The techniques used for repair vary, depending on whether one or two patches are used, the method of treatment of a bridging left superior leaflet, and the technique for avoiding the conduction bundle by staying on the left or right side of the coronary sinus. General principles are described here. Kirklin and Barratt-Boyes (1993) should be consulted for further reading.

Briefly, the two-patch corrective procedure involves inserting a Dacron prosthetic patch to close the ventricular septal defect (Fig. 35–5) and then reconstructing the abnormal left-sided and right-sided AV valvular leaflets, which are attached to the patch at the appropriate level (Fig. 35–6). The atrial septal defect is then closed with pericardium, suturing through the resuspended leaflets into the underlying VSD patch. The VSD patch usually is placed with sutures to the right of the crest of the septum to avoid conduction tissue. The left-to-right orientation and depth of the VSD patch, along with the level of leaflet attachment, determine the size and the competence of the subsequent AV valves.

After the valvular leaflets are reattached to the prosthetic VSD patch and the cleft between the left superior and left inferior leaflets is partially closed, the atrial septal defect is closed, using either a separate patch, as described above (two-patch technique), or a continuation of the ventricular septal defect Dacron patch (single-patch technique). We prefer the two-patch technique because it allows more precise correction of AV valvular insufficiency and is associated with less late leaflet dehiscence. The atrial septal defect patch should be placed either leftward and superficial to the conduction tissue or well rightward around the coronary sinus.

FIGURE 35–5. *A,* Operative photograph of complete atrioventricular canal defect undergoing repair at New York University Medical Center with the two-patch technique. *B,* Dacron patch closure of the ventricular septal defect.

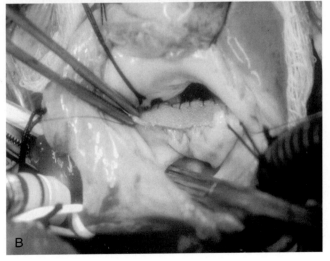

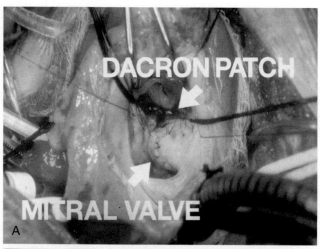

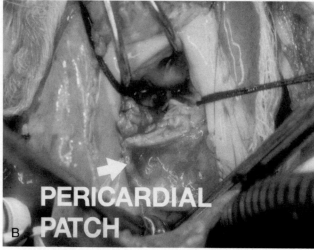

**FIGURE 35–6.** *A,* Operative photograph of a patient at New York University Medical Center with complete atrioventricular canal defect, demonstrating resuspension of leaflet tissue to the underlying Dacron patch. *B,* Completed repair with pericardial patch closure of atrial component.

Operative mortality rates vary with the degree of preoperative left-sided AV valvular incompetence, ranging from 3 to 5% in patients without significant valvular incompetence to 10 to 15% when severe valvular incompetence is present. In our experiences over the past decade, the operative risk has been less than 5% despite significant preoperative pulmonary hypertension in most patients. Late results are excellent unless significant residual left-sided valvular incompetence or irreversible pulmonary vascular disease occurs. Pulmonary hypertension almost always subsides if a large left-to-right shunt is present and surgery is performed in the first year of life. With current techniques, significant residual left-sided valvular incompetence should occur in less than 5 to 10% of patients. Late follow-up of the recent New York University experience with over 50 patients show a 95% rate of freedom of late AV valvular insufficiency at 5 years. Most patients fall into NYHA Class I postoperatively.

## TOTAL ANOMALOUS PULMONARY VENOUS RETURN (TAPVR)

This severe anomaly is rare, occurring in 1 to 3% of patients with congenital heart disease. The natural history of surgically untreated patients is extremely poor, with 50% of infants dying within 3 months and 80% dying before 1 year of age. The 20% who survive beyond 1 year of age without operative treatment usually are those with a concomitant large atrial septal defect.

All patients should undergo surgery promptly after the diagnosis is made. In some infants, surgery is necessary in the first few days of life to prevent death.

The classification suggested by Darling and associates (1957), based on the point of emptying of the anomalous veins into the right side of the heart, generally is used. The four basic types are supracardiac (50%), cardiac (25%), infracardiac (20 to 25%), and mixed (3 to 5%). In the supracardiac type, the most common pattern of entry of the anomalous veins is through a left vertical vein, which in turn drains into the innominate vein. A less frequent type is direct entry of the common venous sinus into the posterior aspect of the right superior cava.

With cardiac drainage, the anomalous veins may enter the right atrium directly or drain into the coronary sinus, either directly or through a common venous sinus. With infracardiac drainage, the pulmonary veins enter a common sinus that travels caudad through the diaphragm to connect with the inferior vena cava. This connection is through the portal vein in approximately two-thirds of the patients and through other veins in the remainder. Infracardiac TAPVR is rapidly fatal because of inherent obstruction in the hepatic and portal venous channels, which often progressively fibrose and obliterate with time, causing severe obstruction to the pulmonary venous return.

## Pathology and Pathophysiology

The anomalous veins usually enter a common venous sinus located behind the posterior pericardium, which connects with the right side of the heart through one of the pathways noted above, producing a significant left-to-right shunt. An atrial septal defect or large foramen ovale must be present to maintain life, although the size varies considerably. Some degree of obstruction to pulmonary venous drainage is common, always present with the infracardiac type. With pulmonary venous obstruction, severe pulmonary congestion and pulmonary hypertension produce rapidly progressive critical respiratory symptoms. In approximately one-third of patients with TAPVR, other major cardiac anomalies are present; a patent ductus is present in most cases.

Because the oxygenated pulmonary venous blood and the systemic venous blood mix in the right atrium, cyanosis always occurs, the degree of which depends on the pulmonary blood flow and the size of the atrial septal defect. The complete mixing of the systemic and pulmonary venous blood in the right atrium makes the findings at cardiac catheterization unique. Oxygen saturations of blood drawn from the right atrium, right ventricle, pulmonary artery, and femoral artery are nearly identical.

A severe physiologic handicap is pulmonary venous obstruction, which results from constriction at the point of entry of the anomalous pulmonary veins into the systemic venous system. This constriction causes severe pulmonary congestion with pulmonary hypertension. A predictable relationship exists between the degree of pulmonary venous obstruction,

the pulmonary vascular resistance, the pulmonary blood flow, and the severity of cyanosis from right to-left shunting across the atrial septal defect. Because of the pulmonary venous obstruction frequently present, balloon septostomy to enlarge an atrial septal defect often has limited value.

In the fortunate infants without pulmonary venous obstruction, but with a large atrial septal defect, the clinical course is similar to that of patients with a large atrial septal defect.

The left atrium and left ventricle usually are small but are physiologically normal. Thus, the left heart may be noncompliant initially, but will enlarge and grow normally after correction.

## Clinical Features

In the first few weeks of life, *severe tachypnea* is the dominant symptom. The clinical picture is easily confused with aspiration pneumonia or primary pulmonary disease. After a few weeks, cyanosis, congestive failure, and progressive cardiac enlargement become more evident. Infants with severe obstruction often have severe pulmonary congestion and hypoxemia, requiring intubation and respiratory support. The cardiac output often is decreased, with poor peripheral perfusion.

The chest film may be diagnostic if there is drainage into a dilated left vertical vein, which creates a well-known double contour, often called a "snowman" configuration (Fig. 35–7). If pulmonary venous obstruction is severe, a diffuse, ground-glass type of pulmonary congestion is present. When cyanosis is prominent, the differential diagnosis includes tetralogy of Fallot, transposition of the great vessels, and tricuspid atresia. The usual differential diagnosis is between TAPVR and transposition, both of which produce cyanosis, cardiac enlargement, and pulmonary congestion.

In the few patients with adequate pulmonary blood flow without pulmonary hypertension, the clinical findings are meager: a mild degree of cyanosis and some enlargement of the right side of the heart.

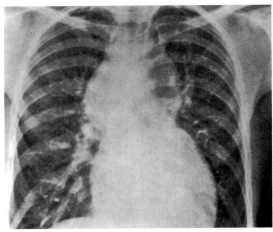

FIGURE 35–7. Chest film of a 24-year-old patient with total anomalous drainage of the pulmonary veins into a left vertical vein. The mediastinal shadow is composed of the dilated left vertical vein and the large superior vena cava. This radiographic appearance is frequently referred to as a "snowman" effect.

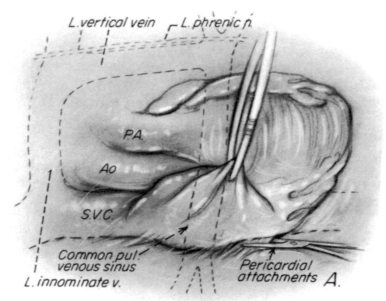

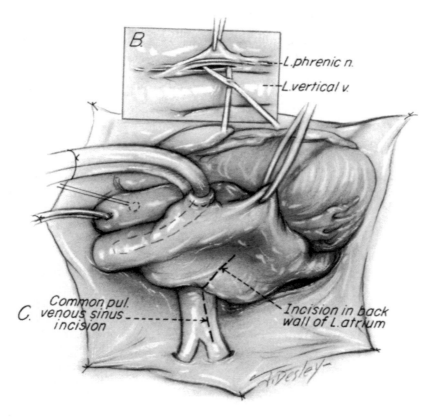

**FIGURE 35–8.** Technique of surgical correction of total anomalous drainage to left innominate vein. *A,* The posterior pericardial attachments are divided to mobilize the heart and expose the common pulmonary venous sinus located behind the pericardium. *B,* The left vertical vein is exposed and mobilized, with the phrenic nerve protected. *C,* The anterior wall of the pulmonary venous sinus is incised parallel to the long axis. The orifices of the left and right pulmonary veins are located and inspected. A corresponding incision is made in the back wall of the left atrium. The incision may have to be carried into the base of the left atrial appendage to the left and over to the atrial septum on the right.

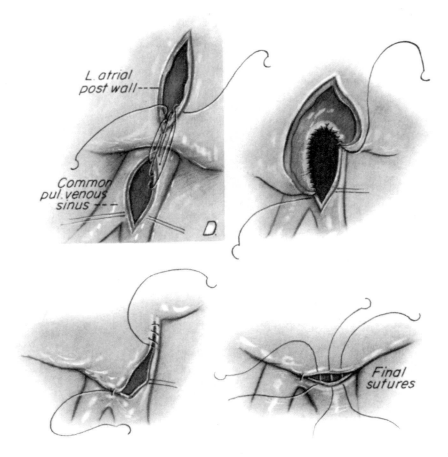

**FIGURE 35–8** *Continued D,* A large anastomosis is constructed with continuous 4-0 or 5-0 polypropylene. (*A–D,* From Kirklin, J. W., and Barratt-Boyes, B. G.: Cardiac Surgery, Churchill Livingstone, New York, 1993.)

Two-dimensional echocardiography is virtually diagnostic, so some centers no longer routinely perform cardiac catheterization. In the 1988 report from London by Lincoln and associates, describing experiences with 83 patients, echocardiography was used without catheterization in 24 of the last 28 patients. If the diagnosis is in doubt, cardiac catheterization and angiography will better define the abnormal venous anatomy, pulmonary blood flow, and associated anomalies. As noted above, the similarity of oxygen saturation in all cardiac chambers and in the femoral artery is diagnostic.

## Treatment

Surgery should take place promptly once the diagnosis is made, often within the first few days of life. Early surgery is recommended even when pulmonary venous obstruction is absent, because operative risk increases significantly once critical obstruction develops. Without surgery, almost 50% of infants die within 3 months. For more than 10 years after the first successful correction with ECC by Kirklin in 1957, the operative mortality rate in infants approached 50%. The outcome improved dramatically with the technique of hypothermia and circulatory arrest, which was developed in 1969 primarily by Barratt-Boyes

and associates in New Zealand. This technique was described in 1973, and is the major reason for the low mortality rate currently reported.

Current results were illustrated well in the 1980a report by Turley and associates, who described experiences with 22 infants undergoing surgery between 1975 and 1978. All 6 undergoing surgery within the first 4 days of life survived. Six others underwent surgery before 1 month of age, and 10 underwent surgery between 1 and 12 months. Of the total group of 22, 19 (87%) survived. Two late deaths occurred from progressive fibrosis of the pulmonary veins, an unsolved problem reported to occur in approximately 10% of infants within 1 year of operation.

The surgical objective is to make a large opening between the anomalous venous sinus and the left atrium, close the atrial septal defect, and ligate any abnormal communications. The operative technique for repair of supracardiac TAPVR is shown in Figure 35–8. Palliative balloon septostomy to enlarge the atrial septal defect has been disappointing because of the frequent presence of pulmonary venous obstruction. With the impressive results of operations in the first few days of life, immediate total correction appears to be the best approach.

When the anomalous veins drain into the coronary sinus, the original method was to excise the common atrial septum between the coronary sinus and the

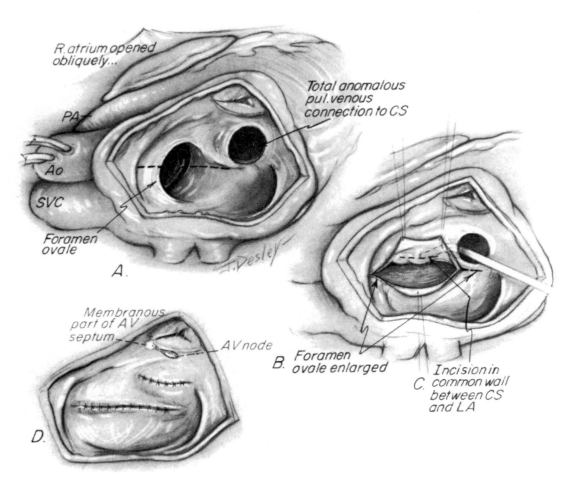

**FIGURE 35–9.** Repair of total anomalous pulmonary venous connection to coronary sinus. *A,* The foramen ovale is enlarged sufficiently to obtain adequate exposure within the left atrium. *B* and *C,* With a clamp placed in the coronary sinus, the coronary is "unroofed" with a long incision between the coronary sinus and the left atrium. *D,* The foramen ovale and the ostium of the coronary sinus are closed. (Ao = aorta; AV = atrioventricular; CS = coronary sinus; LA = left atrium; PA = pulmonary artery; SVC = superior vena cava.) (*A–D,* From Kirklin, J. W., and Barratt-Boyes, B. G.: Cardiac Surgery. Churchill Livingstone, New York, 1993.)

foramen ovale, to unroof the coronary sinus, and to close the newly formed atrial septal defect either primarily or with a pericardial patch. A technique described by Van Praagh and co-workers in 1972 is also commonly used (Fig. 35–9). Both methods have been equally efficacious, with a similar incidence of late arrhythmias.

Surgical approaches for the more uncommon types of anomalous pulmonary veins, such as infracardiac or mixed types, are described well by Kirklin and Barratt-Boyes (1993). Infracardiac drainage is repaired by lifting the heart anteriorly and rightward (Galloway et al., 1985), performing the left atrial anastomosis from outside the heart, or alternately approaching from the right side, and freeing the posterior pericardial structures. The incision in the common vein often is extended into the lobar branches; the vertical vein usually is ligated and divided before it enters the diaphragm.

The hospital mortality rate for operations performed in the first year of life is between 5 and 15%. Kirklin and Barratt-Boyes reported 10 deaths in their experience with a total of 64 patients, a combination of the experiences of the two authors with those reported by Turley and associates. The 1988 report by Lincoln and associates described a total of 12 deaths in 83 patients, with a 14% mortality rate. Operative deaths are related primarily to the presence of preoperative pulmonary venous obstruction, most commonly found with infracardiac type of drainage, and to the preoperative clinical condition of the patient. Operative risk is obviously increased in intubated, acidotic, and hypotensive patients with pulmonary venous obstruction, whereas operative risk is less than 5% in more stable patients. After discharge from the hospital, infants should be monitored for the first year to determine whether late obstruction of the pulmonary venous anastomosis occurs. This serious complication has been reported with a frequency near 10% in all series. Reoperation is indicated when late pulmonary venous obstruction is found and produces mixed results.

In patients who survive the first year of life, the late mortality rate is low. Long-term functional results are excellent.

## SELECTED BIBLIOGRAPHY

Anderson, R. H., Zuberbuhler, J. R., Penkoske, P. A., et al.: Of clefts, commissures, and things. J. Thorac. Cardiovasc. Surg., 90:605, 1985.

Penkoske, P. A., Neches, W. H., Penkoske, P. A., et al.: Further observations on the morphology of atrioventricular septal defects. J. Thorac. Cardiovasc. Surg., 90:611, 1985.

These two papers, published in a series, describe the anatomic findings in 130 hearts with AV septal defects, 50 hearts with ventricular septal defects, 7 hearts with isolated clefts, and 10 normal hearts. All specimens came from the cardiopathologic collection of the Children's Hospital of Pittsburgh.

The studies clearly show that the morphology of hearts with AV septal defects, partial or complete, is different from that of other hearts. The left AV valve is a three-leaflet valve that in no way resembles the normal mitral valve, differing in terms of its chordal support and its papillary muscle.

For more than two decades, it has been debated whether the "cleft" in an ostium primum ("partial atrioventricular canal") defect should be sutured if there were no signs of mitral insufficiency. This reasoning was based on the anatomic fact that the cleft was actually a commissure and was not a true abnormality envisioned as an abnormal separation of the aortic leaflet of the normal mitral valve. Undoubtedly, in some patients without mitral insufficiency, repair has been satisfactory without placing any sutures in the cleft. Nevertheless, most surgeons, including those at New York University, routinely suture the cleft regardless and take care not to distort the valvular anatomy. This is important, because fibrosis and contraction or redundancy around an unsutured cleft has caused recurrent insufficiency and a second operation.

Castaneda, A. R., Mayer, J. E., Jr., and Jonas, R. A.: Repair of complete atrioventricular canal in infancy. World J. Surg., 9:590, 1985.

These data are from the Children's Hospital in Boston. Primary repair of complete AV canal in infancy is strongly recommended to prevent pulmonary venous obstruction. Experiences with 48 patients treated for 5 years are presented (three early deaths and two late deaths). Three patients required reoperation for residual regurgitation; of 20 recatheterized patients, mitral regurgitation was severe in two patients.

King, R. M., Puga, F. J., Danielson, G. K., et al.: Prognostic factors and surgical treatment of partial atrioventricular canal. Circulation, 74(Suppl. I):I–42, 1986.

King and associates describe experiences at the Mayo Clinic with the surgical treatment of 199 patients with partial AV canal treated for 23 years. The 30-day operative mortality rate was almost 5%, less than 3% in the most recent 5 years. The average follow-up was 15 years, making this a valuable source of long-term data. The late survival rate was 91% at 1 year, 96% at 20 years. Reoperation was performed on 18 patients, 15 for mitral insufficiency. No cases of complete heart block have occurred since 1975.

This report is particularly significant because many useful techniques for closure of partial and complete AV canal defects were developed at the Mayo Clinic, especially by McGoon and Kirklin. The authors emphasize that their current practice is to close the cleft in the anterior mitral leaflet regardless of the degree of preoperative valvular insufficiency.

Two patients have been treated in whom insufficiency developed months or years after the initial operation in which the cleft was not sutured. For both patients, a second operation to close the cleft successfully eliminated the regurgitation. Similar experiences have been observed at New York University.

Murphy, J. G., Gersh, B. J., McGoon, M. D., et al.: Long-term outcome after surgical repair of isolated atrial septal defect. Follow-up at 27 to 32 years. N. Engl. J. Med., 323(24):1645, 1990.

These data from the Mayo Clinic report long-term survival rates from surgically treated patients with atrial septal defects. The overall actuarial 30-year survival rate for operative survivors was 74%, as compared with 85% for age- and sex-matched control subjects. Actuarial 27-year survival rates for patients repaired before 11 years of age and between ages 12 and 24 years were 97 and 93%, respectively—not significantly different than survival in the control population. In patients repaired between ages 25 and 41 years and after 41 years of age, the 27-year survival rates were 84 and 40%, respectively, significantly worse than the control population ($p < .001$). Age ($p < .001$) and systolic pulmonary artery pressure ($p < .0027$) were independent predictors of long-term survival by multivariate analysis. Atrial fibrillation, stroke, and cardiac failure were more common in older patients. These data support early operative repair for patients with atrial septal defect, demonstrating survival equal to the control population when repair is performed before 25 years of age.

Pillai, R., Ho, S. Y., Anderson, R. H., and Lincoln, C.: Ostium primum atrioventricular septal defect: An anatomical and surgical review. Ann. Thorac. Surg., 41:458, 1986.

Pillai and colleagues describe a 10-year period of treatment of 84 patients with the ostium primum type of defect at the Brompton Hospital in London. The patch used to close the atrial septal defect is inserted to avoid the AV node and is placed to divert the coronary sinus into the left atrium. The approach taken to the "cleft" mitral valve was selective. In most patients, the cleft was completely sutured. In 11 patients, however, no sutures were inserted because preoperative insufficiency was completely absent.

## BIBLIOGRAPHY

Anderson, R. H., Zuberbuhler, J. R., Penkoske, P. A., et al.: Of clefts, commissures, and things. J. Thorac. Cardiovasc. Surg., 90:605, 1985.

Barratt-Boyes, B. G.: Primary definitive intracardiac operations in infants: Total anomalous pulmonary venous connection. In Kirklin, J. W., (ed): Advances in Cardiovascular Surgery. New York, Grune & Stratton, 1973, p. 127.

Blake, H. A., Hall, R. C., and Manion, W. C.: Anomalous pulmonary venous return. Circulation, 32:406, 1965.

Braunwald, N. S., and Morrow, A. G.: Incomplete persistent atrioventricular canal. J. Thorac. Cardiovasc. Surg., 51:71, 1966.

Campbell, M.: Natural history of atrial septal defect. Br. Heart J., 32:820, 1970.

Castaneda, A. R., Mayer, J. E., Jr., and Jonas, R. A.: Repair of complete atrioventricular canal in infancy. World J. Surg., 9:590, 1985.

Ceithaml, E. L., Midgley, F. M., and Perry, L. W.: Long-term results after surgical repair of incomplete endocardial cushion defects. Ann. Thorac. Surg., 48(3):413, 1989.

Craig, R. J., and Selzer, A.: Natural history and prognosis of atrial septal defect. Circulation, 37:805, 1968.

Darling, R. C., Rothney, W. B., and Craig, J. M.: Total pulmonary venous drainage into the right side of the heart: Report of 17 autopsied cases not associated with other major cardiovascular anomalies. Lab. Invest., 6:44, 1957.

Fiore, A. C., Naunheim, K. S., Kessler, K. A., et al.: Surgical closure of atrial septal defect in patients older than 50 years of age. Arch. Surg., 123:965, 1988.

Galloway, A. C., Campbell, D. N., and Clarke, D. R.: The value of early repair for total anomalous pulmonary venous drainage. Pediatr. Cardiol., 6:77, 1985.

Gibbon, J. H., Jr.: Application of a mechanical heart and lung apparatus to cardiac surgery. Minnesota Med., 37:171, 1954.

Hawe, A., Rastelli, G. C., Brandenburg, R. O., and McGoon, D. C.: Embolic complications following repair of atrial septal defects. Circulation, 39(Suppl. I):I–85, 1969.

King, R. M., Puga, F. J., Danielson, G. K., et al.: Prognostic factors and surgical treatment of partial atrioventricular canal. Circulation, 74(Suppl. I):I–42, 1986.

Kirklin, J. W., and Barratt-Boyes, B. G.: Cardiac Surgery. New York, Churchill Livingstone, 1993.

Lewis, F. J., and Taufic, M.: Closure of atrial septal defects with the aid of hypothermia: Experimental accomplishments and the report of the one successful case. Surgery, 33:52, 1953.

Lincoln, C. R., Rigby, M. L., Mercanti, C., et al.: Surgical risk factors in total anomalous pulmonary venous connection. Am. J. Cardiol., 61:608, 1988.

McMullan, M. H., McGoon, D. C., Wallace, R. B., et al.: Surgical treatment of partial atrioventricular canal. Arch. Surg., 107:705, 1973.

McMullan, M. H., Wallace, R. B., Weidman, W. H., and McGoon, D. C.: Surgical treatment of complete atrioventricular canal. Surgery, 6:905, 1972.

Murphy, J. G., Gersh, B. J., McGoon, M. D., et al.: Long-term outcome after surgical repair of isolated atrial septal defect. Follow-up at 27 to 32 years. N. Engl. J. Med., 323(24):1645, 1990.

Neill, C. A.: Postoperative hemolytic anemia in endocardial cushion defects. Circulation, 30:801, 1964.

Penkoske, P. A., Neches, W. H., Anderson, R. H., et al.: Further observations on the morphology of atrioventricular septal defects. J. Thorac. Cardiovasc. Surg., 90:611, 1985.

Pillai, R., Ho, S. Y., Anderson, R. H., and Lincoln, C.: Ostium primum atrioventricular septal defect: An anatomical and surgical review. Ann. Thorac. Surg., *41*:458, 1986.

Portman, M. A., Beder, S. D., Ankeney, J. L., et al.: A 20-year review of ostium primum defect repair in children. Am. Heart J., *110*:1064, 1985.

Rastelli, G. C., Kirklin, J. W., and Titus, J. L.: Anatomic observations on complete form of persistent common atrioventricular canal with special reference to atrioventricular valves. Mayo Clin. Proc., *41*:296, 1966.

Rastelli, G. C., Weidman, W. H., and Kirklin, J. W.: Surgical repair of the partial form of persistent common atrioventricular canal, with special reference to mitral valve incompetence. Circulation, *31*:31, 1965.

Rastelli, G. C., Rahimtoola, S. H., Ongley, P. A., and McGoon, D. C.: Common atrium: Anatomy, hemodynamics, and surgery. J. Thorac. Cardiovasc. Surg., 55:834, 1968.

Reybrouck, T., Bisschop, A., and van der Hauwaert, L. G.: Cardio-respiratory exercise capacity after surgical closure of atrial septal defect is influenced by the age at surgery. Am. Heart J., *122*:1073, 1991.

Rudolph, A. M.: Congenital Diseases of the Heart. Chicago, Year Book, 1974, p. 259.

Sellers, R. D., Ferlic, R. M., Sterns, L. P., and Lillehei, C. W.: Secundum type atrial septal defects: Results with 275 patients. Surgery, 59:155, 1966.

Spencer, F. C., and Bahnson, H. T.: Intracardiac surgery employing hypothermia and coronary perfusion performed on 100 patients. Surgery, *46*:987, 1959.

Steele, P. M., Fuster, V., Cohen, M., et al.: Isolated atrial septal defect with pulmonary vascular obstructive disease—Long-term follow-up and prediction of outcome after surgical correction. Circulation, *76*:1037, 1987.

Stewart, S., Alexson, C., and Manning, J.: Partial atrioventricular canal defect: The early and late results of operation. Ann. Thorac. Surg., *43*:527, 1987.

Turley, K., Tucker, W. Y., Uhyot, D. J., and Ebert, P. A.: Total anomalous pulmonary venous connection in infancy: Influence of age and type of lesion. Am. J. Cardiol., *45*:92, 1980a.

Turley, K., Wilson, J. M., and Ebert, P. A.: Atrial repairs of infant complex congenital heart lesions: Emphasis on the first three months of life. Arch. Surg., *115*:1335, 1980b.

Van Praagh, R., Harken, A. H., Delisle, G., et al.: Total anomalous pulmonary venous drainage to the coronary sinus: A revised procedure for its correction. J. Thorac. Cardiovasc. Surg., *64*:132, 1972.

# 36

# Major Anomalies of Pulmonary and Thoracic Systemic Veins

John W. Hammon, Jr., and Harvey W. Bender, Jr.

Major anomalies of pulmonary and systemic venous return constitute one of the few forms of congenital heart disease in which the valves and ventricles are usually normal; thus, correction should offer excellent long-term results. Patients with *total anomalous pulmonary venous connection* (TAPVC) rarely survive beyond the first year of life without operative correction, and patients with anomalous systemic venous connections often become symptomatic in infancy and childhood. Operative correction of these conditions usually is successful, and knowledge of this relatively uncommon but important group of congenital anomalies is essential to ensure prompt, accurate diagnosis and therapy. Partial anomalous pulmonary venous connections are considered in Chapter 35.

## EMBRYOLOGY

### Pulmonary Venous System

At approximately 3½ weeks' gestation, the lung bud arises from the primitive foregut and becomes surrounded by a plexus of veins that has been called the pulmonary venous plexus (Los, 1968) (Fig. 36–1A). As differentiation proceeds, this venous system has no direct communication with the heart, but instead shares the routes of drainage of the splanchnic plexus—that is, the cardinal and umbilicovitelline systems of veins (Fig. 36–1B). Normally, this pulmonary venous plexus eventually is connected to the common pulmonary vein (Neill, 1956), a transient structure that arises from the undivided sinus venosus just to the left of the area in which the atrial septal primum develops (Fig. 36–1C). Eventually, connections to the systemic venous system terminate, and the common pulmonary vein is incorporated into the developing left atrium (Fig. 36–1D). Abnormal development of the common pulmonary vein is the embryologic basis for most of the congenital anomalies of the pulmonary veins (Lucas et al., 1962).

If atresia of the common pulmonary vein occurs when systemic communications to the cardinal and umbilicovitelline systems are present, one or several of these collateral channels can enlarge and provide total anomalous pulmonary venous connection to the systemic venous system (Fig. 36–2). If only the right or left portion of the common pulmonary vein is atretic, partial anomalous venous connection occurs.

Persisting segments of the cardinal veins eventually form the superior vena cava, the innominate vein, the coronary sinus, and the azygos vein. The umbilicovitelline system forms the inferior vena cava, the portal vein, and the ductus venosus. The anatomy of the anomalous venous connection is based on the early embryologic connection between the pulmonary venous plexus and the particular splanchnic component that persists. Direct anomalous connections to the right atrium are not explained by such an embryologic accident and are probably due to an abnormality of septation of the two atria, in which the atrial septum forms to the left of the pulmonary veins rather than to the right (Shaner, 1961). Figure 36–3 shows the systemic venous anatomy and the different systemic veins that can become the site of drainage of pulmonary venous blood in patients with TAPVC.

When stenosis of the common pulmonary vein occurs, the result is cor triatriatum (Edwards, 1960). Usually, stenosis occurs late, after systemic venous connections have terminated (Fig. 36–4). Occasionally, cor triatriatum is associated with anomalous pulmonary venous connections to systemic veins, which suggests that significant stenosis of the common pulmonary vein is present while systemic venous connections are still present.

### Systemic Venous System

The first veins to appear in the embryo are the umbilical and vitelline veins (Fig. 36–5A). The cardinal veins are the next to develop (Streeter, 1942). The anterior and posterior cardinal veins unite on each side to form a common cardinal vein. Eventually, the common cardinal, umbilical, and vitelline veins join the right and left horns of the sinus venosus (Fig. 33–5B). By the fourth week of fetal life, the sinus venosus has developed an invagination that separates its left horn from the left atrium and ultimately in which all systemic blood enters the right atrium (Raghib et al., 1965) (Fig. 36–5C).

At this stage, the cardinal systemic veins are symmetric, except for their drainage into the right atrium. During the eighth week of fetal life, the left innominate vein develops and connects the two anterior cardinal veins. As flow through the left innominate vein increases, the left anterior cardinal vein shrinks, so that by the sixth fetal month it has been obliterated and the left common cardinal vein remains to drain

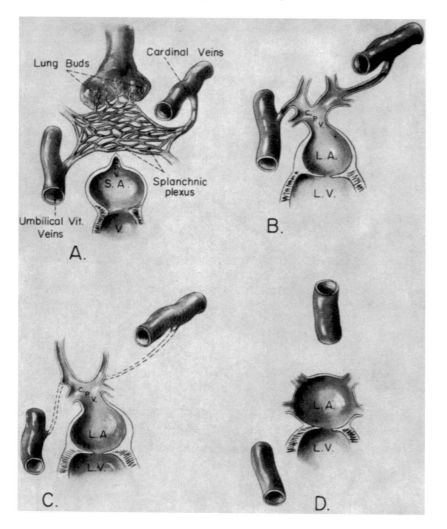

**FIGURE 36–1.** Normal development of the pulmonary venous system. *A,* The splanchnic plexus drains the lung buds and shares connections with the cardinal and umbilicovitelline systems. (S.A. = sinoatrial.) *B,* The common pulmonary vein (C.P.V.) has evaginated from the left atrium (L.A.) and has joined the splanchnic plexus. (L.V. = left ventricle.) *C,* As pulmonary venous blood drains to the left side of the heart, the primitive connections disappear. *D,* Finally, by differential growth, the individual pulmonary veins are incorporated into the left atrium, and the common pulmonary vein disappears. (*A–D,* From Lucas, R. V., Anderson, R. C., Amplatz, K., et al.: Congenital causes of pulmonary venous obstruction. Pediatr. Clin. North Am., *10*:781, 1963.)

only the coronary circulation to the right atrium as the coronary sinus (see Fig. 36–5C). Occasionally, a small portion of the left anterior cardinal vein persists as the oblique ligament or vein of Marshall of the left atrium (Lucas and Schmidt, 1977).

Important abnormalities of the cardinal venous system result from two developmental aberrations: First, failure of obliteration of the left anterior cardinal vein results in persistence of the left superior vena cava. If invagination between the left horn of the sinus venosus has occurred, a coronary sinus is formed, which serves as an outlet for the left superior vena cava. Second, failure of invagination between the left sinus horn and the left atrium and failure of obliteration of the left anterior cardinal vein cause the left superior vena cava to drain directly into the left atrium.

The venous return of the caudal portion of the body drains via the posterior cardinal veins until the sixth week of fetal life. The inferior vena cava develops in the next two weeks (McClure and Butler, 1925).

Development of the inferior vena cava depends on the formation of two centrally located systems. The subcardinal system develops ventral and medial to the posterior cardinal veins. The supracardinal system forms dorsal and medial to the posterior cardinal

veins, and anastomoses develop between the cardinal veins and both systems. The cardinal system atrophies, and no cardinal remnants persist between the iliac veins and the diaphragm. Anastomoses develop between the right and left supracardinal and subcardinal systems. Flow is preferentially directed to the right system, and the left system atrophies; the left supracardinal vein becomes the hemiazygos vein, which joins the right supracardinal (azygos) vein. The right subcardinal vein and hepatic veins join and form the inferior vena cava, which joins the right atrium at the junction of the right common cardinal vein and the atrium.

If the right subcardinal vein and the hepatic vein do not connect, the venous blood from the lower half of the body is directed into the left subcardinal system and produces the common anomaly of interruption of the inferior vena cava with azygos continuation. The normal development of the inferior vena cava and the formation of interrupted inferior vena cava are detailed in Figure 36–6.

Direct connection of the inferior vena cava to the left atrium is not well defined embryologically (Meadows et al., 1961). The more common situation, in which the inferior vena cava drains into the left

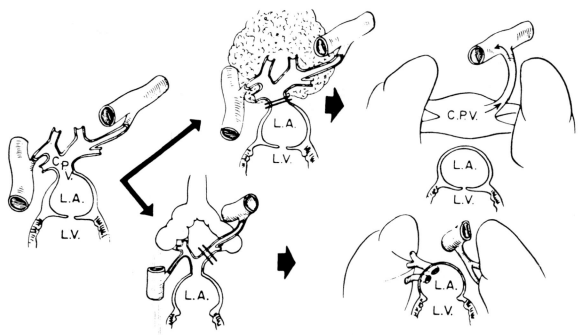

**FIGURE 36–2.** The embryologic explanation for anomalous pulmonary venous connections. *Upper,* If atresia of the common pulmonary vein occurs when systemic connections are still present, total anomalous pulmonary venous connection (TAPVC) results. *Lower,* Atresia of a branch of the common pulmonary veins results in partial anomalous pulmonary venous connection. (C.P.V. = common pulmonary vein; L.A. = left atrium; L.V. = left ventricle.) (Adapted from Lucas, R. V., and Schmidt, R. E.: Anomalous venous connections, pulmonary and systemic. *In* Moss, A. J., Adams, F. H., and Emmanouilides, G. C. [eds]: Heart Disease in Infants, Children and Adolescents. 2nd ed. Copyright 1977, The Williams & Wilkins Company, Baltimore. Reproduced by permission.)

**FIGURE 36–3.** The systemic veins that can be the routes of drainage in TAPVC.

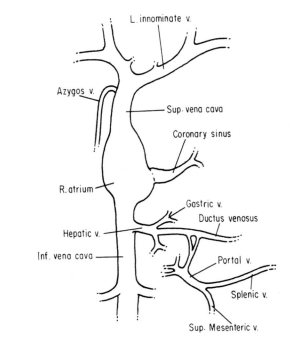

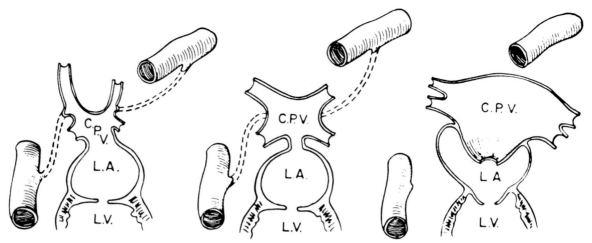

**FIGURE 36–4.** When stenosis of the common pulmonary vein occurs, the result is cor triatriatum. (C.P.V. = common pulmonary vein; L.A. = left atrium; L.V. = left ventricle.) (Adapted from Lucas, R. V., and Schmidt, R. E.: Anomalous venous connections, pulmonary and systemic. *In* Moss, A. J., Adams, F. H., and Emmanouilides, G. C. [eds]: Heart Disease in Infants, Children and Adolescents. 2nd ed. Copyright 1977, The Williams & Wilkins Company, Baltimore. Reproduced by permission.)

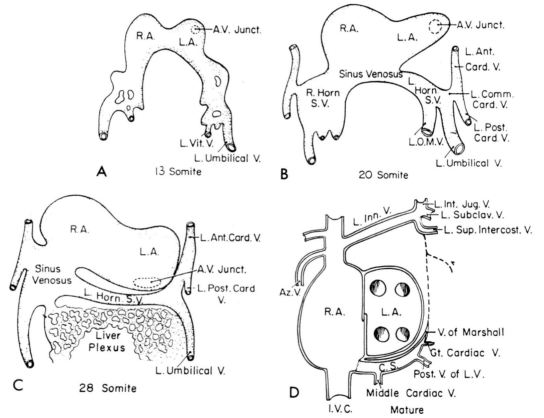

**FIGURE 36–5.** Normal embryology of the cardinal venous system. *A,* Bilaterally symmetric umbilical and vitelline veins drain into the common atrium. Asymmetry begins with the atrioventricular junction (A. V. Junct.) to the left. *B,* The cardinal system develops with continuing asymmetric development of the atrium. *C,* The left (L. Horn S. V.) and right (R. Horn S. V.) horns of the sinus venosus are completely separated, and all systemic blood drains to the right atrium (R. A.). *D,* The left innominate vein (L. Inn. V.) develops, and the left anterior cardinal vein (L. Ant. Card. V.) disappears. The left common cardinal vein (L. Comm. Card. V.) becomes the coronary sinus (C.S.). (L. Post. Card. V. = left posterior cardinal vein; L. Umbilical V. = left umbilical vein; L.A. = left atrium; L. Int. Jug. V. = left internal jugular vein; L. Subclav. V. = left subclavian vein; L. Sup. Intercost. V. = left superior intercostal vein; V. of Marshall = vein of Marshall; Gt. Cardiac V. = great cardiac vein; Post. V. of L.V. = posterior vein of the left ventricle; Middle Cardiac V. = middle cardiac vein; I.V.C. = inferior vena cava; Az. V. = azygos vein; L. Vit. V. = left vitelline vein; L.O.M.V. = left omphalomesenteric vein.) (*A–D,* Adapted from Lucas, R. V., and Schmidt, R. E.: Anomalous venous connections, pulmonary and systemic. *In* Moss, A. J., Adams, F. H., and Emmanouilides, G. C. [eds]: Heart Disease in Infants, Children and Adolescents. 2nd ed. Copyright 1977, The Williams & Wilkins Company, Baltimore. Reproduced by permission.)

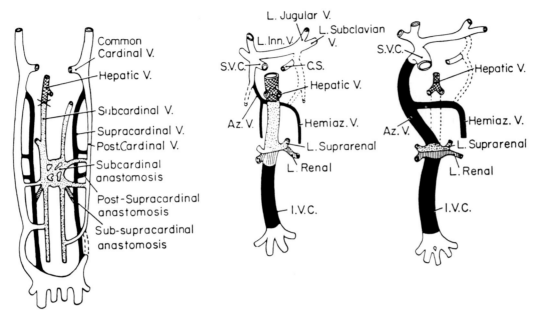

**FIGURE 36–6.** Embryology of the inferior vena cava (I.V.C.). *Left,* In early stages of development, blood can reach the heart by way of the posterior cardinal veins (Post. Cardinal V.), supracardinal veins, and the upper portion of the I.V.C. Multiple anastomotic sites exist in the renal area, as shown. *Center,* Normal development of the I.V.C. The I.V.C. is derived, from below upward, from the posterior cardinal system *(white),* the supracardinal system *(black),* the renal veins *(lined),* the subcardinal system *(strippled),* and the hepatic veins *(cross-hatched).* The supracardinal veins persist as the hemiazygos and azygos veins. *Right,* Interruption of the I.V.C. with azygos continuation. Absence of the I.V.C. above the renal veins occurs when the right subcardinal vein fails to join the hepatic vein. The hepatic veins drain directly into the right atrium. All other blood from the lower body drains via the dilated azygos and hemiazygos systems. (Adapted from Lucas, R. V., and Schmidt, R. E.: Anomalous venous connections, pulmonary and systemic. *In* Moss, A. J., Adams, F. H., and Emmanouilides, G. C. [eds]: Heart Disease in Infants, Children and Adolescents. 2nd ed. Copyright 1977, The Williams & Wilkins Company, Baltimore. Reproduced by permission.)

atrium via an atrial septal defect, can be explained embryologically by persistence and overgrowth of the valves of the sinus venosus that usually form the eustachian and thebesian valves. Rarely, the right valve persists as a membrane that directs all systemic venous blood to the left atrium (Doucette and Knoblich, 1963).

## TOTAL ANOMALOUS PULMONARY VENOUS CONNECTION

The term TAPVC describes the anomaly in which the pulmonary veins have no direct communication with the left atrium. Instead, they connect to the right atrium or to one of the systemic veins.

### Historical Aspects

In 1798, Wilson reported the first known case of TAPVC, a patient whose entire pulmonary venous return entered the coronary sinus. Additional reports were uncommon until 1942, when Brody reviewed the subject with 37 autopsied cases from the literature. In 1957, Darling, Rothney, and Craig added 17 cases and classified the variants of this anomaly. The first clinical diagnosis was made in 1950 by Friedlich and associates, who used cardiac catheterization. In 1951, the first successful operation was reported by Muller,

who provided palliation for the patient by anastomosing the left atrial appendage to anomalous veins from the left lung. In 1956, Lewis and associates reported the first successful open heart correction of the cardiac type of TAPVC in a 5-year-old patient by using hypothermia and inflow occlusion. Cooley and Ochsner (1957) reported the first open heart correction using cardiopulmonary bypass in a patient with a supracardiac anomaly. The first infracardiac anomaly was corrected in 1961 by Sloan, who used deep hypothermia, cardiopulmonary bypass, and a period of circulatory arrest (Sloan et al., 1962).

### Anatomy

The anatomic prerequisite for TAPVC is an absence of connection between any pulmonary veins and the left atrium. The left atrium has no tributaries and receives all blood by an atrial septal defect. The term total anomalous pulmonary venous *connection* describes this anatomic abnormality and should not be confused with total anomalous pulmonary venous *drainage,* in which the pulmonary veins terminate in the left atrium, but blood passes through an interatrial communication into the right atrium because of atresia of the mitral or aortic valves or a combination of both with total left heart atresia. In 1957, Darling and associates divided the anomaly into four subtypes that describe the anatomic connections of the pulmonary venous to the systemic venous circulation.

**Type I—Supracardiac Connection.** The anatomic site of anomalous venous connection in this type aids communications to the remnants of the right or left cardinal venous system. The most common form, in which pulmonary venous drainage is to a common pulmonary vein posterior to the left atrium, is shown in Figure 36–7. A left vertical vein connects this chamber with the innominate vein, and this vessel usually lies anterior to the left pulmonary artery. When the common pulmonary venous chamber connects with remnants of the right cardinal venous system, the connection may be to the superior vena cava or azygos vein or by an additional right vertical vein draining directly into the innominate vein. Occasionally, pulmonary veins separately enter the superior vena cava, azygos, or innominate vein; this type is associated with major cardiac anomalies (Ruttenberg et al., 1964).

**Type II—Cardiac Connection.** Cardiac connections are divided into two major subtypes. In the more common type, the left and right common pulmonary veins join to form a common venous sinus posterior to the left atrium, which then connects to an enlarged coronary sinus in the atrioventricular groove (Fig. 36–8). In the second group, the pulmonary veins drain individually or collectively into a sinus in the posterior right atrium (Fig. 36–9).

**Type III—Infracardiac Connection.** In this group, a common venous chamber posterior to the heart

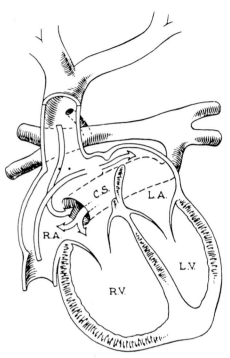

**FIGURE 36–8.** The anatomy and blood flow patterns in TAPVC when the pulmonary venous confluence connects to the coronary sinus (C.S.). (R.A. = right atrium; L.A. = left atrium; R.V. = right ventricle; L.V. = left ventricle.)

connects to an inferior vein that passes through the diaphragm anterior to the esophagus and then to the portal vein or one of its branches or with the ductus venosus (Fig. 36–10). Occasionally, the anomalous descending vein passes through an accessory hiatus in

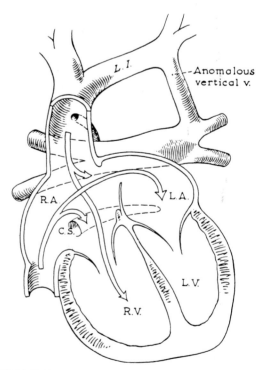

**FIGURE 36–7.** Representation of the most common type of supracardiac TAPVC. (L.I. = left innominate vein; R.A. = right atrium; L.A. = left atrium; C.S. = coronary sinus; R.V. = right ventricle; L.V. = left ventricle.)

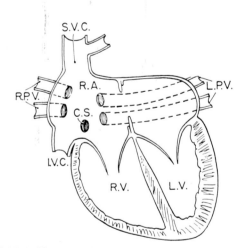

**FIGURE 36–9.** The type of TAPVC in which the pulmonary veins directly connect with the right atrium. (C.S. = coronary sinus; I.V.C. = inferior vena cava; L.P.V. = left pulmonary vein; L.V. = left ventricle; R.A. = right atrium; R.P.V. = right pulmonary vein; R.V. = right ventricle; S.V.C. = superior vena cava.) (Redrawn from Lucas, R. C., and Schmidt, R. E.: Anomalous venous connections, pulmonary and systemic. *In* Moss, A. J., Adams, F. H., and Emmanouilides, G. C. [eds]: Heart Disease in Infants, Children and Adolescents. 2nd ed. Copyright 1977, The Williams & Wilkins Company, Baltimore. Reproduced by permission.)

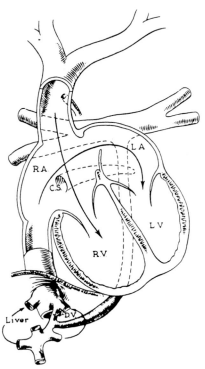

FIGURE 36–10. The most common type of infracardiac TAPVC in which the anomalous descending vein connects the pulmonary venous confluence with the ductus venosus (D.V.).

the diaphragm and joins one of the systemic venous channels, usually the inferior vena cava or one of its branches.

**Type IV—Mixed Connection.** In this uncommon group, the pulmonary venous connections are divided so that one lung drains to one of the systemic veins, and pulmonary veins from the opposite side usually join one of the cardiac chambers, generally the coronary sinus.

## Associated Cardiac Defects

An interatrial communication is required for life to persist beyond the early neonatal period in patients with TAPVC and is present in nearly all cases. The communication varies from a probe–patent foramen ovale to complete absence of the interatrial septum. *Patent ductus arteriosus* (PDA) is present in 25 to 50% of patients with this defect (Burroughs and Edwards, 1960). Infants with pulmonary venous obstruction have a high incidence of PDA, which is the physiologic means of decompressing obstructed pulmonary blood flow into the descending thoracic aorta. A very high incidence of TAPVC and severe congenital cardiac defects is associated with the asplenia syndrome (Ivemark, 1955).

## Incidence

Approximately 1% of infants born with congenital heart disease have TAPVC (Jensen and Blount, 1971).

There is no known genetic predisposition to this lesion. Male infants are affected almost twice as often as female infants. The incidences of the various anatomic types of TAPVC are shown in Table 36–1. These data are taken from several collected series in the literature. The earlier series represent autopsy reports, and the later series are surgical. Supracardiac defects are the most common and affect 50% of patients. The most common supracardiac anomaly is the connection of the pulmonary venous chamber to a left anomalous vertical vein draining to the innominate vein. Type II defects are the second most common anomaly, with pulmonary venous connection to the coronary sinus most prevalent in this group.

Type III and IV defects are the least common, and Type III defects are reported more frequently in surgical series, because these infants survive to diagnosis and treatment. Patients with Type IV anomaly are not common in surgical series because most have major intracardiac defects that preclude correction.

## Pathophysiology

The factors that influence the pathophysiology of TAPVC include obligatory mixing of pulmonary and systemic blood upstream of or at the right atrium, obstruction of the anomalous connection, the size of the atrial septal defect, and associated anomalies. The presence or absence of obstruction of the anomalous connection is the most significant factor in the patient's clinical condition.

Unlike that in atrial septal defects, the mixing of systemic and pulmonary venous blood in TAPVC is obligatory and is not influenced by the compliance of the two ventricles and the end-diastolic pressure in both chambers. In theory, the oxygen saturation should be equal in all four cardiac chambers. The oxygen saturation may not be equal in patients with small atrial septal defects in which streaming of blood occurs, with most of the inferior vena caval blood directed through the patent foramen ovale or small atrial septal defect and with superior vena caval blood entering the right ventricle through the triscupid valve. If the interatrial communication is large and the anomalous connection is not obstructed, flow to the left atrium is adequate, and oxygen saturation will be similar in both the right and left heart chambers. In this condition, blood flow through the lungs is high, and systemic oxygen saturation is only slightly decreased.

In the patient with unobstructed TAPVC, the entire cardiac output is presented to the right ventricle, which accepts its maximal end-diastolic volume from the beginning of life. As the patient grows and exercises vigorously, cyanosis increases only when the pulmonary vascular resistance rises and a high pulmonary/systemic flow ratio cannot be maintained. Not all of these patients develop hyperkinetic pulmonary hypertension, but the incidence of this complication is higher in patients with TAPVC than in other high-flow, low-pressure lesions such as atrial septal

■ **Table 36–1.** COLLECTED CASES OF TAPVC CLASSIFIED BY TYPE

| Types | Burroughs and Edwards (1960) | Bonham-Carter et al. (1969) | Jensen and Blount (1971) | Snellen and Bruins (1968) | Cooley et al. (1966) | Gathman and Nadas (1971) | Breckenridge et al. (1973) | Applebaum et al. (1975) | Turley et al. (1980) | Hammon et al. (1980) | Total | Incidence (%) |
|---|---|---|---|---|---|---|---|---|---|---|---|---|
| **I** *Supracardiac* | | | | | | | | | | | | |
|   Left anomalous vertical vein | 56 | 34 | 12 | 12 | 28 | 26 | 11 | 21 | | | | |
|   Right superior vena cava | 31 | 9 | 2 | 1 | 7 | 8 | 3 | 2 | 9 | 12 | 284 | 51 |
| **II** *Cardiac* | | | | | | | | | | | | |
|   Coronary sinus | 18 | 18 | 5 | 11 | 12 | 14 | 2 | 3 | 6 | 6 | | |
|   Right atrium | 30 | 3 | 6 | 7 | 8 | 3 | 1 | 3 | | | 156 | 28 |
| **III** *Infracardiac* | 28 | 8 | 2 | 4 | 3 | 16 | 3 | 4 | 6 | 5 | 79 | 14 |
| **IV** *Mixed* | 16 | 3 | 0 | 3 | 4 | 8 | 1 | 2 | 1 | 2 | 40 | 7 |
| Totals | 179 | 75 | 27 | 38 | 62 | 75 | 21 | 35 | 22 | 25 | 559 | 100 |

defect (Gathman and Nadas, 1970; Newfield et al., 1980). Heart failure is more common in patients with hyperkinetic pulmonary hypertension but is not uncommon in patients with low pulmonary artery pressure and large left-to-right shunts.

The interatrial communication in patients with TAPVC is usually large, but in very few patients this communication is small and obstructs flow to the left ventricle. In these patients, a gradient of 3 mm Hg or more between the right and left atrium can indicate an obstructing atrial septal defect (Behrendt et al., 1972). The flow to the left side of the heart and thus the cardiac output is improved after a balloon atrial septostomy (Miller and Rashkind, 1968).

Anatomic obstruction of the anomalous connection is common in infants and can occur at several sites (Burroughs and Edwards, 1960). In patients with Type I anomalies, the left vertical vein can be constricted as it passes through the pericardial reflection or, rarely, between the left pulmonary artery and left mainstem bronchus. In Type III lesions, obstruction most commonly occurs when the venous duct closes if the connection attaches at this level. If the anomalous inferior vein communicates with the portal vein, obstruction is a prerequisite, because pulmonary venous blood must pass through the liver capillary bed before returning to the right side of the heart. Occasionally, anatomic obstruction occurs in infracardiac connections in which the vertical vein passes through the diaphragm and is constricted during tidal ventilation. In Type IV connections, obstruction usually occurs because the sites of communication between the pulmonary veins and the right side of the heart are inadequate. Type II connections are rarely obstructed and increase chances of long-term survival.

The pathophysiologic consequences of an obstructed anomalous pulmonary venous connection are pulmonary edema and poor myocardial function. During the first few hours or days of extrauterine life, pulmonary blood flow increases. Pulmonary venous obstruction then causes elevation of pulmonary capillary hydrostatic pressure. When this pressure exceeds the net forces that retain fluid in the vascular space, interstitial pulmonary edema occurs. A vicious cycle ensues; interstitial edema causes decreased pulmonary compliance and increases the work of breathing.

Ventilation and perfusion are not balanced, and arterial oxygen desaturation further compromises the heart's ability to meet the body's oxygen demand. The result is alveolar flooding and perivascular hemorrhage, which ends in frank pulmonary collapse.

The combination of tachycardia, low coronary perfusion pressure, and cyanosis predisposes the myocardium to subendocardial ischemia. This is especially true in the right ventricle, which in this condition encounters an excessive afterload and in most cases has elevated end-diastolic pressure, which further increases oxygen demand and decreases subendocardial coronary blood flow. The low cardiac output that results promotes anaerobic metabolism, which creates a metabolic acidosis with an increase in plasma lactate. Because of these related events, infants with obstructed TAPVC rarely survive the first few weeks of life.

Infants born with obstructed connections often retain ductal patency, which decompresses the pulmonary artery and helps to unload the right ventricle. With ductal closure, severe right-sided heart failure and pulmonary and cardiovascular collapse can occur.

## Diagnosis

**Clinical Manifestations.** The severity of the clinical manifestations of TAPVC are directly related to the presence of obstruction of the anomalous connection. With an obstructed connection, the infant usually becomes symptomatic in the first hours or days after birth. Mild to moderate cyanosis is evident, and the respiratory rate is rapid, with evidence of decreased pulmonary compliance: intercostal retractions, nasal flaring, and sweating. Cardiac output usually is low, shown by decreased pulses and in some cases acidosis. In most of these infants, the obstruction accompanies infradiaphragmatic connections, but it can be seen with supracardiac or mixed connections. It is uncommon for these infants to present after 3 to 6 months of age, because most have expired from complications of pulmonary congestion and low cardiac output.

Children with partially obstructed connections or

hyperkinetic pulmonary hypertension usually present in the first 1 to 2 years of life. These infants have all the hallmarks of pulmonary hypertension and right ventricular dysfunction, with dyspnea on exertion, poor feeding, lack of weight gain, and cyanosis on crying or exercise. A history of frequent respiratory infections is often evident. On physical examination, the right ventricular impulse is prominent, and a left parasternal flow murmur is usually audible. The second heart sound is widely split and fixed and has a loud pulmonary component. Occasionally, there is a continuous murmur in the vicinity of the anomalous vertical vein.

Approximately 10 to 20% of infants with TAPVC have no component of obstruction and do not develop pulmonary hypertension. These children can survive into adulthood, although with some restriction. These patients usually have Type I or II anomalous connections. Except for slight cyanosis, symptoms and signs are similar to those in patients with ostium secundum atrial septal defects, but they usually develop sooner. Dyspnea on exertion and fatigue at the end of the day with inability to keep up with their peers are the hallmark symptoms of these patients. Cyanosis is usually slight and is not visible to the untrained eye. Respiratory infections may be more common than normal. The diagnosis in unobstructed connections may be delayed until the child is seen for a preschool examination. On physical examination, the right ventricle is prominent and hyperactive. The second cardiac sound is split and fixed, but the pulmonary component is not loud. The parasternal systolic flow murmur is present and is similar to that in patients with atrial septal defects.

**Chest Film.** In infants with obstructed TAPVC, the heart is often not enlarged or only mildly enlarged. Normally, after a day or two, the typical appearance of pulmonary venous congestion is seen on the plain chest film (Fig. 36–11). A fine reticular pattern with haziness of the entire area of the lung is the hallmark of the diagnosis, and should be considered pathognomonic of the condition when seen in the very sick infant. In patients with partially obstructed connections or hyperkinetic pulmonary hypertension, the plain chest film shows increased pulmonary vascularity with cardiomegaly due to enlargement of the right atrium and ventricle. In some older children, the mediastinal component of the anomalous connection, the dilated left vertical vein, or coronary sinus may be seen on the chest film and can be used to diagnose the condition (Fig. 36–12). In patients with no pulmonary hypertension, the chest films show an increase in pulmonary vascularity and can show some right atrial and ventricular enlargement. Occasionally, pathognomonic mediastinal silhouettes can be recognized.

**Electrocardiogram.** The electrocardiogram is least helpful in diagnosing TAPVC. Generally, all infants and children with TAPVC have deviation of the right axis and other electrocardiographic changes that indicate right ventricular hypertrophy. If the condition persists beyond 1 to 2 months, the signs of right atrial

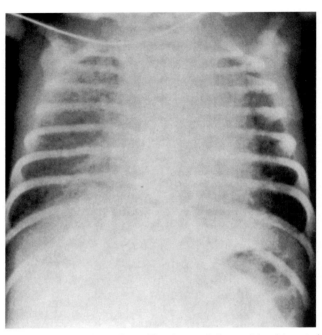

FIGURE 36–11. Plain chest film in an infant with obstructed TAPVC. Note the fine, reticular pulmonary markings and lack of cardiomegaly.

enlargement are present, and the condition persists for some years, first-degree heart block may be evident, with prolongation of the PR interval.

**Echocardiogram.** Echocardiographic signs of right ventricular diastolic volume overload predominate in TAPVC. These are increased right ventricular dimension index and paradoxic ventricular septal movement. An echo-free space posterior to the left atrium

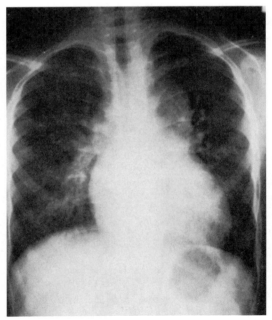

FIGURE 36–12. Typical chest film in an older child with nonobstructed supracardiac TAPVC. The prominent left upper mediastinal silhouette represents the dilated anomalous left vertical vein.

represents the pulmonary venous confluence and is a reliable sign (Paquet and Gutgesell, 1975). Improvements in echocardiographic equipment have enabled physicians to evaluate infants and children with TAPVC more precisely (Fig. 36–13). In a 1991 series, the preoperative diagnosis, including the type of connection, was made in over 90% of patients (Van Der Velde et al., 1991). Thus, it is often possible to avoid preoperative cardiac catheterization in most infants with TAPVC, which has substantial benefits, especially if pulmonary venous return is obstructed.

**Cardiac Catheterization.** Cardiac catheterization is necessary as soon as the diagnosis of TAPVC is considered in an infant. In infants with obstructed connections, oxygen determinations may not be as helpful as anticipated because of the severe degree of pulmonary vascular obstruction and the degree of shunting, which may not be excessive. Severe pulmonary hypertension is present, usually with a right-to-left ductal shunt. Right ventricular cineangiocardiography may show such a large right-to-left ductal shunt that sluggish and insufficient pulmonary blood flow does not allow visualization of the pulmonary veins and their drainage. Visualization may be possible only with injection of contrast medium into individual pulmonary arteries or occlusion of the ductus arteriosus with a balloon catheter and injection of contrast material through a proximal port or separate catheter (Fig. 36–14). Left ventricular cineangiocardiography usually shows a small to normal-sized ventricle and a left atrium that is generally 50% of normal size (Graham and Bender, 1980).

Cardiac catheterization and cineangiocardiography in patients with TAPVC and only mild obstruction or hyperkinetic pulmonary hypertension show findings similar to those in infants with pulmonary venous obstruction, except that pulmonary blood flow is usually more than twice the systemic flow, and pulmonary capillary wedge pressures and pulmonary vascular resistance are low. Cineangiocardiography

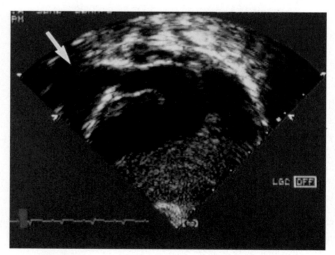

**FIGURE 36–13.** A two-dimensional echocardiogram shows a patient with TAPVC with drainage to the coronary sinus. The *arrow* delineates the pulmonary venous confluence prior to entering the dilated coronary sinus.

shows a greatly dilated right ventricle, and the anomalous connection can be easily seen when contrast material is injected into a pulmonary artery. In Type I connections, it is often possible to delineate the connection by passing the catheter through the innominate vein to the anomalous connection and injecting contrast material at this point.

In patients without pulmonary hypertension, the cardiac catheterization findings are similar to those of atrial septal defect, except that systemic oxygen saturations are slightly lower than normal and the anomalous connection is usually seen without difficulty after injection of contrast material into the pulmonary artery (Fig. 36–15).

## Indications for Operation

More than 80% of infants born with TAPVC die before reaching 1 year of age (Burroughs and Edwards, 1980). The one variable that influences longevity is the presence or absence of significant pulmonary venous obstruction (Gathman and Nadas, 1970). The anomalous pulmonary venous pathway is obstructed in approximately 60 to 75% of infants with TAPVC. Without surgery, it is unusual for these children to survive after 1 year, and most die within 3 months after birth (Gathman and Nadas, 1970). Hyperkinetic pulmonary hypertension develops in a significant number of the remaining 25 to 40% of children with unobstructed TAPVC, and it does so more rapidly than in atrial septal defect (Jensen and Blount, 1971). Approximately 50% of these infants die within their first year, and few survive infancy, despite optimal medical management.

Only 10 to 20% of all patients with TAPVC have no pulmonary hypertension. Although heart failure often develops during infancy, most of these patients survive with proper medical management. The incidence of heart failure or other complications, such as hyperkinetic pulmonary hypertension, becomes obvious over the succeeding years, for very few reach adolescence and young adulthood without symptoms.

Because of the poor survival rate of the patient with TAPVC, the diagnosis is in itself the indication for surgery. In infants with pulmonary venous obstruction, surgery should be prompt because progressive pulmonary insufficiency, low cardiac output, and acidosis are refractory to conventional medical therapy. In infants with hyperkinetic pulmonary hypertension, surgery can be scheduled at a convenient time but soon after cardiac catheterization. Children with unobstructed connections should undergo surgery within the first 5 years of life, and it is reasonable to repair these connections early to prevent damage to the distended right-sided cardiac chambers. In patients with small atrial septal defects and a large pressure gradient between the right and left atrium, balloon atrial septostomy is theoretically effective in increasing cardiac output while the infants are being prepared for surgery. In one series, this procedure

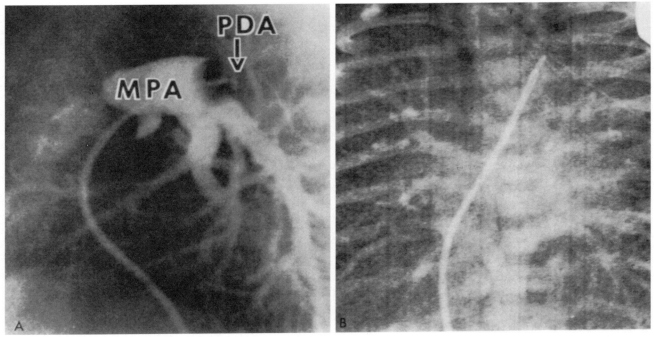

**FIGURE 36–14.** *A,* Cine-angiocardiogram shows occlusion of the ductus arteriosus with a balloon catheter in an infant with infradiaphragmatic TAPVC. (MPA = main pulmonary artery; posterior descending artery.) *B,* Subsequent contrast injection into the pulmonary artery reveals the pulmonary venous confluence and anomalous descending vertical vein.

was not used, and it is rarely necessary (Hammon et al., 1980).

Surgery is contraindicated only when irreversible changes of pulmonary vascular obstruction disease

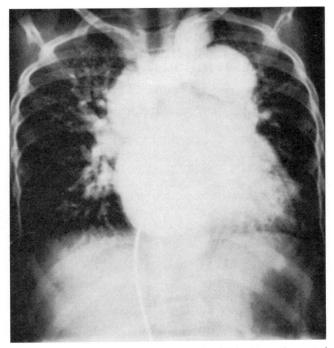

**FIGURE 36–15.** Pulmonary angiogram of a child with unobstructed TAPVC. During the venous phase of the study, the greatly dilated anomalous vertical vein that connects to a similarly large left innominate vein is seen.

have developed. In these patients, intimal hyperplasia and muscular hypertrophy have increased pulmonary vascular resistance to more than 75% of the systemic level. This situation is rare in modern medical practice, and contraindication to operation in TAPVC is unusual.

## Surgical Treatment

Cardiopulmonary bypass is used for all operations involving the correction of TAPVC. The defect is approached best through a median sternotomy, and the type of perfusion support depends on the age of the patient. Children under 1 year of age should undergo either surface-induced hypothermia with cardiopulmonary bypass support (Barratt-Boyes, 1973) or cardiopulmonary bypass with profound hypothermia and low-flow perfusion (Turley et al., 1980). In small infants and children, circulatory arrest or low-flow perfusion helps prevent intraoperative pulmonary venous distention and construct an adequate anastomosis. Cardiopulmonary bypass assists with rapid cooling and rewarming and control of the circulation. Surgical management of infants with profound hypothermia and circulatory arrest has been described (Bender et al., 1979).

Infants are anesthetized with a narcotic-based mixture and cutdowns are done to permit monitoring of arterial and venous pressures. The infants are then transferred to a hypothermia chamber, where surface cooling to 30° C is established. Control of arterial oxygen concentration and acid-base balance is essential during this period, because many infants with obstructive TAPVC have low cardiac output and require buffering to maintain pH at normal levels. Acidosis that develops during the cooling period can predispose to serious arrhythmias, including ventricular fibrillation, and should be avoided at all cost. The infant is then transferred to the operating table, where a standard median sternotomy incision is made. After heparin is administered, the ascending aorta is cannulated, and the right atrium is cannulated through the right atrial appendage. Cardiopulmonary bypass is initiated, and the infant is further cooled to a nasopharyngeal temperature of 18° C. During this time, ventilation is continued, and the ductus is exposed by careful dissection and ligated. At 18° C, the ascending aorta is clamped and the blood drained into the oxygenator. The venous cannula is removed, and the operative repair is made during a period of circulatory arrest. After repair, the venous cannula is reinserted, and the patient's blood volume is re-established. Air is vented from the left ventricular apex and ascending aorta, cardiopulmonary bypass is resumed, and the infant is rewarmed to an esophageal temperature of 35 to 37° C and cardiopulmonary bypass discontinued.

In infants weighing more than 10 kg or children more than 1 year of age, standard cardiopulmonary bypass techniques are used. A median sternotomy incision is made and the thymus is divided or one lobe is resected. After heparinization, the ascending aorta is cannulated, and venous cannulas are placed in the superior and inferior venae cavae after tapes are passed around these structures. Cardiopulmonary bypass is instituted, and moderate hypothermia to 25 to 28° C is established. The aorta is then cross-clamped, and hyperkalemic cardioplegic solution (10 ml/kg) is instilled through the aortic root. Topical hypothermic solution is poured over the heart to help reduce the intramyocardial temperature to 15° C. Cardiopulmonary bypass flows are reduced at this time to less than the calculated arterial flow. The repair is then performed and the cardiac chambers closed. The aortic cross-clamp is then removed, and before the heart is defibrillated, air is vented from the apex of the left ventricle and the aorta.

Supracardiac connections can be repaired by dissecting the right atrium and superior vena cava from their pericardial attachments (Fig. 36–16). With this method, the anastomosis between the left atrium and the posterior venous chamber can be constructed by a combination of lifting the heart upward and completing the anastomosis on the right side of the cava. Pulmonary veins that have directly entered the right atrium or right superior vena cava are repaired through a right-sided atriotomy (Fig. 36–17). The atrial septal defect is enlarged, and a large pericardial patch is used to form a baffle that directs the pulmonary venous flow through the atrial septal defect. Intracardiac connections that drain into the right atrium via the coronary sinus are repaired similarly (Fig. 36–18).

In patients with Type II TAPVC draining to the coronary sinus, an oblique right atriotomy should be done so that the crista terminalis is not divided. The coronary sinus is then incised into the foramen ovale or atrial septal defect. The atrial septal defect or foramen ovale is then enlarged, and a pericardial patch is used to direct the coronary sinus blood into the left atrium. Incising the coronary sinus and removing a portion of the atrial septum may injure one or more of the internodal conduction tracts between the sinus and atrioventricular nodes. Preservation of the crista terminalis usually ensures sinus rhythm.

For Type III, or intracardiac, connections, the heart is elevated superiorly, and a large anastomosis is created between the posterior venous chamber and the left atrium (Fig. 36–19). In some patients, the posterior venous chamber is not a transverse structure but is a tree-like structure with the only large point of communication at the confluence of the descending anomalous vein (Kawashima et al., 1977). In these patients, it is necessary to make a Y-shaped incision in the anomalous venous chamber and connect this to a similarly shaped incision in the posterior left atrium. If ligating the descending anomalous vein compromises the size of the left atrium, this can be left open, because these connections are in all cases obstructed. Mixed (Type IV) TAPVC is repaired by using techniques described for this combination of lesions.

Enlargement of the usually small left atrium may be necessary (Bonham-Carter et al., 1969; Parr et al., 1974). On preoperative cineangiography (Graham and Bender, 1980), at operation (Goor et al., 1976), and following surgery (Parr et al., 1974), the left atrium is small, and reservoir function may be compromised because of poor compliance. Despite these reasons for using a pericardial patch to enlarge the left atrium, several authors have noted that these maneuvers do not appreciably increase survival (Hammon et al., 1980; Katz et al., 1978). There is no convincing evidence that the additional time and the construction of another suture line that may impair internodal conduction are necessary.

Postoperative care may be difficult in patients with TAPVC, especially infants. Stiff, wet lungs are difficult to ventilate, and excessive inspiratory pressure further decreases the function of a heart already compromised by preoperative and intraoperative ischemia. Positive end-expiratory pressure, used judiciously, can increase arterial oxygen concentration by better matching ventilation and perfusion and preventing atelectasis. Many infants require the infusion of catecholamines postoperatively. Isoproterenol in low to moderate doses (0.01 to 0.06 μg/kg/min) has a positive myocardial inotropic and chronotropic effect and dilates both systemic and pulmonary arteries and thus decreases myocardial oxygen demands. Many infants are edematous, and administration of diuretics encourages the return to normal hydration. However, attention to blood and fluid replacement, arterial blood gases, and acid-base balance and maintenance of adequate cardiac output are essential for success.

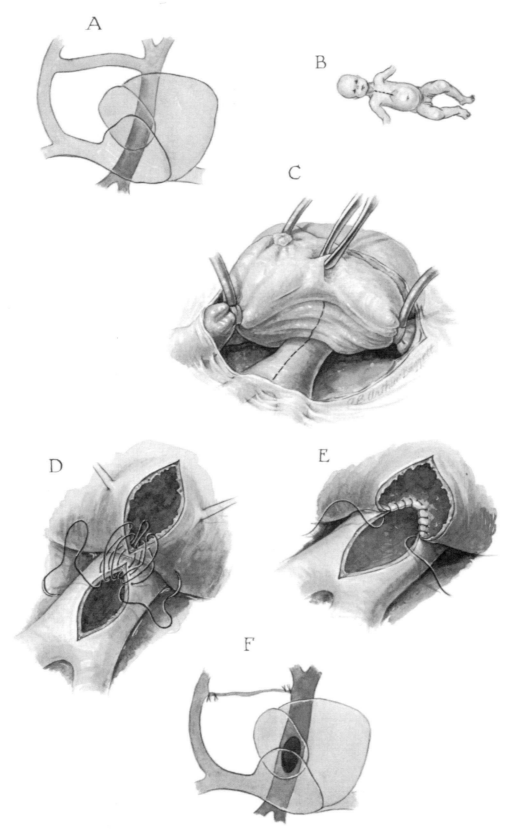

**FIGURE 36–16.** Steps in the repair of supracardiac TAPVC. *A,* Schematic anatomy as seen from the surgeon's view. *B,* Median sternotomy incision. *C,* After dissection of pericardial attachments, proposed incisions on the posterior left atrium and pulmonary venous confluence are shown. *D,* Generous incisions are made, and the first few stitches of a double-armed monofilament suture are shown. *E,* After the sutures are pulled tight, they should be interrupted in several places to avoid constricting the anastomosis. *F,* The final result. (*A–F,* From Kirklin, J. W.: Surgical treatment for total anomalous pulmonary venous connection in infancy. *In* Barratt-Boyes, B. G., Neutz, J. M., and Harris, E. A. [eds]: Heart Disease in Infancy: Diagnosis and Surgical Treatment. Edinburgh and London, Churchill Livingstone, 1973.)

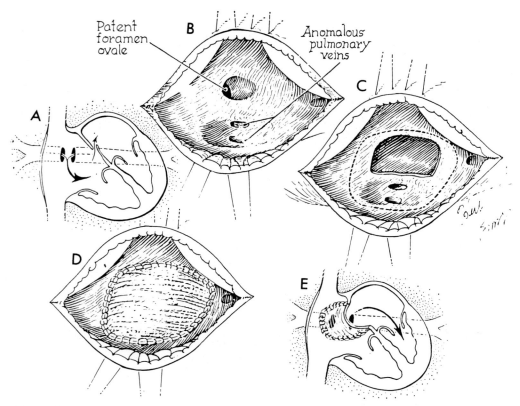

**FIGURE 36–17.** Repair of cardiac type of TAPVC in which the pulmonary veins drain directly to the right atrium. *A*, Anatomic representation. *B*, After right-sided atriotomy. *C*, A generous portion of the atrial septum is excised. *D*, A large pericardial patch is used to direct pulmonary venous blood into the left atrium. *E*, The final result. (*A–E*, From Cooley, D. A., Hallman, G. L., Leachman, R. D., et al.: Total anomalous pulmonary venous drainage: Correction with the use of cardiopulmonary bypass in 62 cases. J. Thorac. Cardiovasc. Surg., *51*:88, 1966.)

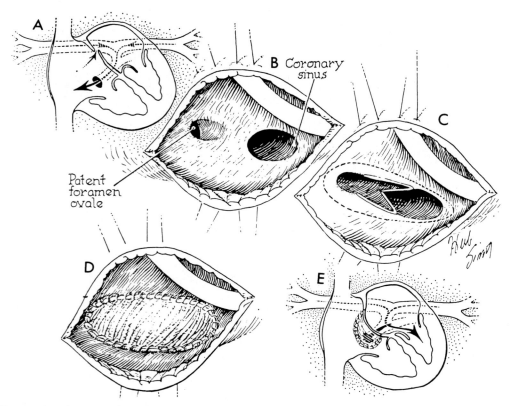

**FIGURE 36–18.** Repair of cardiac type of TAPVC in which the pulmonary veins connect with the coronary sinus. *A*, The surgical anatomy. *B*, A view of the dilated coronary sinus ostium after right-sided atriotomy. *C*, The coronary sinus is incised into the left atrial wall and patent foramen ovale. *D*, A large pericardial patch is used to direct coronary sinus blood into the left atrium. *E*, The final result. (*A–E*, From Cooley, D. A., Hallman, G. L., Leachman, R. D., et al.: Total anomalous pulmonary venous drainage: Correction with the use of cardiopulmonary bypass in 62 cases. J. Thorac. Cardiovasc. Surg., *51*:88, 1966.)

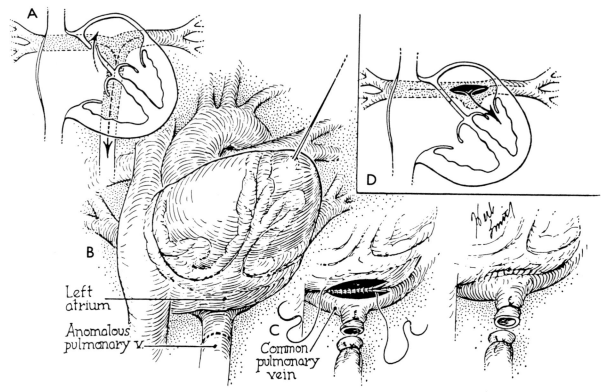

**FIGURE 36–19.** Repair of intracardiac TAPVC. *A,* The anatomy. *B,* The heart is deviated superiorly, and the anomalous descending vein is ligated. *C,* Generous incisions are made in the venous confluence and the left atrium. These are anastomosed with a fine monofilament suture. *D,* The final result after closing the atrial septal defect or patent foramen ovale. (*A–D,* From Cooley, D. A., Hollman, G. L., Leachman, R. D., et al.: Total anomalous pulmonary venous drainage: Correction with the use of cardiopulmonary bypass in 62 cases. J. Thorac. Cardiovasc. Surg., *51:*88, 1966.)

## Results

The results of operations for TAPVC are related directly to the presence of obstruction and thus related indirectly to the type of connection. Infants with obstructed connections usually present in extremis with very low cardiac output and are at great risk of subendocardial necrosis. They are often very difficult to ventilate because of very poor pulmonary compliance, and they suffer the complications of mechanical ventilation that occur in infants with stiff lungs. Cardiac catheterization and surgery in this group usually are done on an emergent basis, and mortality complication rates have been high. The operative mortality rate in infants has decreased from nearly 50% in series reported in the 1960s to less than 30% in the modern era (Hammon et al., 1980; Sano et al., 1989; Turley et al., 1980). More of these infants survive to diagnosis and treatment—a marked improvement in the therapy of this condition. With more prompt diagnosis and therapy, the operative mortality rate should improve in these infants.

The operative mortality rate is even lower in patients between 3 and 12 months of age (Behrendt et al., 1972). In older children and adults, this rate is probably less than 5% (Gomes et al., 1971). In most of these patients, the operative mortality rate is related to the presence of increased pulmonary vascular resistance from long-standing left-to-right intracardiac shunts.

Thus, the presence of obstruction in the anomalous connection most affects the patient's survival both with and without operation. In a series of infants who underwent surgery at Vanderbilt University Hospital between 1970 and 1980, the age of the patient did not directly affect the operative mortality rate (Hammon et al., 1980). In all surgical series, there have been more deaths in Types I and III TAPVC; in these two groups, the presence of anatomic obstruction to the anomalous connection is much more prevalent, especially in Type III.

With successful operation, late complications and mortality are rare. In patients with severe pulmonary hypertension and impaired left ventricular function, normal pulmonary artery pressure (Fig. 36–20) and left ventricular function (Fig. 36–21) can be expected (Hammon et al., 1980; Mathew et al., 1977). Postoperative pulmonary venous obstruction due to a hypertrophic lesion in individual pulmonary veins after repair of various types of TAPVC in infancy has been reported (Behrendt et al., 1972; Breckenridge et al., 1973; Fleming et al., 1979; Turley et al., 1980; Whight et al., 1978). Although this complication is rare, it usually causes severe morbidity or death. The etiology of this problem is not clear; stenosis of individual pulmonary veins and TAPVC have a common embry-

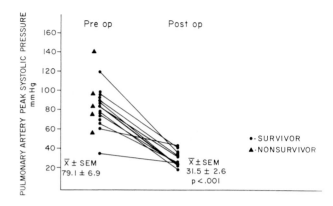

**FIGURE 36–20.** Preoperative and postoperative peak pulmonary artery pressures from a group of infants undergoing repair of TAPVC. Note the marked reduction in survivors. (From Hammon, J. W., Bender, H. W., Graham, T. P., et al.: Total anomalous pulmonary venous connection in infancy. J. Thorac. Cardiovasc. Surg., *80*:544, 1980.)

ologic etiology (Lucas et al., 1962), and affected infants may have a combination of the two lesions. For older children and adults, late complication is rare and is usually due to an arrhythmia (Gomes et al., 1971). Also of concern is a report of a small group of patients studied for more than 5 years after repair of TAPVC using 24-hour electrocardiography and treadmill exercise testing (Saxena et al., 1991). Significant but asymptomatic arrhythmias were seen in over one-third of patients, and one-fourth showed an inappropriate chronotropic exercise response. This study emphasizes the importance of long-term follow-up of all patients with TAPVC, even if they are asymptomatic.

Because repair of TAPVC involves a circumferential suture line, late postoperative stenosis may occur after significant growth. In more than 50 patients who underwent surgery at Vanderbilt University Hospital, two cases of late postoperative pulmonary venous stenosis at the suture line occurred, both more than 10 years postoperatively. The stenotic suture line obstruction is shown in Figure 36–22, which also shows distended pulmonary veins. Operation consists simply of enlarging the suture line by using a triangular pericardial or prosthetic patch. The risk is low, and a good result can be expected.

## COR TRIATRIATUM

In cor triatriatum, the pulmonary veins enter a chamber superior to the left atrium that then joins the left atrium through a narrow opening. Alternatively, the accessory chamber is separate from the left atrium

and directly communicates with the right atrium or indirectly communicates with the right atrium by way of an anomalous channel.

## Historical Aspects

The classic form of cor triatriatum was described clearly in 1868 by Church. Anatomic classifications of cor triatriatum were given by Loeffler in 1949 and further subdivided by Edwards in 1960. The first successful operation for total correction of cor triatriatum was reported by Vineberg and Gialloreto in 1956.

## Incidence

Cor triatriatum is rare; the incidence of cor triatriatum in all patients with congenital heart disease has been reported to be 0.1 to 0.4% (Jegier et al., 1963; Niwayama, 1960). The male/female incidence is approximately equal in most series. Although the etiology is unknown, the accepted embryologic explanation is that the accessory atrium is a common pulmonary vein that has not been incorporated normally into the left atrium (Edwards, 1960).

## Anatomy

The many subtypes of cor triatriatum requires a more inclusive classification than that proposed by Loeffler. The following classification is based on con-

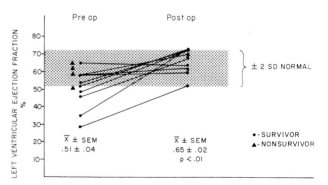

**FIGURE 36–21.** Preoperative and postoperative left ventricular ejection fraction calculated from left ventricular volume data obtained at cardiac catheterization. Note the postoperative return to normal function in survivors. (From Hammon, J. W., Bender, H. W., Graham, T. P., et al.: Total anomalous pulmonary venous connection in infancy. J. Thorac. Cardiovasc. Surg., *80*:544, 1980.)

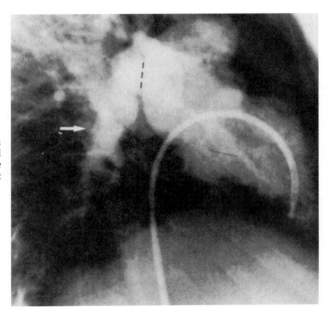

**FIGURE 36–22.** The venous phase of a pulmonary arteriogram in a patient with late postoperative suture line stenosis after repair of total anomalous pulmonary venous connection. The *broken line* shows the stenotic orifice between the pulmonary venous chamber and the left atrium. The *arrow* indicates an engorged pulmonary vein.

tributions of a number of individuals interested in this unusual anomaly (Edwards, 1960; Grondin et al., 1964; Loeffler, 1949; Niwayama, 1960).

**Accessory Left Atrial Chamber Receives All Pulmonary Veins and Communicates with the Left Atrium.** This type is the classic cor triatriatum in which a membranous partition with the shape of a windsock separates the more proximal chamber, which receives the pulmonary veins, from the more distal left atrium, which communicates with the mitral valve (Fig. 36–23A). The partition is usually directed toward the mitral valve and may have one or more orifices. This anomalous septum contains cardiac muscle fibers and is occasionally calcified. The true left atrium communicates with the left atrial appendage and contains a fossa ovalis. In most patients, there is no communication between the right and left atria; occasionally, however, a patent foramen ovale or secundum atrial septal defect allows the lower left atrial chamber to communicate with the right atrium (Niwayama, 1960).

In a few patients, the accessory atrial chamber communicates directly with the left atrium through a stenotic opening and with the right atrium directly (Fig. 36–23B) or via an anomalous venous connection (Fig. 36–23C). The anatomy of complete cor triatriatum communicating with the left atrium was reported in 20 patients (Marin-Garcia et al., 1975). In 12 of these patients, a classic diaphragm divided the left atrium and contained one or more stenotic orifices. In 6 patients, the accessory venous chamber was obstructed by either an hourglass configuration or a tubular narrowing that obstructed flow into the normal left atrium. These obstructions invariably were associated with complex cardiac lesions. The remaining 2 patients demonstrated other anomalous connections to the right atrium.

**Accessory Atrial Chamber Receives All Pulmonary Veins and Does Not Communicate with the Left Atrium.** In this anomaly, the diaphragm separating the common venous chamber from the left atrium is complete and prevents the direct flow of pulmonary venous blood to the left atrium. For the patient to survive, there is a direct communication from the common pulmonary venous chamber to the right atrium (Fig. 36–23D) or via an anomalous channel either to the innominate vein or to the portal vein, as in the supracardiac and infracardiac types of TAPVC (Fig. 36–23E).

## Pathophysiology

In classic cor triatriatum, in which there is no alternative pathway for pulmonary venous blood, the stenotic opening in the membranous partition between the accessory atrial chamber from the true left atrium creates supravalvular mitral stenosis with the features of elevated pulmonary venous pressure transmitted to the lungs, which causes pulmonary edema. The clinical condition of the patient is determined by the size of the opening in the membrane. If the opening is 3 mm or less in diameter, the symptoms occur in infancy and are similar to those of TAPVC with obstruction. If the opening is larger, the symptoms occur later in infancy, in childhood, or occasionally later in life.

In other forms of cor triatriatum, the features of unobstructed TAPVC are found, with hyperkinetic pulmonary hypertension and communications of the pulmonary venous system with the right atrium either directly or through an anomalous channel.

## Diagnosis

**Clinical Manifestations.** Most patients with cor triatriatum present with symptoms within the first few

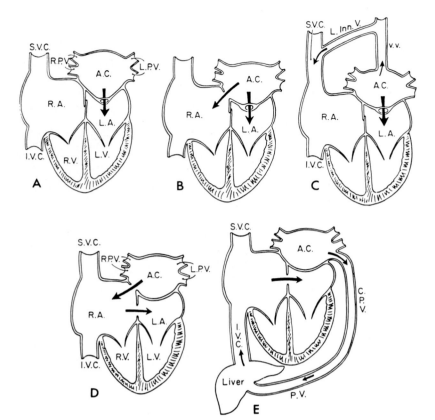

**FIGURE 36–23.** The various types of cor triatriatum. *A,* Classic cor triatriatum in which the accessory chamber (A.C.) receives the pulmonary veins (L.P.V. and R.P.V.) and communicates with the left atrium (L.A.). *B,* Classic cor triatriatum in which the accessory chamber communicates with both the left atrium and the right atrium (R.A.) or *C,* the systemic venous circulation via an anomalous venous connection. *D,* Cor triatriatum in which the accessory chamber communicates with only the right atrium or *E,* the systemic venous circulation via an anomalous vein. (I.V.C. = inferior vena cava; S.V.C. = superior vena cava; L. Inn. V. = left innominate vein.) (*A–E,* Adapted from Lucas, R. V., and Schmidt, R. E.: Anomalous venous connections, pulmonary and systemic. *In* Moss, A. J., Adams, F. H., and Emmanouilides, G. C. [eds]: Heart Disease in Infants, Children and Adolescents, 2nd ed. Copyright 1977, Williams & Wilkins, Baltimore. Reproduced by permission.)

years of life (Niwayama, 1960). In these patients, signs of pulmonary venous obstruction are always prevalent, with bouts of pulmonary edema, extreme feeding difficulties, and poor weight gain. On physical examination, the predominant features are moist rales in the lower fields of the lung associated with a loud pulmonary second sound compatible with pulmonary hypertension. If there is a communication with the right atrium, there is a flow murmur at the left sternal border associated with the large left-to-right intracardiac shunt.

The occasional patient who is discovered with this condition later in life has a history of breathlessness, frequent respiratory infections, and, in some cases, peripheral embolization. As with mitral stenosis, many patients are mistaken to have primary pulmonary disease. The physical examination in these patients reflects severe pulmonary hypertension: a loud pulmonary second sound, right ventricular lift, and pulmonary rales. In many patients, the signs of right-sided heart failure are prominent, with distended peripheral veins and an enlarged liver. The usual cardiac murmur is a soft, blowing, systolic murmur along the left sternal border. In some cases, a diastolic murmur is heard in the mitral area.

**Chest Film.** The plain chest film in cor triatriatum usually reflects pulmonary venous obstruction. Fine, diffuse, reticular pulmonary markings extend from the pulmonary hilus to involve the lower lung fields. In older patients, Kerley's B lines may be present, combined with prominent venous engorgement of the upper pulmonary vessels. There are also signs of left atrial enlargement produced by the dilated accessory chamber (Fig. 36–24).

**Electrocardiogram.** The electrocardiographic findings reflect right ventricular systolic overload. In many cases, there are tall peaked P waves, which suggest right atrial enlargement. Rarely, notched P waves are present, presumably because of the dilated accessory atrial chamber.

**Echocardiogram.** The echocardiographic features vary in cor triatriatum. When the membrane that separates the accessory chamber from the true left atrium is thick and prominent, it is sometimes localized with the echocardiogram. In most cases, however, it is impossible to differentiate the large dilated accessory chamber from TAPVC draining to the coronary sinus or persistent left superior vena cava connecting to the coronary sinus.

**Magnetic Resonance Imaging.** Magnetic resonance imaging (MRI) is a relatively new imaging modality that can be used to diagnose certain conditions, such as cor triatriatum. It can be obtained in patients of any size; however, the limitations involve patient sedation and the removal of all metal objects from the patient during imaging. It is probably not a technique that can be used for the very sick neonate. It is possible to obtain accurate images of intracardiac structures such as the membrane in cor triatriatum (Fig. 36–25). The use of MRI in congenital heart disease is beginning to evolve, and it is not yet known whether it will supplant echocardiography or cardiac catheterization

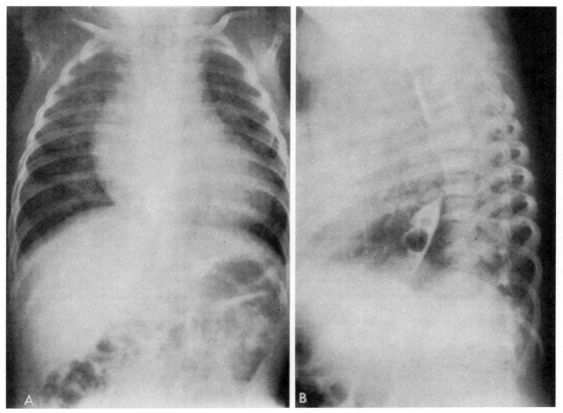

FIGURE 36–24. Plain chest film of a child with cor triatriatum. *A,* Posteroanterior view shows pulmonary venous engorgement and left atrial enlargement. *B,* Lateral view confirms atrial enlargement produced by the dilated accessory chamber, which causes posterior displacement of the barium-filled esophagus.

for the diagnosis of some or all congenital heart lesions.

**Cardiac Catheterization.** The hallmark of hemodynamic findings in cor triatriatum is a pressure gradient between the pulmonary capillary wedge pressure and the left atrial pressure. In most cases, oximetry excludes a left-to-right shunt, and significant pulmonary hypertension is the rule. Selective pulmonary arteriography usually shows cor triatriatum in the

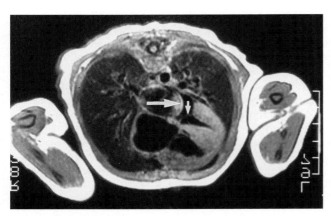

FIGURE 36–25. Coronal magnetic resonance image of a 1-month-old child with cor triatriatum. The *large arrow* points to the thick and highly visible membrane bulging toward the mitral valve *(small arrow).*

venous phase. Pulmonary transit time is prolonged. As the pulmonary veins are opacified, they drain into an accessory left atrial chamber. In most cases, a delay occurs between the opacification of this chamber and the visualization of the true left atrium and left ventricle. With a high-quality study, the interatrial diaphragm can be identified as a linear or windsock-shaped filling defect between the accessory atrial chamber and the true left atrium (Fig. 36–26). The accessory atrial chamber usually remains opacified for some time and does not contract as does the normal left atrial chamber.

## Surgical Treatment

The only successful therapy for cor triatriatum has been surgical. The indications for operation and preoperative preparation are similar to those for patients with TAPVC. Open correction is preferred in all patients. In infants, open correction is facilitated by hypothermia and circulatory arrest. In most cases, the membrane can be resected between the accessory venous chamber and the left atrium through the atrial septum in infants, and in older children by an incision into the true left atrium by developing the interatrial groove. If the preoperative diagnosis suggests TAPVC, exploration of the heart exteriorly usually

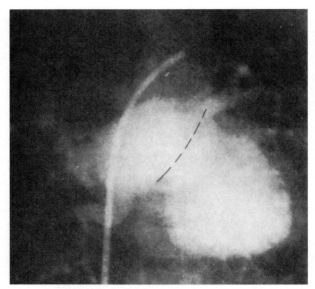

**FIGURE 36–26.** Venous phase of the pulmonary angiogram in a child with cor triatriatum. The *broken line* shows the position of the membrane that separates the dilated accessory chamber from the left atrium.

shows a dilated pulmonary venous chamber, which can be confused with the operative findings in congenital mitral stenosis. When anomalous connections between the accessory chamber and the systemic venous system are present, the operative findings can be confusing, and only a careful and thorough intracardiac and extracardiac examination reveals the true cause of the anomaly, which can then easily be corrected. The number of cases reported in the literature is quite small, so it is difficult to estimate the operative mortality rate. In a surgical series of 11 patients, there were 2 operative deaths, a mortality rate of 17% (Rodefeld et al., 1990). Generally, the mortality rate of very sick infants with pulmonary venous obstruction is higher because of their preoperative condition. Mortality should be rare in older children and adults; however, late complications such as arrhythmias are more common.

## MAJOR ANOMALIES OE THE THORACIC SYSTEMIC VENOUS SYSTEM

Developments in the diagnosis and treatment of cardiovascular disorders have brought anomalies of the thoracic systemic veins to the attention of the cardiologist and thoracic surgeon alike. Consideration of these diverse anomalies requires a simple and practical system classification. A classification based on anatomy tends to be cumbersome, whereas one based on physiology excludes conditions that cause hemodynamic derangement but may provide important information about technical complications of cardiac catheterization and operation. A classification based on embryologic principles is more inclusive and permits practical consideration of the defects (Lucas and Schmidt, 1977). This system of classification includes anomalies of the cardinal venous system, anomalies of the inferior vena cava, and anomalies of the valves of the sinus venosus.

## Anomalies of the Cardinal Venous System

Anomalies of the cardinal venous system involve aberrations in the development of the right and left superior vena cava and abnormalities of the coronary sinus. These anomalies present problems to the cardiac surgeon during repair of other defects or when the anomaly is associated with drainage of desaturated blood into the left atrium.

**Persistent Left Superior Vena Cava.** Persistent left superior vena cava is the most common anomaly of the superior vena caval system. In a series of 4000 unselected autopsies, the prevalence was 0.3% (Geissler and Albert, 1956). The association in patients with additional cardiac defects ranges from 2.8 to 4.3% (Loogen and Rippert, 1958). Generally, persistent left superior vena cava is part of a bilateral superior vena caval system. Left superior vena cava is a normal stage in evolutionary development and in the growth of the human embryo. Its usual anatomic course begins where it arises from the junction of the left subclavian and the left internal jugular veins. It then descends vertically in front of the aortic arch. A short distance from its origin, it receives the superior left intercostal vein. It then passes in front of the left pulmonary artery and left pulmonary veins or in between these vessels (Winter, 1954). It usually receives a hemiazygos vein and then penetrates the pericardium and crosses the posterior wall of the left atrium obliquely to approach the posterior atrial ventricular groove. There it receives the great cardiac vein and becomes the coronary sinus (Fig. 36–27). Rarely, the right superior vena cava is absent, and the entire venous return from the head and arms enters the coronary sinus (see Fig. 36–27). Associated anomalies are common with persistent left superior vena cava; they include sinus venosus atrial septal defect or other congenital syndromes associated with cardiac malposition. The only clinical importance of persistent left superior vena cava is that cardiac catheterization is difficult when done from the left arm. In addition, at open cardiac operations, it is important to recognize the presence of the left superior vena cava and use appropriate cannulation techniques to eliminate the large amount of systemic venous blood that enters the heart through the coronary sinus. It is also important to recognize the absence of collateral vessels between the left and right superior vena cava or, rarely, the absence of the right superior vena cava, in which case ligation of the persistent left superior vena cava would cause venous engorgement in the head and arms.

**Persistent Left Superior Vena Cava Associated with Failure of Coronary Sinus Development (Unroofed Coronary Sinus).** In this defect, the left superior vena cava takes its usual course anterior to the aortic arch and the left pulmonary artery. Then, in-

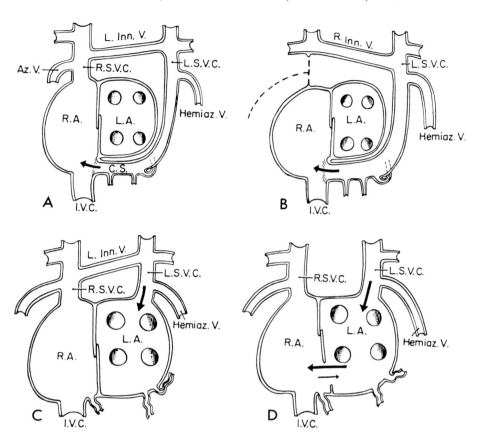

**FIGURE 36-27.** Variation of persistent left superior vena cava (L.S.V.C.). *A,* L.S.V.C. drains via the coronary sinus (C.S.) to the right atrium (R.A.) The sizes of the left innominate vein (L. Inn. V.) and L.S.V.C. vary inversely, and the former is often absent. *B,* Uncommonly, the right superior vena cava (R.S.V.C.) is atretic. *C,* The coronary sinus is absent, and the L.S.V.C. drains directly into the left atrium. Simple ligation of the L.S.V.C. provides a cure. *D,* The coronary sinus is absent, and there is no communication between the two superior venae cavae. A low-lying coronary sinus atrial septal defect is present, and treatment requires baffling the L.S.V.C. into the right atrium and closing the atrial septal defect. (*A–D,* Adapted from Lucas, R. V., and Schmidt, R. E.: Anomalous venous connections, pulmonary and systemic. *In* Moss, A. J., Adams, F. H., and Emmanouilides, G. C. [eds]: Heart Disease in Infants, Children and Adolescents. 2nd ed. Copyright 1977, The Williams & Wilkins Company, Baltimore. Reproduced by permission.)

stead of crossing back to the left atrium to enter the coronary sinus, it connects directly to the upper portion of the left atrium between the atrial appendage and the left superior pulmonary veins (see Fig. 36–27C).

The physiologic consequences of this defect are almost always overshadowed by other major congenital cardiac malformations. The only contribution this defect makes to the overall hemodynamic findings at cardiac catheterization is a small right-to-left shunt at the atrial level.

This defect is almost invariably associated with other anomalies. In a series of eight surgical patients, a coronary sinus atrial septal defect was present in all patients (Quaegebeur et al., 1979) (see Fig 36–27D). This anomaly is also associated with primitive cyanotic congenital heart defects, such as cor biloculare, anomalies of conotruncal development, and the syndrome of splenic agenesis (Campbell and Duechar, 1954).

## Diagnosis

**Clinical Findings.** Features of a complex associated defect usually obscure the clinical effects of left superior vena cava directly connected to the left atrium. When a defect in the atrial septum is associated, the primary manifestations are those found in atrial septal defect. When drainage of the left superior vena cava to the left atrium is an isolated phenomenon, cyanosis is prevalent in early infancy. Although the patient is asymptomatic, clubbing and polycythemia are usual. The heart is normal both on auscultation and on radiographic examination.

**Cardiac Catheterization.** Precise diagnosis of this defect is possible either by following the course of the cardiac catheter through the left superior vena cava or by dye injection in the left arm. These findings in the presence of peripheral cyanosis suggest a systemic vein draining anomalously into the left atrium.

**Surgical Treatment.** The treatment in all cases is surgical. If there are competent bridging veins between the left and right superior vena cava, the surgical treatment is simply ligation of the left superior vena cava and correction of the associated intracardiac defect. If, as in most cases, there are no bridging communications and the coronary sinus septum has not been formed, it is necessary to "roof" the coronary sinus with pericardium or a portion of the left atrium so that the left superior vena cava now drains to the right atrium (Fig. 36–28). Complications are usually related to the magnitude of operation for associated anomalies and not to the operative therapy for this uncommon situation.

## Anomalies of the Inferior Vena Cava

Significant anomalies of the inferior vena cava are those that shunt unsaturated blood into the left

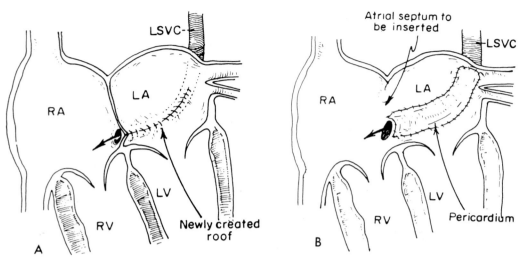

**FIGURE 36–28.** Repair (or roofing) of an unroofed coronary sinus associated with a persistent left superior vena cava (LSVC). *A,* The repair is made by bringing together the posterior left atrial wall to form a channel such that the LSVC communicates with the right atrium (RA). *B,* The same repair is made in a patient with a common atrium by using pericardium. (LA = left atrium; LV = left ventricle; RV = right ventricle.) (*A* and *B,* Quaegebur, J., Kirklin, J. W., Pacifico, A. D., and Bargeron, L.: Surgical experience with unroofed coronary sinus. Reprinted with permission from the Society of Thoracic Surgeons [The Annals of Thoracic Surgery, Vol. 27, 1979, p. 418–425].)

atrium and that can complicate cardiac catheterization and cardiac operations for congenital heart disease. These anomalies are intrahepatic interruption of the inferior vena cava with azygos continuation and anomalous drainage of the inferior vena cava into the left atrium.

**Interrupted Inferior Vena Cava.** Interruption of the inferior vena cava with azygos continuation is more prevalent in patients with congenital heart disease, particularly patients with polysplenia syndrome and with cardiac malpositions (Anderson and Varco, 1961). When interrupted inferior vena cava is an isolated anomaly, it is associated with normal longevity and no physiologic abnormalities. Problems arise when it occurs with other congenital anomalies that require surgical correction. During operations for con-

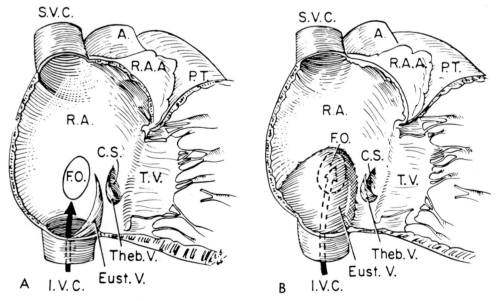

**FIGURE 36–29.** Persistence of the valves of the sinus venosus. *A,* Normal persistence of the valves of the sinus venosus results in the eustachian valve (Eust. V.) and the thebesian valve (Theb. V.). *B,* Abnormal persistence of the eustachian valve has resulted in a membrane that completely diverts inferior vena cava (I.V.C.) blood into the left atrium via the foramen ovale (F.O.). Similarly, the ostium of the coronary sinus (C.S.), the superior vena cava (S.V.C.) orifice, or all three may be isolated from the true right atrium by abnormal persistence of the valves of the sinus venosus. (R.A.A. = right atrial appendage; T.V. = tricuspid valve; P. T. = pulmonary trunk; A. = aorta.) (*A* and *B,* Adapted from Lucas, R. V., and Schmidt, R. E.: Anomalous venous connections, pulmonary and systemic. *In* Moss, A. J., Adams, F. H., and Emmanouilides, G. C. [eds]: Heart Disease in Infants, Children and Adolescents. 2nd ed. Copyright 1977, The Williams and Wilkins Company, Baltimore. Reproduced by permission.)

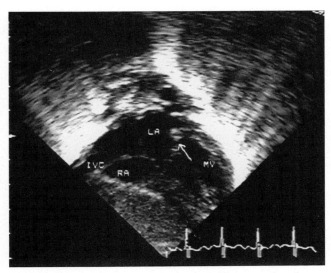

**FIGURE 36–30.** A two-dimensional echocardiogram taken from a child with TAPVC Type I with coexisting *cor triatriatum dexter*. Note the direct communication between the inferior vena cava (IVC) and the left atrium (LA). (MV = mitral valve; RA = right atrium.)

genital heart disease, ligation of the large azygos vein must be recognized, because it can cause death (Effler et al., 1951). The anomaly also leads to difficulties in cannulation for cardiopulmonary bypass; details of this technical problem are given elsewhere (Bosher, 1959).

**Anomalous Drainage of the Inferior Vena Cava into the Left Atrium.** When the inferior vena cava shunts blood directly into the left atrium, a distinction must be made between connection of the inferior vena cava to the left atrium with intact atrial septum and cases in which a low atrial septal defect allows drainage of inferior vena caval blood into the left atrium. Direct connection of the inferior vena cava to the left atrium is uncommon, and the embryology is obscure. The clinical features in these cases are comparable with those of left superior vena cava connections to the left atrium (Gardner and Cole, 1955). Systemic embolization is a risk, and surgery should be performed. The condition is cured via placement of an interatrial baffle to provide normal systemic venous drainage (Black et al., 1964). In some patients, persistence of the valves of the sinus venosus can direct inferior vena caval blood into the left atrium by an atrial septal defect or patent foramen ovale, and this condition has been known as *cor triatriatum dexter* (Doucette and Knoblich, 1963) (Fig. 36–29). Treatment consists of incising the persistent valvular tissue and closing the intertrial communication. This condition can co-exist with pulmonary venous anomalies, as illustrated in Figure 36–30. In some patients with an atrial septal defect, a large eustachian valve may be mistaken for the lower margin of the atrial septal defect. Care must be taken to close the atrial defect itself, because closure of the atrial septum onto the eustachian valve may then divert inferior vena caval blood into the left atrium (Mustard et al., 1964).

## SELECTED BIBLIOGAPHY

Bender, H. W., Fisher, R. D., Walker, W. E., and Graham, T. P.: Reparative cardiac surgery in infants and small children: Five years experience with profound hypothermia and circulatory arrest. Ann. Surg., *190*:437, 1979.

> The authors summarize the results of operations in a large series of infants and children (*n* = 128) using hypothermia and circulatory arrest. The surgical techniques are detailed, and the results are shown.

Darling, R. C., Rothney, W. B., and Craig, J. M.: Total pulmonary venous drainage into the right side of the heart. Lab. Invest., *6*:44, 1957.

> This was the first publication to characterize carefully the types of TAPVC. It contains a beautifully illustrated description of the pathologic anatomy.

Hammon, J. W., Bender, H. W., Graham, T. P., et al.: Total anomalous pulmonary venous connection in infancy. J. Thorac. Cardiovasc. Surg., *80*:544, 1989.

> This article on a series of patients with TAPVC emphasizes preoperative and postoperative hemodynamic and ventricular function studies, and it shows that operative survivors have normal hemodynamic and ventricular function.

Ivemark, B. I.: Implications of agenesis of the spleen on the pathogenesis of conotruncus anomalies in childhood: An analysis of the heart malformations in the splenic agenesis syndrome with fourteen new cases. Acta Paediatr. Scand. Suppl., *104*:1, 1955.

> This is one of the best descriptions of the pathologic anatomy, diagnosis, and surgical treatment of this uncommon anomaly.

Katz, N. M., Kirklin, J. W., and Pacifico, A. D.: Concepts and practices in surgery for total anomalous pulmonary venous connection. Ann. Thorac. Surg., *25*:479, 1978.

> This excellent review article discusses many of the controversial features in the diagnosis and management of TAPVC.

Lucas, R. V., and Schmidt, R. E.: Anomalous venous connection, pulmonary and systemic. *In* Moss, A. J., Adams, F. H., and Emmanouilides, G. G. (eds): Heart Disease in Infants, Children, and Adolescents. Baltimore, Williams & Wilkins, 1977, pp. 437–470.

> This detailed explanation of the embryology of anomalies of pulmonary venous connection to the heart is well illustrated and easily understandable.

Neill, C. A.: Development of the pulmonary veins: With reference to the embryology of anomalies of pulmonary venous return. Pediatrics, *18*:880, 1956.

> This important embryologic study outlines the development of the pulmonary venous system and provides an embryologic explanation for anomalous pulmonary venous connections.

Sano, S., Brawn, W. J., and Mee, R. B. B.: Total anomalous pulmonary venous drainage. J. Thorac. Cardiovasc. Surg., *97*:886, 1989.

> This series from an outstanding clinic illustrates contemporary protocols for preoperative evaluation, operative management, and postoperative care, producing a superb 2.3% (1 of 44 patients) hospital mortality rate, the lowest published to date.

Sloan, H., MacKenzie, J., Morris, J. D., et al.: Open-heart surgery in infancy. J. Thorac. Cardiovasc. Surg., *44*:459, 1962.

> The authors describe the first successful repair of Type III TAPVC in an infant. This work introduced the concept of deep hypothermia induced by surface cooling and cardiopulmonary bypass so that a period of circulatory arrest could be used for operative repair.

## BIBLIOGRAPHY

Anderson, R. C., and Varco, R. L.: Cor triatriatum: Successful diagnosis and surgical correction in a 3-year-old girl. Am. J. Cardiol., *7*:436, 1961.
Barratt-Boyes, B. G.: Primary definitive intracardiac operations in infants: Total anomalous pulmonary venous connection. *In* Kirklin, J. W. (ed): Advances in Cardiovascular Surgery. New York, Grune & Stratton, 1973, pp. 127–140.
Behrendt, D. M., Aberdeen, E., Waterson, D. J., and Bonham-Carter,

R. E.: Total anomalous pulmonary venous drainage in infants. Circulation, 46:347, 1972.

Bender, H. W., Fisher, R. D., Walker, W. E., and Graham, T. P.: Reparative cardiac surgery in infants and small children: Five years experience with profound hypothermia and circulatory arrest. Ann. Surg., 190:437, 1979.

Black, H., Smith, G. T., and Goodale, W. T.: Anomalous inferior vena cava draining into the left atrium associated with intact interatrial septum and multiple pulmonary arteriovenous fistulae. Circulation, 29:258, 1964.

Bonham-Carter, R. E., Capriles, M., and Noe, Y.: Total anomalous pulmonary venous drainage: A clinical and anatomical study of 75 children. Br. Heart J., 31:45, 1969.

Bosher, L. H.: Problems in extracorporeal circulation relating to venous cannulation and drainage. Ann. Surg., 149:652,1959.

Breckenridge, I. M., de Leval, M., Stark, J., and Waterston, D. J.: Correction of total anomalous pulmonary venous drainage in infancy. J. Thorac. Cardiovasc. Surg., 66:447, 1973.

Burroughs, J. T., and Edwards, J. E.: Total anomalous pulmonary venous connection. Am. Heart J., 59:913, 1960.

Campbell, M., and Deuchar, D. C.: The left-sided superior vena cava. Br. Heart J., 423, 1954.

Church, W. S.: Congenital malformation of the heart: Abnormal septum in left auricle. Trans. Pathol. Soc. Lond., 188,1868.

Cooley, D. A., and Ochsner, A.: Correction of total anomalous pulmonary venous drainage. Surgery, 42:1014, 1957.

Darling, R. C., Rothney, W. B., and Craig, J. M.: Total pulmonary venous drainage into the right side of the heart. Lab. Invest., 6:44, 1957.

Doucette, J., and Knoblich, R.: Persistent right valve of the sinus venosus. Arch. Pathol., 75:105, 1963.

Edwards, J. E.: Malformations of the thoracic veins. In Gould, S. E. (ed): Pathology of the Heart. 2nd ed. Springfield, IL, Charles C Thomas, 1960, p. 484.

Effler, D. B., Greer, A. E., and Sifers, E. C.: Anomaly of the vena cava inferior. Report of fatality after ligation. JAMA, 146:1321, 1951.

Fleming, W. H., Clark, E. B., Dooley, K. J., et al.: Late complications following surgical repair of total anomalous pulmonary venous return below the diaphragm. Ann. Thorac. Surg., 27:435, 1979.

Friedlich, A., Bing, R. J., and Blount, S. G.: Physiological studies in congenital heart disease: IX. Circulatory dynamics in the anomalies of venous return to the heart, including pulmonary arteriovenous fistula. Am. Heart J., 86:20, 1950.

Gardner, D. L., and Cole, L.: Long survival with inferior vena cava draining into left atrium. Br. Heart J., 17:93, 1955.

Gathman, G. H., and Nadas, A. S.: Total anomalous pulmonary venous connection: Clinical and physiologic observations of 75 pediatric patients. Circulation, 42:143, 1970.

Geissler, W., and Albert, M.: Persistierende linke obere Hohlvene und Mitralstenose. A. Gesamte Inn. Med., 11:865, 1956.

Gomes, M. M. R., Feldt, R. H., McGoon, D. C., and Danielson, G. K.: Long-term results following correction of total anomalous pulmonary venous connection. J. Thorac. Cardiovasc. Surg., 61:253, 1971.

Goor, D. A., Yellin, A., Frand, M., et al.: The operative problem of small left atrium in total anomalous pulmonary venous connection: Report of 5 patients. Ann. Thorac. Surg., 22:254, 1976.

Graham, T. P., and Bender, H. W.: Preoperative diagnosis and management of infants with critical congenital heart disease. Ann. Thorac. Surg., 29:272, 1980.

Grondin, C., Leonard, A. S., Anderson, R. C., et al.: Cor triatriatum: A diagnostic surgical enigma. J. Thorac. Cardiovasc. Surg., 48:527, 1964.

Hammon, J. W., Bender, H. W., Graham, T. P., et al.: Total anomalous pulmonary venous connection in infancy. J. Thorac. Cardiovasc. Surg., 80:544, 1980.

Ivemark, B. I.: Implications of agenesis of the spleen on the pathogenesis of conotruncus anomalies in childhood: An analysis of the heart malformations in the splenic agenesis syndrome with fourteen new cases. Acta Paediatr. Scand. Suppl., 104:1, 1955.

Jegier, W., Gibbons, J. E., and Wigglesworth, F. W.: Cor triatriatum: Clinical, hemodynamic, and pathologic studies: Surgical correction in early life. Pediatrics, 31:255, 1963.

Jensen, J. B., and Blount, S. G.: Total anomalous pulmonary venous return: A review and report of the oldest surviving patient. Am. Heart J., 82:387, 1971.

Katz, N. M., Kirklin, J. W., and Pacifico, A. D.: Concepts and practices in surgery for total anomalous pulmonary venous connection. Ann. Thorac. Surg., 25:479, 1978.

Kawashima, Y., Matsuda, H., Hakano, S., et al.: Tree-shaped pulmonary veins in infracardiac total anomalous pulmonary venous drainage. Ann. Thorac. Surg., 23:436, 1977.

Lewis, J., Varco, R. L., Taufic, M., and Niazi, S. A.: Direct vision repair of triatrial heart and total anomalous pulmonary venous drainage. Surg. Gynecol. Obstet., 101:713, 1956.

Loeffler, E.: Unusual malformation of the left atrium: Pulmonary sinus. Arch. Pathol., 48:371, 1949.

Loogen, D., and Rippert, R.: Anomalien der grossen Korper und Lungenvenen. Z. Kreislaufforsch., 47:677, 1958.

Los, J. A.: Embryology. In Watson, H. (ed): Pediatric Cardiology. St. Louis, C. V. Mosby, 1968.

Lucas, R. V., and Schmidt, R. E.: Anomalous venous connection, pulmonary and systemic. In Moss, A. J., Adams, F. H., and Emmanouilides, G. C. (eds): Heart Disease in Infants, Children and Adolescents. Baltimore, Williams & Wilkins, 1977, pp. 437–470.

Lucas, R. V., Woolfrey, B. F., Anderson, R. C., et al.: Atresia of the common pulmonary vein. Pediatrics, 29:729, 1962.

Marin-Garcia, J., Tandon, R., Lucas, R. V., Jr., and Edwards, J. E.: Cor triatriatum: Study of 20 cases. Am. J. Cardiol., 35:59, 1975.

Mathew, R., Thilenius, O. G., Replogle, R. L., and Arcilla, R. A.: Cardiac function in total anomalous pulmonary venous return before and after surgery. Circulation, 55:361, 1977.

McClure, C. F. W., and Butler, E. G.: The development of the vena cava inferior in man. Am. J. Anat., 35:331, 1925.

Meadows, W. R., Bergstrand, I., and Sharp, J. T.: Isolated anomalous connection of a great vein to the left atrium. Circulation, 24:669, 1961.

Miller, W. W., and Rashkind, W. J.: Palliative treatment of total anomalous pulmonary venous drainage by balloon atrial septostomy. Lancet, 2:387, 1968.

Muller, W. H.: The surgical treatment of transposition of the pulmonary veins. Ann. Surg., 134: 683, 1951.

Mustard, W. T., Firor, W. B., and Kidd, L.: Diversion of the venae cavae into the left atrium during closure of atrial septal defects. J. Thorac. Cardiovasc. Surg., 47:317, 1964.

Neill, C. A.: Development of the pulmonary veins: With reference to the embryology of anomalies of pulmonary venous return. Pediatrics, 18:880, 1956.

Newfield, E. A., Wilson, A., Paul, M. H., and Reisch, J. S.: Pulmonary vascular disease in total anomalous venous drainage. Circulation, 61:103, 1980.

Niwayama, G.: Cor triatriatum. Am. Heart J., 59:291, 1960.

Paquet, M., and Gutgesell, H.: Echocardiographic features of total anomalous pulmonary venous connection. Circulation, 51: 599, 1975.

Parr, G. V. S., Kirklin, J. W., Pacifico, A. D., et al.: Cardiac performance in infants after repair of TAPVC. Ann. Thorac. Surg., 17:561, 1974.

Quaegebeur, J., Kirklin, J. W., Pacifico, A. D., and Bargeron, L. M.: Surgical experience with unroofed coronary sinus. Ann. Thorac. Surg., 27:418, 1979.

Raghib, G., Ruttenberg, H. D., Anderson, R. C., et al.: Termination of left superior vena cava in left atrium, atrial septal defect, and absence of coronary sinus. Circulation, 31:906, 1965.

Rodefeld, M. D., Brown, J. W., Heimansohn, D. A., et al.: Cor triatriatum: Clinical presentation and surgical results in 12 patients. Ann. Thorac. Surg., 50:562, 1990.

Ruttenberg, H. D., Neufeld, H. N., Lucas, R. V., et al.: Syndrome of congenital cardiac disease with asplenia: Distinction from other forms of congenital cardiac disease. Am. J. Cardiol., 13:387, 1964.

Sano, S., Brawn, W. J., Mee, R. B. B.: Total anomalous pulmonary venous drainage. J. Thorac. Cardiovasc. Surg., 97:886, 1989.

Saxena, A., Fong, L. V., Lamb, R. K., et al.: Cardiac arrhythmias after surgical correction of total anomalous pulmonary venous connection: Late follow-up. Pediatr. Cardiol., 12:89, 1991.

Shaner, R. F.: The development of the bronchial veins with to special reference to anomalies of the pulmonary veins. Anat. Rec., *140*:159, 1961.

Sloan, H., MacKenzie, J., Morris, J. D., et al.: Open-heart surgery in infancy. J. Thorac. Cardiovasc. Surg., *44*:459, 1962.

Streeter, G. L.: Developmental horizons in human embryos. Description of age group XI, 13 to 20 somites, and age group XII, 21 to 20 somites. Carnegie Inst. Contrib. Embryol., *30*(197): 211, 1942.

Turley, K., Tucker, W. Y., Ullyot, D. J., and Ebert, P. A.: Total anomalous pulmonary venous connection in infancy: Influence of age and type of lesion. Am. J. Cardiol., *45*:92,1980.

Van Der Velde, M. E., Parness, I. A., Colan, S. D., et al.: Two-dimensional echocardiography in the pre- and postoperative management of totally anomalous pulmonary venous connection. J. Am. Coll. Cardiol., *18*:1746, 1991.

Vineberg, A., and Gialloreto, O.: Report of a successful operation for stenosis of common pulmonary vein (cor triatriatum). Can. Med. Assoc. J., *74*:719, 1956.

Whight, C. M., Barratt-Boyes, B. G., Calder, A. L., et al.: Total anomalous pulmonary venous connection. J. Thorac. Cardiovasc. Surg., *75*:52, 1978.

Wilson, J.: On a very unusual formation of the human heart. Philos. Trans. Lond., *88*:332, 1798.

Winter, F. S.: Persistent left superior vena cava: Survey of world literature and report of thirty additional cases. Angiology, *5*:90, 1954.

# 37 Atrioventricular Canal

Gordon K. Danielson and Francisco J. Puga

## EMBRYOLOGY

The various congenital deformities of the atrioventricular canal are conveniently designated *atrioventricular* (AV) *canal defects*. Other terms that have been used include endocardial cushion defect (Baron, 1968), atrioventricular defect (Piccoli et al., 1979), atrioventricular septal defect (Becker and Anderson, 1982), and ostium primum atrial septal defect (when there is no interventricular communication). The common AV canal is not seen in the normal, fully developed human heart, but is encountered only in the embryo. It consists of the slightly narrowed zone between the one atrium and the one ventricle when the embryo is in the early tubular stage of development, and it serves as a broad area of connection and communication between the primitive atrium and the primitive ventricle.

During embryonic development, the ventricular septum ascends from the apex and the atrial septum descends from the cephalad atrial wall, dividing the heart into right and left halves. As these septa converge at the AV junction or canal, "cushions" of endothelium form on the anterior and posterior margins of the canal. The progressive enlargement of these cushions contributes to separation of the common AV canal into right and left AV orifices and, together with delamination of ventricular myocardium, to development of their respective valves. Defective development in this area may cause incomplete septation of the AV canal and deformity of one or both AV valves.

## CLASSIFICATION

When embryonic development of the area of the common AV canal is abnormal, the resultant malformation varies and depends on the extent of involvement of the atrial and ventricular septa as well as of the mitral and tricuspid valves. For the surgeon, a surgically oriented classification is preferable. The first distinction is whether an anomaly includes a fully displayed AV canal septal defect in the center of the heart that involves the ostium primum area of the atrial septum as well as the adjacent basal area of the ventricular septum, or whether the anomaly includes a lesser extent of septal defect or none at all and is therefore an incompletely displayed AV canal septal defect. The classification in Table 37–1 is based on this distinction. This table shows the 15 theoretically possible types of anomalies according to which combination of the 4 potential defects in embryogenesis

of the AV canal has occurred. Note that both the ostium primum atrial (O) and the basal ventricular (V) septal defects are present in each type of fully displayed form, whereas they are never associated in the same heart in any incompletely displayed form.

### Incompletely Displayed Forms

Incompletely displayed forms of the anomaly may result in isolated cleft formation in the anterior (aortic) leaflet of the mitral valve (M), isolated inlet ventricular septal defect (V), isolated atrial septal defect of the ostium primum type (O), or combination inlet ventricular septal defect and cleft mitral valve (VM), and so on. These forms of incompletely displayed AV canal septal defect are best classified with mitral valve deformities, atrial septal defects, or ventricular septal defect, whichever best pertains, and can be found in those respective chapters. This chapter discusses the fully displayed AV canal defect, an anomaly that includes a central septal defect that involves both the ostium primum area of the atrial septum and the basal portion of the ventricular septum. This concept is important for clear appreciation of the anatomic and surgical aspects of this anomaly.

■ **Table 37–1.** THEORETICALLY POSSIBLE FORMS OF ATRIOVENTRICULAR CANAL DEFECT

I. Fully displayed AV canal septal defect (both ostium primum [O] and ventricular [V] septal defects are present)
   1. OVMT
   2. OVM
   3. OVT
   4. OV

II. Incompletely displayed AV canal septal defect (O and V are not present together)
   A. Septal defect is present
      1. VMT
      2. OMT
      3. VM
      4. VT
      5. OM
      6. OT
      7. V
      8. O
   B. No septal defect is present
      1. MT
      2. M
      3. T

*Key*: O = ostium primum atrial septal defect; V = basal (inlet) ventricular septal defect; M = typical mitral defect (cleft of anterior leaflet); T = typical tricuspid defect (cleft or partial absence of septal leaflet).

## Fully Displayed Forms

It has been helpful from the surgical point of view to separate the fully displayed AV canal deformities into three types: partial, intermediate, and complete.

### *Partial AV Canal* (Fig. 37–1)

In this type of deformity, there is a centrally located septal defect with both involvement of the ostium primum area of the atrial septum and a deficiency ("scooping out") in the base of the ventricular septum. The distinctive feature of partial AV canal is that the valvular leaflet tissue superadjacent to the ventricular septum has become fused to the underlying crest of the ventricular septum. This fusion prevents a direct interventricular communication deep to the leaflets, the hallmark of the partial AV canal anomaly. In addition, there is almost always a cleft in the anterior (aortic) leaflet of the mitral valve, and most hearts (85%) show incomplete development of the septal leaflet of the tricuspid valve, particularly in its anterior portion. The deficiency of the basal (inlet) portion of the ventricular septum in partial AV canal defect gives an elongated appearance ("gooseneck") to the outflow tract of the left ventricle (Baron, 1968; Rastelli et al., 1967). The issue of deficiency at the base of the ventricular septum has relevance to the surgeon, particularly if it contributes to subaortic stenosis or if valvular replacement is required, as discussed later.

### *Intermediate AV Canal*

Intermediate AV canal is the rarest of the three types of fully displayed AV canal. Widely varying features have been placed in this category by various authors (Bharati et al., 1980b). In the authors' usage, it is characterized by two features, one of which it has in common with the partial form of AV canal, and one it has in common with the complete form. In the intermediate form, distinct mitral and tricuspid valvular orifices have formed through embryonic fusion between the anterior and the posterior common leaflets of the common AV valve at their centers, just as in partial AV canal. However, as opposed to partial AV canal, this centrally connected leaflet tissue does not fully fuse with the underlying crest of the ventricular septum, allowing a direct interventricular communication, as in the complete form of AV canal. Other authors use a more liberal definition for the intermediate designation, and include hearts that have any of various atypical features of the three basic types (partial, intermediate, and complete) of fully displayed AV canal.

### *Complete AV Canal* (Fig. 37–2)

This type of fully displayed AV canal is characterized by failure of the common leaflets of the common AV valvular orifice to fuse to each other centrally to form two separate mitral and tricuspid orifices. The anterior and posterior common leaflets also are not fused with the crest of the underlying ventricular septum, allowing a direct interventricular communication.

### *Subtypes of Complete AV Canal*

Complete AV canal anomalies were subclassified into three types according to the configuration of the anterior common leaflet of the common AV valve by Rastelli and associates (1966). In Type A (Fig. 37–2A), the anterior common leaflet has a natural division between its mitral and its tricuspid components. There are also chordal attachments from the margins of this division to the crest of the underlying ventricular septum. Approximately 80% of patients with complete AV canal belong to this group. In Type B (Fig. 37–2B), the anterior common leaflet is partially divided but is not attached by chordae directly to the crest of the underlying ventricular septum; instead, the edges of the division are attached by chordae to an abnormal papillary muscle that arises in the right ventricle near the apical portion of the ventricular septum. This form of complete AV canal is rare. In Type C (Fig. 37–2C), the anterior common leaflet is undivided and appears as a single continuous leaflet that floats freely over the crest of the underlying

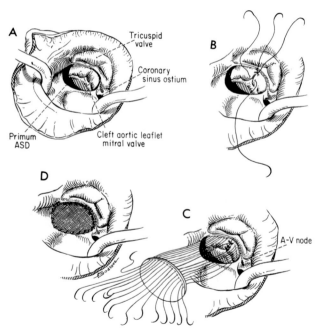

**FIGURE 37–1.** Partial atrioventricular (AV) canal. *A,* Surgical exposure, optimized by long atriotomy from the apex of the appendage to near the inferior caval orifice, and wide mobilization of venous cannulas. (ASD = atrial septal defect.) *B,* Beginning closure of the cleft in the anterior (aortic) mitral leaflet. *C,* Sutures placed between the patch and the mitral valve tissue 1 to 2 mm to the left of the junction of the mitral and the tricuspid valves for closure of the ostium primum atrial septal defect (see also Fig. 37–3). *D,* Repair completed. (*A–D,* From Danielson, G. K.: Endocardial cushion defects. *In* Ravitch, M. M., Welch, K. J., Benson, C. D., et al. [eds]: Pediatric Surgery. 3rd ed. Vol. 1. Copyright © 1979 by Year Book Medical Publishers, Inc., Chicago.)

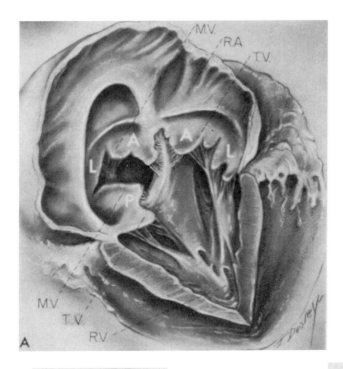

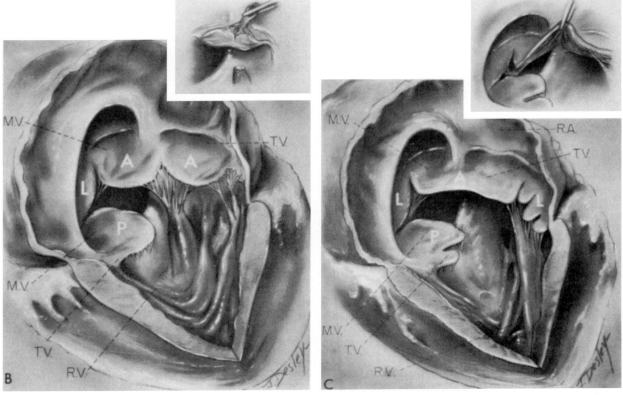

**FIGURE 37–2.** Rastelli classification of complete AV canal. The three types of complete AV canal. *A*, Type A. Anterior common leaflet (A) divided and attached to the crest of the ventricular septum (M.V. = mitral valve; R.A. = right atrium; T.V. = tricuspid valve; P = posterior common leaflet; L = lateral leaflet; R.V. = right ventricle). *B*, Type B. Anterior common leaflet partially divided, with chordae from the central area of the leaflet attached to a single abnormal papillary muscle arising from the right ventricle. *C*, Type C. Anterior common leaflet is undivided and is not attached to the ventricular septum. The insets in *B* and *C* show the extent of the interventricular communication deep to the common anterior leaflet. Note that the ventricular septum below the valvular attachment approximates the position of the anterior rim of the atrial septal defect above the leaflet. Thus, the surgical incision to be made in the common anterior leaflet (see surgical technique) will be made to this area at the base of the common anterior leaflet. (*A–C*, From Rastelli, G. C., Kirklin, J. W., and Titus, J. L.: Anatomic observations on complete form of persistent common atrioventricular canal with special reference to atrioventricular valves. Mayo Cin. Proc., *41*:296, 1966.)

ventricular septum, to which it is not attached. The chordal attachments of the leaflet at its right and left margins are to papillary muscles on the free wall of the right and left ventricles. Down's syndrome and associated cardiac anomalies, especially pulmonary stenosis, are more common in Type C complete AV canal.

No consistent relationship exists between the con-figurations of the anterior and posterior common leaflets. The attachment of the posterior common leaflet to the underlying ventricular septum can vary from sparse chordae to an imperforate membrane, and the division between mitral and tricuspid portions is variable.

Further studies by multiple workers, including important contributions from Piccoli and co-workers

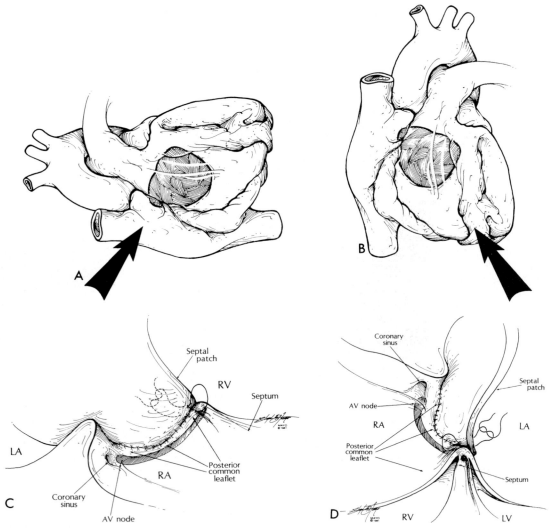

**FIGURE 37–3.** Detail of the positioning and suturing of the septal patch posteroinferiorly (posterocaudally) in partial AV canal. *A* and *B* provide orientation for the points of view of *C* and *D*, respectively. The viewpoint shown in *A* and *C* is that of the surgeon at the operating table, whereas the viewpoint in *B* and *D* is a hypothetical one, as though the viewer were positioned anteroapically within the right ventricle (RV). The central structure shown in *A* and *B* designates the position within the heart of the septal defect typical of the AV canal anomaly. In *C* and *D*, the dark structure coursing along the crest of the ventricular septum, commencing at the AV node, is the bundle of His; its branches are not shown except in *D*, where part of the left bundle branch complex is seen in the cross-section of the ventricular septum. *C* and *D* show only the posterior aspect of the anomaly, the remainder of the heart having been "cut away" by the artist in *C*, a transverse plane just superior to the level of the coronary sinus orifice, with the "cut" slicing through the posterior atrial wall and septum; and *D*, in a coronal plane located toward the posterior part of the ventricular septum, with the "cut" slicing through the posterior common leaflet and through the septal patch. (RA = right atrium; LA = left atrium; LV = left ventricle.)

The patch is attached anteriorly (toward the right in both *C* and *D*) to the line of junction of the mitral and the tricuspid components of the posterior common leaflet, which is fused to the underlying crest of the ventricular septum. As the suturing progresses posteriorly, the line of attachment of the patch is deviated to the left, onto the base of the mitral component of the leaflet; still farther posteriorly after crossing the mitral annulus, the patch attachment remains to the left, away from the conduction tissue and to the left of the rim of the ASD. This provides the widest possible separation between the suture line and the AV node and penetrating portions of the conduction bundle. All sutures shown are placed before lowering the patch into position, allowing optimal exposure for suture placement. (*A–D*, Copyright by Mayo Foundation.)

(1979), have increased understanding of the anatomy of complete AV canal. The divisions in the anterior common leaflet in Rastelli's classification are now recognized as commissures, and the concept of leaflets bridging the ventricular septum is accepted. However, in the authors' surgical experience, the Rastelli classification is still useful in describing this anomaly and in aiding selection of the best techniques of repair, modified according to the individual variations that are common in congenital anomalies.

The location of the AV conduction system in AV canal defects is important to the surgeon. In all types, complete, intermediate, or partial, there is posterior displacement of the AV node compared with its normal relationship to the ostium of the coronary sinus (Fig. 37–3; see also Figs. 37–1 and 37–6). There is also posterior displacement of the common bundle of His, which is intimately related to the posterior rim of the "scooped-out" basal portion of the ventricular septum.

## ANATOMIC TERMINOLOGY

**Anterior and Posterior.** In the normal heart, the septa are not in a true sagittal plane but are obliquely oriented, with the anterior margins to the left and the posterior margins to the right. At operation, when the atrium is opened and the anterior lip of the atriotomy is retracted to the left, the heart rotates and the anterior margins of the septa become situated even more to the left. The crest of the ventricular septum, as seen by the surgeon, appears to be more in the coronal plane than in the sagittal plane, so that which is called anterior becomes more strictly leftward, and vice versa.

**Anterior or Posterior Common Leaflet.** There is only one AV valve in complete AV canal. Anteriorly and posteriorly (called *superiorly* and *inferiorly* in some terminology) in such a valve are leaflets common to the left ventricular and right ventricular inlet orifices. These anterior and posterior common leaflets consist on the left side of tissue that would normally have been incorporated into the anterior leaflet (or *aortic leaflet* in some terminology) of the mitral valve, and on the right side of tissue that would have been incorporated into the septal leaflet of the tricuspid valve. In complete AV canal, this normal differentiation into mitral and tricuspid valves does not occur, and the leaflet tissue anteriorly and posteriorly remains part of the common AV valve. In Figure 37–2, the rudimentary components of the normal mitral valve are present; they consist of the lateral (L) leaflet (which would be called the *posterior* or *mural leaflet* of the normal mitral valve) and the left portion of the anterior common leaflet plus the left portion of the posterior common leaflet, which normally would have fused to form the anterior (*aortic* or *septal*) leaflet of the mitral valve.

Because the leaflet components that would have formed the mitral valve have failed to complete normal fusion, the valve does not have the usual appear-

ance of a mitral valve, and some authors prefer to use the term *left atrioventricular valve*. Similarly, the term *right atrioventricular* valve may be used synonymously with tricuspid valve in AV canal defects.

**Cleft, Division, or Incision.** A clear distinction should be made among the definitions of these three words. *Cleft* refers to the separation that partially persists between the anterior and the posterior components of the anterior leaflet of the mitral valve. The edges of the cleft are thickened where the leaflets meet in systole, and few or no chordae are attached to the cleft. The term *cleft* is best restricted to partial AV canal. A tricuspid counterpart of this cleft seldom exists. *Division* of the anterior common leaflet is found in Type A complete AV canal and refers to the naturally occurring separation, or division, between the mitral and the tricuspid components of the common anterior leaflet. As mentioned previously, this division is now considered a commissure. It may be necessary for the surgeon to make an *incision* in the anterior or posterior common leaflet to expose the underlying crest of the ventricular septum and to place a septal patch between the incised edges of the leaflet, especially in Type C (Figs. 37–4 and 37–5). *Division* therefore refers to a natural separation between the mitral and the tricuspid components of a common leaflet, and *incision* refers to a surgically created separation between the components.

## CLINICAL FEATURES

The partial form of AV canal was more commonly encountered than the complete form in earlier surgical experience, probably because of a greater mortality during infancy for babies born with a complete AV canal. Now that infants seriously ill with congenital heart disease are treated surgically, the complete form has become more commonly encountered.

The symptoms of AV canal are primarily related to increased pulmonary blood flow that results from the septal defect(s) and to the presence of mitral regurgitation that results from mitral deformity. Approximately two-thirds of patients with partial AV canal are asymptomatic at the time of operation, and only one-sixth of patients who are operated on have had severe symptoms, which include dyspnea, fatigue, and frank congestive heart failure. More than two-thirds of patients with complete AV canal have developed heart failure in the first few months of life. Patients with the partial form of AV canal are less likely to develop pulmonary hypertension or pulmonary vascular obstructive disease at any age, whereas in the complete form, pulmonary hypertension is present at birth, and progressive pulmonary vascular disease is common in infancy.

Physical examination shows a systolic ejection murmur at the pulmonary area due to increased flow across the pulmonary valve, and the second heart sound is split. Diastolic flow murmurs across one or both AV valves can be heard in many patients. A holosystolic apical murmur is often present, but the

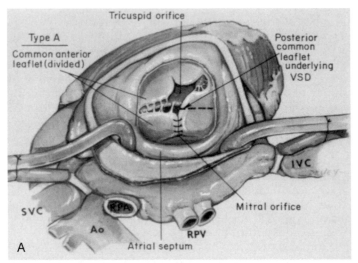

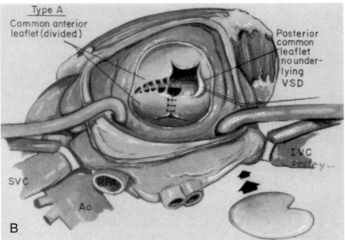

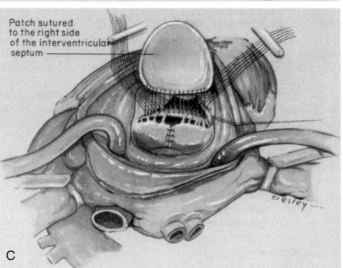

**FIGURE 37–4.** Repair of Type A complete AV canal. *A,* The anterior mitral leaflet has been constructed by approximating the edges of the mitral portions of the anterior and posterior common leaflets. The line for incision of the posterior common leaflet is identified by the *dashed line. B,* In this case, most of the posterior common leaflet is fused to the crest of the ventricular septum, and there is no need to incise the posterior common leaflet; the appropriately shaped patch (bottom right) can be attached to the atrial surface of the posterior common leaflet. *C,* The prosthetic patch is sewn to the right aspect of the ventricular septum with interrupted or pledgeted mattress sutures (see Fig. 37–6 for further detail).

intensity depends on the degree of associated mitral regurgitation.

The vectorcardiogram helps to confirm the diagnosis, because a counterclockwise frontal loop is almost present (Toscano-Barbosa et al., 1956); however, such a configuration may exist in other forms of congenital heart disease. Cardiac catheterization and angiography document the presence and magnitude of intracardiac shunting, help to define the degree of mitral regurgitation, show the classic "gooseneck" configuration of the left ventricular outflow tract (Baron, 1968; Rastelli et al., 1967), and demonstrate the rela-

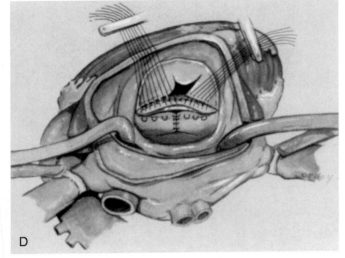

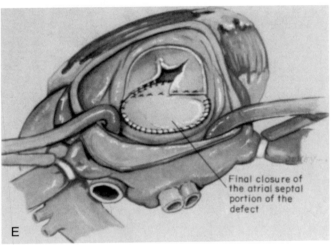

Final closure of the atrial septal portion of the defect

FIGURE 37–4 *Continued D,* The reconstructed anterior leaflet of the mitral valve is attached to the prosthetic patch with interrupted nonabsorbable mattress sutures in the same plane as the annulus of the AV valve. In this case, where the posterior common leaflet was incised, both edges of this incision (tricuspid and mitral) are attached to the respective surface of the patch. The authors usually prefer to use pledgets in these mattress sutures. *E,* The repair is completed by continuous suture approximation to the rim of the atrial septal defect. (SVC = superior vena cava; IVC = inferior vena cava; Ao = aorta; RPA = right pulmonary artery; VSD = ventricular septal defect; RPV = right pulmonary vein.) (*A–E,* From McMullan, M. H., Wallace, R. B., Weidman, W. H., and McGoon, D. C.: Surgical treatment of complete atrioventricular canal. Surgery, *72:*905, 1972.)

tive sizes of the right and left ventricles (balanced or unbalanced ventricles). The echocardiographic display of these lesions in the two-dimensional mode helps distinguish between the complete and the partial forms, assess relative ventricular sizes, and define the anatomic details of the subgroups that are not commonly shown by angiocardiography alone. Doppler echocardiography and color-flow imaging allow excellent assessment of left-to-right shunt flow and of the site and degree of AV valve regurgitation (Reeder et al., 1986).

## INDICATIONS FOR OPERATION

The guidelines for selecting patients for operation in AV canal anomaly are similar to those for patients who have any type of congenital anomaly that increases pulmonary blood flow (Berger et al., 1979). For the symptomatic infant with partial AV canal, the current safety of operation in infancy makes it possible and preferable to operate at whatever age the symptoms develop. For the asymptomatic infant with partial AV canal, elective repair is advised before the

age of 2 to 4 years. Operation is indicated on the basis of the relatively low anticipated hospital mortality for elective correction of partial AV canal (1 to 2%) and on the basis that progressive disability and cardiac failure are common during the second decade of life.

Most infants who have the complete form of AV canal and congestive heart failure respond poorly to medical treatment; early operation is indicated for those infants. Operation is recommended for all patients with complete AV canal by 4 to 6 months of age in order to prevent pulmonary vascular obstructive disease. Irreversible vascular disease has been documented by 4 to 6 months of age, especially in patients with Down's syndrome (Freedom and Smallhorn, 1992; Yamaki et al., 1993).

For surgical teams skilled both in the repair of AV canal defects and in cardiac surgery for infants, correction rather than palliation (pulmonary artery banding) is preferred, and contemporary surgical results support this position (Freedom and Smallhorn, 1992; Gallucci et al., 1986; Hanley et al., 1993; LeBlanc et al., 1986; Studer et al., 1982). Operative mortality in the first 3 months of age can be as low as 5 to 10%, with generally very good results, although a few

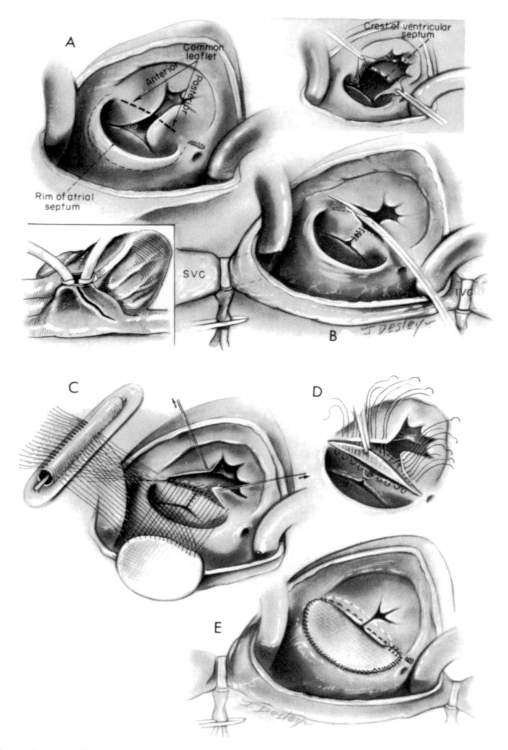

**FIGURE 37–5.** Surgical repair of Type C complete AV canal. *A, Heavy broken line* indicates line of incision of the common AV leaflets. *B,* Incisions are accomplished. *C–E,* The remainder of the repair is similar to that shown in Figure 37–4, except (as seen in *D* and *E*) both the tricuspid and the mitral edges of the incised anterior common leaflet are sutured to the respective sides of the patch. Currently, mattress sutures over felt pledgets are preferred to simple sutures. (*A–E,* From Rastelli, G. C., Ongley, P. A., and McGoon, D. C.: Surgical repair of complete atrioventricular canal with anterior common leaflet undivided and unattached to ventricular septum. Mayo Clin. Proc., *44:*335, 1969.)

patients require further operation to address residual shunts or mitral regurgitation. Alternatively, if surgical repair is not possible for some reason, pulmonary artery banding may be used as an initial operation, followed by debanding and complete repair at a later age.

## OPERATIVE TECHNIQUE

Operation for both the partial and the complete types of AV canal is performed through a median sternotomy and with hypothermic cardiopulmonary bypass. The ascending aorta is cannulated, and both caval lines are either passed through the right atrial appendage so that they can be widely mobilized by the atriotomy to provide optimal intra-atrial exposure or placed directly into each cava via right-angle connectors. Standard techniques of whole-body perfusion are maintained, including use of a slotted-needle air vent in the ascending aorta. The authors prefer moderate hypothermia (25° C) and low flows, as needed, rather than profound hypothermia and circulatory arrest to minimize air embolism and other cerebral problems. Cold blood potassium cardioplegia, supplemented with topical hypothermia, is used for myocardial protection.

### Partial AV Canal

Repair of partial AV canal has two principal objectives: alignment and approximation of the edges of the cleft in the anterior leaflet of the mitral valve and closure of the atrial septal defect with a patch (see Fig. 37–1). Distortion of the mitral leaflet is avoided by suturing the cleft in an alignment that is the same as that during systolic closure of the valve; saline solution is injected into the left ventricle to elevate the leaflets and show the line of closure. Thickened ridges are typically present along the edges of the cleft and are usually identical in length as a result of closure of these edges against each other during systole. A simple suture is first placed to approximate the cleft near the mitral ring. This suture can also be used subsequently to anchor the center of the patch used for closure of the atrial septal defect. Then the thickened edges of the cleft at their farthest margin (closest to the free edge of the leaflet) are temporarily approximated with a traction suture. Chordae are usually absent along the edges of the cleft but are present on the free edge of both leaflet components; their presence can assist in alignment of the edges of the cleft. The first two sutures near the free edge of the leaflet are placed in an inverted manner, so the knots and "ears" are on the ventricular side where they will not injure the opposing surface of the mural leaflet. The first suture can be placed in a mattress style over small pericardial or felt pledgets for additional security of closure. Finally, the intervening sutures are placed.

In the past, if incompetence was minimal or absent before operation, the cleft was often not closed. The authors observed that mitral insufficiency developed later in some of these patients, and now prefer to close the cleft routinely. The authors have not found that mitral stenosis results from accurate repair of the mitral cleft. It is not the authors' practice to transect chordae of the mitral valve, including those attached to the ventricular septum, nor is tissue added to the mitral leaflet in the form of a patch of pericardium or synthetic material. Preoperative mitral regurgitation is usually caused by incomplete closure of the cleft in the mitral valve during systole, and repair of the cleft is effective in reducing or obliterating the regurgitation. In some patients, annular dilatation or, rarely, a deficiency of leaflet length from base to free edge allows regurgitation through the central portion of the valve during systole; this can be controlled by a double purse-string annuloplasty around the free wall of the left ventricle, which reduces the circumference of the valve. Competence of the valve is tested by distending the ventricle with saline solution so that refinements of the repair can be effected as indicated. It is almost never necessary to replace the mitral valve at the time of primary repair.

The interatrial communication is closed by a patch of pericardium that is attached to the mitral side of the junction of the mitral and tricuspid valves along the crest of the ventricular septum with interrupted sutures that are all placed before the patch is lowered into position (see Fig. 37–1). As suture placement continues toward the posterior (right) end of the crest of the ventricular septum, care must be taken to avoid injury to the bundle of His. This is accomplished by carrying the suture line 1 to 2 mm onto the base of the mitral valve leaflet (see Fig. 37–3). Delineation of the line of separation between the right and the left atria along the posterior margin of the defect is facilitated by exerting traction on a suture placed for that purpose in the atrial septal rim of the ostium primum defect. The traction creates a small ridge that demarcates the right atrium from the left atrium. Sutures anchoring the patch should be placed on the left atrial side of that ridge until the suture line reaches the clearly defined septal rim of the ostium primum defect. The cephalad margin of the patch can then be attached to the rim of the atrial septal defect with continuous sutures. This technique precludes the need to carry the suture line to the right of the conduction system, as is required for repair of complete AV canal defects.

### Intermediate AV Canal

If the anatomy permits, two septal patches are placed, one to close the interventricular communication and one to close the interatrial communication. The two patches are separated from each other along their adjacent edges by the midline fused tricuspid and mitral leaflet tissue, but are sutured to each other by stitches that pass through this leaflet substance. More often, exposure of the ventricular septum is inadequate, necessitating transverse division of the fused tissue so that the anterior and posterior common leaflets can be reflected upward. Repair is then carried out as for complete AV canal using either the one-patch or the two-patch technique.

## Complete AV Canal

In the classic, one-patch technique, the first step in the repair of complete AV canal is to identify its anatomic characteristics. After the anatomy of the anterior and posterior common leaflets has been determined and the extent of the underlying interventricular communication has been defined, two or three sutures are placed to approximate the mitral components of the anterior and posterior common leaflets so as to constitute an anterior (or aortic) leaflet of the mitral valve (see Fig. 37–4A). As in partial AV canal, the objective is to avoid distortion of the mitral leaflet tissue as much as possible and to reconstruct the valve in the alignment it would assume during sys-

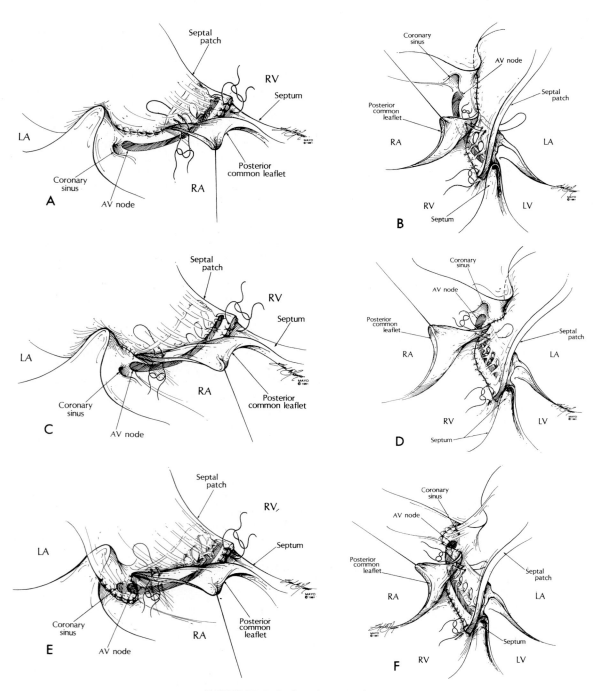

**FIGURE 37–6.** *See legend on opposite page*

tole in the preoperative state. Again, this alignment is often best determined by floating the leaflets into their closed position by instilling saline solution under pressure into the left ventricular cavity. Typically, there are no thickened ridges along the opposing edges of the anterior and posterior components of the anterior mitral leaflet that would correspond to the cleft of the anterior leaflet in the partial form of the defect; this makes it somewhat more difficult to obtain the appropriate alignment of the mitral valve in the complete form. Commissural or central leaks found when the valve is tested are repaired by commissural annuloplasty sutures or double free-wall purse-string sutures, respectively. As noted for repair of partial AV canal, valve replacement at the initial operation is rarely required.

The next step in the one-patch repair is to expose the entire length of the crest of the ventricular septal rim of the interventricular communication. In Type A complete AV canal, the natural division in the anterior common leaflet has already exposed most of the underlying ventricular crest (see Fig. 37–4). In the Type C variant, it is necessary to incise the anterior common leaflet along a line estimated to demarcate the tricuspid from the mitral components of the anterior common leaflet (see Fig. 37–5A and B). The proper site along the free edge for this incision is defined by the line of convergence of chordae from the papillary muscle of the left ventricle with those from the papillary muscle of the right ventricle. The location of the annular end of the incision in the common leaflet is established by the position of the underlying ventricular septum where it joins the annulus of the AV valve. When there is doubt, the authors prefer to err on the side of placing the incision more to the tricuspid aspect than to the mitral aspect of the anterior common leaflet, which is more likely to preserve adequate leaflet area for mitral function. The authors do not agree with the suggestion to incise the common

leaflet far to the tricuspid side in a place remote from the underlying ventricular septum.

In the Type A deformity in which the division of the anterior leaflet is incomplete and in most cases of the Type B deformity (Pacifico and Kirklin, 1973), it is necessary to extend the division in the anterior common leaflet by incising the remaining intact bridging portion of the leaflet all the way to the annulus of the AV valve. A similar incision in the posterior common leaflet is almost always required but extends from the free margin of the leaflet only to the posterior limit of the underlying interventricular communication. Often, this interventricular communication does not reach the true annulus of the AV valve because there is a variable length of fibrous fusion of the base of the posterior common leaflet to the crest of the ventricular septum (Fig. 37–6A and B; see also Fig. 37–4B). The latter is a favorable situation because it provides a buffer area of intact fibrous septum that protects the conduction bundle from the suture line.

The next step is to close the cardiac septum with a patch of knitted synthetic material. The distance from the anterior to the posterior aspect of the annulus of the AV canal—that is, the anteroposterior dimension of the septal defect—is measured and a slightly shorter length is marked off on the patch. It is important not to overestimate the anteroposterior dimension because that would enlarge the circumferences of the AV valve annuli and decrease the possibility of constructing competent valves. The other dimension of the patch is left longer than the apparent distance from the atrial septal rim to the ventricular septal rim of the defect, and is trimmed later to appropriate length. The edge of the patch that will be approximated to the crest of the ventricular septum is then attached with a row of interrupted sutures, which are placed before lowering the patch into position (Figs. 37–4C and 37–5C). The authors

FIGURE 37–6. Detail for anchoring septal patch posterointeriorly in complete AV canal and for reconstructing posterior common leaflet. The view for A, C, and E corresponds to the orientation described for Fig. 37–3A, and that for B, D, and F corresponds to the orientation described for Fig. 37–3B. Illustrated in A and B is the repair used for hearts in which the basilar (or annular) portion of the posterior common leaflet is fused to the underlying ventricular septum by a sheet of fibrous tissue; C and D, and E and F show alternatives for repair where no such fusion has occurred. In both situations, the posterior common leaflet has been incised beginning at its free margin (at the estimated point of junction of its tricuspid and mitral portions) to the posterior limit of any interventricular communication below the valve. In A and B, the incision extends only part way to the annulus, and in C–F, it extends essentially to the annulus. In A and B, the septal patch is attached to the right surface of the ventricular septal crest where the leaflet has been incised, but continuing posteriorly, the suture line then passes along the edge of the fibrous tissue fusing leaflet to septum until it reaches the apex of the incision in the leaflet. The suturing posteriorly from this point proceeds exactly as for partial AV canal, which is described in Fig. 37–3. In reality, all the sutures shown are placed before lowering the patch into position, as in Figs. 37–4C and 37–5C.

In C and D, which was the original technique, the incision in the posterior common leaflet extends posteriorly to the junction of atrium, ventricular septum, and annulus; the patch is again attached along the right surface of the ventricular septal crest, and the sutures become even more superficial and more closely spaced as work proceeds posteriorly. The suture at the apex of the leaflet incision (not shown) grasps only leaflet tissue near the annulus but does not penetrate the annulus; the suture line remains superficial as it crosses right to left to reach the left surface of the rim of the atrial septum, as in Fig. 37–3.

The authors' currently preferred method is shown in E and F, in which the patch is placed entirely to the right of the conduction tissue: The incision in the posterior common leaflet is carried to the right of the plane of the ventricular septum to reach the annulus to the right of the junction of the annulus and ventricular septum, where the conduction tissue lies. The atrial part of the patch, which is cut with an auricular extension, is attached around the right side of the coronary sinus so that it drains into the left atrium. An alternative would be to attach the patch along the inferior lip of the ostium, allowing the coronary sinus to drain to the right atrium. (A–F, Copyright by Mayo Foundation.)

currently prefer to use mattress sutures through pledgets that pass into the right aspect of the ventricular septum below its crest. Care is taken posteriorly to avoid encirclement of the nonbranching and penetrating portions of the conduction tissue.

Where the posterior limit of the interventricular communication is sealed off by a membrane between the ventricular septum and the overlying leaflet, the incision in the posterior common leaflet is extended posteriorly only to the limit of the interventricular communication (see Fig. 37–6A and B). From this point on, in a posterosuperior direction, the patch is sutured to the atrial surface of the posterior common leaflet, then to the posterior atrial wall as far to the left as possible, and finally to the atrial septum (see Fig. 37–6A and B) in the same manner as for repair of partial AV canal described earlier (see Fig. 37–3C and D).

In hearts in which the interventricular communication (or perforating communications) extends all the way to the posterior valvular annulus (see Fig. 37–6C–F), there are two options for placement of the patch to achieve the least risk of heart block. Formerly, the incision was carried in the posterior common leaflet directly to the junction of ventricular septum and AV valvular annulus, with the intent of placing sutures for the patch superficially and close together in this area (see Fig. 37–6C and D). The authors now prefer to carry the incision in the posterior common leaflet toward the annulus to the right of the plane of the ventricular septum, so that the patch crosses the annulus to the right of the junction of annulus and ventricular septum and thus to the right of the conduction tissue (see Fig. 37–6E and F). The atrial part of the patch, which is cut with an auricular extension, is attached around the right side of the coronary sinus so that it drains into the left atrium (Thiene et al., 1981).

The next step is to anchor the incised edges of the mitral and tricuspid components of the anterior and posterior common leaflets to their respective left and right sides of the prosthetic septal patch. This is done with a single row of interrupted mattress sutures (see Figs. 37–4D and 37–5D). These sutures may be buttressed by fine pericardial or felt pledgets, especially in infants, in whom the valve tissues are thin and friable. This attachment of the mitral and tricuspid leaflets should be at a level on the patch that corresponds to the ideal plane of the orifice of the mitral and tricuspid valves, that is, the plane to which the leaflets reach during systole when their retaining chordae are fully stretched (this is also the same plane as the annulus of the common AV valve). For the Type A deformity, the authors attach the mitral but not the corresponding tricuspid edge of the naturally divided anterior common leaflet to the patch (see Fig. 37–4D and E). There is a complete deficiency of the anterior portion of the septal leaflet of the tricuspid valve in the Type A deformity (which corresponds to the usual situation in partial AV canal). Tricuspid regurgitation does not typically occur, despite this deficiency. In Type C deformity, the incised edges of

both the tricuspid and the mitral components of the anterior and posterior common leaflets are attached to the patch (see Fig. 37–5D and E). The tricuspid valve is tested by injecting saline solution into the right ventricle in a manner similar to that used in testing of the mitral valve.

The final step of the repair is the attachment of the cephalad edge of the septal patch to the rim of the atrial septal defect with a continuous suture (see Figs. 37–4E and 37–5E).

Another excellent method for repair of complete AV canal, which was used in some of the earlier operations and is now gaining popularity, is the two-patch technique (Levy et al., 1964; Studer et al., 1982). The authors have also used this technique successfully and find it especially appropriate for infants because it may minimize shortening of the reconstructed valve leaflets and decrease the chance for dehiscence of the delicate valve tissue from the prosthetic patch. A Dacron or Teflon patch is used to close the ventricular septal defect, and the atrial patch is made from autologous pericardium.

A trifoliate repair of the mitral (left AV) valve has been advocated in which the anterior and posterior portions of the bridging leaflets are not approximated by sutures (Carpentier and Chauvaud, 1988). Although this gives satisfactory results in many cases, the authors and others (Starr, 1982) have observed that this repair may be associated with an increased incidence of reoperation for mitral insufficiency. Whether this problem represents lack of understanding of the procedure recommended or is inherent in the concept must still be determined. Leaving the anterior and posterior portions of the bridging leaflet unsutured may be analogous to leaving the cleft of the anterior leaflet of the mitral valve of partial AV canal unsutured, which can cause late mitral insufficiency. In any event, the area of apposition of the mitral components of the common anterior and posterior leaflets is a weak point, and this area must be made completely competent at the time of initial repair. Late (10- to 20-year) results of the trifoliate repair are awaited.

After completion of the repair in both the partial and the complete forms, the right atriotomy is closed, air is evacuated from the heart, continous aspiration is applied to a slotted-needle vent in the ascending aorta, and extracorporeal circulation is gradually discontinued.

For many years, the authors have used double-sampling dye curves to assess competence of the reconstructed mitral valve (Danielson, 1984); this is an excellent method for quantitating the amount of mitral insufficiency. More recently, intraoperative transesophageal echocardiography has provided semi-quantitative estimates of valvular insufficiency and additionally has supplied important information regarding function of the valve (leaflet motion, stenosis, location of regurgitant jets), completeness of closure of the atrial and ventricular septa, ventricular function, and left ventricular outflow tract anatomy (O'Leary et al., 1995). The authors believe that intraoperative transesophageal echocardiographic evaluation of the repair is an important part of all operations for AV canal defects.

The postoperative care of these patients is similar to that of other patients who have had repair of other forms of complex congenital cardiac defects. Arterial pressure and right and (when indicated) left atrial pressures are monitored continuously for the first few days after operation. For partial AV canal, the postoperative course is typically uncomplicated. When a complication occurs, it is usually an arrhythmia of supraventricular type or reduced cardiac output, which may be exacerbated by the presence of residual mitral regurgitation. For complete AV canal, the same considerations pertain, but there is an additional potential complication of pulmonary hypertensive crisis caused by a sudden increase in pulmonary vascular resistance. This produces severe pulmonary hypertension, reduced cardiac output, and systemic hypotension. Hypertensive crises are managed by sedation of the patient, hyperventilation with a high inspired oxygen concentration, maintenance of an alkaline pH, and use of pulmonary vasodilators, especially (most recently) controlled low concentrations of nitric oxide. The incidence of heart block has been low (1 to 3%) with use of the intraoperative precautions (King et al., 1986a; McMullan et al., 1972; Studer et al., 1982).

The difficult surgical treatment of AV canal defect associated with anomalies such as tetralogy of Fallot and other conotruncal malformations has been increasingly successful (Bharati et al., 1980a; Pacifico et al., 1980; Sridaromont et al., 1975; Thiene et al., 1979; Uretzky et al., 1984; Vargas et al., 1986). Surgeons are also having increasing success with repair of AV canal anomalies combined with double-orifice mitral valve, common ventricle, atrial isomerism, AV discordance, and anomalies of cardiac situs and systemic and pulmonary venous return (Danielson, 1984; Lee et al., 1985; Pacifico et al., 1988).

## MITRAL VALVE REPLACEMENT

When it is decided that mitral valve replacement is required, whether at the initial (rarely) or at the subsequent operation, an important anatomic feature bears reemphasis: A deficiency of the basilar portion of the ventricular septum exists in both partial and complete AV canal lesions, and the patch that is placed to close the septal defect has a ventricular septal portion as well as an atrial septal portion. Stated differently, the plane of the mitral annulus lies at a level that does not follow the crest of the ventricular septum; rather, it crosses the patch at a level that centrally on the patch is about 1 or 2 cm superior (or atrialward) from the crest of the scooped-out portion of the ventricular septum. This is the same level that is represented by the superior aspect of the ventricular septal defect patch of a two-patch repair. The mitral valve prosthesis should be secured to the mural aspect of the mitral annulus as always, but on the septal aspect, the line of attachment follows the left

surface of the septal patch corresponding to the true plane of the mitral orifice. Because the bundle of His courses along the ventricular septal crest, the only area in which the bundle of His is vulnerable in this technique is at the junction of the posterior annulus and the septal patch; suturing in this area should be done superficially or in the leaflet remnant.

Left-sided obstructive lesions are common in AV canal anomalies (Piccoli et al., 1982), and the left ventricular outflow tract is typically long and narrow in both the partial and the complete forms. Left ventricular outflow tract obstruction can become a significant problem at the time of repair of AV canal defects or at any later time, requiring additional operations of varying complexity to relieve the subaortic stenosis (DeLeon et al., 1991; Reeder et al., 1992). When mitral valve replacement is required, the prosthetic valve may further narrow the left ventricular outflow tract and obstruct blood flow, produce ventricular arrhythmias by impingement on the ventricular septum, or malfunction from restriction of poppet or disk motion; accordingly, low-profile valve prostheses are preferred. These risks are increased if the prosthesis is attached too high on the septal patch.

## RESULT OF OPERATION

An important factor in the early and late results of repair of partial or complete AV canal deformities is the degree of residual mitral valve regurgitation. In the authors' experience, intraoperative postrepair double-sampling dye dilution studies showed absent or trivial mitral regurgitation in 67% of patients, mild mitral regurgitation (less than 15% regurgitant fraction) in 23%, and moderate regurgitation (15 to 25%) in 6% of patients. Five per cent of patients were left with severe mitral insufficiency (greater than 25%), all early in the series. The overall incidence of reoperation for severe mitral regurgitation is less than 1% per year, but appears to be slightly higher for infants, possibly because valve deformity may be more severe in the infant group. As expected, actuarial freedom from reoperation is predicted by the degree of postrepair mitral regurgitation (Hanley et al., 1993; King et al., 1986a).

In the authors' entire early experience with repair of partial AV canal, the hospital mortality rate was 5.5% (King et al., 1986a). Mortality is now lower with more frequent operation for infants and children who are diagnosed or become symptomatic early in life, and is currently 1 to 2% for those patients without other significant risk factors. Repair of partial AV canal in 52 adults up to 75 years of age (average age, 37 years) has been performed with a 6% risk (Hynes et al., 1981). The actuarial freedom from reoperation is 86% at 20 years, and the incidence of late deaths, which are usually related to arrhythmias or the necessity for mitral valve replacement, is a small fraction of 1% per year; actuarial survival is 96% at 20 years (King et al., 1986a). Most surviving patients with native valves are free of disability; approximately 25% show mild symptoms on strenuous exertion.

The results of operation for complete AV canal were unsatisfactory before current techniques of repair were developed (McGoon et al., 1959). Since the mid-1960s, the hospital mortality rate has progressively decreased from 60% to less than 10% (McMullan et al., 1972). As more patients in the infant age group were operated on, the mortality rate initially increased, but current mortality rate for infants is down to 5 to 10% at the authors' institution and elsewhere (Freedom and Smallhorn, 1992; Gallucci et al., 1986; Hanley et al., 1993; LeBlanc et al., 1986; Studer et al., 1982). Few data are available regarding actuarial survival of patients following repair of complete AV canal, but it is known that survival is decreased compared with that for partial AV canal, due in part to the presence of severe pulmonary vascular obstructive disease in some patients who underwent operation in the early experience. As in the case of partial AV canal, late mortality is also due to arrhythmias and the need for reoperation. In a review of 195 patients at the authors' institution, 10-year survival was 90%, and 78% of the patients were in New York Heart Association Class I or II (King et al., 1986b).

## SELECTED BIBLIOGRAPHY

Hanley, F. L., Fenton, K. N., Jonas, R. A., et al.: Surgical repair of complete atrioventricular canal defects in infancy. J. Thorac Cardiovasc. Surg., 106:387, 1993.

This is a contemporary review of a 20-year experience with 301 patients with complete atrioventricular (AV) canal who presented to the authors' institution. A comprehensive analysis was made of patient-related morphologic, procedure-related, and postoperative variables for associations with perioperative death and reoperation. Current surgical management is discussed.

Studer, M., Blackstone, E. H., Kirklin, J. W., et al.: Determinants of early and late results of repair of atrioventricular septal (canal) defects. J. Thorac. Cardiovasc. Surg., 84:523, 1982.

This report is a thorough review of a large series of patients with partial and complete AV canal who underwent surgical correction. Surgical methods, hospital mortality, risk factors, and late results are analyzed.

Thiene, G., Wenink, A. C. G., Frescura, C., et al.: The surgical anatomy and pathology of the conduction tissues in atrioventricular defects. J. Thorac. Cardiovasc. Surg., 82:928, 1981.

These authors examined in detail the hearts of 16 patients with AV defects and described their findings from the surgeon's viewpoint. Ten hearts had complete defects and 6 had partial ones, and the disposition of the conduction tissue was the same in both groups. The anatomy of the triangle of Koch was found to be distorted, and the authors defined a "nodal triangle" lying between the coronary sinus ostium and the annulus that contained the AV node. Techniques for avoiding injury to the node and bundle are suggested.

## BIBLIOGRAPHY

Baron, M. G.: Endocardial cushion defect. Radiol. Clin. North Am., 6:343, 1968.

Becker, A. E., and Anderson, R. H.: Atrioventricular septal defects: What's in a name? J. Thorac. Cardiovasc. Surg., 83:461, 1982.

Berger, T. J., Blackstone, E. H., Kirklin, J. W., et al.: Survival and probability of cure without and with operation in complete atrioventricular canal. Ann. Thorac. Surg., 27:104, 1979.

Bharati, S., Kirklin, J. W., McAllister, H. A., Jr., and Lev, M.: The surgical anatomy of common atrioventricular orifice associated with tetralogy of Fallot, double outlet right ventricle and complete regular transposition. Circulation, 61:1142, 1980a.

Bharati, S., Lev, M., McAllister, H. A., Jr., and Kirklin, J. W.: Surgical anatomy of the atrioventricular valve in the intermediate type of common atrioventricular orifice. J. Thorac. Cardiovasc. Surg., 79:884, 1980b.

Carpentier, A., and Chauvaud, S.: Repair of the mitral valve in atrioventricular defects. In Dunn, J. M. (ed): Cardiac Valve Disease in Children. New York, Elsevier Science, 1988, p. 254.

Danielson, G. K.: Repair of atrioventricular canal: The "classic" (one-patch) operative approach. In Moulton, A. L. (ed): Congenital Heart Surgery—Current Techniques and Controversies. Pasadena, CA, Appleton Davies, 1984, pp. 317–329.

DeLeon, S. Y., Ilbawi, M. N., Wilson, W. R., Jr., et al.: Surgical options in subaortic stenosis associated with endocardial cushion defects. Ann. Thorac. Surg., 52:1076, 1991.

Freedom, R. M., and Smallhorn, J. F.: Atrioventricular septal defect. In Freedom, R. M., Benson, L. N., and Smallhorn, J. F. (eds): Neonatal Heart Disease. London, Springer-Verlag, 1992, p. 611.

Gallucci, V., Mazzucco, A., Stellin, G., et al.: Repair of complete atrioventricular canal: 1975–1985. J. Cardiac Surg., 1:261, 1986.

Hanley, F. L., Fenton, K. N., Jonas, R. A., et al.: Surgical repair of complete atrioventricular canal defects in infancy. J. Thorac Cardiovasc. Surg., 106:387, 1993.

Hynes, J. K., Tajik, A. J., Seward, J. B., et al.: Partial atrioventricular canal defect in adults. Am. J. Cardiol., 47:466, 1981.

King, R. M., Puga, F. J., Danielson, G. K., et al.: Prognostic factors and surgical treatment of partial atrioventricular canal. Circulation, 74:42, 1986a.

King, R. M., Puga, F. J., Danielson, G. K., et al.: Prognostic factors in the surgical treatment of complete atrioventricular canal [Abstract]. Circulation, 74(Suppl. II):II-248, 1986b.

LeBlanc, J. G., Williams, W. G., Freedom, R. M., et al.: Results of total correction in complete atrioventricular septal defects with congenital or surgically induced right ventricular outflow tract obstruction. Ann. Thorac. Surg., 41:387, 1986.

Lee, C. N., Danielson, G. K., Schaff, H. V., et al.: Surgical treatment of double-orifice mitral valve in atrioventricular canal defects: Experience in 25 patients. J. Thorac. Cardiovasc. Surg., 90:700, 1985.

Levy, M. J., Cuello, L., Tuna, N., et al.: Atrioventricularis communis: Clinical aspects and surgical treatment. Am. J. Cardiol. 14:587, 1964.

McGoon, D. C., DuShane, J. W., and Kirklin, J. W.: The surgical treatment of endocardial cushion defects. Surgery, 46:185, 1959.

McMullan, M. H., Wallace, R. B., Weidman, W. H., and McGoon, D. C.: Surgical treatment of complete atrioventricular canal. Surgery, 72:905, 1972.

O'Leary, P. W., Hagler, D. J., Seward, J. B., et al.: Biplane intraoperative transesophageal echocardiography in congenital heart disease. Mayo Clin. Proc., 70:317, 1995.

Pacifico, A. D., and Kirklin, J. W.: Surgical repair of complete atrioventricular canal with anterior common leaflet attached to an anomalous right ventricular papillary muscle. J. Thorac. Cardiovasc. Surg., 65:727, 1973.

Pacifico, A. D., Kirklin, J. W., and Bargeron, L. M., Jr.: Repair of complete atrioventricular canal associated with tetralogy of Fallot or double outlet right ventricle: Report of 10 patients. Ann. Thorac. Surg., 29:351, 1980.

Pacifico, A. D., Ricchi, A., Bargeron, L. M., Jr., et al.: Corrective repair of complete atrioventricular canal defects and major associated cardiac anomalies. Ann. Thorac. Surg., 46:645, 1988.

Piccoli, G. P., Ho, S. Y., Wilkinson, J. L., et al.: Left-sided obstructive lesions in atrioventricular septal defects: An anatomical study. J. Thorac. Cardiovasc. Surg., 83:453, 1982.

Piccoli, G. P., Wilkinson, J. L., Macartney, F. J., et al.: Morphology and classification of complete atrioventricular defects. Br. Heart J., 42:633, 1979.

Rastelli, G. C., Kirklin, J. W., and Kincaid, O. W.: Angiocardiography of persistent common atrioventricular canal. Mayo Clin. Proc., 42:200, 1967.

Rastelli, G. C., Kirklin, J. W., and Titus, J. L.: Anatomic observations on complete form of persistent common atrioventricular canal with special reference to atrioventricular valves. Mayo Clin. Proc., *41*:296, 1966.

Reeder, G. S., Currie, P. J., Hagler, D. J., et al.: Use of Doppler techniques (continuous-wave, pulsed-wave, and color-flow imaging) in the noninvasive hemodynamic assessment of congenital heart disease. Mayo Clin. Proc., *61*:725, 1986.

Reeder, G. S., Danielson, G. K., Seward, J. B., et al.: Fixed subaortic stenosis in atrioventricular canal defect: A Doppler echocardiographic study. J. Am. Coll. Cardiol., *20*:386, 1992.

Sridaromont, S., Feldt, R. H., Ritter, D. C., et al.: Double-outlet right ventricle associated with persistent common atrioventricular canal. Circulation, *52*:933, 1975.

Starr, A.: Discussion of Bender H. W., Jr., Hammon, J. W., Jr., Hubbard, S. G., et al.: Repair of atrioventricular canal malformation in the first year of life. J. Thorac. Cardiovasc. Surg., *84*:515, 1982.

Studer, M., Blackstone, E. H., Kirklin, J. W., et al.: Determinants of early and late results of repair of atrioventricular septal (canal) defects. J. Thorac. Cardiovasc. Surg., 84:523, 1982.

Thiene, G., Frescura, C., Di Donato, R., and Gallucci, R.: Complete atrioventricular canal associated with conotruncal malformations: Anatomical observations in 13 specimens. Eur. J. Cardiol., *9*:199, 1979.

Thiene, G., Wenink, A. C. G., Frescura, C., et al.: The surgical anatomy and pathology of the conduction tissues in atrioventricular defects. J. Thorac. Cardiovasc. Surg., *82*:928, 1981.

Toscano-Barbosa, E., Brandenburg, R. O., and Burchell, H. B.: Electrocardiographic studies of cases with intracardiac malformations of the atrioventricular canal. Mayo Clin. Proc., *31*:513, 1956.

Uretzky, G., Puga, F. J., Danielson, G. K., et al.: Complete atrioventricular canal associated with tetralogy of Fallot: Morphologic and surgical considerations. J. Thorac. Cardiovasc. Surg., *87*:756, 1984.

Vargas, F. J., Otero Coto, E., Mayer, J. E., Jr., et al.: Complete atrioventricular canal and tetralogy of Fallot: Surgical considerations. Ann. Thorac. Surg., *42*:258, 1986.

Yamaki, S., Yasui, H., Kado, H., et al.: Pulmonary vascular disease and operative indications in complete atrioventricular canal defect in early infancy. J. Thorac. Cardiovasc. Surg., *106*:398, 1993.

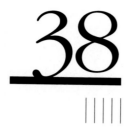

# 38 Surgical Treatment of Ventricular Septal Defect

A. D. Pacifico and James K. Kirklin

A ventricular septal defect (VSD) is a hole in the interventricular septum that can occur as a primary anomaly with or without additional major associated cardiac defects. A VSD may occur as a single component of a wide variety of intracardiac anomalies that include the tetralogy of Fallot, complete atrioventricular canal defects, transposition of the great arteries, corrected transposition, and other anomalies. The defect in its isolated form is considered in this chapter.

## HISTORICAL ASPECTS

A VSD was first repaired in 1954 by Lillehei and associates (1955) at the University of Minnesota. They described an experience with eight patients, five in their first year of life, who had VSD closure by using controlled cross-circulation with an adult as the pump oxygenator. Cardiac ischemia was avoided because the aorta was not cross-clamped, and six of the eight patients survived. This dramatic and spectacular experience was the beginning of the era of intracardiac surgery and is a great tribute to the skill and courage of these surgeons.

In 1956, an experience was reported from the Mayo Clinic with 20 patients who had intracardiac closure of large VSDs by using a mechanical pump oxygenator beginning in March 1955 (DuShane et al., 1956). The duration of cardiopulmonary bypass was from 10 to 45 minutes by using normothermic flow rates of 70 ml/kg/min or approximately 2.1 l/min/m². A pump sucker system was used to return intracardiac blood to the pump oxygenator. Four patients (20%) died in the hospital.

The feasibility of a transatrial approach to VSD closure was shown by Lillehei in 1957 (Stirling et al., 1957). Kirklin and associates (1961) reported an experience of primary repair of VSD in infants, as well as Sloan and associates (Sigmann et al., 1967). The technique of profound hypothermia with surface cooling, total circulatory arrest, and rewarming by a pump oxygenator was applied successfully to infants with VSD by Okamoto and associates (1969). Barratt-Boyes reported an experience commencing in 1969 which showed that routine primary repair of VSD in six small infants was superior to pulmonary artery banding (Barratt-Boyes et al., 1976).

## MORPHOLOGY

The interventricular septum can be considered as having three muscular components that are called the inlet septum, the apical trabecular septum, and the outlet (or infundibular) septum. In addition, there is a fourth component that is fibrous and is called the membranous septum (Fig. 38–1). In the normal heart, the tricuspid valve and mitral valves are attached to the ventricular septum at different levels so that the tricuspid valve attachment is apically displaced compared with that of the mitral valve. Thus, a portion of the ventricular septum is left and is placed between the right atrium and the left ventricle, which is called the atrioventricular muscular septum. It is usually present in most hearts with an isolated VSD. More anteriorly, the tricuspid valve attachment divides the area of the membranous septum into an interventricular component between the left and right ventricles and an atrioventricular component between the left ventricle and the right atrium. When VSD is isolated, the atrioventricular component of the membranous septum is usually intact.

Soto and associates (1980) proposed a classification of VSDs that is surgically useful (Fig. 38–2). Defects were classified as perimembranous when they were in the general area of the membranous septum, as muscular defects when they were completely surrounded by muscular tissue, and as sub-arterial defects when either the aortic or pulmonary valves formed part of the rim of the defect within the infundibular or outlet septum. Perimembranous defects can extend into the inlet, trabecular, or outlet septa

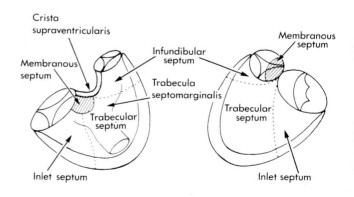

**FIGURE 38–1.** The components of the ventricular septum as seen from the right ventricle (A) and left ventricle (B). (A and B, From Soto, B., Becker, A. E., Moulaert, A. J., et al.: Classification of ventricular septal defects. Br. Heart J., 43:332, 1980.)

1446

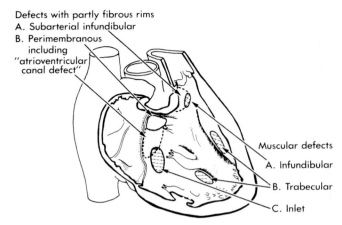

**FIGURE 38–2.** Classification of ventricular septal defects (VSDs) according to their location within the septum. (From Soto, B., Becker, A. E., Moulaert, A. J., et al.: Classification of ventricular septal defects. Br. Heart J., 43:332, 1980.)

and make them confluent with these areas (Fig. 38–3). The atrioventricular canal type of VSD is a perimembranous defect that extends into the inlet septum; the septal leaflet of the tricuspid valve forms its border on the right side. Perimembranous VSDs are related to the anteroseptal commissure of the tricuspid valve and also to the aortic valve. The annulus of these valves often forms part of the rim of the defect, but in some cases it is separated from the VSD by a thin rim of muscular tissue.

Approximately 10% of VSDs are located in the infundibulum or outlet septum. When the aortic and pulmonary valve annuli form part of the rim of the defect, they are called subarterial and form the majority of defects in this location. A few defects in the infundibular septum are surrounded completely

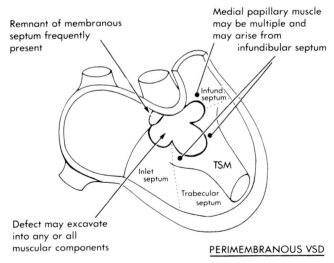

**FIGURE 38–3.** The types of perimembranous VSDs are shown with excavation into the inlet, trabecular, and outlet septa. (TSM = trabecula septomarginalis; Infund. = infundibular.) (From Soto, B., Becker, A. E., Moulaert, A. J., et al.: Classification of ventricular septal defects. Br. Heart J., 43:332, 1980.)

by muscle and are called infundibular muscular defects. Most muscular defects are located in the trabecular portion of the ventricular septum, where they may be single or multiple. When they are multiple, they are usually located in the anterior portion of the trabecular septum.

VSDs vary widely in size, and their division into groups is arbitrary. A large VSD is approximately the size of the aortic orifice or larger and results in systemic right ventricular pressure. Small VSDs have insufficient size to raise right ventricular systolic pressure, and the pulmonary-systemic flow ratio ($Q_P/Q_S$) does not increase above 1.75. Moderate-sized VSDs are "restrictive" but have sufficient size to raise the right ventricular systolic pressure to approximately half of the left ventricular pressure and may result in a $Q_P/Q_S$ of 2 to 3.5. Several small defects may together behave as a large defect.

## ASSOCIATED LESIONS IN "PRIMARY" VENTRICULAR SEPTAL DEFECT

Almost half of patients who undergo surgical treatment for "primary" VSD have an associated lesion (Barratt-Boyes et al., 1976; Blackstone et al., 1976). A *moderate- or large-sized patent ductus arteriosus* is present in approximately 6% of the patients of all ages, but in infants in heart failure, approximately 25% have an associated significant ductus (Barratt-Boyes et al., 1976). A VSD occurs in combination with *severe coarctation* in approximately 12% of patients. However, this combination is also more common among infants with a large VSD coming to operation when less than 3 months old.

Congenital *valvar or subvalvar aortic stenosis* occurs in approximately 4% of patients requiring operation for VSD. Subvalvar stenosis is more common (Lauer et al., 1960) and may also occur in association with VSD and infundibular pulmonary stenosis. It may also develop after pulmonary artery banding (Freed et al., 1973). This subvalvar stenosis is of two types. One type is in the form of a discrete fibromuscular bar that lies inferior (caudad or upstream) to the VSD. The other is distal (downstream) to the VSD and often consists of a displacement of infundibular septal muscle into the left ventricular outflow tract. This latter type is often associated with aortic arch anomalies (Dirksen et al., 1978; Moulaert et al., 1976; Van Praagh et al., 1971). Significant *congenital mitral valve disease* occurs in approximately 2% of patients. One or the other pulmonary artery may be absent or severely stenotic. Severe peripheral pulmonary artery stenoses rarely occur. Severe positional cardiac anomalies, such as isolated dextrocardia or situs inversus totalis, are uncommon in patients with simple VSD.

A number of minor anomalies may also be present in patients coming to operation for VSD (Table 38–1). In small infants, a large atrial septal defect coexisting with a large VSD may be a significant lesion (Barratt-Boyes et al., 1976).

■ **Table 38–1.** ASSOCIATED CONDITIONS OF MINOR ANATOMIC OR FUNCTIONAL SIGNIFICANCE IN 138 PATIENTS WITH LARGE "PRIMARY" VENTRICULAR SEPTAL DEFECTS AND WITHOUT ASSOCIATED CONDITIONS OF MAJOR ANATOMIC OR FUNCTIONAL SIGNIFICANCE AT THE UNIVERSITY OF ALABAMA AT BIRMINGHAM (1967–1976)

| Condition | No. and % of Patients* |
|---|---|
| None | 73 (53%) |
| Mild or moderate pulmonary stenosis | 27 (20%) |
| Atrial septal defect† | 24 (17%) |
| Persistent left superior vena cava | 12 (9%) |
| Dextroposition of the aorta | 7 (5%) |
| Aneurysm of membranous septum | 2 (1%) |
| Mild or moderate coarctation of aorta | 2 (1%) |
| Vascular ring | 1 (0.7%) |
| Tricuspid incompetence, mild | 2 (1%) |
| Mitral incompetence, mild | — |
| Pulmonary valve incompetence | 1 (0.7%) |
| Hepatic veins entering right atrium directly | 1 (0.7%) |
| Anomalous right ventricular muscle band without pulmonary stenosis | 1 (0.7%) |

Modified from Blackstone, E. H., Kirklin, J. W., Bradley, E. L., et al.: Optimal age and results in repair of large ventricular septal defects. J. Thorac Cardiovasc Surg., 72:661, 1976.

*Sum of percentages is >100%, because some patients had more than one minor associated condition.

†Exclusive of simple patent foramen ovale.

## PULMONARY VASCULAR DISEASE

The classic description of the pathology of hypertensive pulmonary vascular disease is that of Heath and Edwards (1958). They defined Grade 1 changes as being characterized by medial hypertrophy without intimal proliferation; Grade 2 by medial hypertrophy with cellular intimal reaction; Grade 3 by intimal fibrosis as well as medial hypertrophy, and possibly with early generalized vascular dilation; Grade 4 by generalized vascular dilation, an area of vascular occlusion by intimal fibrosis, and plexiform lesions; Grade 5 by other "dilatation lesions" such as cavernous and angiomatoid lesions; and Grade 6 by, in addition, necrotizing arteritis.

The pulmonary resistance in patients with a large VSD (and those with a large patent ductus arteriosus) has been correlated positively with the histologic severity of the hypertensive pulmonary vascular disease by Heath and colleagues (1958). However, the authors have reanalyzed their data and find that the "confidence bands" are rather wide around the probability of severe pulmonary vascular disease as predicted from the pulmonary resistance. This is not unexpected, because the Heath-Edwards classification is based on the most severe lesion seen, regardless of its frequency. Furthermore, as emphasized by Wagenvoort (Wagenvoort et al., 1961; Wagenvoort and Wagenvoort, 1970) and by Yamaki and Tezuka (1976), the grading should include an assessment of the number of vessels affected. Moreover, the calculation of pulmonary vascular resistance is open to many errors.

A slightly different view of hypertensive pulmonary vascular disease in infants with large VSD has been provided by Reid and colleagues (Hislop et al., 1975). Other physicians had emphasized earlier that intimal proliferation (and thus Heath-Edwards changes of Grade 2 or more) rarely develops in infants with large VSD until 1 or 2 years of age (Wagenvoort et al., 1961), and yet, infants occasionally do have severely elevated pulmonary resistance. Reid and associates found that infants dying at 3 to 6 months of age with a large VSD and high pulmonary vascular resistance (>8 units/m²) with intermittent right-to-left shunting have marked medial hypertrophy affecting both large and small pulmonary arteries, including those less than 200 μm in diameter (Hislop et al., 1975). The usual number of intra-acinar vessels was present. However, they found that infants (3 to 10 months old) with large VSD, dying with a history of large pulmonary blood flow and congestive heart failure and normal or slightly raised pulmonary vascular resistance, have medial hypertrophy affecting mainly arteries with diameters larger than 200 μm. The intra-acinar vessels were smaller than usual.

The histologic reversibility of pulmonary vascular disease after closure of the VSD has not been documented. The favorable results in infants may be from an increased number of arterioles and capillaries as growth proceeds. Presumably, pulmonary vascular disease of Heath-Edwards Grade 3 or greater severity is not reversible.

## PATHOPHYSIOLOGY

**Determinants of Size and Direction of Shunt.** The magnitude and direction of the shunt across a VSD depend on the size of the defect and the pressure gradient across it during the various phases of the cardiac cycle. The authors have observed these relations with biplane cineangiocardiograms in a large number of patients. Jarmakani and colleagues (1968) and Levin and associates (1966) have studied them with special techniques.

When the VSD is small, it offers considerable resistance to flow, and slight variations in the size of the defect are accompanied by large variations in the rate of flow (or shunting). Across small defects, only a large pressure difference, such as that which occurs during mid and late systole, results in significant flow. When the defect is large, it offers little resistance to flow, and small pressure differences between the left and right ventricle result in shunting. The pressure relations during the entire cardiac cycle must therefore be considered in patients with large defects.

The pressure relations late in systole appear mainly related to the output resistance to left and right ventricular ejection. The determinants of those during diastole and early systole are more complicated. They include the relative compliance of the two ventricles and the relative pressures in the two atria. Asynchronous systole of the two ventricles relates to the pressure relations in the early portion of systole and diastole.

The size of the VSD itself may vary during various

phases of the cardiac cycle. Also, an apparently large VSD may be partially closed during ventricular systole by a flap of muscle or tissue. It is possible that defects in the muscular septum are considerably smaller during systole than during diastole or when seen at operation or autopsy.

**Sequelae of Left-to-Right Shunting.** When a left-to-right shunt is present at ventricular level, pulmonary blood flow is increased above normal and systemic blood flow. Thus, flow through the left atrium and the mitral valve orifice is similarly increased, and greater work is done by both the left and the right ventricles. The left atrium is enlarged to a degree corresponding to the magnitude of increase in pulmonary blood flow, and a diastolic murmur may be heard over the apex of the heart, reflecting the increase in the blood flow across the mitral valve. Left atrial pressure becomes raised relative both to normal and to right atrial pressure as the result of a natural adaptive process related to the Starling-Frank mechanism. The left ventricle is larger than normal, and the right ventricle is dilated.

The raised left atrial (and pulmonary venous) pressure causes many infants with VSD to have an increased amount of interstitial fluid in the lungs. As a result, they tend to have repeated pulmonary infections. The lungs are relatively noncompliant, and the work of breathing is increased. This increases energy expenditure, which, along with the relatively low systemic blood flow, causes these infants to have striking growth failure. These sequelae are well reflected in the physical findings, chest films, and electrocardiograms of patients with a VSD and large pulmonary blood flow (DuShane and Kirklin, 1960).

When pulmonary resistance rises in patients with a large VSD as a result of the development of pulmonary vascular disease, pulmonary blood flow is re-duced, left atrial pressure lessens, and the sequelae of left-to-right shunting lessen. The infant or child appears to improve: as pulmonary infections subside, the work of breathing decreases, and growth improves. Unfortunately, further increases in pulmonary vascular resistance occur slowly, and the classic Eisenmenger complex results. In these patients with severe pulmonary hypertension and bidirectional shunting of equal magnitude in the two directions, the left ventricle is not enlarged and the right ventricle is hypertrophied, but its volume does not increase.

## NATURAL HISTORY

**Spontaneous Closure.** VSDs have a tendency to close spontaneously, and this fact is relevant to decisions about operation (Collins et al., 1972). Spontaneous closure can be complete by 1 year of age, or the defect may have only narrowed by then. Complete closure takes considerably longer. The phenomenon of spontaneous closure or narrowing of VSDs explains the infrequency with which large VSDs are encountered in adults. An inverse relationship exists between the probability of eventual spontaneous closure and the age at which the patient is observed (Blackstone et al., 1976; Hoffman and Rudolph, 1965; Keith et al., 1971) (Fig. 38–4). This is highly relevant to clinical decisions about individual patients. According to these data, approximately 80% of individuals seen at 1 month of age with large VSDs have eventual spontaneous closure, as do approximately 60% of those seen at 3 months of age, approximately 50% of those seen at 6 months of age, and 25% of those seen at 12 months of age.

**Pulmonary Vascular Disease.** A large VSD predisposes the patient to the development of an increased

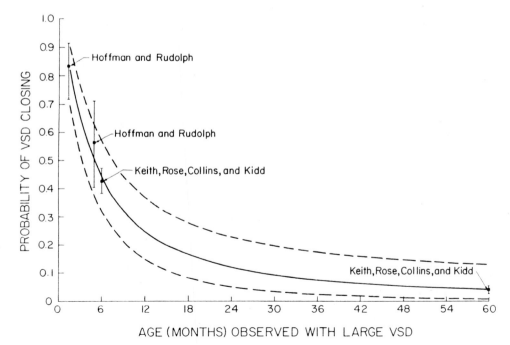

FIGURE 38–4. Probability of eventual spontaneous closure of a large VSD according to the age at which the patient is observed. The *broken lines* enclose the 70% confidence limits (CLs) around the *solid* probability line. The specific ratios, with the 70% CLs reported by Hoffman and Rudolph (1966) and Keith and associates (1971), are shown centered on the mean or assumed ages of patients in their reports. (*p* < .0001.) (From Blackstone, E. H., Kirklin, J. W., Bradley, E. L., et al.: Optimal age and results in repair of large ventricular septal defects. J. Thorac. Cardiovasc. Surg., 72:661, 1976.)

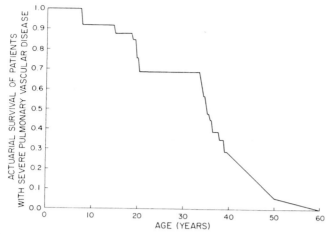

FIGURE 38–5. Actuarial survival of patients with large VSDs who had proven elevation of pulmonary vascular resistance to a level that made them inoperable (≥ 10 units/m²) demonstrated at cardiac catheterization done at various ages. Note that fatalities begin to occur in the second decade of life, that about one-half of the patients are dead by 35 years of age, and that a few survive until 50 years of age. (Modified from Clarkson, P. M., Frye, R. L., Du-Shane, J. W., et al.: Prognosis for patients with ventricular septal defect and severe pulmonary vascular obstructive disease. Circulation, 38:129, 1968. By permission of the American Heart Association, Inc.)

pulmonary vascular resistance from hypertensive pulmonary vascular disease, which tends to grow worse as the individual gets older (Auld et al., 1963; Lucas et al., 1961). Thus, the proportion of patients with a large VSD who have a severely raised pulmonary vascular resistance is related directly to the age of the patient. Patients with severe pulmonary vascular disease are usually dead by 40 years of age (Fig. 38–5).

The statement that some infants less than 2 years of age with large VSD have severely raised pulmonary vascular resistance is doubted by some physicians, but its occurrence is well documented (Barratt-Boyes et al., 1976). It is, however, uncommon. It occurs in some infants because they do not have the usual fall in pulmonary vascular resistance a few weeks to a few months after birth. Others do have this but later, in the first 2 years of life, develop a rapid increase in pulmonary vascular resistance (Hoffman and Rudolph, 1966). Some infants who have a large VSD have normal or mildly raised resistance. They retain this through the first decade of life, and then, if their VSD is still large, later on develop more severe changes (Keith et al., 1971; Kirklin et al., 1963).

**Bacterial Endocarditis.** This is rare and occurs at a rate of approximately 0.3% per year in individuals with VSD (Campbell, 1971; Corone et al., 1977; Shah et al., 1966). Often, a pulmonary process is the presenting feature, presumably developing from emboli secondary to right-sided bacterial vegetations. Prognosis with treatment is excellent.

**Premature Death.** Previous experience and reports in the literature indicate that without surgical treatment some infants (approximately 9% of those with large VSD) die of their disease in the first year of life

(Ash, 1964; Keith et al., 1971). Death may result from congestive heart failure, which may develop very early but usually occurs at approximately 2 to 3 months of age, presumably because at about this time the left-to-right shunt becomes larger as the medial hypertrophy present in the small pulmonary arteries at birth regresses. Death may also result from recurrent pulmonary infections secondary to pulmonary edema from the high pulmonary venous pressure. Death is most likely to occur in those infants with large VSD who have associated conditions of major anatomic or functional significance, such as patent ductus arteriosus, coarctation of the aorta, or a large atrial septal defect (Barratt-Boyes et al., 1976).

After the age of 1 year, few if any patients die because of their VSD until the second decade of life. By then, most patients whose VSDs have remained large have developed pulmonary vascular disease and in subsequent years die from complications of Eisenmenger complex (Clarkson et al., 1968) (see Fig. 38–5). These include hemoptysis, polycythemia, cerebral abscess or infarction, and right-sided heart failure.

Patients with *small* VSDs do not develop pulmonary vascular disease and are unlikely to die prematurely. Their only real risk is bacterial endocarditis, the incidence of which is low (estimated to occur once in 500 patient years [Shah et al., 1966]). It is generally well treated by antibiotics.

**Symptoms.** Patients with small VSDs rarely have symptoms related to the defect. Patients with large VSDs may have symptoms of intractable heart failure in the first few months of life, with poor peripheral pulses, inability to feed, sweating, and chronic pulmonary edema. Approximately one-half of the patients coming to operation in the first 2 years of life do so because of this (Barratt-Boyes et al., 1976) (Table 38–2). During early life, rapid and labored respiration and recurrent pulmonary infections may occur secondary to high pulmonary venous pressure and chronic pulmonary edema. At any time in the first year of life, lobes of the lung may become chronically hyperinflated because of pressure of the large and

■ **Table 38–2.** INDICATIONS FOR REPAIR OF VENTRICULAR SEPTAL DEFECT IN PATIENTS UNDERGOING SURGERY IN THE FIRST 2 YEARS OF LIFE

| Indication for VSD Repair | No. | % of Total | Age in Months Average | (Range) |
|---|---|---|---|---|
| Intractable congestive heart failure | 30 | 53 | 2.9 | (1 to 7) |
| Recurrent respiratory infections | 3 | 5 | 8 | (6 to 9) |
| Controlled congestive heart failure and failure to thrive | 17 | 30 | 11.4 | (4 to 21) |
| Increased pulmonary vascular resistance | 7 | 12 | 14.6 | (10 to 19) |

Modified from Barratt-Boyes, B. G., Neutze, J. M., Clarkson, P. M., et al.: Repair of ventricular septal defect in the first two years of life using profound hypothermia-circulatory arrest techniques. Ann. Surg., 184:376, 1976.

tense pulmonary arteries on the bronchi, preventing complete escape of air during expiration (Oh et al., 1978). As a result of all this, many babies with large VSDs are small and physically underdeveloped. It is these symptomatic patients who fail to respond well to medical management who are at particular risk of dying in the first year of life. Some babies who survive through the first year of life with large VSDs have controlled heart failure and failure to thrive in the second year of life as well.

Children and young adults with large VSDs are usually symptomatic and tend to be small both in height and weight. As pulmonary vascular disease develops, symptoms may regress.

**Development of Aortic Incompetence.** A small proportion of patients (probably approximately 5% in white and black races) develop aortic valve incompetence as a complication of VSD. The incompetence is not present at birth but develops during the first decade of life. It gradually worsens so that by the end of the second decade, it is usually severe. As the incompetence increases, the shunt often decreases, owing to occlusion of the VSD by the prolapsed aortic cusp.

**Development of Infundibular Pulmonary Stenosis.** A small proportion (perhaps 5 to 10%) of patients with a large VSD and large left-to-right shunt in infancy develop infundibular pulmonary stenosis (Gasul et al., 1957; Hoffman and Rudolph, 1970; Keith et al., 1971). The mild and moderate infundibular pulmonary stenoses in patients undergoing surgery for "primary" VSD (see Table 38–1) as well as the more important stenoses probably develop in this way. The stenosis may become sufficiently severe to produce shunt reversal and cyanosis, and the condition can then properly be termed tetralogy of Fallot. Somerville's data (1970) indicate that this transformation occurs in approximately 6% of infants with isolated VSD. Those who have the transformation probably are born with some anterior displacement of the infundibular septum and its extensions.

## DIAGNOSIS

### Examination

The infant with a large VSD and increased pulmonary blood flow presents a particular and highly characteristic clinical picture. Tachypnea with marked subcostal retraction, severe growth failure, and lack of subcutaneous tissue are evident. A waxen complexion and evidence of profuse sweating such as hair that is damp or matted from recently dried perspiration may be noted. The external jugular venous pulses are usually prominent when the infant is supine and often even when he or she is held erect. A bulging precordium is a common finding. On palpation, a rapid, overactive heart is apparent. A thrill is maximal in the third to fifth intercostal spaces on the left. The loud pansystolic murmur is also maximal in the third to fifth intercostal spaces on the left. A short mid-

diastolic murmur is usually appreciated at the apex and gives the entire cardiac cycle a gallop quality. The second sound at the base is usually loud and may be slightly split. The liver and spleen are usually enlarged, and the peripheral pulses are rapid and thready. These infants obviously have heart failure, and many are actually in shock.

In older patients with large VSDs, a protruding sternum, or so-called pigeon breast deformity, is common. Presumably, this is due to the large right ventricle pushing the sternum anteriorly during the period of growth. A systolic thrill over the left precordium is often present. The characteristic murmur of VSD is a pansystolic harsh murmur heard in the second, third, and maximally in the fourth left interspace in the midclavicular line (Leatham and Segal, 1962). In patients with a large pulmonary blood flow, there may be a superimposed systolic ejection murmur originating in the area of the pulmonary valve. Characteristically, an early diastolic filling murmur is heard at the apex, indicating a large flow across the mitral valve. The first heart sound at the base is normal; the second sound at the base is abnormally split, owing both to shortened left ventricular ejection time and to prolonged right ventricular ejection time. The splitting is accentuated in inspiration.

These classic physical findings are altered by the size of the VSD and the magnitude of the pulmonary vascular resistance. Patients with small VSDs and small left-to-right shunts have only a systolic murmur. The heart is not hyperactive, and on palpation, there is no enlargement of the left ventricle and no right ventricular lift. Not only do patients with large VSD, mild elevation of pulmonary vascular resistance, and large pulmonary blood flow have the characteristic systolic murmur, but in addition, the heart is hyperactive, the left ventricle is enlarged on palpation, there is a right ventricular lift, there is an apical diastolic rumble, and the second sound at the base is moderately accentuated. In patients with a large VSD and high pulmonary vascular resistance, and consequently with a net left-to-right shunt that is small or with shunts that are bidirectional and of approximately equal magnitude in the two directions, the heart is quiet on examination. There is no evidence on palpation of left ventricular enlargement, but the right ventricular lift is prominent. The systolic murmur is soft and short, or may almost be absent. There is no apical diastolic rumble. The second sound at the base is greatly accentuated. Patients in whom the pulmonary vascular resistance has become higher than systemic resistance are, of course, cyanotic.

### Chest Film

The chest film in a patient with a VSD reflects the pathophysiology. Patients with small VSDs and small left-to-right shunts usually have normal chest films; those with large VSDs, mild elevation of pulmonary vascular resistance, and large left-to-right shunts have characteristic chest films (Fig. 38–6). In the latter, pul-

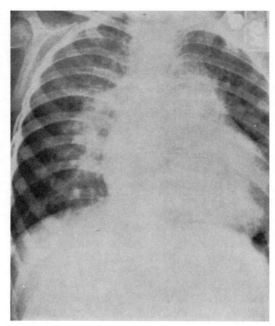

FIGURE 38–6. Chest film of a child with a large VSD, large pulmonary blood flow, and pulmonary hypertension, but only mild elevation of pulmonary vascular resistance. This is reflected in the evidence of left and right ventricular enlargement, enlargement of the main pulmonary artery, and sharp increase in pulmonary blood flow.

monary arteries, both centrally and peripherally, are large, indicating large pulmonary blood flow. There may be evidence of some enlargement of the left atrium; the left ventricle is abnormally large; and the right ventricle appears dilated. When the physician sees *marked* enlargement of the left atrium in a patient suspected of having a VSD, the coexistence of significant mitral valvular incompetence should be suspected.

When the patient has a large VSD and severe rise in pulmonary vascular resistance, the appearance of the chest film is different. The peripheral pulmonary arteries are normal in size, and there is no evidence of increased pulmonary blood flow. The main pulmonary artery is often greatly enlarged. There is no evidence of left atrial or left ventricular enlargement. The right ventricle may appear slightly enlarged, but often the cardiac silhouette, other than the large pulmonary artery, is essentially normal (Fig. 38–7).

## Electrocardiogram

If the defect is large and the pulmonary vascular resistance is only mildly raised, there is evidence of overload of both ventricles. The R wave from the right precordial leads is tall, and when right ventricular peak pressure is similar to left ventricular peak pressure, it is notched on the upstroke. The left precordial leads in this situation have the pattern of ventricular overload previously described, although here there may also be a deeper S wave. As long as

evidence of left ventricular enlargement exists in these leads, the patient probably has a pulmonary-systemic flow more than approximately 1.8 and a pulmonary-systemic resistance less than approximately 0.6 and can undergo surgery. Absence of this pattern by itself is not clear evidence of a higher resistance ratio and inoperability.

## Cardiac Catheterization and Cineangiography

Although clinical findings and the chest film usually allow estimation of the pulmonary blood flow and $Q_P/Q_S$, Doppler echocardiography with color flow mapping provides more precise information concerning the presence of a VSD. This noninvasive technique is useful in defining the status of the atrioventricular valves and left ventricular outflow tract. This technique, however, does not yet permit accurate identification of multiple VSDs, and therefore the authors continue to advise cardiac catheterization studies and angled left ventriculography in projections designed to profile the ventricular septum (Bargeron et al., 1977). This technique also permits definition of the location of the defect and usually allows differentiation of perimembranous from muscular and subarterial defects.

## INDICATIONS FOR OPERATION

When *infants* with *large VSDs* have severe intractable heart failure or intractable, severe respiratory

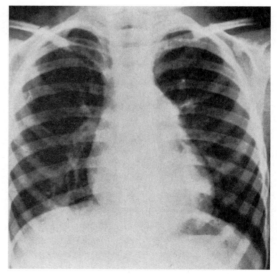

FIGURE 38–7. This chest film is in contrast to that shown in Figure 38–6. The heart is not enlarged overall. The main pulmonary artery is enlarged; there is no evidence of increased pulmonary blood flow. This patient has a large VSD, pulmonary hypertension, severe elevation of pulmonary vascular resistance, and pulmonary blood flow that is less than systemic blood flow. The condition is inoperable. (From DuShane, J. W., and Kirklin, J. W.: Selection for surgery of patients with ventricular septal defect and pulmonary hypertension. Circulation, *21:*13, 1960. By permission of the American Heart Association, Inc.)

symptoms at any time during the first 3 months of life, prompt primary repair is indicated. Operation is not advised *electively* in the first 3 months of life in the hope that spontaneous closure or narrowing of the defect may occur.

When severe symptoms, significant growth failure, or rising pulmonary vascular resistance is present in infants 3 months of age or older, prompt primary repair is advised.

When infants reach 6 months of age with a single large VSD, they are rarely thriving. The probability of cure by spontaneous closure of the VSD has decreased significantly (see Fig. 38–4). Operation generally should be advised at this time because the risk of repair is not demonstrably less for older patients. If the pulmonary vascular resistance is high (e.g., approximately 8 units $\cdot$ m$^2$ or more), repair is advisable without undue delay because further delay reduces the infant's chances of having a "surgical cure."

Patients with *large VSDs* who are first *seen after infancy* must be considered primarily on the basis of the *extent of their pulmonary vascular disease* (Kirklin and DuShane, 1963). When the pulmonary vascular resistance is more than 10 units $\cdot$ m$^2$, in which circumstance the ratio of pulmonary to systemic blood flow ($Q_P/Q_S$) is usually less than 1.5 (with the patient at rest and breathing air), and when the clinical data are also consistent with this hemodynamic state (the systolic murmur is soft or absent; no apical diastolic flow murmur is present; the pulmonary fields on chest films are not plethoric; the left ventricle is normal or almost normal in size; and the electrocardiogram shows at least moderate right ventricular hypertrophy), operation is not advisable. Closure of the defect under these circumstances precludes right-to-left shunting during exercise; thus, exercise capacity and life expectancy are not as good with the defect closed as with it open. When pulmonary vascular resistance is elevated but within the "operable range" (5 to 10 units $\cdot$ m$^2$), operation is generally advisable, with the knowledge that the long-term results may be compromised by persisting and possibly increasing pulmonary vascular disease. However, some patients with resistance values in this range at rest have rather fixed pulmonary vascular resistance, which does not fall during stress. Therefore, when the operability of a defect is borderline and patients are old enough to cooperate, measurement of pulmonary and systemic blood flow and resistances during moderate exercise is helpful; even if $Q_P/Q_S$ is 1.5 or 1.8 at rest, if it becomes 1.0 or less during moderate exercise (from systemic peripheral vasodilation and increased systemic blood flow, and a fixed and high pulmonary vascular resistance preventing increased pulmonary blood flow), operation is not indicated. The simple finding of a significant fall in arterial oxygen saturation during exercise (from right-to-left shunting across the VSD for the reasons described) suggests inoperability. The response of the pulmonary vascular resistance to inhalation of high oxygen mixtures is not useful in determining operability in borderline situations.

In patients with a resting pulmonary vascular resistance of more than 7 units $\cdot$ m$^2$, the response to isoproterenol infusion (0.14 mg/kg/min) may be useful in predicting the postoperative course. A fall in resistance with isoproterenol infusion to less than 7 units $\cdot$ m$^2$ predicts a good postoperative evaluation (Neutze et al., 1989).

A considerable number of children have a *moderate-sized VSD*, which is not sufficient to raise pulmonary artery pressure above 40 to 50 mm Hg systolic and which will not result in later rise in pulmonary vascular resistance and yet produces a $Q_P/Q_S$ of up to 3, moderate cardiomegaly, and significant pulmonary plethora. There are usually few if any symptoms. These patients should be kept under observation for about 5 years in the hope that there will be spontaneous reduction in the size of the VSD. If there is no change on subsequent recatheterization, closure is indicated.

It is not advised that young patients with *small VSDs* undergo repair, because they are suffering no significant ill effects and the defect will probably close.

*Subpulmonary defects* are a special situation. Even though apparently small, they should not be left untreated beyond 5 years of age, because aortic incompetence may develop, and they should be repaired promptly at an earlier age if an aortic diastolic murmur develops.

## SURGICAL TECHNIQUE

The right atrial approach is preferred for most perimembranous and midmuscular VSDs and for some apical and subarterial defects. The right ventricular approach provides good exposure through a transverse infundibular incision for subarterial and infundibular defects, through an apical ventriculotomy for apical muscular defects, and through a longitudinal anterior right ventriculotomy for some multiple muscular defects. Rarely, a left ventriculotomy is used for multiple muscular VSDs in the trabecular septum.

Operations are done through a median sternotomy incision by using standard cardiopulmonary bypass methods with hypothermia to 24 to 28° C. During the procedure, periods of low flow (0.5 to 1 l/min/m$^2$) or in rare circumstances, total circulatory arrest may be used. Ascending aortic cannulation is first accomplished by using a thin-walled, short-tip arterial cannula sized to result in a trans-cannula gradient $\leqslant$ 100 mm Hg at full flow (2.5 l/min/m$^2$). Separate cannulation of each vena cava with appropriately sized thin-walled angled cannulas reduces the clutter in the surgical field and provides superb access for intracardiac exposure through the right atrium (Pacifico, 1988). The inferior vena cava (IVC) purse-string suture is placed directly on the IVC or at the caval-atrial junction and connected to a tourniquet. It is placed slightly to the right of the midline that reduces its interference with the right atriotomy. The superior vena cava (SVC) purse-string suture is placed directly on the SVC as an oval in its longitudinal axis and similarly connected to a tourniquet. The SVC snare is placed before establishing cardiopulmonary bypass (CPB) by mobilizing the SVC at the site of the right pulmonary artery, using a 0 silk ligature that is connected to a tourniquet. The IVC snare is placed after establishing CPB in an effort to avoid prebypass hypotension.

It is important to externally examine the cardiac chambers, making mental note of their size and position, and to determine the possible presence of anomalies of pulmonary or systemic venous return. The presence of a left SVC connecting to the coronary sinus in a small infant usually does not alter the cannulation regimen unless the right SVC is too small to cannulate. In this case, the left and right SVC return can be collected by an intracardiac sump sucker after opening the right atrium, and with periods of low flow or total circulatory arrest, the procedure is usually unhampered. Alternatively, CPB can be used with a single right atrial cannula for venous return, profound hypothermia induced and repair done during total circulatory arrest at 20° C (Barratt-Boyes et al., 1976; Rein et al., 1977). When a left SVC connects directly to the left atrium (unroofed coronary sinus syndrome), repair is more complicated and is best accomplished by using a period of total circulatory arrest in infants or by placing a third venous cannula into the anomalous left SVC in older subjects (Sand et al., 1986).

The patency of the ductus arteriosus should be known from preoperative studies. This detail is important because an open ductus combined with an open cardiotomy allows air to enter the aortic arch and later to go to the brain, if total circulatory arrest is used. Moreover, during CPB it results in increased intracardiac return and overdistends the pulmonary circulation causing potentially serious capillary damage to the lung. When a patent ductus arteriosus is present or suspected, it is ligated from the anterior approach.

CPB is established initially with only the IVC cannula in place, at a maximal flow rate of 1.6 l/min/m² at 25° C; the SVC cannula is inserted and "full flow" is established at 2 to 2.5 l/min/m². The water bath is then adjusted to "coldest temperature" to permit initial cooling of the myocardium by the perfusate. During this period, the IVC snare is placed, and a fine polyvinyl tube is passed into the left atrium through the right superior pulmonary vein for intraoperative and postoperative left atrial pressure monitoring. The action of the heart is usually ineffective by this time, and the right atrium is opened obliquely (Fig. 38–8) and a disposable sump tip sucker is introduced into the left atrium through the foramen ovale or a small intra-atrial defect created in the fossa ovalis. Traction sutures are placed from the edges of the atriotomy to secure the atrial flaps to the subcutaneous tissue.

The aorta is cross-clamped, and cold cardioplegic solution is injected into the aortic root. The temperature is now selected and is usually between 24 and 28° C. Colder temperatures are used for longer, more complex procedures and when the pulmonary venous return is large to provide "safe" periods of low flow. Generally, a flow rate of 0.5 l/min/m² or total circulatory arrest is "safe" for 45 minutes at a nasopharyngeal temperature of 22° C, 30 minutes at 26° C, and 20 minutes at 28° C. Usually, a flow rate of 1.6 l/min/m² is used during the intracardiac repair and until rewarming is commenced, when "full flow" is restored.

The heart is now soft and quiet from the cardioplegic solution infusion. Fine sutures are placed on the tricuspid valve leaflets, and traction is maintained by the weight of shodded clamps. This use and intermittent use of small eyelid or right-angled retractors provide excellent exposure for closure of most VSDs.

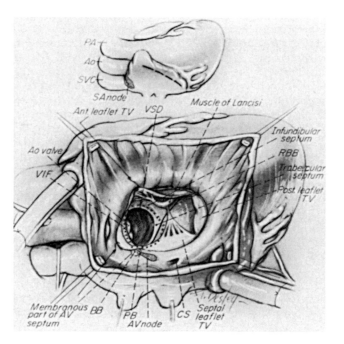

**FIGURE 38–8.** The sinus node and position of the right atriotomy is shown above. Transatrial exposure of a perimembranous VSD is shown below looking through the retracted tricuspid valve (TV) leaflets. The coronary sinus (CS) and the nearby atrioventricular (AV) node with the penetrating portion of the bundle of His (PB) and its branching portion (BB) as well as the right bundle branch (RBB) are shown in relation to the VSD. The pathway of the suture line that will secure the patch used to close the VSD is indicated by the x's along the muscular portion of the ventricular septum as well as the ventriculoinfundibular fold (VIF) and the *dots* shown in the base of the septal leaflet of the TV. The suture line remains well away from the inferior free edge of the VSD and on the tricuspid leaflet near its base to avoid the surgical creation of heart block. (Ao = aorta; PA = pulmonary artery; SVC = superior vena cava; SA = sinoatrial.) (From Bharati, S., Lev, M., Kirklin, J. W.: Cardiac Surgery and the Conduction System. Churchill Livingstone, New York, 1983.)

All VSDs are repaired with a patch. Although various methods of suturing are available, the authors prefer a continuous suturing technique with 4-0 polypropylene suture. The location of the specialized conduction tissue and its relation to the VSD must be understood.

The right atriotomy used for transatrial repair and the view of a perimembranous VSD through the tricuspid valve are shown in Figure 38–8. The sinus node is shown in the intact heart above and the AV node, penetrating portion of the bundle of His as well as its branching portion and right bundle in relation to the tricuspid valve and VSD are shown below (see Fig. 38–8). The precise method of suturing the patch in place is shown in Figure 38–9.

In some cases, a perimembranous VSD is associated with an inlet muscular VSD, leaving an intact muscle bar between them (Fig. 38–10). Usually, they can be nicely exposed by tricuspid valve leaflet retraction, but where the chordal pattern is particularly complicated, exposure is facilitated by incising the anterior and septal leaflets near their base and retracting the leaflets anteriorly (see Fig. 38–10). In this particular defect, the conduction tissue courses in the muscle bar and separates the two defects; its injury is avoided by using a single patch to cover both defects, leaving the muscle bar intact and placing the sutures in the path indicated.

The "atrioventricular canal type" of VSD and the course of the conduction tissue in relation to it are shown in Figure 38–11. No muscle tissue is present between the defect and the base of the septal tricuspid leaflet that is contiguous with the anterior mitral leaflet and usually with part of the aortic valve annulus superiorly. The conduction tissue is related to the inferior border of the defect, and the suture line used to attach the patch in this area is placed approximately 10 mm inferior to the free edge of the VSD.

The specialized conduction tissue is not related directly to a muscular VSD in the trabecular septum (Fig. 38–12). In this case, the patch suture line is placed circumferentially on the free edge of the defect.

Subarterial and muscular defects in the infundibular septum can sometimes be approached through the right atrium. They can always be nicely exposed through a transverse incision in the right ventricular infundibulum and sometimes through a pulmonary arteriotomy working through the retracted pulmonary valve and annulus.

Multiple anterior VSDs can be closed by mattress sutures placed over felt pledgets or strips working transatrially through the tricuspid valve or through a vertical right ventriculotomy incision made near the septum (Breckenridge et al., 1972). A left ventriculotomy also provides excellent exposure (Aaron and Lower, 1975; Singh et al., 1977), but the authors prefer not to use it routinely in infants because it has been associated with left ventricular dysfunction early and late postoperatively in some of the small patients. In older patients, avoidance of a left ventriculotomy appears to be less important.

The rare "Swiss-cheese" septum usually requires a left ventricular approach. An associated perimembranous defect should be repaired through the right atrium, because its repair from the left ventricular side increases the risk of heart block.

When VSD closure is completed, rewarming is commenced, the vent is removed, and the atrial septal defect is closed after inflating the lungs to expel air from the left atrium. Air is aspirated from the ascending aorta, the aortic cross-clamp is released, and the right atriotomy is closed. De-airing is accomplished, and CPB is gradually discontinued. Decannulation is effected, and the incision is closed leaving temporary atrial and ventricular pacing electrodes.

## POSTOPERATIVE CARE

Most infants convalesce normally after VSD repair, and special treatment is usually not required. Generally, the patients are extubated within 24 hours of operation and recover rapidly.

In the unusual case of low cardiac output after operation, in addition to the usual supportive treatment (Kirklin and Kirklin, 1981), consideration should be given to the possibility of an overlooked or incompletely closed VSD. This possibility must especially be considered if the left atrial pressure is considerably higher than the right atrial pressure. If recovery from the low output state does not occur within a few hours and in the absence of secure information from an indicator-dilution study or a Doppler examination with color flow mapping that a residual shunt is not present, urgent recatheterization and possible reoperation are indicated.

Pulmonary hypertensive crisis is a severe postoperative complication that may occur in patients with a reactive pulmonary vasculature. Although this event is more common in patients with complex malformations (e.g., transposition of the great arteries with VSD, truncus arteriosus, atrioventricular septal defects), it may occur in a small number of patients with isolated VSD. Major crises include elevation of pulmonary arterial pressure to suprasystemic levels, increase in right atrial pressure, reduction in left atrial pressure, and systemic arterial hypotension (Hopkins et al., 1991). Minor crises are less severe. Precipitating factors include tracheal suctioning, hypercapnia, metabolic acidosis, hypoxemia, restlessness, epinephrine, high-dose dopamine, and morphine. Patients at risk for this event may benefit from muscular paralysis, hyperventilation with high-inspired oxygen, and continuous anesthesia with fentanyl for 24 to 48 hours postoperatively. The partial pressure of carbon dioxide ($PaCO_2$) should be kept less than 25 mm Hg. The use of phenoxybenzamine (1 mg/kg) to produce alpha-adrenergic blockade, before CPB and during rewarming, as well as 0.5 mg/kg every 8 to 12 hours postoperatively may be beneficial. Prostacyclin infused at a rate of 5 to 15 mg/kg/min initially and increased to 20 mg/kg/min is probably the best agent to treat a major crisis. Other agents used to treat

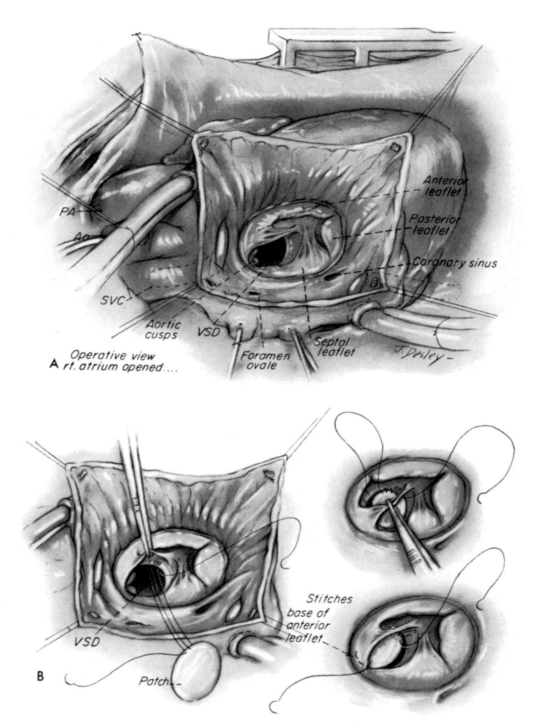

**FIGURE 38–9.** *A,* Right atrial incision and exposure of perimembranous VSD in the region of the tricuspid anteroseptal commissure. Stay sutures have been placed to slightly evert the atrial wall. Note that initially the superior edge of this typical perimembranous defect is not visible. The atrioventricular (AV) node is in the muscular portion of the AV septum, just on the atrial side of the commissure between the tricuspid septal and the tricuspid anterior leaflets. The bundle of His thus penetrates at the posterior angle of the VSD, where it is vulnerable to injury. *B,* The repair of the perimembranous VSD. This is begun by placing a mattress suture of 4-0 Prolene with a small pledget at the 12 o'clock position in the defect as seen by the surgeon through the tricuspid valve. A piece of knitted Dacron velour is trimmed to be slightly larger than the approximate size of the defect, and one arm of the suture is passed through the Dacron patch, back through the septum, and again through the patch. Either now or after placing several more stitches, the sutures are snugged up as the patch is lowered into place. The suture line between the cephalad rim of the defect and the patch is continued. The traction on the suture exposes the next areas to be stitched and provides good visibility. When the junction of the superior muscular rim (ventriculoinfundibular fold) and tricuspid annulus has been reached, the suture is passed through the base of the contiguous portion of the tricuspid valve (usually the anterior leaflet) from the ventricular to the atrial side, then back from the atrial to the ventricular side of the valve and through the patch. After passing the stitch back through the leaflet, the suture is tagged.

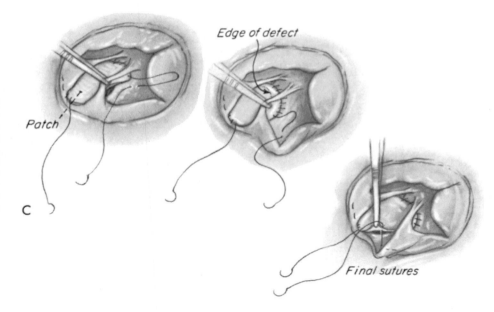

FIGURE 38–9 *Continued C,* Working now with the other limb of the suture, stitches are taken between the ventricular septum and the patch along the caudad side of the defect. These stitches are placed 3 to 5 mm away from the edge of the defect *to avoid the area most probably occupied by the bundle of His* and more posteriorly 5 to 7 mm back from the edge.

pulmonary hypertensive crises include nitroglycerine, sodium nitroprusside, aminophyllin, and tolazoline.

Nitric oxide, administered by inhalation at a dose of 15 ppm, has been shown to be particularly effective in managing postoperative pulmonary hypertension (Berner et al., 1993), and may become the preferred agent.

If complete atrioventricular dissociation was present for a time after CPB, but sinus rhythm reappeared, a demand pacemaker attached to ventricular wires should be in place for 1 week postoperatively, because, rarely, the atrioventricular dissociation recurs temporarily in the early postoperative period.

# RESULTS OF SURGICAL TREATMENT

## Early Results of Primary Repair

The hospital mortality rate for repair of VSD now approaches 0% in most centers properly prepared for this type of procedure, even in very small infants (Barratt-Boyes et al., 1976; Lincoln et al., 1977; Rein et al., 1977; Rizzoli et al., 1980). However, in earlier times, deaths did occur, and a number of incremental risk factors could be identified. The current very low hospital mortality rate is the result of the neutraliza-

FIGURE 38–10. Transatrial exposure for closure of a perimembranous VSD associated with an inlet muscular VSD. The coronary sinus (CS) and atrioventricular (AV) node, as well as an incision in the base of the anterior and septal tricuspid valve (TV) leaflets are shown. The leaflets are retracted anteriorly in the lower part of the figure to expose the two VSDs. The penetrating portion of the bundle of His (PB), its branching portion (BB), and the right bundle branch (RBB) are shown in relation to the VSDs. The pathway of the suture line used to attach the Dacron patch along the muscular portion of the septum is indicated by x's and along the base of the tricuspid valve leaflet by *dots*. When repair is completed, the tricuspid leaflets are reattached to their basilar remnant by a continuous suture of fine polypropylene. (PA = pulmonary artery; Ao = aorta; SVC = superior vena cava.) (From Bharati, S., Lev, M., Kirklin, J. W.: Cardiac Surgery and the Conduction System. Churchill Livingstone, New York, 1983.)

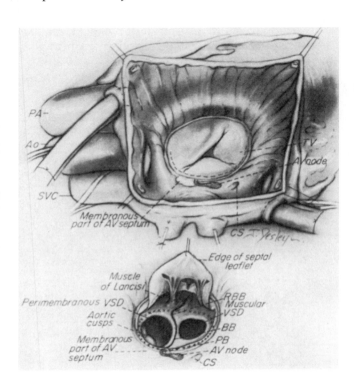

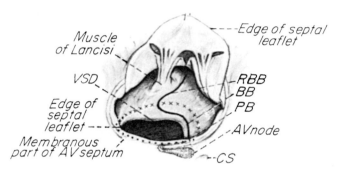

**Figure 38–11.** Transatrial exposure for repair of an "atrioventricular canal type" of VSD is shown after incision of the base of the tricuspid valve and anterior traction as in Figure 38–9. The coronary sinus (CS), atrioventricular (AV) node and its penetrating portion (PB), branching portion (BB), and the right bundle branch (RBB) are shown in relation to the VSD. The x's indicate the path of the suture line used to attach the patch to the muscular portion of the septum and the *dots* along the base of the tricuspid leaflet. Most defects of this type can be closed without incision of the tricuspid leaflets; however, when the chordal pattern is complex, this maneuver aids in exposure. (From Bharati, S., Lev, M., Kirklin, J. W.: Cardiac Surgery and the Conduction System. Churchill Livingstone, New York, 1983.)

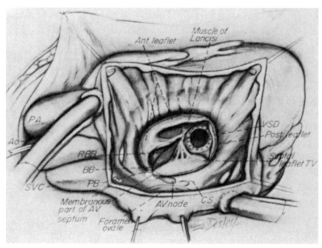

**FIGURE 38–12.** Transatrial exposure of a muscular defect in the trabecular portion of the septum. The pathway of the suture line used to attach the patch to close the defect is along its free edge and indicated by the x's. (CS = coronary sinus; AV = atrioventricular; PB = penetrating portion of the bundle of His; BB = branching portion of the bundle of His; RBB = right bundle branch; Ao = aorta; SVC = superior vena cava; PA = pulmonary artery; Ant. = anterior; TV = tricuspid valve.) (From Bharati, S., Lev, M., Kirklin, J. W.: Cardiac Surgery and the Conduction System. Churchill Livingstone, New York, 1983.)

tion of most of these risk factors by scientific progress and by minimization of human error.

**Type of VSD.** The location of the *single large VSD* is not an incremental risk factor with regard to early or late results of repair. In the past, *multiple VSDs* were an important incremental risk factor (Blackstone et al., 1976; Kirklin et al, 1980). The authors more recent experience indicates that it is only a weak one (Rizzoli et al., 1980) (Table 38–3). This improvement is in part related to the general improvements in infant intracardiac operations, but is also related in a major way to a now higher proportion of patients with complete or almost complete repair and little or no residual shunting. This improvement can be attributed primarily to better preoperative cineangiographic identification of the presence, size, and location of the multiple VSDs.

**Age at Repair.** There have been no deaths at the University of Alabama at Birmingham (UAB) among patients operated on at 24 months of age or older for repair of isolated large VSD in the last decade, and thus, for a long time, the risk of operation under these circumstances has approached 0%.

The incremental risk of young age was clearly apparent in the authors' early experience, as it was in many centers (Binet et al., 1970; Ching et al., 1971; Cooley et al., 1962; Johnson et al., 1974). However, a steady decrease in hospital mortality has occurred with time and affects infants particularly. As a result, the previously apparent incremental risk of young age has been neutralized in more recent experiences

■ **Table 38–3.** HOSPITAL MORTALITY IN 29 PATIENTS (*p* = 0.22) UNDERGOING PRIMARY REPAIR OF MULTIPLE VENTRICULAR SEPTAL DEFECTS WITHOUT MAJOR ASSOCIATED LESIONS AT THE UNIVERSITY OF ALABAMA AT BIRMINGHAM (1967–1979)

| Age (Months) | Total | | | | 1974–1979* | | | |
|---|---|---|---|---|---|---|---|---|
| | | Hospital Deaths | | | | Hospital Deaths | | |
| | *No.* | No. | % | 70% CL (%) | *No.* | No. | % | 70% CL (%) |
| <3 | 1 | 0 | 0 | 0–85 | 1 | 0 | 0 | 0–85 |
| ≥3 <6 | 4 | 2 | 50 | 18–82 | 2 | 0 | 0 | 0–61 |
| ≥6 <12 | 5 | 1 | 20 | 3–53 | 3 | 0 | 0 | 0–47 |
| ≥12 <24 | 7 | 3 | 43 | 20–68 | 4 | 1 | 25 | 3–63 |
| ≥24 <48 | 5 | 3 | 60 | 29–86 | 1 | 0 | 0 | 0–85 |
| ≥48 | 7 | 0 | 0 | 0–24 | 3 | 0 | 0 | 0–47 |
| *Total* | 29 | 9 | 31 | 21–42 | 14 | 1 | 7 | 1–22 |
| | (15 | 8 | 53 | 37–69)† | | | | |

From Rizzoli, G., Blackstone, E. H., Kirklin, J. W., et al.: Incremental risk factors in hospital mortality after repair of ventricular septal defect. J. Thorac. Cardiovasc. Surg., *80*:494, 1980.
*Note the greatly lowered mortality rate in this period.
†Numbers in parentheses are for the period from 1967 to 1974.

**■ Table 38–4.** EFFECT OF AGE ON HOSPITAL MORTALITY* IN 166 PATIENTS UNDERGOING PRIMARY REPAIR OF SINGLE LARGE VENTRICULAR SEPTAL DEFECT WITHOUT MAJOR ASSOCIATED LESIONS AT THE UNIVERSITY OF ALABAMA AT BIRMINGHAM (1967–1979)

| Age (Months) | Total | | | | | 1974–1979 | | | | |
| | | | *Hospital Deaths* | | | | | *Hospital Deaths* | | |
| | *No.* | % | No. | % | 70% CL (%) | *No.* | % | No. | % | 70% CL (%) |
|---|---|---|---|---|---|---|---|---|---|---|
| <3 | 14 | 8.4 | 2 | 14 | 5–31 | 11 | 11.7 | 1† | 9 | 1–28 |
| ≥3  <6 | 12 | 7.2 | 0 | 0 | 0–15 | 10 | 10.6 | 0 | 0 | 0–17 |
| ≥6  <12 | 23 | 13.9 | 3 | 13 | 6–25 | 14 | 14.9 | 0 | 0 | 0–13 |
| ≥12 <24 | 21 | 12.7 | 1 | 5 | 1–15 | 11 | 11.7 | 0 | 0 | 0–16 |
| ≥24 <48 | 27 | 16.3 | 0 | 0 | 0–7 | 15 | 16.0 | 0 | 0 | 0–12 |
| ≥48 | 69 | 41.6 | 0 | 0 | 0–3 | 33 | 35.1 | 0 | 0 | 0–6 |
| *Total* | 166 | | 6 | 3.6 | 2.1–5.8 | 94 | | 1 | 1.1 | 0.1–3.6 |
| | (72 | | 5 | 6.9 | 3.9–11.5)‡ | | | | | |

From Rizzoli, G., Blackstone, E. H., Kirklin, J. W., et al.: Incremental risk factors in hospital mortality after repair of ventricular septal defect. J. Thorac. Cardiovasc. Surg., *80*:494, 1980.

*The *p* value (*n* = 166) = 0.01.

†A 1.2-month-old baby with preoperative seizures was admitted to surgery, intubated, and ventilated; the baby died on third postoperative day with acute cardiac failure.

‡Numbers in parentheses are for the period from 1967 to 1974.

(Barratt-Boyes et al., 1976; Rein et al., 1977; Rizzoli et al., 1980) (Table 38–4 and Fig. 38–13). This has resulted in part from scientific progress, with improved preoperative diagnostic accuracy, improved surgical and support techniques, and improved myocardial preservation. It has also resulted in part from a demonstrated decrease in fatal human surgical and management errors as institutions have increased their experience and expertise with infant intracardiac surgery.

**Pulmonary Artery Pressure and Pulmonary Vascular Resistance.** At present, these are not determinants of hospital mortality, although they do affect late results (Blackstone et al., 1976). This is different from the earlier Mayo Clinic experiences (Cartmill et al., 1966), probably because the upper limit of acceptable ("operable") pulmonary vascular resistance is better understood and management has improved.

**Major Associated Lesions.** The frequency of major associated lesions, particularly in symptomatic infants

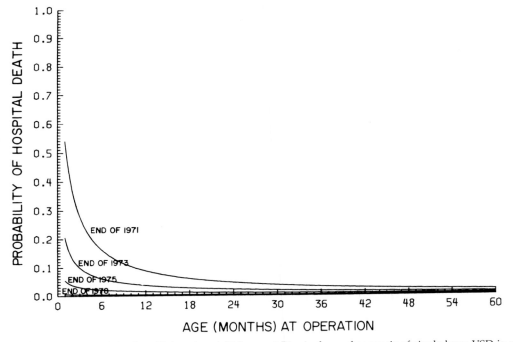

**FIGURE 38–13.** Probability of hospital death at University of Alabama at Birmingham after repair of single large VSD in patients without major associated cardiac anomalies. Note that in 1971 and 1973, the risk was considerably increased in very young patients. By 1979, not only was the risk of hospital death less than 1%, but an incremental risk in patients of young age was no longer apparent. (From Rizzoli, G., Blackstone, E. H., Kirklin, J. W., et al.: Incremental risk factors in hospital mortality after repair of ventricular septal defect. J. Thorac. Cardiovasc. Surg., *80*:494, 1980.)

with large VSDs, has already been emphasized. These do have, even currently, an incremental risk effect on hospital mortality. At the UAB, among 312 patients undergoing surgery for VSD from 1967 to 1979, 16 hospital deaths (6.3%; confidence limits [CL] 4.7 to 8.3%) occurred among 254 patients with single or multiple VSDs but no major associated lesion, whereas 14 (24%; CL 18 to 31%) occurred among 58 patients with major associated lesions ($p < 0.0001$) (Rizzoli et al., 1980). Additional technical and scientific progress will probably improve this situation.

**Surgical Approach.** The surgical approach for repair of the VSD (through the right atrium, through the right ventricle, or through both) has not been a determinant of hospital mortality after repair of single VSDs (Table 38–5). Neither has it been after the repair of muscular or multiple VSDs through a left ventriculotomy, an experience also reported by surgeons at the Boston Children's Hospital (Kirklin et al., 1980). However, concern continues about the long-term functional results of left ventriculotomy in infants.

## Late Results

Repair of VSD in the first year or two of life cures most patients and results in full functional activity and normal or almost normal life expectancy.

**Improved Physical Development.** This is a prominent feature of the late postoperative course after repair of large VSDs in infants (Rein et al., 1977). Lillehei and colleagues first showed an impressive increase in weight after VSD repair in 1955. There is a less impressive increase in length and in head circumference (Clarkson et al., 1973). This improved physical development is usually associated with complete relief of symptoms. The authors have also reported increase in weight postoperatively in children in whom a large VSD had been repaired later in the first decade of life (Cartmill et al., 1966).

Early surgical closure of a large VSD results in near normal long-term growth in most patients (Weintraub et al., 1991).

**Permanent Heart Block** (complete atrioventricular dissociation with independent atrial activity not conducted to the ventricles). This is uncommon with present techniques. For example, heart block was present at death or hospital dismissal in 1.5% (CL 0.5 to 3%) of patients with large VSDs without associated lesions of major anatomic or functional significance in the UAB experience between 1967 and 1976 (Blackstone et al., 1976). The two patients were both unusual. One patient had multiple muscular defects and the other patient had Down syndrome and a large perimembranous defect. In the earlier report from the Mayo Clinic, no such case occurred among the 146 patients with large VSDs undergoing surgery between 1962 and 1966.

**Cardiac Function.** Cardiac function late postoperatively is essentially normal when repair is done in the first 2 years of life by modern techniques through the right atrium or right ventricle. Graham and colleagues found that left ventricular end-diastolic volume, left ventricular systolic output, left ventricular mass, and left ventricular ejection fraction were all normal approximately 1 year after operation in a group of these patients (Cordell et al., 1976). Others have found persistent abnormalities of left ventricular size and function after repair of large VSDs at an older age, although all patients were asymptomatic (Jarmakani et al., 1971, 1972). This information lends support to the idea that, in general, patients with large VSDs should undergo surgery before they are 2 years old.

**Residual Shunting.** Postoperative left-to-right shunts of such magnitude as to indicate reoperation are uncommon when proper techniques are used. One of 138 patients (0.7%; CL 0.1 to 2%) undergoing surgery at UAB for repair of a large VSD has required reoperation (and this was for overlooked multiple muscular defects) (Blackstone et al., 1976). A report from Castaneda's group (Rein et al., 1977) stated that only 1 patient of 48 hospital survivors (2%; CL 0 to 7%) required reoperation for residual VSD.

**Premature Late Deaths.** Late death occurs rarely (<2.5% of patients) when pulmonary vascular resistance is low preoperatively. Presumably, these deaths are from arrhythmias, either ventricular fibrillation or the sudden late development of heart block.

■ **Table 38–5.** EFFECT OF SURGICAL APPROACH ON HOSPITAL MORTALITY* IN 166 PATIENTS UNDERGOING PRIMARY REPAIR OF SINGLE LARGE VENTRICULAR SEPTAL DEFECTS WITHOUT MAJOR ASSOCIATED LESIONS AT THE UNIVERSITY OF ALABAMA AT BIRMINGHAM (1967–1979)

| Surgical Approach | Total | | | | 1974–1979 | | | |
|---|---|---|---|---|---|---|---|---|
| | | Hospital Deaths | | | | Hospital Deaths | | |
| | No. | No. | % | 70% CL (%) | No. | No. | % | 70% CL (%) |
| RA† | 105 | 2 | 1.9 | 0.6–4.5 | 65 | 1 | 1.5 | 0.2–5.1 |
| RA → RV‡ | 4 | 0 | 0 | 0–38 | 2 | 0 | 0 | 0–61 |
| RV | 57 | 4 | 7 | 4–12 | 27 | 0 | 0 | 0–7 |
| Total | 166 | 6 | 3.6 | 2.1–5.8 | 94 | 1 | 1.1 | 0.1–3.6 |

From Rizzoli, G., Blackstone, E. H., Kirklin, J. W., et al.: Incremental risk factors in hospital mortality after repair of ventricular septal defect. J. Thorac. Cardiovasc. Surg., *80*:494, 1980.

*The $p$ value ($n = 166$) = 0.23.

†RA = right atrium.

‡RV = right ventricle.

Patients with a high pulmonary vascular resistance preoperatively have a tendency for this to progress and cause premature death; this becomes of some magnitude ($\pm$ 25% dying within 5 years of operation) when the resistance preoperatively is more than 10 units $\cdot$ m$^2$.

In a study of 296 surviving patients after VSD closure followed for 30 to 35 years postoperatively, higher late mortality was observed in those undergoing surgery after the age of 5 years, those with pulmonary vascular resistance greater than 7 units $\cdot$ m$^2$, and those with transient or permanent complete heart block (Moller et al., 1991).

**Pulmonary Hypertension.** Generally, the younger the child is at the time of repair, the better his or her chances are of having an essentially normal pulmonary artery pressure 5 years later, and thus, presumably, for the rest of the child's life (Barratt-Boyes et al., 1976; Castaneda et al., 1971; DuShane and Kirklin, 1973; Hoffman and Rudolph, 1966; Lillehei et al., 1968; Maron et al., 1973; Sigmann et al., 1977; Yacoub et al., 1978). The lower the pulmonary vascular resistance or the pulmonary artery pressure at the time of repair, the better are the patient's chances of having normal pulmonary artery pressure postoperatively.

Severe pulmonary hypertension postoperatively can increase with time (Friedli et al., 1974) and cause premature late death, usually within 3 to 10 years of operation (DuShane and Kirklin, 1973; Friedli et al., 1974; Hallidie-Smith et al., 1969). However, some patients with pulmonary hypertension and elevated pulmonary vascular resistance late postoperatively have neither progression nor regression of their disease for as long as 20 years, although with some limitation in exercise tolerance (DuShane and Kirklin, 1973; Hallidie-Smith et al., 1975). Their life expectancy, however, is probably not normal.

## SPECIAL SITUATIONS

**VSD Plus Coarctation of the Aorta.** Although there has been controversy as to the management of young infants in congestive heart failure because of this combination, most centers, including the authors', now practice prompt repair of the coarctation (Bergdahl et al., 1982) *without* concomitant pulmonary artery banding. If the baby remains ventilator-dependent for 72 hours, the VSD is then closed. Usually, this is not the case, and prompt improvement occurs after repair of the coarctation. The VSD may then require repair 3 to 12 months later. Often, however, spontaneous reduction in size and eventual closure occur.

**VSD Plus Patent Ductus Arteriosus.** When a young infant with severe congestive heart failure has a large VSD and a patent ductus arteriosus of any size, operation is advisable, and both are repaired at operation through a median sternotomy incision.

When the VSD is small or a moderate size and the patent ductus arteriosus is large and the infant is in the first few months of life, the ductus arteriosus is closed by way of a simple operation through a left-sided thoracotomy incision. The VSD will usually become narrow and will close spontaneously.

## SELECTED BIBLIOGRAPHY

Barratt-Boyes, B. G., Neutze, J. M., Clarkson, P. M., et al.: Repair of ventricular septal defect in the first two years of life using profound hypothermia—Circulatory arrest techniques. Ann. Surg., *184*:376, 1976.

This classic paper describes the results of primary repair of VSD in 57 patients less than 2 years of age, with many of the patients being less than 6 months old. The hospital mortality rate was 4% in the patients without associated coarctation—A remarkable achievement. The late postoperative results are excellent. The method of profound hypothermia and total circulatory arrest and these superb results have had an important and worldwide impact on cardiac operations.

Hoffman, J. I. E., and Rudolph, A. M.: The natural history of ventricular septal defects in infancy. Am. J. Cardiol., *16*:634, 1965.

This classic paper reports data on 62 infants with VSD who were first catheterized under 1 year of age and were followed for 1 to 5 years after that. Forty were recatheterized. Fifty per cent of the infants had congestive heart failure. Spontaneous closure of the VSD occurred in 36% of the patients, and in an additional 28%, marked decrease in the size of the defect occurred. In this series, complete spontaneous closure occurred between 7 and 12 months of age. Sixteen per cent of the group studied did not do well. Five had severe and unrelenting congestive heart failure. One baby had a high pulmonary vascular resistance from birth that never regressed. Four babies had low pulmonary vascular resistance when first catheterized at less than 1 year of age, with significant rises of resistance to pathologic levels when recatheterized subsequently. These data form a rational basis for surgical patient management programs.

Lillehei, C. W., Cohen, M., Warden, H. E., et al.: The results of direct vision closure of ventricular septal defects in eight patients by means of controlled cross-circulation. Surg. Gynecol. Obstet., *101*:446, 1955.

This classic article, reporting the first successful closures of VSDs, still makes superb and informative reading. Although cross-circulation is no longer used, it obviously was a superb support system for these small patients.

Neutze, J. M., Ishikawa, T., Clarkson, P. M., et al.: Assessment and follow-up of patients with ventricular septal defect and elevated pulmonary vascular resistance. Am. J. Cardiol., *63*:327, 1989.

This paper describes in detail the response of patients with elevated pulmonary vascular resistance to infusion of isoproterenol during cardiac catheterization and compares this with their response to surgical closure of VSD. The data indicate that a fall in resistance to less than 7 U·m$^2$ with isoproterenol predicts a good postoperative course.

Rein, J. G., Freed, M. D., Norwood, W. I., and Castaneda, A. R.: Early and late results of closure of ventricular septal defect in infancy. Ann. Thorac. Surg., *24*:19, 1977.

The superb results obtained by Castaneda and colleagues in the operation of primary repair of VSD in the first year of life in 50 infants are reported here. The Kyoto–Barratt-Boyes technique of profound hypothermia and total circulatory arrest was used. The hospital mortality rate was 6%, no late death occurred, and the late functional status was excellent. This paper gave strong supportive evidence for the excellence of the results that can be obtained from primary repair of VSD, even in very young infants.

Rizzoli, G., Blackstone, E. H., Kirklin, J. W., et al.: Incremental risk factors in hospital mortality after repair of ventricular septal defect. J. Thorac. Cardiovasc. Surg., *80*:494, 1980.

This paper describes the incremental risk (degree of difficulty, if you will) of numerous factors in 312 patients undergoing repair of VSD from 1967 to 1979. More important, it describes how these incremental risk factors have gradually been neutralized by scientific advances and minimization of human errors. Thus, in the era beginning in 1978, the hospital mortality rate of repair of single large VSDs is less than 1%, no matter how young the patient (neutralization of the previous incremental risk of young age), and is approximately 5% for multiple VSDs, again without an incremental risk of young age. Major associated cardiac anomalies or procedures (large patent ductus arteriosus, simultaneous repair of coarctation or interrupted arch, and important mitral valve abnormalities) still increase risk.

Soto, B., Becker, A. E., Moulaert, A. J., et al.: Classification of ventricular septal defects. Br. Heart J., *43*:332, 1980.

Many anatomic studies of VSD have been reported through the years, but this study by Anderson and colleagues has been particularly helpful to surgeons. Their work, described in this paper, forms the basis for the description of morphology used in this chapter. The ventricular septum is divided into a membranous and muscular portion, and the latter is divided into an inlet, trabecular, and infundibular (outlet) portion. This paper introduces the advisable phrase *perimembranous VSD* for those defects in the region of the membranous septum, right up against the tricuspid annulus. It also clarifies the fact that the so-called atrioventricular canal *type* of VSD is really a perimembranous one and extends particularly beneath the septal tricuspid leaflet. Beautiful anatomic and cineangiographic plates clarify the description.

## BIBLIOGRAPHY

Aaron, B. L., and Lower, R. R.: Muscular ventricular septal defect repair made easy. Ann. Thorac. Surg., 19:568, 1975.

Ash, R.: Natural history of ventricular septal defects in childhood lesions with predominant arteriovenous shunts. J. Pediatr., 64:45, 1964.

Auld, P. A. M., Johnson, A. L., Gibbons, J. E., and McGregor, M.: Changes in pulmonary vascular resistance in infants and children with intracardiac left-to-right shunts. Circulation, 27:257, 1963.

Bargeron, L. M., Jr., Elliott, L. P., Soto, B., et al.: Axial angiocardiography in congenital heart disease. I: Concept, technical and anatomic considerations. Circulation, 56:1075, 1977.

Barratt-Boyes, B. G., Neutze, J. M., Clarkson, P. M., et al.: Repair of ventricular septal defect in the first two years of life using profound hypothermia—Circulatory arrest techniques. Ann. Surg., 184:376, 1976.

Bergdahl, L. A. L., Blackstone, E. H., Kirklin, J. W., et al.: Determinants of early success in repair of aortic coarctation in infants. J. Thorac. Cardiovasc. Surg., 83:736, 1982.

Berner, M., Behetti, M., Ricou, B., et al.: Relief of severe pulmonary hypertension after closure of a large ventricular septal defect using low dose inhaled nitric oxide. Intensive Care Med., 19:75, 1993.

Binet, J. P., Conso, J. F., Langlois, J., et al.: Fermeture de certaines communications interventriculaires congénitales basses par le ventricule gauche. Arch. Mal. Coeur, 63:1345, 1970.

Blackstone, E. H., Kirklin, J. W., Bradley, E. L., et al.: Optimal age and results in repair of large ventricular septal defects. J. Thorac. Cardiovasc. Surg., 72:661, 1976.

Breckenridge, I. M., Stark, J., Waterston, D. J., and Bonham-Carter, R. E.: Multiple ventricular septal defects. Ann. Thorac. Surg., 13:128, 1972.

Campbell, M.: Natural history of ventricular septal defect. Br. Heart J., 33:246, 1971.

Cartmill, T. B., DuShane, J. W., McGoon, D. C., and Kirklin, J. W.: Results of repair of ventricular septal defect. J. Thorac. Cardiovasc. Surg., 52:486, 1966.

Castaneda, A. R., Zamora, R., Nicoloff, D. M., et al.: High-pressure, high-resistance ventricular septal defect. Surgical results of closure through right atrium. Ann. Thorac. Surg., 12:29, 1971.

Ching, E., DuShane, J. W., McGoon, D. C., and Danielson, G. K.: Total correction of ventricular septal defect in infancy using extracorporeal circulation: Surgical considerations and results of operation. Ann. Thorac. Surg., 12:1, 1971.

Clarkson, P. M.: Growth following corrective cardiac operation in early infancy. In Barratt-Boyes, B. G., Neutze, J. M., and Harris, E. A. (eds): Heart Disease in Infancy: Diagnosis and Surgical Treatment. London, Churchill Livingstone, 1973, p. 75.

Clarkson, P. M., Frye, R. L., DuShane, J. W., et al.: Prognosis for patients with ventricular septal defect and severe pulmonary vascular obstructive disease. Circulation, 38:129, 1968.

Collins, G., Calder, L., Rose, V., Kidd, L., and Keith, J.: Ventricular septal defect: Clinical and hemodynamic changes in the first five years of life. Am. Heart J., 84:695, 1972.

Cooley, D. A., Garrett, H. E., and Howard, H. S.: The surgical treatment of ventricular septal defect: An analysis of 300 consecutive surgical cases. Prog. Cardiovasc. Dis., 4:312, 1962.

Cordell, D., Graham, T. P., Jr., Atwood, G. F., et al.: Left heart volume characteristics following ventricular septal defect closure in infancy. Circulation, 54:294, 1976.

Corone, P., Doyan, F., Gaudeau, S., et al.: Natural history of ventricular septal defect: A study involving 790 cases. Circulation, 55:908, 1977.

Dirksen, T., Moulaert, A. J., Buis-Liem, T. N., and Brom, A. G.: Ventricular septal defect associated with left ventricular outflow tract obstruction below the defect. J. Thorac. Cardiovasc. Surg., 75:688, 1978.

DuShane, J. W., and Kirklin, J. W.: Late results of the repair of ventricular septal defect on pulmonary vascular disease. In Kirklin, J. W. (ed): Advances in Cardiovascular Surgery. New York, Grune & Stratton, 1973, p. 9.

DuShane, J. W., and Kirklin, J. W.: Selection for surgery of patients with ventricular septal defect and pulmonary hypertension. Circulation, 21:13, 1960.

DuShane, J. W., Kirklin, J. W., Patrick, R. T., et al.: Ventricular septal defects with pulmonary hypertension: Surgical treatment by means of a mechanical pump-oxygenator. J. A. M. A., 160:950, 1956.

Freed, M. D., Rosenthal, A., Plauth, W. H., Jr., and Nadas, A. S.: Development of subaortic stenosis after pulmonary artery banding. Circulation, 47, 48(Suppl. III):7, 1973.

Friedli, B., Kidd, B. S. L., Mustard, W. T., and Keith, J. D.: Ventricular septal defect with increased pulmonary vascular resistance. Late results of surgical closure. Am. J. Cardiol., 33:403, 1974.

Gasul, B. M., Dillon, R. F., Vrla, V., and Hait, G.: Ventricular septal defects. Their natural transformation into those with infundibular stenosis or into the cyanotic or non-cyanotic type of tetralogy of Fallot. J. A. M. A., 164:847, 1957.

Hallidie-Smith, K. A., Edwards, R. E., Wilson, R., and Zeidifard, E.: Long-term cardiorespiratory assessment after surgical closure of ventricular septal defect in childhood [Abstract.] Proc. Br. Cardiac Soc., 37:553, 1975.

Hallidie-Smith, K. A., Hollman, A., Cleland, W. P., et al.: Effects of surgical closure of ventricular septal defects upon pulmonary vascular disease. Br. Heart J., 31:246, 1969.

Heath, D., and Edwards, J. E.: The pathology of hypertensive pulmonary vascular disease: A description of six grades of structural changes in the pulmonary arteries with special reference to congenital cardiac septal defects. Circulation, 18:533, 1958.

Heath, D., Helmholtz, H. F., Jr., Burchell, H. B., et al.: Relation between structural changes in the small pulmonary arteries and the immediate reversibility of pulmonary hypertension following closure of ventricular and atrial septal defects. Circulation, 18:1167, 1958.

Hislop, A., Haworth, S. G., Shinebourne, E. A., and Reid, L.: Quantitative structural analysis of pulmonary vessels in isolated ventricular septal defects in infancy. Br. Heart J., 37:1014, 1975.

Hoffman, J. I. E.: Diagnosis and treatment of pulmonary vascular disease. Birth Defects (original article series), 8:9, 1972.

Hoffman, J. I. E., and Rudolph, A. M.: Increasing pulmonary vascular resistance during infancy in association with ventricular septal defect. Pediatrics, 38:220, 1966.

Hoffman, J. I. E., and Rudolph, A. M.: The natural history of isolated ventricular septal defect, with special references to selection of patients for surgery. In Schulman, I. (ed): Advances in Pediatrics. Chicago, Year Book, 1970, p. 57.

Hoffman, J. I. E., and Rudolph, A. M.: The natural history of ventricular septal defects in infancy. Am. J. Cardiol., 16:634, 1965.

Hopkins, R. A., Bull, C., Haworth, S. G., et al.: Pulmonary hypertensive crises following surgery for congenital heart defects in young children. Eur. J. Cardiothorac. Surg., 5:628, 1991.

Jarmakani, J. M., Edwards, S. B., Spach, M. S., et al.: Left ventricular pressure volume characteristics in congenital heart disease. Circulation, 37:879, 1968.

Jarmakani, J. M., Graham, T. P., Jr., and Canent, R. V., Jr.: Left ventricular contractile state in children with successfully corrected ventricular septal defect. Circulation, 45, 46(Suppl. I):102, 1972.

Jarmakani, J. M., Graham, T. P., Jr., Canent, R. V., et al.: The effect of corrective surgery on left heart volume and mass in children with ventricular septal defect. Am. J. Cardiol., 27:254, 1971.

Johnson, D. C., Cartmill, T. B., Celermajer, J. M., et al.: Intracardiac repair of large ventricular septal defect in the first year of life. Med. J. Aust., 2:193, 1974.

Keith, J. D., Rose, V., Collins, G., and Kidd, B. S. L.: Ventricular septal defect: Incidence, morbidity, and mortality in various age groups. Br. Heart. J., 33(Suppl.):81, 1971.

Kirklin, J. K., and Kirklin, J. W.: Management of the cardiovascular subsystem after cardiac surgery. Ann. Thorac. Surg., 32:311, 1981.

Kirklin, J. K., Castaneda, A. R., Keane, J. F., et al.: Surgical management of multiple ventricular septal defects. J. Thorac. Cardiovasc. Surg., 80:485, 1980.

Kirklin, J. W., and DuShane, J. W.: Indications for repair of ventricular septal defects. Am. J. Cardiol., 12:79, 1963.

Kirklin, J. W., and DuShane, J. W.: Repair of ventricular septal defect in infancy. Pediatrics, 27:961, 1961.

Lauer, R. M., DuShane, J. W., and Edwards, J. E.: Obstruction of left ventricular outlet in association with ventricular septal defect. Circulation, 22:110, 1960.

Leatham, A., and Segal, B.: Auscultatory and phonocardiographic signs of ventricular septal defect with left-to-right shunt. Circulation, 25:318, 1962.

Levin, A. R., Boineau, J. P., Spach, M. S., et al.: Ventricular pressure flow-dynamics in tetralogy of Fallot. Circulation, 34:4, 1966.

Lillehei, C. W., Anderson, R. C., Eliot, R. S., et al.: Pre- and postoperative cardiac catheterization in 200 patients undergoing closure of ventricular septal defects. Surgery, 63:69, 1968.

Lillehei, C. W., Cohen, M., Warden, H. E., et al.: The results of direct vision closure of ventricular septal defects in eight patients by means of controlled cross circulation. Surg. Gynecol. Obstet., 101:446, 1955.

Lincoln, C., Jamieson, S., Joseph, M., et al.: Transatrial repair of ventricular septal defects with reference to their anatomic classification. J. Thorac. Cardiovasc. Surg., 74:183, 1977.

Lucas, R. V., Jr., Adams, P., Jr., Anderson, R. C., et al.: The natural history of isolated ventricular septal defect: A serial physiologic study. Circulation, 24:1372, 1961.

Maron, B. J., Redwood, D. R., Hirschfeld, J. W., Jr., et al.: Postoperative assessment of patients with ventricular septal defect and pulmonary hypertension: Response to intense upright exercise. Circulation, 48:864, 1973.

Moller, J. H., Patton, C., Varco, R. L., et al.: Late results (30 to 35 years) after operative closure of isolated ventricular septal defect from 1954 to 1960. Am. J. Cardiol., 68:1491, 1991.

Moulaert, A. J., Bruins, C. G., and Oppenheimer-Dekker, A.: Anomalies of the aortic arch and ventricular septal defects. Circulation, 53:1011, 1976.

Neutze, J. M., Ishikawa, T., Clarkson, P. M., et al.: Assessment and follow-up of patients with ventricular septal defect and elevated pulmonary vascular resistance. Am. J. Cardiol., 63:327, 1989.

Oh, K. S., Park, S. C., Galvis, A. G., et al.: Pulmonary hyperinflation in ventricular septal defect. J. Thorac. Cardiovasc. Surg., 76:706, 1978.

Okamoto, Y.: Clinical studies for open heart surgery in infants with profound hypothermia. Arch. Jpn. Chir., 38:188, 1969.

Pacifico, A. D.: Cardiopulmonary bypass and hypothermic circulatory arrest in congenital heart surgery. In Grillo, H. C., et al. (eds): Current Therapy in Cardiothoracic Surgery. Toronto, B. C. Decker, 1988.

Rein, J. G., Freed, M. D., Norwood, W. I., and Castaneda, A. R.: Early and late results of closure of ventricular septal defect in infancy. Ann. Thorac. Surg., 24:19, 1977.

Rizzoli, G., Blackstone, E. H., Kirklin, J. W., et al.: Incremental risk factors in hospital mortality after repair of ventricular septal defect. J. Thorac. Cardiovasc. Surg., 80:494, 1980.

Sand, M. E., McGrath, L. B., Pacifico, A. D., and Mandke, N. V.: Repair of left superior vena cava entering the left atrium. Ann. Thorac. Surg., 42:560, 1986.

Shah, P., Singh, W. S. A., Rose, V., and Keith, J. D.: Incidence of bacterial endocarditis in ventricular septal defects. Circulation, 34:127, 1966.

Sigmann, J. M., Perry, B. L., Behrendt, D. M., et al.: Ventricular septal defect: Results after repair in infancy. Am. J. Cardiol., 39:66, 1977.

Sigmann, J. M., Stern, A. M., and Sloan, H. E.: Early surgical correction of large ventricular septal defects. Pediatrics, 39:4, 1967.

Singh, A. K., de Leval, M. R., and Stark, J.: Left ventriculotomy for closure of muscular ventricular septal defects. Ann. Surg., 186:577, 1977.

Somerville, J.: Personal communication, 1970.

Soto, B., Becker, A. E., Moulaert, A. J., et al.: Classification of ventricular septal defects. Br. Heart J., 43:332, 1980.

Stirling, G. R., Stanley, P. H., and Lillehei, C. W.: Effect of cardiac bypass and ventriculotomy upon right ventricular function. Surg. Forum, 8:433, 1957.

Van Praagh, R., Bernhard, W. F., Rosenthal, A., et al.: Interrupted aortic arch: Surgical treatment. Am. J. Cardiol., 27:200, 1971.

Wagenvoort, C. A., and Wagenvoort, N.: Primary pulmonary hypertension: A pathological study of the lung vessels in 156 clinically diagnosed cases. Circulation, 42:1163, 1970.

Wagenvoort, C. A., Neufeld, H. N., DuShane, J. W., and Edwards, J. E.: The pulmonary arterial tree in ventricular septal defect. A quantitative study of anatomic features in fetuses, infants, and children. Circulation, 23:740, 1961.

Weintraub, R. G., and Menahem, S.: Early surgical closure of a large ventricular septal defect: Influence on long-term growth. J. Am. Coll. Cardiol., 18:552, 1991.

Yacoub, M. H., Radley-Smith, R., and deGasperis, C.: Primary repair of large ventricular septal defects in the first year of life. G. Ital. Cardiol., 8:827, 1978.

Yamaki, S., and Tezuka, F.: Quantitative analysis of pulmonary vascular disease in complete transposition of the great arteries. Circulation, 54:805, 1976.

# 39

# Tetralogy of Fallot and Pulmonary Atresia or Stenosis with Intact Ventricular Septum

## ■ I Tetralogy of Fallot

Ross M. Ungerleider

*Tetralogy of Fallot* (TOF) is one of the most common congenital heart malformations. Depending on the criteria used to define this entity, it can be present in 3 to 6 infants for every 10,000 births (Mitchell et al., 1971). It is probably proper to consider TOF within the spectrum of pulmonary stenosis (or atresia) with an accompanying *ventricular septal defect* (VSD). The condition usually presents with cyanosis shortly after birth, attracting early medical attention. Diagnosis can be made with two-dimensional echocardiography or cardiac catheterization. Nearly all patients are candidates for surgery, and several options exist that can provide excellent immediate and long-term outcomes for many of these children.

## HISTORICAL ASPECTS

Although Stensen deserves credit for the first description (1672) of what is now termed the *tetralogy of Fallot*, it is Etienne-Louis Arthur Fallot (1888) of Marseilles, France, whose name is characteristically attached to this congenital cardiac disorder. There were others prior to Fallot who described the malformation, including Sandifort (1777), John Hunter (1784), William Hunter (1784), Farre (1814), Gintrac (1824), Hope (1839), and Peacock (1866). Most of these descriptions were case reports of comical curiosities. However, in his description of the disorder, Fallot was the first to accurately describe the clinical and complete pathologic manifestations of this deformity. He emphasized that with a knowledge of the clinical manifestations, the malformation could be diagnosed accurately during life.

In the original description of this congenital anomaly, Fallot (1888) stated, "This malformation consists of a true anatomopathological type represented by the following tetralogy: (1) stenosis of the pulmonary artery; (2) interventricular communication; (3) deviation of the origin of the aorta to the right; (4) hypertrophy, almost always concentric, of the right ventricle. Failure of obliteration of the foramen ovale may occasionally be added in a wholly accessory manner." Fallot reported 55 patients with congenital heart disease, of whom most had the TOF malformation. In retrospect, it is remarkable that such a large number

of patients could have been reported by a single author in that early time.

Despite the fact that accurate clinical diagnosis could often be established after these contributions by Fallot, many years passed before definitive treatment of the condition became available. In 1944, Blalock operated on a critically ill infant with TOF who weighed only 4.5 kg. The child was severely cyanotic and had had multiple episodes of unconsciousness owing to marked hypoxemia. A systemic-pulmonary anastomosis was achieved by joining the subclavian artery to the pulmonary artery, and the child was greatly benefited. Several months later, Blalock and Taussig (1945) reported this patient together with two others, and a new era opened in the field of cardiac surgery. The first successful open repair was performed by Lillehei and Varco at the University of Minnesota in 1954, using "controlled cross circulation" with another patient serving as oxygenator and blood reservoir (Lillehei et al., 1955b, 1986)! The following year, Lillehei and associates (1955a) replaced this technique with the use of cardiopulmonary bypass and described repair of TOF using this technology. Since that time, several advances with life-support technology as well as surgical methodology have evolved that have made surgical treatment of TOF one of the most interesting and often satisfying procedures that congenital heart surgeons can perform.

## ANATOMY

There is wide morphologic variability in the spectrum of TOF. This can encompass the size of the right ventricle, the size and distribution of the pulmonary arteries, the location of the pulmonary stenosis (i.e., subvalvular, valvular, or peripheral), and additional sources of pulmonary blood flow (e.g., systemic-pulmonary collaterals) (Figs. 39–1 and 39–2).

Fallot believed that the lesion consisted of four major defects: infundibular pulmonary stenosis, a VSD, dextroposition of the aorta, and hypertrophy of the right ventricle. It is now recognized by most authorities that the two most important features of TOF are: the right ventricular outflow tract (RVOT) obstruction, which is nearly always infundibular

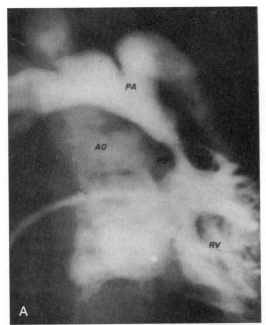

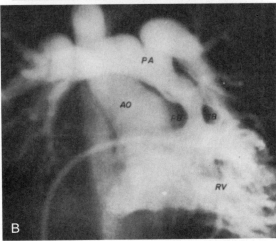

**Figure 39–1.** Obstruction in the region of the infundibulum. *A,* Frame made in systole. *B,* Frame made in diastole. The negative shadows of the hypertrophied parietal bands (PB) and septal bands (SB) are particularly well demonstrated. The pulmonary valve appears domed and at operation was bicuspid but not stenotic. The aorta (AO) is opacified by this right ventricular injection, and its diameter is three times that of the pulmonary artery. The underdevelopment of the infundibulum of the right ventricle, a basic characteristic of tetralogy of Fallot (TOF), is apparent in this angiocardiogram. This patient has anatomy suitable for total correction. (RV, right ventricle; PA, pulmonary artery.) (*A* and *B*, From Kirklin, J. W., and Karp, R. B.: The Tetralogy of Fallot from a Surgical Viewpoint. Philadelphia, W. B. Saunders, 1970.)

and/or valvular in location (Anderson et al., 1981; Arciniegas et al., 1980b; Lev and Eckner, 1964; Kirklin and Barratt-Boyes, 1993; Zerbini et al., 1965); and the VSD, which is usually large, subaortic, adjacent to the membranous septum (perimembranous), and associated with malalignment of the conal septum (Kirklin and Barratt-Boyes, 1993; Lev and Eckner, 1964). A working definition of TOF includes the basic principle that it is a congenital cardiac malformation with a

large VSD (usually as large as the aortic valve orifice, although unusual variants with small and restrictive VSDs have been described) (Flanagan et al., 1988), and with significant pulmonary stenosis (that may be valvular, subvalvular, or supravalvular) that can severely restrict pulmonary blood flow.

These anatomic features nicely explain the basic physiology of the lesion. Shunting across the VSD is determined by the degree of RVOT obstruction. Those patients with severe pulmonary stenosis (regardless of the level of the RVOT obstruction) will shunt right to left across the VSD and will have a degree of cyanosis that reflects the volume of their shunt. When the pulmonary stenosis is less severe, bidirectional shunting may occur. In some patients, the infundibular stenosis is minimal and the predominant shunt is from left to right, producing what is termed the *pink tetralogy.* Although such patients may not appear cyanotic, they often have oxygen desaturation in the systemic arterial blood. Changes in systemic vascular resistance as well as in the pulmonary outflow resistance (which can vary in some patients owing to the tone of the infundibular—or subvalvular—muscle) can produce sudden alterations in the amount of right-to-left shunting and in some patients can produce a hypercyanotic (or "tet") spell. These spells are reversed by the patient (if the patient is old enough) by squatting (to increase systemic vascular resistance and thereby decrease the right-to-left shunt across the VSD), by the pediatrician, who may place these patients on propranolol (to decrease infundibular muscle tone in the hopes of increasing left-to-right shunting across the VSD and into the pulmonary arteries), and by the anesthesiologist, by infusing an alpha-agonist to increase systemic resistance (Greeley et al., 1989) (Fig. 39–3).

The pulmonary arteries can also vary in size and distribution. Occasionally, the left pulmonary artery may be absent (3%), although this is rare for the right pulmonary artery (Fig. 39–4). Many patients have some degree of stenosis of the peripheral pulmonary arteries, which further restricts pulmonary blood flow. There may be no communication between the right ventricle and the main pulmonary artery (pulmonary atresia), and in this case, pulmonary blood flow is maintained by a ductus arteriosus or some other form of bronchopulmonary collateral (Fig. 39–5).

Aortic overriding is caused by true dextroposition and abnormal rotation of the aortic root, creating an aorta that arises from the right ventricle to a varying degree. The aorta itself may have a right arch in as many as 25 to 30% of patients with TOF, and in these situations, the branching pattern of the arch vessels may be abnormal. Occasionally, the ductus arteriosus persists on the side opposite the arch, or it may be completely absent. An aberrant subclavian artery running in a retroesophageal location may be present (5 to 10%), although it is quite rare for the retroesophageal subclavian vessels to cause dysphagia. A persistent left superior vena cava occurs with about the same incidence (Nagao et al., 1967).

Coronary artery anatomy may vary significantly.

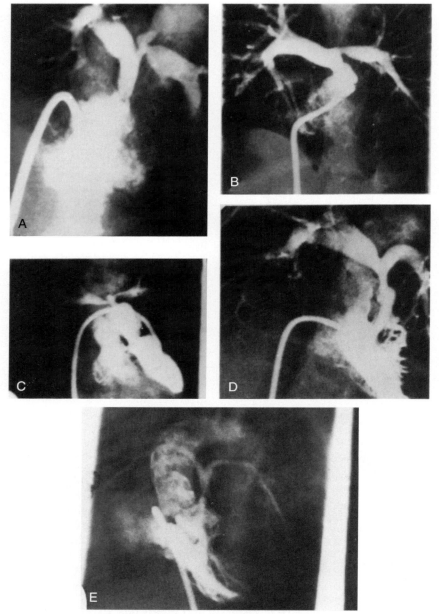

**Figure 39–2.** Angiograms obtained from five different patients with TOF demonstrate the wide variability in pulmonary artery anatomy that can be found. Patient *a* demonstrates stenosis of the proximal left pulmonary artery and a narrowing of the junction between the right ventricle and the main pulmonary artery (RV–PT trunk). There also appears to be persistent flow through a ductus arteriosus at the site of narrowing in the left pulmonary artery. Patient *b* has narrowing of the left pulmonary artery but no evidence of a ductus arteriosus. For Patient *c*, the main pulmonary artery is extremely small, as is the proximal left pulmonary artery. In addition, there appears to be some stenosis at the origin of the right pulmonary artery. Patient *d* has good-caliber right and left pulmonary arteries, but a narrowed main pulmonary artery with a small pulmonary annulus. In addition, there is marked hypertrophy of the infundibular septum. Patient *e* demonstrates an extremely small pulmonary annulus and markedly hypoplastic pulmonary arteries. (*e*, From Kirklin, J. W., and Barratt-Boyes, B. G.: Cardiac Surgery. Copyright © 1986 by John Wiley & Sons, New York.)

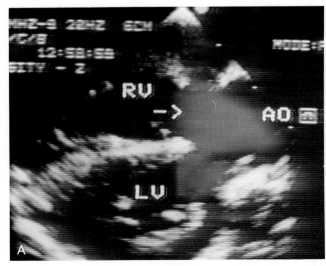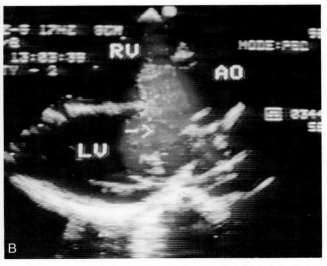

**Figure 39–3.** *A,* Intraoperative Doppler color flow image obtained during a hypercyanotic episode. There is increased right-to-left shunting across the ventricular septal defect (VSD) as demonstrated by blue blood *(arrow)* flowing from the right ventricle (RV) into the aorta (AO). (LV = left ventricle.) *B,* With increase of systemic vascular resistance, this right-to-left shunt is reversed, thus improving systemic arterial oxygen saturation. (LA = left atrium.) (*A* and *B,* From Greeley, W. J., Stanley, T. E., Ungerleider, R. M., and Kisslo, J. A.: Intraoperative hypoxemic spells in tetralogy of Fallot: An echocardiographic analysis of diagnosis and treatment. Anesth. Analg., *68*:815–819, 1989.)

Most notable is the origin of the left anterior descending coronary artery from the proximal right coronary artery, which causes the RVOT to be crossed by this important coronary at variable distances from the pulmonary valve annulus (Dabizzi et al., 1980; Fellows et al., 1975, 1981). Occasionally, all coronaries may arise from a single main coronary ostium (usually the left), or the left coronary may arise from the pulmonary artery (Akasaka et al., 1981).

Associated defects are not uncommon with TOF. The existence of an atrial septal defect (ASD) is frequent enough to prompt its inclusion as "pentalogy" of Fallot. Other defects of importance include atrioventricular (AV) septal defects (Vargas et al., 1986; Westerman et al., 1986), muscular VSDs (Fellows et al., 1981), anomalous pulmonary venous return (Kirklin and Barratt-Boyes, 1993), and aortic incompetence (Matsuda et al., 1980).

## DIAGNOSIS

### Clinical Manifestations

The clinical presentation depends on the severity of the anatomic malformation. Infants with pulmonary atresia may become intensely cyanotic as the ductus arteriosus closes unless they have numerous bronchopulmonary collaterals. Heart failure is usually not a feature unless collaterals are extensive. Patients with right ventricle-to-pulmonary continuity are cyanotic in relation to their degree of stenosis and consequent pulmonary blood flow. This balance is also affected by flow through a ductus arteriosus, and symptoms usually increase when the ductus begins to close shortly after birth. Occasionally, a child will have enough pulmonary blood flow that he or she does not appear cyanotic; the lesion may go undetected until these children begin to outgrow their pulmonary blood flow (Bonchek et al., 1973; Gotsman, 1966). A common way for these older children to increase pulmonary flow is to "squat," thus increasing peripheral vascular resistance and decreasing the size of their right-to-left shunt across the VSD. This position had diagnostic significance and was highly characteristic of TOF in a previous era. Because it is now distinctly unusual for children to remain unrepaired beyond infancy, this "important" descriptive sign of TOF will be less frequently, if ever, observed in the future. Nevertheless, this same physiology is the basis for hypercyanotic or "tet" spells that can be observed in any patient with unrepaired TOF and constitutes the rationale for flexing affected infants into a tight "ball" to increase systemic vascular resistance and break the spell.

The natural history of unrepaired TOF is heavily influenced by the severity of the anatomic defect (Kirklin and Barratt-Boyes, 1993; McCord et al., 1957). Statistics demonstrate a 30% mortality by age 6 months, which increases to 50% by 2 years. Only 20% of patients can be expected to reach 10 years of age, and not more than 5 to 10% live to reach 21 years (Bertranou et al., 1978; Garson et al., 1987; Kirklin and Barratt-Boyes, 1993) (Fig. 39–6). Interestingly, there are rare instances of patients whose shunts are so well balanced that they achieve a normal life span. One example is the American composer, Gilbert, who

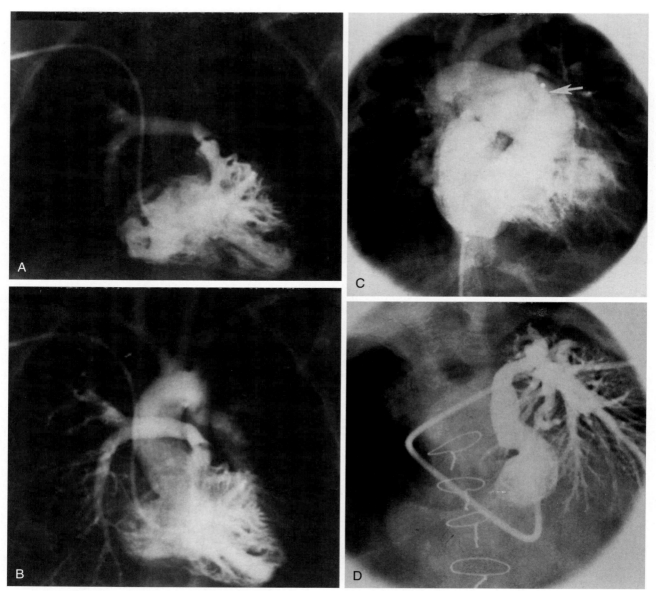

**Figure 39–4.** Pulmonary artery anomalies can be seen in patients with TOF. *A,* A patient demonstrates no evidence of a left pulmonary artery. *B,* An aortagram in the same patient demonstrates that the left pulmonary artery arises as a continuation of the ductus arteriosus off the underside of the aorta. This is repairable anatomy, but requires reconstruction of the pulmonary artery at the time of total correction. *C,* A patient demonstrates absence of the right pulmonary artery, but a small left pulmonary artery *(arrow)* can be seen. The right pulmonary artery was not visible on any study, including pulmonary vein wedge angiograms of the right lung. This patient was treated with an RV outflow tract patch, and a repeat angiogram *(D)* obtained 2 months later demonstrates progressive growth of the left pulmonary artery system and disclosed distal pulmonary artery stenosis (not well appreciated in this view). These stenotic areas underwent balloon angioplasty in the cardiac catheterization laboratory, and the patient eventually came to total correction of her defect (e.g., VSD closure). (*A* and *B*, From Kirklin, J. W., and Barratt-Boyes, B. G.: Cardiac Surgery. Copyright © 1986 by John Wiley & Sons, New York.)

lived to the age of 60 years with TOF and led a relatively productive life without therapy (White and Sprague, 1929). Patients with pulmonary atresia and VSD (TOF with pulmonary atresia) have an even worse prognosis for survival without surgical intervention (Kirklin and Barratt-Boyes, 1993), with a mortality that approaches 50% in the first year of life and can be as high as 84% by 5 years of age. The greatest risks that all TOF patients face (if left unrepaired) is of paradoxical emboli (leading to stroke or end-organ failure), cerebral or pulmonary thrombosis (from in-

creasing polycythemia), and subacute bacterial endocarditis (Arciniegas, 1985). Heart failure is uncommon in surgically untreated patients but does pose a greater risk after creation of a systemic-to-pulmonary artery shunt, especially if preexisting collaterals are not dealt with (Garson et al., 1987).

## Physical Examination

Infants with TOF may appear to be normal in size and otherwise healthy except for a mild to moderate

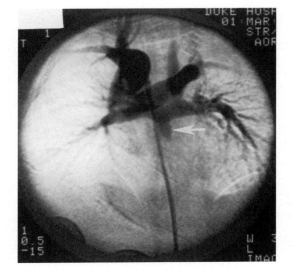

**Figure 39–5.** A digital subtraction angiogram obtained from a patient with a right aortic arch and pulmonary atresia plus VSD ("tet" atresia). In this patient, the pulmonary arteries are of good caliber and there is an excellent main pulmonary artery *(arrow)*. This patient was able to undergo total repair in infancy.

duskiness related to their degree of cyanosis. Older patients may appear to be smaller than expected for their age, and cyanosis of the lips and nail beds is generally apparent. The fingers and toes usually show clubbing (hypertrophic pulmonary osteoarthropathy). On palpation of the chest, a thrill is usually present anteriorly. A harsh systolic murmur is audible over the pulmonary area and along the left sternal border. Absence of a murmur in a patient suspected of having TOF suggests pulmonary atresia. In fact, the harsher the murmur, the more likely that the patient has substantial pulmonary blood flow (and the murmur reflects this flow across the stenotic outflow tract). A murmur that has dissipated in intensity may reflect deficient antegrade flow across the pulmonary outflow tract, and may be accompanied by intense cyanosis unless pulmonary blood flow is provided by a patent ductus arteriosus (PDA) (or by a previously

placed aortopulmonary shunt). The second heart sound is usually single and rarely increased in intensity. During cyanotic spells, murmurs may diminish, reflecting less right ventricular outflow to the pulmonary arteries. A continuous murmur suggests a collateral source of pulmonary blood flow (a PDA, a significant bronchopulmonary collateral, or a surgically created shunt).

## Laboratory Studies

The laboratory studies for infants are ordinarily unremarkable for the age, except for systemic arterial oxygen desaturation. In older patients who have remained cyanotic for some time, the hemoglobin, hematocrit, and erythrocyte count are usually elevated. The magnitude of the increase is generally propor-

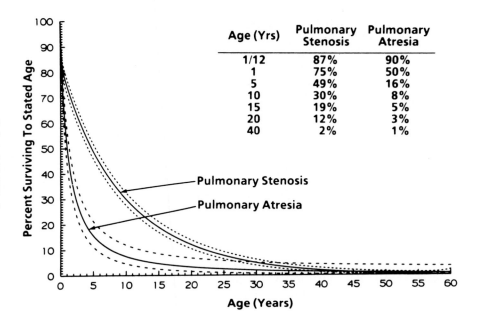

**Figure 39–6.** Nomogram depicting the survival of surgically untreated patients with TOF. The *smooth lines* represent survival of each group and the *dashed lines* enclose the 70% confidence limits around each of these. (From Kirklin, J. W., and Barratt-Boyes, B. G.: Cardiac Surgery. 2nd ed. Churchill Livingstone, New York, 1993.)

| Age (Yrs) | Pulmonary Stenosis | Pulmonary Atresia |
|---|---|---|
| 1/12 | 87% | 90% |
| 1 | 75% | 50% |
| 5 | 49% | 16% |
| 10 | 30% | 8% |
| 15 | 19% | 5% |
| 20 | 12% | 3% |
| 40 | 2% | 1% |

tional to the cyanosis, with hematocrit values varying from normal to as high as 90% (in extreme cases). Similarly, the oxygen saturation in the systemic arterial blood is variable, usually between 65 and 70%. However, in severe forms of the malformation, the arterial oxygen saturation during exercise may fall to as low as 25%. A bleeding tendency is present in some patients with TOF, especially those in whom cyanosis is marked. The usual finding is a diminution in a variety of the factors responsible for blood coagulation, but none of the factors is reduced to critical levels. The platelet count and total blood fibrinogen are frequently diminished slightly, and clot retraction is sometimes poor and associated with prolonged prothrombin and coagulation times. Despite the defects in the clotting mechanism in some patients, the changes are usually insufficient to explain the hemorrhagic tendency noted at the time of operation (Hartmann, 1952; Porter and Silver, 1968).

## Diagnostic Evaluation

In the early stages, the chest film may be normal, but as the ductus arteriosus closes shortly after birth, the chest film in TOF usually shows diminished vascularity in the lungs and absence of prominence of the pulmonary artery. The shadow of the great vessels in the superior mediastinum is narrow, owing to the diminished caliber of the pulmonary artery. If cyanosis and dyspnea are quite prominent, the pulmonary vascular markings are usually markedly diminished. Later, the classic boot-shaped heart (coeur en sabot), which is recognized as a hallmark of TOF, may develop (Fig. 39–7A). Right ventricular enlargement is present and is best demonstrated in the left anterior oblique position. Approximately one-fourth of the patients with TOF have a *right* aortic arch (Fig. 39–7B), and although this can be demonstrated with a barium swallow, it is now common practice to diagnose most anatomic features of the lesion with echocardiography (Silverman, 1993). In fact, the presence of a right aortic arch with cyanosis is strong evidence that the malformation is indeed TOF. Occasionally, there is asymmetric pulmonary vasculature with unilateral oligemia compared with the opposite lung. This suggests absent pulmonary valve syndrome with unilateral pulmonary artery agenesis or anomalous origin of one pulmonary artery from the aorta.

The electrocardiogram shows right ventricular hypertrophy, usually apparent in the standard leads and most consistently found in the unipolar leads. The more commonly encountered findings include tall and peaked T waves, reversal of the RS ratio, and a normal PR interval and QRS duration. If right ventricular hypertrophy is absent, a diagnosis of TOF should be seriously questioned and pulmonary atresia with hypoplastic right ventricle should be considered.

Advances in two-dimensional echocardiography with color-flow Doppler have elevated the diagnostic capabilities of this technology (Kisslo, 1988; Silverman, 1993). It is not uncommon for infants and children to be accurately diagnosed by echocardiogra-

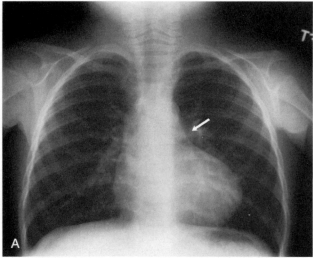

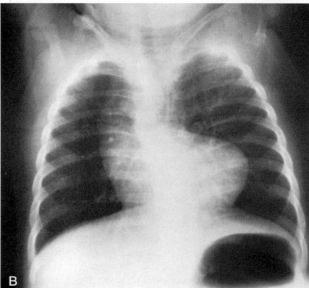

**Figure 39–7.** *A,* Chest film of a patient with TOF and a left aortic arch. The absence of the pulmonary artery shadow *(arrow)* gives the heart a characteristic "boot-shaped" appearance. *B,* In this patient, the boot-shaped appearance of the heart is made even more prominent because of the right aortic arch accentuating the absence of pulmonary arterial shadow.

phy before the performance of any laboratory tests, x-rays, electrocardiograms, or angiograms (Fig. 39–8). Color-flow mapping can sensitively detect the presence of a PDA, an additional muscular VSD, or a small ASD. Echocardiographic documentation of the physiology of a cyanotic spell with right-to-left shunting across a VSD that is reversed by elevation of peripheral vascular resistance has been demonstrated (Greeley et al., 1989) (Fig. 39–3). The coronary anatomy can be revealed with remarkable accuracy, and abnormalities of valvular apparatus (e.g., straddling chords) may be best delineated with this technology. It is not uncommon to take patients to the operating room for palliation or correction based on preoperative echocardiographic data alone (Marino et al., 1987;

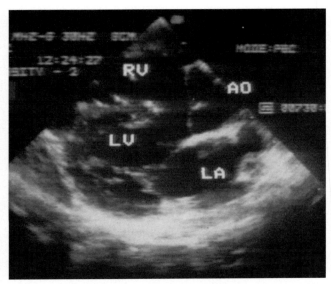

**Figure 39–8.** Long-axis echocardiogram demonstrating the typical features of TOF with a subaortic VSD *(arrow)* and overriding of the aorta so that it appears to arise partially from the right ventricle. (RV = right ventricle; LV = left ventricle; LA = left atrium; AO = aorta.)

Silverman, 1993; Ungerleider et al., 1989, 1990). In many centers, cardiac catheterization is performed only for those patients who have had an echocardiogram that produced inconclusive results regarding the coronary anatomy, the pulmonary artery anatomy, or other sources of pulmonary blood flow.

Cardiac catheterization provides angiographic demonstration of ventricular size, pulmonary artery size, and with aortic root injection, sources of pulmonary blood flow as well as anomalies of coronary artery anatomy. Some authors base prediction of the postrepair right ventricle/left ventricle (RV/LV) pressure ratio on data obtained from catheterization, thus enabling them to plan the type of repair that should be performed (Blackstone et al., 1979a). Other pressure measurements should demonstrate equal pressures in both ventricles (distinguishing this condition from isolated pulmonary stenosis with intact ventricular septum, in which the right ventricular pressure may be considerably greater than that in the left ventricle). Angiograms are especially helpful before complete repair in those patients who have received palliative shunt procedures. These pictures define the anatomy of the pulmonary arteries as well as any iatrogenic distortion caused by the shunt that might need attention. If pressure data (e.g., cardiac catheterization) are not needed, digital subtraction techniques can provide excellent views with minimal invasion—a worthwhile consideration because it is not unusual for cyanotic spells and seizures to occur in these children during intracardiac catheter manipulation.

## INDICATIONS FOR OPERATION

As suggested by the natural history of this lesion, most patients require surgical intervention. Current trends are to provide surgical correction as soon as possible (often electively before the end of the first year of life) and generally by the time the patient has reached the age of 2 years. The urgency with which surgery is performed is affected by numerous variables, including the symptoms at presentation, age at presentation, and associated lesions. The use of prostaglandins, such as prostaglandin E$_1$ (PGE$_1$), to stabilize patients with diminished pulmonary blood flow has greatly influenced the emergent care of these patients (Donahoo et al., 1981; Freed et al., 1981). Rather than performing emergency systemic-to-pulmonary artery shunts on critically ill, hypoxemic, and acidotic neonates, surgeons have the luxury of more fully evaluating the patient's anatomy while prostaglandins maintain ductal patency (and thus pulmonary blood flow). This grants the surgical team time to arrive at the most appropriate decision for each patient and to plan a procedure to correct the underlying lesion, rather than mere palliation. Although controversy continues concerning the prefered operation during infancy, there has been a general trend toward open correction in early infancy (Calder et al., 1979; Castaneda, 1993; Castaneda et al., 1977; Di Donato et al., 1991; Gustafson et al., 1988; Groh et al., 1991; Ilbawi, 1989; Kirklin et al., 1992; Kirklin and Barratt-Boyes, 1993; Norwood and Pigott, 1985; Tucker et al., 1979; Turley et al., 1980). The groups that urge early total correction at any time emphasize that it prevents the need for a second operation and that the current results are sufficiently good to support this judgment. Furthermore, palliation has its own inherent risks, which include death following the procedure or before the patient can return for complete repair (Castaneda, 1993; Kirklin et al., 1992; Vobecky et al., 1993). Palliation, in the form of aortopulmonary shunts, can also significantly distort the pulmonary arteries, complicating and increasing the risk of subsequent complete repair (Vobecky et al., 1993). Therefore, some groups currently believe that corrective surgery should be performed in all patients with TOF regardless of age or weight, including those with TOF with pulmonary atresia (Castaneda, 1993; Di Donato et al., 1991; Kirklin et al., 1992). Opposed to this group are those who feel that palliation is preferable in infancy because the overall mortality is lower (Arciniegas et al., 1980a, 1980b; Hammon et al., 1985; Karl et al., 1992; Kirklin et al., 1979, 1992; Rittenhouse et al., 1985; Vobecky et al., 1993). In addition, these observers are concerned about whether the small heart in infancy will remain corrected as growth continues, feeling perhaps that outflow tract obstruction of the right ventricle may recur (Kirklin et al., 1988).

Two articles have addressed the issue of palliation versus repair (Kirklin et al., 1992; Vobecky et al., 1993) by examining the outcome for patients with TOF from the time they are diagnosed as opposed to from the time they have surgical intervention. The information reported by these studies is important to understanding the natural history of the disease in the first years of life using various treatment protocols. Risk factors

for death (for all patients diagnosed with TOF) include the presence of multiple VSDs, Down's syndrome, large aortopulmonary collateral vessels, complete AV canal defects (especially if the patient is also
trisomy 21), and early age at presentation (Kirklin et
al., 1992). Significant mortality can occur before surgical repair, especially in infants chosen for palliation.
For 237 patients diagnosed with TOF at Toronto Sick
Children's Hospital (Vobecky et al., 1993), there were
8 deaths in 216 patients undergoing complete repair
(3.7%). This very acceptable surgical rate mortality
seems to support a protocol of early shunting followed by subsequent complete repair (in this study,
patients received aortopulmonary shunts if they were
diagnosed and were symptomatic prior to 18 months
of age). However, an additional 15 patients died before complete repair, either as a direct result of attempted palliation or as a result of waiting for surgery
following palliation. This brings the total mortality to
23 out of 231 patients (10%), considerably higher than
mortality of early repair in infancy without previous
palliation (0 to 6%) (Castaneda, 1993; Groh et al.,
1991; Kirklin et al., 1992; Touati et al., 1990). In one
series (Kirklin et al., 1992), it appeared that surgical
repair following previous palliation carried a slightly
higher mortality (12%) than primary repair (6%), and
this might be due to identified risk factors for operative mortality, which include pulmonary artery distortion from previous shunts (Fig. 39–9) and more than
one previous palliative procedure. Other risk factors
for operative mortality include need for a transannular patch, high postrepair (measured in the intensive
care unit) RV/LV pressure ratios (greater than 0.65)
(Kirklin et al., 1992), and persistent, uncontrollable
"tet" spells at the time of repair.

Although "comparative study has shown primary
one-stage repair to be preferable to the two-stage

approach" (Kirklin and Barratt-Boyes, 1993), good results with this protocol, especially in small infants
(under 6 months old), require a team and institution
experienced with and dedicated to all aspects of neonatal and infant congenital heart surgery, including
pediatric cardiac anesthesia and pediatric critical care
medicine. Although the institutions that are properly
"equipped" for specialized neonatal cardiac surgery
can obtain good results with early, one-stage repair of
TOF, the occasional application of primary palliative
procedures may be warranted—for example, palla-
tion may be considered in unusual circumstances,
such as in patients with an anomalous coronary artery
crossing the RVOT, in patients with extremely small
pulmonary arteries, in patients who have been having
severe, unrelenting "tet" spells for several hours, or
in patients with significant and severe associated lesions that may preclude total repair. Therefore, it is
important for surgical teams to be familiar with current options for palliation as well as with the techniques for complete repair.

## SURGICAL TECHNIQUES

### Palliative Procedures

Various factors that increase the risk for early repair
include pulmonary artery problems, major associated
anomalies, more than one previous operation, and
absent pulmonary valve syndrome (Kirklin et al.,
1983). Small size and young age, which at one time
was also felt to be a risk factor for early repair, may
not be a true risk factor when patients are examined
with multivariate analysis that corrects for other anatomic risks (Castaneda, 1993; Kirklin et al., 1992;
Kirklin and Barratt-Boyes, 1993).

The type of palliation offered to infants is variable
and controversial. Although the Blalock-Taussig
shunt has for years been the most popular palliative
procedure, several groups now employ a modification
of the Blalock-Taussig shunt using polytetrafluoroethylene (PTFE) interposition between the subclavian
artery and the pulmonary artery (de Leval et al., 1981)
or between the aorta and the main pulmonary artery
(central shunt) (Amato et al., 1988; Ebert, 1979). In
selected cases, right ventricular outflow patching to
promote right ventricular-to-pulmonary artery continuity and symmetric pulmonary artery growth has
also been advocated (Ebert, 1980; Piehler et al., 1980;
Tucker et al., 1979). Regardless of the type of palliation chosen, the goal is simply to increase pulmonary
blood flow, independent of ductal patency, to allow
for pulmonary artery growth and eventual total correction.

The presence of pulmonary atresia or an anomalous
left anterior descending coronary artery across the
RVOT may preclude the possibility of establishing
transannular right ventricle-to-pulmonary artery continuity, if it is needed, and require placement of a
conduit. Although conduits can be used in infants
(Ebert et al., 1976), some surgeons prefer to defer

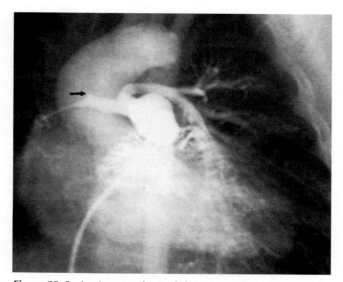

**Figure 39–9.** Angiogram obtained from a patient with TOF who
has severe stenosis of the right pulmonary artery at the site of a
previously placed Blalock-Taussig shunt. This patient presented
with extreme cyanosis from thrombosis of the shunt (arrow). The
right pulmonary artery distal to the shunt is virtually obliterated.

conduit placement until the infant is older and large enough to permit placement of a larger conduit. Nevertheless, the availability of cryopreserved homografts has made conduit placement in infants safer. Likewise, patients with small left ventricular volumes (less than 60% of normal) may do better with initial palliation (Nomoto et al., 1984). Each case must be individualized, but these considerations can adequately justify performing a palliative rather than a corrective procedure when the patient is first diagnosed (Sabiston, 1976).

There are a number of systemic-to-pulmonary artery shunts being performed by various surgeons (Fig. 39–10) but the most common shunts include: the classic Blalock-Taussig shunt, the modified Blalock-Taussig shunt, and a central aortopulmonary shunt using prosthetic graft material. In addition, there seem to be advantages to performing a right ventricular outflow patch instead of a shunt in properly selected patients, such as those with extremely small pulmonary arteries (Tucker et al., 1979; Vobecky et al., 1993). The shunts popularized by Potts and co-workers (1950), Waterston (1962), and Glenn and Patino (1954) are no longer used widely in this setting, because the Waterston anastomosis (ascending aorta-to-right pulmonary artery) can cause kinking and stenosis at the anastomotic site, which may make subsequent open correction difficult (Gay and Ebert, 1973;

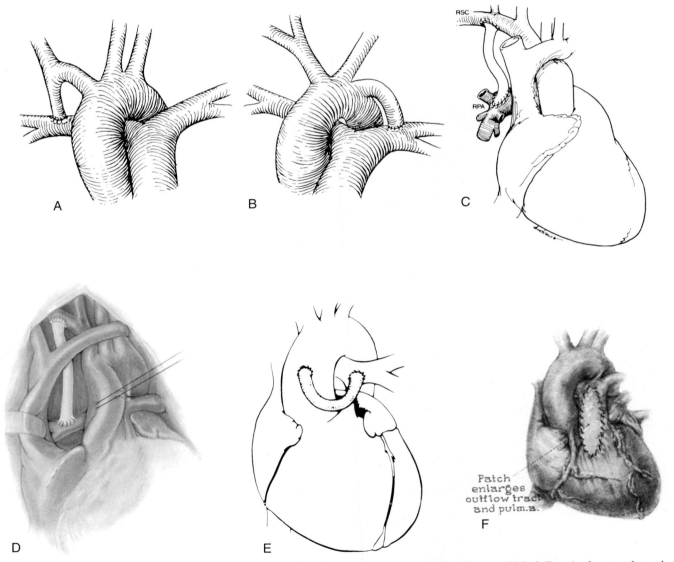

**Figure 39–10.** The most commonly used palliative procedures in 1993 for patients with TOF. *A,* A native Blalock-Taussig shunt performed on the side opposite the aortic arch. *B,* A native Blalock-Taussig shunt performed on the side of the aortic arch. *C,* A modified (Great Ormond Street) Blalock-Taussig shunt with prosthetic material performed through a thoracotomy. *D,* A Gore-Tex interposition shunt between the innominate artery and the pulmonary artery performed through a median sternotomy. *E,* A central aortopulmonary shunt. *F,* A right ventricular outflow tract patch. (*C,* From Cooley, D. A.: Techniques in Cardiac Surgery. 2nd ed. Philadelphia, W. B. Saunders, 1984; *E,* From Turley, K., Tucker, W. Y., and Ebert, P. A.: The changing role of palliative procedures in the treatment of infants with congenital heart disease. J. Thorac. Cardiovasc. Surg., *79,*194, 1980. *F,* From Ebert, P. A.: Past, present, and future of palliative shunts. Adv. Cardiol., *26:*127, 1979.)

Wilson et al., 1981), and the Potts anastomosis (descending aorta-to-left pulmonary artery) can enlarge with time, producing an excessive shunt with pulmonary hypertension and often aneurysm formation at the site of the anastomosis (Ross et al., 1958; Stephens, 1967). Moreover, a Potts anastomosis is more difficult to close at the time of subsequent correction. The Glenn anastomosis (which is between the superior vena cava and the right pulmonary artery) can produce good results initially, but more difficulty is experienced in the subsequent total correction. Most patients now receive one of the palliative procedures mentioned at the beginning of this paragraph, which are described in more detail later.

## Blalock-Taussig Operation

In performance of a subclavian artery-to-pulmonary artery anastomosis, the incision is generally made on the side opposite that on which the aorta descends (Blalock, 1948) (Fig. 39–11; see also Fig. 39–10A). Ideally, the subclavian branch of the innominate artery is used for the anastomosis because the angle produced at its origin from its parent vessel is better than that formed when the subclavian artery is used (Sabiston and Blalock, 1959). The latter arises directly from the aorta and is apt to kink at its origin when deflected inferiorly for an anastomosis to the pulmonary artery (Fig. 39–12; see also Fig. 39–10B). If it is

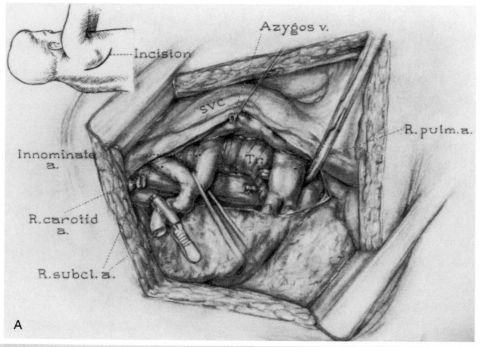

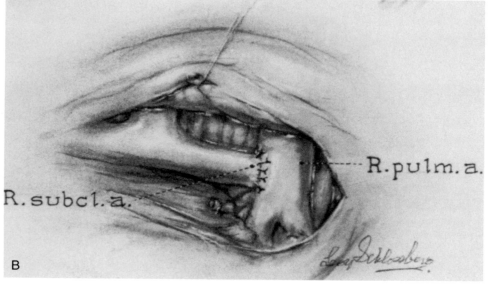

**Figure 39–11.** *A,* A native Blalock-Taussig shunt is usually performed on the side opposite the aortic arch. For most patients with TOF, this shunt is performed through a right thoracotomy. After the azygos vein has been divided, the subclavian artery is dissected as far distally as possible. It is then divided so that it can be turned down onto the right pulmonary artery and anastomosed *(B)* with careful suture technique. It is important to use interrupted sutures for part of this suture line to prevent "purse-stringing" of the anastomosis. (*A* and *B,* From Ebert, P. A.: Atlas of Congenital Cardiac Surgery. Churchill Livingstone, New York, 1989.)

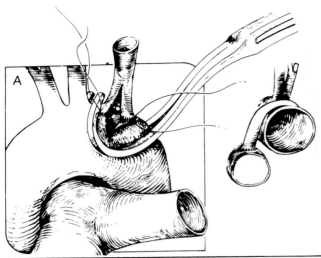

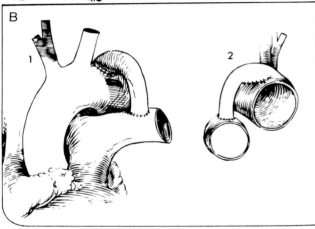

**Figure 39–12.** Subclavian arterioplasty. *A,* To prevent kinking of the ipsilateral subclavian artery when stretched over the prominence of the aorta *(inset),* the aorta at the base of the subclavian artery is partially excluded with a C-type vascular clamp. A vertical incision is made approximately 1.5 cm in length, half on the aorta and half on the subclavian artery. The incision is closed transversely. *B,* This both enlarges the takeoff of the subclavian artery *(1)* and brings its orifice more anterior on the aorta arch *(2). (A* and *B,* From Laks, H., and Castaneda, A. R.: Subclavian arterioplasty for the ipsilateral Blalock-Taussig shunt. Reprinted with permission from the Society of Thoracic Surgeons [The Annals of Thoracic Surgery, 1975, Vol. 19, p. 319].)

necessary to use the subclavian artery on the side of the arch, then the modification introduced by Laks and Castaneda (1975) should be considered (Fig. 39–12). Experimental studies have shown that approximately three-quarters of the blood passing through a subclavian pulmonary shunt is directed to the lung on the side of the anastomosis (Fort et al., 1965). There is evidence to suggest that growth of the pulmonary arteries after shunting is influenced by their structural composition and proportion of elastin as well as by differential blood flow (Rosenberg et al., 1987). Detailed attention must be given in performing the Blalock-Tauissig shunt, especially in the construction of the anastomosis. Every effort must be made to prevent constriction of the anastomosis, and meticulous

technique is essential. In infants, it is preferable to use interrupted sutures to avoid a purse-string effect on the anastomosis. The advantages of the Blalock-Taussig shunt are that it produces a reliable shunt with excellent flow characteristics and shunt flow that is ordinarily well matched to the size of the patient. Significant complications from transection of the subclavian artery are unusual, occurring in less than 1% of patients (Arciniegas et al., 1979; Kirklin and Barratt-Boyes, 1993), but numerous reports (Arciniegas et al., 1979; Harris et al., 1964; Lodge et al., 1983; Zahka et al., 1988) have suggested that subtle changes in arm strength and growth do occur in these patients with regularity. The shunt employs no prosthetic material and is fairly easy to take down at the time of total correction.

Disadvantages are that the shunt requires meticulous and time-consuming dissection, which may be difficult to justify in a severely ill infant. In addition, a Blalock-Taussig shunt can distort the peripheral pulmonary artery even if no technical difficulty is encountered during the procedure. This tendency for the normal healing and scarring process to produce pulmonary artery distortion significant enough to require pulmonary angioplasty at the time of subsequent TOF repair has been approximately 15% (Vobecky et al., 1993) and reaches 50% in patients who receive two palliative shunts before repair. As patients grow, one pulmonary artery may develop better than the other owing to flow characteristics, especially if there is anastomotic distortion. This pulmonary artery distortion may make subsequent total correction more hazardous (Kirklin et al., 1983). After creation of a Blalock-Taussig shunt, progression of the infundibular pulmonary stenosis has been encountered (Sabiston et al., 1964), which can also influence the future operative approach (i.e., transatrial vs. transventricular). Despite these features, the classic Blalock-Taussig shunt remains an excellent, time-proven option for increasing pulmonary blood flow in these patients.

### Modified Blalock-Taussig Shunt

With the advent of reliable prosthetic graft material, technically easier forms of systemic-to-pulmonary artery shunting as means of palliation have become popular. In addition, because most patients return within 2 years for total correction, the temporary nature of "palliation" justifies the use of an artificial conduit that may not have optimal longevity but that does preserve the subclavian arterial supply to the arm (Arciniegas et al., 1979; Lodge et al., 1983; Webb and Burford, 1952). The "Great Ormond Street" shunt (de Leval et al., 1981) or "modified" Blalock-Taussig shunt, requires interposition of a segment of PTFE graft material (usually 4 or 5 mm in diameter) between the subclavian artery and the pulmonary artery (Fig. 39–13; see also Fig. 39–10C and D). Each anastomosis can be performed with a partial occlusion clamp and continuous monofilament suture. The shunts can be easily constructed on either side because kinking of the subclavian artery is no longer a

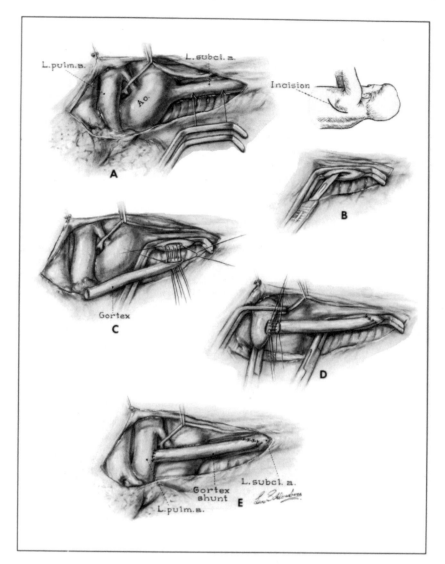

**Figure 39–13.** Performance of a modified left Blalock-Taussig shunt. *A,* The left subclavian artery and left pulmonary artery are isolated through a left thoracotomy incision *(inset). B,* An occluding clamp is placed on the left subclavian artery, and a longitudinal incision is made. *C,* A beveled piece of 4- or 5-mm Gore-Tex is sutured to the subclavian artery with fine, continuous sutures. With the Gore-Tex in place, occluding clamps are placed on the left pulmonary artery. *D,* A longitudinal incision is made in the left pulmonary artery, and the distal anastomosis is performed. *E,* The clamps are removed, and the graft lies in place without kinking either the graft or the left pulmonary artery. The left subclavian artery is preserved by this technique. *(A–E,* From Ebert, P. A.: Atlas of Congenital Cardiac Surgery. New York, Churchill Livingstone, 1989.)

problem. Placement on the side of the aortic arch descent through a thoracotomy may be technically easier, although interposition of graft material between the innominate artery and the ipsilateral pulmonary artery (usually right) through a median sternotomy is also technically feasible (see Fig. 39–10*D*). Although flow through this shunt is still controlled by the size of the subclavian artery, a long segment of prosthetic graft nevertheless supplies its own unique amount of resistance, so flow through these shunts can be more variable. Furthermore, because the graft is fixed in size, distortion of the pulmonary artery by the shunt can be anticipated as the patient grows, although this has not been a universal experience (Lamberti et al., 1984; Ullom et al., 1987). These shunts can be slightly more difficult to take down than a classic Blalock-Taussig shunt, and probably should be divided rather than ligated at the time of total correction. Shunts performed on the left (in patients with a normal left aortic arch) are most diffi-

cult to take down, and some surgeons recommend "wrapping" these shunts in a small envelope of Gore-Tex membrane to prevent the shunt from adhering to adjacent pulmonary parenchyma and to facilitate its identification through the subsequent median sternotomy. Placement of a modified Blalock-Taussig shunt through a median sternotomy (see Fig. 39–10*D*) is gaining increasing favor because it enables the shunt to be placed more centrally on the right pulmonary artery, so that it may be less likely to cause distortion and its location will make eventual shunt takedown quite simple. Regardless of the surgical approach employed, Gore-Tex interposition shunts have become the shunt of choice for some groups in infants less than 1 month of age (Ilbawi et al., 1984).

### Central Aortopulmonary Shunt

Several groups have supported interposing a short segment of prosthetic graft material between the ascending aorta and the main pulmonary artery (Barragry et al., 1987; Ebert, 1979). This is an easy shunt to construct and, in older children, can usually be performed without cardiopulmonary bypass (using partial occlusion clamps while pulmonary blood flow is maintained by the ductus arteriosus) (see Fig. 39–10E). Shunt flow is generally controlled by the size of prosthetic material used, and although there have been numerous suggestions as to how to construct the proper size graft, in most instances a 4-mm graft is appropriate for infants (less than 5 kg) and a 5-mm graft works well for larger children. These grafts have the advantage of creating symmetric pulmonary blood flow and growth without distorting peripheral pulmonary arteries. Although subsequent total correction requires a repeat sternotomy, this is not usually a problem and the shunts are easy to take down because of their anterior location. In patients who are surviving from antegrade blood flow across the RVOT, occlusion of the main pulmonary artery may not be tolerated and placement of a central shunt in these patients requires cardiopulmonary bypass. Nevertheless, even if cardiopulmonary bypass support is necessary, these shunts usually work well and provide symmetric pulmonary artery growth while preventing distortion of the branch pulmonary arteries.

### RVOT Patch

An alternative method for increasing pulmonary blood flow and palliating patients with TOF is to relieve the pulmonary stenosis but leave the VSD open. This is usually done by a combination of infundibular muscle division and then placement of a patch (pericardium or PTFE) across the pulmonary valve annulus (see Fig. 39–10F). This converts the physiology to that of a VSD alone. Most infants with TOF can tolerate this physiology without going into uncontrollable heart failure because their "small" pulmonary arteries offer some resistance to limit the left-to-right shunt across the VSD. However, it is this left-to-right shunt across the VSD that provides increased pulmonary blood flow and that palliates the cyanosis of severe TOF. This "intracardiac" shunt (as opposed to the "extracardiac" shunts described previously) offers the theoretical advantage of symmetric pulmonary artery blood flow with excellent potential for pulmonary artery growth and no risk of shunt thrombosis. Furthermore, in light of the poor experiences with conventional shunts in infants with very small pulmonary arteries (Vobecky et al., 1993)—the very infants who might best benefit from palliation to prepare them for eventual total correction—RVOT patches may be the palliation of choice (Tucker et al., 1979). This procedure must be performed through a median sternotomy and on cardiopulmonary bypass. However, it does not require long cardiopulmonary bypass times and can be performed during aortic cross-clamping or electrical fibrillation with the use of moderate hypothermia (28° C). The surgeon should carefully inspect the anatomy and note the presence of any important anatomic anomalies, such as persistent left superior vena cava. If an anomalous coronary artery is identified (e.g., left anterior descending coronary artery arising from the right coronary artery and crossing across the RVOT), then the procedure must be abandoned and, if palliation (vs. total correction) is still desired, a more conventional aortopulmonary shunt should be performed. In order to achieve adequate palliation with an RVOT patch, the ventricular incision should extend far enough onto the proximal portion of the infundibulum so that after transection of the parietal bands, the right ventricular chamber is easily viewed. The distal extent of the patch should extend to the pulmonary artery bifurcation and the shape of the patch distally should be "squared" or "blunt," not "tapered," to limit the likelihood of late stenosis (Kirklin and Barratt-Boyes, 1993). In patients who receive a good outcome from this procedure, the produced physiology dramatically increases pulmonary blood flow (see Fig. 39–4D). Over time, and with growth of the pulmonary arteries, these patients gradually experience increased congestive heart failure from excessive left-to-right shunting across the VSD. They are then returned to the operating room where the VSD is closed (either through the atrium or by making an incision in the lower portion of the outflow patch).

### Balloon Angioplasty of RVOT

Recent experience and enthusiasm for balloon angioplasty techniques has encouraged some groups to experiment with balloon angioplasty of the RVOT in symptomatic infants with TOF (Boucek et al., 1988; Kvelselis et al., 1985; Sreeram et al., 1990). Although these procedures risk stimulating a severe hypercyanotic spell when the catheter is manipulated across the narrowed outflow tract, and although the anatomy of TOF (with hypoplasia of the muscular infundibulum) would not seem to be amenable to balloon angioplasty, initial results with this technique in properly selected patients have been encouraging; the technique may have a role in the treatment of patients who present a high surgical risk or in those in whom it might be preferable to delay surgical correction. The advantage of these techniques is that they can increase pulmonary blood flow (and thereby relieve cyanotic symptoms) without distorting the anatomy in a way that might interfere with an eventual optimal repair.

The goal of all of these palliative procedures is to increase blood flow to the lungs. The decision of which procedure to use can be based on many factors, including the experience and comfort that a particular surgeon has with each procedure. It must also be recognized today that these procedures in most cases are temporizing and that eventually total correction will be performed. Therefore the shunt should be chosen that gives the best preparation for repair. Individual problems with anatomy (such as proximal stenosis of the right or left pulmonary artery) should be considered, for in such an instance, it may be more

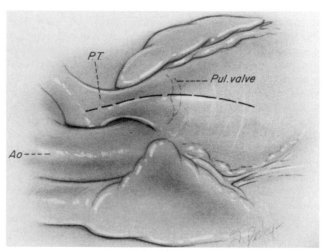

**Figure 39–14.** The most common ventricular incision used for repair of TOF is vertical so that it can be extended as shown from the right ventricle across the pulmonary valve annulus and on to the main pulmonary artery. (PT = pulmonary trunk.) (From Kirklin, J. W., and Barratt-Boyes, B. G.: Cardiac Surgery. 2nd ed. Churchill Livingstone, New York, 1993.)

advantageous to perform a central aortopulmonary shunt or an RVOT patch (even if cardiopulmonary bypass is necessary) to enable concomitant enlargement of the area of pulmonary artery stenosis. Creation of a peripheral subclavian artery-to-pulmonary artery shunt in such a setting might otherwise reduce flow to the contralateral pulmonary artery.

## Total Correction

Total correction is the ideal operation for treatment of TOF, and is accomplished with extracorporeal circulation. Before cardiopulmonary bypass, previously placed systemic-to-pulmonary artery shunts should be identified so that they can be easily controlled. The patients are placed on cardiopulmonary bypass and usually cooled to 25° C (unless a period of deep hypothermic circulatory arrest is anticipated, such as might be the case in infants; in these instances, patients are usually cooled to 18° C). During this time, previously placed shunts are divided or ligated. The goals of operation once cardiopulmonary bypass has been established are to close the VSD, to relieve RVOT obstruction, and to repair any stenoses in the pulmonary arteries.

### VSD Closure

Several methods have been employed for closing the VSD in patients with TOF, and these reflect the variety of choices available for closure of any perimembranous VSD (Kirklin and Barratt-Boyes, 1993). The most time-honored approach has been to close the VSD through the incision that is commonly made in the RVOT to relieve the infundibular stenosis. VSD closure through this incision is similar to closure of any VSD through a transventricular approach, except that the presence of hypertrophied muscle in the infundibulum and the desire to limit the extent of the incision add some difficulty to exposure. The incision should be vertical so that it can be extended across the valve annulus if necessary to relieve pulmonary stenosis (Fig. 39–14). In neonates and young infants, the parietal extension of the infundibular septum can be divided to expose the underlying VSD (Fig. 39–15). It is usually not necessary to resect very much muscle, if any, when performing repair through the RVOT in infants (Groh et al., 1991). It is also possible to perform this part of the procedure through a much more limited ventricular incision than has been described in earlier reports (Ebert, 1989; Kirklin and Karp, 1970; Sabiston et al., 1964) (Fig. 39–16). The VSD should be closed with a patch because it is usually large and unrestrictive. A few cases of TOF with restrictive VSD have been described (Flanagan et al., 1988). The VSD can also be closed through a transatrial approach by exposing it through a right atriotomy (Fig. 39–17) and either by retracting the tricuspid valve leaflets (Kirklin and Barratt-Boyes, 1993; Pacifico et al., 1987)

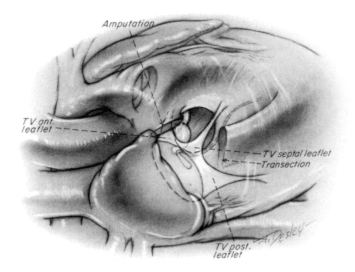

**Figure 39–15.** As viewed through the ventricular approach, the VSD is best exposed by dividing the parietal extension of the infundibular septum. Although this figure demonstrates "amputation" of this area, it is possible to achieve exposure of the VSD by simply dividing this parietal band, especially when this procedure is performed in patients less than 6 months old. (TV = tricuspid valve.) (From Kirklin, J. W., and Barratt-Boyes, B. G.: Cardiac Surgery. 2nd ed. Churchill Livingstone, New York, 1993.)

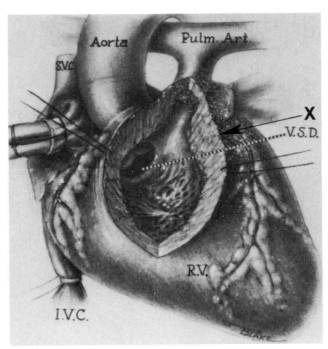

**Figure 39–16.** Although older illustrations describe a long ventricular incision for exposure of the VSD, it is possible to gain adequate exposure to the VSD by extending the incision barely beyond the infundibular septum (X). The resulting incision is less than half the length of the incision diagrammed and yet still enables adequate completion of the procedure. This more "limited ventriculotomy" may help to preserve late right ventricular function yet still enable adequate enlargement of the hypoplastic area in the right ventricle (R.V.) outflow tract. (S.V.C. = superior vena cava; I.V.C. = inferior vena cava.)

or by incising the tricuspid valve annulus to lift the tricuspid valve out of the way (Pridjian et al., 1993). Personal preference of the surgeon determines whether the patch is placed with continuous or with interrupted sutures. The suture line can be inspected and buttressed where necessary with additional sutures, but the best way to evaluate the VSD closure is to use intraoperative echocardiography at the end of the procedure after the patient has been removed from cardiopulmonary bypass (Papagiannis et al., 1993; Ungerleider et al., 1990).

Proponents of the transatrial approach indicate that the entire repair (including relief of RVOT obstruction) can often be performed through the right atrial incision and that this will limit the extent of any incision—if one is needed at all—in the right ventricle, thus preserving long-term right ventricular function and limiting the chance for future ventricular dysrhythmias (Garson et al., 1979; Kirklin and Barratt-Boyes, 1993; Miura et al., 1992; Pacifico et al., 1987; Ungerleider, 1992). Furthermore, the transatrial approach to the VSD also gives the surgeon access to the atrial septum and the ability to close the frequently associated ASD at the same time as VSD closure. Those who prefer the ventricular incision claim that VSD closure is possible through a very limited ventriculotomy, and that the nature of the anatomy of TOF with hypoplasia of the infundibular septum usually

requires patch enlargement in the infundibulum immediately subjacent to the pulmonary valve in any case. Furthermore, this type of repair does not usually require resection of any muscle (unlike the transatrial repair, where muscle in the RVOT must be excised in order to relieve the obstruction). In infants, most surgeons have found it advantageous to leave a small ASD (see "Postoperative Management," later in this chapter), thereby reducing the advantage of using a transatrial incision in these patients. Closure of the VSD can be safely and easily performed by either approach, and selection probably depends on the surgeon's preference and the unique anatomic features of each defect. Knowledge of the location of the conduction tissue (Fig. 39–18) is important, and sutures placed along the posteroinferior border of the defect should take this anatomy into account (Bharati et al., 1983; Kirklin and Barratt-Boyes, 1993; Tamiya et al., 1985).

### Relief of RVOT Obstruction

As mentioned previously, RVOT obstruction can occur at several levels. Hypoplasia of the infundibular septum almost invariably produces some element of subpulmonic stenosis that must be relieved. This is done by dividing the parietal and septal bands (see Figs. 39–15 and 39–17) that bind the infundibular septum to the lateral and septal boundaries of the RVOT. The extremely restricted dimensions of the subpulmonic outflow area make it often desirable to place a patch (pericardium or PTFE) to "raise the roof" over the subvalvular area and to enlarge the outflow from the right ventricular chamber (Fig. 39–19). Initial attempts to perform complete repair were

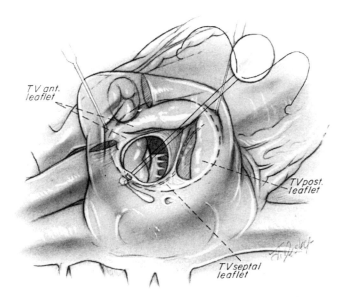

**Figure 39–17.** The VSD can be closed through an atrial approach. From this approach, the parietal band (which is shown amputated) is along the superior aspect of the region exposed and must be resected to provide unobstructed RV outflow. (From Kirklin, J. W., and Barratt-Boyes, B. G.: Cardiac Surgery. 2nd ed. Churchill Livingstone, New York, 1993.)

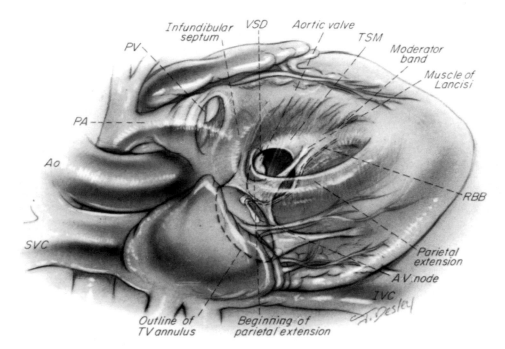

**Figure 39–18.** The location of the conduction tissue in relation to the VSD is such that the atrioventricular (AV) node and the penetrating bundle course along the inferior and posterior border of the VSD. It is in this region that sutures must be placed superficially through the muscle, and special care must be taken in placing sutures around the tricuspid valve annulus. The relation of the VSD to the parietal extension of the infundibular septum can be appreciated. (SVC = superior vena cava; Ao = aorta; IVC = inferior vena cava; PA = pulmonary artery; PV = pulmonary vein; TSM = trabecula septal marginalis; TV = tricuspid valve; RBB = right bundle branch.) (From Kirklin, J. W., and Barratt-Boyes, B. G.: Cardiac Surgery. 2nd ed. Churchill Livingstone, New York, 1993.)

often described in older patients and included considerable resection of muscle from the RVOT (Kirklin and Karp, 1970). Furthermore, these procedures were performed through fairly extensive incisions in the right ventricle, and the combination of extensive muscle resection and long ventriculotomies has raised concern about the long-term outcome of patients undergoing transventricular repair (Garson et al., 1979; Kirklin and Barratt-Boyes, 1993; Miura et al., 1992; Pacifico et al., 1987; Ungerleider, 1992). Therefore, some surgeons now favor a transatrial approach to

muscle resection for relief of the outflow obstruction in TOF repair (Coles et al., 1988; Hudspeth et al., 1963; Karl et al., 1992; Kawashima et al., 1985; Kirklin and Barratt-Boyes, 1993; Pacifico et al., 1987). This approach can be very successful as long as muscle is actually removed from the RVOT so that the intracardiac outflow chamber is enlarged. In some patients, a small ventricular incision is still necessary to allow patch enlargement of the hypoplastic infundibular outflow area, but proponents of the transatrial repair claim that the extent of the ventricular incision is less

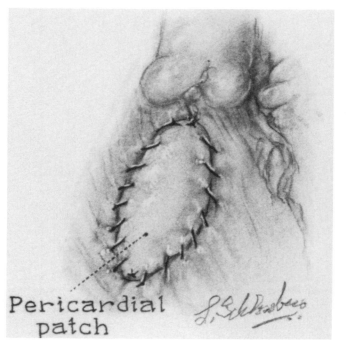

**Figure 39–19.** If the VSD is closed through a "limited" ventricular incision, which is made below the pulmonary valve, it is possible to relieve the RV outflow obstruction by simply dividing the parietal band and then enlarging the outflow chamber with a patch. (From Ebert, P. A.: Atlas of Congenital Cardiac Surgery. Churchill Livingstone, New York, 1989.)

than if it is also used for exposure of the VSD. In actuality, the ventricular incision can be kept quite small even if used for VSD closure (see Fig. 39–16) and the advantages of transatrial over transventricular repair may not appear to be as great if patients from the current era are compared with one another, instead of comparing current transatrial repairs with older transventricular repairs (Ungerleider, 1992).

Despite the methods and approach used to enlarge the subvalvar outflow area, the pulmonary valve and annulus should also be inspected and enlarged if necessary. Severe narrowing of the *right ventricle-pulmonary trunk* (RV-PT) junction seems to correlate with risk of mortality as well as with likelihood for elevated postrepair RV/LV ratios, despite generous patch enlargement (Kirklin et al., 1989, 1992; Kirklin and Barratt-Boyes, 1993) (Fig. 39–20). Many patients with TOF have bicuspid valves, and an incision in the main pulmonary artery provides excellent exposure of the pulmonary valve to enable valvotomy (Fig. 39–21). The pulmonary valve annulus should be sized (Blackstone et al., 1979a, 1979b). If it is too small, the surgeon should not hesitate to perform a transannular incision with enlargement of the RVOT out onto the pulmonary artery (Kirklin et al., 1989; Pacifico et al., 1977) (see Fig. 39–14). Although transannular patches have not been previously considered to be an incremental risk factor for late surgical failure, more recent evidence suggests that the need to place a transannular patch identifies a higher-risk anatomy that does tend to correlate with higher long-term mortality (Kirklin et al., 1989, 1992; Kirklin and Barratt-Boyes, 1993). This may be due to geometric limitations to pulmonary blood flow found in patients with small RV-PT junctions that cannot be corrected simply by performing an adequate transannular patch (Kirklin et al., 1989, 1992; Shimazaki et al., 1992). Thus, the risk imposed by placement of a transannu-

lar patch may be related to the risk of elevated postrepair RV/LV pressures (which can persist despite transannular patches in many of these patients) and not necessarily to the transannular patch itself. Nevertheless, there is also concern that transannular patches can increase long-term risk by causing progressive right ventricular dysfunction (Bove and Byrum, 1983; Graham et al., 1976; Ilbawi et al., 1981; Kirklin et al., 1989, 1992; Kirklin and Barratt-Boyes, 1993), and it is clear that the likelihood of requiring reoperation in the future (e.g., for important pulmonary insufficiency) is significantly greater in patients with transannular patches (Kirklin et al., 1989; Horneffer et al., 1990; Vobecky et al., 1993; Zhao et al., 1985) (Fig. 39–22). Current practice is that transannular patching should not be employed unless necessary to provide adequate right ventricular outflow, and when performed, it should be constructed so as to limit the degree of pulmonary insufficiency in order to preserve long-term right ventricular dynamics (Guo-Wei and Chia-Chiang, 1986; Ilbawi et al., 1987; Kurosawa et al., 1986; Misbach et al., 1983). When performing a transannular patch, many surgeons create a monocusp valve (out of pericardium) to limit pulmonary insufficiency in the short term. Pulmonary homografts have provided excellent long-term pulmonary valve function for many patients who are limited by significant pulmonary insufficiency (Albert et al., 1993).

### Relief of Pulmonary Artery Stenoses

Important obstructions in the main pulmonary artery branches should also be recognized and dealt with at the time of complete repair. These stenoses may be from previous shunts (Vobecky et al., 1993), they may be related to tissue from the ductus arteriosus (Elzenga et al., 1990), or they may be part of the

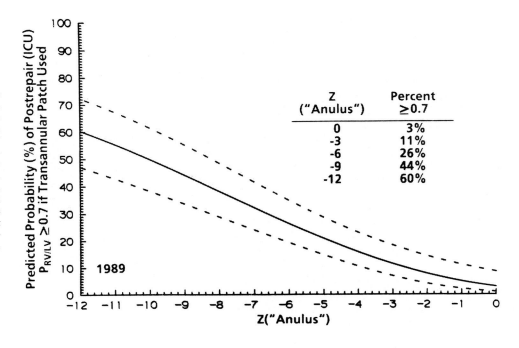

**Figure 39–20.** Despite placement of a transannular patch, patients with small right ventricle–pulmonary trunk (RV–PT) junctions (Z value of pulmonary "anulus" < −5) are at risk for having elevated RV/LV pressures postoperatively. (From Kirklin, J. W., Blackstone, E. H., Jonas, R. A., et al.: Morphologic and surgical determinants of outcome events after repair of tetralogy of Fallot and pulmonary stenosis: A two-institution study. J. Thorac. Cardiovasc. Surg., *103*:706, 1992.)

| Z ("Anulus") | Percent ≥0.7 |
|---|---|
| 0 | 3% |
| -3 | 11% |
| -6 | 26% |
| -9 | 44% |
| -12 | 60% |

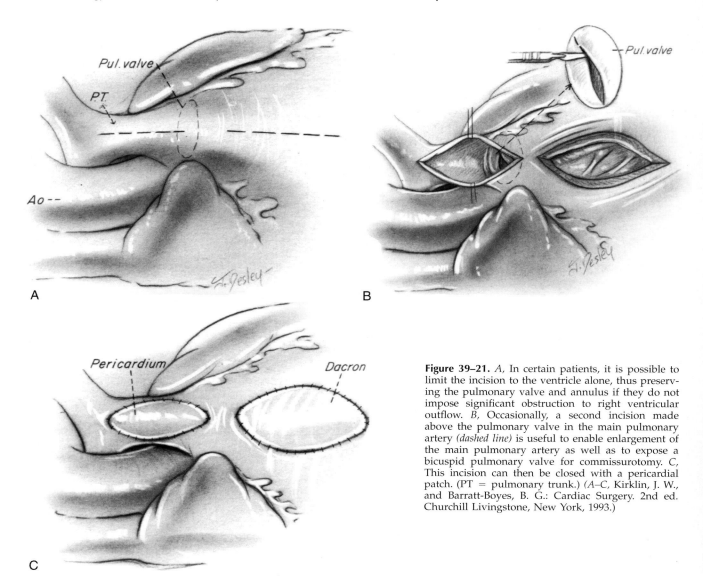

Figure 39–21. *A,* In certain patients, it is possible to limit the incision to the ventricle alone, thus preserving the pulmonary valve and annulus if they do not impose significant obstruction to right ventricular outflow. *B,* Occasionally, a second incision made above the pulmonary valve in the main pulmonary artery *(dashed line)* is useful to enable enlargement of the main pulmonary artery as well as to expose a bicuspid pulmonary valve for commissurotomy. *C,* This incision can then be closed with a pericardial patch. (PT = pulmonary trunk.) *(A–C,* Kirklin, J. W., and Barratt-Boyes, B. G.: Cardiac Surgery. 2nd ed. Churchill Livingstone, New York, 1993.)

spectrum of the anatomy of the defect. Most often, extending the transannular patch past the pulmonary artery bifurcation and onto the left pulmonary artery is sufficient to relieve most significant obstruction. It is important that the distal aspect of the transannular patch be "blunt" and not "tapered" (Kirklin and Barratt-Boyes, 1993) to limit the likelihood of recurrent stenosis at the distal patch site (Fig. 39–23). Obstruction in the main pulmonary arteries can sometimes be treated by local angioplasty at the time of surgical correction, but if the stenosis is more distal in the pulmonary artery (especially the left pulmonary artery, which is difficult to expose at surgery), excellent results have been obtained with the placement of intravascular stents at the time of surgical correction (Mendelsohn et al., 1993; O'Laughlin et al., 1993).

Several groups prefer to perform the procedure under conditions of moderate hypothermia (25° C) with cold potassium cardioplegic arrest, although the procedure can also be accomplished on the cold, non-

cross-clamped, electrically fibrillating heart, or during a period of total circulatory arrest under profound hypothermic conditions (18° C). The optimal method of myocardial protection remains controversial and probably depends on numerous factors related to the anatomy and physiology of each patient's lesion, as well as the patient's age at repair and the conduct of the operation itself (del Nido et al., 1988; Groh et al., 1991; Kirklin and Barratt-Boyes, 1993; Touati et al., 1990; Yamaguchi et al., 1986). Once all levels of obstruction have been relieved and the incision is patched (usually with pericardium, although prosthetic material is acceptable), the patient is rewarmed and removed from cardiopulmonary bypass. Even if conduction problems are not present, it is recommended that temporary atrial and ventricular pacing wires be left in place for the perioperative period. After the patient has been successfully weaned from cardiopulmonary bypass and cannulae have been removed, several methods are available to test for resid-

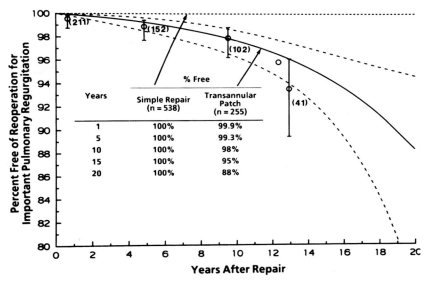

| Years | % Free | |
| --- | --- | --- |
| | Simple Repair (n = 538) | Transannular Patch (n = 255) |
| 1 | 100% | 99.9% |
| 5 | 100% | 99.3% |
| 10 | 100% | 98% |
| 15 | 100% | 95% |
| 20 | 100% | 88% |

**Figure 39–22.** The likelihood of a patient undergoing reoperation for significant pulmonary regurgitation if the repair included a transannular patch instead of simply preserving the pulmonary annulus. Depending on the indications for pulmonary valve replacement, the outcome for patients with transannular patch may be even less favorable than shown. (From Kirklin, J. K., Kirklin, J. W., Blackstone, E. H., et al.: Effect of transannular patching on outcome after repair of tetralogy of Fallot. Reprinted with permission from the Society of Thoracic Surgeons [The Annals of Thoracic Surgery, 1989, Vol. 48, pp. 783–791].)

ual ventricular septal shunting, including selective atrial, ventricular, and pulmonary artery oxygen saturation or pressure measurements. Green dye curves have also been used. Recent experience with intraoperative color-flow Doppler, however, suggests that this technique may provide a more sensitive and accurate ability to assess the quality of the intracardiac repair (Fig. 39–24), especially in relation to long-term outcome (Muhiudeen et al., 1990; Papagiannis et al.,

1993; Ungerleider et al., 1989, 1990). When the surgeon is satisfied with the results of the repair, the chest is closed and the patient is returned to an intensive care setting.

### Special Situations

Because the anatomy varies in patients with TOF, numerous special situations deserve comment. When

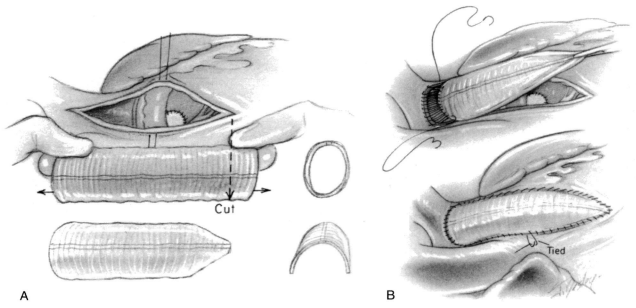

A                                                                                          B

**Figure 39–23.** *A,* When constructing a transannular patch, it is important for the incision to extend on to the left pulmonary artery and for the patch to be tapered at its most distal extent. *B,* This allows the distal pulmonary artery to be "squared off" with the repair and less likely to stenose with time. (*A* and *B,* Kirklin, J. W., and Barratt-Boyes, B. G.: Cardiac Surgery. 2nd ed. Churchill Livingstone, New York, 1993.)

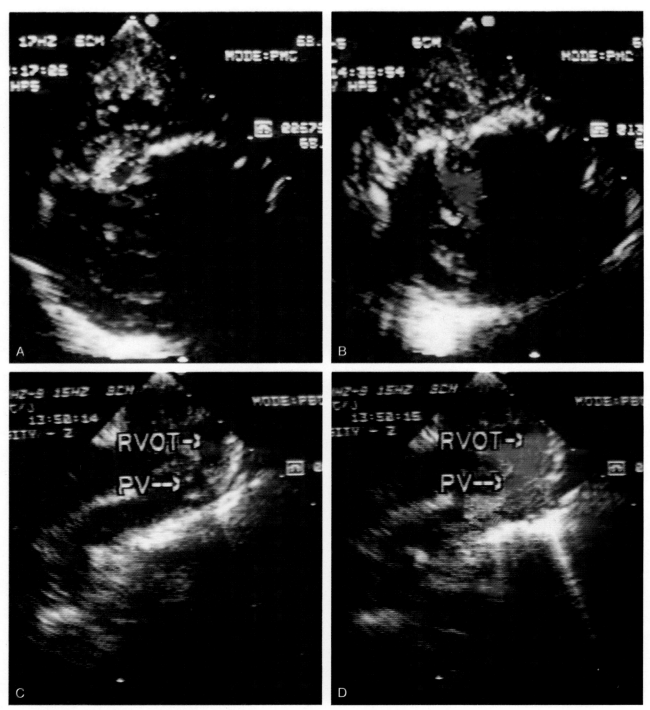

**Figure 39–24.** *A,* This intraoperative echocardiogram obtained from a patient following repair of TOF demonstrates a second, previously unappreciated, VSD in the inlet septum. The patch used for VSD closure is more than a centimeter removed from this second VSD and there is no residual VSD associated with this patch. *B,* The patient was replaced on bypass and this second VSD was closed with an additional patch. The repeat echocardiogram demonstrated a good repair and the patient has had an excellent outcome subsequent to surgery. *C,* Narrowing of the pulmonary valve annulus (PV) can be appreciated in a patient with near-systemic right ventricular pressures. (RVOT = right ventricular outflow tract). *D,* Color-flow demonstrates the turbulence occurring at the pulmonary valve annulus, and this patient responded well to replacement on bypass and creation of a transannular patch.

the left anterior descending coronary artery crosses the RVOT, a standard transannular enlargement is not feasible because this would cause transection of that coronary artery. In these instances (depending on the location of the stenosis), it may be possible to perform a transverse incision in the infundibulum below the coronary artery for closure of the VSD and resection of the infundibular stenosis (Fig. 39–25A). If the pulmonary valve requires commissurotomy or the pulmonary artery requires additional enlarging, this can be performed through a separate incision above the pulmonary annulus with patching of the pulmonary artery after valvotomy has been performed (Humes et al., 1987; Hurwitz et al., 1980) (Fig. 39–25B). These two separate incisions are preferable to dissecting the coronary artery off the outflow tract with placement of the patch beneath the coronary artery as described by Bonchek and colleagues (1973), because right ven-

tricular distention can cause coronary ischemia by stretching the overlying coronary artery. Another alternative in patients with coronary anomalies that prohibit transannular patching is to place a systemic-to-pulmonary artery shunt and to allow the patient to grow until such a time that the patient can accept a large enough conduit between the right ventricle and the pulmonary artery that total correction by this method can be achieved (Fig. 39–25C). However, the availability of cryopreserved homografts, which provide excellent conduits for infants, has encouraged most groups to perform complete repair in infancy, even if a conduit is required.

Patients with pulmonary atresia and VSD who have otherwise normal pulmonary arteries can also be repaired in infancy. In the author's experience, as well as that of others (Castaneda, 1993; Kirklin et al., 1992; Kirklin and Barratt-Boyes, 1993), these patients can

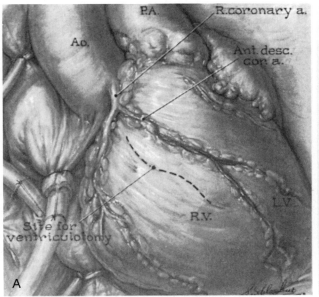

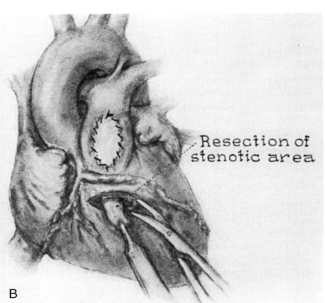

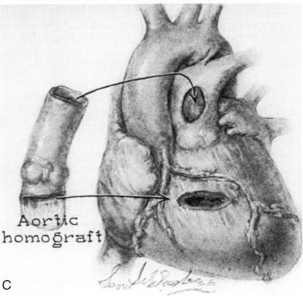

Figure 39–25. A, In patients with an anomalous left coronary artery crossing the RV outflow tract, it is sometimes possible to repair the defect with a ventricular incision placed below the coronary artery. This enables exposure and closure of the VSD as well as resection of obstructive muscle from the subpulmonary region and then simple patch closure of the ventricular incision. B, Occasionally, a second incision must be made in the main pulmonary artery so that a pulmonary valve stenosis can be opened. Between the two incisions, it may be possible to transect all obstructing muscle bands. If this does not provide adequate relief of the pulmonary outflow obstruction, then repair will need to include a conduit (C) to provide additional unobstructed outflow between the right ventricle and the pulmonary artery. The presence of the anomalous coronary prohibits a transannular patch in these patients. (B and C, From Ebert, P. A.: Atlas of Congenital Cardiac Surgery. Churchill Livingstone, New York, 1989.)

receive total correction in infancy following initial stabilization with prostaglandins to enable accurate diagnosis. In many instances (personal experience), correction of "tet atresia" in infancy can be performed without the need for a conduit merely by creating right ventricle-to-pulmonary artery continuity with an RVOT patch. This is possible when there is a main pulmonary artery segment proximal to the atretic RVOT. If this procedure is not performed in infancy, it is doubtful that repair without a conduit would be possible at a later time. The author's group prefers to use a monocusp valve in the RVOT patch in these patients. Although it is acceptable to perform initial palliation (in the form of an aortopulmonary shunt) for patients born with "tet atresia," total repair in infancy can be safely performed with very low mortality and constitutes an excellent option that avoids the long-term problems associated with staged correction.

Following correction and before the surgeon leaves the operating room, right ventricular pressure can be measured and compared with left ventricular (systemic) pressure. Ratios measured in the operating room are usually 10 points higher than those measured 24 hours later in the intensive care unit. There is a greater statistical likelihood of poor outcome for those patients whose postrepair RV/LV ratio (in the intensive care unit) is above 0.65 (Kirklin et al., 1989, 1992; Kirklin and Barratt-Boyes, 1993), and if a transannular patch has not been included as part of the reconstruction, it should be considered in these patients, especially if the obstruction is isolated to the region of the pulmonary valve annulus or immediately subjacent area. All potential levels of obstruction should be evaluated by serial pressure determinations. Occasionally, intraoperative echocardiography can provide useful information about the level of obstruction (Papagiannis et al., 1993) (see Fig. 39–24C and D, color plate). This is an especially important practice because most surgeons try to avoid using a transannular patch whenever possible, and those patients who may benefit from extension of an outflow incision across the pulmonary valve annulus must be recognized and dealt with. Unlike historical descriptions of using large transannular patches for all patients receiving repair of TOF (Kirklin and Karp, 1970), the current rate of transannular patching (in more recent reviews) is approximately 33% (31 to 36%) (Groh et al., 1991; Kirklin et al., 1989; Zhao et al., 1985).

Infants who present with intractable "tet" spells that cannot be controlled despite aggressive intensive care unit care (with sedation, intubation, and neosynephrine) may constitute a high-risk group of patients who warrant consideration for palliation. In a series of 73 patients (Duke University, unpublished) (Table 39–1), the mortality rate for repair of TOF in 28 patients less than 5 months of age who were operated on electively before the "tet" spells began was 0%. This excludes 5 infants with "tet atresia" who were also repaired in infancy with 0% mortality. In 45 patients older than 6 months, the mortality rate was

■ **Table 39–1.** REPAIR OF TETRALOGY OF FALLOT 1987–1993

| Age | Hospital Mortality Rate (%) |
| --- | --- |
| 0–5 mos | 0/28 (0) |
| >6 mos | 3/45 (6.6) |
| Overall | 3/73 (4.1) |

Data from Duke University Pediatric Cardiac Surgery Department.

6.6% (3 in 45). Two of these patients experienced intractable hypercyanotic episodes for several hours preceding surgery, and despite a technically excellent repair and initial good postoperative period, they died before hospital discharge from severe ventricular diastolic dysfunction. The third death in this group was in a patient with severe distortion of the right pulmonary artery (from an aortopulmonary shunt) who had been intensely cyanotic for weeks before referral. This experience suggests that there may be an increased risk to recovery for those patients who have severe cyanosis for several hours before correction. Interestingly, in three patients with TOF who have received palliation at the author's group's institution in the past 6 years, one hospital mortality has occurred, which also was in a patient (9 months old) who experienced prolonged severe cyanotic spells before operation. At the time of operation (planned correction), this patient's heart appeared contracted with severely depressed function, and despite palliation he expired postoperatively. Therefore, this experience suggests that early repair is advantageous, before patients have an opportunity to have hypercyanotic spells, and that those patients who present with spells constitute a very high risk population for whom no management strategy has a distinct advantage. Some authors have suggested placing these patients on extracorporeal membrane oxygenation (ECMO) for 24 to 48 hours before operative correction.

Overall, it appears that, in 1994, the following technical considerations should be emphasized regarding repair of TOF. Patients should receive early correction. Further, there is no advantage and a possible disadvantage to strategies that employ initial palliation (or delay of repair past 12 months of age), except in specific circumstances (e.g., patients with intractable "tet" spells or patients with severely hypoplastic pulmonary arteries and multiple associated defects). Repair should be performed through limited ventricular incisions or through the right atrium. Minimal, if any, right ventricular muscle should be resected, especially if the procedure is being performed through a limited ventriculotomy. Indiscriminate use of a transannular patch should be avoided and the pulmonary valve preserved whenever possible. When a transannular patch is used, it should not be overly abundant (to limit the amount of pulmonary insufficiency) and a monocusp valve can be useful in some cases. The distal portion of the patch should extend onto the left pulmonary artery and should not be tapered. Repair quality should be assessed before leaving the operating room with intraoperative echocardiography or measures of RV/LV pressure ratios, or both.

## POSTOPERATIVE MANAGEMENT

Many variables must be followed postoperatively. Pulmonary function is maintained through an endotracheal tube and respirator until the patient's cardiac and respiratory status is stable, maintaining relatively normal values for the arterial $PO_2$, $PCO_2$, and pH. Maintenance of an adequate cardiac output is also crucial. In small children, cardiac output may be difficult to measure, although techniques are evolving to make this easier (Keagy et al., 1987). It is essential that peripheral perfusion be followed, as well as urine output and acid-base status. Because it is not uncommon for these patients to have elevated right ventricular pressures postoperatively, some inotropic support may be necessary. Patients with this disease have small right ventricular volumes and their cardiac output can be improved more effectively by increasing heart rate rather than stroke volume. Therefore, atrial pacing to improve heart rate or the use of dopamine or dobutamine may be useful. The patients should be maintained on a ventilator until they are hemodynamically stable and show good evidence that they no longer require ventilatory support. Poor peripheral perfusion, indicating low cardiac output, should be treated aggressively. Mechanical causes such as cardiac tamponade should be ruled out, and if necessary, echocardiography performed in the intensive care unit can immediately assess ventricular function or the presence of pericardial fluid. Central venous pressure should be adequate, and in patients with poor right ventricular compliance, central venous pressure may be maintained at slightly higher than normal values. In infants and small children, palpation of the liver edge can be a useful indicator of volume status. Following acid-base status is an excellent way to monitor the clinical convalescence of patients after repair of TOF. Patients who continue to produce lactic acid can be considered to have a cardiac output that is too low to meet tissue oxygen demands, and these patients require aggressive intervention to improve their clinical state. If the patient is adequately volume-loaded, there should be no hesitation about using an inotropic agent such as dobutamine or dopamine to improve cardiac function. Echocardiography performed in the intensive care unit can be very useful in disclosing the nature of the patient's problem. If ventricular function appears depressed, an increase in inotropic support may be warranted. Occasionally, these patients may benefit from a short period of support with extracorporeal life support (Klein et al., 1990).

If echocardiography demonstrates a significant residual defect, this may need to be addressed by the surgical team. If intraoperative echocardiography is performed before the surgeon leaves the operating room, the presence of a residual defect that requires reoperation should occur in less than 2% of patients (Ungerleider et al., 1992). However, occasionally a suture may tear, causing a residual VSD, or RVOT obstruction may become more apparent in the hours following repair. The critical care team should not hesitate to recommend urgent cardiac catheterization or return to the operating room if appropriate for the patient whose convalesence is abnormal. In some patients, stenosis of distal pulmonary artery branches can be treated with placement of intravascular stents in the catheterization laboratory, which avoids return to the operating room (O'Laughlin et al., 1993). If a patient whose recovery is not normal has a documented high RV/LV ratio 24 hours following repair, and if a transannular patch was not part of the repair, it may be prudent to return the patient to the operating room for this procedure (Kirklin et al., 1989; Kirklin and Barratt-Boyes, 1993). In infants, it is advisable to leave the foramen ovale open, and these infants may exhibit some degree of systemic arterial oxygen desaturation in the days immediately following repair. This provides them with physiology similar to that for a fenestrated Fontan operation and enables them to maintain their cardiac output (by right-to-left shunting across the foramen) until the right ventricle becomes more normal and the foramen closes. Although this may take several days following repair, it keeps the patient from having high central venous pressures and low cardiac output because of poor right ventricular compliance.

It is not uncommon for these patients to increase their need for inotropic support throughout the course of their first postoperative night. Daily weights of the patient should be obtained to help follow volume status. These patients retain fluid, so diuretics may be useful. Because prosthetic materials are routinely employed for palliation or correction of this lesion, the use of perioperative broad-spectrum antibiotics should be commonplace. Arrhythmias, when they occur, can often be diagnosed by temporary pacing wires to allow treatment directed specifically at each individual arryhthmia. Patients in heartblock should be AV-sequentially paced until conduction returns in 7 to 10 days. The patient will likely require placement of a permanent pacemaker. However, with properly performed surgical closure of the VSD, the incidence of conduction disturbances requiring permanent pacing should approach 1% (Kirklin et al., 1992; Kirklin and Barratt-Boyes, 1993).

The hemodynamic results after intracardiac repair of TOF have been assessed in several series. Surgical repair of infants under deep hypothermia has been compared hemodynamically with correction by conventional cardiopulmonary bypass, with results that are equal or better with deep hypothermia (Murphy et al., 1980). In a companion study, left ventricular dysfunction as determined after an afterload stress was found to be present postoperatively for those patients who had open correction at an older age but not in patients who underwent repair during infancy. This raises the possibility that early definitive repair may help to preserve postoperative left ventricular function (Borow et al., 1980). Ventricular function in the immediate postoperative period is probably related to several factors, including the myocardial preservation, the surgical technique used, and the ability of the heart to adapt to sudden changes in loading conditions. Neurologic injury is uncommon following correction of TOF, but seizures and major motor impairment can be seen in any patient who has had an operation with the left side of the circulation open (as in TOF), and these findings may occur regardless of whether deep hypothermic circulatory arrest was used during the repair.

## OUTCOME

TOF is now being corrected with an ever-diminishing mortality rate. Results with open correction have been impressive. Nevertheless, it is important to realize that the spectrum of this disease, with respect to the age at presentation as well as the severity of the anatomic derangements, can greatly affect the outcome. Overall, the mortality rate in most series is less than 6% when the repair is performed primarily or after a single systemic-to-pulmonary artery shunt (Castaneda, 1993; Castaneda and Mayer, 1994; Groh et al., 1991; Gustafson et al., 1988; Hammon et al., 1985; Karl et al., 1992; Kawashima et al., 1985; Kirklin et al., 1992; Kirklin and Barratt-Boyes, 1993; Papagiannis et al., 1993; Touati et al., 1990; Vobecky et al., 1993). Improved techniques of myocardial protection with hypothermia, cold cardioplegia, and even total circulatory arrest are enabling more precise anatomic repairs in younger infants with excellent results.

Late outcome is reasonably good, with 85 to 94% of patients living 16 to 28 years after repair (Horneffer et al., 1990; Kirklin and Barratt-Boyes, 1993; Zhao et al., 1985). One study evaluated a group of patients with surgical correction of TOF who survived through adulthood to assess their current state as adults. Among 233 studied, it was concluded that clinical assessment alone is not predictive of the hemodynamic result and that cardiac catheterization should be performed in all patients for objective follow-up. The combination of persistent elevation of right ventricular systolic pressure above 60 mm Hg and ventricular premature depolarizations place the patient at risk of sudden death. However, 80% of the patients lived a normal life without impairment of intellect, exercise tolerance, or fertility (Garson et al., 1979).

With regard to the incidence of sudden death following correction of TOF, in a study of 243 patients evaluated with special emphasis on postoperative conduction disturbances, sudden death occurred in 7 patients, with an average follow-up of 12 years (range, 6.5 to 16.5 years). Among these patients, 4 deaths were in those with right bundle-branch block, and 3 of these 4 patients had premature ventricular contractions for more than 1 month postoperatively. Premature ventricular contractions were documented in 10 of the 158 patients with right bundle-branch block, and sudden death occurred in 3. Three of the 10 patients with trifascicular block pattern died sud-

denly, but no deaths occurred in 24 patients with bifascicular block pattern. The authors of this study concluded that the risk of sudden death in patients with right bundle-branch block and premature ventricular contractions following TOF repair is high and warrants consideration of suppressive therapy (Quattlebaum et al., 1976). The advances in detection and surgical treatment of recurrent sustained ventricular tachycardia have produced a new approach to the therapy of these problems. Ventricular tachyarrhythmias are estimated to occur in 0.3 to 3% of patients following complete repair and have not appeared to be related to the hemodynamic success of the repair. A report in patients experiencing from 30 to 150 documented episodes of sustained ventricular tachycardia with failure of pharmacologic and pacing regimens indicated that the source of the arrhythmia was localized to the right ventriculotomy scar by electrophysiologic mapping (Harken et al., 1980). The scar was surgically excised, and ventricular tachycardia was not inducible following operation and has not recurred following surgical excision of the scar in these patients. These data support the enthusiasm for transatrial repair of TOF when possible, although it remains to be proved whether this will provide long-term protection from dysrhythmias. In the current era, success with radiofrequency ablation of sites of ventricular tachycardia has been reported. Contrary to these data are the findings by Garson and associates (1987) that ventricular arrhythmias after repair of TOF are primarily related to persistent RVOT obstruction, suggesting that ventriculotomy with adequate patching to completely relieve the infundibular obstruction should provide (and has done so, in their series) excellent long-term results with respect to freedom from ventricular ectopy. Long-term success of repair is based on many factors that will mandate continued investigation (Zhao et al., 1985).

## SELECTED BIBLIOGRAPHY

Blalock, A., and Taussig, H. B.: The surgical treatment of malformations of the heart in which there is pulmonary stenosis or pulmonary atresia. J. A. M. A., *128*:189, 1945.

Blalock reports his first three operations for creation of a systemic-pulmonary anastomosis. The first patient, a 15-month-old infant with severe cyanosis, had a history of multiple episodes of loss of consciousness. An anastomosis of the left subclavian artery to the left pulmonary artery was made, and the clinical improvement was striking. Two additional patients with successful results are also described. It is of interest that Blalock refers to earlier experimental work in which subclavian pulmonary anastomoses were performed in the dog in an effort to produce pulmonary hypertension. Although these experiments did not produce an elevated pulmonary arterial pressure, the operation was subsequently used for an entirely different purpose. This procedure was the first of many additional cardiac surgical advances.

Groh, M. A., Meliones, J. N., Bove, E. L., et al.: Repair of tetralogy of Fallot in infancy: Effect of pulmonary artery size on outcome. Circulation, *84*(Suppl. III):206, 1991.

This series reviewed 58 infants less than 1 year old with tetralogy of Fallot (TOF) and pulmonary stenosis or atresia and without important pulmonary artery collaterals. Hospital mortality was 0% despite several patients with pulmonary artery McGoon ratios less than 1.0. The authors also remark that transannular patching was used in only 36% of patients, and in 50% of patients, muscle resection was avoided (whereas it was minimal in the remaining 29 patients). The authors conclude that repair of TOF should not be denied to infants solely on the basis of small pulmonary arteries.

Karl, T. R., Sano, S., Pornviliwan, S., and Mee, R. B. B.: Tetralogy of Fallot: Favorable outcome of nonneonatal transatrial, transpulmonary repair. Ann. Thorac. Surg., *54*:903, 1992.

This excellent series of patients from Royal Children's Hospital in Melbourne, Australia, suggests that early aortopulmonary shunts can be performed with extremely low risk, to allow patients to grow until they are large enough to undergo repair of TOF without ventriculotomy. The authors suggest that the long-term outcome from this protocol will be favorable.

Kirklin, J. W., and Barratt-Boyes, B. G.: Ventricular septal defect and pulmonary stenosis or atresia. *In* Kirklin, J. W., and Barratt-Boyes, B. G. (eds): Cardiac Surgery. 2nd ed. New York, Churchill Livingstone, 1993.

This remarkable book catalogs the extraordinary experience of these two well-known figures in the field of congenital heart surgery. The material included in this chapter is among the most up-to-date, comprehensive, and well-organized presentations available and should be read by anyone who desires in-depth reading in this field.

Kirklin, J. W., Blackstone, E. H., Jonas, R. A., et al.: Morphologic and surgical determinants of outcome events after repair of tetralogy of Fallot and pulmonary stenosis: A two-institution study. J. Thorac. Cardiovasc. Surg., *103*:706, 1992.

This outstanding report compares two different protocols for the management of TOF (with pulmonary stenosis) in infants: a strategy of early infant repair (100 patients from Boston Children's Hospital) and a strategy of initial palliation and delay of complete correction until the patient is older than 6 months (or more) (100 patients from the University of Alabama at Birmingham). The findings from this study demonstrated no advantage and a possible disadvantage to initial palliation as opposed to early repair.

Kirklin, J. K., Kirklin, J. W., Blackstone, E. H., et al.: Effect of transannular patching on outcome after repair of tetralogy of Fallot. Ann. Thorac. Surg., *48*:783, 1989.

This report evaluated 814 patients undergoing repair of TOF with pulmonary stenosis between 1967 and 1986. In this large series, transannular patching was a weak risk factor for death in the early postoperative period, but not late postoperatively. Transannular patching was a risk factor for reoperation for pulmonary regurgitation late postoperatively. This very large and well analyzed series provides an important perspective on the effects of transannular patching in repair of TOF.

Lillehei, C. W., Varco, R. L., Cohen, M., et al.: The first open heart repairs of ventricular septal defect, atrioventricular communis and tetralogy of Fallot using extracorporeal circulation by cross-circulation. A thirty-year follow-up. Ann. Thorac. Surg., *41*:4, 1986.

More than just a 30-year follow-up of the first patients to receive successful open cardiac correction of complex cardiac lesions, this article provides a poignant recapitulation of the early days of open heart surgery. Lillehei's historical account of the frustrations and ingenious attempts by the intrepid individuals who began the era of open heart surgery should be read by all interested in the field. Of equal impact are the thoughts offered by the discussants, who include some of the more prominent figures in cardiac surgery. Reading this article will provide a better understanding of the historical debt that is owed to those individuals with the insight and creativity to tackle the problems of open cardiac surgery.

Vobecky, S. J., Williams, W. G., Trusler, G. A., et al.: Survival analysis of infants under age 18 months presenting with tetralogy of Fallot. Ann. Thorac. Surg., *56*:944, 1993.

This article reports results for 270 patients presenting with TOF over a 10-year period to the Hospital for Sick Children in Toronto. Patients were treated by a protocol of palliation (with aortopulmonary shunts) if they were less than 18 months old and with total correction if they were 18 months or older. Survival was tracked from the time of diagnosis, and the authors provide outstanding outcome data for patients born with TOF who were treated by a protocol of early palliation. Although they found that the surgical mortality rate for those patients who eventually came to surgery was only 3.2%, 15 patients died before surgical correction, either as a result of palliation or as an outcome following palliation. Along with an excellent "companion" invited commentary from Aldo Castaneda (Boston Children's Hospital), this study demonstrates the risks of palliation versus early total correction. The authors also found that palliation, in the form of aortopulmonary shunts, was particularly hazardous for those infants with small (<2 mm) pulmonary arteries—the very patients who might most require a palliative procedure to increase pulmonary blood flow.

# BIBLIOGRAPHY

Akaska, T., Itoh, K., Nakayama, S., et al.: Surgical treatment of anomalous origin of the left coronary artery from the pulmonary artery associated with tetralogy of Fallot. Ann. Thorac. Surg., *31*:469, 1981.

Albert, J. D., Bishop, D. A., Fullerton, D. A., et al.: Conduit reconstruction of the right ventricular outflow tract. Lessons learned in a twelve-year experience. J. Thorac. Cardiovasc. Surg., *106*:228, 1993.

Amato, J. J., Marbey, M. L., and Bush, C.: Systemic-pulmonary polytetrafluoroethylene shunts in palliative operations for congenital heart disease: Revival of the central shunt. J. Thorac. Cardiovasc. Surg., *95*:62, 1988.

Anderson, R. H., Path, M. R. C., and Allwork, S. P.: Surgical anatomy of tetralogy of Fallot. J. Thorac. Cardiovasc. Surg., *81*:887, 1981.

Arciniegas, E.: Tetralogy of Fallot. *In* Arciniegas, E. (ed): Pediatric Cardiac Surgery. 1st ed. Chicago, Year Book Medical, 1985.

Arciniegas, E., Blackstone, E. H., Pacifico, A. D., and Kirklin, J. W.: Classic shunting operations as part of two-stage repair for tetralogy of Fallot. Ann. Thorac. Surg., *27*:514, 1979.

Arciniegas, E., Farooki, Z. Q., and Hakimi, M.: Early and late results of total correction of tetralogy of Fallot. J. Thorac. Cardiovasc. Surg., *80*:770, 1980a.

Arciniegas, E., Farooki, Z. Q., and Hakimi, M.: Results of two-stage surgical treatment of tetralogy of Fallot. J. Thorac. Cardiovasc. Surg., *79*:876, 1980b.

Barragry, T. P., Ring, W. S., and Blatchford, J. W.: Central aortopulmonary artery shunts in neonates with complex cyanotic congenital heart disease. J. Thorac. Cardiovasc. Surg., *93*:767, 1987.

Bertranou, E. G., Blackstone, E. H., and Hazelrig, J. B.: Life expectancy without surgery in tetralogy of Fallot. Am. J. Cardiol., *42*:458, 1978.

Bharati, S., Lev, M., and Kirklin, J. W.: Cardiac Surgery and Conduction System. New York, John Wiley & Sons, 1983.

Blackstone, E. H., Kirklin, J. W., Bertranou, E. G., et al.: Preoperative prediction from cineangiograms of postrepair right ventricular pressure in tetralogy of Fallot. J. Thorac. Cardiovasc. Surg., *78*:542, 1979a.

Blackstone, E. H., Kirklin, J. W., and Pacifico, A. D.: Decision-making in repair of tetralogy of Fallot based on intraoperative measurements of pulmonary arterial outflow tract. J. Thorac. Cardiovasc. Surg., *77*:526, 1979b.

Blalock, A.: Surgical procedures employed and anatomical variations encountered in the treatment of congenital pulmonic stenosis. Surg. Gynecol. Obstet., *87*:385, 1948.

Blalock, A., and Taussig, H. B.: The surgical treatment of malformations of the heart in which there is pulmonary stenosis or pulmonary atresia. J. A. M. A., *128*:189, 1945.

Bonchek, L. I., Starr, A., and Sunderland, C. O.: Natural history of tetralogy of Fallot. Circulation, *48*:392, 1973.

Borow, K. M., Green, L. H., Castaneda, A. R., and Keane, J. F.: Left ventricular function after repair of tetralogy of Fallot and its relationship to age at surgery. Circulation, *61*:1150, 1980.

Boucek, M. M., Webster, H. E., Orsmond, G. S., and Ruttenberg, H. D.: Balloon pulmonary valvotomy: Palliation for cyanotic heart disease. Am. Heart J., *115*:318, 1988.

Bove, E. L., and Byrum, C. J.: The influence of pulmonary insufficiency on ventricular function following repair of tetralogy of Fallot. Evaluation using radionuclide ventriculography. J. Thorac. Cardiovasc. Surg., *85*:691, 1983.

Calder, A. L., Barratt-Boyes, B. G., and Brandt, P. W. T.: Postoperative evaluation of patients with tetralogy of Fallot repaired in infancy. J. Thorac. Cardiovasc. Surg., *77*:704, 1979.

Castaneda, A. R.: Invited commentary to article by Vobecky S. J., Williams, W. G., Trusler, G. A., et al.: Survival analysis of infants under age 18 months presenting with tetralogy of Fallot. Ann. Thorac. Surg., *56*:944, 1993.

Castaneda, A. R., Freed, M. D., Williams, R. G., and Norwood, W. I.: Repair of tetralogy of Fallot in infancy: Early and late results. J. Thorac. Cardiovasc. Surg., *74*:372, 1977.

Castaneda, A. R., and Mayer, J.: Tetralogy of Fallot. *In* Stark, J., and de Leval, M. (eds): Surgery for Congenital Heart Defects. 2nd ed. Philadelphia, W. B. Saunders, 1994, pp. 405–416.

Coles, J. G., Kirklin, J. W., and Pacifico, A. D.: The relief of pulmonary stenosis by a transatrial versus a transventricular approach to the repair of tetralogy of Fallot. Ann. Thorac. Surg., 45:7, 1988.

Dabizzi, R. P., Caprioli, G., and Alazzi, L.: Distribution and anomalies of coronary arteries in tetralogy of Fallot. Circulation, 61:84, 1980.

de Leval, M. R., McKay, R., and Jones, M.: Modified Blalock-Taussig shunt. Use of subclavian artery orifice as flow regulator in prosthetic systemic pulmonary artery shunts. J. Thorac. Cardiovasc. Surg., 81:112, 1981.

del Nido, P. J., Mickle, D. A., and Wilson, G. J.: Inadequate myocardial protection with cold cardioplegic arrest during repair of tetralogy of Fallot. J. Thorac. Cardiovasc. Surg., 95:223, 1988.

Di Donato, R. M., Jonas, R. A., Lang, P., et al.: Neonatal repair of tetralogy of Fallot with and without pulmonary atresia. J. Thorac. Cardiovasc. Surg., 101:126, 1991.

Donahoo, J. S., Roland, J. M., Kan, J., et al.: Prostaglandin E₁ as an adjunct to emergency cardiac operations in neonates. J. Thorac. Cardiovasc. Surg., 81:227, 1981.

Ebert, P. A.: Atlas of Congenital Cardiac Surgery. New York, Churchill Livingstone, 1989.

Ebert, P. A.: Discussion of Piehler, J. M., Danielson, G. K., McGoon, D. C., et al.: Management of pulmonary atresia with ventricular septal defect and hypoplastic pulmonary arteries by right ventricular outflow construction. J. Thorac. Cardiovasc. Surg., 80:552, 1980.

Ebert, P. A.: Past, present, and future of palliative shunts. Adv. Cardiol., 26:127, 1979.

Ebert, P. A., Robinson, S. J., Stanger, P., and Engle, M. A.: Pulmonary artery conduits in infants younger than six months of age. J. Thorac. Cardiovasc. Surg., 72:351, 1976.

Elzenga, N. J., von Suylen, R. J., Frohn-Mulder, I., et al.: Juxtaductal pulmonary artery coarctation. An underestimated cause of branch pulmonary artery stenosis in patients with pulmonary atresia or stenosis and a ventricular septal defect. J. Thorac. Cardiovasc. Surg., 100:416, l990.

Fallot, E. L. A.: Contribution à l'anatomie pathologique de la maladie bleue (cyanose cardiaque). Marseilles Med., 25:77, 138, 207, 270, 341, 403, 1888.

Farre, J. R.: Pathological researches. SA I. On malformations of the human heart: Illustrated by numerous cases, and preceded by some observations on the method of improving the diagnostic part of medicine. London, Longmans, Green, 1814.

Fellows, K. E., Freed, M. K., and Keane, J. R.: Results of routine preoperative coronary angiography in tetralogy of Fallot. Circulation, 51:561, 1975.

Fellows, K. E., Smith, J., and King, J. F.: Preoperative angiocardiography in infants with tetralogy of Fallot. Review of 36 cases. Am. J. Cardiol., 47:1279. 1981.

Flanagan, M. F., Foran, R. B., Van Praagh, R., and Jonas, R. A.: Tetralogy of Fallot with obstruction of the ventricular septal defect: Spectrum of echocardiographic findings. J. Am. Coll. Cardiol., 11:386, 1988.

Fort, L., III, Morrow, A. G., Pierce, G. E., et al.: The distribution of pulmonary blood flow after subclavian-pulmonary anastomosis: An experimental study. J. Thorac. Cardiovasc. Surg., 50:671, 1965.

Freed, M. D., Heymann, M. A., and Lewis, A. B.: Prostaglandin E₁ in infants with ductus arteriosus–dependent congenital heart disease. Circulation, 64:899, 1981.

Garson, A., Jr., McNamara, D. G., and Cooley, D. A.: Tetralogy of Fallot In Roberts, W. C. (ed): Adult Congenital Heart Disease.- Philadelphia, F. A. Davis, 1987, pp. 493–519.

Garson, A., Nihill, M. R., McNamara, D. G., and Cooley, D. A.: Status of the adult and adolescent after repair of tetralogy of Fallot. Circulation, 59:1232, 1979.

Gay, W. A., Jr., and Ebert, P. A.: Aorta-to-right pulmonary anastomosis causing obstruction to the right pulmonary artery. Ann. Thorac. Surg., 16:402, 1973.

Gintrac, E.: Observations et Recherches sur la Cyanose ou Maladie Bleue. Paris, J. Pinard, 1824.

Glenn, W. W. L., and Patino, J. F.: Circulatory bypass of the right heart. I. Preliminary observation on direct delivery of vena caval blood into pulmonary arterial circulation. Azygos vein–pulmonary artery shunt. Yale J. Biol. Med., 27:147, 1954.

Gotsman, M. S.: Increasing obstruction to the outflow tract in Fallot's tetralogy. Br. Heart J., 28:615, 1966.

Graham, T. P., Jr., Cordell, D., and Atwood, G. F.: Right ventricular volume characteristics before and after palliative and reparative operation in tetralogy of Fallot. Circulation, 54:417, 1976.

Greeley, W. J., Stanley, T. E., Ungerleider, R. M., and Kisslo, J. A.: Intraoperative hypoxemic spells in tetralogy of Fallot: An echocardiographic analysis of diagnosis and treatment. Anesth. Analg., 68:815, 1989.

Groh, M. A., Meliones, J. N., Bove, E. L., et al.: Repair of tetralogy of Fallot in infancy: Effect of pulmonary artery size on outcome. Circulation, 84(Suppl. III):206, 1991.

Guo-Wei, H., and Chia-Chiang, K.: Pulmonic regurgitation and reconstruction of right ventricular outflow tract with patch. J. Thorac. Cardiovasc. Surg., 92:128, 1986.

Gustafson, R. A., Murray, G. F., and Warden, H. E.: Early primary repair of tetralogy of Fallot. Ann. Thorac. Surg., 45:235, 1988.

Hammon, J. W., Henry, C. L., and Merrill, W. H.: Tetralogy of Fallot: Selective surgical management can minimize operative mortality. Ann. Thorac. Surg., 40:280, 1985.

Harken, A. H., Horowitz, L. N., and Josephson, M. E.: Surgical correction of recurrent sustained ventricular tachycardia following complete repair of tetralogy of Fallot. J. Thorac. Cardiovasc. Surg., 80:779, 1980.

Harris, A. M., Segel, N., Biship, J. M.: Blalock-Taussig anastomosis for tetralogy of Fallot. A ten- to fifteen-year follow-up. Br. Heart J., 26:266, 1964.

Hartmann, R. C.: Hemorrhagic disorder occurring in patients with cyanotic congenital heart disease. Bull. Johns Hopkins Hosp., 91:49, 1952.

Hope, J.: A Treatise on the Disease of the Heart and Great Vessels, and On the Affections which May Be Mistaken for Them. London, J. Churchill & Sons, 1839.

Horneffer, P. J., Zahka, K. G., Rowe, S. A., et al.: Long-term results of total repair of tetralogy of Fallot in childhood. Ann. Thorac. Surg., 50:179, 1990.

Hudspeth, A. S., Cordell, A. R., and Johnston, F. R.: Transatrial approach to total correction of tetralogy of Fallot. Circulation, 27:796, 1963.

Humes, R. A., Driscoll, D. J., and Daniel, G. K.: Tetralogy of Fallot with anomalous origin or left anterior descending coronary artery: Surgical options. J. Thorac. Cardiovasc. Surg., 94:784, 1987.

Hunder, J.: Medical observations and inquiries by a society of physicians of London. London, 1757–1784.

Hunter, W.: Three cases of malformation of the heart: Case II. Medical Observations and Inquiries by a Society of Physicians in London, 6:291, 1784.

Hurwitz, R. A., Smith, W., and King, H.: Tetralogy of Fallot with abnormal coronary artery: 1967 to 1977. J. Thorac. Cardiovasc. Surg., 80:129, 1980.

Ilbawi, M. N.: Current status of surgery for congenital heart diseases. Clin. Perinatol., 16:157, 1989.

Ilbawi, M. N., Grieco, J., DeLeon, S. Y., et al.: Modified Blalock-Taussig shunt in newborn infants. J. Thorac. Cardiovasc. Surg., 88:770, 1984.

Ilbawi, M. N., Idriss, F. S., and DeLeon, S. Y.: Factors that exaggerate the deleterious effects of pulmonary insufficiency on the right ventricle after tetralogy repair: Surgical implications. J. Thorac. Cardiovasc. Surg., 93:36, 1987.

Ilbawi, M. N., Idriss, F. S., and Muster, A. J.: Tetralogy of Fallot with absent pulmonary valve: Should valve insertion be part of the intracardiac repair? J. Thorac. Cardiovasc. Surg., 81:906, 1981.

Karl, T. R., Sano, S., Pornviliwan, S., and Mee, R. B. B.: Tetralogy of Fallot: Favorable outcome of nonneonatal transatrial, transpulmonary repair. Ann. Thorac. Surg., 54:903, 1992.

Kawashima, Y., Matsuda, H., and Hirose, H.: Ninety consecutive corrective operations for tetralogy of Fallot with or without minimal right ventriculotomy. J. Thorac. Cardiovasc. Surg., 90:856, 1985.

Keagy, B. A., Wilcox, B. R., and Lucus, C. L.: Constant postoperative monitoring of cardiac output after correction of congenital heart defects. J. Thorac. Cardiovasc. Surg., 93:658, 1987.

Kirklin, J. W., and Barratt-Boyes, B. G.: Cardiac Surgery. 2nd ed. New York, Churchill Livingstone, 1993.

Kirklin, J. W., Blackstone, E. H., Colvin, E. V., and McConnell, M. E.: Early primary correction of tetralogy of Fallot. Ann. Thorac. Surg., 45:231, 1988.

Kirklin, J. W., Blackstone, E. H., Jonas, R. A., et al.: Morphologic and surgical determinants of outcome events after repair of tetralogy of Fallot and pulmonary stenosis: A two-institution study. J. Thorac. Cardiovasc. Surg., 103:706, 1992.

Kirklin, J. W., Blackstone, E. H., and Kirklin, J. K.: Surgical results and protocols in the spectrum of tetralogy of Fallot. Ann. Surg., 198:251, 1983.

Kirklin, J. W., Blackstone, E. H., and Pacifico, A. D.: Routine primary repair vs. two-stage repair of tetralogy of Fallot. Circulation, 60:373, 1979.

Kirklin, J. W., and Karp, R. B.: The Tetralogy of Fallot. Philadelphia, W. B. Saunders, 1970.

Kirklin, J. K., Kirklin, J. W., Blackstone, E. H., et al.: Effect of transannular patching on outcome after repair of tetralogy of Fallot. Ann. Thorac. Surg., 48:783, 1989.

Kisslo, J. A.: Doppler color-flow imaging. In Kisslo, J. A., Adams, D. V., and Belkin, R. N. (eds): Doppler Color Flow Imaging. New York, Churchill Livingstone, 1988.

Klein, M. D., Shaheen, K. W., Whittlesey, G. C., et al.: Extracorporeal membrane oxygenation for the circulatory support of children after repair of congenital heart disease. J. Thorac. Cardiovasc. Surg., 100:498, 1990.

Kurosawa, H., Imai, Y., and Nakazawa, M.: Standardized patch for infundibuloplasty for tetralogy of Fallot. J. Thorac. Cardiovasc. Surg., 92:396, 1986.

Kvelselis, D. A., Rocchini, A. P., Snider, A. R., and Rosenthal, A.: Results of balloon valvuloplasty in the treatment of congenital valvar pulmonary stenosis in children. Am. J. Cardiol., 56:527, 1985.

Laks, H., and Castaneda, A. R.: Subclavian arterioplasty for the ipsilateral Blalock-Taussig shunt. Ann. Thorac. Surg., 19:319, 1975.

Lamberti, J., Carlisle, J., and Waldman, J. D.: Systemic-pulmonary shunts in infants and children. J. Thorac. Cardiovasc. Surg., 88:76, 1984.

Lev, M., and Eckner, F. A. Q.: The pathologic anatomy of tetralogy of Fallot and its variations. Dis. Chest., 45:251, 1964.

Lillehei, C. W., Cohen, M., and Warden, H. E.: Direct-vision intracardiac surgical correction of the tetralogy of Fallot, pentalogy of Fallot, and pulmonary atresia defects: Report of first ten cases. Ann. Surg., 142:418, 1955a.

Lillehei, C. W., Cohen, M., Warden, H. E., and Varco, R. L.: The direct-vision intracardiac correction of congenital anomalies by controlled cross-circulation: Results in 32 patients with ventricular septal defects, tetralogy of Fallot, and atrioventricular communis defects. Surgery, 38:11, 1955b.

Lillehei, C. W., Varco, R. L., and Cohen, M.: The first open-heart repairs of ventricular septal defect, atrioventricular communis, and tetralogy of Fallot using extracorporeal circulation by cross-circulation: A thirty-year follow-up. Ann. Thorac. Surg., 41:4, 1986.

Lodge, F. A., Lamberti, J. J., and Goodman, A. H.: Vascular consequences of subclavian artery transection for the treatment of congenital heart disease. J. Thorac. Cardiovasc. Surg., 86:18, 1983.

Marino, B., Corno, A., and Pasquini, L.: Indication for systemic pulmonary artery shunts guided by two-dimensional and Doppler echocardiography: Criteria for patient selection. Ann. Thorac. Surg., 44:495, 1987.

Matsuda, H., Ihara, K., and Mori, T.: Tetralogy of Fallot associated with aortic insufficiency. Ann. Thorac. Surg., 29:529, 1980.

McCord, M. C., van Elk, J., and Blount, G., Jr.: Tetralogy of Fallot: Clinical and hemodynamic spectrum of combined pulmonary stenosis and ventricular septal defects. Circulation, 16:736, 1957.

Mendelsohn, A. M., Bove, E. L., Lupinetti, F. M., et al.: Intraoperative and percutaneous stenting of congenital pulmonary artery and vein stenosis. Circulation, 88:II-210, 1993.

Misbach, G. A., Turley, K., and Ebert, P. A.: Pulmonary valve replacement for regurgitation after repair of tetralogy of Fallot. Ann. Thorac. Surg., 36:684, 1983.

Mitchell, S. C., Korones, S. B., and Berendes, H. W.: Congenital heart disease in 56,109 births: Incidence and natural history. Circulation, 43:323, 1971.

Miura, T., Nakano, S., Shimazaki, Y., et al.: Evaluation of right ventricular function by regional wall motion analysis in patients after correction of tetralogy of Fallot: Comparison of transventricular and nontransventricular repairs. J. Thorac. Cardiovasc. Surg., 104:917, 1992.

Muhiudeen, I. A., Roberson, D. A., Silverman, N. H., et al.: Intraoperative echocardiography in infants and children with congenital cardiac shunt lesions: Transesophageal versus epicardial echocardiography. J. Am. Coll. Cardiol., 16:1687, 1990.

Murphy, J. D., Freed, M. D., and Keane, J. F.: Hemodynamic results after intracardiac repair of tetralogy of Fallot by deep hypothermia and cardiopulmonary bypass. Circulation, 62(Suppl. I):168, 1980.

Nagao, G. I., Daoud, G. I., and McAdams, A. J.: Cardiovascular anomalies associated with tetralogy of Fallot. Am. J. Cardiol., 20:206, 1967.

Nomoto, S., Muraoka, R., and Yokota, M.: Left ventricular volume as a predictor of postoperative hemodynamics and a criterion for total correction of tetralogy of Fallot. J. Thorac. Cardiovasc. Surg., 80:389, 1984.

Norwood, W. I., and Pigott, J. D.: Recent advances in cardiac surgery. Pediatr. Clin. North Am., 32:1117, 1985.

O'Laughlin, M. P., Slack, M. C., Grifka, R. G., et al.: Implantation and intermediate-term follow-up of stents in congenital heart disease. Circulation, 88:605, 1993.

Pacifico, A. D., Kirklin, J. W., and Blackstone, E. H.: Surgical management of pulmonary stenosis in tetralogy of Fallot. J. Thorac. Cardiovasc. Surg., 74:382, 1977.

Pacifico, A. D., Sand, M. E., Bargeron, L. M., Jr., and Colvin, E. C.: Transatrial transpulmonary repair of tetralogy of Fallot. J. Thorac. Cardiovasc. Surg., 93:919, 1987.

Papagiannis, J., Kanter, R. J., Armstrong, B. E., et al.: Intraoperative epicardial echocardiography during repair of tetralogy of Fallot. J. Am. Soc. Echocardiogr., 6:366, 1993.

Peacock, T. B.: On Malformations of the Human Heart. Etc. with Original Cases and Illustrations. 2nd ed. London, J. Churchill and Sons, 1866.

Piehler, J. M., Danielson, G. K., McGoon, D. C., et al.: Management of pulmonary atresia with ventricular septal defect and hypoplastic pulmonary arteries by right ventricular outflow construction. J. Thorac. Cardiovasc. Surg., 80:552, 1980.

Porter, J. M., and Silver, D.: Alterations in fibrinolysis and coagulation associated with cardiopulmonary bypass. J. Thorac. Cardiovasc. Surg., 56:869, 1968.

Potts, W. J., Gibson, S., Riker, W. L., and Leninger, C. R.: Congenital pulmonary stenosis with intact ventricular septum. J. A. M. A., 144:8, 1950.

Pridjian, A. K., Pearce, F. B., Culpepper W. S., et al.: Atrioventricular valve competence after takedown to improve exposure during ventricular septal defect repair. J. Thorac. Cardiovasc. Surg., 106:1122, 1993.

Quattlebaum, T. G., Varghese, P. J., and Neill, C. A.: Sudden death among postoperative patients with tetralogy of Fallot: A follow-up study of 243 patients for an average of twelve years. Circulation, 54:289, 1976.

Rittenhouse, E. A., Mansfield, P. B., and Hall, D. G.: Tetralogy of Fallot: Selective staged management. J. Thorac. Cardiovasc. Surg., 89:772, 1985.

Rosenberg, H. G., Williams, W. G., and Trusler, G. A.: Structural composition of central pulmonary arteries: Growth potential after surgical shunts. J. Thorac. Cardiovasc. Surg., 94:498, 1987.

Ross, R. S., Taussig, H. B., and Evans, M. H.: Late hemodynamic complications of anastomotic surgery for treatment of the tetralogy of Fallot. Circulation, 18:553, 1958.

Sabiston, D. C., Jr.: Role of the Blalock-Taussig operation in the hypoxic infant with tetralogy of Fallot. Ann. Thorac. Surg., 22:303, 1976.

Sabiston, D. C., Jr., and Blalock, A.: The tetralogy of Fallot, tricuspid atresia, transposition of the great vessels and associated disorders. In Derra, E. (ed): Encyclopedia of Thoracic Surgery. Heidelberg, Springer-Verlag, 1959.

Sabiston, D. C., Jr., Cornell, W. P., and Criley, J. M.: The diagnosis and surgical correction of total obstruction of the right ventricle: An acquired condition developing after systemic-pulmonary artery anastomosis for tetralogy of Fallot. J. Thorac. Cardiovasc. Surg., 48:577, 1964.

Sandifort, E.: Observationes Anatomico-Pathologicae. Chap. 1, Fig. 1. Lugdunum Batavorum, P.v.d. Eyk et D. Vygh, 1777.

Shimazaki, Y., Blackstone, E. H., Kirklin, J. W., et al.: The dimensions of the right ventricular outflow tract and pulmonary arteries in tetralogy of Fallot and pulmonary stenosis. J. Thorac. Cardiovasc. Surg., 103:692, 1992.

Silverman, N. H.: Pediatric Echocardiography. Baltimore, Williams & Wilkins, 1993.

Sreeram, N., Saleem, M., Jackson, M., et al.: Results of balloon pulmonary valvuloplasty as a palliative procedure in tetralogy of Fallot. J. Am. Coll. Cardiol., 18:159, 1990.

Stensen, N. (Nicholaus Steno): In Bartholin, T.: Acta Medica et Philosophica Hafnienca, 1671–1972. Vol. 1, p. 302. Reprinted in Stenosis, N.: Opera Philosophica. Vol. 2. Copenhagen, Vilhelm Maar, 1910, pp. 49–53.

Stephens, H. B.: Aneurysm of the pulmonary artery following a Pott's shunt operation. J. Thorac. Cardiovasc. Surg., 53:642, 1967.

Tamiya, T., Yamashiro, T., Matsumoto, T., et al.: A histological study of surgical landmarks for the specialized atrioventricular conduction system, with particular reference to the papillary muscle. Ann. Thorac. Surg., 40:599, 1985.

Touati, G. D., Vouhe, P. R., Amodeo, A., et al.: Primary repair of tetralogy of Fallot in infancy. J. Thorac. Cardiovasc. Surg., 99:396, 1990.

Tucker, W. Y., Turley, K., and Ullyot, D. J.: Management of symptomatic tetralogy of Fallot in the first year of life. J. Thorac. Cardiovasc. Surg., 78:494, 1979.

Turley, K., Tucker, W. Y., and Ebert, P. A.: The changing role of palliative procedures in the treatment of infants with congenital heart disease. J. Thorac. Cardiovasc. Surg., 79:194, 1980.

Ullom, R. L., Sade, R. M., and Crawford, F. A.: The Blalock-Taussig shunt in infants: Standard versus modified. Ann. Thorac. Surg., 44:539, 1987.

Ungerleider, R. M.: Right ventricular function after transatrial versus transventricular repair of tetralogy of Fallot [Invited letter]. J. Thorac. Cardiovasc. Surg., 104:1173, 1992.

Ungerleider, R. M., Greeley, W. J., Kanter, R. J., and Kisslo, J. A.: The learning curve for intraoperative echocardiography during congenital heart surgery. Ann. Thorac. Surg., 54:691, 1992.

Ungerleider, R. M., Greeley, W. J., Sheikh, K. H., et al.: Routine use of intraoperative epicardial echo and Doppler color-flow imaging to guide and evaluate repair of congenital heart lesions: A prospective study. J. Thorac. Cardiovasc. Surg., 100:297, l990.

Ungerleider, R. M., Greeley, W. J., Sheikh, K. H., et al.: The use of intraoperative echo with Doppler color-flow imaging to predict outcome after repair of congenital cardiac defects. Ann. Surg., 210:526, 1989.

Vargas, F. J., Coto, E. O., and Mayer, J. E., Jr.: Complete atrioventricular canal and tetralogy of Fallot: Surgical considerations. Ann. Thorac. Surg., 42:258, 1986.

Vobecky, S. J., Williams, W. G., Trusler, G. A., et al.: Survival analysis of infants under age 18 months presenting with tetralogy of Fallot. Ann. Thorac. Surg., 56:944, 1993.

Waterson, J. D.: Treatment of Fallot's tetralogy in children under 1 year of age. Rozhl. Chir., 41:181, 1962.

Webb, W. R., and Burford, T. H.: Gangrene of the arm following use of the subclavian artery in a pulmonosystemic (Blalock) anastomosis. J. Thorac. Surg., 23:199, 1952.

Westerman, G. R., Norton, J. V., and Van Devanter, S. H.: A double-outlet right atrium associated with Tetralogy of Fallot and common atrioventricular valve. J. Thorac. Cardiovasc. Surg., 91:205, 1986.

White, P. D., and Sprague, H. B.: The tetralogy of Fallot: Report of a case in a noted musician who lived to his sixtieth year. J. A. M. A., 92:787, 1929.

Wilson, J. M., Mack, J. W., Turley, K., and Ebert, P. A.: Persistent stenosis and deformity of the right pulmonary artery after correction of the Waterston anastomosis. J. Thorac. Cardiovasc. Surg., 82:169, 1981.

Yamaguchi, M., Imai, M., and Ohashi, H.: Enhanced myocardial protection by systemic hypothermia in children undergoing total correction of tetralogy of Fallot. Ann. Thorac. Surg., 41:639, 1986.

Zahka, K. G., Manolio, T. A., Rykiel, M. J. F., et al.: Handgrip strength after the Blalock-Taussig shunt: 14- to 34-year follow-up. Clin. Cardiol., 11:627, 1988.

Zerbini, E. J., MacCruz, R., and Bittencourt, D.: Total correction of complex of Fallot under extracorporeal circulation: Immediate results in a group of 221 patients. J. Thorac. Cardiovasc. Surg., 49:430, 1965.

Zhao, H. X., Miller, D. C., Reitz, B. A., and Shumway, N. E.: Surgical repair of tetralogy of Fallot: Long-term follow-up with particular emphasis on late death and reoperation. J. Thorac. Cardiovasc. Surg., 89:204, 1985.

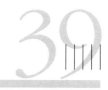

# ■ II Pulmonary Atresia or Stenosis with Intact Ventricular Septum

Ross M. Ungerleider and J. William Gaynor

## HISTORY

Dr. Thomas Peacock described seven patients with pulmonary atresia and intact ventricular septum in 1839, but credited John Hunter with the first case report in 1783 (Hunter, 1783; Peacock, 1869). Hunter's index case was born prematurely (8 months) and died in convulsions on the 13th day of life. Hunter's anatomic description beautifully describes the reasons this lesion is potentially so devastating:

The pulmonary artery, which, at its beginning from the right ventricle, was contracted into a solid substance or cord, and absolutely and completely impervious; so that the lungs had not received one drop of blood from the heart by the trunk of the pulmonary artery. The right ventricle, therefore, had been of no use in transmitting the blood, and had scarcely any cavity left. The blood which was brought to the right auricle, by the two cavae and the coronary veins, had passed through the foramen ovale, which was very large, into the left side of the heart, and so into the aorta, without passing through the lungs, and of course without receiving the benefit of respiration. The pulmonary artery, except just at its beginning, was every where pervious; and the canalis arteriosus had supplied it with a scanty share of blood, which was derived, in a retrograde way, from the aorta. . . . The right auriculoventricular aperture was especially small. . . . The left ventricle was large and powerful. (Hunter, 1783)

## INCIDENCE, EMBRYOLOGY, AND ANATOMY

*Pulmonary atresia with intact ventricular septum* (PA/ IVS) is a rare form of congenital heart disease representing 1 to 3% of all cases or 0.01 to 0.03% of all live births (Kirklin and Barratt-Boyes, 1993; Perloff, 1987). Familial PA/IVS has been occasionally reported, but the condition is usually sporadic. There is a slight predilection toward male predominance. The defect is characterized by absence of continuity between the right ventricle and the main pulmonary artery. Unlike pulmonary atresia with a ventricular septal defect (PA/VSD; tetralogy of Fallot with pulmonary atresia), which is associated with a normal-sized right ventricle, PA/IVS is associated with significant variation in right ventricular size. The size of the right ventricle (and tricuspid valve) largely determines the natural history of patients born with this defect. The defect is highly lethal if untreated, with a 50% mortality rate at 2 weeks of age, increasing to 85% at 6 months (Fig. 39–26). Death occurs secondary to progressive severe

hypoxemia and metabolic acidosis following closure of the ductus arteriosus (Kirklin and Barratt-Boyes, 1993).

The embryologic origin of PA/IVS has been difficult to determine. Kutsche and Van Mierop (1983) propose that atresia of the pulmonary valve occurs after cardiac septation has been completed. The cause of PA/IVS may be secondary to an inflammatory process. Rubella infections have been associated with pulmonary artery obstruction (Perloff, 1987; Wagner, 1981).

The major site of obstruction is the pulmonary valve. Typically, commissural ridges fuse and converge at the center of an imperforate valve. In the vast majority of patients, the pulmonary valve is tricuspid in appearance with fused cusps. Less commonly, the commissural ridges are present only peripherally with a smooth dome-like center (Kutsche and Van Mierop, 1983; Oka and Angrist, 1967; Wagner, 1981). Quadracusp valves have been described. Muscular subvalvular or infundibular obstruction may be present and may be obliterative (Perloff, 1987; Pawade et al., 1993). More than 90% of patients have normal or nearly normal pulmonary arteries, with moderate to severe hypoplasia of either pulmonary artery seen in only 6% of patients (Hanley et al., 1993; Zuberbuhler and Anderson, 1979). Because flow is completely obstructed from the right ventricle to the pulmonary artery and the ventricular septum is intact, survival depends on a patent ductus arteriosus (PDA) to provide pulmonary blood flow, and an atrial septal defect (ASD) or patent foramen ovale to enable systemic venous return to reach the left atrium.

The normal right ventricle consists of three parts: a sinus (or inlet) portion, a trabecular region, and a conus (or infundibulum) (Fig. 39–27). In patients with

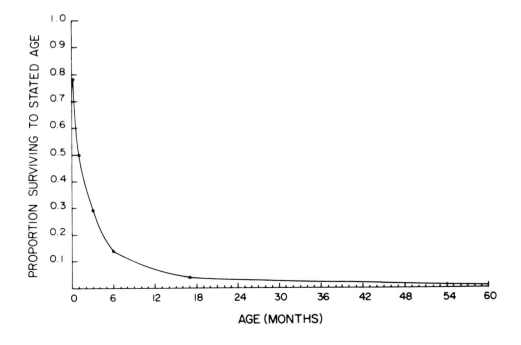

**FIGURE 39–26.** Free-hand estimate of the survival of surgically *untreated* patients with pulmonary atresia and intact ventricular septum (PA/IVS), based on reports in the literature. (From Kirklin, J. W., and Barratt-Boyes, B. G.: Cardiac Surgery. 2nd ed. New York, Churchill Livingstone, 1993.)

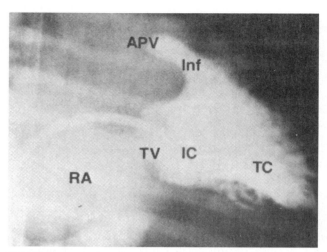

FIGURE 39–27. Right-sided heart angiogram of a patient with PA/IVS. The right ventricle has an atretic pulmonary valve (APV) so that the right ventricle has no outlet and the tricuspid valve (TV) is insufficient, resulting in considerable contrast in the right atrium (RA). The right ventricle in this patient is well formed and "tripartite" demonstrating an inlet component (IC), a trabecular component (TC), and an infundibulum (Inf). There are no sinusoidal connections to the coronary arteries. (From Williams, W. G., Burrows, P., Freedom, F. M., et al.: Thromboexclusion of the right ventricle in children with pulmonary atresia and intact ventricular septum. J. Thorac. Cardiovasc. Surg., 101:222, 1991.)

PA/IVS, the right ventricular size is extremely variable, from very small and hypertrophied with a tiny cavity to dilated and thin-walled with a huge cavity. In 90% of patients, the right ventricle is small, and in 60%, the right ventricle is diminutive (Hanley et al., 1993; Perloff, 1987). The right ventricle is of normal size in only 5% of these patients and is larger than normal in the remaining 5%. In the small right ventricle with pulmonary atresia, all three portions of the right ventricle are represented. The severely small (diminutive) right ventricle is associated with a reduced and sometimes nearly obliterated trabecular and infundibular portion, a thick ventricular wall, and endocardial fibroelastosis (Bharati et al., 1977; Bull et al., 1982) At the other end of the spectrum, the ventricle may be severely dilated with a thin wall similar to that found in Uhl's anomaly (Coté et al., 1973; Patel et al., 1980).

Functionally and morphologically, the tricuspid valve varies with right ventricular size (Becker et al., 1971). Small right ventricular size is correlated with a small tricuspid valve that is thickened with hypoplastic papillary muscles (Davignon et al., 1961; Paul and Lev, 1960; Perloff, 1987). If the right ventricle and therefore the tricuspid valve are large, the leaflets are usually abnormal and have characteristics of Ebstein's malformation, e.g., a large anterior leaflet and downward displacement onto the ventricular wall of the septal leaflet. These large valves are almost always severely insufficient and the right atrium may be massively dilated (Bharati et al., 1977; Kutsche and Van Mierop, 1983). The morphology of the PDA in PA/IVS is usually normal, unlike the sigmoid and downward course of the PDA in patients with PA/

VSD, indicating that fetal pulmonary blood flow was normal at one time and that the anomaly probably developed later in gestation (Santos et al., 1980; Kutsche and Van Mierop, 1983). The bronchial arterial circulation is generally normal without significant associated aortopulmonary collaterals, except in rare patients with absent PDA and large mediastinal collateralization (Kirklin and Barratt-Boyes, 1993).

The left ventricle is hypertrophied and often demonstrates mild fibroelastosis. Septal convex bulging into the left ventricular cavity has been seen and may cause left ventricular outflow obstruction (Zuberbuhler and Anderson, 1979). The ascending aorta is larger in diameter than normal, with a normal-sized descending aorta.

Coronary artery sinusoids or fistulas (Fig. 39–28) occur in 45 to 50% of patients and are more common in hearts with small right ventricles and competent tricuspid valves. The prevalence of sinusoids correlates with tricuspid valve size, and they are most frequently seen in patients with small tricuspid valves (Calder et al., 1987; Coles et al., 1989; Hanley et al., 1993) (Fig. 39–29). Coronary artery fistulas are seen much less commonly in patients with pulmonary stenosis and intact ventricular septum. Early in development, myocardial blood supply is derived from the lumen of the heart through embryologic myocardial lacunae. The coronary arteries communicate with these intramyocardial trabecular spaces, which normally involute to form the microcirculation. If the pulmonary valve fuses before the sinusoids close,

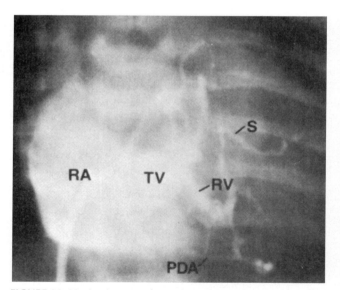

FIGURE 39–28. Angiogram of a patient with diminutive right ventricle (RV) and sinusoidal (S) connections between the small RV cavity and the coronary arteries. The posterior descending coronary artery (PDA) is filled with contrast from this right-sided injection, demonstrating that it receives perfusion, in part, from the desaturated blood in the right ventricle. Decompression of this right ventricle could theoretically produce diastolic flow into the right ventricular chamber instead of the distal coronary beds. (RA = right atrium; TV = tricuspid valve.) (From Williams, W. G., Burrows, P., Freedom, F. M., et al.: Thromboexclusion of the right ventricle in children with pulmonary atresia and intact ventricular septum. J. Thorac. Cardiovasc. Surg., 101:222, 1991.)

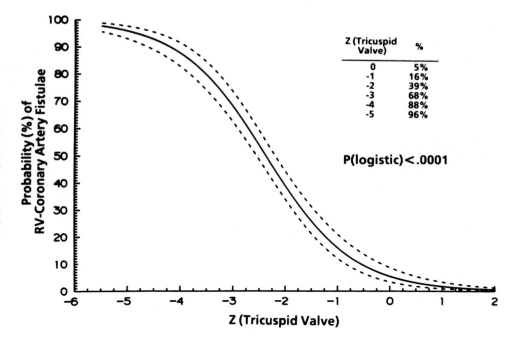

FIGURE 39–29. Nomogram of a regression equation (univariate) expressing the relation between the dimensions of the tricuspid valve and the probability of the presence of right ventricular–coronary artery fistulas in PA/IVS. (From Hanley, F. L., Sade, R. M., Blackstone, E. H., et al.: Outcomes in neonatal pulmonary atresia with intact ventricular septum. J. Thorac. Cardiovasc. Surg., *105*:406, 1993.)

| Z (Tricuspid Valve) | % |
|---|---|
| 0 | 5% |
| -1 | 16% |
| -2 | 39% |
| -3 | 68% |
| -4 | 88% |
| -5 | 96% |

P(logistic) < .0001

flow into the sinusoids may be maintained by elevated right ventricular systolic pressure (Anderson et al., 1991; Bull et al., 1982). Although coronary fistulas may develop in many patients, left ventricular myocardial perfusion depends only on flow through the sinusoids in approximately 10% of patients. Persistence of these embryologic structures is thought to be secondary to a hemodynamic phenomenon (suprasystemic RV pressure) rather than a primary process, unlike defects in which left ventricle sinusoids are present (Rhagib et al., 1965).

Coronary fistulas are associated with two potential problems. Diastolic runoff from the myocardium to the right ventricular chamber (which can occur when the suprasystemic right ventricular chamber is decompressed by a transannular patch) may create a steal phenomenon and cause ischemia to the distal left ventricular myocardial beds. Also, proximal stenoses of the coronary arteries do occur, and then distal myocardial perfusion is dependent on the right ventricle-coronary connection (Fig. 39–30). Depending on the number and locations of fistulas and coronary obstructions, some regions of the myocardium may be perfused during systole (via fistulas) with desaturated blood from the right ventricle, while other regions receive normal, antegrade diastolic flow with saturated blood from the aorta. Decompression of the right ventricle in patients with significant fistulas can result in severe ischemia of the affected regions, so the presence of a fistula is a major consideration in planning surgical intervention (Freedom and Harrington, 1974; Fyfe et al., 1986; Gittenberger-de Groot et al., 1988; Hanley et al., 1993; Williams et al., 1991).

## DIAGNOSIS

Newborn infants with PA/IVS usually appear well developed, but cyanosis is present at or immediately after birth and may range from mild to severe. The pulses are usually normal but may be decreased if congestive heart failure is present. The left ventricular impulse is found in the normal position. When the right ventricle is diminutive, the right ventricular impulse is absent, and if the right ventricle is normal or enlarged, the right ventricular impulse is palpable. A thrill at the lower left sternal border may be found if there is significant tricuspid regurgitation (Perloff, 1987). If the right ventricle and tricuspid valve are small, the first heart sound will be single. There is not usually a prominent murmur, and even the continuous murmur of a PDA is infrequently appreciated (Kirklin and Barratt-Boyes, 1993; Perloff, 1987). Tricuspid regurgitation generally produces a systolic murmur along the left sternal border radiating to the right side and right axilla.

The chest film is not helpful at birth (or later) in distinguishing among small, normal, or large right ventricles. The cardiac silhouette is usually normal at birth, but it soon increases in size secondary to enlargement of the right atrium and left ventricle. Oligemia of the lung fields is generally pronounced, but the pulmonary arteries appear normal because the branch pulmonary arteries in PA/IVS are usually well developed. The right atrial shadow may be large, especially in the presence of tricuspid insufficiency. The cardiac silhouette may fill the entire chest in the case of a dilated right ventricle with tricuspid regurgitation (associated with Ebstein's malformation). The electrocardiogram is rarely normal, even in the neonate. In some patients, criteria for right ventricular hypertrophy may be met even when the right ventricular cavity is small, precluding its use in predicting right ventricular cavity size (Kirklin and Barratt-Boyes, 1993; Perloff, 1987).

Two-dimensional echocardiography is the optimal method to evaluate cardiac anatomy in cyanotic pa-

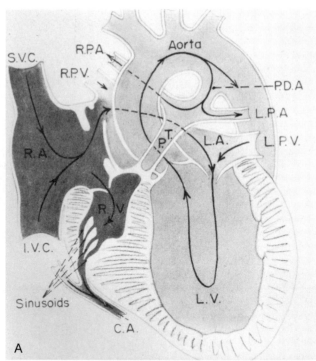

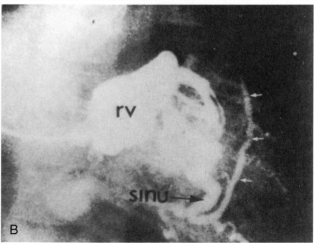

**FIGURE 39–30.** *A,* Schematic demonstrating the physiology of PA/ IVS with RV-coronary sinusoids. The coronary arteries are filled with desaturated blood from the RV. This coronary perfusion occurs throughout the cardiac cycle, since the RV pressure is suprasystemic. Decompression of the RV pressure risks retrograde coronary flow into the RV (coronary steal) with ischemia of the distal myocardial beds. (S.V.C. = superior vena cava; R.A. = right atrium; I.V.C. = inferior vena cava; R.P.A. = right pulmonary artery; R.P.V. = right pulmonary vein; C.A. = coronary artery; P.T. = pulmonary trunk; L.A. = left atrium; L.V. = left ventricle; P.D.A. = posterior descending coronary artery; L.P.A. = left pulmonary artery; L.P.V. = left pulmonary vein.) *B,* In this patient, there is a small right ventricle (rv) with numerous sinusoidal connections (sinu) which eventually connect to the left anterior descending coronary artery (LAD). The LAD has numerous areas of stenosis *(arrows)* and the distal myocardium supplied by the LAD in all likelihood depends on flow of desaturated blood through the sinusoid from the RV. Decompression of the RV in such a patient can have devastating consequences. (*B,* From Williams, W. G., Burrows, P., Freedom, F. M., et al.: Thromboexclusion of the right ventricle in children with pulmonary atresia and intact ventricular septum. J. Thorac. Cardiovasc. Surg., *101*:222, 1991.)

tients. Cavity size, valvular dimensions and function, and the nature of pulmonary artery obstruction (membranous or muscular) can be determined. Coronary artery fistulas are readily identified using pulsed Doppler and color-flow imaging. The presence of restrictive flow across the foramen ovale can be identified, as well as the patency of the ductus arteriosus (Kirklin and Barratt-Boyes, 1993; Perloff, 1987).

Cardiac catheterization with coronary angiography is recommended to document the coronary arterial anatomy and the presence of coronary stenoses (Kirklin and Barratt-Boyes, 1993). Furthermore, myocardial dependence on coronary flow from the right ventricle can be identified. Pressure measurements may reveal a right atrial pressure that is greater than the left atrial pressure, suggesting a restrictive interatrial defect. The right ventricular systolic pressure may be suprasystemic. The systemic arterial oxygen

saturation is variable depending on the amount of flow through the ductus arteriosus. The dimensions of the right ventricular chamber and pulmonary arteries can be evaluated as well, and are important in designing the appropriate right ventricular outflow procedure. Right ventricular function is almost always abnormal, whereas left ventricular function may be normal or impaired (Scognamilgio et al., 1986).

## PREOPERATIVE MANAGEMENT

Infants with PA/IVS have ductal-dependent pulmonary blood flow and require infusion of prostaglandin $E_1$ (PGE$_1$) to maintain ductal patency. PGE$_1$ is frequently started in cyanotic infants before diagnosis has been confirmed and often before the infant arrives in the critical care unit. Once the diagnosis of a ductal-dependent cardiac lesion has been made, the intensive care team must ensure a reliable and dedicated site for administration of PGE$_1$ (Meliones et al., 1994). Following institution of prostaglandin therapy, the ductus arteriosus should open and arterial oxygen saturations improve into the 80% range (or higher) within hours. Because of a 15 to 25% risk of apnea from prostaglandins, the infant may need to be electively intubated and ventilated, or at least carefully observed in an environment where inadequate ventilatory effort can be rapidly recognized and treated. Failure to achieve adequate oxygenation (arterial oxygen saturations greater than 80%) should prompt careful investigation. Oligemia of the lung fields on chest film suggests inadequate pulmonary blood flow either from a ductus arteriosus that has not opened in response to PGE$_1$ or from inadequate pulmonary arteries. Pulmonary hypertension is rarely a problem for these infants, so hyperventilation is not often necessary. Once the diagnosis of PA/IVS has been established and the specifics of the anatomy have been determined, surgical intervention is indicated because of the condition's dismal natural history.

## SURGICAL MANAGEMENT

Surgical decision making for patients with PA/IVS is complex and the initial surgical intervention depends on the anatomic findings. Optimal surgical intervention restores right ventricle-to-pulmonary artery continuity and incorporates the right ventricle into a two-ventricle heart, with the systemic and pulmonary circulations completely separated. However, in many patients, the right ventricle is small and will never provide adequate pulmonary blood flow. Complete primary neonatal repair is almost never possible and most patients require at least one palliative procedure before definitive repair. Several authors have suggested criteria for selection of appropriate therapy based on tricuspid valve size (Hanley et al., 1993), right ventricular morphology (Billingsley et al., 1989; de Leval et al., 1982, 1985), or development of the infundibulum (Pawade et al., 1993). The goal is to safely take as many of these patients as possible to a two-ventricle repair, and stage the remainder toward a single-ventricle repair. In order to achieve this goal, the potential for the tricuspid valve and right ventricle to function as important components of the circulation must be predicted. Patients with extremely small tricuspid valves and tiny right ventricular chambers are unlikely ever to develop an adequate right ventricle and should be staged toward an eventual Fontan-type operation. Patients with larger tricuspid valves and right ventricular chambers should undergo a procedure that provides the right side of the heart with an opportunity to grow. Patients with relatively normal-sized tricuspid valves and right ventricles should have a procedure designed to place the right ventricle in continuity with the pulmonary vascular bed in anticipation of normal function as the child grows. These decisions are fur-

ther influenced by the presence of coronary fistulas. Substantial controversy exists as to which procedures constitute the optimal initial attempt to achieve the stated goals (Billingsley et al., 1989; de Leval et al., 1982, 1985; Pawade et al., 1993; Williams et al., 1991).

Unlike for the left ventricle, a satisfactory geometric model to estimate right ventricular size has not been established. Volumetric estimation based on angiographically or echocardiographically derived data continues to be controversial (Freedom and Harrington, 1974; Patel et al., 1980; Schmidt et al., 1992). Several systems have been proposed to determine initial and subsequent therapy:

1. A relationship between tricuspid valve size and right ventricular cavity has been described (Bull et al., 1982; de Leval et al., 1982; Patel et al., 1980; Zuberbuhler and Anderson, 1979). Hanley and associates (1993), analyzing data from the Congenital Heart Surgeons Society, have reported tricuspid valve size as the only specific risk factor complicating eventual achievement of two-ventricle repair.

2. Presence of all three components (inlet, trabecular, and infundibular) of the right ventricle has also been reported to be important. De Leval and colleagues (1985) suggested that if the diameter of the tricuspid valve in a tripartite ventricle is greater than the lower 99% confidence level to the normal mean tricuspid valve based on the patient's size, the right ventricle can be safely incorporated into a two-ventricle repair, if the major tricuspid insufficiency is not present.

3. Pawade and co-workers (1993) determined suitability for two-ventricle repairs based on echocardiographic assessment of the infundibulum alone. If the infundibulum is well developed, regardless of initial tricuspid valve size or presence of tripartite right ventricular anatomy, the patient is staged toward a two-ventricle repair. If the infundibulum is poorly formed, the patient is staged to a Fontan procedure.

4. Billingsley and associates (1989) classified right ventricular hypoplasia as mild, moderate, or severe, and argued that the overall degree of right ventricular hypoplasia more accurately indicates the appropriate surgical intervention than does the presence or absence of the tripartite components.

## Initial Procedures

A systemic-to-pulmonary artery shunt is usually necessary in infants and is a safe and effective method for short- or long-term palliation. The type of shunt is not critical, although classic or modified (Gore-Tex interposition) Blalock-Taussig shunts or central Gore-Tex shunts are most practical and are routinely used. A systemic-to-pulmonary artery shunt alone is associated with a very low operative and short-term mortality. A shunt alone, without a concomitant procedure to encourage blood flow through the right side of the heart, provides little stimulus for growth of the tricuspid valve and right ventricle, compromising chances for a subsequent two-ventricle repair. There-fore, a shunt alone as initial palliation is indicated only when any additional procedure would carry excessive risk or if eventual two-ventricle repair is considered impossible (Hanley et al., 1993).

There is evidence that pulmonary valvotomy, or a transannular patch, increases forward flow from the right ventricle to the pulmonary artery. This promotes growth of the tricuspid valve and right ventricle and can be performed in conjunction with a systemic-to-pulmonary artery shunt (Kirklin and Barratt-Boyes, 1993). At least half of these patients, undergoing a valvotomy or outflow patch, will require a systemic-to-pulmonary artery shunt to provide adequate pulmonary blood flow because right ventricular compliance may be poor and may not allow adequate antegrade flow to the pulmonary arteries. As an alternative, Foker and colleagues (1986) have recommended maintaining patency of the ductus arteriosus by infusing $PGE_1$ postoperatively, and weaning the patient from prostaglandins as the right ventricle recovers and begins providing adequate pulmonary blood flow (as reflected by improved systemic oxygen saturations and increased antegrade right ventricular outflow by echocardiography). This technique provides the patient with a "natural" systemic-to-pulmonary artery shunt that will obliterate spontaneously when the prostaglandins are discontinued. However, such patients must remain on intravenous therapy in the intensive care unit instead of recovering on the ward and going home, as would be the case if they received a standard shunt. Occasionally, right ventricular compliance does not improve quickly, and reoperation to place a systemic-to-pulmonary artery shunt is required. When this method is properly selected, patients are discharged with essentially normal circulation, and no further intervention is required.

As many as 45 to 50% of patients with PA/IVS have some communication between the right ventricle and the coronary arteries. In some patients (usually those with obstructions in the proximal coronary arteries), the right ventricle-to-coronary connection provides a significant portion of the blood supply to the distal coronary bed. The coronary supply from these fistulous connections is desaturated blood from the right ventricular chamber provided during systole (as opposed to normal diastolic coronary supply) by the suprasystemic right ventricular pressures. Performance of a right ventricular outflow procedure (transannular patch or pulmonary valvotomy) in these patients may decompress the right ventricular pressure so that it will no longer supply the distal coronary bed, and the ischemia produced may be fatal. Therefore, consideration of a right ventricular outflow procedure needs to include the recognition of coronary fistulas and whether they provide important coronary perfusion. Fortunately, many patients with coronary fistulas also have small tricuspid valves (see Fig. 39–29) and severely hypoplastic right ventricles. Such patients are usually staged to a single-ventricle repair without right ventricular decompression (Hanley et al., 1993).

A report of 82 patients with PA/IVS found right ventricle-to-coronary artery fistulas in 26 patients (32%) (Giglia et al., 1992). Retrospective review suggested that the presence of a fistula without associated coronary artery stenosis does not preclude successful right ventricular decompression. Death after right ventricular decompression depended on the amount of left ventricular myocardium at risk for ischemia (i.e., distal to a coronary artery stenosis or occlusion). Stenosis of a single coronary artery proximal to a fistula does not necessarily preclude successful right ventricular decompression, but attempts at decompression should be avoided if both coronary artery systems have proximal stenosis or occlusion (Giglia et al., 1992).

There has also been increased enthusiasm for percutaneous transcatheter methods for dilatation of the atretic pulmonary valve in patients with PA/IVS, either as initial therapy or after previous palliative procedures. Several techniques have used either laser or radiofrequency energy to perforate the valve, which is then dilated with a balloon. These techniques are experimental and the short- and long-term results are unknown (Hausdorf et al., 1993; Rosenthal et al., 1993a, 1993b).

The initial procedure must be highly individualized for each patient. A pulmonary outflow patch (or valvotomy) with or without a shunt is the procedure of choice for patients with potential to develop a functional right ventricle. Patients with little likelihood of developing a right ventricle are well palliated with a shunt alone and staged toward a single-ventricle repair (a Fontan-type procedure). In some patients with severe myopathy from underlying coronary artery abnormalities, cardiac transplantation may be the best long-term therapy.

## Subsequent Procedures

A range of success in obtaining two-ventricle repairs has been reported (32 to 80%), and may be due in part to the variation in the incidence of the very small right ventricles (Billingsley et al., 1989; Hanley et al., 1993; Pawade et al., 1993). If the initial procedure is successful, growth of the right ventricle, tricuspid valve, and pulmonary artery determines the choice of subsequent procedure. Following valvotomy or transannular patching, growth of the structures of the right side of the heart should be evaluated frequently by echocardiography. If growth appears to be adequate, cardiac catheterization best determines whether two-ventricle repair is suitable (Bass et al., 1983; Hanley et al., 1993). Balloon occlusion of the ASD is performed to assess right ventricular compliance and presence of physiologic obstruction. Right atrial pressures of more than 12 mm Hg during balloon occlusion are unacceptable. Systemic arterial oxygen saturations are also measured. If occlusion of the interatrial communication is tolerated, the systemic-to-pulmonary artery shunt is occluded with a second balloon while systemic arterial oxygen saturations are monitored (these will decline if pulmonary blood flow is inadequate). With the ASD and shunt temporarily occluded, right ventricular dimensions, pressure, and compliance are determined. If the catheterization data reveal anatomic and physiologic parameters acceptable for two-ventricle repair, the patient may undergo takedown of the shunt and closure of the ASD. If the catheterization reveals unfavorable parameters, a decision must be made either to wait for further growth or to perform a single-ventricle repair. In some centers, the ASD and the shunt can be occluded with devices in the catheterization laboratory.

## Technical Aspects

### Initial Procedures

**Systemic-to-Pulmonary Artery Shunt.** The most commonly performed shunts are of the Blalock-Taussig type, which supply blood from the subclavian artery to the pulmonary artery and can be performed through either a left or a right thoracotomy. A modified Blalock-Taussig shunt (using an interposition graft of polytetrafluoroethylene [PTFE] between the subclavian artery and the pulmonary artery) can also be performed easily through a median sternotomy (Fig. 39–31). Other options include a central shunt connecting the ascending aorta to the main pulmonary artery with prosthetic material. The ideal shunt should be easy to construct, should not tend to develop excessive pulmonary blood flow, should not cause pulmonary artery distortion, and should be easily closed at subsequent operation. Cardiopulmonary bypass (CPB) is not usually required if a shunt procedure is performed alone, because pulmonary blood flow can be maintained through the ductus arteriosus during construction of the shunt.

**Pulmonary Valvotomy.** Pulmonary valvotomy is generally performed through a median sternotomy, using CPB or inflow occlusion (Fig. 39–32). However, valvotomy can also be performed via a left thoracotomy without CPB (Pawade et al., 1993) (Fig. 39–33). After the pulmonary artery is opened, the pulmonary valve is inspected for size and suitability for valvotomy. If the size is adequate, the commissures are incised to the annulus with a scalpel. Some surgeons prefer to excise the valve leaflets. The pulmonary artery is then closed primarily, or a shunt is placed to the pulmonary artery incision. If the valve is not acceptable for valvotomy, or if the infundibular muscle is narrow and restrictive to right ventricular outflow, a transannular patch may be necessary.

**Right Ventricular (Transannular) Outflow Patch.** If the right ventricular outflow tract (RVOT) is small, the pulmonary annulus is inadequate, or the main pulmonary artery is small, a transannular patch may be required to allow maximal flow through the right ventricle. This should be performed through a median sternotomy on CPB. Although placement of transannular patches without CPB has been described (Chia-

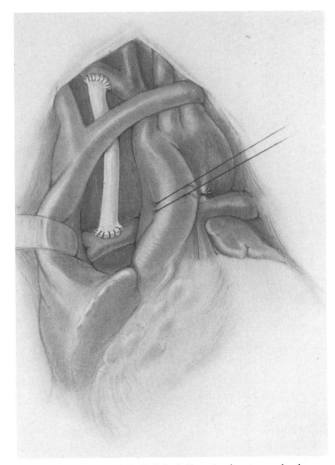

**FIGURE 39–31.** A modified Blalock-Taussig shunt can also be performed through a median sternotomy approach. An interposition graft of Gore-Tex can be easily anastomosed from the right innominate or subclavian artery, brought behind the innominate vein, to an end-to-side connection with the right pulmonary artery. This can be performed with or without cardiopulmonary bypass. A shunt placed in this manner is easily accessible for takedown at future sternotomy.

varelli et al., 1987), it is not recommended. CPB is initiated with an arterial inflow cannula in the ascending aorta and a single venous return cannula in the right atrium. The ductus arteriosus should be occluded with a snare after CPB is begun to prevent pulmonary overcirculation and systemic hypoperfusion during the procedure. The heart can be electrically fibrillated or arrested with aortic cross-clamping and infusion of cardioplegia. The RVOT is then opened and the incision extended through the pulmonary annulus onto the main pulmonary artery to the bifurcation or to a point where the pulmonary artery is normal in diameter. The incision should be extended into the right ventricular cavity proximal to any obstruction (Fig. 39–34). A pericardial patch is used as a roof to enlarge the transannular incision (Fig. 39–35). A systemic-to-pulmonary artery shunt is often required to maintain adequate pulmonary blood flow even if substantial enlargement of the RVOT is accomplished (Fig. 39–36). It is needed because anatomic enlargement of the RVOT does not improve

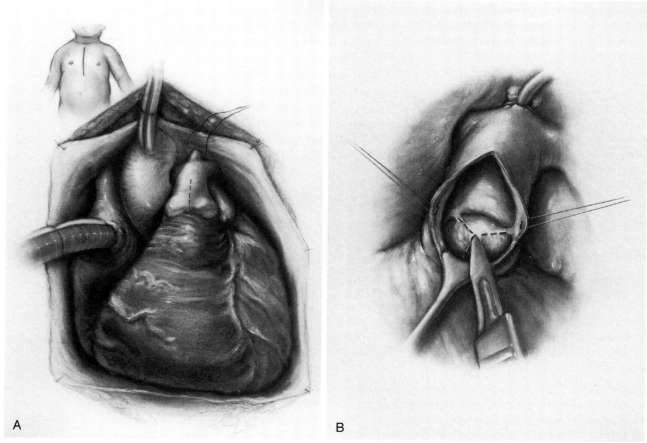

**FIGURE 39–32.** *A,* A patient with PA/IVS. The RV is hypoplastic but the pulmonary artery anatomy is relatively normal. The ductus arteriosus is usually large and must be encircled with a snare so that it can be controlled once cardiopulmonary bypass is begun. *B,* The patient is placed on cardiopulmonary bypass using a single venous cannula and the ductus arteriosus is controlled. An incision is made in the main pulmonary artery and the pulmonary valve is inspected. If the valve is suitable for valvotomy, its leaflets are carefully incised along the lines of commissural fusion. The subvalvar area is inspected through the valve to ensure that it is not potentially obstructive to flow. If there is concern about the subvalvar area, the incision is extended across the top of the pulmonary valve annulus so that a transannular patch can be placed.

the compliance of this abnormal muscle, and poor right ventricular diastolic filling, as well as the pulmonary insufficiency created by the outflow patch, produces inadequate net antegrade flow into the pulmonary arteries. Systemic venous return, in part, crosses the atrial septum and is ejected by the left ventricle. This creates systemic desaturation, which can be reduced by placement of a systemic-to-pulmonary artery shunt.

Some patients with PA/IVS have a large ASD in addition to their other anatomic findings. The need for atrial-level shunting is determined by relative compliance of the ventricles, and the poor right ventricular compliance that accompanies PA/IVS creates a right-to-left shunt across the atrial septum in the initial postoperative period. Closure of the ASD may result in extremely high central venous pressures (reflecting high right ventricular end-diastolic pressure) with fluid retention and edema. Furthermore, if the patient has inadequate antegrade right ventricular outflow that decreases preload of the left ventricle (secondary to failure of systemic venous return to cross the pulmonary vascular bed to the left ventri-

cle), cardiac output may be significantly reduced. Shunting across the ASD maintains system perfusion at the cost of some systemic desaturation. Patients with large ASDs can have the defect size "reduced," but some atrial communication following initial surgery is beneficial, and the ASD should not be completely closed in the infant, despite a favorable appearance after RVOT patching.

## Definitive Procedures

**Conversion to Two-Ventricle Anatomy.** If the patient develops suitability for a two-ventricle repair, closure of the ASD and shunt is straightforward using CPB. The ASD is closed easily through the right atrium. The shunt can be divided and oversewn, or securely ligated with metal clips. Occasionally, pulmonary valve replacement is necessary if right ventricular dysfunction develops secondary to long-term pulmonary valve insufficiency. Pawade and co-workers (1993) reported enlargement of the right ventricular cavity size by excising hypertrophic muscle from

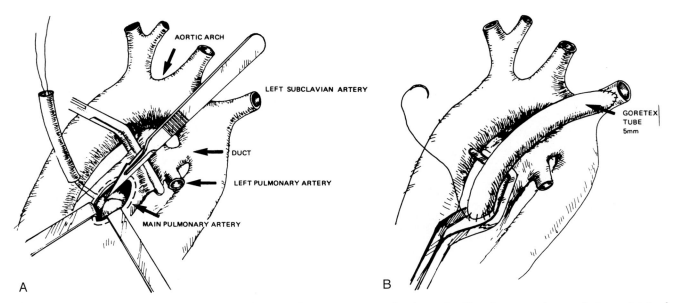

**FIGURE 39–33.** *A,* Via a left thoracotomy, the distal main pulmonary artery can be clamped with pulmonary artery perfusion maintained by a patent ductus arteriosus. Purse-string suture control of the main pulmonary artery enables exposure of the atretic pulmonary valve. In this illustration, the pulmonary valve is depicted as having "imperforate" but well-defined commissures. A valve with this type of anatomy is well-suited for valvotomy by incision of the commissures. The purse-string suture is then tightened to control blood loss. *B,* When a shunt is necessary, the pulmonary artery is controlled with a partial occlusion clamp and an interposition graft of polytetrafluoro-ethylene (PTFE) is placed in a standard manner between the left subclavian artery and the pulmonary arteriotomy that was created for performance of the valvotomy. During placement of this shunt, pulmonary artery blood supply is provided through the patent ductus arteriosus. *(A* and *B,* From Pawade, A., Capuni, A., Penny, D. J., et al.: Pulmonary atresia with intact ventricular septum: Surgical management based on right ventricular infundibulum. J. Card. Surg., *8:*371, 1993.)

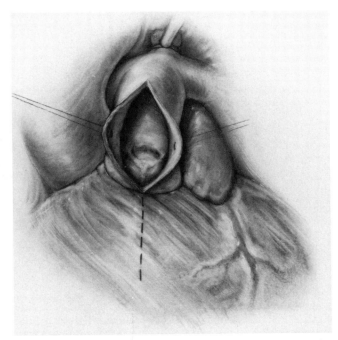

**FIGURE 39–34.** When it is clear that the pulmonary valve annulus is attenuated or if the right ventricular infundibulum is hypoplastic, an incision should be carried proximally from the main pulmonary artery across the pulmonary valve annulus and far enough into the right ventricular chamber to produce an unobstructive opening between the right ventricle and the pulmonary artery.

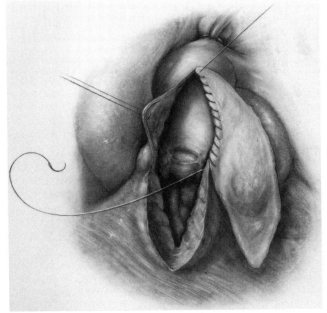

**FIGURE 39–35.** The transannular incision is repaired with a patch of pericardium placed with continuous suture material. Because the right ventricular outflow tract can be very narrow in these patients, care must be exercised to avoid injury to the coronary arteries, which can be extremely close to this suture line. If these patients have clearly recognizable RV–coronary artery communications, these should be obliterated. During the placement of the transannular patch, it is safest to have the heart mechanically arrested or electrically fibrillated.

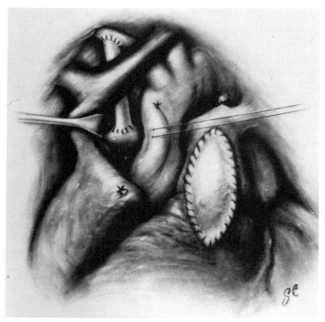

FIGURE 39–36. Following placement of the transannular patch, a Gore-Tex shunt can be placed between the right innominate artery and the right pulmonary artery. This is easily performed on bypass during a period of warming. The patient can then be weaned from bypass and should have excellent oxygen saturation ensured by the systemic-to-pulmonary artery shunt. The ductus arteriosus can be ligated to limit pulmonary artery blood supply, or it can be allowed to close spontaneously by removal of prostaglandins.

the trabecular and infundibular regions of the right ventricle. In some cases where the transannular patch has caused significant pulmonary insufficiency, placement of a pulmonary valve (usually homograft) at the time of this procedure is advised.

**Conversion to Fontan Physiology.** A right side of the heart deemed unsuitable for two-ventricle repair may require single-ventricle repair, which may range from creation of a bidirectional superior vena cava (SVC)-to-pulmonary artery anastomosis (bidirectional Glenn shunt) with concurrent takedown of any previously placed systemic-to-pulmonary artery shunt to performance of a complete Fontan procedure with all the systemic venous return directed into the pulmonary circulation. The decision is made based on the patient's age, anatomy, and physiology.

Patients with marginal right side of the heart anatomy who do not tolerate balloon occlusion of their ASD and shunt may be candidates for a "one and one-half ventricle repair." The goal in these patients is to reduce the volume of blood that must be handled by the right-sided structures, but to retain the right ventricle in some form to assist in the circulation to the pulmonary bed. This is accomplished by dismantling the patient's systemic-to-pulmonary artery shunt and creating a bidirectional SVC-to-pulmonary artery anastomosis (Fig. 39–37). This should be done on cardiopulmonary bypass, and the SVC-to-pulmonary artery anastomosis should be constructed carefully to ensure that it is large and unobstructed. The azygos vein should be ligated as part of this procedure. At

the conclusion of this, the right atrium is opened and the ASD is closed. SVC blood flow returns directly to the pulmonary vascular bed and the right ventricle is responsible only for inferior vena cava (IVC) venous return.

In some patients, there is uncertainty as to whether the right ventricle will be able to contribute in any meaningful way to the circulation. For these patients, a bidirectional SVC-to-pulmonary artery anastomosis without ASD closure is recommended. In this way, the inferior vena cava return can still shunt right to left across the ASD, but pulmonary blood flow is provided by the SVC return instead of a systemic shunt, removing a substantial volume load from the left ventricle (which no longer has to pump the pulmonary circulation in parallel with the systemic circulation). In essence, this procedure creates "partial" Fontan physiology and enables the patient to adjust to this change in the circulation. Many surgeons use this procedure as a first stage toward a complete Fontan procedure, especially in patients with risk factors that increase the risk of Fontan physiology (Bridges et al., 1990a). Patients with substantial pulmonary insufficiency secondary to a previous transannular patch may be ineffectively palliated from a bidirectional SVC-to-pulmonary artery shunt, and a decision must be made regarding potential for the right ventricle. One option is to place a (homograft) valve in the RVOT at the time of bidirectional caval pulmonary shunt, which would allow conversion to a one and one-half ventricle repair by occluding the ASD with a device in the catherization lab. Following creation of a successful bidirectional SVC-to-pulmonary artery anastomosis, patients should be expected to have oxygen saturations in the high 70% to low 80% range and a reduction in their heart size.

In some patients, the structures of the right side of the heart remain unusable and conversion to complete Fontan physiology is necessary. The procedure is performed through a median sternotomy on CPB. The SVC is disconnected from the right atrium and anastomosed to the superior aspect of the right pulmonary artery in an end-to-side manner. The main pulmonary artery is divided and the cardiac end is oversewn. The proximal end of the right atrium, or the right atrial appendage, is connected to the inferior aspect of the right pulmonary artery or to the severed end of the distal main pulmonary artery. The most frequently used modification is the "lateral tunnel" connection between the IVC and the pulmonary artery (*total caval pulmonary connection* [TCPC]) (de Leval et al., 1988). The SVC is divided and a bidirectional Glenn shunt constructed. The IVC return is channeled through an interatrial baffle that leads along the lateral aspect of the right atrium to the proximal SVC, which is subsequently connected to the inferior aspect of the right pulmonary artery. A small fenestration in the lateral tunnel may be created (Fig. 39–38) which will allow a right-to-left shunt at the atrial level to maintain cardiac output at the expense of oxygenation in the presence of any condition

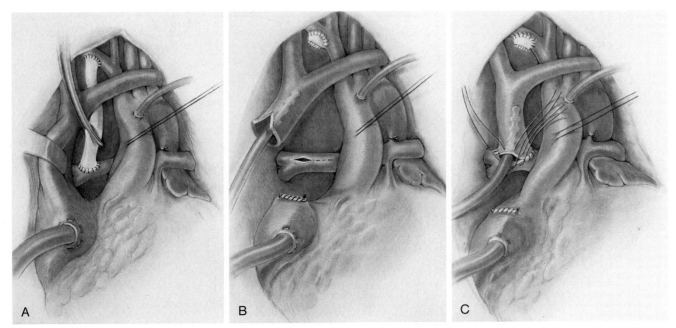

**FIGURE 39–37.** Creation of an SVC-pulmonary anastomosis is performed by reopening the previous sternotomy incision and placing the patient on cardiopulmonary bypass using a single atrial cannula. *A,* The previously placed systemic-to-pulmonary artery shunt is clamped and removed. *B,* Incision in the right pulmonary artery is made through the old shunt site, and the SVC is divided with its proximal (cardiac) end oversewn. The cephalad portion of the SVC is then ready for end-to-side anastomosis with the right pulmonary artery. The azygos vein should be identified and ligated. A separate venous cannula can be placed in the SVC, or alternatively, venous return from the SVC can be controlled with a cardiotomy sucker as shown. *C,* The SVC-pulmonary anastomosis is performed with a continuous posterior suture line but with interrupted sutures for the anterior suture line to prevent "purse-stringing" of this important anastomosis.

that transiently retards pulmonary blood flow during the early postoperative period (Bridges et al., 1990b).

The small right ventricle can be excluded from the circulation by oversewing the tricuspid valve (Williams et al., 1991). This technique is particularly attractive for patients with small right ventricles who have non–right ventricle–dependent fistulous connections to the coronary circulation; it reduces the risk of producing a steal of coronary blood supply. If coronary fistulas are present and there is no myocardial dependence, they can also be ligated at the time of definitive repair (Fyfe et al., 1986). Alternatively, in patients without coronary connections to the right ventricle, the tricuspid valve can be "avulsed" to decompress the right ventricle into the pulmonary circulation. In this manner, all systemic venous return bypasses the right ventricle and flows directly into the pulmonary arteries.

Right ventricular coronary dependence usually occurs in patients with small right ventricles who are generally staged toward a single-ventricle repair. Fully saturated blood must be allowed to enter the right ventricle across the tricuspid valve to deliver sufficient oxygen to the myocardium at risk. Thromboexclusion or right ventricular decompression techniques are not appropriate and may cause myocardial ischemia. Cardiac transplantation may be the best option in these patients (Kirklin and Barratt-Boyes, 1993). When Ebstein's anomaly occurs in combination with PA/IVS, most patients are staged toward a single-ventricle repair. These patients are difficult to

manage and the 1-year mortality rate is 85% (Hanley et al., 1993).

## POSTOPERATIVE CRITICAL CARE

### Management Following Initial Procedure

All patients can be expected to exhibit some degree of cyanosis after operation because of right-to-left shunting across the ASD secondary to poor right ventricular compliance. However, all patients should have a reliable source of pulmonary blood supply that will produce systemic arterial oxygen saturations at least into the high 70% or low 80% range. As is true of any right-to-left shunt, the hypoxemia will not respond to oxygen therapy, and inspired oxygen levels should be reduced as quickly as feasible to limit the risk of oxygen-induced pulmonary injury. Except for those patients who are being maintained on prostaglandins to maintain patency of the ductus arteriosus, $PGE_1$ should be discontinued. The increase in pulmonary blood flow created by a systemic-to-pulmonary artery shunt, in conjunction with the concomitant volume load to the left ventricle, may require inotropic support and diuretic therapy. The need for inotropes, however, should not be great, and escalating need for inotropes warrants further investigation. A fall in systemic oxygen saturation should initiate concern regarding patency or adequacy of the shunt. Although shunt thrombosis is uncommon, it does

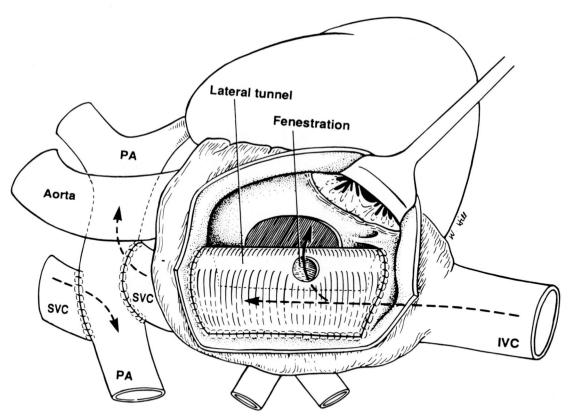

**FIGURE 39–38.** A lateral tunnel modification of the Fontan procedure baffles systemic venous return from the IVC below a patch of prosthetic material (usually Gore-Tex) to the orifice of the SVC, which is then connected to the pulmonary artery (PA). In this illustration, a small fenestration has been left in the prosthetic portion of the lateral tunnel. (From Kopf, G. S., Kleinman, C. S., Hijazi, Z. M., et al.: Fenestrated Fontan operation with delayed transcatheter closure of atrial septal defect: Improved results in high-risk patients. J. Thorac. Cardiovasc. Surg., *103*:1039, 1992.)

occur, and in patients who truly depend on the shunts for pulmonary blood flow, infusion of heparin may be indicated. Changes in the electrocardiogram (suggestive of myocardial ischemia), especially in patients with a requirement for increasing inotropic support, should raise concern about the coronary artery anatomy and supply to the distal myocardial beds. Patients should be able to be rapidly weaned from mechanical ventilation. Following extubation, they may require chronic diuretics and digoxin. As antegrade flow across a surgically created RVOT improves, the systemic oxygen saturation may increase and the patient may gradually begin to exhibit signs of volume overload and congestive heart failure. This usually indicates that the right ventricle is functioning well and the patient is ready for a definitive procedure with takedown of the systemic-to-pulmonary artery shunt.

## Management Following Definitive Procedure

Patients who are able to adapt to a two-ventricle repair can be cared for in a manner similar to that for any postoperative cardiac patient and should exhibit normal circulatory physiology. In some patients, a small ASD may be retained to enable some degree of right-to-left shunt to decompress the right ventricle until its compliance has fully recovered. These patients exhibit mild systemic oxygen desaturation (90 to 95%) and may have slightly increased (12 to 15 mm Hg) central venous pressures.

Patients who receive a bidirectional SVC-to-pulmonary artery anastomosis require postoperative management similar to that given to patients with Fontan physiology. Patients who receive a complete Fontan procedure will likely have a more protracted convalescence in the intensive care unit. All of their systemic venous return must cross the pulmonary vascular bed before it can enter the left ventricle and be available for systemic cardiac output. This has the advantage that these patients eject normally saturated (93 to 98%) blood into their systemic circulation but the disadvantage that this blood is only available to the left ventricle if it can traverse the pulmonary vascular bed. Any factor that reduces pulmonary flow (e.g., transient elevation of the pulmonary vascular resistance following CPB) will affect low cardiac output.

## RISK FACTORS AND OUTCOME

Risk factors that have been identified in PA/IVS include small birth weight, right ventricular dependent coronary flow, and small tricuspid valve (Hanley et al., 1993). The overall 30-day mortality rate is 20%; however, the Hazard function does not plateau until 3 to 6 months, with 72% alive at 6 months (Hanley et al., 1993). Mortality is most often secondary to acute heart failure or hypoxia (Kirklin and Barratt-Boyes, 1993).

Mortality and outcome are related to underlying anatomy and to the type of repair that the patient ultimately receives (Fig. 39–39). The most favorable anatomic subtypes, with adequate tricuspid valves and right ventricles, respond nicely to outflow procedures (valvotomy or transannular patch) and a concomitant shunt. Patients who have unfavorable anatomy for eventual two-ventricle repair and who undergo palliation with a shunt alone have a higher mortality. Patients with favorable anatomy who tolerate two-ventricle repair can live a relatively normal, high-quality life. Patients with unfavorable anatomy have shortened life expectancy with a quality of life that is affected by their suitability for Fontan physiology. The spectrum of variability in PA/IVS mandates that each patient be treated individually with careful consideration of the options available to optimize their survival.

## PULMONARY STENOSIS WITH INTACT VENTRICULAR SEPTUM

*Pulmonary stenosis with intact ventricular septum* (PS/IVS) may present in infancy or in later childhood, depending on the severity of the stenosis. Infants with critical pulmonary stenosis demonstrate cyanosis and ductal-dependent pulmonary blood flow. Valvar pulmonary stenosis usually consists of a dome-shaped pulmonary valve and a small central orifice. Two or three ridges may outline the leaflets (Kirklin and Barratt-Boyes, 1993). The valve may be severely dysplastic. The right ventricle is usually normal in size, although secondary infundibular hypertrophy may occur. Associated anomalies are rare, although PS/IVS may occur in patients with Noonan's syndrome.

### Diagnosis

PS/IVS is usually very amenable to treatment. However, it can be a highly lethal lesion with a dismal prognosis. The outcome depends on the size of the right ventricular chamber as well as the age of the patient at presentation. Infants with critical pulmonary stenosis require valvotomy as an emergency procedure, but in most children, the symptoms develop slowly. The foramen ovale is usually patent, and when increased pressure and decreased compliance develop in the right ventricle, blood is shunted right to left causing cyanosis. Poststenotic dilatation of the main pulmonary artery often develops, and in many cases, infundibular stenosis may also be present. The clinical findings depend mainly on the severity of the valve or pulmonary stenosis and the patency of the foramen ovale. In older children, dypsnea on exertion is the most common complaint, and cyanosis is present if there is a patent foramen ovale or an ASD. Physical examination reveals a harsh systolic murmur and thrill over the pulmonic area. The second pulmonary sound is usually weak or absent. The chest film usually shows prominence of the main pulmonary artery due to postcyanotic dilatation. The diagnosis can be made easily by echocardiogram; cardiac catheterization is performed more often for balloon dilatation of the valve (treatment) than for diagnosis. When it is performed, cardiac catherization reveals a pres-

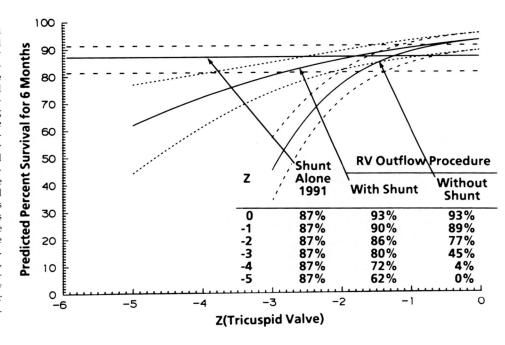

**FIGURE 39–39.** This nomogram summarizes the 6-month survival for neonates with PA/IVS by demonstrating the effect of tricuspid valve dimension versus type of initial procedure. Tricuspid valve size is represented as Z *values*, with 1 Z value representing a standard deviation from the mean (SD). Patients with tricuspid valves within 2 SD below normal had acceptable survival regardless of the initial procedure. As the tricuspid valve size becomes smaller, better survival is achieved with those procedures that include a shunt. Patients with extremely small (Z value less than −4) tricuspid valves are best treated with shunt alone. (From Hanley, F. L., Sade, R. M., Blackstone, E. H., et al.: Outcomes in neonatal pulmonary atresia with intact ventricular septum. J. Thorac. Cardiovasc. Surg., *105*:406, 1993.)

| Z | Shunt Alone 1991 | RV Outflow Procedure With Shunt | RV Outflow Procedure Without Shunt |
|---|---|---|---|
| 0 | 87% | 93% | 93% |
| -1 | 87% | 90% | 89% |
| -2 | 87% | 86% | 77% |
| -3 | 87% | 80% | 45% |
| -4 | 87% | 72% | 4% |
| -5 | 87% | 62% | 0% |

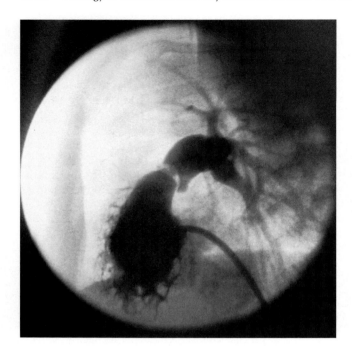

**FIGURE 39–40.** Lateral view of RV angiogram in a patient with pulmonary stenosis. The narrowed and "doming" pulmonary valve can be appreciated as well as the poststenotic dilatation of the otherwise normal main pulmonary artery. The RV is essentially normal in size.

sure gradient between right ventricle and pulmonary artery without evidence of a shunt at the ventricular level. The angiocardiogram usually shows a classic dome-shaped pulmonary valve with a small opening and poststenotic dilatation (Fig. 39–40). In severe cases, a pressure gradient of greater than 200 mm Hg may be present between the right ventricle and the pulmonary artery.

## Treatment

Intervention is indicated when patients are symptomatic or there is a significant pressure gradient between the right ventricle and the pulmonary artery. Valvotomy (either open or by transcatheter techniques) is the standard treatment. Transventricular pulmonary valvotomy, introduced by Brock (1948), used a valvulotome passed through the wall of the

right ventricle into the pulmonary artery to open the stenotic valve. After CPB was introduced, open valvotomy under direct vision using CPB became the standard surgical repair (Fig. 39–41). However, some groups still recommend valvotomy under inflow occlusion (de Leval, 1994). CPB stabilizes critically ill neonates and affords the time necessary for careful valvotomy (Polansky et al., 1984).

In most patients, including critically ill infants, percutaneous balloon valvuloplasty has become the initial therapy of choice, and surgical repair is reserved for children in whom balloon valvuloplasty fails (Kvelselis et al., 1985; Lababidi and Wu, 1983; Lock et al., 1987). Valvotomy for pulmonary stenosis (either open or balloon) yields excellent results and recurrence is rare. The compensatory infundibular hypertrophy that frequently accompanies valvular stenosis usually regresses over time. Although the gradient between the right ventricle and the pulmonary artery

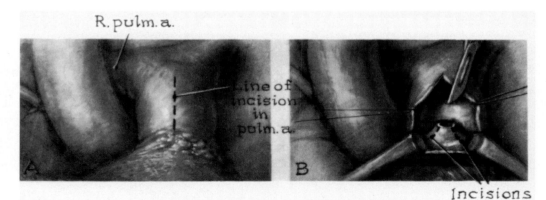

**FIGURE 39–41.** *A, Dashed line* demonstrates line of incision in main pulmonary artery required to perform valvotomy in a patient with pulmonary stenosis. The patient should be maintained on cardiopulmonary bypass for this procedure. *B,* When the main pulmonary artery is opened, the stenotic pulmonary valve can be viewed and incised along its natural commissures to open the outflow area.

may not be totally abolished immediately after operation, regression of the secondary hypertrophy occurs and later catherization shows a sharp reduction in the gradient (Engle et al., 1958). The long-term outcome is excellent for patients with PS/IVS who undergo either balloon valvuloplasty or surgical valvotomy.

## SELECTED BIBLIOGRAPHY

de Leval, M. R., Kilner, P., Gewilling, M., et al.: Total cavopulmonary connection: A logical alternative to atriopulmonary connection for complex Fontan operations. J. Thorac. Cardiovasc. Surg., 96:682, 1988.

This modification of the Fontan operation has become a standard connection for most patients who receive this procedure. For patients with pulmonary atresia with intact ventricular septem (PA/IVS), total cavopulmonary connection (TCPC) provides excellent flow characteristics and an ability to fenestrate the intra-atrial baffle.

Foker, J. E., Braunlin, E. A., St. Cyr, J. A., et al.: Management of pulmonary atresia with intact ventricular septum. J. Thorac. Cardiovasc. Surg., 92:706, 1986.

The authors review a management protocol for neonates with PA/IVS that includes right ventricular outflow tract (RVOT) patching and continuation of prostaglandin $E_1$ (PGE$_1$) infusion postoperatively (to maintain ductal patency) until the need for a shunt can be determined. They suggest that, in many cases, the PGE$_1$ can be stopped in the postoperative period (allowing the ductus to close) and these patients will not have a need for placement of a more permanent systemic-to-pulmonary artery shunt to maintain pulmonary blood flow. Patients who do not tolerate cessation of the prostaglandin infusion can be returned to the operating room for a shunt at a later time. Of concern is the fact that 3 deaths (in 15 patients) are reported to be due to premature cessation of the prostaglandin infusion. This raises an issue regarding the safety of this strategy, especially in patients who have small right ventricles who may depend on a shunt for pulmonary blood flow for several weeks or months following RVOT patching.

Hanley, F. L., Sade, R. M., Blackstone, E. H., et al.: Outcomes in neonatal pulmonary atresia with intact ventricular septum. J. Thorac. Cardiovasc. Surg., 105:406, 1993.

This outstanding article reviews Congenital Heart Surgeons' Society (CHSS) prospective multi-institutional study consisting of 171 neonates with PA/IVS. Multivariate analysis showed small diameter of the tricuspid valve, severe right ventricular coronary dependency, birth weight, and the date and type of initial procedure to be risk factors for time-related death. Eighteen per cent of living patients had received a one-ventricle repair within 3 years, and 32% had received a two-ventricle repair; the remainder (50%) had incompletely separated pulmonary and systemic circulations. The only patient-specific risk factor for not receiving a two-ventricle repair was the Z-value of the tricuspid valve.

Kirklin, J. W., and Barratt-Boyes, B. G. (eds): Cardiac Surgery. 2nd ed. New York, Churchill Livingstone, 1993.

This textbook provides a comprehensive and well-organized review of this defect from all aspects. It is strongly recommended to those readers who wish to study in depth the surgical aspects of this disease. The chapters on pulmonary stenosis and intact ventricular septum and on PA/IVS provide extraordinary overviews of pertinent anatomy, clinical manifestations, and surgical options. Outcome data are cogently presented with ample tables and graphs.

Lababidi, Z., and Wu, J. R.: Percutaneous balloon pulmonary valvuloplasty. Am. J. Cardiol., 52:560, 1983.

This article heralded the interventional catheterization approach to valvular stenosis. The ability for cardiologists to safely open stenotic pulmonary valves with angioplasty balloons has virtually eliminated pulmonary valvotomy as a surgical procedure for patients with pulmonary stenosis.

## BIBLIOGRAPHY

Anderson, R. H., Anderson, C., and Zuberbuhler, J. R.: Further morphologic studies on hearts with pulmonary atresia and intact ventricular septum. Cardiol. Young., 1:105, 1991.

Bass, J. L., Fuhrman, B. P., and Lock, J. E.: Balloon occlusion of atrial septal defect to assess right ventricular capacity in hypoplastic right heart syndrome. Circulation, 68:1081, 1983.

Becker, A. E., Becker, M. J., and Edwards, J. E.: Pathologic spectrum of dysplasia of the tricuspid valve. Arch. Pathol., 91:167, 1971.

Bharati, S., McAllister, H. A., and Chiemmongkoltip, P.: Congenital pulmonary atresia with tricuspid insufficiency: Morphologic study. Am. J. Cardiol., 40:70, 1977.

Billingsley, A. M., Laks, H., Boyce S. W., et al.: Definitive repair in patients with pulmonary atresia and intact ventricular septum. J. Thorac. Cardiocasc. Surg., 97:746, 1989.

Bridges, N. D., Jonas, R. A., and Mayer, J. E. J., et al.: Bidirectional cavopulmonary anastomosis as interim palliation for high-risk Fontan candidates. Circulation, 82(Pt. 2):170, 1990a.

Bridges, N. D., Lock, J. E., and Castaneda, A. R.: Baffle fenestration with subsequent transcatheter closure: Modification of the Fontan operation for patients at increased risk. Circulation, 82:1681, 1990b.

Brock, R. C.: Pulmonary valvulotomy for the relief of congenital pulmonary stenosis: Report of 3 cases. Br. Med. J., 1:1121, 1948.

Bull, C., de Leval, M. R., Mercanti, C., et al.: Pulmonary atresia and intact ventricular septum. Circulation, 66:266, 1982.

Calder, A. L., Co, E. E., and Sage, M. D.: Coronary arterial abnormalities in pulmonary atresia with intact ventricular septum. Am. J. Cardiol., 59:436, 1987.

Chiavarelli, M., Puga, F. J., and Julsrud, P. R.: Right ventricular outflow construction without cardiopulmonary bypass. Circulation, 76(3 Pt. 2):III-34, 1987.

Coles, J. G., Freedom, R. M., Lightfoot, N. E., et al.: Long-term results in neonates with pulmonary atresia and intact ventricular septum. Ann. Thorac. Surg., 47:213, 1989.

Coté, M., Davignon, A., and Fouron, J. C.: Congenital hypoplasia of right ventricular myocardium (Uhl's anomaly) associated with pulmonary atresia in the newborn. Am. J. Cardiol., 31:658, 1973.

Davignon, A. L., Greenwold, W. E., DuShane, J. W., et al.: Congenital pulmonary atresia with intact ventricular septum: Clinicopathologic correlation of two anatomic types. Am. Heart J., 52:591, 1961.

de Leval, M.: Pulmonary stenosis and pulmonary atresia with intact ventricular septum. In Stark, J., and de Leval, M. (eds): Surgery for Congenital Heart Defects. 2nd ed. Philadelphia, W. B. Saunders, 1994, pp. 389–404.

de Leval, M. R., Bull, C., Hopkins, R., et al.: Decision making in the definitive repair of the heart with a small right ventricle. Circulation, 72(Suppl. II):52, 1985.

de Leval, M. R., Bull, C., Stark, J., et al.: Pulmonary atresia and intact ventricular septum: Surgical management based on a revised classification. Circulation, 66:272, 1982.

de Leval, M. R., Kilner, P., Gewilling, M., et al.: Total cavopulmonary connection: A logical alternative to atriopulmonary connection for complex Fontan operations. J. Thorac. Cardiovasc. Surg., 96:682, 1988.

Engle, M. A., Holswade, G. R., Goldberg, H. P., et al.: Regression after open valvotomy of infundibular stenosis accompanying severe valvular pulmonic stenosis. Circulation, 17:862, 1958.

Foker, J. E., Braunlin, E. A., St. Cyr, J. A., et al.: Management of pulmonary atresia with intact ventricular septum. J. Thorac. Cardiovasc. Surg., 92:706, 1986.

Freedom, R. M., and Harrington, D. P.: Contributions of intramyocardial sinusoids in pulmonary atresia and intact ventricular septum. Br. Heart J., 33:892, 1974.

Fyfe, D. A., Edwards, W. D., and Driscoll, D. J.: Myocardial ischemia in patients with pulmonary atresia and intact ventricular septum. J. Am. Coll. Cardiol., 8:402, 1986.

Giglia, T. M., Mandell, V. S., Connor, A. R., et al.: Diagnosis and management of right ventricle–dependent coronary circulation in pulmonary atresia with intact ventricular septum. Circulation, 86:1516, 1992.

Gittenberger-de Groot, A. C., Sauer, U., Bindl, L., et al.: Competition of coronary arteries and ventriculo-coronary arterial communications in pulmonary atresia with intact ventricular septum. Int. J. Surg., 18:243, 1988.

Hanley, F. L., Sade, R. M., Blackstone, E. H., et al.: Outcomes in neonatal pulmonary atresia with intact ventricular septum. J. Thorac. Cardiovasc. Surg., 105:406, 1993.

Hausdorf, G., Schulze-Neick, I., and Lange, P. E.: Radiofrequency-assisted "reconstruction" of the right ventricular outflow tract in muscular pulmonary atresia with ventricular septal defect. Br. Heart J., *69*:343, 1993.

Hunter, W.: Three cases of malconformation in the heart. Med. Obs. Inquiries, *6*:291, 1783.

Kirklin, J. W., and Barratt-Boyes, B. G.: Cardiac Surgery. 2nd ed. New York, Churchill Livingstone, 1993.

Kutsche, L. M., and Van Mierop, L. H. S.: Pulmonary atresia with and without ventricular septal defect: A different etiology and pathogenesis for the atresia in the two types? Am. J. Cardiol., *51*:932, 1983.

Kvelselis, D. A., Rocchini, A. P., Snider, A. R., et al.: Results of balloon valvuloplasty in the treatment of congenital valvar pulmonary stenosis in children. Am. J. Cardiol., *56*:527, 1985.

Lababidi, Z., and Wu, J. R.: Percutaneous balloon pulmonary valvuloplasty. Am. J. Cardiol., *52*:560, 1983.

Lock, J. E., Keane, J. F., and Fellows, K. E.: Diagnostic and Interventional Catheterization in Congenital Heart Disease. Boston, Martinus Nijhoff, 1987.

Meliones, J. N., Ungerleider, R. M., Kern, F. H., et al.: Perioperative management of patients with congenital heart disease: An approach based on physiology. *In* Moylan, J. (ed): Surgical Critical Care. Philadelphia, J. B. Lippincott, 1994.

Oka, M., and Angrist, A.: Mechanism of cardiac valvular fusion and stenosis. Am. Heart J., *74*:37, 1967.

Patel, R. G., Freedom, R. M., Moes, C. A. F, et al.: Right ventricular volume determinations in 18 patients with pulmonary atresia and intact ventricular septum. Circulation, *61*:428, 1980.

Paul, M. H., and Lev, M.: Tricuspid stenosis with pulmonary atresia. Circulation, *12*:198, 1960.

Pawade, A., Capuni, A., Penny, D. J., et al.: Pulmonary atresia with intact ventricular septum: Surgical management based on right ventricular infundibulum. J. Card. Surg., *8*:371, 1993.

Peacock, T. B.: Malformation of the heart: Atresia of the orifice of the pulmonary artery. Trans. Pathol. Soc. Lond., *20*:61, 1869.

Perloff, J.: Pulmonary Atresia with Intact Ventricular Septum. Philadelphia, W. B. Saunders, 1987.

Polansky, D. B., Clark, E. B., and Doty, D. B.: Pulmonary stenosis in infants and young children. Ann. Thorac. Surg., *39*:159, 1984.

Rhagib, G., Bloemendall, R. D., Kanjuh, V. I., et al.: Aortic atresia and premature closure of foramen ovale. Am. Heart J., *70*:476, 1965.

Rosenthal, E., Qureshi, S. A., Chan, K. C., et al.: Radiofrequency-assisted balloon dilatation in patients with pulmonary valve atresia and an intact ventricular septum. Br. Heart J., *69*:347, 1993a.

Rosenthal, E., Qureshi, S. A., Kakadekar, A. P., et al.: Technique of percutaneous laser-assisted valve dilatation for valvar atresia in congenital heart disease. Br. Heart J., *69*:556, 1993b.

Santos, M. A., Moll, J. N., Drumond, C., et al.: Development of the ductus arteriosus in right ventricular outflow obstructions. Circulation, *62*:818, 1980.

Schmidt, K. G., Cloez, J. L., and Silverman, N. H.: Changes of right ventricular size and function in neonates after valvotomy for pulmonary atresia or critical pulmonary stenosis and intact ventricular septum. J. Am. Coll. Cardiol., *19*:1032, 1992.

Scognamilgio, R., Daliento, L., Razzolini, R., et al.: Pulmonary atresia with intact ventricular septum: A quantitative cineventriculographic study of the right and left ventricular function. Pediatr. Cardiol., *7*:183, 1986.

Wagner, H.: Cardiac disease in congenital infections. Clin. Perinatol., *8*:481, 1981.

Williams, W. G., Burrows, P., Freedom, F. M., et al.: Thromboexclusion of the right ventricle in children with pulmonary atresia and intact ventricular septum. J. Thorac. Cardiovasc. Surg., *101*:222, 1991.

Zuberbuhler, J. R., and Anderson, R. H.: Morphologic variations in pulmonary atresia with intact ventricular septum. Br. Heart J., *41*:281, 1979.

# 40

# Truncus Arteriosus

Gary K. Lofland

Truncus arteriosus (persistent truncus arteriosus, truncus arteriosus communis, common aorticopulmonary trunk) is a congenital heart malformation that involves the ventriculoarterial connection in which a single outlet is present. It is characterized by the presence of a single semilunar valve annulus as the only exit from the heart, a subarterial ventricular septal defect, and absence or severe deficiency of the aortopulmonary septum. Two related but different malformations are aortopulmonary window and subarterial ventricular septal defect. The truncus provides the orifices of the coronary and pulmonary arteries before continuing as the aorta. This definition thus excludes hearts that have no true pulmonary arteries, in which case the lung is supplied by aortopulmonary collateral vessels (Type IV of Collett and Edwards, 1949).

Truncus arteriosus constitutes less than 3% of all congenital heart defects (de Leval, 1983).

## HISTORICAL ASPECTS

The first well-documented case of truncus arteriosus was reported in 1798 (Wilson, 1798). In 1864, the entity was confirmed in a clinical and autopsy report on a 6-month-old infant (Buchanan, 1864). Taruffi (1875) reported a similar case, and other reports followed (Lev and Saphir, 1943; Shapiro, 1930; Victoria, 1969). In 1949, after reviewing all published cases, Collett and Edwards proposed a classification system (Fig. 40–1). An alternative system was proposed by Van Praagh and Van Praagh (1965).

The first successful correction of truncus arteriosus was done in 1962 but was not reported until 12 years later (Behrendt et al., 1974). The first report of a successful repair was by McGoon and associates (1968), and an additional case was reported by Weldon and Cameron (1968). The first successful conduit repair in an infant was done by Barratt-Boyes in 1971 (Girinath, 1973). With some technical modifications, the technique described by McGoon (1983) for complete correction is used currently.

## ANATOMY AND CLASSIFICATION

The classification system proposed by Collett and Edwards (1949) is based on the arrangement of the origins of the pulmonary arteries from the truncal artery (see Fig. 40–1). The classification system proposed by Van Praagh and Van Praagh (1965) also

includes cases with a single pulmonary artery and various degrees of development of the ascending aorta and ductus arteriosus. In the Collett and Edwards Type I truncus, the pulmonary arteries arise from a common pulmonary trunk that originates from the truncus. In Type II, the right and left pulmonary arteries arise close together from the dorsal wall of the truncus arteriosus. In Type III, the pulmonary arteries arise separately from the lateral aspects of the truncus. In Type IV, the proximal pulmonary arteries are absent and pulmonary blood flow originates from the multiple aorticopulmonary collateral vessels.

In practice, the distinction among Types I, II, and III truncus is imprecise, and the actual existence of Type III truncus with lateral origins of the pulmonary arteries is questioned (McGoon, 1983) (Fig. 40–2). The Type IV classification of Collett and Edwards should be replaced by the more precise designation *pulmonary atresia with ventricular septal defect*. Also, the term *pseudotruncus* should be replaced by a more descriptive designation of a condition characterized by pulmonary atresia and patent ductus arteriosus (McGoon, 1983).

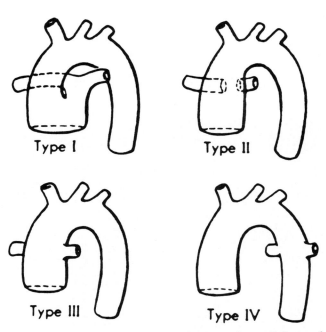

**FIGURE 40–1.** Anatomic types of truncus arteriosus. Collett and Edwards' classification. (From Heart Disease in Infancy and Childhood, by John D. Keith, Richard D. Rowe, and Peter Vlad. Copyright 1958 The Macmillan Company; copyright renewed. Reprinted by permission of Macmillan Publishing Company, a division of Macmillan, Inc.)

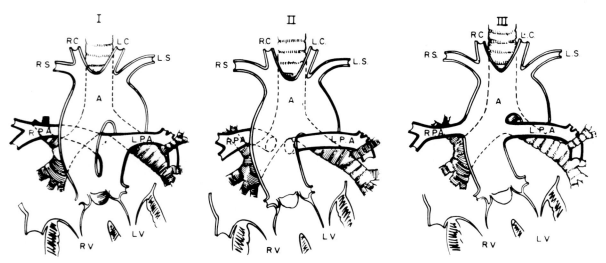

**FIGURE 40-2.** The three most common types of truncus arteriosus. The relationship of the truncal artery to the ventricular septal defect, coronary arteries (RC and LC), pulmonary arteries (RPA and LPA), and aortic arch is shown. The features have been exaggerated for purposes of illustration. The existence of Type III truncus, as shown here and in the Collett and Edwards' classification, is legitimately questioned. (A = aorta; RV = right ventricle; LV = left ventricle; RS = right subclavian artery; LS = left subclavian artery.)

Morphologically, the arterial trunk or truncus is larger than a normal aorta and arises as a solitary vessel from the base of the heart. The truncus originates from both ventricles but usually overrides the septum to lie more over the right than over the left ventricle (Bharati et al., 1974; Crupi et al., 1977; Thiene et al., 1976). Although the ventricular septal defect usually is directly subarterial, in our own series we have seen several patients with a marked degree of override of the ventricular septal defect, such that the truncal artery emerges predominantly from the right ventricle. The coronary and pulmonary arteries arise from this truncus (Fig. 40–3).

In general, the ventricular septal defect associated with truncus arteriosus is in the anterior septum, confluent with the truncus, and the atrioventricular bundle is posterior and unrelated to the rim of the ventricular septal defect. If the ventricular septal defect is related to the membranous septum, the atrioventricular bundle may be close to the ventricular septal defect and susceptible to surgical injury. In truncus, the conduction system varies in its course and is related to the location of the ventricular septal defect and its relationship to the membranous septum. The ventricular septal defect may be close to or related to the membranous septum, and the atrioventricular bundle and the beginning of the bundle branches may be vulnerable to surgical injury (Bharati et al., 1974, 1992).

Although coronary arteries usually arise from orifices in the truncal valve sinuses of Valsalva in a position close to the normal one (left arising posteriorly into the left and right arising anteriorly), variations in coronary anatomy have been reported (An-

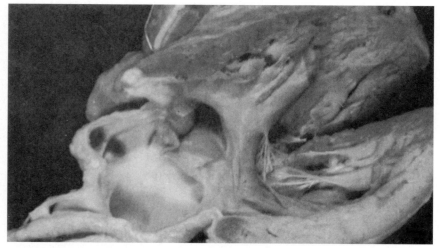

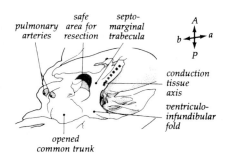

**FIGURE 40-3.** Opened anterior part of the right ventricle in surgical orientation shows the morphology of a subarterial defect with a muscular posterior inferior rim and a common trunk. The origin of both pulmonary arteries is from the left and posterior aspect of the trunk. (From Wilcox, B. R., and Anderson, R. H.: Surgical Anatomy of the Heart. New York, Raven Press, 1985, p. 7.20.)

derson et al., 1978; Bharati et al., 1974; Bove et al., 1993; Crupi et al., 1977; Shrivastava and Edwards, 1977; Van Praagh and Van Praagh, 1965).

The pulmonary arteries usually originate just downstream from the truncal valve, on the left posterolateral aspect of the truncus, although true lateral, true posterior, and true anterior origins have been described (Anderson et al., 1978). There is often a single orifice that soon divides into right and left pulmonary arteries (Type I of Collett and Edwards) (see Fig. 40–3). Less commonly, the pulmonary arteries have separate orifices (Type II of Collett and Edwards). These two types account for 86% of cases in the Barratt-Boyes series (Barratt-Boyes, 1986).

The pulmonary arteries may also be nonconfluent, and one or more branch pulmonary arteries may arise from the ascending aorta, the descending aorta, the innominate artery, or the ductus arteriosus (Fig. 40–4).

The morphology of great arteries varies in both the pulmonary and aortic pathways, and the pattern of the aortic arch has considerable surgical significance. The aortic arch is interrupted (Calder et al., 1976), usually at the level of the isthmus, but sometimes proximal to the origin of the left subclavian artery. In either case, the descending aorta is supplied by the ductus arteriosus. Truncus arteriosus with aortic arch interruption is found in up to one-fifth of autopsy series (Bharati et al., 1974; Calder et al., 1976; Crupi et al., 1977; Van Praagh and Van Praagh, 1965). More recently, Bove and associates found interrupted aortic arch in 5 of 46 patients, and Hanley and associates found interrupted aortic arch in 6 of 63 patients (Bove et al., 1993; Hanley et al., 1993).

The truncal valve is posterior and inferior in position but still points more anteriorly than the normal aortic valve (Calder et al., 1976). There is fibrous continuity between the posterior leaflet and the anterior mitral valve leaflet (Calder et al., 1976) (Fig. 40–5). The truncal valve usually has three cusps but may have two to six cusps. In one series, truncal valve incompetence was severe in 6%, moderate in 31%, and absent to minimal in 63% of cases (Di Donato et al., 1985). Although dysplastic truncal valves have been seen with some frequency in autopsy series

(Becker et al., 1971), it was formerly felt that they did not pose a major problem in surgical repair in infancy (Anderson, 1985). More recently, however, one series showed truncal valve regurgitation severe enough to require truncal valve replacement in 5 of 46 patients, 3 of whom also had significant systolic pressure gradients (Bove et al., 1993).

The pathophysiology of truncus arteriosus is that of a large left-to-right shunt at a ventricular or great artery level, with a high ratio of pulmonary to systemic blood flow ($\dot{Q}_P/\dot{Q}_S$). Systemic pressures usually exist in the right ventricle and pulmonary arteries. There is an increased pulmonary vascular resistance (2 to 4 Wood units/m$^2$) from birth. Rarely does truncal valve stenosis or a restrictive ventricular septal defect modify this hemodynamic pattern. Through infancy, pulmonary vascular resistance increases progressively, with a gradual decrease in arterial oxygen saturation.

## CLINICAL PRESENTATION AND DIAGNOSIS

The clinical symptoms of truncus arteriosus are those of severe congestive heart failure from infancy onward, and they include tachypnea ("breathlessness"), tachydardia, irritability, poor feeding, respiratory infections, and ultimately failure to thrive. Cyanosis is not common in infants but can affect older children as Eisenmenger's physiology develops.

Physical examination reveals tachydardia and collapsing arterial pulses secondary to a runoff of systemic blood into the lower-pressure pulmonary circuit. The precordium is active, and a prominent systolic murmur is present. There may be an ejection click coincident with opening of the truncal valve. Truncal valve incompetence is associated with a coexistent diastolic murmur and is of concern, because an incompetent truncal valve is associated with a poorer prognosis than a competent valve.

The chest film shows pulmonary plethora and cardiomegaly and may demonstrate other abnormalities of the pulmonary arteries (Calder et al., 1976). Pulmo-

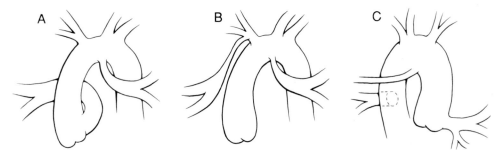

**FIGURE 40–4.** Pulmonary artery anatomy in four patients with nonconfluent pulmonary vessels. In two patients (A), the right pulmonary artery arose from the usual position on the ascending aorta and the left pulmonary artery from the ductus arteriosus. In one patient (B), the right pulmonary artery arose from the innominate artery and the left from the ductus arteriosus. In the final patient (C), the right upper lobe pulmonary artery arose from an occluded ductus arteriosus and the right lower lobe from a right-sided descending thoracic aorta. The left pulmonary artery arose directly from the proximal left coronary sinus of Valsalva, and the left coronary artery branched from the pulmonary artery. (A–C, From Bove, E. L., Lupinetti, F. N., Pridjian, A. K., et al.: Results of a policy of primary repair of truncus arteriosus in the neonate. J. Thorac. Cardiovasc. Surg., 105:1057, 1993.)

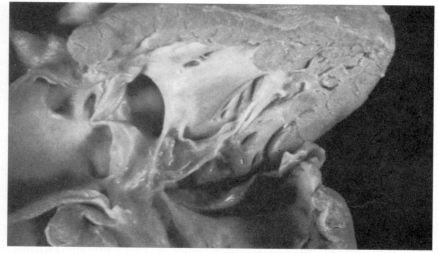

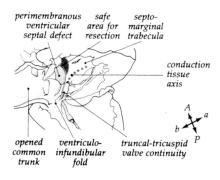

**FIGURE 40–5.** Common trunk with a perimembranous defect. The conduction axis is much closer to the posterior inferior rim than that shown in Figure 40–3. The safe area for surgical resection or placement of sutures is in a similar position. (From Wilcox, B. R., and Anderson, R. H.: Surgical Anatomy of the Heart. New York, Raven Press, 1985, p. 7.20.)

nary vascularity gradually decreases in patients who survive into childhood. Electrocardiographic findings are nonspecific but usually include left ventricular or biventricular hypertrophy and P-pulmonale. Echocardiography is diagnostic and shows a single great vessel, the subarterial ventricular septal defect, the origin of the pulmonary arteries, and the leaflets of the truncal valve (Marin-Garcia and Tonkin, 1982; Riggs and Paul, 1982). Echocardiography may even show the coronary artery distribution. Two-dimensional echocardiography combined with color-flow Doppler is an excellent technique for evaluating truncal valve incompetence or stenosis and blood flow patterns and gradients across the ventricular septal defect.

Cardiac catheterization and angiocardiography are still used to define the pulmonary arteries, the aortic arch, and the hemodynamic state (Barratt-Boyes, 1986). Cineangiography with contrast injection shows the site of origin of both pulmonary arteries and, if a pulmonary artery is absent, enables determination of the blood supply to the affected lung. Cardiac catheterization is also important in defining pulmonary vascular resistance.

## SURGICAL CORRECTION

Total surgical correction involves closure of the ventricular septal defect and establishment of continuity between the right ventricle and pulmonary artery by using an extracardiac conduit. The basis of this repair was first described by two groups independently (McGoon et al., 1968; Weldon and Cameron, 1968). The complete procedure is shown in Figure 40–6.

The operation is done through a median sternotomy incision. After entry into the pericardium and creation of a pericardial cradle, the aorta and the pulmonary artery are dissected. The patient is cannulated for cardiopulmonary bypass, with the aortic cannula placed just proximal to the innominate origin.

In infants in whom circulatory arrest is anticipated, a single atrial cannula is used. Otherwise, dual caval cannulation with maintenance of flow is preferred. Venting of the left ventricle is desirable to prevent overdistention as the patient is cooled.

After bypass is begun, the patient is cooled to a rectal temperature of 20° C, which provides latitude for further cooling if circulatory arrest becomes necessary. During cooling, it is desirable to occlude blood

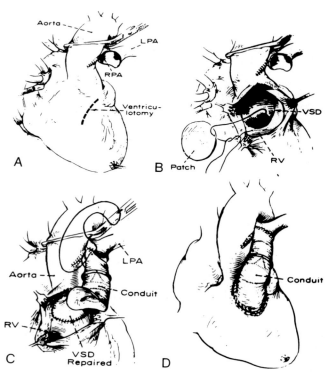

**FIGURE 40–6.** *A–D,* The complete procedure. (LPA = left pulmonary artery; RPA = right pulmonary artery; RV = right ventricle; VSD = ventricular septal defect.)

flow to the pulmonary arteries partially or totally to prevent flooding of the lungs and overdistention of the left atrium and ventricle. It is also necessary to occlude flow to the pulmonary arteries during instillation of cardioplegic solution.

After the aorta is cross-clamped, the pulmonary arteries are detached from the truncal artery, and the defect in the truncal artery is closed (Fig. 40–7). Closure must be done so that distortion of the truncal valve is avoided. Placement of a patch rather than a primary closure may be necessary. It is desirable to leave intact as much proximal length of the truncal artery as possible to prevent distortion of the left coronary ostium.

When the coronary artery pattern over the right and left epicardium has been defined, a longitudinal or transverse incision is made in the right ventricular infundibulum. It is not necessary to excise any right ventricular free wall to accommodate the anastomosis between the right ventricle and the extracardiac conduit. After creation of the ventriculotomy, the ventricular septal defect is usually easily seen, because it involves the infundibular septum. The defect is closed with a synthetic patch, using either a continuous running or interrupted technique. A continuous 4-0, 5-0, or 6-0 polypropylene suture with a tightly curved needle is preferred. Alternatively, a 5-0 braided polyester suture with small pledgets may be placed in an interrupted mattress manner. The cephalad margin of the suture line may be anchored to the epicardium and myocardium at the cephalad margin of the ventriculotomy (Fig. 40–8).

After closure of the ventricular septal defect, an extracardiac conduit is selected. Because of the increased pulmonary vascular resistance, a valved conduit usually is necessary, although correction of trun-

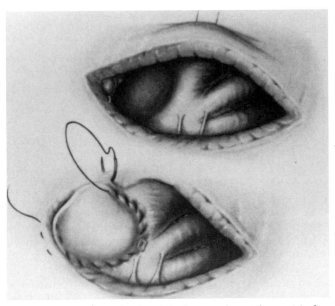

**FIGURE 40–8.** Longitudinal ventriculotomy shows the ventricular septal defect *(top)* and closure of the ventricular septal defect *(bottom)* using a synthetic patch and continuous suture technique. (From de Leval, M.: Persistent truncus arteriosus. *In* Stark, J., and de Leval, M. [eds]: Surgery for Congenital Heart Defects. London, Grune & Stratton, 1983, p. 421.)

cus arteriosus in neonates with nonvalved conduits has been reported (Peetz et al., 1982; Spicer et al., 1984). Valved conduits became commercially available in the 1970s and are supplied by several manufacturers in sizes ranging from 12 to 30 mm. These conduits usually give an excellent early result, but the valve component of the conduit degenerates rapidly and must be replaced within 2 years in approximately 50% of patients (Ebert et al., 1984).

Aortic and pulmonary homografts preserved with various techniques have been used, even before the advent of commercially available conduits. With earlier preservation techniques, homografts tended to calcify, and their use was abandoned in most institutions (Moodie et al., 1976). Other groups who use homografts have remained enthusiastic about them (Shabbo et al., 1980).

Unlike the disappointing results with synthetic valved conduits, those for cryopreservation techniques have improved, thus reinforcing the viability of fibroblasts within a conduit. There has been a resurgence of interest in cryopreserved human aortic and pulmonary homografts, although the long-term durability of these conduits remains to be seen. In a recent report, small pulmonary allografts (7 to 9 mm in diameter) were found to last longer than comparably sized aortic allografts (Heinemann et al., 1993).

The conduit that is selected should be trimmed to an appropriate length by estimating the distance from the ventriculotomy to the transected pulmonary arteries. The length should be such that the conduit is neither redundant nor subject to compression by the sternum. The anastomosis should also be under no

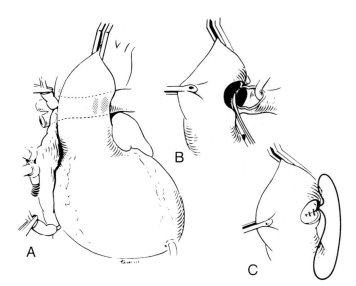

**FIGURE 40–7.** First step of surgical repair. *A*, Cardiopulmonary bypass is instituted and the ascending aorta is clamped. *B*, Excision of pulmonary arteries from the truncus. *C*, The defect in the truncus (aorta) is repaired. (*A–C*, From Wallace, R. B., Rastelli, G. C., Ongley, P. A., et al.: Complete repair of truncus arteriosus defects. J. Thorac. Cardiovasc. Surg., 57:96, 1969.)

tension and should not compress the left coronary artery.

The pulmonary anastomosis should be done first; I use a continuous technique with fine polypropylene suture (Fig. 40–9). The origins of the pulmonary arteries may be enlarged with pericardial patches (Fig. 40–10) or by spatulating the pulmonary end of the valved conduit (Fig. 40–11).

The ventricular anastomosis is accomplished by a similar technique. Care must be taken to avoid distortion of the conduit, and synthetic conduits may be beveled for this purpose (Fig. 40–12). If an aortic homograft is used, the anterior mitral valve leaflet may be used as a gusset. The ventricular anastomosis may be done with the aorta still cross-clamped or may be done during rewarming with the aorta unclamped and the heart beating. The completed procedure is shown in Figure 40–13.

A surgical technique for treating the combination of interrupted aortic arch and truncus arteriosus is illustrated in Figure 40–14. Because of the need to reconstruct the aortic arch, this procedure would be performed using profound hypothermia and circulatory arrest.

The presence of truncal valve insufficiency complicates the surgical procedure and should be assessed. Mild insufficiency may be tolerated, but the ventricle should be well vented and should not be allowed to overdistend. More severe truncal valve insufficiency may be amenable to valvuloplasty, but this usually

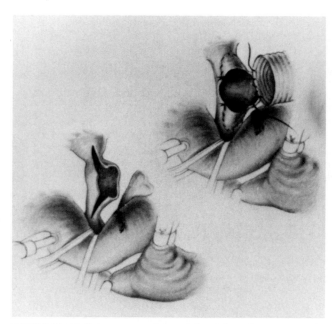

**FIGURE 40–10.** Enlargement of the origin of the pulmonary arteries with pericardium and anastomosis of the conduit to the enlarged pulmonary arteries. (From de Leval, M.: Persistent truncus arteriosus. *In* Stark, J., and de Leval, M. [eds]: Surgery for Congenital Heart Defects. London, Grune & Stratton, 1983, p. 423.)

extends the operation and requires replacement of the valve (Bove et al., 1993; de Leval et al., 1974). Good results may be achieved with an aggressive approach. Pulmonary artery banding was previously attempted as a palliative procedure (Muller and Dammann, 1952). The mortality rate with this approach varied

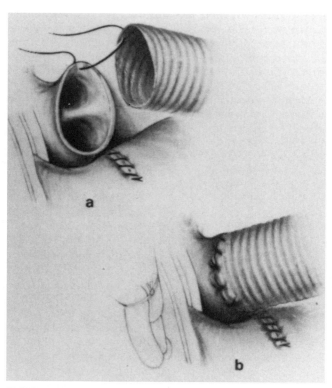

**FIGURE 40–9.** *a* and *b*, Anastomosis of the conduit to the pulmonary arteries. (*a* and *b*, From de Leval, M.: Persistent truncus arteriosus. *In* Stark, J., and de Leval, M. [eds]: Surgery for Congenital Heart Defects. London, Grune & Stratton, 1983, p. 421.)

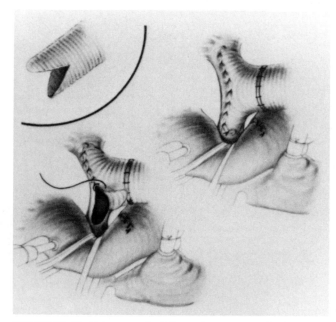

**FIGURE 40–11.** Enlargement of the pulmonary arteries by spatulating the pulmonary end of the conduit. (From de Leval, M.: Persistent truncus arteriosus. *In* Stark, J., and de Leval, M. [eds]: Surgery for Congenital Heart Defects. London, Grune & Stratton, 1983, p. 423.)

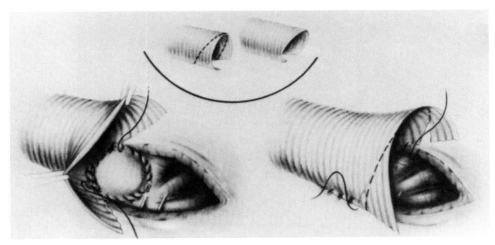

FIGURE 40–12. Completion of the ventriclar septal defect closure; the ventricular end of the conduit is beveled to prevent distortion or kinking of the conduit. (From de Leval, M.: Persistent truncus arteriosus. *In* Stark, J., and de Leval, M. [eds]: Surgery for Congenital Heart Defects. London, Grune & Stratton, 1983, p. 422.)

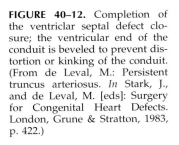

from 33 to 100% in a review by Poirier and associates (1975). Definitive correction in infancy has entirely replaced this approach.

## RESULTS

Because truncus arteriosus is relatively rare, few large series of patients have been described. One must be aware of the age of patients included in the series reports as well as the inclusion of patients who have coexistent anomalies or extracardiac valve conduits for other reasons.

A large review of results of surgical repair for truncus arteriosus as a discrete entity was provided by Marceletti and associates (1977) at the Mayo Clinic. The initial report of 92 patients was later expanded to 100 patients (McGoon et al., 1982) and then to 167 patients (Di Donato et al., 1985). Marceletti's report

described a 25% mortality rate within 30 days of operation and noted that mortality was correlated with the age of the patient at the time of repair; patients younger than 2 years had a higher risk.

A more recent and encouraging experience was described by Ebert and associates (Ebert, 1981; Ebert et al., 1984; Stanger et al., 1977), who reported an 11% mortality rate for repair of truncus arteriosus in 56 infants younger than 6 months. They also reported that 50% of the conduits were replaced within 2 years after operation, but no mortality was associated with conduit replacement. This series demonstrated the value of early corrective operation. Excellent results have been reported with neonatal correction by two groups (Bove et al., 1993; Hanley et al., 1993). Repair should be accomplished once the diagnosis has been established in the neonatal period. The results of several more recent series are shown in Table 40–1.

Incremental risk factors identified in the combined

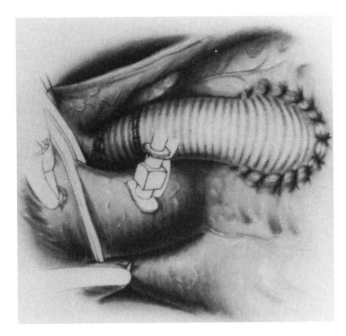

FIGURE 40–13. The completed repair. (From de Leval, M.: Persistent truncus arteriosus. *In* Stark, J., and de Leval, M. [eds]: Surgery for Congenital Heart Defects. London, Grune & Stratton, 1983, p. 422.)

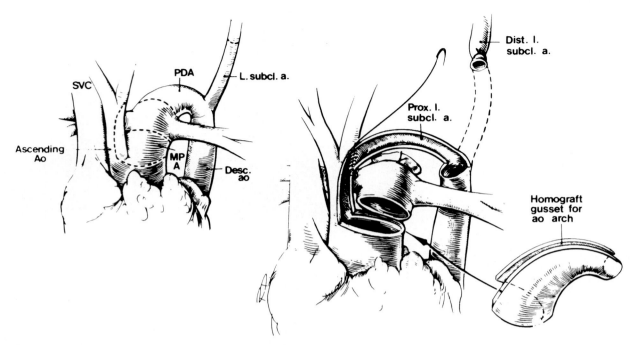

**FIGURE 40–14.** Reconstruction of aortic arch in truncus arteriosus with interrupted aortic arch. (SCV = superior vena cava; PDA = patent ductus arteriosus; MPA = main pulmonary artery.) (From Hanley, F. L., Heinemann, M. K., Jones, R. A., et al.: Repair of truncus arteriosus in the neonate. J. Thorac. Cardiovasc. Surg., *105*:1047, 1993.)

experience of the University of Alabama in Birmingham and Green Lane Hospital, Auckland, New Zealand, included the following (Barratt-Boyes, 1986):

1. Poor preoperative clinical status
2. Important truncal valve incompetence
3. A previously placed pulmonary artery band
4. Younger age
5. Pulmonary vascular disease
6. Earlier date of operation
7. Major coexisting cardiac anomalies (this is not supported by multivariate statistical analysis)

In a more recent series, according to both univariate and multivariate techniques, severe truncal valve regurgitation, interrupted aortic arch, coronary artery anomalies, and age at repair greater than 100 days were important risk factors for perioperative death. In the 33 patients without these risk factors, early survival was 100%. In the 30 patients with one or more of these risk factors, survival was 63%. Pulmonary hypertensive episodes were fewer, and duration of ventilator dependence and pulmonary artery pressure were significantly less in patients undergoing the operation before 30 days of age. Advances in surgical technique and better understanding of neonatal pulmonary physiology mean that young age at repair is no longer an incremental risk factor for death. Repair in the early neonatal period clearly reduces the prevalence of postoperative pulmonary vascular morbidity (Hanley et al., 1993).

The pulmonary vascular structure in a large group of children with various congenital anomalies, including a large group with truncus arteriosus, was studied by Juaneda and Haworth (1984) by using quantitative morphometric techniques. These studies showed abnormal extension of muscle, increased pulmonary arterial medial thickness, and intimal proliferation even in infants less than 1 year of age with truncus arteriosus. Even in the presence of increased pulmonary vascular resistance ($\geq$ 8 units/m$^2$), the changes were potentially reversible in infants. These studies strongly support early intracardiac repair.

The natural history of truncus arteriosus is such that only approximately 10% of patients born with truncus survive to 1 year of age without operative intervention. Early definitive correction as described

■ **Table 40–1.** MORTALITY FOR SURGICAL REPAIR OF TRUNCUS ARTERIOSUS

| Authors | Period | Total No. of Patients | Age at Correction | Late Mortality (%) | Early Mortality (%) |
|---|---|---|---|---|---|
| Ebert et al., 1984 | 1974–1981 | 106 | <6 months | 11 | 0 |
| Di Donato et al., 1985 | 1965–1982 | 167 | 18 days–33 years | 28.7 | 15.6 |
| Sharma et al., 1985 | 1979–1983 | 23 | 1 month–2 years | 13 | 0 |
| Hanley et al., 1993 | 1986–1991 | 63 | 3–216 days | 17 | 0 |
| Bove et al., 1993 | 1986–1992 | 46 | 1 day–7 months | 11 | 6 |

by Ebert and associates and more recently confirmed by Bove and associates and Hanley and associates is clearly the approach of choice.

## SELECTED BIBLIOGRAPHY

Bove, E. L., Lupinetti, F. M., Pridjian, A. K., et al.: Results of a policy of primary repair of truncus arteriosus in the neonate. J. Thorac. Cardiovasc. Surg., *105*:1057, 1993.

Forty-six neonates and infants ranging in age from 1 day to 7 months underwent complete repair of truncus arteriosus. Four patients had non-confluent pulmonary arteries, five patients had interrupted aortic arch, and five patients had truncal valve pathology severe enough to warrant valve replacement. In spite of the complex anomalies encountered in the patients in this series, the hospital mortality rate was only 11%, with a late mortality rate of 6%. This paper illustrates the excellent results that can be achieved with early definitive correction, even in a complex group of patients.

Di Donato, R. M., Fyfe, D. A., Puga, F. J., et al.: Fifteen-year experience with surgical repair of truncus arteriosus. J. Thorac. Cardiovasc. Surg., *89*:414, 1985.

This paper discusses 167 patients 18 days to 33 years of age with a mean age of 6 years. There were 48 hospital deaths (28.7%). The 119 hospital survivors had a 5-year survival rate of 84.4% and a 10-year survival rate of 68.8%. Reoperation was necessary for 36 patients (30%) during the follow-up period, primarily for right ventricular pulmonary arterial conduit replacement or for truncal valve replacement. This is the largest and most extensive experience in the literature.

Ebert, P. A., Turley, K., Stanger, P. E., et al.: Surgical treatment of truncus arteriosus in the first 6 months of life. Ann. Surg., *200*:451, 1984.

One hundred infants underwent physiologic correction before 6 months of age. There were 11 operative deaths (a mortality rate of 11%). Of the 86 long-term survivors, 55 returned for conduit change within 2 years. This paper showed the feasibility of physiologic correction in the first 6 months of life, with a low operative mortality rate and no mortality associated with conduit replacement. The low operative mortality rate indicated that corrective operation is the best method of intervention to control failure and reduce the likelihood of pulmonary vascular disease, even though reoperation for enlargement of the conduit will be required.

Hanley, F. L., Heinemann, M. K., Jonas, R. A., et al.: Repair of truncus arteriosus in the neonate. J. Thorac. Cardiovasc. Surg., *105*:1047, 1993.

In this group of 63 patients, 30 variables were examined as potential risk factors for the outcome events of death, reoperation, and presence of pulmonary vascular morbidity. According to both univariate and multivariate techniques, severe truncal valve regurgitation, interrupted aortic arch, coronary artery anomalies, and age at repair greater than 100 days were important risk factors for perioperative death. In the absence of these factors, truncus arteriosus can be repaired with excellent surgical outcome in the neonatal and early infancy period. Furthermore, repair in the early neonatal period was found to reduce the prevalence of postoperative pulmonary vascular morbidity.

Juaneda, E., and Haworth, S. G.: Pulmonary vascular disease in children with truncus arteriosus. Am. J. Cardiol., *54*:1314, 1984.

Pulmonary vascular structure was analyzed with quantitative morphometric techniques in lung biopsy specimens from 23 patients 18 days to 13 years of age with truncus arteriosus Type I or II. The paper showed that pulmonary vascular obstructive disease begins very early in this group of patients, but even in infants with increased pulmonary arteriolar resistance, the changes were potentially reversible. The paper shows the type of in-depth morphometric analysis of pulmonary arteriolar structure that has increased our understanding of conditions involving large left-to-right shunts (increased $\dot{Q}_P/\dot{Q}_S$). The results strongly support early intracardiac repair to prevent development of permanent pulmonary vascular disease.

## BIBLIOGRAPHY

Anderson, K. R., McGoon, D. C., and Lie, J. T.: Surgical significance of the coronary arterial anatomy in truncus arteriosus communis. Am. J. Cardiol., *41*:76, 1978.

Anderson, R. H.: Common arterial trunk. *In* Wilcox, B. R., and Anderson, R. H. (eds): Surgical Anatomy of the Heart. New York, Raven Press, 1985.

Barratt-Boyes, B. G.: Truncus arteriosus. *In* Kirklin, J. W., and Barratt-Boyes, B. G. (eds): Cardiac Surgery. New York, John Wiley & Sons, 1986.

Becker, A. E., Becker, M. J., and Edwards, J. E.: Pathology of the semi-lunar valve in persistent truncus arteriosus. J. Thorac. Cardiovasc. Surg., *62*:16, 1971.

Behrendt, D. M., Kirsch, M. M., Stern, A., et al.: The surgical therapy for pulmonary artery–right ventricular discontinuity. Ann. Thorac. Surg., *18*:122, 1974.

Bharati, S., Karp, R., and Lev, M.: The conduction system in truncus arteriosus and its surgical significance. J. Thorac. Cardiovasc. Surg., *104*:954, 1992.

Bharati, S., McAllister, H. A., Rosenquist, G. C., et al.: The surgical anatomy of truncus arteriosus communis. J. Thorac. Cardiovasc. Surg., *67*:501, 1974.

Bove, E. L., Lupinetti, F. M., Pridjian, A. K., et al.: Results of a policy of primary repair of truncus arteriosus in the neonate. J. Thorac. Cardiovasc. Surg., *105*:1057, 1993.

Buchanan, A.: Malformation of the heart: Undivided truncus arteriosus. Heart otherwise double. Trans. Path. Soc. Lond., *15*:89, 1864.

Calder, L., Van Praagh, R., Van Praagh, S., et al.: Truncus arteriosus communis: Clinical, angiographic, and pathologic findings in 100 patients. Am. Heart J., *92*:23, 1976.

Collett, R. W., and Edwards, J. E.: Persistent truncus arteriosus: A classification according to anatomic types. Surg. Clin. North Am., *29*:1245, 1949.

Crupi, G., Macartney, F. J., and Anderson, R. H.: Persistent truncus arteriosus: A study of 66 autopsy cases with special reference to definition and morphogenesis. Am. J. Cardiol., *40*:569, 1977.

de Leval, M. R., McGoon, D. C., Wallace, R. B., et al.: Management of truncal valvular regurgitation. Ann. Surg., *180*:427, 1974.

de Leval, M.: Persistent truncus arteriosus. *In* Stark, J., and de Leval, M. (eds): Surgery for Congenital Heart Defects. New York, Grune & Stratton, 1983.

Di Donato, R. M., Fyfe, D. A., Puga F. J., et al.: Fifteen year experience with surgical repair of truncus arteriosus. J. Thorac. Cardiovasc. Surg., *89*:414, 1985.

Ebert, P. A.: Truncus arteriosus. *In* Parenzan, L., Crupi, G., and Graham, G. (eds): Congenital Heart Disease in the First Three Months of Life, Medical and Surgical Aspects. Bologna, Patron Editore, 1981, p. 439.

Ebert, P. A., Turley, K., Stranger, P., et al.: Surgical treatment of truncus arteriosus in the first 6 months of life. Ann. Surg., *200*:451, 1984.

Girinath, M. R.: Case presentation: Truncus arteriosus: Repair with homograft reconstruction in infancy. *In* Barratt-Boyes, B. G., Neutze, J. M., and Harris, E. A. (eds): Heart Disease in Infancy. Diagnosis and Surgical Treatment. Edinburgh, Churchill Livingstone, 1973, p. 234.

Hanley, F. L., Heinemann, M. K., Jonas, R. A., et al.: Repair of truncus arteriosus in the neonate. J. Thorac. Cardiovasc. Surg., *105*:1047, 1993.

Heinemann, M. K., Hanley, F. L., Fenton, K. N., et al.: Fate of small homograft conduits after early repair of truncus arteriosus. Ann. Thorac. Surg., *55*:1409, 1993

Juaneda, E., and Haworth, S. G.: Pulmonary vascular disease in children with truncus arteriosus. Am. J. Cardiol., *54*:1314, 1984.

Lev, M., and Saphir, O.: Truncus arteriosus communis persistens. J. Pediatr., *20*:74, 1943.

Marceletti, C., McGoon, D. C., Danielson, G. K., et al.: Early and late results of surgical repair of truncus arteriosus. Circulation, *55*:636, 1977.

Marin-Garcia, J., and Tonkin, L. D.: Two-dimensional echocardiographic evaluation of persistent truncus arteriosus. Am. J. Cardiol., *50*:1376, 1982.

McGoon, D. C.: Truncus arteriosus. *In* Sabiston, D. C., Jr., and Spencer, F. C. (eds): Gibbons's Surgery of the Chest. Philadelphia, W. B. Saunders, 1983.

McGoon, D. C., Danielson, G. K., Puga, F. J., et al.: Late results after extracardiac conduit repair for congenital cardiac defects. Am. J. Cardiol., *49*:1741, 1982.

McGoon, D. C., Rastelli, G. C., and Ongley, P. A.: An operation for the correction of truncus arteriosus. J. A. M. A., *205*:59, 1968.

Moodie, D. S., Mair, D. D., Fulton, R. E., et al.: Aortic homograft obstruction. J. Thorac. Cardiovasc. Surg., 72:553, 1976.

Muller, W. H., Jr., and Dammann, J. F., Jr.: The treatment of certain congenital malformations of the heart by the creation of pulmonic stenosis to reduce pulmonary hypertension and excessive pulmonary blood flow: A preliminary report. Surg. Gynecol. Obstet., 95:213, 1952.

Peetz, D. J., Jr., Spicer, R. L., Crowley, D. C., et al.: Correction of truncus arteriosus in the neonate using a nonvalved conduit. J. Thorac. Cardiovasc. Surg., 83:743, 1982.

Poirier, R. A., Berman, M. A., and Stansel, H. C., Jr.: Current status of the surgical treatment of truncus arteriosus. J. Thorac. Cardiovasc. Surg., 69:169, 1975.

Riggs, T. W., and Paul, M. H.: Two-dimensional echocardiographic prospective diagnosis of common truncus arteriosus in infants. Am. J. Cardiol., 50:1380, 1982.

Shabbo, F. P., Wain, W. H., and Ross, D. N.: Right ventricular outflow reconstruction with aortic homograft conduit: Analysis of the long-term results. Thorac. Cardiovasc. Surg., 28:21, 1980.

Shapiro, P. F.: Truncus solitarus pulmonalis: A rare type of congenital cardiac anomaly. Arch. Pathol., 10:671, 1930.

Sharma, A. K., Brawn, W. J., and Mee, R. B. B.: Truncus arteriosus: Surgical approach. J. Thorac. Cardiovasc. Surg., 90:45, 1985.

Shrivastava, S., and Edwards, J. E.: Coronary arterial origin in persistent truncus arteriosus. Circulation, 55:551, 1977.

Spicer, R. L., Behrendt, D. M., Crowley, D. C., et al.: Repair of truncus arteriosus in neonates with the use of a valveless conduit. Circulation, 70:1, 1984.

Stanger, P., Robinson, S. J., Engle, M. A., and Ebert, P. A.: "Corrective" surgery for truncus arteriosus in the first year of life [Abstract]. Am. J. Cardiol., 39:293, 1977.

Taruffi, C.: Sulle malattie congenite e sulle anomalie del cuore. Mem. Soc. Med. Chir. Bologna, 8:215, 1875.

Thiene, G., Bortolotti, A., Gallucci, V., et al.: Anatomical study of truncus arteriosus communis with embryological and surgical considerations. Br. Heart J., 38:1109, 1976.

Van Praagh, R., and Van Praagh, S.: The anatomy of common aorticopulmonary trunk (truncus arteriosus communis) and its embryonic implications: A study of 57 necropsy cases. Am. J. Cardiol., 16:406, 1965.

Victoria, B. E., Krovetz, L. J., Elliott, C. P., et al.: Persistent truncus arteriosus in infancy. Am. Heart J., 77:13, 1969.

Weldon, C. S., and Cameron, J. L.: Correction of persistent truncus arteriosus. J. Cardiovasc. Surg., 9:463, 1968.

Wilson, J.: A description of a very unusual malformation of the human heart. Philos. Trans. R. Soc. London (Biol.), 18:346, 1798.

# 41

# Congenital Aortic Stenosis

Ross M. Ungerleider

Congenital aortic stenosis may be caused by a spectrum of lesions that obstruct the flow of blood from the left ventricle into the aorta. Aortic stenosis may be congenital in 3 to 10% of cases (Nadas and Fyler, 1972; Olley et al., 1978; Trinkle et al., 1975) and is associated with various other cardiovascular anomalies in 8 to 30% of patients (Bernhard et al., 1973; Mulder et al., 1968), including coarctation of the aorta, patent ductus arteriosus, *endocardial fibroelastosis* (EFE), *ventricular septal defects* (VSDs), pulmonary stenosis, and mitral stenosis (Trinkle et al., 1975). Certain forms of congenital aortic stenosis are frequently associated with predictable anomalies (Shone et al., 1963). The site of obstruction is classified anatomically as valvular, subvalvular, or supravalvular (Fig. 41–1). A fourth form, caused by hypertrophy of the interventricular muscular septum, presents a unique variety of subvalvular obstruction that varies physiologically from the other forms of stenotic lesions and is therefore considered a separate entity. Although these lesions usually occur separately, patients can present with combinations of the anatomic varieties (Kirklin and Barratt Boyes, 1993), and *left ventricular outflow tract obstruction* (LVOTO) is perhaps a more descriptive term for this spectrum of congenital anomalies.

## HISTORICAL ASPECTS

Stenosis of the aortic valve was described as early as 1646 by Riverius and was further expanded on by Bonetti in 1700 and Morgagni in 1769 (Hallman and Cooley, 1983). However, it was not until 1844 that the congenital etiology of this form of stenosis was appreciated from Paget's description of bicuspid aortic valves (Paget, 1844). The potential clinical significance of this anomaly was recognized 42 years later when Osler described a patient with endocarditis on a bicuspid aortic valve (Osler, 1886). Even more devastating implications were documented by Thursfield and Scott in 1913 when they described the sudden death of a 14-year-old boy with subaortic stenosis (Thursfield and Scott, 1913). Around the same time Carrel (Carrel, 1910) and Jeger (Jeger, 1913) were independently experimenting with the use of conduits between the left ventricle and aorta to bypass aortic valvular obstruction. Concurrently, Tuffier (Tuffier, 1914) first successfully dilated a calcific aortic valve, thus demonstrating that flow could be restored through the normal anatomic route. Initial therapeutic approaches centered around aortic valvular dilatation, but in 1955 Swan and Kortz performed the first open aortic valvotomy under direct vision using systemic hypothermia with caval occlusion (Swan and Kortz, 1956). Success with this technique was also reported by others (Lewis et al., 1956), but it quickly gave way in popularity to extracorporeal circulation, which allowed for the performance of open aortic valvotomy using *cardiopulmonary bypass* (CPB), as reported by Spencer in 1958 (Spencer et al., 1958). Since that time, the treatment of the spectrum of lesions causing LVOTO has expanded rapidly.

## NATURAL HISTORY, CLINICAL PRESENTATION, AND DIAGNOSIS

Stenosis of the aortic valve may occur at any age, from infancy to old age. In most patients it worsens progressively with growth (Ankeney et al., 1983; El-Said et al., 1972; Friedman et al., 1979). Few patients survive through the sixth decade of life without developing serious unfavorable signs or symptoms; initially asymptomatic patients should be followed routinely, because the untreated mortality rate can be 60% or more by the age of 40 (Campbell, 1968). Infants who present with symptoms have a 23% mortality rate if untreated in the first year of life, and the mean age of death for patients with untreated lesions is 35 years (Campbell, 1968). Congenital valvular aortic stenosis is 3 to 4 times more common in males than in females, and the natural history is greatly influenced by the age at presentation. There now seems to be little argument that when this lesion presents in infancy, the prognosis is considerably worse than when it presents later in life (Kirklin and Barratt-Boyes, 1993). Numerous studies have demonstrated that whereas infants with critical aortic stenosis often present in New York Heart Association (NYHA) Class IV or V, with an urgent need for surgical relief, the natural history for infants is greatly affected by the presence of associated lesions, especially those which also involve the left side of the heart/aorta complex (Karl et al., 1990; Kirklin and Barratt-Boyes, 1993; Leung et al., 1991). In particular, critically ill neonates may also have severe (usually stenotic) anomalies of the mitral valve, endocardial firbroelastosis, hypoplasia of the left ventricular cavity, hypoplasia of the subaortic left ventricular outflow tract, and coarctation of the aorta. In addition, many patients may have atrial defects and VSDs. Patients with a mitral valve annulus of less than 9 mm (or mitral valve area $< 4.75$ cm$^2 \cdot$ m$^{-2}$), a left ventricular volume of less than 20 ml/m$^2$, left ventric-

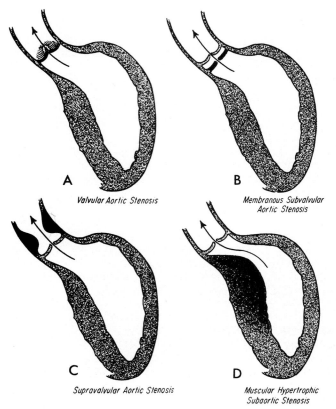

A   *Valvular Aortic Stenosis*

B   *Membranous Subvalvular Aortic Stenosis*

C   *Supravalvular Aortic Stenosis*

D   *Muscular Hypertrophic Subaortic Stenosis*

**FIGURE 41–1.** *A–D,* The various levels at which left ventricular outflow tract obstruction can occur. (*A–D,* From Oldham, H. N. Jr.: Congenital aortic stenosis. *In* Sabiston, D. C., Jr. [ed]: Textbook of Surgery, The Biological Basis of Modern Surgical Practice. 13th ed. Philadelphia, W. B. Saunders, 1986.)

ular inflow dimension less than 25 mm, EFE, or an aortic valve annulus of less than 5 mm have a particularly poor prognosis (Leung et al., 1991; Rhodes et al., 1991).

In these patients, the ability of the left side of the heart ever to participate adequately in the circulation is sometimes arguable; many of these patients, if they are to survive, may need to be staged toward a univentricular repair (Rhodes et al., 1991). Children who present after 1 year of age may have few symptoms, and their greatest risk appears to be more from the development of *subacute bacterial endocarditis* (SBE) or the ongoing risk of sudden death (Braverman and Gibson, 1957; Campbell, 1968; Glew et al., 1969). Although critically ill infants may need emergent aortic valvotomy, children who are discovered to have stenotic aortic valves later in life may live for many years with slowly progressive left ventricular outflow gradients before they require surgical intervention. The degree of stenosis in children at the time of diagnosis predicts the likelihood of developing severe obstruction; only 20% of mild lesions become severe within 10 years, although 60% of moderate lesions become severe within that same time frame (Friedman et al., 1979; Hossack et al., 1980; Mills et al., 1978). When valvular stenosis presents in neonates and infants, the lesion is almost always severe, and

most of these patients will die within days to weeks without therapy (Kirklin and Barratt-Boyes, 1993).

Symptoms vary greatly with the severity of the lesion and the age at presentation. Infants with critical aortic stenosis usually appear to be in rampant congestive heart failure with poor peripheral perfusion, acidosis, tachypnea, pallor, perspiration, and inability to feed. Left ventricular forward output may be extremely restricted, and patency of the ductus arteriosus is often mandatory to support systemic perfusion. If the ductus is closed, the infant demonstrates all signs of severe low cardiac output: cold extremities, diminished pulses, and pulmonary edema. These infants are critically ill and can present in a moribund condition. In infants who are not so critically ill, physical examination demonstrates a systolic ejection murmur with narrow pulse volume. However, in severe lesions, the diminished flow across the aortic valve combined with a depressed cardiac output may make the cardiac examination relatively unimpressive. Laboratory examination will reveal hypoxemia with acidosis due to congested pulmonary vasculature and poor peripheral perfusion. Hypoxemia is caused by the pulmonary congestion associated with left ventricular outflow obstruction, but these infants also have reduced systemic arterial oxygen saturation distal to the left subclavian artery (e.g., in an umbilical artery catheter) from the right-to-left shunt across a patent ductus. Acidosis is a sign of severely compromised circulation and indicates inadequate cardiac output to supply tissue oxygen demands. It is not necessarily related to the hypoxemia. In fact, in infants who can support systemic perfusion across a ductus arteriosus, acidosis may correct itself, despite failure to improve systemic arterial oxygenation. The chest film should reveal cardiomegaly and pulmonary edema. Electrocardiographic findings may demonstrate left ventricular strain. Older children and adults may be entirely asymptomatic or may have fatigue, dyspnea, angina, or syncope with exercise. Because older patients (including infants who are not critically ill and who have not been diagnosed in the neonatal period) are usually able to maintain adequate cardiac output across the left ventricular outflow area to supply tissue oxygen demands, they usually demonstrate a prominent systolic ejection murmur on physical examination. Older patients, particularly, may also have a prominent left ventricular lift over the precordium. Laboratory parameters are usually normal, and the chest film may show mild left ventricular hypertrophy with prominence of the ascending aorta.

The primary symptoms attributable to left ventricular outflow tract obstruction are expected from increasing ventricular work. As the systolic pressure gradient across the outflow tract increases, flow can be maintained only by increasing left ventricular pressure. In the neonate this may not be possible, and acute cardiac decompensation results. Peripheral perfusion can then be maintained by left-to-right shunting across a patent foramen ovale and right-to-left shunting across a patent ductus arteriosus. This explains the importance of maintaining ductal patency with prostaglandins in newborns with critical aortic stenosis (Jonas et al., 1985).

In patients who survive infancy and have persistent aortic stenosis, the left ventricular muscle undergoes concentric hypertrophy, thereby altering myocardial mechanics. This larger muscle mass creates greater systolic wall tension, which increases myocardial oxygen consumption—in other words, it increases the amount of oxygen necessary to adequately meet the metabolic demands of the myocardium. Unfortunately, the hypertrophied left ventricle is also somewhat stiffer than the normal ventricle (less compliant), and the end-diastolic pressure necessary to adequately volume-load the ventricular chamber is increased. This higher end-diastolic pressure occurs while the myocardium receives its coronary blood flow and probably prevents an adequate supply to the subendocardial layer. This produces ischemia, because oxygen demand is increasing but supply is decreasing; for this reason, severe stenosis eventually leads to heart failure (Spann et al., 1980). If the pressure gradient between the left ventricle and the aorta is less than 50 mm Hg and aortic valve orifice size is greater than 0.7 cm$^2$/m$^2$ of body surface area, the heart can usually adapt to its increased demands without clinical evidence of failure (Oldham, 1986). Nevertheless, exercise necessitates an increase in the cardiac outflow and therefore the flow per minute across the obstruction. This augments the severity of the lesion and demonstrates that the measured gradient must be correlated to the cardiac index to ensure a reasonable degree of accuracy in gauging its severity. The inability to increase forward flow to meet the metabolic demands of the body explains why most patients experience initial symptoms with exercise. As the stenosis becomes more severe with growth, these symptoms may become more prominent and are thought to reflect hemodynamically severe obstruction that requires appropriate treatment to prevent death.

A major issue is the proper time for therapeutic intervention, and periodic re-evaluation of children with suspicious murmurs is advised. These children may show little more than a harsh systolic ejection murmur most prominent over the second right intercostal space radiating to the neck and often associated with a thrill. As many as 22% of patients may have a diastolic murmur of aortic insufficiency, and there may also be a precordial lift (Braunwald et al., 1963). Several criteria have been evaluated as indicators of more severe obstruction, because these children would be at greater risk. Symptoms rarely occur except with severe stenosis. In addition, a systolic precordial thrill usually suggests a gradient greater than 30 mm Hg. Likewise, narrowing of the peripheral pulse pressure (indicating obstructed forward flow) suggests severe stenosis. It is now well recognized that the chest film may appear normal despite significant stenosis. Aortic valves rarely calcify until the fourth decade of life, but calcification in this location is evidence of an abnormal aortic valve. Although an electrocardiographic pattern of left ventricular strain

(ST segment and T-wave abnormalities) often suggests advanced disease, this correlation is not absolute, and children have died suddenly with aortic stenosis with previously documented normal electroencephalogram (ECG) results (Glew et al., 1969; Hossack et al., 1980).

When significant stenosis is suspected, the diagnosis can be established by cardiac ultrasonography or cardiac catheterization. Two-dimensional echocardiography with Doppler color-flow imaging provides a sensitive and specific indicator of both the anatomy and the severity of the obstruction (Kisslo et al., 1988; Silverman, 1993). Additionally, color-flow imaging enables detection of even trivial amounts of aortic insufficiency, as well as associated small VSDs and other associated lesions. Doppler shifts can allow measurement of the velocity across areas of stenosis (in meters per second), and by employing a simplification of Bernoulli's equation, one can predict gradients with superb accuracy ($P = 4 \cdot V^2$, where P = the peak instantaneous pressure gradient across the area of stenosis and V = the measured Doppler shift obtained by echo. For example, a velocity across a stenotic valve of 5 m/sec creates a peak instantaneous pressure gradient of 100 mm Hg). Although the peak instantaneous pressure may overestimate the peak-to-peak gradient, especially in conditions of severe aortic stenosis, this technology has nevertheless been very useful for noninvasively following the progression of aortic stenosis before, during, and after surgery (Kisslo et al., 1988; Silverman, 1993). Echocardiography is now so good at providing anatomic and physiologic information that the role of cardiac catheterization has become more limited. Two-dimensional echocardiography can reliably demonstrate the anatomy of the aortic valve (e.g., number of cusps and how well they function); associated intracardiac lesions such as VSDs, mitral valve stenosis, and EFE; and important extracardiac lesions such as aortic coarctation and the presence (as well as the shunt direction) of a patent ductus arteriosus. Two-dimensional echocardiography thereby provides the surgeon with all the anatomic information necessary to perform the proper operation. Critically ill infants can be diagnosed, resuscitated, and sent to the operating room with the information obtained by echocardiography. For older children, echocardiography is an excellent means of following the progression of the aortic outflow gradient.

Although cardiac catheterization is now primarily used for balloon angioplasty treatment (discussed later), it is still a reasonable (and time-honored) method of delineating the various types of aortic stenosis and quantitating their severity. It must be recognized that gradients are altered significantly by the hemodynamic state (which is not normal in the cardiac catheterization laboratory or in the operating room, especially after CPB). Therefore, any measurement of gradient across an area of stenosis must consider the cardiac output at the time of measurement. Withdrawal of the catheter from the left ventricle into the ascending aorta can provide critical pressure measurements delineating the area of obstruction as well as quantitating the gradient across it at a given cardiac index. A gradient greater than 75 mm Hg or a valve area less than 0.5 cm$^2$/m$^2$ indicates severe stenosis. In addition, elevation of the left ventricular end-diastolic pressure may correlate with left ventricular failure. With the various modalities available, the aortic valve gradient can be quantified somewhat. Gradients less than 40 mm Hg at rest suggest mild stenosis, whereas gradients less than 75 mm Hg and usually with a mean of 50 mm Hg reflect moderate stenosis. Patients with severe stenosis not only have pressure gradients in excess of 75 mm Hg but may have a mean calculated aortic valve area of 0.38 ± 0.15 cm$^2$/m$^2$ (Hossack et al., 1980).

## INDICATIONS FOR OPERATIONS AND TREATMENT

### Valvular Stenosis

In most cases (70 to 80%), LVOTO is caused by valvular lesions (Nadas and Fyler, 1972) and usually entails thickening of the valve leaflets and some degree of fusion of the commissures (Leung et al., 1991; McKay et al., 1992). This creates valves that appear bicuspid, unicuspid, or, rarely, quadricuspid (Peretz et al., 1969; Robicshek et al., 1969) (see Fig. 41–1). Seventy-six per cent of hearts with unicuspid valves have associated EFE, whereas only 14% of hearts with bicuspid valves have EFE (Van Praagh, personal communication). In critically ill infants, the precise features of valve abnormality may be difficult to discern. Bicuspid valves occur in 0.7 to 2% of human hearts and in 70% of hearts with valvular aortic stenosis (Roberts, 1970). Although they may function normally, many calcify and become stenotic in later life. These valves are abnormal because of commissural fusion, whereas the valve annulus and coronary arteries are normal (McKay et al., 1992). No surgical procedure can restore a stenotic valve to a completely normal one, so the goal of operation is to relieve stenosis. This is usually performed by an incision (valvotomy) separating the fused commissures (Fig. 41–2). It is important to restrict this incision so that it does not extend to the annulus, because the support mechanism of the leaflet could be destroyed, causing severe aortic insufficiency. This goal is more easily accomplished in some anomalies than in others (Dobell et al., 1981) (Fig. 41–3). Along with the relief of obstruction, some element of aortic insufficiency may be created. Infants may tolerate some aortic regurgitation better than they did the previous stenosis (Hallman and Cooley, 1983). Because these valves remain abnormal after relief of the stenosis, valvotomy is a palliative procedure. Thus, the surgical goal of valvotomy should be to increase the orifice size as much as possible within the limit of each individual valve. A recently suggested technique (Ilbawi et al., 1991) includes release of the cusps at their hinge points by incising them from the circumference of the annulus

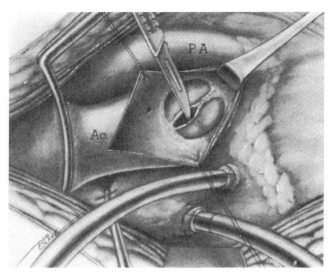

**FIGURE 41–2.** A bicuspid aortic valve is exposed through an aortotomy with the patient on cardiopulmonary bypass and the aorta (Ao) cross-clamped. The heart has been arrested with cardioplegia solution. The fused commissure is incised to the annulus as shown by the *dashed line*. (P.A. = pulmonary artery.)

for a few millimeters. This may enhance aortic valve opening following valvotomy (Fig. 41–4), but long-term results of this procedure are not available. Others (McKay, 1993) have suggested opening raphes in the hopes of creating valves that are more trileaflet in their function.

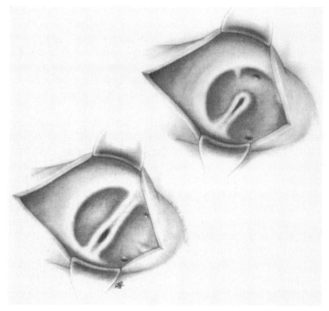

**FIGURE 41–3.** The *lower illustration* depicts a bicuspid aortic valve with a fused commissure in the anterior region. This valve can be opened relatively easily with a valvotomy. The *upper illustration* shows a unicuspid valve with only minimal fusion of the commissure. It is difficult to open this valve significantly with valvotomy, and balloon valvuloplasty by catheter techniques can cause devastating aortic insufficiency. (From de Leval, M.: Surgery of the left ventricular outflow tract. *In* Stark, J., and de Leval, M. [eds]: Surgery for Congenital Heart Defects. 2nd ed. Philadelphia, W. B. Saunders, 1994, pp. 511–538.)

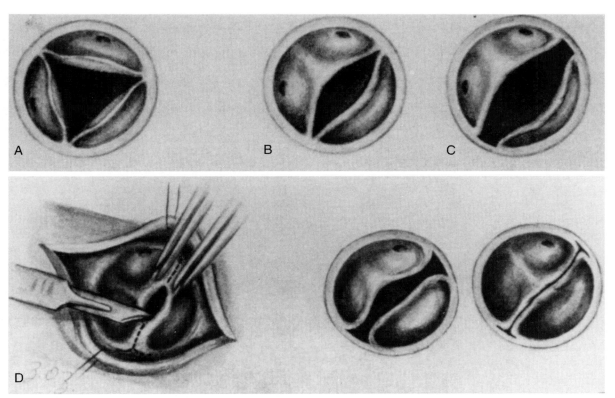

**FIGURE 41–4.** *A,* The degree of opening that can be expected from a normal tricuspid aortic valve compared with limited opening in a bicuspid aortic valve *(B)* and improved opening in a bicuspid aortic valve *(C)* when an extended aortic valvotomy is performed as shown in *D.* In this operation, the aortic valve is opened along the fused commissures and around the circumference of the annulus for a short way to improve the opening of the cusps. (*A–D,* From Ilbawi, M. N., DeLeon, S. Y., Wison, W. R. J., et al.: Extended aortic valvuloplasty: A new approach for the management of congenital valvular aortic stenosis. Reprinted with permission from the Society of Thoracic Surgeons [The Annals of Thoracic Surgery, 1991, Vol. 52, pp. 663–668].)

The approach to aortic stenosis, as well as the urgency with which the lesion is treated, depends on the location of the obstruction and the age and condition of the patient at presentation. Infants in congestive heart failure who respond poorly to medical management require urgent intervention (Hallman and Cooley 1983; Kirklin and Barratt-Boyes, 1993; Turley et al., 1990). Older children and young adults with severe stenosis also should undergo surgical correction because they have a higher risk of sudden death (de Leval, 1994; Hossack et al., 1980). A peak systolic gradient across the obstruction of 50 to 75 mm Hg during normal cardiac output or a valve surface area of less than 0.5 cm²/m² body surface area suggests a need for operation.

## Neonates

Critically ill neonates require urgent intervention. After diagnosis, prostaglandin $E_1$ should be started via a centrally located intravenous line, to provide reasonable resuscitation from the poor systemic perfusion and acidosis. These infants often require endotracheal intubation and mechanical ventilation. Hyperventilation (to lower $PCO_2$) with 100% inspired oxygen may lower the pulmonary artery hypertension that usually accompanies this defect and possibly improve left ventricular outflow (as the anatomy allows). Furthermore, inotropic agents such as dopamine are often helpful during resuscitation. The use of prostaglandins to open the ductus arteriosus has been an important benefit. Restoring the ability of these critically ill infants to shunt right to left across the ductus decompresses pulmonary hypertension and maintains systemic perfusion even in the face of marked left ventricular dysfunction and severe left ventricular outflow tract obstruction (Jonas et al., 1985).

There has been increasing enthusiasm for treating certain patients nonoperatively by percutaneous balloon valvuloplasty (Lock et al., 1987; Zeevi et al., 1989, 1992). This technique was first reported in 1983 (Lababidi, 1983) and is now employed by numerous pediatric cardiologists using various guidelines (Choy et al., 1987; Walls et al., 1984). Extensive experience with this approach by Lock and his colleagues (Lock et al., 1987; Zeevi et al., 1989, 1992) has guided this approach to its current status and has enabled interventional cardiology to significantly affect the treatment of critical aortic stenosis. Short-term results of balloon aortic valvotomy appear comparable with surgical valvotomy for congenital aortic stenosis. Neonates, who present the most difficult challenge to this technique, may obtain the greatest benefit as technology provides for safer application with smaller catheters and low-profile balloons. Aortic insufficiency remains a contraindication to this option. In addition, patients with aortic stenosis who also present with severe aortic coarctation or interruption of the aortic arch would not be candidates for balloon valvuloplasty.

Aortic valvotomy also has been attempted through a closed transventricular approach, with dilators or balloons introduced through the left ventricular apex (Duncan et al., 1987; Neish et al., 1991; Pelech et al., 1987). This has been particularly useful in infants with co-existing aortic coarctation because this approach is available during left-sided thoracotomy for repair of the coarctation (Trinkle et al., 1975). Others have described combined repair of coarctation with aortic valvotomy through a median sternotomy approach on CPB (Ungerleider and Ebert, 1987). Although closed transventricular valvotomy may be useful occasionally, most centers today employ an open transaortic valvotomy for patients with this disease.

Although some groups have advocated direct-vision repair of valvular aortic stenosis in infants, using venous occlusion with varying degrees of hypothermia (Castañeda and Norwood, 1985; de Leval, 1994; Sink et al., 1984), this technique is now applied only in the exceptional case. Caval occlusion has some attractiveness because it avoids bypass, but during this procedure neither the body nor the heart receives any blood flow and repair must be performed in less than 2 to 3 minutes. This technique has been criticized by others experienced in this procedure (Messina et al., 1984) because these infants often cannot tolerate the additional hemodynamic insult of this technique. Furthermore, the long-term adequacy of valvotomy performed in this manner is questionable (Stewart et al., 1978). Most surgeons now perform transaortic valvotomy on CPB. The use of CPB, which provides resuscitation and support for infants during the valvotomy, has improved surgical results (Turley et al., 1990). Techniques for CPB vary among different institutions. We use a median sternotomy, and in critically ill infants the pump prime is cooled to 7° C so that the heart is perfused with cold blood as soon as CPB is begun. Before establishing CPB, intraoperative color-flow Doppler can be performed using a hand-held epicardial probe. Placement of the probe directly on the epicardial surface eliminates all chest wall attenuation and provides superb anatomic delineation of the LVOTO. In this manner, before the aorta is cross-clamped, the anatomy of the aortic valve and any subvalvular pathology can be identified (Ungerleider et al., 1990).

The ascending aorta is cannulated near the innominate artery; a single venous cannula is employed (Fig. 41–5). After CPB is initiated, the ductus arteriosus is snared. The ascending aorta is cross-clamped, but no cardioplegia is administered if only aortic valvotomy is planned. A standard transverse aortotomy is performed. The aortic valve is inspected carefully so that the most direct and specific procedure can be performed. Because rewarming is begun almost immediately, CPB time is limited. The aortotomy is closed after completion of the procedure, and de-airing is performed prior to release of the cross-clamp. In patients with significant pulmonary artery hypertension, it is occasionally reasonable to unsnare the ductus and leave it patent with prostaglandin infusion for the first few postoperative days (Ungerleider, 1991). In these patients, a patent ductus in the immediate postoperative period helps to maintain systemic perfusion and to decompress pulmonary artery hypertension while the left ventricular compliance improves. However, if ductal patency is still required beyond 3 to 5 days, the adequacy of the left ventricular outflow tract to sustain a systemic function should be questioned. A pulmonary artery line and left atrial line are advisable to assist in postoperative management. The patient is always placed in an intensive care unit postoperatively.

## Older Infants and Children

Patients who present beyond the neonatal period with valvular aortic stenosis are usually not as critically ill, and the goal of operation is to reduce the left ventricular outflow gradient. The use of percutaneously introduced balloons for dilitation of valvular aortic stenosis may hold promise in older children, because the balloon opens valves along the areas of commissural fusion and, when properly used, produces minimal, if any, regurgitation and good long-

FIGURE 41–5. *A*, The physiology of critical aortic stenosis in infancy is benefited by patency of the ductus arteriosus. This allows right ventricular outflow to assist with perfusion of the aorta and permits decompression of the pulmonary hypertension that is often associated with this defect. It is for this reason that these patients often require infusion of prostaglandin $E_1$ ($PGE_1$) until more definitive therapy is available. *B*, In neonates with critical aortic stenosis who require valvotomy, the heart is approached through a median sternotomy (*inset*), and the patient is cannulated for cardiopulmonary bypass using a single atrial cannula. Bypass is begun with a cold (7° C) prime, and immediately after inception of bypass, the ductus arteriosus is occluded with a snare. An aortic cross-clamp is placed, and the transverse incision is made in the ascending aorta. It is not necessary to provide cardioplegia solution in infants. Rewarming on bypass is begun immediately after the aorta is cross-clamped. *C*, The stenotic aortic valve is inspected through the aortotomy incision, and the areas of commissural fusion are identified. *D*, The fused commissures are usually opened with a knife blade; the incision should be extended toward the annulus at either extreme. It is important, however, to keep the incision from extending into the annulus so that postvalvotomy aortic insufficiency is minimized. *E*, In some patients with dysplastic but tricommissural aortic valves, it is helpful to insert a cardiotomy sucker through the valve to enable careful incision of all fused commissures. *F*, The aortotomy is then repaired with a double line of continuous suture, and the patient is weaned from cardiopulmonary bypass. The ductus arteriosus should be ligated if the patient is stable; if the patient has persistent pulmonary hypertension and low cardiac output, however, the ductus can be left open and the patient can be maintained on prostaglandin infusion during the initial postoperative course until left ventricular compliance and forward cardiac output through the left ventricle improves. (*A–F*, From Sabiston, D. C., Jr.: Atlas of Cardiothoracic Surgery. Philadelphia, W. B. Saunders, 1995.)

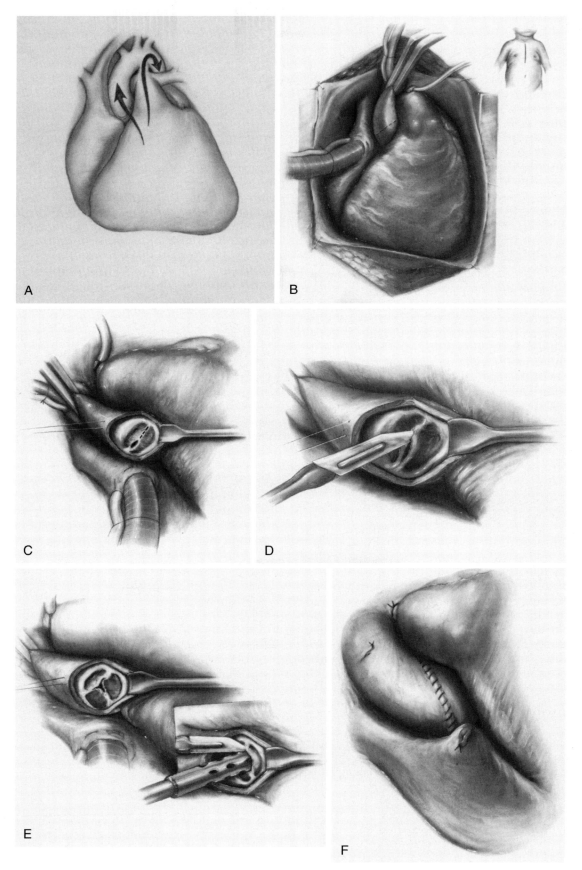

**FIGURE 41–5.** *See legend on opposite page*

term relief of the left ventricular outflow obstruction. Several techniques, including the use of double balloons in larger children, provide excellent results. For this reason, surgical valvotomy is less commonly employed at many centers. Nevertheless, balloon valvotomy is contraindicated in children with significant aortic insufficiency, and some practitioners prefer the more exacting technique of direct surgical valvotomy, especially when the valve anatomy (seen through echocardiography) appears to be unicuspid or potentially tricuspid. Currently, no prospective studies compare the outcomes of balloon and surgical valvotomy in any age group (Freedom, 1990).

The techniques of surgical valvotomy for older children are different from those used in neonates. These procedures are always performed with CPB, using an asanguinous prime if possible. Unless the patient has an associated cardiac defect that is being repaired and that requires bicaval cannulation, a single venous return cannula is sufficient for straightforward aortic valvotomy. The aortic valve is visualized through a transaortic incision after the heart is arrested with cold cardioplegic solution. Moderate systemic hypothermia is employed (30 to 32°C), and rewarming is begun early to limit CPB time. In older patients (beyond the neonatal age group), the anatomy of the aortic valve should be inspected carefully and the valve should be incised along lines of commissural fusion that extend all the way to the annulus. Raphes (which do not extend to the annulus) should not be incised, because this will create unacceptable aortic insufficiency. The aorta and the left side of the heart should then be carefully de-aired, and the aortotomy should be closed. Although there is some value in measuring the left ventricular/aorta gradient using a direct transseptal puncture in the operating room following completion of the procedure (Mavroudis et al., 1984), this pressure gradient must be interpreted in relation to the cardiac output across the valve. Patients are often hyperdynamic after being weaned from CPB (and their hematocrits often change significantly compared with preoperative values), and the cardiac output across the valve can be increased compared with the preoperative state. Intraoperative Doppler imaging can also predict the gradient of the repaired valve and demonstrate the degree of aortic insufficiency that is left after valvotomy.

## Results of Valvotomy

Unfortunately, because EFE is associated with aortic valve stenosis in neonates, the success of even the best procedures has been limited, and the mortality rate in infants has been 9 to 33% (Gundry and Behrendt, 1986; Karl et al., 1990; Kugler et al., 1979; Messina et al., 1984; Pelech et al., 1987; Turley et al., 1990). This rate is highly affected by associated lesions and preoperative condition. Young age appears to be a risk factor only in that it correlates with worse preoperative functional status and associated lesions that propel early presentation (Kirklin and Barratt-Boyes,

1993). Older children respond better, and the mortality rate of valvotomy in children older than 1 year should approach zero (Kirklin and Barratt-Boyes, 1993).

## Aortic Valve Replacement

It is hoped that valvotomy will reduce the aortic valve gradient and enable children to grow until such a time that, if their left ventricular outflow obstruction persists, they can accommodate placement of an adult-size prosthetic valve. It can be predicted that within 10 to 20 years of valvotomy, 35% of children will require a repeat aortic valve operation (Fig. 41–6). Reasons for repeat operation range from recurrent stenosis to progressive aortic insufficiency, and they cannot always be dealt with by repeat valvotomy. The need for eventual reoperation apparently is unrelated to age at initial valvotomy, although the likelihood that the second operation will be limited to repeat valvotomy seems to increase if the initial valvotomy was performed in infancy (Fulton et al., 1983). The usual interval until reoperation in those patients who will require one is 7 years (Johnson et al., 1985). If a second valvotomy can be performed, it usually will last the patient for 34 years before further aortic valve surgery may be required. Given these data, it is not surprising that only 70% of patients surviving an initial valvotomy are able to retain their own valve

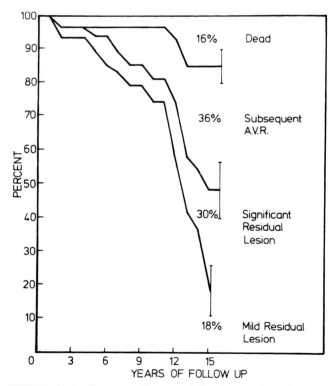

**FIGURE 41–6.** Outcome 15 years following aortic valvotomy. (A.V.R. = aortic valve replacement.) (From Hossack, K. F., Neutze, J. M., Lowe, J. B., et al.: Congenital valvar aortic stenosis: Natural history and assessment for operation. Br. Heart J., 43:561, 1980.)

for more than 10 years (Kirklin and Barratt-Boyes, 1993). The smallest available prosthesis (16 to 17 mm) may be smaller than desirable, and in many cases of aortic valve replacement in children, annular enlarging procedures should be considered. Placement of an aortic valve too small to accommodate the patient's predicted growth can produce short-term successes doomed to eventual failure (Pugliese et al., 1984).

Several types of annular enlarging procedures are available (Fig. 41–7). The simplest technique is to secure the prosthetic valve in a supra-annular position along the noncoronary sinus (David and Uden, 1983; Olin et al., 1983). This sinus can even be enlarged with graft material to allow placement of a larger valve (Najafi et al., 1969; Piehler et al., 1983). The aortic annulus also can be enlarged by incising through the annulus in various locations (Manouguian and Seybold-Epting, 1979; Nicks et al., 1970; Rittenhouse et al., 1979). Most of these procedures allow placement of a valve that is 3 to 5 mm larger at most than what could be accepted by the native annulus. For small children who require more radical enlargement of the aortic annulus, or for children who require relief of subaortic obstruction, the technique of aortoventriculoplasty has been well described and can be performed with a low mortality rate (Konno et al., 1975; Misback et al., 1982; Rastan and Koncz, 1975) (Fig. 41–8). For the safe conduct of any of these procedures, the surgeon must have a clear appreciation of the complex anatomic relationships of the aortic root to important cardiac morphologic and conduction structures (Sud et al., 1984) (Fig. 41–9).

Pulmonary autograft has become increasingly popular, because the autograft may grow with the patient (Elkins, 1992; Elkins et al., 1992; Matsuki et al., 1988; Ross, 1991; Ross et al., 1991). This procedure transfers the patient's normal pulmonary valve to the aortic position (Fig. 41–10) and replaces the pulmonary valve with a cryopreserved homograft. The pulmonary autograft gives young patients a semilunar valve composed of their own normal living tissue. Unlike prosthetic valves, the pulmonary autograft can grow and may represent a dynamic "living annular enlargement" (Elkins, 1992; Ross et al., 1991). This procedure requires caution, because the homograft valve in the pulmonary position will need to be replaced in the future, and the long-term outcome for the transplanted pulmonary valve is still unknown.

The type of valve selected for children is important. Despite initial enthusiasm for their use (Sade et al., 1979), it is now well demonstrated that bioprosthetic valves may undergo early degeneration in children and young adults (Thandroyen et al., 1980; Williams et al., 1982). Therefore, mechanical valves are preferred. Concerns about long-term anticoagulation in children have been raised, and although several groups report excellent results using antiplatelet therapy for children with mechanical aortic prostheses (Verrier et al., 1986), carefully monitored long-term anticoagulation with warfarin (Coumadin) probably

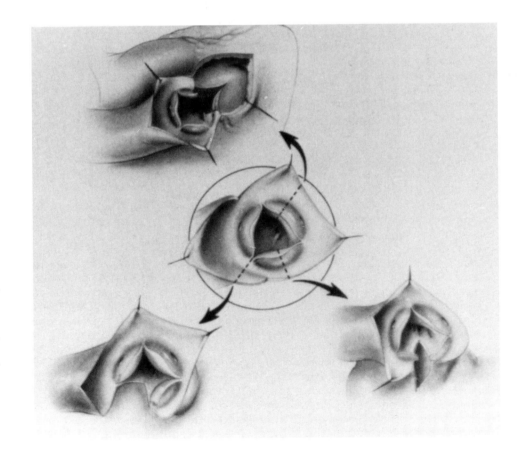

FIGURE 41–7. The various options for enlarging the aortic annulus. Counterclockwise from the lower left, (1) the Rittenhouse-Manouguian procedure, (2) the Nicks (or the Nunez) procedure, and (3) the Konno-Rastan procedure. The Manouguian incision (through the left coronary-noncoronary commissure) can be extended onto the leaflet of the mitral valve, as shown. This area is then patched and can enlarge the aortic annulus by approximately 3 to 5 mm. The Nicks procedure extends through the noncoronary sinus and may or may not enter the roof of the left atrium. The Konno-Rastan aortoventriculoplasty provides the largest increase in aortic annular size and is the method of choice when there is associated subaortic fibromuscular stenosis. (From Doty, D. B.: Replacement of the aortic valve allograft: Considerations and techniques in children. J. Thorac. Cardiovasc. Surg., 2:129, 1987.)

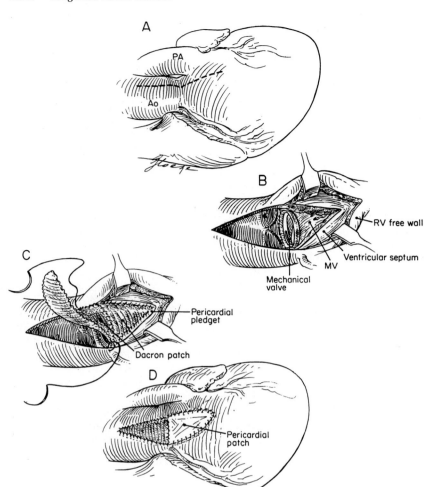

**FIGURE 41–8.** The incision for an aortoventriculoplasty operation *(A)*. This incision is begun on the anterior aspect of the aorta (Ao) and connected to a second incision on the anterior aspect of the right ventricle such that the incisions meet to the left side of the right coronary ostium, where they are extended through the aortic valve annulus onto the interventricular septum *(B)*. (PA = pulmonary artery; MV = mitral valve; RV = right ventricle.) An aortic valve prosthesis can then be placed, and the left ventricular outflow tract can be enlarged *(C)* with a Dacron or Gore-Tex patch. The right ventricle is then repaired *(D)* with a pericardial or Gore-Tex patch. *(A–D,* From Drinkwater, D. C. J., and Laks, H.: The management of subaortic stenosis in children. *In* Jacobs, M. L., and Norwood, W. I. [eds]: Pediatric Cardiac Surgery. Stoneham, MA, Butterworth-Heinemann, 1992, pp. 123–134.)

constitutes standard therapy (Jaklitsch and Leyland, 1988; McGrath et al., 1987; Stewart et al., 1978). Some authors have recommended adding aspirin to warfarin therapy (Turpie et al., 1993). More recently, cryopreserved homografts placed into the aortic position have become another option for valve replacement in children (Angell et al., 1987). Further, homografts may provide viable donor cells that enable growth of the implanted valve (O'Brien et al., 1987). Although only long-term follow-up will support the validity of this concept, homografts often are an excellent option for children and young adults. These valves can be placed in the normal annular position using a freehand technique (Doty et al., 1987, 1993), but more recent data suggest that long-term valve function is better if these valves are placed using aortic root replacement (O'Brien et al., 1991). This technique involves reimplantation of the coronary arteries into the wall of the homograft, but it usually poses no problem to surgeons accustomed to performing arterial switch procedures in neonates (Fig. 41–11). Replacement of the aortic valve using this "miniroot" technique has become the preferred method for homograft aortic valve replacement in infants and children, especially those with underlying congenital aortic ste-

nosis, because the orientation of the commissures increases the likelihood that the homograft valve will become distorted when it is sewn into place using the freehand technique.

## SUBVALVULAR STENOSIS

Discrete subvalvular stenosis was first described by Chevers in 1842. In 1956, Brock and Fleming described five cases of subvalvular aortic stenosis diagnosed in living patients. Initial treatment was by transventricular dilatation (Brock, 1954), but in 1960 Spencer and colleagues (1960) described the surgical therapy of this lesion using CPB. A more severe form of muscular obstruction of the left ventricular outflow tract was described by Spencer and associates (1960) and Reis and associates (1971). Various attempts at resection of this form of subaortic stenosis via the left atrium (Lillehei and Levy, 1963), left ventricle (Kirklin and Ellis, 1961), right side of the ventricular septum (Cooley et al., 1967), or aorta (Morrow, 1978) have been reported. Currently, the preferred approach for resection of most forms of subaortic stenosis is through the aorta. Some (Newfeld et al., 1976) believe

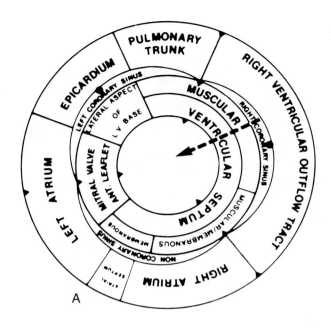

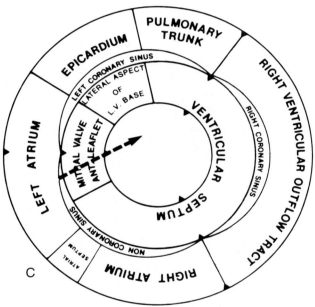

**FIGURE 41–9.** Relationship of various structures at the base of the heart to incisions that can be made for annular enlargement. *A,* The incision that is made for a Manouguian procedure at the commissure between the left coronary and the noncoronary sinus. *B,* The incision made through the noncoronary sinus for a Nicks annular enlargement. *C,* The incision into the muscular ventricular septum used for an aortoventriculoplasty (Konno) procedure. (*A–C,* From Sud, A., Parker, F., and Magilligan, D. J. J.: Anatomy of the aortic root. Reprinted with permission from the Society of Thoracic Surgeons [The Annals of Thoracic Surgery, 1984, Vol. 38, pp. 76–79].)

that subvalvular stenosis requires early repair (i.e., gradient 40 mm Hg) to prevent progression of the lesion to a subaortic fibromuscular tunnel that can be more difficult to repair later (de Leval, 1994). Sudden death from arrhythmias (presumably due to progressive involvement of the His bundle tissue) has evolved from initially mild subaortic stenosis (James et al., 1988).

Subvalvular aortic stenosis occurs in 8 to 20% of cases of LVOTO. It may present as either a thin discrete membrane located anteriorly, immediately below the aortic valve or, less commonly, as a diffuse fibromuscular "tunnel" beneath the aortic leaflets. Unusual variants caused by accessory endocardial cushion tissue (Nanton et al., 1979) (Fig. 41–12) and

by tethering of the anterior leaflet of the mitral valve to the interventricular septum (Wright and Wittner, 1983) have been described. Discrete subvalvular aortic stenosis presents rarely in infancy but more often in young children or young adults (Kirklin and Barratt-Boyes, 1993). It may commonly be associated with a VSD and can be seen after spontaneous closure of a VSD. Once present, the lesion can progress rapidly, and frequent follow-up is advised (Mody and Mody, 1975). This can be done with serial two-dimensional echocardiography with Doppler shift analysis. Indications for operative intervention are similar to those for valvular aortic stenosis, but the variability in the anatomy and the age at presentation make the decision more complex. Correction of the membranous

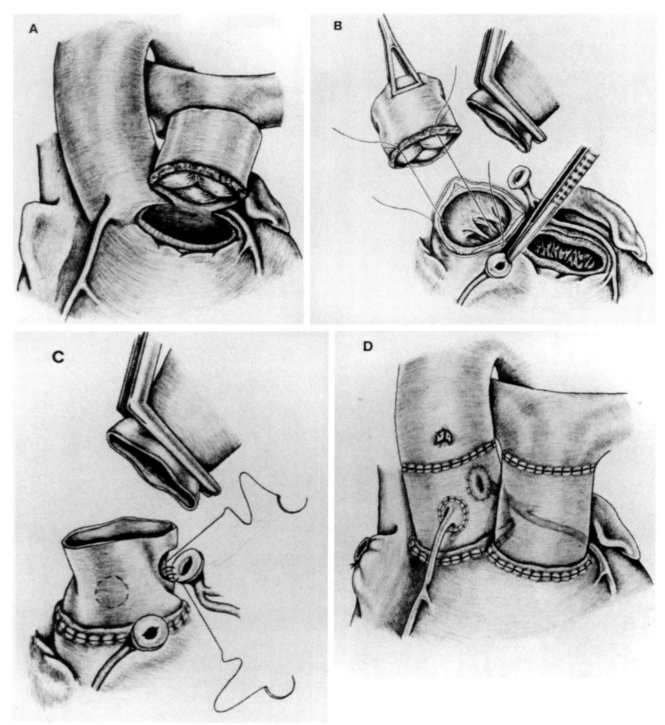

**FIGURE 41–10.** *A,* The pulmonary autograft operation transfers the pulmonary valve, which is carefully excised, especially in its posterior aspect to avoid injury to the first septal perforating branch of the left anterior descending coronary artery (LAD). The patient's native aorta and aortic valve are excised, leaving only the coronary arteries with generous-sized buttons of sinus material. *B,* The pulmonary autograft is then secured to the root of the aorta. This suture line can be continuous or interrupted. *C,* After the pulmonary autograft is secured to the root of the aorta, the left coronary artery is sutured in place on the posterior wall of the autograft. Next, the distal anastomosis between the autograft and the distal aorta is performed. *D,* Then the right coronary artery is sutured to the anterior aspect of the autograft in an appropriate location. The completed autograft procedure utilizes a pulmonary homograft to reconstruct continuity between the right ventricle and the distal pulmonary artery. (*A–D,* From Elkins, R. C.: Autografts and cryopreserved allografts for valve replacement in children. *In* Jacobs, M. L., and Norwood, W. I. [eds]: Pediatric Cardiac Surgery. Stoneham, MA, Butterworth-Heinemann, 1992, pp. 168–181.)

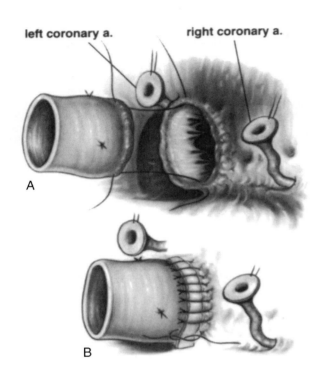

left coronary a.    right coronary a.

A

B

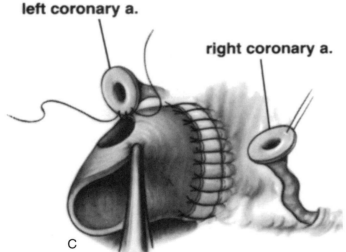

left coronary a.

right coronary a.

C

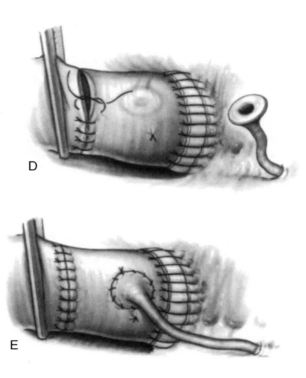

D

E

**FIGURE 41–11.** The aortic valve can be replaced with aortic homograft. *A,* In this case, the patient's native aortic valve and aorta have been removed except for large sinuses of aortic wall, which contain the right and left coronary arteries. *B,* A cryopreserved aortic homograft is then secured to the aortic annulus using interrupted or continuous suture technique. A Teflon felt pledget can be used to reduce the incidence of bleeding. *C,* The left coronary artery is then anastomosed to the posterior wall of the homograft using continuous suture. *D,* Next, the distal anastomosis between the homograft and the distal aorta is performed. This can be done with continuous or interrupted sutures. *E,* Finally, the right coronary artery is secured to the anterior wall of the homograft in a manner that prevents distortion of the coronary artery. (*A–E,* From de Leval, M.: Surgery of the left ventricular outflow tract. *In* Stark, J., and de Leval, M. [eds]: Surgery for Congenital Heart Defects. 2nd ed. Philadelphia, W. B. Saunders, 1994, pp. 511–538.)

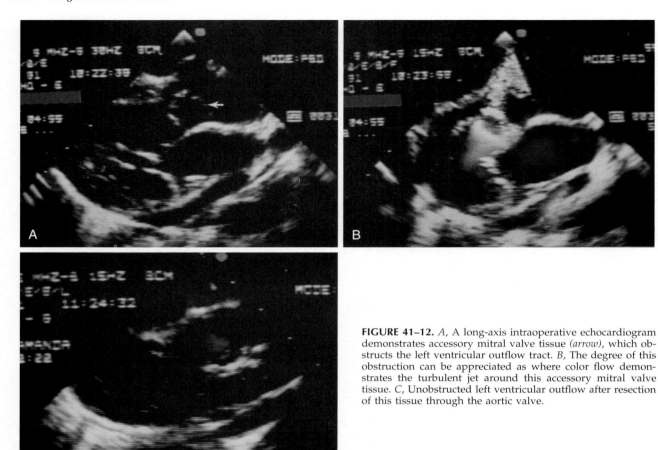

**FIGURE 41–12.** *A,* A long-axis intraoperative echocardiogram demonstrates accessory mitral valve tissue *(arrow),* which obstructs the left ventricular outflow tract. *B,* The degree of this obstruction can be appreciated as where color flow demonstrates the turbulent jet around this accessory mitral valve tissue. *C,* Unobstructed left ventricular outflow after resection of this tissue through the aortic valve.

form necessitates an incision in the aorta, retraction of the usually normal aortic valve leaflets, and careful resection of the membrane; care must be taken not to injure the conduction system, the sinus portion of the right aortic valve cusp, or the anterior leaflet of the mitral valve (which is usually subjacent to the lesion) (de Leval, 1994; Spencer et al., 1960; Sud et al., 1984) (Fig. 41–13). Most surgeons now recommend resection of a portion of the muscle in the interventricular septum at the same time that the subaortic membrane is resected in order to reduce residual obstruction from hypertrophied septal muscle (Gallotti et al., 1981) and to limit the likelihood of early recurrence (Drinkwater and Laks, 1992; Lupinetti et al., 1992) (Fig. 41–14). Early resection may prevent progression to the more severe fibromuscular variety (Oldham, 1986).

Repair of the LVOTO caused by the more diffuse, fibromuscular lesions may be amenable to resection of enough obstructing tissue to relieve the stenosis, although there is an increased danger of damaging the integrity of the interventricular septum, the mitral valve, or the conduction system. Some obstructions cannot be relieved safely by transaortic resection and require more complicated procedures, such as aorto-ventriculoplasty using prosthetic (mechanical) valves or cryopreserved homograft (Konn et al., 1975; Mis-

back et al., 1982; Rastan and Koncz, 1975; Schaffer et al., 1986) (Figs. 41–8 to 41–15) or implantation of a valved conduit between the left ventricle and the aorta, thus bypassing the normal outflow tract (Behrendt and Rocchini, 1987; Brown et al., 1984; Norwood et al., 1983). The indications for a left ventricular/aorta conduit are debatable, and in any case this option is rarely used because it does not provide good long-term solutions (Kirklin and Barratt Boyes, 1993). When the aortic valve and annulus are normal and elongated subaortic fibrous obstruction occurs, a modified septoplasty to enlarge the subaortic area is warranted (Cooley and Garrett, 1986) (Fig. 41–16). Expectations for good outcome depend heavily on the extent of the lesion and the age of the patient. Patients with discrete subvalvular stenosis can respond nicely to simple excision of the obstructing membrane, with a mortality rate that approaches 0%. The rate of recurrent stenosis varies but is in the range of 15 to 20% and probably warrants continued follow-up, although recurrence may reflect inadequate initial resection, especially if no muscle is resected from the interventricular septum below the right/left coronary commissure (Katz et al., 1977; Kirklin and Barratt-Boyes, 1993; Lupinetti et al., 1992). The results are not quite as good in patients with more severe forms of tunnel stenosis (Moses et al.,

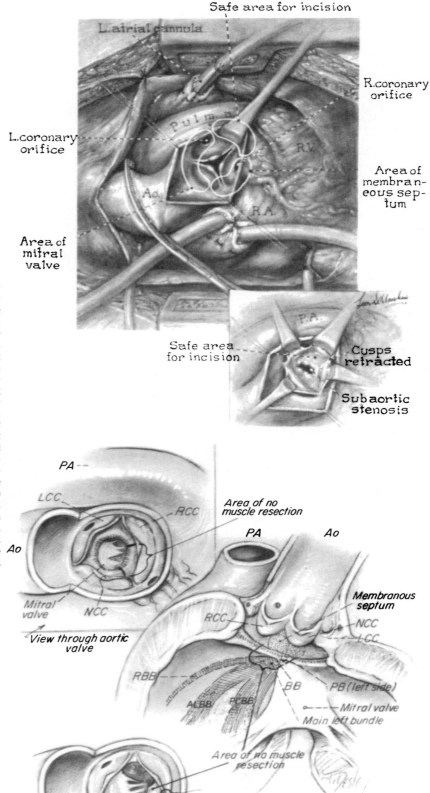

**FIGURE 41–13.** *A*, The areas that must be understood before resection of discrete subaortic stenosis. With the valve cusps retracted, the area of subaortic stenosis can be visualized *(inset)*. It is important to preserve tissue in the area of the membranous septum. The mitral valve must be protected from damage during resection of the membrane in this region. *B*, Appearance of the subvalvular area after resection of the membrane. Note that muscle along the region of the membranous septum is preserved to protect the conduction system. (Ao. = aorta; R.V. = right ventricle; R.A. = right atrium; P.A. = pulmonary artery; LCC = left coronary cusp; RCC = right coronary cusp; NCC = noncoronary cusp; RBB = right bundle branch; BB = bundle branch; PB = penetrating bundle; ALBB = anterior left bundle branch; PLBB = posterior left bundle branch.) (*A*, From Spencer, F. C., Neill, C. A., Sank, L., and Bahnson, H. I.: Anatomical variations in 46 patients with congenital aortic stenosis. Am. Surg., *26*:204, 1960; *B*, From Bharati, S., Lev, M., and Kirklin, J. W.: Cardiac Surgery and the Conduction System. Churchill Livingstone, New York, 1983.)

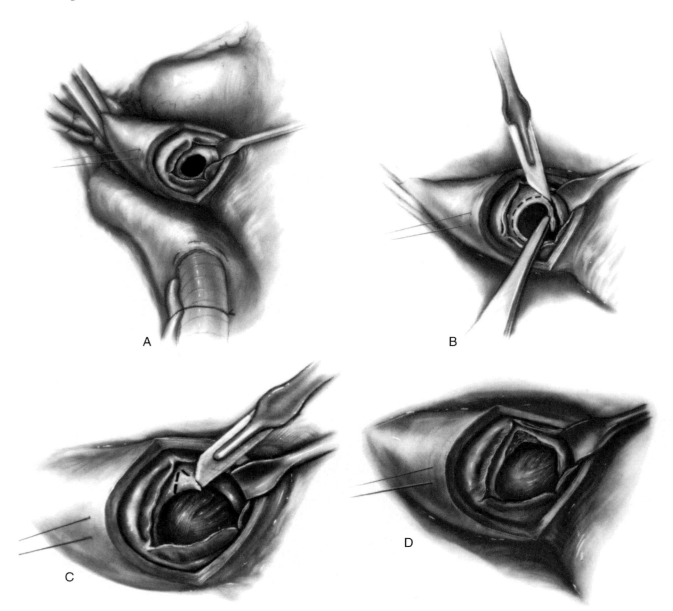

**FIGURE 41–14.** *A,* Subaortic stenosis that is discrete is approached through an aortotomy after the aorta is clamped. Because these patients are usually older and well beyond the neonatal period, it is convenient and helpful to protect the heart with cardioplegia solution. The aortic valve leaflets are carefully retracted, and the fibromuscular shelf can usually be identified below the right and left coronary leaflets. *B,* This membrane is carefully excised with a combination of sharp and blunt dissection. It is important to appreciate the location of the conduction tissue between the noncoronary and the right coronary cusp and to avoid deep incision into the interventricular septum in this region. *C,* After the "membrane" has been completely excised, it is beneficial to remove a wedge of muscle from the interventricular septum below the right and left coronary leaflets. This is a safe region for muscle excision that does not risk the conduction tissue and that produces further disruption of the fibromuscular ridge. This optimizes relief of the subaortic outflow obstruction, as shown in *D.* (*A–D,* From Sabiston, D. C., Jr.: Atlas of Cardiothoracic Surgery. Philadelphia, W. B. Saunders, 1995.)

1984), especially if simple resection is performed, and more extensive procedures such as aortoventriculoplasty should be included in the ultimate plan for these patients. Aortoventriculoplasty has been reported in a 5-day-old infant (Guyton et al., 1986), but is generally deferred until patients are at least 2 years old. It may be more appropriate to consider pulmonary autografts in young patients because of their growth potential (Elkins, 1992; Ross et al., 1991). Because it is unusual for subaortic stenosis to present in

infancy, patients who present with severe subvalvular LVOTO in infancy may have serious deformity of the entire left side of the heart-aorta complex and might be better staged to a Fontan procedure (Kirklin and Barratt-Boyes, 1993; Rhodes et al., 1991).

A variant of subaortic stenosis is created by asymmetric septal hypertrophy. It has been well described by Braunwald and colleagues (1964) and Morrow and colleagues (1975) and is called *idiopathic hypertrophic subaortic stenosis* or *hypertrophic obstructive cardiomyop-*

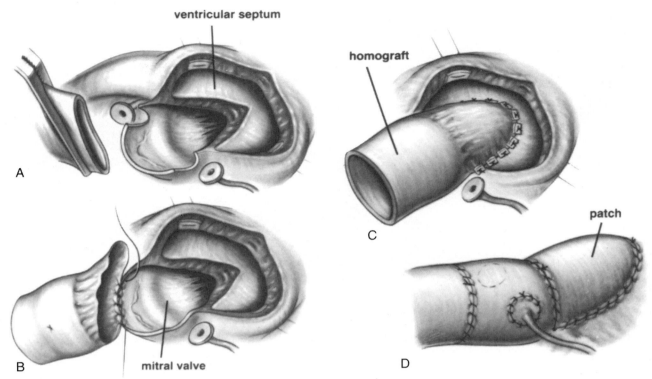

**FIGURE 41–15.** An aortoventriculoplasty can be performed with cryopreserved homograft. *A,* The native aorta and aortic valve have been excised except for buttons of tissue that contain the coronary arteries. An incision in the right ventricle, which is to the left of the right coronary artery, is then performed to expose the interventricular septum, which is incised into the left ventricular outflow tract to enlarge the subaortic area. *B,* A cryopreserved aortic valve homograft is secured to this opening by first placing the posterior portion of the homograft to the native aortic root. *C,* The mitral valve tissue of the aortic valve homograft is used to patch enlarge the incision in the interventricular septum. Coronary arteries are then placed into the homograft, and the homograft is anastomosed to the distal aorta. Finally, *D,* the incision in the right ventricular outflow tract is closed with a patch (usually Gore-Tex, homograft, or pericardium). (*A–D,* From de Leval, M.: Surgery of the left ventricular outflow tract. *In* Stark, J., and de Leval, M. [eds]: Surgery for Congenital Heart Defects. 2nd ed. Philadelphia, W. B. Saunders, 1994, pp. 511–538.)

*athy* (HOCM). Unlike the other forms of fixed LVOTO, this appears to be a dynamic obstruction in which the hypertrophied septum interferes with outflow and depends on the contractile state of the heart and the left ventricular systolic volume. The obstruction is exacerbated by anterior motion of the anterior leaflet of the mitral valve during systole so that it anatomically approaches the hypertrophied septum and obstructs the left ventricular outflow tract. This obstruction is increased by inotropic agents, by diminished blood volume, by the Valsalva maneuver, or by nitroglycerin (Braunwald et al., 1964). The gradient is reduced by propranolol or adrenergic blockage, by increased blood volume, or by general anesthesia (Oldham, 1986). These patients can be treated medically with propranolol or they may be managed surgically by myectomy with excision of a portion of the hypertrophied septum (through the aortic valve) (Morrow, 1978) (Fig. 41–17). Some surgeons favor mitral valve replacement with a low-profile mitral valve, because this also removes part of the anatomic obstruction. This approach may be most useful in patients with pronounced *systolic anterior motion* of the mitral valve or in those with substantial mitral insufficiency. A surgical approach is indicated when the

patient remains symptomatic despite appropriate medical management.

## SUPRAVALVULAR STENOSIS

Supravalvular aortic stenosis was first described by Mencarelli in 1930. In 1958, Dennie and Verhuegt demonstrated how this form of LVOTO could be recognized by retrograde arterial catheterization with pull-back pressures at various locations. In 1961, Williams and colleagues described the association of supravalvular aortic stenosis, mental retardation, and "elfin" facies (Fig. 41–18), a syndrome that now bears his name and that has been substantiated by others (Cornell et al., 1966). Subsequently, the presence of severe infantile hypercalcemia (Garcia et al., 1964; Hooft et al., 1963) or peripheral pulmonary stenosis (Beuren et al., 1964) has been associated with this syndrome. Also, a form of supravalvular aortic stenosis occurs without the characteristic facies (Sissman et al., 1959). The first successful surgical correction of supravalvular aortic stenosis by patch graft enlargement was reported by McGoon and associates at the Mayo Clinic in 1961. The first patient in this series

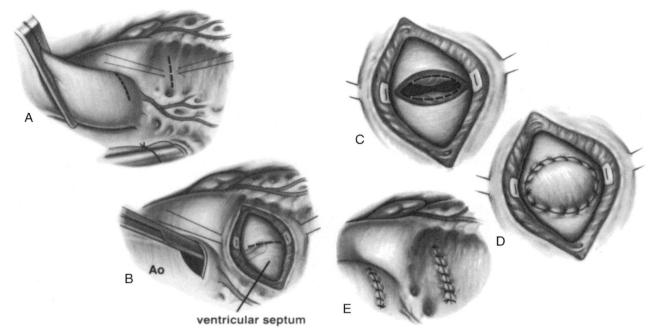

ventricular septum

FIGURE 41–16. Patients who have obstruction of the left ventricular outflow tract but a normal aortic valve can undergo a modified aortoventriculoplasty. *A,* An incision is made in the aorta (Ao) and in the right ventricular outflow tract. A right-angle clamp *(B)* is then placed through the aortic valve and against the interventricular septum so that its location can be identified through the incision in the right ventricular outflow tract. *C,* An incision is made over the clamp, and the obstructing tissue in the left ventricular outflow tract *(dashed line)* can be excised. The ventricular septal defect is then repaired with a patch *(D)*, and both incisions are closed *(E)*. (*A–E,* From de Leval, M.: Surgery of the left ventricular outflow tract. *In* Stark, J., and de Leval, M. [eds]: Surgery for Congenital Heart Defects. 2nd ed. Philadelphia, W. B. Saunders, 1994, pp. 511–538.)

actually underwent surgery in 1956. Reports of treatment for this lesion with resection and end-to-end anastomosis (Hara et al., 1962) as well as by excision of the intimal ridge without patch enlargement (Hancock, 1961) also appeared. Currently, patch aortoplasty is the recommended treatment.

This form of stenosis can also present as either localized or diffuse (Fig. 41–19). The lesion is actually a coarctation or hypoplasia of the ascending aorta with varying degrees of intimal hyperplasia. The disease is uncommon in adults, and untreated patients with supravalvular stenosis probably die before reaching adult life (Pasengrau et al., 1973). Presentation is similar to that in other forms of LVOTO,

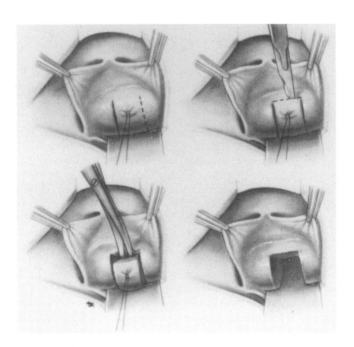

FIGURE 41–17. For patients with muscular subaortic stenosis (as in idiopathic hypertrophic subaortic stenosis), a wedge of muscle in the outflow septum can be safely excised between the right and the left aortic cusps. (From de Leval, M.: Left ventricular outflow tract obstruction. *In* Stark, J., and de Leval, M. [eds]: Surgery for Congenital Heart Defects. New York, Grune & Stratton, 1983.)

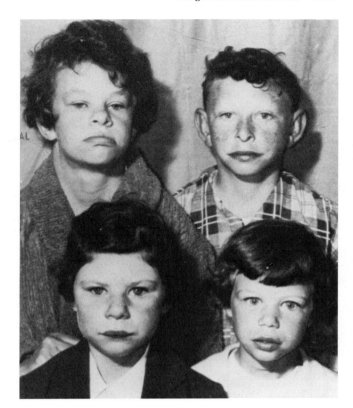

**FIGURE 41–18.** The "elfin" facies prominent in patients with supravalvular stenosis. Note the features of the ears, nose, and lips in these patients. (From Williams, J. C. P., Barratt-Boyes, B. G., and Lowe, J. B.: Supravalvular aortic stenosis. Circulation, 24:1311, 1961. By permission of the American Heart Association.)

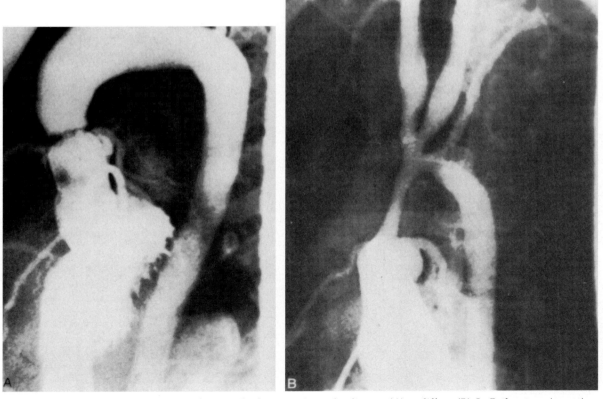

**FIGURE 41–19.** The angiographic appearance of supravalvular stenosis can be discrete (A) or diffuse (B). In B, the stenosis continues onto the innominate, carotid, and subclavian arteries. (A and B, From Kirklin, J. W., and Barratt-Boyes, B. G.: Cardiac Surgery. Churchill Livingstone, New York, 1986.)

although associated anomalies such as peripheral pulmonary stenosis may complicate the clinical course.

Surgical treatment for the discrete form of this lesion is performed on CPB with moderate hypothermia. After the aorta has been cross-clamped and the heart protected with cardioplegia, the proximal aorta is opened through the area of stenosis with an incision that extends into both the right and noncoronary sinus of Valsalva (Fig. 41–20). A Y-shaped patch of prosthetic material is then used to enlarge the ascending aorta (Doty et al., 1977). Resection of an intimal ridge opposite prosthetic patch aortoplasty increases the risk of aneurysm formation, so this part of the procedure should be omitted (DeSanto et al., 1987; Hehrlein et al., 1986). Alternative procedures include a single-patch (Fig. 41–21) or end-to-end aortic anastomosis after excision of the narrowed area (Fig. 41–22). It is important to relieve constriction of the sinus area of the aortic valve (Doty et al., 1977; Myers et al., 1993). Because the area of narrowing can be fairly proximal and diffuse, excision with end-to-end anastomosis may be difficult and may risk injury to the aortic valve leaflets and the coronary arteries.

When the stenosis is diffuse, with generalized hypoplasia of the ascending aorta, arterial cannulation may need to be accomplished through the femoral route. The patient is cooled to 18° C, and the repair is accomplished under total circulatory arrest. A longitudinal incision is made through the area of stenosis; this can be patched with prosthetic material or with a piece of homograft. During this procedure, the head vessels should be clamped and the incision should be carried onto the proximal portion of these vessels if stenosis exists at this level. Some groups suggest treating this form of stenosis with a left ventricular apical-to-aortic bypass shunt (Keane et al., 1976).

Repair of the localized form of congenital supravalvular aortic stenosis carries a lower hospital mortality rate and better long-term prognosis than its diffuse counterpart. The operative mortality rate in the localized form approaches 0%, whereas it can be as high as 40% in the diffuse form. Similarly, late survival is good, and the reoperation rate is low (Kirklin and Barratt-Boyes, 1993; Myers et al., 1993). Because this is a form of left ventricular outflow tract obstruction, indications for surgery are similar to those for valvular or subvalvular stenosis.

## OVERALL RESULTS

In the evaluation of any procedure on young patients for congenital lesions, it is crucial to assess the long-term benefits of the surgical intervention. The complications of LVOTO include sudden death, SBE, and heart failure (from chronic left ventricular systolic overload or aortic insufficiency). Most procedures performed on infants or young children are palliative, relieving the stenosis and reducing the chance of early death. Many patients with valvular lesions eventually require valve replacement when they are larger. The incidence of sudden death among patients with congenital aortic stenosis varies between 1 and 19%, and in untreated patients the risk has been estimated at

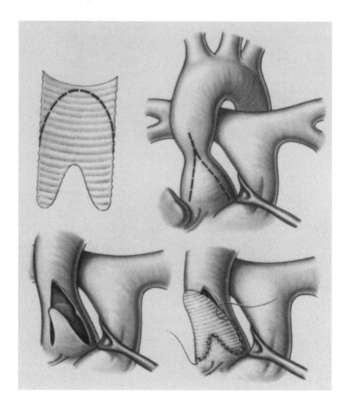

FIGURE 41–20. A patient with discrete supravalvular aortic stenosis can be repaired by making a Y incision through the area of narrowing and into the noncoronary and right coronary sinus. A patch is then fashioned (out of Gore-Tex or Dacron) and sutured into this incision such that it enlarges the aorta and the subjacent sinuses. (From Myers, J. L., Waldhausen, J. A., Cyran, S. E., et al.: Results of surgical repair of congenital supravalvular aortic stenosis. J. Thorac. Cardiovasc. Surg., *105*:281–288, 1993.)

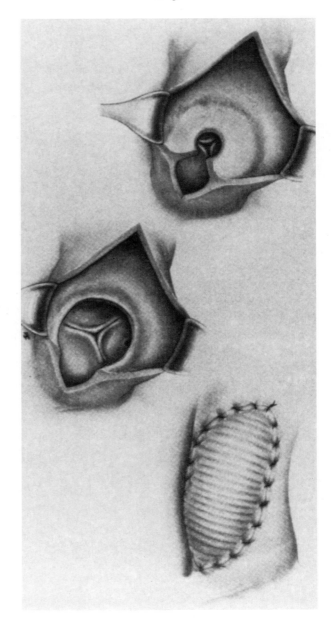

**FIGURE 41–21.** A patient with discrete supravalvular aortic stenosis can be repaired with a single patch after the obstructing ridge has been incised and the excess tissue has been excised. The aorta is then repaired with a single patch. (From Myers, J. L., Waldhausen, J. A., Cyran, S. E., et al.: Results of surgical repair of congenital supravalvular aortic stenosis. J. Thorac. Cardiovasc. Surg., *105*:281–288, 1993.)

0.9% per annum (Campbell, 1968; Glew et al., 1969; Kirklin and Barratt-Boyes, 1993). Those with more severe lesions, as evidenced by symptoms, pertinent physical findings, or objective pressure data, appear to be at greatest risk for sudden death (Braunwald et al., 1963; Glew et al., 1969; Hossack et al., 1980). Valvotomy does not eliminate this risk, but it does reduce it to an estimated 0.29% per annum (Stewart et al., 1978). SBE is always a risk in the presence of turbulence across abnormal anatomy. Without operation, approximately 3.1 episodes of SBE will occur for every 1000 patient-years with aortic stenosis—in other words, there is a 1.4% chance of endocarditis in the first 30 years of life. This incidence increases after operation, with a 7.4% risk of SBE in the first 30 years of life (Stewart et al., 1978). Although the chance of heart failure from systolic overload is reduced by an adequate procedure, the incidence of aortic insuffi-

ciency probably triples in patients with primary valvular lesions from 11% preoperatively to 30 to 40% postoperatively (Stewart et al., 1978). Twenty per cent of these patients may be symptomatic.

Despite these figures, the survival of patients with significant stenotic lesions is enhanced by surgery. However, because the procedures for valvular aortic stenosis are palliative and increase the risk of SBE and aortic regurgitation, they should probably be performed only in children with severe lesions who are at high risk of sudden death (Olley et al., 1978). Correction of subvalvular and supravalvular forms of LVOTO can lead to a better long-term result, depending on the nature of the lesion. The palliative nature of these procedures requires proper timing in patient selection so that the current clinical condition is not replaced by new problems of equal or greater concern.

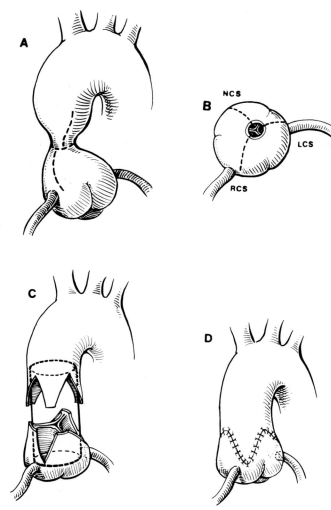

**FIGURE 41–22.** End-to-end reconstruction of the aorta in a patient with supravalvular narrowing can be performed without prosthetic material. *A*, The aorta is transected at the level of narrowing, and incisions are made *(B)* into each coronary sinus. (NCS = noncoronary sinus; RCS = right coronary sinus; LCS = left coronary sinus.) *C*, The distal aorta is then anastomosed to the aortic root by making counter incisions to provide flaps of aortic tissue. *D*, This provides excision of the area of the discrete narrowing and aortic reconstruction without the use of prosthetic material. (*A–D*, From Myers, J. L., Waldhausen, J. A., Cyran, S. E., et al.: Results of surgical repair of congenital supravalvular aortic stenosis. J. Thorac. Cardiovasc. Surg., *105*:281–288, 1993.)

## SELECTED BIBLIOGRAPHY

Campbell, M.: The natural history of congenital aortic stenosis. Br. Heart J., *30*:514, 1968.

In order to make proper therapeutic decisions it is essential that one have an understanding of the natural history of a disease. This paper nicely depicts the expectations for various forms of aortic stenosis. It is based on these data that current surgical decisions can be made.

de Leval, M.: Surgery of the Left Ventricular Outflow Tract. *In* Stark, J., and de Leval, M. (eds): Surgery for Congenital Heart Defects. 2nd ed. Philadelphia, W. B. Saunders, 1994, pp. 511–538.

This newly revised edition of the experience from Great Ormond Street Hospital for Sick Children in London, England, is a beautifully illustrated work that provides up-to-date information regarding the variety of procedures used to treat the various forms of aortic stenosis. This book is especially helpful for the practicing surgeon because it emphasizes the technical aspects of congenital heart surgery.

Kirklin, J. W., Barratt-Boyes, B. G.: Cardiac Surgery. 2nd ed. New York, Churchill Livingstone, 1993.

These two authors share their extraordinary experience in the field of congenital heart surgery and supply a comprehensive and beautifully organized document that discusses all aspects of the presentation and treatment of the various forms of congenital aortic stenosis. This chapter is must reading for anyone who desires in-depth knowledge of this field.

Sud, A., Parker, F., and Magilligan, D. J., Jr.: Anatomy of the aortic root. Ann. Thorac. Surg., *38*:76–79, 1984.

The authors provide beautiful, precise anatomic illustrations of the anatomy of the aortic root. Clear understanding of this anatomy is essential for safe surgical therapy for the various forms of congenital aortic stenosis.

Turley, K., Bove, E. L., Amato, J. J., et al.: Neonatal aortic stenosis. J. Thorac. Cardiovasc. Surg., *99*:679–684, 1990.

In this article the authors maintain that aortic valvotomy can be performed more safely in critically ill newborns with the technique of cardiopulmonary bypass. Forty infants (from 3 institutions) requiring aortic valvotomy in the first 30 days of life had an overall hospital survival of 87.5% (35/40). Although multiple methods of perfusion and valvotomy were used, the single unifying factor of cardiopulmonary bypass stabilization was present in all 40 patients. The authors suggest that these are the results against which balloon aortic valvotomy should be compared and that this technique should be considered the standard form of therapy in the modern era.

## BIBLIOGRAPHY

Angell, W. W., Angell, J. D., and Oury, J. H.: Long-term follow-up of viable frozen aortic homografts. A viable homograft valve bank. J. Thorac. Cardiovasc. Surg., *93*:815–822, 1987.

Ankeney, J. L., Tzena, T. S., and Liebman J.: Surgical therapy for congenital aortic valvular stenosis. J. Thorac. Cardiovasc. Surg., *85*:41, 1983.

Behrendt, D. M., Rocchini M.: Relief of the left ventricular outflow tract obstruction in infants and small children with valved extracardiac conduits. Ann. Thorac. Surg., *43*:82–86, 1987.

Bernhard, W. F., Kean, J. F., Fellows, K. E., et al.: Progress and problems in the surgical management of congenital aortic stenosis. J. Thorac. Cardiovasc. Surg., *66*:404, 1973.

Beuren, A. J., Schulze C., Eberlet P., et al.: The syndrome of supravalvular aortic stenosis, peripheral pulmonary stenosis, mental retardation and similar facial appearance. Am. J. Cardiol., *13*:471, 1964.

Braunwald, E., Goldblatt, A., Augen, M. M., et al.: Congenital aortic stenosis. I: Clinical and hemodynamic findings in 100 patients. Circulation., *27*:426, 1963.

Braunwald, E., Oldham, H. N., and Ross, J.: The circulatory response of patients with idiopathic hypertrophic subaortic stenosis to nitroglycerin and to the Valsalva maneuver. Circulation., *29*:422, 1964.

Braverman, I. B., and Gibson S.: The outlook for children with congenital aortic stenosis. Am. Heart J., *53*:487, 1957.

Brock, R. C.: Valvotomy for aortic stenosis. Br. Heart J., *16*:471, 1954.

Brown, L. W., Girod, D. A., Hurwitz, R. A., et al.: Apicoaortic valved conduits for complex left ventricular outflow obstruction. Technical considerations and current status. Ann. Thorac. Surg., *38*:162-168, 1984.

Campbell, M.: The natural history of congenital aortic stenosis. Br. Heart J., *30*:514, 1968.

Carrel, A.: On the experimental surgery of the thoracic aorta and the heart. Ann. Surg., *52*:83, 1910.

Castaneda, A., Norwood, W.: Left ventricular outflow tract obstruction. *In* Arciniegas, E. (ed): Pediatric Cardiac Surgery. Chicago, Year Book, 1985.

Choy, N., Beekman, R. H., Rocchini, A. P., et al.: Percutaneous balloon valvuloplasty for valvular aortic stenosis in infants and children. Am. J. Cardiol., *59*:1010–1013, 1987.

Cooley, D. A., Bloodwell, R. D., Hallman, G. L., et al.: Surgical treatment of muscular subaortic stenosis: Results from septectomy in twenty-six patients. Circulation, *35*:124, 1967.

Cooley, D. A., and Garrett, J. R.: Septoplasty for left ventricular outflow obstruction without aortic valve replacement: A new technique. Ann. Thorac. Surg., *42*:445–448, 1986.

Cornell, W. P., Elkins, R. C., Criley, J. M., and Sabiston, D. C., Jr.: Supravalvular aortic stenosis. J. Thorac. Cardiovasc. Surg., 51:484, 1966.

David, T. E., and Uden, R. C.: Aortic valve replacement in adult patients with small aortic annuli. Ann. Thorac. Surg., 51:484, 1983.

de Leval, M.: Surgery of the left ventricular outflow tract. In Stark, J., and de Leval, M. (eds): Surgery for Congenital Heart Defects. 2nd ed. Philadelphia, W. B. Saunders, 1994, pp. 511–538.

DeSanto, A., Bills, R. G., and King, H.: Pathogenesis of aneurysm formation opposite prosthetic patches used for coarctation repair. An experimental study. J. Thorac. Cardiovasc. Surg., 94:720–723, 1987.

Dobell, A. R. C., Bloss, R. S., Gibbons, J. E., Collins, G. F.: Congenital valvular aortic stenosis. J. Thorac. Cardiovasc. Surg., 81:916, 1981.

Doty, D. B., Michielon, G., Wang, N. D., et al.: Replacement of the aortic valve with cryopreserved aortic allograft. Ann. Thorac. Surg., 56:228–236, 1993.

Doty, D. B., Polansky, D. B., Jenson, C. B.: Supravalvular aortic stenosis: Repair by external aortoplasty. J. Thorac. Cardiac Surg., 74:362, 1977.

Doty, D. B., Polansky, D. B., Jenson, C. B.: Replacement of the aortic valve with cryopreserved aortic valve allograft: Considerations and techniques in children. J. Cardiac Surg. 2(1):129, 1987.

Drinkwater, D. C. J., and Laks, H.: The management of subaortic stenosis in children. In Jacobs, M. L., and Norwood, W. I. (eds): Pediatric Cardiac Surgery. Stoneham, MA, Butterworth Heinemann, 1992, pp. 123–134.

Duncan, K., Sullivan, I., Robinson, P., et al.: Transventricular aortic valvotomy for critical aortic stenosis in infants. J. Thorac. Cardiovasc. Surg., 93:546–50, 1987.

El-Said, G., Galioto, F. M., Mullins, C. E., et al.: Natural hemodynamic history of congenital aortic stenosis in childhood. Am. J. Cardiol., 30:6, 1972.

Elkins, R. C.: Autografts and cryopreserved allografts for valve replacement in children. In Jacobs, M. L., and Norwood, W. I. (eds): Pediatric Cardiac Surgery. Stoneham, MA, Butterworth Heinemann, 1992, pp. 168–181.

Elkins, R. C., Santangelo, K., Stelzer, P., et al.: Pulmonary autograft replacement of the aortic valve: An evolution of technique. J. Cardiac Surg., 7:108–116, 1992.

Freedom, R. M.: Neonatal aortic stenosis–The balloon deflated? J. Thorac. Cardiovasc. Surg., 100:927–928, 1990.

Friedman, W. F., Modlinger, J., and Morgan, J. R.: Serial hemodynamic observations in asymptomatic children with valvular aortic stenosis. Circulation, 43:91–97, 1979.

Fulton, D. R., Hougen, T. J., Keane, J. F., et al.: Repeat aortic valvotomy in children. Am. Heart J., 1067:60, 1983.

Gallotti, R., Wain, W. H., and Ross, D. N.: Surgical enucleation of discrete sub-aortic stenosis. Thorac. Cardiovasc. Surg., 29:312, 1981.

Garcia, R. E., Friedman, W. F., Kaback, M. M., and Rowe, R. D.: Idiopathic hypercalcaemia and supravalvular aortic stenosis: Documentation of a new syndrome. N. Engl. J. Med., 271:117, 1964.

Glew, R. H., Varghese, P. J., Krovetz, L. J., et al.: Sudden death in congenital aortic stenosis: A review of eight cases with an evaluation of premonitory clinical features. Am. Heart J., 78:615, 1969.

Gundry, S. R., Behrendt, D. M.: Prognostic factors in valvotomy for critical aortic stenosis in infancy. J. Thorac. Cardiovasc. Surg., 92:747–754, 1986.

Guyton, R. A., Michalik, R. E., McIntyre, A. B., et al.: Aortic atresia and aortico-left ventricular tunnel: Successful surgical management by Konno aortoventriculoplasty in a neonate. J. Thorac. Cardiovasc. Surg., 92:1099–1105, 1986.

Hallman, G. L., and Cooley, D. A.: Congenital aortic stenosis. In Sabiston, D. C., Jr. and Spencer, F. C. (eds): Gibbon's Surgery of the Chest. Philadelphia, W. B. Saunders, 1983, pp. 1109–1115.

Hancock, E.: Differentiation of valvular, subvalvular and supravalvular aortic stenosis. Guy's Hosp. Rep., 110:1, 1961.

Hara, M., Duncan, T., and Lincoln, B.: Supravalvular aortic stenosis: Report of successful excision and aortic re-anastomosis. J. Thorac. Cardiovasc. Surg., 43:212, 1962.

Hehrlein, F. W., Mulch, J., Rautenburg, H. W., et al.: Incidence and pathogenesis of late aneurysms after patch graft aortoplasty for coarctation. J. Thorac. Cardiovasc. Surg., 92:226–230, 1986.

Hooft, C., Vermassen, A., and Blancquaert, A.: Observation concerning the evolution of the chronic form of idiopathic hypercalcaemia in children. Helv. Paediatr. Acta, 18:138, 1963.

Hossack, K. F., Neutze, J. M., Lowe, J. B., et al.: Congenital valvular aortic stenosis: Natural history and assessment for operation. Br. Heart J., 43:561, 1980.

Ilbawi, M. N., DeLeon, S. Y., Wison, W. R. J., et al.: Extended aortic valvuloplasty: A new approach for the management of congenital valvular aortic stenosis. Ann. Thorac. Surg., 52:663–668, 1991.

Jaklitsch, M., and Leyland, S.: Aspirin anticoagulation for mechanical heart valves and Reye's syndrome. J. Thorac. Cardiovasc. Surg., 95:146–147, 1988.

James, T. N., Jordan, J. D., Riddick, L., and Bargeron, L. M.: Subaortic stenosis and sudden death. J. Thorac. Cardiovasc. Surg., 95:247–254, 1988.

Jeger, E.: Die Chirurgie der Blutgafassen und des Herzens. Berlin, August Hirchwald, 1913.

Johnson, R. G., Williams, G. R., Razook, J. D., et al.: Reoperation in congenital aortic stenosis. Ann. Thorac. Surg., 40(2):156–162, 1985.

Jonas, R. A., Lang, P., Mayer, J. E., and Castañeda, A. R.: The importance of prostaglandin $E_1$ in resuscitation of the neonate with critical aortic stenosis. J. Thorac. Cardiovasc. Surg., 89:314, 1985.

Karl, T. R., Sano, S., Brawn, W., and Mee, R.: Critical aortic stenosis in the first month of life: Surgical results in 26 infants. Ann. Thorac. Surg., 50:105–109, 1990.

Katz, N. M., Mortimer, J. B., and Liberthson, R. R.: Discrete membranous subaortic stenosis: Report of 31 patients, review of the literature, and delineation of management. Circulation, 56(6):1034–1038, 1977.

Keane, J. F., Fellows, K. E., LaFarge, C. G., et al.: The surgical management of discrete and diffuse supravalvular aortic stenosis. Circulation, 54(1):112–117, 1976.

Kirklin, J. W., and Ellis, F. H.: Surgical relief of diffuse subvalvular aortic stenosis. Circulation, 24:739, 1961.

Kirklin, L. W., and Barratt-Boyes, B. G.: Cardiac Surgery. 2nd ed. New York, Churchill Livingstone, 1993.

Kisslo, J. A., Adams, D. B., and Belkin, R. N. (eds): Doppler Color Flow Imaging. New York, Churchill Livingstone, 1988.

Konno, S., Yasuharu, I., Yoshinau, I., et al.: A new method for prosthetic valve replacement in congenital aortic stenosis associated with hypoplasia of the aortic valve ring. J. Thorac. Cardiovasc. Surg., 70:909, 1975.

Kugler, J. D., Campbell, E., Vargo, T. A., et al.: Results of aortic valvotomy in infants with isolated aortic valvular stenosis. J. Thorac. Cardiovasc. Surg., 78:553–558, 1979.

Lababidi, A.: Aortic balloon valvuloplasty. Am. Heart J. 106:751, 1983.

Leung, M. P., McKay, R., Smith, A., et al.: Critical aortic stenosis in early infancy: Anatomic and echocardiographic substrates of successful open valvotomy. J. Thorac. Cardiovasc. Surg., 101:526–535, 1991.

Lewis, F. J., Shumway, N. E., and Niazi, S. A.: Aortic valvulotomy under direct vision during hypothermia. J. Thorac. Cardiovasc. Surg., 32:481, 1956.

Lillehei, C. W., and Levy, M. J.: Transatrial exposure for correction of subaortic stenosis. J. A. M. A., 186:8, 1963.

Lock, J. E., Keane, J. F., and Fellows, K. E.: Diagnostic and Interventional Catheterization in Congenital Heart Disease. Boston, Martinus Nijhoff, 1987.

Lupinetti, F. M., Pridjian, A. K., Callow, L. B., et al.: Optimum treatment of discrete subaortic stenosis. Ann. Thorac. Surg., 54:467–471, 1992.

Manouguian S., Seybold-Epting, W.: Patch enlargement of the aortic valve ring by extending the aortic incision into the anterior mitral leaflet: New operative technique. J. Thorac. Cardiovasc. Surg., 78:402, 1979.

Matsuki, O., Okita, Y., Almeida, R. S., et al.: Two decades' experience with aortic valve replacement with pulmonary autograft. J. Thorac. Cardiovasc. Surg., 95:705–711, 1988.

Mavroudis, C., Rees, A., Solinger, R., and Elbl, F. The prognostic value of intraoperative pressure gradients with congenital aortic stenosis. Ann. Thorac. Surg., 38(3):237–241, 1984.

McGoon, D. C., Mankin, H. T., Vlad, P., and Kirklin, J. W.: The surgical treatment of supravalvular aortic stenosis. J. Thorac. Cardiovasc. Surg., 41:125, 1961.

McGrath, L. B., Gonzalez-Lavin, L., Eldredge, W. J., et al.: Thromboembolic and other events following valve replacement in a pediatric population treated with antiplatelet agents. Ann. Thorac. Surg., 43:285–287, 1987.

McKay, R.: Invited letter concerning critical aortic stenosis. J. Thorac. Cardiovasc. Surg., 105:365–367, 1993.

McKay, R., Smith, A., Leung, M. P., et al.: Morphology of the ventriculoaortic junction in critical aortic stenosis: Implications for hemodynamic function and clinical management. J. Thorac. Cardiovasc. Surg., 104:434–442, 1992.

Messina, L. M., Turley, K., Stanger, P., et al.: Successful aortic valvotomy for severe congenital valvular aortic stenosis in the newborn infant. J. Thorac. Cardiovasc. Surg., 88:92, 1984.

Mills, P., Leech, G., Davies, M., and Leatham, A.: The natural history of a non-stenotic bicuspid aortic valve. Br. Heart J., 40:951, 1978.

Misback, G. A., Turley, K., Ullyot, D. J., and Ebert, P. A.: Left ventricular outflow enlargement by the Konno procedure. J. Thorac. Cardiovasc. Surg., 84:696–703, 1982.

Mody, M. R., and Mody, G. T.: Serial hemodynamic observations in congenital valvular and subvalvular aortic stenosis. Am. Heart J., 89:137, 1975.

Morrow, A. G.: Hypertrophic subaortic stenosis: Operative methods utilized to relieve left ventricular outflow obstruction. J. Thorac. Cardiovasc. Surg., 76(4):423–430, 1978.

Morrow, A. G., Reitz, B. A., Epstein, S. E., et al.: Operative treatment in hypertrophic subaortic stenosis: Techniques and the results of pre- and post-operative assessments in 83 patients. Circulation, 52:88, 1975.

Moses, R. D., Barnhart, G. R., and Jones, M.: The late prognosis after localized resection for fixed (discrete and tunnel) left ventricular outflow tract obstruction. J. Thorac. Cardiovasc. Surg., 87:410, 1984.

Mulder, D. G., Katz, R. D., Moss, A. J., et al.: The surgical treatment of congenital aortic stenosis. J. Thorac. Cardiovasc. Surg., 88:786, 1968.

Myers, J. L., Waldhausen, J. A., Cyran, S. E., et al.: Results of surgical repair of congenital supravalvular aortic stenosis. J. Thorac. Cardiovasc. Surg., 105:281–288, 1993.

Nadas, A. S., and Fyler, D.: Pediatric Cardiology. Philadelphia, W. B. Saunders, 1972.

Najafi, H., Ostermiller, W. E., and Hushang, J.: Narrow aortic root complicating aortic valve replacement. Arch. Surg., 99:690, 1969.

Nanton, M. A., Belcourt, C. L., and Gillis, D. A.: Left ventricular outflow tract obstruction owing to accessory endocardial cushion tissue. J. Thorac. Cardiovasc. Surg., 78:537–541, 1979.

Neish, S. R., O'Laughlin, M. P., Nihill, M. R., et al: Intraoperative balloon valvuloplasty for critical aortic valvular stenosis in neonates. Am. J. Cardiol., 68:807–810, 1991.

Newfeld, E. A., Muster, A. J., Paul, M. H., et al.: Discrete subvalvular aortic stenosis in childhood: Study of 51 patients. Am. J. Cardiol. Vol., 38:53–61, 1976.

Nicks, R., Cartmill, T., Bernstein, L.: Hypoplasia of the aortic root. Thorax, 25:339, 1970.

Norwood, W. I., Lang, P., Castañeda, A. R., and Murphy, J. D.: Management of infants with left ventricular outflow obstruction by conduit interposition between the ventricular apex and thoracic aorta. J. Thorac. Cardiovasc. Surg., 86:771–776, 1983.

O'Brien, M. F., McGriffin, D. C., Stafford, E. G., et al.: Allograft aortic valve replacement: Long-term comparative clinical analysis of the viable cryopreserved and antibiotic 4° C stored valves. J. Cardiac Surg., 6(Suppl. 4):534–543, 1991.

O'Brien, M. F., Stafford, E. G., Gardner, M. A., et al.: A comparison of aortic valve replacement with viable cryopreserved and fresh allograft valves, with a note on chromosomal studies. J. Thorac. Cardiovasc. Surg., 94:812–823, 1987.

Oldham, H. N., Jr.: Congenital aortic stenosis. In Sabiston, D. C., Jr. (ed): Davis-Christopher Textbook of Surgery: The Biologic Basis of Modern Surgical Practice. 13th ed. Philadelphia, W. B. Saunders, 1986, pp. 2261–2279.

Olin, C. L., Bomfim, V., Halvazulis, V., et al.: Optimal insertion technique for the Bjork Shiley valve in the narrow aortic ostium. Ann. Thorac. Surg., 36(5):567–576, 1983.

Olley, P. M., Bloom, K. R., and Rowe, R. D.: Aortic stenosis: Valvular, subaortic, and supravalvular. In Keith, J. D., Rowe, R. D., and Vlad, P. (eds): Heart Disease in Infancy and Childhood. 3rd ed. New York, Macmillan, 1978, pp. 698–727.

Osler, W.: The bicuspid condition of the aortic valves. Trans. Assoc. Am. Physicians, 2:185, 1886.

Paget, J.: On obstruction of the branches of the pulmonary artery. Med. Chir. Trans., 27:162, 1844.

Pasengrau, D. G., Kioshos, J. M., Durnin, R. E., and Kroetz, F. W.: Supravalvular aortic stenosis in adults. Am. J. Cardiol., 31:635, 1973.

Pelech, A. N., Trusler, G. A., Olley, P. M., et al.: Critical aortic stenosis. J. Thorac. Cardiovasc. Surg., 94:510–517, 1987.

Peretz, D. I., Changfoot, G. H., and Gourlay, R. H.: Four-cusped aortic valve with significant hemodynamic abnormality. Am. J. Cardiol. Vol., 23:291–293, 1969.

Piehler, J. M., Danielson, G. K., Pluth, J. R., et al.: Enlargement of the aortic root or anulus with autogenous pericardial patch during aortic valve replacement. J. Thorac. Cardiovasc. Surg., 86:350, 1983.

Pugliese, P., Bernabei, M., Santi, C., et al.: Posterior enlargement of the small annulus during aortic valve replacement versus implantation of a small prosthesis. Ann. Thorac. Surg., 38(1):31–36, 1984.

Rastan, H., Koncz, J.: Plastische erweiterung der linken ausflussbahn: Eine neue operations methode. Thorax-chirurgie, 23:169, 1975.

Reis, R. L., Peterson, L. M., Mason, D. T., et al.: Congenital fixed subvalvular aortic stenosis: An anatomical classification and correlations with operative results. Circulation, 43(Suppl. I):I–II, 1971.

Rhodes, L. A., Colan, S. D., Perry, S. B., et al.: Predictors of survival in neonates with critical aortic stenosis. Circulation, 84:2325–2333, 1991.

Rittenhouse, E. A., Sauvage, L. R., Stamm, S. J., et al.: Radical enlargement of the aortic root and outflow tract to allow valve replacement. Ann. Thorac. Surg., 27:367, 1979.

Roberts, W. C.: The congenitally bicuspid aortic valve: A study of 85 autopsy cases. Am. J. Cardiol., 26:72–83, 1970.

Robicshek, F., Sanger, P. W., Daugherty, H. K., and Montgomery, C. C.: Congenital quadricuspid aortic valve with displacement of the left coronary orifice. Am. J. Cardiol., 23:288–290, 1969.

Ross, D.: Replacement of the aortic valve with a pulmonary autograft: The Switch operation. Ann. Thorac. Surg., 52:1346–1350, 1991.

Ross, D., Jackson, M., and Davies, J.: Pulmonary autograft aortic valve replacement: Long term results. J. Cardiac Surg., 6(Suppl. 4):529–533, 1991.

Sade, R. M., Ballenger, J. F., Hohn, A. R., et al.: Cardiac valve replacement in children: Comparison of tissue with mechanical prostheses. J. Thorac. Cardiovasc. Surg., 78(1):123–127, 1979.

Schaffer, M. S., Campbell, D. N., Clarke, D. R., et al.: Aortoventriculoplasty in children. J. Thorac. Cardiovasc. Surg., 92:391–395, 1986.

Shone, J. D., Sellars, R. D., Anderson, R. C., et al.: The developmental complex of parachute mitral valve, supravalvular ring of left atrium, subaortic stenosis, and coarctation of aorta. Am. J. Cardiol., 11:715, 1963.

Silverman, N. H.: Pediatric Echocardiography. Baltimore, Williams & Wilkins, 1993, p. 111.

Sink, J. D., Smallhorn, J. F., Macartney, F. J., et al.: Management of critical aortic stenosis in infancy. J. Thorac. Cardiovasc. Surg., 887:82, 1984.

Sissman, N. J., Neill, C. A., Spencer, F. C., and Taussig, H. B.: Congenital aortic stenosis. Circulation, 19:458, 1959.

Spann, J. F., Bove, A. A., Natarajan, G., et al.: Ventricular performance, pump function and compensatory mechanisms in patients with aortic stenosis. Circulation, 62:576, 1980.

Spencer, F. C., Neill, C. A., and Bahnson, H. T.: The treatment of congenital aortic stenosis with valvotomy during cardiopulmonary bypass. Surgery, 44:109, 1958.

Spencer, F. C., Neill, C. A., Sank, L., and Bahnson, H. T.: Anatomical variations in 46 patients with congenital aortic stenosis. Am. Surg., *26*:204, 1960.

Stewart, J. R., Paton, B. C., Blount, S. G., et al.: Congenital aortic stenosis: Ten to 22 years after valvulotomy. Arch. Surg., *113*:1248, 1978.

Sud, A., Parker, F., and Magilligan, D. J. J.: Anatomy of the aortic root. Ann. Thorac. Surg. *38*(1):76–79, 1984.

Swan, H., and Kortz, A. B.: Direct vision trans-aortic approach to the aortic valve during hypothermia. Experimental observations and report of successful clinical case. Ann. Surg., *144*:205, 1956.

Thandroyen, F. T., Witthon, I. N., Pirie, D., et al.: Severe calcification of glutaraldehyde preserved porcine xenografts in children. Am. J. Cardiol., *45*:690–696, 1980.

Thursfield, H., and Scott, H. W.: Sub-aortic stenosis. Br. J. Child. Dis., *10*:104, 1913.

Trinkle, J. K., Norton, J. B., Richardson, J. D., et al.: Closed aortic valvotomy and simultaneous correction of associated anomalies in infants. J. Thorac. Cardiovasc. Surg., *69*:758, 1975.

Tuffier, T.: Etat actuel de la chirurgie intrathoracique. Trans. Int. Cong. Med., London, 1914.

Turley, K., Bove, E. L., Amato, J. J., et al.: Neonatal aortic stenosis. J. Thorac. Cardiovasc. Surg., *99*:679–684, 1990.

Turpie, A. G. G., Gent, M., Laupacis, A., et al.: A comparison of aspirin with placebo in patients treated with warfarin after heart-valve replacement. N. Engl. J. Med., *329*:524–529, 1993.

Ungerleider, R. M., and Ebert, P. A.: Indications and techniques for midline approach to aortic coarctation in infants and children. Ann. Thorac. Surg., *44*(5):517–522, 1987.

Ungerleider, R. M., Greeley, W. J., Sheikh, K. H., et al.: Routine use of intraoperative epicardial echocardiography and Doppler color flow imaging to guide and evaluate repair of congenital heart defects: A prospective study. J. Thorac. Cardiovasc. Surg., *100*:297–309, 1990.

Ungerleider, R. M.: Is there a role for prosthetic patch aortoplasty in the repair of coarctation? Ann. Thorac. Surg., *52*:601–603, 1991.

Verrier, E. D., Tranbaugh, R. F., Soifer, S. J., et al.: Aspirin anticoagulation in children with mechanical aortic valves. J. Thorac. Cardiovasc. Surg., *92*:1013–1020, 1986.

Walls, J. T., Lababidi, Z., Curtis, J. J., and Silver, D.: Assessment of percutaneous balloon pulmonary and aortic valvuloplasty. J. Thorac. Cardiovasc. Surg., *88*:352–356, 1984.

Williams, D. B., Danielson, G. K., McGoon, D. C., et al.: Porcine heterograft valve replacement in children. J. Thorac. Cardiovasc. Surg., *84*:446–450, 1982.

Williams, J. C. P., Barratt-Boyes, B. G., and Lowe, J. B.: Supravalvular aortic stenosis. Circulation, *24*:1311, 1961.

Wright, P. W., and Wittner, R. S.: Obstruction of the left ventricular outflow tract by the mitral valve due to a muscle band. J. Thorac. Cardiovasc. Surg., *85*(6):938–940, 1983.

Zeevi, B., Keane, J. F., Castañeda, A. R., et al.: Neonatal critical valvular aortic stenosis: A comparison of surgical and balloon dilatation therapy. Circulation, *80*:831–839, 1989.

Zeevi, B., Keane, J. F., Perry, S. B., and Lock J. E.: Invasive catheter techniques in the management of critical aortic stenosis in infants. *In* Jacobs, M. L., and Norwood, W. I. (eds): Pediatric Cardiac Surgery. Stoneham, MA, Butterworth-Heinemann, 1992, pp. 115–122.

# 42

# Congenital Malformations of the Mitral Valve

Alon S. Aharon, Hillel Laks, and Eli Milgalter

Congenital lesions of the mitral valve are rare, occurring in 0.6% of autopsied patients with congenital heart disease and in 0.21 to 0.42% of clinical series (Baker et al., 1962; Collins-Nakai et al., 1977). Mitral valve lesions are diverse and are frequently associated with other complex intracardiac abnormalities, including atrioventricular septal defects, univentricular heart, hypoplastic left ventricle, forms of atrioventricular discordant connection, transposition of the great vessels, pulmonary outflow tract obstruction, and double-inlet left ventricle. Mitral valve lesions frequently are complex and may involve multiple components of the mitral valve apparatus, including the supravalvular area, the contiguous atrium, the annulus, the leaflets, and the subvalvular apparatus, with the chordae papillary muscles and ventricular septum. The clinical presentation of mitral stenosis or insufficiency depends on the severity of the mitral valve lesion and the associated intracardiac defects. Technique and timing of surgical repair depend on the age of the patient, clinical status, severity of the mitral valve lesion, and associated congenital cardiac defects. This chapter reviews isolated congenital mitral valve lesions as well as those associated with other congenital cardiac defects. The UCLA experience is also included when pertinent.

## HISTORY

The first description of congenital mitral valve disease was made by Smith in 1846, who provided an early description of congenital mitral valve stenosis (Smith, 1846). In 1902, Fisher described two cases of congenital mitral valve disease of the heart. These cases included supravalvular mitral ring and parachute mitral valve. Early contemporary descriptions of mitral valve pathology were made by Vlad in 1954 and Shone and colleagues (1963); the latter described the Shone heart. Carpentier and coworkers (1976), Duran (1991), Devachi and colleagues (1971), Ruchman and colleagues (1971), and Van Praagh (1978) all made important contributions to our understanding of the morphologic spectrum and pathophysiology of congenital mitral valve lesions.

Surgical repair of congenital mitral lesions was reported by Bower and Gerrardi in 1953, who described a successful closed mitral commissurotomy in a 5½-year-old child. Starkey, in 1959, described treatment of congenital mitral valve lesions using both closed and open methods, and Creech and associates in 1962 reported successful repair of cleft posterior leaflet in a 2-year-old girl. Results of mitral valve repair in children were initially poor; Collins-Nakai and colleagues (1977) reported a late survival rate of only 18%. Functional classification of congenital mitral valve lesions and innovative surgical techniques of mitral valve repair described by Carpentier and coworkers (1976) have enabled the surgeon to analyze and repair multiple components of the abnormal mitral valve.

## EMBRYOLOGY

The mitral valve is formed from the endocardial cushions and from trabeculations of the primitive left ventricle (Van Mierap et al., 1962). During the fourth week of embryonic life, the dorsal and ventral endocardial cushions, along with lateral infolds from the adjacent canal wall, partition the atrioventricular canal into atria and ventricles. After completion of ventricular and atrial septation during the fifth and sixth weeks, the future mitral and tricuspid valves are separated.

During the sixth and seventh weeks, the mitral leaflets are formed from the endocardial cushions and lateral projection tissue; at the same time the papillary muscles and chordae are shaped from primitive muscular trabeculations of the left ventricle. Until the 24th week, the ventricular trabeculations slowly fuse into two distinct papillary muscles. The leaflets and chordae of the valve gradually change their muscular character into a thin, delicate, collagenous tissue.

## ANATOMY

The normal mitral valve complex is composed of the fibrous annulus, two leaflets, two commissures, multiple chordae tendineae, and two papillary muscles (Fig. 42–1).

The annulus is a fibrous structure that is part of the fibrous skeleton of the heart. It separates the left atrium from the left ventricle and includes the mitral and aortic orifices. Anteriorly, the annulus merges with the aortic valve annulus beneath the left and noncoronary aortic valve cusps. Laterally and posteri-

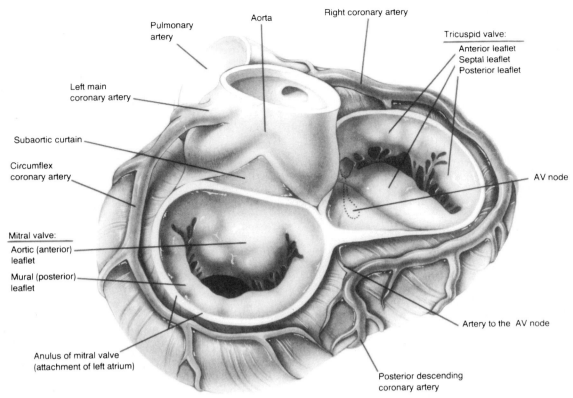

**FIGURE 42–1.** Cross-section of the heart showing the anatomic relations of the normal mitral valve. (AV = atrioventricular.) (From Khonsari, S.: Cardiac Surgery. Safeguards and Pitfalls in Operative Technique. Gaithersburg, MD, Aspen, 1988.)

orly, it lies deep in the atrioventricular groove beneath the coronary sinus and circumflex coronary artery. Medially, it joins the tricuspid valve annulus and membranous interventricular septum. The mitral valve is surrounded by a triangular portion of fibrous annulus, with its apices forming the thickened portion of the right and left fibrous trigones of the heart and its anterior leg dividing the aortic and mitral valves. The fibrous annulus is a dynamic structure with attachments to the base of the left ventricle and left

ventricular outflow tract—a factor important in effective valve repair. The diameter of the mitral valve in children ranges from 11.2 to 24.2 mm, depending on body surface area and the size of the child (Table 42–1).

The two leaflets of the mitral valve are separated by anterolateral and posteromedial commissures and insert at their bases along the entire length of the mitral orifice. The anterior leaflet is wider than the posterior leaflet and attaches to 150 degrees of the annulus. The

■ **Table 42–1.** MEAN NORMAL VALVE DIAMETERS IN CHILDREN

| Body Surface Area (m²) | Mitral (mm)* | Tricuspid (mm)* | Aortic (mm) | Pulmonary (mm) |
|---|---|---|---|---|
| 0.25 | 11.2 | 13.4 | 7.4 | 8.4 |
| 0.3 | 12.6 | 14.9 | 8.1 | 9.3 |
| 0.35 | 13.6 | 16.2 | 8.9 | 10.1 |
| 0.4 | 14.4 | 17.3 | 9.5 | 10.7 |
| 0.45 | 15.2 | 18.2 | 10.1 | 11.3 |
| 0.5 | 15.8 | 19.2 | 10.7 | 11.9 |
| 0.6 | 16.9 | 20.7 | 11.5 | 12.8 |
| 0.7 | 17.9 | 21.9 | 12.3 | 13.5 |
| 0.8 | 18.8 | 23.0 | 13.0 | 14.2 |
| 0.9 | 19.7 | 24.0 | 13.4 | 14.8 |
| 1.0 | 20.2 | 24.9 | 14.0 | 15.3 |
| 1.2 | 21.4 | 26.2 | 14.8 | 16.2 |
| 1.4 | 22.3 | 27.7 | 15.5 | 17.0 |
| 1.6 | 23.1 | 28.9 | 16.1 | 17.6 |
| 1.8 | 23.8 | 29.1 | 16.5 | 18.2 |
| 2.0 | 24.2 | 30.0 | 17.2 | 18.0 |

Modified from Rowlatt, U. F., Rimoldi, H. J. A., and Lev, M.: The quantitative anatomy of the normal child's heart. Pediatr. Clin. North Am., 10:499, 1963.
*The approximate standard deviations (±) are: mitral <0.3 m² = 1.9 mm; >0.3 m² = 1.6 mm; tricuspid <1 m² = 1.7 mm, >1 m² = 1.5 mm.

1546 Congenital Malformations of the Mitral Valve

anterior leaflet has less redundant tissue and a larger surface area than the posterior leaflet, which is attached to approximately 210 degrees of the annular circumference. The posterior leaflet often is subdivided into a large central scallop and two or more smaller lateral scallops. The geometric configuration of the anterior and posterior leaflets is important in repair of leaflet prolapse. The leaflets usually are thin and flexible, and they have smooth surfaces. They also have a line of co-aptation that parallels the posterior part of the annulus and is a few millimeters proximal to the free margin of the leaflets and their left atrial surface.

## Chordae

Normal chordae are thin, pliable structures that arise from the anterior and posterior papillary muscles and insert in an arcade-like manner into the anterolateral and posteromedial commissures areas. These chordae further extend circumferentially from the commissures along both leaflets. Several main strut chordae arise from each papillary muscle and are supported by smaller, finer accessory chordae. Prolapse of the anterior or posterior leaflet is due to elongation or rupture of these main strut chordae. There are three generations of chordae tendineae. The first-order chordae fuse with the free margins of the leaflets. Four to six chordae connect adjacent halves of the two leaflets to a papillary muscle. The second-generation chordae are attached to the undersurface of the leaflets, a few millimeters away from the free margin. The third-order chordae are attached to the leaflets close to the annulus and originate either from the papillary muscle or the left ventricular free wall close to the annulus. Anomalous and/or redundant chordae, when present, may alter leaflet coaptation or impede inflow into the left ventricle, causing mitral insufficiency stenosis or mixed lesions.

## Papillary Muscles

The two papillary muscles are separate structures whose bases originate from the middle one-third of the ventricular free wall. The anterolateral papillary muscle is attached to the lateral wall of the left ventricle and supports the anterolateral commissure. The chordae arise from the apex of the papillary muscle and support the anterolateral commissure and proximal one-half of the anterior and posterior leaflets. Blood supply to the anterolateral papillary muscle originates either from the left anterior descending or circumflex coronary arteries or from the diagonal, or marginal, branches. The anterior papillary muscle usually has one head, but chordae can originate from two or more heads in both normal and diseased mitral valves. The posteromedial papillary muscle is attached to the interventricular septum and posterior ventricular wall. It supports the posteromedial commissure and one-half of the anterior and posterior

leaflets. Its blood supply is derived from branches of the posterior descending or circumflex coronary arteries. During systole, the subvalvular apparatus formed by the anterolateral and posteromedial papillary muscles arrests the upward motion of the leaflets so that the line of coaptation of the two leaflets parallels the level of the valve annulus. During diastole, the leaflets collapse into the ventricle. The gap between the two leaflets is called the primary orifice. In congenital malformations of the mitral valve, the secondary mitral valve orifice is the sum of the multiple gaps between the chordal network, papillary muscles, and left ventricular wall. In congenital mitral disease, the papillary muscles may be absent, hypoplastic, hypertrophied, or fused, or they may form a subvalvular arcade causing stenotic, insufficient, or mixed mitral lesions.

## MORPHOLOGY

Early classification of mitral valve lesions was based on autopsy specimens of congenital mitral stenosis. A more surgically oriented classification system was suggested by Carpentier and co-workers (1976), based on a large series of autopsy specimens and clinical experience.

Malformations of the mitral valve may involve one or more levels of the mitral valve apparatus: adjacent left atrium (as in supravalvular mitral ring), valve annulus, leaflets, commissures, chordae tendinae, papillary muscles, and adjacent left ventricle (as in fibroelastosis and dilated left ventricle). These lesions are classified as producing either insufficiency or stenosis. Lesions causing insufficiency are classified as occurring in association with normal leaflet motion (Type I), excessive leaflet motion as seen in prolapse (Type II), or restricted leaflet motion (Type III) with either normal or abnormal papillary muscles. Lesions causing mitral stenosis are classfied as occurring with normal papillary muscles or abnormal papillary muscles (Table 42–2). This pathophysiologic classification has proved important in the application of techniques of mitral valve reconstruction. The purpose of this functional classification system is to restore normal valve function rather than normal valve anatomy.

### Morphology of Congenital Mitral Incompetence

#### Type I: With Normal Leaflet Motion

Mitral insufficiency may be caused by pathology of either the mitral valve annulus, the leaflets, or the subvalvular apparatus. Congenital primary annular dilatation of the mitral valve is rare and is more often secondary to functional left ventricular dilatation or to ischemia or myocardial infarction.

ANNULAR DILATATION

Rarely, primary annular dilatation is the only congenital defect; more often it is found in patients with

■ **Table 42–2.** PATHOPHYSIOLOGIC CLASSIFICATION OF CONGENITAL MALFORMATIONS OF THE MITRAL VALVE AND BREAKDOWN OF THE DIFFERENT SUBTYPES IN 107 AUTOPSY SPECIMENS AND 70 SURGICAL CASES

| Malformation | Clinical | Autopsy |
|---|---|---|
| *Mitral Valve Incompetence* | | |
| Type I: Normal Leaflet Motion | 15 | 16 |
|   1. Isolated annulus dilatation | 8 | 7 |
|   2. Cleft leaflet | 6 | 4 |
|     a. True cleft leaflet | | 3 |
|     b. Three-leaflet valve | | 1 |
|   3. Leaflet defect | 1 | 1 |
| Type II: Prolapsed Leaflet | 27 | 17 |
|   1. Absent chordae | 5 | 6 |
|   2. Elongated chordae | 14 | 11 |
|   3. Elongated papillary muscle | 8 | 0 |
| Type III: Restricted Leaflet Motion | 10 | 51 |
|   A. Normal papillary muscles | | |
|     1. Commissure fusion | 2 | 4 |
|     2. Short chordae | 1 | 18 |
|     3. Ebstein type mitral valve | 0 | 0 |
|   B. Abnormal papillary muscles | | |
|     1. Parachute valve | 2 | 5 |
|     2. Hammock valve | 2 | 5 |
|     3. Papillary hypoplasia | 3 | 19 |
| *Mitral Stenosis* | | |
| Type A: Normal Papillary Muscles | 10 | 18 |
|   1. Commissure fusion | 7 | 11 |
|   2. Excess valvular tissue | 1 | 2 |
|   3. Annulus hypoplasia | 0 | 4 |
|   4. Supravalvular ring | 2 | 1 |
| Type B: Abnormal Papillary Muscles | 8 | 5 |
|   1. Parachute valve | 3 | 1 |
|   2. Hammock valve | 5 | 3 |
|   3. Absent papillary muscles | 0 | 1 |

From Carpentier, A., Branchini, B., Cour, J. C., et al.: Congenital malformations of the mitral valve in children. J. Thorac. Cardiovasc. Surg., 72:854, 1976.

univentricular heart. The infrequency of isolated annular dilatation is due to the structure of the mitral valve annulus. The mitral annulus is contiguous with the aortic valve annulus and the fibrous trigone and thus is partially protected from dilatation. Dilatation, when it occurs, is found mainly in the posterior leaflet. An ostium secundum atrial septal defect is associated with 50% of cases of primary annular dilatation of the mitral valve.

CLEFT LEAFLET

Mitral valve insufficiency also may be secondary to a cleft in the anterior or posterior leaflets, three-leaflet valves, or leaflet defects. Clefts usually occur in the anterior leaflet, and they are most often associated with primum atrial septal defect and incomplete atrioventricular canal. Posterior cleft leaflets are rare and should not be mistaken for the normal deep indentations that are common between the scallops of the posterior leaflet. True three-leaflet mitral valves are similar to the left-sided atrioventricular valve seen in atrioventricular canal defects. The papillary muscles in this subtype are displaced laterally, and there

is a separate, distinct third triangular lateral mitral leaflet.

LEAFLET DEFECTS

Leaflet defects are holes created by localized agenesis of the leaflet tissue, and are seen particularly in the posterior leaflet. In the absence of prior surgical therapy or infection, these defects are presumed to be congenital malformations.

### Type II: With Prolapsed Leaflet

Lesions that cause leaflet prolapse include absent or elongated chordae, elongated or ruptured papillary muscles, and abnormal implantation of the papillary muscles. Prolapse of the anterior and/or posterior leaflet secondary to elongated chordae may occur in patients with univentricular heart, incomplete atrioventricular canal, Marfan's syndrome, and isolated mitral defects. Elongation or rupture of the papillary muscles most often occurs secondary to infarction of the papillary muscle in the context of anomalous origin of the left coronary artery from the pulmonary artery.

### Type III: Mitral Regurgitation with Restricted Leaflet Motion

Restricted leaflet motion may occur with either normal or abnormal papillary muscles and may prevent co-aptation, thus causing regurgitation.

RESTRICTED LEAFLET MOTION WITH NORMAL PAPILLARY MUSCLES

Commissural fusion in which the commissures are obliterated and the papillary muscles adhere to the commissures, causing central failure of co-aptation, may cause significant mitral regurgitation. Shortened chordae and/or thickened chordae limiting leaflet motion may cause both mitral regurgitation and stenosis secondary to restricted leaflet motion and subvalvular restriction to flow. Ebstein's anomaly of the mitral valve, in which there is downward displacement of the septal and posterior leaflets, may also produce restriction of the leaflets and mitral regurgitation (Ruschaupt et al., 1976).

RESTRICTED LEAFLET MOTION WITH ABNORMAL PAPILLARY MUSCLES

Subvalvular mitral lesions with restriction of leaflet motion may be caused by mixed insufficient and stenotic pathology. Parachute mitral valve deformity occurs when all of the chordae originate from a single large papillary muscle that is formed either from fusion of the two papillary muscles or from the presence of one dominant papillary muscle with the other being hypoplastic and without chordal connections. Hammock mitral valve is another deformity that frequently causes both mitral regurgitation and stenosis.

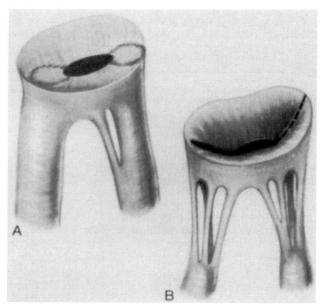

**FIGURE 42–2.** Congenital mitral stenosis. *A*, Papillary commissural fusion. Note the insertion of papillary muscles directly onto the fused commissures. *B*, After repair by commissurotomy and papillary splitting. (*A* and *B*, From Stark, J., and de Leval, M. [eds]: Surgery for Congenital Heart Defects. Orlando, FL, Grune & Stratton, 1983.)

In this malformation, the two normal papillary muscles are absent and are replaced by numerous papillary muscles and fibrous bands, which are inserted high on the posterior wall of the ventricle, just below the mitral valve leaflets. As a consequence, restricted leaflet motion is accompanied by stenosis at the secondary orifice because the interchordal spaces are obliterated by excessive valve tissue.

### ABSENT PAPILLARY MUSCLES

In this condition, there are no papillary muscles, and the chordae attach to the ventricular wall. There are variable imperforate interchordal spaces.

### MORPHOLOGY OF CONGENITAL MITRAL STENOSIS

Congenital mitral stenosis may occur at the supravalvular, annular, or subvalvular levels and is classified as occurring with normal or with abnormal papillary muscles.

### Type A: Mitral Stenosis with Normal Papillary Muscles

This group contains four subtypes: commissural fusion, excessive valve tissue, annular hypoplasia, and supravalvular ring.

### COMMISSURAL FUSION

The commissures and the two papillary muscles are fused, producing both valvular and subvalvular

stenosis. The two papillary muscles most often are fused directly with the valve leaflets, and an arcade of thickened papillary muscles often is present, causing further subvalvular stenosis (Fig. 42–2).

### EXCESSIVE VALVE TISSUE

The major malformation is excessive tissue that bridges and obliterates the interchordal spaces. The leaflets, papillary muscles, and valve motion are all normal. A large bridge of valvular tissue may join the two leaflets, creating a double-orifice mitral valve (Fig. 42–3).

### ANNULAR HYPOPLASIA

Mitral valve hypoplasia with a hypoplastic annulus represents a series of lesions in which may involve varying degrees of valve development, ranging from an almost completely absent mitral valve to isolated annular hypoplasia. These lesions usually occur in association with the spectrum of hypoplastic left heart syndrome (Ruckman and Van Praagh, 1978). Rarely, isolated annular hypoplasia occurs (Carpentier et al., 1976) and may be associated with a normally developed left ventricle.

### SUPRAVALVULAR RING

Mitral stenosis may result from a fibrous ring located on the left atrial side of the mitral valve annulus. The size and the degree of obstruction can vary from mild to severe, causing left atrial hypertension and pulmonary edema in the first few days of life (Shone et al., 1963). Supravalvular ring may occur

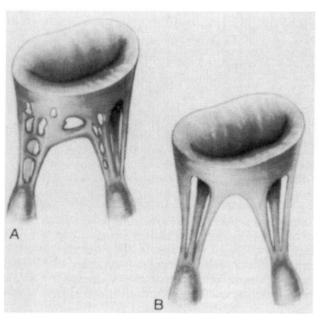

**FIGURE 42–3.** Congenital mitral stenosis. *A*, Excessive mitral valve tissue. Note the obstruction of secondary orifice. *B*, After repair. (*A* and *B*, From Stark, J., and de Leval, M. [eds]: Surgery for Congenital Heart Defects. Orlando, FL, Grune & Stratton, 1983.)

as an isolated defect, but more frequently it co-exists with other cardiac anomalies—especially Shone syndrome, which includes supramitral ring, parachute mitral valve, left ventricular outflow tract obstruction, and co-arctation of the aorta. Supravalvular ring must be differentiated from cor triatrum, in which the fibrous diaphragm is closer to the pulmonary veins and lies proximal to the left atrial appendage, and the mitral valve is normal.

## Co-Existent Cardiac Anomalies

Cardiac anomalies often co-exist with congenital mitral valve disease. In the combined Greenlane Hospital and University of Alabama series (Kirklin and Barrett-Boyes, 1986), only 25% of patients had isolated congenital mitral stenosis. In 30% there was also a ventricular septal defect, and in 40% there was some form of left ventricular outflow tract obstruction. Carpentier and associates (1976) noted a 60% incidence, and Ruckman and Van Praagh (1978) found a 96% incidence of associated lesions. In the UCLA experience, 94% of patients with congenital mitral valve disease had other associated intracardiac anomalies, including pulmonary atresia, tricuspid atresia or insufficiency, left ventricular ouflow tract obstruction, and ventricular septal defect. The left ventricular outflow tract obstruction occurred either as a discrete subvalvular lesion or as a combined valvular and subvalvular aortic stenosis.

Co-existing intracardiac lesions may mask or unmask mitral valve pathology, may frequently increase the complexity of surgical repair, and may require staged surgical procedures before mitral valve repair can be performed. As a consequence, associated malformations should be searched for and diagnosed before operation, and they should be treated at the time of mitral valve repair. In the very young, associated patent ductus arteriosus or coarctation of the aorta may be better treated as a first stage before mitral valve repair (Carpentier et al., 1976).

## CLINICAL PRESENTATION

The clinical presentation of mitral regurgitation or stenosis in infants and children depends on the age, severity, and type of mitral valve lesion, as well as the type of co-existing congenital cardiac pathology. Children generally present with signs and symptoms of pulmonary venous congestion and decreased pulmonary compliance, which may increase susceptibility to pneumonia, central cyanosis, orthopnea, dyspnea, tachypnea, growth retardation, and failure to thrive. Without appropriate surgical intervention, pulmonary hypertension often progresses to biventricular failure and death.

Mitral insufficiency presents with an overactive precordium secondary to left ventricular volume overload, a pansystolic murmur that may radiate to the axilla, and often a third heart sound. An increased

second heart sound with an overactive precordium may indicate pulmonary hypertension. In chronic regurgitant lesions, progressively increasing left atrial size without significant increases in pressure may delay symptoms and progression to congestive heart failure and cyanosis. In contrast, children with acute rupture of a major strut chorda may present with sudden pulmonary edema and acute cardiac failure.

In isolated mitral stenosis, children present with an increased pulmonary second heart sound, secondary to increased pulmonary artery pressure, and a late diastolic murmur with presystolic accentuation at the apex. Compared with acquired mitral stenosis, an opening snap usually is not present. The symptoms are those of pulmonary venous hypertension, including dyspnea, cough, orthopnea, failure to thrive, and recurrent pneumonia. Reactive pulmonary hypertension is progressive and fatal without surgical intervention. The age at presentation depends on the severity of the mitral valve lesion and co-existing intracardiac pathology. Generally, mitral regurgitation is tolerated better than stenosis. The age of presentation also varies in medical and surgical series: Van der Horst (Van der Horst and Hartreister, 1967) reported the onset of symptoms during the first month of life in 33% of their patients and in 75% by 1 year of age. Once symptoms appeared, deterioration was rapid, and the mortality rate was 50% at 6 months.

In a surgical series from Boston's Children's Hospital (Collins-Nakai et al., 1977), the mean age of onset of symptoms was 1.6 years. In the University of Alabama series (Kirklin and Barratt-Boyes, 1976), 39% of patients with mitral insufficiency and 62% of patients with mitral stenosis underwent mitral valve replacement or repair by 4 years of age. The mean age at operation in the Carpentier series was 3 years for mitral stenosis and 6 years, 4 months for mitral insufficiency (Carpentier et al., 1976). Okita and co-workers (1988) reported a mean age at operation of 5.5 years for patients with mitral regurgitation. In the UCLA experience, the mean age at operation in patients with congenital mitral lesions was 4.9 years (5.5 to 17 years).

## LABORATORY FINDINGS

### Electrocardiogram

Left atrial enlargement and right ventricular hypertrophy are usually present. In mitral regurgitation or with co-existing left ventricular outflow tract obstruction, signs of left ventricular hypertrophy and dilatation may be present. Compared with acquired mitral valve disease, atrial fibrillation is rare.

### Chest Film

The chest film usually shows cardiomegaly that is more pronounced with mitral incompetence. Signs of left atrial enlargement and pulmonary venous hypertension usually are present. Massive enlargement of the left atrium compresses the bronchus and may cause the left lung to collapse. Co-existing cardiac anomalies usually increase the severity of radiologic findings.

## Echocardiogram

Two-dimensional and M-mode echocardiography provides essential information in the evaluation of congenital mitral valve disease and other congenital cardiac pathology. Echocardiography can accurately delineate supramitral ring, annular and leaflet size, leaflet motion, morphology of the subvalvular apparatus and papillary muscles, and ventricular function. Echocardiography with color flow mapping can quantify the extent of the regurgitant volume, valve area, and pressure gradients. Echocardiography may also provide nonquantitative information about the degree of pulmonary hypertension based on the velocity of a regurgitant tricuspid jet and pulmonary flow pattern. Echocardiography may be crucial in assessing the various components of the mitral valve and in predicting the likelihood of valve repair rather than replacement. This assessment may influence the timing of surgery.

## Cardiac Catheterization

Cardiac catheterization helps one evaluate and treat children with mitral valve disease. Catheterization provides essential information concerning the severity of pulmonary vascular disease, intracardiac pressure measurements, and delineation of co-existing congenital cardiac lesions.

## TREATMENT

Because the repair of a valve is not always possible and replacement may be required, the timing of operation is important. Because of the poor prognosis once symptoms and pulmonary hypertension develop, these patients should be followed closely and intervention should be seriously considered.

Medical management is based on controlling heart failure and preventing and treating pulmonary edema or infection. Salt restriction, digitalis, and diuretics are effective initially, but once episodes of pulmonary edema occur or signs of severe pulmonary hypertension develop, surgical intervention usually is indicated. Chest films, echocardiography, and repeated cardiac catheterization are necessary to evaluate the progression of mitral regurgitation and pulmonary hypertension.

## INDICATIONS FOR SURGERY

Those planning surgical repair of mitral stenosis in children must consider the natural history of the dis-

ease and aim to preserve ventricular function and prevent progression of pulmonary vascular disease. Early repair may be advised in order to minimize long-term distortion of the valve components, myocardial dysfunction, and progressive hypertension. Most patients with congenital mitral valve lesions require an operation in infancy or early childhood. It is sometimes advisable to correct associated extracardiac lesions first, such as patent ductus arteriosis or coarctation of the aorta, in the hope that the child will improve and mitral valve surgical therapy can be delayed. If operation on the mitral valve or associated intracardiac anomalies is indicated, every effort should be made to repair the mitral valve rather than replace it. Repair may result in better left ventricular function due to preservation of the chordal attachments (Carpentier et al., 1976; Kirklin and Barratt-Boyes, 1986). Insertion of a mitral prosthesis in an infant or small child requires reoperation as the child outgrows the prosthesis. Anticoagulation, which is required for a mechanical valve, is difficult to control in children. The porcine bioprosthesis, which does not require anticoagulation, has an accelerated rate of calcification and early failure in children (Geha et al., 1979). Thus, even a functionally imperfect mitral valve repair may be superior to a prosthesis, as long as the child can grow and does not have severe congestive heart failure or pulmonary hypertension.

## SURGICAL TECHNIQUES

The classification system based on the pathologic malformation of the separate components of the mitral valve apparatus has allowed the surgeon to address more completely each specific lesion of the mitral valve. The goal of valve repair is to restore a *functional valve* rather than normal mitral valve anatomy. Every attempt should be made to repair rather than replace the mitral valve in children. Mitral valve replacement in children has a relatively high early and late mortality rate and rate of reoperation when compared with mitral valve repair. Early surgical intervention may decrease the need for mitral valve replacement and improve the postoperative results.

## Preparation for Repair, Conduct of Bypass, and Myocardial Protection

The operation is performed through a median sternotomy. The ascending aorta and both venae cavae are cannulated, and the blood is cooled on bypass to 24° C. The method of myocardial protection at UCLA is intermittent cold blood cardioplegia given in an antegrade and retrograde manner with monitoring of pressure and flow rate. At the conclusion of the procedure, controlled reperfusion with substrate-enhanced warm blood cardioplegia is given prior to release of the cross-clamp.

The mitral valve is exposed via the right atrium and atrial septum or directly via the left atrium, de-

**■ Table 42–3.** FUNCTIONAL CLASSIFICATION OF MITRAL VALVE LESIONS AND TYPE OF REPAIR

| Type of Lesion | n | Technique of Repair | n |
|---|---|---|---|
| Annular dilatation | 68 | Modified De Vega annuloplasty | 65 |
|  |  | Gluteraldehyde-preserved pericardial strip annuloplasty | 2 |
|  |  | Carpentier-Edwards ring | 1 |
| Cleft anterior leaflet | 39 | Primary repair | 39 |
| Prolapsed anterior leaflet | 16 | Chordal shortening | 9 |
|  |  | Triangular resection | 6 |
|  |  | Chordal substitution | 1 |
| Prolapsed posterior leaflet | 5 | Triangular resection | 3 |
|  |  | Chordal shortening | 2 |
| Restricted leaflet motion | 7 | Splitting of papillary muscles with resection of subvalvular apparatus | 7 |
| Common atrioventricular valve | 2 | Closure of cleft and repair of leaflets | 2 |

pending on the size of the left and right atria and the associated procedures. The morphologic abnormalities of the mitral valve are then assessed systematically. First, the left atrium should be searched for clots, septal defects, or the presence of a supramitral ring. Valve function may be assessed in a cold perfused fibrillating heart (Carpentier et al., 1976) or a beating perfused heart with the aorta cross-clamped (Yacoub et al., 1981). We prefer to assess valve function after cardioplegic arrest by injection of cold St. Thomas solution into the left ventricle with a syringe and fine catheter. This technique, first reported by Kirklin and Barratt-Boyes in 1986, uses a cold crystalloid solution injection into the left ventricle. The degree of stenosis and/or insufficiency is assessed, and the valve apparatus is inspected in both open and closed positions. Annular size, leaflets, commissures, chordae, and papillary muscles are assessed. Leaflet motion is classified as normal, prolapsed, or restricted, and commissural fusion, clefts, or leaflet defects should be sought. Evaluation of the chordae and papillary muscles is the final step in valve assessment. The functional classification and techniques of repair of mitral valve lesions used at UCLA are presented in Table 42–3. We presently use transesophageal and transthoracic echocardiography in all children and adults to assess final repair (Fig. 42–4).

## Repair of Mitral Valve Insufficiency

### Annular Dilatation

Annular dilatation in children occurs most frequently with other congenital lesions of the mitral valve and primarily affects the region of the posterior leaflet. These children usually come to operation after 5 to 6 years of age with cardiomegaly and ventricular failure. Techniques of annuloplasty include modified De Vega (De Vega, 1976) or Reed (Reed et al., 1974) annuloplasty, in which annuloplasty is performed in two or more sections using a continuous suture with Teflon, felt, or pericardial pledgets placed at both commissures. We have used gluteraldehyde-treated pericardial strip annuloplasty, which is also performed in two or more sections to allow for annular growth (Fig. 42–5). Other techniques include Wooler annuloplasty, in which heavy sutures anchored by

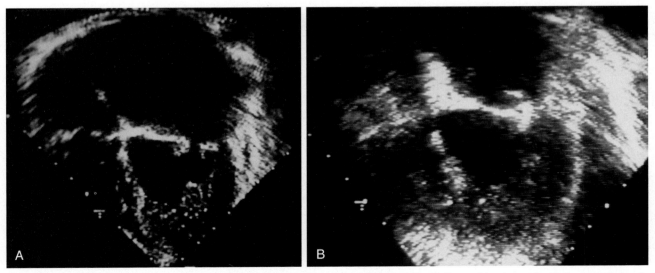

**FIGURE 42–4.** Preoperative and postoperative apical four-chambered transthoracic echocardiographic views. *A,* An incompetent mitral valve with prolapse of the anterior leaflet. *B,* A competent mitral valve following resection of the anterior leaflet, shortening of chordae to the anterior leaflet, and modified De Vega annuloplasty.

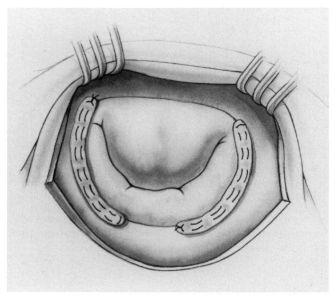

**FIGURE 42–5.** Technique of gluteraldehyde-preserved pericardial strip annuloplasty. Two strips of gluteraldehyde-preserved pericardium are used to reinforce the modified De Vega annuloplasty, also allowing for growth.

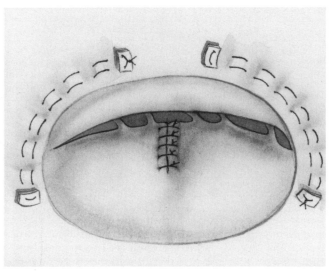

**FIGURE 42–6.** Technique of primary repair of cleft anterior leaflet. Modified De Vega annuloplasty is also shown.

pledgets are placed at each commissure to plicate the adjacent annulus of the posterior leaflet (Wooler et al., 1962). Carpentier-Edwards ring annuloplasty should be avoided in young children because it prevents growth of the mitral annulus. The modified annuloplasty has had good results, with a low early mortality rate and excellent long-term valve function. In the UCLA experience, 13 patients underwent modified De Vega annuloplasty for isolated annular dilatation with no early or late mortality, and all patients had no or minimal postoperative mitral regurgitation. We prefer not to use Prolene for the annuloplasty suture because it tends to straighten out and lose its effect. We prefer a polyfilament suture and a pericardial strip or multiple pledgets.

### Cleft Leaflet

True cleft anterior leaflet may be repaired by closing the cleft with interrupted sutures, with care taken not to incorporate excessive valve tissue (Fig. 42–6). If the mitral annulus is dilated, an annuloplasty at each lateral commissure also may be necessary. A pericardial patch reconstruction can be performed when the leaflets are severely rolled or retracted. In some patients with an intermediate form of complete atrioventricular canal or unbalanced atrioventricular canal, the lateral commissures may be poorly developed, with a small triangular posterior leaflet. In such a case, closure of the cleft will cause stenosis of the valve. For this reason, only two or three sutures may be placed in the anterior part of the cleft. Complete atrioventricular canal with a hypoplastic left or right ventricle and regurgitation of the common valve can present a difficult challenge. We find that annuloplasty alone for the common atrioventricular valve is

inadequate, and that support of the central portion of the valve by suture of the cleft and of the central components of the right-sided portions of the valve is necessary to achieve a competent valve (Fig. 42–7). True cleft of the posterior leaflet can be treated with suture of the cleft and plication of the annulus. Leaflet defects can be treated by direct suture or pericardial patch repair.

### Leaflet Prolapse

Prolapse of the anterior leaflet secondary to chordal elongation may be repaired by shortening of the

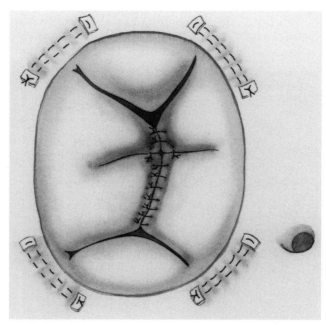

**FIGURE 42–7.** Regurgitation through the central position of the atrioventricular valve was repaired by supporting the central portion of the common atrioventricular valve by closure of the cleft and suture of the adjacent central portion of the leaflets.

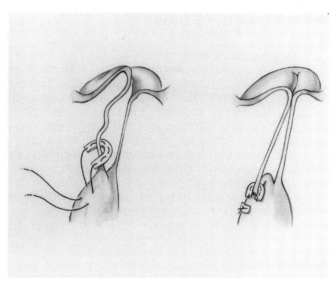

FIGURE 42–8. Technique of chordal shortening for prolapsed anterior leaflet. Pericardial pledgeted Tevdek suture is used to plicate the elongated chordae to the anterior papillary muscle.

chordae using several techniques. In a technique developed by Carpentier and co-workers (1976), the elongated portion of the chordae is buried in the depth of a groove made at the base of the corresponding papillary muscle. We prefer to suture the elongated chordae to the adjacent papillary muscle with a pericardial pledgeted Tevdek suture (Fig. 42–8). Prolapse of the posterior leaflet may be treated with shortening of the elongated chordae, as described above, or by quadrangular resection of the flail portion of the posterior leaflet and plication of the annulus. Absent or ruptured chordae to the free margin of the anterior or posterior leaflet may be treated with chordal transposition (Lessana et al., 1985), resection, or chordal replacement (Revuelta et al., 1985). Gore-Tex 2.0 sutures make an excellent artificial cord; they are attached to the free edge of the leaflet and the papillary muscle. We have performed chordal replacement and transposition with good functional results and minimal postoperative mitral regurgitation. Triangular resection of the anterior leaflet, unlike the posterior leaflet, does not create a good functional repair, so we prefer resuspension of the flail segment with a false or an accessory cord. Papillary muscle elongation causing leaflet prolapse may be treated with chordal shortening or by burying the elongated portion of the papillary muscle in a trench created in the adjacent left ventricular wall (Carpentier et al., 1976).

### Restricted Leaflet Motion

Mitral insufficiency with restricted leaflet motion can in occur two types: with normal and with abnormal papillary muscles. With normal papillary muscles, the restricted leaflet motion results from commissural fusion, short chordae, or (rarely) Ebstein's anomaly of the mitral valve. Repair can be achieved

by commissurotomy, papillary muscle splitting, fenestration, and resection of secondary chordae with remodeling of the mitral annulus. The left-sided systemic Ebstein's valve in corrected transposition can be difficult to repair and may require valve replacement. When restricted leaflet motion is caused by abnormal papillary muscles, the lesions usually are complex and involve all levels of the mitral apparatus; both stenosis and insufficiency are present. Lesions with abnormal papillary muscles include parachute valve, hammock valve, and absent papillary muscles. In parachute mitral valve, all chordae originate from a single papillary muscle, which is formed either from fusion of the two papillary muscles or from the presence of only one papillary muscle with the other being hypoplastic without chordal connections (Fig. 42–9). The stenotic component usually is found at the secondary orifice and occurs when excessive valve tissue obliterates the interchordal space. In hammock mitral valve, the two papillary muscles are replaced by numerous papillary muscles and muscular fibrous bands, which insert high on the posterior wall of the ventricle, just below the mitral valve leaflets. This subvalvular arcade causes obstruction at the secondary orifice, often producing both stenotic and regurgitant lesions. Repair of parachute or hammock valves is difficult; it is based on resecting some of the obstructing chordae, thinning and splitting the papillary muscles, and excising bands that are not attached to the free leaflet margins. Valve replacement may be necessary if valve support is lost in the course of the

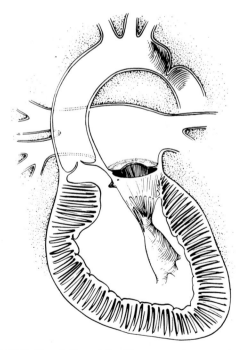

FIGURE 42–9. Description of the Shone complex: parachute mitral valve, supramitral ring, subaortic stenosis, and coarctation of the aorta. (From Shone, J. D., Sellers, R. D., Anderson, R. C., et al.: The developmental complex of "parachute mitral valve," supravalvular ring of left atrium, subaortic stenosis and coarctation of the aorta. Am. J. Cardiol., *11*:714, 1963.)

resection. Mitral valves with absent or hypoplastic papillary muscles also are difficult to repair, and they frequently require valve replacement. In the UCLA experience, 22% of congenital lesions with restricted leaflet motion and abnormal papillary muscles were not amenable to repair and required a mitral valve replacement.

## Repair of Congenital Mitral Stenosis

Congenital mitral stenosis is divided into two main groups according to the anatomy of the papillary muscles.

### Mitral Stenosis with Normal Papillary Muscles

Papillary muscle commissural fusion is treated by commissurotomy, fenestration, splitting of papillary muscles, and resection of secondary chordae. The secondary orifice usually is affected and is treated by resection of unnecessary chordae, fenestration of matted chordae, and thinning and splitting of the papillary muscles. In infancy, there are rare severe forms of isolated annular hypoplasia associated with an adequately sized left ventricle. Valve replacement may be difficult even in the supracardiac position in a small infant. An extracardiac valved conduit between the left atrium and left ventricle has been used in this case (Laks et al., 1980; Mazzer et al., 1988). A supraannular ring is treated by resection; the ring may extend onto the valve leaflets. The abnormal tissue next must be separated from the valve tissue without causing holes in the valve. The underlying valve is then carefully inspected for additional defects.

### Mitral Stenosis with Abnormal Papillary Muscles

As previously described, parachute or hammock valves may cause subvalvular obstruction as well as insufficiency, and they are treated with thinning and splitting of the papillary muscles, fenestration of the interchordal spaces, and resection of all the chordae and bands that are not attached to the free leaflet margins. Repair is difficult, and mitral valve replacement may be necessary.

### Assessment of Valve Repair

Assessment of valve function is done by injection of cold St. Thomas solution into the left ventricle with a syringe before closure of the left atrium, and by transesophageal echocardiography after termination of cardiopulmonary bypass. Transesophageal echocardiography allows excellent visualization of the entire mitral valve apparatus and thus provides essential information concerning the adequacy of repair. If severe mitral regurgitation persists, it is probably necessary to re-establish cardiopulmonary bypass and to make additional repairs to the valve or consider valve replacement.

## POSTOPERATIVE COURSE

Early postoperative complications include low cardiac output, neurologic sequelae from intraoperative air emboli, bleeding, arrhythmias, pulmonary failure, and infection. Low cardiac output is frequent; contributing factors are preoperative ventricular dysfunction, high pulmonary resistance, and incomplete valve repair. Therefore, left and right atrial pressure monitoring and frequent echocardiographic assessment of ventricular function and adequacy of repair are necessary. In the immediate postoperative period, careful volume replacement, inotropic support, and afterload-reducing agents usually are necessary.

## RESULTS

### Early Mortality

The early mortality rate in patients following repair of congenital mitral valve lesions has decreased substantially since the early era of mitral valve repair, when the hospital mortality rate reportedly exceeded 50% in children who underwent repair of mitral stenosis. Kirklin and Barratt-Boyes (1976) reported a 21% early mortality rate in patients with congenital mitral regurgitation or stenosis, Collins-Nakai and associates (1977) reported a 38% early mortality rate, and Carpentier and co-workers (1976) reported a 13% early mortality rate in 47 patients undergoing mitral valve repair. In the UCLA experience of eight patients undergoing repair for isolated congenital mitral regurgitation or stenosis, the early mortality rate was 6% (1 of 18 patients), with the only death occurring in a 4½-year-old patient with minimal postoperative mitral regurgitation. In patients with intracardiac congenital defects requiring concomitant repair at UCLA, the early mortality rate was 6% (1 of 17) in patients with univentricular heart who underwent Fontan procedure, 8% (1 of 13) in patients with prior repair of atrioventricular canal and persistent postoperative mitral regurgitation, and 0% (0 of 25) in patients with primum atrial septal defect. The two early deaths occurred secondary to low-output cardiac failure in patients with minimal postoperative mitral regurgitation.

According to Kirklin and Barratt-Boyes (1986), incremental risk factors for hospital death were young age at operation, functional status of the child before operation, and the presence of major associated cardiac anomalies. The results were not influenced by the nature of the lesion (stenosis or incompetence) or whether repair or replacement was done. Edmunds and Wagner (1985) found better results in operation for mitral regurgitation than for mitral stenosis. In the UCLA experience, age, type of mitral valve lesion, concomitant intracardiac pathology, preoperative cardiac status, and type of mitral valve repair were not statistically significant predictors of early mortality.

## Late Results

The long-term results of mitral valve repair in children are significantly better than those of replacement. Kirklin and Barratt-Boyes (1986) reported a 63% 10-year survival rate for mitral valve repair, compared with a 30% 10-year survival rate for replacement. Okita and colleagues (1988) reported an actuarial survival rate of 93% at 7 years and 88% at 17 years in children undergoing repair. Carpentier and his co-workers reported a 90% 10-year survival rate in children undergoing repair for mitral insufficiency (Chauvaud et al., 1986). In the UCLA experience, the actuarial survival rate was 94% at 1 year and 92% at 8 years in the repair group, as compared with 82% at 1 year and 76% at 8 years in the replacement group in children with congenital mitral regurgitation or stenosis (Fig. 42–10). Freedom from reoperation is also improved in children with mitral valve repair when compared with replacement. Kirklin and Barratt-Boyes (1986) reported a freedom from reoperation rate of 75% at 10 years, Carpentier and co-workers (1976) reported an actuarial risk of reoperation of 21% at 10 years, and Okita and co-workers (1988) reported a freedom from reoperation rate of 89% at 10 years. In the UCLA experience, the actuarial freedom from reoperation rate in children undergoing mitral valve repair was 97% after 2 years, 92% after 4 years, and 83% at 8 years. The actuarial freedom from reoperation rate in children undergoing mitral valve replacement during a similar period at UCLA was 84% at 2 years, 75% at 4 years, and 63% at 8 years (Fig. 42–11). The actuarial rate of freedom from valve failure (defined as need for mitral valve replacement or re-repair, valve-related death, or persistent moderate or severe postoperative mitral regurgitation seen on echocardiography) was 96% at 2 years, 91% at 4 years, and 80% at 8 years in the UCLA experience. Func-

tional long-term results also have been better in the repair group when compared with children undergoing mitral valve replacement (Carpentier et al., 1976). In the UCLA experience, 89% of the patients had minimal to no postoperative mitral regurgitation, and 9% had moderate regurgitation. Further, 98% of long-term survivors were asymptomatic or had only minimal to mild exercise intolerance.

## Mitral Valve Replacement

Patients with severe congenital abnormalities of the mitral valve not amenable to repair may require mitral valve replacement for treatment of pulmonary edema or heart failure and to prevent pulmonary and ventricular dysfunction. Lesions difficult to repair include those affecting the subvalvular area, with abnormal papillary muscles (including parachute and hammock valves) and papillary muscle agenesis. These lesions are frequently stenotic. The increased early and late mortality and morbidity in children undergoing mitral valve replacement is thus partially due to their impaired preoperative ventricular function and pulmonary hypertension. Mitral valve replacement should be performed using the largest possible low-profile prosthetic valve, such as the St. Jude mechanical valve. Technique for implantation is similar to that in adults, with nonabsorbable pledgeted mattress sutures placed through the sewing ring and annulus of the resected valve. We prefer a series of continuous Prolene sutures with a strip of pericardium to reinforce the annulus. The valve is then lowered into the appropriate position, and the sutures are tied. Supra-annular placement of the bioprosthesis may be necessary in the presence of a small annulus. Preservation of the chordal apparatus during replace-

**FIGURE 42–10.** Actuarial survival after initial mitral valve repair (dotted line) versus replacement (solid line) for congenital mitral valve disease. (From Laks, H., and Aharon, A.: Personal communication, 1993.)

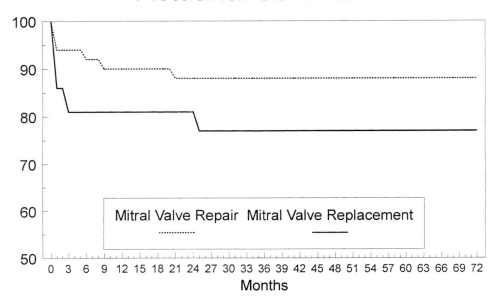

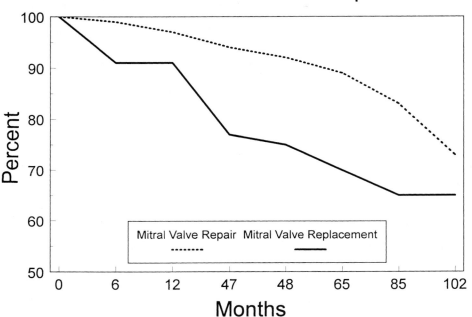

**FIGURE 42–11.** Actuarial freedom from reoperation after initial mitral valve repair (*dotted line*) versus replacement (*solid line*) for congenital mitral valve disease. (From Laks, H., and Aharon, A.: Personal communication, 1993.)

ment may improve postoperative ventricular hemodynamics (David et al., 1982; Hennein et al., 1989).

The early mortality rate associated with mitral valve replacement in young children has been relatively high, with low-output cardiac failure as a major contributing factor. However, recent reports of mitral valve replacement in older children have been encouraging, with decreased morbidity and early and late mortality (Craver et al., 1990). Boston's Children's Hospital reported an actuarial survival rate of 52% at 1 year and 43% at 5 years following mechanical valve replacement or porcine bioprosthesis in children under 1 year of age. In our 10-year experience of mitral valve replacement in children at a mean age of 6 years (range 2 weeks to 18 years), the early mortality rate was 29% (7 of 24). The early mortality rate was 14% (1 of 7) in children under 1 year and 15% (2 of 13) in children under 2 years. The late mortality rate was 4% (1 of 24) and 25% (6 of 24) in the patients who required late re-replacement of the mitral valve. In infants, mitral valve replacement using bioprosthetic xenograft valves has not improved early survival, as compared with mechanical valves. Further, bioprosthetic valves in children suffer from an accelerated rate of tissue degeneration as reported by Geha and associates (1979), Silver and colleagues (1980), and others (Kutsche et al., 1979; Kopf et al., 1986).

In general, factors contributing to the high rate of failure include the continued growth of the child, tissue overgrowth of the prosthesis orifice causing stenosis, and the early calcific degeneration of bioprosthetic valves, reported to be 9% per patient-year (Kutsche et al., 1979). The late mortality rate has also been high in infants and young children undergoing mitral valve replacement with mechanical and bio-

prosthetic valves. The 10-year survival rate was reported as 76% after mitral valve replacement with Starr-Edwards valve prosthesis (Attie et al., 1981), and a 5-year survival rate of 53% was reported by Williams and co-workers (1982) after mitral valve replacement with the St. Jude Medical valve. Currently, mitral valve replacement with mechanical or bioprosthetic valves should be avoided if possible; mitral valve repair is the treatment of choice for congenital mitral regurgitation or stenosis.

Besides repair or replacement, few other therapeutic measures can be added to the treatment of congenital mitral valve disease in infancy. Alday and Juaneda (1987) and Kveselis and associates (1986) reported successful percutaneous balloon dilatation for congenital mitral stenosis in infants. The valve area could be doubled in some patients. This modality is suitable only for isolated cases of commissural stenosis and cannot be used for most other lesions. Laks and associates (1980) and others (Lansing et al., 1983; Mazzar et al., 1988; Midgely et al., 1985) described bypass of the left atria to left ventricle using external valved conduits. The early and late mortality rates following this type of reconstruction have been high.

Mitral valve repair in children is a safe procedure with low early and late mortality rates, and it has the advantage of avoiding many of the well-described complications of prosthetic valve replacement. Repair of the valve at an early age is important in avoiding the pulmonary hypertension and ventricular dysfunction that may occur when surgical therapy is delayed. Good results require careful functional assessment of the valve lesion. When possible, mitral valve repair is the procedure of choice for correction of both mitral insufficiency and stenosis in children.

# BIBLIOGRAPHY

Alday, L. E, and Juaneda, E.: Percutaneous balloon dilatation in congenital mitral stenosis. Br. Heart J., 57(5):479–482, 1987.

Attie, F., Kurt, J., Zanoniani, C., et al.: Mitral valve replacement in children with rheumatic heart disease. Circulation, 64:812, 1981.

Baker, C. G., Benson, P. F., Joseph, M. C., et al.: Congenital mitral stenosis. Br. Heart J., 24:498, 1962.

Bower, B. D., and Gerrardi, J. W.: Two cases of congenital mitral stenosis treated by valvotomy. Arch. Dis. Child., 28:91, 1953.

Carpentier, A., Branchini, B., Cour, J. C., et al.: Congenital malformations of the mitral valve in children. J. Thorac. Cardiovasc. Surg., 72:854, 1976.

Chauvaud, S., Perier, P., Touati, G., et al.: Long-term results of valve repair in children with acquired mitral valve incompetence. Circulation, 74(Suppl. 1):1–104, 1986.

Collins-Nakai, R. L., Rosenthal, A., Castañeda, A. R., et al.: Congenital mitral stenosis—A review of 20 years' experience. Circulation, 56:1039, 1977.

Craver, J. M., Cohen, C., and Weintraub, W. S.: Case-matched comparison of mitral valve replacement and repair. Ann Thorac. Surg., 49:964–969, 1990.

Creech, O., Ledbetter, M. K., and Reemtsma, K.: Congenital mitral insufficiency with cleft posterior leaflet. Circulation, 25:390, 1962.

David, L., Castañeda, A. R., and Van Praagh, R.: Potentially parachute mitral valve in common atrioventricular canal: Pathological anatomy and surgical importance. J. Thorac. Cardiovasc. Surg., 84:178–186, 1982.

De Vega, N. G.: La annuloplastica selectiva. Rev. Esp. Cardiol., 25:555, 1977.

Devachi, F., Moller, J. H., and Edwards, J. E.: Diseases of the mitral valve in infancy. Circulation, 43:565, 1971.

Duran, C. M. G., Gometza, B., Balasundaram, S., and Al Halees, Z.: A feasibility study of valve repair in rheumatic mitral regurgitation. Eur. Heart. J., 12(Suppl. B):34–38, 1991.

Edmunds, L. H., and Wagner, H. R.: Congenital anomalies of the mitral valve. In Arciniegas, E. (ed): Pediatric Cardiac Surgery. Chicago, Year Book, 1985.

Geha, A. S., Laks, H., Stansel, H. C., et al.: Late failure of porcine valve heterografts in children. J. Thorac. Cardiovasc. Surg., 78:351–364, 1979.

Hennein, H. A., Swain, J. A., McIntosh, C. L., et al.: Comparative clinical assessment of mitral valve repair with and without chordal preservation. Abstract Program of the American Association for Thoracic Surgery, 69th Annual Meeting, Boston, May 1989.

Kirklin, J. W., and Barratt-Boyes, B. G.: Cardiac Surgery. New York, John Wiley and Sons, 1986, pp. 1091–1106.

Kopf, G. S., and Geha, A. S., Hellenbrand, W. E., Kleinman, C. S.: Fate of leftsided cardiac bioprosthesis valves in children. Arch. Surg., 121(4):488–490, 1986.

Kutsche, L., Oyer, P., Shumway, N., and Baum, D.: An important complication of Hancock mitral valve replacement in children. Circulation, 58(Suppl. 11):11–148, 1979.

Kveselis, D. A., Rocchini, A. P., Beekman, R., et al.: Balloon dilatation for congenital and rheumatic mitral stenosis. Am. J. Cardiol., 57:348, 1986.

Laks, H., Hellenbrand, W. E., Kleinman, C., and Talner, N. S.: Left atrial to left ventricular conduit for relief of congenital mitral stenosis in infancy. J. Thorac. Cardiovasc. Surg., 80:782, 1980.

Lansing, A. M., Elbe, F., Solinger, R. E.: Left atrial to left ventricular bypass for congenital mitral stenosis. Ann. Thorac. Surg., 35:667, 1983.

Lessana, A., Escorsin, M., Romano, M., et al.: Transposition of posterior leaflet for treatment of ruptured main chordae of the anterior mitral leaflet. J. Thorac. Cardiovasc. Surg., 89:804, 1985.

Mazzer, E., Corno, A., Didonato, J., et al.: Surgical bypass of the systemic A-V valve in children by means of a valved conduit. J. Thorac. Cardiovasc. Surg., 96:321, 1988.

Midgley, F. M., Perry, L. W., and Potter, B. M.: Conduit bypass of the mitral valve. Am. J. Cardiol., 56:493, 1985.

Okita, Y., Miki, S., Kusuhara, K., et al.: Early and late results of reconstructive operation for congenital mitral regurgitation in pediatric age group. J. Thorac. Cardiovasc. Surg., 96:294–298, 1988.

Reed, G. E., Pooley, R. W., and Moggio, R. A.: Durability of measured mitral annuloplasty. J. Thorac. Cardiovasc. Surg., 79:321–325, 1980.

Revuelta, J. M., Garcia-Rinaldi, R., and Duran, C. M.: Tricuspid commissurotomy. Ann. Thorac. Surg., 39:489–491, 1985.

Rowlatt, U. F., Rimoldi, H. J. A., and Lev, M.: The quantitative anatomy of the normal child's heart. Pediatr. Clin. North Am., 10:499, 1963.

Ruckman, R. N., and Van Praagh, R.: Anatomic types of congenital mitral stenosis: Report on 49 autopsy cases. Am. J. Cardiol., 42:592, 1978.

Ruschaupt, D. G., Bharati, S., and Lev, M.: Mitral valve malformations of Ebstein's type in the absence of corrected transposition. Am. J. Cardiol., 38:109, 1976.

Shone, J. D., Sellers, R. D., Anderson, R. D., et al: The developmental complex of "parachute mitral valve," supravalular ring of left atrium, subaortic stenosis and coarctation of the aorta. Am. J. Cardiol., 11:714, 1963.

Silver, K. M., Polbck, J., Silver, D., et al.: Calcification in porcine xenograft valves in children. Am. J. Cardiol., 45:685, 1980.

Smith, E.: Premature occlusion of the foramen ovale, large pulmonary artery, and contracted left heart. Trans. Pathol. Soc. London, 1:52, 1846. (Cited by Ferencz, C., et al.: Congenital mitral stenosis. Circulation, 9:161, 1954.)

Starkey, G. W. B.: Surgical experience in the treatment of congenital mitral stenosis and insufficiency. J. Thorac. Cardiovasc. Surg., 38:336, 1959.

Van der Horst, R. L., and Hartreister, A. R.: Congenital mitral stenosis. Am. J. Cardiol., 20:773, 1967.

Van Mierap, L. H. S., Alley, R. D., Kaasel, H. W., et al.: The anatomy and embryology of endocardial cushion defects. J. Thorac. Cardiovasc. Surg., 43:71, 1962.

Vlad, P.: Mitral valve anomalies in children. Circulation, 9:161, 1954.

Williams, D. B., Danielson, G. K., McGoon, D. C., et al.: Porcine heterograft valve replacement in children. J. Thorac. Cardiovasc. Surg., 84:446, 1982.

Wooler, G. H., Nixon, P. G. F., and Grimshaw, V. A.: Experience with the repair of the mitral valve in mitral incompetence. Thorax, 17:49, 1962.

Yacoub, M., Halim, M., Radley-Smith, R., et al.: Surgical treatment of mitral regurgitation caused by floppy valves. Repair versus replacement. Circulation, 64(Suppl. 11):210–216, 1981.

# 43 Transposition of the Great Arteries

## ■ I The Mustard Procedure

George A. Trusler and Robert M. Freedom

*Transposition of the great arteries* (TGA) is a severe cardiac malformation in which the aorta arises from the right ventricle and the pulmonary artery arises from the left ventricle. With a concordant atrioventricular connection (whether in situs solitus or inversus), the physiologic effects are acute, and cyanosis and distress are usually obvious soon after birth. Survival depends on the mixing of blood between pulmonary and systemic circulations, mainly through a patent foramen ovale and assisted by a *patent ductus arteriosus* (PDA) and sometimes a co-existent *ventricular septal defect* (VSD). If left untreated, many infants die in the first week of life, and most die by 1 year of age. Survival is extended by procedures that increase mixing, mainly by enlarging the atrioseptal communication. Techniques for repair have advanced dramatically over the last few decades, and the outlook for infants with TGA has improved greatly.

## HISTORICAL ASPECTS

In 1797, Matthew Baillie first described the pathologic anatomy of TGA. The first palliative operation, an ingenious closed technique for creating an *atrial septal defect* (ASD), was performed by Blalock and Hanlon in 1948. Lillehei and Varco (1953) tried to transfer the *inferior vena cava* (IVC) to the left atrium and the right pulmonary veins to the right atrium. In 1956, Baffes described a palliative procedure, which was a partial repair, that consisted of suturing the right pulmonary veins to the right atrium and connecting the inferior vena cava to the left atrium with a graft. For some years, this procedure provided effective palliation for many children. A very important advance in palliation was the development of balloon atrial septostomy (Rashkind and Miller, 1966).

The first attempts at repair of TGA were directed toward the great arteries. In 1954, Mustard and associates described a technique for switching the great arteries plus one coronary artery. They were unsuccessful, as were Bailey and co-workers (1954), Björk and Bouckaert (1954), Kay and Cross (1955), Senning (1959), Idriss and colleagues (1961), and Baffes and associates (1961). It was not until 1975 that the first successful arterial repair was reported by Jatene and co-workers (1975, 1976). This encouraged other surgeons to attempt this operation, but the mortality rate was high. Since then the risk of arterial repair has

decreased owing to better selection and technical management of patients.

A technique for complete repair by rearranging venous inflow at the atrial level was first suggested by Albert (1955), who later attempted an intra-atrial repair with a patch of plastic material. Later trials by Merendino and colleagues (1957), Kay and Cross (1955, 1957), Creech and associates (1958), Shumacker (1961), and Wilson and associates (1962) using various materials and techniques were all unsuccessful. Senning performed the first successful intra-atrial repair in 1959 with a clever but complicated procedure involving flaps of atrial wall and septum. Kirklin and colleagues (1961) used Senning's technique with success, but the mortality rate was high. In 1961, Barnard and co-workers performed a successful intra-atrial repair using a large crimped tube made of Teflon to connect the pulmonary veins to the tricuspid valve. In 1963, Mustard applied Albert's principle by using a patch or baffle of pericardium to partition the atria and redirect venous inflow to match the transposed arteries. This operation was not only relatively simple but could be reproduced safely; its success stimulated an immediate and widespread awakening of interest in the repair of TGA.

Other historical highlights include the development of Rastelli's procedure in 1969 for TGA with VSD and *pulmonary stenosis* (PS) and of intraventricular repair by McGoon in 1972 for patients with large and suitably positioned VSDs.

## PATHOLOGIC ANATOMY

TGA refers to that condition in which the aorta originates from the morphologic right ventricle and the pulmonary artery is supported by the morphologic left ventricle. When complete TGA is present, the atrioventricular connections are concordant—that is, the morphologic right atrium connects with the morphologic right ventricle, and the left atrium connects with the morphologic left ventricle. This definition of "transposition" excludes the concept of spatial relationships between the two great arteries because they vary so much and, because it concerns "connections," is independent of infundibular anatomy. Complete TGA can occur in hearts with dextrocardia or mesocardia, but our experience indicates that levocardia is evident in more than 95% of pa-

1558

tients. Similarly, more than 95% of patients with complete transposition show visceroatrial situs solitus, and only a few patients show visceroatrial situs inversus. A few patients with isomeric left atria, but with the right-sided atrium receiving the entire systemic venous return and the left-sided atrium receiving the pulmonary venous connections, have been identified. In this situation, the presence of normal or noninverted ventricles and discordant ventriculoarterial connections creates the physiology of complete TGA. Among most patients with complete TGA and visceroatrial situs solitus, the ventricular relationship is that of a noninverted pattern—the so-called d-loop or right-hand pattern. In this pattern, the inlet-apical trabecular-outlet axis of the morphologic right ventricle is from right to left, and the outlet or infundibular component of the right ventricle is to the left of the inlet zone. With rare exceptions, concordant atrioventricular connections implies a d-ventricular loop. Hearts with superoinferior ventricles or cross-atrioventricular connections can have discordant ventriculoarterial connections (Freedom et al., 1978). Approximately 70% of patients with complete TGA have an intact ventricular septum, absence of *left ventricular outflow tract obstruction* (LVOTO), a small and inadequate interatrial communication, and a small PDA. The morphology of the ventricular mass in hearts with TGA differs considerably from that of the normal heart (Smith et al., 1986a). In hearts with transposition, the ventricular septum is a straight structure, and thus the ventricles have a side-by-side relationship. The entire atrioventricular septal area is reduced, and there is less wedging of the pulmonary outflow tract between the atrioventricular valves than in the deeply wedged aortic valve in the normal heart. Significant anomalies of the tricuspid valve and in the structure of the trabecula septomarginalis were observed in hearts with simple TGA. In addition, the inlet-outlet dimensions of the right ventricle in hearts with transposition are abnormal when compared with those of the normal heart, and the outlet/inlet ratio is increased.

## Major Anomalies Associated with Transposition

The most common associated anomalies among patients with complete TGA include VSD and LVOTO (Rowe et al., 1981). VSDs can occur in any portion of the ventricular septum and may occur as a single defect or as multiple defects. With a tripartite schema of the ventricular septum, which was advocated by Soto and associates (1980), the septum can be seen as having an inlet component, an apical trabecular component, and an infundibular or subarterial component. In most patients, the VSD involves either the infundibular septum or the perimembranous septum (Oppenheimer-Dekker, 1978). As might be anticipated, a defect of one zone may be confluent with that of another zone. The infundibular (or subarterial) VSD can result from an isolated defect or deficiency of the infundibular septum (analogous to the isolated supracristal VSD in the otherwise normal heart), or it can result from a malalignment between the infundibular septum (the portion of interventricular septum that separates the aorta from the pulmonary artery) and the trabecula septomarginalis. With malalignment, the infundibular septum is almost always deviated posteriorly, encroaching on the left ventricular outflow tract and producing a muscular subpulmonary stenosis. Anterosuperior deviation of the infundibular septum is infrequently identified in these patients. This deviation encroaches on the right ventricular subaortic outflow tract and may be seen in the patient with complete TGA, VSD, and an obstructive anomaly of the aortic arch.

The complete form of atrioventricular defect rarely occurs in the patient with complete TGA, but it is identified more frequently in the patient with isomeric right or left atria and thus an ambiguous atrioventricular connection. The isolated defect of the inlet component of the ventricular septum is also uncommon. This defect can be accompanied by straddling of the tricuspid valve. Moene and colleagues (1985, 1986) have characterized the VSD in 50 hearts with TGA and have compared these findings with those of 105 hearts with VSD and normally connected great arteries. The most common forms of VSD found in the normally connected group—the central muscular VSD, the perimembranous VSD with left-sided malalignment of the outlet septum, and perimembranous VSD with overriding posterior artery—were not found in hearts with VSD and transposition. Chiu and colleagues (1984) reviewed morphologic features of an intact ventricular septum that are susceptible to subpulmonary obstruction in complete transposition. This autopsy study focused on the "bulging" or "nonbulging" of the ventricular septum. A fibrous ridge was observed on the ventricular septum in 82% of those with the bulging ventricular septum, but no fibrous ridge was noted in those without a bulging ventricular septum. These authors suggest that the subpulmonary outflow tract is more susceptible to obstruction if the aorta lies anterior and to the left of the pulmonary trunk rather than side by side and to the left.

It is difficult to consider the morphologic basis of LVOTO without first considering the basic pattern of infundibular anatomy among patients with complete TGA. Approximately 95% of patients have a subaortic infundibulum; thus, the aortic valve is separated from the tricuspid valve, whereas the pulmonary and mitral valves are in fibrous continuity. Approximately 4% of patients have bilateral muscular infundibula with neither semilunar valve in fibrous continuity with the atrioventricular valve. A rare patient will have bilaterally deficient infundibula, with both semilunar valves in continuity with the atrioventricular valves (Van Praagh et al., 1980). The conal anatomy in 119 patients with d-loop transposition of the great arteries and ventricular septal defect has been assessed in an echocardiographic and pathologic study (Pasquini et al., 1993). One hundred five patients

(88.2%) had only a subaortic infundibulum; infundibula were present beneath each great artery in eight patients (6.7%); four patients had only a subpulmonary infundibulum, including one with so-called posterior transposition (3.4%); and two patients (1.7%) had bilaterally deficient infundibula.

LVOTO can result from one or more pathologic mechanisms (Aziz et al., 1979; Idriss et al., 1977; Jiminez and Martinez, 1974; Sansa et al., 1979; Shrivastava et al., 1976; Van Gils, 1978; Van Gils et al., 1978). These mechanisms include (1) posterior malalignment of the infundibular septum, (2) fibrous subpulmonary membrane, (3) accessory tissue tags, often pendunculated and mobile, originating from an atrioventricular valve and contiguous structures, (4) a muscular or tunnel form of subpulmonary obstruction, (5) aneurysm of the membranous or perimembranous interventricular septum, (6) straddling atrioventricular valve tissue, (7) pulmonary valve stenosis, (8) maladherent anterior leaflet of the mitral valve, (9) dynamic subvalvular obstruction due to posterior systolic bulging of the ventricular septum, and (10) combinations of these mechanisms. The most common mechanism results from the left-sided and posterior deviation of a malaligned infundibular septum (Van Gils et al., 1978), which is consistent with the observation that most patients with LVOTO complicating complete TGA have an associated VSD. The spatial relationships between the great arteries at the semilunar level in hearts with atrioventricular concordance and ventriculoarterial discordance vary, and the relative positions of the great arteries are at least partly predicated on the infundibular anatomy. The most common relationship is the location of the aorta to the right of and anterior to the pulmonary valve, but side-by-side, left anterior, right anterior, and left posterior relationships have all been described. Thus, "transposition" should not be defined in terms of the relative position of the great arteries but should be seen instead in terms of the ventriculoarterial connection.

## Less Common Anomalies Associated with Transposition

Left juxtaposition of the right atrial appendage (Rosenquist et al., 1974) has been identified in approximately 1 to 2% of our patients with complete transposition. These patients have had dextrocardia or mesocardia and often have an unusual spatial ventricular relationship. Almost any anomaly of the atrioventricular valve can complicate complete transposition (Layman and Edwards, 1967). Straddling of the tricuspid valve can be identified in some patients. It is particularly important to exclude an abnormality of the right atrioventricular junction in the patient with right ventricular hypoplasia (Riemenschneider et al., 1968). Structural anomalies of the mitral valve are common in patients with complete transposition (Rosenquist et al., 1975), but, fortunately, functional disturbances appear to be less frequent. Thus, although mitral stenosis or straddling of the anterior

leaflet of the mitral valve has been recorded, these cases are uncommon. Tricuspid atresia may be more common than mitral atresia. Huhta and colleagues from the Mayo clinic (1982) addressed structural anomalies of the tricuspid valve and identified these anomalies in 38 of 121 autopsied specimens. In addition to straddling and overriding of the tricuspid valve, abnormal chordal insertions often were found. These abnormal chordal insertions to the infundibular septum could compromise the potential for the Rastelli operation and others. Obstructive anomalies of the aortic arch, including coarctation, atresia, and complete interruption of the aortic arch, have been identified in approximately 6% of our patients. Although severe coarctation can be found when the ventricular septum is intact and when the right ventricle is of normal size, these aortic arch anomalies are more frequently identified when a VSD is present or when the morphologic right ventricle is underdeveloped. Finally, aortic valve atresia rarely complicates the condition of the patient with complete TGA and an intact ventricular septum (McGarry et al., 1980). Thirty-two patients with complete TGA and coarctation of the aorta were identified at the Hospital for Sick Children, Toronto, between 1963 and 1983 (Vogel et al., 1984a, 1984b). More than two-thirds of patients had an associated VSD. Less than 20% had significant hypoplasia of the morphologic right ventricle. Subaortic stenosis resulting from a malaligned infundibular septum, anomalous right ventricular muscle bundles, a prominent right-sided ventriculoinfundibular fold, or combinations of these, was identified in several of these 32 patients. In a postmortem study, Moene and colleagues (1983) addressed the morphologic substrates responsible for anatomic obstruction of the right ventricular outflow tract in TGA. Seventy-one of the 126 patients in this study had an intact ventricular septum, and only 2 of 71 patients had *right ventricular outflow tract obstruction* (RVOTO). However, of the 55 specimens with VSD, 15 (27%) had distinct RVOTO, which resulted from wedging of the subaortic outflow tract between an anteriorly malaligned infundibular septum and a prominent right-sided ventriculoinfundibular fold in 75% of these cases.

## Laterality of the Aortic Arch

A left-sided aortic arch is found in approximately 90 to 92% of patients with complete TGA; the aortic arch is right-sided in 8 to 10%. The lowest frequency of right-sided aortic arch (approximately 4%) is found in patients with an intact ventricular septum, and the highest incidence (approximately 16%) is seen among those with VSD and left ventricular outflow tract stenosis (Mathew et al., 1974).

## Coronary Arteries

Knowledge of the aortic origin of the coronary arteries and their epicardial distribution is necessary for the operative management of some forms of transposition. The epicardial distribution must be defined before interposition of a right-ventricular pulmonary artery conduit. Because the anterior descending coronary artery can cross the right ventricular outflow tract, this distribution may prevent or make difficult interposition of a right ventricular conduit in the young or small patient. Since 1975, when Jatene and colleagues successfully performed an anatomic repair with coronary artery reimplantation, there has been a resurgence of interest in the anatomy and variations of the origin of the coronary artery in these patients. Kurosawa and colleagues (1986) did a morphometric study of the coronary arterioles in newborns, infants, and children, and compared findings from normal patients with those from patients with aortic atresia and TGA. Among patients with TGA, the number of arterioles per surface area from birth to 1 year of age is below that anticipated in normal hearts. This difference was even more pronounced in the morphologic right ventricle than in the left ventricle. Moreover, the average medial thickness of the arterioles seems to be less than anticipated from the normal. The functional implications of these observations are unclear.

The specific origin of the left and right coronary arteries from sinus 1 or sinus 2 of the aortic valve, the specific anatomic relationship between the coronary artery and the commissure of the aortic valve, and the presence or absence of an intramural course is certainly less relevant to the atrial repair than to the arterial repair. The importance of the coronary anatomy in the arterial switch operation is discussed later.

## Wall Thickness of Ventricular Chambers in Transposition

Bano-Rodrigo and colleagues (1980) examined the wall thickness of ventricular chambers in TGA. The surgical implications of these findings with regard to the arterial switch are obvious. Among their patients with TGA and an intact ventricular septum, the left ventricular/right ventricular ratio was decreased after the neonatal period, and after 8 months of age the thickness of the left ventricular wall in this group was under 95% confidence limits for normalcy. The same was true for patients with an associated large VSD after 18 months of age. Because of their findings, these authors could not recommend anatomic correction after 8 months of age for the patients with an intact ventricular septum or after 18 months of age for the patient with a large VSD.

## Pulmonary Arteries

Among patients with complete TGA and an intact ventricular septum, the main and branch pulmonary arteries are usually dilated, especially after the newborn period. In addition, after the newborn period,

the surgeon can recognize asymmetric distribution of the pulmonary blood flow between the right and left lungs (Muster et al., 1976). The inclination of geometry of the left ventricular outflow tract favors blood flow from the main pulmonary artery to the right pulmonary artery. This maldistribution of flow may increase when there is LVOTO or when there are anatomic stenoses in the left pulmonary artery. The disparity in perfusion between the two lungs may be progressive. Patients with associated VSD and left ventricular outflow tract stenosis can have all of the anomalies of pulmonary arteries anticipated in patients with tetralogy of Fallot. Among patients with pulmonary atresia and VSD (but posterior pulmonary artery), it is necessary to define the site(s) or origin of the pulmonary arteries (e.g., single ductus, ascending aorta, aortopulmonary collaterals, and bilateral homologous ducts when the right and left pulmonary arteries are not confluent).

## Left Pulmonary Vein Stenosis

Pulmonary vein stenosis has been described both as a sequela and as a complication of Mustard's operation, but unilateral left-sided pulmonary vein stenosis may also be a congenital anomaly that complicates complete TGA. Moreover, the degree of obstruction may become progressive as a result of the topography of the left ventricular outflow tract in hearts with transposition, which, postnatally, mandates preferential blood flow to the right lung (Vogel et al., 1984a).

### Fetal Course of Transposition of the Great Arteries

Fermont from Paris has addressed the impact of prenatal detection on outcome in patients with transposition of the great arteries (Fermont, 1992). Among 819 fetuses identified with congenital heart disease, 34 had isolated TGA, one VSD, or coarctation of the aorta. The mean age of arrival at a specialized cardiac center of a neonate in whom transposition had been recognized prenatally was 4.2 hours, compared with 14.5 hours for neonates who had not benefited from prenatal recognition. Two false-negative diagnoses were encountered, but no false-positive diagnoses. Simple transposition was not associated with aneuploidy.

## PATHOPHYSIOLOGY

The neonate with complete TGA, an intact ventricular septum, a small ASD, and a closing PDA can be seen to have two parallel circulations: a systemic circulation and a pulmonary circulation. Survival in this group of patients for even a short time is predicated on adequate mixing between the two parallel circulations. The presence of a large VSD or a large

PDA affords some mixing between the two circulations. Thus, intense cyanosis is less common, and frequently these patients are only mildly to moderately cyanotic. However, in this group, congestive heart failure may be conspicuous and may not respond to anticongestive therapy.

The natural history of the patient with associated VSD and LVOTO is similar to that of the patient with tetralogy of Fallot. An increased severity of LVOTO causes inadequate pulmonary blood flow, so hypoxia and polycythemia may become progressive. When the pulmonary arteries are not continuous with the heart, pulmonary blood flow may be duct-dependent, or, depending on the site or origin of the pulmonary arteries, saturation may be reasonable in the aorta.

## CLINICAL MANIFESTATIONS

Data from the New England Regional Infant Cardiac Program reveal an incidence of 0.218 per 1000 live births (Fyler, 1980). This study showed that 59% of infants with simple transposition were hospitalized before the third day of life, compared with 34% of those with large associated VSD. Two-thirds of patients with complete transposition are males (Fyler, 1980). Although 9% of patients with complete transposition included in the New England Regional Infant Cardiac Program had extracardiac congenital anomalies, most of these anomalies were minor. Reviewing 140 clinical and autopsy cases of complete transposition, Landtman and colleagues (1975) found extracardiac malformations in 39 patients, which were thought to be responsible for the death of 22 of these patients. Low birth weight was not a consistent feature. The clinical manifestation depends on whether there are associated cardiovascular anomalies. Because circulatory mixing is usually inadequate in patients with complete transposition, these patients inevitably present in the newborn period. The most striking physical sign of TGA is persistent cyanosis that does not respond to an increased oxygen concentration (Goldman et al., 1973; Jones et al., 1976; Shannon et al., 1972; Tooley and Stanger, 1972). Cyanosis, which is usually progressive, may be intense, especially when the neonate is also relatively polycythemic. Cyanosis may be less intense, or even equivocal, in the patient with good circulatory mixing. When ductal patency is responsible for only equivocal cyanosis, the reprieve may be transient, and ductal closure may cause rapid clinical deterioration (Rowe et al., 1981). Differential cyanosis with relatively pink lower extremities and deeper cyanosis of the upper extremities may be found in patients with associated severe thoracic coarctation or interruption of the aortic arch.

After cyanosis, the next most conspicuous finding in these patients is congestive heart failure, with tachycardia, tachypnea, dyspnea, and an enlarged liver. Signs of heart failure are distinctly uncommon in the patient with severe LVOTO. Conversely, the patient with a large VSD or ductus arteriosus or severe obstructive anomaly of the aortic arch may present in severe cardiorespiratory distress and may have relatively mild to moderate hypoxia and cyanosis. The profoundly acidotic infant may present in extremis. The heart is usually overactive and has a prominent left parasternal lift. The heart sounds are usually loud and crisp; the second sound is single. When the ventricular septum is intact, there may be no murmur, or a soft systolic ejection murmur may be audible along the left sternal border. A soft pansystolic murmur may indicate the presence of a small or moderate VSD. It is uncommon to appreciate the typical "machinery" murmur of a PDA in the immediate newborn period. The caliber and timing of the femoral pulses may indicate an obstructive anomaly of the aortic arch.

## LABORATORY FINDINGS

### Radiologic Features

The typical radiographic appearance of TGA is that of an enlarged heart with the appearance of an egg on its side (Fig. 43–1). Pulmonary plethora may be conspicuous; beyond the first 1 or 2 months of life, a disparity in the pulmonary perfusion may be apparent, and the right lung may be more plethoric than the left lung. Characteristically, the cardiac pedicle is narrow (Guerin et al., 1970; Kurlander et al., 1968; Moes, 1975; Nogrady and Dunbar, 1969; Tonkin et al., 1980). Although these features can be seen in the first few days of life, there are numerous exceptions to the classic appearance. Counahan and colleagues (1973)

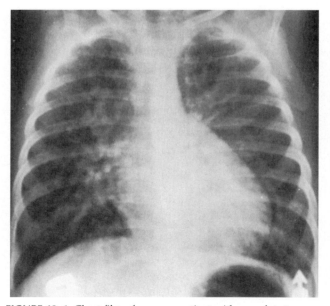

**FIGURE 43–1.** Chest film of a young patient with complete transposition of the great arteries (TGA). The cardiac pedicle is narrow, and the configuration is egg-shaped. Pulmonary plethora is conspicuous. (Courtesy of C. A. F. Moes, M.D., Department of Radiology, The Hospital for Sick Children, Toronto.)

suggested that 10% of plain chest films obtained from infants less than 1 month of age with complete TGA were interpreted as normal.

## Electrocardiography

Most patients have normal sinus rhythm or a sinus tachycardia. Approximately 2% have the so-called coronary sinus rhythm with a negative P wave in leads 2, 3, and aVF, and a normal PR interval. The mean QRS axis congregates around 100 degrees to more than 120 degrees, although some patients have profound right-axis deviation of 150 degrees to more than 240 degrees. It is uncommon to identify left-axis deviation in patients with uncomplicated TGA.

There is no clear-cut relationship between the pattern of ventricular hypertrophy and the presence or absence of a VSD or LVOTO. Most patients, especially hypoxic neonates, show a pattern of right ventricular hypertrophy of dominance, and our data indicate that left ventricular hypertrophy or combined ventricular hypertrophy is uncommon in the neonate. Even in the patient with severe LVOTO with or without a VSD, it is unusual for the electrocardiogram to show severe left ventricular hypertrophy. ST-T wave changes are common and may reflect some degree of myocardial ischemia, especially in the severely hypoxic and acidotic neonate.

## Echocardiography

Both M-mode and two-dimensional echocardiographic examinations have had a major impact on the noninvasive diagnosis of complete TGA. The two-dimensional technique can demonstrate the abnormal spatial relationship between the aorta and the pulmonary artery (when compared with the normal relationship) and their respective origins from the discordant ventricle in only a few minutes (Bierman and Williams, 1979a; Houston et al., 1978). But what is the relevance of the echocardiographic examination to the surgeon? When the diagnosis of complete transposition has been unequivocally confirmed, two-dimensional echocardiographic techniques should allow (1) visualization of the atrial septum and the adequacy of balloon atrial septostomy, (2) longitudinal assessment of ventricular contractility and wall motion, (3) assessment of the atrioventricular junction in the patient with complex transposition, (4) recognition of the type of LVOTO when left ventricular angiography is unsatisfactory (Aziz et al., 1978, 1979), (5) imaging of the ventricular septum and quantitation of the number and type of VSDs, and (6) imaging of the aortic isthmus and juxtaductal or juxtaligamental level with regard to the question of coarctation. After the Mustard operation, echocardiographic techniques allow visualization of the baffle and serial assessment of right ventricular function. Microcavitation facilitates postoperative recognition of baffle leaks or residual shunting at the ventricular level.

## Angiocardiography

An extensive literature is devoted to angiocardiography of patients with complete TGA (Barcia et al., 1967; Deutsch et al., 1970; Fisher et al., 1970; Freedom et al., 1974; Paul, 1977; Sansa et al., 1979; Silove and Taylor, 1973). Selective right ventriculography is usually done in frontal and lateral projections, and most institutions perform selective angiocardiography in the biplane mode. Frontal and lateral ventriculograms are most common; they show the discordant ventriculoarterial connection, the subaortic infundibulum, the size and function (when using cine technique) of the right ventricle, and the presence or absence of tricuspid regurgitation, as well as when the ventricular septum is intact (or when only a small VSD is present), the status of the aortic isthmus, ductus arteriosus, and the presence or absence of a juxtaductal coarctation or other obstructive anomaly of the aortic arch (Figs. 43-2 and 43-3). With a significant VSD, opacification of the main and left pulmonary arteries may obscure the aortic isthmus. Thus, selective aortography may be necessary to more completely define the caliber of the aortic isthmus and to exclude obstructive anomalies of the aortic arch (Fig. 43-4). In addition, the origin of the coronary arteries is best seen by aortography filmed in the biplane mode.

Selective biplane left ventriculography is best filmed using axial cineangiography. These projections, which were advocated initially by Bargeron and colleagues (1977) and Elliott and associates (1977), elongate the left ventricular outflow tract and give two immediate advantages. First, axial cineangiography allows precise definition of the left ventricular outflow tract without the "shoulder" of the left ventricle compromising the immediate subpulmonary area (Fig. 43-5). Second, the left long axial oblique projection should profile most of the VSD involving the infundibular or perimembranous septum. When a more posteriorly positioned VSD is suspected, the hepatoclavicular four-chamber projection is better. This profiles more adequately show the inlet and posterior aspects of the ventricular septum.

As mentioned earlier, the anatomic causes of LVOTO are diverse. The left long axial oblique projection is ideal to show posterior malalignment of the infundibular septum and the resultant VSD. The presence of associated pulmonary valve stenosis, fibrous diaphragm, fibromuscular tunnel form of subpulmonary stenosis, and accessory tissue tags is usually profiled best with this projection, but the exact degree of obliqueness must be individualized for every patient (Figs. 43-6 to 43-8).

Atrial angiography may be useful in evaluating the atrioventricular junction when the concordant ventricle is underdeveloped. In addition, when mesocardia or dextrocardia is present, a selective right atrial angiogram excludes left juxtaposition of the right atrial appendage, a condition that makes Blalock-Hanlon's atrial septectomy or intra-atrial repair more difficult, especially in the very young and small patient (Rosenquist et al., 1975; Urban et al., 1976).

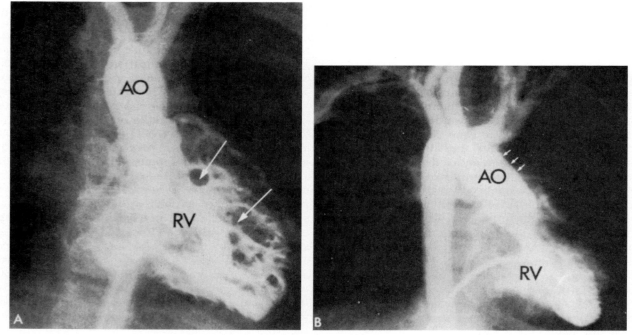

**FIGURE 43–2.** Complete TGA. *A,* Frontal right ventriculogram with opacification of aorta (AO). The right ventricle (RV) is heavily trabeculated *(arrows).* The ascending aorta is in the usual position. *B,* In this patient with complete transposition, the aorta is relatively levopositioned, and the ascending aorta *(arrows)* forms the left border of the cardiac silhouette.

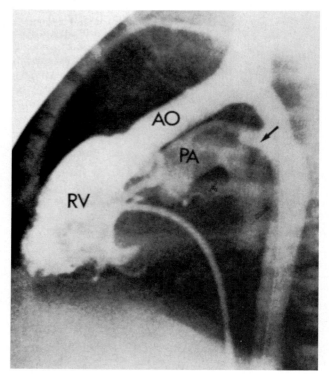

**FIGURE 43–3.** Complete transposition with patent ductus arteriosus (PDA). Lateral right ventriculogram shows an anteriorly positioned, discordantly connected aorta (AO). The larger and posteriorly positioned pulmonary artery (PA) is opacified via a moderate-sized PDA *(arrow).* (RV = right ventricle.)

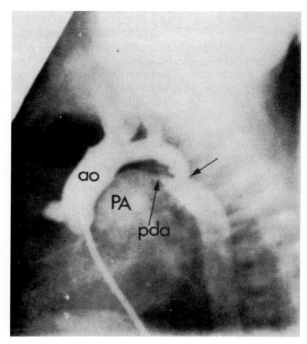

**FIGURE 43–4.** Coarctation of the aorta *(arrow on right)* complicating complete TGA. This aortogram shows a relatively small ascending aorta (ao), a small aortic isthmus, and a discrete coarctation of aorta with a posterior shelf. The small patent ductus arteriosus (pda) opacifies the pulmonary artery (PA).

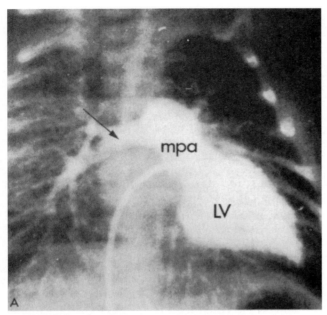

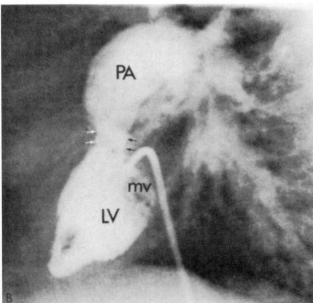

**FIGURE 43–5.** Left ventriculogram in a patient with complete TGA and an intact ventricular septum. *A,* Frontal left ventriculogram opacifies the discordantly connected pulmonary artery (mpa). There is preferential flow into the right pulmonary artery *(arrow)* because of the inclination of the left ventricular outflow tract. (LV = left ventricle.) *B,* An intact ventricular septum and absence of left ventricular outflow tract obstruction (LVOTO) *(between white and black arrows).* (PA = pulmonary artery; mv = mitral valve.)

## NATURAL HISTORY OF THE PATIENT WITH COMPLETE TRANSPOSITION OF THE GREAT ARTERIES

Before the introduction of balloon atrial septostomy by Rashkind and Miller in 1966, the natural history for these patients was clear: 90% of patients with TGA would not survive to their first birthday, and almost half of all these patients would die by 1 month of age

(Liebman et al., 1969). Although nonoperative atrial septostomy has irrevocably altered the natural history, a substantial number of patients with transposition still die before reaching 1 year of age. Data compiled from the New England Infant Cardiac Program (Fyler, 1980) show a crude first-year mortality rate of 39% for patients with complete transposition. Reviewing 112 consecutive neonates with complete transposition seen at the Texas Children's Hospital from 1967 to 1977, Gutgesell and colleagues (1979) found that the first month of life was the period of greatest risk, with an 8% mortality rate. Between the balloon atrial septostomy and baffle repair, 14 of 103 patients at risk either died or sustained a cerebrovascular accident. The mortality rate at baffle repair in their series was 14%, and there were three late postoperative deaths. Actuarial analysis suggested that approximately 50% of newborns with TGA survive for 5 years with excellent function, and that an additional 15 to 20% survive with one or more medical handicaps. Plauth and associates (1968) reviewed serial hemodynamic studies among patients with complete TGA. Like a small VSD in a patient with an otherwise

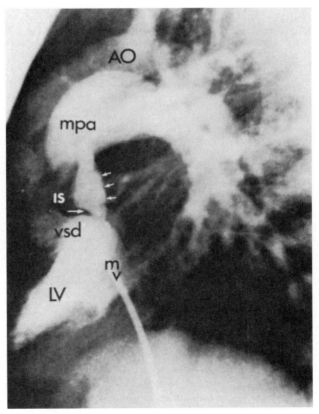

**FIGURE 43–6.** LVOTO at several sites in a child with complete TGA and malalignment type of ventricular septal defect (vsd). This long-axial oblique left ventriculogram shows that the pulmonary artery (mpa) is supported by the left ventricle (LV). The infundibular septum (IS) is deviated posteriorly *(solitary white arrow)* and is seen superior to the large vsd. The subpulmonary infundibulum is an elongated muscular structure *(small white arrows),* and because it is well developed but poorly expanded, there is discontinuity between the pulmonary valve and the anterior leaflet of the mitral valve (mv). (AO = aorta.)

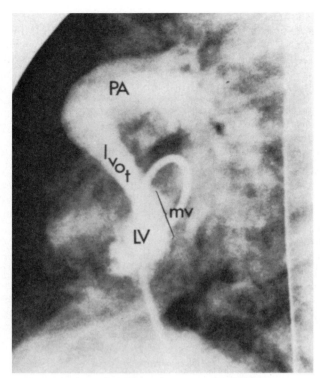

**FIGURE 43–7.** Muscular tunnel form of subpulmonary stenosis in a patient with complete TGA and multiple small VSDs. This lateral left ventriculogram shows the greatly elongated left ventricular outflow tract (lvot). The main pulmonary trunk (PA) has good caliber. Clearly, the mitral valve (mv) is not in continuity with the pulmonary valve. (LV = left ventricle.)

normal heart, the small VSD in the patient with complete TGA can decrease spontaneously in size or can close spontaneously. Reduction in size may be accompanied by aneurysmal transformation. Because the aneurysm protrudes into the left ventricular outflow tract, subpulmonary stenosis may occur (Vidne et al., 1976). The spontaneous closure rate of a small VSD in the patient with complete transposition is assumed to be almost the same as that in the individual with an otherwise normal heart. LVOTO can develop or may become increasingly likely with time in the patient with an associated VSD or in the patient with an intact ventricular septum. Our data indicate that the incidence of LVOTO in the individual with an intact ventricular septum is in the range of 2 to 3% and is slightly higher in the patient with an associated VSD. Tonkin and co-workers (1980) provided excellent angiographic verification of developing LVOTO in patients with complete TGA and an intact ventricular septum. Pulmonary vascular obstructive disease is uncommon within the first few years of life in the patient with complete TGA and an intact ventricular septum. However, Lakier and colleagues (1975) and Newfeld and associates (1974) described early onset of pulmonary vascular obstruction in a few patients. More common is the development of pulmonary vascular arteriopathy in patients with an associated large VSD or large PDA (Newfeld et al., 1974; Waldman et al., 1977). Although it is difficult and unwise to

generalize, many patients with complete transposition and an unrestrictive VSD or ductus arteriosus may develop severe pulmonary vascular obstruction by 1 year of age (Yamaki and Tezuka, 1976).

## MEDICAL TREATMENT

The initial medical therapy of the severely hypoxic neonate should correct metabolic acidosis, treat congestive heart failure with parenteral digoxin and diuretics, maintain normothermia, treat hypoglycemia, and provide adequate ventilation for the profoundly distressed infant. Echocardiographic examination should be as expeditious as possible, and the neonate should be transferred to the cardiac catheterization laboratory. If the clinical and echocardiographic features of complete transposition are unequivocal in the critically ill neonate, we perform balloon atrial septostomy before hemodynamic and angiocardiographic investigations. Balloon atrial septostomy should be performed with the largest balloon catheter that can be safely introduced. This is possible through a saphenofemoral venous cutdown, by the percutaneous approach, through the umbilical vein. We perform the septostomy maneuver several times until no

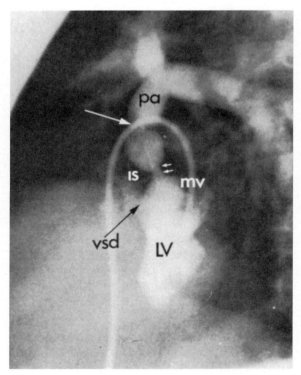

**FIGURE 43–8.** A relatively small ventricular septal defect (vsd) and severe subpulmonary obstruction are shown by this long-axial oblique left ventriculogram done via the mitral valve (mv). The vsd is inferior to the posteriorly malaligned infundibular septum (IS). There is concentric stenosis (two *small white arrows*) of the left ventricular outflow tract. The severely stenotic pulmonary valve (*long white arrow*) is partially obscured by the catheter. The muscular subpulmonary infundibulum prevents pulmonary valve–mitral valve fibrous continuity. (LV = left ventricle; pa = pulmonary artery.)

further resistance is met at the atrial septum. When hemodynamic recordings are obtained before balloon atrial septostomy, a withdrawal pressure tracing is routinely recorded from the left to the right atrium after balloon septostomy, and arterial oxygen tension and saturation data are obtained before and after the procedure.

With the diagnosis of transposition of the great arteries readily confirmed by cross-sectional echocardiography, there is less emphasis on hemodynamics. Indeed, much of the anatomic information in the patient with simple transposition of the great arteries and an intact ventricular septum can be defined by echocardiographic examination, including definition of the origin of the coronary arteries.

There is no unanimous definition of an adequate response to balloon atrial septostomy (the pertinent literature is summarized in Rowe et al., 1981). Some neonates remain hypoxic despite apparently adequate balloon atrial septostomy. The adequacy of the balloon atrial septostomy can be seen in terms of abolishing the interatrial pressure gradient and visualization of the atrial septum after septostomy to quantitate the adequacy of the tear (Bierman and Williams, 1979b; Clark et al., 1977; Korns et al., 1972).

We have tried two maneuvers to facilitate atrial mixing in neonates in whom a better response to balloon atrial septostomy was anticipated. If congestive heart failure is not a feature, hypertransfusion with 5 to 10 ml/kg of whole blood by increasing atrial filling may substantially improve arterial oxygen saturation. However, when an adequate tear of the atrial septum is obvious, the administration of an E type of prostaglandin may improve systemic oxygenation (Benson et al., 1979; Driscoll et al., 1979; Henry et al., 1981; Lang et al., 1979). The E type of prostaglandin maintains patency of the ductus arteriosus (Coceani and Olley, 1973; Olley et al., 1978). The increase in pulmonary venous blood to the left atrium facilitated by the prostaglandin may alter the compliance of the left atrium; if interatrial communication is adequate, the result may be increased mixing. We urge care in the use of prostaglandin when the interatrial communication is marginal (Benson et al., 1979). When the interatrial defect is restrictive, the E type of prostaglandins, by increasing pulmonary blood flow, may actually precipitate or increase congestive heart failure. Despite an "adequate" balloon atrial septostomy, hypertransfusion, and administration of an E type of prostaglandin, some infants—fortunately, few—remain severely hypoxic. These infants may appear reasonably comfortable despite an arterial oxygen tension of 20 to 25 mm Hg.

For institutions performing the arterial switch operation, these concerns are less important, because the arterial switch with coronary transfer may be conducted within 1 to 3 days of initially stabilizing the baby with an urgent balloon septostomy. In institutions continuing to perform an atrial-type repair, persistent hypoxemia after balloon septostomy can be treated with an early Mustard or Senning repair. Cen-

ters in which neonatal repair cannot be achieved should consider a Blalock-Hanlon atrial septectomy.

The medical management of the neonate with an associated small or moderate VSD is the same as that for the patient with an intact ventricular septum.

The management of the patient with TGA and large PDA when placed on a Mustard or Senning tract may be particularly hazardous. The patient with large PDA risks pulmonary vascular obstruction even in the first months of life. One is tempted to deal with the PDA, but abrupt surgical closure may make the patient quite cyanotic and hypoxemic. Thus, balloon septostomy is always advocated before PDA division in these patients. These concerns are obviated by the arterial switch operation in the neonate when the PDA is surgically addressed.

Similarly, the infant with transposition of the great arteries and large VSD will require surgical intervention in the first months of life to prevent pulmonary vascular obstruction and/or the ravages of congestive heart failure. Again, the concerns of pulmonary vascular disease are lessened by an early arterial switch operation with closure of the ventricular septal defect.

## TREATMENT

### Palliative Procedures

The basic principle of palliation is to improve mixing between the pulmonary and systemic circulations by creating or enlarging an ASD. Enlargement of an ASD by balloon atrial septostomy (Rashkind and Miller, 1966) is performed at initial cardiac catheterization in almost all infants with TGA.

Before balloon septostomy was devised, some type of surgical atrial septectomy was essential to management of infants with TGA and *intact ventricular septum* (IVS). Although closed techniques using various ingenious instruments or open excision of the septum with inflow caval occlusion were often effective, the resultant ASD was relatively small, and the palliation was sometimes barely adequate. The original operation by Blalock and Hanlon (1950) created a large ASD and remained the surgical procedure of choice for palliation (Fig. 43–9). The technique is demanding but, if it is done carefully, the operative risk is about 5% and the results are excellent. Conduction disturbances may occur, and it is important to leave the superior margin of the atrial septum to preserve the artery to the *sinoatrial* (SA) node (Trusler et al., 1980).

Improved techniques and management have reduced the mortality of TGA repair, particularly arterial repair. Five to 10 years ago, many surgeons recommended primary repair at an early age whenever the protection given by balloon septostomy was no longer adequate (de Begona et al., 1992; Turley et al., 1982), whereas other surgeons recommended surgical septectomy for infants who required operation in the first 1 to 2 months of life in the belief that repair at this age was associated with a slightly higher risk of operative death and postoperative complications.

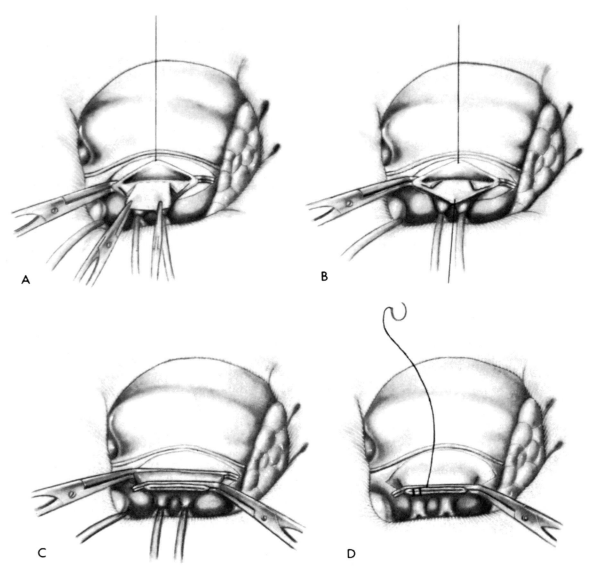

**FIGURE 43–9.** Approach by a right lateral thoracotomy through the fifth interspace with snares around the right pulmonary artery and the upper and lower right pulmonary veins, and a partial-occlusion clamp with one jaw posterior to the pulmonary veins and the other anterior so that a portion of the right and left atria has been included. The pericardium has been opened posterior to the right phrenic nerve, and the right and left atria have been opened by an incision parallel to the atrial septum. The atrial septum has been incised with scissors, the free edges have been grasped with hemostats, and an extra portion of atrial septum has been withdrawn from the heart while the partial occlusion clamp was gently released *(A)*. The mobilized flap of atrial septum is then cut through its pedicle *(B)*, and a smaller partial-occlusion clamp is applied to the free edges of the incision in the left and right atria and lies anterior to the right pulmonary veins *(C)*. The larger occlusion clamp is then released, as are the snares on the pulmonary veins and the pulmonary artery. The incision in the atrium can then be closed at leisure *(D)*. *(A–D,* From Aberdeen, E.: Blalock-Hanlon operation and Rashkind procedure. *In* Rob, C., and Smith, R. [eds]: Operative Surgery. 2nd ed., Vol. 2. London, Butterworth, 1968, pp. 193–199.)

Now arterial repair is generally recommended and carried out soon after the diagnosis is confirmed, preferably within 2 weeks of birth and seldom later than 1 month.

Infants with TGA and large VSDs require treatment before the age of 6 months to prevent pulmonary vascular disease and often earlier to relieve congestive heart failure. Balloon atrial septostomy, soon after birth, helps by eliminating left atrial hypertension and improving oxygen saturation. Pulmonary artery banding, once the main form of palliation, is now seldom used; early arterial repair is preferred. Occa-

sionally in the presence of some complicating feature, such as a large apical muscular VSD or hypoplastic ventricle, pulmonary artery banding rather than repair is advisable. To apply an adequate band in these patients, one must be sure of a satisfactory ASD. If not, a Blalock-Hanlon septectomy should be performed with the banding. Both procedures can be performed through a right-sided anterolateral thoracotomy. Edwards described a modification of the Blalock-Hanlon operation (Edwards et al., 1964) in which the atrial septum is not resected but is sutured to the posterior wall of the left atrium medial to the right pulmonary venous orifices. This produces obligatory mixing of the right pulmonary venous return in the right atrium, and, in infants with TGA and VSD, it appears to provide better palliation than the Blalock-Hanlon procedure when associated with pulmonary artery banding.

In infants with TGA plus VSD and LVOTO in whom the VSD is large and the LVOTO cannot be relieved directly, the best treatment is a Rastelli operation, but the risk is lessened if this is delayed until after the child's fifth birthday. If treatment is needed earlier, a Blalock-Taussig shunt is implemented to improve oxygen saturation. The most common modification involves a prosthesis from the subclavian artery to the pulmonary artery, as described by de Leval and associates (1981).

In infants with TGA and LVOTO without a VSD, creation of a large ASD usually provides adequate palliation until repair is possible. If the LVOTO is severe and cannot be relieved directly, it may be advisable to palliate the condition for some years with a Blalock-Taussig shunt as well as with the Blalock-Hanlon septectomy. Patients who undergo such palliation may risk early onset of pulmonary vascular obstructive disease and should be observed closely. Because early arterial repair has become routine, fixed LVOTO, with or without VSD, seems to be encountered much less frequently than before, suggesting that the LVOTO is often an acquired malformation.

## Surgical Repair

Various repair procedures are now available, and the choice is in part dictated by the anatomy. Arterial repair is used by most surgeons for TGA and IVS and for TGA with VSD. Rastelli's repair is used for TGA, VSD, and LVOTO, and intraventricular repair is used for exceptional cases with large VSDs. For atrial repair, either the Senning operation or the Mustard operation is still used in special situations. The Senning operation is discussed in a separate section. A description of the Mustard operation follows.

### Technique of the Mustard Repair

Through a median sternotomy, the anterior aspect of the pericardial sac is cleared for a width of 5 to 6 cm and superiorly to the great arteries, where the thymus is reflected. The pericardium is incised along the diaphragm and an approximately rectangular patch of pericardium is taken for the atrial baffle (Fig. 43–10). The patch is hollowed or made concave on both sides to create a waist 2.5 to 3 cm wide. Both ends are rounded for adequate caval channels. The IVC end (5 cm) is slightly larger than the *superior vena cava* (SVC) end (4 cm) and is more rounded to allow flexibility of choice in the position of the suture line. The long side of the patch is 7 cm long and is taken some distance from, but almost parallel to, the right phrenic nerve. It extends from the diaphragm below to the most prominent point on the ascending aorta

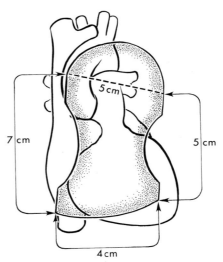

FIGURE 43–10. The pericardial patch *(stippled area)* for the intra-atrial baffle. Basic dimensions are 7 × 4 cm for a 10-kg child, 0.5 cm less for a 5-kg child. The slightly convex superior vena cava portion is taken along the diaphragm. The long border is on the right atrium and extends up to the ascending aorta. The other two borders are basically 5 cm long, but the superior border is fully rounded to allow flexibility in choosing the suture line position around the inferior vena cava.

above. The opposite side is 5 cm long. This size fits a child who weighs 10 kg. In an infant who weighs 5 kg, the dimensions are 0.5 to 1 cm less on all sides. The size and shape of the pericardial baffle differs for each surgeon; the trouser-shaped baffle advocated by Brom (1975) is preferred by some surgeons. Synthetic materials such as Dacron or Gore-Tex have also been used for the baffle.

Most Mustard operations are performed in the first year of life using deep hypothermia and circulatory arrest. Older children who weigh more than 10 kg are repaired with cardiopulmonary bypass and moderate hypothermia. Low-flow bypass and aortic cross-clamping are useful adjuncts to improve exposure for short periods.

Infants are allowed to cool moderately during the early part of the operation. After the pericardial baffle is prepared, cannulas are inserted into the ascending aorta and right atrial appendage, and bypass is begun with core-cooling to a rectal temperature of 16 to 18° C and esophageal temperature of approximately 12° C. During cooling, tourniquets are placed around the cavae and the aorta, the thin cooling device pad is positioned to surround the ventricles, and the cardioplegia line is filled and inserted into the ascending aorta.

During bypass cooling, the rectal temperature falls more slowly than the esophageal temperature and is thus likely to be a safer guide to brain temperature. At 16 to 18° C (rectal), the pump is stopped and the aorta cross-clamped. Cold (4° C) potassium blood cardioplegia is injected into the aorta root. The caval tourniquets are snugged, the venous cannula is removed, and the right atrium is opened with a longitudinal incision well away from the SA node (Fig. 43–11).

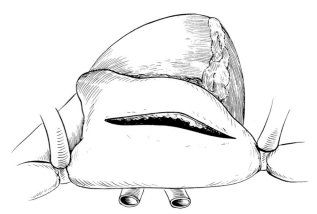

FIGURE 43–11. With circulatory arrest and the venous cannula removed, the caval tourniquets are tightened and a longitudinal incision is made in the right atrium.

After cardioplegia is begun, the interior of the right atrium is examined, as are the pulmonary venous orifices, left atrial appendage, and mitral valve (Fig. 43–12). The remaining atrial septum is partly excised. The first incision is made from the superior border of the ASD up to the middle of the SVC orifice. The ridge of septum to the left of this incision is preserved because it often contains the artery to the SA node and may also act as a conduction pathway between the SA node and the atrioventricular node. The atrial septum to the right of the incision is excised completely. This excision is extended to include any septal remnant near the IVC. The coronary sinus is incised back into the left atrium for approximately 1.5 cm, and any residual septum between the IVC and coronary sinus is excised. The raw incised margins left by excising septum are oversewn with a 5-0 suture; relatively small bites are taken to avoid a purse-string effect (Fig. 43–13).

The intra-atrial baffle is now sutured into the common atrium by using a double-armed continuous 3–0 braided synthetic suture (Fig. 43–14). The midpoint of the long side of the baffle is sutured and tied to the anterior margin of the internal orifice of the left

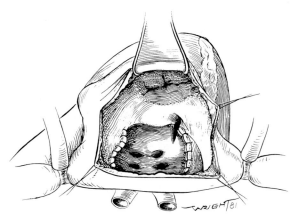

FIGURE 43–13. The first incision is made from the superior border of the ASD up to the middle of the superior vena cava (SVC) orifice. The ridge of septum to the left of this incision is preserved, because it often contains the artery to the sinoatrial (SA) node and may act as a conduction pathway between the SA node and the atrioventricular (AV) node. The atrial septum to the right of this incision is excised completely. This excision is extended to include any septal remnant near the inferior vena cava (IVC). The coronary sinus is incised back into the left atrium for a distance of approximately 1.5 cm, and any residual septum between the IVC and the coronary sinus is excised. The raw cut margins left by the excision of septum are oversewn with 5-0 suture material, taking relatively small bites to avoid a purse-string effect.

pulmonary veins. The continuous suture line then passes around the orifice of the left superior pulmonary vein to reach the posterior wall of the left atrium, crosses that wall curving inferiorly for a short distance to create a larger SVC channel, and then passes between the right superior pulmonary vein and the SVC orifice. The first corner of the baffle, which is one end of the long border, should reach the lateral wall of the right atrium. The short SVC border of the baffle is sutured around the internal orifice of the SVC, and the second corner of the baffle reaches partially across the roof of the right atrium between

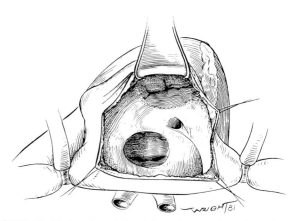

FIGURE 43–12. Interior of the right atrium with moderately large atrial septal defect (ASD).

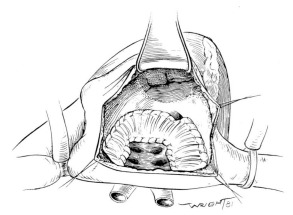

FIGURE 43–14. The intra-atrial baffle is sutured into the common atrial chamber with a double-armed continuous 3-0 braided synthetic suture. The IVC tourniquet is loosened to improve exposure for choice of suture line position. At the coronary sinus, which has been cut back, the suture line runs 5 to 8 mm to the left of the original coronary sinus orifice.

the SVC and the residual ridge of atrial septum. Initially, on this border, relatively large bites of baffle and small bites of SVC orifice are taken to increase ballooning of the channel and to avoid flattening of the baffle across the SVC orifice. The SA node, approximately 1 cm away from this orifice, should be carefully avoided. This suture line continues onto the third border of the baffle, which, like the first, is made slightly concave. Part of this border is sutured to the roof of the right atrium and then to the residual atrial septum near the tricuspid valve; it stops at the middle of the septum.

The second end of the original 3–0 suture is now used to suture the remainder of the long border of the baffle around the internal orifice of the left inferior pulmonary vein and across the posterior wall of the left atrium to the right atrium. In crossing, the suture line curves up slightly to enlarge the IVC channel, but should not be too close to the previous superior suture line, because future baffle contraction may obstruct the left pulmonary veins. The corner of the baffle between the long border and the fully curved IVC border reaches the lateral wall of the right atrium between the right inferior pulmonary vein and the IVC in a position that allows ample flow through both pulmonary and caval venous channels.

At this point, if there is circulatory arrest, it is expedient to remove the IVC tourniquet. With the IVC open, anatomic details can be distinguished easily and an appropriate path for the baffle suture line can be selected. If the eustachian valve is well formed and sturdy, the baffle may be sutured to it directly. If it is not, then either the base of the eustachian valve or some ridge nearby on the right atrial wall will serve. The last corner of baffle marking the end of the IVC border should reach a point approximately midway along the ridge that extends from the eustachian valve to the coronary sinus. The final border of the baffle is then sutured to this ridge. At the coronary sinus, the suture line extends down one cut edge of coronary sinus for 5 to 8 mm, across the sinus, and then back up the other cut edge and along the atrial septum a short distance to meet the first suture and complete the baffle. Before the suture is tied, the left side of the heart is filled gently with saline to reduce the amount of trapped air. When completed, the baffle is inspected briefly, and then the right atrial incision is closed.

The venous cannula is reinserted into the right atrium, and the infant is placed back on bypass to rewarm. The cardioplegia line is placed on suction to evacuate any air that may have been trapped in the heart and reached the aortic root. The tip of the venous cannula is inserted gently through the tricuspid valve for a few seconds to remove any major amount of air in the right ventricle. Reinsertion of the venous cannula into the right atrial appendage is simple and convenient. Because this is now the pulmonary venous atrium, there is some reduction in venous return to the pump for 2 to 3 minutes. Gentle cardiac massage and ventilation of the lungs move blood from the systemic venous side through the lungs to the

cannula. The venous return becomes stable once the heart starts to beat spontaneously. During rewarming, two atrial and two ventricular temporary pacemaker wires are inserted for postoperative support and monitoring. When the infant's rectal temperature has returned to 34° C, bypass is terminated. The venous cannula is removed from the right atrial appendage, and a small plastic tube is inserted for postoperative monitoring of pulmonary venous pressure.

## Variations in Surgical Repair

When there is left juxtaposition of the right atrial appendage, repair leaves the right appendage as part of the systemic venous atrium. The new pulmonary venous atrium is smaller than usual and should be enlarged with a patch of pericardium. Mesocardia or dextrocardia with situs solitus makes access to the right atrium difficult from an anterior approach. A right lateral thoracotomy provides better exposure. Here, too, the right atrium may be small and may require enlargement with a pericardial patch.

Moderate to large VSDs are closed from the right atrium through the tricuspid valve. Very small VSDs are left untouched, not only to save time, but to avoid the danger of causing right bundle-branch block. LVOTO is usually approached through the pulmonary artery and valve but is accessible through the mitral valve. When repair of one of these conditions is necessary in conjunction with a Mustard procedure, the time required may exceed the limits of safety for a single period of circulatory arrest. To avoid excessive ischemia, at least part of the repair is done on bypass by switching to two acutely curved cannulas that are inserted into the cavae through the open atriotomy.

When pulmonary vascular disease has become severe, patients can still benefit from a Mustard repair in which the VSD is left open (Humes et al., 1988; Lindesmith et al., 1972). Occasionally, severe pulmonary vascular disease develops in children with TGA and IVS. These conditions can be palliated with a Mustard operation and creation of an apical VSD (Byrne et al., 1978).

A few infants with TGA and intact septum have a severe form of LVOTO that cannot be relieved directly. They should be treated palliatively with a Blalock-Taussig shunt with or without a Blalock-Hanlon atrial septectomy, and repair should be delayed until the child is older. With intra-atrial repair, the LVOTO should be relieved directly as completely as possible and, as necessary, the balance of the obstruction should be bypassed with a valved conduit between the left ventricle and pulmonary artery (Crupi et al., 1985).

If there is a large and high VSD, an option in some patients is the intraventricular repair described originally by McGoon (1972). The VSD is exposed through a right ventriculotomy. Excision of infundibular muscle and enlargement of the VSD are often necessary. A large patch directs blood from the left ventricle across the VSD to the aorta while leaving a

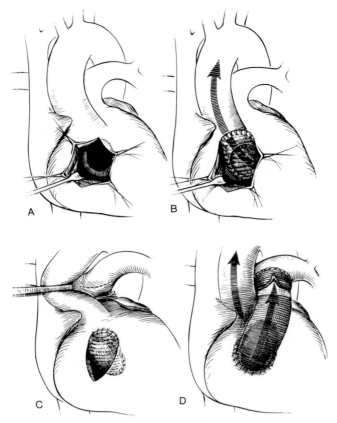

**FIGURE 43–15.** *A,* The right ventricle is incised with due regard for the position of the VSD, the distribution of the coronary arteries, and the desired placing of the conduit. *B,* The VSD is closed with a large patch that extends to cover the aortic root. *C,* The main pulmonary artery is securely ligated or divided and oversewn, and an incision is made near the bifurcation. *D,* The distal end of a valved conduit is sutured to the pulmonary artery bifurcation and the proximal end to the right ventricular incision. (*A–D,* From Trusler, G. A., and Freedom, R. M.: Complete transposition of the great arteries. *In* Arciniegas, E. [ed]: Pediatric Cardiac Surgery. Chicago, Year Book Medical, 1985.)

channel for right ventricular blood to cross the VSD and reach the pulmonary artery. Increased knowledge of this complex anatomy is leading to more aggressive resection and repair (Smolinsky et al., 1988).

Rastelli and associates (1969) devised a repair for children with substantial VSD and LVOTO (Fig. 43–15). The VSD is closed with a patch that extends to

include the aortic root, thus diverting flow from the left ventricle to the aorta. The pulmonary artery channel is closed, either within the ventricle through the VSD or by closing the pulmonary valve or artery or both outside the heart. A valved conduit, either a homograft aorta with aortic valve or one of the commercially available Dacron tubes with porcine valves, is then interposed between the ventricular incision and the distal pulmonary artery. This repair is particularly appropriate in patients in whom the LVOTO cannot be relieved surgically. It requires a VSD that is the same size as the aortic root or at least one that can be enlarged to that size. As an alternative to the valved conduit, the distal pulmonary artery may be transposed anterior to the aorta and sutured directly to the right ventricle (LeCompte, 1991; Vouhe et al., 1992).

In arterial repair, the great arteries are divided and switched and the coronary arteries are transferred to the new aorta. After the first successful arterial repair by Jatene in 1975, this operation was attempted widely although originally with high mortality. It is best suited to patients with TGA with a normal left ventricular outflow tract, low pulmonary vascular resistance, and a left ventricle that can generate systemic pressures. Thus, the first major application of this operation was for infants with TGA and VSD in the first 6 months of life before pulmonary vascular resistance increased. In this group of children, the results of atrial repair were poorest, with relatively high early and late mortality and a high incidence of late problems. Subsequently, the arterial switch procedure was employed in newborn infants with TGA and IVS. As results improved, this operation became increasingly competitive with atrial repair and is now the procedure of choice in most centers (Castañeda et al., 1984; Idriss et al., 1988; Norwood et al., 1988; Quagebeur et al., 1986). If there is diminished right ventricular function, arterial repair should be considered even in older infants who require preliminary pulmonary artery banding and a shunt to condition the left ventricle.

## RESULTS

### Early Mortality

The overall early and late results with the Mustard operation at the Hospital for Sick Children, Toronto,

■ **Table 43–1.** MUSTARD OPERATION FOR TGA

| | May '63–Dec '73 | | | Jan '74–Dec '92 | | |
|---|---|---|---|---|---|---|
| | No. | Late Death | Early Death | No. | Late Death | Early Death |
| With intact ventricular septum | 106 | 11 | 23 | 249 | 2 | 13 |
| With VSD | 35 | 14 | 7 | 41 | 8 | 5 |
| VSD + LVOTO | 13 | 6 | 4 | 32 | 0 | 6 |
| IVS + LVOTO | 9 | 3 | 1 | 38 | 5 | 3 |
| *Total* | 163 | 34 | 35 | 362 | 15 | 27 |

*Key:* IVS = intact ventricular septum; LVOTO = left ventricular outflow tract obstruction; TGA = transposition of the great arteries; VSD = ventricular septal defect.

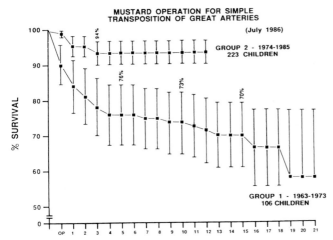

**FIGURE 43–16.** Actuarial survival in two groups of patients with simple transposition. Group 1 patients, who underwent surgery from 1963 to 1973, had 5-year and 10-year survival rates of 75.4 and 73.4%, respectively. However, Group 2 patients, who underwent surgery from 1974 to 1985, had 5-year and 10-year survival rates of 93.7%. (From Trusler, G. A., Williams, W. G., Duncan, K. F., et al.: Results with the Mustard operation in simple transposition of the great arteries 1963–1985. Ann. Surg., *206*:251, 1987.)

are shown in Table 43–1, which simplifies classification into four groups and compares the first decade with the last 19 years. There were 525 patients with 49 early hospital deaths. This early mortality (within 30 days of operation) has gradually decreased for all groups. The patients with TGA and intact ventricular septum were reviewed in 1986. The early mortality rate decreased from 11% in those undergoing repair before 1974 to 0.8% in the 239 patients since that time. This is shown in Figure 43–16, which provides an actuarial comparison of the two groups of patients with simple TGA. The overall results of the treatment protocol from the time that infants with simple TGA were first admitted to the hosptial are shown in Figure 43–17 and include the effect of death related to cardiac catheterization and surgical septectomy as well as the atrial repair. Survival at 1 month, 1 year, 10 years, and 20 years is 95%, 90%, 83%, and 80%, respectively. Mortality was higher in patients with complex TGA. Other surgeons have reported similar results (Castañeda et al., 1988; de Begona et al., 1992).

The results reflect changing patterns of treatment. For example, in TGA with VSD, mortality was high initially because most children were older when they underwent surgery, when they had pulmonary hypertension. Mortality was later reduced by preliminary palliation with pulmonary artery banding and surgical septectomy, and it was decreased further when primary repair in the first 6 months of life became routine. Most infants in this group now undergo arterial repair.

Similarly, the mortality rate for children with transposition with VSD and LVOTO changed when selected cases were treated by Rastelli's procedure. Atrial repair is now reserved for those with relatively small VSDs and an obstruction that can be relieved

surgically. In this particular subset, there has been no early mortality recently in our series.

The most common causes of early mortality in the whole series were low-output myocardial failure (26 patients), pulmonary vascular disease (10 patients), and dysrhythmias (4 patients). Pulmonary vascular disease is now prevented mainly by early repair, but myocardial failure is still the chief cause of death, particularly in infants with complex TGA. Other causes were bleeding (2 patients), other cardiac malformations (4 patients), and miscellaneous causes (3 patients).

## Late Mortality

From May 1963 to December 31, 1992, in our series, there were 476 early survivors, among whom there were 62 late deaths, which occurred in all groups but more commonly in those with complex TGA. Five-, 10-, and 15-year actuarial survival rates after Mustard repair in patients with simple TGA since 1973 were 94%, 93%, and 91%, respectively.

Cardiac failure, the most common cause of death (19 patients), was likely related in part to the conduct of operation and has been reduced in recent years by improved myocardial protection by using lower temperatures, cardioplegia, shorter periods of myocardial ischemia, and local myocardial cooling. Inexplicable failure still occurs, and continued refinement of methods of myocardial protection in infants is necessary. Perhaps myocardial damage can result from postoperative low-output failure or dysrhythmias.

Dysrhythmia caused death in 13 patients and was the possible cause in another 9 patients who died

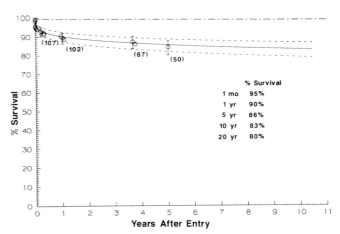

**FIGURE 43–17.** Survival after entry of 115 consecutive patients with simple TGA from 1976 to 1985. Each *circle* represents a death (*n* = 16) positioned along the horizontal axis according to the time of death and actuarially along the vertical axis. The *solid line* is the parametrically determined present survival rate, and the *dashed lines* are the 70% confidence intervals (limits). The *dashed and dotted line* shows the survival of a general population matched for age, sex, and race. (From Williams, W. G., Trusler, G. A., Kirklin, J. W., et al.: Early and late results of a protocol for simple transposition leading to an atrial switch [Mustard] repair. J. Thorac. Cardiovasc. Surg., *95*:717, 1988.)

■ **Table 43–2.** BAFFLE COMPLICATIONS (476 SURVIVORS; 205 CATHETERIZATIONS)

| Complication | Total | Major | Repaired | Died |
|---|---|---|---|---|
| Baffle leaks | 48 | 8 | 7 | 1 |
| SVC stenosis | 37 | 12 | 5 | 0 |
| IVC stenosis | 6 | 2 | 2 | 1 |
| PV stenosis | 13 | 13 | 11 | 8 |
| *Total* | 104 | 35 | 25 | 10 |

*Key:* IVC = inferior vena cava; PV = pulmonary venous; SVC = superior vena cava.

suddenly. Pulmonary venous obstruction was responsible in 8 patients but seldom occurs now. Pulmonary vascular disease was responsible for 5 late deaths early in the series. Other isolated causes were baffle detachment, congenital respiratory problems, pulmonary venous thrombosis, septicemia, and inferior vena caval obstruction. In 2 patients, the cause of death was not clear.

## COMPLICATIONS

Many of the complications of atrial repair for TGA are identical to those that follow any major cardiac repair. Postoperative bleeding, hemothorax, and cardiac tamponade may occur, particularly if there are pericardial adhesions from earlier palliative procedures, but these complications can be prevented by meticulous hemostasis and maintenance of blood coagulability with appropriate blood clotting factors. Low-output cardiac failure may occur after repair, especially in complicated cases, and cause early death or residual impairment of right ventricular contractility. This is likely due to inadequate myocardial protection and can be prevented mainly by the appropriate use of hypothermia and cardioplegia and by avoiding prolonged myocardial ischemia. Air embolism is not a common problem if appropriate preventive measures are taken but is a constant danger, and we believe that transient and sometimes permanent neurologic problems are seen more often after repair of TGA than after other heart malformations.

Phrenic nerve paralysis occurred in approximately 7% of operations, probably from dissection of the large pericardial patch. The incidence of paralysis rose to 10% in the presence of adhesions from previous palliative surgery (Watanabe et al., 1987). Nerve injury may be related to local mechanical trauma or cautery, particular superiorly near the level of the great vessels, where the space between the two phrenic nerves is narrower; alternatively, perhaps strong traction on the pericardial stay sutures near a phrenic nerve causes injury.

### Baffle Complications

Because many complications are related to changes in the atrial partition, it is useful to consider what happens to it after operation. Mohri and associates

(1970) found that the partition, regardless of the material used, was soon covered by a layer of fibrin that later fibrosed and formed a neoendocardium that, with the underlying graft material, gradually contracted to approximately 50% of its original area. The neoendocardium that formed over Dacron was thicker than over pericardium. They concluded that adequate atrial volume would be maintained by growth of normal atrial wall. With a pericardial baffle, the fibrous layer gradually matures and becomes thinner, so that many years later the baffle is reasonably thin and supple.

Our observations at reoperation and necropsy indicate that baffle shrinkage is limited or restricted by tension, both from sutures and blood flow. Where the pericardium partially encircles a venous orifice, the appropriate channel is maintained if the sutures are secure. If several sutures pull out, the pericardium contracts between the remaining points of fixation, partly obstructing the venous channel and creating a leak between the atrial chambers. With pericardium, a relatively large patch can be used, and the final shape is determined by the relative pressures and flow within the two atria as well as the security and position of the suture line. Soon after insertion, the mobile pericardium, covered by fibrin, may adhere to itself or to other raw areas, so a redundant baffle should be avoided, and raw areas of atrial wall should be oversewn.

Synthetic materials do not conform as easily as pericardium does and must be tailored precisely to avoid ridges or narrow channels. Excessive shrinkage or an error in the line of suture is more critical,

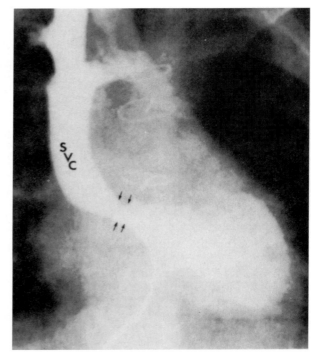

**FIGURE 43–18.** Mild narrowing *(arrows)* of the superior limb of the baffle after the Mustard operation. (SVC = superior vena cava.)

especially in infants in whom all the venous orifices and channels are smaller, and there is less margin for error. This does not mean that synthetic materials should not be used, but pericardium appears to be safer, particularly in infants.

Although baffle complications are identified fairly frequently, most are mild and have no consequence (Table 43–2). Thirty-five (7.4%) of the 476 children who were early survivors of the Mustard repair had major complications. A repair was attempted in 25 (5.3%) of the early survivors, and 10 (2.1%) died of the baffle complications.

### Baffle Leaks

The most common late complication is a leak around the baffle. By the end of 1992, 205 of 476 early survivors had undergone one or more cardiac catherizations after the Mustard repair. Forty-eight of these children had leaks. Fortunately, 40 were small and only 8 were significant, 6 with left-to-right shunts exceeding 1.5:1 and 2 with a right to-left shunt. Leaks were easily repaired, but when they were associated with caval obstruction, it was necessary to patch the baffle to relieve the associated venous obstruction.

### Superior Vena Cava Obstruction

This obstruction may cause symptoms and signs of increased SVC pressure soon after operation, al-

though many patients are asymptomatic and are only identified at late cardiac catheterization. Occasionally, paraspinal densities reflecting venous collateralization may reflect SVC obstruction (Polansky et al., 1980). Sometimes there is persistent bilateral or right-sided pleural effusion or chylothorax. Communicating hydrocephalus has been described (Markowitz et al., 1984; Sweeney et al., 1982). The obstruction usually occurs where the new SVC channel crosses the plane of the atrial septum and may be due to a residual ridge of atrial septum or to flattening of the baffle (Figs. 43–18 and 43–19). If several sutures disengage, the baffle may contract across the caval orifice and cause obstruction. A change in our technique of atrial septal excision increased with mild-to-moderate SVC narrowing resulting from the residual ridge of atrial septum between the SVC and the tricuspid valve. This was partly avoided by using a slightly larger and redundant baffle in this area. There have been 37 known cases of SVC stenosis among the 476 early survivors, an incidence of 8%. However, it is really not a major problem because only 5 (1% overall) required repair, 2 in association with baffle leaks. The incidence of SVC obstruction was increased when Dacron was used for the baffle material (Hagler et al., 1978; Kron et al., 1985; Stark et al., 1974).

Wyse and associates (1979) found that the echocardiographic jugular venous flow profile recording was

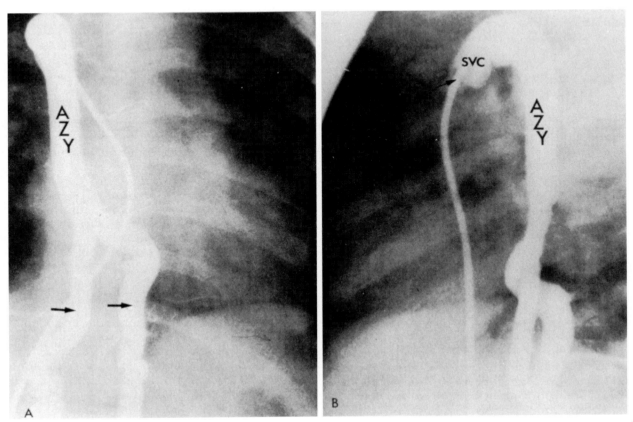

FIGURE 43–19. *A* and *B*, Severe stenosis of the superior limb of the baffle after the Mustard operation. This asymptomatic patient had paravertebral densities that proved to be venous in origin (Castellino et al., 1968; Polansky and Culham, 1980). Although the SVC could be probed from the venous route, most of the SVC blood passed via large azygos (AZY) and hemiazygos collaterals *(arrows)* and through the inferior limb of the baffle.

an effective method of screening for SVC obstruction. Two-dimensional echocardiography with Doppler ultrasound or contrast is useful in assessing the status of the SVC pathway (Aziz et al., 1981; Silverman et al., 1981). Transeophageal echocardiography provided a more detailed and accurate assessment of atrial baffle morphology and function (Kaulitz et al., 1990; Stumper et al., 1991).

In most cases, the SVC stenosis has been relieved directly through a median sternotomy incision or a right-sided thoracotomy (Stark, 1993). Patching the narrow area of the baffle may be sufficient, but a more extensive revision may be necessary (e.g., revising the whole SVC end of the baffle and sometimes patching the adjacent wall of the atrium). A number of surgeons have relieved the SVC obstruction by anastomosing the innominate vein to the left atrial appendage either directly (Coulson et al., 1984) or with a graft (Abbruzzese et al., 1984; Danilowicz et al., 1981). Balloon dilatation has been used but has been more permanently successful when self-expanding metallic stents are used (Chatelaine et al., 1991; Waldman et al., 1983).

### Inferior Vena Cava Obstruction

Although uncommon, this may occur either at the plane of the atrial septum by the coronary sinus from a tight baffle or at the IVC orifice if several sutures dislodge. Severe obstruction is associated with increased IVC pressure and causes hepatomegaly and ascites or even low cardiac output failure. Protein-losing enteropathy has been reported (Kirk et al., 1988; Moodie et al., 1976).

IVC obstruction was identified in 6 of our 476 early survivors. In 2 children, it was associated with a baffle leak that required repair, and in 1 child the obstruction was identified at autopsy. The other 3 children are asymptomatic with partial obstruction that has not been repaired. Stark and associates (1974) described an increased incidence of IVC obstruction when Dacron was used as a baffle material in infants. Diagnosis and treatment is similar to that for SVC obstruction. Cutting back the coronary sinus into the left atrium, if not done at the initial repair, may be an important part of the reoperation.

### Pulmonary Venous Obstruction

This most serious baffle complication was identified in 13 (2.7%) of the 476 early surviving patients. All four pulmonary veins were involved in 7 of the 13 patients. The obstruction occurred where the new pulmonary venous channel crossed the plane of the atrial septum, just anterior to the entrance of the right pulmonary veins, and appeared to be due to progressive adherence and fibrous stenosis between the baffle and adjacent margin of residual atrial septum by the right lateral atrial wall. This appears to occur more often if the raw cut margin of the atrial septum is not oversewn, and there is a large redundant baffle that can make contact with the wall of

the atrium. Routine patching of the right atrial wall extending down between the two right pulmonary veins or performance of a V-Y atrioplasty to accomplish this objective has been advocated to prevent pulmonary venous obstruction (Barratt-Boyes, 1986). Several series report high incidence of pulmonary venous obstruction, which appears to be more common when repair is done in early infancy and when Dacron is used (Driscoll et al., 1977; Hagler et al., 1978). It has also been described as a result of using bovine pericardium for atrial augmentation (Cochrane and McGough, 1987).

Children with pulmonary venous obstruction usually present within 3 to 6 months of operation with respiratory distress and pulmonary edema. Delayed presentation up to 10 years after operation also has been described (Campbell et al., 1987). Pulsed Doppler echocardiography has proven useful in the detection of pulmonary venous obstruction (Smallhorn et al., 1986). If diagnosed early, the condition can be treated successfully by patching both the baffle and the atrial wall between the two right pulmonary veins. Corno and associates (1987) suggested patching with pericardium in situ to allow for growth. Some relief of obstruction can be achieved with balloon angioplasty (Cooper et al., 1989; Coulson et al., 1990). With delayed diagnosis, severe pulmonary vascular disease progresses rapidly and mortality is high.

An uncommon variation that we and others (Pappas, 1986) have encountered is isolated obstruction of the left pulmonary venous channel, which appears to result from excessive contraction of the baffle when the upper and lower suture lines between right and left pulmonary veins are brought too close together on the posterior wall of the left atrium. The orifices of the left pulmonary veins may also be involved in the stenosis, so the suture line should not venture too close to these orifices. Affected children may present with chronic left pulmonary edema, pleural effusion, or hemoptysis. Pulsed Doppler echocardiography is useful for diagnosis, and on angiocardiography, there is a sharp reduction in pulmonary blood flow to the left lung. Repair, which requires patching of both the posterior left atrial wall and the baffle itself at the site of obstruction, is often unsatisfactory because of the frequently associated stenosis of the left pulmonary venous orifices, which is difficult to relieve.

### Other Complications

Some degree of LVOTO appears to be common in children with TGA following atrial repair (Dasmahapatra et al., 1989; Gomes et al., 1980; Idriss et al., 1977; Vidne, 1976). We identified pressure gradient of 10 mm Hg or more across the left ventricular outflow tract in 54 children in our series. Most stenoses were minor and derived from bulging of the muscular septum into the outflow tract; only 20 patients had gradients over 25 mm Hg. Although some stenoses represented residual obstruction incompletely relieved by operation, most were in children who were considered to have uncomplicated TGA. Fortunately, only one child has required operative intervention.

Other complications that have been identified include small persistent VSDs. Most of these are small defects that were recognized originally but were not treated because they had no physiologic significance. Moderate or severe pulmonary vascular disease occurred in a few children after repair, sometimes secondary to pulmonary problems and sometimes without obvious cause. Mitral incompetence has developed in some children.

## Dysrhythmias

Dysrhythmia, a relatively common and potentially serious complication, is generally considered to stem from interference with function of the SA node either directly or from injury to the SA node artery (El-Said et al., 1976; Gillette et al., 1980). The wide excision of the atrial septum and the long atrial suture line must also play a part. The significance of obliterating or excising the pathways of impulse transmission from the SA node to the atrioventricular node is less clear, but it is possible that preservation of at least part of the atrial septum for internodal conduction is important.

In the early years of the Mustard operation, the atrial septum was excised widely and there was a relatively high incidence of dysrhythmia. Some dysrhythmias were responsible for both early and late deaths, including a number of sudden unexpected deaths that were probably due to this cause. Temporary atrial and ventricular pacemaker wires were inserted routinely at operation and monitored carefully to maintain sinus rhythm and avoid serious dysrhythmias that are common for a few days after operation.

In recent years, with knowledge of the problem and attention to detail, the incidence of dysrhythmias is lower, and sinus rhythm is maintained in most children (Lincoln and Southall, 1983). From 1973 to 1986, sinus rhythm was maintained at discharge in 92% of children with simple TGA who underwent a Mustard operation in Toronto. Of 180 patients available for review, 72% maintained sinus rhythm by last electrocardiogram, whereas 18% showed junctional rhythm, 3% had sick sinus syndrome, 4% a wandering pacemaker, 2% atrial flutter, and 1% SA-atrioventricular dysfunction (Trusler et al., 1987b). Three children required pacemakers. These results showed an improvement over the experience of the first 10 years.

The true incidence of abnormal rhythm, however, can be identified only by exercise studies and 24-hour monitoring. Our experience with Holter recordings after Mustard repair in 126 patients showed that although sinus rhythm was observed in 91%, the predominant cardiac rhythm was a junctional bradycardia or atrial flutter. Multicatheter electrophysiologic studies at an average of 52.5 months after operation showed frequent suppression of sinus node function and sometimes subtle abnormalities of atrioventricular node function.

It is now generally accepted that the incidence of dysrhythmia increases with time (Clarkson et al., 1976; Duster et al., 1985; Flinn et al., 1984; Hayes and Gersony, 1986). In a series that included complex TGA, Deanfield and colleagues (1991) and Bierman and associates (1983) reported only 30% of patients free of arrhythmias 9 years after repair, but symptoms from rhythm or conduction disturbances were rare. Our experience shows that although only about one-quarter of children with abnormal rhythms are symptomatic, the need for pacemakers increases with time; 23 of 327 patients (7%) with isolated TGA repaired before 1986 required pacemakers up to the end of 1992. The dysrhythmia problem is one of the main factors indicating arterial over atrial repair.

## Right Ventricular Dysfunction

Another major concern is the recognition of some diminution of right ventricular contractility. In our patients this is often a subjective assessment made by the radiologist or the cardiologist, mainly from the angiocardiogram but also by echocardiography, and it was recognized in 69 children (34%) who had undergone postrepair cardiac catheterization. Although most are mild changes, 11% of children with simple TGA show a definite decrease in function. Some children also have a degree, usually mild, of tricuspid incompetence, and occasionally the incompetence occurs alone. A few of these children died later from cardiac failure, usually within 4 years of operation, and have been discussed as late deaths. Progressive right ventricular failure beyond 4 years postoperatively is uncommon, and most children are asymptomatic. The incidence of right ventricular dysfunction is higher in the complicated forms of transposition where there has been repair of a VSD. Right ventricular contractility at cardiac catheterization was reduced in 43 of 149 children (29%) with simple transposition and in 18 of 26 children (69%) who also underwent VSD repair. The incidence of accompanying tricuspid incompetence was higher in the latter group and suggests that the VSD repair may lead to tricuspid incompetence in some patients. In other patients, the incompetence may be related to pre-existing valve abnormalities, arrhythmia, or, more commonly, right ventricular dysfunction itself (Deal et al., 1985; Huhta et al., 1982; Smith et al., 1986b).

There have been many studies of right ventricular function after atrial repair of TGA, and the ultimate significance is still not clear. Abnormal size and ejection fraction of the right ventricle after atrial repair were noted (Buch et al., 1988; Graham et al., 1975; Hagler et al., 1979; Jarmakani et al., 1974; Redington et al., 1989). By using gated equilibrium nuclear angiography, Benson and associates (1982) found an abnormal response to exercise with a decrease or at least no increase in right ventricular ejection fraction. Similar results were obtained by others (Baker et al., 1986; Borow et al., 1981; Murphy et al., 1986). Parrish and associates (1983) also noted an abnormal left ventricular response to exercise in 10 of 11 children tested after a Mustard repair and concluded that biventricular dysfunction was frequently present. In each study, some children had normal right ventricular function at rest and during exercise, which suggests that the right ventricular problem may not be inevitable. Benson and associates (1986) reported normal systemic ventricular function in patients with congenitally corrected TGA. Graham and co-workers (1985), comparing groups of patients after atrial repair of simple TGA, found an improvement in the postoperative right ventricular ejection fraction in patients undergoing surgery after 1974, whether by Mustard or Senning technique, compared with patients undergoing surgery earlier. They suggest that this improvement may be due to a younger age at operation or changes in operative technique, particularly myocardial protection. Smith and associates (1986b), however, warn that the general architecture of the ventricular mass and the atrioventricular valves is not normal, so the function of the normal heart may not always be an approriate yardstick for comparison.

Likely, some of the right ventricular problems originate at operation, and the right ventricle in transposition is more susceptible to ischemic damage than the left ventricle is in a normal heart (Shuhaiber et al., 1990). Every effort should be made to protect the myocardium during repair. Postoperative low-output failure and dysrhythmias may harm the myocardium and should be avoided if possible. Some cases of poor right ventricular function, however, occur in children whose operation and postoperative course appear to have been good, thus causing concern about the long-term fate of the right ventricle in transposition.

Staged conversion to an arterial switch repair has been advocated for late right ventricular failure (Mee, 1986). The pulmonary artery is banded as an initial first stage to prepare the left ventricle for systemic arterial pressures. At last report, 23 patients had been entered in this program (Cochrane et al., 1993). The mortality rate for the actual switch conversion was 2 of 16 patients, with 2 late deaths. Actuarial survival probability for all patients was 78% (confidence limits 42 to 92%) at 5 years. In our experience, relatively few patients with late severe right ventricular dysfunction would be clear candidates for this procedure.

## CLINICAL STATUS

The quality of life in the surviving children is good, and most are asymptomatic. Infants and children grow at a more normal rate and regain their birth-weight percentile after TGA repair, which is considered an indication for early repair (Levy et al., 1978; Sholler and Celermajer, 1986; Takahashi et al., 1977). Stark and co-workers (1980) did not find a significant difference between patients repaired in infancy and later. Newberger and associates (1984) found evidence to suggest that postponing repair to an older age was associated with progressive impairment of cognitive

function; only 6 of 38 children studied had undergone repair when younger than 1 year of age.

In the infants and children with simple TGA undergoing surgery from May 1963 to December 1985, late follow-up indicated that 76% were in New York Hospital Association (NYHA) Class I and 24% in NYHA Class II. No children were in Classes III or IV. Only 21% were taking medication, which was almost all for management of dysrhythmias. Most of the children were unrestricted in their activities, and some children participated in athletic events. Stark and associates (1980) found that exercise performance of asymptomatic patients who appeared to be living normal lives 6 to 13 years after the Mustard operation was slightly diminished compared with a group of normal children, and this finding has also been shown by cardiopulmonary exercise testing (Mathews et al., 1983). Musewe and associates (1988) found that although patients who remained asymptomatic 10 years or more after a Mustard operation had reduced maximal aerobic capacity, cardiac output and stroke volume response to submaximal exercise were normal, in part explaining the lack of symptoms with daily activity.

Of a group of 24 patients followed at the adult clinic who underwent a Mustard operation in the first decade (1963 to 1972), 11 are in functional Class I, 12 in Class II, and 1 in Class III. Dysrhythmias account for most of the symptoms, and only 6 patients (25%) maintain sinus rhythm. Sixty-three per cent achieved a college education, and 18 (75%) are employed. Two have children.

## SENNING OPERATION

In an attempt to reduce the incidence of complications, many surgeons changed to another form of atrial repair, the Senning operation. In this operation, flaps of atrial wall are used to divert venous return, and because there is no pericardial baffle, there is less nonliving tissue and the new atrial walls are more likely to contract and grow (Bjornstad et al., 1984). When growth is most important, such as in infants less than 2 months old, there is likely to be an advantage to the Senning procedure, with less chance of caval obstruction. When the incidence of obstruction has been high, it has often been related to the use of Dacron for the baffle (Cobanoglu et al., 1984). However, most complications that may occur after the Mustard operation have also been encountered after the Senning procedure, with a similar incidence (Bender et al., 1980). In addition, the results from the multi-institutional series indicate better survival with the Mustard operation (Castañeda et al., 1988).

## INDICATIONS FOR ATRIAL REPAIR VERSUS ARTERIAL REPAIR

In complex TGA, for many years, procedures other than atrial repair have been preferred, such as the

Rastelli operation for children with a large VSD and severe LVOTO and arterial repair for infants with associated large VSDs. Although arterial repair has become the procedure of choice for infants with simple TGA, there are a few indications for atrial repair, but even these are not universally agreed on. It is generally conceded that the risk of arterial repair increases with age, and by the time an infant with simple TGA reaches the age of 4 weeks, the left ventricle is less capable of supporting the systemic circulation. Although many surgeons would then consider atrial repair in an infant older than 4 weeks, others suggest preparation of the left ventricle by pulmonary arterial banding and a shunt followed by arterial repair (Jonas, 1991). The Melbourne group extend the time for arterial repair to the end of the second month of life (Davis et al., 1993). Certain coronary artery patterns, particularly single coronary arteries with intramural courses, have been associated with a higher mortality and might be considered for atrial repair, although improved techniques are reducing this risk. Fixed LVOTO is an indication for atrial repair, but this occurs infrequently, and it is now apparent that most LVOTO is acquired and avoided by early arterial repair. Other uncommon indications for atrial repair over arterial repair include isolated atrioventricular discordance and the presence of a moderately hypoplastic left ventricle, in which instance a bidirectional cavopulmonary shunt is placed along with the Mustard operation and as part of an Ilbawi procedure (Ilbawi et al., 1990).

## Isolated Atrioventricular Discordance

The Mustard atrial repair has been applied to patients with isolated atrioventricular discordance. In this uncommon condition, the morphologic right atrium connects through a mitral valve with the left ventricle, which in turn supports the aorta; the left atrium receiving the pulmonary veins connects through the tricuspid valve with the right ventricle, which supports the pulmonary artery (Abbott and Beattie, 1921; Anderson and Wilkinson, 1975; Calabro et al., 1982; Freedom et al., 1984; Van Praagh and Van Praagh, 1966). Thus, despite the fact that the great arteries are not anatomically transposed, the physiology is that of transposition.

Most patients do not have atrioventricular discordance in isolation. Rather, there are frequently associated abnormalities, including hypoplasia of the morphologically right ventricle, ventricular septal defect, and abnormalities of the tricuspid valve. Some of these patients will not have complicating associated anomalies, however, and the Mustard atrial repair has been applied (Arciprete et al., 1985; Leijala et al., 1981; Ostermeyer et al., 1983; Park et al., 1984; Ranjit et al., 1991).

There are still many parts of the world in which infants with TGA are not identified until after 1 month of age and the expertise and experience for safe arterial repair are not available. In such circum-

stances, atrial repair is indicated. The early mortality rate for either the Mustard or the Senning operation approaches zero with experience. We prefer the Mustard procedure for its simplicity and reliable early results. Both forms of atrial repair share the significant disadvantages of late dysrhythmias and possible late ventricular dysfunction.

## SELECTED BIBLIOGRAPHY

Castañeda, A. R., Trusler, G. A., Paul, M. H., et al.: The early results of treatment of simple transposition in the current era. J. Thorac. Cardiovasc. Surg., 95:14, 1988.

This article reports a 20-institution study of 187 neonates with simple TGA, all of whom initially entered the study when less than 15 days old. Results with the Mustard, Senning, and arterial switch procedures are compared. Overall survival rate was 81% at 1 year. The only risk factors for death were birth weight, date of entry in the study, and an arterial switch protocol in the group of institutions at high risk for arterial switch repair. The preliminary data suggested that the early (1-year) survival rate after the Mustard operation was better than either the Senning or the arterial switch procedure. Since then, the mortality rate with arterial repair has improved.

Flinn, C. J., Wolff, G. S., Dick, M., II, et al.: Cardiac rhythm after the Mustard operation for complete transposition of the great arteries. N. Engl. J. Med., 310:1635, 1984.

In this multi-institutional review from eight pediatric cardiac centers, 372 patients, who survived a Mustard operation for repair of TGA, were followed for 0.4 to 15.9 (mean 4.5) years to determine the effect on cardiac rhythm. Mean resting heart rates were consistently lower than in age-matched normal children. Normal sinus rhythm was present in 76% at 1 year and 57% by the end of the eighth postoperative year. Twenty-five patients died during the follow-up period, and nine died suddenly. This paper clearly indicates that the incidence of abnormal rhythm increases with time.

Gewillig, M., Cullen, S., Mertens, B., et al.: Risk factors for arrhythmia and death after Mustard operation for simple transposition of the great arteries. Circulation, 84:III-187, 1991.

This is an excellent review of the late results in 249 patients who underwent a Mustard operation from 1965 to 1980 at Great Ormond Street, London. The 20-year survival rate was 67%. Dysrhythmia incidence increased with time.

Graham, T. P., Burger, J., Bender, H. W., et al.: Improved right ventricular function after intra-atrial repair of transposition of the great arteries. Circulation, 72:II-45, 1985.

This report is an extension of Graham's earlier studies evaluating right ventricular function after atrial repair and compares 32 patients after a Senning operation with 26 patients after a Mustard procedure. The authors documented a decrease in right ventricular ejection fraction after both procedures. Of particular interest was the observation that ventricular performance was significantly better in both the Senning group and the later Mustard group (1975 to 1978) than in the earlier Mustard patients (1971 to 1974). They speculated that this resulted from younger patients at operation, better preoperative function, and, possibly, improved intraoperative myocardial protection. They also suggested that the earlier evidence indicating severe right ventricular dysfunction may not be a valid reason for the use of the arterial switch operation in patients with simple transposition.

Williams, W. G., Trusler, G. A., Kirklin, J. W., et al.: Early and late results of a protocol for simple transposition leading to an atrial switch (Mustard) repair. J. Thorac. Cardiovasc. Surg., 95:717, 1988.

This paper reports the early and intermediate (20 years) results of patient management protocol in 115 consecutive newborn infants leading to a Mustard operation at the Hospital for Sick Children, Toronto. The prevalence of junctional rhythm progressively increased with time. The 20-year survival rate was 80% (95%—CL 70 to 88%).

## BIBLIOGRAPHY

Abbott, M. E., and Beattie, W. W.: Rare cardiac anomaly. Am. J. Dis. Child., 22:508, 1921.

Abbruzzese, P. S., Issenberg, H., Cobanoglu, A., et al.: Superior vena cava obstruction after Mustard repair of d-transposition of the great arteries. Scand. J. Thorac. Cardiovasc. Surg., 18:5, 1984.

Albert, H. M.: Surgical correction of transposition of the great vessels. Surg. Forum, 5:74, 1955.

Anderson, R. H., and Wilkinson, J. L.: Isolated ventricular inversion with situs solitus. Br. Heart J., 37:1202, 1975.

Arciprete, P., Macartney, F. J., De Leval, M., and Stark J.: Mustard's operation for patients with ventriculoarterial concordance: Report of two cases and a cautionary tale. Br. Heart J., 53:443, 1985.

Aziz, K. U., Paul, M. H., Bharati, S., et al.: Two dimensional echocardiographic evaluation of Mustard operation for d-transposition of the great arteries. Am. J. Cardiol., 47:654, 1981.

Aziz, K. U., Paul, M. H., Idriss, F. S., et al.: Clinical manifestations of dynamic left ventricular outflow tract stenosis in infants with d transposition of the great arteries with intact ventricular septum. Am. J. Cardiol., 44:290, 1979.

Aziz, K. U., Paul, M. H., and Muster, A. J.: Echocardiographic assessment of left ventricular outflow tract in d-transposition of the great arteries. Am. J. Cardiol., 41:543, 1978.

Baffes, T. G.: A new method for surgical correction of transposition of the aorta and pulmonary artery. Surg. Gynecol. Obstet., 102:227, 1956.

Baffes, T. G., Ketola, F. H., and Tatooles, C. J.: Transfer of coronary ostia by "triangulation" in transposition of the great vessels and anomalous coronary arteries: A preliminary report. Dis. Chest, 39:648, 1961.

Bailey, C. P., Cookson, B. A., Downing, D. F., and Neptune, W. B.: Cardiac surgery under hypothermia. J. Thorac. Surg., 27:73, 1954.

Baillie, M.: The Morbid Anatomy of Some of the Important Parts of the Human Body. London, Johnson and Nicol, 1797, p. 38.

Baker, E. J., Shubao, C., Clarke, S. E., et al.: Radionuclide measurement of right ventricular function in atrial septal defect, ventricular septal defect and complete transposition of the great arteries. Am. J. Cardiol., 57:1142, 1986.

Bano-Rodrigo, A., Quero-Jiminez, M., Moreno-Granado, F., and Gamallo-Amat, C.: Wall thickness of ventricular chamber in transposition of the great arteries. Surgical implications. J. Thorac. Cardiovasc. Surg., 79:592, 1980.

Barcia, A., Kincaid, O. W., Davis, G. D., et al.: Transposition of the great arteries. An angiocardiographic study. Am. J. Roentgenol., 100:249, 1967.

Bargeron, L. M., Jr., Elliott, L. P., Soto, B., et al.: Axial cineangiography in congenital heart disease. Section I. Concept, technical and anatomical considerations. Circulation, 56:1075, 1977.

Barnard, C. N., Schrire, V., and Beck, W.: Complete transposition of the great vessels: A successful complete correction. J. Thorac. Cardiovasc. Surg., 43:768, 1962.

Barratt-Boyes, B. G.: Complete transposition of the great arteries. In Kirklin and Barratt-Boyes (eds): Cardiac Surgery. New York, John Wiley & Sons, 1986, p. 1129.

Bender, H. W., Jr., Graham, T. P., Jr., Boucek, R. J., Jr., et al.: Comparative operative results of the Senning and Mustard procedures for transposition of the great arteries. Circulation, 62:I-197, 1980.

Benson, L. N., Bonet, J., McLaughlin, P., et al.: Assessment of right ventricular function during supine bicycle exercise after Mustard's operation. Circulation, 65:1052, 1982.

Benson, L. N., Burns, R., Schwaiger, M., et al.: Radionuclide angiographic evaluation of ventricular function in isolated congenitally corrected transposition of the great arteries. Am. J. Cardiol., 58:319, 1986.

Benson, L. N., Olley, P. M., Patel, R. G., et al.: Role of prostaglandin E₁ infusion in the management of transposition of the great arteries. Am. J. Cardiol., 44:691, 1979.

Bierman, F. Z., and Williams, R. G.: Prospective diagnosis of d-transposition of the great arteries in neonates by subxiphoid two-dimensional echocardiography. Circulation, 60:1496, 1979a.

Bierman, F. Z., and Williams, R. G.: Subxiphoid two-dimensional imaging of the interatrial septum in infants and neonates with congenital heart disease. Circulation, 60:80, 1979b.

Bierman, L. B., Neches, W. H., Fricker, F. J., et al.: Arrhythmias in

transposition of the great arteries after the operation. Am. J. Cardiol., 51:1530, 1983.

Björk, V. O., and Bouckaert, L.: Complete transposition of the aorta and the pulmonary artery: An experimental study of the surgical possibilities for its treatment. J. Thorac. Surg., 28:632, 1954.

Bjornstad, P. G., Tjonnedland, S., and Semb, B. K. H.: Echocardiographic evaluation of atrial function after Senning and Mustard correction for transposition of the great arteries. Thorax, 39:114, 1984.

Blalock, A., and Hanlon, C. R.: The surgical treatment of complete transposition of the aorta and the pulmonary artery. Surg. Gynecol. Obstet., 90:1, 1950.

Borow, K. M., Keane, J. F., Castañeda, A. R., and Freed, M. D.: Systemic ventricular function in patients with tetralogy of Fallot, ventricular septal defect and transposition of the great arteries repair during infancy. Circulation, 64:878, 1981.

Brom, G. A.: Technique of Mustard operation. In Hahn, C. (ed) Thorax Chirurgie. Lieden 1950–75. Leiden, Netherlands Drukkerij Bedrijf BC, 1975.

Buch, J., Wennevold, A., Jacobsen, J. R., et al.: Long-term followup of right ventricular function after Mustard operation for transposition of the great arteries. Scand. J. Thorac. Cardiovasc. Surg., 22:197, 1988.

Byrne, J., Clarke, D., Taylor, J. F. N., et al.: Treatment of patients with transposition of the great arteries and pulmonary vascular obstructive disease. Br. Heart J., 40:221, 1978.

Calabro, R., Marino, B., and Marsico, F.: A case of isolated atrioventricular discordance. Br. Heart J., 47:400, 1982.

Campbell, R. M., Moreau, G. A., Graham, T. P., Jr., and Bender, H. W.: Symptomatic pulmonary venous obstruction in adolescence after Mustard's repair of transposition in infancy. Am. J. Cardiol., 59:1218, 1987.

Castañeda, A. R., Norwood, W. I., Jonas, R. A., et al.: Transposition of the great arteries and intact ventricular septum: Anatomical repair in the neonate. Ann. Thorac. Surg., 38:438, 1984.

Castañeda, A. R., Trusler, G. A., Paul, M. H., et al.: The early results of treatment of simple transposition in the current era. J. Thorac. Cardiovasc. Surg., 95:14, 1988.

Castellino, R. A., Blank, N., and Adams, D. F.: Dilated azygos and hemiazygos veins presenting as paravertebral intrathoracic masses. N. Engl. J. Med., 278:1087, 1968.

Chatelaine, P., Meier, B., and Friedli, B.: Stenting of superior vena cava and inferior vena cava for symptomatic narrowing after repeated atrial surgery for d-transposition of the great vessels. Br. Heart J., 66:466, 1991.

Chiu, I. S., Anderson, R. H., Macartney, F. J., et al.: Morphologic features of an intact ventricular septum susceptible to subpulmonary obstruction in complete transposition of the great arteries. Am. J. Cardiol., 53:1633, 1984.

Clark, E. B., Sweeny, L. J., and Rosenquist, G. C.: Atrial defect size after Blalock-Hanlon atrioseptectomy. Am. J. Cardiol., 40:405, 1977.

Clarkson, P. M., Barratt-Boyes, B. G., and Neutze, J. M.: Late dysrhythmias and disturbances of conduction following Mustard operation for complete transposition of the great arteries. Circulation, 53:519, 1976.

Cobanoglu, A., Abbruzzese, P. A., Freimanis, I., et al.: Pericardial baffle complications following the Mustard operation. J. Thorac. Cardiovasc. Surg., 87:371, 1984.

Coceani, F., and Olley, P. M.: The response of the ductus arteriosus in prostaglandins. Can. J. Physiol. Pharmacol., 51:220, 1973.

Cochrane, A. D., Karl, T. R., and Mee, R. B.: Staged conversion to arterial switch for late failure of the systemic right ventricle. Ann. Thorac. Surg., 56:854, 1993.

Cochrane, R. P., and McGough, E. C.: Bovine pericardium: A source of pulmonary venous obstruction in the Mustard procedure. Ann. Thorac. Surg., 44:552, 1987.

Cooper, S. G., Sullivan, I. D., Bull, C., and Taylor, J. F. N.: Balloon dilatation of pulmonary venous pathway obstruction after Mustard repair for transposition of the great arteries. J. Am. Coll. Cardiol., 14:194, 1989.

Corno, A. F., Laks, H., George, B., and Williams, R. G.: Use of in-situ pericardium for surgical relief of pulmonary venous obstruction following Mustard's operation. Ann. Thorac. Surg., 43:443, 1987.

Coulson, J. D., Jennings, R. B., Jr., and Johnson, D. H.: Pulmonary venous atrial obstruction after the Senning procedure: Relief by catheter balloon dilatation. Br. Heart J., 64:160, 1990.

Coulson, J. D., Pitlick, P. T., Miller, C., et al.: Severe superior vena caval syndrome and hydrocephalus after the Mustard procedure: Findings and a new surgical approach. Circulation, 70:147, 1984.

Counahan, R., Simon, G., and Joseph, M.: The plain chest radiograph in d-transposition of the great arteries in the first month of life. Pediatr. Radiol., 1:217, 1973.

Creech, O., Jr., Maffey, D. E., Sayegh, S. F., and Sailors, E. L.: Complete transposition of the great vessels: A technique for intracardiac correction. Surgery, 43:349, 1958.

Crupi, G., Pillai, R., Parenzan, L., and Lincoln, C.: Surgical treatment of subpulmonary obstruction in transposition of the great arteries by means of a left ventricular-pulmonary arterial conduit. J. Thorac. Cardiovasc. Surg., 89:907, 1985.

Danilowicz, D., Isom, A. W., and Whiddon, L.: Superior vena caval syndrome after Mustard repair: Surgical decompression using a saphenous vein homograft. Am. Heart J., 101:862, 1981.

Dasmahapatra, H. K., Freedom, R. M., Moes, C. A. F., et al.: Surgical experience with left ventricular outflow tract obstruction in patients with complete transposition of the great arteries and essentially intact ventricular septum undergoing the Mustard operation. Eur. J. Cardiothorac. Surg., 3:241, 1989.

Davis, A. M., Wilkinson, J. L., Karl, T. R., and Mee, R. B.: Transposition of the great arteries with intact ventricular septum: Arterial switch repair in patients 21 days of age or older. J. Thorac. Cardiovasc. Surg., 106:111, 1993.

Deal, B. J., Chin, A. J., Sanders, S. P., et al.: Subxiphoid two-dimensional echocardiographic identification of tricuspid valve abnormalities in transposition of the great arteries with ventricular septal defect. Am. J. Cardiol., 55:1146, 1985.

Deanfield, J. E., Cullen, S., and Gewillig, M.: Arrhythmias after surgery for complete transposition: Do they matter? Cardiol. Young, 1:91, 1991.

de Begona, J. A., Kawauchi, M., Fullerton, D., et al.: The Mustard procedure for correction of simple transposition of the great arteries before 1 month of age. J. Thorac. Cardiovasc. Surg., 104:1218, 1992.

DeLeval, M. R., McKay, R., Jones, M., et al.: Modified Blalock-Taussig shunt. J. Thorac. Cardiovasc. Surg., 81:112, 1981.

Deutsch, V., Shem-Tov, A., Yahini, J. H., and Neufeld, H. N.: Cardioangiographic evaluation of the relationship between atrioventricular and semilunar valves. Its diagnostic importance in congenital heart disease. Am. J. Roentgenol., 110:474, 1970.

Driscoll, D. J., Kugler, J. D., Nihill, M. R., and McNamara, D. G.: The use of prostaglandin $E_1$ in a critically ill infant with transposition of the great arteries. J. Pediatr., 95:259, 1979.

Driscoll, D. J., Nihill, M. R., Vargo, T. A., et al.: Late development of pulmonary venous obstruction following Mustard's operation using a Dacron baffle. Circulation, 55:484, 1977.

Duster, M. C., Bink-Boelkens, M. T. E., Wampler, D., et al.: Long term followup of dysrhythmias following the Mustard procedure. Am. Heart J., 109:1323, 1985.

Edwards, W. S., Bargeron, L. M., Jr., and Lyons, C.: Reposition of right pulmonary veins in transposition of the great vessels. J.A.M.A., 188:522, 1964.

Elliott, L. P., Bargeron, L. M., Jr., Bream, P. R., et al.: Axial cineangiography in congenital heart disease. Section II. Specific lesions. Circulation, 56:1084, 1977.

El-Said, G. M., Gillette, P. C., Cooley, D. A., et al.: Protection of the sinus node in Mustard's operation. Circulation, 53:788, 1976.

Fermont, L.: Transposition of the great arteries: Advantages and results of prospective fetal detection. Experience from 1983–1990. In Vogel, M., and Buhlmeyer, K. (eds): Transposition of the Great Arteries 25 Years after Rashkind Balloon Septostomy. New York, Springer-Verlag, 1992, p. 39.

Fisher, E. H. R., Muster, A. J., Lev, M., and Paul, M. H.: Angiocardiographic and anatomic findings in transposition of the great arteries with left ventricular outflow tract gradients. Am. J. Cardiol., 25:95, 1970.

Flinn, C. J., Wolff, G. S., Dick, M., II, et al.: Cardiac rhythm after Mustard operation for complete transposition of the great arteries. N. Engl. J. Med., 310:1635, 1984.

Freedom, R. M., Culham, J. A. G., and Moes, C. A. F.: Angiocardiography of Congenital Heart Disease. New York, Macmillan, 1984, pp. 575.

Freedom, R. M., Culham, G., and Rowe, R. D.: The criss-cross and supero-inferior ventricular heart: An angiocardiographic study. Am. J. Cardiol., 42:620, 1978.

Freedom, R. M., Harrington, D. P., and White, R. I., Jr.: The differential diagnosis of levo transposed or malposed aorta: An angiocardiographic study. Circulation, 50:1040, 1974.

Fyler, D. C.: Report of the New England Regional Infant Cardiac Program. Pediatrics, 65(Suppl):422, 1980.

Gillette, P. C., Kugler, J. D., Garson, A., Jr., et al.: Mechanisms of cardiac arrhythmias after the Mustard operation for transposition of the great arteries. Am. J. Cardiol., 45:1225, 1980.

Goldman, H. E., Maralit, A., Sun, S., and Lanzkowsky, P.: Neonatal cyanosis and arterial oxygen saturation. J. Pediatr., 82:319, 1973.

Gomes, A. S., Nath, P. H., Singh, A., et al.: Accessory flaplike tissue causing ventricular outflow obstruction. J. Thorac. Cardiovasc. Surg., 80:211, 1980.

Graham, T. P., Jr., Atwood, G. F., Boucek, R. J., Jr., et al.: Abnormalities of right ventricular function following Mustard's operation for transposition of the great arteries. Circulation, 52:678, 1975.

Graham, T. P., Jr., Burgery, J., Bender, H. W., et al.: Improved right ventricular function after intra-atrial repair of transposition of the great arteries. Circulation, 72(II):45, 1985.

Guerin, R., Soto, B., Karp, R. B., et al.: Transposition of the great arteries: Determination of the position of the great arteries in conventional chest roentgenograms. Am. J. Roentgenol., 110:747, 1970.

Gutgesell, H. P., Garson, A., and McNamara, D. G.: Prognosis for the newborn with transposition of the great arteries. Am. J. Cardiol., 44:96, 1979.

Hagler, D. J., Ritter, D. G., Mair, D. D., et al.: Clinical angiographic and hemodynamic assessment of late results after the Mustard operation. Circulation, 57:1214, 1978.

Hagler, D. J., Ritter, D. G., Mair, D. D., et al.: Right and left ventricular function after the Mustard procedure in transposition of the great arteries. Am. J. Cardiol., 44:276, 1979.

Hayes, C. J., and Gersony, W. M.: Arrhythmias after the Mustard operation for transposition of the great arteries. A long term study. J. Am. Coll. Cardiol., 7:133, 1986.

Henry, C. G., Goldring, D., Hartman, A. F., et al.: Treatment of d-transposition of the great arteries. Management of hypoxemia after balloon atrial septostomy. Am. J. Cardiol., 47:299, 1981.

Houston, A. B., Gregory, N. L., and Coleman, E. N.: Echocardiographic identification of aorta and main pulmonary artery in complete transposition. Br. Heart J., 40:377, 1978.

Huhta, J. C., Edwards, W. D., Danielson, G. K., and Feldt, R. H.: Abnormalities of the tricuspid valve in complete transposition of the great arteries with ventricular septal defect. J. Thorac. Cardiovasc. Surg., 83:569, 1982.

Humes, R. A., Driscoll, D. J., Mair, D. D., et al.: Palliative transposition of venous return. J. Thorac. Cardiovasc. Surg., 96:364, 1988.

Idriss, F. S., DeLeon, S. Y., Nikaidoh, H., et al.: Resection of left ventricular outflow obstruction in d-transposition of the great arteries. J. Thorac. Cardiovasc. Surg., 74:343, 1977.

Idriss, F. S., Goldstein, I. R., Grana, L., et al.: A new technique for complete correction of transposition of the great vessels: An experimental study with preliminary clinical report. Circulation, 24:5, 1961.

Idriss, F. S., Ilbawi, M. N., De Leon, S. Y., et al.: Arterial switch in simple and complex transposition of the great arteries. J. Thorac. Cardiovasc. Surg., 95:29, 1988.

Ilbawi, M. N., DeLeon, S. Y., Backer, C. L., et al.: An alternative approach to the surgical management of physiologically corrected transposition with ventricular septal defect and pulmonary stenosis or atresia. J. Thorac. Cardiovasc. Surg., 100:410, 1990.

Jarmakani, J. M. M., and Canent, R. V., Jr.: Preoperative and postoperative right ventricular function in children with transposition of the great vessels. Circulation, 49, 50(II):39, 1974.

Jatene, A. D., Fontes, V. F., Paulista, P. P., et al.: Anatomic correction of transposition of the great vessels. J. Thorac. Cardiovasc. Surg., 72:364, 1976.

Jatene, A. D., Fontes, V. F., Paulista, P. P., et al.: Successful anatomic correction of transposition of the great vessels. A preliminary report. Arq. Bras. Cardiol., 28:461, 1975.

Jiminez, M. Q., and Martinez, V. P.: Uncommon conal pathology in complete dextro transposition of the great arteries with ventricular septal defect. Chest, 66:411, 1974.

Jonas, R. A.: Update on the rapid two-stage arterial switch procedure. Cardiol. Young, 1:99, 1991.

Jones, R. W. A., Baumer, J. H., Joseph, M. C., and Shinebourne, E. A.: Arterial oxygen tension and response to oxygen breathing in differential diagnosis of congenital heart disease in infancy. Arch. Dis. Child., 51:667, 1976.

Kaulitz, R., Stumper, O. F. W., Geuskens, R., et al.: Comparative values of the precordial and transesophageal approaches in the echocardiographic evaluation of atrial baffle function after an atrial correction procedure. J. Am. Coll. Cardiol., 16:686, 1990.

Kay, E. B., and Cross, F. S.: Surgical treatment of transposition of the great vessels. Surgery, 38:712, 1955.

Kay, E. B., and Cross, F. S.: Transposition of the great vessels corrected by means of atrial transposition. Surgery, 41:938, 1957.

Kirk, C. R., Gibbs, J. L., Wilkinson, J. L., et al.: Protein losing enteropathy caused by baffle obstruction after Mustard's operation. Br. Heart J., 59:69, 1988.

Kirklin, J. W., Devloo, R. A., and Weldman, W. H.: Open intracardiac repair for transposition of the great vessels: 11 cases. Surgery, 50:58, 1961.

Korns, M. E., Garabedian, H. A., and Lauer, R. M.: Anatomic limitation of balloon atrial septostomy. Hum. Pathol., 3:345, 1972.

Kron, I. L., Rheuban, K. S., Koob, A. W., et al.: Baffle obstruction following the Mustard operation: Cause and treatment. Ann. Thorac. Surg., 29:112, 1985.

Kurlander, G. J., Petry, E. L., and Girod, D. A.: Plain film diagnosis of congenital heart disease in the newborn period. Am. J. Roentgenol., 103:566, 1968.

Kurosawa, S., Kurosawa, H., and Becker, A. E.: The coronary arterioles in newborns, infants and children. A morphometric study of normal hearts and hearts with aortic atresia and complete transposition. Int. J. Cardiol., 10:43, 1986.

Lakier, J. B., Stanger, P., Heymann, M. A., et al.: Early onset of pulmonary vascular obstruction in patients with aortopulmonary transposition and intact ventricular septum. Circulation, 51:875, 1975.

Landtman, B., Louhimo, I., Rapola, J., and Tuuteri, L.: Causes of death in transposition of the great arteries. A clinical and autopsy study of 140 cases. Acta Paediatr. Scand., 64:785, 1975.

Lang, P., Freed, M. D., Bierman, F. Z., et al.: Use of prostaglandin E₁ in infants with d-transposition of the great arteries and intact ventricular septum. Am. J. Cardiol., 44:76, 1979.

Layman, T. E., and Edwards, J. E.: Anomalies of the cardiac valves associated with complete transposition of the great vessels. Am. J. Cardiol., 19:247, 1967.

LeCompte, Y.: Reparation a l'etage ventriculaire—The REV procedure: Technique and clinical results. Cardiol. Young, 1:63, 1991.

Leijala, M. A., Lincoln, C. R., Shinebourne, E. A., and Nellen, M.: A rare congenital cardiac malformation with situs inversus and discordant atrioventricular and concordant ventriculoarterial connections: Diagnosis and surgical treatment. Am. Heart J., 101:355, 1981.

Levy, R. J., Rosenthal, A., Castañeda, A. R., and Nadas, N. S.: Growth after surgical repair of simple d-transposition of the great arteries. Ann. Thorac. Surg., 25:225, 1978.

Liebman, J., Cullum, L., and Belloc, N. B.: Natural history of transposition of the great arteries. Anatomy and birth and death characteristics. Circulation, 40:237, 1969.

Lillehei, C. W., and Varco, R. L.: Certain physiologic, pathologic and surgical features of complete transposition of the great vessels. Surgery, 34:376, 1953.

Lincoln, C. R., and Southall, D.: Cardiac rhythm and conduction before and after Mustard's operation for complete transposition of the great arteries. Pediatr. Cardiol., 4(1):165, 1983.

Lindesmith, G. G., Stiles, Q. R., Tucker, B. L., et al.: The Mustard operation as a palliative procedure. J. Thorac. Cardiovasc. Surg., 64:75, 1972.

Markowitz, R. I., Kleinman, C. S., Hellenbrand, W. E., et al.: Communicating hydrocephalus secondary to superior vena caval obstruction. Am. J. Dis. Child., 138:638, 1984.

Mathew, R., Rosethal, A., and Fellows, K.: The significance of the right aortic arch in d-transposition of the great arteries. Am. Heart J., 87:314, 1974.

Mathews, R. A., Fricker, F. J., Beerman, L. B., et al.: Exercise studies after the Mustard operation in transposition of the great arteries. Am. J. Cardiol., 51:1526, 1983.

McGarry, K. M., Taylor, J. F. N., and Macartney, F. J.: Aortic atresia occurring with complete transposition of the great arteries. Br. Heart J., 44:711, 1980.

McGoon, D. C.: Intraventricular repair of transposition of the great arteries. J. Thorac. Cardiovasc. Surg., 64:430, 1972.

Mee, R. B. B.: Severe right ventricular failure after Mustard or Senning operation. J. Thorac. Cardiovasc. Surg., 92:385, 1986.

Merendino, K. A., Jesseph, J. E., Herron, P. W., et al.: Interatrial venous transposition—A one stage intracardiac operation for the conversion of complete transposition of the aorta and pulmonary artery to corrected transposition: Theory and clinical experience. Surgery, 42:898, 1957.

Moene, R. J., Oppenheimer-Dekker, A., and Bartelings, M. M.: Anatomic obstruction of the right ventricular outflow tract in transposition of the great arteries. Am. J. Cardiol., 51:1701, 1983.

Moene, R. J., Oppenheimer-Dekker, A., Bartelings, M. M., et al.: Morphology of ventricular septal defect in complete transposition of the great arteries. Am. J. Cardiol., 55:1566, 1985.

Moene, R. J., Oppenheimer-Dekker, A., Bartelings, M. M., et al.: Ventricular septal defect with normally connected great arteries and with transposed great arteries. Am. J. Cardiol., 58:627, 1986.

Moes, C. A. F.: Analysis of the chest in the neonate with congenital heart disease. Radiol. Clin. North Am., 13:251, 1975.

Mohri, H., Barnes, R. W., Rittenhouse, E. A., et al.: Fate of autologous pericardium and Dacron fabric used as substitutes for total atrial septum in growing animals. J. Thorac. Cardiovasc. Surg., 59:501, 1970.

Moodie, D. S., Feldt, R. H., and Wallace, R. B.: Transient protein-losing enteropathy secondary to elevated caval pressures and caval obstruction after the Mustard procedure. J. Thorac. Cardiovasc. Surg., 72:379, 1976.

Murphy, J. H., Barlai-Kovach, M. M., Mathews, R. A., et al.: Rest and exercise right and left ventricular function late after the Mustard operation: Assessment by radionuclide ventriculography. Am. J. Cardiol., 57:1142, 1986.

Musewe, N. N., Reisman, J., Benson, L. N., et al.: Cardiopulmonary adaptation at rest and during exercise 10 years after Mustard atrial repair for transposition of the great arteries. Circulation, 77:1055, 1988.

Mustard, W. T.: Successful two-stage correction of transposition of the great vessels. Surgery, 55:469, 1964.

Mustard, W. T., Chute, A. L., Keith, J. D., et al.: A surgical approach to transposition of the great vessels with extracorporeal circuit. Surgery, 36:39, 1954.

Muster, A. J., Paul, M. H., Van Grondelle, A., and Conway, J. J.: Asymmetric distribution of the pulmonary blood flow between the right and left lungs in d-transposition of the great arteries. Am. J. Cardiol., 38:352, 1976.

Newberger, J. W., Silvert, A. R., Buckley, L. P., and Fyler, D. C.: Cognitive function and age at repair of transposition of the great arteries in children. N. Engl. J. Med., 310:1495, 1984.

Newfeld, E. A., Paul, M. H., Muster, A. J., and Idriss, F. S.: Pulmonary vascular disease in complete transposition of the great arteries. A study of 200 patients. Am. J. Cardiol., 34:75, 1974.

Nogrady, M. B., and Dunbar, J. S.: Complete transposition of the great vessels. Re-evaluation of the so-called "typical configuration" on plain films of the chest. J. Can. Assoc. Radiol., 20:124, 1969.

Norwood, W. I., Dobell, A. R., Freedom, M. D., et al.: Intermediate results of the arterial switch repair. J. Thorac. Cardiovasc. Surg., 96:854, 1988.

Olley, P. M., Coceani, F., and Rowe, R. D.: Role of prostaglandin E₁ and E₂ in the management of neonatal heart disease. Adv. Prostaglandin Thromboxane Res., 4:345, 1978.

Oppenheimer-Dekker, A.: Interventricular communications in transposition of the great arteries. *In* Van Mierop, L. H. S. (ed): Embryology and Teratology of the Heart. Leiden, Ledien University Press, 1978, p. 136.

Ostermeyer, J., Bircks, W., Krain, A., et al.: Isolated atrioventricular discordance. J. Thorac. Cardiovasc. Surg., 86:926, 1983.

Pappas, G.: Left pulmonary vein stenosis associated with transposition of the great arteries. Ann. Thorac. Surg., 41:208, 1986.

Park, S. C., Siewers, R. D., Neches, W. H., et al.: Ventricular inversion with normal ventriculoarterial connection and left atrial isomerism: Correction by the Mustard operation. J. Am. Coll. Cardiol., 4:136, 1984.

Parrish, M. D., Graham, T. P., Jr., Bender, H. W., et al.: Radionuclide angiographic evaluation of right and left ventricular function during exercise after repair of transposition of the great arteries. Circulation, 67(1):178, 1983.

Pasquini, L., Sanders, S. P., Parness, I. A., et al.: Conal anatomy in 119 patients with d-loop transposition of the great arteries and ventricular septal defect: An echocardiographic and pathologic study. J. Am. Coll. Cardiol., 21:1712, 1993.

Paul, M. H.: D-transposition of the great arteries. *In* Moss, A. J., Adams, F. H., and Emmanoulides, G. S. (eds): Heart Disease in Infants, Children and Adolescents. Baltimore, Williams & Wilkins, 1977, p. 301.

Plauth, H. W., Jr., Nadas, A. S., Bernhard, W. F., and Gross, R. E.: Transposition of the great arteries: Clinical and physiological observations on 74 patients treated by palliative surgery. Circulation, 37:316, 1968.

Polansky, S. M., and Culham, J. A. G.: Paraspinal densities developing after repair of transposition of the great arteries. Am. J. Roentgenol., 134:394, 1980.

Quaegebeur, J. M., Rohmer, J., Ottenkamp, J., et al.: The arterial switch operation: An 8 year experience. J. Thorac. Cardiovasc. Surg., 92:361, 1986.

Ranjit, M. S., Wilkinson, J. L., and Mee, R. B.: Discordant atrioventricular connexion with concordant ventriculo-arterial connexion (so-called "isolated ventricular inversion") with usual atrial arrangement (situs solitus). Int. J. Cardiol., 31(1):114, 1991.

Rashkind, W. J., and Miller, W. W.: Creation of an atrial septal defect without thoracotomy: A palliative approach to complete transposition of the great arteries. J.A.M.A., 196:991, 1966.

Rastelli, G. C., McGoon, D. C., and Wallace, R. B.: Anatomic correction of transposition of the great arteries with ventricular septal defect and subpulmonary stenosis. J. Thorac. Cardiovasc. Surg., 58:545, 1969.

Redington, A., Rigby, M. L., Oldershaw, P., et al.: Right ventricular function 10 years after the Mustard operation for transposition of the great arteries: Analysis of size, shape, and wall motion. Br. Heart J., 62:455, 1989.

Riemenschneider, T. A., Vincent, W. R., Ruttenberg, H. D., and Desilets, D. T.: Transposition of the great vessels with hypoplasia of the right ventricle. Circulation, 38:386, 1968.

Rosenquist, G. C., Stark, J., and Taylore, J. F. N.: Congenital mitral valve disease in transposition of the great arteries. Circulation, 51:731, 1974.

Rowe, R. D., Freedom, R. M., Mehrizi, A., and Bloom, K. R.: The neonate with congenital heart disease. Major Probl. Clin. Pediatr., 5:3, 1981.

Sansa, M., Tonkin, I. L., Bargeron, L. M., Jr., and Elliott, L. P.: Left ventricular outflow tract obstruction in transposition of the great arteries: An angiographic study of 74 cases. Am. J. Cardiol., 44:88, 1979.

Senning, A.: Surgical correction of transposition of the great vessels. Surgery, 45:966, 1959.

Shannon, D. C., Lusser, M., Goldblatt, A., and Bunnell, J. B.: The cyanotic infant—Heart disease or lung disease? N. Engl. J. Med., 287:951, 1972.

Sholler, G. F., and Celermajer, J. M.: Cardiac surgery in the first year of life. The effect on weight gain of infants with congenital heart disease. Aust. Paediatr. J., 22:305, 1986.

Shrivastava, S., Tadavarthy, S. M., Fukuda, T., and Edwards, J. E.: Anatomic causes of pulmonary stenosis in complete transposition. Circulation, 54:154, 1976.

Shuhaiber, H. J., Juggi, J. S., John, V., et al.: Differences in the recovery of right and left ventricular function after ischemic arrest and cardioplegia. Eur. J. Cardiothorac. Surg., 4:435, 1990.

Shumacker, H. H. B., Jr.: A new operation for transposition of the great vessels. Surgery, 50:733, 1961.

Silove, E. D., and Taylor, J. F. N.: Angiographic anatomical features of subvalvular left ventricular outflow obstruction in transposition of the great arteries. The possible role of the anterior mitral valve leaflet. Pediatr. Radiol., 1:87, 1973.

Silverman, N. H., Snider, A. R., Colo, J., et al.: Superior vena caval obstruction after Mustard's operation by two-dimensional contrast echocardiography. Circulation, 64:392, 1981.

Smallhorn, J. F., Gow, R., Freedom, R. M., et al.: Pulsed Doppler echocardiographic assessment of the pulmonary venous pathway after the Mustard or Senning procedure for transposition of the great arteries. Circulation, 73:765, 1986.

Smith, A., Wilkinson, J. L., Anderson, R. H., et al.: Architecture of the ventricular mass and atrioventricular valves in complete transposition with intact septum compared with the normal. I. The left ventricle, mitral valve and interventricular septum. Pediatr. Cardiol., 6:253, 1986a.

Smith, A., Wilkinson, J. L., Anderson, R. H., et al.: Architecture of the ventricular mass and atrioventricular valves in complete transposition with intact septum compared with the normal. II. The right ventricle and tricuspid valve. Pediatr. Cardiol., 6:299, 1986b.

Smolinsky, A., Castaneda, A. R., and Van Praagh, R.: Infundibular septal resection: Surgical anatomy of the superior approach. J. Thorac. Cardiovasc. Surg., 95:486, 1988.

Soto, B., Becker, A. E., Moulaert, A. J., et al.: Classification of ventricular septal defects. Br. Heart J., 43:332, 1980.

Stark, J.: Concordant transposition—Mustard operation. *In* Stark, J., and DeLeval, M. R. (eds): Surgery for Congenital Heart Defects. Philadelphia, W. B. Saunders, 1993.

Stark, J., Silove, E. D., Taylor, J. F. N., and Graham, G. R. L.: Obstruction to systemic venous return following the Mustard operation for transposition of the great arteries. J. Thorac. Cardiovasc. Surg., 68:742, 1974.

Stark, J., Weller, P., Leanage, R., et al.: Late results of surgical treatment of transposition of the great arteries. Adv. Cardiol., 27:254, 1980.

Stumper, O., Witsenburg, M., Sutherland, G. R., et al.: Transesophageal echocardiographic monitoring of interventional cardiac catheterization in children. J. Am. Coll. Cardiol., 18:1506, 1991.

Sweeney, M. F., Bell, W. E., Doty, D. B., and Schieken, R. M.: Communicating hydrocephalus secondary to venous complications following intra-atrial baffle operation (Mustard procedure) for d-transposition of the great arteries. Pediatr. Cardiol., 3237, 1982.

Takahashi, M., Lindesmith, G. G., Lewis, A. B., et al.: Long term results of the Mustard procedure. Circulation, 56(2):85, 1977.

Tonkin, I. L., Sansa, M., Elliott, L. P., and Bargeron, L. M., Jr.: Recognition of developing left ventricular outflow tract obstruction in complete transposition of the great arteries. Radiology, 134:53, 1980.

Tooley, W. H., and Stanger, P.: The blue baby—Circulation or ventilation or both? N. Engl. J. Med., 287:983, 1972.

Trusler, G. A., Castañeda, A. R., Rosenthal, A., et al.: Current results of management in transposition of the great arteries with special emphasis on patients with associated ventricular septal defect. J. Am. Coll. Cardiol., 10:1061, 1987a.

Trusler, G. A., Williams, W. G., Duncan, K. F., et al.: Results with the Mustard operation in simple transposition of the great arteries 1963–1985. Ann. Surg., 206:251, 1987b.

Trusler, G. A., Williams, W. G., Izukawa, T., and Olley, P. M.: Current results with the Mustard operation in isolated transposition of the great arteries. J. Thorac. Cardiovasc. Surg., 80:381, 1980.

Turley, K., Mavroudis, C., and Ebert, P. A.: Repair of congenital cardiac lesions during the first week of life. Circulation, 66:1, 1982.

Urban, A. E., Stark, J., and Waterston, D. J.: Mustard's operation for transposition of the great arteries complicated by juxtaposition of the atrial appendages. Ann. Thorac. Surg., 21:304, 1976.

Van Gils, F. A. W.: Left ventricular outflow tract obstruction in transposition with interventricular communication: Anatomical aspects. *In* Van Mierop, L. H. S., Oppenheimer-Dekker, A., and Bruins, C. L. D. (eds): Embryology and Teratology of the Heart. Leiden, Leiden University Press, 1978, p. 160.

Van Gils, F. A. W., Moulaert, A. J., Oppenheimer-Dekker, A., and Wenink, A. C. G.: Transposition of the great arteries with ventricular septal defect and pulmonary stenosis. Br. Heart J., 40:494, 1978.

Van Praagh, R., Layton, W. M., and Van Praagh, S.: The morphogenesis of normal and abnormal relationship between the great arteries and the ventricle: Pathologic and experimental data. *In* Van Praagh, R., and Takao, A. (eds): Etiology and Morphogenesis of Congenital Heart Disease. Mt. Kisco, NY, Futura, 1980, p. 271.

Van Praagh, R., and Van Praagh, S.: Isolated ventricular inversion. Am. J. Cardiol., 17:395, 1966.

Vidne, B. A., Subramanian, S., and Wagner, H. R.: Aneurysm of the membranous ventricular septum in transposition of the great arteries. Circulation, 53(1):157, 1976.

Vogel, M., Ash, J., Rowe, R. D., et al.: Congenital unilateral pulmonary vein stenosis complicating transposition of the great arteries. Am. J. Cardiol., 54:166, 1984a.

Vogel, M., Freedom, R. M., Smallhorn, J. F., et al.: Complete transposition of the great arteries and coarctation of the aorta. Am. J. Cardiol., 53:1627, 1984b.

Vouhe, P. R., Tamisiers, D., Leca, F., et al.: Transposition of the great

arteries, ventricular septal defect, and pulmonary outflow tract obstruction. J. Thorac. Cardiovasc. Surg., 103:428, 1992.

Waldman, J. D., Paul, M. H., Newfeld, E. A., et al.: Transposition of the great arteries with intact ventricular septum and patent ductus arteriosus. Am. J. Cardiol., 39:232, 1977.

Waldman, J. D., Waldman, J., and Jones, M. C.: Failure of balloon dilatation in mid cavity obstruction of the systemic venous atrium after Mustard operation. Pediatr. Cardiol., 4:151, 1983.

Watanabe, T., Trusler, G. A., Williams, W. G., et al.: Phrenic nerve paralysis after pediatric cardiac surgery. J. Thorac. Cardiovasc. Surg., 94:383, 1987.

Williams, W. G., Trusler, G. A., Kirklin, J. W., et al.: Early and late results of a protocol for simple transposition leading to an atrial switch (Mustard) repair. J. Thorac. Cardiovasc. Surg., 95:717, 1988.

Wilson, H. E., Nafrawi, A. G., Cardozo, R. H., and Aguillon, A.: Rational approach to surgery for complete transposition of the great vessels. Ann. Thorac. Surg., 155:258, 1962.

Wyse, R. K. H., Hawroth, S. G., Taylor, J. F. N., and Macartney, F. J.: Obstruction of superior vena caval pathway after Mustard's repair. Reliable diagnosis by transcutaneous Doppler ultrasound. Br. Heart J., 42:162, 1979.

Yamaki, S., and Tezuka, F. L.: Quantitative analysis of pulmonary vascular disease in complete transposition of the great arteries. Circulation, 54:805, 1976.

# ■ II  The Senning Procedure for Transposition of the Great Vessels

A. D. Pacifico

The operations described by Senning in 1959 and by Mustard in 1964 are the most common types of procedures used to accomplish venous switching. The arterial switch operation, first successfully accomplished by Jatene and associates in 1975, has become the procedure of choice for patients with transposition of the great arteries and similar malformations in most medical centers (Castañeda et al., 1988). Nevertheless, venous switching continues to be used infrequently in some centers, is of historical interest, and is applicable to the repair of certain complex defects.

Although the Senning operation was described 5 years earlier than the Mustard operation, the latter became the procedure of choice soon after it was introduced for patients with transposition of the great arteries. The probable reasons for this included the reported high early mortality for the Senning operation done as a single-stage procedure (Kirklin et al., 1961), which actually was related more to the selection of patients than to the operative procedure itself, and the belief that the Mustard procedure was simpler to do. The Mustard operation was done after a preliminary Blalock-Hanlon atrial septectomy and, therefore, the patients were older and larger and were often in the second to fourth year of life. As time

passed, balloon atrial septostomy at the time of neonatal catheterization was described (Rashkind and Miller, 1966) and supplanted the initial Blalock-Hanlon operation in many centers. The improvement resulting from balloon septostomy was not maintained as long as that from surgical septectomy, and this led to earlier performance of the Mustard operation with many groups advising that it be performed electively during the first year of life (Stark et al., 1974). Earlier performance of the Mustard procedure led to increased reports of pulmonary and systemic venous pathway obstructive complications that were reduced by various technical modifications.

In an attempt to reduce the obstructive complications after the Mustard procedure, Brom reintroduced the Senning operation (Quaegebeur et al., 1977), and it soon became the venous switching procedure of choice.

The Senning and Mustard operations both accomplish intra-atrial transposition of venous return by using living autologous atrial tissue in the former and a baffle tailored from autologous pericardium or synthetic material in the latter. At least theoretically, the intra-atrial venous pathways after the Senning procedure have greater potential for future growth

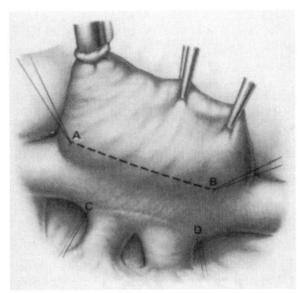

**FIGURE 43–20.** A marking suture (A) is placed 1 cm anterior to the crista terminalis at the superior extent of the right atriotomy incision. Marking suture B is placed a few millimeters cephalad from the junction of the inferior vena cava (IVC) and right atrium, at a measured point from the caudal marking suture (D) on the interatrial groove, equal to two-thirds the circumference of the IVC or a minimal distance of 15 mm. The *dashed line* shows the extent of the longitudinal right atrial incision. Points C and D are placed on the interatrial groove to define the cephalic and caudal extent of the left atrial incision. (From Pacifico, A. D.: Concordant transposition—Senning operation. *In* Stark, J., and DeLeval, M. [eds]: Surgery for Congenital Heart Defects. London, Grune & Stratton, 1983.)

because they are composed entirely of living atrial tissue. However, only part of the venous pathways of the Mustard operation consists of living tissue. A possible additional advantage of the Senning operation is that atrial function may be better preserved than after the Mustard procedure (Parenzan et al., 1978), although the incidence of atrial dysrhythmias remains similar to that of the Mustard procedure.

## TECHNIQUE

The technique that follows is the one fundamentally described by Senning in 1959 and modified by myself (Pacifico, 1983). It can be applied in infants and older children, and the use of nonviable material is usually avoided.

The standard incision is a median sternotomy to expose the heart and great vessels. Purse-string sutures are placed in the ascending aorta for arterial cannulation and directly on each vena cava for venous cannulation. The purse-string on the superior vena cava (SVC) is made oval to minimize narrowing of this structure when it is later tied. If the SVC is particularly small, the purse-string is used solely to secure the cannula in place, and later the defect in the SVC is closed directly with a continuous fine monofilament suture. Separate caval cannulation, with thin-walled angled metal cannulas, provides ex-

cellent intracardiac exposure for this procedure and others and avoids the need for long periods of total circulatory arrest (Pacifico, 1988).

Before cardiopulmonary bypass is established, the circumferences of the SVC and inferior vena cava (IVC) are each measured and recorded. Marking sutures are placed on the interatrial groove to define the cephalic (C) and caudal (D) extent of the left atriotomy (Fig. 43–20). Care is taken to place these marking sutures on the lateral margin of each vena cava and not posterior to them. A marking suture (A) may be placed 1 cm anterior to the crista terminalis at the superior extent of the right atrium. An additional marking suture (B) is placed a few millimeters cephalad from the junction of the IVC and right atrium, at a point measured from the caudal marking suture (D) on the interatrial groove, equal to two-thirds of the circumference of the IVC or a minimal distance of 15 mm (see Fig. 43–20). Points A and B define the superior and inferior extent of the longitudinal right atrial incision.

Cardiopulmonary bypass is established initially with the arterial and IVC cannulas in place, and later on the SVC cannula is inserted. The temperature of the perfusate is progressively reduced to cool the patient to 24° C. Ligatures are placed about each vena cava for later occlusion around each caval cannula, and the midportion of the interatrial groove is dissected about 1 cm to the left (Fig. 43–21). This dissection is limited by the previously placed marking sutures and must not extend beneath either vena cava, or it may later contribute to caval obstruction and distortion by the suture line used to construct the

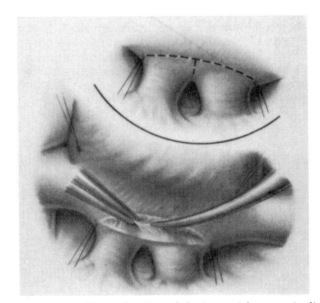

**FIGURE 43–21.** The midportion of the interatrial groove is dissected approximately 1 cm to the left. The dissection is limited by the previously placed marking sutures and must not extend beneath either vena cava. The *dashed line* indicates the extent of the left atrial incision. (From Pacifico, A. D.: Concordant transposition—Senning operation. *In* Stark, J., and DeLeval, M. [eds]: Surgery for Congenital Heart Defects. London, Grune & Stratton, 1983.)

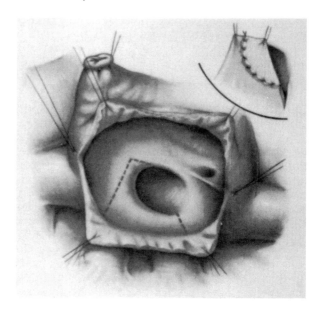

**FIGURE 43–22.** A view through the right atrial incision shows the atrial septum and its fossa ovalis defect. The coronary sinus can be seen to the right and anteriorly as well as the edge of the tricuspid valve annulus. The *dashed line* indicates the extent of the atrial septal incision to develop the septal flap. The incision is directed toward the superior aspect of the right superior pulmonary vein as well as the inferior aspect of the right inferior pulmonary vein. Formerly, a small patch of Dacron or pericardium *(inset)* was used to create a trapezoid configuration of the septal flap (see Fig. 43–23). (From Pacifico, A. D.: Concordant transposition—Senning operation. *In* Stark, J., and DeLeval, M. [eds]: Surgery for Congenital Heart Defects. London, Grune & Stratton, 1983.)

anterior wall of the pulmonary venous pathway. When cardiac ejections cease, a small incision is made into the left atrium at the right interatrial groove between points C and D, and a disposable sump tip vent is inserted. The aorta is cross-clamped, and cold cardioplegic solution is infused into the aortic root.

The right atrium is opened between points A and B (see Fig. 43–20), and the left margin of the atriotomy is sutured to the subcutaneous tissue for traction. The right margin is retracted by two sutures placed over the right chest wall and is held by the weight of a curved clamp. The atrial septum is inspected, and a flap is developed from the limbic tissue anteriorly toward the superior and inferior aspects of each respective right pulmonary vein. This flap remains attached at the right interatrial groove (Fig. 43–22). The flap has a trapezoid shape with a defect created by the existing interatrial communication. Formerly, a small patch of Dacron or pericardium was sutured to the septal flap to accommodate this deficiency, leaving a trapezoid configuration (see Fig. 43–22).

Currently, however, the coronary sinus is incised on its anterior margin, which is shown in Figure 43–23, to create a triangular-shaped coronary sinus flap. The tissue at the left apex of the coronary sinus flap and the left wall of the left atrium just above the left pulmonary veins is imbricated with a mattress suture to create a small roof above the left pulmonary veins. The coronary sinus flap is then combined with the atrial septal flap to form the roof of the left pulmonary venous pathway (Fig. 43–24). If the atrial septal defect (ASD) is small and centrally positioned, it is closed primarily before creating the septal flap, and the coronary sinus flap is not used. If a surgical atrial septectomy was performed earlier, a synthetic or pericardial patch may be required to reconstruct the atrial septum, although in some cases the coronary sinus flap and remaining atrial septal tissue suffice. The roof of the left pulmonary venous pathway is constructed as shown in Figures 43–24 and 43–25 by using continuous 4-0 polypropylene suture. The superior portion of the suture line lies above the left pul-

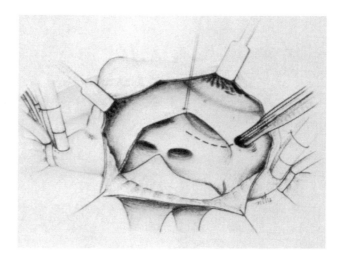

**FIGURE 43–23.** The coronary sinus is incised on its anterior margin to create a triangular-shaped coronary sinus flap. The tissue at the left apex of the coronary sinus flap and the left wall of the left atrium just above the left pulmonary veins is imbricated with a mattress suture to create a small roof above the left pulmonary veins.

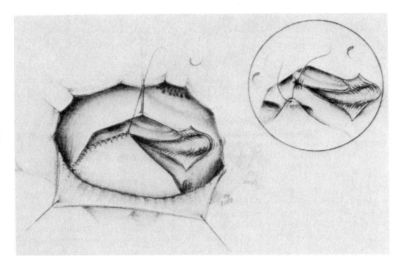

FIGURE 43–24. The coronary sinus flap is combined with the atrial septal flap to form the roof of the left pulmonary venous pathway.

monary veins and courses within the left atrium to the origin of the septal flap near the SVC junction. Similarly, the inferior border of the flap courses back to its origin near the IVC junction. These divergent suture lines are shown in Figure 43–25.

All of these maneuvers have been accomplished during standard cardiopulmonary bypass methods with core cooling. In some patients, suturing of the atrial septal flap above the left pulmonary veins is facilitated by the use of circulatory arrest. When this is used, the arrest time is usually between 5 and 10 minutes. If temporary total circulatory arrest had been established, cardiopulmonary bypass is reinstituted at 24° C when the septal flap suture lines have been completed.

The roof of the vena cava pathway is constructed with continuous 4-0 polypropylene suture. The inferior aspect of the right side of the free right atrial wall is sutured to the atrial tissue about the IVC orifice that continues superiorly to the coronary sinus (Fig. 43–26). If the coronary sinus has not been in-

cised, it is left to drain with the pulmonary venous blood. When a coronary sinus flap has been used, care is taken to place this suture line slightly posterior to the remaining rim of the coronary sinus to avoid the area of the specialized conduction tissue. A second suture is used to complete the superior attachment of the right side of the free right atrial wall, attaching this about the SVC and along the limbic tissue. The completed suture line is shown in Figure 43–27.

The incision in the left atrium that is used initially for the left atrial vent is extended between the marking sutures (C and D) on the interatrial groove (see Fig. 43–20), and the perimeter of the left atriotomy is lengthened by incising onto the right superior pulmonary vein for a distance of about 1 cm, which is shown in Figure 43–28. When the right superior and inferior pulmonary veins are oriented more horizontally, the incision is made between them (Fig. 43–29). The original right atrial incision is extended anteriorly at each end, from A to A' and from B to B', which is

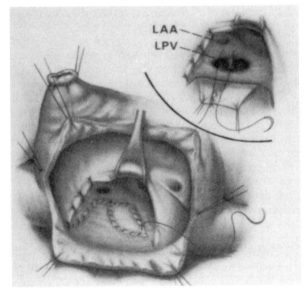

FIGURE 43–25. The roof of the left pulmonary venous pathway has been constructed with a continuous suture of 4-0 polypropylene. The superior portion of the suture line is above the left pulmonary veins (LPV) (see inset) and posterior to the origin of the left atrial appendage (LAA). (From Pacifico, A. D.: Concordant transposition—Senning operation. In Stark, J., and DeLeval, M. [eds]: Surgery for Congenital Heart Defects. London, Grune & Stratton, 1983.)

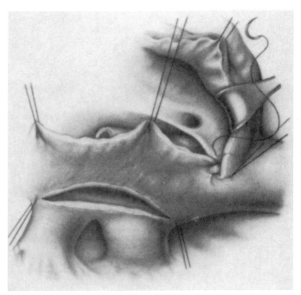

FIGURE 43–26. The roof of the caval pathway is formed by using the right side of the free right atrial wall beginning the suture line near the inferior vena cava and continuing beyond the area cephalad of the coronary sinus. A second suture is used to form this pathway near the superior vena cava. (From Pacifico, A. D.: Concordant transposition—Senning operation. *In* Stark, J., and DeLeval, M. [eds]: Surgery for Congenital Heart Defects. London, Grune & Stratton, 1983.)

shown in Figure 43–29. The length of each extension is almost one-quarter of the circumference of SVC and IVC, respectively, which will increase the perimeter of this flap by half the circumference of each vena cava, and leave additional length for attachment above the right pulmonary veins. These incisions permit the development of an advancement flap similar to that

used in plastic surgical procedures. When properly made, they allow point A″ to reach point C without constricting or use of a purse-string to the circumference of the superior vena cava pathway (see Fig. 43–29). Similarly, point B″ is brought to point D without compromising the IVC circumference. Initially, a 6-0 polypropylene suture attaches point A″ to point C, and this suture is tied. A second suture is placed at point A and is tied and retracted. The perimeter of the right atrial flap from A to A″ is then sutured superficially along the SVC pathway by using interrupted 6-0 polypropylene sutures (Fig. 43–30). Traction in opposite directions from points A through C permits the placement of accurate and superficial sutures, which avoids the area of the sinus node. Similarly, interrupted sutures placed at points B and D are tensed in opposite directions, and multiple interrupted 6-0 polypropylene sutures are used to attach this portion of the right atrial wall to the IVC pathway (Fig. 43–31). The use of interrupted sutures (compared with the continuous suture shown in Figure 43–30) obviates the potential purse-string effect of a continuous suture line that would reduce the circumference of each vena cava. Point E is then attached to point F with an interrupted 6-0 polypropylene suture, which is shown in Figure 43–31. Multiple interrupted sutures are placed to complete the attachment of the remaining segment of this flap to the right edge of the left atriotomy to complete the pulmonary venous pathway (Fig. 43–32). Rewarming is accomplished, air is removed from the heart and aorta, and the cross-clamp is removed.

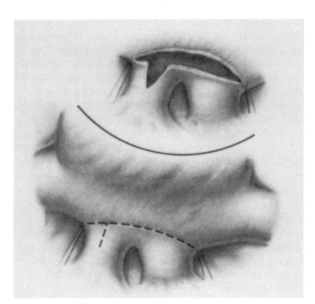

FIGURE 43–28. The extent of the left atrial incision is defined by the *dashed line.* The perimeter is enlarged by incising the right superior pulmonary vein, and the resultant atriotomy is shown above. When the right superior and inferior pulmonary veins are oriented horizontally, it is sometimes advantageous to enlarge the perimeter by incising between the right superior and the right inferior veins, which is shown in Figures 43–29 and 43–31. (From Pacifico, A. D.: Concordant transposition—Senning operation. *In* Stark, J., and DeLeval, M. [eds]: Surgery for Congenital Heart Defects. London, Grune & Stratton, 1983.)

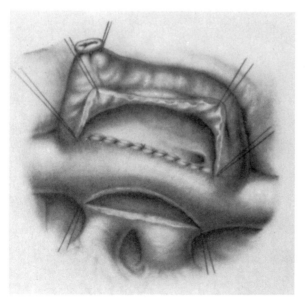

FIGURE 43–27. The completed caval pathway. (From Pacifico, A. D.: Concordant transposition—Senning operation. *In* Stark, J., and DeLeval, M. [eds]: Surgery for Congenital Heart Defects. London, Grune & Stratton, 1983.)

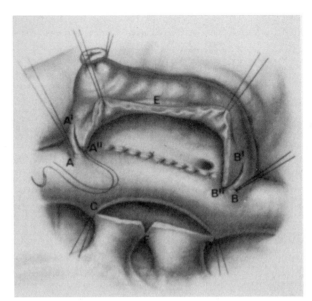

**FIGURE 43–29.** The original right atrial incision is extended anteriorly at each end, from A to A′ and from B to B′. The length of each extension is almost one-quarter the circumference of the superior and inferior vena cava, respectively. An advancement flap has been created permitting point A″ to reach point C, and point B″ to reach point D. (From Pacifico, A. D.: Concordant transposition—Senning operation. *In* Stark, J., and DeLeval, M. [eds]: Surgery for Congenital Heart Defects. London, Grune & Stratton, 1983.)

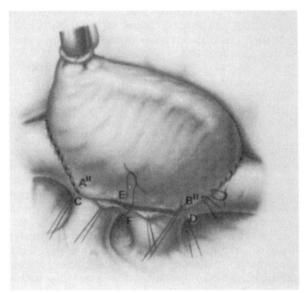

**FIGURE 43–31.** The perimeter of the right atrial flap from B to B″ is sutured along the inferior vena cava–right atrial junction. Interrupted sutures of 6-0 polypropylene are preferred. (From Pacifico, A. D.: Concordant transposition—Senning operation. *In* Stark, J., and DeLeval, M. [eds]: Surgery for Congenital Heart Defects. London, Grune & Stratton, 1983.)

The technique described differs from that reported by Quaegebeur and associates (1977) primarily by the method of venous cannulation and by not using the eustachian valve in construction of the inferior vena cava pathway. The eustachian valve may be well developed in some patients and essentially nonexistent in others, and therefore I prefer not to rely on it. In addition, direct inferior vena cava cannulation sometimes results in injury of the eustachian valve. Avoiding the use of the eustachian valve, however, requires that the caudal aspect of the right atriotomy

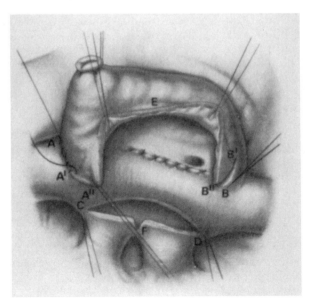

**FIGURE 43–30.** The perimeter of the right atrial flap from A to A″ is sutured superficially along the SVC pathway to point C. Interrupted 6-0 polypropylene sutures are preferred to avoid the purse-string effect of a continuous suture. (From Pacifico, A. D.: Concordant transposition—Senning operation. *In* Stark, J., and DeLeval, M. [eds]: Surgery for Congenital Heart Defect. London, Grune & Stratton, 1983.)

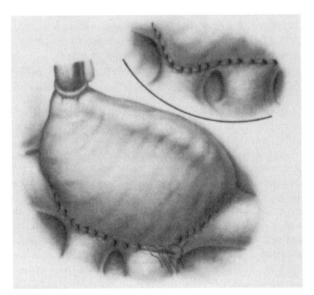

**FIGURE 43–32.** Point E is attached to point F with an interrupted 6-0 polypropylene suture and multiple similar interrupted sutures are used to complete the pulmonary venous pathway. (From Pacifico, A. D.: Concordant transposition—Senning operation. *In* Stark, J., and DeLeval, M. [eds]: Surgery for Congenital Heart Defects. London, Grune & Stratton, 1983.)

incision be directed more anteriorly (i.e., farther to the left or anterior from the interatrial groove) to leave sufficient right atrial tissue for construction of this segment of the caval pathway. The atriotomy incision presented here is similar to that used originally by Senning in 1959 but does require a greater perimeter of the remaining free right atrial wall for proper construction of the roof of the pulmonary venous pathway, which is achieved by using the advancement flap technique (see Fig. 43–29).

The combination of the coronary sinus flap with the atrial septal flap avoids the use of a nonviable patch to fill in the ASD.

## RESULTS

The hospital mortality rate after the Senning procedure in 146 patients with various forms of transposition of the great arteries, collected from three institutions, was 2.7% (Pacifico, 1983). This procedure included 58 patients undergoing surgery in Leiden, Holland (Brom, 1982), 53 patients undergoing surgery at the Hospital for Sick Children at Great Ormond Street, London, England (Stark et al, 1984), and 35 patients undergoing surgery in Bergamo, Italy (Locatelli et al., 1979). This reflected the early experience with the Senning operation after its revival in 1977 by Quaegebeur and associates from Leiden, Holland.

The results of the Mustard and Senning operations were reviewed in 123 consecutive patients with transposition of the great arteries and intact ventricular septum who had atrial switching between 1972 and 1980 at the Children's Hospital Medical Center in Boston (Marx et al., 1983). A Mustard operation was performed in 66 patients at a mean age of 15.5 months between 1972 and 1978. There were 7 deaths (11%) within 30 days of operation and 5 deaths (8%) during the follow-up period that extended to 43.5 months. However, 57 patients underwent a Senning operation between 1978 and 1980 at a mean age of 6.6 months. There were 3 deaths (5%) within 30 days of operation and 2 late deaths (4%) during the follow-up period that extended to 13.6 months.

In a more recent experience with 35 patients with transposition of the great arteries and intact ventricular septum undergoing surgery between 1982 and 1985, there was 1 hospital death (2.9%) and no late mortality among 29 of 33 patients who were followed between 2 and 36 months postoperatively (mean = 14 ± 10 months) (George et al., 1987).

Some neonates with transposition of the great arteries and intact ventricular septum continue to be hypoxic despite an adequate balloon atrial septostomy. It was formerly believed that the atrial switch operation in the neonatal period was associated with high hospital mortality. DeLeon and associates (1984) reviewed their experience with the Senning operation in 19 patients who underwent surgery between 2 and 24 days of age (mean = 12 days). There were 2 early deaths (10%) and 1 late death (5%) during the follow-up interval that ranged between 7 and 40 months.

The three deaths occurred in the first 3 infants who underwent surgery in the series, and the subsequent 16 patients were all alive and well at follow-up. This experience and others support the conclusion that the Senning operation can be done at low risk even in the sick hypoxemic neonate (Fortune et al., 1983; Matherne et al., 1985; Rubay et al., 1987; Turley et al., 1985).

In general, the early and late results of the Senning operation combined with closure of a large ventricular septal defect in infants with transposition are worse than for the group with intact ventricular septum. In one series of 46 infants ranging from 12 days to 12 months of age at operation (median = 5.1 ± 3.2 months), the hospital mortality rate was 15.2% and the late mortality rate was 5.1% (Penkoske et al., 1983). In another experience, there were no early (< 30 days) deaths but 3 late deaths among 10 patients with various forms of complex transposition whose repair included a Senning operation (George et al., 1987).

Various complications that can occur after the Senning operation include systemic or pulmonary venous obstruction, baffle suture line leaks, tricuspid valve incompetence, residual or recurrent ventricular septal defect, left ventricular outflow tract obstruction, arrhythmias, and reduction of systemic (right) ventricular function.

The incidence of superior vena caval obstruction ranges from 0 to 13% after the Senning operation (George et al., 1987; Marx et al., 1983). This obstruction has been implicated as a cause of early mortality, but its incidence appears to be no higher when the operation is performed in younger and smaller subjects (DeLeon et al., 1984). This complication can result from a technical error during the initial construction of the systemic venous pathways and can also be related to narrowing of the perimeter of the superior vena cava by the suture line for the roof of the pulmonary venous pathway. Reoperation to repair systemic venous obstruction is uncommonly required, and in some patients it may be managed effectively by percutaneous catheter balloon dilatation. The living autologous tissue used in the Senning procedure may result in a lesser incidence of late baffle obstructive complications than that observed in patients after the Mustard type of repair.

Pulmonary venous obstruction in most series is rare after the Senning operation. It developed in 6 of 57 patients (11%) who underwent the Senning operation at a mean age of 6.6 months (Marx et al., 1983). This obstruction has not occurred in most series reported in the literature.

Baffle leaks can occur after the Senning operation but are uncommon. Such a leak occurred in 1 of 54 survivors (1.9%) of the Senning operation in one series (Marx et al., 1983).

Tricuspid valve incompetence and systemic ventricular dysfunction can occur after atrial switch operations. In the Boston experience, mild and severe tricuspid valve incompetence was reported in 3 patients among 39 survivors of the Senning operation and

VSD closure (Penkoske et al., 1983). Tricuspid valve replacement was required in the 3 patients with severe incompetence. Graham and associates (1985) studied right ventricular function after intra-atrial repair of transposition of the great arteries. Postoperative right ventricular ejection fraction was below normal (< 0.49) in 16 of 32 patients who underwent the Senning procedure. Mean postoperative right ventricular ejection fraction was lower for patients undergoing surgery between 1971 and 1974 (0.39 ± 0.11) than for patients in either the Mustard group from 1975 to 1978 (0.47 ± 0.13, $p < 0.03$) or the Senning group (0.48 ± 0.09). Improved postoperative right ventricular performance was shown in patients who had a more recent intra-atrial repair, which leads to the speculation that younger age at operation, better preoperative function, and improved methods of myocardial protection may be responsible for improved postoperative ventricular performance.

The incidence of rhythm disturbances is similar for both the Mustard and the Senning operations. The incidence of sinus rhythm after the Senning operation varies between 88 and 100% with follow-ups ranging from 10 to 25 months. Rhythm disturbances are likely to be similar to those occurring after the Mustard procedure, and the incidence will probably increase progressively with time.

Although the quality of life and overall results after the Senning operation are very good, the current trend to advise the arterial switch operation as the procedure of choice for patients with transposition of the great arteries will probably continue. Careful early and late follow-up after each type of procedure is necessary to provide a proper comparison of results.

## SELECTED BIBLIOGRAPHY

Castañeda, A. R., Trusler, G. A., Paul, M. H., et al.: The early results of treatment of simple transposition in the current era. J. Thorac. Cardiovasc. Surg., 95:14, 1988.

This paper reports the early results in the modern era from 20 institutions in North America consisting the Congenital Heart Surgeon's Society. A total of 187 neonates within the first 2 weeks of life were admitted into this cooperative study between January 1, 1985 and June 1, 1986. Seventy-six patients were initially entered into a protocol leading to an arterial switch repair, 45 into one leading to a Mustard type of repair, and 49 into one leading to a Senning repair. The risk factors for death were low birth weight, earlier date of entry into the study, and an arterial switch protocol in the group of institutions at high risk for arterial switch repair. A detailed analysis of these patients is given and leads to the conclusion that the arterial and atrial switch repairs can have similar early results.

Quaegebeur, J. M., Rohmer, J., Brom, A. G., and Tinkelenberg, J.: Revival of the Senning operation in the treatment of transposition of the great arteries. Thorax, 32:517, 1977.

Although the Senning operation was used in a few institutions soon after it was introduced in 1959, it was abandoned in favor of the Mustard operation for many years. This paper was responsible for the revival of the Senning operation as a commonly performed procedure for transposition of the great arteries. The technique, which is used by the authors, is clearly detailed, and the results are nicely analyzed.

Senning, A.: Surgical correction of transposition of the great vessels. Surgery, 45:966, 1959.

This paper describes the original surgical procedures performed by Senning for patients with transposition of the great arteries and forms the basis of the current Senning procedure.

## BIBLIOGRAPHY

Bender, H. W., Jr., Graham, T. P., Jr., Boucek, R. J., Jr., et al.: Comparative operative results of the Senning and Mustard procedures for transposition of the great arteries. Circulation, 62(Suppl. I):197, 1980.

Brom, G.: The Senning procedure. In Moulton, A. (ed): Current Controversies and Techniques in Congenital Heart Disease. Pasadena, Appleton Davis, 1982.

Castaneda, A. R., Trusler, G. A., Paul, M. H., et al.: The early results of treatment of simple transposition in the current era. J. Thorac. Cardiovasc. Surg., 95:14, 1988.

DeLeon, V. H., Hougen, T. J., Norwood, W. I., et al.: Results of the Senning operation for transposition of the great arteries with intact ventricular septum in neonates. Circulation, 70(Suppl. I):21, 1984.

Fortune, R. L., Pacquet, M., Collins-Nakai, R. L., and Duncan, N. F.: Intracardiac repair of dextro-transposition of the great arteries in the newborn period. J. Thorac. Cardiovasc. Surg., 85:371, 1983.

George, B. L., Laks, H., Klitzner, T. S., et al.: Results of the Senning procedure in infants with simple and complex transposition of the great arteries. Am. J. Cardiol., 59:426, 1987.

Graham, T. P., Burger, J., Bender, H. W., et al.: Improved right ventricular function after intraatrial repair of transposition of the great arteries. Circulation, 72(Suppl. II):45, 1985.

Jatene, A. D., Fontes, V. F., Paulista, P. P., et al.: Successful anatomic correction of transposition of the great vessels: A preliminary report. Arg. Braz. Cardiol., 28:461, 1975.

Kirklin, J. W., Devloo, R. A., and Weidman, W. H.: Open intracardiac repair for transposition of the great vessels: 11 cases. Surgery, 50:68, 1961.

Locatelli, G., DiBenedetto, G., Villani, M., et al.: Transposition of the great arteries: Successful Senning's operation in 35 consecutive patients. Thorac. Cardiovasc. Surg., 27:120, 1979.

Marx, G. R., Hougen, T. J., Norwood, W. I., et al.: Transposition of the great arteries with intact ventricular septum: Results of Mustard and Senning operations in 123 consecutive patients. J. Am. Coll. Cardiol., 1:476, 1983.

Matherne, G. P., Razook, J. D., Thompson, W. M., Jr., et al.: Senning repair for transposition of the great arteries in the first week of life. Circulation, 72:840, 1985.

Mustard, W. T.: Successful two-stage correction of transposition of the great vessels. Surgery, 55:469, 1964.

Pacifico, A. D.: Cardiopulmonary bypass and hypothermic circulatory arrest in congenital heart surgery. In Grillo, H. C., Austen, W. G., Wilkins, E. W., Jr., et al. (eds): Current Therapy in Cardiothoracic Surgery. Toronto, B. C. Decker, 1988.

Pacifico, A. D.: Concordant transposition—Senning operation. In Stark, J., and DeLeval, M. (eds): Surgery for Congenital Heart Defects. London, Grune & Stratton, 1983, p. 345.

Parenzan, L., Locatelli, G., Alfieri, O., et al.: The Senning operation for transposition of the great arteries. J. Thorac. Cardiovasc. Surg., 76:305, 1978.

Penkoske, P. A., Westerman, G. R., Marx, G. R., et al.: Transposition of the great arteries and ventricular septal defect: Results with the Senning operation and closure of the ventricular septal defect in infants. Ann. Thorac. Surg., 36:281, 1983.

Quaegebeur, J. M., and Brom, A. G.: The trousers-shaped baffle for use in the Mustard operation. Ann. Thorac. Surg., 25:240, 1978.

Quaegebeur, J. M., Rohmer, J., Brom, A. G., and Tinkelenberg, J.: Revival of the Senning operation in the treatment of transposition of the great arteries. Thorax, 32:517, 1977.

Rashkind, W. J., and Miller, W. W.: Creation of an atrial septal defect without thoracotomy: A palliative approach to complete transposition of the great arteries. J. A. M. A., 196:173, 1966.

Rubay, J. E., de Halleux, C., Moulin, D., et al.: Long-term follow-up of the Senning operation for transposition of the great arteries in children under 3 months of age. J. Thorac. Cardiovasc. Surg., 94:75, 1987.

Senning, A.: Surgical correction of transposition of the great vessels. Surgery, 45:966, 1959.

Stark, J.: Current operative approach to transposition of the great arteries with left ventricular outflow tract obstruction. *In* Moulton, A. L. (ed): Congenital Heart Surgery: Current Techniques and Controversies. Pasadena, Appleton Davies, 1984, p. 47.

Stark, J., de Leval, M. R., Waterston, D. J., et al.: Corrective surgery of transposition of the great arteries in the first year of life:

Results in 63 infants. J. Thorac. Cardiovasc. Surg., *67*:673, 1974.

Turley, K., and Ebert, P. A.: Transposition of the great arteries in the neonate: Failed balloon atrial septostomy. J. Cardiovasc. Surg., *26*:564, 1985.

# ■ III Anatomic Correction of Transposition of the Great Arteries at the Arterial Level

Roberto M. Di Donato and Aldo R. Castañeda

The term *anatomic* correction of *transposition of the great arteries* (TGA) applies to all repairs connecting the right ventricle (RV) with the pulmonary artery and the left ventricle (LV) with the aorta. This can be accomplished at the ventricular level (Lecompte et al., 1981; McGoon, 1972; Rastelli et al., 1969) or at the arterial level, either with coronary transfer (Jatene et al., 1975) or without coronary transfer (Aubert et al., 1978; Damus, 1975; Kaye, 1975; Stansel, 1975). This chapter part reviews the procedure that is now called the *arterial switch operation* (ASO)—that is, anatomic repair of TGA at the arterial level with coronary transfer.

## HISTORICAL ASPECTS

The ASO, as first attempted in 1954 by Mustard and colleagues, included the use of a monkey lung as an oxygenator and the transfer of only the left coronary artery. None of the patients survived. Before the widespread use of cardiopulmonary bypass, attempts to switch the great arteries without coronary transfer failed, both experimentally (Björk and Boukaert, 1954) and clinically (Bailey et al., 1954; Kay and Cross, 1955).

Despite the impressive results with the atrial inversion operation, or *physiologic* repair (Mustard, 1964; Senning, 1959), a few investigators continued to explore the possibility of switching the great arteries along with the coronary arteries. Senning (1959) reported three patients with TGA treated by a technique involving en-bloc transfer of the pulmonary valve and artery and diversion of the LV to the aorta through a *ventricular septal defect* (VSD). Idriss and colleagues (1961) translocated a segment of ascending aorta, including both coronary arteries, onto the proximal pulmonary artery. Other experimental techniques were reported by Baffes and colleagues (1961) and by Anagnostopoulos (1973).

Jatene and colleagues (1975), in an epic report, described the first successful ASO in a patient with TGA and a large VSD. Many of the technical advances learned from coronary artery bypass and, more important, a clearer understanding of the need for an LV capable of supporting the systemic circulation contributed to the success of this first operation. In fact, this operation was restricted to patients with TGA and VSD, large *patent ductus arteriosus* (PDA), or *left ventricular outflow tract obstruction* (LVOTO) whose left ventricular pressure was at or close to systemic levels after birth.

Because the high early operative mortality rate of the ASO was in part attributed to technical difficulties related to transfer of the coronary arteries, alternative techniques, avoiding mobilization of the coronary arteries, were developed. These techniques included (1) baffling of the coronary arteries to a surgically created aortic-pulmonary window (Aubert et al., 1978), (2) translocation of the entire aortic root including the proximal coronary arteries (Bex et al., 1980), and (3) end-to-side anastomosis of the proximal pulmonary artery to the ascending aorta with placement of a conduit from the RV to the distal pulmonary artery (Damus, 1975; Kaye, 1975; Stansel, 1975). However, the ASO with coronary artery transfer retained its original appeal. Lecompte and colleagues (1981) added an important technical modification by transferring the distal pulmonary artery anterior to the ascending aorta, thus facilitating direct anastomosis of the neopulmonary artery without conduit interposition.

Because approximately 75% of the patients with TGA have an intact ventricular septum (TGA/IVS), the application of the ASO to this largest subset of patients with TGA interested several investigators. In addition to sporadic reports of successful primary ASO in infants (Abe et al., 1978; Mauck et al., 1977), most of the earlier attempts to use this approach failed, primarily because of left ventricular dysfunction. To prepare the LV for systemic pressure work, Yacoub and colleagues (1977) introduced a two-stage approach for TGA-IVS by first banding the main pulmonary artery (with or without systemic-pulmonary shunt) to stimulate the development of left ventricular muscle mass, followed by an ASO several months later. The principle of performing the ASO as a primary repair in neonates with TGA while the LV is still capable of systemic pressure work was successfully introduced at the Children's Hospital in Boston in 1983 (Castañeda et al., 1984). In 1988, in the same institution, the concept of a "rapid two-stage ASO" for TGA-IVS was also introduced; this procedure consists of banding of the pulmonary artery along with a systemic-to-pulmonary shunt in preparation for the ASO, limiting the interval between the first and second operation to an average of 7 days (Jonas et al., 1989).

## REASONS FOR ASO

The fact that the LV and the mitral valve are more suitable than the RV and the tricuspid valve to serve the systemic circulation is supported by several anatomic, functional, and clinical considerations.

From an *anatomic-functional* point of view (Van Praagh and Jung, 1991), the LV is the ancient "professional" pump with a well-represented stratum compactum, a prevalence of the sinus or pumping portion over the distal infundibular component, and double coronary and conduction tissue systems. Because of its cylindrical shape, its concentric contraction pattern, and the location of both the inlet and the outlet orifices within its base, the LV appears to be ideally adapted to work as a *pressure pump* (Mayer et al., 1986). By contrast the RV, which is a comparatively recent modification of the bulbus cordis, has a much less well-represented stratum compactum and a more prominent infundibular component, which is better suited to prevent regurgitation than to pump. Furthermore, it is a one-coronary and one-bundle-branch ventricle. Because of its crescent-shaped cavity, its large internal surface area–to-volume ratio, its bellows-like contraction pattern, and its more separated inlet and outlet segments, the RV appears to serve better as a *volume pump*.

The *mitral valve* leaflets seem better designed to occlude a circular systemic atrioventricular orifice than are the *tricuspid valve* leaflets. In addition, the papillary muscles of the LV are large, paired, and well balanced, both arising from the left ventricular free wall. By contrast, the papillary muscles of the RV are comparatively small, numerous, and unbalanced, and they arise from both right ventricular septal and free walls. Hence, dilatation of the RV is more prone to pull the papillary muscles apart, favoring the development or exacerbation of tricuspid regurgitation.

From a *clinical* point of view, the fate of the atrial or "physiologic" type of repairs is of increasing concern. Although the hospital mortality rate of both the Mustard and the Senning operations is extremely low, the long-term outcome of these procedures is affected by several complications, the most important being a high incidence of atrial dysrhythmias (more than 50% by 10 years) (Gewillig et al., 1991; Paul, 1989; Vetter et al., 1987, 1988; Williams et al., 1988), and a less clearly established incidence of late RV (systemic ventricle) dysfunction (approximately 10%) (Graham et al., 1975; Kato et al., 1989; Trowitzsch et al., 1985; Turina et al., 1989; Williams et al., 1988).

Furthermore, in patients with isolated congenitally corrected TGA, a progressive deterioration of the right (systemic) ventricular function, affecting long-term survival, has been suggested by clinical (Masden and Franch, 1980) and functional studies (Graham et al., 1983; Peterson et al., 1988).

The ASO recruits the LV as the systemic pump, and because atrial manipulation is essentially limited to closure of an atrial communication, it was anticipated and has already been partly demonstrated that atrial dysrhythmias are significantly reduced after the ASO.

## ANATOMIC CLUES AND PREOPERATIVE DIAGNOSIS

Anatomic features of TGA and its associated cardiovascular defects are described in the first part of this chapter. Diagnostic clues relevant to an ASO are coronary arterial anatomy, position of great arteries, and presence of associated defects (e.g., VSD, left and/or right ventricular outflow tract obstruction [LVOTO, RVOTO], aortic arch obstruction, and atrioventricular valve anomalies) (Fig. 43–33).

Currently, two-dimensional echocardiography provides sufficient anatomic and physiologic information for an ASO in cases of TGA. In particular, two-dimensional echocardiography appears extremely accurate in outlining the origin and the epicardial course of the coronary arteries, including the less-common variants of distribution patterns (Pasquini et al., 1987) (Fig. 43–34). In addition, intramural coronary arteries, present in approximately 5% of cases (Mayer et al., 1990), also appear to be more accurately defined by two-dimensional echocardiography (Pasquini et al., 1993a) than by aortic root injections (Mandell et al., 1990; Vairo et al., 1991). Intramural coronary arteries are characterized by juxtacommissural ostia, acute angulation at the origin, and lack of adventitial separation between ascending aorta and proximal coronary arterial segment (Gittenberger-de Groot et al., 1986). A typical two-dimensional echocardiographic finding is detection of a coronary artery coursing between the arterial roots within the posterior aortic wall, creating a "double border" appearance (Pasquini et al., 1993a). Cardiac catheterization is now mainly used to assess left ventricular suitability for systemic work in patients with TGA/IVS requiring surgery beyond the neonatal period.

## INDICATIONS AND TIMING FOR ASO

Proper timing for ASO varies with the type of TGA. The management of TGA/IVS is concerned with the

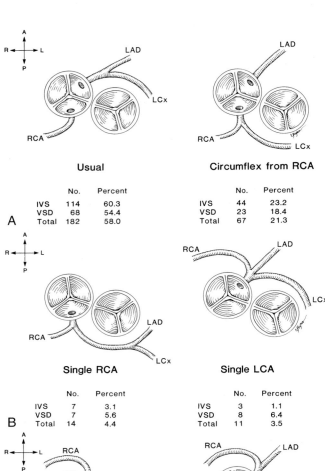

**Usual**

|  | No. | Percent |
|---|---|---|
| IVS | 114 | 60.3 |
| VSD | 68 | 54.4 |
| Total | 182 | 58.0 |

A

**Circumflex from RCA**

|  | No. | Percent |
|---|---|---|
| IVS | 44 | 23.2 |
| VSD | 23 | 18.4 |
| Total | 67 | 21.3 |

**Single RCA**

|  | No. | Percent |
|---|---|---|
| IVS | 7 | 3.1 |
| VSD | 7 | 5.6 |
| Total | 14 | 4.4 |

B

**Single LCA**

|  | No. | Percent |
|---|---|---|
| IVS | 3 | 1.1 |
| VSD | 8 | 6.4 |
| Total | 11 | 3.5 |

**Inverted Coronaries**

|  | No. | Percent |
|---|---|---|
| IVS | 2 | 1.1 |
| VSD | 8 | 6.4 |
| Total | 10 | 3.2 |

C

**Inverted Circumflex and RCA**

|  | No. | Percent |
|---|---|---|
| IVS | 7 | 3.7 |
| VSD | 8 | 6.4 |
| Total | 15 | 4.8 |

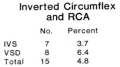

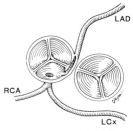

**Intramural LCA**

|  | No. | Percent |
|---|---|---|
| IVS | 11 | 5.8 |
| VSD | 3 | 2.4 |
| Total | 14 | 4.4 |

D

**Intramural LAD**

|  | No. | Percent |
|---|---|---|
| IVS | 1 | 0.5 |
| VSD | 0 | 0 |
| Total | 1 | 0.3 |

**FIGURE 43–33.** Coronary Arterial Anatomy. At the Boston Children's Hospital, a descriptive terminology is used. The six most common types of coronary anatomy in transposition of the great arteries (TGA) and two examples of intramural coronary arteries are shown in parts *A* through *D*. Incidence: *usual coronary anatomy*, about 60%; *left circumflex (LCx) from right coronary artery (RCA)*, about 20%; *single RCA*, about 4%; *single left coronary artery (LCA)*, about 3%; *other types*, about 13%. In TGA/IVS, the coronary arteries tend to be of the more common varieties compared with TGA/VSD. (LAD = left anterior descending coronary artery; IVS = intact ventricular septum; VSD = ventricular septal defect.) (*A–D,* From Mayer, J. E., Jr., Sanders, S. P., Jonas, R. A., et al.: Coronary artery pattern and outcome of arterial switch operation for transposition of the great arteries. Circulation, *82*IV:139, 1990.)

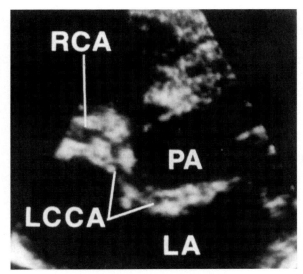

FIGURE 43–34. Two-dimensional echocardiogram of a newborn with TGA. Parasternal short-axis view showing the left circumflex coronary artery (LCCA) originating from the right coronary artery (RCA) and passing leftward posterior to the pulmonary artery (PA) root to reach the base of the left atrium (LA). (From Pasquini, L., Sanders, S. P., Parness, I. A., and Colan, S. D.: Diagnosis of coronary artery anatomy by two-dimensional echocardiography in patients with transposition of the great arteries. Circulation, 75:557, 1987.)

issue of suitability of the LV for systemic work, whereas the management of TGA/VSD mainly deals with the problem of accelerated *pulmonary vascular obstructive disease* (PVOD). Other conditions, such as combined LVOTO or a large PDA, further compound the pathophysiologic arrangement.

## Suitability of the LV for ASO

Most anatomic and functional features of a ventricle depend on the following three factors: (1) type of hemodynamic load (pressure versus volume load) to which the ventricle is subjected (Hood et al., 1968; Van Doesburg et al., 1983), (2) degree of ventricular wall stress (Gaasch, 1979), and (3) age at which the hemodynamic load is imposed (fetal/neonatal vs. later in life) (Di Donato et al., 1992). As a general rule, only a pressure overload can elicit ventricular hypertrophy. When applied in neonatal hearts, this pressure-induced myocardial hypertrophy is characterized by myocyte hyperplasia and hypertrophy and by capillary proliferation. In older hearts, a pressure overload induces only myocyte hypertrophy without hyperplasia and no capillary proliferation (Fig. 43–35).

In TGA, the LV works under different hemodynamic conditions, depending on the presence of a VSD or LVOTO, and its anatomic and functional features vary accordingly. In TGA/IVS, the pathophysiology is mostly that of a volume overload placed on the LV; in TGA with VSD or large PDA, there is both left ventricular volume and pressure overload; and in TGA/LVOTO with or without a VSD, there is predominantly left ventricular pressure overload

(Danford et al., 1985). In TGA/IVS, the left ventricular wall thickness is normal at birth. However, the rapidly decreasing pulmonary vascular resistance causes a drop of peak left ventricular pressure and, hence, decreased development of left ventricular muscle mass (Baño-Rodrigo et al., 1980; Danford, 1985; Huhta et al., 1982; Maroto et al., 1983). By 1 month of age, many patients with TGA/IVS have a peak left ventricular/right ventricular pressure ratio equal to or less than 65%. The leftward displacement of the ventricular septum, secondary to the transseptal pressure difference, causes a crescent-shaped transverse configuration of the left ventricular cavity and may also cause dynamic LVOTO (Chiu et al., 1984; Van Doesburg et al., 1983). Furthermore, increased left ventricular volume load due to augmented pulmonary blood flow leads to progressive left ventricular dilatation (Smith, 1982). Therefore, the general policy in cases of TGA/IVS is to perform the ASO during the neonatal period (within the first 2 to 3 weeks of life), when the LV is still "prepared" to support the systemic circulation by the intrauterine physiology. Because this is not always practically possible, we have developed some criteria for predicting postoperative left ventricular performance similar to those elaborated by Yasui and associates (1989). Before 2 weeks of age, all patients with TGA/IVS are repaired regardless of preoperative left ventricular pressure measurements. After this age, we have arbitrarily chosen a left ventricular/right ventricular pressure ratio of 0.6 as the lowest limit of acceptable left ventricular pressure. Two-dimensional echocardiographic indices of LV suitable for ASO include ventricular septal position, degree of left ventricular wall thickness, left ventricu-

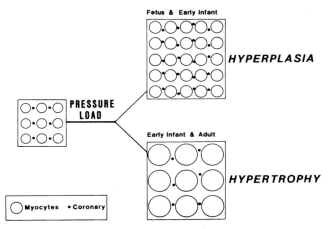

FIGURE 43–35. Age-dependent ventricular response to pressure overload. Cross-sectional schema of a fragment of ventricular myocardium before *(left quadrant)* and after (two *right quadrants)* imposition of a pressure overload. In the neonate or in early infancy *(upper right quadrant),* the increase in myocardial mass (myocardial hypertrophy) is due to myocyte hyperplasia plus moderate hypertrophy and is characterized by increased angiogenesis. In late infancy or adulthood *(lower right quadrant),* myocardial hypertrophy is due only to massive myocyte hypertrophy, and there is no capillary proliferation. (From Di Donato, R. M., Fujii, A. M., Jonas, R. A., and Castañeda, A. R.: Age-dependent ventricular response to pressure overload. Considerations for the arterial switch operation. J. Thorac. Cardiovasc. Surg., 104:713, 1992.)

lar volume, and left ventricular muscle mass. If criteria for a "prepared" LV are not fulfilled, we proceed with a *rapid two-stage ASO*. Interestingly, however, Karl and colleagues demonstrated that primary ASO can be safely performed at up to 4 to 8 weeks of age, provided there is intensive perioperative management with the alpha-blocker phenoxybenzamine (unpublished data, 1993).

## PVOD

Patients with TGA typically develop early and rapidly progressive PVOD (Haworth et al., 1987; Newfeld et al., 1979). In the group of infants with TGA/VSD, Heath-Edwards Grade 3 lesions were found in 19% of patients less than 3 months of age, in 24% of those 3 to 11 months of age, and in close to 80% of patients over 1 year of age. In infants with TGA/IVS, Grade 3 lesions occur in less than 1% under 3 months of age and remain below 17% within the first year of life (Clarkson, 1976). Awareness of the accelerated PVOD in TGA is essential because of the unreliability of pulmonary blood flow and pulmonary vascular resistance calculations in this disease. Therefore, in patients with TGA-VSD or TGA and a large PDA, we also recommend closure of the VSD or PDA and an ASO within the first month of life (Di Donato et al., 1989).

## PDA

Ductal patency is essential to keep adequate oxygenation in the first few days of life. Occasionally, a large PDA may cause a low cardiac output syndrome and pulmonary edema. In these cases, the ASO should be accomplished as soon as possible unless the patient is significantly premature, in which case an emergency PDA ligation may prove the safest course.

## PREOPERATIVE MANAGEMENT

Only in critically ill neonates is preoperative *balloon atrial septostomy* (BAS) indicated (Baylen et al., 1992), and often it can be accomplished at the patient's bedside under two-dimensional echocardiographic guidance (Ward et al., 1992). When severe hypoxia and/or metabolic acidosis are present, prostaglandin $E_1$ may be added to maintain ductal patency and improve oxygenation (Lang et al., 1979). In occasional newborns with TGA, persistence of a fetal pattern of pulmonary circulation imposes an increased therapeutic challenge (Chang et al., 1991).

## OPERATIVE TECHNIQUE

### Surgical Approach

The operation is performed through a midline sternotomy. A segment of pericardium is harvested and prepared with 0.6% glutaraldehyde solution. The ascending aorta and main pulmonary artery are then dissected free. After heparinization (2 mg/kg body weight), the aorta is cannulated as far distally as possible to allow adequate length for the aortic anastomosis. A single venous cannula is inserted through the right atrial appendage, and core cooling to profound hypothermia is initiated. During the cooling period, the ductus arteriosus is divided. Both pulmonary arteries are dissected peripherally until the first pulmonary artery branches become visible. This maneuver allows eventual anastomosis of the pulmonary artery under no or minimal tension (Fig. 43–36A). At 18° C rectal temperature, the distal ascending aorta is clamped, and cold cardioplegic solution is instilled into the aortic root. Additional doses of cardioplegia may be provided by retrograde infusion (Yonenaga et al., 1990). Most often, in cases of TGA/IVS, continuous deep hypothermic perfusion at low flows (20 to 50 ml/kg/min) is used, limiting the period of circulatory arrest to the closure of the atrial communication. In the presence of a VSD or of an aortic arch obstruction, deep hypothermic circulatory arrest is preferentially used, sometimes alternated with a period of 10 to 15 minutes of hypothermic reperfusion.

The aorta is transected approximately 1 cm distal to the origin of the coronary arteries. The coronary ostia are inspected from within and gently probed to identify anomalies of origin and branching. The pulmonary artery is then divided proximal to its bifurcation, and the native pulmonary valve is carefully explored (Fig. 43–36B).

---

FIGURE 43–36. Surgical technique of arterial switch operation (ASO) as seen by the surgeon. *A*, After instituting cardiopulmonary bypass, the ductus arteriosus is divided between suture ligatures, and the branch pulmonary arteries are thoroughly dissected. The *broken lines* represent the levels of transection of the aorta and the main pulmonary artery. Marking sutures are placed in the predicted sites of the coronary anastomoses. The *inset* shows the details of ductal division. *B*, Transection of the great arteries. Retraction sutures are placed at the level of the pulmonary valve commissures. *C*, The coronary arterial flaps are excised from the free edge of the aorta to the base of the sinus of Valsalva. The *insets* show details of the coronary flap excision in the tangential *(above)* and frontal *(below)* views. *D*, The coronary arterial flaps are anastomosed to V-shaped excisions made in the pulmonary (neoaortic) wall. *E*, The pulmonary artery is brought anterior to the aorta (Lecompte's maneuver). Anastomosis of the proximal neoaorta to the distal aorta is shown. *F*, Filling of the coronary donor sites with a single, long, inverted bifurcated pericardial patch. *G*, Anastomosis of the proximal neopulmonary artery and the distal pulmonary artery.

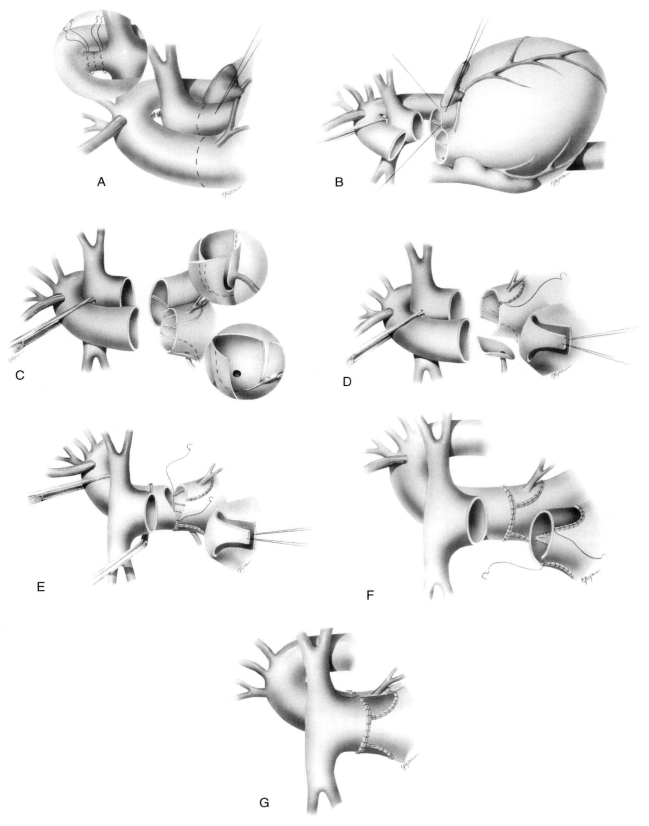

**FIGURE 43–36** *See legend on opposite page*

## Coronary Transfer

The left and right coronary ostia are then explanted along with a generous portion of surrounding aortic wall. Only minimal dissection of the proximal segment of the coronary arteries is necessary, and rarely it may be necessary to sacrifice small conal branches as they are encountered (Fig. 43–36C). An equivalent V-shaped excision of the pulmonary arterial wall is excised from both the left and right anterior sinuses of the neoaorta. The coronary flaps are then sewn into these incisions with continuous 7-0 absorbable or nonabsorbable monofilament sutures (Fig. 43–36D).

Although most coronary arterial patterns in TGA lend themselves to the ASO, there are few instances, particularly when the great arteries are side-by-side, in which the coronary transfer may be at risk for tension, torsion, or kinking. Single right coronary artery and "inverted" coronary artery pattern increase the mortality rate (25%) (Mayer et al., 1990).

When the circumflex coronary artery arises from the right coronary artery, the site of implantation must be kept slightly higher to avoid kinking of the circumflex coronary artery. This often requires adequate mobilization of the right coronary artery. If the two coronary arteries arise from the same sinus, they can often be mobilized in a single bloc, except in the presence of an intramural coronary artery.

If the ostium of an intramural coronary artery is juxtacommissural, excision of the posterior commissure of the native aortic valve may be necessary: the resultant neopulmonary regurgitation is generally mild and well tolerated.

Occasionally, with either single or intramural coronary arteries, the aortocoronary flap is left in situ after excision from the proximal aorta. The cephalad border of the flap is sutured to an abutting incision in the anterior wall of the proximal neoaorta, and a glutaraldehyde-tanned pericardial patch is sutured to the remaining caudal free edge of the flap and to the opening made within the distal ascending aorta, a technique also adopted by Day and associates (1992) (Fig. 43–37). Sometimes, the coronary-neoaortic anastomosis requires interposition of a segment of pericardium to avoid kinking. In other cases, especially in the presence of bilateral intramural coronary arteries with a common ostium, an Aubert operation (1978) or one of its modifications (Moat et al., 1992; Takeuchi and Katogi, 1990) may be considered. A Damus-Stansel-Kaye operation (di Carlo et al., 1991) or an internal mammary artery graft can also be used in these patients (Rheuban et al., 1990). Alternatively, a diversion to an atrial switch repair may be considered.

## Reconstruction of the Great Arteries

The distal pulmonary artery is usually brought anterior to the aorta (*Lecompte's maneuver*). However, with side-by-side great arteries or the more rare posterior aorta, a Lecompte maneuver is not usually per-

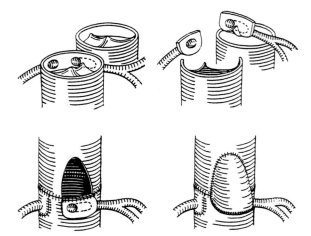

**FIGURE 43–37.** Technique for reimplantation of an intramural coronary segment between the great arteries. *Top left,* Surgical anatomy of a typical intramural left coronary artery. *Top right,* Separate coronary buttons may be excised when distance between the left and the right ostia is adequate. The entire intramural segment and the superior portion of the aortic valve commissure are included in the large coronary button. *Bottom left,* The button of the intramural segment is left facing anteriorly, and the superior margin is sewn to the native pulmonary trunk to avoid potential torsion or kinking of proximal coronary branches. The anastomosis of the ascending aorta and the pulmonary trunk is performed with an aortic window adjacent to the intramural button. *Bottom right,* A pericardial patch is then sewn from the aortic window to the lateral and inferior margins of the button to complete the conduit. (From Day, R. W., Laks, H., and Drinkwater, D. C.: The influence of coronary anatomy on the arterial switch operation in neonates. J. Thorac. Cardiovasc. Surg., *104*:706, 1992.)

formed, and the central stoma in the transverse pulmonary artery is moved to the right pulmonary artery. The distal aorta is anastomosed to the proximal neoaorta with 6-0 continuous absorbable monofilament suture (polydioxanone [PDS]). Portions of the aortic flaps are incorporated into this anastomosis to compensate for discrepancies in size (Fig. 43–36E). The right atrial communication is then closed through a right atriotomy. After closure of the right atriotomy, the venous cannula is reinserted and cardiopulmonary bypass is restarted. The aortic cross-clamp can be removed at this point, provided the left side of the heart is fully vented through a stab incision in the ascending aorta.

The coronary donor sites in the neopulmonary artery can be filled with either two separate patches of glutaraldehyde-pretreated autologous pericardium or, as currently preferred, with a single, long, inverted bifurcated patch. An incision is made into this pericardial patch to fit into the posterior commissure (Fig. 43–36F). Finally, the distal pulmonary artery is sewn to the proximal neopulmonary artery. Discrepancies in caliber of the two ends of the neopulmonary artery are easily reconciled with the pericardial addition (Fig. 43–36G).

## Completion of the Operation

Rewarming, usually started when the aortic clamp is released, is completed on bypass to a rectal temperature of 36° C. Weaning from cardiopulmonary by-pass relies on close monitoring of heart rate and left atrial pressure. The systemic blood pressure is maintained at about 60 mm Hg, adding calcium and inotropic agents, usually dopamine, if necessary. Abnormalities of cardiac rhythm or of myocardial performance suggest a coronary perfusion problem that, once identified, requires aggressive treatment (Quaegebeur et al., 1991). In approximately 5 to 6% of patients, marked myocardial edema imposes secondary closure of the sternotomy, preceded by temporary coverage with a silastic sheet sutured to the skin edges for a median of 4 days postoperatively.

## Additional Surgical Problems

### VSD Closure

A VSD is present in about 25% of patients with TGA. All of the possible different locations of VSD have been encountered in TGA: perimembranous with or without malalignment, muscular subaortic, subarterial, atrioventricular canal type, and multiple (Hoyer et al., 1992).

Usually the VSD is closed through the right atrium. Some of the perimembranous or malalignment defects, especially if associated with multiple muscular defects, can also be closed through the neopulmonary (anterior semilunar) valve or by a combined trans-atrial and transneoaortic (posterior semilunar) valvar approach (Di Donato et al., 1989). Approach through a right ventriculotomy may be necessary in patients with right ventricular infundibular hypoplasia and a VSD (often associated with aortic arch obstruction). All large defects are closed with a patch. Apical muscular defects are preferably closed with a clamshell device applied either in the catheterization laboratory or in the operating room under direct vision (Bridges et al., 1991). In patients with established PVOD, a so called *palliative ASO* (i.e., without VSD closure) may be performed (Pridjian et al., 1992).

### Posterior Aorta

This variant of TGA, first recognized by Van Praagh and colleagues in 1971, is present in 3 to 4% of cases of TGA/VSD (Pasquini et al., 1993b). Tam and associates (1990) demonstrated that this anatomic arrangement does not preclude coronary transfer or an adequate pulmonary arterial reconstruction.

### Management of Atrioventricular Valve Anomalies

Important abnormalities of the tricuspid or mitral valve are rare and include anomalous chordal attachments, overriding annulus, and straddling tensor apparatus (Deal et al., 1985; Huhta, 1982). Neither straddling of an atrioventricular valve (if not associated with hypoplasia of the respective ventricle) (Wernovsky, 1990) nor complete atrioventricular canal

(Kumar et al., 1992) precludes a successful ASO. Preoperative tricuspid regurgitation is a strong indication for an ASO rather than a physiologic repair.

### Management of LVOTO

LVOTO is present in approximately 20% of TGA/IVS and 30 to 35% of TGA/VSD cases. No surgery on the left ventricular outflow tract is indicated in cases of "dynamic" subpulmonary (neoaortic) obstruction (Chiu et al., 1984). In all cases of anatomic LVOTO, the transpulmonary approach allows easy and safe resection of not only a discrete subpulmonary membrane or endocardial cushion excrescence but often also of a posteriorly deviated infundibular septum in cases of tunnel subpulmonary obstruction (Wernovsky et al., 1990).

### Aortic Arch Repair

Aortic coarctation or even aortic arch interruption is found in about 5% of patients with TGA/VSD. We currently prefer to treat the arch obstruction during the ASO, an approach shared by many others (Karl et al., 1992; Pigott et al., 1987; Planché et al., 1993). Notably, subaortic obstruction often co-exists (Akiba et al., 1993; Moene et al., 1985; Schneeweiss et al., 1981), and liberal use of a patch on the right ventricular outflow tract is recommended in these patients (Fig. 43–38). Alternatively, a Damus-Stansel-Kaye approach may be considered.

## TWO–STAGE ASO

In a *two-stage ASO*, repair is performed after a preliminary procedure to "prepare" the LV—that is, a pulmonary artery banding with or without a combined systemic-pulmonary shunt (Yacoub et al., 1977). Experimentally, LV preparation by placement of an adjustable balloon catheter in the main pulmonary artery has also been achieved (Bonhoeffer et al., 1992). Current indications for this staged approach are limited (1) to cases of TGA/IVS presenting beyond the first month of age, with a left ventricular/right ventricular pressure ratio of less than 0.6, and (2) to instances of right ventricular failure occurring late after an atrial inversion operation.

## Rapid Two-Stage ASO

Recent laboratory studies have demonstrated surprisingly rapid induction (within 48 hours) of the genes responsible for the isozyme adaptation response of rat myocardial myosin, actin, and tropomyosin to an acute pressure load. Furthermore, various proto-oncogenes involved in cell growth regulation accumulate in rat cardiac cells within 1 hour of an acute pressure load. Stress protein (HSP-70) is also seen in high levels within 2 to 3 hours of an acute pressure load (Izumo et al., 1988). We have developed

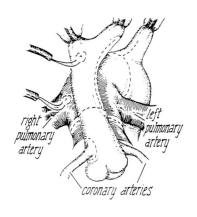

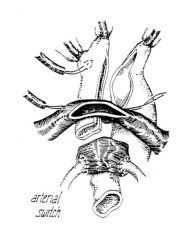

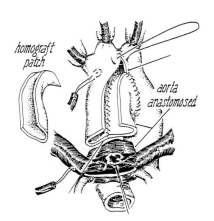

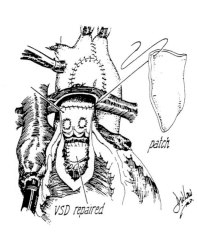

**FIGURE 43–38.** Technique of combined ASO, ventricular septal defect (VSD) closure and interrupted aortic arch repair. The ASO is performed in the usual fashion, the VSD is patch-closed through a right infundibulotomy, and the interrupted aortic arch is repaired with patch augmentation of the inner curvature. Because of the frequent native subaortic stenosis and infundibular narrowing, the infundibulotomy is often extended across the annulus of the neopulmonary valve, and the right ventricular outflow tract is reconstructed with a transannular patch. (From Edmunds, L. H., Norwood, W. I., and Low, D. W.: Atlas of Cardiothoracic Surgery. Philadelphia, Lea & Febiger, 1990, p. 155.)

and successfully performed an ASO consistent with these laboratory findings an average of 7 days after pulmonary artery banding in over 30 patients (Jonas et al., 1989). The most common indications for this approach were late referral from a geographically distant center and elective postponement of ASO (e.g., in premature patients or in neonates with multiorgan failure).

Technically, the *first stage* is accomplished either through a right-sided thoracotomy or a midline sternotomy. A modified right Blalock-Taussig shunt is placed, using a 3.5- or 4-mm polytetrafluoroethylene (PTFE) graft, and then a silastic band is tightened around the main pulmonary artery to achieve a left ventricular pressure that is approximately 75% of systemic pressure. The pericardium is irrigated with heparinized saline before being loosely reapproximated. During the *interval period*, serial two-dimensional echocardiographic examinations are used to monitor changes in left ventricular mass, volume, and ejection fraction; in most patients, a cardiac catheterization is also performed to assess the left ventricular/right ventricular pressure ratio. At the *second stage*, adhesions do not usually present a problem. The shunt and the pulmonary band are taken down, and the ASO is performed.

## Two-Stage ASO for Late Right Ventricular Failure after Atrial Inversion Operation

The possibility of "retraining" the LV by placing a pulmonary artery banding in patients in whom severe right ventricular dysfunction has developed late after a Mustard or Senning operation was first described by Mee in 1986. At the Boston Children's Hospital, this approach has been applied in about 50% of these patients; the remaining patients, characterized by biventricular failure, have been treated with cardiac transplantation (Chang et al., 1992). Interestingly, a two-stage ASO in this condition does not require the addition of a systemic-pulmonary shunt because of the physiologically corrected (in series) circulations. However, because of the greater age at which the pressure load is imposed on the LV, the myocardial response is limited to myocyte hypertrophy without increased angiogenesis, causing reduced functionl reserve (Di Donato et al., 1992) (see Fig. 43–33), and the optimal interval before ASO is less predictable (Chang et al., 1992).

## POSTOPERATIVE MANAGEMENT

Postoperative management after a primary ASO is similar to that following repair of complex cardiac lesions. Mechanical ventilation, sedation, and moderate inotropic support are provided during the first 24 to 48 hours or until hemodynamic stability is achieved.

With rapid two-stage ASO, the initial postoperative period after pulmonary artery banding is frequently complicated by low cardiac output syndrome, requiring prolonged mechanical ventilation and intensive inotropic support (Wernovsky et al., 1992). Cardiac dysfunction in these patients is probably sustained by a combination of acute (fixed) right ventricular volume overload from the shunt and acute (transient) left ventricular pressure overload from the band.

## RESULTS

Of the 500 patients who underwent ASO at the Boston Children's Hospital for TGA from January 1983 through December 1992, 294 (58.8%) had TGA/IVS and 206 (41.2%) had TGA/VSD, including 14 patients with double-outlet RV and subpulmonary VSD. In the TGA/IVS group, 30 patients (9.6%) underwent rapid two-stage ASO. In the TGA/VSD group, 150 patients (74.5%) underwent primary ASOs. Of the 45 patients with an aortic arch obstruction, 30 received the arch repair before the ASO, 15 during the ASO.

**Hospital Mortality.** Twenty-six patients died in the hospital following an ASO (5.2%). In the low-risk group (TGA/IVS, TGA with single VSD, normal arch, normal atrioventricular valves, and the two most common coronary artery patterns), the hospital mortality rate was 2.4% (8 of 334) and only 0.5% among the last 208 consecutive patients. Fifteen of the 26 hospital deaths were attributed to coronary artery obstruction.

**Late Mortality.** Among the 474 hospital survivors, there were 10 late deaths (2.1%). Five were related to coronary problems, two to PVOD, one to aspiration, one to residual VSD and aortic regurgitation, and one to severe aortic regurgitation after balloon valvotomy.

**Postoperative Hemodynamic Studies.** Control cardiac catheterization was performed in 244 of the 474 late survivors (51.3%), a mean of 11.9 ± 6.7 months after the ASO.

**Supravalvular Pulmonary Stenosis.** Supravalvular pulmonary stenosis was the most frequent postoperative hemodynamic abnormality. Three mechanisms were identified: (1) tension of the anastomosis with anteroposterior flattening of the main pulmonary artery and its branches, (2) circumferential cicatricial narrowing at the suture line, and (3) isolated branch stenosis. In 22 patients, the gradient exceeded 40 mm Hg at rest and the right ventricular pressure was either systemic or suprasystemic. Reinterventions included balloon angioplasty in 7, patch plasty in 13, and conduit interposition in the remaining 2 patients.

**Semilunar Valve Regurgitation.** Aortic root angiography revealed trivial aortic incompetence in 20% of the patients. Severe aortic incompetence is an occasional finding (Jenkins et al., 1991) and may require aortic valve replacement (Ungerleider et al., 1992).

**Coronary Anastomosis.** Proximal occlusion of the left coronary artery was found in four patients, all of whom were asymptomatic, with normal electrocardiogram tracings, ventricular end-diastolic pressures, ejection fractions, and two-dimensional echocardiographic indices of ventricular function.

**Intracardiac Shunting.** Four patients had residual left-to-right shunt at the ventricular level with a $\dot{Q}_P/\dot{Q}_S$ (pulmonary/systemic flow) ratio greater than 1.5 : 1.0. The residual VSD was closed surgically in two patients and with clamshell device in the other two.

**PVOD.** Five patients who had TGA/VSD had persistent pulmonary hypertension and progression to PVOD. Their age at operation ranged from 6 to 28 months (mean 16 months). Three of these patients had not undergone pulmonary artery banding, and in the other two the banding was ineffective. An additional patient, who had TGA/IVS and a large nonrestrictive PDA, developed PVOD despite an ASO at 7 weeks of age.

**Systemic-to-Pulmonary Collaterals.** Among 119 patients with suitable postoperative angiographic study results, 55 (46%) had significantly enlarged bronchial collateral vessels. Some of these patients presented with cardiomegaly, continuous murmurs, and hemodynamic evidence of left ventricular volume overload. Five patients were managed by coil embolization of the enlarged collateral vessels. This finding remains unexplained.

**Echocardiographic Examination.** Patients evaluated as late as 4 years after repair were found to have normal regional wall motion with no evidence of regional dysfunction. Ventricular size, wall thickness, systolic function, afterload, preload, contractility, and early diastolic function were also normal (Colan et al., 1988).

**Arrhythmias and Conduction Disturbances.** Sinus rhythm was present in 98% of patients on the most recent electrocardiograms or Holter records. Electrophysiologic studies of 114 patients revealed normal sinus node recovery times in 96%. The A-H and H-V intervals and atrioventricular node response to rapid atrial pacing were also normal in all patients. Five patients with TGA/VSD had permanent postoperative complete heart block (2.5%).

**Results of the Rapid Two-Stage ASO.** Among the 31 patients undergoing a preparatory procedure, one died of associated severe stenosis of the left pulmonary veins. One other child required emergency takedown of the pulmonary band and the shunt (which were replaced within days).

Twenty-four of 28 patients required intensive inotropic support. The echocardiographically determined left ventricular ejection fraction before the preparatory procedure averaged 77 ± 11%, decreased to 55 ± 19% on the first postoperative day, to again increase to 73 ± 14% prior to the ASO. The left ventricular mass index increased from a pre-preparatory 46 ± 17 g/m² (range 24 to 87) to 72 ± 23 g/m² (range 36 to 122) prior to the ASO ($p < .001$). Cardiac catheterization performed at a median of 6 days after pulmonary artery banding and shunting revealed a mean left ventricular/right ventricular ratio of 98 ± 19%, compared with values of 48 ± 8% before the pulmonary artery banding (Jonas et al., 1989; Takahashi et al., 1991).

Two of the 28 patients who received secondary ASO died, one of aortic thrombosis and one of severe pneumonia. In all other children, the second-stage ASO was well tolerated, the mean hospital stay after the operation being 12 ± 5 days.

## SUMMARY

Until today, it has been premature to establish a definitive superiority of the ASO over the atrial inversion operation for the treatment of TGA (Castañeda et al., 1989). Although the different lengths of the respective follow-ups do not allow adequate comparison, it seems that the hazard function for death in the long run favors the ASO (Castañeda et al., 1988; Norwood et al., 1988; Trusler et al., 1987). The ASO presents a single phase of rapidly declining risk approaching zero by 12 months after surgery, whereas the atrial repair, in addition to an early phase of declining risk, shows a constant hazard phase extending indefinitely. This difference becomes even more striking if one compares the hazard function per death in a protocol of routine early ASO versus a protocol of initial BAS and atrial inversion operation at 2 months (Quaegebeur et al., 1986).

According to the most recent report of a multicenter analysis, the 1-month, 1-year, and 5-year survival rates after ASO in patients less than 15 days of age are 84%, 82%, and 82%, respectively. Certain coronary artery patterns, presence of multiple VSDs, and certain institutions were proven to be risk factors for death (Kirklin et al., 1992).

The early and intermediate results of ASO have been progressively improving and, currently, an optimal midterm outcome is achievable in many centers (Lupinetti et al., 1992; Serraf et al., 1991; Yamaguchi et al., 1990). This reflects technical improvement (e.g., for coronary anastomoses) and better timing (e.g., for prevention of PVOD). We are encouraged by the favorable intermediate echocardiographic and hemodynamic results of left ventricular function and by the electrocardiographic and electrophysiologic data showing a 98% incidence of regular sinus mechanism 55 months after the ASO in patients with TGA/IVS (Wernovsky et al., 1988, 1989). However, the potential hazard of late coronary insufficiency (Mayer et al., 1990) and aortic valve (anatomic pulmonary valve) dysfunction (Jenkins et al., 1991) demand continued monitoring of these patients.

## SELECTED BIBLIOGRAPHY

Di Donato, R. M., Fujii, A. M., Jonas, R. A., and Castañeda, A. R.: Age-dependent ventricular response to pressure overload. Considerations for the arterial switch operation. J. Thorac. Cardiovasc. Surg., 104:713, 1992.

This is an extensive review of the experimental literature on the effect of maturation on the development of pressure-overload hypertrophy in nor-mal hearts and in those with TGA. This information supports the current use of primary ASO in neonates with TGA/IVS and of rapid two-stage ASO in infants older than 3 to 4 weeks. It also fosters some concern about the practice of late LV retraining in cases of failed atrial inversion operation.

Jonas, R. A., Giglia, T. M., Sanders, S. P., et al.: Rapid two-stage arterial switch for transposition of the great arteries and intact ventricular septum beyond the neonatal period. Circulation, 80(Suppl. I):203, 1989.

This is the original report on the *rapid two-stage ASO* for infants with TGA/IVS no longer suitable for a primary ASO. Serial two-dimensional echocardiography showed that the left ventricular mass increases by 85% over a median period of 9 days following pulmonary artery banding. Ten of 11 patients underwent successful ASOs, whereas the remaining patient underwent a Senning operation because of a left intramural coronary artery.

Kirklin, J. W., Blackstone, E. H., Tchervenkov, C. I., and Castañeda, A. R.: Clinical outcomes after the arterial switch operation for transposition. Patient, support, procedural, and institutional risk factors. Congenital Heart Surgeons Society. Circulation, 86:1501, 1992.

This is the most recent annual report of an ongoing multi-institutional prospective study on neonates with TGA/IVS or TGA/VSD enrolled for diagnosis and treatment at less than 15 days of age and undergoing an ASO. Good early and midterm clinical results can be achieved with this approach. The outcomes, however, are worse in certain high-risk institutions and in cases of origin of the left main coronary artery or only the left anterior descending or the left circumflex artery from the right posterior sinus.

Planché, C., Serraf, A., Comas, J. V., et al.: Anatomic repair of transposition of great arteries with ventricular septal defect and aortic arch obstruction. One-stage versus two-stage procedure. J. Thorac. Cardiovasc. Surg., 105:925, 1993.

The combination of TGA/VSD and aortic arch obstruction is a challenging therapeutic problem. In a era in which excellent results are achieved with isolated primary ASO in many institutions, this is the most comprehensive report regarding the applicability of ASO in these uncommon and difficult cases.

## BIBLIOGRAPHY

Abe, T., Kuribayashi, R., Sato, M., et al.: Successful Jatene operation for transposition of the great arteries with intact ventricular septum. A case report. J. Thorac. Cardiovasc. Surg., 75:64, 1978.

Akiba, T., Neirotti, R., and Becker, A. E.: Is there an anatomic basis for subvalvular right ventricular outflow tract obstruction after an arterial switch repair for complete transposition? A morphometric study and review. J. Thorac. Cardiovasc. Surg., 105:142, 1993.

Anagnostopoulos, C. E.: A proposed new technique for correction of transposition of the great arteries. Ann. Thorac. Surg., 15:565, 1973.

Aubert, J., Pannetier, A., Couvelly, J. P., et al.: Transposition of the great arteries: New technique for anatomical correction. Br. Heart J., 40:204, 1978.

Baffes, T. G., Ketola, F. H., and Tatooles, T. J.: Transfer of coronary ostia by "triangulation" in transposition of the great vessels and anomalous coronary arteries: A preliminary report. Dis. Chest., 39:648, 1961.

Bailey, C. P., Cookson, B. A., Downing, D. F., and Neptune, W. B.: Cardiac surgery under hypothermia. J. Thorac. Surg., 27:73, 1954.

Bano-Rodrigo, A., Quero-Jimenez, M., Moreno-Granado, F., and Gamallo-Amat, C.: Wall thickness of ventricular chambers in transposition of the great arteries: Surgical implications. J. Thorac. Cardiovasc. Surg., 79:592, 1980.

Baylen, B. G., Grzeszczak, M., Gleason, M. E., et al.: Role of balloon atrial septostomy before early arterial switch repair of transposition of the great arteries. J. Am. Coll. Cardiol., 19:1025, 1992.

Bex, J. P., Lecompte, Y., Baillot, F., and Hazan, E.: Anatomical correction of transposition of the great arteries. Ann. Thorac. Surg., 29:86, 1980.

Björk, V. O., and Bouckaert, L.: Complete transposition of the aorta and the pulmonary artery. J. Thorac. Surg., 28:632, 1954.

Bonhoeffer, P., Carminati, M., Parenzan, L., and Tynan, M.: Nonsurgical left ventricular preparation for arterial switch in transposition of the great arteries [Letter]. Lancet, 340:549, 1992.

Bridges, N. D., Perry, S. B., Keane, J. F., et al.: Preoperative transcatheter closure of congenital muscular ventricular septal defects. N. Engl. J. Med., 324:1312, 1991.

Castañeda, A. R., Mayer, J. E., Jr., Jonas, R. A., et al.: Transposition of the great arteries: The arterial switch operation. Cardiol. Clin., 7:369, 1989.

Castañeda, A. R., Norwood, W. I., Jonas, R. A., et al.: Transposition of the great arteries and intact ventricular septum: Anatomical repair in the neonate. Ann. Thorac. Surg., 38:438, 1984.

Castañeda, A. R., Trusler, G. A., Paul, M. H., et al.: The early results of treatment of simple transposition in the current era. J. Thorac. Cardiovasc. Surg., 95(1):14, 1988.

Chang, A. C., Wernovsky, G., Kulik, T. J., et al.: Management of the neonate with transposition of the great arteries and persistent pulmonary hypertension. Am. J. Cardiol., 68:1253, 1991.

Chang, A. C., Wernovsky, G., Wessel, D. L., et al.: Surgical management of late right ventricular failure after Mustard or Senning repair. Circulation, 86(Suppl. II):140, 1992.

Chiu, I., Anderson, R. H., Macartney, F. J., et al.: Morphologic features of an intact ventricular septum susceptible to subpulmonary obstruction in complete transposition. Am. J. Cardiol., 53:1633, 1984.

Clarkson, P. M., Neutze, J. M., Wardill, J. C., and Barratt-Boyes, B. G.: The pulmonary vascular bed in patients with complete transposition of the great arteries. Circulation, 53(III):539, 1976.

Colan, S. D., Trowitzsch, E., Wernovsky, G., et al.: Myocardial performance after arterial switch operation for transposition of the great arteries with intact ventricular septum. Circulation, 78:132, 1988.

Damus, P.: [Letter]. Ann. Thorac. Surg., 20:724, 1975.

Danford, D. A., Huhta, J. C., and Gutgesell, H. P.: Left ventricular wall stress and thickness in complete transposition of the great arteries. Implications for surgical intervention. J. Thorac. Cardiovasc. Surg., 89:610, 1985.

Day, R. W., Laks, H., and Drinkwater, D. C.: The influence of coronary anatomy on the arterial switch operation in neonates. J. Thorac. Cardiovasc. Surg., 104:706, 1992.

Deal, B. J., Chin, A. J., Sanders, S. P., et al.: Subxiphoid two-dimensional echocardiographic identification of tricuspid valve abnormalities in transposition of the great arteries with ventricular septal defect. Am. J. Cardiol., 55:1146, 1985.

di Carlo, D., Di Donato, R., Carotti, A., et al.: The Damus-Kaye-Stansel operation in infancy: Critical review. Ann. Thorac. Surg., 52:1148, 1991.

Di Donato, R. M., Wernovsky, G., Walsh, E. P., et al.: Results of the arterial switch operation for transposition of the great arteries with ventricular septal defect. Surgical considerations and midterm follow-up data. Circulation, 80:1689, 1989.

Gaasch, W. H.: Left ventricular radius to wall thickness ratio. Am. J. Cardiol., 43:1189, 1979.

Gewillig, M., Cullen, S., Mertens, B., et al.: Risk factors for arrhythmia and death after Mustard operation for simple transposition of the great arteries. Circulation, 84:187, 1991.

Gittenberger-de Groot, A. C., Sauer, U., and Quaegebeur, J. M.: Aortic intramural coronary artery in three hearts with transposition of the great arteries. J. Thorac. Cardiovasc. Surg., 91:566, 1986.

Graham, J., Atwood, G. F., Boucek, J., et al.: Abnormalities of right ventricular function following Mustard's operation for transposition of the great arteries. Circulation, 52:678, 1975.

Graham, T. P., Jr., Parrish, M. D., Boucek, R. J., Jr., et al.: Assessment of ventricular size and function in congenitally corrected transposition of the great arteries. Am. J. Cardiol., 51:245, 1983.

Haworth, S. G., Radley-Smith, R., and Yacoub, M. H.: Lung biopsy findings in transposition of the great arteries with ventricular septal defect: Potentially reversible pulmonary vascular disease is not always synonymous with operability. J. Am. Coll. Cardiol., 9:327, 1987.

Hood, W. P., Jr., Rackley, C. E., and Rolett, E. L.: Wall stress in the normal and hypertrophied human left ventricle. Am. J. Cardiol., 22:550, 1968.

Hoyer, M. H., Zuberbuhler, J. R., Anderson, R. H., and del Nido, P.: Morphology of ventricular septal defects in complete transposition. Surgical implications. J. Thorac. Cardiovasc. Surg., 104:1203, 1992.

Huhta, J. C., Edwards, W. D., Danielson, G. K., and Feldt, R. H.: Abnormalities of the tricuspid valve in complete transposition of the great arteries with ventricular septal defect. J. Thorac. Cardiovasc. Surg., 83:569, 1982.

Idriss, F. S., Goldstein, I. R., Grana, L., et al.: A new technique for complete correction of transposition of the great vessels: An experimental study with a preliminary clinical report. Circulation, 24:5, 1961.

Izumo, S., Nadal-Ginard, B., and Mahdavi, V.: Protooncogene induction and reprogramming of cardiac gene expression produced by pressure overload. Proc. Natl. Acad. Sci. U. S. A., 85:339, 1988.

Jatene, A. D., Fontes, V. F., Paulista, P. P., et al.: Successful anatomic correction of transposition of the great vessels. A preliminary report. Arg. Braz. Cardiol., 28:461, 1975.

Jenkins, K. J., Hanley, F. L., Colan, S. D., et al.: Function of the anatomic pulmonary valve in the systemic circulation. Circulation, 84(Suppl. III):173, 1991.

Karl, T. R., Sano, S., Brawn, W. J., and Mee, R. B. B.: Repair of hypoplastic or interrupted aortic arch via sternotomy. J. Thorac. Cardiovasc. Surg., 104:688, 1992.

Kato, H., Nakano, S., Matsuda, H., et al.: Right ventricular myocardial function after the atrial switch operation for transposition of the great arteries. Am. J. Cardiol., 63:226, 1989.

Kay, E. B., and Cross, F. S.: Surgical treatment of transposition of the great vessels. Surgery, 39:712, 1955.

Kaye, M. P.: Anatomic correction of transposition of the great arteries. Mayo Clin. Proc., 50:638, 1975.

Kumar, N., Prabhakar, G., Wilson, N., et al.: Total correction of transposition of great arteries with atrioventricular septal defect. Ann. Thorac. Surg., 54:989, 1992.

Lang, P., Freed, M. D., Bierman, F. Z., et al.: Use of prostaglandin E1 in infants with D-transposition of the great arteries and intact ventricular septum. Am. J. Cardiol., 44:76, 1979.

Lecompte, Y., Zannini, L., Hazan, E., et al.: Anatomic correction of transposition of the great arteries: New technique without use of a prosthetic conduit. J. Thorac. Cardiovasc. Surg., 82:629, 1981.

Lupinetti, F. M., Bove, E. L., Minich, L. L., et al.: Intermediate-term survival and functional results after arterial repair for transposition of the great arteries. J. Thorac. Cardiovasc. Surg., 103:421, 1992.

Mandell, V. S., Lock, J. E., Mayer, J. E., et al.: The "laid-back" aortogram: An improved angiographic view for demonstration of coronary arteries in transposition of the great arteries. Am. J. Cardiol., 65:1379, 1990.

Maroto, E., Fouron, J. C., Douste-Blazy, M. Y., et al.: Influence of age on wall thickness, cavity dimensions and myocardial contractility of the left ventricle in simple transposition of the great arteries. Circulation, 67:1311, 1983.

Masden, R. R., and Franch, R. H.: Isolated congenitally corrected transposition of the great arteries. In Hurst, J. W. (ed): The Heart—Update III. New York, McGraw-Hill, 1980, p. 59.

Mauck, H. P., Jr., Robertson, L. W., Parr, E. L., and Lower, R. R.: Anatomic correction of transposition of the great arteries without significant ventricular septal defect or patent ductus arteriosus. J. Thorac. Cardiovasc. Surg., 74:631, 1977.

Mayer, J. E., Jr., Jonas, R. A., and Castañeda, A. R.: Arterial switch operation for transposition of the great arteries with intact ventricular septum. J. Cardiac. Surg., 1(II):97, 1986.

Mayer J. E., Jr., Sanders, S. P., Jonas, R. A., et al.: Coronary artery pattern and outcome of arterial switch operation for transposition of the great arteries. Circulation, 82(IV):139, 1990.

McGoon, D. C.: Intraventricular repair of transposition of the great arteries. J. Thorac. Cardiovasc. Surg., 64:430, 1972.

Mee, R. B. B.: Severe right ventricular failure after Mustard or Senning operation. Two-stage repair: Pulmonary artery banding and switch. J. Thorac. Cardiovasc. Surg., 92:385, 1986.

Moat, N. E., Pawade, A., Lamb, R. K.: Complex coronary arterial anatomy in transposition of the great arteries. Arterial switch procedure without coronary relocation. J. Thorac. Cardiovasc. Surg., 103:872, 1992.

Moene, R. J., Ottenkamp, J., Oppenheimer-Dekker, A., and Bartelings, M. M.: Transposition of the great arteries and narrowing of the aortic arch. Emphasis on right ventricular characteristics. Br. Heart J., 53:58, 1985.

Mustard, W. T., Chute, A. L., Keith, J. D., et al.: A surgical approach to transposition of the great vessels with extracorporeal circuit. Surgery, 36(I):39, 1954.

Mustard, W. T.: Successful two-stage correction of transposition of the great vessels. Surgery, *55*(III):469, 1964.

Newfeld, E. A., Paul, M. H., Muster, A. J., and Idriss, F. S.: Pulmonary vascular disease in transposition of the great vessels and intact ventricular septum. Circulation, *59*(III):525, 1979.

Norwood, W. I., Dobell, A. R., Freed, M. D., et al.: Intermediate results of the arterial switch repair. A 20-institution study. J. Thorac. Cardiovasc. Surg., *96*:854, 1988.

Pasquini, L., Parness, I. A., Colan, S. D., et al.: Echocardiographic diagnosis of intramural coronary artery in transposition of the great arteries [Abstract]. J. Am. Coll. Cardiol., *21*:367A, 1993a.

Pasquini, L., Sanders, S. P., Parness, I. A., and Colan, S. D.: Diagnosis of coronary artery anatomy by two-dimensional echocardiography in patients with transposition of the great arteries. Circulation, *75*(III):557, 1987.

Pasquini, L., Sanders, S. P., Parness, I. A., et al.: Conal anatomy in 119 patients with D-loop transposition of the great arteries and ventricular septal defect: An echocardiographic and pathologic study. J. Am. Coll. Cardiol., *21*:1712, 1993b.

Paul, M. H.: Complete transposition of the great arteries. *In* Adams, F. H., Emmanouilides, G. C., Riemenschneider, T. A. (eds): Heart Disease in Infants, Children and Adolescents. Baltimore, Williams & Wilkins, 1989, p. 371.

Peterson, R. J., Franch, R. H., Fajman, W. A., and Jones, R. H.: Comparison of cardiac function in surgically corrected and congenitally corrected transposition of the great arteries. J. Thorac. Cardiovasc. Surg., *96*:227, 1988.

Pigott, J. D., Chin, A. J., Weinberg, P. M., et al.: Transposition of the great arteries with aortic arch obstruction. Anatomical review and report of surgical management. J. Thorac. Cardiovasc. Surg., *94*:82, 1987.

Pridjian, A. K., Tacy, T. A., Teske, D., and Bove, E. L.: Palliative arterial repair for transposition, ventricular septal defect, and pulmonary vascular disease. Ann. Thorac. Surg., *54*:355, 1992.

Quaegebeur, J. M., Rohmer, J., Ottenkamp, J., et al.: The arterial switch operation: An eight-year experience. J. Thorac. Cardiovasc. Surg., *92*:361, 1986.

Quaegebeur, J., van Daele, M., Stumper, O., and Sutherland, G. R.: Intraoperative ultrasonographic identification of coronary artery compression after an arterial switch procedure. J. Thorac. Cardiovasc. Surg., *102*:837, 1991.

Rastelli, G. C., Wallace, R. B., and Ongley, P. A.: Complete repair of transposition of the great arteries with pulmonary stenosis. A review and report of a case corrected by using a new surgical technique. Circulation, *39*:83, 1969.

Rheuban, K. S., Kron, I. L., and Bulatovic, A.: Internal mammary artery bypass after the arterial switch operation. Ann. Thorac. Surg., *50*:125, 1990.

Schneeweiss, A., Motro, M., Shem-Tov, A., and Neufeld, H. N.: Subaortic stenosis: An unrecognized problem in transposition of the great arteries. Am. J. Cardiol., *48*:336, 1981.

Senning, A.: Surgical correction of transposition of the great vessels. Surgery, *45*(VI):966, 1959.

Serraf, A., Bruniaux, J., Lacour-Gayet, F., et al.: Anatomic correction of transposition of the great arteries with ventricular septal defect. Experience with 118 cases. J. Thorac. Cardiovasc. Surg., *102*:140, 1991.

Stansel, H. C.: A new operation for D-loop transposition of the great vessels. Ann. Thorac. Surg., *19*:565, 1975.

Takahashi, Y., Nakano, S., Shimazaki, Y., et al.: Echocardiographic comparison of postoperative left ventricular contractile state between one- and two-stage arterial switch operation for simple transposition of the great arteries. Circulation, *84*(III):180, 1991.

Takeuchi, S., and Katogi, T.: New technique for the arterial switch operation in difficult situations. Ann. Thorac. Surg., *50*:1000, 1990.

Tam, S., Murphy, J. D., and Norwood, W. I.: Transposition of the great arteries with posterior aorta. Anatomic repair. J. Thorac. Cardiovasc. Surg., *100*:441, 1990.

Trowitzsch, E., Colan, S. D., and Sanders, S. P.: Global and regional right ventricular function in normal infants and infants with transposition of the great arteries after Senning operation. Circulation, *72*(V):1008, 1985.

Trusler, G. A., Castañeda, A. R., Rosenthal, A., et al.: Current results of management in transposition of the great arteries, with special emphasis on patients with associated ventricular septal defect. J. Am. Coll. Cardiol., *10*(V):1061, 1987.

Turina, M. I., Siebenmann, R., von Segesser, L., et al.: Late functional deterioration after atrial correction for transposition of the great arteries. Circulation, *80*(Suppl. I):162, 1989.

Ungerleider, R. M., Gaynor, J. W., Israel, P., et al.: Report of neoaortic valve replacement in a ten-year-old girl after an arterial switch procedure for transposition [Letter]. J. Thorac. Cardiovasc. Surg., *104*:213, 1992.

Vairo, U., Di Donato, R. M., Marino, B., et al.: Balloon occlusion of the ascending aorta for angiographic visualization of the coronary arteries in neonates with transposition of the great arteries. Am. Heart J., *121*:917, 1991.

van Doesburg, N. H., Bierman, F. Z., and Williams, R. G.: Left ventricular geometry in infants with D-transposition of the great arteries and intact ventricular septum. Circulation, *68*:733, 1983.

Van Praagh, R., Perez-Trevino, C., Lopez-Cuellar, M., et al.: Transposition of the great arteries with posterior aorta, anterior pulmonary artery, subpulmonary conus and fibrous continuity between aortic and atrioventricular valves. Am. J. Cardiol., *28*:621, 1971.

Van Praagh, R., and Jung, W. K.: The arterial switch operation in transposition of the great arteries: Anatomic indications and contraindications. Thorac. Cardiovasc. Surg., *39*(Suppl. II):138, 1991.

Vetter, V. L., Tanner, C. S., and Horowitz, L. N.: Electrophysiologic consequences of the Mustard repair of d-transposition of the great arteries. J. Am. Coll. Cardiol., *10*:1265, 1987.

Vetter, V. L., Tanner, C. S., and Horowitz, L. N.: Inducible atrial flutter after the Mustard repair of complete transposition of the great arteries. Am. J. Cardiol., *61*:428, 1988.

Ward, C. J., Hawker, R. E., Cooper, S. G., et al.: Minimally invasive management of transposition of the great arteries in the newborn period. Am. J. Cardiol., *69*:1321, 1992.

Wernovsky, G., Di Donato, R., Lang, P., et al.: Early results of the arterial switch operation in 195 consecutive patients. *In* Crupi, G., Anderson, R. H., Parenzan, L. (eds): Perspectives in Pediatric Cardiology. Pediatric Cardiac Surgery. Vol. 2, Part 2. Mount Kisko, NY, Futura, 1989, p. 20.

Wernovsky, G., Giglia, T. M., Jonas, R. A., et al.: Course in the intensive care unit after "preparatory" pulmonary artery banding and aortopulmonary shunt placement for transposition of the great arteries with low left ventricular pressure. Circulation, *86*(II):133, 1992.

Wernovsky, G., Hougen, T. J., Walsh, E. P., et al.: Midterm results after the arterial switch operation for transposition of the great arteries with intact ventricular septum: Clinical, hemodynamic, echocardiographic and electrophysiologic data. Circulation, *77*:1333, 1988.

Wernovsky, G., Jonas, R. A., Colan, S. D., et al.: Results of the arterial switch operation in patients with transposition of the great arteries and abnormalities of the mitral valve or left ventricular outflow tract. J. Am. Coll. Cardiol., *16*:1446, 1990.

Williams, W. G., Trusler, G. A., Kirklin, J. W., et al.: Early and late results of a protocol for simple transposition leading to an atrial switch (Mustard) repair. J. Thorac. Cardiovasc. Surg., *95*:717, 1988.

Yacoub, M. H., Radley-Smith, R., and MacLaurin, R.: Two-stage operation for anatomical correction of transposition of the great arteries with intact ventricular septum. Lancet, *1*:1275, 1977.

Yamaguchi, M., Hosokawa, Y., Imai, Y., et al.: Early and midterm results of the arterial switch operation for transposition of the great arteries in Japan. J. Thorac. Cardiovasc. Surg., *100*:261, 1990.

Yasui, H., Kado, H., Yonenaga, K., et al.: Arterial switch operation for transposition of the great arteries, with special reference to left ventricular function. J. Thorac. Cardiovasc. Surg., *98*:601, 1989.

Yonenaga, K., Yasui, H., Kado, H., et al.: Myocardial protection by retrograde cardioplegia in arterial switch operation. Ann. Thorac. Surg., *50*:238, 1990.

# 44

# Pulmonary Atresia with Intact Ventricular Septum

Erle H. Austin III

Pulmonary atresia with intact ventricular septum (PA/IVS) is an uncommon cardiac anomaly occurring in less than 1% of infants born with congenital heart disease (Freedom, 1989). This malformation is characterized by a variably sized right ventricle that has no exit, failing to provide pulmonary blood flow and unable to decompress itself through the interventricular septum. Blood flow through the ductus arteriosus permits survival at birth, but within hours, hypoxemia progresses to death as the ductus closes. Thus, without early diagnosis and treatment, PA/IVS is uniformly fatal. Before 1970, reported survival to 3 years of age was less than 3% (Gersony et al., 1967). Improvements in diagnosis and management have increased the 3-year survival rate to greater than 60% (Hanley et al., 1993), but the defect remains lethal for a significant portion of these infants.

Despite much success in the surgical treatment of PA/IVS, uncertainty and controversy exists regarding many details in its management. Because this anomaly is uncommon and its morphology is heterogeneous, reports and recommendations from individual institutions have been based on small series with variable morphologic compositions. Although a great deal has been learned from the experiences of these individual centers (Alboliras et al., 1987; Coles et al., 1989; DeLeval et al., 1985; Hawkins et al., 1990; McCaffrey et al., 1991; Milliken et al., 1985; Pawade et al., 1993; Steinberger et al., 1992), much more is now being derived from a prospective multi-institutional study initiated by the Congenital Heart Surgeons Society in 1987 (Hanley et al., 1993). Data acquired from this study are providing important new insights into the spectrum of morphology as well as the outcome of surgical treatment of this malformation.

## HISTORY

PA/IVS was first described pathologically by John Hunter in 1783, and Novelo and associates, in 1951, were the first to report the clinical diagnosis of this lesion. The broad spectrum of right ventricular morphology was first described by Greenwold and colleagues in 1956. Although the presence of right ventricular sinusoids and right ventricle–to–coronary artery fistulas was described by Grant in 1926, it was not until 1975 that Essed and co-workers recognized that in some cases the coronary circulation is derived

solely from the right ventricle. Although isolated reports of successful surgery appeared as early as 1962 (Benton et al, 1962; Ziegler and Taber, 1962), consistent surgical results did not appear until 1971, when Bowman and colleagues described their experience combining pulmonary valvotomy with the creation of a systemic-to-pulmonary shunt.

## ANATOMY

Characteristically, PA/IVS occurs in hearts with situs solitus and atrioventricular and ventriculoarterial concordance. The essential feature of this lesion is an absent communication between the right ventricle and the pulmonary trunk (Fig. 44–1). The fibrous diaphragm at this junction often exhibits commissural ridges that meet in the center, but this tissue may appear as a smooth membrane. In contrast to pulmonary atresia with ventricular septal defect, the pulmonary trunk and branch pulmonary arteries are near

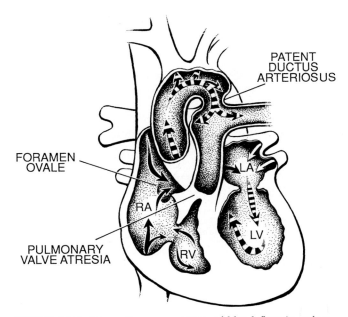

FIGURE 44–1. Schematic representation of blood flow in pulmonary atresia with intact ventricular septum (PA/IVS). An obligatory right-to-left shunt occurs at the atrial level. Peripheral oxygenation is dependent on flow through the ductus arteriosus. (RA = right atrium; RV = right ventricle; LA = left atrium; LV = left ventricle.)

1605

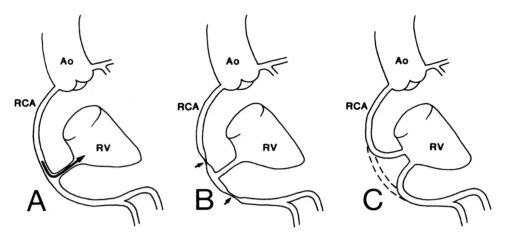

FIGURE 44–2. Right ventricular–coronary artery fistulas in PA/IVS. *A*, Without coronary stenosis: Potential RV "steal" phenomenon. *B*, With proximal or distal coronary stenosis: Potential "steal" or ischemia. *C*, With coronary occlusion/atresia: Potential isolation and myocardial infarction. (RV = right ventricle; RCA = right coronary artery; Ao = aorta.) (*A–C*, From Giglia, T. M., Mandell, S., Connor, A. R., et al.: Diagnosis and management of right ventricle–dependent coronary circulation in pulmonary atresia with intact ventricular septum. Circulation, *86*:1516, 1992.)

normal in size and configuration. The size and morphology of the right ventricle varies significantly in this condition, and in most patients, the right ventricular cavity is reduced in size. There is a continuum from tiny "unipartite" chambers that have only an inlet component to larger than normal "tripartite" ventricles that have well-defined inlet, trabecular, and infundibular portions. The rare patients with enlarged right ventricular cavities often also have Ebstein's anomaly with severe tricuspid regurgitation. Marked hypertrophy of the right ventricular wall is present, often contributing to obliteration of the outflow portion of the cavity. The tricuspid valve is usually small in size with thickened leaflets and abnormal chordae. The diameter of the tricuspid valve correlates with the size of the right ventricular cavity and provides a useful index of right ventricular size. The right atrium is enlarged, and an interatrial communication, usually a patent foramen ovale, is present. At birth, the ductus arteriosus is patent, providing the only blood flow to the lungs. Significant aortopulmonary collateral arteries are uncommon.

An important anatomic feature of PA/IVS is the presence in some patients of connections between the right ventricle and the coronary circulation (Figs. 44–2 and 44–3). Sinusoids or "intermuscular spaces" in the right ventricular myocardium occur in about 50% of

patients (Hanley et al., 1993). In 90% of these patients, the sinusoids communicate with the coronary arteries. The smaller the tricuspid valve (and thus the right ventricular cavity), the more likely that right ventricular–coronary arterial fistulas are present. In 20% of patients with these fistulas, significant proximal coronary artery stenoses exist, making myocardial blood flow dependent on blood from the right ventricle (Hanley et al., 1993). Knowledge of the presence of a right ventricular–dependent coronary circulation is important in deciding on surgical therapy, because in these cases decompression of the right ventricle may cause myocardial ischemia or infarction (Giglia et al., 1992).

## PATHOPHYSIOLOGY

In PA/IVS, desaturated systemic venous blood is obliged to cross the interatrial septum to mix with saturated pulmonary venous blood in the left atrium (see Fig. 44–1). The resultant admixture is ejected into the systemic arterial circulation, and the systemic arterial saturation is dependent on adequate pulmonary blood flow. Closure of the ductus arteriosus soon after birth markedly reduces pulmonary blood flow, and progressive hypoxemia and tissue acidosis leads

■ **Table 44–1.** EFFECT OF DEGREE OF RIGHT VENTRICULAR HYPOPLASIA ON SURGICAL MANAGEMENT OF PULMONARY ATRESIA WITH INTACT VENTRICULAR SEPTUM

| Parameter/Surgical Management | Degree of Right Ventricular Hypoplasia | | |
|---|---|---|---|
| | *Mild* | *Moderate* | *Severe* |
| Tricuspid Z-value | $\geq -2$ | $-2$ to $-4$ | $< -4$ |
| Right ventricular morphology | Tripartite | Bipartite | Unipartite |
| Infundibular cavity | Present | Intermediate | Absent |
| Right ventricular–dependent coronary circulation | Rare | Possible | Common |
| Surgical palliation | Transannular patch ± shunt | Transannular patch + shunt (no right ventricular decompression if right ventricular–dependent coronary circulation) | Shunt only |
| Definitive operation | Two-ventricle repair | Two-ventricle repair; mixed circulations; Fontan if right ventricular–dependent coronary circulation | Fontan |

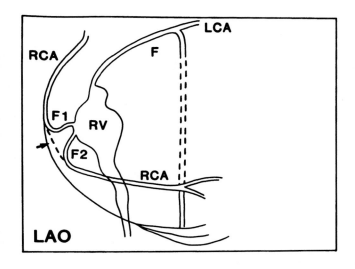

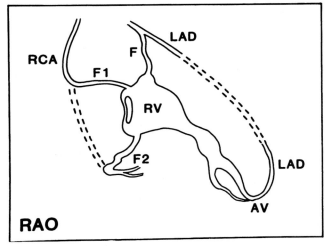

**FIGURE 44–3.** Outlines of right ventricular cine-angiograms in a patient with right ventricular–dependent coronary circulation. (RCA = right coronary artery; LCA = left coronary artery; RV = right ventricle; LAD = left anterior descending artery; RAO = right anterior oblique; LAO = left anterior oblique; AV = apical vessels; F = fistula locations. The *dashed lines* indicate coronary occlusion.) (From Giglia, T. M., Mandell, S., Connor, A. R., et al.: Diagnosis and management of right ventricle–dependent coronary circulation in pulmonary atresia with intact ventricular septum. Circulation, 86:1516, 1992.)

to death. Expeditious administration of prostaglandin E₁ can temporarily reverse ductal closure until a surgical procedure to increase pulmonary blood flow can be performed.

## CLINICAL FEATURES

Infants with PA/IVS are typically full-term, well-developed babies without other anomalies. Delivery is usually uncomplicated, but cyanosis develops on the first day of life and rapidly progresses to respiratory distress and metabolic acidosis. A murmur is unusual unless significant tricuspid regurgitation exists. There is no splitting of the second heart sound. Chest radiography demonstrates clear lung fields

with decreased vascular markings. The electrocardiogram is often normal, although the typical neonatal pattern of right ventricular hypertrophy may be absent. Definitive diagnosis is made using two-dimensional echocardiography, which reveals the right ventricular outflow obstruction and the size of the right ventricle and tricuspid valve, and combined with color-flow Doppler techniques, can identify right ventricular–coronary artery fistulas (Leung et al., 1988; Sanders et al., 1989).

Cardiac catheterization and cineangiography are not required before initial surgical therapy in patients with nearly normal-sized tricuspid valves and tripartite right ventricular chambers. However, these studies are imperative in patients at the other end of the spectrum to identify the presence of a right ventricular–dependent coronary circulation (see Figs. 44–2 and 44–3).

## MANAGEMENT

As soon as the diagnosis of PA/IVS is suspected, an infusion of prostaglandin E₁ is begun. Elective intubation and controlled ventilation may be advisable, especially if the infant is to be transported to a tertiary treatment center, because apnea is a common complication of prostaglandin E₁ infusion.

The surgical management of PA/IVS is best undertaken in two stages, the first for palliation and the second for definitive repair. The approach for each stage must take into account the degree of right ventricular hypoplasia.

In the neonate, it is useful to classify right ventricular hypoplasia into mild, moderate, and severe degrees (Table 44–1). Echocardiographic measurement of the diameter of the tricuspid valve with conversion to a Z-value provides a quantitative measurement to facilitate classification (Kirklin and Barrett-Boyes, 1993) (Fig. 44–4). Patients with mild right ventricular hypoplasia have tricuspid valve Z-values of −2 or greater. Tricuspid Z-values between −4 and −2 indicate moderate right ventricular hypoplasia, and Z-values of −4 or less are seen in patients with severe right ventricular hypoplasia. Tripartite right ventricles with a well-developed right ventricular outflow tract fall into the mild group, whereas unipartite right ventricles without a definable infundibular or trabecular portion are classified as severe (Bull et al., 1982). Patients with mild right ventricular hypoplasia have definite potential for conversion to a two-ventricle system at the time of definitive repair, whereas those with severe right ventricular hypoplasia can only achieve separation of systemic and pulmonary circulations with a one-ventricle repair (a Fontan operation). Patients with moderate right ventricular hypoplasia are also potential candidates for biventricular repair provided they do not have a right ventricular–dependent coronary circulation.

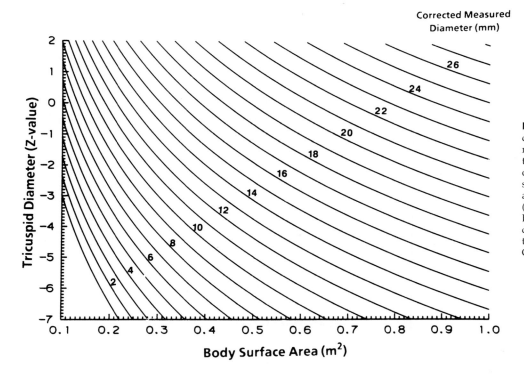

**FIGURE 44–4.** Nomogram for converting echocardiographically measured tricuspid valve diameters to the Z-value. Knowledge of the tricuspid Z-value may help select initial surgical management and predict long-term outcome. (From Hanley, F. L., Sade, R. M., Blackstone, E. H., et al.: Outcomes in neonatal atresia with intact ventricular septum. J. Thorac. Cardiovasc. Surg., *105*:406, 1993.)

## Initial Surgical Management for Neonates with Mild to Moderate Right Ventricular Hypoplasia

To encourage ventricular growth and provide adequate pulmonary blood flow, these infants are best served by relieving the right ventricle–to–pulmonary artery obstruction and creating a systemic-to-pulmonary shunt. This may be accomplished with or without cardiopulmonary bypass. Without bypass, a pulmonary valvotomy can be performed blindly with a transventricular dilator or under direct vision through the main pulmonary artery (Kanter et al., 1987) (Fig. 44–5). A systemic-to-pulmonary artery shunt is performed concomitantly with a 5-mm polytetrafluoroethylene (PTFE) tube graft. The use of cardiopulmonary bypass allows safe access into the right ventricular outflow tract so that obstructing infundibular muscle can be excised and a transannular outflow patch placed (Fig. 44–6). By maximizing unobstructed forward flow, transannular patching provides the greatest possibility for right ventricular growth (Foker et al., 1986; Hanley et al., 1993). Because early postoperative right ventricular failure may cause increased right-to-left shunting across the patent foramen ovale, a systemic-to-pulmonary artery shunt should also be created to prevent life-threatening hypoxia. Initial results from the Congenital Heart Surgeons Society's study suggest that concomitant insertion of a transannular patch and placement of a systemic-to-pulmonary artery shunt is the optimal initial treatment for neonates with tricuspid valve Z-values between −1.5 and −4 (Hanley et al., 1993).

However, any form of right ventricular decompression is contraindicated if a right ventricular–dependent coronary circulation exists. Initial therapy in these patients should be limited to the placement of a systemic-to-pulmonary artery shunt.

## Initial Surgical Management for Neonates with Severe Right Ventricular Hypoplasia and/or Right Ventricular–Dependent Coronary Circulation

As the potential for a definitive two-ventricle repair is low and the risk of a right ventricular outflow procedure is increased in these patients (Fig. 44–7), initial surgical therapy should be limited to a systemic-to-pulmonary artery shunt (Hanley et al., 1993). A 4- or 5-mm PTFE tube graft placed via a right thoracotomy from the right subclavian artery to the right pulmonary artery provides adequate pulmonary blood flow and facilitates shunt access at the time of definitive one-ventricle repair.

## Definitive Surgical Management for Infants with Mild to Moderate Right Ventricular Hypoplasia

Patients with mild to moderate right ventricular hypoplasia should be followed closely after the initial procedure. Those infants treated originally with valvotomy rather than transannular patching are especially vulnerable to residual or recurrent right ventric-

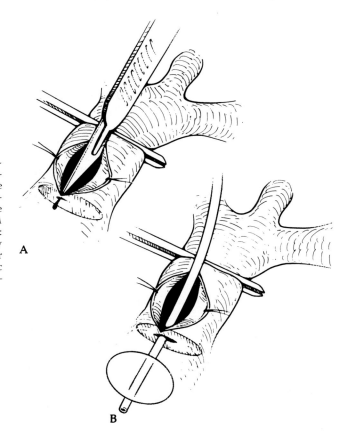

**FIGURE 44–5.** Open pulmonary valvotomy without cardiopulmonary bypass can be performed via median sternotomy or left thoracotomy. *A,* After clamping the pulmonary trunk just proximal to the bifurcation, the pulmonary artery is opened and the atretic pulmonary valve is opened sharply. *B,* A Fogarty catheter positioned in the infundibulum provides hemostasis as the atretic valve is excised. (*A* and *B,* From Kanter, K. R., Pennington, D. G., Nouri, S., et al.: Concomitant valvotomy and subclavian–main pulmonary artery shunt in neonates with pulmonary atresia and intact ventricular septum. Reprinted with permission from the Society of Thoracic Surgeons [The Annals of Thoracic Surgery, 1987, Vol. 43, pp. 490–494].)

ular outflow tract obstruction (Hanley et al., 1993). Follow-up cardiac catheterization should be performed between 6 and 12 months of age. At catheterization, the systemic-to-pulmonary artery shunt is temporarily occluded. If arterial saturations remain high, the atrial septal defect (patent foramen ovale) is occluded as well. If right atrial pressure remains below 15 mm Hg and cardiac output is adequate, the shunt and atrial communication can be closed permanently and a two-ventricle circulation achieved. At

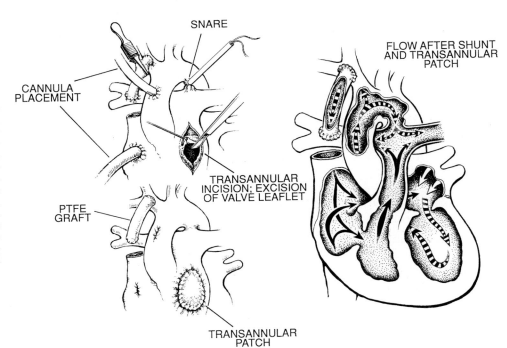

**FIGURE 44–6.** Concomitant placement of a transannular patch and a systemic–pulmonary artery shunt. A 4-mm polytetrafluoroethylene (PTFE) tube graft is placed from the innominate artery to the right pulmonary artery. Cardiopulmonary bypass is established, and the shunt and ductus are temporarily occluded. A pulmonary artery incision is extended into the right ventricular outflow tract. Obstructing tissue is excised, and a pericardial patch is sewn in place.

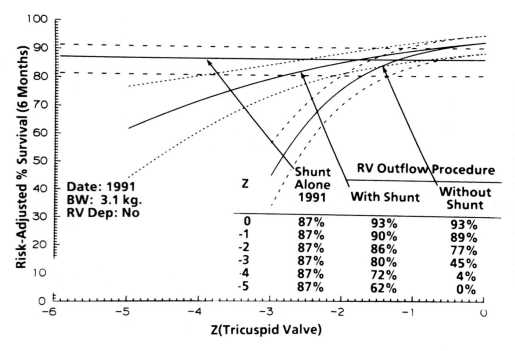

FIGURE 44–7. The effect of tricuspid valve diameter (Z-value) and type of initial procedure on 6-month survival in neonates with PA/IVS. This nomogram was derived after analyzing 171 neonates and solving a multivariable equation setting birth weight (BW) at "3.1 kg," right ventricular–dependent (RV Dep) circulation at "no," and date of shunt operation at "1991." RV outflow procedure includes valvotomy and transannular patch. (From Hanley, F. L., Sade, R. M., Blackstone, E. H., et al.: Outcomes in neonatal atresia and intact ventricular septum. J. Thorac. Cardiovasc. Surg., 105:406, 1993.)

Within figure:

Date: 1991
BW: 3.1 kg.
RV Dep: No

| Z | Shunt Alone 1991 | RV Outflow Procedure | |
|---|---|---|---|
| | | With Shunt | Without Shunt |
| 0 | 87% | 93% | 93% |
| -1 | 87% | 90% | 89% |
| -2 | 87% | 86% | 77% |
| -3 | 87% | 80% | 45% |
| -4 | 87% | 72% | 4% |
| -5 | 87% | 62% | 0% |

some centers, the shunt and atrial defect can be closed using percutaneous techniques (Rome et al., 1990).

Patients who do not tolerate temporary occlusion of the systemic-to-pulmonary artery shunt are unlikely to achieve two-ventricle repair and should be considered candidates for a modified Fontan procedure. Those who tolerate shunt occlusion but not atrial septal defect closure are best followed with repeat evaluation at 6- to 12-month intervals.

Many patients with moderate right ventricular hypoplasia may achieve definitive two-ventricle repair with a policy employed by Laks and colleagues that includes enlargement of the right ventricular outflow tract, creation of a bidirectional superior cavopulmo-

nary anastomosis (a bidirectional Glenn procedure), and placement of an adjustable snare around the atrial septal defect (Billingsley et al., 1989; Laks et al., 1992) (Fig. 44–8). The bidirectional superior cavopulmonary anastomosis reduces the volume load on the right ventricle, and the adjustable atrial septal defect permits controlled right-to-left shunting and adequate cardiac output during the early postoperative period. When right atrial pressure falls with improvement in pulmonary vascular resistance and right ventricular function, the atrial septal defect can be narrowed or closed in the intensive care unit without the need for thoracotomy or cardiopulmonary bypass. In some cases, right ventricular function may be further en-

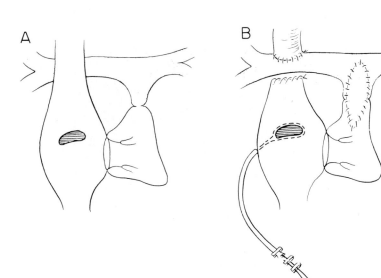

FIGURE 44–8. A and B, A form of definitive two-ventricle repair for patients with moderate right ventricular hypoplasia. In addition to right ventricular outflow patching, a bidirectional cavopulmonary anastomosis is performed to relieve the right ventricle of the superior vena caval blood flow. Placement of an adjustable snare around the atrial septal defect permits incremental closure in the postoperative period. (A and B, From Billingsley, A. M., Laks, H., Boyce, S. W., et al.: Definitive repair in patients with pulmonary atresia and intact ventricular septum. J. Thorac. Cardiovasc. Surg., 97:746, 1989.)

hanced by the insertion of an appropriately sized homograft valve in the right ventricular outflow tract (Billingsley et al., 1989; Laks et al., 1992).

## Definitive Surgical Management for Infants with Severe Right Ventricular Hypoplasia and/or Right Ventricular–Dependent Coronary Circulation

These patients are considered candidates for the Fontan repair at 12 to 24 months of age. Cardiac catheterization is essential to ensure adequate left ventricular function and low pulmonary vascular resistance. Poor left ventricular function would leave cardiac transplantation as the only alternative therapy. Heart-lung transplantation would be the only alternative if pulmonary vascular resistance is elevated. When relative contraindications such as mitral insufficiency or pulmonary artery distortion are identified, these abnormalities are best corrected and combined with a bidirectional superior cavopulmonary anastomosis as an interim procedure before proceeding to the Fontan operation.

When the Fontan procedure is performed, a lateral atrial tunnel technique is employed to direct inferior vena caval blood flow to the pulmonary artery (Pearl et al., 1991) (Fig. 44–9). If the coronary circulation is not dependent on the right ventricle, the right ventricle is decompressed by incising the tricuspid valve. Conversely, if a right ventricular–dependent coronary circulation exists, tricuspid valve competence must be preserved. The interatrial septum is opened widely, and the coronary sinus is unroofed to ensure that the blood entering the right ventricle is well oxygenated.

## RESULTS

Until recently, reports of early and late results in PA/IVS have been limited to studies of 20 to 30 patients often enrolled over a long period of time (Milliken et al., 1985; Alboliras et al., 1987; Hawkins et al., 1990; McCaffrey et al., 1991; Steinberger et al., 1992). In 1987, the Congenital Heart Surgeons Society initiated a prospective multi-institutional study at 31 centers and, within 4 years, enrolled 171 unselected neonates with this diagnosis. The initial right ventricular morphology and tricuspid valve size (Z-value) were known for all patients, and follow-up through 1991 was complete. Techniques for surgical management were not randomized but left to the discretion of each institution. The first report from this ambitious ongoing study provides an unbiased evaluation of

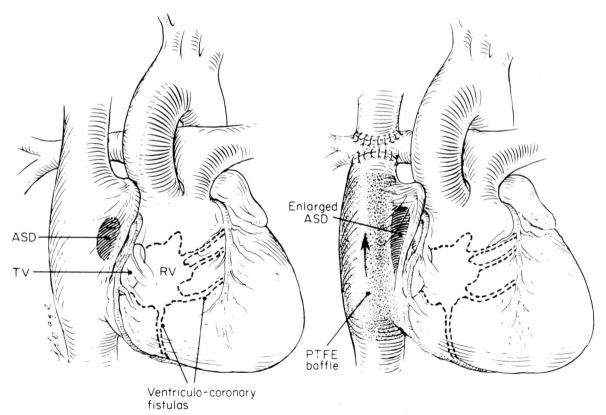

**FIGURE 44–9.** Lateral tunnel Fontan procedure in a patient with right ventricular–dependent coronary circulation. Inferior vena caval flow is directed to superior vena cava by PTFE baffle. The atrial septal defect (ASD) is enlarged, allowing fully saturated pulmonary venous blood to enter the right ventricle (RV). (TV = tricuspid valve.) (From Pearl, J. M., Laks, H., Stein, D. G., et al.: Total cavopulmonary anastomosis versus conventional modified Fontan procedure. Reprinted with permission from the Society of Thoracic Surgeons [The Annals of Thoracic Surgery, 1991, Vol. 52, pp. 189–195].)

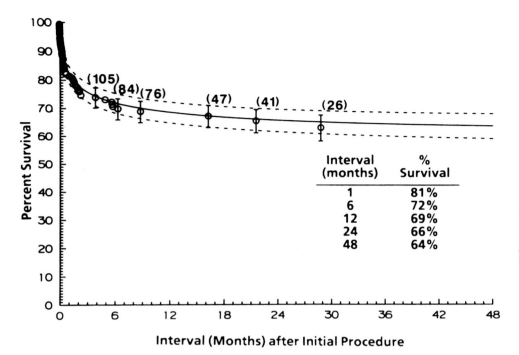

FIGURE 44–10. Survival (derived from life-table and parametric methods) after initial procedure of neonates with PA/IVS. *Circles* represent individual deaths. *Vertical bars* and *dotted lines* represent 70% confidence intervals. (From Hanley, F. L., Sade, R. M., Blackstone, E. H., et al.: Outcomes in neonatal pulmonary atresia with intact ventricular septum. J. Thorac. Cardiovasc. Surg., *105:* 406, 1993.)

| Interval (months) | % Survival |
|---|---|
| 1 | 81% |
| 6 | 72% |
| 12 | 69% |
| 24 | 66% |
| 48 | 64% |

current surgical management of this lesion (Hanley et al., 1993).

In this unselected group, 54% of patients were found to have severe right ventricular hypoplasia (right ventricular cavity size −4 or −5) and 29% had moderate right ventricular hypoplasia (right ventricular cavity size −2 to −3). Survival at 1 month after the first intervention was 81%, with survival at 4 years of 64% (Fig. 44–10). Multivariable analysis indicated that small size (Z-value) of the tricuspid valve, right ventricular–dependent coronary circulation, and low birth weight were the strongest risk factors for death. Patients who initially underwent transannular patching with a systemic-to-pulmonary artery shunt were less likely to require an interim procedure before definitive correction. When a valvotomy or transannular patch was performed without a concomitant systemic-to-pulmonary shunt, approximately 50% of the patients required shunt placement within the first 4 weeks following the initial procedure. In addition, approximately 40% of patients treated initially with pulmonary valvotomy required a transannular patch at a subsequent operation (Hanley et al., 1993). Of patients alive 24 months after entry, 11% had undergone a definitive one-ventricle repair (the Fontan operation) with an operative mortality of 12.5% (1 out of 8). Twenty-four per cent had received a complete two-ventricle repair with an operative mortality of 5% (1 out of 21) (Hanley et al., 1993). The long-term survival of these two groups, as well as the fate of those patients still in a mixed circulation state, must await further time and analysis.

## SELECTED BIBLIOGRAPHY

Freedom, R. M. (ed): Pulmonary Atresia with Intact Ventricular Septum. Mount Kisco, NY, Futura, 1989.

This comprehensive text is devoted solely to the subject of pulmonary atresia and intact ventricular septum (PA/IVS). The many facets of this disorder are thoroughly discussed, including the heterogeneity in morphology and the effects of right ventricular–coronary artery connections. The extensive institutional experience of the Hospital for Sick Children, Toronto, Canada, is described and analyzed.

Hanley, F. L., Sade, R. M., Blackstone, E. H., et al.: Outcomes in neonatal pulmonary atresia with intact ventricular septum: A multi-institutional study. J. Thorac. Cardiovasc. Surg., *105:*406, 1993.

This is the first report by the Congenital Heart Surgeons Society of its multi-institutional study of PA/IVS. Over a 4-year period, 171 consecutive unselected infants were enrolled in this study, and follow-up has been complete. The morphologic spectrum of the malformation is demonstrated clearly and the effects of risk factors and initial surgical management on survival and suitability for definitive repair are described. This landmark paper should be read and studied by all pediatric cardiologists and cardiovascular surgeons.

Kirklin, J. W., and Barratt-Boyes, B. G.: Pulmonary atresia and intact ventricular septum. *In* Kirklin, J. W., and Barratt-Boyes, B. G. (eds): Cardiac Surgery. 2nd ed. New York, Churchill Livingstone, 1993.

This chapter on PA/IVS succinctly but comprehensively describes the morphology, natural history, and treatment of this disorder. Data from the Congenital Heart Surgeons Society multi-institutional study are discussed and analyzed.

## BIBLIOGRAPHY

Alboliras, E. T., Julsrud, P. R., Danielson, G. K., et al.: Definitive operation for pulmonary atresia with intact ventricular septum. J. Thorac. Cardiovasc. Surg., *93:*454, 1987.

Benton, J. W., Jr., Elliot, L. P., Adams, P., Jr., et al.: Pulmonary atresia and stenosis with intact ventricular septum. Am. J. Dis. Child., *104:*83, 1962.

Billingsley, A. M., Laks, H., Boyce, S. W., et al.: Definitive repair in patients with pulmonary atresia and intact ventricular septum. J. Thorac. Cardiovasc. Surg., *97:*746, 1989.

Bowman, F. O., Malm, J. R., Hayes, C. J., et al.: Pulmonary atresia with intact ventricular septum. J. Thorac. Cardiovasc. Surg., *61:*85, 1971.

Bull, C., DeLeval, M. R., Mercanti, C., et al.: Pulmonary atresia and intact ventricular septum: A revised classification. Circulation, *66:*266., 1982.

Coles, J. G., Freedom, R. M., Lightfoot, N. E., et al.: Long-term results in neonates with pulmonary atresia and intact ventricular septum. Ann. Thorac. Surg., 47:213, 1989.

DeLeval, M., Bull, C., Hopkins, R., et al.: Decision making in the definitive repair of the heart with a small right ventricle. Circulation, 72(Suppl. II):II-52, 1985.

Essed, C. E., Klein, H. W., Krediet, P., and Vorst, E. J.: Coronary and endocardial fibroelastosis of the ventricles in the hypoplastic left and right heart syndromes. Virchows Arch. A. Pathol. Anat. Histol., 368:87, 1975.

Foker, J. E., Braunlin, A., St. Cyr, J. A., et al.: Management of pulmonary atresia with intact ventricular septum. J. Thorac. Cardiovasc. Surg., 92:706, 1986.

Freedom, R. M. (ed): Pulmonary Atresia with Intact Ventricular Septum. Mount Kisco, NY, Futura, 1989.

Gersony, W. M., Bernhard, W. F., Nadas, A., and Gross, R. E.: Diagnosis and surgical treatment of infants with critical pulmonary outflow obstruction: Study of 34 infants with pulmonary stenosis or atresia, and intact ventricular septum. Circulation, 35:765, 1967.

Giglia, T. M., Mandell, S., Connor, A. R., et al.: Diagnosis and management of right ventricle–dependent coronary circulation in pulmonary atresia with intact ventricular septum. Circulation, 86:1516, 1992.

Grant, R. T.: Unusual anomaly of coronary vessels in malformed heart of a child. Heart, 13:273, 1926.

Greenwold, W. E., Dushane, J. W., Burchell, H. B., et al.: Congenital pulmonary atresia with intact ventricular septum: Two anatomic types [Abstract]. Circulation, 14:945, 1956.

Hanley, F. L., Sade, R. M., Blackstone, E. H., et al.: Outcomes in neonatal pulmonary atresia with intact ventricular septum: A multi-institutional study. J. Thorac. Cardiovasc. Surg., 105:406, 1993.

Hawkins, J. A., Thorne, J. K., Boucek, M. M., et al.: Early and late results in pulmonary atresia and intact ventricular septum. J. Thorac. Cardiovasc. Surg., 100:492, 1990.

Hunter, J.: Observations and Enquiries 6:291, 1783. Cited in Peacock, T. B.: Malformations of the heart; atresia of the orifice of the pulmonary artery; aorta communicating with both ventricles. Trans. Pathol. Soc. Lond., 20:61, 1869.

Kanter, K. R., Pennington, D. G., Nouri, S., et al.: Concomitant valvotomy and subclavian–main pulmonary artery shunt in neonates with pulmonary atresia and intact ventricular septum. Ann. Thorac. Surg., 43:490, 1987.

Kirklin, J. W., and Barratt-Boyes, B. G.: Anatomy, dimensions, and terminology. In Kirklin, J. W., and Barratt-Boyes, B. G. (eds): Cardiac Surgery. 2nd ed. New York, Churchill Livingstone, 1993.

Laks, H., Pearl, J. M., Drinkwater, D. C., et al.: Partial biventricular repair of pulmonary atresia with intact ventricular septum: Use of an adjustable atrial septal defect. Circulation, 86(Suppl. II):II-159, 1992.

Leung, M. P., Mok, C., and Hue P.: Echocardiographic assessment of neonates with pulmonary atresia and intact ventricular septum. J. Am. Coll. Cardiol., 12:719, 1988.

Mccaffrey, F. M., Leatherbury, L., and Moore, H. V.: Pulmonary atresia and intact ventricular septum. J. Thorac. Cardiovasc. Surg., 102:617, 1991.

Milliken, J. C., Laks, H., Hellenbrand, W., et al.: Early and late results in the treatment of patients with pulmonary atresia and intact ventricular septum. Circulation, 72(Suppl. II):II-61, 1985.

Novelo, S., Chait, L. O., Zapata-Diaz, J., and Valasquez, T.: Atresia pulmonaria estenosis tricuspidea sin comunicaciones interventricular. Arch. Inst. Cardiol. Mex., 21:325, 1951.

Pawade, A., Capuani, A., Penny, D. J., et al.: Pulmonary atresia with intact ventricular septum: Surgical management based on right ventricular infundibulum. J. Card. Surg., 8:371, 1993.

Pearl, J. M., Laks, H., Stein, D. G., et al.: Total cavopulmonary anastomosis versus conventional modified Fontan procedure. Ann. Thorac. Surg., 52:189, 1991.

Rome, J. J., Keane, J. F., Perry, S. B., et al.: Double-umbrella closure of atrial defects. Circulation, 82:751, 1990.

Sanders, S. P., Parness, I. A., and Colan, S. D.: Recognition of abnormal connections of coronary arteries with the use of Doppler color-flow mapping. J. Am. Coll. Cardiol., 13:922, 1989.

Steinberger, J., Berry, J. M., Bass, J. L., et al.: Results of a right ventricular outflow patch for pulmonary atresia with intact ventricular septum. Circulation, 86(Suppl. II):II-167, 1992.

Ziegler, R. F., and Taber, R. E.: Diagnostic criteria and successful surgery in an operable form of complete pulmonary valve atresia [Abstract]. Circulation, 26:807, 1962.

# 45

# Univentricular Heart

Erle H. Austin III

The term *univentricular heart* applies to a group of cardiac morphologies in which both the right and the left atria connect to a single ventricular chamber. In most cases, this *univentricular connection* is by two separate *atrioventricular* (AV) valves or one common AV valve. These hearts are most accurately described as *double-inlet ventricles* (Anderson et al., 1979). The remaining univentricular hearts are those with right- or left-sided AV valve atresia. Although the atrioventricular connection is univentricular, the term *single ventricle* may be misleading because in most cases the ventricular mass consists of two chambers: a dominant ventricle connected to the atria and a "rudimentary" ventricle that often serves as an outlet chamber or occasionally as a trabecular pouch (Anderson, 1983).

Since the early 1950s, surgical techniques have been available to palliate patients with univentricular heart by either increasing (systemic–pulmonary artery shunting) or decreasing (pulmonary artery banding) pulmonary blood flow. Definitive correction is now possible in many patients using the techniques of ventricular septation or the Fontan operation, but preliminary palliation is necessary in most of these patients. Selection of the appropriate palliative procedure is important in optimizing the results of subsequent definitive repair.

## HISTORY

The earliest pathologic description of a heart with a solitary ventricle is attributed to Holmes (1824). In 1936, Abbott reported 27 cases of single ventricle with associated cardiac anomalies. Van Praagh and colleagues (1964) were the first to emphasize that the connection of both AV valves to the same ventricle was the distinctive feature of these hearts. Anderson and associates (1979, 1983, 1985, 1987) have done much to accurately describe the morphologic variants and clarify terminology.

Surgical palliation of single ventricles with pulmonary stenosis was made possible by the introduction of the Blalock-Taussig shunt in 1945. Similarly, the report of pulmonary artery banding by Muller and Damman (1952) described a palliative technique that would be applied to single ventricles without pulmonary stenosis. Atrial septectomy, originally described by Blalock and Hanlon (1950) for transposition of the great arteries, was applied to patients with left-sided AV valve atresia by Redo and co-workers (1967).

The first septation of a single ventricle was performed at the Mayo Clinic in 1956 on a patient thought preoperatively to have corrected transposition with ventricular septal defect (VSD) (McGoon et al., 1977). Sakakibara and colleagues (1972) and Edie and associates (1973) deserve credit for the first series of septation procedures.

The concept of separating the pulmonary and systemic venous returns at the atrial level and relying on elevated systemic venous pressure and low pulmonary vascular resistance to achieve satisfactory pulmonary blood flow is attributed to Fontan and Baudet (1971). A 1971 report by this group describes the first successes of this procedure in patients with tricuspid atresia. Application of the Fontan concept for definitive correction of univentricular heart was first reported by Yacoub and Radley-Smith (1976).

## ANATOMY

### General Features

Connection of both atrial chambers to a single ventricle is the common feature of all univentricular hearts and includes double-inlet ventricles and those with absent right or left AV connections. Tricuspid atresia is a univentricular heart with absent right connection, and is discussed fully in Chapter 46. Excluding tricuspid atresia, the majority of univentricular hearts are double-inlet ventricles.

The internal architecture of the dominant ventricle may reflect left ventricular (finely trabeculated) or right ventricular (coarsely trabeculated) morphology. The ventricular pattern of the nondominant (rudimentary) ventricle is always complementary to that of the dominant chamber. The rudimentary chamber is connected to the dominant ventricle by a VSD often referred to as an outlet or bulboventricular foramen. In a small proportion of patients, the ventricular mass is made up of a single indeterminate ventricle that lacks a rudimentary chamber (Fig. 45–1).

Any type of atrial situs can exist, but situs solitus occurs most commonly with double-inlet left ventricle. An isomeric atrial pattern is more common with double-inlet right or indeterminate ventricle. Two patent AV valves are positioned entirely in the dominant chamber, although occasionally a portion of the tension apparatus of one of the valves will attach within the nondominant chamber. In some patients, a common AV valve connects the two atria to the dominant ventricle. Any connection between the ventricular mass and the great vessels is possible (concordant,

1614

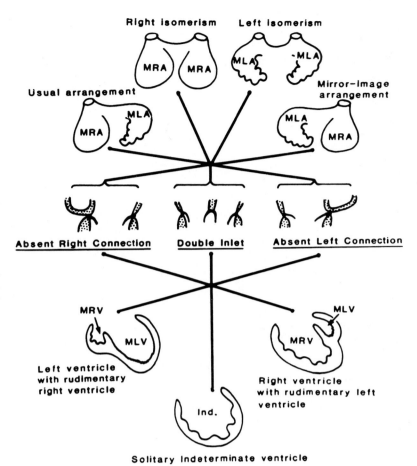

**FIGURE 45–1.** Any combination of four atrial arrangements, three atrioventricular connections, and three ventricular morphologies is possible in univentricular atrioventricular connection. (MRA = morphologic right atrium; MLA = morphologic left atrium; MRV = morphologic right ventricle; MLV = morphologic left ventricle; Ind. = indeterminate.) (From Anderson, R. H., Becker, A. E., Tynan, M., and Wilkinson, J. L.: Definitions and terminology—The significance of sequential segmental analysis. *In* Anderson, R. H., Crupi, G., and Parenzan, L. [eds]: Double-Inlet Ventricle. New York, Elsevier, 1987.)

discordant, double-outlet, single-outlet) (Fig. 45–2), although a discordant ventriculoarterial (VA) connection is most common.

The position of the AV node and conduction tissue is abnormal in most double-inlet ventricles. In double-inlet left ventricle, the AV node is located not at the apex of the triangle of Koch but along the anterior quadrant of the right AV valve. The penetrating bundle then extends to the right margin of the VSD, where it branches on the left ventricular aspect several millimeters from the crest of the septum. Viewed through the right AV valve, the conduction bundle runs anterior to the pulmonary valve and extends just above the superior border of the VSD.

## Types of Univentricular Heart

### Double-Inlet Left Ventricle

The most common type of univentricular heart is double-inlet left ventricle, representing 60 to 70% of double-inlet ventricles. Eighty per cent of double-inlet left ventricles exhibit a discordant VA connection (transposition) with a right-sided pulmonary artery arising posteriorly from a dominant right-sided left ventricular chamber and a left-sided aorta arising from a small right ventricular outlet chamber (Figs.

45–3A and 45–4). Double-inlet left ventricle with VA concordance, the *Holmes heart*, represents about 20% of double-inlet left ventricles. These hearts resemble a normal heart, with the aorta arising from a dominant left ventricle and the pulmonary artery arising from a small right-sided right ventricular outlet chamber (Fig. 45–3B). Pulmonary stenosis is common in these hearts.

### Double-Inlet Right and Indeterminate Ventricles

Double-inlet right ventricle and double-inlet indeterminate ventricle are the other less common types of double-inlet ventricle. In the former, the incomplete left ventricle is always positioned posteriorly and inferiorly and usually exists only as a trabecular pouch without connection to a great vessel. Double-inlet indeterminate ventricles are similar to double-inlet right ventricles except that an accessory ventricular chamber cannot be found (Fig. 45–3C). Situs ambiguus and situs inversus are common in these hearts. Connection to the great vessels is usually double or single (pulmonary atresia) outlet. Pulmonary stenosis or atresia is common.

### Mitral Atresia

Hearts with mitral valve atresia make up an important group of hearts with univentricular AV con-

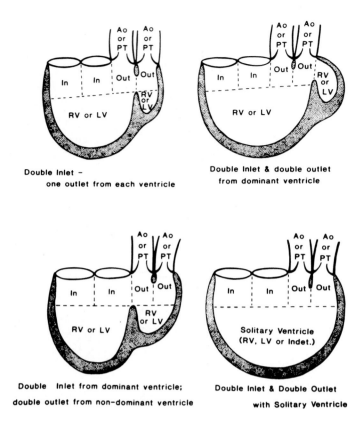

Double Inlet –
one outlet from each ventricle

Double Inlet & double outlet
from dominant ventricle

Double Inlet from dominant ventricle;
double outlet from non-dominant ventricle

Double Inlet & Double Outlet
with Solitary Ventricle

FIGURE 45–2. A variety of ventriculoarterial connections may occur in univentricular atrioventricular connection. (Ao = aorta; PT = pulmonary trunk; RV = right ventricle; LV = left ventricle; Indet. = indeterminate.) (From Anderson, R. H., Becker, A. E., Tynan, M., and Wilkinson, J. L.: Definitions and terminology—The significance of sequential segmental analysis. *In* Anderson, R. H., Crupi, G., and Parenzan L. [eds]: Double-Inlet Ventricle. New York, Elsevier, 1987.)

nection. This group should be recognized separately from hearts with combined mitral and aortic atresia (hypoplastic left-sided heart syndrome). Although the morphology of this defect may vary significantly, the typical arrangement is atrial situs solitus with a dominant right-sided right ventricle connected to the right atrium through a patent tricuspid valve. A small left ventricle is connected to the right ventricle by a VSD

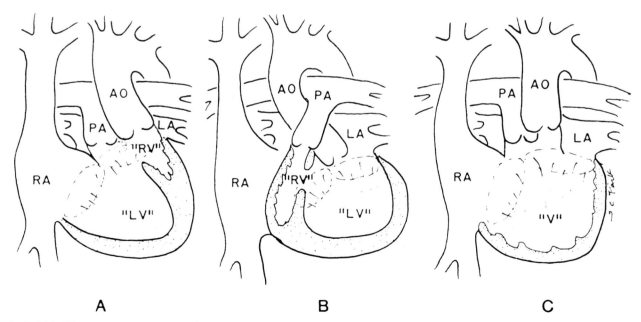

FIGURE 45–3. The most common types of univentricular heart. *A*, Double-inlet left ventricle (LV) with ventriculoarterial discordance. *B*, Double-inlet LV with ventriculoarterial concordance (Holmes' heart). *C*, Double-inlet indeterminate ventricle. (AO = aorta; PA = pulmonary artery; RV = right ventricle; RA = right atrium; V = ventricle.) (*A–C*, From Zuberbuhler, J. R.: Double-inlet ventricle. *In* Neches, W. M., Park, S. C., and Zuberbuhler, J. R. [eds]: Pediatric Cardiac Catheterization. Volume 3 of the series Perspectives in Pediatric Cardiology. Mount Kisco, NY, Futura, 1991.)

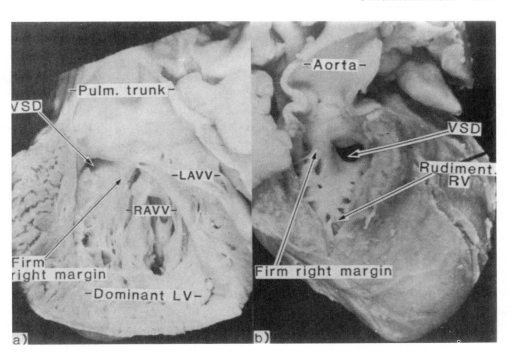

FIGURE 45–4. Specimen of double-inlet left ventricle (LV) with ventriculoarterial discordance. *a,* View into dominant LV shows both atrioventricular valves (RAVV and LAVV), the pulmonary trunk and the ventricular septal defect (VSD) or outlet foramen. The firm right margin is the area that carries the conduction tissue. *b,* View into rudimentary right ventricle (RV) shows the systemic outflow tract. A restrictive VSD causes subaortic stenosis. (*a* and *b,* From Becker, A. E., Anderson, R. H., Penkoske, P. A., and Zuberbuhler, J. R.: Morphology of double-inlet ventricle. *In* Anderson, R. H., Crupi, G., and Parenzan, L. [eds]: Double-Inlet Ventricle. New York, Elsevier, 1987.)

and gives rise to the aorta. Obstruction to flow may exist at several levels, including the interatrial septum, the VSD, and the aortic arch.

## Associated Cardiac Anomalies

Associated cardiac anomalies occur in approximately one-third of patients with univentricular AV connection (Kirklin and Barratt-Boyes, 1993). Those that have the most significant effect on clinical presentation and natural history include pulmonary stenosis or atresia, subaortic stenosis, and coarctation of the aorta. Subaortic stenosis is most commonly secondary to a restrictive VSD in the setting of double-inlet left ventricle or mitral atresia, and is commonly associated with coarctation or interrupted aortic arch. Anomalous pulmonary venous connection may be seen in some patients with right atrial isomerism.

## PATHOPHYSIOLOGY

### Mixing of Venous Returns

The principal effect of a univentricular AV connection on circulatory physiology is the obligatory mixing of systemic and pulmonary venous blood within the dominant ventricular chamber. The relative contributions of saturated and desaturated blood depend on anatomic and physiologic factors that determine what proportion of cardiac output goes to each circulation. In a perfectly balanced situation, pulmonary and systemic blood flow are equal. In such a case,

there is usually an element of pulmonary stenosis to offset the normally lower vascular resistance present in the pulmonary arterial bed. More commonly, systemic and pulmonary blood flow are unequal, creating hypoxia at one end of the spectrum or congestive heart failure at the other. Marked cyanosis progressing to metabolic acidosis can be expected in univentricular hearts with severe pulmonary stenosis or atresia. At the other extreme, pulmonary edema, inadequate tissue perfusion, and metabolic acidosis may be caused by a univentricular heart with a restrictive VSD, hypoplastic aortic arch, coarctation, and an unrestricted pathway to the pulmonary arteries.

### Pulmonary Vascular Resistance

Time-related changes in pulmonary vascular resistance may also affect the balance between pulmonary and systemic blood flow. The relatively high pulmonary vascular resistance at birth decreases to a low point between 3 and 6 months of age. Without an anatomic obstruction to limit pulmonary blood flow, congestive heart failure is likely to worsen as pulmonary vascular resistance decreases. As further time passes, pulmonary vascular beds unprotected from systemic pressure and high pulmonary blood flow will increase vascular resistance as pulmonary vascular disease develops.

Obstruction to pulmonary venous return may occur in some hearts with univentricular AV connection (mitral atresia with restrictive interatrial septum and double-inlet ventricles with anomalous pulmonary venous connection). A combined clinical picture of cyanosis and congestive heart failure is the result of limited pulmonary venous blood for mixing and increased hydrostatic pressure in the pulmonary vascular bed.

## NATURAL HISTORY

Overall survival rates for patients with double-inlet ventricle are 57% at 1 year, 40% at 5 years, and 35% at 10 years (Franklin et al., 1991a) (Fig. 45–5). However, survival is significantly affected by the presence or absence of risk factors. Figure 45–6 demonstrates the dramatic effect these risk factors have on estimated survival. A typical patient with atrial situs solitus, double-inlet left ventricle, discordant VA connection, pulmonary stenosis, balanced pulmonary blood flow, and presenting between 14 and 60 days of age has an estimated 10-year survival rate of greater than 90% (Curve A). At the other extreme, a patient with right atrial isomerism, double-inlet and double-outlet right ventricle, a common AV orifice, anomalous pulmonary venous connection, low pulmonary blood flow, and presenting before 14 days of age has a predicted 1-year survival rate of only 3% (Curve D). Using multivariate analysis, Franklin and colleagues (1991a) derived an additive index of relative risks (Table 45–1) that permits stratification of patients into risk groups. As one might expect, infants that present with severe acidosis and low cardiac output are at highest risk for early death.

Subaortic stenosis is an important risk factor when the aorta arises from an outlet chamber, as in double-inlet left ventricle with VA discordance and in mitral atresia with VA concordance. This subaortic stenosis derives primarily from restriction at the outlet foramen and may be evident soon after birth, when it is

**■ Table 45–1.** SIMPLE ADDITIVE INDEX FOR PATIENTS WITH DOUBLE-INLET VENTRICLE, CALCULATED FROM MULTIVARIATE-DERIVED RELATIVE RISKS*

| Variable | Rounded-Off Cox Coefficient |
|---|---|
| Pulmonary valvular or subvalvular stenosis | −2 |
| Presentation at age greater than 2 months | −2 |
| Presentation at age 2 weeks to 2 months | −1 |
| Balanced pulmonary blood flow | −1 |
| Double-inlet right ventricle | −1 |
| Mirror-image arrangement (situs inversus) | −1 |
| Left atrial isomerism | −1 |
| Right atrial isomerism | +1 |
| Concordant ventriculoatrial connection | +1 |
| Pulmonary atresia | +1 |
| Systemic outflow obstruction at any level | +1 |
| Presentation before 1980 | +1 |
| Double-outlet dominant ventricle | +2 |
| Aortic atresia or common arterial trunk | +2 |
| Anomalous pulmonary venous connection | +2 |
| Presentation with severe low output and acidosis | +4 |

*A total score is derived for each patient by adding together the rounded Cox coefficient for 11 variables, which include atrial arrangement, dominant ventricular morphology, and presence or absence of systemic outflow obstruction. The more positive the total score, the less favorable is the predicted outcome.

From Franklin, R. C. G., Spiegelhalter, D. J., Anderson, R. H., et al.: Double-inlet ventricle presenting in infancy. I. Survival without definitive repair. J. Thorac. Cardiovasc. Surg., *101*:767, 1991.

commonly associated with aortic arch obstruction. The VSD may be large at birth causing no obstruction, but may narrow with time. Pulmonary artery banding appears to accelerate this process (Franklin et al., 1990; Freed et al., 1971; Freedom et al., 1977, 1986). Furthermore, subaortic stenosis may develop after a Fontan procedure when the VSD narrows secondary to the acute decrease in ventricular volume. In some

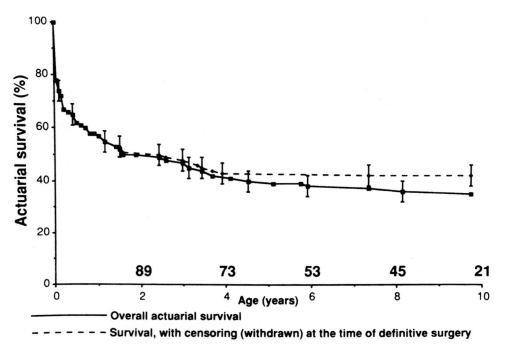

**FIGURE 45–5.** Actuarial survival of patients born with double-inlet ventricle. Kaplan-Meier life-table analysis of 191 patients. *Dashed line* refers to survival before definitive surgery. *Vertical bars* represent 70% confidence limits. (From Franklin, R. C. G., Spiegelhalter, D. J., Anderson, R. H., et al.: Double-inlet ventricle presenting in infancy. I. Survival without definitive repair. J. Thorac. Cardiovasc. Surg., *101*: 767, 1991.)

——————— Overall actuarial survival

– – – – – – Survival, with censoring (withdrawn) at the time of definitive surgery

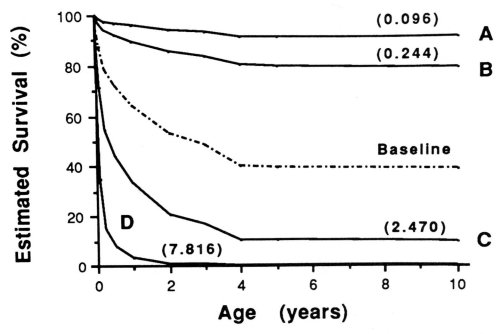

**FIGURE 45–6.** Curves of estimated survival before definitive surgery in patients with double-inlet ventricle. The effect of risk factors: *A,* Patients born with double-inlet LV, discordant ventriculoarterial (VA) connection, moderate pulmonary stenosis with balanced pulmonary blood flow presenting between 14 and 60 days of age. *B,* Same morphology with low pulmonary blood flow ($Q_P/Q_S < 1$). *C,* Same morphology with pulmonary atresia presenting at less than 14 days of age, *D,* Right atrial isomerism, double-inlet and double-outlet RV, a common AV valve, extracardiac anomalous pulmonary venous connection presenting with low pulmonary blood flow at less than 14 days of age. *Numbers in parenthesis* are the total calculated relative risk compared with the fictitious baseline patient *(dotted curve). (A–D,* From Franklin, R. C. G., Spiegelhalter, D. J., Anderson, R. H., et al.: Double-inlet ventricle presenting in infancy. I. Survival without definitive repair. J. Thorac. Cardiovasc. Surg., *101:*767, 1991.)

cases, it may take 1 to 2 years to become evident (Razzouk et al., 1992). Subaortic stenosis, therefore, may become manifest at any stage. Recognition of its presence or potential is important in planning both palliative and definitive surgery.

## CLINICAL FEATURES

Univentricular AV connection affects approximately 3% of infants born with congenital heart disease and is slightly more common in males. Its clinical presentation is determined primarily by associated lesions that affect the balance between pulmonary and systemic blood flow. Patients with mild to moderate pulmonary stenosis and balanced blood flow may be asymptomatic; the condition may be discovered only when a murmur is detected on routine physical examination. More commonly, pulmonary blood flow is either insufficient or excessive. If severe pulmonary stenosis or atresia exists, the infant presents on the first day of life with marked cyanosis. On the other hand, if there is no pulmonary stenosis, the patient is likely to present at 1 to 2 months of age with severe heart failure and little or no cyanosis. The presence of systemic outflow obstruction at any level severely unbalances the circulation, causing early presentation of heart failure that may progress to metabolic acidosis and death.

Physical findings and routine investigations also reflect the balance of pulmonary and systemic blood flow. Cyanosis is the key feature in those with obstructed pulmonary blood flow, whereas an active precordium, tachypnea, and hepatomegaly indicate the presence of excessive pulmonary blood flow. Peripheral pulses are normal except in those patients with subaortic stenosis or arch obstruction. A systolic murmur is present in most patients.

Chest radiography also reveals the amount of pulmonary blood flow. Decreased vascular markings and a normal or small cardiac silhouette are seen when pulmonary blood flow is limited; cardiomegaly and plethoric lung fields are noted when pulmonary blood flow is excessive. Radiographic appearance of pulmonary venous hypertension may indicate the presence of mitral atresia with a restrictive foramen ovale.

In most patients, definitive diagnosis is made initially with two-dimensional echocardiography. The presence of two AV valves or one common valve opening into a single ventricular chamber is diagnostic. The VA connection, size of the outlet foramen, and the presence of important associated lesions, such as coarctation, can be assessed echocardiographically.

Although not always required, cardiac catheterization and cineangiography may be performed to confirm or enhance the echocardiographic diagnosis. In older patients who are potential candidates for ventricular septation or the Fontan procedure, cardiac catheterization is required to measure pulmonary vascular resistance and ventricular end-diastolic pressure and to angiographically assess the pulmonary arteries.

## TREATMENT

### Initial Management

Initial management of patients with univentricular heart is tailored to the pathophysiology at presentation. Infants that present in the first days of life with severe cyanosis are stabilized with prostaglandin $E_1$ to maintain ductal patency until a systemic–pulmonary artery shunt can be constructed. Prostaglandin $E_1$ is also indicated for newborns with subaortic and aortic arch obstructions to improve systemic blood flow by allowing antegrade flow across the ductus arteriosus. The pathophysiology in this critically ill subgroup is similar to that seen in hypoplastic left-sided heart syndrome. Thus, supplemental inspired oxygen should be avoided to prevent overwhelming pulmo-

nary blood flow. Patients with little or no pulmonary stenosis who present after the newborn period with congestive heart failure can be managed initially with routine medications, including digoxin and diuretics. Patients with balanced blood flow require no initial treatment, but should be followed closely and considered candidates for definitive repair.

### Palliative Surgery

The aim of surgical palliation in patients with univentricular heart is to optimize pulmonary blood flow and pressure. Inherent in the selection of technique is the desire to establish and maintain suitable anatomy and hemodynamics for eventual correction with either ventricular septation or a modified Fontan operation.

#### Systemic–Pulmonary Artery Shunt

Patients with inadequate pulmonary blood flow undergo the creation of a systemic–pulmonary artery

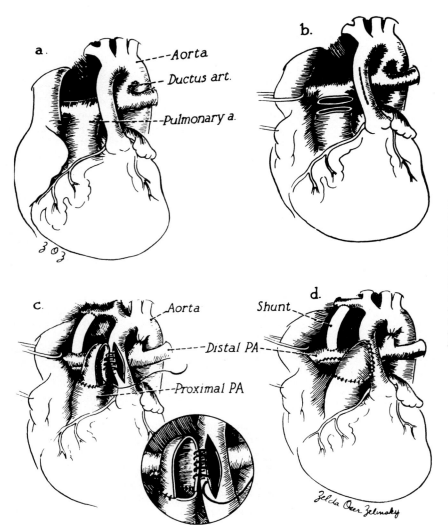

**FIGURE 45–7.** *a–d,* Damus-Kaye-Stansel anastomosis with systemic–pulmonary artery (PA) shunt for subaortic stenosis in the neonate. Transected pulmonary artery is anastomosed to the side of the ascending aorta with a hood of pericardium or polytetrafluoroethylene (PTFE). *(a–d,* From Ilbawi, M. N., DeLeon, S. Y., Wilson, W. R., et al.: Advantages of early relief of subaortic stenosis in single-ventricle equivalents. Reprinted with permission from the Society of Thoracic Surgeons [The Annals of Thoracic Surgery, 1991, Vol. 52, pp. 842–849].)

shunt. This is commonly performed through a right thoracotomy with placement of a 4- or 5-mm polytetrafluoroethylene (PTFE) tube graft from the right subclavian artery to the right pulmonary artery.

### Pulmonary Artery Banding

This procedure is indicated for those patients with an unprotected pulmonary vascular bed who are at risk of developing irreversible pulmonary vascular disease. The band is tightened to decrease pulmonary artery pressure to less than half of systemic arterial pressure, while a peripheral oxygen saturation of 75% or more is maintained on an inspired fractional oxygen content of 50%. The tendency for subaortic stenosis to develop after pulmonary artery banding has discouraged some authors from applying this technique (Freedom, 1987). However, this approach appears to have a low risk if applied to patients without aortic arch obstruction and with an outlet foramen greater than $2 \text{ cm}^2/\text{M}^2$ (Matitiau et al., 1992).

### Other Palliative Procedures

For patients who present with subaortic stenosis or obstruction of the aortic arch, several alternative, although high-risk, procedures are available. The objective of these techniques is to bypass the subaortic stenosis by bringing the aorta into direct communication with the dominant ventricle. The Damus-Kaye-Stansel procedure involves dividing the main pulmonary artery just proximal to the bifurcation and anastomosing the proximal pulmonary trunk to the side of the aorta. Flow to the pulmonary arteries is provided by a PTFE systemic–pulmonary artery shunt (Ilbawi et al., 1991; Jonas et al., 1985; Rychik et al., 1991) (Fig. 45–7). When aortic arch hypoplasia, coarctation, or arch interruption coexists with subaortic stenosis, a more extensive procedure is required. The Norwood procedure combines the Damus-Kaye-Stansel approach with an augmentation of the arch and ascending aorta (Tchervenkov et al., 1990; Rychik et al., 1991) (Fig. 45–8). The arterial switch procedure has also been applied to this group of patients, transferring the obstructed outflow to the pulmonary circulation while establishing unrestricted flow to the aorta (Freedom and Trusler, 1991; Karl et al., 1991; Lacour-Gayet et al., 1992).

Atrial septectomy is an important palliative procedure for patients with mitral atresia and a restrictive interatrial septum. It can be performed using the closed technique of Blalock and Hanlon (1950) or under direct vision with inflow occlusion or a short period of cardiopulmonary bypass.

### Interim Procedures

Should subaortic stenosis develop after initial palliation, an interim procedure is warranted to relieve this obstruction. The VSD can be directly enlarged by incising the outlet chamber and removing a wedge of muscle from the superior edge of the VSD. When

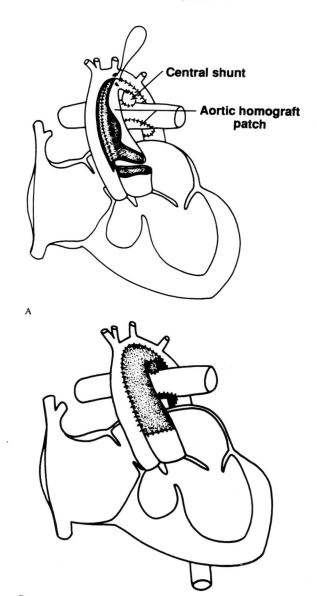

**FIGURE 45–8.** *A* and *B*, The Norwood procedure for neonates with univentricular heart, subaortic stenosis, and aortic arch obstruction. An aortic homograft is used to reconstruct the ascending aorta and aortic arch and to patch the divided main pulmonary artery. (*A* and *B*, From Tchervenkov, C. I., Beland, M. J., Latter, D. A., and Dobell, A. R. C.: Norwood operation for univentricular heart with subaortic stenosis in the neonate. Reprinted with permission from the Society of Thoracic Surgeons [The Annals of Thoracic Surgery, 1990, Vol. 50, pp. 822–825].)

visualized through the outlet chamber, the conduction tissue runs along the inferior edge of the defect (Anderson et al., 1987; Cheung et al., 1990) (Fig. 45–9). Alternatively, the subaortic stenosis can be left alone and bypassed with the Damus-Kaye-Stansel technique (Jonas et al., 1985; Laks et al., 1992; Lin et al., 1986).

When patients with univentricular heart have one or more risk factors for the Fontan procedure, such as subaortic stenosis, elevated pulmonary vascular

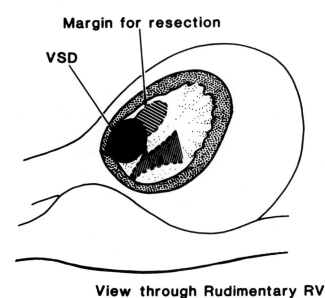

**Margin for resection**

**VSD**

**View through Rudimentary RV**

**FIGURE 45–9.** Operative technique for enlarging a restrictive VSD through the outlet chamber. From this perspective, the conduction axis runs along the inferior border of the VSD. (From Anderson, R. H., Becker, A. E., Ho, S. Y., et al.: Disposition of the conduction tissues. *In* Anderson, R. H., Crupi, G., and Parenzan, L. [eds]: Double-Inlet Ventricle. New York, Elsevier, 1987.)

resistance, or pulmonary artery distortion, a policy of staged reconstruction is advisable. As an intermediate step to a Fontan procedure, a bidirectional superior cavopulmonary anastomosis (bidirectional Glenn procedure) is performed in combination with relief of the subaortic stenosis (Fig. 45–10) or reconstruction of the pulmonary arteries (Bridges et al., 1990a; Douville et al., 1991; Lamberti et al., 1990; Pridjian et al., 1993).

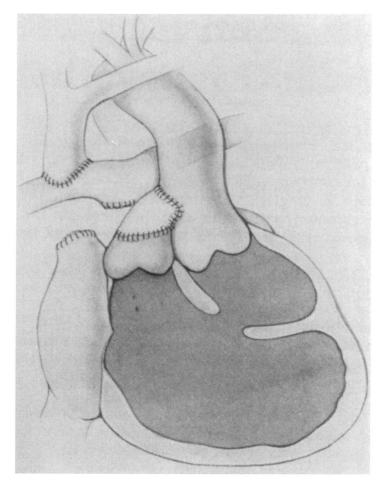

**FIGURE 45–10.** Damus-Kaye-Stansel procedure with bidirectional superior cavopulmonary Glenn anastomosis for acquired subaortic stenosis in univentricular heart. (From Laks, H., Gates, R. N., Elami, A., and Pearl, J. M.: Damus-Stansel-Kaye procedure: Technical modifications. Reprinted with permission from the Society of Thoracic Surgeons [The Annals of Thoracic Surgery, 1992, Vol. 54, pp. 169–172].)

## Definitive Repair

The objective of definitive repair is to separate the systemic and pulmonary circulations and place them in series so that ventricular demand is normalized and pulmonary and systemic blood flow balanced. It is assumed that this improvement in circulatory physiology will improve survival and functional capacity. The earliest definitive repairs in univentricular hearts employed the technique of ventricular septation. Anatomic constraints, however, have prevented its application in many cases. Variations in intraventricular anatomy, however, do not preclude application of the Fontan procedure.

Suitability for definitive repair must be determined preoperatively by cardiac catheterization and cineangiography. Normal ventricular function with a ventricular end-diastolic pressure of 15 mm Hg or less and low pulmonary vascular resistance must be ensured. For the Fontan procedure, pulmonary vascular resistance must not exceed 2 Woods units/M$^2$. Slightly higher resistance (up to 6 Woods units/M$^2$) is acceptable for septation. Severe distortion of the pulmonary arteries, moderate or severe AV valve regurgitation, and systemic outflow obstruction must be ruled out or repaired before definitive correction is undertaken.

### Ventricular Septation

Candidates for ventricular septation are limited to those with double-inlet ventricle with left or indeterminate ventricular morphology, two normal AV valves, a discordant or double outlet from the dominant ventricle, VA connection with the aorta anterior and to the left of the pulmonary artery, mild or absent pulmonary outflow obstruction, and no other intracardiac anomalies. The chordal attachments of the two AV valves, assessed intraoperatively, must also permit separation into two chambers (Pacifico, 1986).

The procedure is performed through a median sternotomy with cardiopulmonary bypass, moderate hypothermia, and cardioplegic myocardial protection. The intracardiac anatomy is first examined through a right atriotomy and the right-sided AV valve. The area beneath the pulmonary valve, the VSD, and the left AV valve and its chordal attachments are all examined. A fishmouth incision in the main ventricular chamber provides improved exposure of the intracardiac anatomy but may adversely affect postoperative ventricular function. A line of septation is identified that separates the right and left AV valves directing inflow from the left AV valve to the outlet foramen (Fig. 45–11). Numerous interrupted pledgeted Dacron mattress sutures are placed, and a piece of knitted Dacron velour backed with pericardium is cut into the appropriate size and shape and inserted. The need to place sutures along the anterior border of the outlet foramen places the conduction axis at significant risk. Thus, permanent epicardial atrial and ventricular pacing wires are placed at the conclusion of the operation (Pacifico et al., 1985).

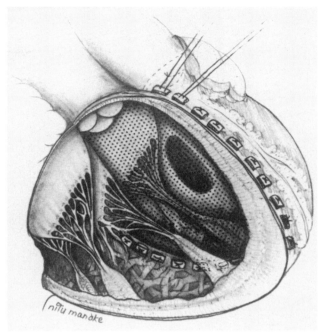

**FIGURE 45–11.** Ventricular septation divides the dominant ventricle into two separate compartments, placing the right AV valve and PA to the right and the left AV valve, VSD, and outlet chamber to the left. (From Pacifico, A. D., Kirklin, J. W., and Kirklin, J. K.: Single ventricle with double-inlet atrioventricular connection. *In* Arciniegas, E. [ed]: Pediatric Cardiac Surgery. Chicago, Year Book Medical, 1985.)

### The Fontan Procedure

The Fontan procedure is applicable to a greater proportion of patients with univentricular heart than is ventricular septation. Optimal timing of this procedure appears to be between 18 and 36 months of age (Franklin et al., 1991c; Kirklin and Barratt-Boyes, 1993). Earlier methods of atriopulmonary anastomosis have evolved into a favored technique of total cavopulmonary connection using a lateral intra-atrial tunnel to direct inferior vena caval blood to the pulmonary arteries (Jonas and Castañeda, 1988; Pearl et al., 1991) (Fig. 45–12).

As with ventricular septation, the Fontan procedure is performed using cardiopulmonary bypass with bicaval cannulation, moderate hypothermia, and cardioplegic myocardial protection. The main pulmonary artery is divided and oversewn at both ends. The superior vena cava is divided and both ends are anastomosed end-to-side into the right pulmonary artery. Through a right atriotomy, a tunnel is created with a PTFE patch connecting the orifices of the superior and inferior venae cavae and leaving the coronary sinus on the pulmonary venous side. Any residual atrial septum is excised. Right and left atrial pressures are measured as cardiopulmonary bypass is weaned. If satisfactory arterial blood pressure and cardiac output are achieved with right atrial pressures of 15 mm Hg or less, a good result is to be expected.

In patients in whom pulmonary vascular resistance may be elevated or other factors appear to compro-

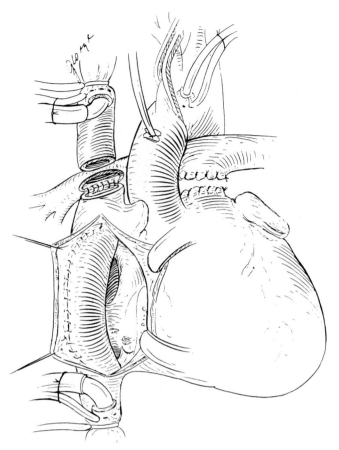

**FIGURE 45–12.** The Fontan procedure using the lateral tunnel technique. A partial tube of PTFE directs inferior vena caval flow to the superior vena cava, which is anastomosed to the right pulmonary artery. The main pulmonary artery has been divided and oversewn. (From Pearl, J. M., Laks, H., Stein, D. G., et al.: Total cavopulmonary anastomosis versus conventional modified Fontan procedure. Reprinted with permission from the Society of Thoracic Surgeons [The Annals of Thoracic Surgery, 1991, Vol. 52, pp. 189–196].)

mise cardiac output, a fenestration of 4 to 5 mm may be placed in the PTFE baffle to permit controlled right-to-left shunting and improve cardiac output at the expense of a small decrease in arterial oxygen saturation (Bridges et al., 1990b; Kopf et al, 1992; Laks, 1990; Mavroudis et al., 1992) (Fig. 45–13) Laks and colleagues (1991) encircle the fenestration with a snare that can be tightened in the intensive care unit. Other centers rely on transvenous techniques to close the fenestration after recovery from the operation (Bridges et al., 1990b; Kopf et al., 1992).

## RESULTS

### Palliative Operations

Franklin and associates (1991b) evaluated the effect of palliation on 191 consecutive infants with double-inlet ventricle. Survival rates after a systemic-pulmonary artery shunt were 84% at 1 year and 62% at 5

years. After pulmonary artery banding, survival rates were 77% at 1 year and 45% at 5 years. Survival rates after repair of aortic arch obstruction in addition to banding of the pulmonary trunk were significantly worse, with a 1-year survival of 44% and a 5-year survival of 22% (Fig. 45–14).

Of 136 infants considered at the time of presentation to be potential Fontan candidates, only 78 (57%) were alive and suitable candidates at 2 years of age. Sixty per cent of patients who received an initial systemic–pulmonary artery shunt and 42% of patients who underwent isolated pulmonary artery banding were still alive and suitable for a Fontan procedure at 2 years of age. Only 1 of the 12 patients (8%) who required coarctation repair and pulmonary artery banding remained alive and suitable for a Fontan procedure at the same interval. Other than death, the most common causes of unsuitability for a Fontan procedure were the development of subaortic stenosis (7 patients) and pulmonary vascular disease (5 patients) (Franklin et al., 1991c).

The poor prognosis of patients requiring aortic arch repair in addition to pulmonary artery banding is the rationale for applying the Norwood procedure or the arterial switch in these neonates. Early mortality for these procedures, however, is 20 to 30% (Rychik et al., 1991), and subsequent suitability for a Fontan procedure is not assured.

## Definitive Procedures

### Ventricular Septation

The major limitation with ventricular septation has been its stringent anatomic requirements. In the study

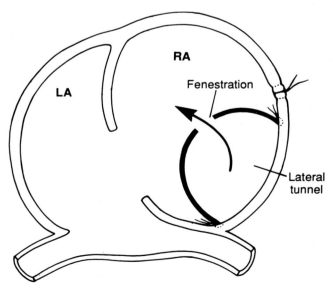

**FIGURE 45–13.** Cross-sectional view of lateral tunnel in which fenestration has been made to permit controlled right-to-left shunting. (From Kopf, G. S., Kleinman, C. S., Hijazi, Z. M., et al.: Fenestrated Fontan operation with delayed transcatheter closure of atrial septal defect. J. Thorac. Cardiovasc. Surg., *103*:1039, 1992.)

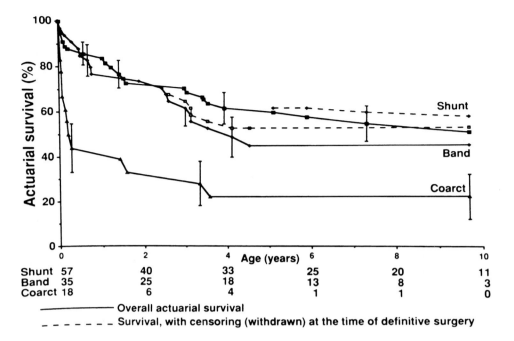

**FIGURE 45–14.** Actuarial survival of patients with double-inlet ventricle after initial systemic-PA shunt, PA banding, or repair of coarctation (or aortic interruption) plus PA banding. (From Franklin, R. C. G., Spiegelhalter, D. J., Anderson, R. H., et al.: Double-inlet ventricle presenting in infancy. II. Results of palliative operations. J. Thorac. Cardiovasc. Surg., *101*:917, 1991.)

by Franklin and co-workers (1991c), only 23% of patients had suitable morphology for septation at the time of presentation. By 2 years of age, only 70% of this group (16% of the initial group) were still alive and candidates for septation.

The hospital mortality rate after ventricular septation is 30 to 40%, and surgical heart block develops in over 80% of patients (Pacifico, 1986). Given the limited number of suitable patients, the high hospital mortality, and the high incidence of complete heart block, very little enthusiasm currently exists for this procedure.

### Fontan Procedure

The early and late results of the Fontan procedure have been less favorable for patients with univentricular heart than for those with tricuspid atresia. Nevertheless, Mayer and colleagues (1992), describing their results in 225 patients with functional single ventricle, demonstrated an overall failure rate (death or Fontan takedown) of 13.3%. In the last 2 years of the study, failure rates had decreased to 6.5 and 3.4%. A Mayo Clinic study of long-term follow-up after a Fontan procedure in patients with univentricular heart demonstrated a 1-year survival of 81%, a 5-year survival of 73%, and a somewhat disappointing 10-year survival of 57% (Driscoll et al., 1992). A similar study in 124 patients at the Hospital for Sick Children in Toronto, Canada, revealed actuarial survival of 77% at 1 year, 66% at 5 years, and 49% at 10 years (Cohen et al., 1991). The declining survival late postoperatively is similar to what has been seen in patients with tricuspid atresia (Driscoll et al., 1992; Fontan et al., 1990). Despite this decline in late survival, the functional status of long-term survivors of the Fontan

procedure for univentricular heart has been good to excellent in most patients (Mair et al., 1992).

## SELECTED BIBLIOGRAPHY

Anderson, R. H., Crupi, G., and Parenzan, L. (eds): Double-Inlet Ventricle: Anatomy, Diagnosis and Surgical Management. New York, Elsevier, 1987.

This text is probably the most comprehensive treatise on the univentricular heart that exists. Because of the date of its publication, the surgical section does not discuss some more recent techniques. The chapters on anatomy and terminology, however, clarify a confusing subject.

Driscoll, D. J., Offord, K. P., Feldt, R. H., et al.: Five- to fifteen-year follow-up after Fontan operation. Circulation, *85*:469, 1992.

This monumental study describes the results of the Fontan procedure in 352 patients operated on between 1973 and 1984 at the Mayo Clinic. Unsurpassed in terms of number of patients followed and length of follow-up, this paper provides an accurate assessment of the long-term results of the Fontan operation in patients with tricuspid atresia and those with univentricular heart.

Franklin, R. C. G., Spiegelhalter, D. J., Anderson, R. H., et al.: Double-inlet ventricle presenting in infancy. I. Survival without definitive repair. J. Thorac. Cardiovasc. Surg., *101*:767, 1991a.

This study of 191 consecutive infants with double-inlet ventricle presenting in the first year of life examines the "natural history" of this lesion before definitive repair. The effect of risk factors on survival is identified and illustrated.

Franklin, R. C. G., Spiegelhalter, D. J., Anderson, R. H., et al.: Double-inlet ventricle presenting in infancy. II. Results of palliative operations. J. Thorac. Cardiovasc. Surg., *101*:917, 1991.

The effect of palliative operations on natural history is investigated in this study of 191 consecutive patients with double-inlet ventricle.

Franklin, R. C. G., Spiegelhalter, D. J., Filho, R. I. R., et al.: Double-inlet ventricle presenting in infancy. III. Outcome and potential for definitive repair. J. Thorac. Cardiovasc. Surg., *101*:924, 1991.

The suitability for definitive repair with either ventricular septation or the Fontan operation is examined in 191 consecutive infants with double-inlet ventricle.

Franklin, R. C. G., Sullivan, I. D., Anderson, R. H., et al.: Is banding of the pulmonary trunk obsolete for infants with tricuspid atresia and double-inlet ventricle with a discordant ventriculoarterial connection? Role of aortic arch obstruction and subaortic stenosis. J. Am. Coll. Cardiol., 16:1455, 1990.

This analysis of 102 patients demonstrates that the presence of aortic arch obstruction is associated with the rapid development of subaortic stenosis after pulmonary artery banding.

Kirklin, J. W., and Barratt-Boyes, B. G.: Double-inlet ventricle and atretic atrioventricular valve. In Kirklin, J. W., and Barratt-Boyes, B. G. (eds): Cardiac Surgery. 2nd ed. Chap. 44. New York, Churchill Livingstone, 1993.

This chapter presents a comprehensive and up-to-date review of the morphology and natural history of these defects. The technical details of the surgical procedures are well described and illustrated. Results of surgical management of these complex lesions are thoroughly analyzed.

# BIBLIOGRAPHY

Abbott, M. E.: Atlas of Congenital Cardiac Disease. New York, American Heart Association, 1936.

Anderson, R. H.: Weasel words in pediatric cardiology: Single ventricle. Int. J. Cardiol., 2:425, 1983.

Anderson, R. H., Crupi, G., and Parenzan, L. (eds): Double-Inlet Ventricle: Anatomy, Diagnosis and Surgical Management. New York, Elsevier, 1987.

Anderson, R. H., Penkoske, P. A., and Zuberbuhler, J. R.: Variable morphology of ventricular septal defect in double-inlet left ventricle. Am. J. Cardiol., 55:1560, 1985.

Anderson, R. H., Tynan, M., Freedom, R. M., et al.: Ventricular morphology in the univentricular heart. Herz, 4:194, 1979.

Blalock, A., and Hanlon, C. R.: The surgical treatment of complete transposition of the aorta and the pulmonary artery. Surg. Gynecol. Obstet., 90:1, 1950.

Blalock, A., and Taussig, H. B.: The surgical treatment of malformations of the heart in which there is pulmonary stenosis or pulmonary atresia. J. A. M. A., 128:189, 1945.

Bridges, N. D., Jones, R. A., Mayer, J. E., et al.: Bidirectional cavopulmonary anastomosis as interim palliation for high-risk Fontan candidates: Early results. Circulation, 82(Suppl. IV):IV-70, 1990a.

Bridges, N. D., Lock, J. E., and Castañeda, A. R.: Baffle fenestration with subsequent transcatheter closure: Modification of the Fontan operation for patients at increased risk. Circulation, 82:1681, 1990b.

Cheung, H. C., Lincoln, C., Anderson, R. H., et al.: Options for surgical repair in hearts with univentricular atrioventricular connection and subaortic stenosis. J. Thorac. Cardiovasc. Surg., 100:672, 1990.

Cohen, A. J., Cleveland, D. C., Dyck, J., et al.: Results of the Fontan procedure for patients with univentricular heart. Ann. Thorac. Surg., 52:266, 1991.

Douville, E. C., Sade, R. M., and Fyfe, D. A.: Hemi-Fontan operation in surgery for single ventricle: A preliminary report. Ann. Thorac. Surg., 51:893, 1991.

Driscoll, D. J., Offord, K. P., Feldt, R. H., et al.: Five- to fifteen-year follow-up after Fontan operation. Circulation, 85:469, 1992.

Edie, R. N., Ellis, K., Gersony, W. M., et al.: Surgical repair of single ventricle. J. Thorac. Cardiovasc. Surg., 66:350, 1973.

Fontan, F., and Baudet, E.: Surgical repair of tricuspid atresia. Thorax, 26:240, 1971.

Fontan, F., Kirklin, J. W., Fernandez, G., et al.: Outcome after a "perfect" Fontan operation. Circulation, 81:1520, 1990.

Franklin, R. C. G., Spiegelhalter, D. J., Anderson, R. H., et al.: Double-inlet ventricle presenting in infancy. I. Survival without definitive repair. J. Thorac. Cardiovasc. Surg., 101:767, 1991a.

Franklin, R. C. G., Spiegelhalter, D. J., Anderson, R. H., et al.: Double-inlet ventricle presenting in infancy. II. Results of palliative operations. J. Thorac. Cardiovasc. Surg., 101:917, 1991b.

Franklin, R. C. G., Spiegelhalter, D. J., Filho, R. I. R., et al.: Double-inlet ventricle presenting in infancy. III. Outcome and potential for definitive repair. J. Thorac. Cardiovasc. Surg., 101:924, 1991c.

Franklin, R. C. G., Sullivan, I. D., Anderson, R. H., et al.: Is banding of the pulmonary trunk obsolete for infants with tricuspid atresia and double-inlet ventricle with a discordant ventriculoarterial connection? Role of aortic arch obstruction and subaortic stenosis. J. Am. Coll. Cardiol., 16:1455, 1990.

Freed, M., Rosenthal, A., Plauth, W. J. J., Jr., and Nadas, A. S.: Development of subaortic stenosis after pulmonary artery banding. Circulation, 43:83, 1971.

Freedom, R. M.: The dinosaur and banding of the main pulmonary trunk in the heart with functionally one ventricle and transposition of the great arteries: A saga of evolution and caution. J. Am. Coll. Cardiol., 10:427, 1987.

Freedom, R. M., and Trusler, G. A.: Arterial switch for palliation of subaortic stenosis in single ventricle and transposition: No mean feat? Ann. Thorac. Surg., 52:415, 1991.

Freedom, R. M., Benson, L. N., Smallhorn, J. F., et al.: Subaortic stenosis, the univentricular heart, and banding of the pulmonary artery: An analysis of the courses of 43 patients with univentricular heart palliated by pulmonary artery banding. Circulation, 43:758, 1986.

Freedom, R. M., Sondheimer, H., Dische, R., and Rowe, R. D.: Development of "subaortic stenosis" after pulmonary arterial banding for common ventricle. Am. J. Cardiol. 39:78, 1977.

Holmes, A. F.: Case of malformation of the heart. Trans. Med. Chir. Soc. Edinb., 1:252, 1824.

Ilbawi, M. N., Deleon, S. Y., Wilson, W. R., et al.: Advantages of early relief of subaortic stenosis in single-ventricle equivalents. Ann. Thorac. Surg., 52:842, 1991.

Jonas, R. A., and Castañeda, A. R.: Modified Fontan procedure: Atrial baffle and systemic venous to pulmonary artery anastomotic techniques. J. Card. Surg., 3:91, 1988.

Jonas, R. A., Castañeda, A. R., and Lang, P.: Single ventricle (single- or double-inlet) complicated by subaortic stenosis: Surgical options in infancy. Ann. Thorac. Surg., 39:361, 1985.

Karl, T. R., Watterson, K. G., Sano, S., and Mee, R. B. B.: Operations for subaortic stenosis in univentricular hearts. Ann. Thorac. Surg. 52:420, 1991.

Kirklin, J. W., and Barratt-Boyes, B. G.: Cardiac Surgery. 2nd ed. New York, Churchill Livingstone, 1993.

Kopf, G. S., Kleinman, C. S., Hijazi, Z. M., et al.: Fenestrated Fontan operation with delayed transcatheter closure of atrial septal defect. J. Thorac. Cardiovasc. Surg., 103:1039, 1992.

Lacour-Gayet, F., Serraf, A., Fermont, L., et al.: Early palliation of univentricular hearts with subaortic stenosis and ventriculoarterial discordance. J. Thorac. Cardiovasc. Surg., 104:1238, 1992.

Laks, H.: The partial Fontan procedure: A new concept and its clinical application [Editorial]. Circulation, 82:1866, 1990.

Laks, H., Gates, R. N., Elami, A., and Pearl, J. M.: Damus-Stansel-Kaye procedure: Technical modifications. Ann. Thorac. Surg., 54:169, 1992.

Laks, H., Pearl, J. M., Haas, G. S., et al.: Partial Fontan: Advantages of an adjustable interatrial communication. Ann. Thorac. Surg., 52:1084, 1991.

Lamberti, J. J., Spicer, R. L., Waldman, J. D., et al.: The bidirectional cavopulmonary shunt. J. Thorac. Cardiovasc. Surg., 100:22, 1990.

Lin, A. E., Laks, H., Barber, G., et al.: Subaortic obstruction in complex congenital heart disease: Management by proximal artery to ascending aorta end-to-side anastomosis. J. Am. Coll. Cardiol., 7:617, 1986.

Mair, D. D., Puga, F. J., and Danielson, G. K.: Late functional status of survivors of the Fontan procedure performed during the 1970s. Circulation, 86(Suppl. II):II-106, 1992.

Matitiau, A., Geva, T., Colan, S. D., et al.: Bulboventricular foramen size in infants with double-inlet left ventricle or tricuspid atresia with transposed great arteries: Influence on initial palliative operation and rate of growth. J. Am. Coll. Cardiol., 19:142, 1992.

Mavroudis, C., Zales, V. R., Backer, C. L., et al.: Fenestrated Fontan with delayed catheter closure. Circulation, 86(Suppl. II):II-85, 1992.

Mayer, J. E., Bridges, N. D., Lock, J. E., et al.: Factors associated with marked reduction in mortality for Fontan operations in patients with single ventricle. J. Thorac. Cardiovasc. Surg., 103:444, 1992.

McGoon, D. C., Danielson, G. K., Ritter, D. G., et al.: Correction of the univentricular heart having two atrioventricular valves. J. Thorac. Cardiovasc. Surg., 74:218, 1977.

Muller, W. H., Jr., and Damman, J. F., Jr.: Treatment of certain congenital malformations of the heart by the creation of pulmonic stenosis to reduce pulmonary hypertension and excessive pulmonary blood flow: A preliminary report. Surg. Gynecol. Obstet., *95*:213, 1952.

Pacifico, A. D.: Surgical treatment of double-inlet ventricle ("single ventricle"). J. Card. Surg., *1*:105, 1986.

Pacifico, A. D., Kirklin, J. W., and Kirklin, J. K.: Single ventricle with double-inlet atrioventricular connection. *In* Arciniegas, E. (ed): Pediatric Cardiac Surgery. Chicago, Year Book Medical, 1985.

Pearl, J. M., Laks, H., Stein, D. G., et al.: Total cavopulmonary anastomosis versus conventional modified Fontan procedure. Ann. Thorac. Surg., *52*:189, 1991.

Pridjian, A. K., Mendelsohn, A. M., Lupinetti, F. M., et al.: Usefulness of the bidirectional Glenn procedure as staged reconstruction for the functional single ventricle. Am. J. Cardiol., *71*:959, 1993.

Razzouk, A. J., Freedom, R. M., Cohen, A. J., et al.: The recognition, identification of morphological substrate, and therapy of subaortic stenosis after a Fontan operation: An analysis of 12 patients. J. Thorac. Cardiovasc. Surg., *104*:938, 1992.

Redo, S. F., Engle, M. A., Ehlers, K. H., and Farnsworth, P. B.: Palliative surgery for mitral atresia. Arch. Surg., *95*:717, 1967.

Rychik, J., Mundison, K. A., Chin, A. J., and Norwood, W. I.: Surgical management of severe aortic outflow obstruction in lesions other than the hypoplastic left heart syndrome: Use of a pulmonary artery to aorta anastomosis. J. Am. Coll. Cardiol., *18*:809, 1991.

Sakakibara, S., Tomimaga, S., Imai, Y., et al.: Successful total correction of common ventricle. Chest, *61*:192, 1972.

Tchervenkov, C. I., Beland, M. J., Latter, D. A., and Dobell, A. R. C.: Norwood operation for univentricular heart with subaortic stenosis in the neonate. Ann. Thorac. Surg. *50*:822, 1990.

Van Praagh, R., Ongley, P. A., and Swan, H. J. C.: Anatomic types of single or common ventricle in man. Morphologic and geometric aspects of 60 necropsied cases. Am. J. Cardiol., *13*:367, 1964.

Yacoub, M. H., and Radley-Smith, R.: Use of a valved conduit from right atrium to pulmonary artery for "correction" of single ventricle. Circulation, *54*(Suppl. III):III-63, 1976.

# 46 Tricuspid Atresia

John R. Handy, Jr., and Robert M. Sade

The hallmark of tricuspid atresia is the absence of direct communication between the right atrium and the right ventricle. It is the third most common congenital heart malformation, after tetralogy of Fallot and transposition of the great arteries.

The special importance of tricuspid atresia is that it served as the focal point for the development of a corrective operation for children with only one functional ventricle: the Fontan operation. The concept underlying this procedure, that a pump is not needed for the pulmonary circuit, was startling when introduced in 1971 (Fontan and Baudet, 1971). Few new cardiac operations have proved to apply to such various pathologies and to accommodate such a multitude of technical modifications (Cowgill, 1991).

## HISTORICAL NOTE

The first clear description of a heart with the anatomic features of tricuspid atresia was that of Kreysig in 1817 (Rashkind, 1982). Schuberg (1861) first applied the term *atresia* to this malformation. Although several cases were described in the 19th-century English language literature, the first use of the term *atresia* did not appear in that literature until 1917 (Hess). Kuhne (1906) recognized that patients with tricuspid atresia may have either normally related or transposed great arteries.

Surgical treatment for tricuspid atresia began in 1945 when Blalock performed a subclavian artery–to–pulmonary artery anastomosis in a patient with tricuspid atresia only a few months after he first used the operation in tetralogy of Fallot (Taussig et al., 1973). Subsequently, Potts and associates (1946) introduced the descending aortopulmonary shunt and Waterston (1962) developed the ascending aortopulmonary shunt. A different kind of palliative shunt, connecting a systemic vein directly to a pulmonary artery, was investigated experimentally by Carlon and colleagues (1951) and was clinically applied by Glenn (1958) and Bakulev and Kolesnikov (1959).

Surgical palliation of tricuspid atresia may include enlargement of a restrictive *atrial septal defect* (ASD): a surgical method was first described by Blalock and Hanlon in 1950 and a cardiac catheterization technique, balloon atrioseptostomy, by Rashkind and Miller in 1966. Occasionally, a patient with tricuspid atresia with excessive pulmonary blood flow has benefited from the technique of pulmonary artery banding, first described by Muller and Dammann (1952).

Surgical correction of tricuspid atresia was first performed by Fontan in 1968 and reported by Fontan and Baudet in 1971. Their revolutionary procedure rested on the observation, first made by Carlon and colleagues (1951), that pulmonary vascular resistance (PVR) is so low that a pumping chamber is not needed for the pulmonary circuit. A wide variety of techniques to connect the systemic venous return to the pulmonary artery in various malformations have been developed, and are called *modified Fontan operations*.

## CLASSIFICATION AND ANATOMY

The term *tricuspid atresia* is likely to remain in widespread use, although its embryologic, morphologic, and anatomic accuracy has been the object of debate (Anderson and Rigby, 1987). Tricuspid atresia is the largest subgroup of a collection of anomalies referred to as *univentricular atrioventricular connection* (Anderson et al., 1984), which includes double-inlet left ventricle, mitral atresia, and other lesions. The logic of this grouping is reinforced by the fact that coronary artery distribution and ventricular morphology of hearts with tricuspid atresia and those with double-inlet left ventricle are nearly identical (Deanfield et al., 1982).

Edwards and Burchell's (1949) classification by associated malformations is still widely used in modified form (Fig. 46–1), although it does not accommodate some examples of tricuspid atresia by the definition given earlier (Anderson and Rigby, 1987). In the most common type of tricuspid atresia, Edwards and Burchell's Type Ib, the atria are normally related and the tricuspid valve is represented by a dimple in the muscular floor of the right atrium.

An atrial septal communication is always present. It is a patent foramen ovale in 60% of patients, and in the remainder, it is an ASD, usually ostium secundum. The communication is generally widely patent, but may be restrictive, especially when the ventriculoarterial connection is discordant (Weinberg, 1980).

The atresia of the right atrioventricular connection may take many morphologic forms (Van Praagh et al., 1971). Most commonly, there is a dimple in the floor of the right atrium directly overlying the left ventricle (Rosenquist et al., 1970), suggesting total absence of any relation between right atrium and right ventricle. Rarely, a normally formed right atrium and right ventricle are separated by an imperforate membrane in the tricuspid orifice (Crupi et al., 1984).

The relation of the right atrium to the ventricles is

1628

TRICUSPID ATRESIA WITH NORMALLY RELATED GREAT ARTERIES

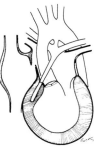 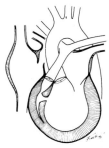 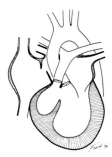

Ia PULMONARY ATRESIA          Ib PULMONARY HYPOPLASIA, SMALL          Ic NO PULMONARY HYPOPLASIA, LARGE
                                 VENTRICULAR SEPTAL DEFECT                 VENTRICULAR SEPTAL DEFECT

TRICUSPID ATRESIA WITH *d*-TRANSPOSITION

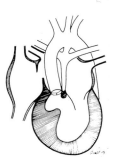 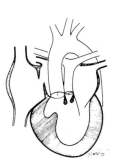 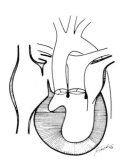

IIa PULMONARY ATRESIA          IIb PULMONARY STENOSIS          IIc LARGE PULMONARY ARTERY

TRICUSPID ATRESIA WITH *l*-TRANSPOSITION

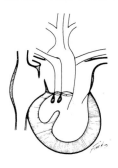

III SUBPULMONARY OR SUBAORTIC STENOSIS

**FIGURE 46–1.** Classification of tricuspid atresia according to associated lesions. *Type I* refers to normally related great arteries, *Type II* to *d*-transposition, and *Type III* to *l*-transposition. *Subtype a* refers to pulmonary atresia, *Subtype b* to pulmonary stenosis, and *Type c* to unobstructed pulmonary outflow tract. (From Keith, J. D., Rowe, R. D., and Vlad, P.: Heart Disease in Infancy and Childhood. New York, Macmillan, 1967.)

not constant. In the case of imperforate valve, the valve membrane is usually committed entirely to the right ventricle, but it may override an intact ventricular septum, relating to both the right ventricle and the left ventricle (Ottenkamp et al., 1984). A similar spectrum in cases of absent valve was postulated by Wenink and Ottenkamp (1987) when they found that the dimple in the right atrial floor may connect by way of a fibrous strand with the right ventricle rather than the left. Thus, the relation of the right atrium to the right ventricle may be concordant, discordant, or biventricular (Anderson and Rigby, 1987).

The morphology of the right ventricle is different in cases of ventriculoarterial concordance from those with discordance (Ottenkamp et al., 1985). In both situations, the inlet portion of the right ventricle is usually absent. In *ventriculoarterial concordance,* the

outlet foramen (ventricular septal defect [VSD]) separates the inferior trabeculated portion of the right ventricle from the superior infundibular portion. Obstruction to pulmonary blood flow is common (80% of patients), and is usually due to a small outlet foramen, often accompanied by infundibular stenosis, and occasionally by valvular stenosis. In contrast, in *ventriculoarterial discordance,* the right ventricle not only lacks an inlet portion but also an infundibular outlet, so the outlet foramen is immediately subjacent to the aortic valve, and the outlet chamber (right ventricle) is completely trabeculated. Malalignment of the outlet septum lying between the pulmonary artery and the aorta reciprocally affects the size of the subpulmonary and subaortic regions. Restricted pulmonary blood flow is seen in only 40% of patients with ventriculoarterial discordance, and subaortic stenosis rarely occurs; in cases of unrestricted pulmonary blood flow, subaortic stenosis is often seen, and may be associated with aortic anomalies such as coarctation, isthmic hypoplasia or atresia, interruption of the aortic arch, or aortic valve atresia.

Other lesions of the heart and great vessels associated with tricuspid atresia may have important implications for surgical management. A left superior vena cava is present in 22% of patients (Weinberg, 1980), usually draining to the coronary sinus. Unusual interatrial communications may confound complete separation of the right from the left atrium. Coronary sinus septal defect (Lee and Sade, 1979) may occur in as many as 2.5% of patients with tricuspid atresia and, if not recognized, may leave a residual right-to-left shunt after the Fontan procedure (Coles et al., 1987; Rumisek et al., 1986). The same physiology may occur owing to cardiac veins connecting the coronary sinus to the left atrium (Westerman et al., 1985). Anomalous pulmonary venous return (Scalia, 1984) and coronary artery anomalies (Voci et al., 1987) rarely occur.

Congenital absence of the pulmonary valve (pulmonary orifice unguarded by a valve) may be associated with tricuspid atresia of the imperforate membrane type, usually with ventriculoarterial concordance, aortic dilatation, and intact ventricular septum (Marin-Garcia et al., 1973). Unlike absence of the pulmonary valve in tetralogy of Fallot, the pulmonary arteries are not large and bronchial compression does not occur (Forrest et al., 1987).

Juxtaposition of the atrial appendages may occur in tricuspid atresia in as many as 20% of patients with ventriculoarterial discordance (Scalia et al., 1984; Weinberg, 1980). The smallness and inaccessibility of the right atrial appendage may affect the options for atriopulmonary anastomosis, and in addition, the volume of the right atrium itself is reduced (Scalia et al., 1984).

## PATHOPHYSIOLOGY

The systemic venous return cannot reach the ventricular cavity directly, so it must cross an atrial septal communication from the right atrium to the left atrium where it mixes with the pulmonary venous return. The mixed blood reaches the ventricular cavity by traversing the mitral valve, which is larger than normal, and enters a hyperplastic left ventricle. The mixed blood exits the left ventricle through a normally connected aortic valve and aorta. Blood reaches the lungs from the left ventricle through an outlet foramen, into the hypoplastic right ventricle, which connects normally to a pulmonary valve and pulmonary artery. Additional pulmonary blood flow may come from a *patent ductus arteriosus* (PDA).

Certain hemodynamic characteristics are shared among all subtypes of tricuspid atresia. The atrial septal communication is usually large and nonobstructive, but in some patients with ventriculoarterial discordance, it may be obstructively small. The systemic and the pulmonary venous returns are totally mixed in the pulmonary venous atrium. The oxygen saturations in the chambers and vessels downstream from the mitral valve are the same.

Patients with a restrictive subpulmonary pathway have reduced pulmonary blood flow and pulmonary venous return is reduced, so they are moderately to severely hypoxemic (71% of patients) (Keith et al., 1978). The small additional volume load on the left ventricle usually does not cause congestive heart failure (CHF).

Patients without subpulmonary obstruction have excessive pulmonary blood flow. The increased pulmonary venous return produces a highly oxygenated mixture of blood in the left atrium and systemic circulation, so these patients are frequently acyanotic. The left ventricle must do the work of pumping a large pulmonary blood flow, and this overload often leads to CHF. Severe CHF is usually seen in patients with ventriculoarterial discordance. They may develop pulmonary vascular obstructive disease owing to increased pulmonary blood flow, and may continue to have a significant increase in pulmonary arterial smooth muscle despite banding of the pulmonary artery (Juaneda and Haworth, 1984).

Patients with ventriculoarterial concordance and unrestricted pulmonary blood flow usually have mild or moderate CHF that responds well to anticongestive medications. The outlet foramen, however, often decreases in size over time, and this may lead to progressively increasing pulmonary outflow obstruction, increasing cyanosis, and the eventual need for a systemic-to–pulmonary artery shunt (Gallaher and Fyler, 1967).

## CLINICAL FEATURES AND NATURAL HISTORY

Tricuspid atresia afflicts boys and girls about equally, although there is a slight male predominance among the patients with ventriculoarterial discordance (Dick et al., 1975). Its incidence ranges from 1% of all children with heart malformations in clinical series (Nadas and Fyler, 1972) to 3% in autopsy series (Keith et al., 1978). Of all infants with a heart malformation who were hospitalized or died in the first year of life, 2.5% had tricuspid atresia (Rosenthal, 1980).

Cyanosis or a heart murmur is found in 50% of patients on the first day of life, and 85% are recognized within the first 2 months. Cyanosis is the most constant clinical finding (Nadas and Fyler, 1972). Squatting occurs rarely, and clubbing is usually present in cyanotic patients over the age of 2 years. Hypoxic spells, comprising hyperpnea, increased cyanosis, and occasionally loss of consciousness, may be seen in half the patients.

CHF occurs in 12% of patients (Dick et al., 1975), frequently during infancy. Mild CHF may remain stable for many years but, if severe, may produce a high mortality rate. Right-sided heart failure may be manifested by systemic venous congestion, hepatomegaly, liver and jugular pulsation, and peripheral edema. It may be consequent to left-sided heart failure, or may occur because of obstruction to right side of the heart emptying by a small atrial septal communication. Cerebral vascular accidents and brain abscess may occur, but are relatively uncommon (less than 5% of patients). Infective endocarditis occurs in less than 5% of patients without previous operations.

The electrocardiogram demonstrates left axis deviation in almost 90% of patients: Its presence in a cyanotic child should raise a strong suspicion of tricuspid atresia. Right axis deviation may be seen with patients with ventriculoarterial discordance and unrestricted pulmonary blood flow. Left ventricular hypertrophy is almost always present, and may progress over time. The P wave may indicate right, left, or combined atrial hypertrophy.

The appearance of the chest x-ray is extremely variable (Wittenborg et al., 1951). The heart size is usually normal or only slightly increased. Cardiomegaly may become quite marked, however, when pulmonary blood flow is large. The cardiac silhouette is not characteristic. A right aortic arch is seen in 8% of patients.

Pulmonary vascular markings are usually reduced in patients with decreased pulmonary blood flow. Pulmonary plethora may be seen in patients with increased pulmonary blood flow associated with large outlet foramen, a large PDA, or a large systemic-to–pulmonary artery shunt (Keith et al., 1978). The natural history of tricuspid atresia is one of early death for most patients. Fifty per cent die within the first 6 months of life, and about 66% within 1 year. By 10 years, 90% of patients are dead.

Patients with extremes of pulmonary blood flow usually die before the age of 3 months. Survival for several decades is associated with adequate but not excessive pulmonary blood flow, low PVR, and no associated congenital heart malformations (Patterson et al., 1982). In one large series, 6 of 18 patients age 15 to 45 years had no previous surgery. The longest survivor without surgery died at the age of 65 years (Beaver et al., 1988): He had tricuspid and pulmonic valve atresia, a secundum ASD with pulmonary perfusion supplied by aortopulmonary collateral vessels.

Certain anatomic and physiologic changes may occur with increasing age. Progressive cyanosis may occur in association with decreasing size of outlet foramen (Gallaher and Fyler, 1967; Rao, 1983b), and this may advance to complete closure. In cases of markedly increased pulmonary blood flow, initial lack of cyanosis may replaced by progressive cyanosis with the development and advancement of pulmonary vascular obstructive disease (Patterson et al., 1982). Declining left ventricular function may occur with increasing age in unoperated patients and in those with aortopulmonary shunts (LaCorte et al., 1975).

The grim prognosis of tricuspid atresia is reflected in life insurance practices in the United States. Although patients with many types of congenital heart disease are considered insurable at standard or in-creased rates, patients diagnosed as having tricuspid atresia are considered completely uninsurable by 89% of insurance companies (Truesdell et al., 1986).

## DIAGNOSTIC STUDIES

### Echocardiography

Echocardiography has become the primary diagnostic test for tricuspid atresia (Fig. 46–2). Two-dimensional and M-mode echocardiography can define all the anatomic features of tricuspid atresia: the size and location of cardiac chambers, great arteries, cardiac valves, ASDs, outlet foramen, and PDAs. It can also detect and define associated malformations, such as subaortic stenosis, coarctation of the aorta, left superior vena cava, and juxtaposition of the atrial appendages. Echocardiography can clarify the relation of the right atrium to the ventricular mass, and can distinguish among the several types of tricuspid atresia (absent atrioventricular connection, imperforate tricuspid valve, Ebstein's malformation with imperforate valve, and double-chamber right ventricle with complete intraventricular septum).

Doppler echocardiography provides additional physiologic information. It can assess pressure gradients across septal defects and cardiac valves and can detect and quantitate valvular regurgitation. Echocardiography cannot accurately assess the size of branch pulmonary arteries outside the pericardium or the amount of pulmonary blood flow.

### Magnetic Resonance Imaging

The place of magnetic resonance imaging (MRI) in the evaluation of tricuspid atresia is not established.

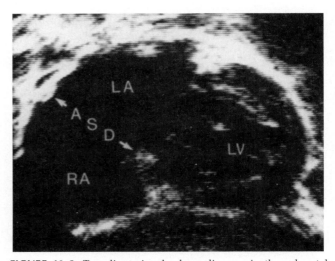

**FIGURE 46–2.** Two-dimensional echocardiogram in the subcostal view showing features of tricuspid atresia. A large atrial septal defect (ASD) is noted. The right atrium (RA) does not communicate with a ventricle. The left atrium (LA) and left ventricle (LV) appear to be normal.

In general, it provides anatomic information similar to that provided by echocardiography, but is less useful in providing physiologic data. MRI has been successful in determining the size of the cardiac chambers, the appearance of the great arteries, the visceroatrial situs, the type of ventricular loop, and the relations of the great arteries (Didier et al., 1986). MRI may be helpful in distinguishing types of tricuspid atresia: The right atrioventricular sulcus in typical tricuspid atresia is very deep and is filled with fat (Fletcher et al., 1987), appearing as a bright linear or triangular structure replacing the tricuspid valve. In cases of tricuspid atresia owing to imperforate valve or Ebstein's anomaly, the right atrioventricular sulcus is shallow, as it is in the normal heart. In a rare patient with an imperforate tricuspid valve, this information may be important in planning surgery (Crupi et al., 1984).

## Cardiac Catheterization

The hazards of cardiac catheterization are small, but greatest in the newborn. The completeness and accuracy of the diagnostic information provided by echocardiography now permits making therapeutic decisions, including those relating to palliative surgery, without cardiac catheterization. Catheterization is always required, however, before corrective operation is undertaken because of information it provides beyond that obtained at echocardiography. Size of pulmonary arteries, particularly those lying outside the pericardium, can be accurately determined by

angiocardiography. Estimation of severity of valve regurgitation can supplement that determined at echocardiography, and pressure gradients across septal defects and cardiac valves can confirm those determined by echocardiography. In particular, significant but low pressure gradients sometimes found across the atrial septal communication (on the order of 2 to 5 torr) are more accurately determined at cardiac catheterization than at echocardiography.

If blood pressure and oxygen data can be obtained in the systemic and pulmonary veins, both atria, and the great arteries, then accurate pressure, flow, and resistance calculations can be made that are obtainable in no other way. It is often not possible to obtain all this information at cardiac catheterization, particularly measurements in the right ventricle and pulmonary artery, so angiocardiographic information must be used to make inferences regarding pulmonary flow and resistance. Right atrial angiocardiography may show the size and location of the ASD, and also confirm the absence of a connection between the right atrium and the ventricles (Fig. 46–3). Selective left ventricular angiography perhaps provides the most valuable information: It delineates outlet foramen size, right ventricular size, and the degree and location of pulmonary stenosis. The systemic arterial oxygen saturation is directly related to the magnitude of pulmonary blood flow.

Pressure data are characteristic. The right ventricle cannot be entered through the tricuspid valve. There is a prominent A wave in the right atrium and a right-to-left shunt at the atrial level. A large pressure gradient across the atrial septum may be associated

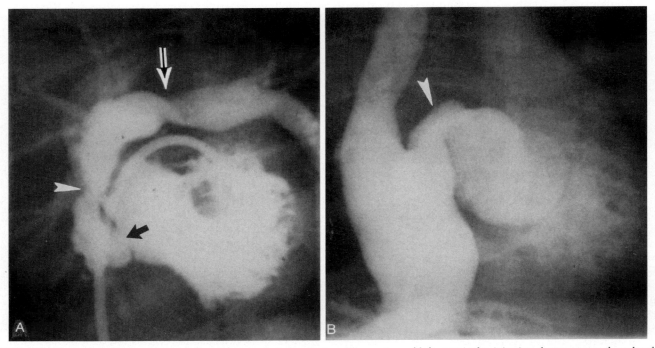

**FIGURE 46–3.** Angiocardiography in tricuspid atresia. *A*, Left anterior oblique view of left ventricular injection demonstrates three levels of obstruction to pulmonary blood flow: small ventricular septal defect (VSD) *(black arrow)*, obstructive infundibulum *(white arrowhead)*, and pulmonary annular stenosis *(white arrow)*. *B*, Left anterior oblique view of right atrial injection shows the flow of contrast material directly into the left atrium (LA) through an atrial septal defect (ASD) *(arrowhead)* and no flow into right ventricle (RV).

with a small ASD. Identical oxygen saturations are found in the left atrium, left ventricle, right ventricle, and great arteries.

## PALLIATIVE TREATMENT

The corrective operation for tricuspid atresia, the Fontan operation, cannot be performed safely in infants, so palliative operations are needed when insufficient pulmonary blood flow, excessive pulmonary blood flow, or an inadequate interatrial communication is present.

### Insufficient Pulmonary Blood Flow

#### Systemic-to–Pulmonary Artery Shunt

Newborns who become severely cyanotic can be resuscitated by continuous infusion of prostaglandin $E_1$ to restore patency of the ductus arteriosus (Elliott et al., 1975; Hatem et al., 1980). Use of this drug has dramatically improved the results of surgery for cyanotic newborns requiring a shunt operation. Ductal patency maintains pulmonary blood flow, and allows an elective operation on a stable patient. The infusion of prostaglandin $E_1$ may be continued if necessary for a week or longer (Teixeira et al., 1984).

The Blalock-Taussig shunt, in either its classic (direct anastomosis of the subclavian artery to a pulmonary artery) or its modified (interposition of a *polytetrafluoroethylene* [PTFE] graft between a subclavian artery and a pulmonary artery) form is now the most widely used systemic-to–pulmonary artery anastomosis. The current operative mortality risk of performing such a shunt in patients with tricuspid atresia is under 10% (Tam et al., 1989). The advantage of the Blalock-Taussig shunt, both classic and modified, is that the lumen of the subclavian artery limits pulmonary blood flow, so CHF due to excessive pulmonary blood flow and left ventricular volume overload is very infrequent (Deverall et al., 1969), but systemic oxygen saturation is adequate. Disadvantages of this shunt include decreased growth of the ipsilateral arm (Currarino and Engle, 1965), phrenic nerve injury (Smith et al., 1986), and rarely, tissue loss owing to gangrene (Geiss et al., 1980).

Two series in which the classic was compared with the modified Blalock-Taussig shunt (Moulton et al., 1985; Ullom et al., 1987) found the modified shunt to be superior to the classic shunt, especially in newborns, because it provides better immediate patency and arterial oxygen saturation, greater longevity of the shunt, better growth of the pulmonary arteries, and less distortion of the pulmonary arteries. Patients with tricuspid atresia who undergo systemic-to–pulmonary artery shunt have survival at 10 years of about 80% (Kirklin and Barratt-Boyes, 1986).

Several adverse anatomic and physiologic sequelae of systemic-to–pulmonary artery anastomoses militate against a successful future Fontan operation. Such shunts may lead to distortion of the pulmonary arterial tree or to pulmonary artery hypertension with increased pulmonary arterial resistance, high left ventricular end-diastolic volume and pressure owing to high pulmonary blood flow. These effects are most likely to occur after Potts' or Waterston's anastomoses because of difficulty in achieving appropriate shunt size (Arciniegas et al., 1980). In addition, distortion of the pulmonary arteries after such shunts may require reconstruction at the time of corrective surgery (Gay and Ebert, 1973). Nearly 25% of patients with tricuspid atresia who undergo an aortopulmonary shunt after the age of 1 year may develop a contraindication to the Fontan operation owing to adverse anatomic and physiologic effects of the shunt (Mietus-Snyder et al., 1987), so systemic-to–pulmonary artery anastomosis should probably be reserved for children who cannot safely undergo a bidirectional cavopulmonary anastomosis (those under 3 to 4 months of age), a Fontan operation (those under 10 to 12 months of age), or older children with substantial contraindications to such surgery.

#### Cavopulmonary Anastomosis

Cavopulmonary anastomosis has certain theoretical advantages over systemic-to–pulmonary artery anastomosis: The lung is supplied with pure systemic venous blood, the systemic venous pressure rises only slightly and remains in physiologic range, and there is no volume load on the ventricles. Pulmonary artery hypertension seldom occurs and endocarditis is rare (Robicsek et al., 1966).

Two important problems have been found to be associated with the classic cavopulmonary anastomosis: Superior vena cava syndrome may occur early postoperatively, and failure of palliation owing to increasing cyanosis and rising hematocrit may occur late. Superior vena cava syndrome results from too high a pressure in the superior vena cava and can be anatomically related to inadequate size of the pulmonary artery, so cavopulmonary anastomosis should not be performed unless the right pulmonary artery is at least the same diameter as the superior vena cava.

Late clinical deterioration after cavopulmonary anastomosis may be related to progressive subvalvular obstruction to pulmonary blood flow into the left lung, ventilation-perfusion imbalance as bronchiolar collateral vessels displace caval flow from the upper and middle lobes to the lower lobe (Mathur and Glenn, 1973), development of pulmonary arteriovenous fistulas (McFaul et al., 1977), decreasing right pulmonary artery flow owing to development of collateral vessels from the superior vena cava to the inferior vena cava (Laks et al., 1977), or increasing PVR because of the high viscosity associated with rising hematocrit (Mathur and Glenn, 1973). When clinical deterioration occurs, the treatment may be a Fontan operation, if that operation is not contraindicated, or a contralateral aortopulmonary shunt (DiCarlo et al., 1982).

A variant of cavopulmonary anastomosis that has

been found useful prior to an ultimate Fontan repair is the bidirectional cavopulmonary shunt, in which the proximal end of the divided superior vena cava is connected to the side of the right pulmonary artery, permitting superior vena caval flow into both lungs. The physiologic benefits of this procedure are the same as for the classic shunt, but in addition, disproportional commitment of 33% of the systemic venous return (superior vena cava) to 55% of the pulmonary capillary bed (right lung) is avoided, and the pulmonary arteries remain in continuity. In a series of 12 such operations prior to a Fontan procedure, there was excellent relief of cyanosis, and no deaths, shunt failures, pulmonary artery deformities, or arteriovenous fistulas (Hopkins et al., 1985).

The mortality associated with the Fontan operation after initial palliation in hypoplastic left-sided heart syndrome led to the development of a staged approach, wherein first a *hemi-Fontan* operation, dedicating the superior vena caval return to both pulmonary arteries, was established to allow the chronically volume-overloaded ventricle to resolve its hypertrophy. The operation is essentially a complete Fontan operation, except that a patch separating the atriocavopulmonary anastomosis from the right atrium commits the inferior vena cava to the systemic rather than the pulmonary circulation (Douville et al., 1991). Subsequent conversion to a total cavopulmonary connection is associated with improvement in survival (Norwood et al., 1992).

The physiology of the hemi-Fontan operation is that of a bidirectional cavopulmonary shunt, but all aortopulmonary shunts and ventriculopulmonary connections have been interrupted, thus relieving the ventricle of all pulmonary work. Additionally, cardiac output is not limited by pulmonary blood flow, as it is after the Fontan operation, because the inferior vena caval blood goes directly to the ventricle.

The hemi-Fontan has proved useful in patients who are candidates for the Fontan operation but are at high risk, patients whose physiology may benefit from early unloading of ventricular volume, and patients who develop low cardiac output and high pulmonary artery pressure after a Fontan operation (Douville et al., 1991). Technical and physiologic aspects of this procedure are illustrated in "Technique of Corrective Operation," later in this chapter.

### Current Management of Decreased Pulmonary Blood Flow

Newborns with tricuspid atresia associated with decreased pulmonary blood flow are placed on prostaglandin $E_1$ to stabilize them and to permit resuscitation if necessary. This is followed within a day or two by a modified Blalock-Taussig shunt using a 5-mm PTFE graft. Patients beyond the early newborn period up to 3 to 4 months of age also undergo a modified Blalock-Taussig shunt. If a patient in need of palliation is over 3 to 4 months of age or if an early shunt fails before the patient is 1 year old, a bidirectional cavopulmonary anastomosis or hemi-Fontan is per-

formed. Patients older than 1 year who require surgical intervention undergo a Fontan operation. If correction is contraindicated, then a bidirectional cavopulmonary anastomosis is performed.

### Enlargement of Atrial Septal Communication

If the obligatory interatrial communication is obstructively small, peripheral edema, pulsatile and distended neck veins, and hepatomegaly may denote right-sided heart failure. Echocardiography is usually able to define the diameter of the ASD, and Doppler echocardiography can estimate the interatrial pressure gradient (Fyfe et al., 1987). Cardiac catheterization may demonstrate a pressure difference between the atria of 3 torr or more.

If the atrial septal communication is inadequate, a balloon septostomy can be performed at cardiac catheterization if the patient is under 1 month of age (Rashkind and Miller, 1966). In older children, increased septal thickness may require blade septostomy at cardiac catheterization (Park et al., 1982). If these measures fail, an ASD can be surgically created by the closed technique of Blalock and Hanlon (1950), by open atrial septectomy under either inflow occlusion (Hallman et al., 1968) or cardiopulmonary bypass.

### Reduction of Excessive Pulmonary Blood Flow

Fortunately, fewer than 20% of all patients with tricuspid atresia (Keith et al., 1978) have unrestricted pulmonary blood flow, and only a fraction of them have CHF severe enough to need surgical treatment. Patients with tricuspid atresia and CHF due to increased pulmonary blood flow usually have ventriculoarterial discordance and little or no pulmonary stenosis. Pulmonary artery banding, as originally suggested by Muller and Dammann (1952), increases resistance to flow from the right ventricle to the pulmonary artery, pulmonary blood flow decreases, and the consequent decreased volume overload of the left ventricle alleviates CHF. Reduced pulmonary blood flow and pulmonary artery pressure decreases the possibility of later pulmonary vascular obstructive disease. The mortality rate of pulmonary artery banding for patients with tricuspid atresia has been about 30%, but survivors usually have good resolution of CHF (Sade, 1983).

Although pulmonary artery banding successfully palliates survivors by decreasing pulmonary blood flow and CHF, it does not completely protect against the development of pulmonary vascular obstructive disease. Even when the PVR after banding is less than 4 units m², significant pulmonary vascular abnormalities may remain: increased pulmonary vascular smooth muscle and occlusive organized pulmonary arterial thrombi (Juaneda and Haworth, 1984). The pulmonary artery band also frequently produces branch pulmonary arterial stenosis, more often on the right than on the left, increasing the risk of a later Fontan procedure.

In tricuspid atresia with ventriculoarterial discordance, as in other types of univentricular atrioventricular connection, there is a reciprocal relation between the size of the systemic and the pulmonary ventricular outlet flow pathways, so patients with large pulmonary blood flow are likely to have some degree of subaortic obstruction (Ottenkamp et al., 1985). Furthermore, when subaortic stenosis is clearly demonstrable anatomically, there may be no pressure gradient at rest, but a gradient can often be elicited with isoprenaline infusion at cardiac catheterization (Freedom et al., 1986). The outlet foramen in as many as 40% of patients with tricuspid atresia with ventriculoarterial discordance may decrease in size over time (Rao, 1983a), and this process may be accelerated by the presence of a pulmonary artery band (Freed et al., 1973). Because the outlet chamber is subaortic, decreasing size of the outlet foramen produces subaortic stenosis, ventricular hypertrophy, and a consequent decrease in ventricular diastolic compliance. Poor diastolic ventricular compliance and excessive left ventricular hypertrophy are important mortality risk factors after the Fontan operation (Caspi et al., 1990). Pulmonary artery banding itself has been implicated as a risk factor for death after a modified Fontan procedure.

For these reasons, the role for pulmonary artery banding in the surgical management of tricuspid atresia (and other kinds of univentricular atrioventricular connection) with increased pulmonary blood flow may be diminishing (Freedom, 1987). Subaortic stenosis may be resected or bypassed with a valve-bearing conduit from the left ventricular apex to the descending aorta (Penkoske et al., 1984; Rothman et al., 1987a), but neither procedure has had noteworthy success. Reasonable results have been achieved by creating an aortopulmonary window proximal to a pulmonary artery band (Park, 1982; Penkoske et al., 1984). The disadvantages of the pulmonary artery band itself, however, are not avoided with this procedure.

Several groups have used with success an alternative operation that employs the principle of the Norwood operation (Pigott et al., 1988) in this clinical situation, completely avoiding the use of a pulmonary artery band. The main pulmonary artery is divided, and its proximal end is sutured to the side of the ascending aorta, thus bypassing the subaortic obstruction. The procedure is completed with a palliative shunt to the pulmonary artery or a corrective Fontan operation (Jonas et al., 1985; Freedom, 1987; Lin et al., 1986) or a bidirectional cavopulmonary anastomosis (Di Donato et al., 1993).

Many uncertainties remain, but considering all the currently available information, certain recommendations can be made for patients with tricuspid atresia with unrestricted pulmonary blood flow. Anatomic and physiologic evaluation for subaortic obstruction should be done with two-dimensional and Doppler echocardiography and by cardiac catheterization, using exercise or catecholamines if no gradient can be demonstrated at rest. If there is no evidence of subaortic stenosis in young infants, the pulmonary artery may be banded. In patients with evidence of subaortic stenosis, the pulmonary artery may be divided, its proximal end anastomosed to the ascending aorta, and a Blalock-Taussig shunt (in patients under 3 to 4 months of age), or bidirectional cavopulmonary anastomosis (in patients over 3 to 4 months) constructed. All patients with a pulmonary artery band need surveillance for the development of subaortic obstruction. At the first appearance of anatomic evidence of subaortic stenosis with or without a gradient, the Norwood variant described previously should be performed in patients under about 1 year of age, or in patients over about 1 year, enlargement of the outlet foramen preceding or simultaneously with a Fontan operation.

## THE FONTAN OPERATION

Surgical correction of tricuspid atresia was made possible by a radical conceptual shift: the recognition that a ventricle is not needed for the pulmonary circulation (Fontan and Baudet, 1971; Sade and Castañeda, 1975), because PVR is normally so low that a minor rise in caval pressure is needed to create a transpulmonary vascular pressure gradient sufficient to move the systemic venous return across the pulmonary capillary bed. The development of the concept is illustrated in Figure 46–4.

### Selection of Candidates

On the basis of their early experience, Fontan and co-workers developed a list of specific anatomic and physiologic criteria that would permit a Fontan procedure to be performed safely by optimizing postoperative pulmonary blood flow and assuring low caval pressures (Choussat et al., 1978). Most of these risk factors have now been found to be relative rather than absolute contraindications to correction. Based on current information, the authors have modified Fontan's original list (Table 46–1).

**Age.** Age over 15 years is not a risk factor for operative survival (Mair et al., 1985; Mayer et al., 1986), although late survival may be adversely affected by deteriorating left ventricular function in some patients (Mair et al., 1985), and good operative survival in older patients may require more rigid adherence to selection criteria (Warnes and Somerville, 1987). Age under 4 years was a risk factor in earlier series (Cleveland et al., 1984; Fontan et al., 1983; Mair et al., 1985), but this appears no longer to be true (Kirklin et al., 1986; Mayer et al., 1986). The lower age limit for safe operation is not known, but operation is known to be dangerous during early infancy. It is likely that, at very young ages, the influ-

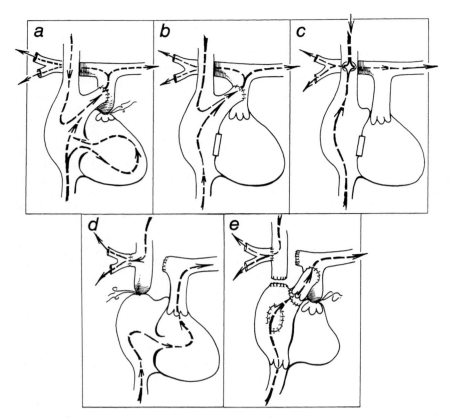

**FIGURE 46–4.** The development of procedures to bypass the RV. *a*, Rodbard and Wagner (1949) ligated the main pulmonary artery (MPA) and anastomosed the right atrial appendage to the distal MPA. *b*, Warden and associates (1954) did the same procedure but ligated the tricuspid instead of the pulmonary valve (PV). *c*, Haller and co-workers (1966) ligated the tricuspid valve, anastomosed the superior vena cava (SVC) to the right pulmonary artery (RPA), side to side. *d*, Carlon and colleagues (1951) ligated the cavoatrial junction and sutured the cut distal end of the RPA to the caval origin of the azygos vein. *e*, Fontan and Baudet (1971) corrected tricuspid atresia by constructing a cavopulmonary shunt, inserting an allograft valve in the inferior vena cava (IVC), interposing an allograft valve between the right atrial appendage and the pulmonary artery (PA), closing the ASD, and ligating the proximal MPA.

ence of other risk factors becomes more critical, particularly PVR more than 2 units m² and pulmonary artery distortion owing to preexisting shunts (Mayer et al., 1986). Age-related decreases in exercise performance (Driscoll et al., 1986) and increases in ventricular hypertrophy (Kirklin et al., 1986) have suggested that the best age for a Fontan operation is under 6 years, and may be as low as 6 to 7 months (Pearl et al., 1992; Weber et al., 1992). Performance of a Fontan procedure at a young age avoids the theoretical risks of chronic hypoxemia and the demonstrated risks of chronic ventricular volume overload, the mortality associated with palliative procedures, and the risk of developing pulmonary vascular obstructive disease.

**Rhythm.** Normal sinus rhythm is not required be-

### Table 46–1. CONTRAINDICATIONS TO THE FONTAN PROCEDURE

#### Absolute Contraindications

Early infancy (age <6–10 months)
Severe hypoplasia of parenchymal pulmonary arteries
Pulmonary vascular resistance >4 clinical units

#### Relative Contraindications

Age <1–2 years
Pulmonary artery pressure >15 mm Hg
Ventricular end-diastolic pressure >15 mm Hg
Pulmonary vascular resistance 2–4 clinical units
Previous pulmonary artery band
Substantial ventricular hypertrophy
Mitral or aortic valve insufficiency > mild

fore operation. Preexisting atrial flutter-fibrillation may be easier to control after the Fontan repair than before (Alboliras et al., 1985). Preoperative heart block can be treated with a pacemaker after corrective operation. Atrial contraction has even been found to be detrimental by creating turbulence and impeding pulmonary flow (DeLeval et al., 1988).

**Venous Drainage Pathways.** Abnormal systemic and pulmonary venous connections can usually be accommodated during corrective operation (King et al., 1985; Mair et al., 1985; Mayer et al., 1986; Vargas et al, 1987b), so they do not contraindicate the Fontan operations.

**Pulmonary Artery Pressure.** The mean pulmonary artery pressure need not be less than 15 torr (Mair et al., 1985; Mayer et al., 1986), and may be acceptable up to 25 torr, if associated with increased pulmonary blood flow and a low calculated PVR.

**Pulmonary Vascular Resistance.** Pulmonary vascular obstruction remains an absolute contraindication to the Fontan repair: This may be indicated by a PVR more than 4 units m² (Mair et al., 1985) or by incomplete arborization of the peripheral pulmonary arteries (Kirklin et al., 1986). There is a nearly linear relation between PVR and survival after corrective operation (Mair et al., 1985). Operative survival is likely to be good if the resistance is less than 2 units m² (Mayer et al., 1986), but may still be satisfactory when it is 2 to 4 units m² in selected patients (Mair et al., 1985).

**Pulmonary Artery Anatomy.** Very small pulmonary arteries contraindicate the Fontan repair. The pulmonary artery index (cross-sectional area of the branch pulmonary arteries normalized for body surface area) predicts survival if greater than 250 mm m⁻² becomes $m^{-2}$ (Nakata et al., 1984). However, staging the repair with a bidirectional cavopulmonary anastomosis or hemi-Fontan operation allows an eventual Fontan reconstruction with much smaller pulmonary arteries (Douville et al., 1991). Local stenoses of the branch pulmonary arteries may be amenable to balloon dilatation at preoperative cardiac catheterization (Lock et al., 1983; Ring et al., 1985), but if this cannot be performed, corrective operation may still be possible if the pulmonary artery deformity can be repaired at the time of corrective operation. Pulmonary artery deformities produced by a pulmonary artery band may be correctable at a Fontan operation (Mair et al., 1985; Kirklin et al., 1986), but such deformities may contribute to a high operative mortality rate (Mayer et al., 1986). Pulmonary artery deformities associated with systemic-to–pulmonary artery shunts may be particularly difficult to deal with (Franklin et al., 1993). Correction of even severe central pulmonary artery hypoplasia is now routinely possible with a staged approach (Douville et al., 1991).

**Left Ventricular Function.** Elevated left ventricular end-diastolic pressure and ventricular hypertrophy are markers for diastolic dysfunction (lack of ventricular compliance), the prime pathophysiologic lesion behind this risk factor (Seliem et al., 1989). Left ventricular end-diastolic pressure appears not to be a risk factor unless over 25 torr (Mair et al., 1985), if associated with ventricular volume overload owing to correctable causes like increased pulmonary blood flow or atrioventricular valve insufficiency (Graham et al., 1986). Relief of volume overload and of myocardial hypoxia may lead to improved left ventricular function postoperatively.

Ventricular hypertrophy is a significant risk factor, both early and late (Cohen et al., 1991; Freedom, 1987; Kirklin et al., 1986). It may be associated with increased pulmonary blood flow with or without a pulmonary artery band, subaortic obstruction, especially in transposition of the great arteries (Freedom et al., 1986; Rothman et al., 1987b), and increasing age (Kirklin et al., 1986; Mair et al., 1985). Subaortic obstruction is associated with a high mortality rate at corrective operation and may require a preliminary operation to relieve the obstruction (see "Reduction of Excessive Pulmonary Blood Flow," earlier in this chapter).

## TECHNIQUE OF CORRECTIVE OPERATION

The goal of corrective surgery for tricuspid atresia is to separate the systemic and pulmonary circuits by connecting the systemic venous return directly to the pulmonary artery without obstruction, and closing all communications between the right side and the left side of the heart. Success depends primarily on a widely patent connection of the systemic venous return to the pulmonary circuit, sufficient cross-sec-

tional area of pulmonary arteries, and low pulmonary venous and left atrial pressures. The operation requires the correction of all anatomic abnormalities that militate against these requirements.

Fontan and Baudet's successful application of these principles in three patients (1971) was achieved against a background of considerable experimental and clinical work (Sade, 1992), including several unsuccessful clinical attempts to bypass the right ventricle (Harrison, 1962; Hurwitt et al., 1955; Shumacker, 1955). Fontan and Baudet's approach included a cavopulmonary anastomosis and homograft valves in the inferior vena cava and the atriopulmonary anastomosis. Subsequent techniques simplified the operation by omitting the cavopulmonary shunt while connecting the right atrium to the main pulmonary artery with a homograft (Ross and Somerville, 1973) and, in addition, deleting the inferior vena caval valve (Kreutzer et al., 1973). Many other modifications have been described (Cowgill, 1991).

The most critical technical factor in determining the outcome of Fontan and Baudet's procedure is the size of the atriopulmonary connection. Even minor degrees of obstruction are not well tolerated. Because Dacron grafts tend to become obstructed late postoperatively, they have largely been abandoned (DeLeon et al., 1984; Girod et al., 1987; Kreutzer et al., 1982). When a conduit is needed, homografts serve well for periods that now extend to 16 years (Girod et al., 1987). Externally supported PTFE grafts may also work well as conduits (Nawa et al., 1987). Anastomotic narrowing may perhaps be best avoided by doing the atriopulmonary anastomosis behind the aorta. The posterior anastomosis can be performed in cases of ventriculoarterial concordance or discordance (Kreutzer et al., 1982). The authors' technique of accomplishing cavoatriopulmonary anastomosis is illustrated in Figure 46–5, and another widely used method is shown in Figure 46–6.

Early postoperatively, there is no functional pump for the pulmonary circuit, regardless of the type of atriopulmonary connection, so there is no early advantage to connecting the right atrium to the right ventricle rather than the pulmonary artery (DiSessa et al., 1984; Kreutzer et al., 1982; Lee et al., 1986), although agreement on this question is not universal (Coles et al., 1987). Late postoperatively, however, the type of connection may have some importance. There is now little doubt that connecting the right atrium to the right ventricle with a valve-bearing conduit can lead to growth and function of the right ventricle as a pump, producing normally low right atrial pressures and a normal pulmonary artery pressure curve and pulmonary blood flow (Bowman et al., 1978; Bull et al., 1983; Fontan et al., 1983; Gussenhoven et al., 1986; Laks et al., 1984). Atrioventricular connection with a nonvalved conduit has been found by most authors to confer no long-term advantage over atriopulmonary connection. Exercise capacity has been shown not to be improved (Rhodes et al., 1990). However, one report has shown better long-term survival in atrioventricular connection (Coles et al., 1987) and

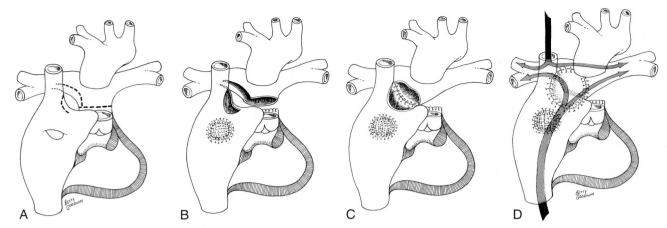

**FIGURE 46–5.** The authors' preferred method of the Fontan operation. *A*, Tricuspid atresia shown diagrammatically with a cutaway view through the aorta. Sites to be incised are indicated. *B*, The MPA is divided and oversewn proximally, the MPA is incised extending into the RPA, the posteromedial SVC is incised extending onto the anterior right atrial appendage, and the ASD is closed. *C*, The posterior cavoatrial incision is sewn to the posterior PA incision. *D*, The anterior cavoatrial PA anastomosis is completed with homograft material. The arrows demonstrate the flow of systemic venous return to the lungs.

another has shown better left ventricular function (Del Torso et al., 1985). Although no clear disadvantage of atrioventricular connection has been found, regurgitation from right ventricle to right atrium may rarely increase with time, leading to the need for valve interposition (Fontan et al., 1983; Laks et al., 1984). There appears to be little advantage to interposing a valve between the right atrium and the right pulmonary artery (Laks et al., 1984), although Fontan and colleagues (1983) have shown a slightly lower right atrial pressure when a valve is present.

Simple ligation of the pulmonary artery has been used during atriopulmonary anastomosis (Humes et al., 1987); a residual left-to-right shunt may occur through the ligature, so division of the main pulmo-

nary artery with oversewing of the proximal stump has been advocated (Girod et al., 1987).

To separate the systemic from the pulmonary venous return, the atrial septal communication need only be closed with a patch. Simple suture closure is not sufficient because occurrence of right-to-left shunt is common owing to suture line tension. The technique of total cavopulmonary connection (DeLeval et al., 1989; Matsuda et al., 1987; Puga et al., 1986) is now widely used for lesions other than tricuspid atresia, and its application in tricuspid atresia may be increasing. The superior vena cava is divided and the upstream end anastomosed to the cephalic side of the right pulmonary artery, and the downstream end either to the opposite side of the right pulmonary

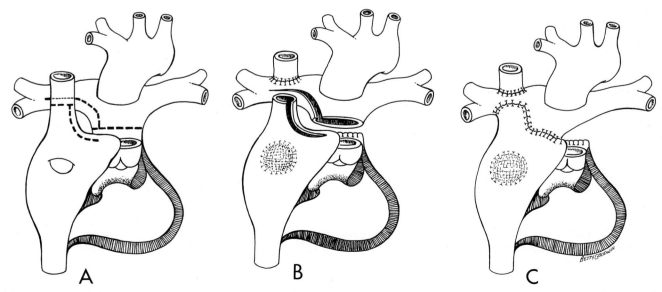

**FIGURE 46–6.** An alternative method of the Fontan operation. *A*, Tricuspid atresia with a cutaway view through the aorta. The sites to be incised are indicated. *B*, The MPA is divided and oversewn proximally and then incised extending into the RPA; the SVC is transected and anastomosed end to side to the RPA; the transected proximal SVC is incised onto the right atrial appendage. The ASD is closed. *C*, The cavoatriotomy is anastomosed to the distal PA providing systemic venous return to the pulmonary circulation.

The mortality and poor postoperative ventricular function associated with the Fontan operation in high-risk groups led to the development of the hemi-Fontan operation (Fig. 46–7), as discussed in "Cavopulmonary Anastomosis," earlier in this chapter. The high risk for some patients also stimulated the development of the "partial Fontan" operation, fenestration of the interatrial patch allowing right-to-left shunting postoperatively (Bridges et al., 1990; Laks and Billingsley, 1989) (Fig. 46–8). This is used in patients with important risk factors: high pulmonary artery pressure with increased PVR, small size of the pulmonary arteries, diminished ventricular function, and infancy (because of infants' poor tolerance for venous hypertension). The fenestrated Fontan operation theoretically would decrease mortality due to low cardiac output and the morbidity associated with systemic venous hypertension (Laks, 1990) by allowing the increased systemic venous pressure to decompress into the systemic circulation. This would reduce the systemic venous pressure and support cardiac output by allowing the ventricular preload to be relatively independent of pulmonary blood flow. The concept has been extended to include the use of an adjustable interatrial communication (Laks et al., 1991), allowing closure of the fenestration at a simple subcutaneous procedure sometime after the operation. The defect

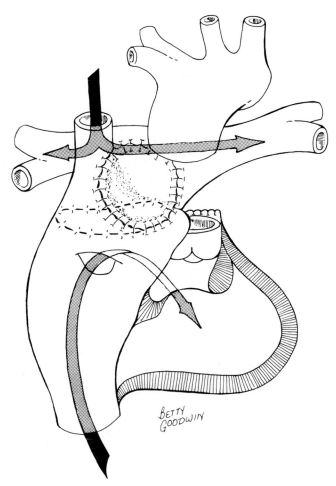

**FIGURE 46–7.** Hemi-Fontan's operation shown diagrammatically. The performance is the same as that of the Fontan operation indicated in Figure 46–5, differing in two important aspects. The ASD is not closed and the cavoatrial-pulmonary anastomosis is isolated from the right atrium (RA) by a patch closure of the superior RA. This allows inferior vena caval blood to cross the ASD into the LA and then into the left ventricle (LV). Thus the ventricular preload is partially independent of the pulmonary venous return. This assures that the ventricle that had been chronically volume-overloaded and therefore has diastolic dysfunction is not acutely unloaded due to pulmonary vasospasm. The SVC return flows bidirectionally to both lungs.

artery or to the open end of the divided main pulmonary artery. In an effort to reduce turbulence and stasis, the inferior vena cava has been connected to the superior vena caval anastomosis with an intracardiac baffle, creating a nearly straight conduit. This procedure commits the ASD, the coronary sinus, and the majority of the right atrium to the systemic circulation. Additionally, reduced turbulence may prevent energy loss as blood flows from cava to pulmonary artery, and may lower the likelihood of right atrial thrombosis because of reduced stasis (DeLeval et al., 1989). Early mortality has been reported as improved (Balaji et al., 1991) or the same (Pearl et al., 1991) following total cavopulmonary connection versus atriopulmonary connection, but a definite decrease in arrhythmias has been confirmed in total cavopulmonary connection (Balaji et al., 1991; Pearl et al., 1991).

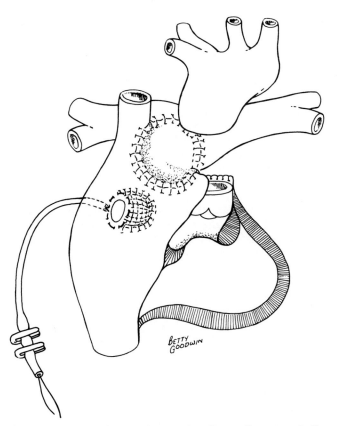

**FIGURE 46–8.** Partial Fontan's operation shown diagrammatically. The ASD closure has an adjustable fenestration, allowing for either increasing or decreasing right-to-left shunting depending on the patient's physiologic requirements.

has also been closed at cardiac catheterization with a clamshell device (Bridges et al., 1990).

Although associated cardiac anomalies are not as commonly seen with tricuspid atresia as with other forms of univentricular atrioventricular connection, some must be dealt with at the time of corrective surgery. A moderately or severely insufficient mitral valve may be repaired or replaced (Mair et al., 1985; Vargas et al., 1987a). Deformities of the pulmonary artery may be directly repaired by patch reconstruction or, in some cases, may be dilated intraoperatively by balloon angioplasty (Ring et al., 1985). A right pulmonary artery deformed by a preexisting Waterston shunt can be divided distal to the deformity and anastomosed to the side of the superior vena cava (Uretzky et al., 1983). Anomalies of the venous drainage can usually be dealt with by an intra-atrial baffle, but a left superior vena cava is best handled by division and anastomosis to the left pulmonary artery (Vargas et al., 1987b).

The patch closing the atrial septal communication should encircle the coronary sinus, leaving it to drain into the low-pressure left atrium. When the right atrial pressure exceeds 15 torr, coronary sinus drainage and left ventricular function may be impaired (Ilbawi et al., 1986), although there is some evidence that such impairment may not be important (Ward et al., 1988). Leaving the coronary sinus in the left atrium has the additional advantage of obviating the possibility of a residual right-to-left shunt in the 2% of tricuspid atresia patients who have a coronary sinus septal defect (Coles et al., 1987; Girod et al., 1987; Rumisek et al., 1986).

All preexisting palliative shunts should be closed at the time of corrective surgery, except for classical cavopulmonary anastomoses, which are usually left intact. In order to prevent commitment of a third of the systemic venous return to more than half of the pulmonary capillary bed, the authors have reconstructed the cavoatrial junction with a patch at a Fontan repair in patients with a previous cavopulmonary shunt to make the entire pulmonary capillary bed available to all the systemic venous return.

Many of the uncertainties of the early experience with the Fontan operation have been clarified, so specific recommendations for operative management of patients with tricuspid atresia are possible. A two-ventricle repair may be achieved in patients with ventriculoarterial concordance, normal pulmonary artery and valve, mild to moderate hypoplasia of the right ventricle, and adequate retrosternal space. These patients may undergo patch repair of both the outlet foramen and the atrial septal communication at the same time as a valved allograft is placed from the right atrium to the right ventricle, with a high expectation of growth of the right ventricle. Patients with severe right ventricular hypoplasia, the majority of tricuspid atresia patients, should undergo cavoatriopulmonary anastomosis with ligation or division of the main pulmonary artery and patch closure of the atrial septal communication. Patients with important risk factors should have fenestration of the interatrial

patch. Correction of associated anatomic abnormalities should accompany the repair.

## POSTOPERATIVE MANAGEMENT

The immediate postoperative period is a time of dramatic hemodynamic adjustment to new circulatory physiology. There is no pump in the pulmonary circuit and already impaired left ventricular function has been compromised further by recent operation. Since the two circulations are now separated and in series, cardiac output is limited by the pulmonary blood flow, which in turn varies directly with the transpulmonary pressure gradient. Cardiac output may be increased by increasing right atrial pressure, decreasing PVR, and decreasing left atrial pressure (Sade, 1992). Right atrial pressure can be increased by colloid transfusion. PVR can be decreased by hyperventilation to achieve hypocarbia as low as 20 torr and respiratory alkalosis to a pH of 7.45 to 7.50. Maintaining a relatively low hematocrit (30 to 35%) decreases resistance by decreasing blood viscosity. Left atrial pressure can be reduced by improving left ventricular function with the use of inotropic drugs and systemic arteriolar dilators.

In the immediate postoperative period, the requirement of a right atrial pressure of 18 to 20 torr or higher predicts a high morbidity and mortality rate (Cohen et al., 1991; Mair et al., 1990) (Fig. 46–9). When the cardiac output remains low despite the measures described previously, intermittent abdominal compression may be used to good advantage (Heilberg et al., 1977; Milliken et al., 1986). Several techniques of compression have been described. An adult arm or thigh blood pressure cuff may be wrapped loosely around the abdomen and connected to a ventilator or

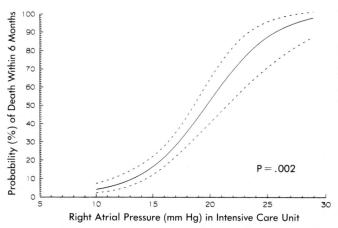

**FIGURE 46–9.** Right atrial pressure in the intensive care unit is an important predictor of mortality. The probability of death within 6 months of a Fontan operation, according to right atrial pressure about 2 hours after the operation, rises sharply when the pressure is greater than 16 to 17 mm Hg. The *broken lines* enclose the 70% confidence limits. (From Kirklin, J. K., Kirklin, J. W., Pacifico, A. D., and Bargeron, L. M., Jr.: The Fontan operation: Ventricular hypertrophy, age and date of operation as risk factors. J. Thorac. Cardiovasc. Surg., *92*:1049, 1986.)

a pneumatic pressure–cycled extremity pump (Jobst Institute). The cuff is inflated to a sufficient pressure (usually 30 to 45 torr) to keep the left atrial pressure at 20 to 25 torr. The cuff is inflated for 30 to 40 seconds, and deflated for 15 to 30 seconds. The device is usually needed for 12 to 36 hours. The use of medical antishock trousers (MAST) suits has also been described (Tobias et al., 1990).

If cardiac output remains low despite all these measures, a specific cause should be sought, like atriopulmonary obstruction, pulmonary hypertension, or left ventricular failure. If no correctable cause is found, the patient should undergo reoperation and the Fontan converted to hemi-Fontan anatomy. This approach has afforded a marked improvement in survival in a dire situation (Douville et al., 1991). If an adjustable fenestrated Fontan was constructed, the fenestration could be opened as widely as possible while the hemodynamic effect is observed.

Arterial hypoxemia in the immediate postoperative period may be caused by intrapulmonary shunting owing to atelectasis or interstitial edema, and may respond to pulmonary toilet or addition of positive end-expiratory pressure. The latter should be used with caution because more than 6 torr may be associated with substantial decreases in cardiac output (Williams et al., 1984). Persistent hypoxemia despite adequate ventilation may be related to pulmonary venous collateral vessels or arteriovenous fistulas, especially in patients with a previous cavopulmonary anastomosis. Other anatomic causes of hypoxemia may be dehiscence of the atrial septal closure, small ASDs that escaped detection at operation, unusual coronary vein connections between right atrium and left atrium, or coronary sinus septal defect (Girod et al., 1987; Rumisek et al., 1986; Westerman et al., 1985). In these patients, early reoperation may be needed.

Atrioventricular sequential pacing early postoperatively is often helpful when rhythm is not sinus and cardiac output is marginal.

Nearly all patients after a Fontan operation retain fluid for reasons that are not entirely clear. There is a general inflammatory response to cardiopulmonary bypass resulting in elevated complement levels (Kirklin et al., 1983), and atrial natriuretic peptide and antidiuretic hormone are abnormally elevated in patients after the Fontan operation (Stewart et al., 1991). Fluid retention is associated with pleural effusions, usually bilateral, requiring chest tube drainage for 1 to 3 weeks or longer after operation. Chest tubes placed laterally may be required in addition to mediastinal tubes.

## RESULTS OF CORRECTIVE OPERATION

Results of the Fontan operations are often reported without differentiation among anatomic types of univentricular atrioventricular connection. This is reasonable because there are few differences in morbidity and mortality among hospital survivors with tricuspid atresia or other kinds of univentricular atrioventricular connection (Coles et al., 1987; Humes et al., 1987). Therefore, the following discussions of results will not distinguish between Fontan operations performed for tricuspid atresia and for other malformations, unless specifically stated.

### Early Mortality

The hospital mortality rate for the Fontan operation in tricuspid atresia in the cited reports is 51 of 373 patients (14%) (Annecchino et al., 1988; de Vivie and Rupprath, 1986; Girod et al., 1987; Mair et al., 1990; Stellin et al., 1988; Pearl et al., 1992; Tam et al., 1989). Mortality is clearly related to preoperative risk factors. When Fontan and colleagues' criteria are strictly observed, operative risk is very low, on the order of 0 to 7% (Fontan et al., 1983; Humes et al., 1987; Laks et al., 1984). Most of the criteria, however, are relative risk factors. In the Mayo Clinic series, the operative mortality for all patients with tricuspid atresia was only 10%, yet 76% of the patients violated one to eight of the criteria (Humes et al., 1987). The mortality risk increases when more than two (Mayer et al., 1986) or three (Mair et al., 1985) risk factors are present, but these rates may still be acceptable in view of the long-term poor outcome of palliative surgery (Dick et al., 1975). Patch fenestration may reduce this low mortality rate lower still.

### Functional Results

Exercise capacity improves substantially from preoperative levels after a Fontan operation (Driscoll et al., 1986), and ranges from 50 to 100% of normal (Fontan et al., 1983; Kreutzer et al., 1982). The ventilatory response to exercise also decreases toward normal after operation compared with the preoperative response (Driscoll et al., 1986). However, both peak work load and oxygen consumption are approximately 65% of normal, compared, for example, with postrepair tetralogy of Fallot patients at 83% of normal (Rhodes et al., 1990).

At postoperative cardiac catheterization, the cardiac index is usually in the low normal range, 2.2 to 3.2 l/min$^{-1}$/m$^{-2}$, the right atrial pressure is about 15 torr, the oxygen saturation is 91 to 98%, and the left ventricular end-diastolic pressure is normal, averaging 8 torr (Driscoll et al., 1986; Kreutzer et al., 1982; Laks et al., 1984; Mair et al., 1985; Nakazawa et al., 1984).

The hemodynamic response to exercise is not normal. The cardiac index increases only 50 to 100% during exercise (Laks et al., 1984; Shachar et al., 1982), although one study found a nearly normal response to exercise (Peterson et al., 1984). The left ventricular ejection fraction during exercise is abnormally low in most clinically well patients, and correlates poorly both with resting ejection fraction measurements and with exercise capacity (Del Torso et al., 1985). Stroke volume may rise or fall slightly during exercise (Driscoll et al., 1986; Shachar et al, 1982); much of the

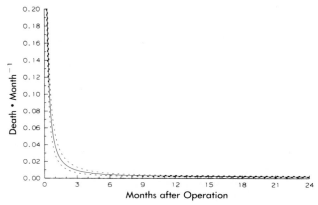

**FIGURE 46–10.** The hazard function (instantaneous risk of death in patients still living) after a Fontan operation (102 patients: 32 deaths). The *broken lines* enclose the 70% confidence limits. The greatest danger is within the first 2 to 3 months after operation. (From Kirklin, J. K., Kirklin, J. W., Pacifico, A. D., and Bargeron, L. M., Jr.: The Fontan operation: Ventricular hypertrophy, age and date of operation as risk factors. J. Thorac. Cardiovasc. Surg., 92:1049, 1986.)

increase in cardiac index with exercise in post-Fontan patients is due to an increase in heart rate that falls short of normal (Driscoll et al., 1986; Laks et al., 1984). During exercise, there is a sharp rise in right atrial pressure that may (Shachar et al., 1982) or may not (Laks et al., 1984) be associated with atriopulmonary obstruction. When there is obstruction to atriopulmonary flow, a pressure gradient not demonstrable at rest may appear with exercise (Shachar et al., 1982).

Left ventricular ejection fraction is near the low range of normal, changing little from preoperative to postoperative determinations (Fontan et al., 1983; Sanders et al., 1982). Serial studies have shown that low ejection fraction early after a Fontan operation does not deteriorate, but either remains stable or improves over 1 to 3 years (Hurwitz et al., 1986). There is a substantial (about two-thirds) decrease in left ventricular end-diastolic volume from preoperative to postoperative measurements, mostly due to closing of shunts and improvement in myocardial oxygen supply (Graham et al., 1986; Mair et al., 1985; Sanders et al., 1982), as well as a concomitant decrease in left ventricular end-diastolic pressure by as much as 50% (Mair et al., 1985). There is a decrease in ventricular dimensions and improved contractility from preoperatively to as early as 10 days after a Fontan operation (Gewillig et al., 1990).

## Late Results

The following analysis combines the late follow-up of all patients undergoing Fontan operations from the cited reports. Among 624 patients undergoing a Fontan operation, 51 (8%) died after leaving the hospital (Cohen et al., 1991; Girod et al., 1987; Mair et al., 1990, 1991; Pearl et al., 1992; Weber et al., 1992). Among the 28 deaths for which data are available, 6 were related to failure of the dominant ventricle

(21%), 5 to sudden death or arrhythmias (18%), 1 to right-sided heart failure (4%), 10 occurred during reoperation (36%), and 6 were due to other causes (21%). Instantaneous hazard analysis suggests that most of the late mortality occurs within the first 6 months (Fig. 46–10) after the Fontan operation (Coles et al., 1987; Fontan et al., 1983; Humes et al., 1987; Kirklin et al., 1986; Stefanelli et al., 1984), and there may be a 1% annual mortality rate up to 16 years after operation (Girod et al, 1987).

Among 500 patients, 60 (12%) underwent reoperation—residual shunt at the atrial or ventricular level (13%); obstruction of the atriopulmonary connection (15%) including 1 clotting episode; Fontan takedown (3%); pacemaker placement (12%); heart transplantation (1%); and other operations (16%) (Girod et al., 1987; Mair et al., 1990, 1991; Pearl et al., 1992; Weber et al., 1992). The need for reoperation may be most frequent in the first 5 years after operation (Fig. 46–11). Technical modifications such as total cavopulmonary anastomosis (lateral tunnel), abandonment of the use of Dacron conduits, and large atriopulmonary anastomosis may decrease this reoperation rate. Moreover, new techniques of therapeutic catheterization may allow treatment of some residual abnormalities that formerly would have required reoperation: for example, devices to close atrial communications, balloons to dilate vascular narrowing, and stents to hold open vascular strictures (Rao, 1991).

Protein-losing enteropathy was a contributing factor in 8 of 23 late deaths in one large series (Humes et al., 1987) and may be associated with a high diastolic right atrial pressure (Hess et al., 1984), leading to *increased lymph production* because of high inferior vena cava and portal pressure, and to *obstruction to lymph drainage* owing to high pressure in the superior vena cava. Loss of protein into the gut may lead to hypoalbuminemia and consequent generalized edema and immunologic abnormalities. The possibility of atriopulmonary obstruction must be investigated because operative correction may cure protein-losing enteropathy (Girod et al., 1987). Otherwise, treatment is with a low-fat, medium-chain triglyceride diet,

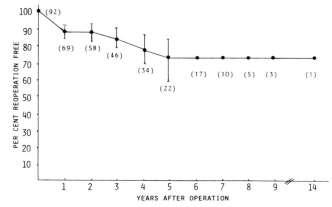

**FIGURE 46–11.** Reoperation-free actuarial curve in Fontan's first 100 patients shows a reoperation-free rate of 75% at 5 years after operation that persists.

which may take several weeks or months to be effective. Treatment with corticosteroids has been successful (Rychik et al., 1991). If all of the foregoing fail, inflow valves in the venae cavae may dramatically reverse this condition (Crupi et al., 1980).

Chronic pleural and pericardial effusions occur rarely, may be associated with high right atrial pressure, and are difficult to treat. Treatment with prednisone followed by slow tapering has been successful in a few patients (Rothman et al., 1987b). Placement of pleuroperitoneal shunts has also been successful (Sade and Wiles, 1990). High right atrial pressure may lead to cardiac cirrhosis (Lemmer et al., 1983), but this complication remains rare, although many patients may have mild abnormalities of liver function (Girod et al., 1987).

Arrhythmias may require a pacemaker in as many as 5% of patients (Taliercio et al., 1985). Pacemakers in patients with a Fontan operation pose special anatomic problems, but can be managed quite safely. There is a linear increase with time postoperatively in the incidence of supraventricular tachycardia, reaching at least 20% of followed patients 5 years postoperatively (Danielson, 1988). The availability of antitachycardia pacemakers allows better control than that afforded by drugs in some patients after Fontan operations, so the use of pacing devices is likely to increase in the future in these patients (Balaji et al., 1994).

Thrombus formation in the right side of the heart is an uncommon event, but it is often fatal when it occurs. When recognized during life, thrombus may be surgically excised or may be treated successfully with streptokinase (Fyfe et al., 1991). Some centers treat patients for a few months or indefinitely after a Fontan operation with warfarin in an effort to prevent this problem.

Late functional status is excellent in long-term survivors of the Fontan operation. In a combined group of 366 reported patients (Girod et al., 1987; Mair et al., 1990, 1991; Cohen et al., 1991), 203 (56%) were in New York Heart Association Class I, 124 (34%) were in Class II, 37 (10%) were in Class III, and 2 (0.5%) were in Class IV. Almost all patients (97%) are able to work or attend school, and the majority (55%) are on no medications (Humes et al., 1987).

The longest follow-up available is that of Fontan's earliest patients, 32 of whom survived at least 1 year and were followed for 7 to 16 years (mean, 9 years). There were 5 late deaths (16%), 3 at reoperation, and 2 sudden unexplained or arrhythmias. The most frequent problem in this group has been conduit obstruction, both of synthetic grafts and of homografts, but 26 of the 27 survivors remain in Class I or II (Girod et al, 1987). Fontan's first patient, operated in 1968, is still alive, is married, and engages in the normal activities of a housewife (Fontan, unpublished).

## BIBLIOGRAPHY

Alboliras, E. T., Porter, C. J., Danielson, G. K., et al.: Results of the modified Fontan operation for congenital heart lesions in patients without preoperative sinus rhythm. J. Am. Coll. Cardiol., 6:228, 1985.

Anderson, R. H., Becker, A. E., Tynan, M., et al.: The univentricular atrioventricular connection: Getting to the root of a thorny problem. Am. J. Cardiol. 54:822, 1984.

Anderson, R. H., and Rigby, M. L.: The morphological heterogeneity of "tricuspid atresia." Int. J. Cardiol. 16:67, 1987.

Annecchino, F. P., Brunelli, F., Borghi, A., et al.: Fontan repair for tricuspid atresia: Experience with 50 consecutive patients. Ann. Thorac. Surg., 45:43, 1988.

Arciniegas, E., Farooki, Z. Q., Hakimi, M., and Green, E. W.: Results of two-stage surgical treatment of tetralogy of Fallot. J. Thorac. Cardiovasc. Surg., 79:876, 1980.

Bakulev, A. N., and Kolesnikov, S. A.: Anastomosis of superior vena cava and pulmonary artery in the surgical treatment of certain congenital defects of the heart. J. Thorac. Surg., 37:693, 1959.

Balaji, S., Gewillig, M., Bull, C., et al.: Arrhythmias after the Fontan procedure: Comparison of total cavopulmonary connection and atriopulmonary connection. Circulation, 84(Suppl. III): 162, 1991.

Balaji, S., Johnson, T. B., Sade, R. M., et al.: Management of atrial tachyarrhythmias after the Fontan procedure. J. Am. Coll. Cardiol., 23:1209, 1994.

Beaver, T. R, Shroyer, K. R, Muro-Cacho, C. A., et al.: Survival to age 65 years with tricuspid and pulmonic valve atresia. Am. J. Cardiol., 62:165, 1988.

Blalock, A., and Hanlon, C. R.: The surgical treatment of transposition of the aorta and the pulmonary artery. Surg. Gynecol. Obstet., 90:1, 1950.

Bowman, F. O., Jr., Malm, J. R., Hayes, C. J., and Gersony, W. M.: Physiological approach to surgery for tricuspid atresia. Circulation, 58(Suppl. I):83, 1978.

Bridges, N. D., Lock, J. E., and Castaneda, A. R.: Fontan repair with baffle fenestration and subsequent transcatheter closure in high-risk patients. J. Am. Coll. Cardiol. 15:203A, 1990.

Bull, C., DeLeval, M. R., Stark, J., et al.: Use of a subpulmonary ventricular chamber in the Fontan circulation. J. Thorac. Cardiovasc. Surg., 85:21, 1983.

Carlon, C. A., Mondini, P. G., and DeMarchi, R.: Surgical treatment of some cadiovascular diseases (a new vascular anastomosis). J. Int. Coll. Surg., 16:1, 1951.

Caspi, J., Rabinovitch, M., Cohen, D., et al.: Morphological findings contributing to a failed Fontan procedure. Circulation, 82:177, 1990.

Choussat, A., Fontan, F., Besse, P., et al.: Selection criteria for Fontan's procedure. In Anderson, R. H., and Shinebourne, E. A. (eds): Pediatric Cardiology. Edinburgh, Churchill Livingstone, 1978, pp. 559–566.

Cleveland, D. C., Kirklin, J. K., Naftel, D. C., et al.: Surgical treatment of tricuspid atresia. Ann. Thorac. Surg., 38:447, 1984.

Cohen, A. J., Cleveland, D. C., Dyck, J., et al.: Results of the Fontan procedure for patients with univentricular heart. Ann. Thorac. Surg., 52:1266, 1991.

Coles, J. G., Kielmanowicz, S., Freedom, R. M., et al.: Surgical experience with the modified Fontan procedure. Circulation, 76(Suppl. 3):61, 1987.

Cowgill, L. D.: The Fontan procedure: A historical review. Ann. Thorac. Surg., 51:1026, 1991.

Crupi, G., Locatelli, R., Tiraboschi, M., et al.: Protein-losing enteropathy after Fontan operation for tricuspid atresia (imperforate tricuspid valve). J. Thorac. Cardiovasc. Surg., 28:359, 1980.

Crupi, G., Villani, M., Di Benedetto, G., et al.: Tricuspid atresia with imperforate valve: Angiographic findings and surgical implications in two cases with AV concordance and normally related great arteries. Cardiology, 5:49, 1984.

Currarino, G., and Engle, M. A.: The effects of ligation of the subclavian artery on the bones and soft tissues of the arms. J. Pediatr., 67:808, 1965.

Danielson, G. K.: Personal communication, 1988.

Deanfield, J. E., Tommasini, G., Anderson, R. H., and Macartney, F. J.: Tricuspid atresia: Analysis of coronary artery distribution and ventricular morphology. Br. Heart J., 48:485, 1982.

DeLeon, S. Y., Koopot, R., Mair, D. D., et al.: Surgical management of occluded conduits after the Fontan operation in patients with Glenn shunts. J. Thorac. Cardiovasc. Surg., 88:601, 1984.

DeLeval, M. R., Bull, C., and Kilner, P. Total cavopulmonary connection: A logical alternative to atriopulmonary connection for complex Fontan operations—Experimental studies and early clinical experience. J. Thorac. Cardiovasc. Surg., 97:636, 1989.

DeLeval, M. R, Kilner, P., Gewillig, M., and Bull, C.: Total cavopulmonary connection: A logical alternative to atriopulmonary connection for complex Fontan operations. J. Thorac. Cardiovasc. Surg., 96:682, 1988.

Del Torso, S., Kelly, M. J., Kaliff, V., and Venables, A. W.: Radionuclide assessment of ventricular contraction at rest and during exercise following the Fontan procedure for either tricuspid atresia or single ventricle. Am. J. Cardiol., 55:1127, 1985.

Deverall, P. B., Lincoln, J. C., Aberdeen, E., et al.: Surgical management of tricuspid atresia. Thorax, 24:239, 1969.

de Vivie, E. R., and Rupprath, G.: Long-term results after Fontan procedure and its modifications. J. Thorac. Cardiovasc. Surg., 91:690, 1986.

DiCarlo, D., Williams, W. G., Freedom, R. M., et al.: The role of cava-pulmonary (Glenn) anastomosis in the palliative treatment of congenital heart disease. J. Thorac. Cardiovasc. Surg., 83:437, 1982.

Dick, M., Fyler, D. C., and Nadas, A. S.: Tricuspid atresia: Clinical course in 101 patients. Am. J. Cardiol., 36:327, 1975.

Didier, D., Higgins, C. B., Fisher, M. R., et al.: Congenital heart disease: Gated MR imaging in 72 patients. Radiology 158:227, 1986.

Di Donato, R. M., Amodeo, A., di Carlo, D. D., et al.: Staged Fontan operation for complex cardiac anomalies with subaortic obstruction. J. Thorac. Cardiovasc. Surg., 105:398, 1993.

DiSessa, T. G., Child, J. S., Perloff, J. K., et al.: Systemic venous and pulmonary arterial flow patterns after Fontan's procedure for tricuspid atresia or single ventricle. Circulation, 70:898, 1984.

Douville, E. C., Sade, R. M., and Fyfe, D. A.: Hemi-Fontan operation in surgery for single ventricle: A preliminary report. Ann. Thorac. Surg., 51:893, 1991.

Driscoll, D. J., Danielson, G. K., Puga, F. J., et al.: Exercise tolerance and cardiorespiratory response to exercise after the Fontan operation for tricuspid atresia or functional single ventricle. J. Am. Coll. Cardiol., 7:1087, 1986.

Edwards, J. E., and Burchell, H. B.: Congenital tricuspid atresia: A classification. Med. Clin. North Am., 33:1177, 1949.

Elliott, R. B., Starling, M. B., and Neutze, J. M.: Medical manipulation of ductus arteriosus. Lancet, 1:140, 1975.

Fletcher, B. D., Jacobstein, M. D., Abramowsky, C. R., and Anderson, R. H.: Right atrioventricular valve atresia: Anatomic evaluation with MR imaging. Am. J. Roentgenol., 148:671, 1987.

Fontan, F.: Unpublished discussion of Lee, C. N., Schaff, H. V., Danielson, G. K., et al.: Comparison of atriopulmonary versus atrioventricular connections for modified Fontan/Kreutzer repair of tricuspid valve atresia. J. Thorac. Cardiovasc. Surg., 92:1038, 1986.

Fontan, F., and Baudet, E.: Surgical repair of tricuspid atresia. Thorax, 26:240, 1971.

Fontan, F., Deville, C., Quaegebeur, J., et al.: Repair of tricuspid atresia in 100 patients. J. Thorac. Cardiovasc. Surg., 85:647, 1983.

Forrest, P., Bini, R. M., Wilkinson, J. L., et al.: Congenital absence of the pulmonic valve and tricuspid valve atresia with intact ventricular septum. Am. J. Cardiol., 59:482, 1987.

Franklin, R. C. G., Spiegelhalter, D. J., Sullivan, I. D., et al.: Tricuspid atresia presenting in infancy: Survival and suitability for the Fontan operation. Circulation, 87:427, 1993.

Freed, M., Rosenthal, A., Planth, W. H., Jr., and Nadas, A. S.: Development of subaortic stenosis after pulmonary artery banding. Circulation, 47(Suppl. VI):7, 1973.

Freedom, R. M.: The dinosaur and banding of the main pulmonary trunk in the heart with functionally one ventricle and transposition of the great arteries: A saga of evolution and caution. J. Am. Coll. Cardiol., 10:427, 1987.

Freedom, R. M., Lee, N. B., Smallhorn, J. F., et al.: Subaortic stenosis, the univentricular heart, and banding of the pulmonary artery: An analysis of the courses of 43 patients with univentricular heart palliated by pulmonary artery banding. Circulation, 73:758, 1986.

Fyfe, D. A., Kline, C. H., Sade, R. M., and Gillette, P. C.: Transesoph-

ageal echocardiography detects thrombus formation not identified by routine echocardiography after the Fontan operation. J. Am. Coll. Cardiol., 18:1733, 1991.

Fyfe, D. A., Taylor, A. B., Gillette, P. C., et al.: Doppler echocardiographic confirmation of recurrent atrial septal defect stenosis in infants with mitral valve atresia. Am. J. Cardiol., 60:410, 1987.

Gallaher, M. E., and Fyler, D. C.: Observations on changing hemodynamics in tricuspid atresia without associated transposition of the great vessels. Circulation, 35:381, 1967.

Gay, W. A., Jr., and Ebert, P. A.: Aorta-to-right pulmonary artery anastomosis causing obstruction of the right pulmonary artery. Management during correction of tetralogy of Fallot. Ann. Thorac. Surg., 16:402, 1973.

Geiss, D., Williams, W. G., Lindsay, W. K., and Rowe, R. D.: Upper extremity gangrene: A complication of subclavian artery division. Ann. Thorac. Surg., 30:487, 1980.

Gewillig, M. H., Lundstrom, U. R., Deanfield, J. E., et al.: Impact of Fontan operation on left ventricular size and contractility in tricuspid atresia. Circulation, 81:118, 1990.

Girod, D. A., Fontan, F., Deville, C., et al.: Long-term results after the Fontan operation for tricuspid atresia. Circulation, 75:605, 1987.

Glenn, W. W. L.: Circulatory bypass of the right side of the heart. II. Shunt between superior vena cava and distal right pulmonary artery—Report of a clinical application. N. Engl. J. Med., 259:117, 1958.

Graham, T. P., Jr., Franklin, R. C. G., Wyse, R. K. H., et al.: Left ventricular wall stress and contractile function in childhood: Normal values and comparison of Fontan repair versus palliation only in patients with tricuspid atresia. Circulation, 74(Suppl. I):61, 1986.

Gussenhoven, W. J., The, H. K., Schippers, L., et al.: Growth and function of the right ventricular outflow tract after Fontan's procedure for tricuspid atresia: A two-dimensional echocardiographic study. J. Thorac. Cardiovasc. Surg., 34:236, 1986.

Haller, J. A., Adkins, J. C., Worthington, J., et al.: Experimental studies on permanent bypass of the right heart. Surgery, 59:1128, 1966.

Hallman, G. L., Stasney, C. R., and Cooley, D. A.: Surgical treatment of tricuspid atresia. J. Cardiovasc. Surg., 9:154, 1968.

Harrison, R.: Discussion of Bopp, R. K., Larsen, P. B., Caddell, J. L., et al.: Surgical considerations for treatment of congenital tricuspid atresia and stenosis: With particular reference to vena cava-pulmonary artery anastomosis. J. Thorac. Cardiovasc. Surg., 43:97, 1962.

Hatem, J., Sade, R. M., Upshur, J. K., and Hohn, A. R.: Maintaining patency of the ductus arteriosus for palliation of cyanotic congenital cardiac malformations. Ann. Surg., 192:124, 1980.

Heilberg, K., Kirchoff, P. G., Orellano, L. E., et al.: Supporting the pump function of the right atrium. A new therapeutic concept after physiological repair of tricuspid atresia. Thoraxchir. Vasc. Chir., 25:400, 1977.

Hess, J. H.: Congenital atresia of the right auriculoventricular orifice with complete absence of tricuspid valves. Am. J. Dis. Child., 13:167, 1917.

Hess, J. H., Kruizinga, K., Bijleveld, C. M. A., et al.: Protein-losing enteropathy after Fontan operation. J. Thorac. Cardiovasc. Surg., 88:606, 1984.

Hopkins, R. A., Armstrong, B. E., Serwer, G. A., et al.: Physiological rationale for a bidirectional cavopulmonary shunt: A versatile complement to the Fontan principle. J. Thorac. Cardiovasc. Surg., 90:391, 1985.

Humes, R. A., Porter, C. J., Mair, D. D., et al.: Intermediate follow-up and predicted survival after the modified Fontan procedure for tricuspid atresia and double-inlet ventricle. Circulation, 76(Suppl. III):67, 1987.

Hurwitt, E. S., Young, D., and Escher, D. J. W.: The rationale of anastomosis of the right auricular appendage to the pulmonary artery in the treatment of tricuspid atresia. J. Thorac. Surg., 30:503, 1955.

Hurwitz, R. A., Caldwell, R. L., Girod, D. A., and Wellman, H.: Left ventricular function in tricuspid atresia: A radionuclide study. J. Am. Coll. Cardiol., 8:916, 1986.

Ilbawi, M. N., Idriss, F. S., Muster, A. J., et al.: Effects of elevated coronary sinus pressure on left ventricular function after the Fontan operation. J. Thorac. Cardiovasc. Surg., 92:231, 1986.

Jonas, R. A., Castañeda, A. R., and Lang, P.: Single ventricle (single- or double-inlet) complicated by subaortic stenosis: Surgical options in infancy. Ann. Thorac. Surg., 39:361, 1985.

Juaneda, E., and Haworth, S. G.: Pulmonary vascular structure in patients dying after a Fontan procedure. The lung as a risk factor. Br. Heart J., 52:575, 1984.

Keith, J. D., Rowe, R. D., and Vlad, P.: Heart Disease in Infancy and Childhood. 3rd ed. New York, Macmillan, 1978.

King, R. M. J., Puga, F. J., Danielson, G. K., and Julsrud, P. R.: Extended indications for the modified Fontan procedure in patients with anomalous systemic and pulmonary venous return. Pediatric Cardiology: Proceedings of the Second World Congress. New York, Springer-Verlag, 1985, pp. 1–523.

Kirklin, J. K., Blackstone, E. H., Kirklin, J. W., et al.: The Fontan operation. Ventricular hypertrophy, age, and date of operation as risk factors. J. Thorac. Cardiovasc. Surg., 92:1049, 1986.

Kirklin, J. K., Westaby, S., Blackstone, E. H., et al.: Complement and the damaging effects of cardiopulmonary bypass. J. Thorac. Cardiovasc. Surg., 86:845, 1983.

Kirklin, J. W., and Barratt-Boyes, B. G.: Tricuspid atresia. In Kirklin, J. W., and Barratt-Boyes, B. G. (eds): Cardiac Surgery. New York, Churchill Livingstone, 1986, pp. 857–888.

Kreutzer, G. O., Galindez, E., Bono, H., et al.: An operation for the correction of tricuspid atresia. J. Thorac. Cardiovasc. Surg., 663:613, 1973.

Kreutzer, G. O., Vargas, F. J., Schlichter, A. J., et al.: Atriopulmonary anastomosis. J. Thorac. Cardiovasc. Surg., 83:427, 1982.

Kuhne, M.: Uber zwei Falle kongenitaler atresie des ostium venosum dextrum. Jahrbuch Kinderheildkunde Physiche Erziehung, 63:235, 1906.

LaCorte, M. A., Dick, M., Scheer, G., et al.: Left ventricular function in tricuspid atresia. Angiographic analysis in 28 patients. Circulation, 52:996, 1975.

Laks, H.: The partial Fontan procedure. Circulation, 82:1681, 1990.

Laks, H., and Billingsley, A. M.: Advances in the treatment of pulmonary atresia with intact ventricular septum: Palliative and definitive repair. Cardiol. Clin., 7:387, 1989.

Laks, H., Milliken, J. C., Perloff, J. K., et al.: Experience with the Fontan procedure. J. Thorac. Cardiovasc. Surg., 88:939, 1984.

Laks, H., Mudd, J. G., Standeven, J. W., et al.: Long-term effect of the superior vena cava-pulmonary artery anastomosis on pulmonary blood flow. J. Thorac. Cardiovasc. Surg., 74:253, 1977.

Laks, H., Pearl, J. M., Haas, G. S., et al.: Partial Fontan: Advantages of an adjustable interatrial communication. Ann. Thorac. Surg., 52:1084, 1991.

Lee, C. N., Schaff, H. V., Danielson, G. K., et al.: Comparison of atriopulmonary versus atrioventricular connections for modified Fontan/Kreutzer repair of tricuspid valve atresia. J. Thorac. Cardiovasc. Surg., 92:1038, 1986.

Lee, M. E., and Sade, R. M.: Coronary sinus septal defect. Surgical considerations. J. Thorac. Cardiovasc. Surg., 78:563, 1979.

Lemmer, J. H., Coran, A. G., Behrendt, D. M., et al.: Liver fibrosis (cardiac cirrhosis) five years after modified Fontan operation for tricuspid atresia. J. Thorac. Cardiovasc. Surg., 86:757, 1983.

Lin, A. E., Laks, H., Barber, G., et al.: Subaortic obstruction in complex congenital heart disease: Management by proximal pulmonary artery-to-ascending aorta end-to-side anastomosis. J. Am. Coll. Cardiol., 7:617, 1986.

Lock, J. E., Castañeda-Zuniga, W. R., Fuhrman, B. P., and Bass, J. L.: Balloon dilation angioplasty of hypoplastic and stenotic pulmonary arteries. Circulation, 67:962, 1983.

Mair, D. D., Hagler, D. J., Julsrud, P. R., et al.: Early and late results of the modified Fontan procedure for double-inlet left ventricle: The Mayo Clinic experience. J. Am. Coll. Cardiol., 18:1727, 1991.

Mair, D. D., Hagler, D. J., Puga, F. J., et al.: Fontan operation in 176 patients with tricuspid atresia: Results and a proposed new index for patient selection. Circulation, 82(Suppl. IV):164, 1990.

Mair, D. D., Rice, M. J., Hagler, D. J., et al.: Outcome of the Fontan procedure in patients with tricuspid atresia. Circulation, 72(Suppl. II):88, 1985.

Marin-Garcia, J., Roca, J., Blieden, L. C., et al.: Congenital absence of the pulmonary valve associated with tricuspid atresia and intact ventricular septum. Chest, 64:658, 1973.

Mathur, M., and Glenn, W. W. L.: Long-term evaluation of cava-pulmonary artery anastomosis. Surgery, 74:899, 1973.

Matsuda, H., Kawashima, Y., Hirose, H., et al.: Modified Fontan operation for single ventricle with common atrium and abnormal systemic venous drainage: Usefulness of an additional superior vena cava-to-pulmonary artery anastomosis. Pediatr. Cardiol., 8:43, 1987.

Mayer, J. E., Jr., Helgason, H., Jonas, R. A., et al.: Extending the limits for modified Fontan procedures. J. Thorac. Cardiovasc. Surg., 92:1021, 1986.

McFaul, R. C., Tajik, A. J., Mair, D. D., et al.: Development of pulmonary arteriovenous shunt after superior vena cava-right pulmonary artery (Glenn) anastomosis. Circulation, 55:212, 1977.

Mietus-Snyder, M., Lang, P., Mayer, J. E., et al.: Childhood systemic-pulmonary shunts: Subsequent suitability for Fontan operation. Circulation, 76(Suppl. III, Pt. 2):39, 1987.

Milliken, J. C., Laks, H., and George, B.: Use of a venous assist device after repair of complex lesions of the right heart. J. Am. Coll. Cardiol., 8:922, 1986.

Moulton, A. L., Brenner, J. I., Ringel, R., et al.: Classic versus modified Blalock-Taussig shunts in neonates and infants. Circulation, 72(Suppl. II):35, 1985.

Muller, W. H., Jr., and Dammann, J. F., Jr.: The treatment of certain congenital malformations of the heart by the creation of pulmonary stenosis to reduce pulmonary hypertension and excessive pulmonary blood flow. Surg. Gynecol. Obstet., 95:213, 1952.

Nadas, A. S., and Fyler, D. C.: Pediatric Cardiology. 3rd ed. Philadelphia, W. B. Saunders, 1972.

Nakata, S., Imai, Y., Takanashi, Y., et al.: A new method for the quantitative standardization of cross-sectional areas of the pulmonary arteries in congenital heart diseases with decreased pulmonary blood flow. J. Thorac. Cardiovasc. Surg., 88:610, 1984.

Nakazawa, M., Nakanishi, T., Okuda, H., et al.: Dynamics of right heart flow in patients after Fontan procedure. Circulation, 69:306, 1984.

Nawa, S., Matsuki, T., Shimizu, A., et al.: Pulmonary artery connection in the Fontan procedure. Flexible polytetrafluoroethylene conduit for expansion. Chest, 91:552, 1987.

Norwood, W. I., Jacobs, M. L., and Murphy, J. D.: Fontan procedure for hypoplastic left heart syndrome. Ann. Thorac. Surg., 54:1025, 1992.

Ottenkamp, J., Wenink, A. C. G., Quaegebeur, J. M., et al.: Tricuspid atresia. Morphology of the outlet chamber with special emphasis on surgical implications. J. Thorac. Cardiovasc. Surg., 89:597, 1985.

Ottenkamp, J., Wenink, A. C. G., Rohmer, J., and Gittenberger-de Groot, A.: Tricuspid atresia with overriding imperforate tricuspid membrane: An anatomic variant. Int. J. Cardiol., 6:599, 1984.

Park, S. C., Neches, W. H., Mullins, C. E., et al.: Blade atrial septostomy: Collaborative study. Circulation, 66:258, 1982.

Patterson, W., Baxley, W. A., Karp, R. B., et al.: Tricuspid atresia in adults. Am. J. Cardiol., 49:141, 1982.

Pearl, J. M., Laks, H., Drinkwater, D. C., et al.: Modified Fontan procedure in patients less than 4 years of age. Circulation, 86(Suppl. II):100, 1992.

Pearl, J. M., Laks, H., Stein, D. G., et al.: Total cavopulmonary anastomosis versus conventional modified Fontan procedure. Ann. Thorac. Surg., 52:189, 1991.

Penkoske, P. A., Freedom, R. M., Williams, W. G., et al.: Surgical palliation of subaortic stenosis in the univentricular heart. J. Thorac. Cardiovasc. Surg., 87:767, 1984.

Peterson, R. J., Franch, R. H., Fajman, W. A., et al.: Noninvasive determination of exercise cardiac function following Fontan operation. J. Thorac. Cardiovasc. Surg., 88:263, 1984.

Pigott, J. D., Murphy, J. D., Barber, G., and Norwood, W. I.: Palliative reconstructive surgery for hypoplastic left heart snydrome. Ann. Thorac. Surg., 45:122, 1988.

Potts, W. J., Smith, S., and Gibson, S.: Anastomosis of the aorta to a pulmonary artery. J. A. M. A., 132:627, 1946.

Puga, F. J., Chiavarelli, M., and Hagler, D. J.: The Fontan operation for patients with left atrioventricular valve atresia. Circulation 74(Suppl. II):49, 1986.

Rao, P. S.: Further observations on the spontaneous closure of physiologically advantageous ventricular septal defects in tricuspid atresia: Surgical implications. Ann. Thorac. Surg., 35:121, 1983a.

Rao, P. S.: Left to right atrial shunting in tricuspid atresia. Br. Heart J., 49:345, 1983b.

Rao, P. S.: Percutaneous balloon valvotomy/angioplasty in congential heart disease. In Bashore, T. M., and Davidson, C. J. (eds): Percutaneous Balloon Valvuloplasty and Related Techniques. Baltimore, Williams & Wilkins, 1991, pp. 251–334.

Rashkind, W. J.: Tricuspid atresia: A historical review. Pediatr. Cardiol., 2:85, 1982.

Rashkind, W. J., and Miller, W. W.: Creation of an atrial septal defect without thoracotomy. A palliative approach to complete transposition of the great arteries. J. A. M. A., 196:991, 1966.

Rhodes, J., Garofano, R. P., Bowman, F. O., et al.: Effect of right ventricular anatomy on the cardiopulmonary response to exercise: Implications for the Fontan procedure. Circulation, 81:1811, 1990.

Ring, J. C., Bass, J. L., Marvin, W., et al.: Management of congenital stenosis of a branch pulmonary artery with balloon dilation angioplasty. J. Thorac. Cardiovasc. Surg., 90:35, 1985.

Robicsek, F., Sanger, P. W., Gollucci, V., and Daugherty, H. K.: Long-term circulatory exclusion of the right heart. Surgery, 59:431, 1966.

Rodbard, S., and Wagner, D.: Bypassing the right ventricle. Proc. Soc. Exp. Biol. Med., 71:69, 1949.

Rosenquist, G. C., Levy, R. J., and Rose, R. D.: Right atrial–left ventricular relationships in tricuspid atresia: Position of the presumed site of the atretic valve as determined by transillumination. Am. Heart J., 80:493, 1970.

Rosenthal, A.: Current status of treatment for tricuspid atresia. Introduction to symposium. Ann. Thorac. Surg., 29:304, 1980.

Ross, D. N., and Somerville, J.: Surgical correction of tricuspid atresia. Lancet, 1:845, 1973.

Rothman, A., Lang, P., Lodk, J. E., et al.: Surgical management of subaortic obstruction in single left ventricle and tricuspid atresia. J. Am. Coll. Cardiol., 10:421, 1987a.

Rothman, A., Mayer, J. E., and Freed, M. D.: Treatment of chronic pleural effusions after the Fontan procedure with prednisone. Am. J. Cardiol., 60:408, 1987b.

Rumisek, J. D., Pigott, J. D., Weinberg, P. M., and Norwood, W. I.: Coronary sinus septal defect associated with tricuspid atresia. J. Thorac. Cardiovasc. Surg., 92:142, 1986.

Rychik, J., Piccoli, D. A., and Barber, G.: Usefulness of corticosteroid therapy for protein-losing enteropathy after the Fontan procedure. Am. J. Cardiol., 68:819, 1991.

Sade, R. M.: Experimental observations on the physiology of the pulmonary circulation after right heart bypass. In Rao P. S., (ed): Tricuspid Atresia. Mt. Kisco, NY, Futura, 1992, pp. 321–340.

Sade, R. M.: Tricuspid atresia. In Sabiston, D. C., Jr., and Spencer, F. C. (eds): Surgery of the Chest. 4th ed. Philadelphia, W. B. Saunders, 1983, pp. 1186–1203.

Sade, R. M., and Castañeda, A. R.: The dispensable right ventricle. Surgery, 77:624, 1975.

Sade, R. M., and Wiles, H. B.: Pleuroperitoneal shunt for persistent pleural drainage after Fontan procedure. J. Thorac. Cardiovasc. Surg., 100:621, 1990.

Sanders, S. P., Wright, G. B., Keane, J. F., et al.: Clinical and hemodynamic results of the Fontan operation for tricuspid atresia. Am. J. Cardiol., 49:1733, 1982.

Scalia, D., Russo, P., Anderson, R. H., et al.: The surgical anatomy of hearts with no direct communication between the right atrium and the ventricular mass: So-called tricuspid atresia. J. Thorac. Cardiovasc. Surg., 87:743, 1984.

Schuberg, W.: Beobachtung von Verkummergung des rechten Herzventrikels in Folge von Atresie des Ost. venos. dextr.: Perforation des Herzscheidewand und dadurch Bildung eines Canales, der durch den rudimentaren rechtaen Ventrikel in die Art. pulmon. fuhrt. Virchows Arch. Pathol. Anat., 20:294, 1861.

Seliem, M., Muster, A. J., Paul, M. H., and Benson, D. W.: Relation between preoperative left ventricular muscle mass and outcome of the Fontan procedure in patients with tricuspid atresia. J. Am. Coll. Cardiol., 14:750, 1989.

Shachar, G. B., Fuhrman, B. P., Wayny, Y., et al.: Rest and exercise hemodynamics after the Fontan procedure. Circulation, 65:1043, 1982.

Smith, C. D., Sade, R. M., Crawford, F. A., Jr., and Othersen, H. B.: Diaphragmatic eventration in infants. J. Thorac. Cardiovasc. Surg., 91:490, 1986.

Stefanelli, G., Kirklin, J. W., Naftel, D. C., et al.: Early and intermediate-term (10-year) results of surgery for univentricular atrioventricular connection ("single ventricle"). Am. J. Cardiol. 54:811, 1984.

Stellin, G., Mazzucco, A., Bortolotti, U., et al.: Tricuspid atresia versus other complex lesions: Comparison of results with a modified Fontan procedure. J. Thorac. Cardiovasc. Surg., 96:204, 1988.

Stewart, J. M., Gewitz, M. H., Clark, B. J., et al.: The role of vasopressin and atrial natriuretic factor in postoperative fluid retention after the Fontan procedure. J. Thorac. Cardiovasc. Surg., 102:821, 1991.

Taliercio, C. P., Vlietstra, R. E., McGoon, M. D., et al.: Permanent cardiac pacing after the Fontan procedure. J. Thorac. Cardiovasc. Surg., 90:414, 1985.

Tam, C. K. H., Lightfoot, N. E., Finlay, C. D., et al.: Course of tricuspid atresia in the Fontan era. Am. J. Cardiol., 63:589, 1989.

Taussig, H. B., Keinonen, R., Momberger, H., and Kirk, H.: Long-time observations on the Blalock-Taussig operation. IV. Tricuspid atresia. Johns Hopkins Med. J., 132:135, 1973.

Teixeira, O. H., Carpenter, B., MacMurray, S. B., and Vlad, P.: Long-term prostaglandin $E_1$ therapy in congenital heart defects. J. Am. Coll. Cardiol., 3:838, 1984.

Tobias, J. D., Schleien, C. L., and Reitz, B. A.: Use of the MAST suit in the postoperative care of patients after the Fontan procedure. Crit. Care Med., 18:781, 1990.

Truesdell, S. C., Skorton, D. J., and Lauer, R. M.: Life insurance for children with cardiovascular disease. Pediatrics 77:687, 1986.

Ullom, R. L., Sade, R. M., Crawford, F. A., Jr., et al.: The Blalock-Taussig shunt in infants: Standard versus modified. Ann. Thorac. Surg., 44:539, 1987.

Uretzky, G., Puga, F. J., and Danielson, G. K.: Modified Fontan procedure in patients with previous ascending aorta-pulmonary artery anastomosis. J. Thorac. Cardiovasc. Surg., 85:447, 1983.

Van Praagh, R., Ando, M., and Dungan, W. T.: Anatomic types of tricuspid atresia: Clinical and developmental implications. Circulation, 44(Suppl. II):115, 1971.

Vargas, F. J., Mayer, J. E., Jr., Jonas, R. A., and Castañeda, A. R.: Anomalous systemic and pulmonary venous connections in conjunction with atriopulmonary anastomosis (Fontan-Kreutzer). Technical considerations. J. Thorac. Cardiovasc. Surg., 93:523, 1987a.

Vargas, F. J., Mayer, J. E., Jr., Jonas, R. A., and Castañeda, A. R.: Atrioventricular valve repair or replacement in atriopulmonary anastomosis: Surgical considerations. Ann. Thorac. Surg., 43:403, 1987b.

Voci, G., Diego, J. N., Shafie, H., et al.: Type Ia tricuspid atresia with extensive coronary artery abnormalities in a living 22-year-old woman. J. Am. Coll. Cardiol., 10:1100, 1987.

Ward, K. E., Fisher, D. J., and Michael, L.: Elevated coronary sinus pressure does not alter myocardial blood flow or left ventricular contractile function in mature sheep. J. Thorac. Cardiovasc. Surg., 95:511, 1988.

Warden, H. E., DeWall, R. A., and Varco, R. L.: Use of the right auricle as a pump for the pulmonary circuit. Surg. Forum, 5:16, 1954.

Warnes, C. A., and Somerville, J.: Tricuspid atresia with transposition of the great arteries in adolescents and adults: Current state and late complications. Br. Heart J., 57:543, 1987.

Waterston, D. J.: The treatment of Fallot's tetralogy in children under one year of age. Rozhl. Chir., 41:181, 1962.

Weber, H. S., Gleason, M. M., Myers, J. L., et al.: The Fontan operation in infants less than 2 years of age. J. Am. Coll. Cardiol., 19:828, 1992.

Weinberg, P. M.: Anatomy of tricuspid atresia and its relevance to current forms of surgical therapy. Ann. Thorac. Surg., 29:306, 1980.

Wenink, A. C. G., and Ottenkamp, J.: Tricuspid atresia. Microscopic findings in relation to "absence" of the atrioventricular connexion. Int. J. Cardiol., *16*:57, 1987.

Westerman, G. R., Readinger, R. I., and Van Devanter, S. H.: Unusual interatrial communication after the Fontan procedure. J. Thorac. Cardiovasc. Surg., *90*:627, 1985.

Williams, D. B., Kiernan, P. D., Metke, M. P., et al.: Hemodynamic response to positive end-expiratory pressure following right atrium-pulmonary artery bypass (Fontan procedure). J. Thorac. Cardiovasc. Surg., *87*:856, 1984.

Wittenborg, M. H., Neuhauser, E. B. D., and Sprunt, W. H.: Roentgenographic findings in congenital tricuspid atresia with hypoplasia of the right ventricle. Am. J. Roentgenol., *66*:712, 1951.

# 47

# Ebstein's Anomaly

Gordon K. Danielson

## HISTORICAL ASPECTS

In 1866, Dr. Wilhelm Ebstein, a young physician in Breslau, Poland, described the unusual cardiac findings in a 19-year-old laborer who had died of cyanotic heart disease. The anterior leaflet of the tricuspid valve was enlarged and fenestrated. There was a downward displacement of the posterior and septal leaflets in a spiral manner below the true annulus; the leaflets were hypoplastic, thickened, and adherent to the wall of the right ventricle. The atrialized portion of the ventricle was thinned and dilated, the right atrium was enlarged, and an open foramen ovale was present (Mann and Lie, 1979; Schiebler et al., 1968).

In addition to describing the characteristic anatomic findings in this anomaly, Ebstein accurately described the hemodynamic abnormalities and correlated them with the patient's cardiomegaly, pulsating jugular veins, and cardiac murmurs. His comprehensive report included two excellent full-sized illustrations. During his lifetime, Ebstein was praised for other contributions he made to pathology and medicine, but his students and colleagues overlooked his classic description of the congenital cardiac anomaly with which his name is identified today (Mann and Lie, 1979).

## EMBRYOLOGY AND PATHOLOGIC ANATOMY

The exact embryology of Ebstein's anomaly is unknown. The leaflets and the tensor apparatus of the tricuspid valve are thought to be formed at a relatively late stage in cardiac development by a process of delamination of the inner layers of the inlet zone of the right ventricle (Netter and Van Mierop, 1969). In Ebstein's anomaly, the insertions of the septal and posterior leaflets (and occasionally the right lateral aspect of the anterior leaflet) are displaced to the junction of the inlet and trabecular components of the ventricle, suggesting failure of delamination of these leaflets (Anderson et al., 1979). In some hearts, the endocardium is thickened and white, suggesting that formation of the valve leaflets had begun but then ceased before full leaflet development and delamination had occurred. The broad spectrum of pathologic changes seen in Ebstein's anomaly suggests that the mechanisms responsible for leaflet formation and right ventricular development are complex and probably related, in part, to hemodynamic forces (Anderson et al., 1979).

Ebstein's anomaly is characterized by a deformity of the valve in which the posterior and septal leaflets are displaced downward in a spiral manner below the true annulus (Fig. 47–1). The displaced leaflets are hypoplastic and thickened and often adhere to the wall of the right ventricle. Their displacement leaves a portion of the ventricle above the valve as an integral part of the right atrium; this is called the *atrialized ventricle*.

The anterior leaflet of the tricuspid valve in Ebstein's anomaly is typically larger than normal and has been described as sail-like. It may be fenestrated, and various portions of the leading edge may be attached to the right ventricular endocardium. The chordae tendineae and papillary muscles of the tricuspid valve are anomalous and abnormally positioned. The malformed tricuspid valve usually is incompetent, but occasionally, it may be stenotic or, rarely, imperforate.

The atrialized ventricle is thinned and dilated, but careful observation shows that the entire wall of the right ventricle, both proximal and distal to the abnormal insertion of the tricuspid leaflets, including the infundibulum, is also dilated. Dilatation of the right ventricular wall is associated not only with thinning of the wall but also with an absolute decrease in the number of myocardial fibers (Anderson and Lie, 1979). The atrioventricular node is located at the apex

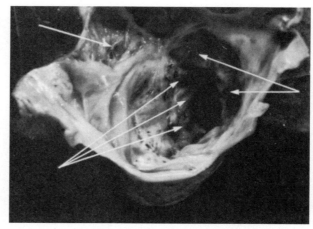

**FIGURE 47–1.** Ebstein's anomaly in a 9-day-old infant. View from the right atrium. The pathology is very similar to the original heart described by Ebstein. The *single arrow* indicates a patent foramen ovale. The anterior leaflet is enlarged and hooded (*double arrow*). The posterior and septal leaflets are dysplastic and displaced in a spiral manner toward the apex of the right ventricle (*triple arrow*). (Courtesy of William D. Edwards, M.D.)

of the triangle of Koch, and the conduction system is normally situated. Atrial septal defect and other associated anomalies are common.

In those congenital cardiac anomalies in which there is atrioventricular discordance with ventriculo-arterial discordance (corrected transposition), Ebstein's anomaly of the left atrioventricular valve is common. The displacement of the septal and posterior leaflets in left-sided Ebstein's anomaly is similar to that in the right-sided form, but the anterior leaflet is smaller and anatomically different (Anderson et al., 1978). Other differences relate to the functional portion of the morphologically right ventricle, which is rarely dilated, and the atrialized portion of the ventricle, which has less thinning of the wall. The atrioventricular conduction tissue in corrected transposition is right-sided and anterior, at a distance from the left-sided tricuspid valve (Anderson et al., 1974).

## PATHOLOGIC PHYSIOLOGY

The functional impairment of the right ventricle and the incompetence of the deformed tricuspid valve retard forward flow of blood through the right side of the heart. Moreover, during contraction of the atrium, the atrialized portion of the right ventricle is in diastole and balloons out (if very thin) or acts as a passive reservoir, decreasing the volume to be ejected; during ventricular systole, it contracts, creating a pressure wave that impedes venous filling of the right atrium, which is in the diastolic phase. In most cases, there is a communication between the left and the right atria, either because the foramen ovale is patent, caused by stretching of the atrial septum, or because a distinct secundum atrial septal defect is present. The movement of blood through the septal opening is generally from right to left but may be from left to right in some patients. The overall effect of these structural abnormalities on the right atrium is to produce gross dilatation, which may reach enormous proportions, even in infancy. This dilatation leads to further incompetence of the tricuspid valve and further widening of the interatrial communication. In older children and adults, significant hypertrophy of the right atrial wall is also usually present.

## CLINICAL FEATURES

Ebstein's anomaly is a rare cardiac anomaly that accounts for less than 1% of all congenital heart disease. It involves both sexes equally. Although a few patients reach advanced age, life expectancy for most is limited. The most common causes of death are congestive heart failure, hypoxia, and cardiac arrhythmias. When the diagnosis of Ebstein's anomaly is made in infancy, the prognosis is worse; one-third to one-half of these patients will die before 2 years of age (Giuliani et al., 1979; Kumar et al., 1971). Because a broad spectrum of pathologic changes occurs in Ebstein's anomaly, the hemodynamic alter-

ations vary. Symptoms are related to the severity of the incompetence of the tricuspid valve, the presence or absence of an associated atrial septal defect, the impairment of right ventricular function, and the presence of associated cardiac anomalies.

In the early neonatal period, any tricuspid incompetence is accentuated by the normally occurring elevated pulmonary arteriolar resistance, and infants with Ebstein's anomaly may develop severe congestive heart failure. Because the foramen ovale is patent in early infancy, severe tricuspid incompetence, with its resultant elevation of right atrial pressure, will produce a right-to-left atrial level shunt, and afflicted infants may be deeply cyanotic. If the infant survives this critical period, the degree of cyanosis and the symptoms often diminish as the fetal pulmonary hypertension regresses.

In older patients, the predominant symptoms are fatigability, dyspnea on exertion, and cyanosis. Palpitations in the form of paroxysmal atrial arrhythmias and premature ventricular beats are common. Less frequently, ascites and peripheral edema are present.

In an experience with 67 patients who had a mean follow-up of 12 years, Giuliani and associates (1979) found that 39% remained in functional New York Heart Association (NYHA) Class I or II and 61% progressed at some time into Class III or IV. Death occurred in 21% of the patients, who were characterized by one or more of the following features: They were functional Class III or IV; the cardiothoracic ratio was greater than 0.65; they had cyanosis or an arterial oxygen saturation of less than 90%; or they were infants when the diagnosis was made.

The physical signs vary. Heart sounds are usually soft, and a multiplicity of sounds and murmurs is often heard, all originating from the right side of the heart. A systolic murmur of tricuspid regurgitation may be heard along the left sternal border. Low-intensity diastolic and presystolic murmurs that result from anatomic or functional tricuspid stenosis may be present; they characteristically become louder with inspiration. There is wide splitting of both the first and the second heart sounds. Atrial and ventricular filling sounds are relatively common and they contribute to the cadence quality that is so often found in patients with Ebstein's anomaly. Summation of these gallop sounds may result from prolongation of atrioventricular conduction.

The arterial and jugular venous pulse forms usually are normal. A large V wave sometimes can be seen in the jugular venous pulse, but this is not usually prominent. The liver may be palpably enlarged, but it is almost never pulsatile.

## DIAGNOSIS

**Electrocardiography.** The electrocardiogram usually is abnormal, but it is not diagnostic. Complete or incomplete right bundle-branch block and right-axis deviation are typically present. The P waves are large, and the R waves in leads $V_1$ to $V_2$ are small. The PR interval is often prolonged, and the QRS complex is slurred. Arrhythmias are common. Ventricular preexcitation (Wolff-Parkinson-White syndrome) is encountered in approximately 15% of patients and is almost always of the right ventricular free wall or posterior septal type; a broad band or multiple pathways may be identified at intraoperative electrophysiologic mapping.

**Roentgenography.** The cardiac silhouette may vary from almost normal to the typical configuration, which consists of a globular-shaped heart with a narrow waist similar to that seen with pericardial effusion. This appearance is produced by enlargement of the right atrium and displacement of the right ventricular outflow tract outward and upward. Vascularity of the pulmonary fields is either normal or decreased.

**Echocardiography.** Two-dimensional echocardiography has revolutionized the diagnosis of Ebstein's anomaly. Enough anatomic and hemodynamic details can be obtained by an experienced echocardiographer that cardiac catheterization and angiography are usually unnecessary. Echocardiography allows an accurate evaluation of the tricuspid leaflets (displacement, tethering, dysplasia, absence), the size of the right atrium (including the atrialized portion of the right ventricle), and the size and function of the right and left ventricles. Doppler echocardiography and color-flow imaging allow detection of an atrial septal defect and the direction of shunt flow. In addition, color-flow imaging allows assessment of the site and degree of tricuspid valve regurgitation (Reeder et al., 1986).

Echocardiography provides the best method for assessing which patients are amenable to a valve reconstruction procedure and which require tricuspid valve replacement (Shiina et al., 1983) (Fig. 47–2).

**Cardiac Catheterization.** The right atrial pressure is usually moderately elevated, and the pulse contour may show a dominant V wave with a steep Y descent. However, in patients with a greatly dilated right atrium, the atrial pressure pulse may be normal despite the presence of severe tricuspid incompetence. Right ventricular pressure is most often normal, although the end-diastolic pressure may be elevated. Pulmonary artery pressure is normal or decreased. In patients with an associated atrial septal defect and right-to-left shunt, oximetry shows systemic arterial desaturation, and intracardiac dye-dilution curves from the venae cavae confirm the shunt. In the few patients who have a left-to-right shunt through an atrial septal defect, this is also shown by oximetry and dye-dilution curves.

**Angiography.** Injection of contrast medium into the right atrium shows enlargement of this chamber and normal position of the tricuspid annulus. An indentation on the inferior wall of the right ventricle some distance to the left of the tricuspid annulus represents the site of origin of the displaced leaflets of the tricuspid valve. The leaflets sometimes appear as radiolucent lines laterally and superiorly within the body of the right ventricle. Contrast medium often moves back and forth between the right atrium and the right ventricle, and right-to-left shunting at the atrial level may be found in the presence of an atrial septal defect

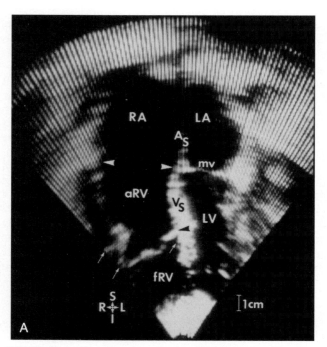
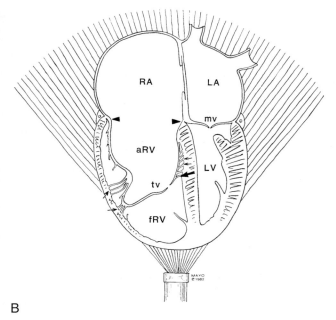

**FIGURE 47–2.** Two-dimensional echocardiogram (four-chamber view) *(A)* and interpretive diagram *(B)*, showing features typical of Ebstein's anomaly. (RA = right atrium; LA = left atrium; mv = mitral valve; LV = left ventricle; fRV = functional right ventricle; tv = tricuspid valve; aRV = atrialized right ventricle; $A_S$ = atrial septum; $V_S$ = ventricular septum; *arrows* = tethering of leaflets.) *(A,* From Shiina, A., Seward, J. B., Edwards, W. D., et al.: Two-dimensional echocardiographic spectrum of Ebstein's anomaly: Detailed anatomic assessment. Reprinted with permission from the American College of Cardiology [Journal of the American College of Cardiology, 1984, Vol. 3, pp. 356–370]; *B,* Courtesy of Mayo Foundation.)

or a patent foramen ovale. Flow through the right side of the heart and lungs is slow. Currently, cardiac catheterization is rarely done unless associated lesions are present or a previous shunt has been performed. In the latter case, angiography is desirable to define areas of pulmonary artery distortion, and may also be helpful in assessing patients with suspected pulmonary artery hypoplasia.

## ELECTROPHYSIOLOGIC EVALUATION

Atrial and ventricular arrhythmias are common in patients with Ebstein's malformation; they often present therapeutic problems and may cause sudden death. Twenty-four-hour ambulatory electrocardiographic monitoring is suggested for rhythm assessment in patients with palpitation or tachycardia. Invasive electrophysiologic study is performed for all patients with Ebstein's anomaly who have preexcitation on their electrocardiogram or who have a history of recurrent supraventricular tachycardia, undefined "wide-complex" tachycardia, or syncope as aspects of their clinical presentation.

## TREATMENT

Medical management has little to offer patients with Ebstein's anomaly, except for management of fluid retention and some arrhythmias. The prognosis is poorest for NYHA Classes III and IV patients and for those who have congestive heart failure, marked cyanosis, associated cardiac anomalies, extreme cardiomegaly (cardiothoracic ratio greater than 0.65), and diagnosis of the condition in infancy (Giuliani et al., 1979; Kumar et al., 1971). Serious cardiac arrhythmias without congestive failure or hypoxemia may also be life-threatening.

Observation alone is advised for only mildly symptomatic patients. Those patients who have survived infancy generally do well for a number of years, and correction can be postponed in such cases until deterioration is evident. However, since all patients with Ebstein's anomaly ultimately will show progressive deterioration, all will sooner or later become possible candidates for operation. Correction is usually possible, but in some patients with advanced cardiomyopathic changes, especially when the left ventricle is also involved, cardiac transplantation is the only option.

Surgical attempts to treat Ebstein's anomaly began in the 1950s with the use of systemic-to-pulmonary artery shunts for relief of cyanosis. For the few patients with obstruction of blood flow through the right side of the heart caused by pulmonary valvular or subvalvular stenosis or a stenotic or imperforate tricuspid valve, a shunt in infancy could be lifesaving. In the absence of obstructing lesions, systemic-pulmonary shunts have not usually benefited patients or have ended fatally.

A superior vena cava–pulmonary artery (Glenn) shunt was proposed as a more physiologic means of improving oxygenation; with this, approximately one-third of the unoxygenated venous return would be diverted away from the right side of the heart and directly into the pulmonary circulation. However, the caval shunt is of limited usefulness in Ebstein's anomaly. In a collected series of 36 cases of vena cava–pulmonary artery shunts performed for this anomaly, 17 patients survived the operation and 14 benefited from it (Glenn et al., 1966).

Reconstruction of the deformed tricuspid valve, directed toward total correction of the hemodynamic abnormality, began in 1958, when Hunter and Lillehei attempted to create a competent valve by repositioning the displaced posterior and septal leaflets. Their method, employed in two patients, also entailed excluding the atrialized ventricular chamber. Both patients developed heart block, and neither survived (Lillehei et al., 1967). Later, Hardy and co-workers (1964) revived and modified the Hunter-Lillehei operation. They placed interrupted sutures close together on the spiral line of the displaced posterior and septal cusp bases and wider apart at the annulus. Tying of the sutures created multiple tucks in the leaflets, narrowed the tricuspid orifice somewhat, and pulled the displaced leaflets back to the tricuspid annulus. The technique was employed in six patients, four of whom survived; one of the survivors had complete heart block (Hardy and Roe, 1969). Although some good early results have been reported with this procedure, it has not been generally effective in establishing a competent valve in the moderate and severe forms of Ebstein's anomaly. With suture placement in the septum as originally shown, heart block may occur. Moreover, it is not possible to transpose the septal leaflet and medial portions of the posterior leaflet to the tricuspid annulus because the ventricular septum cannot be plicated in the same way as the free wall of the right ventricle. Finally, direct approximation of the displaced leaflet to the tricuspid annulus along the free wall does not obliterate the atrialized ventricle, which protrudes below the heart as an aneurysmal sac and, despite efforts to the contrary, usually remains in communication with the right ventricle.

In 1963, Barnard and Schrire successfully replaced the deformed tricuspid valve with a mechanical prosthetic valve in two patients. In their technique, the sutures anchoring the prosthesis were deviated cephalad to the coronary sinus and atrioventricular node in order to avoid injuring the conduction system. With the sutures thus placed, blood from the coronary sinus drained directly into the right ventricle. The atrialized portion of the ventricle was not obliterated.

In 1967, Lillehei and associates replaced the tricuspid valve with a Starr-Edwards ball valve in five patients. In two patients, the prosthetic valve was sutured to the true annulus, causing complete atrioventricular dissociation. One of the two died; in the remaining three patients, attachment of the prosthesis according to the Barnard and Schrire technique prevented heart block.

Other surgical techniques used for Ebstein's anomaly include atrioventricular plication combined with tricuspid valve replacement (Timmis et al., 1967) and replacement of the tricuspid valve with a tissue valve together with obliteration of the atrialized portion of the right ventricle and closure of the atrial septal defect (Ross and Somerville, 1970). For selected neonates, closure of the tricuspid valve, atrial septectomy, and an aortopulmonary shunt have been advocated (Starnes et al., 1991).

Although it remains the most popular way to repair Ebstein's anomaly, prosthetic valve replacement has given less-than-ideal results for some patients. Mechanical valves in the tricuspid position are associated with a higher frequency of valve malfunction and thrombotic complications than they are in other cardiac positions (Sanfelippo et al., 1976). Tissue valves do not have the thromboembolic complications of mechanical valves, but they do have a limited life expectancy, particularly in infants and children. In the author's group's experience, the overall failure-free rate of porcine heterograft valves in children is only 58.5% at 5 years (Williams et al., 1982), although current results show that the longevity of porcine valves is more favorable in the tricuspid position. Prosthetic valves are also undesirable in the small patient because reoperation may be required for replacement of the valve owing to somatic growth.

In 1972, the author's group developed a repair that consists of plication of the free wall of the atrialized portion of the right ventricle, posterior tricuspid annuloplasty, and excision of redundant right atrial wall (right reduction atrioplasty) (Danielson et al., 1979). The repair is based on the construction of a monocuspid valve by the use of the anterior leaflet of the tricuspid valve, which usually is enlarged in this anomaly. The early and late (up to 19 years follow-up) results of the author's experience have been reported (Danielson et al., 1992). The author's group believes repair is preferable to valve replacement whenever it is feasible because it avoids the problems of prosthetic valve dysfunction, anticoagulation, and in children, outgrowth. Other types of valve reconstruction have been proposed (Carpentier et al., 1988; Quaegebeur et al., 1991; Schmidt-Habelmann et al., 1981), but late results of these procedures in significant numbers of patients have not yet been reported.

## INDICATIONS FOR OPERATION

The indications for surgical intervention in Ebstein's anomaly are still incompletely defined. Most patients in functional Classes I and II can be managed medically, as was done for most patients diagnosed with Ebstein's anomaly who were seen at the author's institution during the interval covered by this surgical experience. Operative correction is offered when progressive deterioration is evident. Exceptions that would prompt earlier surgical intervention include moderately severe or progressive cyanosis, paradoxical emboli, and right ventricular outflow tract obstruction. In borderline situations, the ability to re-

construct the tricuspid valve, as determined by echocardiography, makes the decision to operate easier. The presence of atrial arrhythmias related to accessory conduction pathways and the observation of progressive cardiomegaly are relative indications for operation. Once symptoms develop and progress to Classes III and IV, medical management has little to offer and operation is advised.

## OPERATIVE MANAGEMENT

The author's operative management of patients with Ebstein's anomaly consists of (1) electrophysiologic mapping for localization of accessory conduction pathways in patients with ventricular preexcitation; (2) excision of any attenuated atrial septum and pericardial patch closure of the defect for patients with an atrial septal defect or patent foramen ovale; (3) plication of the atrialized portion of the right ventricle; (4) reconstruction of the tricuspid valve, when feasible, or valve replacement; (5) correction of associated anomalies such as relief of pulmonary stenosis, ablation of accessory conduction pathways, or perinodal cryoablation for atrioventricular nodal reentry tachycardia; and (6) right reduction atrioplasty.

After a median sternotomy is performed, adhesions are freed and the external cardiac anatomy is confirmed. Electrophysiologic mapping is performed if preexcitation has been diagnosed on preoperative electrophysiologic study. Mapping of the ventricles is performed with a multielectrode sock during sinus rhythm and atrial pacing; mapping of the atria is performed during ventricular pacing and reciprocating tachycardia. Immediate results are available through computer analysis of the recorded data (CR, Bard, Inc., Murray Hill, NJ).

Cannulation is accomplished by using the ascending aorta for arterial inflow and separate caval cannulae inserted through the right atrial appendage for venous outflow to the pump. Cardiopulmonary bypass is instituted at 2.4 l/min/M² and the perfusate temperature is lowered to 25° C. The left side of the heart is vented with a catheter inserted through the right superior pulmonary vein and an aortic tack vent is placed. The aorta is temporarily cross-clamped and the myocardium is protected with multidose cold blood cardioplegia and topical hypothermia. The myocardial temperature is kept between 15 and 20° C. The right atrium is opened from the appendage to the inferior vena cava and repair is performed as shown in Figure 47–3. The author prefers to excise all attenuated atrial septal tissue and to patch the resulting atrial septal defect. This preference is based on experience that an atrial septal defect closed by suture in patients with a high-pressure right atrium (as in Ebstein's anomaly or a modified Fontan procedure) may reopen either early or late because of the sutures pulling through the septal tissue.

The ventricular plication sutures are placed in the atrialized right ventricle so as to avoid large branches of the right coronary artery and the posterior de-

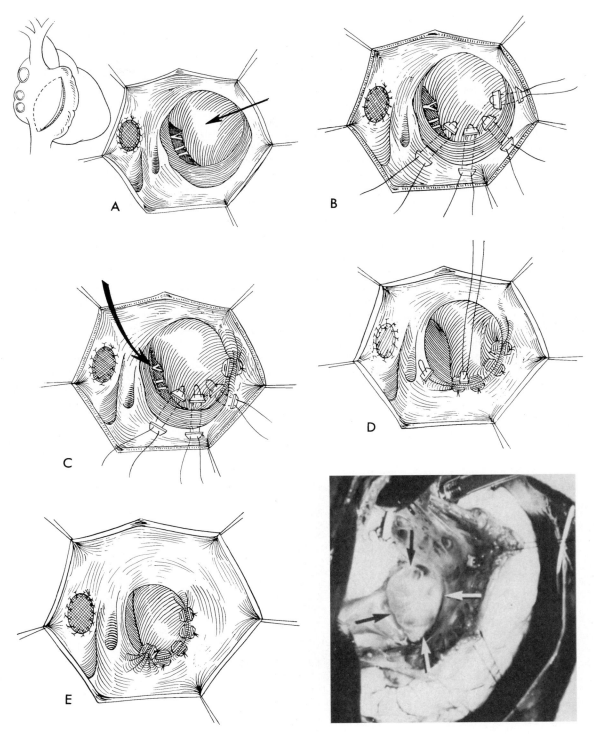

**FIGURE 47–3.** Diagram of repair. *A, Left,* The right atrium is incised from the atrial appendage to the inferior vena cava. The redundant portion of the right atrium is excised *(dotted line)* so that the final size of the right atrium is normal. *Right,* The atrial septal defect is closed with a patch. The large anterior leaflet is indicated by the *arrow.* The posterior leaflet is displaced down from the annulus and the septal leaflet is hypoplastic and not visible in this view. *B,* Mattress sutures passed through pledgets of Teflon felt are used to pull the tricuspid annulus and tricuspid valve together. Sutures are placed in the atrialized portion of the right ventricle as shown so that when they are subsequently tied, the atrialized ventricle is plicated and the aneurysmal cavity is obliterated. *C,* The sutures are tied down sequentially. The hypoplastic, markedly displaced septal leaflet is now visible *(arrow).* *D,* A posterior annuloplasty is performed to narrow the diameter of the tricuspid annulus. The coronary sinus marks the posterior and leftward extent of the annuloplasty, which is terminated there to avoid injury to the conduction bundle. One or more additional sutures may be required to obliterate the posterior aspect of the annuloplasty repair to render the valve totally competent. At this time, the tricuspid annulus will admit two or more fingers in the adult. *E,* Completed repair that allows the anterior leaflet to function as a monocusp valve. *F,* Operative photograph of completed repair. The large anterior leaflet forms a competent monocusp valve *(arrows).* (*A–F,* From Danielson, G. K., Maloney, J. D., Devloo, R. A. E.: Surgical repair of Ebstein's anomaly. Mayo Clin. Proc., *54:*185, 192, 1979.)

scending coronary artery. The epicardial arteries are inspected after each plication suture is placed; the suture is removed and relocated if an important coronary artery branch has been compromised. The posterior annuloplasty (Fig. 47–3D and E) is a critical part of the procedure. The posterior aspect of the annulus is first narrowed with the annuloplasty suture and then further obliterated by additional interrupted mattress sutures passed through felt pledgets from the free wall annulus to the septum as needed to provide complete competence of the reconstructed valve.

Because this repair is based on the presence of a satisfactory anterior leaflet, significant abnormalities of the leaflet may compromise the result. For most patients with fenestrations or perforations in the anterior leaflet, the defects can be satisfactorily repaired with fine running sutures. Small anterior leaflets may permit construction of a competent tricuspid valve, but at the expense of creating some (usually acceptable) degree of tricuspid stenosis. Anterior leaflets with linear or hyphenated attachment of the leading edge to the right ventricular endocardium—a condition associated with absence of the papillary muscles and chordae—are not appropriate for reconstruction. The presence of short papillary muscles and chordae does not necessarily preclude a satisfactory repair, if the remaining leaflet tissue is well formed. A few patients will have enough posterior leaflet tissue present to permit a bileaflet repair; and rarely, all three leaflets will be moderately well formed but displaced, permitting a trileaflet repair.

After the reconstruction is completed, the tricuspid valve is tested by temporarily clamping the pulmonary artery and injecting saline solution under pressure into the right ventricle with a bulb syringe and large catheter. Following venous decannulation, the surgeon's finger is introduced into the right atrium for direct palpation of the tricuspid valve in the beating heart. The results have also been assessed by intraoperative transesophageal echocardiography since 1985. Temporary pacemaker wires are attached to the right atrium and right ventricle for postoperative monitoring of rhythm and for pacing in selected cases. The basic techniques of repair have not changed since the original successful case in 1972. However, because the anatomy in no two patients is exactly alike, each repair is tailored appropriately until the valve is competent.

When the tricuspid valve cannot be reconstructed, the valve is excised and a prosthetic valve is inserted. The suture line is deviated to the atrial side of the coronary sinus and atrioventricular node to avoid injury to the conduction mechanism (Fig. 47–4). In patients with normal hearts, mechanical prostheses in the tricuspid position have a higher incidence of malfunction and thrombotic complications than they do in either the aortic or the mitral position. However, mechanical valves have functioned better in patients with Ebstein's anomaly, perhaps because the right ventricles are larger and there is less tendency for fibrous tissue ingrowth into the prostheses. In the author's group's experience, bioprosthetic valves also last longer in the tricuspid position in Ebstein's anom-

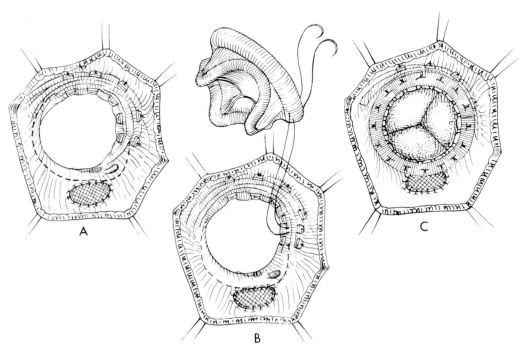

**FIGURE 47–4.** Diagram of technique for tricuspid valve replacement in Ebstein's anomaly. *A*, If the atrialized right ventricle is dilated, thin, and noncontractile, it is plicated. *B*, Medially, the suture line is deviated to the atrial side of the coronary sinus and atrioventricular node *(dotted line)* to avoid injury to the conduction mechanism. *C*, The sutures are tied with the heart perfused and beating to assure that a conducted rhythm is preserved. (*A–C*, From Danielson, G. K.: Ebstein's anomaly of the tricuspid valve. *In* Mavroudis, C. and Backer, C. L. (eds): Pediatric Cardiac Surgery. 2nd ed. Chap. 28. Mosby–Year Book, St. Louis, 1994, pp. 413–424.)

■ **Table 47–1.** ASSOCIATED CARDIAC DEFECTS

| Defects | Number of Patients |
|---|---|
| Atrial septal defect | 169 |
| Accessory conduction pathway(s) | 28 |
| Pulmonary stenosis | 16 |
| Ventricular septal defect | 7 |
| Atrioventricular nodal reentry tachycardia | 4 |
| Partial atrioventricular canal | 4 |
| Absent coronary sinus | 3 |
| Anomalous pulmonary venous connection | 2 |
| Bilateral superior venae cavae | 2 |
| Pericarditis | 2 |
| Patent ductus arteriosus | 2 |
| Other | 10 |

■ **Table 47–3.** CONCOMITANT CARDIAC PROCEDURES

| Procedures | Number of Patients |
|---|---|
| Closure of atrial septal defect | 169 |
| Ablation accessory pathway(s) | 28 |
| Repair of pulmonary stenosis | 16 |
| Closure shunt | 13 |
| Repair of ventricular septal defect | 7 |
| Repair of partial atrioventricular canal | 4 |
| Ablation atrioventricular nodal reentry tachycardia | 4 |
| Closure of patent ductus arteriosus | 2 |
| Repair of partial anomalous pulmonary venous connection | 2 |
| Other | 9 |

aly compared with their performance in hearts with normal ventricular anatomy.

## CLINICAL DATA

Between April 1972 and December 31, 1993, 253 consecutive patients with Ebstein's anomaly have undergone operation on the author's surgical service. The results from the first 189 patients have been analyzed (Danielson et al., 1992). Patients ranged in age from 11 months to 64 years (median, 16 years; mean, 19.1 years). Hemoglobin values ranged between 10.8 and 23.4 g/dl, cardiothoracic ratios ranged between 0.49 and 0.96, and arterial oxygen saturations ranged between 65 and 98%.

Associated cardiac defects are shown in Table 47–1, and previous cardiovascular operations are shown in Table 47–2.

## RESULTS

Valve repair by plication of the atrialized right ventricle and valvuloplasty was accomplished in 110 of the 189 consecutive patients (58.2%). Tricuspid valve replacement was required in 69 patients (36.5%). Right ventricular plication was added to the valve replacement if the atrialized ventricle was dilated, thin, and noncontractile. Porcine bioprostheses were used in 50 patients; 19 received mechanical prosthe-

ses. Two patients (1.1%) with a prior Glenn anastomosis who had unrepairable valves underwent plication of the atrialized right ventricle and resection of their tricuspid valves without valve replacement—a type of modified Fontan procedure. Eight other patients (4.2%) who had hemodynamically mild tricuspid insufficiency underwent repair of other significant anomalies without a procedure on the tricuspid valve.

Concomitant cardiac procedures are shown in Table 47–3. In all 28 patients, the accessory conduction pathways were successfully ablated; no patient sustained permanent complete heart block. The four patients with atrioventricular nodal reentry tachycardia underwent successful ablation of their arrhythmias without production of heart block. One patient who had paroxysmal atrial flutter and atrial fibrillation underwent cryoablation of the atrioventricular node and implantation of a permanent pacemaker for control of the arrhythmias.

Twelve deaths (6.3%) occurred within 30 days or during the initial hospitalization (Table 47–4). Four deaths were caused by sudden ventricular fibrillation in patients who were otherwise doing well but who had massive cardiomegaly. Other causes of death included low cardiac output ($n = 5$), postoperative hemorrhage ($n = 1$), respiratory arrest ($n = 1$), and coagulopathy ($n = 1$).

When two-dimensional echocardiography and Doppler and color-flow imaging became available, all patients were studied by these modalities before hospital discharge. Most patients had tricuspid insufficiency rated as trivial or mild. The atrial septum was intact in all patients.

To date, follow-up has been obtained in 151 of the 177 operative survivors (85.3%). Ten late deaths have occurred; causes of death were sudden (presumably

■ **Table 47–2.** PREVIOUS CARDIOVASCULAR OPERATIONS

| Operations | Number of Patients |
|---|---|
| Blalock-Taussig shunt | 10 |
| Closure of atrial septal defect | 8 |
| Glenn anastomosis | 6 |
| Pacemaker | 6 |
| Attempted repair* | 5 |
| Waterston shunt | 5 |
| Partial pericardiectomy | 2 |
| Other | 7 |

*All performed elsewhere with various surgical techniques including the use of a rigid tricuspid ring.

■ **Table 47–4.** EARLY POSTOPERATIVE DEATHS

| Procedures | Number of Patients | Number of Early Deaths (%) |
|---|---|---|
| Plication and valvuloplasty | 110 | 8 (7.3) |
| Tricuspid valve replacement | 69 | 4 (5.8) |
| Plication and Fontan | 2 | — |
| Other | 8 | — |
| Total | 189 | 12 (6.3) |

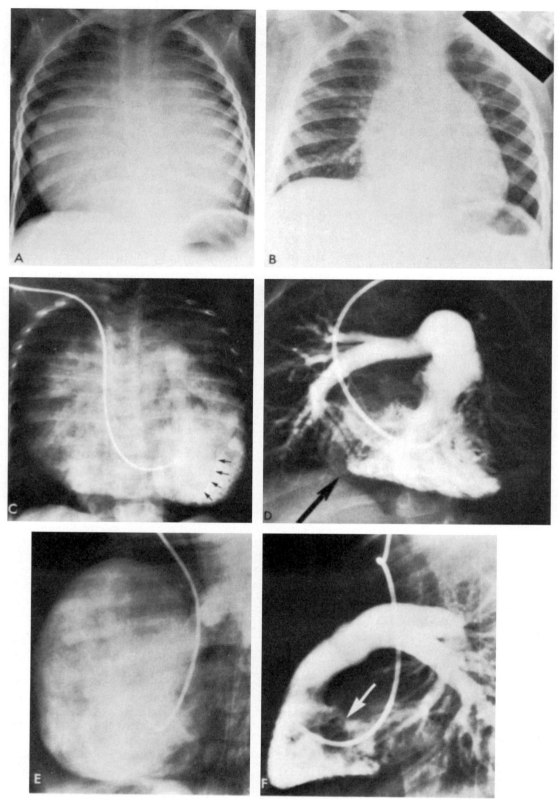

**FIGURE 47–5.** The patient was a 2-year-old girl with Ebstein's anomaly and history of pneumonia, cardiorespiratory arrest, and failure to thrive. *Chest films: A,* Preoperative (cardiothoracic ratio–0.9). *B,* Thirteen days postoperatively (cardiothoracic ratio–0.55). *Right ventricular angiogram, anteroposterior view: C,* Preoperative. The contrast medium refluxes through the tricuspid valve to fill the entire cardiac silhouette. A radiolucent line within the cavity of the ventricle shows the location of the displaced tricuspid leaflets *(arrows). D,* Postoperative. There is rapid transit of contrast medium from the right ventricle to the pulmonary arteries with only a trace of tricuspid insufficiency. The *arrow* indicates the new plane of the tricuspid valve. *Right ventricular angiogram, lateral view: E,* Preoperative. *F,* Postoperative. The tricuspid valve is competent. The *arrow* points to filling defect created by the anterior leaflet. This patient is now 19 years old. She is asymptomatic, is taking no cardiac medications, and is an "A" student. (*A–F,* From Danielson, G. K., Maloney, J. D., and Devloo, R. A. E.: Surgical repair of Ebstein's anomaly. Mayo Clin. Proc., *54:*185, 1979.)

1656

arrhythmic) in 4 patients, congestive heart failure in 3, automobile accident (passenger) in 1, abdominal abscess in 1, and unknown in 1. Because of the high incidence of both early and late sudden deaths in the initial experience, presumably related to ventricular arrhythmias, the author's group now administers intravenous lidocaine prophylactically for the first 48 hours and then changes to procainamide with an initial intravenous loading dose and subsequent oral doses. The author's group advises the continuation of procainamide administration for 3 months, at which time its use can be tapered and discontinued if no further tendency to develop ventricular ectopy is seen in the patient. Twenty-four-hour ambulatory monitoring is then suggested for rhythm assessment.

Reoperations for tricuspid valve replacement were required in 4 of the 110 patients who had undergone tricuspid valve repair. This represents a total incidence of 3.6% in a follow-up extending to 19 years. In the first patient, who was 1 year old, a less-than-ideal repair was accepted as an alternative to valve replacement, in the hope that the child would grow further before a valve prosthesis would be required. The child developed for 6½ years before valve replacement was necessary, at which time she received a 31-mm (adult size) porcine bioprosthesis. The second patient sustained an inferior wall myocardial infarction from kinking of the distal right coronary artery at the time of operation. This produced enough distortion of the right ventricle that the valve became insufficient and required replacement 1 year later. The other 2 patients required valve replacement 6 and 14 years after initial repair, respectively, because of progressive dilatation of the tricuspid annulus and right ventricle. All 4 patients survived reoperation and are now in NYHA Class I or II. Two additional patients required reoperation for replacement of a mechanical valve, and both survived. There have been no operations yet for replacement of a porcine valve.

Of survivors more than 1 year after surgery, 92.9% were in NYHA Class I or II. Postoperative reduction in heart size was usual and occasionally considerable (Fig. 47–5). Nine female patients have undergone a total of 12 successful pregnancies with delivery of normal children.

In a study of cardiac arrhythmias in some of these patients, Oh and co-workers (1985) found that, of patients with preoperative paroxysmal supraventricular tachycardia and paroxysmal atrial fibrillation or flutter, only 33% continued to have symptomatic tachycardia after operation.

Maximal exercise testing shows a significant increase in work performance, exercise duration, and maximal oxygen uptake after operation (Driscoll et al., 1988). Maximal oxygen consumption in the author's group's patients increased from a mean of 47% of predicted value before operation to a mean of 72% of predicted value after operation. Operative treatment of Ebstein's anomaly also favorably affects cardiac output, particularly in response to exercise,

normalizes systemic arterial oxygen saturation, and reduces excess ventilation at rest and during exercise.

In summary, operation is indicated for those patients with Ebstein's anomaly who are in NYHA Class III or IV and for selected other patients who show clinical deterioration. Whenever possible, the author's group prefers a valve repair that is based on available usable valve leaflet tissue, usually the anterior tricuspid leaflet. Occasionally, a bileaflet or trileaflet repair can be accomplished. Operation eliminates right-to-left intracardiac shunting with its attendant risks, improves exercise tolerance, and reduces supraventricular arrhythmias. In addition, longevity is increased in those patients who are improved to functional NYHA Class I or II status.

## SELECTED BIBLIOGRAPHY

Special review of Ebstein's anomaly. Mayo Clin. Proc., 54:163, 1979.

This monograph describes the historical, clinical, and morphologic aspects of Ebstein's anomaly. The clinical features and natural history of 67 consecutive patients with Ebstein's anomaly who were monitored for a mean of 12 years are described. This monograph gives a good overview of the present knowledge of Ebstein's anomaly.

Danielson, G. K., Driscoll, D. J., Mair, D. D., et al.: Operative treatment of Ebstein's anomaly. J. Thorac. Cardiovasc. Surg., 104:1195, 1992.

This article presents the largest surgical series of patients operated on for Ebstein's anomaly. Valve repair by plication of the atrialized right ventricle and valvuloplasty was accomplished in 58.2% of the 189 patients.

Ebstein's anomaly. Prog. Pediatr. Cardiol., 2:1, 1993.

This monograph is an excellent current review of Ebstein's anomaly and includes a chapter on the neonatal expression of Ebstein's anomaly.

## BIBLIOGRAPHY

Anderson, K. R., Danielson, G. K., McGoon, D. C., and Lie, J. T.: Ebstein's anomaly of the left-sided tricuspid valve: Pathological anatomy of the valvular malformation. Circulation (Suppl. I), 58:87, 1978.
Anderson, K. R., and Lie, J. T.: The right ventricular myocardium in Ebstein's anomaly. A morphometric histopathologic study. Mayo Clin. Proc., 54:181, 1979.
Anderson, K. R., Zuberbuhler, J. R., Anderson, R. H., et al.: Morphologic spectrum of Ebstein's anomaly of the heart: A review. Mayo Clin. Proc., 54:174, 1979.
Anderson, R. H., Becker, A. E., Arnold, R., and Wilkinson, J. L.: The conducting tissues in congenitally corrected transposition. Circulation, 50:911, 1974.
Barnard, C. N., and Schrire, V.: Surgical correction of Ebstein's malformation with prosthetic tricuspid valve. Surgery, 54:302, 1963.
Carpentier, A., Chauvaud, S., Mace, L., et al.: A new reconstructive operation for Ebstein's anomaly of the tricuspid valve. J. Thorac. Cardiovasc. Surg., 96:92, 1988.
Danielson, G. K., Driscoll, D. J., Mair, D. D., et al.: Operative treatment of Ebstein's anomaly. J. Thorac. Cardiovasc. Surg., 104:1195, 1992.
Danielson, G. K., Maloney, J. D., and Devloo, R. E. A.: Surgical repair of Ebstein's anomaly. Mayo Clin. Proc., 54:185, 1979.
Driscoll, D. J., Mottram, C. D., and Danielson, G. K.: Spectrum of exercise intolerance in 45 patients with Ebstein's anomaly and observations on exercise tolerance in 11 patients after surgical repair. J. Am. Coll. Cardiol., 11:831, 1988.
Ebstein, W.: Ueber einen sehr seltenen Fall von Insufficienz der Valvula Tricuspidalis, bedingt durch eine angeborene hochgradige Missbildung derselben. Arch. Anat. Physiol., 1866, p. 238.
Giuliani, E. R., Fuster, V., Brandenburg, R. O., and Mair, D. D.: The

clinical features and natural history of Ebstein's anomaly of the tricuspid valve. Mayo Clin. Proc., 54:163, 1979.

Glenn, W. W. L., Browne, M., and Whittemore, R.: Circulatory bypass of the right side of the heart: Cava-pulmonary artery shunt–Indications and results (report of a collected series of 537 cases). In Cassels, D. E. (ed): The Heart and Circulation in the Newborn and Infant. New York, Grune & Stratton, 1966, pp. 345–357.

Hardy, K. L., May, I. A., Webster, C. A., and Kimball, K. G.: Ebstein's anomaly: A functional concept and successful definitive repair. J. Thorac. Cardiovasc. Surg., 48:927, 1964.

Hardy, K. L., and Roe, B. B.: Ebstein's anomaly: Further experience with definitive repair. J. Thorac. Cardiovasc. Surg., 58:553, 1969.

Hunter, S. W., and Lillehei, C. W.: Ebstein's malformation of the tricuspid valve: Study of a case together with suggestion of a new form of surgical therapy. Dis. Chest, 33:297, 1958.

Kumar, A. E., Fyler, D. C., Miettinen, O. S., and Nadas, A. S.: Ebstein's anomaly: Clinical profile and natural history. Am. J. Cardiol., 28:84, 1971.

Lillehei, C. W., Kalke, B. R., and Carlson, R. G.: Evolution of corrective surgery for Ebstein's anomaly. Circulation, 35, 36(Suppl. I):111, 1967.

Mann, R. J., and Lie, J. T.: The life story of Wilhelm Ebstein (1836–1912) and his almost overlooked description of a congenital heart disease. Mayo Clin. Proc., 54:197, 1979.

Netter, F. H., and Van Mierop, L. H. S.: Embryology. In Yonkman, F. F. (ed): The Ciba Collection of Medical Illustrations. Vol. 5. Summit, NJ, Ciba Pharmaceutical Company, 1969, p. 125.

Oh, J. K., Holmes, D. R., Jr., Hayes, D. L., et al.: Cardiac arrhythmias in patients with surgical repair of Ebstein's anomaly. J. Am. Coll. Cardiol., 6:1351, 1985.

Quaegebeur, J. M., Sreeram, N., Fraser, A. G., et al.: Surgery for Ebstein's anomaly: The clinical and echocardiographic evaluation of a new technique. J. Am. Coll. Cardiol., 17:722, 1991.

Reeder, G. S., Currie, P. J., Hagler, D. J., et al.: Use of Doppler techniques (continuous-wave, pulsed-wave, and color-flow imaging) in the noninvasive hemodynamic assessment of congenital heart disease. Mayo Clin. Proc., 61:725, 1986.

Ross, D., and Somerville, J.: Surgical correction of Ebstein's anomaly. Lancet, 2:280, 1970.

Sanfelippo, P. M., Giuliani, E. R., Danielson, G. K., et al.: Tricuspid valve prosthetic replacement: Early and late results with the Starr-Edwards prosthesis. J. Thorac. Cardiovasc. Surg., 71:441, 1976.

Schiebler, G. L., Gravenstein, J. S., and Van Mierop, L. H. S.: Ebstein's anomaly of the tricuspid valve: Translation of original description with comments. Am. J. Cardiol., 22:867, 1968.

Schmidt-Habelmann, P., Meisner, H., Struck, E., and Sebening, F.: Results of valvuloplasty for Ebstein's anomaly. Thorac. Cardiovasc. Surg., 29:155, 1981.

Shiina, A., Seward, J. B., and Tajik, A. J., et al.: Two-dimensional echocardiographic-surgical correlation in Ebstein's anomaly: Preoperative determination of patients requiring tricuspid valve plication vs. replacement. Circulation, 68:534, 1983.

Starnes, V. A., Pitlick, P. T., Bernstein, D., et al.: Ebstein's anomaly appearing in the neonate. J. Thorac. Cardiovasc. Surg., 101:1082, 1991.

Timmis, H. H., Hardy, J. D., and Watson, D. G.: The surgical management of Ebstein's anomaly. The combined use of tricuspid valve replacement, atrioventricular plication, and atrioplasty. J. Thorac. Cardiovasc. Surg., 53:385, 1967.

Williams, D. B., Danielson, G. K., McGoon, D. C., et al.: Porcine heterograft valve replacement in children. J. Thorac. Cardiovasc. Surg., 84:446, 1982.

# 48 Hypoplastic Left Heart Syndrome

William I. Norwood

Among congenital cardiac malformations that present in the first year of life, hypoplastic left heart syndrome is the fourth most common and is found in approximately 2500 babies born in the United States each year. This malformation also is by far the most common of the abnormalities that share the feature of only one well-developed ventricle. Lev (1952) initially described the constellation of abnormalities including isolated hypoplasia of the aorta, hypoplasia of the left ventricle with ventricular septal defect, and hypoplasia of the aorta with aortic stenosis or atresia with or without mitral stenosis or atresia, and named these abnormalities "hypoplasia of the aortic tract complexes." Noonan and Nadas (1958) subsequently referred to these lesions as hypoplastic left heart syndrome, now the widely accepted term. As attention has been drawn to this category of malformations, the anatomic definition has increased in precision.

## DEFINITION AND ANATOMY

Hypoplastic left heart syndrome is a collective term describing a group of cardiac malformations in which aortic valve hypoplasia, stenosis, or atresia occurs with either hypoplasia or absence of the left ventricle. As a consequence of limited blood flow in the ascending aorta, the left ventricle is correspondingly hypoplastic. Associated severe mitral hypoplasia or mitral atresia is also present. A less common variation includes malalignment of the common atrioventricular canal over the right ventricle. Finally, 10% of patients with hypoplastic left heart syndrome have a double-outlet right ventricle rather than the usual normally related great arteries. However, cases involving transposition of the great arteries with hypoplasia of the left ventricle and pulmonary artery or hypoplasia of the right ventricle and aorta are not considered hypoplastic left heart syndrome. The anatomy of patients with aortic stenosis/atresia has been thoroughly described (Bharati and Lev, 1984; Bjerregaard and Laursen, 1980; Bulkley et al., 1983; Elzenga and Gittenberger de Grott, 1985; Hawkins and Doty, 1984; Jonas et al., 1986; Kanjuh et al., 1965; Lev, 1952; Moodie et al., 1986; Noonan and Nadas, 1958; O'Connor et al., 1982; Roberts et al., 1976; Sinha et al., 1968; van der Horst et al., 1983; von Reuden et al., 1975; Watson and Rowe, 1962; Weinberg et al., 1985, 1986). The inferior vena cava and right superior vena cava empty into the right atrium normally. In 2.5 to 4.3% of patients, there is a persistent left superior vena cava (Bharati et al., 1984; Roberts et al., 1976). The right atrium usually is dilated, and the tricuspid valve orifices are enlarged (Barber et al., 1988; Bharati and Lev, 1984; Hawkins and Doty, 1984; van der Horst et al., 1983). The right ventricle is larger than normal, as are the pulmonary orifice and main pulmonary artery (Bharati and Lev, 1984; Ehrlich et al., 1986; Kanjuh et al., 1965; van der Horst et al., 1983; von Reuden et al., 1975). Several patients have been reported with aortic atresia with pulmonary valve abnormalities (thickened nodular leaflets) (Bharati and Lev, 1984). This represents an extremely small portion of patients with hypoplastic left heart syndrome, compared with the large number at Children's Hospital of Philadelphia.

In patients dying before 2 weeks of age, there is no significant difference in the size and character of the small and medium pulmonary artery branches (Sinha et al., 1968). Pulmonary venous connection usually is normal, but occasionally there is anomalous or accessory pulmonary venous connection, usually through a persistent left vertical vein to the left innominate vein (Watson and Rowe, 1962). The left atrium is usually small and frequently hypertrophied (Bharati and Lev, 1984; Elliot et al., 1965; Kanjuh et al., 1965; Roberts et al., 1976; van der Horst et al., 1983; Watson and Rowe, 1962). Interatrial communication is common, although there may be a congenitally small foramen ovale (Bharati and Lev, 1984; Elliot et al., 1965; Watson and Rowe, 1962; Weinberg et al., 1986). In an autopsy series, 65% of patients had a posterior and leftward displacement of the superior attachment of the septum primum vis-à-vis septum secundum (Weinberg et al., 1986).

Mitral stenosis or hypoplasia is present in approximately 60% of the patients; the remaining 40% have mitral atresia (Bharati and Lev, 1984; Roberts et al., 1976). When there is mitral stenosis, the mitral valve leaflets are thickened with short thick chordae attached to short papillary muscles (Bharati and Lev, 1984). In patients with mitral atresia, there may be a blind dimple in the floor of the left atrium at the usual site of the mitral valve, with no grossly recognizable mitral valve tissue, or there may be atretic mitral valve tissue (Elliot et al., 1965; Kanjuh et al., 1965). The left ventricle does not form the apex of the heart in patients with mitral hypoplasia or stenosis (patent left ventricular inflow), and there is often prominent endocardial fibroelastosis with myofiber disarray (Bharati and Lev, 1984; Bulkley et al., 1983; Lev, 1952; O'Connor et al., 1982; Roberts et al., 1976; Sinha et al., 1968).

1659

In a study by Bharati and Lev (1984), 87% of patients had aortic atresia, and 13% had aortic valve hypoplasia. The coronary arteries originate normally from the aortic root and are normally distributed (Bharati and Lev, 1984). The ascending and transverse aorta are hypoplastic. With aortic atresia, the ascending aorta size is usually 1 to 3 mm. In rare cases with aortic hypoplasia, the mean size of the ascending aorta has been reported to be as large as 5 to 6 mm. True coarctation of the aorta is not a common finding. There is, however, a posterolateral intimal ridge at the junction of the aortic isthmus, the ductus arteriosus, and the thoracic aorta in most patients.

## EPIDEMIOLOGY

Hypoplastic left heart syndrome has been reported to occur in at least 0.016 to 0.036% of live births, making it the most common defect in which there is only one ventricle (Bridges et al., 1992; Fyler, 1980). In pathologic series, it accounts for 1.4 to 3.8% of congenital heart disease and has been reported to cause 23% of the deaths due to congenital heart disease in newborns (Abbott, 1936; Elliot et al., 1965; Watson and Rowe, 1962). There is a slight male predominance in hypoplastic left heart syndrome. Currently, 57% of patients with hypoplastic left heart syndrome observed at the Children's Hospital of Philadelphia are male. The recurrence risk for siblings of patients with hypoplastic left heart syndrome has been reported as 0.5% with a 2.2% risk for other forms of congenital heart disease (Bridges et al., 1992; Holmes et al., 1974; Nora and Nora, 1978).

## ETIOLOGY

The abnormal development of the left-sided cardiac structures primarily follows atresia or marked hypoplasia of the aortic valve. When there is left ventricular outflow obstruction with an intact ventricular septum, the left ventricle is not induced to reach normal size. In the rare case in which left ventricular outflow obstruction co-exists with an unrestrictive ventricular septal defect, left ventricular development is normal. Thus, a primary myocardial abnormality is an unlikely cause of hypoplastic left heart syndrome. The resultant elevation in left ventricular pressure that occurs with obstructed left ventricular outflow in the absence of ventricular septal defect probably causes the endocardial fibroelastosis observed in some patients. Whereas a congenitally small or absent foramen ovale has been suggested as a possible cause for hypoplastic left heart syndrome (Benner, 1939; Bharati and Lev, 1984; Lev et al., 1963), this is more likely the result of increased left atrial pressure secondary to the left ventricular outflow obstruction.

## PHYSIOLOGY

The left ventricle in hypoplastic left heart syndrome cannot function as a systemic ventricle. Pulmonary venous return must therefore be to the right atrium. This occurs through an atrial septal defect, a foramen ovale, or rarely, an anomalous pulmonary venous connection. In the right atrium, systemic and pulmonary venous return mix and fill the right ventricle during diastole. The right ventricle must provide output to both the pulmonary and the systemic circulation. Systemic output passes through the ductus arteriosus, which must remain patent for systemic perfusion. In utero oxygenation occurs via the placenta. Normally, the right ventricle manages 60% of the systemic output through the ductus arteriosus. In the fetus with hypoplastic left heart syndrome, the right ventricle accommodates to maintain total systemic output, and the child develops normally in utero. Perfusion is retrograde through the transverse arch and ascending aorta to the carotid and coronary arteries. At birth, the right ventricle must take on the additional volume work of the pulmonary circulation as the pulmonary vascular resistance suddenly falls and pulmonary perfusion increases during the first hours of newborn life. As long as the ductus arteriosus remains patent, however, systemic perfusion generally meets metabolic demands; but with the pulmonary arteries connected in parallel with the ductus arteriosus and descending aorta, the relative ratio of pulmonary to systemic blood flow depends on a delicate balance between the pulmonary and systemic vascular resistances. In some, a low pulmonary-to-systemic resistance ratio develops, causing excessive pulmonary blood flow relative to systemic blood flow. Although arterial oxygen saturation may be greater than 90% secondary to the high pulmonary-to-systemic blood flow ratio, systemic perfusion becomes marginal and the child may develop metabolic acidosis. In rare cases, a very restrictive interatrial communication produces a high pulmonary-to-systemic resistance ratio. These patients appear markedly cyanotic at birth with $Pa_{O_2}$ less than 20 mm Hg, which does not meet metabolic demands for oxygen. Anaerobic metabolism thus results in metabolic acidosis.

## CLINICAL FEATURES

When hypoplastic left heart syndrome presents within 24 hours of birth, it usually is secondary to severe obstruction to pulmonary blood flow at the interatrial level (congenitally smaller absent foramen ovale). More typically, however, Apgar scores are normal at birth. Within 24 to 48 hours, most patients with hypoplastic left heart syndrome develop a dusky cyanosis and evidence of tachypnea and respiratory distress (Elliot et al., 1965; Noonan and Nadas, 1958; Roberts et al., 1976; Watson and Rowe, 1962). When the ductus arteriosus begins to close, the patient develops metabolic acidosis. Prostaglandins have proved very effective in reestablishing or maintaining patency of the ductus arteriosus. Both intravenously administered prostaglandin $E_1$ and orally administered prostaglandin $E_2$ have proved effective (Fujiseki et al., 1983; Lewis et al., 1981; Schlemmer et al., 1982;

Yabek and Mann, 1979). Physical examination typically reveals a mildly cyanotic infant with tachypnea and tachycardia. Depending on the degree of patency of the ductus arteriosus at the time of evaluation, peripheral pulses may be normal, diminished, or absent. Rales may be auscultated, although generally the lung fields are clear. Cardiac examination revealed a dominant right ventricular impulse on palpation with a decreased left ventricular (apical) impulse. The S1 heart sound is normal, and S2 is usually single and increased in intensity (Watson and Rowe, 1962). The electrocardiogram frequently reflects the underlying pathologic process. Right atrial enlargement is observed in 30 to 41% of patients, and right ventricular hypertrophy is found in 78 to 92% of patients (Elliot et al., 1965; Noonan and Nadas, 1958; Sinha et al., 1968). Approximately 56% of patients have a QR pattern in lead $V_1$ (Sinha et al., 1968; Watson and Rowe, 1962). In patients with malaligned common atrioventricular canal, the QRS axis is leftward and superior.

The findings on chest film of patients with hypoplastic left heart syndrome are nonspecific. Cardiomegaly is reported in 75 to 85% of patients, and pulmonary vascular markings are increased in 68 to 82% (Roberts et al., 1976; Sinha et al., 1968).

Two-dimensional echocardiography diagnoses this lesion (Bash et al., 1986; Bass et al., 1980; Bierman, 1984; Farooki et al., 1976; Helton et al., 1986; Jonas et al., 1986; Mandorla et al., 1984; Mortera and Leon, 1980; Sahn et al., 1975, 1982; Skovranek et al., 1981; Suzuki et al., 1982). The intracardiac anatomy should be examined with subcostal frontal sagittal left oblique and right oblique sweeps (Chin et al., 1985; Isaaz et al., 1985; Marino et al., 1985). With accurate diagnosis, made possible by two-dimensional and Doppler echocardiography, cardiac catheterization no longer is routinely necessary or advisable in hypoplastic left heart syndrome. Moreover, because some obstruction of pulmonary venous return limits pulmonary overcirculation of patients with hypoplastic left heart syndrome, balloon atrial septotomy during cardiac catheterization may cause hemodynamic deterioration and should be avoided.

## NATURAL HISTORY

Untreated, over 95% of patients with hypoplastic left heart syndrome die within the first month of life (Fyler et al., 1981). Hypoplastic left heart syndrome accounts for approximately 25% of cardiac deaths during the first month of life (Noonan and Nadas, 1958). Rarely does the ductus arteriosus remain persistently patent. If pulmonary and systemic resistances are similar, survival for 4 to 6 years has been reported sporadically (Ehrlich et al., 1986; Moodie et al., 1986). These patients all have expired secondary to the development and progression of pulmonary vascular obstructive disease in childhood.

## RATIONALE OF MANAGEMENT

This malformation is difficult to ignore because it is one of the most common congenital cardiac malformations. All patients die without surgical therapy, and most patients are otherwise healthy, well-developed babies, free of associated congenital abnormalities. Observations made since the introduction of Fontan's operation to treat tricuspid atresia make it clear that normal systemic ventricular work and efficiency can be achieved in patients with only one effective ventricle by diverting systemic venous return to the pulmonary arteries and the low-resistance mature pulmonary vascular bed. Moreover, experience with congenitally corrected transposition of the great arteries and transposition of the great arteries (S,D,D) managed by atrial inversion surgery supports the concept that the right ventricle can be an effective systemic ventricle.

Thus, beginning in 1978, the development of reconstructive surgical therapy was approached systematically, resulting in the adaptation of Fontan's operation for the treatment of hypoplastic left heart syndrome, the most common of a group of cardiac malformations in which there is only one effective ventricle. At that time, it was well understood that the pulmonary vascular resistance of the newborn is naturally near systemic levels and decreases to normal low pulmonary vascular resistance over the first year of life with maturation of the pulmonary vasculature. Thus, a staged operative approach was deemed necessary. Although prostaglandins effectively maintain patency of the ductus arteriosus, high pressure and flow during the first months of life to the pulmonary vasculature impede normal development. The pulmonary vascular resistance decreases in the first weeks and months of life to levels far less than systemic, and the volume demands on the right ventricle increase to four and five times normal, abrogating long-term survival with prostaglandins alone.

In 1979, initial palliation included three components: (1) association of the ascending aorta to the right ventricle using proximal main pulmonary artery along with patch augmentation of the sides of the ascending aorta and transverse aortic arch, (2) atrial septectomy to provide unrestricted pulmonary venous return to the right atrium and right ventricle, and (3) interposition of a 4-mm tube graft between the innominate artery and the right pulmonary artery to provide and regulate pulmonary blood flow to allow for normal pulmonary vascular maturation. The results of initial palliation for hypoplastic left heart syndrome at the Children's Hospital of Philadelphia from January 1984 through May 1993 included 406 patients. There were 125 (27%) early deaths and 35 (10%) late deaths. Early in this experience, it became clear that survival depended not solely on a surgical exercise but most critically on management of the physiology of a single ventricle, managing combined systemic and pulmonary circulations connected in parallel. Feedback loops match systemic output and demand, but total cardiac output (pressure-volume work) depends on $\dot{Q}_P{:}\dot{Q}_S$ ratio. It was discovered that a $\dot{Q}_P{:}\dot{Q}_S$ ratio of 1 produces an adequate oxygen saturation on the order of 80% to meet metabolic demands with some reserve, without excessively volume loading the single ventricle. A $\dot{Q}_P{:}\dot{Q}_S$ ratio of 1, of course, causes an extra-volume work demand twice normal, which can be accommodated without marked ventricular dilatation and failure for some time.

In the early postoperative period, systemic and pulmonary vascular resistances are very dynamic, producing wide fluctuations of systemic arterial oxygenation and systemic perfusion. This physiologic lability was thought to account for a considerable proportion of the early mortality, so attenuation of the dynamics of the pulmonary vascular resistance was pursued. It was obvious that pulmonary vascular tone is extremely sensitive to carbon dioxide, with tone increasing as $P_{CO_2}$ increases. In the mid-1980s, hypoventilation was used routinely to adjust the $\dot{Q}_P{:}\dot{Q}_S$ ratio to slightly less than 1 and attenuate pulmonary vascular tone fluctuation. It became apparent that marginal ventilation also accounted for a considerable proportion of early mortality, so an alternative means of controlling the dynamics of systemic and pulmonary perfusion was sought. Ventilatory management of the patient in the early postoperative period now includes positive pressure ventilation with a volume preset ventilator set at a rate of 20, a tidal volume of 30 ml/kg and $F_{I_{O_2}}$ of 0.30, and a $P_{CO_2}$ of 14 mm Hg. Anticipated effects of the addition of carbon dioxide to inspired gases on arterial blood gases are illustrated by increasing pH from 7.39 to 7.52, increasing $P_{CO_2}$ from 38 to 41 mm Hg, decreasing $P_{O_2}$ from 47 to 39 mm Hg, and increasing base excess from $-1$ to 8 on the average in 10 patients. This systematic use of carbon dioxide as inspired gas in the early postoperative period is reflected in experience with 63 patients from May 1992 to May 1993 undergoing initial palliative operation for hypoplastic left heart syndrome. The early mortality rate was 10%, and the late mortality rate was 3%, a substantial improvement over the overall experience beginning in 1984. In conclusion, the management of patients with hypoplastic left heart syndrome in the newborn period has evolved in its surgical details, but the remaining complexities of management are largely physiologic. The addition of carbon dioxide to inspired gases has been shown to limit pulmonary blood flow while avoiding the risks of hypoventilation and may be an important tool in the management of neonates with parallel systemic and pulmonary circulations.

Following sufficient maturation of the pulmonary vasculature, usually complete by 6 months of age, one can take advantage of the low pulmonary vascular resistance to surgically divert superior and inferior vena cava return directly to the branch pulmonary arteries. This procedure induces low-pressure passive flow through the pulmonary vascular bed for oxygenation of systemic venous return to the right ventricle, which, after closure of the systemic to pulmonary arterial shunt, manages only the systemic circulation. The hemodynamic advantage of such an operation is

decrease in the volume work of the systemic ventricle to normal, allowing for diminution in end-diastolic volume to normal. In the initial group of patients undergoing Fontan's operation, however, the mortality rate was substantial, and there was no predictive value of preoperative cardiac catheterization in terms of hemodynamic parameters identifying risks of mortality. Echocardiograhic and pathologic examination showed that all patients who became hemodynamically unstable and/or died in the early postoperative period after Fontan's operation for hypoplastic left heart syndrome exhibited similar characteristics of a markedly decreased end-diastolic volume, a hyperactive systolic component of the cardiac cycle, and marked increased in wall thickness, presumably caused by the natural sudden decrease in volume demands by the systemic circulation. However, the resulting diminution in end-diastolic volume and increase in apparent wall thickness, while maintaining the same muscle mass, caused marked impairment of diastolic performance and thus an increase in ventricular filling pressure, pulmonary artery pressure, and systemic venous pressure to nonviable levels. With an inability to predict which patients would undergo rapid changes in geometry with impairment of diastolic function by any preoperative information, it was concluded that separation of the Fontan procedure into two parts—namely, associating the superior vena cava directly to the pulmonary arteries initially, followed months later by association of the inferior vena cava with pulmonary arteries—could attenuate the morbid effects of diastolic impairment in some patients.

Thus, in 1989, what we termed the *hemi Fontan operation* was introduced to systematically manage hypoplastic left heart syndrome as a component of staged surgery. The goals were to attenuate the adverse effects of geometric changes in the early postoperative period, to allow the volume load on the systemic right ventricle to decrease very early in life, and to minimize late mortality from first-stage operation. In a study of 117 patients undergoing hemi Fontan operation at various ages for various malformations, the 18-month actuarial survival rate was 92%. A comparison of malformations with a dominant right ventricle with those with a dominant left ventricle showed no difference in actuarial survival, suggesting that the right ventricle is indeed equivalent to the left ventricle in managing the systemic circulation in this time frame. All deaths occurred in patients who underwent the hemi Fontan operation at less than 6 months of age. Thus, the systematic protocol was developed in May 1989 to interpose the hemi Fontan operation at age 6 months as a component of staged management of hypoplastic left heart syndrome. From May 1989 to May 1993, 200 patients have undergone hemi Fontan operation in the management of hypoplastic left heart syndrome, with 21 early deaths (10%) and 6 late deaths (3%). From May 1992 to May 1993, 45 patients underwent the hemi Fontan operation in the management of hypoplastic left heart syndrome, with 1 early death and no late deaths.

Since January 1984, 201 patients have undergone Fontan's operation with or without a preceding hemi Fontan operation. Among the 201 patients, there were 28 early deaths (14%) and 10 late deaths (6%). The late deaths were from respiratorial syncytial virus infection in 2 patients and complications associated with massive effusions in 8 patients. In a retrospective study of all patients undergoing Fontan's operation with or without preceding hemi Fontan, effusions occurred in approximately 50% of patients. No preoperative or postoperative hemodynamic information predicted effusions. Moreover, because effusions are extremely rare after the hemi Fontan operation despite the fact that superior vena caval pressure increases similarly after hemi Fontan operation, thus inducing lymphatic pressure to drain into the junction of the jugular and innominate veins, an increase in central venous pressure alone probably cannot account for development of effusions. Furthermore, there is a low incidence of effusions in patients undergoing superior vena caval pulmonary arterial anastomosis for the treatment of the heterotaxy syndrome, wherein there is an interruption of inferior vena cava with azygous continuation to a superior vena cava. This leaves only the hepatic veins draining directly into the atrium and bypassing the pulmonary vasculature. This suggests that hepatic venous drainage patterns may influence the development of effusions.

Given this hypothesis, 44 patients underwent Fontan's operation by a technique that allows one of several hepatic veins to bypass the lungs and return under low pressure to the systemic ventricle atrial system. These patients showed a marked diminution in effusions: There were four deaths, and only three patients developed effusions. Of those three, all were found to have occlusion of the excluded hepatic vein, thus supporting the concept that partial hepatic venous exclusion from the pulmonary circulation can abrogate development of effusive complications following Fontan's operation. Among the 44 patients, two underwent revision for effusions, at which time the hepatic vein was found to be occluded, and two patients underwent revision surgery for significant and progressive hypoxemia with oxygen saturations of less than 80%. The long-term effects of partial exclusion of hepatic veins as a form of Fontan's operation remain to be seen. There is, of course, the hypothetic consideration that intrahepatic venous collaterals can develop eventually, shunting systemic venous return away from the lungs through hepatic collaterals to the low-pressure systemic atrial and ventricular systems. From May 1992 to May 1993, 21 patients underwent the partial exclusion of hepatic vein type of Fontan's operation, with no deaths and no effusions.

Laks, Castañeda, and others (Bridges et al., 1992; Pearl et al., 1992) have advanced the concept of creating a fenestration in the systemic venous interatrial systemic venous channel to attenuate the potential adverse effects of all systemic venous return passing through the additional resistor of the pulmonary vascular circuit in the early postoperative period of the Fontan operation. Later closure of the fenestration has been proposed: Two invasive techniques use a tourniquet system or plugging the fenestration at catheterization. The concept that multiple small fenestrations could close spontaneously in the first weeks after Fontan's operation, thus avoiding the necessity for further invasive procedures, was applied to 23 patients undergoing completion of Fontan's operation for hypoplastic left heart syndrome. In these patients, four holes, 2 mm in diameter, were created in the interatrial systemic channel. $PA_{O_2}$ averaged 58 mm Hg in the early postoperative period, and the oxygen saturation rose to 92% mean by 2 postoperative months. Among the 23 patients so treated, however, 15 developed effusions. Fenestration alone does not seem to influence the development of effusions. Finally, from May 1992 to May 1993, 40 patients underwent various forms of completion Fontan for hypoplastic left heart syndrome, and they have experienced no early or late mortality.

Our management of hypoplastic left heart syndrome has evolved dramatically over the last 15 years with the establishment of reconstructive surgical therapeutic techniques in three stages: initial palliation shortly after birth, a hemi Fontan procedure planned at age 6 months, and a completion Fontan operation at age 1 year. It is now clear that with an increased understanding of the physiology of the various circulations created by structural reorganization for hypoplastic left heart syndrome, one can reduce mortality and create a systemic ventricular system that functions at normal geometry and output, with normal systemic arterial oxygen saturation and concomitant normal growth and development of the patient (Baffa et al., 1992; Farrell et al., 1992; Jacobs and Norwood, 1992; Norwood, 1991; Qazi et al., 1981; Seliem et al., 1992). Further refinements may increase the safety of each operation and eliminate morbidity, such as effusions from the perioperative state.

## SELECTED REFERENCES

Bailey, L., Concepcion, W., Shattuck, H., and Huang, L.: Method of heart transplantation for treatment of hypoplastic left heart syndrome. J. Thorac. Cardiovasc. Surg., 92:1, 1986.

Technical details of the investigational orthotopic cardiac transplantation for management of hypoplastic left heart syndrome in the neonate are presented. A technique of extracorporeal perfusion and the need for extensive aortic arch reconstruction are emphasized. The source of donor graft in this case report was a subhuman primate, but it is emphasized that the donor graft makes little difference with regard to the unique technical aspects of cardiac transplantation in a ductus-dependent newborn infant with a diminutive aortic arch.

Bailey, L. L., et al.: Cardiac allotransplantation in newborns as therapy for hypoplastic left heart syndrome. N. Engl. J. Med., 315:949, 1986.

These authors present the initial Loma Linda experience with heart replacement therapy for hypoplastic left heart syndrome. This report not only demonstrates the feasibility of heart replacement in patients with the aortic arch anatomy of hypoplastic left heart syndrome but also illustrates the complex circumstances surrounding procurement within a limited time frame of a heart sufficiently small to fit in the mediastinum of the newborn. Short-term results suggest that immunosuppressive management of the newborn and small infant is no more complicated than in the adult population.

Jonas, R. A., et al.: First-stage palliation of hypoplastic left heart syndrome: The importance of coarctation and shunt size. J. Thorac. Cardiovasc. Surg., 92:6, 1986.

This report describes the experience with palliative surgery for 25 neonates between January 1984 and July 1985. During this time there were six deaths. The authors emphasize the importance of a posterior shelf at the junction of the isthmus of the aorta with the thoracic aorta, which can cause late coarctation of the aorta. Moreover, they emphasize the fact that careful ventilatory and pharmacologic management of the ratio of pulmonary to systemic vascular resistance is an essential part of the perioperative management of these neonates with two parallel competing circulations.

Norwood, W. I., Lang, P., and Hansen, D.: Physiologic repair of aortic atresia—Hypoplastic left heart syndrome. N. Engl. J. Med., 308:23, 1983.

This report outlines early experience with reconstructive surgical management of hypoplastic left heart syndrome beginning in 1979. This case report is of one patient in that series who underwent physiologic correction by modification of Fontan's operative procedure demonstrating the feasibility of reconstructive surgical management of hypoplastic left heart syndrome. The patient underwent physiologic correction at age 16 months, at which time the pulmonary vascular resistance was calculated to be 2 Woods units. The child was reported as clinically well during 6 months of follow-up after physiologically corrective surgery. In fact, the patient remains clinically well with a right atrial pressure of 11 mm Hg determined by cardiac catheterization at age 7 years.

Noonan, J. A., and Nadas, A. S.: The hypoplastic left heart syndrome. Pediatr. Clin. North Am., 5:1029, 1958.

This seminal paper coins the term *hypoplastic left heart syndrome* and outlines the anatomic-physiologic and natural historical features of this constellation of anatomic abnormalities in the development of the structures of the left side of the heart. Although the modern concepts of hypoplastic left heart syndrome are somewhat more focused today, this report represents the initial specific categorization.

Pigott, J. D., Murphy, J. D., Barber, G., and Norwood, W. I.: Palliative reconstructive surgery for hypoplastic left heart syndrome. Ann. Thorac. Surg., 45:122, 1988.

This report constitutes the experience from August 1985 through August 1987 with 104 consecutive nonselected neonates who underwent palliative surgery as newborns for hypoplastic left heart syndrome at the Children's Hospital of Philadelphia. It presents an evolution in technique to optimize pulmonary vascular development, minimize late aortic arch obstruction, and achieve a balanced pulmonary and systemic flow ratio. Such techniques were developed to achieve the best possible preparation for application of Fontan's procedure for the treatment of hypoplastic left heart syndrome.

# REFERENCES

Abbott, M. E.: Atlas of Congenital Cardiac Diseases. New York, American Heart Association, 1936, pp. 48 and 61.

Anderson, R. H., Ho, S. Y., Zuberbuhler, J. R., et al.: Surgery for hypoplastic left heart syndrome: A fiction? Surgical anatomy and definition. *In* Marcelletti, C., Anderson, R. H., Becker, A. E., et al. (eds): Pediatric Cardiology. New York, Churchill Livingstone, 1986, pp. 111–121.

Baffa, J. M., Chen, S.-L., Guttenburg, M. E., et al.: Coronary arteries and right ventricular histology in hypoplastic left heart syndrome. J. Am. Coll. Cardiol., 20:350–358, 1992.

Bailey, L., Concepcion, W., Shattuck, H., and Huang, L.: Method of heart transplantation for treatment of hypoplastic left heart syndrome. J. Thorac. Cardiovasc. Surg., 92:1, 1986.

Bailey, L. L., et al.: Cardiac allotransplantation in newborns as therapy for hypoplastic left heart syndrome. N. Engl. J. Med., 315:949, 1986.

Bailey, L. L., Nehlsen-Cannarella, S. L., Concepcion, W., and Jolley, W. B.: Baboon-to-human cardiac xenotransplantation in a neonate. J. A. M. A., 254:3321, 1985.

Barber, G., Helton, J. G., Aglira, B. A., et al.: The significance of tricuspid regurgitation in hypoplastic left heart syndrome. Am. Heart J., 116:1563, 1988.

Barber, G., Murphy, J. D., Pigott, J. D., and Norwood, W. I.: The evolving pattern of surgical following palliative surgery for hypoplastic left heart syndrome. J. Am. Coll. Cardiol., 2:139A, 1988.

Bash, S. E., Huhta, J. C., Vick, G. W., III, et al.: Hypoplastic left heart syndrome: Is echocardiography accurate enough to guide surgical palliation. J. Am. Coll. Cardiol., 7:610, 1986.

Bass, J. L., Ben-Shachar, G., and Edwards, J. E.: Comparison of M-mode echocardiography and pathologic findings in the hypoplastic left heart syndrome. Am. J. Cardiol., 45:79, 1980.

Benner, M. C.: Premature closure of the foramen ovale. Am. Heart J., 17:437, 1939.

Bharati, S., and Lev., M.: The spectrum of common atrioventricular orifice (canal). Am. Heart J., 86:553, 1973.

Bharati, S., and Lev, M.: The surgical anatomy of hypoplasia of aortic tract complex. J. Thorac. Cardiovasc. Surg., 88:97, 1984.

Bharati, S., Nordenberg, A., Brock, R. R., and Lev, M.: Hypoplastic left heart syndrome with dysplastic pulmonary valve with stenosis. Pediatr. Cardiol., 5:127, 1984.

Bidot-Lopez, P., Matisoff, D., Talner, N. S., et al.: Hypoplastic left heart in a patient with 45,X/46,XX/47,XXX mosaicism. Am. J. Med. Genet., 2:341, 1978.

Bierman, F. Z.: Two-dimensional echocardiography and its influence on cardiac catheterization. Cardiovasc. Intervent. Radiol., 7:140, 1984.

Bjerregaard, P., and Laursen, H. B.: Persistent left superior vena cava. Acta Paediatr. Scand., 69:105, 1980.

Bridges, N. D., Mayer, J. E., Jr., Lock, J. E., et al.: Effect of baffle fenestration on outcome of the modified Fontan operation. Circulation, 86:1762, 1992.

Brownell, L. G., and Shokeir, M. H.: Inheritance of hypoplastic left heart syndrome. Clin. Genet., 9:245, 1976.

Bulkley, B. H., D'Amico, B., and Taylor, A. L.: Extensive myocardial fiber disarray in aortic and pulmonary atresia. Circulation, 67:191, 1983.

Chin, A. J., Sanders, S. P., Sherman, F., et al.: Accuracy of subcostal two-dimensional echocardiography in prospective diagnosis of total anomalous pulmonary venous connection. Am. Heart. J., 113:1153, 1987.

Chin, A. J., Yeager, S. B., Sanders, S. P., et al.: Accuracy of prospective two-dimensional echocardiographic evaluation of left ventricular outflow tract in complete transposition of the great arteries. Am. J. Cardiol., 55:759, 1985.

Cloez, J. L., Isaaz, K., and Pernot, C.: Pulsed Doppler flow characteristics of ductus arteriosus in infants with associated congenital anomalies of the heart or great arteries. Am. J. Cardiol., 57:845, 1986.

Cobanoglu, A., Metzdorff, M. T., Pinson, C. W., et al.: Valvotomy for pulmonary atresia with intact ventricular septum. J. Thorac. Cardiovasc. Surg., 89:482, 1985.

DiDonato, R. M., Fyfe, D. A., Puga, F. I., et al.: Fifteen-year experience with surgical repair of truncus arteriosus. J. Thorac. Cardiovasc. Surg., 89:414, 1985.

Doty, D. B., and Knott, H. W.: Hypoplastic left heart syndrome. Experience with an operation to establish functionally normal circulation. J. Thorac. Cardiovasc. Surg., 74:624, 1977.

Edwards, J. E.: Congenital malformation of the heart and great vessel. *In* Gould, S. E. (ed): Pathology of the Heart. Springfield, IL, Charles C Thomas, 1953, p. 407.

Ehrlich, M., Bierman, F. Z., Ellis, K., and Gersony, W. M.: Hypoplastic left heart syndrome: Report of a unique survivor. J. Am. Coll. Cardiol., 7:361, 1986.

Elliot, R. S., et al.: Mitral atresia. A study of 32 cases. Am. Heart J., 71:6, 1965.

Elzenga, N. J., and Gittenberger de Grott, A. C.: Coarctation and related aortic arch anomalies in hypoplastic left heart syndrome. Int. J. Cardiol., 8:379, 1985.

Farooki, Z. Q., Henry, J. G., and Green, E. W.: Echocardiographic spectrum of the hypoplastic left heart syndrome: A clinicopathologic correlation in 19 newborns. Am. J. Cardiol., 38:337, 1976.

Farrell, P. E., Change, A. C., Murdisoll, K. A., et al.: Outcome and assessment after the modified Fontan procedure for hypoplastic left heart syndrome. Circulation, 85:116–122, 1992.

Fontan, F., and Baudet, E.: Surgical repair of tricuspid atresia. Thorax, 26:240, 1971.

Friedman, S., Murphy, L., and Ash, R.: Congenital mitral atresia with hypoplastic nonfunctioning left heart. J. Dis. Child., 90:176, 1955.

Fujiseki, Y., Yamamoto, H., Hattori, M., et al.: Oral administration of prostaglandin E$_2$ in hypoplastic left heart syndrome. Jpn. Heart J., 24:481, 1983.

Fyler, D. C.: Report of the New England Regional Infant Cardiac Program. Pediatrics, 65(Suppl.):463, 1980.

Fyler, D. C., Rothman, K. J., Buckley, L. P., et al.: The determinants of five year survival of infants with critical congenital heart disease. In Engle, M. A. (ed): Pediatric Cardiovascular Disease. (Cardiovascular Clinics.) Philadelphia, F. A. Davis, 1981, pp. 393–405.

Harh, J. Y., Paul, M. H., Gallen, W. J., et al.: Experimental production of hypoplastic left heart syndrome in the chick embryo. Am. J. Cardiol., 31:51, 1973.

Hastreiter, A. R., van der Horst, R. L., Dubrow, I. W., and Eckner, F. O.: Quantitative angiographic and morphologic aspects of aortic valve atresia. Am. J. Cardiol., 51:1705, 1983.

Hawkins, J. A., and Doty, D. B.: Aortic atresia: Morphologic characteristics affecting survival and operative palliation. J. Thorac. Cardiovasc. Surg., 88:620, 1984.

Helton, J. G., Aglira, B. A., Chin, A. J., et al.: Analysis of potential anatomic or physiologic determinants of outcome of palliative surgery for hypoplastic left heart syndrome. Circulation, 74(Suppl. I):70, 1986.

Holmes, L. B., Rose, V., and Child, A. H.: Comment on hypoplastic left heart syndrome. Birth Defects Original Article Series. In Bergsma, D. (ed): Clinical Delineation of Birth Defects. XVI: Urinary System and Others. Baltimore, Williams & Wilkins, 1974, pp. 228–230.

Hutchins, G. M.: Coarctation of the aorta explained as a branch point of the ductus arteriosus. Am. J. Pathol., 63:203, 1971.

Isaaz, K., Cloez, J. L., Danchin, N., et al.: Assessment of right ventricular outflow tract in children by two-dimensional echocardiography using a new subcostal view. Am. J. Cardiol., 56:539, 1985.

Jacobs, M. I., and Norwood, W. I. (eds): Hypoplastic left heart syndrome. In Pediatric Cardiac Surgery: Current Issues. Butterworth-Heinemann, 1992, pp. 182–192.

Jonas, R. A., et al.: First-stage palliation of hypoplastic left heart syndrome: The importance of coarctation and shunt size. J. Thorac. Cardiovasc. Surg., 92:6, 1986.

Kanjuh, V. I., Elliot, R. S., and Edwards, J. E.: Coexistent mitral and aortic valvular atresia. A pathologic study of 14 cases. Am. J. Cardiol., 15:611, 1965.

Kirklin, J. W., and Barratt-Boyes, B. G.: Cardiac Surgery, Morphology, Diagnostic Criteria, Natural History, Techniques, Results, and Indications. New York, John Wiley & Sons, 1986, pp. 843–856.

Lehman, E.: Congenital atresia of the foramen ovale. Am. J. Dis. Child., 33:585, 1927.

Lev, M.: Pathologic anatomy and interrelationship of hypoplasia of the aortic tract complexes. Lab. Invest., 1:61, 1952.

Lev, M., Arcilla, R., Remoldi, H. J. A., et al.: Premature narrowing or closure of the foramen ovale. Am. Heart J., 65:638, 1963.

Lewis, A. B., Freed, M., Heymann, M. A., et al.: Side effects of therapy with prostaglandin E$_1$ in infants with critical congenital heart disease. Circulation, 64:893, 1981.

Lumb, G., and Dawkins, W. A.: Congenital atresia of mitral and aortic valves with vestigial left ventricle (three cases). Am. Heart J., 60:378, 1960.

Mandorla, S., Narducci, P. L., Migliozzi, L., et al.: Fetal echocardiography. Prenatal diagnosis of hypoplastic left heart syndrome. G. Ital. Cardiol., 14:517, 1984.

Marino, B., Ballerini, L., Marcelletti, C., et al.: Complete transposition of the great arteries: Visualization of left and right outflow tract obstruction by oblique subcostal two-dimensional echocardiography. Am. J. Cardiol., 55:1140, 1985.

Milo, S., Ho, S. Y., and Anderson, R. H.: Hypoplastic left heart syndrome. Can this malformation be treated surgically? Thorax, 35:351, 1980.

Moodie, D. S., Gallen, W. J., and Friedberg, D. Z.: Congenital aortic atresia. Report of long survival and some speculation about surgical approaches. J. Thorac. Cardiovasc. Surg., 63:726, 1972.

Moodie, D. S., Gill, C. C., Sterba, R., et al.: The hypoplastic left heart syndrome: Evidence of preoperative myocardial and hepatic infarction in spite of prostaglandin therapy. Ann. Thorac. Surg., 42:307, 1986.

Mortera, C., and Leon, G.: Detection of persistent ductus in hypoplastic left heart syndrome by contrast echocardiography. Br. Heart J., 44:596, 1980.

Natowicz, M., and Kelley, R. I.: Association of Turner syndrome with hypoplastic left heart syndrome. Am. J. Dis. Child., 141:218, 1987.

Noonan, J. A., and Nadas, A. S.: The hypoplastic left heart syndrome. Pediatr. Clin. North Am., 5:1029, 1958.

Nora, J. J., and Nora, A. H.: Genetics and counseling in cardiovascular diseases. Springfield, IL, Charles C Thomas, 1978, p. 181.

Norwood, W. I.: Hypoplastic left heart syndrome. In Balle, Geha, A. S., Hammond, G. L., Laks, H., and Naunheim, K. S. (eds): Glenn's Thoracic and Cardiovascular Surgery. 5th ed. Vol. II. Norwalk, CT, Appleton & Lange, 1991, pp. 1123–1130.

Norwood, W. I., Jacobs, M. L., and Murphy, J. D.: Fontan procedure for hypoplastic left heart syndrome. Ann. Thorac. Surg., 54:1025–1030, 1992.

Norwood, W. I., Kirklin, J. K., and Sanders, S. P.: Hypoplastic left heart syndrome. Experience with palliative surgery. Am. J. Cardiol., 45:87, 1980.

Norwood, W. I., Lang, P., Castañeda, A. R., and Campbell, D. N.: Experience with operations for hypoplastic left heart syndrome. J. Thorac. Cardiovasc. Surg., 82:511, 1981.

Norwood, W. I., Lang, P., and Hansen, D.: Physiologic repair of aortic atresia–hypoplastic left heart syndrome. N. Engl. J. Med., 308:23, 1983.

O'Connor, W. N., Cash, J. B., Cottrill, C. M., et al.: Ventriculocoronary connections in hypoplastic left hearts: An autopsy microscopic study. Circulation, 66:1078, 1982.

Pearl, J. M., Laks, H., Barthel, S. W., et al.: Quantification of flow through an internal communication. J. Thorac. Cardiovasc. Surg., 104:1702, 1992.

Qazi, Q. H., Kanchanapoomi, R., Cooper, R., et al.: Brief clinical report: Dup(12p) and hypoplastic left heart. Am. J. Med. Genet., 9:195, 1981.

Roberts, W. C., Perry, L. W., Chandra, R. S., et al.: Aortic valve atresia: A new classification based on necropsy study of 73 cases. Am. J. Cardiol., 37:753, 1976.

Sade, R. M., Fyfe, D., and Alpert, C. C.: Hypoplastic left heart syndrome: A simplified palliative operation. Ann. Thorac. Surg., 43:309, 1987.

Sahn, D. J., Allen, H. D., Goldberg, S. J., et al.: Pediatric echocardiography: A review of its clinical utility. J. Pediatr., 87:335, 1975.

Sahn, D. J., Shenker, L., Reed, K. L., et al.: Prenatal ultrasound diagnosis of hypoplastic left heart syndrome in utero associated with hydrops fetalis. Am. Heart J., 104:1368, 1982.

Schall, S. A., and Dalldorf, F. G.: Premature closure of the foramen ovale and hypoplasia of the left heart. Int. J. Cardiol., 5:103, 1984.

Schlemmer, M., Khoss, A., Salzer, H. R., and Wimmer, M.: Prostaglandin E$_2$ in newborns with congenital heart disease. Z. Kardiol., 71:452, 1982.

Seliem, M. A., Chin, A. J., and Norwood, W. I.: Patterns of anomalous pulmonary venous connection/drainage in hypoplastic left heart syndrome: Diagnostic role of Doppler color flow mapping and surgical implications. J. Am. Coll. Cardiol., 19(1):135–141, 1992.

Silverberg, B.: Coexistent aortic and mitral atresia associated with persistent common atrioventricular canal. Am. J. Cardiol., 16:754, 1965.

Sinha, S. N., Rusnak, S. L., Sommers, H. M., et al.: Hypoplastic left ventricle syndrome. Analysis of thirty autopsy cases in infants with surgical consideration. Am. J. Cardiol., 21:166, 1968.

Skovranek, J., First, T., and Samanek, M.: Contribution of pulsed Doppler echocardiography to ultrasound diagnosis of congenital heart disease. Cor Vasa, 23:34, 1981.

Snider, A. R., and Silverman, N. H.: Suprasternal notch echocardiography: A two-dimensional technique for evaluating congenital heart disease. Circulation, 63:165, 1981.

Suzuki, K., Hitata, K., Eto, Y., et al.: Echocardiographic assessment of anatomical detail in patients with hypoplastic left heart syndrome. J. Cardiogr., 12:991, 1982.

Tuma, S., Samanek, M., Benesova, D., and Voriskova, M.: Premature closure of the foramen ovale with levoatriocardinal vein. Eur. J. Pediatr., *129*:205, 1978.

van der Horst, R. L., Hastreiter, A. R., DuBrow, I. W., and Eckner, F. A. O.: Pathologic measurements in aortic atresia. Am. Heart J., *106*:1411, 1983.

Von Reuden, T. J., Knight, L., Moller, J. H., and Edwards, J. E.: Coarctation of the aorta associated with aortic valve atresia. Circulation, *52*:951, 1975.

Watson, D. G., and Rowe, R. D.: Aortic-valve atresia: Report of 43 cases. J. A. M. A., *179*:14, 1962.

Weinberg, P. M., et al.: Postmortem echocardiography and tomographic anatomy of hypoplastic left heart syndrome after palliative surgery. Am. J. Cardiol., *58*:1228, 1986.

Weinberg, P. M., Peyser, K., and Hackney, J. R.: Fetal hydrops in a newborn with hypoplastic left heart syndrome: Tricuspid valve stopper. J. Am. Coll. Cardiol., *6*:1365, 1985.

Weldon, C. S., Hartman, A. F., and McKnight, R. C.: Surgical management of hypoplastic right ventricle with pulmonary atresia or critical pulmonic stenosis and intact ventricular septum. Ann. Thorac. Surg., *37*:12, 1984.

Yabek, S. M., and Mann, J. S.: Prostaglandin $E_1$ infusion in the hypoplastic left heart syndrome. Chest, *76*:330, 1979.

# 49

## Acquired Disease of the Tricuspid Valve

Robert B. Karp

Acquired tricuspid valve disease is classified surgically as either functional or organic. The physiology of the circulation and the surgical results are each related to the situation on the left side of the heart. Thus, functional tricuspid insufficiency results from left-sided mitral stenosis or regurgitation much more frequently than from isolated aortic valve disease. The degree of functional impairment is related to the severity of the left-sided lesion, the duration of aortic or mitral valve dysfunction and the resultant severity of the pulmonary vascular resistance, the degree of pulmonary artery hypertension, and the degree of right ventricular dilatation.

The causative factor most often associated with organic disease of the tricuspid valve is *rheumatic fever*. Organic disease of the tricuspid valve is also related to the left-sided disease, because rheumatic involvement rarely occurs on the tricuspid valve without also affecting the mitral or aortic valve.

Infrequent causes of organic tricuspid valve disease include trauma (penetrating or blunt) leading to incompetence, carcinoid syndrome, and nonbacterial endocarditis such as Libman-Sacks, eosinophilic leukemia, and diffuse collagen disorders. An increasingly frequent cause of organic tricuspid valve disease is infective endocarditis.

### ANATOMY

The tricuspid orifice is the largest of the four cardiac valves, and in normal adults the valve area is approximately 10.5 cm$^2$ and the diameter is 36 ± 4.5 mm. In congestive heart failure, the tricuspid annulus may be 40 to 45 mm in diameter. The three tricuspid leaflets are supported by a tensor apparatus composed of chordae tendineae (primary, secondary, and tertiary) and papillary muscles (usually a single major anterior papillary muscle and several accessory papillary muscles). There is no tricuspid annulus, but the bases of the three leaflets are attached to the heart at the atrioventricular junction. In normal situs and connection, this "ring" is related to the base of the aortic valve, the membranous septum, the central fibrous body, the right coronary artery, the lateral atrioventricular junction, the coronary sinus, and the bundle of His (clockwise from medially). With its tensor apparatus, the tricuspid valve in part defines the morphologic right ventricle. Of the three more or less well-defined tricuspid leaflets, the anterior is the largest, and the chordae are attached to the dominant papillary muscle. It is separated from the septal leaflet by the anterior septal commissure and from the small posterior leaflet by the posterior commissure. The base of the septal leaflet harbors the penetrating portion of the conducting system. Both the septal and posterior leaflets have chordae attaching directly to the right ventricular myocardium in the septal and parietal walls (Figs. 49–1 and 49–2).

The anterior commissure lies adjacent to the atrioventricular septum, and the tricuspid valve lies in a plane caudad to the mitral valve. Thus, a needle passed horizontally from the atrial side of the septal leaflet will exit into the left ventricle.

With right ventricular dilatation, the tricuspid annulus enlarges along the major portion of the attachment of the anterior leaflet, the posterior leaflet, and the lateral third of the septal leaflet.

### PHYSIOLOGY

Disease of the tricuspid valve causes circulatory depression in several ways. Organic stenosis may limit flow into the pulmonary circulation and into the left side of the heart. With decreased preload to the left side of the heart, left ventricular stroke volume decreases, causing salt and water retention via the renin-aldosterone-angiotensin mechanism (forward heart failure). Tricuspid stenosis also may cause "backward heart failure," with hepatic congestion, ascites, and peripheral edema.

Tricuspid incompetence, organic or functional, also may limit preload to the left side of the heart. In addition, tricuspid incompetence leads to right ventricular dilatation. Right ventricular enlargement may also result from tricuspid regurgitation secondary to lesions in the left side of the heart.

The clinical signs of tricuspid valve disease are shown in Figure 49–3. Hepatojugular reflux is encountered in tricuspid regurgitation only, and increased intensity of murmurs with inspiration aids in distinguishing tricuspid murmurs from mitral murmurs.

Hepatic dysfunction often accompanies tricuspid valve disease and must be defined before surgical intervention.

### INDICATIONS FOR OPERATION

Surgical indications in all but a few cases (of isolated tricuspid valve disease) are those related to the

1667

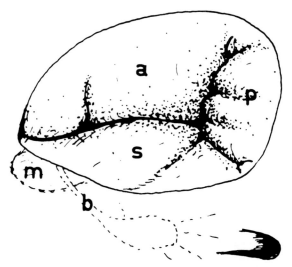

**FIGURE 49–1.** Normal tricuspid orifice. (a = anterior leaflet; p = posterior leaflet; s = septal leaflet; b = bundle of His; m = membranous septum.) (From Carpentier, A., Deloche, A., Hanania, G., et al.: Surgical management of acquired tricuspid valve disease. J. Thorac. Cardiovasc. Surg., 67:53, 1974.)

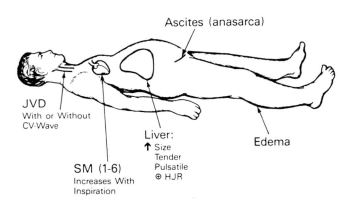

**FIGURE 49–3.** Signs of tricuspid insufficiency. (JVD = jugular venous distention; SM = systolic murmur; HJR = hepatojugular reflux.) (From Cohen, S. R., Sell, J. E., McIntosh, C. L., and Clark, R. E.: Tricuspid regurgitation in patients with acquired, chronic, pure mitral regurgitation. I: Prevalence, diagnosis, and comparison of preoperative clinical and hemodynamic features in patients with and without tricuspid regurgitation. J. Thorac. Cardiovasc. Surg., 94:481, 1987.)

left-sided valvular dysfunction. Tricuspid valve dysfunction, both functional and organic, usually occurs in the late stages of left-sided valve problems. Thus, the results of tricuspid valve surgery must be interpreted with regard to early and late results of mitral and double-valve procedures. Also, it follows that tricuspid valve repair or replacement is almost always done in patients with New York Heart Association (NYHA) functional Classes III and IV.

## RESULTS OF OPERATION

In 1974, Stephenson and colleagues (Stephenson et al., 1977) reported a 24% operative mortality rate (30-

day) in 38 patients undergoing triple-valve replacement (aortic, mitral, and tricuspid). The operative risk was influenced by NYHA functional class (18% for NYHA Class III and 40% for Class IV) (Fig. 49–4). The 5-year survival rate for the entire group was 53%. Triple-valve replacement is seldom done now. Instead, tricuspid valve repair is used almost uniformly when tricuspid valve involvement is associated with important left-sided valve stenosis or incompetence. For example, Duran and colleagues (1980) reported 150 patients who underwent tricuspid valve involvement and in whom left-sided repair or replacement was done. Seventy-eight patients had organic disease, and 72 patients had functional tricuspid incompetence. One hundred nineteen patients had tricuspid valve repair (46 commissurotomies and 115 annuloplasties), and in 31 patients the tricuspid disease was surgically ignored. Postoperatively, 97% of

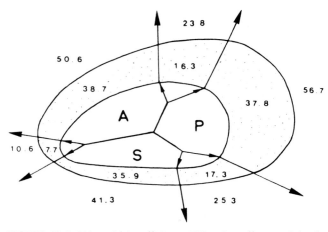

**FIGURE 49–2.** Tricuspid insufficiency. Dilatation affects mainly the posterior (P) and the anterior (A) leaflets. Numbers indicate the average lengths (in millimeters) of the attachment of the leaflets in a normal (central numbers) and a dilated (peripheral numbers) orifice. Most annuloplasties shorten the annulus at the anterior and posterior leaflets. (s = septal leaflet.) (From Carpentier, A., Deloche, A., Hanania, G., et al.: Surgical management of acquired tricuspid valve disease. J. Thorac. Cardiovasc. Surg., 67:53, 1974.)

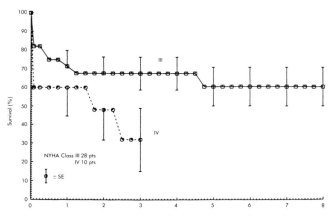

**FIGURE 49–4.** Actuarial survival after triple valve replacement in 38 patients according to preoperative functional class. (From Stephenson, L. W., Kouchoukos, N. T., and Kirklin, J. W.: Triple-valve replacement: An analysis of eight years' experience. Reprinted with permission from The Society of Thoracic Surgeons [The Annals of Thoracic Surgery, Vol. 23, 1977, pp. 327–332].)

patients with hemodynamically corrected left-sided lesions were NYHA functional Class I or II. In addition, appropriate repair of left-sided valve dysfunction determined the postoperative cardiac index. The operative mortality rate in that series was 8.4%. Residual tricuspid incompetence was present when pulmonary vascular resistance remained elevated. Eighty per cent of patients with preoperative tricuspid incompetence did not have postoperative regurgitation when pulmonary vascular resistance fell below 500 dyn-sec/cm$^3$, compared with 47% of patients with pulmonary vascular resistance greater than 500 dyn postoperatively (i.e., 53% had residual tricuspid incompetence). Approximately 30% of patients have small or moderate postoperative tricuspid gradients after repair. Most residual gradients and incompetence are not clinically important if hemodynamic correction of the left-sided heart disease is adequate.

Baughman and colleagues (1984) at Massachusetts General Hospital reported on 74 patients who underwent multiple valve surgery including procedures on the tricuspid valve. This report represents contemporary data—for example, congestive heart failure systems, Classes III and IV, were present preoperatively in 82%. Fifty-five of the 74 patients had undergone one or two previous cardiac operations. The 30-day mortality rate was 22%, and the survival rate continued to decrease minimally to plateau at 70%. Male sex, NYHA functional Class IV, ascites or pulmonary edema, elevated preoperative bilirubin, mean pulmonary artery pressure greater than 40 mm Hg, and pulmonary vascular resistance greater than 6 Wood's units all were associated with increased risk of death after operation. Multivariate risk analysis identified severity of peripheral edema and level of pulmonary artery pressure as the most predictive combination of those independent variables.

Indications for tricuspid valve surgery cannot be dissociated from operations on left-sided lesions. Results of tricuspid valve operations depend on the appropriate procedure for aortic or mitral valve lesions, the degree and reversibility of left ventricular dysfunction, the degree and reversibility of pulmonary vascular resistance, and the severity of right ventricular dysfunction. Therefore, better results occur if patients present for operation early in the course of congestive heart failure.

Although it cannot be documented, most surgeons believe that tricuspid valve repair is preferable to valve replacement. The hemodynamics are comparable: There is a higher incidence of mild incompetence with repair versus a higher gradient after replacement. The complications associated with replacement (e.g., thromboembolism, thrombosis, and anticoagulant-related problems) do not occur with reparative procedures. These facts alone favor use of repair as often as possible.

## TECHNIQUE OF OPERATION

Because most tricuspid valve operative procedures are associated with surgical therapy for aortic or mi-tral disease, the usual approach is through a median sternotomy. Infrequently, a right anterior thoracotomy approach can be used for isolated tricuspid valve operations or mitral and tricuspid valve procedures. Before cardiopulmonary bypass, the right atrial size is assessed and the thrill of tricuspid incompetence is palpated on the right atrial wall and, more definitively, by the index finger inserted through the right atrial appendage. At this time, organic changes in the tricuspid valve are determined. Scarring of the leaflets and thickening and adhesions or closure at the commissures, most frequently at the anterior commissure, are characteristic of organic valve disease. Shortening of the anterior leaflet and occasionally thickening of the chordae may also be present. Functional tricuspid incompetence exists in the absence of scarring and commissural changes. The annulus is dilated. The jet of tricuspid incompetence is graded I through VI. Generally, functional tricuspid incompetence, Grades I or II, is ignored. Repair is done when there are organic changes or when tricuspid incompetence is Grade III to VI.

A single period of aortic cross-clamping is used, and myocardial protection is afforded by oxygenated potassium blood cardioplegia and external myocardial cooling. The perfusate is stabilized at 26° C. The aortic or mitral valve or both are repaired or replaced.

## TECHNIQUE OF TRICUSPID VALVE REPAIR

Commissurotomy for tricuspid stenosis is relatively straightforward. The anterior and occasionally posterior commissures are incised with a scapel. A suture or two is occasionally necessary to obliterate a cleft or to shorten the annulus posterolaterally.

Tricuspid annuloplasty can be accomplished by various techniques. The three basic methods are directed to narrowing the dilated tricuspid annulus while maintaining leaflet length and function and preserving the course of the conduction fibers as they penetrate from the right atrium to the membranous ventricular septum, posteromedially. The Kay or Wooler annuloplasty uses mattress or figure-of-eight sutures to obliterate the commissure and most of the annulus between the anterior and posterior leaflets (Fig. 49–5). The DeVega technique uses a double purse-string suture to narrow the annulus from the anterior commissure to the posterior septal commissure. A valve sizer is often inserted to gauge correctly the degree to which the annuloplasty suture is tightened (Fig. 49–6). A slightly more complex but perhaps more definitive procedure uses a Carpentier ring, which has actually evolved to an interrupted C-shaped configuration open at the area of the penetrating bundle of His. This ring is inserted at the level of the annulus to narrow and stabilize it. The tissue of the annulus is gathered by interrupted or continuous sutures to the slightly flexible Dacron-covered metal prosthetic annulus. A reproducible reduction in the circumference of the tricuspid annulus is achieved. This repair may be more durable and more effective

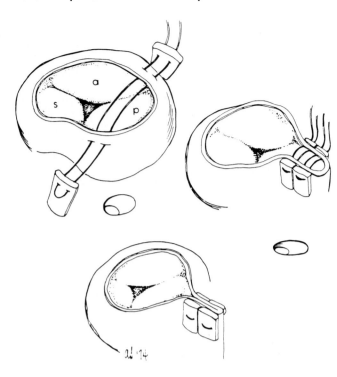

**FIGURE 49–5.** Basic commissural annuloplasty according to Kay or Wooler. (s = septal leaflet; a = anterior leaflet; p = posterior leaflet.) (From Boyd, A. D., Engleman, R. M., Isom, O. W., et al.: Tricuspid annuloplasty, five and one-half years' experience with 78 patients. J. Thorac. Cardiovasc. Surg., *68*:344, 1974.)

than either the Kay-Wooler or the DeVega technique (Fig. 49–7).

## TRICUSPID VALVE REPLACEMENT

For severe organic tricuspid valve disease, valve replacement is occasionally necessary. In the tricuspid position, a tissue valve is used most often. Mechanical valves on the right side of the heart have a very high incidence of thromboembolism and thrombosis. Thus,

a porcine xenograft or a pericardial valve is preferred. The bioprosthesis is inserted within the tricuspid annulus, where special care is taken in suturing near the bundle of His. The sutures are placed at the redundant septal leaflet and its base; otherwise, the needle bites pass through the annulus. A valve is occasionally placed supra-annularly—that is, on the atrial side of the tricuspid ring—with the coronary sinus draining into the right ventricle. This technique avoids the conduction system altogether.

In a nonconcurrent analysis, a study from the Mayo

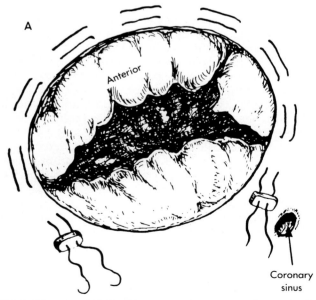

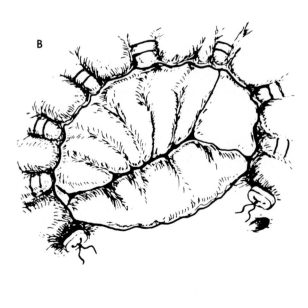

**FIGURE 49–6.** *A* and *B*, Double purse-string suture technique in DeVega's annuloplasty. (*A* and *B*, From Rabago, G., Fraile, J., Martinell, J., and Artiz, V.: Technique and results of tricuspid annuloplasty. J. Cardiovasc. Surg., *1*:247, 1986.)

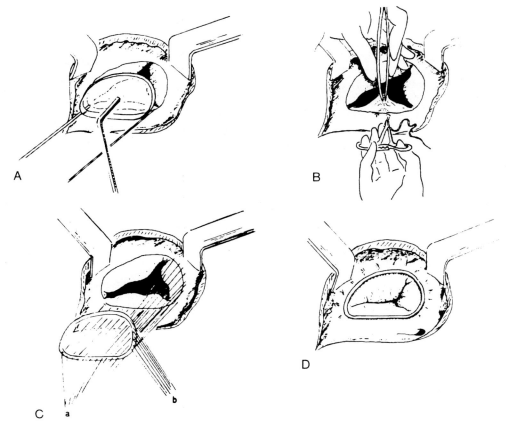

**FIGURE 49–7.** *A–D,* Carpentier's ring annuloplasty. The sutures at the base of the septal leaflet are passed through the corresponding segment of the prosthetic ring at the same intervals between them. The intervals are reduced to purse-string the anterior and septal annulus. (*A–D,* From Carpentier, A., Deloche, A., Hanania, G., et al.: Surgical management of acquired tricuspid valve disease. J. Thorac. Cardiovasc. Surg., *67*:53, 1974.)

Clinic (Fig. 49–8) compares long-term survival in patients undergoing tricuspid valve replacement versus those undergoing repair. The groups are not strictly similar, but repair resulted in better survival.

## INFECTIVE ENDOCARDITIS

An increasing indication for tricuspid valve surgical intervention is infective endocarditis, which has be-come more widespread because of the rising incidence of intravenous drug abuse. Some tricuspid endocarditis can be controlled effectively with specific antibiotic treatment. However, surgical intervention is necessary in the presence of continued sepsis, moderate or severe heart failure (secondary to tricuspid insufficiency), and multiple pulmonary emboli. Arbulu and Asfaw (1981) described tricuspid valvulectomy without replacement for this condition. The in-

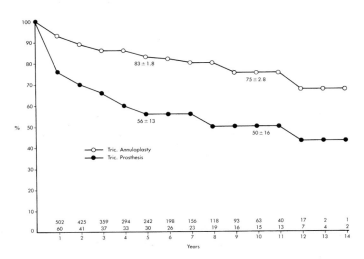

**FIGURE 49–8.** Comparative survival curves of patients with tricuspid (Tric.) prostheses or annuloplasty. (From Rabago, G., Fraile, J., Martinell, J., and Artiz, V.: Technique and results of tricuspid annuloplasty. J. Cardiovasc. Surg., *1*:247, 1986.)

fected focus is removed, and sepsis is controlled. Valve replacement is not done because of the high incidence of recidivism. In most cases, congestive heart failure is present postoperatively but can be controlled. This valvulectomy approach is not favored. The incidence and severity of hepatic congestion are manifestly high, and reoperation for subsequent valve replacement is tedious, with considerable blood loss. For initial tricuspid valve endocarditis, intensive medical therapy is advocated. If operative intervention is necessary, valve replacement is done and aggressive counseling is offered to prevent further drug abuse.

## SELECTED BIBLIOGRAPHY

Abe, T., Tukamoto, M., Yanagiya, M., et al.: DeVega's annuloplasty for acquired tricuspid disease: Early and late results in 110 patients. Ann. Thorac. Surg., 46:670, 1989.

DeVega's annuloplasty is a simple, reliable procedure. The procedure results in marked decrease of tricuspid regurgitation early after operation. There has been some question as to the durability of this procedure. Abe and colleagues assessed 110 tricuspid annuloplasties done with DeVega's procedure in association with mitral or combined mitral and aortic valve disease. There were seven early deaths (6.3%). Twenty-three (62%) of 37 randomly selected patients evaluated by echocardiography and 14 (70%) of 20 patients evaluated by right ventricular angiography showed complete disappearance of tricuspid regurgitation 1 to 18 months after annuloplasty. The actuarial rate of freedom from reoperation on the tricuspid valve was 96.7% ± 1.4%. In this relatively large group of patients, intermediate-term follow-up suggests that the DeVega annuloplasty is indeed a reliable and durable method to reduce or eliminate tricuspid regurgitation.

Boyd, A. D., Engelman, R. M., Isom, O. W., et al.: Tricuspid annuloplasty: Five and one-half years' experience with 78 patients. J. Thorac. Cardiovasc. Surg., 68:344, 1974.

Boyd and colleagues at New York University Hospitals reported 78 tricuspid annuloplasties and 90 tricuspid valve replacements done in association with mitral or mitral and aortic valve procedures. Tricuspid insufficiency was not recognized preoperatively, either clinically or by cardiac catheterization, in 35% of these patients. This finding emphasizes the importance of routine digital palpation of the tricuspid valve. The hospital mortality rate was 14% in the group undergoing annuloplasty and 34% in the group undergoing replacement. Late survival of the patients undergoing annuloplasty was perhaps slightly better than in those undergoing tricuspid valve replacement.

Braunwald, N. S., Ross, J., and Morrow, A. G.: Conservative management of tricuspid regurgitation in patients undergoing mitral valve replacement. Circulation, 35 and 36(Suppl. I):63, 69, 1966.

Braunwald and colleagues at the National Institutes of Health were perhaps among the first to characterize functional tricuspid regurgitation. They reported 28 patients undergoing mitral valve replacement. Twenty-five patients had no operative procedure on the tricuspid valve, and three had a tricuspid annuloplasty. Four patients died. Of the 24 survivors, 21 patients were asymptomatic and functional Class I or II. Mean right atrial pressures averaged 5 mm Hg, and systolic pulmonary artery pressures averaged 39 mm Hg postoperatively. The authors concluded that in many patients who undergo a satisfactory left-sided heart procedure, functional tricuspid regurgitation of mild, moderate, or even severe degree regresses postoperatively.

Kawachi, Y., Tominaga, R., Hisahara, M., et al.: Excellent durability of the Hancock porcine bioprosthesis in the tricuspid position. A sixteen-year follow-up study. J. Thorac. Cardiovasc. Surg., 104:1561, 1992.

In the aortic or mitral position, young age is an incremental risk factor for structural valve failure of glutaraldehyde-preserved porcine bioprostheses. Kawachi and colleagues studied 23 consecutive patients who underwent tricuspid valve replacement with the Hancock porcine bioprosthesis. Their ages ranged from 9 to 53 years (mean 36.2); mean follow-up was 9.1 years. Structural valve failure of the tricuspid bioprosthesis was noted in two patients, a 9-year-old boy and a 13-year-old girl, 3.4 and 16.5 years after implantation. The rate of actuarial freedom from structural valve failure at 10 years was 94 ± 6%. Five patients with double or triple valve replacement with porcine bioprostheses underwent reoperation 11.4 years postoperatively. Examination showed no valve dysfunction in the explants from the tricuspid position but degenerative changes with valve dysfunction with those in the mitral and aortic position. The authors conclude that selection of a Hancock bioprosthesis in the tricuspid position is acceptable because of the low incidence of prosthesis-related complications and excellent durability in these patients in their second, third, and fourth decades.

McGrath, L. B., Chen, C., Bailey, B. M., et al.: Early and late phase events following bioprosthetic tricuspid valve replacement. J. Cardiovasc. Surg., 7:245, 1992.

At Deborah Heart Center, over 26 years, 2% of 9247 patients underwent tricuspid valve replacement, of whom 154 also underwent bioprosthetic valve implantation. The authors reviewed those patients. There were 27 males and 127 females, and age ranged from 10 to 75 years. Log rank test indicated that incremental risk factors for late death were longer cross-clamp time at repair, higher pulmonary artery systolic pressure preoperatively, earlier date of surgery, and larger tricuspid prosthesis size. Structural failure of the bioprosthesis in the tricuspid position occurred in 17 patients (12.7%). The rate of actuarial freedom from tricuspid valve re-replacement was 70% at 10 years. The authors conclude that the bioprostheses in the tricuspid position are at relatively low risk of valve-related events. Risk factors for premature late death ·· related to earlier date of surgery, more complex repairs requiring prolonged aortic occlusion, and signs of increasing failure of the right side of the heart.

## BIBLIOGRAPHY

Arbulu, A., and Asfaw, I.: Tricuspid valvulectomy without prosthetic replacement: Ten years of clinical experience. J. Thorac. Cardiovasc. Surg., 82:684, 1981.

Baughman, K. L., Kallman, C. H., Yurchak, P. M., et al.: Predictors of survival after tricuspid valve surgery. Am. J. Cardiol., 54:137, 1984.

Duran, C. M. G., Pomar, J. L., Colman, T., et al.: Is tricuspid valve repair necessary? J. Thorac. Cardiovasc. Surg., 80:849, 1980.

Stephenson, L. W., Kouchoukos, N. T., and Kirklin, J. W.: Triple-valve replacement: An analysis of eight years' experience. Ann. Thorac. Surg., 23:327, 1977.

# 50 Acquired Disease of the Mitral Valve

Frank C. Spencer, Aubrey C. Galloway, and Stephen B. Colvin

## HISTORICAL ASPECTS

In 1923, Cutler and Levine, after detailed studies of diseased mitral valves, made a pioneering effort to perform mitral valvulotomy for mitral stenosis. Unfortunately, they reasoned incorrectly that part of the diseased valve must be excised. Although the first patient survived, the next several died; thus, the procedure was abandoned for over 20 years. In England, in 1925, Souttar performed a digital commissurotomy on one patient who survived, but for unknown reasons Souttar performed no further operations.

Over 20 years later, Harken and associates and Bailey independently demonstrated the feasibility and value of digital commissurotomy (Bailey, 1949; Harken et al., 1948). The results were dramatic. Hundreds of patients soon underwent surgery because mitral stenosis was a common, inevitably fatal disease from cerebral emboli or pulmonary edema. This launched the modern era of cardiac surgery. The previous concern had been that simply touching the heart might cause cardiac arrest or fibrillation.

Because the stenosed valve often could not be opened completely by digital commissurotomy, the stenosis recurred in as many as 50% of patients within 4 to 5 years. Hence, numerous mechanical mitral valve dilators were developed, the most popular of which was developed in England by Tubbs (Logan and Turner, 1959). This produced a more extensive commissurotomy, although mitral insufficiency resulted in a significant percentage of patients.

Open heart surgery had become feasible by this time, for Gibbon's first successful operation in 1953 was soon followed by independent important achievements by Lillehei and Kirklin in 1955. Initially, the complications of cardiopulmonary bypass made closed digital commissurotomy a safer procedure, but improvements in cardiopulmonary bypass technology enabled open valvulotomy during bypass to be adopted by most centers by 1970 to 1972. Today, digital commissurotomy is still done with any frequency only in areas of the world where a heart-lung machine is not available. In 1990, John and co-workers reported experiences from Southern India with over 4000 closed valvulotomies, usually using the Tubbs dilator. An open heart procedure was employed in only 109 patients.

For mitral insufficiency, a number of ingenious closed techniques were attempted before 1955, but none proved durable. When cardiopulmonary bypass developed, different forms of annuloplasty were tried. Lillehei and Merendino independently developed a selective form of posterior leaflet annuloplasty in 1957 (Lillehei et al., 1957; Merendino and Bruce, 1957). Subsequently, in 1960, McGoon described an effective technique of localized plication for a flail segment of mitral valve from ruptured chordae, which was applicable in selected patients. However, nothing could be done for most patients.

Following a few years of intensive research on development of cardiac prostheses throughout the United States, the Starr-Edwards ball valve prosthesis became clinically available in 1961. This valve firmly launched the modern era of prosthetic valve replacement. This remarkable prosthesis evolved from the combined work of Starr, a cardiac surgeon at the medical school in Portland, Oregon, and Edwards, a mechanical engineer.

It was immediately found that all mechanical prostheses required permanent anticoagulation with warfarin to prevent catastrophic thromboembolism. In the last 30 years, a wide variety of both ball and disk valves have been developed, but a mechanical prosthesis still does not exist that does not require anticoagulants. The original ball valve prostheses had some problems with the durability of the Silastic ball, but these were corrected by 1966. Disk prostheses, which have a larger cross-sectional area and less hemolysis than ball valves, were subsequently developed, but many were abandoned because of mechanical failure or thromboembolism. The most successful was the Björk-Shiley valve developed by Björk in Stockholm working with the Shiley Company in California. In 1979, Björk reported that more than 200,000 disk prostheses had been implanted. Unfortunately, a later model, the concave-convex disk, developed strut fracture in a few patients, causing medicolegal problems and withdrawal of the Björk prosthesis from the market.

Several disk prostheses are currently in use. The two most popular are the St. Jude bileaflet prosthesis (Fig. 50–1), introduced in 1977, and the Medtronic-Hall disk prosthesis. There seems to be little physiologic difference among the different disk prostheses available. The disk prostheses are currently more popular than ball valve prostheses because they have better flow characteristics.

All mechanical prostheses require permanent anti-

1673

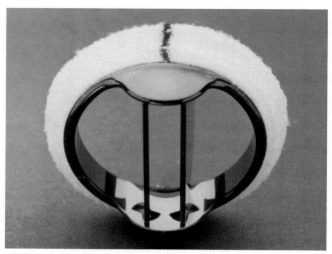

**FIGURE 50–1.** Leaflet mechanical mitral valve. (Courtesy of St. Jude Medical.)

coagulation to minimize thromboembolism; thus, the twin hazards with any prosthetic valve are thromboembolism and hemorrhage from anticoagulant therapy. Even with conservative anticoagulant therapy, maintaining the prothrombin time 1.5 to 2 times normal, there is still a small but definite danger of either thromboembolism or hemorrhage. These two hazards clearly show the importance of careful permanent medical supervision of patients with prosthetic valves. A collective review by Edmunds in 1987 ably summarized the frequency of thrombotic and bleeding complications with prosthetic valves.

Because of thromboembolic problems with mechanical prostheses, different types of tissue valves have been investigated since the late 1960s. It was quickly noted that bioprosthetic valves have a much lower frequency of thromboembolism and often do not require anticoagulant therapy. Valves constructed from autogenous fascia lata or homologous dura mater were used for several years, principally in the aortic valve, but all have been discarded because they frequently deteriorate within a few years. Various heterograft valves were evaluated in the 1960s, but all soon failed from fibrosis and calcification until the glutaraldehyde-preserved porcine prosthesis was developed in the late 1960s, principally by Carpentier in Paris and Hancock in the United States. The durability 5 years following implantation was found to be nearly 95%, so the prosthesis was quickly adopted throughout the world. Unfortunately, long-term durability has now been found to be disappointing: 15 to 20% of prostheses fail within 10 years, after which the rate of deterioration accelerates. In 1988, Magilligan reported that the 15-year failure rate exceeded 50%.

Ionescu in Leeds, England, developed glutaraldehyde-preserved valves constructed from bovine pericardium, which subsequently were widely used. A high frequency of calcification and disruption within a few years led to abandonment of the prosthesis. Recently, good results for over 5 years have been reported with a pericardial prosthesis preserved with "low-pressure fixation" which, thus far, has given excellent results, but at least 10 years of observation will be required for a final decision.

With the initial availability of prosthetic valves, interest in mitral reconstruction decreased sharply in the United States for more than 20 years. Fortunately, a few groups continued reconstructive techniques in selective patients. The leaflet plication reported in 1960 by McGoon was used in select patients at the Mayo Clinic. In 1963, Kay and Edgerton described posterior leaflet suture annuloplasty combined with repair of ruptured chordae. At New York University (NYU), Reed and associates (1965) described the technique of asymmetric mitral annuloplasty.

During the 1970s, major contributions to mitral valve reconstruction were made by Carpentier in France and Duran in Spain. An important step was the development of a method of quadrangular excision of a diseased segment of the posterior leaflet. Techniques of chordal shortening, chordal reimplantation, and leaflet transposition were developed to correct anterior leaflet prolapse. The reconstruction technique was combined with an annuloplasty ring to correct annular dilatation. Carpentier favored a rigid annuloplasty ring, but Duran later developed a flexible annuloplasty ring (Duran et al., 1978). The different methods are well described in the report by Carpentier in 1983 in his "Honored Guest Address" to the American Association for Thoracic Surgery.

The Carpentier and Duran techniques were used to a limited extent in the United States in the 1970s by only a few investigators. In 1979, Colvin at NYU began to apply the Carpentier technique in selected patients. Excellent results were obtained; since then, mitral reconstruction has been performed with increasing frequency. Experiences at NYU now include over 560 patients. At the Cleveland Clinic, Cosgrove and associates (1986) popularized the concept of mitral valve reconstruction with excellent results in a large number of patients. By 1994, several reports of 10-year data following reconstruction had been reported, and the technique is becoming more widely adopted as the primary treatment for mitral insufficiency.

## MITRAL STENOSIS

### Etiology and Pathology

Rheumatic fever is the only known cause of mitral stenosis, although a definite clinical history can be obtained in only about 50% of patients. In an extensive report describing pathologic changes in cardiac valves, Roberts (1992) concluded that the dominant cause was rheumatic heart disease. Aschoff bodies, the only anatomic lesion pathognomonic of rheumatic heart disease, have never been found in hearts without mitral valve disease. Congenital mitral stenosis is rare.

With the widespread effective prophylaxis of rheumatic fever over the past decades, the frequency of mitral stenosis has decreased markedly in the United States. In many areas of the world, however, especially India and South Africa, mitral stenosis is common. In 1990, John estimated that there were probably 400,000 patients in India with mitral stenosis!

Although the rheumatic inflammatory process is a pancarditis involving the endocardium, myocardium, and pericardium, permanent injury is predominantly in the cardiac valves, especially the mitral valve. If valves other than the mitral valve are diseased, the mitral valve apparently is always involved. Roberts, following his extensive pathologic studies, concluded that isolated aortic valve disease is never rheumatic in origin (1992). Permanent injury from rheumatic myocarditis has not been recognized, but Carabello in 1991 stated that studies found some left ventricular abnormality in 25 to 50% of patients. The exact cause is uncertain.

Rheumatic valvulitis produces at least three distinct pathologic changes, the degree varying widely among different patients: fusion of the valve leaflets at the commissures; fusion and shortening of the chordae tendineae; and fibrosis of the leaflets with subsequent stiffening, contraction, and calcification. The most extensive changes usually are seen in patients with recurrent attacks of rheumatic fever.

Commissural fusion is the most common result because the inflamed endocardium ulcerates where the two leaflets normally appose in systole. If commissural fusion alone is present, excellent results can be obtained by commissurotomy, either by the surgical or by the balloon dilatation method. However, if the valve leaflets have become fibrotic and calcified, restoration of normal mobility is usually impossible, so prosthetic replacement is required. Shortening and fusion of the underlying chordae tendineae occurs in probably 25 to 30% of patients. This important fact is why surgical commissurotomy is superior to balloon dilatation, for these fused chordae can be surgically divided, and mobility can be restored.

After an initial attack of rheumatic fever, the pathologic changes often progress slowly, evolving over decades. Carabello (1991) estimated from different reports that 85% of patients with Class I mitral stenosis, but only 50% of those in the Class II category, survived 10 years. The pathologic process apparently is an initial fusion of the commissures, followed by progressive fibrosing and stiffening of the commissures, chordae, and valve leaflets. It is remarkable to see patients in the fifth, sixth, or seventh decade of life with severe mitral stenosis apparently resulting from rheumatic fever as a child. Seltzer in 1972 proposed that this slow evolution was due to stiffening and fibrosis from turbulent flow of blood. This is a strong reason for *early* operation, even in asymptomatic patients.

If recurrent episodes of untreated rheumatic fever occur, however, the course is far more virulent. Severe valvular destruction and calcification may develop by 10 to 12 years of age. This is rare in the United States but common in Africa and India.

## Pathophysiology

The cross-sectional area of the mitral valve is 4 to 6 cm$^2$, varying with body size. Significant hemodynamic changes from mitral stenosis do not appear, however, until the cross-sectional area is reduced to less than 2 to 2.5 cm$^2$. Patients with this mild degree of mitral stenosis may have classic physical findings but are asymptomatic (Class I). With more severe reduction in cross-sectional area to 1 to 2 cm$^2$, symptoms appear initially with moderate exertion and then with mild degrees of exertion (Classes II and III). A patient with a mitral valve opening as small as 1 cm$^2$ is usually symptomatic with minimal effort. An opening near 0.5 cm$^2$ is said to be about the smallest size compatible with life. Stenosis of this severity produces symptoms despite complete bed rest (Class IV).

The dominant physiologic change with mitral stenosis is a chronic increase in mean left atrial pressure above the normal limit of 10 to 12 mm Hg. Many of the symptoms of mitral stenosis result from this chronic elevation in left atrial pressure. The decreased flow of blood into the left ventricle also reduces cardiac output, with resulting fatigue and muscular wasting. The chronically elevated left atrial pressure sequentially produces left atrial hypertrophy, atrial fibrillation, and eventually mural thrombi and systemic embolism. As discussed in later paragraphs, some patients also develop pulmonary hypertension from an increase in pulmonary vascular resistance.

The degree of increase in left atrial pressure above 10 to 12 mm Hg varies with at least three factors: the severity of the mitral stenosis, the cardiac output, and the heart rate, which determines the duration of diastolic filling of the left ventricle. Hence, the significance of elevation of left atrial pressure must be correlated with the cardiac output. The most precise physiologic measurement is the cross-sectional area, calculated from the pressure gradient and the cardiac output with a formula developed by Gorlin. Elevation in atrial pressure to levels of 15 to 20 mm Hg occur with moderately severe stenosis. If mean left atrial pressure exceeds 30 mm Hg (which is above the oncotic pressure of plasma), transudation of fluids into the pulmonary interstitial tissues occurs. Pulmonary edema may or may not develop, depending on the transport capacity of the pulmonary lymphatic circulation.

Thus the dominant symptoms of mitral stenosis are those of pulmonary congestion, such as cough, hemoptysis, orthopnea, paroxysmal nocturnal dyspnea, and pulmonary edema. Similarly, when the patient exercises and the cardiac output increases, the left atrial pressure rises, the lungs become congested, and the patient becomes symptomatic. This is the basis of the widely recognized classic symptom of mitral stenosis, "dyspnea on exertion." Such patients quickly learn to avoid exertion. The classic physiologic abnormality found on catheterization is an inability to increase cardiac output with exercise, with a simultaneous rise in the transvalvular gradient.

As mitral stenosis decreases the flow of blood into the left ventricle, there is a decrease in cardiac output with resulting fatigue, weakness, and muscular wasting, eventually producing "cardiac cachexia."

The left atrial hypertension often produces pulmonary vasoconstriction and an increase in pulmonary vascular resistance. Hypertrophy of the intima and media of the pulmonary arterioles may be found on histologic studies of the pulmonary vessels, but permanent organic obstruction probably results principally from thrombosis. There is a great variation among individual patients in the degree of increase in pulmonary vascular resistance. Probably more than 50% of patients never develop any significant increase, whereas a few patients develop an increased resistance 4 to 5 times greater than normal, with a pulmonary artery systolic pressure as high as 100 to 140 mm Hg. Fortunately, in most patients the increased vascular resistance subsides greatly after operation, a marked contrast to the dismal picture in congenital heart disease, where elevated pulmonary vascular resistance often becomes irreversible early in life. A corollary to this fortunate fact is that pulmonary hypertension from mitral stenosis in adults may increase the operative risk, but is seldom a total contraindication to operation.

Camara and associates in 1988 reported experiences with 88 patients with severe pulmonary hypertension treated by operation over a period of 10 years. The average systolic pulmonary artery pressure was 95 mm Hg, ranging from 70 to 180. The operative mortality rate was 5%. On late follow-up, averaging over 4 years, results were excellent. There were only six late deaths. Catheterization in 14 patients later found that there was an average decrease in systolic pressure from a mean value near 100 to about 40 mm Hg.

As noted earlier, chronic elevation in left atrial pressure causes hypertrophy of the smooth muscle in the left atrial wall and eventually atrial fibrillation. This decreases cardiac output 10 to 15% when it develops. The most serious complication from atrial fibrillation is the development of thrombi in the left atrial appendage and in the body of the left atrium from stasis. Rarely, huge thrombi, 5 to 10 cm in diameter, almost fill the left atrial cavity. Systemic emboli are a serious threat, because a high percentage go to the brain. This frequency of cerebral embolism constitutes a major indication for early operation once atrial fibrillation develops. Fortunately, after successful commissurotomy, combined with closure of the atrial appendage, emboli are rare and virtually unknown if a sinus rhythm is present.

## Diagnostic Considerations

The characteristic symptom of mitral stenosis is dyspnea on exertion. This may be the only symptom in early stages of the disease except for general weakness and fatigue. There is some correlation between the severity of the stenosis and the degree of exertion required to produce dyspnea. Because the symptoms of mitral stenosis primarily result from pulmonary congestion, this type of symptom is influenced by the effect of gravity. Dyspnea that appears in a patient in the supine position is called orthopnea. At night there may be paroxysmal nocturnal dyspnea or even pulmonary edema. Hemoptysis, an alarming symptom, is fortunately rarely of great magnitude, but it is occasionally severe enough to require urgent operation to prevent death from asphyxia.

When right-sided failure develops with elevation of right atrial pressure, the familiar findings of chronic congestive failure with hepatomegaly, engorged neck veins, and peripheral edema appear. Physical findings of pulmonary hypertension or tricuspid insufficiency may also be present.

On physical examination, patients with chronic mitral stenosis are often thin and frail from diffuse muscular atrophy, a reflection of long-standing restriction of cardiac output. These chronic metabolic abnormalities may be reflected by anergy to skin tests and a negative nitrogen balance, which increase the susceptibility to infection at the time of operation. The cardiac rhythm in most patients with chronic disease is atrial fibrillation.

Significantly, the size of the heart is usually normal in patients with mitral stenosis, with an apical impulse of normal or decreased intensity. This occurs because the left ventricle is small. A forceful apical impulse immediately suggests that additional valvular disease, such as mitral insufficiency or aortic valvular disease, has produced hypertrophy of the left ventricle. If pulmonary hypertension has produced hypertrophy of the right ventricle, a forceful systolic impulse may be palpable in the left parasternal area.

The three characteristic auscultatory findings of mitral stenosis, called the "auscultatory triad," include an apical diastolic rumble, an increased first sound, and an opening snap. These are sufficiently characteristic to establish the diagnosis with an accuracy approaching 100% on physical examination alone. The apical diastolic rumble, produced by blood flowing through the stenotic orifice, may be sharply localized to an area at the apex no larger than 1 inch in diameter. The intensity varies, usually Grade II or III, but occasionally is loud enough to produce a palpable thrill. The intensity, however, does not correlate with the severity of the stenosis. Rarely, in advanced cases with a calcified, immobile valve, so-called "silent" mitral stenosis is present with no murmur detectable even by phonocardiography.

The increased first sound, which probably results from thickening of the mitral leaflets, is one of the earliest findings. The opening snap can be identified on careful examination but is absent with rigid, mobile leaflets. A short apical systolic murmur is frequent but has little significance. However, a loud pansystolic murmur, transmitted to the axilla, usually indicates mitral insufficiency. A systolic murmur along the left lower sternal border, loudest near the xiphoid process, is commonly seen with tricuspid insufficiency.

Several abnormalities are seen on the chest film.

The earliest change is enlargement of the left atrium, typically seen on the posteroanterior film as a double contour visible behind the right atrial shadow. The overall cardiac size is often normal, but the enlargement of the left atrium and pulmonary artery obliterates the normal concavity between the aorta and the left ventricle, producing a "straight" left border of the heart. Calcification of the mitral valve, occasionally extensive, may be seen. In the lung fields, several abnormalities result from pulmonary congestion with distention of the pulmonary arteries and veins and engorgement of pulmonary lymphatics and pleural effusion. The enlarged pulmonary lymphatics, often called *Kerley's lines*, occur with severe mitral stenosis and can be recognized as distinct horizontal linear opacities in the lower lung fields.

Echocardiography is now well established as a valuable noninvasive technique for evaluating mitral stenosis. This can measure the cross-sectional area of the valve as well as the size of the left atrium and the left ventricle. The electrocardiogram, by contrast, is an inadequate guide to the severity of the stenosis and may even be normal. The accuracy of echocardiography makes cardiac catheterization and angiography frequently unnecessary to establish the diagnosis, but these procedures should be done in older patients or in patients with long-standing disease to evaluate associated factors, such as pulmonary hypertension, mitral insufficiency, coronary disease, or aortic valve disease. This information may help estimate the risk of operation and the likelihood that a prosthetic valve replacement will be required. If significant mitral insufficiency is found in association with severe stenosis, a prosthetic replacement frequently is necessary.

Tricuspid stenosis or insufficiency may be difficult to detect, because echocardiography frequently overestimates the degree of tricuspid insufficiency. Hence, an important routine at operation is always to palpate the tricuspid valve by insertion of a finger through the right atrial wall before the venous cannulas are inserted. This is particularly crucial in patients with preoperative symptoms of right-sided heart failure or with an elevated central venous pressure.

## Operative Treatment

### Indications for Operation

For over 15 years, the senior author has strongly recommended that most patients with hemodynamically significant mitral stenosis (cross-sectional area 1.0 to 1.5 cm²) should undergo surgery, even though they are asymptomatic, unless severe associated diseases create a serious operative risk (Spencer, 1978). Currently, exercise catheterization or exercise echocardiography may be used to help evaluate the need for early operation. If the mitral valve gradient increases significantly with exercise and the pulmonary artery pressure rises, operation is indicated.

The concept of early operation based on hemodynamic abnormalities rather than symptoms, as with coarctation of the aorta in children, is crucial. Two insidious dangers are always present. The risk of cerebral embolism always exists, even though it is small as long as the patient is in sinus rhythm. Nevertheless, in a few patients, a crippling stroke is the first major symptom. A second, more important reason is that the turbulent flow of blood through the stenotic valve produces progressive deterioration from fibrosis and eventual calcification. The valve usually must be replaced once extensive disease is present, but early in the disease process over 90% of stenotic valves can be treated effectively by commissurotomy.

A more conservative approach was recommended in 1991 by Carabello, who usually recommended operation when the stenotic mitral orifice was reduced to near 1.0 cm² or less. When operation is postponed for this length of time, however, atrial fibrillation is present in most patients, many of whom continue to fibrillate postoperatively, and a significant percentage have already had at least one embolic episode.

The concept of basing recommendations for operation on hemodynamic abnormalities in asymptomatic patients is especially important because mitral stenosis often progresses insidiously. Patients may be treated medically for years with few symptoms except for some limitation of activities, quite unaware that progressive destruction of the mitral valve is occurring.

At the other extreme, patients almost never have disease so far advanced that operation is impossible. Even in Class IV patients with cardiac cachexia and ascites, operative risk is now in the range of 5 to 10%. Remarkable improvement can often be obtained by valve replacement in these patients, although long-term results are inferior to those obtained in patients undergoing surgery earlier, before pulmonary hypertension and right-sided heart failure have developed. The ability to operate successfully on most seriously ill patients with mitral stenosis is based on the fact that function of the left ventricle is almost always adequate because the stenotic valve has restricted the inflow of blood into the ventricular cavity.

The risk of operation for Class IV patients can be greatly reduced by intense preoperative therapy with bed rest, nutritional support, and diuresis for days, even weeks, before operation. The time required for effective preoperative therapy varies widely, so a fixed schedule cannot be planned. Similarly, improvement in nutrition will significantly lessen the perioperative risk of infection or multiorgan failure.

The risk of early operation for mitral stenosis is very small, less than 1%, with a probability greater than 90% that commissurotomy is possible. In 1986, Kirklin and Barratt-Boyes reported that only one death occurred after 259 commissurotomies performed over a period of several years. Early commissurotomy, combined with surgical obliteration of the atrial appendage, also provides marked protection from future arterial embolism. Over a decade ago, Gross and associates (1981) reported excellent long-term results in a group of 202 patients treated at NYU.

The ideal operation for mitral stenosis, therefore, is

open mitral commissurotomy combined with obliteration of the atrial appendage. If the patient remains in sinus rhythm, such a procedure is highly effective, and functional results over the next decade are excellent.

### Technique of Open Mitral Commissurotomy

The basic NYU technique for open mitral commissurotomy was described by Mullin 20 years ago (1974). Experiences with techniques of mitral reconstruction for mitral insufficiency have led to even more aggressive commissurotomy, including incision of the fused chordal-papillary muscle apparatus, division of shortened secondary chordae that restrict motion of the mural leaflet, and selective débridement of calcium. In recent years, the frequency of rheumatic fever has declined sharply, so patients with isolated mitral stenosis are rarely seen. A median sternotomy incision is almost always used, although commissurotomy can be performed through either a right-sided anterior thoracotomy or a left-sided posterolateral thoracotomy. The tricuspid valve is examined with a finger introduced through the right atrial appendage to detect insufficiency or stenosis. The thickness of the right atrial wall is a useful guide, because an atrial wall of normal thickness suggests that tricuspid insufficiency is probably of recent origin and will regress significantly with correction of the mitral valve disease. The bypass technique is a standard one with sufficient heparinization to produce an activated clotting time of more than 500 seconds. Arterial cannulation is in the ascending aorta; the venae cavae are cannulated separately. A membrane oxygenator is used, primed with a balanced crystalloid solution, usually 20 to 30 ml/kg of the patient's body weight. The perfusion rate is near 2 to 2.5 $l/m^2/min$ at a temperature of 30° C. Blood is added to the perfusate if the hematocrit decreases below 20%. Following clamping of the aorta, the heart is arrested with cold potassium cardioplegic solution, usually an injection of about 20 ml/kg (1000 to 1500 ml) of cold blood or crystalloid cardioplegic solution. We prefer a blood cardioplegia solution. Either the aortic antegrade or the coronary sinus retrograde technique can be used.

Sufficient cardioplegic solution is infused to cool all areas of the heart below 10 to 12° C; the temperatures of different areas are measured with a needle thermistor. Subsequently, the heart is wrapped in a laparotomy tape, and cold electrolyte solution (4° C) is infused onto the surface of the right ventricle, removing fluid from the operating field through a sump placed at the bottom of the pericardial cavity.

This method of continuous topical hypothermia, a modification of the technique introduced by Shumway at Stanford decades ago, is particularly valuable for patients with hypertrophy of the right ventricle from pulmonary hypertension. Otherwise, the hypertrophied right ventricle is vulnerable to rewarming from lights in the operating room and other factors.

At NYU, cold blood cardioplegic solution is reinfused every 20 to 30 minutes, with myocardial temperature monitored so that it remains below 10 to 15° C. Unless topical hypothermia is used, the myocardium may gradually rewarm because of the aorta lying posteriorly, the diaphragm lying inferiorly, and the operating room lights above. In all probability, this rewarming is the origin of right-sided heart failure reported by some groups.

Once the heart has been arrested and cooled, the left atrium is opened with a longitudinal incision posterior to the interatrial groove, extending the atriotomy beneath and to the left of both the superior and inferior vena cava. The Carpentier mitral retractor (Fig. 50–2) is particularly valuable for providing adequate exposure, because its design permits multiple adjustments of the different blades.

Initially, the atrial cavity is examined for thrombi, especially inside the atrial appendage. If the patient is in atrial fibrillation, the atrial appendage is then excluded from the left atrium by closing the orifice with a continuous suture of 3-0 Prolene. The needle is placed carefully in a horizontal direction, not far beneath the endocardium, so the shaft of the needle is faintly visible. This method has virtually eliminated the hazard of injury to the circumflex coronary artery—no such problems have occurred at NYU in over a decade. Unless the appendage is closed, the patient remains at risk from emboli developing in a fibrillating appendage.

Following closure of the appendage, the mitral valve is exposed by applying horizontal traction to the leaflets adjacent to the commissures, often by placing a right-angle clamp beneath the commissure. The important concept is horizontal rather than vertical traction (Fig. 50–3). This may also be done with a suture inserted in each leaflet, which in turn is grasped with a right-angle clamp. The horizontal traction stretches the leaflets and facilitates identification of the commissures.

The "fused commissure" is actually a scar that develops at the line of commissural closure of the mitral leaflets from ulceration of endocardium. In most patients, this can be readily identified as a "depressed trench" with thickened tissue different in color and texture from the adjacent leaflets. If fibrosis of the leaflets is severe, the exact location of the commissure may be difficult to identify. Examination of the commissural chordae beneath the commissure may provide an additional landmark, for the commissural chordae radiate from the papillary muscle, like spokes in a wheel, to the mitral leaflets.

Once the commissure has been identified, a right-angle clamp is introduced beneath the fused commissure, stretching the adjacent chordae and leaflets, after which the commissure can be carefully incised with a knife, 2 to 3 mm at a time, serially confirming that the separated margins of the commissural leaflet are attached to chordae tendineae. The usual commissurotomy curves slightly anteriorly and does not go directly laterally. Because the "commissure" is a scar, the incised tissue is thicker than the normal leaflet. The incision should stop a few millimeters from the valve annulus, where the leaflet tissue becomes thin.

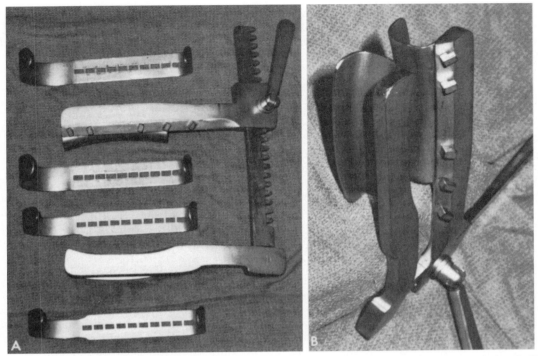

**FIGURE 50–2.** *A,* The sternal retractor developed by Carpentier in Paris with a variety of blades that can be attached to facilitate exposure of the mitral valve, greatly enhancing techniques of reconstruction. The instrument is very useful, with five different areas on the blades where the retractors can be attached with different degrees of tension. Adequate exposure is essential for complex techniques of reconstruction, even more so than for simple prosthetic replacement. *B,* Side view of the same instrument.

This is the normal mitral anatomy, indicating the transition from the fused commissure to the normal commissural leaflet of the mitral valve.

Occasionally landmarks are grossly distorted with fusion of leaflets to the underlying papillary muscle from shortening and fusion of chordae tendineae. In such instances, the commissurotomy may be started laterally by making a short stab wound with a No. 15 knife blade through the commissural tissue. Spreading the margins of the incised commissure with for-

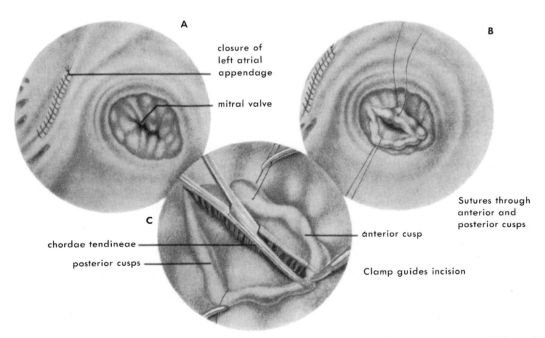

**FIGURE 50–3.** *A,* Closure of left atrial appendage. *B,* Exposure of mitral valve with horizontal traction on sutures. *C,* The right-angle clamp guides incision.

ceps permits extension of the commissurotomy slowly to the free margin of the mitral orifice, identifying and protecting underlying chordae and then incising the fused papillary muscle for 5 to 10 mm (Fig. 50–4).

Following separation of the commissure and the underlying chordae tendineae, leaflet mobility is assessed visually and by injection of fluid with a bulb syringe. Restricted motion of the mural leaflet may be improved by dividing short secondary chordae, originally recommended by Carpentier. Restricted anterior leaflet motion may be improved by splitting both the chordae and the papillary muscle from which the fused chordae arise, which improves leaflet mobility considerably. In a few patients, débridement of calcium from leaflets with rongeurs is feasible, although recurrence is significant in such diseased valves. In over 30% of patients, more than simple incision of the commissure is required to produce an adequate mitral orifice and restore mobility of the valve. This is an additional anatomic reason that open surgical commissurotomy produces a result superior to that feasible by balloon valvuloplasty.

The presence of mitral insufficiency can be visually assessed by inspection of the apposition of the valve leaflets. If localized prolapse exists, a selected annuloplasty can be done, avoiding undue constriction of the mitral orifice. Subsequently, the absence of significant insufficiency is confirmed by digitally palpating the mitral valve with the heart beating before bypass is stopped. Intraoperative transesophageal echocardiography is also a valuable guide for evaluation of mitral insufficiency.

Following open commissurotomy, the incision in the left atrium is sutured with continuous Prolene. After the suture lines are completed, ventricular fibrillation is induced and the aorta unclamped. Air is serially removed from different cardiac chambers, either by applying gentle suction to a catheter in the left ventricle or by needle aspiration. Before the heart is defibrillated, the head is lowered, the aorta may be partly clamped, and the aortic root may be vented. Then the heart is defibrillated, permitting blood from the contracting ventricle to be ejected through the aortic vent site. Alternatively, the cardioplegia catheter in the ascending aorta may be placed on gentle suction, while the heart is defibrillated with the patient in the "head down" position. Signs of air embolism are extremely rare when these techniques are employed.

Following bypass, with normal cardiac contractility and blood pressure, correction of the mitral stenosis should be confirmed by measuring left atrial and left ventricular end-diastolic pressures, demonstrating that the gradient has been satisfactorily corrected. In most patients, the gradient is 0 to 2 mm Hg. A residual gradient of 4 to 5 mm Hg may be tolerated in some patients with thickened stiff leaflets, but prosthetic replacement may be necessary within a few years from progressive fibrosis and calcification of the leaflets. If the residual gradient is more than 4 to 5 mm Hg, commissurotomy should be abandoned and valve replacement performed.

### Technique of Closed Commissurotomy

We have not performed this operation for many years, because better and safer results are obtained with an open technique and cardiopulmonary bypass. Unless a heart-lung machine is not available, almost the only indication for closed commissurotomy is pregnancy, because of the risk to the fetus from heparinization.

The technique of commissurotomy described in previous editions of this book is summarized here. A left-sided posterolateral thoracotomy in the fourth intercostal space, with the patient turned slightly beyond the true lateral position, approximately 110 degrees rather than 90 degrees, is best. The increased rotation facilitates exposure of the posterior aspect of the left atrium. This approach can also be used for mitral valve replacement, and remains useful in certain complicated cases in which the standard anterior approach is not feasible. A left-sided anterolateral thoracotomy can also be used for closed commissurotomy but provides less exposure of the atrium.

The pericardium is incised anterior to the phrenic nerve, after which stay sutures are inserted for traction. The atrial appendage is then examined for possible thrombi. An appendage containing an organized thrombus often has a rubbery consistency, very differ-

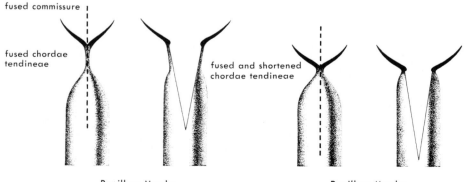

fused commissure

fused chordae tendineae

fused and shortened chordae tendineae

Papillary Muscles

Papillary Muscles

A

B

FIGURE 50–4. *A*, Separation of fused chordae tendineae with incision into papillary muscle. *B*, Deeper incision into papillary muscle when valve leaflets are fused to underlying papillary muscle.

ent from the soft compressible feel of a normal appendage. A fibrotic contracted appendage suggests chronic fibrotic organization of a thrombus over a long time.

Initially, a purse-string suture is placed around the base of the appendage and secured with a snare that can be tightened around the finger to minimize loss of blood. An important adjunct is to have the anesthesiologist identify both carotid pulses at the start of the operation to permit intermittent digital occlusion for 30 to 60 seconds during significant intracardiac manipulations. Cerebral embolism is fortunately rare with this technique.

When the atrial appendage is incised, a jet of blood is allowed to flush from the opening momentarily to dislodge any free-floating thrombi. Rarely, a thrombus as large as 1 to 2 cm in diameter is expelled. Subsequently, the index finger is introduced, with care taken to watch for undue resistance or laceration. If a tear begins, the finger should be withdrawn promptly and the atrial incision extended superiorly toward the left pulmonary vein. Lacerations in this area can be readily controlled, whereas those extending toward the circumflex coronary artery can produce lethal hemorrhage. An alternative approach is to suture a sleeve of Dacron graft or pericardium onto the pericardium, through which a finger can be introduced.

Once the index finger has been introduced into the atrium, the degree of stenosis, insufficiency, and valvular calcification is noted. It is particularly important to detect friable calcific granules along the margins of the valve, because these are associated with a great risk of cerebral embolization. Temporary occlusion of the carotid vessels is particularly important if it is necessary to proceed with the commissurotomy. Consideration should be given to terminating the operation and subsequently performing an open commissurotomy.

If hazardous calcification is not detected, commissurotomy is then performed by pressure with the index finger alternately on the two fused commissures, opening each commissure gradually and noting any mitral insufficiency that results after each manipulation. A variety of digital maneuvers, varying with individual patients, may be necessary when the commissures are densely fused.

Usually, repeated efforts are necessary to open a commissure, gradually weakening and tearing the rigid scar; a mechanical transventricular dilator is often used, which applies more mechanical force than possible with the finger. This, however, has the hazard of producing insufficiency. Rather than resorting to a mechanical dilator, the surgeon should consider stopping the operation if an open commissurotomy can be subsequently performed. Kirklin and Barratt-Boyes, however, frequently use the Tubbs dilator, serially opening the valve from 2.5 to 3.5 or 4.0 cm as long as regurgitation does not develop.

In ideal circumstances, unless mitral insufficiency develops, both commissures should be opened to within a few millimeters of the mitral annulus. Subsequently, after the finger is removed from the atrium, any gradient remaining across the mitral valve can be measured by needle puncture of the left atrium and left ventricle. Ideally, the end-diastolic gradient will have been abolished.

With adequate precautions, surgery carries a small risk, 1 to 2%. As discussed earlier, the main objections to this approach are the inability to open the valve properly if fused chordae are present and the inability to correct any insufficiency produced at operation.

### Open Versus Closed Commissurotomy or Balloon Valvuloplasty

For several reasons, open commissurotomy appears to be the best approach for most patients. Closed commissurotomy is an inferior procedure and should be done only in unusual circumstances, such as pregnancy or the unavailability of a heart-lung machine. The operative risk of open commissurotomy is less than 1%, the same or less than with closed commissurotomy. The risk of cerebral embolism is also less with open commissurotomy, approaching 0%. Also, commissurotomy is more effective when one separates fused chordae tendineae as well as fused commissures. If mitral insufficiency is present, it can often be evaluated and treated with the techniques of mitral valve reconstruction described later in this chapter. In other parts of the world, however, closed commissurotomy is still a viable option. In 1990, John and co-workers reported experiences in India with over 4000 cases of closed commissurotomy, obtaining good results in most.

The choice between surgical commissurotomy and balloon valvuloplasty varies widely among different centers, partly because long-term results (5 to 10 years) following balloon valvuloplasty are not yet available. Certainly, the excellent long-term results with open mitral valve commissurotomy are well documented and provide a standard by which future decisions about the role of balloon valvuloplasty should be made. Nevertheless, excellent short-term results can be obtained in selected patients with balloon valvuloplasty, which is simpler than surgical commissurotomy. Balloon valvuloplasty appears to give excellent hemodynamic results in selected patients who are early in the disease process. Unfortunately, elderly patients who might otherwise be the best candidates for balloon valvuloplasty are usually the worst anatomic candidates, because their calcified valvular lesions are usually more advanced. Failure rates are predictably high in this group. Thus, despite the simplicity and availability of balloon valvuloplasty, available data predict that 5- and 10-year results following treatment will be considerably better in most patients with open commissurotomy. However, balloon valvuloplasty may now be the procedure of choice for mitral stenosis in many parts of the world where open commissurotomy is not readily available. In this country, balloon valvuloplasty has become a viable option for selected patients.

## Technique of Mitral Valve Replacement

The techniques of perfusion and the initial surgical approach are identical to those described earlier for open mitral commissurotomy. The tricuspid valve is routinely palpated at the time of insertion of the venous cannulas. Potassium cardioplegia is induced either by antegrade aortic injection or by retrograde injection through the coronary sinus. The coronary sinus technique is usually used at NYU and is specifically preferred if significant coronary disease is present, because it improves myocardial distribution of the cardioplegia solution.

Topical hypothermia is routinely employed, and the myocardial temperature is monitored, with the temperature kept below 10 to 15° C. With this technique, the duration of aortic clamping has little influence on operative mortality, because ischemia times as long as 2 to 3 hours are well tolerated. Much shorter periods of occlusion, usually between 60 and 90 minutes, are adequate for most patients.

After the left atrium is opened, the diseased mitral valve is removed, preserving as many chordae as possible, particularly posteriorly. In 1964, Lillehei and associates suggested that preservation of mural leaflet chordae preserved left ventricular function. For over 25 years, this concept was intermittently discussed with no conclusive data about the value of chordae preservation. Numerous studies now have found that better ventricular function is obtained if the chordae are preserved. The mural leaflet chordae are easily preserved by imbricating the mural leaflet tissue and placing the sutures, inserting the prosthetic valve through the base of the leaflet. The best technique for preservation of chordae to the aortic leaflet is not yet clear. With disk prostheses, caution is required to be certain that the preserved chordae and leaflet tissue do not impair the motion of the disk.

In 1986, David and Ho reported experiences with 51 consecutive patients treated for mitral regurgitation from myocardial infarction. Fifteen were in cardiogenic shock as surgery began. The chordae were preserved in 32 of the group. Statistical analysis found that chordae excision was an independent risk factor. Actuarial survival at 4 years was 89% for patients with preserved chordae, compared with 59% for patients in whom the chordae were excised.

Subsequently, in 1990, Hennein and associates reported experiences at the National Heart Institute with long-term studies in 69 patients. The chordae were completely excised in 55 patients, whereas the chordae were partly or completely preserved in 14. Much better ventricular function was found in the group in whom the chordae were preserved. In an editorial in 1990, Tyers stated that preservation of the chordae could influence as much as 40% of ventricular function.

In 1992, Carabello reported a study of patients undergoing prosthetic valve replacement, comparing those whose chordae were preserved with those whose chordae were transected. The chordae transection group experienced a rise in left ventricular systolic volume, an increase in end-systolic stress, and a major fall in ejection fraction, often from 60 to 40%. The chordae preservation group, by contrast, experienced a decrease in left ventricular end-diastolic volume, a decrease in left ventricular systolic volume, a decrease in end-systolic stress, and no changes in ejection fraction.

Finally, Miller and associates, in several reports, the most recent in 1993, have demonstrated in a large number of experiments the value of chordae preservation, preserving the "valve ventricular interaction." Thus, several important studies have found that preservation of mitral valve chordae is associated with significantly better ventricular function.

A separate advantage of chordae preservation, discussed in a subsequent section, is that this may protect against rupture of the left ventricle.

After the diseased mitral valve has been partly removed, preserving as many chordae as possible, a prosthetic valve of appropriate size is selected with a plastic sizer. The appropriate size varies with body size. Most prostheses are between 29 and 31 mm in diameter, but sizes as small as 25 to 27 mm are adequate in small patients. With any type of prosthesis, care should be taken that the prosthesis opens freely, without impingement in the ventricular cavity.

Either a porcine or a mechanical prosthesis may be used. The valvular function is similar for virtually all types of mitral prostheses, although larger cross-sectional areas are obtained with the disk prostheses.

The major question in choosing between porcine and mechanical prostheses is the ability of the patient to tolerate anticoagulant therapy with warfarin permanently, with appropriate medical supervision. Mechanical prostheses require permanent anticoagulation, but with tissue prostheses, the need for anticoagulants varies with cardiac rhythm, size of the left atrium, and other factors. In patients with a sinus rhythm and a small left atrium, anticoagulants are sometimes stopped a few months after insertion. Thromboembolic rates are slightly higher for porcine valves in the mitral position when anticoagulants are not used, however.

In choosing the prosthesis, the surgeon should make a recommendation to the patient, who can make the final decision; the patient usually agrees with the surgical recommendation but occasionally disagrees. This important medicolegal point involves informed consent.

The age of the patient is another major consideration, because porcine prostheses function longer in older patients. By contrast, in children, porcine prostheses deteriorate rapidly, so they are virtually never used. Most reports indicate that in adults, about 80% of porcine prostheses are functioning adequately 10 years following operation, but only about 50% do so 15 years after operation. Hence, a patient has the choice between the likely possibility of reoperation within 10 to 15 years with a porcine prosthesis and permanent anticoagulant therapy with a more durable mechanical prosthesis.

Experiences with 1424 mitral valve operations at

NYU were reported by Galloway and co-workers in 1988 (Galloway et al., 1988b). A porcine prosthesis was used in about 975 patients, although in the last few years porcine prostheses have been used much less frequently and are now chosen primarily because of age or inability to tolerate anticoagulant therapy safely. The relative frequency of the use of mechanical prostheses, porcine prostheses, and mitral reconstruction over the past few years at NYU is shown in Table 50–1. Porcine prostheses are now used mainly in elderly patients.

A mechanical prosthesis usually is recommended for patients under 70 years of age, but also in some older patients who are able to take warfarin and who are in otherwise excellent general health. With mechanical prostheses, the type is primarily determined by the preference of the surgeon. The St. Jude disk prosthesis is most commonly used at NYU, though equally good results have been obtained with the Medtronic-Hall disk prosthesis and others. In discussing the paper of Fiore and associates (1992), Arom described a report of over 4000 patients, noting similar results with the St. Jude and Medtronic-Hall prostheses.

Hammermeister and colleagues, in 1993, reported results from a large randomized study of porcine versus mechanical valves in the Veterans Administration. Five hundred seventy-five patients were randomized between aortic and mitral mechanical or tissue valves. An average follow-up of 11 years showed no significant difference between the two groups regarding probability of death. About 5 years following operation, the mortality rate was near 40% with mitral prostheses, 30% with aortic; at 11 years, it was near 60% with both mitral and aortic prostheses. Structural failure and reoperation were more likely in patients receiving bioprosthetic valves, whereas thromboemboli and bleeding complications were more likely in patients with mechanical valves. Overall, the frequency of valve-related complications was equal in the two groups.

The mitral prosthesis is routinely inserted with 12 to 16 mattress sutures of 2-0 Tycron, all buttressed with Teflon pledgets. The mattress suture pledget technique has been used uniformly at NYU for over 20 years because it virtually eliminates perivalvular leakage. Care is taken to insert the sutures precisely in the annulus of the mitral valve, confirmed both by inspection and by the tactile sense of resistance as the needle is inserted. Particular caution is taken to avoid deeper insertion of sutures, which may injure critical structures. Deep sutures may injure the circumflex coronary artery laterally and posteriorly, the atrial ventricular node anteromedially, or the aortic valve anterolaterally.

After the prosthesis is lowered into position, the sutures are tied securely but gently, with only enough tension to create a visible dimple on the surface of the cloth of the prosthesis. Strong upward traction during the tying of the sutures may inadvertently avulse the mitral annulus from the underlying ventricular muscle and rupture the left ventricle. Similarly, following insertion of the prosthesis, undue elevation of the left ventricle is avoided, because the left ventricle may rupture. A rigid prosthetic ring constitutes a fixed point that cannot bend if the apex of the left ventricle is raised. For this reason, a left ventricular vent is avoided in most patients.

As the atriotomy incision is closed, a plastic catheter may be placed across the prosthetic valve into the left ventricle to keep the prosthesis incompetent until air has been removed; alternatively, the left ventricle is de-aired by aspiration with a large needle. Following closure of the atriotomy incision, ventricular fibrillation is induced and the aorta unclamped. Air is removed from the different cardiac chambers with the technique described in the preceding section for open mitral commissurotomy.

Following discontinuation of bypass and neutralization of heparin with protamine, a small plastic catheter is usually left in the atrium to monitor left atrial pressure; a Swan-Ganz catheter in the pulmonary artery can also be used. Pacemaker wires are left on the atrium and ventricle.

### Rupture of Left Ventricle After Mitral Valve Replacement

This rare but usually lethal complication can occur from three typical causes. The most obvious, and most easily avoided, is a pure *atrioventricular* (AV) groove rupture. A true AV groove rupture may be caused from overzealous excision of the annulus, particularly when calcium is débrided from the posterior annulus, or from partial avulsion of the mitral annulus due to excessive traction while removing the valve or tying the sutures. This type of AV groove tear can almost always be prevented by avoiding overly aggressive resection posteriorly and by minimizing upward traction during all parts of the operation. Valvular sutures must be inserted precisely into the annulus, rather than into the underlying ventricular muscle. The most common causes of primary AV groove injury include excessive removal of calcium or fibrotic leaflet tissue, excision of part of the annulus, upward traction during the tying of sutures, and undue elevation of the apex of the left ventricle during de-airing. Constant awareness of these dangers usually is sufficient to prevent this complication in most patients.

A second type of left ventricular rupture can result from direct injury to the muscle, either by excising the papillary muscles too deeply and producing a

■ **Table 50–1.** MITRAL VALVE RECONSTRUCTION VERSUS MITRAL VALVE REPLACEMENT AT NYU, 1989–1992

| Year | Carpentier Repair | Mitral Valve Replacement (Porcine) | Mitral Valve Replacement (Mechanical) | Total Mitral Valve Replacement |
|------|-------------------|-----------------------------------|--------------------------------------|-------------------------------|
| 1989 | 83 | 58 | 68 | 126 |
| 1990 | 84 | 35 | 103 | 138 |
| 1991 | 80 | 56 | 90 | 146 |
| 1992 | 72 | 61 | 89 | 150 |

"buttonhole" injury or by choosing a prosthesis that is too large for the ventricular cavity, which can produce injury from the valve struts. With present knowledge, direct injury to the left ventricular wall during mitral valve replacement is uncommon. Care is taken either to leave a rim of papillary muscle with the ventricle while excising the chordae or to preserve the chordae altogether. With porcine or cage prostheses, the position of the struts in relation to the adjacent ventricular wall is routinely examined.

The third type of ventricular rupture after mitral valve replacement, the midventricular freewall rupture, was designated "Type III" by Miller in 1978. This type is the most puzzling, occurring as a transverse rupture midway between the annulus of the mural leaflet and the posterior papillary muscle. The elegant report by Cobbs and associates from Emory University in 1980 describes seven such fatal ruptures with clear illustrations from autopsy specimens. They hypothesized that these ruptures evolved from strong contractions of the left ventricle after removal of chordae attached to the mural leaflet—the "untethered loop" hypothesis.

This subject was investigated in depth at NYU and was reported in 1985. As the report describes, before 1981 rupture of the left ventricle was recognized in 14 patients after mitral valve replacement over a period of 9 years. True AV groove rupture and traumatic injury were considered the most probable causes until late 1981, when four fatal ruptures occurred over a period of 2 months. In none of the four was undue traction or direct injury recognized, but all patients had undergone total excision of the posterior chordae. This grim experience led to the prospective study described in the 1985 report. In brief, in almost all operations since 1981, some chordae have been preserved to the annulus of the mural leaflet. Since making this technical change, we have not encountered subsequent midventricular freewall rupture after mitral valve replacement. Whether this virtual absence of left ventricular rupture is due to preservation of chordae or simply to a constant awareness of the problem is unknown. It seems plausible that preservation of chordae is the major factor in preventing "Type III" midventricular freewall rupture, because others have stated that with routine preservation of the mural leaflet over a period of 10 to 20 years, rupture of the left ventricle has never been seen. This subject was well analyzed in a collective review by Karlson and associates in 1988.

## Associated Procedures

### Coronary Bypass

If significant obstructive coronary disease is present, concomitant coronary bypass grafting is almost always done. For example, from 1990 through 1994 at NYU, bypass grafts were used in 20 to 40% of the patients undergoing mitral valve repair or replacement.

Virtually all reports of operative mortality describe a higher mortality rate with mitral valve replacement and coronary bypass, a 7 to 10% operative risk, than with isolated mitral valve replacement, which has a 2 to 5% operative risk. This may occur because two diseases are present, or because the coronary patients are generally older and have more impaired ventricular function.

Particular attention should be given to details of the myocardial preservation technique. The coronary sinus method of cardioplegia is preferred at NYU in most patients, because it seems to give better myocardial distribution in the presence of coronary disease. Likewise, a combination of antegrade and retrograde injection may be used. If only antegrade cardioplegia is given, it is important to attach the bypass grafts before the prosthetic valve is inserted in order to assure distribution of cardioplegia to the ischemic areas of myocardium. Cardioplegia can then be injected down the bypass grafts every 20 to 30 minutes.

### Treatment of Tricuspid Insufficiency

If significant tricuspid insufficiency is detected by preoperative evaluation or by intraoperative digital palpation of the tricuspid valve, it is almost always repaired with a posterolateral annuloplasty. The technique used, devised by Reed and reported by Boyd and associates at NYU in 1974, is a modification of the procedure previously described in 1965 by Kay and co-workers. An 8-cm segment of tricuspid annulus behind the septal and anterior leaflets is measured, after which the remaining lateral annulus, principally adjacent to the posterior leaflet, is plicated between Teflon-buttressed mattress sutures. This produces an orifice near 27 mm in diameter. Correction of the insufficiency is then confirmed by injection of saline with a bulb syringe into the ventricular cavity to distend and coapt the tricuspid leaflets.

This technique has been used for almost two decades, and results have been consistently excellent. In the rare instance of severe intrinsic leaflet disease, prosthetic replacement may be required instead of simple annular dilatation. Significant recurrent insufficiency is virtually unknown.

In 1988, Nakano and co-workers in Japan reported almost identical experiences with 133 patients treated by the Kay bicuspidalization procedure over a period of 17 years. During that time, only three tricuspid valve replacements were performed. A repeat operation was necessary in seven patients, six of whom had persistent mitral valve disease.

A different and equally efficacious, but more complex, approach is the Carpentier tricuspid ring annuloplasty, preferred by Kirklin and Barratt-Boyes. This is described in the second edition (1993) of their textbook.

## Operative Results

The operative mortality rate for mitral valve replacement has steadily decreased in recent years, probably from the combination of better techniques of perfusion, better cardioplegia, and improved surgical preoperative and postoperative care. In the 1988 report of experiences at NYU with 1425 mitral valve operations during the preceding decade, the operative mortality rate for mitral valve replacement was approximately 7%, rising to above 10% for patients who had undergone multiple procedures. By multivariate analysis, the major predictors of increased operative risk were age, NYHA functional classification, previous cardiac surgery, and concomitant cardiac surgical procedures. The operative mortality rate is currently 5% for isolated mitral valve replacement.

Kirklin and Barratt-Boyes (1993) reported similar results. They found that the incremental risk factors that increased the risk of premature death (early or late) after mitral valve replacement were age, race, NYHA functional classification, pure mitral insufficiency (as opposed to stenosis), ischemic mitral insufficiency, left ventricular enlargement (decreased ventricular contractility), left atrial enlargement, previous coronary bypass procedures, global myocardial ischemic time, and concomitant tricuspid annuloplasty or coronary bypass grafting.

## Postoperative Care

At operation, intravascular catheters are left in the left atrium, and a Swan-Ganz catheter is usually placed in the pulmonary artery. Temporary pacemaker wires are left on the right ventricle and on the right atrium if the patient is not in atrial fibrillation. In the recovery room, the left atrial pressure, pulmonary artery pressure, systemic arterial pressure, and electrocardiogram are continuously monitored on an oscilloscopic screen. If there are signs of right-sided heart failure, comparison of right atrial pressure and left atrial pressure also may be valuable.

Cardiac output is measured periodically, with the goal of maintaining a cardiac index of 2.3 to 2.5 l/m². This is accomplished by infusing sufficient fluid to maintain an appropriate preload, by treating increased afterload with vasodilators, and by selectively using inotropic agents. Inotropic drugs may include dopamine, dobutamine, amrinone, or epinephrine. Sodium nitroprusside may be infused to decrease peripheral vascular resistance and control postoperative hypertension. If the pulmonary vascular resistance is significantly elevated, vasodilating agents, such as nitroglycerine, nitroprusside, or amrinone, may be given into the central venous circulation; alpha-adrenergic agonists are infused directly into the left atrium to bypass the pulmonary vascular alpha-adrenergic receptors and to maintain peripheral vascular tone. This approach allows a degree of selective manipulation of the pulmonary and peripheral vascular resistances.

Minor arrhythmias are common, especially atrial fibrillation; thus, monitoring of cardiac rhythm, either visually or by telemetry, is particularly important. Pacemaker wires are usually left in place for 5 to 7 days, treating bradycardia with electrical pacing, preferably atrial or atrioventricular, at a rate between 80 and 90 beats per minute. Rapid atrial fibrillation is treated with digitalis and other agents to control the heart rate. If atrial fibrillation is refractory to appropriate drug therapy, cardioversion may be effective, but it seldom has a lasting effect if the left atrial size is over 4.5 to 5 cm. The most frequently used antiarrhythmic drugs are lidocaine, procainamide, quinidine, beta-adrenergic blockers, and calcium channel blockers.

A *postpericardiotomy* syndrome can occur after all types of open heart surgery. Although the syndrome has been recognized for decades, the etiology is somewhat obscure, apparently a reaction associated with surgical manipulation of the pericardial and pleural surfaces. The clinical manifestations vary but include low-grade fever, a white blood cell count usually less than 10,000 cells/mm³, a pericardial or pleural effusion, and an audible pericardial friction rub. Therapy with ibuprofin (Motrin) in appropriate doses for a few days is usually satisfactory. In unusually refractory cases, a short course of steroid therapy may be necessary.

Small pericardial or pleural effusions are common and require no specific treatment except appropriate diuresis. Large pleural effusions are evacuated by aspiration. The hazard of tamponade is present with every cardiac operation. Large asymptomatic pericardial effusions can usually be detected by chest film or with echocardiography and may respond to treatment with anti-inflammatory agents. If symptoms of tamponade develop, surgical drainage is done by the subxiphoid route or by pericardial aspiration.

Prophylactic antibiotics should be selected according to the prevailing bacterial flora found in wound infections in any individual hospital. Both cefamandole (Mandol) or cefazolin (Ancef) have been used at NYU for the past 10 years, with equal success. Generally, 2 g are given before operation and 1 g every 2 hours during the procedure, with the final dose given just as the sternum is closed. Antibiotics are continued postoperatively for 48 to 72 hours, usually until intracardiac and central intravascular catheters have been removed. Fortunately, infection of any type is uncommon. Sternotomy infection, formerly occurring at a rate nearing 1%, has continued to decrease in frequency. Sternal osteomyelitis detected at an early stage usually responds to débridement and closed mediastinal irrigation with appropriate antibiotics. In more advanced cases of osteomyelitis, débridement followed by a muscle flap procedure is employed.

Fortunately, postoperative endocarditis is very rare. If it occurs, it usually reflects bacterial contamination at operation and may require prompt reoperation.

Anticoagulant therapy is begun 2 to 3 days after operation with sodium warfarin (Coumadin), elevating the prothrombin time to near 20 seconds. A greater degree of anticoagulation, elevating the prothrombin time to twice normal levels, was found unnecessary many years ago. Higher levels produced greater frequency of hemorrhage but no greater protection from thromboembolism. Neither dipyridamole (Persantine) nor aspirin is used routinely for long-term platelet inhibition.

With porcine prostheses, anticoagulation with warfarin may be stopped after 3 months if the patient is in a sinus rhythm. When the warfarin is stopped, antiplatelet therapy with aspirin is recommended. In all patients with mechanical prostheses, and in patients with atrial fibrillation, a large left atrium, or chronic congestive failure, warfarin therapy is continued indefinitely.

Patients are usually discharged from the hospital 7 to 10 days following operation and gradually resume normal activities over the next 2 to 3 months. Diuretic therapy is usually necessary for weeks to months in patients with advanced preoperative symptoms or significant ventricular dysfunction. This decision can be made by daily measurements of body weight. Three to 6 months are often required to obtain full benefit from the operation, especially in patients with muscle wasting and weight loss from advanced cardiac failure.

## Long-Term Management and Results

**After Open Commissurotomy.** In 1981, Gross reported results in 202 patients undergoing commissurotomy at NYU between 1967 and 1978, with a 98% complete follow-up. The late mortality rate was only 2.5%. Five years following operation, 87% of patients who had no residual valve dysfunction after commissurotomy were free of any complications. The frequency of thromboembolism was only 0.3% per year in the first 10 years after operation.

Similar results were reported by Halseth in 1980, who described experiences with 222 patients undergoing surgery over 10 years. The operative mortality rate was low, 1.5%; two of the three deaths that occurred were in patients who underwent emergency surgery. Only 7% of the 191 patients surviving commissurotomy later required mitral valve replacement.

Unfortunately, the rheumatic injury to the cardiac valves appears to cause a permanent injury, because fibrosis and degeneration continue to appear even 15 to 20 years after successful commissurotomy, usually producing mitral insufficiency. Recurrent stenosis following a complete commissurotomy is almost unknown except from thickening and stiffening of the leaflets, not fusion of the commissures. Hence, patients following commissurotomy should be evaluated periodically, because it is likely that eventually, perhaps after over two decades, significant recurrent mitral disease will develop.

**After Prosthetic Replacement of the Mitral Valve.** An important principle is that any patient with a prosthetic valve requires lifelong periodic surveillance by a physician, similar to a patient with diabetes. The six most common complications that occur are thromboembolism, anticoagulant hemorrhage, endocarditis, arrhythmias, prosthesis malfunction, and cardiac failure. These are discussed in the following paragraphs. Data from several large series of valve prostheses reported in recent years are summarized in the Selected Bibliography.

**Thromboembolism.** The 1989 report by Galloway and associates from NYU included 169 mechanical mitral prostheses. There was a surprisingly high rate of freedom from thromboembolism at 5 years—94%—much higher than most reports published by others. This surprising finding probably indicates the importance of precise management of anticoagulant therapy by both patient and physician. These patients were carefully selected, because during this time about 975 porcine prostheses were inserted. The rate of freedom from thromboembolism in patients with porcine prostheses was actually less, 87%. Freedom from anticoagulant hemorrhage was about 95% in both groups. Reports by Kirklin and Barratt-Boyes and by Starr's group found about 95% of patients free from thromboemboli 5 years after operation. Starr's group found that the frequency of thromboemboli had sharply decreased from that of previous years. However, a higher frequency of embolism with ball valve prostheses was reported by Miller, who found an event in nearly 45% of patients within a decade following operation. In the excellent 1987 collective review by Edmunds on the frequency of thromboembolic complication, the percentage of patients free from thromboembolism at 5 years ranged from 65 to 89% with mechanical prostheses to 90 to 97% with porcine prostheses.

**Hemorrhage from Anticoagulants.** Bleeding associated with anticoagulants remains a permanent hazard in any patient. This emphasizes the importance of the selective use of prostheses, because some patients are unable to supervise anticoagulant therapy properly, either because of intrinsic problems or socioeconomic factors. The wide range in frequency of bleeding is well tabulated in Edmunds' 1987 collective review, including data from 20 reports. The frequency in five large series reported in recent years ranged from 1.2 to 4.5 per 100 patient-years. Although most episodes are minor, fatal hemorrhage occurs occasionally in almost all series reported. Hence, freedom from anticoagulant therapy is the main attraction of bioprostheses. Judging from different reports, bleeding seems to be significantly less if the prothrombin time is only 1½ times normal, compared with higher levels.

**Endocarditis.** Any patient with a prosthetic valve has a permanent susceptibility to bacterial endocarditis that develops after a period of transient bacteremia. The most common inciting episodes are dental extractions and cystoscopic procedures. Thus, it has long been recognized that appropriate antibiotic therapy must be given briefly before and after any procedure that might produce transient septicemia. Unfortunately, other patients develop endocarditis from unknown causes. Patients with porcine and mechanical prostheses are equally susceptible. In the 1989 NYU report by Galloway and associates, endocarditis occurred with a frequency of about 1% per year. Similar results have been reported by others. For unknown reasons, an extremely low frequency has been reported by Lindblom (1988) in Sweden, near 0.1%. One of the several advantages of mitral valve reconstruction over replacement is that endocarditis is extremely rare following mitral valve reconstruction.

Prosthetic valve endocarditis is a serious complication after valve replacement: Overall mortality rates from different institutions range from 25 to 50%. If appropriate antibiotic therapy does not promptly control signs of sepsis, surgical intervention should be performed promptly. Though it is often stated, this principle has often been neglected. Delaying operation and continuing ineffective antibiotic therapy significantly increases overall mortality. The infection gradually spreads beyond the prosthesis into the annulus and adjacent tissues, creating a more serious problem. What is not often recognized is that operation can be performed safely within as short a time as 2 to 3 days after the onset of endocarditis if the antibiotic sensitivity of the infecting organism is known and appropriate antibiotics are given. Hence, the only reason for delaying operation and continuing antibiotics is that it seems reasonably certain that the antibiotic therapy will be curative.

**Arrhythmias.** A significant percentage of deaths that occur 5 to 10 years after operation are apparently due to arrhythmias, because these often occur suddenly without any warning symptoms. Postmortem examination may find only various degrees of ventricular fibrosis. These episodes of "sudden death" are more common in patients who have serious impairment of ventricular function before operation, which may partly explain the much higher frequency of death in the first 5 years following operation (30 to 40%) in NYHA Class IV patients compared with Class II patients (10%). Postoperative monitoring of patients with known arrhythmias seems to be important, including 24-hour Holter monitoring in patients with poor ventricular function or known arrhythmias. Electrophysiologic studies can be done in selected cases and in all cases with a documented clinical event. Serious ventricular arrhythmias refractory to antiarrhythmic drugs may be treated with the implantable automatic defibrillator. A completely satisfactory solution for this difficult problem has not yet been found. The best of all solutions is probably to operate before severe myocardial injury has become irreversible. This is one of the attractive features of performing mitral valve reconstructive procedures earlier than is classically indicated for prosthetic valve replacement.

**Prosthesis Malfunction.** Late deterioration is the major handicap with porcine prostheses. In general, durability is excellent, approaching 95% in the first 5 years after operation, but subsequently failure increases at a more rapid rate. Only about 80% of porcine prostheses are functioning 10 years after operation, and less than 50% are functioning at 15 years. Thus, periodic evaluation of the patient, combined with echocardiography if new symptoms or murmurs appear, is important.

A 1986 report by Spencer and colleagues from NYU described institutional experiences with 1643 porcine prostheses over a period of 7 years and found that early deterioration was uncommon in the first few years after operation, occurring at a rate of about 1 to 2% per year. In 1988, Jamieson and colleagues reported experiences with over 1300 prostheses implanted over 11 years with an average follow-up near 6 years. The rate of freedom from valve failure at 10 years was about 77%. A most significant point in their report was that age had a major influence: Adult patients less than 30 years of age had only 27% of valves functioning at 10 years, those between 30 and 60 years had 77% functioning, whereas those over 60 had 83% functioning.

Malfunction of current mechanical prostheses is extremely rare. An excellent long-term analysis of 25 years of experience with the Starr-Edwards ball valve prosthesis was reported by Cobanoglu and colleagues in 1985. Likewise, to our knowledge, strut fracture has not occurred with current disk prostheses. The St. Jude valve and other tilting disk prostheses have shown excellent durability for 15 to 20 years.

**Late Cardiac Failure.** Some improvement virtually always occurs following mitral valve replacement but cannot be assessed precisely for 3 to 4 months following operation. Late functional status seems to depend primarily on what degree of preoperative impairment of ventricular function was irreversible. A recent exciting development, as yet unsupported by significant long-term data, is the suggestive evidence that preservation of chordae of the mitral valve apparatus may better preserve ventricular function after operation.

When cardiac function initially improves, but late cardiac failure develops months or years later, four possible causes should be considered: paravalvular leakage, malfunction of the valve repair or prosthesis, additional cardiac disease, and primary failure of left ventricular muscle. A particularly important principle that merits repeated emphasis is that all patients who present with late heart failure after valve replacement should be closely re-evaluated with echocardiography, cardiac catheterization, or both. It can be a serious mistake to treat such patients with increasing amounts of medication on the assumption that failure of the cardiac muscle is the primary cause of symptoms. With cardiac catheterization, the etiology of late heart failure can virtually always be readily established. Primary left ventricular failure is manifested by an elevated end-diastolic pressure, often 20 to 25 mm Hg or higher, without other valvular lesions or ischemic etiology. Other causes such as paravalvular leakage, prosthesis deterioration, or disease in another valve can be readily detected and subsequently corrected surgically.

## Late Mortality

The major factors influencing long-term survival after mitral valve repair or replacement are age, race, preoperative NYHA classification (reflecting the degree of preoperative left ventricular failure), urgency of operation, mitral insufficiency (versus stenosis), ischemic etiology, degree of pulmonary hypertension present preoperatively, and need for concomitant procedures such as tricuspid valve repair or coronary bypass grafting (Galloway et al., 1989; Kirklin and Barratt-Boyes, 1993). The type of valve procedure or the type of prosthesis has not been convincingly found to significantly influence late survival (Galloway et al., 1989; Hammermeister et al., 1993). In general, the 5-year survival rate after mitral valve operation is 60 to 90% and the 10-year survival rate is 40 to 75%, with late survival varying with the number and the severity of the preoperative risk factors present.

## MITRAL INSUFFICIENCY

### Etiology and Pathology

Although mitral stenosis is virtually always due to rheumatic fever, mitral insufficiency can result from several causes. Rheumatic fever was previously the most common one but is now less common in the United States; it remains the major cause in other areas of the world. Degenerative disease of the mitral apparatus (mitral prolapse and ruptured chordae) is probably the most common cause in this country, accounting for 40 to 50% of cases of mitral valve insufficiency. Other causes include ischemic disease, endocarditis, congenital heart disease, and, rarely, cardiomyopathy.

The four major structural components of the mitral valve are the annulus, leaflets, chordae, and papillary muscles. Any one or all of these in different combinations may be injured and create insufficiency. Hence, at operation, the functional integrity of each of these structures must be assessed to determine the type of reconstruction that should be done. The pathologic anatomy found in mitral insufficiency from different causes has been studied in detail by Carpentier and associates (1971, 1977, 1980; Carpentier, 1977).

**Rheumatic Disease.** With rheumatic mitral insufficiency, the valve leaflets are often fibrotic and contracted with focal areas of calcification. The commissures are almost always fused to a varying degree. Valvular stenosis, insufficiency, or both may be present.

The chordae tendineae, especially to the mural leaflet, are often short, thick, and fused. Secondary asymmetric dilatation of the annulus develops, primarily in the posteromedial area, and changes the contour of the mitral valve from an ellipse with a long transverse axis between the commissures to an ellipse with the long axis in the anteroposterior direction. An important point in mitral valve reconstruction is that the annulus of the aortic leaflet does not dilate because it is anchored to the fibrous skeleton of the base of the heart, and virtually all dilatation occurs posteriorly.

**Mitral Valve Prolapse.** Mitral valve prolapse (Barlow's syndrome) has been termed "floppy valve"

or "myxomatous degeneration," emphasizing the leaflet and chordae abnormality. The major histologic abnormality is the replacement of part of the collagen of the leaflets with an acid mucopolysaccharide. Roberts (1992) has studied the pathologic findings in detail. The leaflets, chordae, and annulus are all involved. There is an increase in the transverse dimension of the leaflets so that a scalloping effect is produced with bulging of different areas of the leaflets, an appearance of "excess tissue." The chordae are elongated and thin. These periodically rupture and produce a major increase in insufficiency. Isolated rupture of a chorda is probably a variant of the prolapse syndrome in which the major part of the degeneration is concentrated in certain chordae.

The annulus usually is dilated to a significant degree, again posteriorly. Although the mitral annulus in normal adults is near 9 cm in circumference, with mitral valve prolapse and severe mitral regurgitation the annulus is dilated to 14 to 18 cm, more than 50% above normal.

Insufficiency may result from pure dilatation of the annulus, from ruptured chordae tendineae, from leaflet prolapse secondary to chordal elongation, or from a combination. In 1987, Roberts and colleagues described the pathologic findings in 83 mitral valves that had been excised for severe regurgitation. Fifty-eight per cent had both dilatation of the annulus, above 11 cm in circumference, and ruptured chordae; 19% only had annular dilatation; whereas another 19% had ruptured chordae without dilatation.

Mild degrees of mitral valve prolapse are very common, estimated to occur in at least 5% of the normal female population. In most patients it is of minor physiologic significance, but in some patients years or decades later, severe mitral insufficiency gradually evolves as a result of leaflet fibrosis and chordae elongation. Similarly, acute symptoms can develop from chordal rupture. Before the syndrome of mitral valve prolapse was recognized, the long clinical history of a systolic murmur since childhood led to the erroneous conclusion that the abnormality originated in rheumatic fever, even though there was no evidence that this occurred.

**Ischemic Heart Disease.** The spectrum of pathologic changes may be wide. Some are obvious, resulting from a myocardial infarction with overt rupture of a papillary muscle or chordae or from fibrotic contraction and distortion of the papillary muscle and adjacent ventricular wall.

In 1989, Rankin and associates, analyzing over 300 patients at Duke University, described the pathologic abnormalities with ischemic mitral regurgitation. The least common was papillary muscle rupture, which usually appeared with a new murmur and congestive heart failure a few days after infarction. Most of these patients had a posterior papillary muscle dysfunction in association with a large posterior wall infarction. The structural injury includes a dilatation of the posterior annulus, elongation of the papillary muscle, and loss of the papillary muscle's ability to shorten.

Rankin observed a third category of the disease in

patients who had diffuse ventricular infarctions, low ejection fraction, and generalized annular dilatation, a group with an unusually poor prognosis.

In 1991, Hendren and colleagues reported that 84 patients with ischemic mitral insufficiency were seen over a period of 5 years in a group of 1290 patients treated at the Cleveland Clinic. Sixty-five of these underwent repair of the mitral valve. Eleven underwent surgery during the first 4 weeks after infarction, the remainder at a later date. Valve dysfunction was classified by preoperative echocardiography. Prolapse was found in 40% of patients, resulting from either rupture of a papillary muscle or papillary muscle infarction with elongation. Leaflet motion was restricted in 60% of patients as a result of regional or global ventricular dilatation. Hendren concluded that the most common pathologic abnormality was a papillary muscle annular dysfunction, evidenced by posterior annular dilatation, papillary muscle elongation, and loss of papillary muscle shortening. Experimental studies have found that mitral regurgitation does not develop from fibrosis limited to papillary muscles, but that it requires additional impairment of the function of the adjacent ventricular wall.

Oury and associates (1994), discussing Hendren's report (Hendren et al., 1992), described experiences with 169 patients in the preceding 5 years. Three different types of abnormalities were found: primary annular dilatation, coronary disease with ischemic or infarcted papillary muscles, and coronary disease with leaflet or chordal pathology.

## Pathophysiology

The basic physiologic abnormality with mitral insufficiency is regurgitation of part of the stroke volume of the contracting left ventricle into the left atrium, which reduces systemic blood flow and elevates left atrial pressure. Left atrial pressure tracings show a systolic pressure spike as high as 30 to 40 mm Hg, occasionally even higher, followed by an abrupt decline in diastole. At the end of diastole, the pressure may remain slightly elevated with a small gradient across the mitral valve, even though no organic stenosis is present. This "flow gradient" results from increased flow of blood during diastole. The mean left atrial pressure is usually 15 to 20 mm Hg, but in some patients it is normal. The pulmonary vascular resistance is increased less often than in patients with mitral stenosis, perhaps because left atrial pressure is elevated only intermittently. Similarly, left atrial thrombi and emboli occur less frequently than with mitral stenosis because stasis is absent in the left atrium. Left ventricular function may be adequate for long periods despite massive mitral regurgitation. Eventually, however, the left ventricle gradually fails, manifested by dilatation and hypertrophy. The dilatation of the ventricle can be measured well by echocardiography, because left ventricular diameter at the end of diastole is normally 5.2 to 5.6 cm. Once the end-diastolic diameter rises above 6 cm, symptoms gradually appear.

There is a corresponding gradual increase in size of the left atrium above the normal upper limit of 4 cm. A left atrial dimension of 4.5 to 6 cm is common. As this occurs, atrial arrhythmias, eventually atrial fibrillation, evolve. Concurrent with the dilatation of the left ventricle, there is an initial increase in the stroke volume of the heart, and the ejection fraction is well maintained. Eventually, however, this compensatory mechanism fails, and the ejection fraction decreases. A significant fall in ejection fraction below the normal of 50 to 60% is a relatively late finding, for the ventricle is initially "unloaded" by ejecting some blood through the insufficient valve into the left atrium.

## Diagnostic Considerations

With mild mitral insufficiency, an apical systolic murmur is present without any disability. Such patients may remain well for many years, with the left ventricle adapting adequately to the increased workload. The only significant hazard is an increased susceptibility to bacterial endocarditis. As stated earlier, the adaptation of the left ventricle to an increased workload with mitral insufficiency is by dilatation, increasing stroke volume by increasing the diastolic fiber length. Hence, the principal questions in evaluating the severity of mitral insufficiency are: What is the degree of left ventricular enlargement? And is the systolic function of the heart being affected?

As mitral insufficiency progresses, the most common symptoms are weakness, fatigue, and palpitations, with some dyspnea on exertion. These symptoms arise both from a decrease in left cardiac output and from elevation of left atrial pressure. As left ventricular failure evolves, symptoms of pulmonary congestion become more prominent, similar to those described in the preceding section on mitral stenosis. Right-sided heart failure with hepatic enlargement and peripheral edema develop with far advanced disease, almost always associated with a certain degree of permanent ventricular injury. Ideally, surgical therapy is performed well before this occurs.

On physical examination, the two characteristic findings are an apical systolic murmur and a forceful apical impulse. The apical murmur is harsh and blowing in quality, transmitted to the axilla. However, with certain types of chordae rupture, the murmur is loudest in the aortic area. Rarely, very little murmur is audible with diffuse insufficiency. The severity of the insufficiency does not correlate with the intensity of the murmur, but the pansystolic characteristic does. With mild mitral insufficiency, the systolic murmur does not extend completely through systole, whereas with severe insufficiency, it occupies all of systole.

The most important finding on physical examination is a forceful apical impulse, which reflects the degree of enlargement of the left ventricle. This finding contrasts sharply with the normal or decreased apical impulse with mitral stenosis.

The characteristic change on the chest film is enlargement of the left atrium and the left ventricle (Fig. 50–5). As long as left ventricular size is normal, a nonoperative approach may be acceptable, although current trends favor operation for severe physiologic abnormalities rather than for anatomic changes. Postponing operation until the left ventricle is severely enlarged often produces a suboptimal surgical result because of irreversible left ventricular injury.

Echocardiography, especially by the transesophageal route, has emerged as one of the most valuable diagnostic techniques. The technique can help determine the site of insufficiency, and specifically whether the mural, aortic, or both leaflets are significantly prolapsed. Ruptured chordae tendineae may be visualized.

An important measurement with echocardiography is the size of the cardiac chambers. The size of the left atrium reflects both the chronicity and the severity of the disease. A normal left atrium seldom has an internal diameter larger than 4 cm. With severe insufficiency, dilatation of the left atrium to 5 to 6 cm or more is common. When the left atrium dilates, arrhythmias and eventually atrial fibrillation develop. The upper limit of normal size of the left ventricle is an end-diastolic dimension between 5.2 and 5.6 cm. As previously mentioned, an end-diastolic diameter above 6 cm is a clear indicator of significant decompensation of the ventricle.

A change in ventricular systolic function, often manifested as a drop in ventricular ejection fraction with exercise, is a valuable guide for assessing the physiologic effects of mitral insufficiency. Normally, the ejection fraction rises with exercise; a fall in ejection fraction with exercise is a clear warning of

significant ventricular decompensation, because the resting ejection fraction may remain deceptively "normal" until late in the course of the disease. Reflux of blood into the left atrium decreases "afterload" on the left ventricle, allowing the resting ejection fraction to remain normal until relatively late in the disease process.

The electrocardiogram is not a precise guide; atrial fibrillation is common. Cardiac catheterization and coronary angiography should be done before operation in patients over 45 to 50 years of age or in patients with advanced symptoms, noting the degree of pulmonary hypertension, the ejection fraction, and the presence of associated valvular pathology or coronary artery disease.

## Operative Treatment

### Indications for Operation

Traditionally, operation was not recommended for mitral insufficiency until significant disability was present. The usual clinical abnormalities include exertional dyspnea, congestive heart failure, arrhythmias, and significant cardiac enlargement. However, clinical results have shown that once significant congestive heart failure is present, there is often a certain degree of irreversible ventricular injury. A well-established fact is that the more seriously ill patients, manifested by the NYHA functional status, have a worse prognosis. For example, the 5-year survival rate is over 90% for preoperative NYHA Class II patients but only about 50 to 60% in NYHA Class IV patients. About 50% of the late deaths are from heart failure.

Certainly, the long-term morbidity and mortality from prosthetic valves have been significant considerations when determining the timing of operative intervention. Historically, with the well-known problems from anticoagulation, thromboembolism, and endocarditis after prosthetic valve replacement, operation has been delayed until the patient with mitral valve insufficiency became symptomatic.

The potential advantage of mitral valve reconstruction, as compared with prosthetic valve replacement, is that these prosthetic-related hazards may be greatly diminished. Patients who remain in a sinus rhythm do not need permanent anticoagulants after mitral valve reconstruction; thus, the risks of thromboembolism and anticoagulation are markedly reduced. Endocarditis is rare after valve reconstruction. These facts, combined with the fact that reconstruction is possible in most patients with degenerative valvular disease (approximately 90%, possibly higher), indicates that the proper timing for operation in patients with mitral insufficiency should now be much earlier, based on progressive hemodynamic abnormalities before the development of significant symptoms.

The concept of recommending operation for asymptomatic or minimally symptomatic patients because of hemodynamic abnormalities has been discussed periodically in different reports. Studies of the

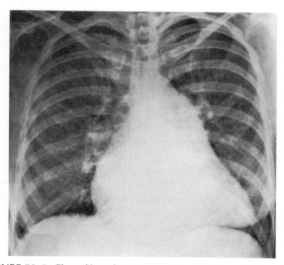

**FIGURE 50–5.** Chest film of a patient with mitral insufficiency. The distinctive features include an enlarged cardiac shadow with a prominent pulmonary artery. The shadow of the left atrium is visible in the right border of the cardiac shadow behind the shadow of the right atrium. The pulmonary vascular markings are prominent.

natural clinical history of mitral insufficiency have found that totally asymptomatic patients with severe mitral insufficiency usually progress to severe disability within 5 years. In 1981, Carabello carefully studied certain indices of ventricular function that correlated with an excellent result after valve replacement. The best results were obtained in patients with an ejection fraction above 70%, combined with sophisticated measurements of ventricular function, including end-systolic wall stress and end-systolic diastolic volume. By contrast, if the ejection fraction was less than 55%, poor results were obtained. These considerations were reviewed in detail by Levine in 1990.

The current guidelines for recommending operation at NYU are as follows: (1) significant mitral valve insufficiency, measured by echocardiography or by cardiac catheterization, along with (2) clinical symptoms, (3) enlargement of the left atrium to over 4.5 to 5.0 cm with recent onset of atrial fibrillation, (4) progressive enlargement of the left ventricular end-diastolic dimension to over 6.0 cm, or (5) a measurable decline in the resting or exercise-induced systolic function of the heart, as indicated by a rise in the echocardiographic left ventricular end-systolic dimension or a drop in radionuclide ejection fraction.

Ideally, operation is performed in the patient with severe but correctable mitral insufficiency, who has well-maintained ventricular function and who is still in sinus rhythm. If sinus rhythm can be maintained, long-term anticoagulants are not necessary; if systolic function is still normal, long-term functional results and survival are improved. Many of these concepts were previously reviewed and reported in 1988 (Galloway et al., 1988a).

## Mitral Valve Repair or Replacement?

Mitral valve repair is theoretically possible as long as a functioning anterior leaflet is present, because the cross-sectional area of the aortic leaflet alone is greater than the orifice area of most prosthetic valves.

If a functioning anterior leaflet can be achieved after repair, extensive calcification or significant disease in the posterior leaflet is seldom a contraindication. When annular or posterior leaflet calcium is present, valve reconstruction is possible if sufficient calcium can be safely removed to permit subsequent annular repair and ring annuloplasty. For example, calcium has now been extensively removed in over 58 cases at NYU with no adverse affect on late results. Reoperation was required in 6.9% of the patients who required calcium débridement and in 6.8% of those who did not. Thus, calcium per se has not adversely affected long-term results in our experience.

If the pathologic anatomy is suitable for mitral valve reconstruction, age has also not been a contraindication to valve repair. Since 1980, more than 146 patients 70 years of age or older have undergone mitral valve reconstruction at NYU. The hospital mortality rate was 4.4% for isolated mitral valve reconstruction in this group of patients, with a 5-year rate

of freedom from cumulative cardiac death and reoperation of 74%.

Mitral valve reconstruction is clearly feasible in most patients with mitral insufficiency from degenerative disease (90 to 95%). With rheumatic valves, feasibility of repair varies with the relative degree of stenosis or insufficiency. If insufficiency is the dominant lesion and the leaflets are mobile, repair appears to be possible in over one-half of rheumatic cases. A significant late recurrence rate is present in rheumatic patients undergoing valve reconstruction, however. In the NYU experience, the 10-year rate of freedom from reoperation after mitral reconstruction was 90% in nonrheumatic patients but only 67% in patients with rheumatic disease ($p < .0001$).

Mitral insufficiency secondary to bacterial endocarditis can be repaired as long as disease is discrete. With insufficiency from coronary disease, however, data are insufficient to permit more than broad guidelines. When the site of insufficiency is localized, repair is often possible. Insufficiency secondary to annular dilatation from any cause is almost always amenable to ring annuloplasty. With more diffuse pathology, involving multiple areas of both leaflets and the annulus, the feasibility of durable valve repair is less certain, but such repair is possible in selected cases.

Long-term survival after operation for mitral insufficiency could theoretically be better with valve repair than with valve replacement, because the hazards of thromboemboli, bleeding, and endocarditis are diminished. A survival advantage has been difficult to demonstrate statistically, however. Ventricular function is probably better with valve repair than with valve replacement, because the chordae are preserved routinely. But this difference may be small, and newer techniques allowing chordal preservation with valve replacement may prove equally beneficial. At present, the influence of the type of valvular procedure on survival remains uncertain because randomized data are not available.

The primary advantage of valve reconstruction seems to be a lower incidence of valve-related complications. In a review by Yun and Miller (1991), which compared valve repair and replacement in 10 large series, virtually every series reported better overall long-term results with valve repair, primarily because of a lower incidence of valve-related morbidity.

## Selected Annuloplasty Techniques

For several years after open heart surgery became clinically possible in 1955, prosthetic valves were not routinely available. Hence, different forms of mitral annuloplasty were explored by several investigators. The most durable techniques were developed independently by Lillehei and Merendino in 1957, and by Wooler in England. Poor results were obtained in many patients. After prosthetic valves became available in 1961 and 1962, interest in annuloplasty, with a few exceptions, virtually ceased.

Three different groups, however, continued to

apply annuloplasty in selected patients. In 1960, McGoon reported a method of treatment for isolated ruptured chordae of the mural leaflet by plicating the flail segment and subsequently performing suture annuloplasty. Twenty-five years later, Orsulak, at the Mayo Clinic, reported cumulative experiences with this technique in 131 patients. About 25% of patients required a subsequent operation within 10 years. In 1963, Kay and Egerton in Los Angeles described selected annuloplasty in the mural leaflet for ruptured chordae and applied suture annuloplasty for patients with mitral insufficiency from coronary disease. Experiences with 101 such patients with ischemic disease were reported by Kay and associates in 1986, about half of whom had ruptured chordae.

At NYU, in 1965, Reed and co-workers reported a technique of asymmetric annuloplasty, plicating a significant part of the annulus of the mural leaflet as well as a small part of the annulus of the aortic leaflet, narrowing the commissures and creating an orifice about 6 cm in circumference. Reed and colleagues summarized their collective experiences with 196 patients in 1980. Only 8% of the patients required a repeat operation. Thromboembolism has been infrequent.

In 1992, Czer and associates reported experiences with 60 patients with coronary disease and mitral insufficiency, comparing results with the Carpentier ring annuloplasty in 27 patients and with the Kay commissure suture annuloplasty in 33. The ring reduced the mitral annulus more than the suture technique but produced much better results with correction of the mitral insufficiency, 96% versus 67%. Nevertheless, 1-year survival was similar in both groups; the improvement in clinical status was similar.

The results reported with suture annuloplasty are good, but limited, because most patients with mitral insufficiency have additional abnormalities of the leaflet and chordae that are not amenable to treatment with simple annuloplasty. For example, only about 10% of patients in the NYU series could be treated by annuloplasty alone. Nevertheless, in patients with mitral insufficiency primarily due to annular dilatation, suture annuloplasty has been a viable and effective method of surgical correction. The suture annuloplasty technique should be considered a viable alternative to ring annuloplasty in selected patients.

## Carpentier Technique of Mitral Valve Reconstruction

The most significant developments in mitral valve reconstruction were made by Carpentier and associates over a period of 10 or more years at the Hôpital Broussais in Paris. These experiences were well summarized by Carpentier in his classic "Honored Guest Address" to the American Association for Thoracic Surgery in 1983. At that time he had performed surgery on more than 1400 patients, most of whom had mitral insufficiency from rheumatic fever. The basic

four techniques include the use of the annuloplasty ring, quadrangular segmental resection of diseased mural leaflet, shortening of elongated chordae, and transposition of mural leaflet chordae to the aortic leaflet. The ring annuloplasty was based on the fact that the anatomic deformity causing mitral insufficiency was principally an asymmetric dilatation of the annulus, occurring primarily in the posterior annulus. A most important point is that the annulus of the aortic leaflet does not dilate, for it is part of the basic fibrous skeleton of the heart. In association with the asymmetric dilatation of the mitral annulus, other anatomic abnormalities include elongation (or rupture) of chordae to produce increased leaflet motion, and localized restrictive disease in the leaflets or chordae to produce decrease leaflet mobility.

During the 1970s, significant contributions were also made by Duran in Spain and later by Paneth and Yacoub in England. The NYU experience began in 1979 after a visit by one of the faculty members, Dr. Stephen Colvin, with Carpentier in Paris. Valve reconstruction at NYU initially was used cautiously until durability was determined, because Carpentier's experience had been primarily with younger rheumatic patients, whereas degenerative disease with prolapse and insufficiency is more common in the United States. Progressive experiences have been serially reported, in 1985, 1988, and 1994, and now total nearly 600 cases. In more than 90% of patients, two or more abnormalities were corrected.

Particularly important is that a surprisingly large amount of the mural leaflet (3 to 4 cm; 40 to 60% of the leaflet) can be safely resected as a quadrangular resection. This astonishing ability to excise most or all of a diseased leaflet is one of the important principles that makes reconstruction feasible.

The basic NYU techniques of mitral valve reconstruction (Fig. 50–6), all developed from the original techniques of Carpentier, are described in the following paragraphs.

### Initial Approach

Standard cardiopulmonary bypass is established, the aorta clamped, and the heart arrested. Cardioplegia is given, preferably by the retrograde coronary sinus technique, especially if concomitant coronary artery disease is present. Alternatively, antegrade or combined antegrade-retrograde techniques may be used. The left atrium is opened with an incision posterior to the interatrial groove, extended superiorly and inferiorly beneath the venae cavae. The Carpentier retractor (see Fig. 50–2) is routinely employed, with the individual blades adjusted to the individual anatomy. Valve exposure is usually good but varies with the size of the atrium and the size of the patient.

Initially, the valve is examined in detail to determine anatomic abnormalities and how these can be corrected. This is naturally a critical part of the operation.

A localized, roughened area of atrial endocardium,

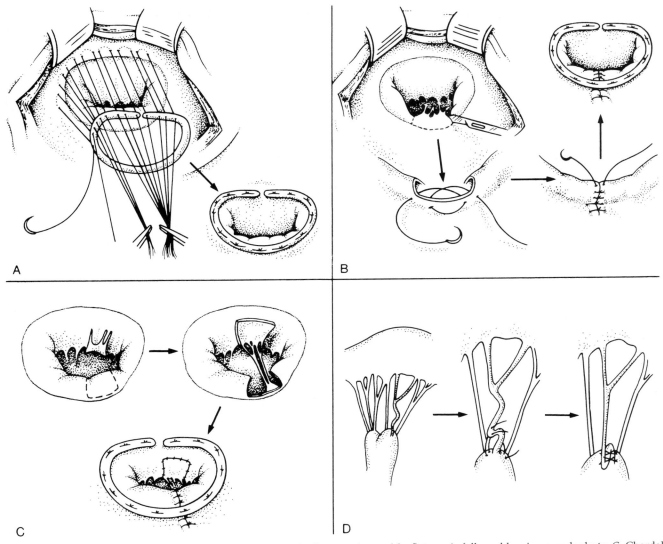

**FIGURE 50–6.** *A*, Insertion of annuloplasty ring. *B*, Posterior leaflet resection and leaflet repair followed by ring annuloplasty. *C*, Chordal transposition. *D*, Chordal shortening plasty. (*A–D*, From Galloway, A. C., Colvin, S. B., Baumann, F. G., et al.: Current concepts of mitral valve reconstruction for mitral insufficiency. Circulation, *78*:1087, 1988. By permission of the American Heart Association, Inc.)

an "atrial jet lesion," may be present from a regurgitant jet from the mitral valve, providing a guide to the location of the most serious insufficiency.

1. The degree of enlargement of the annulus of the posterior leaflet and commissures is noted. As stated earlier, the annulus of the anterior leaflet does not enlarge, a key concept in reconstruction.

2. The commissures are then examined, with attention to whether these are prolapsed, fused, or malformed. The closing plane of the leaflets in the area supported by commissural chordae is determined.

3. The anterior and posterior leaflets are then serially examined in detail; any gross leaflet abnormalities such as perforation, fibrosis, calcification, or clefts are noted.

4. Determining the degree of prolapse of the valve leaflets is one of the most subjective decisions.

The "billowing" mitral valve originally described

by Barlow has excess leaflet tissue but may remain competent if the chordae are not elongated. In such cases, the rough free edge of the leaflet closes at the proper level, even though the midportion of the leaflet may contain excessive tissue.

As emphasized by Carpentier, the anterolateral commissural leaflet is seldom prolapsed; so elevating the commissural leaflet with a nerve hook provides a valuable "reference point" from which the degree of elongation of other chordae can be determined. A particularly important point is that in the arrested heart, the free edge of the valve leaflets may appear to close slightly above the level of the annulus, whereas in the normal contracting heart, the distended left ventricle with the papillary muscles pulls the leaflets down into the proper plane. The most useful guide for deciding the degree of prolapse in individual segments is to compare how many millimeters the valve leaflets rise above the horizontal plane of the annulus with the chordae at the "reference point" described earlier. Normal chordae are seldom over 16 to 19 mm in length. With severe prolapse, however, chordae may be further elongated as much as 0.5 to 1.5 cm. Similarly, total lack of structural integrity from chordal rupture can cause a flail leaflet.

In patients with restrictive disease, the chordae may be contracted and foreshortened, which produces decreased motion of the leaflet, preventing the leaflet from reaching the proper plane of coaptation during systole.

5. Following evaluation of the leaflets and the chordae, the papillary muscles are examined for any anatomic abnormalities. Various unnamed congenital abnormalities are periodically encountered with fusion of the papillary muscles and adjacent chordae. These apparently cause only minimal insufficiency early in life unless the malformation is exceedingly severe. Over time, fibrosis with either elongation or shortening of the chordae may occur, probably from chronic turbulent blood flow, and insufficiency gradually may become more severe. Nevertheless, these grotesque severe abnormalities can usually be effectively repaired.

## Repair Techniques

### Quadrangular Resection of the Posterior Leaflet

Quadrangular resection of the posterior leaflet is one of the key features of mitral valve reconstruction. Diseased leaflet tissue in the posterior leaflet usually is excised with a wide quadrangular excision; 2 to 4 cm of tissue, or over 50% of the leaflet, can be excised if necessary. This technique is shown in Figure 50–6B. Strong chordae are identified on each side of the tissue to be excised and encircled with stay sutures. A rectangular excision is then performed, cutting directly down to the mitral annulus but not excising any of it. It is extremely important that the incision across the valve leaflet be perpendicular to the annulus, not slanting inward. A serious technical error can occur if the excision is angled so that the amount of valve tissue excised is less at the annulus than at the central orifice: Subsequent annuloplasty may not adequately remove the tension on the leaflet margins.

Once the quadrangular excision is done, the annulus of the excised segment of leaflet is plicated with several interrupted 2-0 Tevdek sutures placed about 5 mm apart. These are started centrally and extended to include a few millimeters of annulus adjacent to the remaining leaflets. When these annular sutures are tied, the leaflet margins are automatically brought into apposition without any tension. This is an important point: If tension existed on the leaflet tissues, dehiscence of the subsequent leaflet repair would be a serious hazard.

Once the annular sutures have been tied, the leaflet margins are approximated with simple or figure-of-

eight sutures, usually either 4-0 or 5-0 polypropylene, depending on the thickness of the leaflets.

Because the mural leaflet is often scalloped, usually into three sections, the height of the mural leaflet may vary in different areas. In planning the quadrangular excision, this variation should be considered; otherwise there may be a major difference in the length of the two incised leaflet margins. As the figure-of-eight sutures are placed in the leaflets, wider bites may be taken on the longer side, gaining less than 50% to prevent distortion of the leaflet. The leaflet margins are sutured from the annulus outward to the margin of the intact leaflet, to the point at which the previously identified adjacent support chordae are encircled with stay sutures.

Often the valve appears quite competent at this time. Injecting saline into the ventricle with a bulb syringe and noting both the mobility of the leaflets and their apposition has proved the best visual guide for competency. If localized insufficiency remains in other areas, additional procedures can be done, such as leaflet plication, triangular excision of redundant anterior leaflet, chordal shortening, or chordal reimplantation.

### Anterior Leaflet Reconstruction

Different approaches must be used for the anterior leaflet, and the techniques must be exacting, because a well-functioning anterior leaflet is necessary for valve repair to be successful. Nevertheless, the results of repair requiring anterior leaflet reconstruction have been excellent. In the overall NYU experience, more than 150 patients who underwent valve reconstruction have required significant anterior leaflet repair procedures, with no adverse affect on late valve durability.

Quadrangular excision similar to that done in the posterior leaflet cannot be done on the anterior leaflet because the annulus of the anterior leaflet cannot be plicated. The aortic valve annulus is also continuous with the anterior mitral annulus. Elongated anterior leaflet chordae may be shortened for diffuse prolapse, as described by Carpentier. The degree of chordal elongation is visually estimated, after which the chorda is shortened by imbricating a segment of chorda onto the underlying papillary muscle (see Fig. 50–6D). Ruptured chordae may be sutured to an adjacent intact chorda, if available.

A particularly valuable technique for repair of ruptured chordae, developed by Carpentier, is chordae transposition. A segment of posterior leaflet directly opposite the ruptured chordae in the anterior leaflet is outlined, after which a small quadrangular excision of the posterior leaflet with the attached chordae is performed. The mobilized segment of posterior leaflet and chordae is then transposed onto the anterior leaflet to provide structural support (see Fig. 50–6C). This is somewhat similar to tendon transfer in hand surgery. The quadrangular defect in the posterior leaflet is then repaired by the previously described techniques.

A triangular excision of 8- to 15-mm segments of enlarged aortic leaflets was developed by Carpentier but abandoned over a decade ago because of recurrent insufficiency. In recent years, Colvin at NYU has re-evaluated triangular excision in selected patients with large, redundant anterior leaflets—the "billowing valve" originally described by Barlow. Experiences thus far with over 40 patients have been excellent. Triangular resection has now been used as the primary treatment of mitral insufficiency due to redundant, prolapsing anterior leaflet. The technique seems particularly helpful for prevention of systolic anterior motion (SAM) of the mitral valve and left ventricular outflow obstruction.

### Carpentier Ring Selection and Insertion

The size of the mitral orifice is measured with Carpentier calibrated obturators to determine the size of the annuloplasty ring to be inserted. The goal is to correct the abnormal dilatation of the annulus of the mural leaflet. The annuloplasty rings were developed by measuring the distance between the commissures. The cross-sectional area of the ring should be approximately that of the anterior leaflet.

Once the proper size has been selected, the ring is inserted with a series of 2-0 Tevdek sutures carefully placed tangentially in the mitral valve annulus; between 10 and 14 sutures are usually needed. Particular care is required in inserting these sutures to be certain that the sutures are in the mitral annulus, not peripherally situated in the leaflet tissue. The annulus can be identified by traction on the attached leaflet; tactile resistance as the suture is inserted is another valuable guide. Care must be taken to avoid placing sutures lateral to the annulus, because the aortic valve cusps are only 2 to 3 mm beyond the annulus anteriorly, and the circumflex coronary artery is a similar distance laterally and posteriorly.

After the annuloplasty ring has been tied in position, saline is again injected with a bulb syringe to distend the leaflets and reflect their mobility. An ideal repair can be recognized by apposition of the leaflets about 0.5 cm above the level of the ring in a line parallel to the annuloplasty ring (Fig. 50–7).

If focal insufficiency remains, several ancillary procedures can be considered, beyond the scope of this presentation. These include plication or triangular excision of small prolapsing segments of leaflet. Elongated chordae may be selectively shortened.

Partial dehiscence of the annuloplasty ring from the annulus has occurred a few times. Hence, additional "buttressing" sutures are inserted, either in the valve annulus or in the nearby atrial wall. The most common technique at NYU is to place four pledgeted mattress sutures in four quadrants around the annuloplasty ring. Since the buttressing sutures have been used, dehiscence of the annuloplasty ring has not been observed.

When the atriotomy incision is closed, an opening is left for later insertion of an index finger to palpate the reconstructed valve in the beating heart. After air has been removed and the heart has been defibrillated, the cardiopulmonary bypass machine is slowed or stopped, permitting the left atrium to fill and the left ventricle to eject with a systolic pressure of 100 to 110 mm Hg. The mitral valve can then be palpated and any residual insufficiency noted. This important technique has been highly effective.

Transesophageal echocardiography is used routinely in the operating room, to assess the valve for residual insufficiency and to detect any left ventricular outflow obstruction. If echocardiography shows any outflow tract obstruction, the gradient between the left ventricle and aorta can be measured by needle puncture.

**Systolic Anterior Motion of the Mitral Valve.** Some degree of left ventricular outflow obstruction develops in 5 to 8% of patients following Carpentier annuloplasty with the rigid ring. According to several reports, it seldom, if ever, occurs when a flexible ring is used.

SAM of the anterior mitral leaflet has long been recognized as a major cause of obstruction in *idiopathic hypertrophic subaortic stenosis* (IHSS) cardiomyopathy. The first reports describing SAM following

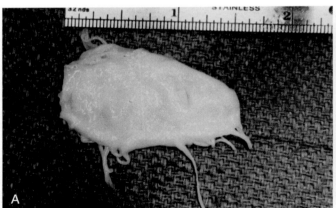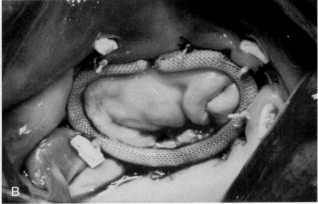

**FIGURE 50–7.** *A*, Flail segment of posterior leaflet mitral valve. *B*, Completed mitral valve reconstruction with Carpentier annuloplasty ring.

complex mitral valve reconstruction appeared in 1983 by Gallerstein and associates and in 1984 by Kronzon and co-workers. In 1992, Grossi and colleagues reported NYU experiences with 28 cases following mitral valve reconstruction in 438 patients, an incidence of 6.4%. Ten of the 28 patients had a resting left ventricular outflow tract gradient, exceeding 50 mm Hg in four patients.

There is no agreement about the cause of the condition except that it is associated with "excess" leaflet tissue, the basic characteristic of the billowing mitral valve. Whether it is due primarily to excessive tissue in the anterior leaflet, to overelevation of the posterior annulus after posterior leaflet resection, to changing the "angle of closure," or to all three is yet uncertain. Carpentier has stated that SAM more commonly occurs after extensive (more than 3 cm) resection of the annulus of the posterior leaflet.

At NYU, the basic treatment for postoperative SAM after mitral valve reconstruction has been medical—primarily avoidance of inotropic drugs such as dobutamine or epinephrine and selective use of beta-adrenergic blockers or calcium channel blockers. Intraoperative and early postoperative treatment has also included maintaining an adequate preload with fluids and using alpha-adrenergic agents, such as metaraminol or neosynephrine, to increase cardiac afterload. This approach is analogous to the medical treatment of IHSS. Valve repair operation has not been abandoned, and mitral valve replacement is performed when postoperative SAM with outflow tract obstruction is found. This option should be considered if severe hemodynamic problems are refractory to the medical treatment outlined earlier.

A particularly significant finding in the report by Grossi and associates (1992) was that the outflow tract gradient, measured by echocardiography, completely resolved after medical treatment in all patients (at a mean postoperative interval of 32 months). Thus, SAM after mitral reconstruction is self-limiting to a certain extent.

Newer techniques that attempt to avoid SAM include linear resection of the base of the posterior leaflet (Carpentier) and triangular excision of redundant anterior leaflet tissue (Colvin). The long-term efficacy of these methods remains to be determined.

## Supplemental Considerations

### Valve Repair and Acute Endocarditis

An impressive report in 1990 by Dreyfus and co-workers from Carpentier's group described experiences with repair of the mitral valve with insufficiency from acute endocarditis, including patients undergoing surgery within 6 weeks of the onset of symptoms, before the normal full course of antibiotic therapy was completed. The time between onset of endocarditis and operation ranged from 12 to 45 days, with a mean of 30 days. The lesions found included cusp perforation in 17, chordae rupture in 22, vegeta-

tions in 13, and an annular abscess in 4. The standard techniques of the Carpentier reconstruction were employed, with some additional specific techniques. Autologous pericardial patching was used for anterior leaflet perforation in 7 patients. Chordae transposition for ruptured chordae was used in 8 patients. A prosthetic ring was considered unnecessary for 16 patients who were free of annular dilatation.

The results were quite remarkable: There were no recurrences of infection. There was one operative death, one early reoperation for recurrent insufficiency, and one late death 2 years later from unknown causes.

In 1992, Hendren and associates reported experiences at the Cleveland Clinic with 22 patients who were less acutely ill—only six underwent surgery while blood culture results were still positive. Active infection was cured by antibiotic therapy in 16 patients. Reconstruction was possible in all members of the group. There were two operative deaths. No insufficiency or recurrences occurred in a follow-up averaging 24 months.

### Artificial Chordae Tendineae (Polytetrafluoroethylene)

Experimental studies by Frater and colleagues (1990) and by Revuelta and associates (1989) found that polytetrafluoroethylene (PTFE, known as Gore-Tex) artificial chordae functioned well for over a year, becoming covered with a fibrous sheath. Sizes near 4-0 or 5-0 seemed best: Larger sizes developed a thick sheath of fibrous tissue. Subsequently in 1990, Zussa and Frater reported experiences with nine patients, most of whom were doing well 18 months later. One required repeat operation because a normal chorda ruptured.

A larger clinical experience was reported by David and co-workers in 1991. Forty-three patients underwent surgery between 1985 and 1990. Sizes 4-0 and 5-0 sutures were used. Two failures occurred, but late rupture of the Gore-Tex chordae was not observed. The major question, of course, is whether the Gore-Tex chordae continue to function satisfactorily for 5 to 10 years or longer, and, if so, how this compares with the chordal reimplantation and chordal transposition techniques described by Carpentier.

### Annuloplasty with Rigid or with Flexible Ring?

All of the experiences at NYU have been with the standard Carpentier rigid prosthetic ring. In 1978, Duran and colleagues reported a flexible annuloplasty ring, designed to more closely resemble the normal mitral annulus, which contracts about 25% in systole. Although NYU has had no experience with the flexible ring, the ability to securely remodel and reconstruct the mitral annulus, as envisioned by Carpentier with his rigid ring, would theoretically seem more difficult. By introducing movement into the repair, the flexible ring could theoretically negatively effect late durability.

Two significant studies have compared the rigid and the flexible ring in more detail. In 1989, David (see also David et al., 1989) evaluated this issue in 25 patients, randomized into two groups, one with a rigid annuloplasty, one with a flexible annuloplasty. Studies conducted 2 to 3 months after operation found that there was a greater decrease in end-systolic volume with the flexible ring. Other measurements were similar in both groups. A year following surgery, however, 11 patients were restudied, and no differences could be demonstrated between those with a flexible or with a rigid ring.

In 1993, Castro and associates reported sophisticated experimental studies in 18 dogs, using multiple tantalum markers to measure left ventricular volume and geometry following a rigid or a flexible ring annuloplasty. Global and regional systolic function were assessed with load-insensitive indices. Studies at both 1 and 6 weeks found that neither type of ring worsened ventricular function, and there were no differences between the two.

Thus, current data suggest that ventricular function is equally well preserved with the rigid and the flexible ring. Several authors have reported that SAM of the anterior leaflet is infrequently seen with a flexible ring, whereas this problem is recognized, to some extent, in 5 to 7% of patients following Carpentier ring annuloplasty. The most durable long-term results have been reported with the use of the rigid ring, however.

## Postoperative and Long-Term Care

Convalescence following operation is usually uneventful. Anticoagulation with warfarin is started approximately 48 hours postoperatively and continued for 2 to 3 months, keeping the prothrombin time 1½ to 2 times normal, usually 18 to 20 seconds. In patients in sinus rhythm, warfarin is stopped after that time, and antiplatelet therapy with aspirin is subsequently given indefinitely. In patients with continued atrial fibrillation or with extremely large left atria (>5.5 to 6 cm), anticoagulant therapy with warfarin is continued, keeping the prothrombin time at 16 to 18 seconds.

Echocardiography usually is obtained before discharge from the hospital. Subsequently, patients are followed at 6-month intervals, with routine annual echocardiography. Standard prophylactic antibiotics are recommended for any invasive procedures, as with valvular prostheses, but late endocarditis is rare. Normal physical activity and sports are allowed if ventricular function is good, although heavy isometric exercises are discouraged.

## Results

Cumulative experiences at NYU have been reported periodically since the first reconstruction in 1979 (Galloway et al., 1988b; Spencer et al., 1985). An analysis of 560 patients treated at NYU between 1979 and 1993 has been completed and is summarized here.

The primary etiology of the mitral insufficiency was degenerative in 46%, rheumatic in 21%, ischemic in 18%, and other in 15% of patients. Concomitant procedures were performed in 51% of patients. The hospital mortality rate was 2.5% for isolated valve reconstruction and 5.9% overall.

Clinical and echocardiographic follow-ups have been 98% complete, with a mean follow-up interval of 3.5 years, ranging from 1 to 14 years. Over 80 patients have been followed for 10 years or longer. The actuarial rates of freedom from complications at 5 and 10 years, respectively, were as follows: thromboembolic = 93 and 86%; anticoagulant-related complications = 97 and 97%; endocarditis = 97 and 95%; and reoperation = 90 and 83% (Table 50–2). The postoperative rate of freedom from reoperation has been significantly better in nonrheumatic patients (93% at 5 years, 90% at 10 years) than in rheumatic patients (82% at 5 years, 67% at 10 years; $p < .0001$) (Fig. 50–8), similar to that in reports by others.

Multivariate analysis of NYU data has identified NYHA functional classification, age, associated coronary disease, concomitant cardiac procedures, and preoperative pulmonary pressure as the risk factors that affect survival after mitral valve reconstruction (Table 50–3), similar to those of patients undergoing mitral valve replacement. In the NYU series, survival from late cardiac death after mitral valve reconstruction was exceedingly good, over 80% at 10 years (Fig. 50–9). These excellent late survival results after mitral reconstruction may be due to the minimal numbers of lethal complications associated with valve repair, such as thromboemboli, and to the improved cardiac function achieved by preserving the subvalvular apparatus.

Comparable long-term results after mitral reconstruction were reported by DeLoche and associates

■ **Table 50–2.** CARPENTIER–TYPE MITRAL VALVE RECONSTRUCTION IN 560 PATIENTS: FREEDOM FROM COMPLICATIONS

| Complication Type | 5 Years | 10 Years |
|---|---|---|
| Thromboembolic | 93% | 86% |
| Anticoagulant | 97% | 97% |
| Endocarditis | 97% | 95% |
| Reoperation | 90% | 83% |

■ **Table 50–3.** RISK FACTORS AFFECTING OVERALL SURVIVAL IN 560 PATIENTS WITH CARPENTIER–TYPE MITRAL VALVE REPAIR

| | |
|---|---|
| Early | NYHA class |
| | Age |
| | Associated coronary disease |
| Late | Concomitant procedure |
| | Associated coronary disease |
| | Pulmonary artery pressure |

# MITRAL VALVE REPAIR IN 560 PATIENTS
## FREEDOM FROM REOPERATION BY ETIOLOGY

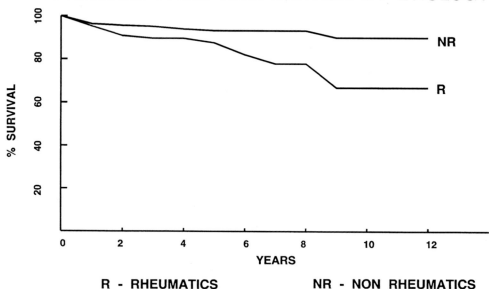

**R - RHEUMATICS**          **NR - NON RHEUMATICS**

**FIGURE 50–8.** Freedom from reoperation after mitral valve reconstruction in 560 patients undergoing mitral valve reconstruction for mitral insufficiency at New York University (NYU) Medical Center.

and by Carpentier in 1990. Among 206 patients undergoing operative repair between 1972 and 1979, 195 survived. Fifteen-year actuarial overall survival and valve-related survival rates were 72 and 83%, respectively. At 15 years, 94% of patients were free from thromboembolism, and 97% were free from endocarditis. Ninety-three per cent of patients with mitral insufficiency from degenerative disease were free from reoperation, as compared with 76% of those with rheumatic disease.

Subsequently, in a short report in 1991, El Asmar and colleagues discussed the cause of 72 failures of reconstruction following 1705 mitral valve repairs performed between 1969 and 1985. The reoperation rate was less than 1% per patient-year for degenerative disease but over 4% for rheumatic disease. Errors in surgical technique were the principal cause of failures in reconstruction for degenerative disease, but progressive disease was the major cause in patients with rheumatic disease.

A review article in 1989 by Cosgrove and Stewart described the Cleveland Clinic's experiences with mitral repair and replacement. Among 1141 mitral valve operations performed over a period of 4 years, 57% were for isolated mitral insufficiency. About 70% of patients with pure insufficiency underwent repair.

# MITRAL VALVE REPAIR IN 560 PATIENTS
## FREEDOM FROM LATE CARDIAC DEATH - ALL PATIENTS

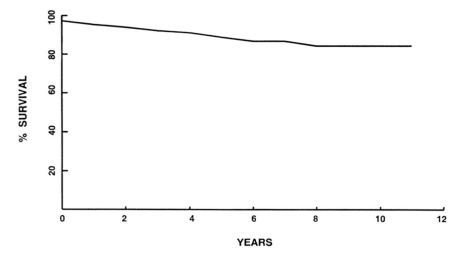

**FIGURE 50–9.** Freedom from late cardiac and valve-related death in 560 patients undergoing mitral valve reconstruction at NYU Medical Center.

In 1991, Duran and associates (1991b) described experiences over the preceding 2 years in Saudi Arabia with 304 patients who had rheumatic mitral insufficiency. Repair was possible in about two-thirds of the group, but within the next 2 years, about 27% of patients under age 20 required reoperation; by contrast, only about 5% of older patients required reoperation during this time. Severe hemolysis required reoperation in 10 young patients; in 8 others, active rheumatic carditis was the principal cause.

In a review article in 1992, Antunes reviewed his 15 years of experience with mitral reconstruction, including over 500 cases. He emphasized the limitations of annuloplasty alone; in a prospective study of 240 patients, 95% had annular dilatation, but 90% of these had additional significant abnormalities such as elongated chordae or diseased leaflets. He concluded that repair was possible in almost all patients with myxomatous disease, probably in about 90% of patients with pure rheumatic regurgitation.

In 1991, Yun and Miller extensively reviewed published data comparing mitral valve repair with replacement, analyzing reports from over 10 large series. Virtually every report found better long-term results with valve repair. Two groups reported experiences in their second decade, including the report by DeLoche and Carpentier discussed earlier and a report by Lassana, who described a 13-year experience with 275 patients.

Current data suggest that valve reconstruction should be seriously considered in patients with mitral insufficiency from degenerative disease. Valve reconstruction in nonrheumatic patients appears to be as durable as mechanical prostheses. Patients undergoing valve reconstruction have a lower risk of thromboembolism, anticoagulant-related complications, and endocarditis, which are known hazards with prosthetic valves, and ventricular function is better preserved than with conventional mitral valve replacement. The best long-term results are obtained when patients undergo surgery early in the physiologic disease process.

## SELECTED BIBLIOGRAPHY

Arom, K. V., Nicoloff, D. M., Kersten, T. E., et al.: St. Jude medical prosthesis: Valve-related deaths and complications. Ann. Thorac. Surg., 43:591, 1987.

The authors describe experiences with 816 patients who were treated for 8 years. Of these patients, 300 underwent mitral valve replacement. There was no malfunction of the valve, but thrombosis occurred in four patients (0.6%). Thromboembolism frequency was 1.8% per patient-year, and anticoagulant hemorrhage frequency was 3.2% per patient-year.

Boyd, A. D., Engelman, R. H., Isom, O. W., et al.: Tricuspid annuloplasty. J. Thorac. Cardiovasc. Surg., 68:344, 1974.

Many types of tricuspid valve reconstruction have been described in recent years. The technique of posterolateral tricuspid annuloplasty using pledget-reinforced mattress sutures, described initially in this report 20 years ago, is simple and reliable. The technique has been used at NYU for more than two decades with satisfactory results except when advanced organic disease of the tricuspid valve requires valvular replacement.

Carpentier, A.: Cardiac valve surgery—The "French Correction." J. Thorac. Cardiovasc. Surg., 86:323, 1983.

This classic paper reviews the Carpentier approach for mitral valve reconstruction, stressing a functional assessment of mitral valvular lesions, regardless of etiology. Carpentier defines three major types of valvular dysfunction. Type I is normal leaflet motion, which can be secondary to endocarditis causing a leaflet perforation, or any disease that causes isolated annular dilatation. Type II is leaflet prolapse secondary to chordal rupture, chordal elongation, papillary muscle rupture, or papillary muscle elongation. Type III includes restricted leaflet motion, secondary to fusion, thickening and foreshortening of the valve, and subvalvular apparatus. The paper describes specific techniques of valvular repair for each pathologic finding and reports follow-up on Carpentier's initial 1421 patients. The reoperation rate was amazingly low: 0.6% per year in nonrheumatic patients and 1.6% per year in rheumatic patients. Thromboembolic rate was 0.6% per year, without the need for long-term anticoagulation. These data, presented in 1983 to the American Association of Thoracic Surgery, launched a resurgence of interest in mitral valve reconstruction in the United States.

Cobbs, B. W., Jr., Hatcher, C. R., Jr., Craver, J. M., et al.: Transverse midventricular disruption after mitral valve replacement. Am. Heart J., 99:33, 1980.

An infrequent but lethal complication of mitral valve replacement is rupture of the posterior wall of the left ventricle. This can occur from at least three areas, as described in detail in this chapter. The most bizarre is a transverse rupture of the muscle of the posterior ventricular wall, between the mitral annulus above and the insertion of the papillary muscles below. This paper is the most extensive report in the English literature of this unusual complication, which is perhaps a result of removal of the posterior papillary muscle in elderly people with small left ventricles.

Deloche, A., Jebara, V. A., Relland, J. Y. M., et al.: Valve repair with Carpentier techniques: The second decade. J. Thorac. Cardiovasc. Surg., 99:990, 1990.

The authors reviewed 206 consecutive patients who underwent mitral valve repair with a prosthetic ring between 1972 and 1979, providing 15-year survival and actuarial data for Carpentier-type valve reconstructions. Mitral insufficiency was secondary to degenerative disease in 58%, to rheumatic disease in 38%, and to ischemic and other causes in 4%. The 15-year actuarial and valve-related survival rates were 72.4 and 82.8%, respectively. Of these patients, 93.9% were free from thromboembolism, 96.6% were free from endocarditis, 95.6% were free from anticoagulant-related hemorrhage, and 87.4% were free from reoperation. The actuarial rate of freedom from reoperation was higher in the degenerative disease group (92.7%) than in the rheumatic group (76.1%). Echocardiography showed normal ventricular contractility in 84.5%, no mitral regurgitation in 74%, mild insufficiency in 17%, and severe insufficiency in 2.5%.

Edmunds, L. H., Jr.: Thrombotic and bleeding complications of prosthetic heart valves: Collective review. Ann. Thorac. Surg., 44:430, 1987.

This extensive review analyzes the reported frequency of thrombotic and bleeding complications with prosthetic valves in more than 20 different institutions. The average linearized rate of thrombotic and bleeding complications for bioprosthesis and mechanical prosthesis in the mitral position was approximately equal (4% per year), but the linearized rates of fatal complications were 2 to 4 times higher for mechanical valves. The report clearly documents the significant incidence of thromboembolic and bleeding complications that are associated with the currently available prosthetic valves.

Fiore, A. C., Naunheim, K. S., D'Orazio, S., et al.: Mitral valve replacement: Randomized trial of St. Jude and Medtronic-Hall prostheses. Ann. Thorac. Surg., 54:68, 1992.

One-hundred two patients were randomized to receive the St. Jude or the Medtronic-Hall mitral valve prosthesis. The linearized rates of valve-related events and the hemodynamic performance of the valves were not different between the two groups. The report suggests that the two prostheses are equally reliable.

Galloway, A. C., Colvin, S. B., Baumann, F. G., et al.: Current concepts of mitral valve reconstruction for mitral insufficiency. Circulation, 78:1087, 1988.

The authors review the literature concerning mitral valve reconstruction and analyze the initial NYU experience. This article reviews various mitral valve repair techniques and gives comparative results from 13 centers from 1980 to 1988. In the NYU experience, significant factors for increased operative risk were ischemic etiology, previous myocardial infarction, age over 70, preoperative NYHA Class IV status, and emergency operation. NYU follow-up results demonstrated a 90% freedom from reoperation rate and a 95% freedom from thromboembolic complications rate at 5 years.

Galloway, A. C., Colvin, S. B., Baumann, F. G., et al.: A comparison of mitral valve reconstruction with mitral valve replacement: Intermediate-term results. Ann. Thorac. Surg., 47:655, 1989.

This retrospective study from NYU compares operative and late results for 975 porcine mitral valve replacements, 169 mechanical mitral valve replacements, and 280 Carpentier type mitral repairs from 1977 to 1987. Actuarial 5-year survival rates from all cardiac and valve-related deaths were 81% for repair, 73.9% for mechanical valves, and 73.1% for porcine valves. The 5-year freedom from reoperation rates were 94.4% for non-rheumatic patients undergoing mitral repair, 77.4% for rheumatic patients, and 96.4% and 96.6% for mechanical and porcine mitral valve replacement, respectively. The paper demonstrates that the 5-year freedom from valve-related morbidity and mortality was significantly better after valve reconstruction than with either form of valve replacement.

Hammermeister, K. E., Sethi, G. K., Henderson, W. G., et al.: A comparison of outcomes in men 11 years after heart-valve replacement with a mechanical valve or bioprosthesis. N. Engl. J. Med., 328:1289, 1993.

Five-hundred seventy-five patients undergoing aortic or mitral valve replacement were randomized to receive either a mechanical or a bioprosthetic valve. During an average follow-up of 11 years, there was no difference in the probability of death or in the probability of valve-related complications. Structural failure was observed only with bioprosthetic valves, whereas bleeding complications were more frequent among patients with mechanical valves. This paper further clarifies that structural failure with reoperation is the primary late risk with bioprostheses, whereas thromboemboli remain the primary risk with mechanical prostheses.

Jamieson, W. R. E., Rosado, L. J., Munro, A. I., et al.: Carpentier-Edwards standard porcine bioprosthesis: Primary tissue failure (structural valve deterioration) by age groups. Ann. Thorac. Surg., 46:155, 1988.

Experiences with 1401 porcine prostheses for 11 years were analyzed, with a mean follow-up of 5.6 years. One-hundred four prostheses failed. The rate of freedom from primary tissue failure at 10 years was almost 80%. The rate of freedom from deterioration increased by decades: 10 years after operation, only 27% of patients under 30 years of age were free of valve failure; of those 30 to 59, 77%; and of those over 60, 83%.

Rankin, J. S., Feneley, M. P., Hickey, M. S. J., et al.: A clinical comparison of mitral valve repair versus valve replacement in ischemic mitral regurgitation. J. Thorac. Cardiovasc. Surg., 95:165, 1988.

A six-year retrospective study from Duke University Medical Center reviewed 611 patients who underwent mitral valve procedures. Fifty-five of these patients were found to have ischemic mitral regurgitation, 37 of whom required emergent procedures. Thirty-one of the 55 had isolated posterior papillary muscle dysfunction, 9 had papillary muscle rupture, and 15 had severe ventricular dysfunction and annular dilatation. Thirty-two patients were treated with primary mitral valve replacement, the remaining 23 with mitral valve repair. Repair and replacement groups were similar in baseline characteristics, but operative survival was improved after repair (p = .03 for the overall group; p = .05 for acute papillary muscle dysfunction).

Sarris, G. E., Fann, J. I., Niczyporuk, M. A., et al.: Global and regional left ventricular systolic performance in the in situ ejecting canine heart: Importance of the mitral apparatus. Circulation, 80(Suppl. 1):24, 1989.

This study addresses the importance of an intact mitral apparatus in left ventricular systolic performance. An open-chested ejecting canine heart preparation was used. Mitral valve replacement was performed preserving the anterior and posterior papillary muscle apparatus. End-systolic/pressure volume and stroke work/end-diastolic volume were used to measure global left ventricular systolic function. The chordae were then divided, and immediate reassessment revealed deterioration of global left ventricular function. End-systolic/pressure volume declined by 72%, and stroke work declined by 34%.

Spencer, F. C., Galloway, A. C., and Colvin, S. B.: A clinical evaluation of the hypothesis that rupture of the left ventricle following mitral valve replacement can be prevented by preservation of the chordae of the mural leaflet. Ann. Surg., 202:673, 1985.

Results from a study at NYU concerning rupture of the left ventricle are described. Fourteen patients experienced rupture of the left ventricle after mitral valve replacement over 9 years, ending in 1981. A prospective study, begun at that time, concentrated on preservation of some chordae to the annulus of the mural leaflet at operation. No additional patients were seen with rupture of the ventricle after this technique was adopted.

Yun, K. L., and Miller, D. C.: Mitral valve repair versus replacement. Cardiol. Clin., 9:315, 1991.

This paper reviews over 10 large clinical series comparing mitral valve repair with mitral valve replacement and reviews experimental and clinical data concerning left ventricular systolic function after valve repair

or replacement. The authors conclude that fewer thromboembolic and endocarditis-related complications and improved left ventricular function are factors that favor valve repair, but they note that there is yet no definitive objective evidence of the superiority of repair over replacement. The results after valve repair appear to greatly depend on the surgeon's experience, whereas uniform results are predictable after valve replacement. Ventricular function is best maintained after valve replacement when the chordae are preserved.

# BIBLIOGRAPHY

Antunes, M. J.: Mitral valve repair into the 1990s. Eur. J. Cardiothorac. Surg., 6:S13, 1992.

Bailey, C. P.: The surgical treatment of mitral stenosis (mitral commissurotomy). Dis. Chest, 15:377, 1949.

Björk, V. O., and Henze, A.: Ten years' experience with the Björk-Shiley tilting disk valve. J. Thorac. Cardiovasc. Surg., 78:331, 1979.

Boyd, A. D., Engelman, R. H., Isom, O. W., et al.: Tricuspid annuloplasty. J. Thorac. Cardiovasc. Surg., 68:344, 1974.

Camara, J. L., Aris, A., Padro, J. M., et al.: Long-term results of mitral valve surgery in patients with severe pulmonary hypertension. Ann. Thorac. Surg., 45:133, 1988.

Carabello, B. A.: Timing of surgery in mitral and aortic stenosis. Cardiol. Clin., 9:229, 1991.

Carpentier, A.: Plastic and reconstructive mitral valve surgery. In Jackson, J. W. (ed): Operative Surgery. Boston, Butterworths, 1977, p. 527.

Carpentier, A.: Cardiac valve surgery—The "French Correction." J. Thorac. Cardiovasc. Surg., 86:323, 1983.

Carpentier, A., Chauvaud, S., Fabiani, J. N., et al.: Reconstructive surgery of mitral valve incompetence: Ten-year appraisal. J. Thorac. Cardiovasc. Surg., 79:338, 1980.

Carpentier, A., Deloche, A., Dauptain, J., et al.: A new reconstructive operation for correction of mitral and tricuspid insufficiency. J. Thorac. Cardiovasc. Surg., 61:1, 1971.

Carpentier, A., Guerinon, J., Deloche, A., et al.: Pathology of the mitral valve. In Jackson, J.W. (ed): Operative Surgery. Boston, Butterworths, 1977, p. 65.

Castro, L. J., Moon, M. R., Rayhill, S. C., et al.: Annuloplasty with flexible or rigid ring does not alter left ventricular systolic performance, energetics, or ventricular-arterial coupling in conscious, closed-chest dogs. J. Thorac. Cardiovasc. Surg., 105:643, 1993.

Cobanoglu, A., Grunkemeier, G. L., Aru, G. M., et al.: Mitral replacement: Clinical experience with a ball-valve prosthesis. Ann. Surg., 202:376, 1985.

Cobbs, B. W., Jr., Hatcher, C. R., Jr., Craver, J. M., et al.: Transverse midventricular disruption after mitral valve replacement. Am. Heart J., 99:33, 1980.

Cosgrove, D. M., Chavez, A. M., Lytle, B. W., et al.: Results of mitral valve reconstruction. Circulation, 74(Suppl. 1):82, 1986.

Cosgrove, D. M., and Stewart, W. J.: Mitral valvuloplasty. Curr. Prob. Cardiol., 14:355, 1989.

Cutler, E. C., and Levine, S. A.: Cardiotomy and valvulotomy for mitral stenosis. Boston Med. Surg. J., 188:1023, 1923.

Czer, L. S. C., Maurer, G., Trento, A., et al.: Comparative efficacy of ring and suture annuloplasty for ischemic mitral regurgitation. Circulation, 86(Suppl. 2):46, 1992.

David, T. E.: Effect of mitral annuloplasty ring in left ventricular function. Semin. Thorac. Cardiovasc. Surg., 1:144, 1989.

David, T. E., Bos, J., and Rakowski, H.: Mitral valve repair by replacement of chordae tendineae with polytetrafluoroethylene sutures. J. Thorac. Cardiovasc. Surg., 101:495, 1991.

David, T. E., and Ho, W. C.: The effect of preservation of chordae tendineae on mitral valve replacement for postinfarction mitral regurgitation. Circulation, 74(Suppl. 1):116, 1986.

David, T. E., Komeda, M., Pollick, C., and Burns, R. J.: Mitral valve annuloplasty: The effect of the type on left ventricular function. Ann. Thorac. Surg., 47:524, 1989.

Deloche, A., Jebara, V. A., Relland, J. Y. M., et al.: Valve repair with Carpentier techniques: The second decade. J. Thorac. Cardiovasc. Surg., 99:990, 1990.

Dreyfus, G., Serraf, A., Jebara, V. A., et al.: Valve repair in acute endocarditis. Ann. Thorac. Surg., 49:706, 1990.

Duran, C. M. G., Pomar, J. L., and Cucchiara, G.: A flexible ring for atrioventricular heart valve reconstruction. J. Cardiovasc. Surg., 19:417, 1978.

Duran, C. M. G., Gometza, B., Balasundaram, S., and Al Halees, Z.: A feasibility study of valve repair in rheumatic mitral regurgitation. Eur. Heart J., 12:34, 1991a.

Duran, C. M. G., Gometza, B., and De Vol, E. B.: Valve repair in rheumatic mitral disease. Circulation, 84(Suppl. 3):125, 1991b.

Edmunds, L. H., Jr.: Thrombotic and bleeding complications of prosthetic heart valves. Ann. Thorac. Surg., 44:430, 1987.

El Asmar, B., Perier, P., Couetil, J. P., and Carpentier, A.: Failures in reconstructive mitral valve surgery. J. Med. Libin., 39:7, 1991.

Fiore, A. C., Naunheim, K. S., D'Orazio, S., et al.: Mitral valve replacement: Randomized trial of St. Jude and Medtronic-Hall prostheses. Ann. Thorac. Surg., 54:68, 1992.

Frater, R. W. M., Vetter, H. O., Zussa, C., et al.: Chordal replacement in mitral valve repair. Circulation, 82(Suppl. 4):125, 1990.

Gallerstein, P. E., Berger, M., Rubenstein, S., et al.: Systolic anterior motion of the mitral valve and outflow obstruction after mitral valve reconstruction. Chest, 83:819, 1983.

Galloway, A. C., Colvin, S. B., Baumann, F. G., et al.: Current concepts of mitral valve reconstruction for mitral insufficiency. Circulation, 78:1087, 1988a.

Galloway, A. C., Colvin, S. B., Slater, J., et al.: Long-term results of mitral valve reconstruction with Carpentier techniques in 148 patients with mitral insufficiency. Circulation, 78(Suppl. 1):97, 1988b.

Galloway, A. C., Colvin, S. B., Baumann, F. G., et al.: A comparison of mitral valve reconstruction with mitral valve replacement: Intermediate-term results. Ann. Thorac. Surg., 47:655, 1989.

Gross, R. I., Cunningham, J. N., Jr., Snively, S. L., et al.: Long-term results of open radical mitral commissurotomy: Ten-year follow-up study of 202 patients. Am. J. Cardiol., 47:821, 1981.

Grossi, E. A., Galloway, A. C., Parish, M. A., et al.: Experience with twenty-eight cases of systolic anterior motion after mitral valve reconstruction by the Carpentier technique. J. Thorac. Cardiovasc. Surg., 103:466, 1992.

Hammermeister, K. E., Sethi, G. K., Henderson, W. G., et al.: A comparison of outcomes in men 11 years after heart-valve replacement with a mechanical valve or bioprosthesis. N. Engl. J. Med., 328:1289, 1993.

Harken, D. E., Ellis, L. B., Ware, P. F., and Norman, L. R.: The surgical treatment of mitral stenosis. N. Engl. J. Med., 239:801, 1948.

Hendren, W. G., Morris, A. S., Rosenkranz, E. R., et al.: Mitral valve repair for bacterial endocarditis. J. Thorac. Cardiovasc. Surg., 103:124, 1992.

Hendren, W. G., Nemec, J. J., Lytle, B. W., et al.: Mitral valve repair for ischemic mitral insufficiency. Ann. Thorac. Surg., 52:1246, 1991.

Hennein, H. A., Swain, J. A., McIntosh, C. L., et al.: Comparative assessment of chordal preservation versus chordal resection during mitral valve replacement. J. Thorac. Cardiovasc. Surg., 99:828, 1990.

Jamieson, W. R., Rosado, L. J., Munro, A. I., et al.: Carpentier-Edward's standard porcine bioprosthesis: Primary tissue failure (structural valve deterioration) by age groups. Ann. Thorac. Surg., 46:155, 1988.

John, S., Bashi, V. V., Ravikumar, E., et al.: Closed mitral valvotomy in the older subject: Results in 367 consecutive patients. J. Cardiovasc. Surg., 31:14, 1990.

Karlson, K. J., Ashraf, M. M., and Berger, R. L.: Rupture of left ventricle following mitral valve replacement. Ann. Thorac. Surg., 46:590, 1988.

Kay, G. L., Kay, J. H., Zubiate, P., et al.: Mitral valve repair for mitral regurgitation secondary to coronary artery disease. Circulation, 74(Suppl. 1):88, 1986.

Kay, J. H., and Egerton, W. S.: The repair of mitral insufficiency associated with ruptured chordae tendineae. Ann. Surg., 157:351, 1963.

Kay, J. H., Maselli-Campagna, C., and Tsuji, H. K.: Surgical treatment of tricuspid insufficiency. Ann. Surg., 53:162, 1965.

Kirklin, J. W., and Barratt-Boyes, B. G.: Cardiac Surgery, 1st ed. New York: John Wiley & Sons, 1986.

Kirklin, J. W., and Barratt-Boyes, B. G.: Cardiac Surgery, 2nd ed. New York, Churchill Livingstone, 1993.

Kronzon, I., Cohen, M. L., Winer, H. E., and Colvin, S. B.: Left ventricular outflow obstruction: A complication of mitral valvuloplasty. J. Am. Coll. Cardiol., 4:825, 1984.

Levine, H. J.: Is valve surgery indicated in patients with severe mitral regurgitation even if they are asymptomatic? Cardiovasc. Clin., 21:161, 1990.

Lillehei, C. W., Gott, V. L., DeWall, R. A., and Varco, R. L.: Surgical correction of pure mitral insufficiency by annuloplasty under direct vision. Lancet, 77:446, 1957.

Lillehei, C. W., Levy, M. J., and Bonnabeau, R. C.: Mitral valve replacement with preservation of papillary muscles and chordae tendineae. J. Thorac. Cardiovasc. Surg., 47:532, 1964.

Lindblom, D.: Long-term clinical results after mitral valve replacement with the Björk-Shiley prosthesis. J. Thorac. Cardiovasc. Surg., 95:321, 1988.

Magilligan, D. J.: The future of bioprosthetic valves. ASAIO Trans., 34:1031, 1988.

McGoon, D. C.: Repair of mitral insufficiency due to ruptured chordae tendineae. J. Thorac. Cardiovasc. Surg., 39:357, 1960.

Merendino, K. A., Bruce, R. A.: One hundred seventeen surgically treated cases of valvular rheumatic heart diseases: With preliminary report of two cases of mitral regurgitation treated under direct vision with aid of a pump-oxygenator. J. A. M. A., 64:749, 1957.

Nakano, S., Kawashima, Y., Nirose, H., et al.: Evaluation of long-term results of bicuspidalization annuloplasty for functional tricuspid regurgitation. J. Thorac. Cardiovasc. Surg., 95:340, 1988.

Oury, J. H., Cleveland, J. C., Duran, C. G., et al.: Ischemic mitral valve disease: Classification and systemic approach to management. J. Card. Surg., 9:262, 1994.

Rankin, J. S., Feneley, M. P., Hickey, M. S. J., et al.: A clinical comparison of mitral valve repair versus valve replacement in ischemic mitral regurgitation. J. Thorac. Cardiovasc. Surg., 95:165, 1988.

Rankin, J. S., Hickey, M. S. J., Smith, R., et al.: Ischemic mitral regurgitation. Circulation, 79(Suppl. 1):116, 1989.

Reed, G. E., Pooley, R. W., and Moggio, R. A.: Durability of measured mitral annuloplasty: Seventeen-year study. J. Thorac. Cardiovasc. Surg., 79:321, 1980.

Reed, G. E., Tice, D. A., and Clauss, R. H.: Asymmetric exaggerated mitral annuloplasty: Repair of mitral insufficiency with hemodynamic predictability. J. Thorac. Cardiovasc. Surg., 49:752, 1965.

Revuelta, J. M., Garcia-Rinaldi, R., Gaite, L., et al.: Generation of chordae tendineae with polytetrafluoroethylene stents. J. Thorac. Cardiovasc. Surg., 97:98, 1989.

Roberts, W. C.: Morphologic aspects of cardiac valve dysfunction. Am. Heart J., 123:1610, 1992.

Roberts, W. C., McIntosh, C. L., and Wallace, R. B.: Mechanisms of severe mitral regurgitation in mitral prolapse determined from analysis of operatively excised valves. Am. Heart J., 113:1316, 1987.

Spencer, F. C.: A plea for early, open mitral commissurotomy. Am. Heart J., 95:668, 1978.

Spencer, F. C., Colvin, S. B., Culliford, A. T., Isom, O. N.: Experiences with the Carpentier techniques of mitral valve reconstruction in 103 patients (1980–1985). J. Thorac. Cardiovasc. Surg., 90:341, 1985.

Spencer, F. C., Grossi, E. A., Baumann, F. G., et al.: Experiences with 1643 porcine prosthetic valves in 1492 patients. Ann. Surg., 203:691, 1986.

Tyers, G. F. O.: Mitral valve replacement: What should be the standard technique? Ann. Thorac. Surg., 49:861, 1990.

Yun, K. L., and Miller, D. C.: Mitral valve repair versus replacement. Cardiol. Clin., 9:315, 1991.

Yun, K. L., and Miller, D. C.: Mitral valve repair: When is it preferable to replacement? Cardiol. Rev., 1:187, 1993.

Zussa, C., Frater, R. W. M., Polesel, E., et al.: Artificial mitral valve chordae: Experimental and clinical experience. Ann. Thorac. Surg., 50:367, 1990.

# 51

# Complications from Cardiac Prostheses

## ■ I Prosthetic Valve Endocarditis

David A. Fullerton and Frederick L. Grover

*Prosthetic valve endocarditis* (PVE) is one of the most devastating complications of valve replacement. In most large series, the incidence of PVE is reported to be 2 to 4% (Cowgill et al., 1986); a range of 1 to 9% is reported in the literature (Calderwood et al., 1986). For unclear reasons, prosthetic valves are more likely to become infected in the aortic position than in the mitral position (Cowgill et al., 1987). This is in contradistinction to native valve endocarditis, wherein the mitral valve is more likely to become infected. In patients undergoing simultaneous aortic and mitral valve replacements, the incidence of prosthetic valve infection is greater, but the likelihood of either prosthesis becoming infected is probably equal (Baumgartner et al., 1983) (Fig. 51–1).

## HISTORICAL NOTE

Not long after the initial reports of valve replacements by Starr and Harken, the first reports of PVE appeared in the literature. Before the routine use of prophylactic antibiotics, Geraci and associates (1963) and Stein and co-workers (1966) reported incidences of early PVE of 10 and 12%, respectively. The incidence of this devastating complication was markedly reduced by routine prophylactic antibiotics. In a consecutive series of 288 patients receiving preoperative antibiotics, the incidence of PVE was reduced to 0.2% (Stein et al., 1963). From the outset, the surgical management of PVE has been a formidable challenge and remains so today. Early reports described débridement and drainage of the infection, which was associated with an extremely high mortality rate. Discouraged by such early surgical experience, cardiac surgeons made strong efforts to avoid operation for PVE. In 1972, Ross successfully performed aortic root replacement for PVE using an aortic homograft (Ross, 1990). His report stressed the importance of complete surgical débridement of all infected tissue, and the use of a homograft for reconstruction offered greater surgical flexibity and the advantage of minimizing

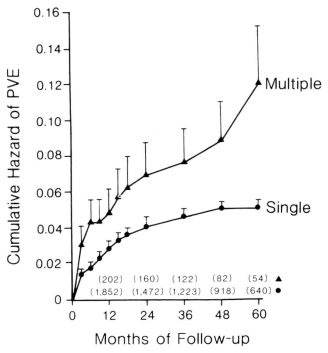

**FIGURE 51–1.** Cumulative hazard curve of prosthetic valve endocarditis (PVE) in single- and multiple-valve recipients. (From Calderwood, S. B., Swinsky, L. A., Waternaux, C. M., et al.: Risk factors for the development of prosthetic valve endocarditis. Circulation, 72:31, 1985. Reproduced with permission. Copyright 1985 American Heart Association.)

the placement of foreign material into the infected area. Olinger and Maloney reported replacement of an infected aortic prosthesis and external felt buttressing for correction of aortic ventricular discontinuity in 1977. The following year, Frantz, Murray, and Wilcox reported repair of ventricular-aortic discontinuity from endocarditis and abscess formation by aortic root replacement using a synthetic valved conduit. Danielson and associates (1974) described a technique for treating extensive periannular abscess formation in native aortic valve endocarditis by translocation of a prosthetic aortic valve into the ascending aorta and saphenous vein coronary artery bypass grafting. In 1981, Reitz and co-workers successfully applied this technique to treatment of prosthetic aortic valve endocarditis. In 1982, Symbas and colleagues combined aortic valve replacement with patch repair of periannular abscess cavity. Over the past decade, the incidence of PVE has remained fairly stable: most series have reported an incidence of 2 to 4% (Cowgill et al., 1986), and PVE continues to be one of the most serious and surgically challenging complications of valve replacement.

## RISK

The risk of prosthetic valve infection to the patient is lifelong. However, as assessed by hazard function analysis, the risk of infection appears to be greatest at approximately 5 weeks following valve implantation and thereafter declines. By 12 months after valve implantation, the risk reaches a low, constant level (Calderwood et al., 1985, 1986; Ivert et al., 1984) (Fig. 51–2). By clinical convention, PVE that is diagnosed within 60 days of valve implantation is called "early" PVE, whereas PVE diagnosed beyond 60 days of

valve implantation is called "late" (Dismukes et al., 1973). The incidence of PVE appears to be evenly distributed between early and late, each occurring with an incidence of approximately 1 to 2% (Cowgill et al., 1986). This distinction of early from late PVE is clinically valuable in providing insight into the acquisition of the infection, the clinical course of the patient, and management of the disease.

## Early Prosthetic Valve Endocarditis

Early PVE is believed to arise from perioperative contamination of the valve. In a review of nearly 1500 consecutive patients undergoing valve replacement, Ivert and co-workers (1984) identified the following as risk factors for early PVE: valve replacement for native valve endocarditis, black race, male gender, and prolonged cardiopulmonary bypass time.

Perioperative bacteremia, perhaps arising from infections such as wound infections, mediastinitis, and pneumonia, all increase the risk of early prosthetic valve contamination. Fortunately, such perioperative bacteremia cause PVE in a relatively small percentage of cases. Parker and co-workers (1983) reported that 32 of 890 patients had documented bacteremia in the early postoperative period following valve replacement. Surprisingly, of these 32 bacteremic patients, only 2 patients (6%) developed PVE, but both died.

The most likely source of infection is intraoperative contamination. Cardiac surgical procedures are extremely complex and entail numerous operating room personnel, multiple intravascular monitoring devices, and the circuit of the heart-lung machine. But even given the complexity of cardiac surgical procedures, the incidence of positive intraoperative cultures is

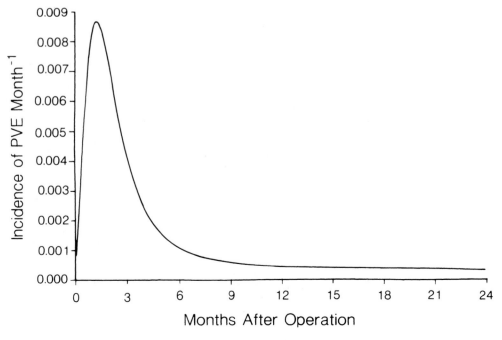

**FIGURE 51–2.** Hazard function curve for prosthetic valve endocarditis (PVE) for patients undergoing single-valve replacement. (From Ivert, T. S., Dismukes, W. E., Cobbs, C. G., et al.: Prosthetic valve endocarditis. Circulation, *69*:223, 1984. Reproduced with permission. Copyright 1984 American Heart Association.)

frighteningly high. Kluge and co-workers (1974) reported that 71% of cardiac surgical patients had positive intraoperative cultures taken from a variety of sampling sites such as intravenous and intra-arterial catheters and urinary bladder drainage catheters. Likewise, Ankeney and Parker (1969) reported that 19% of cardiac surgical patients had positive intraoperative blood cultures. In the latter study, 3 of the 12 patients with positive intraoperative blood cultures who did not receive preoperative prophylactic antibiotics developed early PVE.

The heart-lung bypass circuit has been implicated in several studies as a source of intraoperative contamination. The suction devices of the circuit in particular are believed to return bacteria from the air over the operative field and from the operative field directly into the blood of the pump circuit. Intraoperative use of autologous transfusion via red blood cell recycling devices has increased markedly in recent years. Of particular interest is the very high incidence of positive cultures in these blood recycling circuits. Bland and associates (1992) reported that in 30 of 31 cases (97%), bags of recycled blood yielded positive cultures.

The choice of suture materials used to implant the prosthesis may influence the risk. In a laboratory study designed to examine sutures commonly used to implant valves, Shuhaiber and colleagues (1989) used gram-positive bacteria labeled with (3H)-leucine to demonstrate that adherence of bacteria was least to monofilament polypropylene suture, 3 times higher to braided polyester, and 10 times higher to braided polyester coated with polybutylate. Invasive monitoring devices such as intra-arterial catheters, central venous catheters, pulmonary arterial catheters, thermodilution cardiac output measurement systems, and urinary bladder catheters all carry the risk of perioperative infection. Although difficult to quantitate, the risk clearly rises the longer these devices are in place. In fact, by 72 hours after insertion, the incidence of central venous line infection is estimated to be 12%, and this incidence rises daily thereafter (Corona et al., 1990). Therefore, every effort should be made to remove these monitoring devices as early as possible in the perioperative period.

Considering the high frequency of positive intraoperative cultures, it is surprising that early prosthetic valve infection does not occur more frequently. Prophylactic antibiotic administration is standard practice, although the data supporting the efficacy of such therapy must be inferred from observational studies. These show that use of prophylactic antibiotics has been associated with a significantly lower incidence of PVE than in historical control subjects. Stein and co-workers (1966) noted a reduction in the incidence of early PVE from 12% to nearly 0% with use of preoperative prophylactic antibiotics. Ankeney and Parker (1969) noted that 3 of 12 patients not receiving prophylactic antibiotics but who were bacteremic perioperatively developed PVE, whereas no bacteremic patients receiving antibiotics developed PVE.

## Late Prosthetic Valve Endocarditis

Late PVE is believed to arise either from infection acquired after the perioperative period or from insidious infection acquired during the operation but that is not clinically evident until more than 60 days following valve implantation.

As with any patient with valvular heart disease, patients with prosthetic valves should receive prophylactic antibiotics before any procedure that may produce bacteremia (Bayer et al., 1990). Such bacteremias are common with dental procedures and any procedures involving the genitourinary or gastrointestinal tracts. The prophylactic regimens recommended by the American Heart Association are listed in Table 51–1.

## Type of Prosthesis

Regardless of the specific type of mechanical prosthesis used, most large series have found the incidence of PVE to be the same whether a mechanical or bioprosthetic valve is used (Cowgill et al., 1987). However, the risk of early as opposed to late PVE may differ as a function of the type of prosthesis. Calderwood and colleagues (1985) found that the overall incidence of PVE at 5 years was not different between mechanical and bioprosthetic valves. However, the incidence of early PVE was higher in the mechanical group, whereas the incidence of late PVE was higher in the bioprosthetic group (Fig. 51–3).

The hazard function of PVE for homografts differs from that of other prosthetic devices. Unlike data pertaining to mechanical and bioprosthetic valves, which demonstrate the risk of PVE to be highest in the early postoperative period, data from several series suggest that the incidence of endocarditis following homograft valve implantation is both low and constant (Haydock et al., 1992; McGiffin et al., 1992; O'Brien et al., 1987) (Fig. 51–4).

■ **Table 51–1.** STANDARD PROPHYLACTIC ANTIBIOTIC REGIMEN FOR HEART VALVES

| Antibiotic Administered | Time of Administration |
|---|---|
| **Standard regimen:** Ampicillin, 2.0 g intravenously or intramuscularly, *plus* gentamicin, 1.5 mg/kg intravenously or intramuscularly (not to exceed 80 mg) | 30 minutes before procedure |
| **For patients allergic to amoxicillin/ ampicillin:** Vancomycin, 1.0 g intravenously over 1 hour, *plus* gentamicin, 1.5 mg/kg intravenously or intramuscularly (not to exceed 80 mg); may be repeated once 8 hours after initial dose | 1 hour before procedure |

Modified from the American Heart Association.

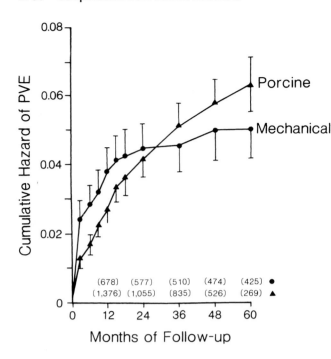

**FIGURE 51–3.** Cumulative hazard of prosthetic valve endocarditis (PVE) in recipients of mechanical prostheses and porcine prostheses. (From Calderwood, S. B., Swinsky, L. A., Waternaux, C. M., et al.: Risk factors for the development of prosthetic valve endocarditis. Circulation, 72:31, 1985. Reproduced with permission. Copyright 1985 American Heart Association.)

## OPERATION FOR NATIVE ENDOCARDITIS

Valve replacement in the setting of native valve endocarditis might be expected to increase the incidence of PVE. Surprisingly, however, most large studies have demonstrated the incidence to be approximately 4%, which is not higher than the overall reported incidence of PVE (Cowgill et al., 1986). An exception is the study by Ivert and associates (1984), which found a 5-fold increase in PVE when valve replacement was performed for active native valve endocarditis.

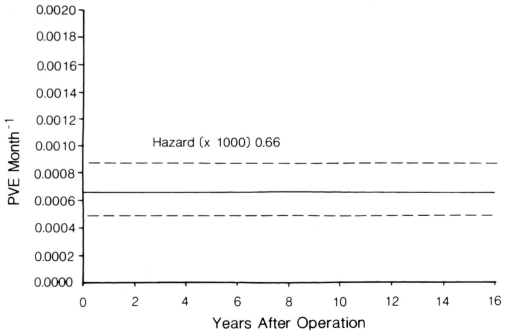

**FIGURE 51–4.** Hazard function curve for homograft endocarditis (PVE). The hazard function is constant. (From O'Brien, M. F., Stafford, E. G., Gardner, M. A., et al.: A comparison of aortic valve replacement with viable cryopreserved and fresh allograft valves, with a note on chromosomal studies. J. Thorac. Cardiovasc. Surg., 94:812, 1987.)

The type of valve used in the setting of active endocarditis might also be expected to influence this risk, although no data from prospective, randomized controlled trials are available to address this question. Use of an aortic homograft offers the theoretical advantage of placing minimal foreign material in the setting of infection. In a series of 78 patients undergoing aortic valve replacement with an aortic homograft for active aortic endocarditis, 8 patients (10%) developed endocarditis in the homograft valve (Haydock et al., 1990). McGiffin and associates (1992) reported a nonrandomized series that examined the influence of replacement valve type for active aortic endocarditis. In this series, the incidence of both early and late endocarditis in the replacement device was 5% (2 of 40 patients) if a homograft was used, 10.8% (4 of 37 patients) if a mechanical prosthesis was used, and 17% (7 of 41 patients) if a bioprosthetic device was used. Finally, Okita and associates (1988) reported a 4.4% reinfection rate with use of aortic homograft for aortic root replacement to treat severe periannular abscess, which is virtually the same as reports of procedures using mechanical bioprostheses.

## MICROBIOLOGY

Early prosthetic valve infections are believed to result from perioperative contamination, and contamination is reflected in the microbiology of early PVE. In most series, staphylococcal species account for at least 50% of early infections, whereas streptococcal and diphtheroid species together account for another 20 to 25% (Table 51–2). A variety of gram-negative organisms account for approximately 20% of early infections; fungal infections are quite rare.

On the other hand, the microbiology of late PVE is quite similar to that of native valve endocarditis. Gram-positive cocci also dominate the microbiology of late PVE. But unlike in early PVE, in which staphylococcal species predominate, streptococci, particularly non–Group D streptococci, are the most prevalent organisms, accounting for at least 30% of cases

of late PVE. *Staphylococcus epidermidis* also accounts for approximately 30% of cases (Cowgill et al., 1986). *S. aureus*, gram-negative bacilli, and fungi each account for only approximately 10% of cases. Thus, the bacteriology of late PVE is more favorable to successful antibiotic treatment than is early PVE.

## PATHOLOGY

A feature common to all prosthetic valves is the sewing ring. This foreign material markedly reduces the inoculum of bacteria required to produce infection, and the valve sewing ring therefore becomes the primary focus of infection. Thus the pathologic hallmark of PVE is the valve ring abscess. Perhaps because PVE is more common in the aortic position than the mitral position, valve ring abscess appears to occur much more frequently in the aortic position than in the mitral position (Mayer and Schownbaum, 1982); the incidence of valve ring abscess is between 50 and 75% (Cowgill et al., 1986). With abscess formation, the surrounding tissue may be progressively destroyed. With such destruction, valve dehiscence begins, and a paravalvular leak is produced.

As the infection progresses, a myocardial abscess may be produced. If the myocardial abscess extends into the conduction system, conduction from the atrium to the ventricle is delayed, and the electrocardiographic (P-R) interval will lengthen. Ultimately, complete atrioventricular block may occur.

The infectious pathology differs somewhat between mechanical and bioprosthetic valves. Mechanical valve infection is centered in the sewing ring, and therefore ring abscess formation occurs in 63% and myocardial abscess occurs in 40% of mechanical valve infections (Arnett and Roberts, 1976). On the other hand, infections of tissue valves commonly involve the valve leaflets. Probably for this reason, valve ring abscess formation occurs in less than 20% of tissue valves, and myocardial abscess formation is more rare (Bortolotti et al., 1981; Calderwood et al., 1986; Cowgill et al., 1987). Infections of the bioprosthetic valve leaflets may also cause stenosis of the infected tissue valve from vegetations in 28% and valve leaflet destruction and perforation in 36% of cases (Cowgill et al., 1986). Because the incidence of abscess formation is lower in tissue valve infection, success of antibiotic therapy has been reported to be greater in treatment of infected tissue valves (Rossiter et al., 1978).

## DIAGNOSIS

### Clinical Findings

PVE, particularly early PVE, may be difficult to diagnose. Fever is the most common clinical finding and is virtually always present (Cowgill et al., 1986). However, in the postoperative period, there are many potential sources of fever, making this a nonspecific finding. Nonetheless, the diagnosis of PVE must be

■ Table 51–2. BACTERIOLOGY OF PVE

| Early PVE | | Late PVE | |
|---|---|---|---|
| *Organism* | *Percentage* | *Organism* | *Percentage* |
| Streptococci | 10 | Streptococci | 40 |
| | | S. viridans | 30 |
| | | Group D, S. pneumoniae | 10 |
| Staphylococci | 45 | Staphylocci | 35 |
| S. epidermidis | 25 | S. epidermidis | 25 |
| S. aureus | 20 | S. aureus | 10 |
| Gram-negative organisms | 20 | Gram-negative organisms | 10 |
| Fungi | 10 | Fungi | 5 |
| Diphtheroids | 10 | Diphtheroids | 5 |
| Other | 5 | Other | 5 |

From Cowgill, L. D., Addonizio, V. P., Hopeman, A. R., and Harken, A. H.: Prosthetic valve endocarditis. *In* O'Rourke, R. A., and Crawford, M. J. (eds): Current Problems in Cardiology. Chicago, Year Book, 9:617, 1986.

considered in any patient with a prosthetic valve and fever.

Other physical findings include a new regurgitant murmur or a changing murmur, frequently causing valve dehiscence. This occurs in approximately 56% of patients (Cowgill et al., 1986) and is therefore not found in close to one-half of patients with PVE.

One of the classic physical findings of native valve endocarditis is splenomegaly, present in 25% of early PVE cases and 44% of late PVE cases (Wantanakunakorn, 1979). However, other physical signs that are classically associated with native valve endocarditis, such as petechiae, Roth's spots, Osler's nodes, and Janeway lesions, are only rarely found with PVE.

Most laboratory data are very nonspecific in the diagnosis of PVE. Despite the presence of fever, leukocytosis with a white blood cell count of greater than 12,000/mm$^3$ is present in only one-half of patients (Cowgill et al., 1986). As in native valve endocarditis, anemia (hematocrit less than 34%) is present in more than 70% of patients, particularly with late PVE (Cowgill et al., 1986). Again, however, anemia is a very nonspecific finding in patients following cardiac surgery. As in native valve endocarditis, hematuria is common and is found in 57% of patients (Cowgill et al., 1986).

The diagnosis of PVE is confirmed by positive blood cultures. Two blood cultures drawn from separate venipuncture sites will be positive in at least 99% of patients with bacterial endocarditis (Weinstein et al., 1983). However, infection by very fastidious organisms or fungus may not create positive cultures for several weeks; cultures should therefore be kept for at least 3 weeks before being considered negative.

## Diagnostic Studies

The electrocardiogram should be followed carefully on a daily basis. A variety of cardiac dysrhythmias may be produced by the infection itself or by the cardiac impairment produced by valvular dysfunction. The electrocardiogram should be specifically scrutinized for an increasing P-R interval, which strongly suggests atrioventricular conduction impairment produced by a myocardial abscess. This may be the harbinger of complete heart block.

Valve sewing ring abscess with destruction of the surrounding tissues causes paravalvular leak and valve dehiscence. In the past, cardiac fluoroscopy routinely was used to look for valve dehiscence. "Rocking" of the prosthetic valve annulus of more than 7 to 10 degrees is consistent with the diagnosis. On the other hand, cardiac catheterization is of limited value in making the diagnosis.

Transesophageal echocardiography has recently become a valuable tool in diagnosing PVE. This technique overcomes the technical limitations of transthoracic echocardiography imposed structurally by lung parenchyma, chest wall deformities, and pericardial adipose tissue. Pederson and colleagues (1991) directly compared transthoracic and transesophageal

echocardiography in the evaluation of PVE. The transthoracic modality was 50% sensitive and 93% specific, whereas the transesophageal modality was 100% sensitive and 100% specific. Transesophageal echocardiography is particularly valuable in visualizing a myocardial abscess (Alton et al., 1992).

## MANAGEMENT

The management of PVE is extremely challenging. Patients should be hospitalized, at least for the initiation of therapy, and monitored for cardiac dysrhythmias. As in the management of native valve endocarditis, the mainstay of medical therapy is antibiotic therapy. As reviewed by Cowgill and co-workers (1986), the following guidelines should be followed: (1) bactericidal antibiotics should be used (Kloster, 1975), (2) therapy should include two drugs that have synergistic bactericidal efficacy against the pathogen (Dismukes et al., 1973; Masur and Johnson, 1980; Watanakunakorn et al., 1974), (3) in vitro susceptibility testing should be performed to ensure that bactericidal drug levels are achieved (Kloster, 1975; Washington, 1982), and (4) antibiotic therapy should be administered for 6 to 8 weeks (Kay et al., 1983; Von Reyn et al., 1981).

The first objective of medical therapy is to sterilize the blood. After antibiotic therapy is initiated, blood cultures should be drawn every 3 to 4 days to ensure blood sterilization (Cowgill et al., 1987). Once cultures are consistently negative, they should be drawn weekly or whenever the patient experiences fever or other clinical change. Blood cultures should become negative within 3 to 5 days of initiation of antibiotic therapy. Blood cultures should continue to be negative for at least 1 month after completion of antibiotic therapy. Failure of blood cultures to become negative after starting antibiotic therapy or relapse during therapy or once therapy has been discontinued is an indication for surgical intervention.

Although the technique is somewhat controversial, anticoagulation should be started in patients with PVE. The infection may serve as a nidus for thrombus formation with subsequent embolization, and cerebral embolization is a major cause of death among these patients (Carpenter and McAllister, 1983). Neurologic complications of PVE are common, and both early and late PVE are associated with a 25 to 40% incidence of neurologic complication (Karchmer et al., 1978; Leport et al., 1987; Madison et al., 1975; Masur and Johnson, 1980). Among patients with PVE who do not undergo anticoagulation, the incidence of embolic stroke has been reported to be 25 to 60% (Karchmer et al., 1978; Wilson et al., 1978), which anticoagulation reduces to 3 to 14% (Davenport and Hart, 1990). Davenport and Hart (1990) estimate that the daily stroke rate is 1 to 9%. Of note, most emboli occur with uncontrolled infection, and their incidence is markedly decreased with initiation of antibiotics. Once control of the infection is achieved with antibiotics, recurrent embolization is rare

(Quenzer et al., 1976; Salgado et al., 1989). Therefore, if recurrent embolization does occur, it should be inferred that the infection is not controlled; recurrent embolization may be considered a relative indication for surgery.

One of the most challenging problems faced by the cardiac surgeon is the surgical management of PVE. As reviewed by Cowgill and associates (1987), the indications for replacement of the infected prosthesis all stem from failure of medical management. They include congestive heart failure, ongoing sepsis or relapse of infection, valve obstruction, new onset of heart block (which implies a myocardial abscess), unstable prosthesis by fluoroscopy, fungal infection, and recurrent systemic embolism. Of these surgical indications, congestive heart failure is probably the most significant prognostic factor. Medical therapy alone produced a 100% mortality rate in patients with significant heart failure, whereas a combined medical and surgical approach produced a 49% mortality rate (Karchmer et al., 1978; Richardson et al., 1978).

## PROGNOSIS

PVE is associated with an extremely high mortality rate. Overall, the reported mortality rate averages 54% (Cowgill et al., 1986). Early PVE is quite lethal and carries a mortality rate of 74%. Although somewhat better, the mortality rate with late PVE is also substantial at 43%. Factors contributing to the higher mortality rate of early PVE include a predominance of nonstreptococcal organisms, postoperative debilitation of patients, and involvement of a freshly implanted, nonendothelialized valve and sewing ring.

The infecting organism has a significant relationship to prognosis. Nonstreptococcal organisms have a significantly higher mortality rate than streptococcal organisms do (Cowgill et al., 1986). The mortality rate associated with fungi is 93%, S. aureus 86%, diphtheroids 64%, and gram-negative bacilli 60%. On the other hand, streptococcal infections have a mortality rate of 32%.

Other factors that significantly affect prognosis include congestive heart failure, which is the leading prognostic factor; its presence is associated with a mortality rate exceeding 75%. Likewise, renal dysfunction and systemic emboli are associated with a significant increase in mortality rate (Mullany et al., 1989).

A review of several major series demonstrates that the overall mortality rate of patients treated medically is approximately 60% (Cowgill et al., 1987). However, late streptococcal PVE is commonly amenable to medical therapy alone. In comparison, the mortality rate of those patients treated by a combination of antibiotics and valve replacement is approximately 40% (Cowgill et al., 1987).

The type of valve infected also is significant. Although PVE appears to occur as often with mechanical as with bioprosthetic valves, antibiotic sterilization of bioprosthetic valves, particularly when infected with *Streptococcus*, is much more frequently successful than is such treatment of mechanical valves (Cowgill et al., 1987). This greater ability to sterilize infected bioprosthetic valves likely stems from infection of the leaflets of bioprosthetic valves and a reduced frequency of perivalvular abscess formation. However, even if the eradication of acute infection of a bioprosthetic valve may be accomplished, Tornos and coworkers (1992) have reported that such valves rapidly deteriorate in follow-up and therefore frequently require replacement.

## SURGICAL THERAPY

The principal surgical objectives are to débride all infected tissue and to replace the involved valve. Because a sewing ring abscess may be present, operation may be extremely difficult and technically challenging.

### Surgery for Annular Abscess

More than one-half of all patients with aortic PVE have periannular abscess formation (Cowgill et al., 1987). Without surgery, most of these patients will die of sepsis or congestive heart failure. Even with surgical therapy, periannular abscess formation has been identified as a significant risk factor for operative death (David et al., 1990).

Extension of the infection into the annular and periannular structures is a major determinant of both early and late surgical results. The presence of periannular destruction relates to both the virulence of the organism and the duration of infection. Varying degrees of annular involvement are a constant feature of PVE. Abscess formation that begins at the sewing ring often extends into the aortic annulus, commonly in the region of aortic-mitral valvar continuity. The spectrum of periannular infection ranges from a simple localized abscess to larger subannular aneurysms, with or without perforation, in the other cardiac chambers. Likewise, the infection may extend into the pericardial space or create total disruption of ventriculo-aortic continuity or disrupt the mitral-aortic trigone.

When operating for periannular abscess, the surgeon must both ensure complete débridement of all grossly infected structures and nonviable tissue and re-establish valve competency with elimination of any external or intracardiac defects in a tension-free manner that excludes attenuated areas from high pressure. These principles sometimes require radical cardiac débridement, but if these principles are not adhered to, the patient is at significant risk for recurrent infection, valvar dehiscence, or both (Ergin et al., 1989).

The choice of surgical reconstruction is determined by the particular situation after complete débridement of the infection. Small abscess cavities may be débrided and then closed primarily or incorporated into the valve placement sutures (Nelson et al., 1984).

Larger abscesses may require reconstruction or exclusion by patch technique. Although Dacron has been used successfully for such patch reconstruction (Fiore et al., 1986), autologous pericardium appears to be the material of choice (Cabrol et al., 1990; David et al., 1989) (Fig. 51–5).

Reconstruction in the setting of extensive periannular destruction or aortic-ventricular disruption is exceptionally challenging. As initially described by Danielson and co-workers (1974) and employed by Reitz and associates (1981), one surgical option is translocation of the aortic valve into the distal ascending aorta and coronary artery bypass grafting (Fig. 51–6). However, because an aneurysm may form subsequently in the attenuated periannular region, and because the technique depends on coronary bypass grafts, this procedure is rarely indicated. It is, however, important for the surgeon to have this technique in his or her armamentarium. Aortic root replacement is currently the procedure of choice in this situation (Cabrol et al., 1990). Initially accomplished by using a synthetic valved conduit (Frantz et al., 1978), this procedure does place synthetic material into the area of infection (Fig. 51–7). Aortic root replacement using

a homograft overcomes this disadvantage by placement of minimal synthetic material into the area of infection (Glazier et al., 1991; Ross, 1990; Zwischenberger et al., 1989). Use of a homograft, whether as a free-sewn valve replacement (Tuna et al., 1990) or as an aortic root replacement, offers additional flexibility in reconstructing the débrided areas, particularly by using the attached anterior leaflet of the mitral valve of an aortic homograft to reconstruct débrided areas (Clarke, 1987; Miller, 1990) (Fig. 51–8). Whether accomplished by synthetic valved conduit or by homograft, aortic root replacement excludes attenuated regions from high pressure and permits suturing to noninfected, viable structures. If necessary, transmural sutures may be used to secure the conduit to the interventricular crest (Borst, 1990). Jault and colleagues (1993) have reported a 6-year survival rate of 54% following surgical reconstruction of aortic periannular abscess in PVE.

Fortunately, destruction of the mitral annular region is much less common than periaortic annular destruction (David et al., 1989); débridement and reconstruction of the mitral annulus is much more difficult here than in the aortic region. The mitral

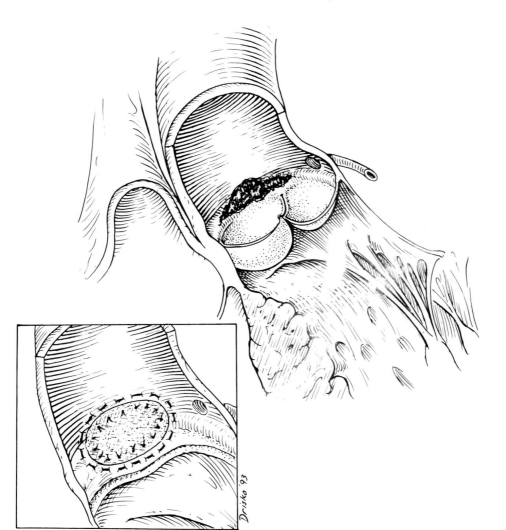

**FIGURE 51–5.** Débridement of localized periannular abscess. *Inset*, Closure with a pericardial patch. (From Cabrol, C., Gandjbakch, I., Pavie, A., et al.: Endocarditis symposium: Approach to advanced aortic root infection. J. Card. Surg., 5:48, 1990.)

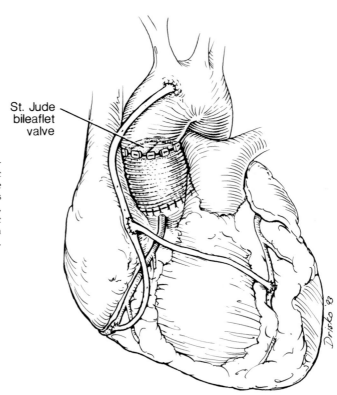

FIGURE 51–6. After removal of the infected valve and annular débridement, the ascending aorta is reconstructed and a new prosthetic valve is placed distal to the coronary ostia, which are oversewn. The coronary circulation is then reestablished with aortocoronary bypass grafts. (Modified from Danielson, G. K., Titus, J. L., and DuShane, J. W.: Successful treatment of aortic valve endocarditis and aortic root abscesses by insertion of prosthetic valve in ascending aorta and placement of bypass grafts to coronary arteries. J. Thorac. Cardiovasc. Surg., *67*:443, 1974.)

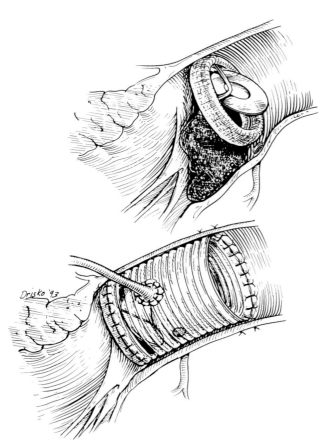

FIGURE 51–7. Extensive periannular abscess associated with prosthetic valve dehiscence. Repair utilizing aortic valved conduit for aortic root replacement. (From Frantz, P. T., Murray, G. F., and Wilcox, B. R.: Surgical management of left ventricular-aortic discontinuity complicating bacterial endocarditis. Reprinted with permission from the Society of Thoracic Surgeons [The Annals of Thoracic Surgery] 1978, Vol. 29, p. 1].)

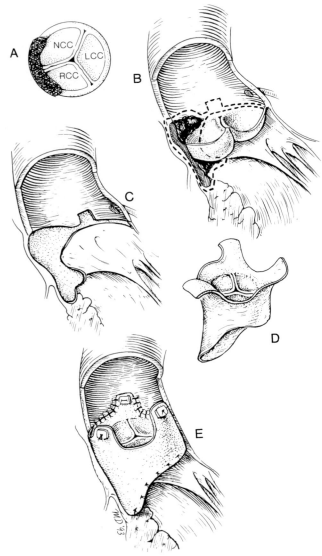

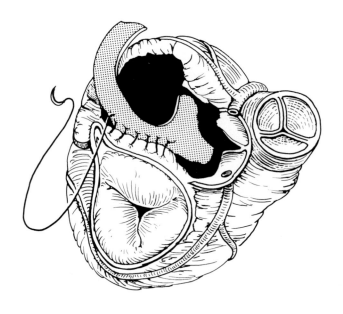

region may be reconstructed using a modification of the technique described by Rastan and associates (1981). The material used in the reconstruction should be a sandwich of pericardium exposed to the blood side and synthetic material for stability (Fig. 51–10).

## Operation with Recent Stroke

As noted earlier, neurologic complications are common with PVE. The mechanisms of neurologic injury include pyogenic arteritis, hemorrhagic transforma-

**FIGURE 51–8.** *A–E,* Aortic homograft offers flexibility in annular reconstruction after periannular débridement. (LCC = left coronary cusp; NCC = noncoronary cusp; RCC = right coronary cusp.) (*A–E,* From Zwischenberger, J. B., Shalaby, T. Z., and Conti, V. R.: Viable cryopreserved aortic homograft for aortic valve endocarditis and annular abscesses. Reprinted with permission from the Society of Thoracic Surgeons [The Annals of Thoracic Surgery, 1989, Vol. 48, pp. 365–370].)

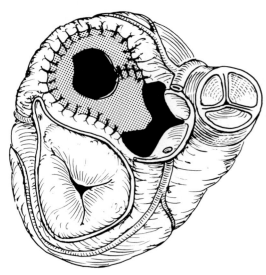

annulus may be reconstructed with autologous pericardium following débridement, as described by David and Feindel (1987) and by David and associates (1987, 1989) (Fig. 51–9). If the posterior mitral annular region requires reconstruction, this may be done using pericardium, following which, if necessary, the new mitral prosthesis may be translocated onto either the atrial or the ventricular side of the annulus. If it is technically possible, ventricular translocation can prevent exposure of the attenuated area to high pressure (Ergin et al., 1989; Rochiccioli et al., 1986). Although uncommon, repair of aortic mitral discontinuity is particularly difficult to reconstruct. This trigonal

**FIGURE 51–9.** Use of pericardium to reconstruct the mitral annulus and central fibrous body of the heart. (From David, T. E., Feindel, C. M., and Ropchan, G. V.: Valvular heart disease: Reconstruction of the left ventricle with autologous pericardium. J. Thorac. Cardiovasc. Surg. *94*:710, 1987.)

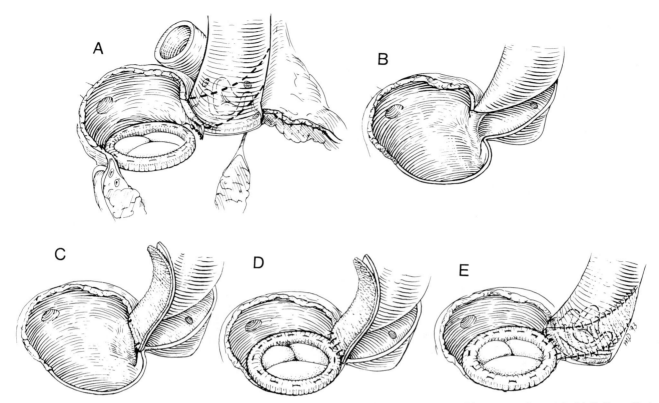

FIGURE 51–10. *A–E*, Steps in reconstruction of extensive destruction of the left fibrous trigone with a composite patch. (*A–E*, From Ergin, M. A., Raissi, S., Follis, F., et al.: Annular destruction in acute bacterial endocarditis: Surgical techniques to meet the challenge. J. Thorac. Cardiovasc. Surg. *97*:755, 1989.)

tion of embolic infarction, rupture of intracranial mycotic aneurysms, and ischemic stroke secondary to embolization of clot or septic material (Hart et al., 1987; Salgado et al., 1989). Such neurologic events are associated with significant morbidity and mortality. Intracranial hemorrhage in the setting of PVE carries a mortality rate as high as 28 to 69% (Davenport and Hart, 1990; Karchmer et al., 1978; Keyser et al., 1990).

The most common neurologic complication is ischemic stroke (Davenport and Hart, 1990). From the surgical perspective, the main concern is the transformation of an ischemic infarct into a hemorrhagic infarct as a consequence of the anticoagulation required during cardiopulmonary bypass. This is particularly important, because in a study by Ting and associates (1991), 32% of cerebral infarctions in patients with endocarditis were asymptomatic. In this study, all patients with intracranial hemorrhage secondary to endocarditis who then underwent valve replacement suffered a perioperative stroke, which was associated with a significantly increased mortality rate. On the other hand, patients with an ischemic infarct (without hemorrhage) secondary to endocarditis who underwent valve replacement had no perioperative strokes. Nonetheless, the risk of transforming an ischemic infarct into a hemorrhagic one has been documented by DiSesa (1991). Thus, before undergoing valve replacement, patients with PVE should undergo a careful neurologic evaluation, including computed to-

mography of the head. If a small ischemic infarct is identified, the risk of making this worse with valve replacement appears to be low. However, if a large ischemic infarct or intracranial hemorrhage is identified, the risk of significant perioperative neurologic event is high. In such patients, the need for valve replacement should be balanced against high neurologic risk. If possible, operation should be delayed as long as possible to allow healing of the brain injury.

## SELECTED BIBLIOGRAPHY

Cowgill, L. D., Addonizio, V. P., Hopeman, A. R., and Harken, A. H.: Prosthetic valve endocarditis. *In* O'Rouke, R. A., and Crawford, M. J. (eds): Current Problems in Cardiology. Chicago, Year Book, *9*:617, 1986.

This outstanding monograph comprehensively discusses all aspects of prosthetic valve endocarditis. From the surgical perspective, it offers excellent guidelines in the surgical treatment of this condition.

David, T. E., Komeda, M., and Brofman, P. R.: Surgical treatment of aortic root abscess. Circulation, *80*(Suppl. 1):269, 1989.

The authors report on 21 patients with aortic root abscess from endocarditis. the article provides illustrations that are extremely helpful in planning surgical reconstruction after debridement of such abscesses.

Glazier, J. J., Verwilghen, J. O., Donaldson, R. M., and Ross, D. N.: Treatment of complicated prosthetic aortic valve endocarditis with annular abscess formation by homograft aortic root replacement. J. Am. Coll. Cardiol., *17*:1177, 1991.

The authors review the outcome of 30 consecutive cases of prosthetic valve endocarditis treated surgically with homograft aortic root replacement. The mortality rate was 30%, and the recurrence rate of endocarditis was 9.5%. The authors stress the importance of wide surgical débridement of all infected tissue.

McGiffin, D. C., Galbraith, A. J., McLachlan, G. J., et al.: Aortic valve infection. Risk factors for death and recurrent endocarditis after valve replacement. J. Thor. Cardiovasc. Surg., *104*:511, 1992.

The authors reviewed the incidence of recurrent aortic endocarditis after operation for native or prosthetic endocarditis in 195 patients undergoing 209 aortic valve replacements over a 22-year period. Seventy-nine per cent of patients were free of recurrent endocarditis at 10 years. Recurrent endocarditis was diagnosed in 5% of patients receiving aortic homografts, in 10% receiving mechanical prostheses, and in 17% receiving bioprostheses.

# BIBLIOGRAPHY

Alton, M. E., Pasierski, T. J., Orsinelli, D. A., et al.: Comparison of transthoracic and transesophageal echocardiography in evaluation of 47 Starr-Edwards prosthetic valves. J. Am. Coll. Cardiol., 20:1503, 1992.

Ankeney, J. L., and Parker, R. F.: Staphylococcal endocarditis following open heart surgery related to positive intraoperative blood cultures. In Brewer, L. (ed): Prosthetic Heart Valves. Springfield, IL, Charles C Thomas, 1969, p. 719.

Arnett, E. N., and Roberts, W. C.: Prosthetic valve endocarditis: Clinicopathologic analysis of 22 necropsy patients. Am. J. Cardiol., 38:281, 1976.

Baumgartner, W. A., Miller, D. C., Rieitz, B. A., et al.: Surgical treatment of prosthetic valve endocarditis. Ann. Thorac. Surg., 35:87, 1983.

Bayer, A. S., Nelson, F. J., and Slama, T. G.: Current concepts in prevention of prosthetic valve endocarditis. Chest, 97:1203, 1990.

Bland, A., Villarino, M. E., Ardnino, J. J., et al.: Bacteriologic and endotoxin analysis of salvaged blood used in autologous transfusions during cardiac operation. J. Thorac. Cardiovasc. Surg., 103:582, 1992.

Borst, H. G.: Repair of septic aortic root defects without conduit. J. Cardiovasc. Surg., 5:44, 1990.

Bortolotti, U., Thiene, G., Milano, A., et al.: Pathological study of infective endocarditis on Hancock porcine bioprosthesis. J. Thorac. Cardiovasc. Surg., 81:94, 1981.

Cabrol, C., Gandjbakhch, L., Pavie, A., et al.: Endocarditis Symposium: Approach to advanced aortic root infection. J. Cardiovasc. Surg., 5:48, 1990.

Calderwood, S. B., Swinski, L. A., Waternaux, C. M., et al.: Risk factors for the development of prosthetic valve endocarditis. Circulation, 72:31, 1985.

Calderwood, S. B., Swinski, L. A., Karchmer, A. W., et al.: Prosthetic valve endocarditis. Analysis of factors affecting outcome of therapy. J. Thorac. Cardiovasc. Surg., 92:776, 1986.

Carpenter, J. L., and McAllister, C. K.: Anticoagulation in prosthetic valve endocarditis. South. Med. J., 76:11372, 1983.

Clarke, D. R.: Extended aortic root replacement for treatment of left ventricular outflow tract obstruction. J. Card. Surg., 1:121, 1987.

Corona, M. L., Peters, S. G., Narr, B. J., and Thompson, R. L.: Infections related to central venous catheters. Mayo Clin. Proc., 65:979, 1990.

Cowgill, L. D., Addonizio, V. P., Hopeman, A. R., and Harken, A. H.: Prosthetic valve endocarditis. In O'Rouke, R. A., and Crawford, M. J. (eds): Current Problems in Cardiology. Chicago, Year Book, 9:617, 1986.

Cowgill, L. D., Addonizio, V. P., Hopeman, A. R., and Harken, A. H.: A practical approach to prosthetic valve endocarditis. Ann. Thorac. Surg., 43:450, 1987.

Danielson, G. K., Titus, J. L., and DuShane, J. W.: Successful treatment of aortic valve endocarditis and aortic root abscesses by insertion of prosthetic valve in ascending aorta and placement of bypass grafts to coronary arteries. J. Thorac. Cardiovasc. Surg., 67:443, 1974.

Davenport, J., and Hart, R. G.: Prosthetic valve endocarditis 1976–1987. Stroke, 21:993, 1990.

David, T. E., Bos, J., Christakis, G. T., et al.: Heart valve operations in patients with active infective endocarditis. Ann. Thorac. Surg., 49:701, 1990.

David, T. E., and Feindel, C. M.: Valvular heart disease: Reconstruction of the mitral anulus. Circulation, 76:111–102, 1987.

David, T. E., Feindel, C. M., and Ropchan, G. V.: Reconstruction of the left ventricle with autologous pericardium. J. Thorac. Cardiovasc. Surg., 94:710, 1987.

David, T. E., Komeda, M., and Brofman, P. R.: Surgical treatment of aortic root abscess. Circulation, 80(Suppl. I):I-269, 1989.

DiSesa, V. J.: Art and science in the management of endocarditis. Ann. Thorac. Surg., 51:6, 1991.

Dismukes, W. E., Karchmer, A. W., Buckley, M. J., et al.: Prosthetic valve endocarditis: An analysis of 38 cases. Circulation, 48:365, 1973.

Ergin, M. A., Raissi, S., Follis, F., et al.: Annular destruction in acute bacterial endocarditis: Surgical techniques to meet the challenge. J. Thorac. Cardiovasc. Surg., 97:755, 1989.

Fiore, A. C., Ivey, T. D., McKeown, P. P., et al.: Patch closure of aortic annulus mycotic aneurysms. Ann. Thorac. Surg., 42:372, 1986.

Frantz, P. T., Murray, G. F., and Wilcox, B. R.: Surgical management of left ventricular-aortic discontinuity complicating bacterial endocarditis. Ann. Thorac. Surg., 29:1, 1978.

Geraci, J. E., Dale, A. J. D, McGoon, D. C., et al.: Bacterial endocarditis and endarteritis following cardiac operations. Wis. Med. J., 62:302, 1963.

Glazier, J. J., Verwilghen, J. O., Donaldson, R. M., and Ross, D. N.: Treatment of complicated prosthetic aortic valve endocarditis with annular abscess formation by homograft aortic root replacement. J. Am. Coll. Cardiol., 17:1177, 1991.

Hart, R. G., Kagan-Hallet, K., and Joerns, S. E.: Mechanisms of intracranial hemorrhage in infective endocarditis. Stroke, 18:1048, 1987.

Haydock, D., Barratt-Boyes, B., Macedo, T., et al.: Aortic valve replacement for active infectious endocarditis in 108 patients. J. Thorac. Cardiovasc. Surg., 103:130, 1992.

Ivert, T. S. A., Dismukes, W. E., Cobbs, C. G., et al.: Prosthetic valve endocarditis. Circulation, 69:223, 1984.

Jault, F., Gandjbakhch, L., Chastre, J. C., et al.: Prosthetic valve endocarditis with ring abscesses: Surgical management and long-term results. J. Thorac. Cardiovasc. Surg., 105:1106, 1993.

Karchmer, A. W., Dismukes, W. E., Buckley, M. J., and Austen, W. G.: Late prosthetic valve endocarditis: Clinical features influencing therapy. Am. J. Med., 64:199, 1978.

Kay, P. H., Oldershaw, P. J., Lincoln, J. C. R., et al.: The management of prosthetic valve endocarditis. J. Cardiovasc. Surg., 224:127, 1983.

Keyser, D. L., Biller, J., Coffman, T. T., and Adams, J. P., Jr.: Neurologic complications of late prosthetic valve endocarditis. Stroke, 21:472, 1990.

Kloster, F. E.: Diagnosis and management of complications of prosthetic heart valves. Am. J. Cardiol. 335:872, 1975.

Kluge, R. M., Calia, F. M., McLaughlin, J. A., et al.: Source of contamination in open heart surgery. J. A. M. A., 230:14115, 1974.

Leport, C. C., Vilde, J. L., Bricaire, F., et al.: Fifty cases of late prosthetic valve endocarditis: Improvement in prognosis over a 15-year period. Br. Heart J., 58:66, 1987.

Madison, J., Wang, K., Gobel, F. L., and Edwards, J. E.: Prosthetic valve endocarditis. Circulation, 51:940, 1975.

Masur, H., and Johnson, W. D., Jr.: Prosthetic valve endocarditis. J. Thorac. Cardiovasc. Surg., 80:31, 1980.

Mayer, K. H., and Schownbaum, S. C.: Evaluation and management of prosthetic valve endocarditis. Prog. Cardiovasc. Dis., 25:43, 1982.

McGiffin, D. C., Galbraith, A. J., McLachlan, G. J., et al.: Aortic valve infection. Risk factors for death and recurrent endocarditis after aortic valve replacement. J. Thorac. Cardiovasc. Surg., 104:511, 1992.

Miller, D. C.: Predictors of outcome in patients with prosthetic valve endocarditis (PVE) and potential advantages of homograft aortic root replacement for prosthetic ascending aortic valve-graft infections. J. Cardiovasc. Surg., 5:53, 1990.

Mullany, C. J., McIsaacs, A. L., Rowe, M. H., and Hale, G. S.: The surgical treatment of infective endocarditis. World J. Surg., 13:132, 1989.

Nelson, R. J., Harley, D. P., French, W. J., and Bayer, A. S.: Favorable ten-year experience with valve procedures for active infective endocarditis. J. Thorac. Cardiovasc. Surg., *87*:493, 1984.

Okita, Y., Franciosi, G., Matsuki, O., et al.: Early and late results of aortic root replacement with antibiotic-sterilized aortic homograft. J. Thorac. Cardiovasc. Surg., *95*:696, 1988.

Olinger, G. N., and Maloney, J. V., Jr.: Repair of left ventricular-aortic discontinuity complicating endocarditis from an aortic valve prosthesis. Ann. Thorac. Surg., *23*:576, 1977.

O'Brien, M. R., Stafford, E. G., Garner, M. A. H, et al.: A comparison of aortic valve replacement with viable cryopreserved and fresh allograft valves, with a note on chromosomal studies. J. Thorac. Cardiovasc. Surg., *94*:812, 1987.

Parker, F. B., Greiner-Hayes, C., Tomar, R. H., et al.: Bacteremia following prosthetic valve replacement. Ann. Surg., *197*:11147, 1983.

Pedersen, W. R., Walker, M., Olson, J. D., et al.: Value of transesophageal echocardiography as an adjunct to transthoracic echocardiography in evaluation of native and prosthetic valve endocarditis. Chest, *100*:351, 1991.

Quenzer, R. W., Edwards, L. D., and Levin, S.: A comparative study of 48 host valve and 24 prosthetic valve endocarditis cases. Am. Heart J., *92*:15, 1976.

Rastan, H., Atai, M., Hadi, H., et al.: Enlargement of mitral valvular ring. New technique for double valve replacement in children or adults with small mitral annulus. J. Thorac. Cardiovasc. Surg., *81*:106, 1981.

Reitz, B. A., Stinson, E. B., Watson, D. C., et al.: Translocation of the aortic valve for prosthetic valve endocarditis. J. Thorac. Cardiovasc. Surg., *81*:212, 1981.

Richardson, J. V., Karp, R. B., Kirklin, J. W., et al.: Treatment of infective endocarditis: A 10-year comparative analysis. Circulation, *58*:589, 1978.

Rochiccioli, C., Chastre, J., Lecompte, Y., et al.: Prosthetic valve endocarditis. J. Thorac. Cardiovasc. Surg., *92*:784, 1986.

Ross, D.: Allograft root replacement for prosthetic endocarditis. J. Cardiovasc. Surg., *5*:68, 1990.

Rossiter, S. J., Stinson, E. B., Oyer, P. E., et al.: Prosthetic valve endocarditis, comparison of heterograft tissue valves and mechanical valves. J. Thorac. Cardiovasc. Surg., *76*:795, 1978.

Salgado, A. V., Furlan, A. J., Keys, T. F., et al.: Neurological complications of endocarditis: A 12 year experience. Neurology, *39*:173, 1989.

Shuhaiber, H., Chugh, T., and Burns, G.: In vitro adherence of bacteria to sutures in cardiac surgery. J. Thorac. Cardiovasc. Surg., *30*:749, 1989.

Stein, P. D., Harken, D. E., and Dexter, L.: The nature and prevention of prosthetic valve endocarditis. Am. Heart J., *71*:393, 1966.

Symbas, P. N., Vlais, S. E., Zacharopuolos, L., and Lutz, J. F.: Acute endocarditis: Surgical treatment of aortic regurgitation and aortic-left ventricular discontinuity. J. Thorac. Cardiovasc. Surg., *84*:291, 1982.

Ting, W., Silverman, N., and Levitsky, S.: Valve replacement in patients with endocarditis and cerebral septic emboli. Ann. Thorac. Surg., *51*:18, 1991.

Tornos, P., Sanz, E., Permanyer-Miralda, G., et al.: Late prosthetic valve endocarditis. Chest, *101*:37, 1992.

Tuna, I. C., Orszulak, T. A., Schaff, H. V., and Danielson, G. K.: Results of homograft aortic valve replacement for active endocarditis. Ann. Thorac. Surg., *49*:619, 1990.

Von Reyn, C. F., Levy, B. S., Arbeit, R. D., et al.: Infective endocarditis: An analysis based on strict case definitions. Ann. Intern. Med., *94*:505, 1981.

Washington, J. A.: The role of the microbiology laboratory in the diagnosis and antimicrobial treatment of infective endocarditis. Mayo Clin. Proc., *57*:22, 1982.

Watanakunakorn, C., and Glotzbecker, C.: Enhancement of the effects of anti-staphylococcal antibiotics by aminoglycosides. Antimicrob. Agents Chemother., *6*:802, 1974.

Watanakunakorn, C.: Prosthetic valve infective endocarditis: A review. Prog. Cardiovasc. Dis., *22*:181, 1979.

Weinstein, M. P., Reller, L. B., Murphy, J. R., et al.: The clinical significance of positive blood cultures: A comprehensive analysis of 500 episodes of bacteremia and fungemia in adults: I. Laboratory and epidemiology observations. Rev. Infect. Dis., *5*:35, 1983.

Wilson, W. R., Geraci, J. E., Danielson, G. K., et al.: Anticoagulant treatment and central nervous system complications in patients with prosthetic valve endocarditis. Circulation, *57*:1004, 1978.

Zwischenberger, J. B., Shalaby, T. Z., and Conti, V. R.: Viable cryopreserved aortic homograft for aortic valve endocarditis and annular abscesses. Ann. Thorac. Surg., *48*:365, 1989.

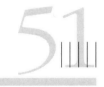

# ■ II Thrombosis and Thromboembolism of Prosthetic Cardiac Valves and Extracardiac Prostheses

David N. Campbell and Frederick L. Grover

## ARTIFICIAL SURFACES, COAGULATION CASCADES, THROMBOSIS, AND LYSIS

Intravascular placement of any foreign body with its nonendothelial surface activates the clotting mechanism and thrombus formation. One possible exception is, of course, an aortic allograft valve or an allograft pulmonary valved conduit. The exposure of blood to the synthetic surface leads rapidly to deposition of a fine layer of plasma components, mostly protein, followed by platelet deposition. The intrinsic coagulation cascade is initiated along with the extrinsic coagulation cascade; the inflammatory response, including leukocyte activation; the complement system; and fibrinolysis.

Fibrinogen is one of the major plasma proteins, often the first, that is deposited on these artificial surfaces. Once the layer of fibrinogen is absorbed onto the surface, platelets can adhere to the fibrinogen. Although surfaces vary greatly in their tendency to promote thrombosis, the reactivity to blood of most materials can be significantly increased if they are

### Surface Activation

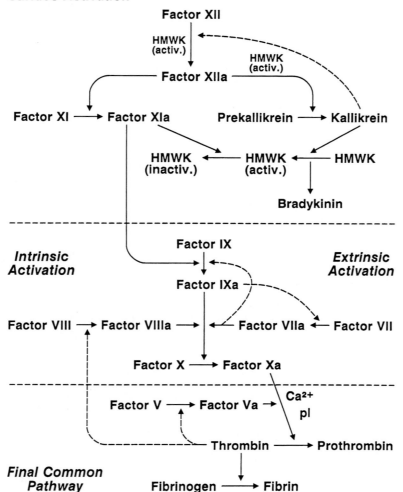

**FIGURE 51–11.** The coagulation cascade from surface activation to the final common pathway. (HMWK = high molecular weight kininogen.) (From Ware, J. A., Lewis, J., and Salzman, E. W.: Antithrombotic therapy. *In* Rutherford, R. B. [ed]: Vascular Surgery. 3rd ed. Philadelphia, W. B. Saunders, 1989.)

first exposed to fibrinogen (Salzman and Merrill, 1987). Other proteins also are deposited, including fibronectin (a surface protein of many cells), von Willebrand's factor (a glycoprotein essential for the adhesion of platelets to subendothelial tissue), thrombospondin (a platelet protein secreted by activated platelets), and Factor XII (Hageman's factor, the primary activator of the intrinsic coagulation system).

Once platelets attach to the protein layer and spread out on the artificial surface, materials present in the platelet intracellular granules are secreted, including beta-thromboglobulin, which inhibits prostacyclin production, platelet Factor IV, which neutralizes heparin sulfate in the endothelium, serotonin, *adenosine triphosphate* (ATP), and *adenosine diphosphate* (ADP). Synthesis of prostaglandins E and F is evident as well, suggesting that endoperoxide metabolism has taken place along with formation of thromboxane $A_2$ from platelet arachidonic acid. Serotonin, thromboxane $A_2$, and endoperoxide are potent vasoconstrictors and platelet stimulatory factors (Mehta and Mehta, 1993). Finally, platelet aggregation follows platelet ad-

hesion, probably by ADP and serotonin secretion from the adherent platelets. Fibrinogen and thromboxane $A_2$ are key in this step.

The coagulation cascade is initiated either by reaction of plasma proteins with the artificial surface to form enzymatically active components such as Factor XII (intrinsic system) or by introduction of thromboplastin via exposure of subendothelial tissue to the surface (extrinsic system). Figure 51–11 is a schematic diagram of the clotting cascade. Activation of Factors XIIa and XIa initiates the intrinsic system leading to activated Factor Xa. Platelets provide the phospholipid surface for this reaction. Activated Factor XIIa also initiates the kininogen-kallikrein system, and kallikrein provides positive feedback for contact activation. Kallikrein cleaves Factor XII to convert it to Factor XIIa, thereby accelerating contact activation. Bradykinin is also released when kallikrein cleaves *high-molecular-weight kininogen* (HMWK). Activated HMWK can then bind more prekallikrein and Factor XI to the activating surface, which further increases the reaction. In the final common pathway, prothrombin is converted to thrombin, and fibrinogen is converted to fibrin. Thrombin recruits more platelets, creating more adhesion and aggregation. A fibrin platelet clot is formed, and thrombosis occurs (Coleman et al., 1987).

Activation of the clotting cascade on the surface of an artificial device occurs similarly whether on a cardiac valve, cardiopulmonary bypass system, vascular graft, *extracorporeal membrane oxygenation* (ECMO) circuit, mechanical assist device, or vascular catheter. It will produce thrombus formation; macroscopic and microscopic platelet-fibrin emboli occur commonly as well (Blauth et al., 1988). Factor XII, kallikrein, and plasmin activate the complement system and activate neutrophils, and kinin formation mediates vasodilatation, vascular permeability, and white blood cell migration. Normally, a delicate balance is maintained between these two systems, so that uncontrolled clotting or hemorrhage does not occur. While the coagulation cascade is initiated, Factor XII and kallikrein initiate clot lysis with conversion of plasminogen to plasmin. Antiplasmins in the circulating blood, particularly alpha$_2$-antiplasmin, rapidly neutralize most of the circulating plasmin; however, plasmin also is incorporated into the clot during clot formation. The fibrin meshwork protects plasmin from antiplasmin once the plasminogen is activated to plasmin, allowing fibrin degradation in the clot. In fact, many natural inhibitors offset activated procoagulant protein. Protein C, heparin, antithrombin III, protein S, thrombomodulin, prostacycline, and plasmin all counter steps in the coagulation cascade (Edmunds, 1987).

## ANTICOAGULATION THERAPY

Clinically useful drugs that block the clotting cascade fall into four primary groups: orally administered vitamin K antagonists, natural anticoagulants such as the heparin–antithrombin III system, antiplatelet drugs, and fibrinolytic agents.

Warfarin sodium is the most popular orally administered vitamin K antagonist used today in the United States. It blocks the formation of the four vitamin K–dependent clotting factors—prothrombin, VII, IX, and X—creating a buildup of their precursors. Warfarin sodium blocks the vitamin K cycle at the regeneration of reduced vitamin K, which is the active form of vitamin K (Fig. 51–12).

Heparin's anticoagulant effect is fairly complex and not completely understood. Heparin sulfate is a glycosaminoglycan that binds to antithrombin III and activates this serine protease inhibitor. Heparin and antithrombin III occur naturally in humans, are secreted by endothelial cells, and are both required to produce their anticoagulant effect. Antithrombin III binds to thrombin and blocks the enzymes of the intrinsic coagulation cascade, including thrombin and Factors IXa, Xa, XIa, and XIIa.

The various antiplatelet drugs have different mechanisms of action, making them more or less useful as therapeutic anticoagulation agents. Figure 51–13 is a schematic diagram of the actions of antiplatelet drugs. Aspirin inhibits platelet aggregation by *irreversible* acetylation of platelet cyclo-oxygenase, hence blocking the synthesis of prostaglandins and thromboxane

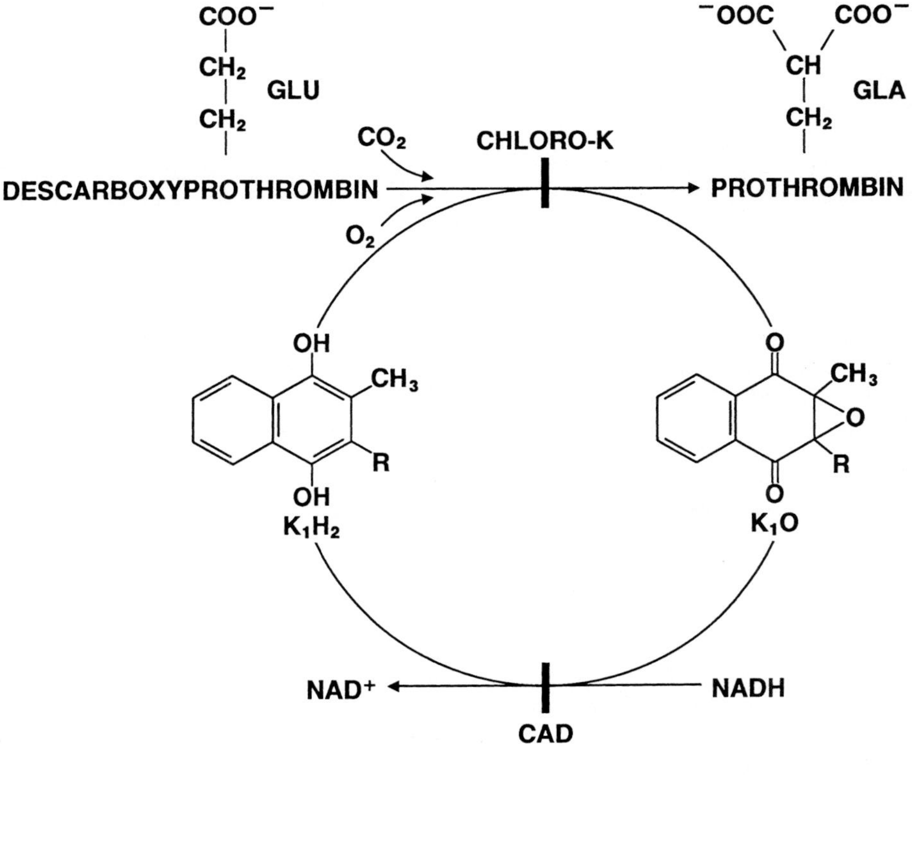

FIGURE 51–12. The vitamin K cycle in the formation of the vitamin K–dependent clotting factors. Vitamin K enters the body and is reduced to vitamin $K_1H_2$. $K_1H_2$ and carboxylase convert vitamin K–dependent clotting factor precursor proteins into active factors, while epoxidase converts vitamin $K_1H_2$ to vitamin $K_1$–epoxide ($K_1O$). Reduced vitamin $K_1H_2$ is regenerated by reduced nicotinamide-adenine dinucleotide (NAD) (NADH) and is the warfarin-sensitive step. (CAD = coumarin-type anticoagulant drugs.) (From O'Reilly, R. A.: Therapeutic modalities for thrombotic disorders: Vitamin K antagonists. *In* Colman, R. W., Hirsh, J., Marder, V. J., and Salzman, E. W. [eds]: Hematosis and Thrombosis. Basic Principles and Clinical Practice. 2nd ed. Philadelphia, J. B. Lippincott, 1987.)

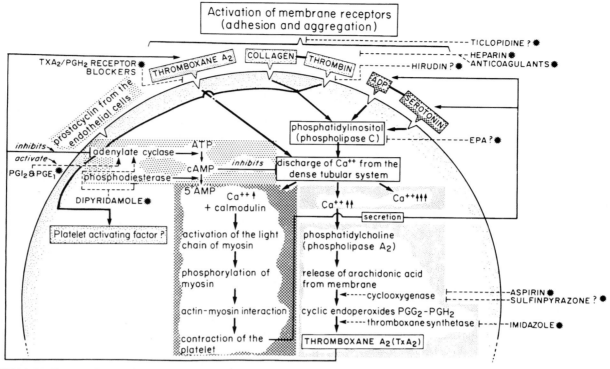

**FIGURE 51–13.** Presumed sites of action of various platelet inhibitors. Cyclic adenosine monophosphate (cAMP) inhibits calcium mobilization from the dense tubular system. *Asterisks* indicate a platelet inhibitor drug. *Dashed lines* indicate the presumed site of action of the drug. (From Stein, B., Fuster, V., Israel, D. H., et al.: Platelet inhibitor agents in cardiovascular disease; An update. Reprinted with permission from the American College of Cardiology [Journal of the American College of Cardiology, 1989, Vol. 14, pp. 813–836].)

$A_2$. Aspirin *will* prolong the bleeding time, and its effect lasts for about 10 days (the life of the platelet). Dipyridamole, on the other hand, is a *reversible* antiplatelet agent, a weak vasodilator, and a weak inhibitor of the enzyme phosphodiesterase, which degrades cyclic adenosine monophosphate (AMP) to 5' AMP. With this block, more cyclic AMP is available to inhibit platelet aggregation. Sulfinpyrazone appears to *reversibly* block platelet prostaglandin synthesis and is another fairly weak anticoagulant. Low-molecular-weight dextran prevents platelet adhesion and aggregation by a mechanism that also is poorly understood. At clinical dosages, neither dipyridamole nor sulfinpyrazone prolongs the bleeding time.

Finally, fibrinolytic therapy has a small but definite place in the management of thrombosis of artificial devices. *Streptokinase* (SK) and *urokinase* (UK) act similarly and induce rapid thrombolysis by activating plasminogen and subsequently forming plasmin. Plasmin causes degradation of the fibrin, reducing thrombus size. Unfortunately, SK and UK also induce a generalized plasma protolytic state as well as local fibrin degradation in the thrombus, and this can lead to uncontrolled hemorrhage. Newer agents (second-generation plasminogen activators) such as recombinant tissue plasminogen activator were developed to prevent induction of this generalized plasma protolytic state by making these agents fibrin-specific. However, this function appears to depend on the dose, and clinical use has not confirmed the decrease

in potential for hemorrhage that was hoped for with these drugs.

In clinical practice, anticoagulant therapy for artificial devices placed in the bloodstream, particularly artificial valves, is based primarily on the orally administered vitamin K antagonists (warfarin sodium). Warfarin therapy is managed by following the prothrombin time and maintaining it in a therapeutic range of 1.5 to 2 times normal or 3 to 4.5 international normalized ratios (Chesebro et al., 1983; Edmunds, 1987; Hirsh et al., 1986; Poller, 1985). However, many things affect the level, including foods high in vitamin K (such as broccoli), liver disease, gut absorption, and albumin binding. Therefore, 30 to 50% of all measured prothrombin times in patients with prosthetic valves are outside the therapeutic range (Chesebro et al., 1983), and close follow-up of any patient is necessary. Several studies with prosthetic valves, including those by Sullivan and co-workers (1971), Altman and colleagues (1976), and Dale and associates (1977), have shown the benefit of adding antiplatelet therapy to warfarin.

It is well recognized that with artificial devices, particularly prosthetic heart valves, platelet survival time is decreased significantly and correlates closely with increased platelet activation and deposition (Weily et al., 1974). Addition of an antiplatelet drug (aspirin, dipyridamole, or sulfinpyrazone) normalizes platelet survival time, indicating a block in the thrombotic process (Harker and Slichter, 1970; Steele et al.,

1975; Weily et al., 1974). Several studies document a decrease in the incidence of thromboembolism in patients receiving both orally administered vitamin K antagonist anticoagulation and aspirin. However, the risk of gastrointestinal bleeding was significantly higher with the concomitant use of aspirin (Chesebro et al., 1981, 1983; Dale et al., 1980). Therefore, aspirin should not be used with warfarin because of excessive bleeding complications.

Use of antiplatelet agents alone is strongly discouraged with mechanical valves, except possibly for a St. Jude valve placed in the aortic position in a child. Verrier and associates (1986) reported that children with mechanical aortic valves and in normal sinus rhythm can be treated safely with antiplatelet agents alone with little or no risk of thrombotic events, including valve thrombosis or valve failure. Rao and colleagues (1989) found that aspirin plus dipyridamole was adequate for mechanical aortic valves in children, but warfarin was necessary with double valves or a valve in the mitral position. Robbins and associates (1988) had similar findings. Sade initially indicated that the St. Jude valve could be placed in children without anticoagulation (Pass et al., 1984) but, after 7 years of follow-up, reported an excessive thromboembolic rate when no anticoagulation was used (Sade et al., 1988). Yet Sade was unable to answer the question of whether it was necessary to provide full anticoagulation with coumadin or whether use of antiplatelet agents alone was adequate. Other studies have suggested that antiplatelet agents alone in adults and children provide adequate anticoagulation (Hartz et al., 1986; Ilbawi et al., 1987; Makhlouf et al., 1987), but most patients with mechanical valves should undergo anticoagulation with warfarin unless they are at high risk for bleeding.

For tissue bioprostheses, the decision of whether to use anticoagulation is more difficult. In the initial 3- to 6-month period following implantation, the risk of thrombus formation on the sewing ring is increased, so anticoagulation is usually recommended. Most centers use warfarin sodium, but aspirin alone has been used if the patients tend to bleed (McGrath et al., 1987; Myers et al., 1989; Ribeiro et al., 1986; Schaffer et al., 1987). Warfarin sodium often is continued indefinitely if the patient is older or has atrial fibrillation, ventricular function, a history of emboli, or a valve placed in the mitral position. Results of a multicenter study suggest that left dimension is not independently related to the development of systemic embolism in patients undergoing valve replacement (Burchfiel et al., 1990). Edmunds (1987) believes that neither warfarin nor antiplatelet drugs are justified from the time of bioprosthetic valve replacement unless *more* than one of the mentioned risk factors for systemic embolization are present.

Full anticoagulation with heparin is used for cardiopulmonary bypass, intra-aortic balloon assist devices, ECMO circuits, and mechanical assist devices. During bypass, *activated clotting times* (ACTs) are employed. The ACT should be maintained above 400 seconds, because clot has been shown to form below this value (Young et al., 1978). If a mechanical assist device is to remain in a patient for a prolonged period, the patient may be switched to orally administered anticoagulation with warfarin sodium. The addition of antiplatelet therapy in this group of patients, particularly those on cardiopulmonary bypass or ECMO circuits, has had significant theoretical support but *no* clear clinical advantage. Cardiopulmonary bypass requires that the blood come into extensive contact with the tubing, heat exchanger, reservoir, and oxygenator, either bubble or membrane. Platelets become activated, form aggregates, and release thromboxane $A_2$. However, membrane oxygenators are much less likely to cause severe damage to the blood than bubble oxygenators, and 20-$\mu$m millipore filters (Ware et al., 1982) are usually employed to remove the platelet aggregates that may form to prevent microemboli, particularly to the brain.

Initially, thrombosis is the major problem, but in time hemorrhage becomes the more significant complication as heparin is continued; platelet function is severely disturbed; thrombocytopenia occurs secondary to dilution, consumption, and sequestration of the platelets in the reticuloendothelial cell system; and fibrinolysis is initiated. For this reason, inhibition of platelet activation while the patient is on cardiopulmonary bypass has been tried with infusion of prostaglandin $E_1$ and *prostacyclin* ($PGE_2$). These agents block platelet adhesion and aggregation by increasing platelet cyclic AMP. However, hypotension from vasodilatation has been a significant problem, and several studies have shown no true benefit (Faichney et al., 1982; Fish et al., 1986; Malpass et al., 1984). New studies using aprotinin with cardiopulmonary bypass are more promising. Aprotinin is a serine protease inhibitor that has been shown to be a powerful antithrombolytic agent, and it is being used with increasing frequency to reduce perioperative and postoperative blood loss during open heart surgery. Aprotinin may also have some antiplatelet effect, which preserves platelet function during cardiopulmonary bypass and adds to the ability to clot postoperatively, thereby decreasing blood loss. Mohr and associates (1992) suggested that aprotinin has a known antifibrinolytic effect and may protect postoperative platelet aggregation by inhibiting the high deleterious plasmin levels. This probably occurs through preservation of the glycoprotein Ib and glycoprotein IIb-IIIa receptors.

Finally, fibrinolytic therapy has been used to declot valves to avoid high-risk emergency operations. All prosthetic valves, including bioprostheses, are subject to thrombosis (Baciewicz et al., 1990; Deviri et al., 1991; Kurzrok et al., 1987; Lesnefsky et al., 1986; Martinell et al., 1987; Prabha et al., 1986). Some authors recommend that patients who are stable and less critically ill undergo surgery to either declot (Deviri et al., 1991) or remove the valve and replace it with another valve (Martinell et al., 1991). In the case of a mechanical valve, this has usually meant replacement with a bioprosthesis. However, fibrinolytic therapy as the primary and sole method of treatment for both left- and right-sided thrombosed valves has gained considerable support (Czer et al., 1985; Graver et al., 1988; Kurzrok et al., 1987; Ledain et al., 1986; Roudaut et al., 1992; Silber et al., 1993; Witchitz et al., 1980).

## Complications of Orally Administered Anticoagulants

### Warfarin Sodium

Bleeding is obviously the most common and most significant complication encountered with the use of warfarin, and therefore close monitoring of the prothrombin time is mandatory. Excessive amounts of warfarin that increase the prothrombin time beyond 2.5 times control will increase bleeding complications 4 to 8 times (Coon and Willis, 1974; Edmunds, 1987; Forfar, 1979; Levine et al., 1986). The gastrointestinal tract is the site of most bleeding complications and is often associated with pre-existing disease states such as peptic ulcer, gastritis, genitourinary lesions, cancer, and hypertension. Another significant complication of *initial* warfarin therapy is skin necrosis. This is secondary to a temporary hypercoagulable state induced in the capillaries when the concentration of protein C (a natural vitamin K–dependent and coumadin-sensitive anticoagulant that circulates in the blood) falls before warfarin's inhibition of factors II, IX, and X becomes effective and the desired hypocoagulable state occurs. The activated form of protein C is a powerful inactivator of Factors V and VIII. Why this is limited to the skin is unknown (Crouse and Comp, 1986). When used in pregnant women, warfarin can cause embryopathy in 4 to 8% of fetuses exposed in the first trimester, and exposure to warfarin in the second and third trimester causes central nervous system abnormalities in 3% of pregnancies. Finally, prematurity, fetal hemorrhage, and stillbirth are increased in babies exposed to warfarin (Edmunds, 1987; Hall et al., 1980; Iturbe-Alessio et al., 1986; Larrea et al., 1983; Lutz et al., 1978; Salazar et al., 1984). For this reason, bioprostheses or allografts should always be placed, when possible, in women of childbearing age.

### Heparin-Sulfate System

Again, the most common complication of heparin therapy is bleeding. Hemorrhagic complications occur in 10 to 20% of patients with normal hemostasis and in up to 50% of patients with thrombocytopenia or uremia (Ware et al., 1989). Thrombocytopenia has been reported in 31% of patients and can cause significant morbidity and mortality when associated with platelet clumping and thrombosis. This thrombocytopenia appears to be immunologic and occurs more commonly with the use of bovine lung heparin. Interestingly, fractions of heparin that display this effect have the least anticoagulant activity, so the use of low-molecular-weight heparin with high anticoagulant effect and low ability to lead to platelet clump-

ing may become clinically important in the future (Ware et al., 1989).

### Antiplatelet Agents: Aspirin

Use of aspirin with orally administered anticoagulants should be avoided because of the reports of excessive bleeding. However, aspirin does not cause a generalized bleeding abnormality except in patients with an underlying hemostatic defect, such as hemophilia or uremia. In fact, aspirin may uncover a mild hemorrhagic disorder or vascular defect by inducing bleeding when used therapeutically (Fuster et al., 1993).

## PROSTHETIC HEART VALVES

McGoon (1984), Edmunds (1982, 1987), Edmunds and co-workers (1988), and Cohn (1990) have detailed the need for standardized reporting of thrombotic complications, including uniform definitions, stratification of the data to include the severity of the event including death, and careful complete long-term follow-up. Without this standardization, it is difficult to make accurate statements about results, complications, and appropriate anticoagulation therapy.

Likewise, it is difficult to compare valves placed in the 1960s and 1970s and their associated complications with valves placed in the 1980s and 1990s and their complications. Today, only four mechanical valves are approved by the Food and Drug Administration for use in the United States (Akins, 1991): the Starr-Edwards Model 1260 Aortic Valve and the 6120 Mitral Valve, the St. Jude Bileaflet Valve, the Hall-Medtronic Tilting Disk Valve, and the Omniscience Tilting Disk Valve.

Through the years, bioengineering advances have led to fewer thrombogenic materials, such as carbon pyrolite for the St. Jude valve, and a better mechanical valve design has decreased the incidence of valve thrombosis and thromboembolism through greater central flow characteristics. However, more effective anticoagulation has been the most important factor for the decreased incidence of thrombotic events in the 1980s and 1990s as compared with the 1960s and 1970s, particularly with mechanical valves. Bioprosthetic valves have less inherent thrombogenicity, but this is due to better central flow characteristics, flexible leaflets, and sinusoidal washout more than to true thromboresistance of the preserved tissue (Magilligan et al., 1984). At present, two porcine xenograft valves are used: the Hancock and the Carpentier Edwards Glutaraldehyde Preserved Valves. Several pericardial valves also have been used. These include the Ionescu-Shiley Pericardial Valve and the Hancock Pericardial Valve, both of which have been withdrawn from use in the United States. The Carpentier Edwards Pericardial Aortic Valve is the only remaining pericardial valve being implanted today. The major problem with the former two pericardial xenograft valves was their durability. Both valves developed tearing of the cusps secondary to stress after only a few years of use (Trowbridge et al., 1988).

Most prosthetic valves have a sewing ring that is covered with a Dacron or Teflon cloth. When this is exposed to the blood, an adherent layer of thrombus is laid down and serves as a blood-compatible coating. It is initially thin and delicate but later becomes invaded by well-vascularized fibrous tissue. This resists further formation of thrombus (Isom et al., 1973). However, if the flow pattern is abnormal, this tissue ingrowth can creep into the orifice from below the valve sewing ring, forming an *obstructive pannus*. Recent reports of "stentless" insertion of xenografts (Angell et al., 1992; David et al., 1990; Hofig et al., 1992; Pillai et al., 1993) have indicted that placement of porcine xenografts in the aortic root with either a cylinder of xenograft tissue or a thin Dacron support cylinder has shown excellent early hemodynamic results without any evidence of thromboembolic events in a small number of patients. These results are encouraging, but a much longer follow-up is needed. Finally, as mentioned earlier, allograft aortic valves and pulmonary valved conduits have almost normal platelet survival time and do not form thrombi.

All prosthetic valves, including bioprostheses, may develop thrombotic occlusion, but the incidence is higher for the mechanical valve, specifically the ball-caged valve and the tilting disk valve. The thrombosis is usually more acute, presenting as "sudden" valve dysfunction with clinical shock, pulmonary edema, and loss of valve click sounds in mechanical valves and muffled sounds in bioprostheses. The diagnosis is made by fluoroscopy or two-dimensional echocardiography, or both. Mortality is high without treatment, either fibrinolytic therapy or reoperation. The incidence of this complication is less than 0.3 per 100 patient-years, except for the Omniscience Tilting Disk Valve placed in the mitral position, which has significantly higher incidence of thrombosis (Edmunds, 1987).

The incidence of all thrombotic complications, including thromboembolic events for a mechanical aortic prosthesis, is about 1 to 2% per patient-year, whereas the rate for bioprosthetic valves in the aortic position is about half that of the mechanical prostheses (Edmunds, 1987). The risk of a bleeding complication is, however, significantly higher for the mechanical valves because of the use of anticoagulants, particularly warfarin sodium.

The incidence of thrombotic complications for a prosthetic mitral valve is similar in mechanical and bioprosthesis, except for the Omniscience valve. There is little difference between the two valve positions (aortic and mitral) and between the use of a mitral prosthesis alone or a combined aortic and mitral prosthesis. However, fatal thrombotic events occur 2 to 4 times more often in patients with mechanical valves (Edmunds, 1987). Hammermeister and the Veterans Affairs Cooperative Study on Valvular Heart Disease (1993) concluded that after 11 years, the rates of survival and freedom from all valve-related complications were similar for patients who received mechanical heart valves and for those who received bioprostheses. Structural failure, however, was observed only with the bioprosthetic valves, and bleeding complications were statistically more frequent among patients who received mechanical valves. Hammond and associates (1987), in another study of 1012 adult patients who underwent placement of either a mechanical valve or a bioprosthesis with a follow-up of 4814 patient-years, found little direct evidence to strongly support the generalized use of one type of valve over another.

Unfortunately, bioprostheses have a very high failure rate in children, probably due to accelerated calcium metabolism, and there is currently a renewed interest in the use of both fresh and commercially available frozen allograft valves for children and young adults to prevent anticoagulation. The risk of thrombotic or thromboembolic events using allograft aortic valves in the subcoronary position, as a free-sewn graft or using the root replacement technique in which a cylinder including the valve is placed by the technique of Ross (Sommerville and Ross, 1982), is nearly zero *without anticoagulation*. Matsuki and co-workers (1988b) reported on 555 consecutive hospital survivors who underwent isolated aortic valve replacement using a free-sewn allograft. The incidence of thromboembolism was 0.034% per patient-year, or 1 patient of the 555 studied. Results with the aortic root replacement in 108 patients reported by Okita and associates (1988) showed no incidence of thromboembolism in 180 patient-years of follow-up. Penta and colleagues (1984) likewise found no incidence of thrombosis or thromboemboli in 140 consecutive patients who underwent homograft replacement of the aortic valve and were followed for a minimum of 10 years. Many of these valves were either fresh or antibiotic-preserved valves. O'Brien and associates (1987) reported on a comparison of aortic valve replacements with viable cryopreserved and fresh allograft valves. The freedom from thromboembolism for both groups was 97% at 10 years and 96% at 15 years, but the reoperation rate for valve failure was much greater in the fresh valves. O'Brien believes that cryopreserved valves are superior because fibroblastic cell viability is preserved, providing durability.

The fate of the aortic valve or pulmonary valve used as a conduit to reconstruct the right ventricular outflow tract is not so clear. Bull and associates (1987) reported on 249 patients who received extracardiac conduits in the right side of the heart. Of the 173 patients who survived 30 days, 72 underwent placement of antibiotic sterilized aortic homografts, 97 underwent placement of xenografts conduits of various types, and 4 underwent placement of valveless tubes. The complication and reoperation rates for both valved conduit groups were similar. Calcification of the allograft tube occurred commonly, but, interestingly, the obstruction tended to be at the proximal portion of the conduit where Dacron extensions, which are circumferential, were commonly placed. The development of a neointimal peel in this position led to the obstruction in over two-thirds of patients.

If a *noncircumferential* proximal hood is used, thrombus and neointimal peel formation is minimal, and obstruction is markedly decreased. Livi and associates (1987) have shown that the valve of choice for right ventricular outflow tract reconstruction is, in fact, the pulmonary allograft rather than the aortic allograft. Finally, Matsuki and associates (1988a) have used the pulmonary autograft valve (the patient's own pulmonary valve) to replace the aortic valve with excellent results (Ross' procedure). However, this requires reconstruction of the right ventricular outflow tract with a pulmonary or aortic allograft, essentially giving the patient disease of two valves rather than the one-valve disease the patient had originally. Despite this, Matsuki and associates (1988a) have shown excellent results with this technique.

Several general rules make some clinically applicable sense out of all of these sometimes conflicting data. For children, aortic valve replacement should be carried out either with a mechanical valve such as the St. Jude Bileaflet Valve, or with aortic root replacement using an aortic allograft, as described by Ross. As more experience is gained with the pulmonary autograft technique to replace the aortic valve, this may become the method of choice for aortic valve replacement in children. For mitral valve replacement in children, mechanical valves are required, and these patients should undergo full anticoagulation with warfarin. Porcine xenograft bioprostheses should not be used because of the rapid calcification and degeneration that occurs with these valves in children. Similar guidelines should be followed for young adults. For women who are of childbearing age or wish to have children, mechanical valves should be strongly *discouraged*. The complications of anticoagulation, particularly with warfarin sodium and heparin, place the young woman and unborn child at too great a risk. For nonchildbearing women and for men under 60, individual differences in the patients and their desired lifestyle following valve replacement should be strongly considered in choosing the valve. Finally, probably for patients over the age of 60 but definitely for those over 70, the use of porcine xenograft bioprostheses or aortic allografts should be strongly considered in view of the decreased degeneration rate of these valves in older patients and the higher risk of anticoagulation in this patient population.

## CARDIOPULMONARY BYPASS CIRCUITS

The harmful effects of cardiopulmonary bypass result from the large surface interface of blood with the artificial materials in the circuitry, including the tubing, the oxygenator, the heat exchanger, the cardiotomy reservoir, and the blood suction system. Although technologic advances such as the hollow-fiber membrane oxygenator have removed a few of these negative effects (van Oeveren et al., 1985), major hemologic complications continue to contribute to major operative and postoperative morbidity and mortality. Respiratory distress, postoperative bleeding, para-

doxic thrombosis, increased susceptibility to infection, and multiorgan failure have been linked to the thrombocytopenia, platelet dysfunction, leukopenia and leukocyte activation, complement activation, and other changes in plasma proteins, particularly during routine periods of hypothermia during cardiopulmonary bypass. All the components of the humoral amplification system are activated by the bypass circuitry, including the coagulation cascade, the fibrinolytic system, the kallikrein system, the complement system, and the leukocyte inflammatory system (Kirklin et al., 1983).

In blood, only Factor XII (Hageman's factor) and platelets are directly activated by initial contact with foreign surfaces. On the other hand, prekallikrein, HMWK, and Factor XI—the three other primary proteins of the contact activation system—are rapidly activated after Factor XII is activated. This system initiates the inflammatory response, which includes the coagulation system, complement activation, fibrinolysis, kinin formation, and neutrophil activation (Edmunds et al., 1991). Blood component trauma occurs throughout the circuitry as the blood passes through the silicon rubber or polyurethane tubing and is exposed to high sheer stress, turbulence, and complex hydrolytic stresses while it is constantly deformed by the passage of the components through the roller pump, the heat exchanger, and the gas exchange device (Coleman et al., 1987). Centrifugal pump devices such as the Medtronic Bio-Medicus are less traumatic to the blood but still lead to hemostatic dysfunction.

Abnormal bleeding after cardiopulmonary bypass is a problem in about 2 to 5% of patients (Harker et al., 1980). This is significantly increased for ECMO because of the greater time the circuitry is required, anywhere from several hours to several weeks in duration. Platelet numbers are reduced, platelet function is markedly impaired, platelet release products from platelet granules appear in the plasma, and excessive fibrinolysis may occur. Platelet numbers are decreased primarily because of hemodilution, but also because some activated platelets are damaged and are removed by the reticuloendothelial system. Other activated platelets adhere to the foreign surfaces through membrane receptor links with fibrinogen, platelet adhesive receptors (glycoprotein Ib), and aggregating receptors (glycoprotein complex IIb/IIIa).

The most important of these platelet factors is platelet dysfunction. Platelet dysfunction occurs very early during the first pass of blood through the cardiopulmonary bypass circuit (van Oeveren et al., 1990). The platelets are activated, and contractile platelet elements cause a sequence of typical morphologic alterations called the "platelet shape change." Interestingly, the platelet morphology returns to normal although the stimulus of cardiopulmonary bypass continues. Most platelets return to the blood milieu, with only a few passing through adhesion to irreversible "secondary" aggregation with release of their specific granules. "Alpha granules" release platelet Factor IV, beta-thromboglobulin, and fibrinogen, whereas "dense granules" release ADP, ATP, serotonin, and calcium (Zilla et al., 1989). During bypass, these platelets become less responsive to soluble agonists with time, which indicates this increased platelet dysfunction (Edmunds and Williams, 1983).

Wenger and associates (1989) have suggested that as bypass begins, platelets are activated by ADP released from hemolyzed red cells or release of human neutrophil elastase by activation of the contact pathway. The *fibrinogen receptors* (glycoprotein IIb/IIIa) of the activated platelets are exposed, and the platelets adhere to the surface of absorbed fibrinogen. Some pull away, have fewer glycoprotein IIb/IIIa receptors, and hence are not fully functional. Van Oeveren and co-workers (1990) found no change in the platelet membrane glycoprotein-aggregating complex IIb/IIIa between a control group and a group given aprotinin. However, there was a significant decrease in the platelet membrane adhesive Ib glycoproteins in the control group, suggesting that this occurs routinely with bypass. *Von Willebrand's factor* (vWF) is required in platelet adhesion, and the platelet glycoprotein Ib receptor is the primary target for vWF. This theory is supported by improvement in hemostasis after bypass with desmopressin acetate, which increases levels of vWF (Czer et al., 1987; Salzman et al., 1986).

Heparin is the primary anticoagulant that blocks formation of thrombin and fibrin deposition, but several other agents have been used during cardiopulmonary bypass along with heparin to decrease the deleterious effects of activation of blood components, particularly platelets. These include the antiplatelet agents dipyridamole and desmopressin acetate, prostanoids including prostaglandin $E_1$, prostacyclin, and iloprost, aprotinin, and epsilon-aminocaproic acid. Interestingly, heparin by itself can inhibit platelet function (John et al., 1993).

Unfortunately, aspirin increases postcardiotomy bleeding in patients undergoing cardiopulmonary bypass when given preoperatively because of its irreversibility (Goldman et al., 1991). However, dipyridamole has been shown to preserve platelet counts by reducing platelet activation, aggregation, and depletion through inhibition of platelet phosphodiesterase activity and increasing cyclic AMP concentration. Clinically, this has reduced postoperative blood loss (Hicks et al., 1985; Teoh et al., 1988). Results of studies with desmopressin acetate, as mentioned earlier, have shown shortened bleeding time and increased plasma levels of vWF.

The results with the use of prostanoids have been mixed. Addonizio and associates (1978, 1979) demonstrated that prostacyclin preserved platelet function during *simulated* cardiopulmonary bypass and ECMO. However, hypotension was a problem. Fish and colleagues (1986) studied prostacyclin in a randomized, double-blind study of patients undergoing coronary bypass operations. Prostacyclin preserved platelet numbers, decreased granule release, reduced the bleeding time, and reduced early blood loss. However, hypotension caused by vasodilatation, a significant side effect, tempered the authors' enthusiasm

for its routine use. Malpass and colleagues (1984), Faichney and co-workers (1982), and DiSesa and associates (1984), however, found no platelet-sparing effect of prostacyclin. More recent studies with cardiopulmonary bypass and ECMO circuits with iloprost, a prostacyclin analogue, have been more encouraging (Addonizio et al., 1985; Cottrell et al., 1988).

Aprotinin is a serum protease inhibitor that is effective against trypsin, chymotrypsin, plasmin, and kallikreins. By blocking plasmin, it blocks a major activator of the fibrinolytic system. Its more important effect, however, may be in blocking kallikreins. Kallikreins act as plasminogen activators leading to plasmin formation and can be activated by Factor XIIa (activated by contact with the artificial tubing in the bypass circuit). They can in turn activate more Factor XII. Kallikrein also accelerates the "cold dependent" activation of Factor VII, leading to activation of the extrinsic pathway during hypothermia used commonly with cardiopulmonary bypass. Finally, kallikrein activates the kinin and complement systems (Havel et al., 1991) and activates leukocytes. Blocking the kallikrein system with aprotinin, therefore, may block all five systems, including the coagulation system, complement system, fibrinolysis system, kinin system, and inflammatory system (Wachtfogel et al., 1993). The primary effect of aprotinin is probably to stabilize platelet function through a preserved adhesive capacity of platelets (Bidstrup et al., 1989; Mohr et al., 1992; van Oeveren et al., 1990). Edmunds and co-workers (1991) have suggested that plasmin, generated during cardiopulmonary bypass, activates platelets and causes changes in the platelet membrane glycoproteins IIb/IIIa and Ib. These activated platelets become nonreactive, and lower temperatures probably enhance this effect. Aprotinin blocks the plasmin and hence adhesion and aggregation of the platelets. A few believe that aprotinin's major effect is on the prevention of hyperfibrinolysis and not on the platelets (Havel et al., 1991; Huang et al., 1993). Concern about renal dysfunction and coronary graft thrombosis has been raised with aprotinin (Cosgrove et al., 1992), but this may be unwarranted, because the incidence of reported renal dysfunction is quite low, and when it occurs it is usually mild (Blauhut et al., 1991). However, care must be taken when aprotinin is used during cardiopulmonary bypass. For now it probably should only be used in high-risk groups, particularly those undergoing reoperation or those with endocarditis. It should be remembered that aprotinin prolongs the ACT independently of heparin and is a procoagulant. Therefore, ACTs need to be maintained around 750 seconds or greater to prevent clotting (Hunt et al., 1992).

It is also clear that excessive fibrinolysis can occur during cardiopulmonary bypass (Lambert et al., 1979), but its occurrence is uncommon with adequate heparinization. Van der Salm and colleagues (1988) have suggested the routine use of *epsilon-aminocaproic acid* (EACA), a clotting agent, following cardiopulmonary bypass, as did Lambert and colleagues (1979). However, consumption coagulopathy (secondary disseminated intravascular coagulation) is more likely to occur than primary fibrinolysis, because platelets aggregate during cardiopulmonary bypass and this may be accelerated by complement activation. Clinically important primary fibrinolysis for which EACA should be used is uncommon following cardiac surgery, and administration of EACA in a routine situation would only make platelet consumption worse. Therefore, its routine use cannot be recommended.

## EXTRACORPOREAL MEMBRANE OXYGENATION SYSTEMS

Use of ECMO circuitry (more appropriately called extracorporeal life support [ECLS]) has had renewed interest over the last decade. Initial reports by Hill and co-workers (1972) and Bartlett and co-workers (1977a) have led to its use in over 6000 patients since 1972. The survival rate is high for infants treated for respiratory failure (80 to 90%), particularly when meconium aspiration or blood aspiration is involved (90 to 100% survival). The results are less impressive for sepsis, persistent primary pulmonary hypertension, and respiratory distress syndrome. Initially, venoarterial access was employed (Bartlett et al., 1977b), but more recently Gattinoni and associates (1986) and Sinard and Bartlett (1990) favored the use of venovenous access if cardiac function is normal. This eliminates the need for constant mechanical ventilation and prevents overventilation and distention of the alveoli by providing low continuous positive pressure inflation.

Following excellent results in neonates, ECLS has been employed in nearly 200 children for respiratory failure and in over 200 pediatric patients for cardiac failure (often secondary to cardiac surgery and the inability bypass). This experience has not been as rewarding, with only 44% of pediatric pulmonary patients successfully weaned off ECMO and 43% successfully weaned off ECMO for cardiac failure (Meliones et al., 1991). More adults are also being placed on ECLS for a variety of indications, including both pulmonary and cardiac failure. Early experience with such use has shown a similar recovery rate of 40% (Anderson et al., 1992).

Complications with ECMO or ECLS are similar to those with cardiopulmonary bypass but are amplified because of the prolonged time required for support. Heparin is required to maintain the ACT at 180 to 200 seconds, though some centers have recommended ACTs as high as 250 to 300 seconds. Platelet counts often are markedly decreased, and significant bleeding complications occur in 10 to 75% of patients. Platelet counts should be maintained well above 50,000, with several centers recommending well above 100,000. If counts drop below 50,000 to 100,000, platelet transfusions should be given. Application of biologic glue to the neck cannula sites has decreased the bleeding in neonates at the surgical site (Moront et al., 1988). However, intracranial bleeding remains a significant problem. Mediastinal hemorrhage in pa-

tients placed on ECLS for cardiac failure is likewise a significant problem (Sell et al., 1986).

Recent reports of the successful clinical use of nitric oxide (endothelial-derived relaxing factor) by Roberts and associates (1991, 1992), and Kinsella and colleagues (1992) have markedly decreased the need for ECMO in neonates in those centers where it is being studied. Nitric oxide directly stimulates cyclic AMP in vascular smooth muscle, causing relaxation. When given by inhalation, it selectively dilates the pulmonary vascular bed.

## VALVED AND NONVALVED VASCULAR PROSTHESES IN THE THORACIC AORTA

Prosthetic vascular grafts used in the thorax are for the most part large-diameter conduits with high-low and low-resistance characteristics. Thrombosis and thromboembolism rarely occur, and 5- to 10-year patency rates of 80 to 90% are common (Claggett, 1987). Smaller conduits using Dacron or *polytetrafluoroethylene* (PTFE), particularly for coronary revascularization wherein the diameter is 4 mm or smaller, have a much poorer patency rate. Most reports indicate less than 67% patency at 1 year (Islam et al., 1981; Molina et al., 1978; Murtra et al., 1985; Yokoyama et al., 1978). Coronary grafts using autologous saphenous vein have a significantly better patency rate than synthetic materials, but because of damage of the endothelium with preparation (high potassium flush, devascularization, rapid distention, arterial pulsatile flow), platelet deposition occurs, followed by thrombus formation. The reported 1-year patency rate is 80%, and the 10-year patency rate is 40%, considerably worse than the internal mammary artery graft, which has a 10-year patency rate of 85 to 90%. This appears to be due to much greater progression of atherosclerosis in the vein graft compared with the arterial graft, because the vein graft is not designed by nature to handle high-pressure flow as well as the artery (Loop et al., 1986).

Large grafts made out of low-porosity woven or velour-knitted Dacron are often preclotted with albumin, platelets, plasma, or unheparinized blood. If a composite valved conduit is used, the mechanical valve is protected from the preclotting solution, and the graft is autoclaved at 270° F for 5 minutes. A knitted graft must be preclotted because the fabric weave is very porous. Woven grafts are much less porous, and preclotting is optional but still a good idea. PTFE grafts are not very low-porous and do not require preclotting. However, both Dacron and PTFE similarly form an internal neointimal layer.

Following implantation of the prosthesis, a fibrin-platelet thrombus is rapidly deposited on the surface, indicated by a rapid decrease in platelet survival time (Harker et al., 1977). Over the first year, the platelet survival normalizes (McCollum et al., 1981; Stratton et al., 1983) but the graft does not become endothelialized at the anastomotic sites (Sauvage et al., 1975), where fibrous intimal hyperplasia may lead to late graft obstruction and thrombosis. Instead, the surface is covered with a compacted fibrin layer overlying a collagenous matrix (Fig. 51–14). With Dacron grafts, fibroblasts are dispersed sporadically throughout this matrix, secondary to ingrowth through the interstices of the porous graft wall. PTFE graft has a similar neointima except that fibroblasts are not present, because the interstices are much less porous. Roughened velour material has been implemented to promote fibroblastic infiltration through the more porous knitted Dacron interstices, enhance growth of the neointima, and decrease thrombogenicity. However, the roughness of the velour surface may, in fact, promote thrombosis because of increased platelet adhesion. Whether the internal velour lining is an advantage to help decrease thrombogenicity is still controversial.

PTFE also has been used intrathoracically for construction of aortopulmonary shunts, right ventricular outflow tract nonvalved conduits, and patch repair and interposition graft replacement for coarctation repairs in children with complex coarctation of the thoracic aorta. Gazzania and colleagues (1976) first described the use of PTFE for construction of aortopulmonary shunts, and since then multiple reports have shown excellent palliation with greater than 89% patency at 2 years (de Leval et al., 1981; Donahoo et al., 1980; McKay et al., 1980; Opie et al., 1986). However, complications such as thrombosis, infection, cardiac failure, shunt stenosis, and deformity of the pulmonary arteries occur with the use of PTFE grafts, particularly the grafts that are 4 mm in diameter. The use of 5-mm and 6-mm grafts is encouraged to decrease thrombosis.

Chronic anticoagulation has not been proved necessary and therefore is not used in large thoracic vascular grafts. Mechanical valve aortic conduits require the same anticoagulation regimen that isolated aortic valve replacement with a mechanical valve requires (usually warfarin alone). However, a review by Peigh and co-workers (1990) reported a significantly higher incidence of neurologic and ophthalmologic phenomena after aortic valve conduit surgery. In that study, 27 patients undergoing valved conduit replacement were compared with 21 patients who underwent combined aortic valve replacement and ascending aortic graft replacement, but not as a combined valved conduit. Among the 20 surviving valved conduit patients, 50% experienced repetitive neurologic and visual signs (felt to be embolic), whereas no patient who underwent aortic valve replacement plus ascending aortic graft experienced any events. These authors recommended the addition of antiplatelet therapy which, in their population, seemed to help decrease the incidence with the addition of dipyridamole.

PTFE should only be used in aortocoronary procedures when no autologous vein or intrinsic arterial graft is available (Sapsford et al., 1981). Antiplatelet therapy is advisable (Harker et al., 1977; Oblath et al., 1978), although Kohler and co-workers (1984), in a double-blind, prospective, randomized study of aspirin (325 mg) and dipyridamole (75 mg) 3 times a day, found no beneficial effect in lower-extremity PTFE grafts. PTFE is used extensively for aortopulmonary shunts without anticoagulation primarily because it is a temporary step. Long-term patency usually is not required, and therefore it is important to avoid the effects of over-anticoagulation. Use of 325 mg of aspirin and 75 mg of dipyridamole 3 times a day has been shown to improve saphenous vein graft patency for aortocoronary conduits (Chesebro et al., 1982, 1984), especially when it is started preoperatively, but it is probably most important in the first year following surgery (McEnany et al., 1982). Orally administered anticoagulants have been recommended by some (McEnany et al., 1982) but are probably not advantageous when the increased bleeding complications are considered.

## VENTRICULAR ASSIST DEVICES

*Ventricular assist devices* (VADs) include (1) systems that can be used for separate left-sided heart assist, right-sided heart assist, or both, and (2) the total artificial heart. These systems include pulsatile *external* pneumatic assist devices, such as the Pierce-Donachy VAD and the Abiomed BVS System 5000; *totally implantable* devices, such as the pneumatically driven Thermo Cardiosystems (HeartMate 1000 IP) LVAD and the electrically driven Novacor LVAD; intravascular continuous flow pumps, such as the hemopump; and nonpulsatile centrifugal VADs, such as the Medtronic Bio-Medicus system. Early experience with these devices included a very high complication rate, particularly with bleeding, mediastinitis, and neurologic deficit (Pennington et al., 1988). However, differences in implantation technique, inexperience with these devices, lack of uniform anticoagulation regimen, poor patient selection, delayed implantation, and lack of biventricular support were primarily responsible for the high complication rate (Adamson et al., 1989; Park et al., 1986). More recently, as experience has been gained, use of VADs, either total or

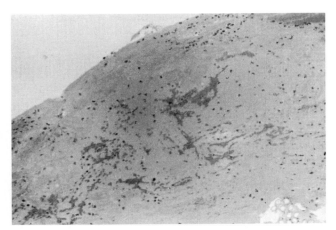

**FIGURE 51–14.** Photomicrograph of thick, compacted fibrin-lined surface of a Dacron double-velour prosthesis after 4 weeks of canine implantation. Note absence of any endothelial cells. (Courtesy of M. B. Herring, M.D.)

partial as a bridge to transplantation, has yielded a much lower incidence of bleeding and thromboembolism (Joyce et al., 1989a; Schoen et al., 1986; Wampler et al., 1991). These patients are all desperately ill and often have some degree of hypotension preimplant. It is thus quite difficult to know whether neurologic complications are due to embolic phenomena or to prolonged hypotension. Walenga and co-workers (1992) studied specific blood markers in patients who underwent placement of the Jarvik 7 total artificial heart and found significant hemostatic abnormalities, including a marked hypercoagulable state, platelet activation even though the platelet count was normal, and excessive fibrinolytic activation. Low levels of protein C and antithrombin III contributed to the hypercoagulable state. It appears that these devices, left in contact with the bloodstream for a long time, disturbed the delicate balance between clotting and lysis. Patients placed on mechanical assist or the total artificial heart should be anticoagulated initially with low-molecular-weight dextran, particularly if they have recently undergone cardiotomy. Then when bleeding is slowed, heparin should be started. Use of an antiplatelet agent, later switching those patients to coumadin, appears to reduce the incidence of thromboembolism, but these patients must be followed closely for excessive bleeding (Joyce et al., 1989b).

Finally, the use of newer biomaterials for the blood sac may decrease thrombus formation even further. A new segmented polyurethane elastomer coated with a 1% concentration of high-molecular-weight polymeric, surface-modifying additive is now being used in the Pierce-Donachy VAD. The surface activity of this additive causes it to migrate to the blood-contacting surface to reduce interfacial energy while still bound to the base polymer (Farrar et al., 1988). Thermo Cardiosystems (HeartMate 1000 IP) has used the design of a textured polyurethane lining rather than the smooth lining in the Pierce-Donachy device. The rationale for this has been to encourage formation of a thin, adherent pseudointima. Initial experience with this lining is encouraging, with no evidence of thromboembolism in 34 patients (Frazier et al., 1992).

## INTRA–AORTIC BALLOON ASSIST DEVICES

Placement of the intra-aortic balloon assist device (known as the IABP, which stands for "intra-aortic balloon pump") remains the first-line therapy for medically refractory angina or cardiac failure either preoperatively or postoperatively, and approximately 70,000 balloons are placed each year (Kantrowitz, 1990). Initially, the intra-aortic balloons were placed directly in the femoral artery with graft extensions, but more recently they have been placed by the femoral or subclavian percutaneous method or with a direct cutdown to the artery and use of the Seldinger technique through the arterial wall, with no graft. A few balloons are placed transthoracically (at the time of open heart surgery) if a balloon cannot be placed

by one of the former techniques (Pappas, 1974). The need for this has decreased with the placement of a guidewire percutaneously, preoperatively in high-risk patients.

The risk of vascular complications, including bleeding, ischemia, thrombosis, and central and peripheral embolism, remains significant, anywhere from 2.5 to 30% in the high-risk patients, particularly females and diabetics. Most reports have found the risk to be greater when the balloon is placed percutaneously (Di Lello et al., 1988; Goldberg et al., 1987; Pennington et al., 1983; Sanfelippo et al., 1986). However, a recent report by Naunheim and co-workers (1992) found no difference overall between the two techniques. Also the vascular complication rate has significantly decreased over the last two decades, probably because of the use of smaller (No. 9.5 French) diameter devices, use of a guidewire, and liberal use of direct visualization of the artery. It is difficult to be sure whether vascular complications are due to pre-existing atherosclerotic vascular disease in these patients, vascular occlusion due to thrombosis, or, more likely, a combination of both. In the report of Naunheim and colleagues, 3.6% of patients required IABP removal, and 3.6% required thrombectomy. Four patients (0.7%) required amputation. Other groups have reported similar thromboembolic complications despite anticoagulation, primarily due to the severity of the atherosclerotic disease. Spinal paralysis, renal failure, and bowel infarction have all been reported (Harris et al., 1986; Jarmolowski and Poirier, 1980; Macoviak et al., 1980). Management of limb ischemia, when it occurs, remains a difficult problem. If the IABP can be removed safely with the patient remaining stable, this should be the procedure of choice. Concomitant thrombectomy may be necessary. Evans (1987) has suggested that simple withdrawal of the sheath from the femoral artery may sometimes be enough to re-establish distal flow, so the balloon does not have to be removed. If an IABP is required, it can be removed after a second is placed in the opposite leg. Other authors have suggested femoral-femoral bypass to relieve the ischemia in the leg receiving the balloon (Alpert et al., 1980b; Gold et al., 1986). More recently, placement of the balloon via the subclavian artery into the thoracic aorta has been suggested so that patients can be mobile while waiting for heart transplantation. Percutaneous removal should be accomplished with temporary manual occlusion of the distal femoral artery while the balloon is removed. The arterial puncture site is not occluded, and blood is allowed to flush out the arterial debris for a few seconds. This will often prevent distal emboli and obviate the need for arterial embolectomy.

Anticoagulation is necessary and is usually accomplished using full-dose heparin or low-molecular-weight dextran if bleeding is a major problem. Clinical reports have shown that endothelial damage occurs secondary to trauma from the balloon, and that platelet counts drop to below 50% of the baseline over several days (Dunkman et al., 1972; McCabe et al., 1978; Weber and Janicki, 1974), probably because of mechanical trauma, adhesion and aggregation, and sequestration. Hoover and associates (1988) have demonstrated that, despite this drop in platelets, prostacyclin levels are significantly elevated, and levels of thromboxane $A_2$ are decreased. The exact significance of this is unknown.

## VASCULAR CATHETERS

Catheters placed for arterial or venous access, including Swan-Ganz catheters, arterial cannulas to monitor blood pressure, central venous lines often for chronic access, and umbilical artery and venous catheters in neonates, all have a high rate of thrombogenicity, approaching 90 to 100%. The major determinants to thrombus formation, however, are size of the vessel in relation to the cannula, flow characteristics of the blood, high flow versus low flow, duration of catheter placement, trauma to the vessel during implantation, and stiffness of the catheter. Microthrombus formation on the catheter may cause infection, which then causes thrombosis of the major vessel.

Radial artery cannulation produces partial or complete thrombosis in up to 25% of patients. However, hand ischemia is uncommon if the ulnar blood supply is adequate (Slogoff et al., 1983). Umbilical artery lines in sick, unstable neonates may lead to aortic thrombosis, visceral ischemia, paraplegia, and lower-extremity ischemia in 1 to 2% of neonates (Alpert et al., 1980a; McFadden and Ochsner, 1983). Local infection occurs in 20% of cases, and sepsis occurs about 4 to 5% of the time (Band and Maki, 1979).

Use of smooth-surface, pliable infusion catheters for chronic indwelling central venous lines, such as the Hickman-Broviac catheters and the Groshong catheters (Broviac et al., 1973; Hickman et al., 1979), has decreased the incidence of major venous thrombosis and thromboembolism, but these conditions still occur in 8% of patients in whom these techniques are used (Thomas et al., 1980). Major venous thrombosis may be tolerated well by children when isolated, but when both superior and inferior venae cavae are occluded (Mulvihill and Fonkalsrud, 1984) or when the occlusion occurs in neonates or infants, major complications may occur, including pulmonary embolus, congestive heart failure, sepsis, and death (Mollitt and Golladay, 1983).

Use of percutaneous placement, careful sterile technique, routine care of the catheters by experienced personnel, and removal of the cannulas and catheters as soon as possible help to keep the thrombus rate low. For chronic indwelling catheters, proper placement in high-flow areas, sterile technique, and careful monitoring for infection are necessary.

Finally, the use of heparin bonding in catheters such as the Swan-Ganz catheter has decreased the incidence of venous thrombosis (Hoar et al., 1981). Reports of successful declotting of infected catheters with thrombolytic therapy may decrease the up to 20% incidence of catheter removal for continued infection and thrombus formation in these often very ill, very small children (Fishbein et al., 1990; Jones et al., 1993; Lacey et al., 1988). In these patients, vascular access is often required for a long period, immunocompromise is common, and repeated implantation of these catheters leads to a higher complication rate.

## THROMBORESISTANT SURFACES

No artificial material today resembles living endothelium in its freedom from activation of the thrombotic process. Research in the past has centered on development of inert materials such as polyurethane and silicone rubber. However, such research may be misdirected, because the role of products of endothelial metabolism, including prostacyclin, the heparin–antithrombin III system, and the thrombomodulin system, in preventing platelet activation on endothelial surface is well known (Salzman and Merril, 1987). Inert materials alone, in vivo, may always require pharmacologic manipulation.

Properties such as surface wettability and surface charge have been thought to be very important. Hydrophilic (wettable) surfaces appear to resist thrombosis better than hydrophobic (nonwettable) surfaces, and materials that combine polyurethane and silicone rubber, taking advantage of this chemical property, appear to be among the most thromboresistant materials made today. Attempts at designing a negatively charged surface that will resist the negatively charged platelets and plasma proteins have not as yet been clinically successful. On the other hand, covalent, heparin-bonded surfaces have been used clinically since Gott first introduced the idea in 1961 (Gott et al., 1961), but the exact mechanism by which the heparin confers thromboresistance to the artificial surface is not clear. One theory is that it is desorbed from the surface and provides a thin film of anticoagulated blood just above the surface. A second theory is that it stays bonded in the material and forms a complex with plasma antithrombin III, providing an anticoagulant effect. However, heparin-bonded surfaces still may not affect platelet deposition, and this whole mechanism of clotting may not be addressed. Despite this, the Gott shunt, which combines a graphite lining with heparin bonding, has been used clinically with great success for many years in repair of thoracic and thoracoabdominal aneurysms. Recent *experimental* work has shown heparin-bonded (Carmeda Bio-Active surface) cardiopulmonary bypass, ventricular assist, and ECMO circuitry to be thromboresistant. This material prevents activation of the complement system and preserves platelet count and function without systemic heparinization (Koul et al., 1992; Saito et al., 1992; Videm et al., 1991; von Segesser and Turina, 1989). Recent *clinical* reports have demonstrated a 45% reduction in complement activation, decreased blood loss, and reduced transfusion requirements, with 25% lower heparin use and with the ACT maintained around 200 seconds (Aranki et al., 1993; Borowiec et al., 1992; Gu et al., 1993; Videm et al., 1992; von Segesser et al., 1992).

It is doubtful that any bioprosthetic material can be made to act like endothelium. Therefore, a major thrust of experimental development of vascular grafts has been to develop truly endothelialized grafts. One approach has been to use selectively *biodegradable* vascular grafts using Dacron coated with either polyethylene oxide polylactic acid (Uretzky et al., 1990) or completely biodegradable grafts of polyurethane and poly-L-lactic acid (van der Lei et al., 1985, 1987). With this technique, a neointima is developed that contains true endothelial cells and smooth muscle cells that migrate from the anastomoses. As the biodegradable lattice disintegrates, fibroblasts migrate inward from the perigraft tissue anchoring the vascular neointima, essentially forming a neoartery.

A second approach has been direct endothelial cell seeding of freshly harvested or cultured cells onto a synthetic graft. Herring and associates (1978) first described a single-stage technique for seeding vascular grafts with autologous endothelium (Fig. 51–15). However, many endothelial cells are necessary to seed the graft, and most patients who require these grafts have little or no saphenous vein. In clinical trials, results were inconclusive. Zilla and co-workers (1987, 1989) and Fasol and colleagues (1989) found no difference in overall results between seeded and nonseeded grafts.

An alternative to the single-stage seeding has been the two-stage approach using the cell culture technique. The advantage of this technique is that it provides a uniformly endothelialized graft immediately after implantation (Zilla et al., 1993). Results of early clinical trials appear favorable (Kadletz et al., 1992; Zilla et al., 1993). This technique also holds great promise for mechanical heart devices, particularly with polyurethane sacks (Zilla et al., 1991) and with bioprosthetic heart valves when the toxic aldehydes

are neutralized by L-glutamic acid and a collagenous precoating is used (Eberl et al., 1992; Eybl et al., 1992).

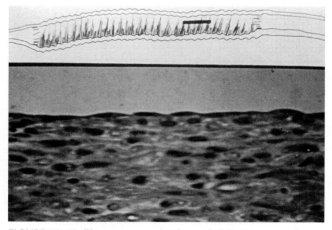

**FIGURE 51–15.** Photomicrograph of a seeded Dacron arterial prosthesis after 4 weeks following implantation in the abdominal aorta of a dog. Distinct lining cells are seen on the luminal surface. These cells have a high nuclear-to-cytoplasmic ratio consistent with endothelium. There is excellent sublining cellularity and organization. The top portion shows where the preparation was obtained from in the graft. (Courtesy of M. B. Herring, M.D.)

## SELECTED BIBLIOGRAPHY

Edmunds, L. H.: Thrombotic and bleeding complications of prosthetic heart valves. Ann. Thorac. Surg., 44:430, 1987.

This is a collective review of articles published between 1979 and 1987 concerning cardiac valve implants. Despite the lack of standardization, this collective review gives a clear, concise evaluation of the different types of valves, the effect of valve position, and their thrombotic and bleeding complications.

Stein, B., Fuster, V., Israel, D. H., et al.: Platelet inhibitor agents in cardiovascular disease: An update. J. Am. Coll. Cardiol., 14:813, 1989.

This article is an excellent clinical review of platelet inhibitor—agents, their mechanism of action, and their use in cardiovascular disease.

Westaby, S.: Aprotinin in perspective. Ann. Thorac. Surg. (Current Review), 55:1033, 1993.

This is a comprehensive review of the recent literature on the use of aprotinin in cardiac surgery, including the mechanism of action and safety in clinical use.

Zilla, P., von Oppell, U., and Deutsch, M.: The endothelium: A key to the future. J. Cardiovasc. Surg., 8:32, 1993.

This excellent clinical review discusses the key position of the endothelium as a modulator in a variety of biologic systems as they relate to cardiac surgery. The role of endothelium and endothelial injury in vein grafts and vascular spasm, surface thrombogenicity of prosthetic grafts, endothelial protection, and the future of endothelialization of prosthetic implants are covered with a good mix of basic and clinical sciences.

## BIBLIOGRAPHY

Adamson, R. M., Dembitsky, W. P., Reichman, R. J., et al.: Mechanical support: Assist or nemesis? J. Thorac. Cardiovasc. Surg., 98:915, 1989.
Addonizio, V. P., Fisher, C. A., Jenkin, B. K., et al.: Iloprost (2K36374), a stable analogue of prostacyclin, preserves platelets during simulated extracorporeal circulation. J. Thorac. Cardiovasc. Surg., 89:926, 1985.
Addonizio, V. P., Jr., Macarak, E. J., Nicolaou, K. C., et al.: Effects of prostacyclin and albumin on platelet loss during in vitro simulation of extracorporeal circulation. Blood, 53:1033, 1979.
Addonizio, V. P., Strauss, J. F., III, Macarak, E. J., et al.: Preservation of platelet number and function with prostaglandin E_1 during total cardiopulmonary bypass in Rhesus monkeys. Surgery, 85:619, 1978.
Akins, C. W.: Mechanical cardiac valvular prostheses: Current review. Ann. Thorac. Surg., 52:161, 1991.
Alpert, J., O'Donnell, J. A., Parsonnet, V., et al.: Clinically recognized limb ischemia in the neonate after umbilical artery catheterization. Am. J. Surg., 140:413, 1980a.
Alpert, J., Parsonnet, V., Goldenkrantz, R. J., et al.: Limb ischemia during intra-aortic balloon pumping: Indication for femorofemoral crossover graft. J. Thorac. Cardiovasc. Surg., 79:729, 1980b.
Altman, R., Boullon, F., Rouvier, J., et al.: Aspirin and prophylaxis of thromboembolic complications in patients with substitute heart valves. J. Thorac. Cardiovasc. Surg., 72:127, 1976.
Anderson, H. L., III, Delius, R. E., Sinard, J. M., et al.: Early experience with adult extracorporeal membrane oxygenation in the modern era. Ann. Thorac. Surg., 53:553, 1992.
Angell, W. W., Pupello, D. F., Bessone, L. N., and Hiro, S. P.: University method for insertion of unstented aortic autografts, homografts, and xenografts. J. Thorac. Cardiovasc. Surg., 103:642, 1992.
Aranki, S. F., Adams, D. H., Rizzo, R. J., et al.: Femoral venoarterial extracorporeal life support with minimal or no heparin. Ann. Thorac. Surg., 56:149, 1993.
Baciewicz, P. A., del Rio, C., Concalves, M. A., et al.: Catastrophic thrombosis of porcine aortic bioprostheses. Ann. Thorac. Surg., 50:817, 1990.

Band, J. D., and Maki, D. G.: Infections caused by arterial catheters used for hemodynamic monitoring. Am. J. Med., 67:735, 1979.

Bartlett, R. H., Gazzaniga, A. B., Fong, S. W., et al.: Extracorporeal membrane oxygenator support for cardiopulmonary failure. Experience in 28 cases. J. Thorac. Cardiovasc. Surg., 73:375, 1977a.

Bartlett, R. H., Gazzaniga, A. B., Huxtable, R. F., et al.: Extracorporeal (ECMO) in neonatal failure. J. Thorac. Cardiovasc. Surg., 74:826, 1977b.

Bidstrup, B. P., Royston, D., Sapsford, R. N., et al.: Reduction in blood loss and blood use after cardiopulmonary bypass with high dose Aprotinin (Trasylol). J. Thorac. Cardiovasc. Surg., 97:364, 1989.

Blauhut, B., Gross, C., Necek, S., et al.: Effects of high-dose Aprotinin on blood loss, platelet function, fibrinolysis, complement, and renal function after cardiopulmonary bypass. J. Thorac. Cardiovasc. Surg., 101:958, 1991.

Blauth, C. I., Arnold, J. V., Schulenberg, W. E., et al.: Cerebral micro-embolism during cardiopulmonary bypass. J. Thorac. Cardiovasc. Surg., 95:668, 1988.

Borowiec, J., Thelin, S., Bagge, L., et al.: Heparin-coated circuits reduce activation of granulocytes during cardiopulmonary bypass. A clinical study. J. Thorac. Cardiovasc. Surg., 104:642, 1992.

Broviac, J. W., Cole, B. S., and Scribner, B. H.: A silicone rubber atrial catheter for prolonged parenteral-alimentation. Surg. Gynecol. Obstet., 136:602, 1973.

Bull, C., Horvath, P., Merrill, W., et al.: Evaluation of long term results of homograft and heterograft valves in extracardiac conduits. J. Thorac. Cardiovasc. Surg., 94:12, 1987.

Burchfiel, C. M., Hammermeister, K. E., Krause-Steinrauf, H., et al.: Left atrial dimension and risk of systemic embolization in patients with a prosthetic heart valve. J. Am. Coll. Cardiol., 15:32, 1990.

Chesebro, J. H., Clements, I. P., Fuster, V., et al.: Platelet-inhibitor-drug trial in coronary artery bypass operations: Benefit of perioperative dipyridamole and aspirin therapy on early post operative vein-graft patency. N. Engl. J. Med., 307:73, 1982.

Chesebro, J. H., Fuster, V., Elveback, L. R., et al.: Effect of dipyridamole and aspirin on late vein-graft patency after coronary bypass operations. N. Engl. J. Med., 310:209, 1984.

Chesebro, J. H., Fuster, V., Elveback, L. R., et al.: Trial of combined warfarin plus dipyridamole or aspirin therapy in prosthetic heart valve replacement: Danger of aspirin compared with dipyridamole. Am. J. Cardiol., 51:1537, 1983.

Chesebro, J. H., Fuster, V., Humphrey, C. W., et al.: Combined warfarin platelet inhibitor antithrombotic therapy in prosthetic heart valve replacement. Circulation, 64(Suppl. IV):76, 1981.

Clagett, G. P.: Artificial devices in clinical practice. In Coleman, R. W., Hirsh, J., Marder, V. J., and Salzman, E. W. (eds): Hemostasis and Thrombosis. 2nd ed. Philadelphia, J. B. Lippincott, 1987.

Cohn, L. H.: Statistical treatment of valve surgery outcomes: An influence on the evaluation of devices as well as practice. J. Am. Coll. Cardiol., 15:574, 1990.

Coleman, R. W., Marder, V. J., Salzman, E. W., and Hirsh, J.: Overview of hemostasis. In Coleman, R. W., Hirsh, J., Marder, V. J., and Salzman, E. W. (eds): Hemostasis and Thrombosis. 2nd ed. Philadelphia, J. B. Lippincott, 1987.

Coon, W. W., and Willis, P. W., III: Hemorrhagic complications of anticoagulant therapy. Arch. Intern. Med., 133:386, 1974.

Cosgrove, D. M., III, Heric, B., Lytle, B. W., et al.: Aprotinin therapy for reoperative myocardial revascularization: A placebo-controlled study. Ann. Thorac. Surg., 54:1031, 1992.

Cottrell, E. D., Icappa, J. R., Stonach, N., et al.: Temporary inhibition of platelet function with iloprost (ZK36374) preserves canine platelets during extracorporeal membrane oxygenation. J. Thorac. Cardiovasc. Surg., 96:535, 1988.

Crouse, L. H., and Comp, P. C.: The regulation of hemostasis: The protein C system. N. Engl. J. Med., 314:1298, 1986.

Czer, L. S. C., Bateman, T. M., Gray, R. J., et al.: Treatment of severe platelet dysfunction and hemorrhage after cardiopulmonary bypass: Reduction in blood product usage with desmopressin. J. Am. Coll. Cardiol., 9:1139, 1987.

Czer, L., Weiss, M., Bateman, T. M., et al.: Fibrinolytic therapy

of St. Jude valve thrombosis under guidance of digital cine-fluoroscopy. J. Am. Coll. Cardiol., 5:1244, 1985.

Dale, J., Myhre, E., and Loew, D.: Bleeding during acetylsalicylic acid and anticoagulant therapy in patients with reduced platelet reactivity after aortic valve replacement. Am. Heart J., 99:746, 1980.

Dale, J., Myhre, E., Storstein, O., et al.: Prevention of arterial thromboembolism with acetylsalicylic acid: A controlled clinical study in patients with aortic ball valves. Am. Heart J., 94:101, 1977.

David, J. E., Pollick, C., Boss, J.: Aortic valve replacement with stentless porcine aortic bioprosthesis. J. Thorac. Cardiovasc. Surg., 99:113, 1990.

de Leval, M. R., McKay, R., Jones, M., et al.: Modified Blalock-Taussig shunt. J. Thorac. Cardiovasc. Surg., 81:112, 1981.

Deviri, E., Sareli, P., Wisenbaugh, T., et al.: Obstruction of mechanical heart valve prostheses: Clinical aspects and surgical management. J. Am. Coll. Cardiol., 17:646, 1991.

Di Lello, F., Mullen, D. C., Flemma, R. J., et al.: Results of intra-aortic balloon pumping after cardiac surgery: Experience with the Percor balloon catheter. Ann. Thorac. Surg., 46:442, 1988.

DiSesa, V. J., Huval, W., Lelcuk, S., et al.: Disadvantages of prostacyclin infusion during cardiopulmonary bypass. A double-blind study of 50 patients having coronary revascularization. Ann. Thorac. Surg., 38:514, 1984.

Donahoo, J. S., Gardner, T. J., Zahka, K., and Kidd, B. S. L.: Systemic pulmonary shunts in neonates and infants using microporous expanded polytetrafluoroethylene: Immediate and late results. Ann. Thorac. Surg., 30:146, 1980.

Eberl, T., Siedler, S., Schumacher, B., et al.: Experimental in vitro endothelialization of cardiac valve leaflets. Ann. Thorac. Surg., 53:487, 1992.

Edmunds, L. H.: Thrombotic and bleeding complications of prosthetic heart valves. Ann. Thorac. Surg., 44:430, 1987.

Edmunds, L. H.: Thromboembolic complications of current cardiac valvular prostheses. Ann. Thorac. Surg., 34:96, 1982.

Edmunds, L. H., and Williams, W.: Microemboli and the use of filters during cardiopulmonary bypass. In Utley, J. R. (ed): Pathophysiology and Techniques in Cardiopulmonary Bypass. Baltimore, Williams & Wilkins, 1983.

Edmunds, L. H., Clark, R. E., Cohn, L. H., et al.: Guidelines for reporting morbidity and mortality after cardiac valvular operations. J. Thorac. Cardiovasc. Surg., 96:351, 1988.

Edmunds, L. H., Niewiarowski, S., Coleman, R. W.: Invited letter concerning Aprotinin. J. Thorac. Cardiovasc. Surg., 101:1103–1104, 1991.

Evans, R. W.: Incidence and management of limb ischemia with percutaneous wire-guided intra-aortic balloon catheters. J. Am. Coll. Cardiol., 9:524, 1987.

Eybl, E., Grimm, M., Grabenwoger, M., et al.: Endothelial cell lining of bioprosthetic heart valve materials. J. Thorac. Cardiovasc. Surg., 104:763, 1992.

Faichney, A., Davidson, K. G., Wheatley, D. J., et al.: Prostacyclin in cardiopulmonary bypass operations. J. Thorac. Cardiovasc. Surg., 84:601, 1982.

Farrar, D. J., Litwak, P., Lawson, J. H., et al.: In vivo evaluations of new thrombo-resistant polyurethane for artificial heart blood pumps. J. Thorac. Cardiovasc. Surg., 95:191, 1988.

Fasol, R., Zilla, P., Deutsch, M., et al.: Human endothelial cell seeding: Evaluation of its effectiveness by platelet parameters after one year. J. Vasc. Surg., 9:432, 1989.

Fish, K. J., Sarnguist, F. H., van Steennis, C., et al.: A prospective, randomized study of the effects of prostacyclin on platelets and blood loss during coronary bypass operations. J. Thorac. Cardiovasc. Surg., 91:436, 1986.

Fishbein, J. D., Friedman, H. S., Bennett, B. B., et al.: Catheter related sepsis. Refractory to antibiotics treated successfully with adjunctive urokinase infusion. Pediatr. Infect. Dis. J., 9:676, 1990.

Forfar, J. C.: A 7 year analysis of hemorrhage in patients on long-term anticoagulant therapy. Br. Heart J., 42:128, 1979.

Frazier, O. H., Rose, E. A., Macmanus, Q., et al.: Multicenter clinical evaluation of the HeartMate 1000 IP left ventricular assist device. Ann. Thorac. Surg., 53:1080, 1992.

Gattinoni, L., Pesenti, A., Mascheroni, D., et al.: Low frequency positive pressure ventilation with extracorporeal $CO_2$ removal in severe acute respiratory failure: Clinical results. J. A. M. A., 256:881, 1986.

Gazzaniga, A. B., Lamberti, J. J., Siewers, R. D., et al.: Arterial prosthesis of microporous expended polytetrafluoroethylene for construction of aorto-pulmonary shunts. J. Thorac. Cardiovasc. Surg., 72:357, 1976.

Gold, J. D., Cohen, J., Shemin, R. J., et al.: Femorofemoral bypass to relieve acute leg ischemia during intra-aortic balloon pump cardiac support. J. Vasc. Surg., 3:351, 1986.

Goldberg, M. J., Rubenfire, M., Kantrowitz, A., et al.: Intra-aortic balloon pump insertion: A randomized study comparing percutaneous and surgical techniques. J. Am. Coll. Cardiol., 9:515, 1987.

Goldman, S., Copeland, J., Murtiz, T., et al.: Starting aspirin therapy after operation: Effects on early graft patency. Circulation, 84:520, 1991.

Gott, V. L., Koepke, D. E., Daggett, R. L., et al.: The coating of intravascular plastic prostheses with colloidal graphite. Surgery, 50:382, 1961.

Graver, L. M., Gelber, P. M., and Tyras, D. H.: The risks and benefits of thrombolytic therapy in acute aortic and mitral valve dysfunction: Report of a case and review of the literature. Ann. Thorac. Surg., 46:85, 1988.

Gu, Y. J., van Oeveren, W., Akkerman, C., et al.: Heparin coated circuits reduce the inflammatory response to cardiopulmonary bypass. Ann. Thorac. Surg., 55:917, 1993.

Hall, J. G., Pauli, R. M., and Wilson, K. M.: Maternal and fetal sequelae of anti-coagulation during pregnancy. Am. J. Med., 68:122, 1980.

Hammermeister, K. E., Sethi, G. K., Henderson, W. G., et al.: A comparison of outcomes in men 11 years after heart-valve replacement with a mechanical valve or bioprosthesis. N. Engl. J. Med., 328:1289, 1993.

Hammond, G. L., Geha, A. S., Kopf, G. S., and Hashim, S. W.: Biological versus mechanical valves. J. Thorac. Cardiovasc. Surg., 93:182, 1987.

Harker, L. A., and Slichter, S. J.: Studies of platelet and fibrinogen kinetics in patients with prosthetic heart valves. N. Engl. J. Med., 283:1302, 1970.

Harker, L. A., Malpass, T. N., Branson, H. E., et al.: Mechanism of abnormal bleeding in patients undergoing cardiopulmonary bypass: Acquired transient platelet dysfunction associated with selective granule release. Blood, 56:824, 1980.

Harker, L. A., Slichter, S. J., and Sauvage, L. R.: Platelet consumption by arterial prostheses: The effects of endothelialization and pharmacologic inhibition of platelet function. Ann. Surg., 186:594, 1977.

Harris, R. E., Reimer, K. A., Crain, B. J., et al.: Spinal cord infarction following intra-aortic balloon support. Ann. Thorac. Surg., 42:206, 1986.

Hartz, R. S., Locicero, J., Kucich, V., et al.: Comparative study of warfarin vs. antiplatelet therapy in patients with a St. Jude Medical valve in the aortic position. J. Thorac. Cardiovasc. Surg., 92:684, 1986.

Havel, M., Teufelsbauer, H., Knobl, P., et al.: Effect of intraoperative Aprotinin administration on postoperative bleeding in patients undergoing cardiopulmonary bypass operation. J. Thorac. Cardiovasc. Surg., 101:968, 1991.

Herring, M., Gardner, A., Glover, J.: A single-staged technique for seeding vascular grafts with autogenous endothelium. Surgery, 84:498, 1978.

Hickman, R. O., Buckner, C. D., Clift, R. A., et al.: A modified right atrial catheter for access to the venous system in marrow transplant recipients. Surg. Gynecol. Obstet., 148:871, 1979.

Hicks, G., Jensen, L. A., Norsen, L. H., et al.: Platelet inhibitors and hydroxyethyl starch: Safe and cost-effective interventions in coronary artery surgery. Ann. Thorac. Surg., 39:422, 1985.

Hill, J. D., O'Brien, J. G., Murray, J. J., et al.: Prolonged extracorporeal oxygenation for acute post-traumatic respiratory failure (shock lung syndrome). N. Engl. J. Med., 286:629, 1972.

Hirsh, J., Deykin, D., and Poller, L.: Theraputic range for oral anticoagulant therapy. Chest, 89:115, 1986.

Hoar, P. F., Wilson, R. M., Mangano, D. T., et al.: Heparin bonding reduces thrombogenicity of pulmonary artery catheters. N. Engl. J. Med., 305:993, 1981.

Hofig, M., Nellessen, U., Mahmoodi, M., et al.: Performance of a stentless xenograft aortic bioprosthesis up to four years after implantation. J. Thorac. Cardiovasc. Surg., 103:1068, 1992.

Hoover, E. L., Kharma, B., Ross, M., et al.: The temporal relationship in arterial and venous prostacyclin and thromboxane activity during 24 hours of IABP in dogs. Ann. Thorac. Surg., 46:661, 1988.

Huang, H., Ding, W., Su, K., et al.: Mechanism of the preserving effect of Aprotinin on platelet function and its use in cardiac surgery. J. Thorac. Cardiovasc. Surg., 106:11, 1993.

Hunt, B. J., Segal, H., and Yacoub, M.: Aprotinin and heparin monitoring during cardiopulmonary bypass. Circulation, 86(Suppl. II):410, 1992.

Ilbawi, M. N., Lockhart, C. G., Idriss, F. S., et al.: Experience with the St. Jude Medical valve prosthesis in children: A word of caution regarding right sided placement. J. Thorac. Cardiovasc. Surg., 93:73, 1987.

Islam, M. N., Zikria, E. A., Sullivan, M. E., et al.: Aortocoronary Goretex graft: 18 month patency. Ann. Thorac. Surg., 31:S69, 1981.

Isom, O. W., Williams, D., Falk, E. A., et al.: Evaluation of anticoagulant therapy in cloth-covered prosthetic valves. Circulation, 48(Suppl. III):48, 1973.

Iturbe-Alessio, I., Fonseca, M., Mutchinik, O., et al.: Risks of anticoagulant therapy in pregnant women with artificial heart valves. N. Engl. J. Med., 315:1390, 1986.

Jarmolowski, C. R., and Poirier, R. L.: Small bowel infarction complicating intra-aortic balloon counterpulsation via the ascending aorta. J. Thorac. Cardiovasc. Surg., 79:735, 1980.

John, L. C. H., Rees, G. M., and Kovacs, I. B.: Inhibition of platelet function by heparin: An etiologic factor in post bypass hemorrhage. J. Thorac. Cardiovasc. Surg., 105:816, 1993.

Jones, G. R., Konsler, G. X., Dunaway, R. P., et al.: Prospective analysis of urokinase in the treatment of catheter sepsis in pediatric hematology-oncology patients. J. Pediatr. Surg., 28:350, 1993.

Joyce, L. D., Emery, R. W., Ealos, F., et al.: Mechanical circulatory support as a bridge to transplantation. J. Thorac. Cardiovasc. Surg, 98:935, 1989a.

Joyce, L. D., Johnson, K. E., Toninato, C. J., et al.: Results of the first 100 patients who received symbion total artificial hearts as a bridge to cardiac transplantation. Circulation, 80(Suppl. III):192, 1989b.

Kadletz, M., Magometschnigg, H., Minar, E., et al.: Implantation of in vitro endothelialized polytetrafluoroethylene grafts in human beings. A preliminary report. J. Thorac. Cardiovasc. Surg., 104:736, 1992.

Kantrowitz, A.: Origins of intra-aortic balloon pumping. Ann. Thorac. Surg., 50:672, 1990.

Kinsella, J. P., Neish, S. R., Shaffer, E., and Abman, S. H.: Low dose inhalational nitric oxide in persistent pulmonary hypertension of the newborn. Lancet, 340:819, 1992.

Kirklin, J. K., Wostaby, S., Blackstone, E. H., et al.: Complement and the damaging effects of cardiopulmonary bypass. J. Thorac. Cardiovasc. Surg., 86:845, 1983.

Kohler, T. R., Kaufman, J. L., Kacoyanis, G., et al.: Effect of aspirin and dipyridamole on the patency of lower extremity bypass grafts. Surgery, 96:461, 1984.

Koul, B., Vesterqvist, O., Egberg, N., and Steen, S.: Twenty-four hour heparin-free veno-right ventricular ECMO: An experimental study. Ann. Thorac. Surg., 53:1046, 1992.

Kurzrok, S., Singh, A. K., Most, A. S., et al.: Thrombolytic therapy for prosthetic cardiac valve thrombosis. J. Am. Coll. Cardiol., 9:592, 1987.

Lacey, S. R., Zaritsky, A. L., and Azizkhan, R. G.: Successful treatment of candida-infected caval thrombosis in critically ill infants by low-dose streptokinase infusion. J. Pediatr. Surg., 23:1204, 1988.

Lambert, C. J., Marengo-Rowe, A. J., Leveson, J. E., et al.: The treatment of post perfusion bleeding using $\epsilon$-aminocaproic acid, cryoprecipitate, fresh frozen plasma, and protamine sulfate. Ann. Thorac. Surg., 28:440, 1979.

Larrea, J. L., Nunez, L., Reque, J. A., et al.: Pregnancy and mechanical valve prostheses: A high risk situation for the mother and fetus. Ann. Thorac. Surg., 36:459, 1983.

Ledain, L. D., Ohayon, J. P., Colle, J. P., et al.: Acute thrombotic obstruction with disc valve prostheses: Diagnostic considerations and fibrinolytic treatment. J. Am. Coll. Cardiol., 7:743, 1986.

Lesnefsky, E., Woelfel, G. F., Dauber, I. M., et al.: Early thrombosis of a porcine aortic valve. Am. J. Cardiol., 5:1120, 1986.

Levine, M. N., Raskob, G., and Hirsh, J.: Hemorrhagic complications of long term anticoagulant therapy. Chest, 89:165, 1986.

Livi, U., Abdulla, A. K., Parker, R., et al.: Viability and morphology of aortic and pulmonary homografts. A comparative study. J. Thorac. Cardiovasc. Surg., 93:755, 1987.

Loop, F. D., Lytle, B. W., Cosgrove, D. M., et al.: Influence of the internal mammary artery graft on 10-year survival and other cardiac events. N. Engl. J. Med., 314:1, 1986.

Lutz, D. J., Noller, K. L., Spittell, J. A., et al.: Pregnancy and its complications following cardiac valve prostheses. Am. J. Obstet. Gynecol., 131:460, 1978.

Macoviak, J., Stephenson, L. W., Edmunds, L. H., et al.: The intraaortic balloon pump: An analysis of five years' experience. Ann. Thorac. Surg., 29:451, 1980.

Magilligan, D. J., Jr., Oyama, C., Klein, S., et al.: Platelet adherence to bioprosthetic cardiac valves. Am. J. Cardiol., 53:945, 1984.

Makhlouf, A. E. L., Friedli, B., Oberhansli, I., et al.: Prosthetic heart valve replacement in children: Results and followup of 273 patients. J. Thorac. Cardiovasc. Surg., 93:80, 1987.

Malpass, T. W., Amory, D. W., Harker, L. A., et al.: The effect of prostacyclin infusion on platelet hemostatic function in patients under going cardiopulmonary bypass. J. Thorac. Cardiovasc. Surg., 87:550, 1984.

Martinell, J., Fraile, J., Artiz, V., et al.: Reoperations for left-sided low profile mechanical prosthetic obstructions. Ann. Thorac. Surg., 43:172, 1987.

Martinell, J., Jimenez, A., Rabago, G., et al.: Mechanical cardiac valve thrombosis: Is thrombectomy justified? Circulation, 84(Suppl. III):70, 1991.

Matsuki, O., Okita, Y., Almoida, R. S., et al.: Two decades experience with aortic valve replacement with pulmonary autograft. J. Thorac. Cardiovasc. Surg., 95:705, 1988a.

Matsuki, O., Robles, A., Gibbs, S., et al.: Long-term performance of 555 aortic homografts in the aortic position. Ann. Thorac. Surg., 46:187, 1988b.

McCabe, J. C., Abel, R. M., Subramanian, V. A., and Gay, W. A.: Complications of intra-aortic balloon insertion and counterpulsation. Circulation, 57:769, 1978.

McCollum, C. N., Kester, R. C., Rajah, S. M., et al.: Arterial graft maturation: The duration of thrombotic activity in dacron aorto bifemoral grafts measured by platelet and fibrinogen kinetics. Br. J. Surg., 68:61, 1981.

McEnany, M. T., Salzman, E. W., Mundth, E. D., et al.: The effect of antithrombotic therapy on patency rates of saphenous vein coronary artery bypass grafts. J. Thorac. Cardiovasc. Surg., 83:81, 1982.

McFadden, P. M., and Ochsner, J. L.: Neonatal aortic thrombosis: Complication of umbilical artery cannulation. J. Cardiovasc. Surg, 24:1., 1983.

McGoon, D. C.: The risk of thromboembolism following valvular operations: How does one know? J. Thorac. Cardiovasc. Surg., 88:782, 1984.

McGrath, L. B., Gonzalez-Lavin, L., Eldredge, W. J., et al.: Thromboembolic and other events following valve replacement in a pediatric population treated with antiplatelet agents. Ann. Thorac. Surg., 43:285, 1987.

McKay, R., de Leval, M. R., Rees, P., et al.: Postoperative angiographic assessment of modified Blalock-Taussig shunts using PTFE (Gore-Tex). Ann. Thorac. Surg., 30:137, 1980.

Mehta, P., and Mehta, J.: Effects of aspirin in arterial thrombosis: Why don't animals behave the way humans do? J. Am. Coll. Cardiol., 21:511, 1993.

Meliones, J. N., Custer, J. R., Snedecor, S., et al.: Extracorporeal life support for cardiac assist in pediatric patients. Review of ELSO registry data. Circulation, 84(Suppl. III):168, 1991.

Mohr, R., Goor, D. A., Lusky, A., and Lavee, J.: Aprotinin prevents cardiopulmonary bypass-induced platelet dysfunction: A scanning electron microscope study. Circulation, 86(Suppl. II):405, 1992.

Molina, J. E., Carr, M., and Yarnoz, M. D.: Coronary artery bypass with Gortex graft. J. Thorac. Cardiovasc. Surg., 75:769, 1978.

Mollitt, D. L., and Golladay, E. S.: Complications of TPN catheter-induced vena caval thrombosis in children less than one year of age. J. Pediatr. Surg., 18:462, 1983.

Moront, M. G., Katz, K., O'Connell, J., et al.: The use of fibrin glue at neonatal ECMO cannulation sites. Surg. Gynecol. Obstet., 166:358, 1988.

Mulvihill, S. J., and Fonkalsrud, E. W.: Complications of superior versus inferior vena cava occlusion in infants receiving central total parenteral nutrition. J. Pediatr. Surg., 19:752, 1984.

Murtra, M., Mostres, C. A., and Igual, A.: Longterm patency of PTFE vascular grafts in coronary artery surgery. Ann. Thorac. Surg., 39:86, 1985.

Myers, M. L., Lawrie, G. M., Crawford, E. S., et al.: The St. Jude valve prostheses: Analysis of the clinical results in 815 implants and the need for systemic anticoagulation. J. Am. Coll. Cardiol., 13:57, 1989.

Naunheim, K. S., Swartz, M. T., Pennington, D. G., et al.: Intra-aortic balloon pumping in patients requiring cardiac operations. Risk analysis and long term followup. J. Thorac. Cardiovasc. Surg., 104:1654, 1992.

O'Brien, M. F., Stafford, E. G., Gardner, M. A. H., et al.: A comparison of aortic valve replacement with viable cryopreserves and fresh allograft valves with a note on chromosome studies. J. Thorac. Cardiovasc. Surg., 94:812, 1987.

Oblath, R. W., Buckley, F. O., Green, R. M., et al.: Prevention of platelet aggregation and adherence to prosthetic vascular grafts by aspirin and dipyridamole. Surgery, 84:37, 1978.

Okita, Y., Franciosi, G., Matsuki, O., et al.: Early and late results of aortic root replacement with antibiotic sterilized aortic homograft. J. Thorac. Cardiovasc. Surg., 95:696, 1988.

Opie, J. C., Traverse, L., Hayden, R. I., et al.: Experience with polytetrafluoroethylene grafts in children with cyanotic congenital heart surgery. Ann. Thorac. Surg., 41:164, 1986.

Pappas, G.: Intrathoracic intra-aortic balloon insertion for pulsatile cardiopulmonary bypass. Arch. Surg., 109:842, 1974.

Park, S. B., Liebler, G. A., Burkholder, J. A., et al.: Mechanical support of the failing heart. Ann. Thorac. Surg., 42:627, 1986.

Pass, H. I., Sade, R. M., Crawford, F. A., and Hohn, A. R.: Cardiac valve prostheses in children without anticoagulation. J. Thorac. Cardiovasc. Surg., 87:832, 1984.

Peigh, P. S., DiSesa, V. J., Cohn, L. H., Collins, J. J., Jr.: Neurological and ophthalmological phenomena after aortic conduit surgery. Circulation, 82(Suppl. IV):47, 1990.

Pennington, D. G., Swartz, M., Codd, J. E., et al.: Intra-aortic balloon pumping in cardiac surgical patients: A nine year experience. Ann. Thorac. Surg., 36:125, 1983.

Pennington, D. G., Kanter, K. R., McBride, L. R., et al.: Seven years' experience with the Pierce-Donachy ventricular assist device. J. Thorac. Cardiovasc. Surg., 96:901, 1988.

Penta, A., Qureshi, S., Radley-Smith, R., and Yacoub, M. H.: Patient status 10 or more years after "fresh" homograft replacement of the aortic valve. Circulation 70(Suppl. I):182, 1984.

Pillai, R., Spriggings, D., Amarasena, N., et al.: Stentless aortic bio prostaesis? The way forward: Early experience with the Edwards valve. Ann. Thorac. Surg., 56:88, 1993.

Poller, L.: Therapeutic ranges In anticoagulant administration. Br. Med. J., 290:1683, 1985.

Prabhu, S., Friday, K. J., Reynolds, D., Elkins, R., et al.: Thrombosis of aortic St. Jude valve. Ann. Thorac. Surg., 41:332, 1986.

Rao, P. S., Solymar, L., Mardini, M. K., et al.: Anticoagulant therapy in children with prosthetic valves. Ann. Thorac. Surg., 47:589, 1989.

Ribeiro, P. A., Zaibag, M. A., Idris, M., et al.: Antiplatelet drugs and the incidence of thromboembolic complications of the St. Jude Medical aortic prosthesis in patients with rheumatic heart disease. J. Thorac. Cardiovasc. Surg., 91:92, 1986.

Robbins, R. C., Bowman, F. O., and Malm, J. R.: Cardiac valve replacement in children: A twenty year series. Ann. Thorac. Surg., 45:56, 1988.

Roberts, J. D., Jr., Polaner, D. M., Todres, I. D., et al.: Inhaled nitric oxide (NO): A selective pulmonary vasodilator for the treatment of persistent pulmonary hypertension of the newborn. Circulation, 84:A-1279, 1991.

Roberts, J. D., Jr., Polaner, D. M., Lane, P., et al.: Inhaled nitric oxide in persistent pulmonary hypertension of the newborn. Lancet, 340:818, 1992.

Roudaut, R., Labbe, T., Lorient-Roudaut, M. F., et al.: Mechanical cardiac valve thrombosis: Is fibrinolysis justified? Circulation, 86(Suppl. II):8, 1992.

Sade, R. M., Crawford, F. A., Jr., Fyfe, D. A., and Stroud, M. R.: Valve prostheses in children: A reassessment of anticoagulation. J. Thorac. Cardiovasc. Surg., 95:553, 1988.

Saito, A., Hayashi, J., and Eguchi, S.: Mechanical circulatory assist using heparin coated tube and roller pump system. Ann. Thorac. Surg., 53:659, 1992.

Salazar, E., Zajarias, A., Gutierrez, N., et al.: The problem of cardiac valve prostheses, anticoagulants, and pregnancy. Circulation, 70:169, 1984.

Salzman, E. W., and Merrill, E. W.: Interaction of blood, with artificial surfaces. In Coleman, R. W., Hirsh, J., Marder, V. J., Salzman, E. W. (eds): Hemostasis and Thrombosis. Philadelphia, J. B. Lippincott, 1987.

Salzman, E. W., Weinstein, M. J., Weintraub, R. M., et al.: Treatment with desmopressin acetate to reduce blood loss after cardiac surgery: A double-blind randomized study. N. Engl. J. Med., 314:1402, 1986.

Sanfelippo, P. M., Baker, N. H., Ewy, H. G., et al.: Experience with intraaortic balloon counterpulsation. Ann. Thorac. Surg., 41:36, 1986.

Sapsford, R. N., Oakley, G. D., and Talbot, S.: Early and late patency of expanded polytetrafluoroethylene vascular grafts in aorto-coronary bypass. J. Thorac. Cardiovasc. Surg., 81:860, 1981.

Sauvage, L. R., Berger, K., Beilin, L. B., et al.: Presence of endothelium in an axillary-femoral graft of knitted dacron with an external velour surface. Ann. Surg., 182:749, 1975.

Schaffer, M. S., Clarke, D. R., Campbell, D. N., et al.: The St. Jude Medical cardiac valve in infants and children: Role of anticoagulant therapy. J. Am. Coll. Cardiol., 9:235, 1987.

Schoen, F. J., Palmer, D. C., Bernard, W. F., et al.: Clinical temporary assist device. J. Thorac. Cardiovasc. Surg., 92:1071, 1986.

Sell, L. L., Cullen, M. L., Whittlesey, G. L., et al.: Hemorrhagic complications during extracorporeal membrane oxygenation: Prevention and treatment. J. Pediatr. Surg., 21:1087, 1986.

Silber, H., Khan, S. S., Matloff, J. M., et al.: The St. Jude valve thrombolysis as the first line of therapy for cardiac valve thrombosis. Circulation, 87:30, 1993.

Sinard, J. M., and Bartlett, R. H.: Extracorporeal life support in critical care medicine. J. Crit. Care, 5:165, 1990.

Slogoff, S., Keats, A. S., and Arlund, C.: On the safety of radial artery cannulation. Anesthesiology, 59:42, 1983.

Sommerville, J., and Ross, D.: Homograft replacement of the aortic root with reimplantation of coronary arteries. Br. Heart J., 47:473, 1982.

Steele, P., Weily, H., Davies, H., et al.: Platelet survival time following aortic valve replacement. Circulation, 51:358, 1975.

Sullivan, J. M., Harker, D. E., and Gorlin, R.: Pharmacologic control of thromboembolic complications of cardiac valve replacement. N. Engl. J. Med., 284:1391, 1971.

Teoh, K. H., Christakis, G. T., Weisel, R. D., et al.: Dipyridamole preserved platelets and reduced blood loss after cardiopulmonary bypass. J. Thorac. Cardiovasc. Surg., 96:332, 1988.

Thomas, J. H., MacArthur, R. I., Pierce, G. E., et al.: Hickman-Broviac catheters: Indications and results. Am. J. Surg., 140:791, 1980.

Trowbridge, E. A., Lanford, P. V., Crofts, C. E., and Roberts, K. M.: Pericardial heterografts: Why do these valves fail? J. Thorac. Cardiovasc. Surg., 95:577, 1988.

Uretzky, G., Appelbaum, Y., Younes, H., et al.: Long term evaluation of a new selectively biodegradable vascular graft coated with polyethylene oxide-polylactic acid for right ventricular conduit: An experimental study. J. Thorac. Cardiovasc. Surg., 100:769, 1990.

van Oeveren, W., Harder, M. P., Roozendaal, K. J., et al.: Aprotinin protects platelets against the initial effect of cardiopulmonary bypass. J. Thorac. Cardiovasc. Surg., 99:788, 1990.

van Oeveren, W., Kazdtchkine, M. D., Descamps-Latscha, B. D., et al.: Deleterious effects of cardiopulmonary bypass: A prospec-tive study of bubble vs. membrane oxygenation. J. Thorac. Cardiovasc. Surg., 89:888, 1985.

van der Lei, B., Darius, H., Schror, K., et al.: Arterial wall regeneration in small-caliber vascular grafts in rats. J. Thorac. Cardiovasc. Surg., 90:378, 1985.

van der Lei, B., Wildevuur, C. R. H., Dijk, F., et al.: Sequential studies of arterial wall regeneration in microporous, compliant, biodegradable small caliber vascular grafts in rats. J. Thorac. Cardiovasc. Surg., 93:695, 1987.

Van der Salm, T. J., Ansell, J. E., Okike, O. N., et al.: The role of epsilon aminocaproic acid in reducing bleeding after cardiac operation: A double-blind randomized study. J. Thorac. Cardiovasc. Surg., 95:538, 1988.

Verrier, E. D., Tranbaugh, R. F., Soifer, S. J., et al.: Aspirin anticoagulation in children with mechanical aortic valves. J. Thorac. Cardiovasc. Surg., 92:1013, 1986.

Videm, V., Mollnes, T. E., Garred, P., and Svennevig, J. L.: Biocompatibility of extracorporeal circulation. J. Thorac. Cardiovasc. Surg., 101:654, 1991.

Videm, V., Svennevig, J. L., Fosse, E., et al.: Reduced complement activation with heparin-coated oxygenator and tubings in coronary bypass operations. J. Thorac. Cardiovasc. Surg., 103:806, 1992.

von Segesser, L. K., Turina, M.: Cardiopulmonary bypass without systemic heparinization. J. Thorac. Cardiovasc. Surg., 98:386, 1989.

von Segesser, L. K., Weiss, B. M., Garcia, E., et al.: Reduction and elimination of systemic heparinization during cardiopulmonary bypass. J. Thorac. Cardiovasc. Surg., 103:790, 1992.

Walenga, J. M., Hopponsteadt, D., Fareed, J., and Pifarre, R.: Hemostatic abnormalities in total artificial heart patients as detected by specific blood markers. Ann. Thorac. Surg., 53:844, 1992.

Wampler, R. K., Frazier, O. H., Lansing, A. M., et al.: Treatment of cardiogenic shock with the hemopump left ventricular assist device. Ann. Thorac. Surg., 52:506, 1991.

Ware, J. A., Scott, M. A., Horak, J. K., et al.: Platelet aggregation during and after cardiopulmonary bypass: Effect of two different cardiotomy filters. Ann. Thorac. Surg., 34:204, 1982.

Ware, J. A., Lewis, J., Salzman, E. W.: Antithrombic Therapy. In Rutherford, R. B. (ed): Vascular Surgery. Philadelphia, W. B. Saunders, 1989.

Wachtfogel, Y. T., Kucick, U., Hack, C. E., et al.: Aprotinin inhibits the contact, neutrophil, and platelet activation systems during simulated extracorporeal perfusion. J. Thorac. Cardiovasc. Surg., 106:1, 1993.

Weber, K. T., and Janicki, J. S.: Intra-aortic balloon counterpulsation: A collective review. Ann. Thorac. Surg., 17:602, 1974.

Weily, H. S., Steele, P. P., Davies, H., et al.: Platelet survival in patients with substitute heart valves. N. Engl. J. Med., 290:534, 1974.

Wenger, R. K., Lukasiewicz, H., Mikuta, B. S., et al.: Loss of platelet fibrinogen receptors during clinical cardiopulmonary bypass. J. Thorac. Cardiovasc. Surg., 97:235, 1989.

Witchitz, S., Veyrat, C., Moisson, P., et al.: Fibrinolytic treatment of thrombus on prosthetic heart valves. Br. Heart J., 44:545, 1980.

Yokoyama, T., Gharavi, M. A., Lee, Y. G., et al.: Aortocoronary revascularization with an expanded polytetrafluoroethylene vascular graft. A preliminary report. J. Thorac. Cardiovasc. Surg., 76:552, 1978.

Young, J. A., Kisker, C. T., and Doty, D. B.: Adequate anticoagulation during cardiopulmonary bypass determined by activated clotting time and the appearance of fibrin monomer. Ann. Thorac. Surg., 26:231, 1978.

Zilla, P., Fasol, R., Deutsch, M., et al.: Endothelial cell seeding of polytetrafluoroethylene vascular grafts in humans: A preliminary report. J. Vasc. Surg., 6:535, 1987.

Zilla, P., Fasol, R., Grimm, M., et al.: Growth properties of cultured human endothelial cells on differently coated artificial heart materials. J. Thorac. Cardiovasc. Surg., 101:671, 1991.

Zilla, P., Fasol, R., Groscurth, P., et al.: Blood, platelets in cardiopulmonary bypass operations recovery occurs after initial stimulation, rather than continued activation. J. Thorac. Cardiovasc. Surg., 97:379, 1989.

Zilla, P., von Oppell, U., and Deutsch, M.: The endothelium: A key to the future. J. Cardiovasc. Surg., 8:32, 1993.

# 52 Acquired Aortic Valve Disease

Donald D. Glower

## HISTORICAL ASPECTS

In 1914, Tuffier first attempted to relieve aortic stenosis by inserting a finger through the aorta to dilate the aortic valve. An experimental study of aortic valvotomy was reported by Smithy and Parker in 1947, yet Smithy himself later died of rheumatic heart disease. Clinical aortic valve dilatation was subsequently performed with a mechanical dilator inserted through the left ventricle (Bailey et al., 1952) or with a finger through a sleeve sewn onto the aorta (Ellis and Kirklin, 1955). The first prosthesis used to treat aortic valve disease was a ball valve inserted into the descending aorta in 1953 by Hufnagel and Harvey in a patient with aortic valve regurgitation. The Hufnagel prosthesis was designed for rapid insertion into the aorta, but left the patient with aortic insufficiency of the upper body.

After the development of cardiopulmonary bypass by Gibbon in 1954, aortic valvotomy for débridement of aortic valvular calcium became possible (Kirklin and Mankin, 1960). Single-leaflet prostheses for partial replacement of the aortic valve (Bahnson et al., 1960; Harken et al., 1960) were followed by single-unit bioprosthetic replacement of the aortic valve in 1961 (Lillehei et al., 1961; McGoon, 1961; Muller et al., 1961). In 1960, Starr and colleagues (1963) and Harken and associates (1960) independently placed a ball valve prosthesis in the subcoronary position. Cartwright and co-workers (1963) first reported simultaneous replacement of the aortic and mitral valves, and Starr and associates (1964) first replaced the aortic, mitral, and tricuspid valves.

An aortic homograft valve was placed in the descending thoracic aorta for aortic insufficiency as early as 1956 (Murray, 1956), and Ross first achieved successful orthotopic placement of an aortic homograft valve in 1962. Combined aortic and aortic valve homografts were later developed by Yacoub (Gula et al., 1977) and Ross and colleagues (1979). Ross initially used pulmonary autografts for clinical aortic valve replacement in 1967. Other biologic aortic valve prostheses included the autologous fascia lata valve introduced by Senning (1967) and porcine aortic valves fixed in formaldehyde (Binet et al., 1965), but these techniques were later abandoned owing to rapid leaflet degeneration. Bovine pericardium with glutaraldehyde fixation was introduced by Ionescu and co-workers in 1971 (Ionescu et al., 1972). Carpentier and associates (1974) developed the glutaraldehyde-preserved porcine valve in Paris in 1967.

## NORMAL AORTIC VALVE ANATOMY

The normal aortic valve is tricuspid, with left coronary, right coronary, and noncoronary leaflets each attached just beneath one of three sinuses of Valsalva (Fig. 52–1). The aortic valve is supported by a fibrous skeleton with a U-shaped configuration at each leaflet, and this fibrous skeleton is continuous with the anterior leaflet of the mitral valve and with the membranous interventricular septum. The atrioventricular conduction system passes through the interventricular septum beneath the noncoronary cusp near the right noncoronary commissure. The valve leaflets themselves consist of fibrous tissue lined with endothelium and without a specific vascular supply; and centrally located along the free edge of each leaflet is a fibrous nodule called the *nodule of Arantius*. During systole, each leaflet retracts toward the aortic wall with eddy currents in the sinuses of Valsalva preventing occlusion of the coronary ostia. In diastole, all three leaflets meet at the central nodules of Arantius, with each leaflet touching the adjoining two leaflets along a 1- to 2-mm leaflet edge. This thin rim of contact between leaflets is narrower than in the mitral valve and may contribute to increased difficulty in aortic versus mitral valve repair.

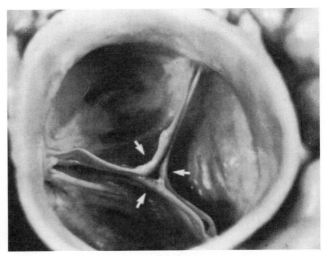

**FIGURE 52–1.** Normal aortic valve with slight thickening of the leaflet edges relative to the remaining leaflets. The three fibrous nodules of Arantius in the middle of the leaflet edges meet near the midpoint of the valve during diastole *(arrows)*. (From Sutton, G. C., and Anderson, R. H. [eds]: Slide Atlas of Cardiology. London, Medi-Cine Productions, 1978.)

■ **Table 52–1.** CAUSES OF NATIVE AORTIC VALVE DISEASE*

| Cause | Aortic Stenosis<br>n (%)<br>(n = 253) | Aortic Regurgitation<br>n (%)<br>(n = 192) |
|---|---|---|
| Calcific | 184 (73) | 56 (29) |
| Rheumatic | 38 (15) | 47 (24) |
| Congenital | 25 (10) | 17 (9) |
| Other degenerative | 6 (3) | 23 (12) |
| Myxomatous | 0 | 26 (14) |
| Endocarditic | 0 | 23 (12) |

*Patients undergoing Carpentier-Edwards aortic valve replacement at Duke University 1975–1990.

## AORTIC STENOSIS

### Cause

The most common cause of clinically evident aortic stenosis is degenerative valve calcification (Table 52–1 and Fig. 52–2). Increasing collagen disruption and small calcific deposits are common in patients without clinically evident aortic valve disease, but significant aortic valve calcification is rarely present before the age of 20 years. Calcification tends to progress with age, generally becoming symptomatic in the fifth and sixth decades of life, often earlier in bicuspid valves and earlier in men than in women. Calcific deposits may become a friable, cauliflower-like mass involving both the leaflets and the aortic valve annulus, with occasional extension into the interventricular septum and with resultant partial or complete block of atrio-ventricular conduction. The calcified aortic valve becomes rigid, has a slit-like orifice, and may be associated with mild aortic insufficiency.

Rheumatic fever remains an important cause of valvular aortic stenosis (see Table 52–1), although the incidence of rheumatic aortic valve disease has declined since the mid-1970s, in the United States and other countries. In the early phases, rheumatic valvulitis may produce edema, lymphocytic infiltration, and neovascularization of the leaflets, followed later by leaflet thickening, commissural fusion, rolling of the leaflet edges, and often, late valvular calcification and aortic insufficiency (see Fig. 52–2). Rheumatic disease of the aortic valve is usually accompanied by clinical or subclinical disease of the mitral or tricuspid valves.

Some degree of congenital aortic valve abnormality is a common contributor to aortic stenosis. Patients may present in infancy with dome-shaped or unicuspid valves that ultimately undergo calcification and fibrotic replacement. Bicuspid aortic valves may be present in as much as 1% of the general population (Fenoglio et al., 1977) (see Fig. 52–2), and bicuspid aortic valves tend to calcify between the ages of 20 and 30 years, followed by the onset of symptomatic aortic stenosis between the ages of 30 and 60 years.

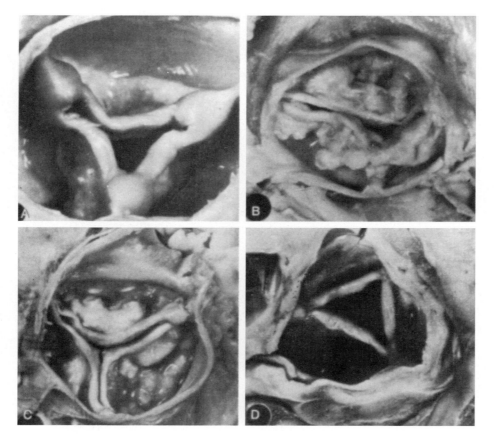

**FIGURE 52–2.** Examples of pathologic aortic valves. *A,* Rheumatic aortic stenosis. *B,* Calcific aortic stenosis in a congenitally bicuspid valve. *C,* Calcific aortic stenosis in a tricuspid valve. *D,* Rheumatic aortic insufficiency. (*A–D,* From Williams, J. M., and Sabiston, D. C., Jr.: Acquired diseases of the aortic valve. *In* Sabiston, D. C., Jr. [ed]: Essentials of Surgery. Philadelphia, W. B. Saunders, 1987, p. 1138; modified from Edwards, J. E.: Pathology of acquired diseases of the heart. Semin. Roentgenol., *14*:108, 1979.)

## Pathophysiology

The primary effect of aortic stenosis is to elevate left ventricular afterload with secondary impairment of left ventricular emptying during systole. Whereas the normal aortic valve has a gradient of less than 5 mm Hg during systole, the stenotic aortic valve may have a systolic gradient of over 100 mm Hg (Fig. 52–3). Aortic stenosis may be quantified by measuring the systolic pressure gradient across the aortic valve or by calculating an effective aortic valve orifice area. Using the Gorlin formula (Gorlin and Gorlin, 1951), *aortic valve area* (AVA) may be estimated as

$$AVA = \frac{AVF}{44.5\sqrt{AVG}}$$

where AVF = mean systolic aortic valve flow and AVG = mean systolic aortic valve gradient. A simpler estimate of aortic valve area may be calculated as

$$AVA = \frac{CO}{\sqrt{AVG}}$$

where CO = cardiac output (l/min). The normal aortic valve cross-sectional area is 2 to 4 cm², and an aortic valve area of 0.8 cm² (0.5 cm²/m² of body surface area) or a mean aortic valve gradient over 50 mm Hg typically corresponds to severe aortic stenosis.

As a result of the pressure gradient across the aortic valve, left ventricular pressure must rise in order to maintain a normal perfusion pressure in the ascending aorta. This increased left ventricular pressure (P) increases left ventricular wall stress (r) during systole by Laplace's law: r = Pr/2h where r = left ventricular radius of curvature and h = left ventricular wall thickness. In turn, increased wall stress is thought to be the stimulus for left ventricular hypertrophy (Grossman et al., 1975), which ultimately may normalize wall stress by increased wall thickness. Severe left ventricular hypertrophy may increase left ventricular mass from 150 g/m² to over 300 g/m² and may produce histologic findings of sarcomere disruption, disarray of myocardial filaments, and disappearance of organelles (Maron et al., 1975). Left ventricular hypertrophy due to aortic stenosis tends to be concentric—i.e., the left ventricular cavitary volume tends to be normal or decreased despite significant increases in left ventricular wall mass (Grossman et al., 1975). More recent studies of patients with aortic stenosis have suggested that concentric hypertrophy is predominant in women, whereas men are more likely than women to develop eccentric left ventricular hypertrophy, some degree of left ventricular dilatation along with increased left ventricular wall mass (Carroll et al., 1992). If left ventricular hypertrophy is insufficient to normalize ventricular wall stress by increased wall thickness (a condition termed *afterload mismatch*), chronic elevation of wall stress may produce left ventricular failure with decreased ventricular contractility and progressive left ventricular dilatation. Ventricular dilatation, in turn, increases wall stress by Laplace's law and may further accentuate left ventricular failure.

The compensated phase of aortic stenosis with progressive left ventricular hypertrophy may leave the patient asymptomatic for decades. As the left ventricle becomes less compliant owing to hypertrophy, atrial systole becomes more important for left ventricular filling and maintaining cardiac output, and the onset of atrial fibrillation in aortic stenosis may suddenly worsen clinical symptoms. In the early phases

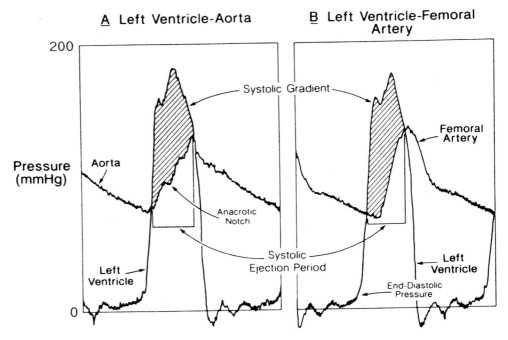

FIGURE 52–3. Hemodynamic tracings in aortic stenosis with simultaneous recordings from the left ventricle and either the ascending aorta (*A*) or the femoral artery (*B*). (*A* and *B*, From Wilson, R. F.: Catheterization of patients with aortic valve disease. *In* Emery, R. W., and Arom, K. V. [eds]: The Aortic Valve. Philadelphia, Hanley & Belfus, 1991.)

of left ventricular decompensation, left ventricular ejection fraction may fall rather markedly, both owing to loss of left ventricular contractility and owing to the fact that ejection fraction falls with elevation of afterload even without any change in contractility (Kass et al., 1987). Thus, the patient with a mildly depressed ejection fraction and severe aortic stenosis may actually have well-preserved left ventricular contractility. Once symptomatic congestive heart failure develops, left ventricular dysfunction may progress rapidly toward death.

Symptoms of congestive heart failure generally reflect elevated pulmonary venous pressure at rest or with exercise. Aortic stenosis may produce pulmonary venous hypertension as a direct effect of afterload elevation or owing to decreased left ventricular diastolic compliance—which, in turn, may result from a combination of left ventricular hypertrophy and dilatation. In addition to congestive heart failure, patients may experience exertional angina related to an impairment of subendocardial blood flow with increased left ventricular pressure (Bache, 1988). Syncope also is common, owing either to arrhythmia or to exercise-induced vasodilatation resulting from abnormal baroreceptor activity and sudden changes in left ventricular pressure (Johnson, 1971).

Correction of aortic stenosis immediately improves left ventricular ejection fraction, left ventricular end-diastolic volume, and capillary wedge pressure owing to reduced left ventricular afterload (Harpole and Jones, 1990; Hwang et al., 1989). Left ventricular hypertrophy from aortic stenosis tends to resolve over 6 to 12 months after aortic valve replacement, but may not totally normalize (Monrad et al., 1988). Factors that correlate with persistent postoperative left ventricular dysfunction include low preoperative ejection fraction, preoperative myocardial infarction, and coronary artery disease without revascularization (Hwang et al., 1989). The relationship between ejection fraction and wall stress has not helped to predict outcome from valve replacement in aortic stenosis because patients with low ejection fraction and low wall stress often do well after valve replacement (Smucker et al., 1989).

## Clinical Findings

Whereas patients with early aortic stenosis may be asymptomatic for many years, those with symptoms generally present with exertional dyspnea, angina, or syncope (Table 52–2). On physical examination, the most prominent finding of aortic stenosis is a systolic ejection murmur best heard in the second intercostal space to the right of the sternum with radiation into both carotid arteries. In severe aortic stenosis, the murmur may peak in late systole, with a palpable thrill often being present, but severe left ventricular failure with decreased cardiac output may actually diminish the systolic murmur of aortic stenosis. The left ventricular impulse may be delayed and sustained by aortic stenosis, and the ventricular impulse may be laterally displaced in patients with left ventricular dilatation. In severe aortic stenosis, the second heart sound may be less prominent, and an associated murmur of aortic insufficiency may also be present.

The electrocardiogram generally shows left ventricular hypertrophy with strain, but may also demonstrate atrial fibrillation or intraventricular conduction defects, such as left or right bundle-branch block or atrioventricular nodal block. Chest radiograph may demonstrate calcification of the aortic valve, left ventricular enlargement, poststenotic dilatation of the ascending aorta, and occasionally, pulmonary edema associated with left ventricular failure.

## Diagnosis

Doppler echocardiography is a valuable noninvasive means to diagnose aortic stenosis. Doppler echocardiography can estimate the peak systolic gradient across the *aortic valve* (AVG) using the modified Bernoulli equation $AVG(mm\ Hg) = 4V^2$ where V = peak blood velocity distal to the valve (m/sec). Doppler echocardiography may also detect aortic regurgitation, and two-dimensional echocardiography may estimate the degree of valve thickening, calcification, and immobility along with left ventricular ejection fraction and volume.

Cardiac catheterization remains the gold standard for the diagnosis of aortic stenosis. The gradient across the aortic valve may be measured directly (see Fig. 52–3), aortic regurgitation may be demonstrated on aortic root injection, and left ventricular function may be assessed from the left ventriculogram. Unlike echocardiography, cardiac catheterization can also evaluate the coronary artery anatomy through coronary arteriography. Given the availability of Doppler echocardiography, the current indications for cardiac catheterization in aortic stenosis are age over 40 years, the presence of risk factors for coronary disease, or borderline degree of stenosis seen through Doppler echocardiography, especially in the presence of impaired left ventricular function.

## Natural History

Patients with mild aortic stenosis may remain asymptomatic for decades owing to compensatory left ventricular hypertrophy. The rate at which mild

■ **Table 52–2.** SYMPTOMS OF NATIVE AORTIC VALVE DISEASE*

| Symptom | Aortic Stenosis n (%) (n = 255) | Aortic Regurgitation n (%) (n = 212) |
|---|---|---|
| Dyspnea | 236 (93) | 191 (90) |
| Angina | 173 (68) | 97 (46) |
| Syncope or presyncope | 83 (33) | 31 (15) |

*Patients undergoing Carpentier-Edwards aortic valve replacement at Duke University 1975–1990.

aortic stenosis progresses to severe stenosis is probably quite variable (Roger et al., 1990). However, most patients with moderate to severe aortic stenosis ultimately do develop symptoms of angina, congestive heart failure, or syncope. Studies by Ross and Braunwald, (1968) and Morrow and colleagues (1968) concluded that the average survival was 3 to 5 years after onset of angina, 3 years after syncope, and 1.5 to 2 years after onset of congestive heart failure. These studies have been updated by Lieberman and co-workers (in press) and others finding survival at 1, 2, and 3 years to be roughly 50%, 30%, and 20%, in patients with symptomatic aortic stenosis managed medically, regardless of whether symptoms were syncope, angina, or congestive heart failure (Fig. 52–4). Most patients with untreated aortic stenosis die from congestive heart failure, but many die from sudden death presumably associated with ventricular arrhythmias.

## Management

Medical therapy has a limited role in the treatment of symptomatic aortic stenosis. Diuretics to minimize symptoms of congestive heart failure and digoxin or antiarrhythmics to control atrial fibrillation may provide some symptomatic benefit, probably without altering the unfavorable natural history of symptomatic aortic stenosis. Afterload reduction therapy may excessively reduce coronary perfusion pressure and is relatively contraindicated in aortic stenosis. Any symptoms of angina, congestive heart failure, or syncope constitute indications for aortic valve replacement. In relatively asymptomatic patients, a mean aortic valve gradient of 50 mm Hg or an aortic valve area of 0.8 cm$^2$ or 1.2 cm$^2$/m$^2$ would indicate the need for aortic valve replacement. Similarly, any evidence of impaired left ventricular function (such as decreased ejection fraction, left ventricular dilatation, or

significantly elevated left ventricular diastolic pressure at rest or with exercise) would be an indication for aortic valve replacement with or without any clinical symptoms. Aortic valve repair for aortic stenosis has yielded relatively poor long-term results in comparison with aortic valve replacement (Craver, 1990).

Percutaneous balloon aortic valvuloplasty has a very limited role to palliate severe aortic stenosis in patients otherwise too ill to undergo aortic valve replacement (Smedira et al., 1993). Studies now show that balloon aortic valvuloplasty may improve aortic valve area by up to 50% with some improvement in symptoms, although most hemodynamic or symptomatic benefits from balloon aortic valvuloplasty are lost 6 months after the procedure (Davidson et al., 1990).

## AORTIC REGURGITATION

### Cause

The cause of aortic regurgitation overlaps significantly with that of aortic stenosis (see Table 52–1), so mixed aortic stenosis and regurgitation occurs frequently. Degenerative calcific aortic valve disease may cause aortic insufficiency owing to leaflet fixation that prevents full closure of the leaflets during diastole. Similarly, rheumatic heart disease may cause fibrosis of the aortic valve leaflets with retraction and rolling of the edges and secondary failure of the leaflets to fully approximate during diastole. Congenital bicuspid aortic valve disease may produce some degree of aortic valve regurgitation owing to progressive fibrosis and calcification of the leaflets or owing to distortion of the leaflets.

Aortic regurgitation may result from annuloaortic ectasia, defined as abnormal dilatation of the aortic valve annulus and aortic root, often with displacement of the right coronary ostium to over 1.5 cm from the aortic valve annulus. Cystic medial necrosis of the aortic wall is a frequent histologic finding in annuloaortic ectasia, and is characterized by degeneration of elastic bands in the aortic wall, abnormal organization of smooth muscle bundles, increased collagen, and cystic vacuoles in the aortic media (Roberts and Honig, 1982). Aortic stenosis or regurgitation may be accompanied by secondary aneurysm of the ascending aorta with or without annuloaortic ectasia.

Other causes of aortic regurgitation include myxoid degeneration of the aortic valve leaflets with progressive leaflet thinning, prolapse, and failure to coapt during diastole (Lakier et al., 1985). Aortic dissection may produce aortic regurgitation owing to detachment of the aortic valve apparatus from the aortic wall with prolapse of the leaflets inward toward the left ventricle. Bacterial endocarditis may account for 12% of patients with aortic regurgitation (see Table 52–1) and typically produces aortic regurgitation by perforation or rupture of the aortic valve leaflets. Although endocarditis can occur on a previously normal valve, endocarditis commonly affects patients

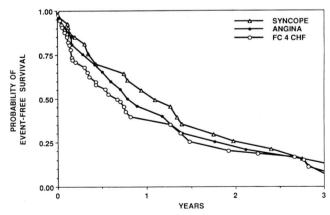

FIGURE 52–4. Event-free survival in patients with aortic stenosis managed medically. Note similar survival whether symptoms were syncope, angina, or functional class IV heart failure (FC 4 CHF). (From Lieberman, E. B., Bashore, T. M., Hermiller, J. B., et al.: Balloon aortic valvuloplasty in the elderly: The final chapter? Circulation, [in press].)

with underlying aortic valve disease. Other inflammatory conditions, such as rheumatoid arthritis, ankylosing spondylitis, and Reiter's syndrome, have been associated with aortitis and aortic regurgitation (Kawasuji et al., 1982). Finally, blunt or penetrating chest trauma may produce aortic regurgitation by either rupture or puncture of the aortic valve leaflets (Ovil et al., 1990).

## Pathophysiology

Aortic regurgitation represents a volume overload of the left ventricle. Although left ventricular hemodynamics are relatively normal during systole in aortic regurgitation, significant aortic regurgitation causes left ventricular diastolic filling from both the left atrium and the ascending aorta. Because a certain fraction of the forward cardiac output during systole returns to the left ventricle during diastole, the left ventricular output during systole is increased by autonomic reflexes to maintain a normal net forward cardiac output (Florenzano and Glantz, 1987). As a result of the increased left ventricular diastolic filling and the increased stroke volume necessary to maintain forward cardiac output, aortic regurgitation immediately increases left ventricular diastolic filling pressure. This increased diastolic filling pressure in turn raises left ventricular diastolic volume and diastolic wall stress, which causes long-term progressive

left ventricular dilatation. The increased left ventricular wall stress due to elevated filling pressure and increased radius of curvature produces eccentric hypertrophy of the left ventricle with both dilatation and increased wall mass, as opposed to the concentric hypertrophy generally seen in aortic stenosis (Grossman et al., 1975). With progressive left ventricular dilatation, massive enlargement of the left ventricle may occur, prompting the term *cor bovinum*.

Although increased circulating catecholamines may maintain ventricular performance in early aortic regurgitation (Florenzano and Glantz, 1987), progressive left ventricular dilatation and increased wall stress subsequently lead to progressive fall in left ventricular contractility and ejection fraction, until forward cardiac output can no longer be maintained and the patient expires from progressive congestive heart failure. Symptoms of congestive heart failure derive from the increased pulmonary venous pressure at rest or with exercise owing to increased left ventricular diastolic pressure. The onset of atrial fibrillation may be highly symptomatic in aortic regurgitation owing to loss of the atrial systole that is normally so critical to filling a dilated, hypertrophied, and noncompliant left ventricle. Subendocardial ischemia may occur owing to decreased diastolic coronary perfusion pressure, increased diastolic ventricular pressure, left ventricular hypertrophy, and increased left ventricular workload (Folts and Rowe, 1974). Left ventricular afterload reduction may significantly improve for-

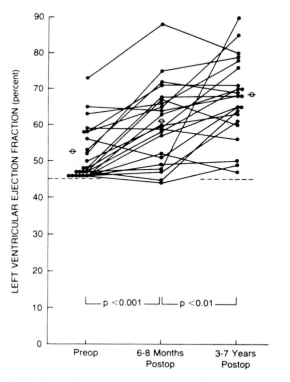
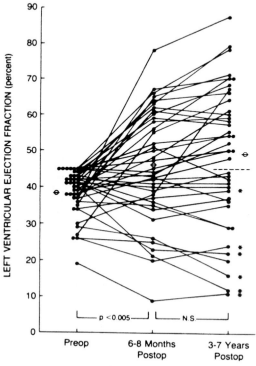

**FIGURE 52–5.** Serial changes in left ventricular ejection fraction in patients with normal *(left panel)* or abnormal *(right panel)* ejection fraction prior to surgical correction of aortic regurgitation. (*Asterisk* = Patients who subsequently died from heart failure. (From Lee, R. T., and St. John Sutton, M.: Left ventricular function after aortic valve surgery. *In* Emery, R. W., and Arom, K. V. [eds]: The Aortic Valve. Philadelphia, Hanley & Belfus, 1991; modified from Bonow, R. O., Dodd, J. T., Maron, B. J., et al.: Long-term serial changes in left ventricular function and reversal of ventricular dilation after valve replacement for chronic aortic regurgitation. Circulation, *78*:1108, 1988.)

ward cardiac output in aortic regurgitation (unlike aortic stenosis) by decreasing the pressure gradient across the aortic valve during diastole and thereby reducing the amount of regurgitation.

Aortic valve replacement has a more variable effect on postoperative left ventricular function in aortic regurgitation than in aortic stenosis. Correction of aortic regurgitation tends to normalize left ventricular ejection fraction, systolic and diastolic volumes, wall stress, and wall mass over a period of weeks to years (Bonow et al., 1988; Borer et al., 1991) (Fig. 52–5). However, a preoperative combination of abnormal ventricular chamber performance and abnormal myocardial function evidenced by the relationship between ejection fraction and end-systolic stress increases the likelihood of persistent or even progressive left ventricular dysfunction postoperatively (Starling et al., 1991) (Fig. 52–6). Patients with persistent left ventricular dilatation 6 months after aortic valve replacement are much more likely to die early from cardiac disease (Bonow et al., 1980).

## Clinical Findings

The most frequent symptoms in aortic regurgitation are those of congestive heart failure: dyspnea, orthop-

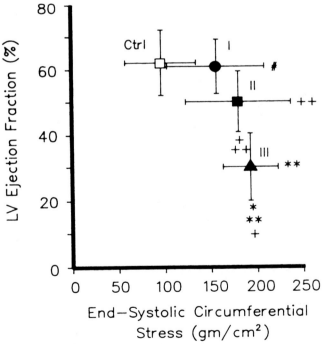

FIGURE 52–6. Relationship between preoperative ejection fraction and end-systolic stress in control patients (Ctrl) and in patients with aortic regurgitation (Groups I, II, and III). Group III patients with abnormal preoperative chamber performance ($E_{max}$) and abnormal ejection fraction versus stress relationship tended to have unfavorable outcome after aortic valve replacement. (From Starling, M. R., Kirsch, M. M., Montgomery, D. G., and Gross, M. D.: Mechanisms for left ventricular systolic dysfunction in aortic regurgitation: Importance for predicting the functional response to aortic valve replacement. College of Cardiology [Journal of the American College of Cardiology, 1991, Vol. 17, pp. 887–897].)

nea, and paroxysmal nocturnal dyspnea (see Table 52–2). Angina may occur in less than half of patients, and syncope is relatively unusual in aortic regurgitation. Physical examination may demonstrate lateral displacement of the left ventricular apical impulse. Because of increased systolic stroke volume and decreased diastolic aortic pressure to 60 mm Hg or less, the aortic pulse pressure may be markedly increased to over 50 mm Hg in aortic regurgitation. As a result, peripheral pulses may be dramatically pulsatile and of a "water hammer" character, often with bobbing of the head and extremities with each cardiac cycle. Cardiac auscultation reveals an early diastolic decrescendo murmur radiating toward the left ventricular apex. In the presence of severe aortic regurgitation, a mid-diastolic Austin-Flint murmur may occur at the left ventricular apex owing to the regurgitant aortic jet fluttering the anterior mitral valve leaflet. A third heart sound may be present in association with left ventricular dilatation, decreased left ventricular compliance, and more rapid diastolic filling of the left ventricle (Glower et al., 1992).

## Diagnosis

The chest radiograph in aortic regurgitation may be normal or may demonstrate left ventricular enlargement, enlargement of the ascending aorta, pulmonary edema, or pulmonary venous engorgement. Left ventricular hypertrophy with strain may be present on electrocardiogram.

Doppler echocardiography readily demonstrates diastolic regurgitation of blood flow across the aortic valve (Fig. 52–7) which may be quantified on a 1+ to 4+ scale (Fig. 52–8). Two-dimensional echocardiography may also detect associated aortic valve pathology, such as leaflet thickening, calcification, or stenosis; left ventricular dilatation or hypertrophy and impaired ejection fraction are also easily visualized.

Cineradiography can quantify diastolic regurgitation of dye across the aortic valve, using a similar scale of 1+ to 4+ (Sellers et al., 1964). Left ventriculography and aortography may demonstrate left ventricular dilatation, impaired left ventricular ejection fraction, and dilatation of the ascending aorta. Coronary arteriography is necessary to delineate coronary anatomy, and this should be performed in patients over the age of 40 years or with risk factors for coronary artery disease. Either echocardiography or cineangiography may demonstrate aortic dissection involving the ascending aorta.

## Natural History

As with aortic stenosis, aortic regurgitation may be present for many years before symptoms develop, and clinical symptoms may appear even 3 to 10 years after onset of severe aortic regurgitation (Spagnuolo et al., 1971). The onset of symptoms correlates with elevation of left ventricular end-diastolic pressure, left

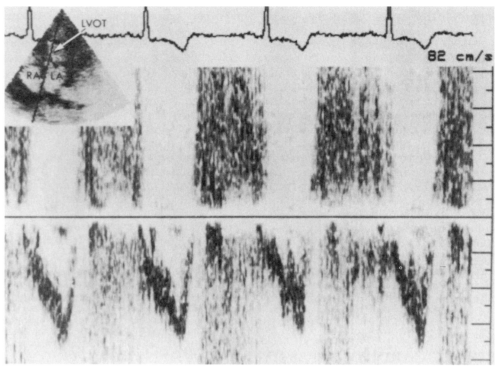

**FIGURE 52–7.** Doppler echocardiogram demonstrating aortic regurgitation as a high-velocity flow during diastole (below the center line) in the left ventricular outflow tract (LVOT). (From Feigenbaum, H.: Echocardiography. 4th ed. Philadelphia, Lea & Febiger, 1986, p. 291.)

ventricular dilatation, and depressed left ventricular contractility, and generally follows within 3 to 6 months of detectable left ventricular dilatation in patients with asymptomatic aortic regurgitation (Bonow et al., 1983). Survival may be 81% at 5 years in medically treated patients with aortic regurgitation, no symptoms, and normal left ventricular function (Bonow et al., 1983). Once symptoms develop, left ventricular performance may fall rapidly; mean survival is 5 years after onset of angina and 2 years after onset of heart failure with medical therapy (Hegglin et al., 1968). Acute onset of severe aortic regurgitation owing to aortic valve endocarditis may accelerate clinical deterioration with decompensated heart failure or even death within days or weeks.

## Management

Because the likelihood of death is small, patients with asymptomatic aortic regurgitation and normal left ventricular function may be managed medically. Diuretics or afterload reduction, or both, may improve early symptoms until surgical correction can be performed. Although the intra-aortic balloon pump may be a useful means of afterload reduction in other critically ill patients, it is relatively contraindicated in patients with aortic regurgitation because the balloon pump will increase aortic diastolic pressure and actually worsen aortic regurgitation.

The indications for aortic valve repair or replacement for 3+ to 4+ aortic regurgitation include the

**LAX**

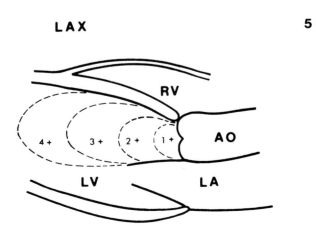

**5 CH**

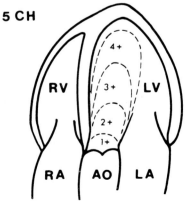

**FIGURE 52–8.** Use of pulsed Doppler mapping to quantify severity of aortic regurgitation on two-dimensional echocardiogram. (LAX = long-axis view; RV = right ventricle; AO = aorta; LA = left atrium; LV = left ventricle; 5 CH = 5-chamber view; RA = right atrium.) (From Feigenbaum, H.: Echocardiography. 4th ed. Philadelphia, Lea & Febiger, 1986, p. 293.)

presence of symptoms or any impairment of left ventricular function, left ventricular dilatation, or significant elevation of left ventricular end-diastolic pressure. Although no single parameter clearly contraindicates aortic valve replacement, impairment of both ventricular and myocardial performance seems to predict poor outcome after aortic valve replacement (Starling et al., 1991) (see Fig. 52–6).

## MIXED AORTIC VALVE DISEASE

In a series of patients undergoing aortic valve replacement at Duke University, 18% of patients (78 of 432) had both significant aortic stenosis and 3+ or more aortic regurgitation. Depending on the relative degree to which stenosis or regurgitation are present, the pathophysiology, clinical findings, and natural history may resemble both aortic stenosis and aortic regurgitation. In patients with balanced stenosis and regurgitation, symptoms of aortic stenosis may predominate. Balanced aortic stenosis and regurgitation results from congenitally abnormal aortic valves in one-half of patients, and rheumatic disease or other

inflammatory disorders are the cause in the remainder (Kirklin and Barratt-Boyes, 1993). Mixed aortic valve disease is diagnosed and treated in the same manner as isolated stenosis or regurgitation, with aortic valve replacement being the treatment of choice for symptomatic patients.

## HYPERTROPHIC CARDIOMYOPATHY

### Cause

Hypertrophic cardiomyopathy, a spectrum of disease characterized by asymmetric septal hypertrophy and microscopic disorganization of muscle bundles (Fig. 52–9), was first described in association with subaortic obstruction by Teare (1958). Importantly, muscle disorganization and septal hypertrophy may each occur alone in patients with disorders other than hypertrophic cardiomyopathy. The cause of hypertrophic cardiomyopathy is thought to be genetic, often with an autosomal dominant pattern of inheritance. Sporadic cases also occur (Maron et al., 1987a), with some studies demonstrating point mutations of the

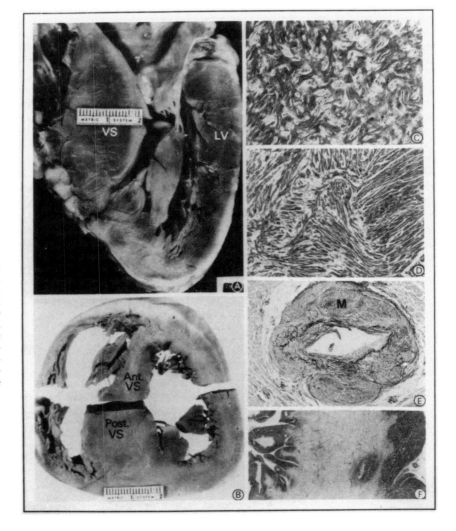

**FIGURE 52–9.** Pathologic features of hypertrophic cardiomyopathy. *A,* Heart specimen sectioned longitudinally demonstrating asymmetric septal hypertrophy with wall thickening primarily in the anterior septum that bulges into the left ventricular outflow tract. (VS = ventricular septum; LV = left ventricle.) *B,* Specimen with hypertrophy primarily in the posterior ventricular septum. (Post. VS). (Ant. VS = anterior ventricular septum.) *C,* Disordered cellular architecture with adjacent myocytes arranged at perpendicular or oblique angles. *D,* Bundles of hypertrophied cells with a disorganized, interwoven arrangement. *E,* Intramural coronary artery with narrowed lumen and medial hypertrophy (M). *F,* Extensive transmural scarring of the septum. (*A–F,* From Maron, B. J., Bonow, R. O., Cannon, R. O., et al.: Hypertrophic cardiomyopathy: Interrelations of clinical manifestations, pathophysiology, and therapy. Part I. Reprinted, by permission of the New England Journal of Medicine *316:*780, 1987.)

myosin protein in some familial forms of hypertrophic cardiomyopathy (Hejtmancik et al., 1991). Histologically, ventricular muscle demonstrates a characteristic whorled, disorganized pattern of muscle bundles with occasional patchy myocardial fibrosis. Grossly, the left ventricular septum tends to be at least 1.3 times the thickness of the left ventricular free wall (Wynne and Braunwald, 1988), although the location of the septal thickening may vary and be more predominant at the subaortic area in some patients or at the left ventricular apex in others (Maron et al., 1987a).

## Pathophysiology

Twenty-five per cent of patients with hypertrophic cardiomyopathy have dynamic systolic subaortic obstruction resulting from contact between the left ventricular septum and the mitral valve leaflets. Anatomically, the narrowing of the left ventricular outflow tract results from increased septal thickness and from abnormal anterior displacement of the mitral valve. The dynamic subaortic obstruction may occur spontaneously and tends to be augmented by increased contractility, decreased arterial pressure, or decreased left ventricular volume. Mitral regurgitation may also occur in a minority of patients owing to increased leaflet area, abnormal papillary muscle insertion, or abnormal systolic anterior motion of the mitral valve leaflets (Klues et al., 1992). Left ventricular diastolic dysfunction evidenced by impaired relaxation, decreased compliance, and impairment of diastolic left ventricular filling is present in most patients with hypertrophic cardiomyopathy (Maron et al., 1987a). Left ventricular diastolic dysfunction may be improved by calcium channel blockers and may be accentuated by atrial fibrillation with the loss of atrial systole. Myocardial ischemia may occur along with chest pain in the absence of coronary artery disease owing to elevated left ventricular pressure, increased myocardial oxygen demand, and abnormalities in small coronary vascular flow.

## Clinical Findings

The symptoms of hypertrophic cardiomyopathy commonly include dyspnea, fatigue, and chest pain, with presyncope and syncope occurring in some patients. The severity of clinical symptoms has correlated poorly with the severity of underlying pathophysiologic mechanisms. On examination, most patients with hypertrophic cardiomyopathy have an S4 gallop, and a minority of patients may have an intermittent or persistent systolic flow murmur. The systolic flow murmur may be accentuated by amyl nitrate administration, Valsalva's maneuver, and standing. Unlike valvular aortic stenosis, hypertrophic cardiomyopathy is characterized by a rapid carotid upstroke.

## Diagnosis

Most patients with symptomatic hypertrophic cardiomyopathy have an abnormal electrocardiogram with such findings as atrial fibrillation, left ventricular hypertrophy, or ST-segment and T-wave abnormalities. The chest radiograph may be relatively normal or may demonstrate left ventricular enlargement.

Echocardiography can detect most anatomic abnormalities in hypertrophic cardiomyopathy, such as asymmetric septal hypertrophy, *systolic anterior motion* of the mitral valve, mitral valve regurgitation, subvalvular aortic stenosis, and impaired diastolic performance (Fig. 52–10). Most of these features may also be demonstrated on cardiac catheterization, along with the presence of any coronary artery disease. Dynamic subvalvular outflow obstruction may be elicited during cardiac catheterization by administering amyl nitrate or during a postextrasystole (Brockenbrough's maneuver). A resting subvalvular aortic gradient over 30 mm Hg or an elicited gradient over 50 mm Hg is considered hemodynamically significant.

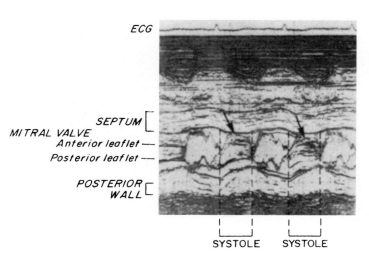

FIGURE 52–10. M-mode echocardiogram from a patient with hypertrophic cardiomyopathy. Note the abnormal systolic anterior motion of the mitral valve *(arrow)*. The thickness of the septum clearly exceeds that of the posterior left ventricular wall. (From Powell, W. J., Jr.: Hypertrophic nondilated cardiomyopathy: Idiopathic hypertrophic subaortic stenosis and its variants. *In* Johnson, R. A., Hobsen, E., and Austen, W. G. [eds]: The Practice of Cardiology. Boston, Little, Brown, 1980, p. 657.)

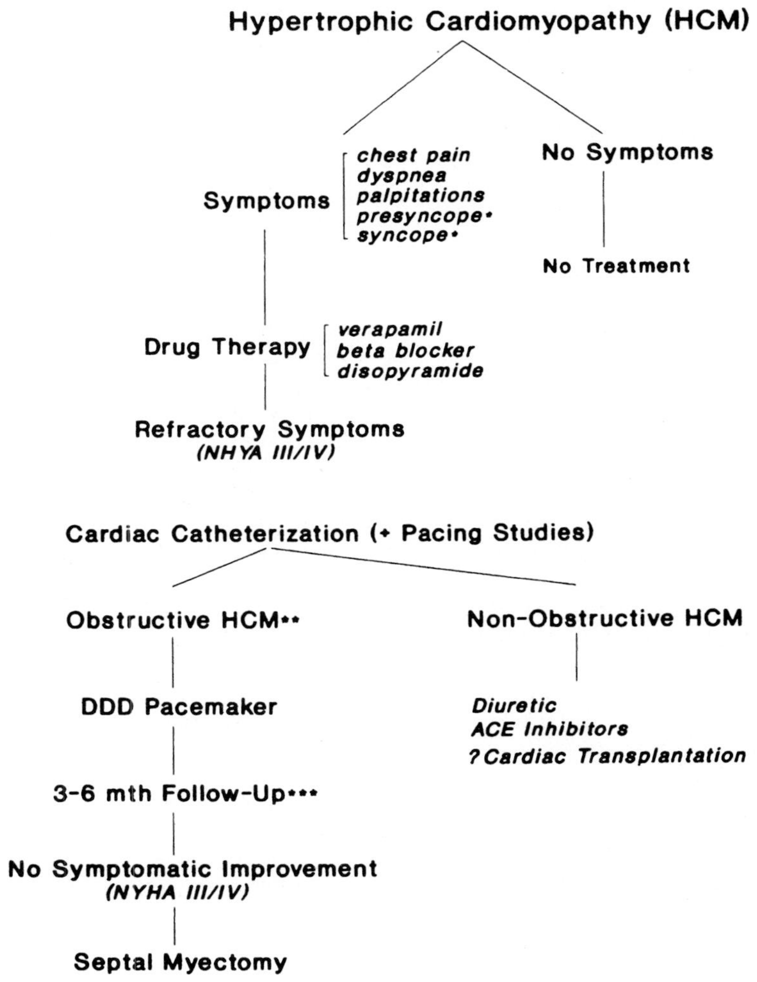

## Hypertrophic Cardiomyopathy (HCM)

Symptoms
- chest pain
- dyspnea
- palpitations
- presyncope•
- syncope•

No Symptoms

No Treatment

Drug Therapy
- verapamil
- beta blocker
- disopyramide

Refractory Symptoms
*(NHYA III/IV)*

Cardiac Catheterization (+ Pacing Studies)

Obstructive HCM••

DDD Pacemaker

3-6 mth Follow-Up•••

No Symptomatic Improvement
*(NYHA III/IV)*

Septal Myectomy

Non-Obstructive HCM

*Diuretic*
*ACE Inhibitors*
*?Cardiac Transplantation*

FIGURE 52–11. Proposed management of patients with hypertrophic cardiomyopathy (HCM). (NYHA = New York Heart Association functional class; DDD = dual-chamber pacing; mth = month; ACE = angiotensin-converting enzyme.) (From Fananapazir, L., Cannon, R. O., Tripodi, D., and Panza, J. A.: Impact of dual-chamber permanent pacing in patients with obstructive hypertrophic cardiomyopathy with symptoms refractory to verapamil and β-adrenergic blocker therapy. Circulation, 85:2149, 1992.)

## Natural History

Although hypertrophic cardiomyopathy is a congenital disorder that has been demonstrated pathologically in all age groups, most patients remain asymptomatic until the third or fourth decade of life. Clinical symptoms are often acutely exacerbated by the onset of atrial fibrillation. Sudden death may occur, with an incidence of 2 to 3% per patient-year in patients with hypertrophic cardiomyopathy (Maron et al., 1987b), and is thought to result from atrial arrhythmias with hypotension, bradyarrhythmias, or ventricular tachycardia (Maron and Fananapazir, 1992). Congestive heart failure or arrhythmias may also cause death in a minority of patients.

## Management

Medical therapy controls symptoms in most patients with hypertrophic cardiomyopathy. The mainstays of medical treatment are beta-blockers and calcium channel blockers, but neither of these classes of

agents appears to decrease the incidence of sudden death (McKenna, 1983). Amiodarone may be used in selected patients with nonsustained ventricular tachycardia or refractory atrial arrhythmias (McKenna et al., 1984). Most patients with symptoms refractory to medical therapy will receive symptomatic improvement with atrioventricular pacing, which has been shown to improve subvalvular gradients, presumably by altered timing of septal contraction (Fananapazir et al., 1992) (Fig. 52–11).

Currently, operative treatment of hypertrophic cardiomyopathy is indicated in patients with a subvalvular gradient of 50 mm Hg or significant mitral regurgitation, and whose symptoms do not respond to medical therapy and atrioventricular pacing. The primary surgical procedure for hypertrophic cardiomyopathy is septal myotomy-myectomy, which involves removing a strip of obstructing septal muscle at the point of contact with the mitral valve. Mitral valve replacement has also relieved symptoms in patients with hypertrophic cardiomyopathy and subvalvular aortic stenosis, particularly in patients with severe mitral valvular disease or previous septal myotomy. Up to 70% of patients gain long-lasting symptomatic relief from operative intervention up to 25 years postoperatively.

## SURGICAL THERAPY FOR AORTIC VALVE DISEASE

### Preoperative Preparation

In addition to the normal preparation for any general anesthetic, several special considerations should be addressed in patients undergoing aortic valve surgery. Before elective aortic valve operation, patients with dental abscesses or severe periodontal disease should have infected teeth removed and any potential source of sepsis corrected. Elective aortic valve operation may then be performed 5 to 10 days later. Patients requiring emergent or urgent aortic valve replacement may need to delay definitive treatment of dental disease until after aortic valve operation. Similarly, other sources of ongoing infection should be sought and corrected before elective aortic valve operation. Such sources include urinary tract infections, respiratory infections, or any potentially septic process in the gastrointestinal tract.

Because of the possibility of postoperative anticoagulation in patients undergoing aortic valve operation, a careful history should be taken regarding any difficulties with bleeding from previous surgical procedures, gastrointestinal bleeding, peptic ulcer disease, or easy bruising or bleeding. Clotting parameters such as the prothrombin time, partial thromboplastin time, and platelet count should be evaluated preoperatively.

### Conduct of Routine Aortic Valve Replacement

After routine preparation for cardiopulmonary bypass (see Chapter 32), a median sternotomy is performed, and the patient is heparinized. The distal ascending aorta is generally cannulated, although cannulation of the femoral artery may be preferable in some redo aortic valve replacements or in the presence of aneurysmal or atherosclerotic disease of the ascending aorta. The right atrium is cannulated either with bicaval cannulae or with a single two-stage cannula, and cardiopulmonary bypass is initiated at 32 to 34° C. If severe aortic regurgitation is present, consideration should be given to initiating cardiopulmonary bypass slowly at normothermia while a left ventricular vent is placed to prevent ventricular fibrillation and distention owing to aortic insufficiency. The left ventricle is vented with a cannula inserted through the right superior pulmonary vein to prevent left ventricular distention, to keep the operative field clear of blood during aortic valve placement, and to evacuate air after removing the aortic cross-clamp. Alternatively, a vent may be inserted through the left ventricular apex, or it may be placed in the proximal pulmonary artery in the absence of significant aortic

regurgitation. Suction is placed on the left ventricular vent, and the bypass perfusion temperature is dropped to 25 to 28° C. The aorta and pulmonary artery are dissected free posteriorly to the area of the left main coronary artery, and the anterior aortic root is exposed, with care taken not to injure the right coronary artery.

Preparations are made for cardioplegic arrest in one of several methods. A combination of anterograde and retrograde cardioplegia is often used because retrograde cardioplegia may be administered easily while continuing operation on the aortic valve. Retrograde cardioplegia also minimizes trauma to the coronary ostia and optimizes left ventricular preservation in the presence of coronary artery disease. Most commonly, retrograde cardioplegia is delivered by a balloon-tipped coronary sinus catheter placed into the coronary sinus through a purse-string in the right atrium prior to right atrial cannulation. An anterograde cardioplegic cannula is placed in the most anterior portion of the ascending aorta to vent air from the aorta after removal of the aortic cross-clamp. Left ventricular septal temperature is generally monitored with a septal thermistor to optimize myocardial preservation in a hypertrophied left ventricle. As soon as the left ventricle fibrillates or when the myocardial temperature reaches 29° C, the ascending aorta is cross-clamped, and anterograde cardioplegia is administered to obtain rapid cardiac arrest. Once adequate cardiac arrest is achieved, subsequent cardioplegic doses are administered through the retrograde coronary sinus catheter to maintain a myocardial temperature of 10° C. The left ventricular vent should be turned off during administration of the anterograde cardioplegic dose, particularly in the presence of aortic regurgitation, which might require massage of the left ventricle to prevent left ventricular distention from regurgitant cardioplegia.

After the initial dose of cardioplegia is administered into the ascending aorta, aortotomy is begun transversely (Fig. 52–12), and suction is reinitiated on the left ventricular vent. Once the location of the aortotomy is ascertained relative to the coronary ostia and the aortic valve commissures, the aortotomy is extended rightward down toward the mid-noncoronary cusp and leftward toward the left-right coronary commissure, taking care that the aortotomy remains at least 10 to 15 mm above the aortic valve commissures and the coronary ostia. Somewhat different aortotomy incisions will be made if pulmonary valve autograft or ascending aortic grafting (see Chapter 33, Part IV) is anticipated. Small traction sutures may be placed transmurally or in the adventitia of the edge of the superior aortic lip to obtain better exposure.

The aortic valve is inspected, and a narrow gauze sponge may be inserted into the left ventricle to trap any valve fragments. To remove the valve, the initial incision into the valve should begin in the most accessible area, often the central portion of the right coronary leaflet or the right noncoronary commissure. With either a scalpel or scissors, each leaflet should be excised, leaving 1 to 2 mm of valve tissue internal

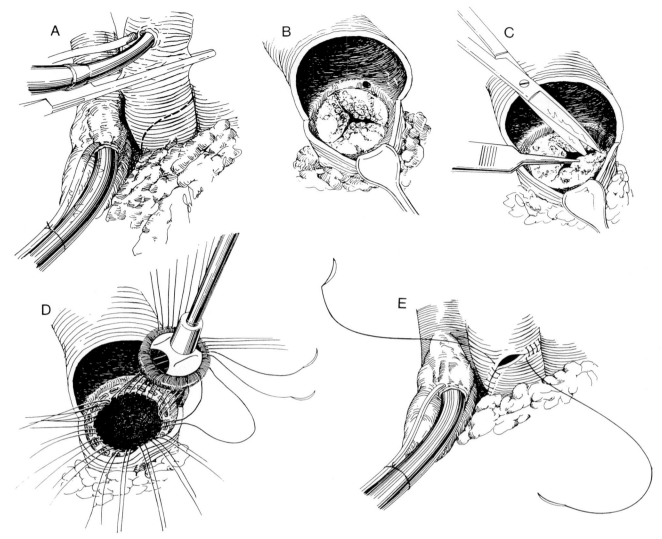

**FIGURE 52–12.** Technique of aortic valve replacement with a mechanical or stented tissue valve prosthesis. *A,* The aortic cross-clamp has been placed proximal to the aortic perfusion cannula. An oblique aortotomy incision is made, as indicated by the *broken line.* To the left, the incision passes into the sulcus between the aorta and the main pulmonary artery. To the right, the extension of the incision is angled obliquely toward the heart, into the center of the noncoronary sinus. *B,* The anterior edge of the proximal aortic wall is gently retracted, which gives excellent exposure of the aortic valve. *C,* Excision of the valve is begun at a point that lends itself most readily to incision. After the valve leaflets have been excised, the annulus is carefully débrided by using rongeurs to remove as much calcium as possible (not shown). *D,* Pledgeted mattress sutures are passed through the aortic annulus and then through the sewing ring of the prosthetic valve. *E,* The aortotomy incision is closed with continuous monofilament sutures.

to the valve annulus, taking care not to incise the annulus or the aortic wall. In the presence of extensive leaflet and annular calcification, attempts to totally decalcify the annulus should be avoided because this might separate the aorta from the left ventricle. Instead, annular calcification should be débrided only to the extent that is necessary to properly seat the replacement valve. Bone ronguers may be useful to crush and remove some of these calcified fragments. The annulus is then carefully inspected to ascertain that all loose fragments have been removed and that the remaining tissue is of adequate quality to seat the valve. The packing sponge may be removed, and the left ventricular cavity may be irrigated to remove any remaining loose debris with the vent turned off. The

left ventricular vent is reactivated, and a second cardioplegic infusion may be administered either retrograde or through direct coronary ostial cannulation.

The aortic annulus is sized using a sizer appropriate for the valve to be inserted. Sutures are placed through the aortic annulus and valve sewing ring using one of several techniques. In an annulus that is not overly narrow or where annular strength is suboptimal, a horizontal mattress of 2-0 polyester multifilament suture with subannular pledgets will provide the greatest strength, with the disadvantage of possibly having to deal with the subannular pledgets at a future reoperation. For the narrow annulus, particularly where the valve is placed in a supra-annular position, simple interrupted sutures of 3-0 polyester might be preferable. Other techniques include a figure-of-eight suture and a horizontal mattress suture with supra-annular pledgets. All sutures may be placed through the annulus first, with all sutures passing in sequence through the valvular sewing ring. Alternatively, each suture may be placed through the annulus and then through the sewing ring in one motion. Suture placement is generally begun in the area of greatest exposure, generally the noncoronary cusp, using each suture to provide exposure of the next suture. A normal aortic annulus requires 12 to 16 horizontal mattress sutures.

The sutures are tied starting at the area where proper valve seating is the most critical and most difficult, typically the left coronary cusp. Rewarming to normothermia is begun as the first valve sutures are being tied. Five to six throws are placed in each polyester multifilament suture, and the sutures are cut, with care taken to see that the knots and suture tags do not interfere with valve motion. The valve is then inspected to ensure that the valve functions freely without danger of leaflet entrapment and that no areas of potential perivalvular leak are evident.

The aortotomy is closed in two layers of continuous 3-0 or 4-0 polypropylene suture. A pledgeted mattress suture is placed at each corner of the aortotomy and brought toward the midaortotomy using a continuous horizontal mattress suture for the first layer. Before the suture is tied, air is expressed from the left atrium, left ventricle, and aorta by discontinuing suction on the left ventricular vent, transfusing volume from the heart-lung machine, having the anesthesiologist ventilate the lungs, and briefly flashing the aortic cross-clamp. The first layer of aortotomy is then closed and the cross-clamp released, at which time a second layer of continuous 3-0 or 4-0 polypropylene suture is then run from each corner as a vertical mattress suture.

When the clamp is removed, suction on the left ventricular vent is begun, and the anterograde cardioplegia site in the ascending aorta is either placed on suction or allowed to bleed freely to vent air from the ascending aorta. Additional air may be released from the left ventricle by aspirating the left ventricular apex with a 21-gauge needle.

The heart is electrically cardioverted as necessary, and temporary right atrial and right ventricular pacing wires are placed. Cardiopulmonary bypass is discontinued in the standard manner after the patient has rewarmed to 36° C. The left ventricular vent generally is removed once the patient reaches 34° C, once the left ventricle is ejecting well without distention, and when air has been sufficiently aspirated from the left ventricle and the left atrium. After discontinuing cardiopulmonary bypass for several minutes, the vent and cardioplegia site in the ascending aorta are repaired with a 4-0 Prolene horizontal mattress suture. Transesophageal echocardiography may be useful postbypass in some patients to assess aortic valve function and left ventricular contractile function (de Bruijn et al., 1987).

## Choice of Valvular Prosthesis

A wide array of valvular prostheses are available for aortic valve replacement (Fig. 52–13). Choice of a particular valve in an individual patient requires consideration of such factors as age, medical co-morbidity, life expectancy, life-style, and ability to comply with chronic anticoagulation therapy. Particular characteristics of the valve that must be considered are durability, thrombogenicity, hemodynamic performance, high versus low profile, availability, failure modes, and even cost.

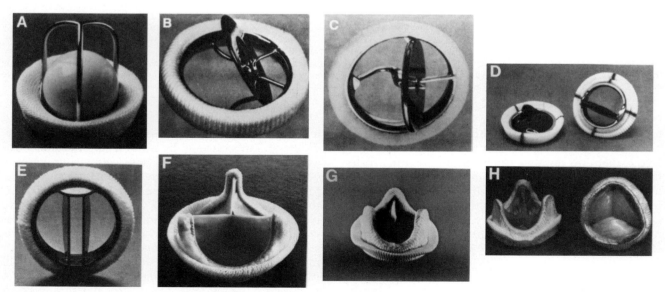

**FIGURE 52–13.** Examples of aortic valve prostheses. *A*, Starr-Edwards. *B*, Björk-Shiley. *C*, Medtronic Hall. *D*, Omniscience aortic *(left)* and mitral *(right)*. *E*, St. Jude Medical. *F*, Carpentier-Edwards pericardial. *G*, Hancock porcine. *H*, Carpentier-Edwards porcine. (Courtesy of: *A*, *F*, and *H*, Baxter Healthcare Corp.; *B*, Shiley Medical; *C* and *G*, Reprinted with permission from Medtronic, Inc., © Medtronic, Inc. 1988; *D*, Medical Incorporated; and *E*, St. Jude Medical.)

All available prostheses fall into the two broad categories of mechanical prostheses and biologic prostheses. Biologic prostheses generally have the advantage of not requiring anticoagulation and the disadvantage of a longevity limited to 10 to 12 years in the aortic position. Porcine bioprostheses and possibly other bioprostheses have been documented to have a shorter life span in younger patients (Williams, 1991), making bioprostheses more ideally suited for patients over the age of 60 years and for patients with a life expectancy of less than 10 to 12 years. Chronic renal failure may be a relative contraindication to bioprostheses, according to case reports of premature calcification of these valves. On the other hand, endocarditis with extensive aortic root abscess may be a relative indication for such stentless bioprostheses as the homograft and pulmonic valve autograft. Young women desiring further pregnancies should undergo placement of a bioprosthesis owing to the teratogenic and hemorrhagic risks associated with anticoagulation during pregnancy.

Mechanical prostheses generally have a greater longevity of 10 to 20 years or more, but require long-term anticoagulation to reduce the incidence of thromboembolism. On warfarin therapy with prothrombin ratios of 1.3 to 1.5 times normal, the thromboembolic rates of mechanical valves have been similar for all prostheses, roughly 2% per patient-year (Table 52–3). Management of mechanical aortic valves with antiplatelet therapy alone increases the thromboembolic rate to roughly 8% per patient-year (Czer et al., 1985). Anticoagulation with warfarin carries a 0.2% per patient-year mortality rate and a 2 to 3% per patient-year rate of anticoagulant-related hemorrhage (Edmunds, 1987; Lytle et al., 1989). The risks of warfarin therapy have decreased recently by lowering anticoagulation levels from prothrombin time ratios of 2.0 (International Ratio [INR] 5 to 6) or more to 1.3 to 1.5 (INR 2.0 to 2.5) today (Saour et al., 1990).

Several randomized trials have compared mechanical valves with biologic valves. Eleven years after aortic valve replacement in the Veterans Affairs Cooperative Study, mechanical and biologic valves did not differ in patient survival, thromboembolism, or freedom from any valve-related complication (Hammermeister et al., 1993). Mechanical valves had a higher incidence of hemorrhage whereas biologic valves had a higher incidence of reoperation (Hammermeister et al., 1993). In patients over 70 years old, bioprostheses may be favored by a low probability of reoperation and by hemorrhage rates as high as 9% per patient-year with mechanical valves (Borkon et al., 1988), although other series have not confirmed a higher rate of hemorrhage in elderly patients (Lytle et al., 1989). For patients over 40 years old in the nonrandomized study of Lytle and associates (1989), biologic valves provided better survival up to 10 years postoperatively, but survivals at 10 years were not different for mechanical and biologic valves.

**Hancock Porcine Valve.** Among the bioprostheses, the most extensively used are the stented bioprostheses generally made from porcine aortic valves fixed with glutaraldehyde. The Hancock model 242 valve became available in 1970 in sizes 19-mm to 31-mm and was subsequently followed by the modified-orifice (model 250) Hancock valve with a larger effective orifice (Cohn et al., 1989). Freedom from prosthetic dysfunction has been 82±3% at 10 years (Cohn et al., 1991) for the modified-orifice valve.

**Carpentier-Edwards Porcine Valve.** The standard Carpentier-Edwards model 2625 porcine valve became available in 1975 in sizes 19-mm to 31-mm (Jamieson et al., 1990) and was followed by the supra-annular model, which incorporated low pressure fixation and slight modification of the sewing ring and stent (Jamieson et al., 1991). Freedom from dysfunction has been 79±5% at 10 years for the standard valve (Jamieson et al., 1990) and 94±1% at 7 years for the supra-annular valve (Jamieson et al., 1991).

**Medtronic Intact Porcine Valve.** The Medtronic intact porcine valve became available in 1983 in sizes 19-mm to 29-mm. The valve is fixed with glutaraldehyde at low pressure and treated with toluidine to inhibit calcium deposition. Freedom from structural deterioration has been 100% at 4 to 6 years (Barratt-Boyes et al., 1991; Jaffe et al., 1989).

**Ionescu-Shiley Bovine Pericardial Valve.** The Ionescu-Shiley bovine pericardial valve became available in 1976 and was used extensively because of better flow dynamics and effective orifice area in small sizes relative to porcine valves (Table 52–4). The Ionescu-Shiley valve was subsequently found to have durability inferior to that of porcine valves, with freedom from prosthetic dysfunction being only 48±7% at 10 years (Masters et al., 1991).

**Carpentier-Edwards Pericardial Valve.** The Carpentier-Edwards pericardial valve became available in Europe in 1980, and preliminary data suggest that the durability of the Carpentier-Edwards pericardial valve may be superior to existing porcine bioprostheses, with freedom from prosthetic dysfunction being 97% at 7 years (Frater et al., 1992). Like other pericardial valves, this valve has a greater effective valve orifice area than do porcine valves, especially in the 19-mm and 21-mm sizes (see Table 52–4).

**Unstented Free Aortic Valve Homograft.** Free aortic

■ **Table 52–3.** THROMBOEMBOLIC RATES FOR AORTIC VALVE PROSTHESES (%/Patient-Year)

| | |
|---|---|
| Free aortic homograft | 0.2 (Daly et al., 1991) |
| Pulmonic valve autograft | <0.2 (Ross et al., 1991b) |
| Hancock porcine valve | 0.8–1.9 (Bortolotti et al., 1991; Cohn et al., 1984) |
| Carpentier-Edwards porcine valve | 1.3 (Jamieson et al., 1990) |
| Carpentier-Edwards pericardial valve | 0.7–1.7 (Frater et al., 1992; Perier et al., 1991) |
| Ionescu-Shiley pericardial valve | 1.2 (Gonzales-Lavin et al., 1991) |
| Standard Björk-Shiley valve | 1.9 (Swanson and Starr, 1989) |
| Starr-Edwards 1260 valve | 2.3 (Swanson and Starr, 1989) |
| St. Jude Medical valve | 1.4 (Swanson and Starr, 1989) |
| Medtronic-Hall valve | 1.8 (Swanson and Starr, 1989) |
| Björk-Shiley monostrut valve | 1.7 (Arts et al., 1992) |
| Omniscience valve | 2.7 (Swanson and Starr, 1989) |

homograft valves have been prepared with numerous techniques, including irradiation, chemical sterilization, fresh antibiotic sterilization, and cryopreservation. Current data suggest that the cryopreserved homograft has the greatest durability, with freedom from valvular degeneration at 10 years being 100% versus 57 to 89% for fresh homografts and considerably less for irradiated and chemically sterilized valves (Matsuki et al., 1988b; O'Brien et al., 1987). Homograft valves have excellent flow characteristics for the small annular sizes and thus might be indicated as a bioprosthesis for annular sizes less than 23 mm. The incidence of thromboembolism is extremely low, 0.2% per patient-year (see Table 52–3).

Relative indications for a homograft valve are a life expectancy greater than 10 years with contraindication for anticoagulation (children, women of childbearing age, young active adults), aortic root replacement, aortic root enlargement, small aortic annulus, bacterial endocarditis, and possibly, reoperation for other failed bioprosthesis (Hopkins, 1989). The primary disadvantages of free aortic homografts are limited availability, the cost of procurement and handling, and the greater technical demands of inserting a free homograft valve as opposed to the stented prostheses. Relative contraindications for homograft placement include severe annular calcification producing inadequate valve seating, unfavorable coronary ostial anatomy, aortic annular diameter larger than 30 mm, other complex cardiac procedures requiring significant cross-clamp time, severe left ventricular dysfunction, and connective tissue disorders such as Marfan's syndrome (Hopkins, 1989). In the event of an aortic valve

size over 30 mm, the aortic root may be reduced in size, a standard stented valve may be used, or any form of aortic root replacement may be employed, including a homograft "miniroot" replacement where only a very short length of homograft ascending aorta is retained (Glazier et al., 1991).

The technique of inserting free aortic valve homografts differs somewhat from that for stented valves. After excision of the aortic valve, the aortic valve is sized in the area from the commissures to the annulus. A homograft should be 2 to 4 mm smaller than the patient's aortic annulus. The homograft is cut straight 5 mm distal to the valve commissures, and scallops are then created in each homograft sinus of Valsalva, taking the scallop no closer than 3 mm to the homograft leaflet (Fig. 52–14A and B). The underside of the homograft is cut straight 2 mm below the lowest insertion of the cusps, and excess muscle is trimmed from the homograft. Three 3-0 braided sutures are then placed from the base of each graft sinus to the underside of the recipient annulus, with care taken to align the right homograft sinus with the left recipient sinus. The homograft valve is inverted, and one arm of each 3-0 suture is sewn to secure the lower edge of the homograft (Fig. 52–14C). The homograft is then everted, and the homograft commissural posts are secured to the aortic wall with nontransmural 4-0 Prolene sutures running from the midportion of each sinus up to the commissural post, where they are brought through the aortic wall and over pledgets (Hopkins, 1989) (Fig. 52–14D). The aortotomy is closed, and the procedure completed in the standard manner.

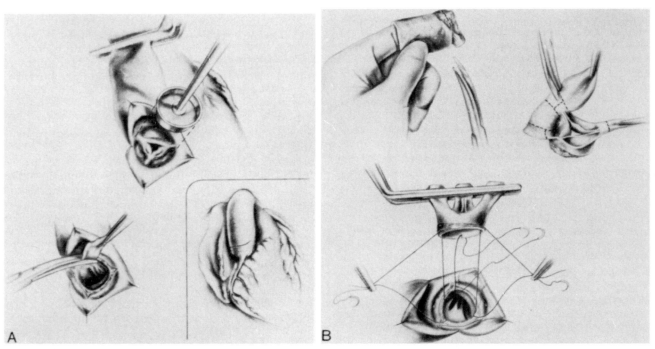

**FIGURE 52–14.** Technique of aortic valve replacement with nonstented homograft. *A,* The aortotomy incision extends into the noncoronary sinus of Valsalva. The annulus is measured and the valve is excised. *B,* Excessive ventricular septal muscle is trimmed from the aortic homograft. Aortic sinus tissue is excised, leaving a rim of 3 to 4 mm of aortic tissue for attachment to the recipient aorta. The valve is oriented within the recipient aortic root by placing three sutures, one beneath each of the commissures.

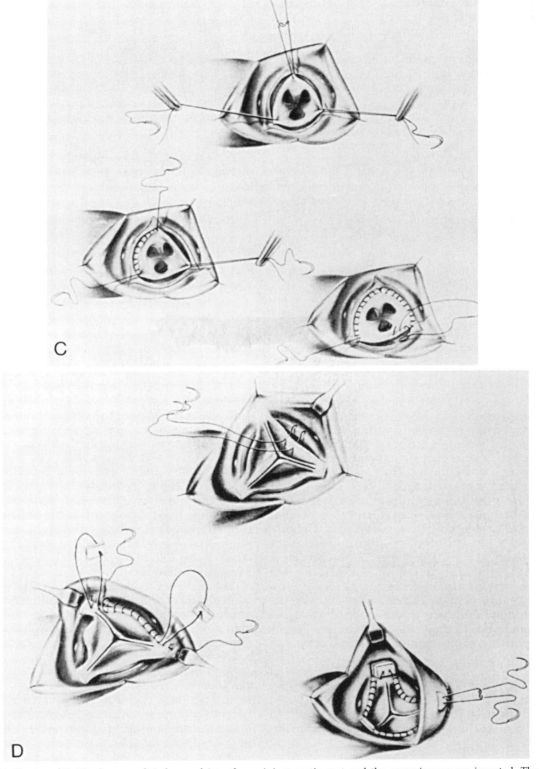

**FIGURE 52–14** *Continued C,* The homograft is lowered into the recipient aortic root and the commissures are inverted. The edge of the graft is sutured to the outflow tract below the aortic annulus with continuous sutures. *D,* The inverted commissures are brought back up into the aortic root. The rim of sinus tissue of the homograft is sutured to the sinus of the recipient aorta with continuous sutures. The tops of the commissures are secured with Teflon pledgets. (*A–D,* From Doty, D. B.: Replacement of the aortic valve with cryopreserved aortic valve allograft: Considerations and techniques in children. J. Cardiac. Surg., *1*[Suppl.]:130, 1987.)

**Aortic Root Homograft.** Aortic root homografts have seen increasing use at certain institutions since the mid-1980s, with durability similar to that of free aortic valve homografts (Okita et al., 1988). Potential advantages of the aortic root homograft include repair of extensive aortic root damage due to endocarditis (Tuna et al., 1990), lesser technical difficulties in valve insertion than with the free aortic homografts, and the ability to enlarge the aortic root. Potential indications for homograft aortic root replacement include tunnel aortic stenosis, valvular aortic stenosis with hypoplastic annulus, aortic stenosis with distorted anatomy precluding freehand homograft, bacterial endocarditis with destruction of aortoventricular continuity, and aortic insufficiency with aortic root dilatation in the absence of Marfan's syndrome or connective tissue disease (Hopkins, 1989). Relative

disadvantages include somewhat greater difficulty in reoperation owing to the greater amount of calcified tissue to be removed. The technique of root replacement is discussed in Chapter 33, Section IV (Hopkins, 1989).

**Pulmonic Valve Autograft.** The pulmonic valve autograft has been used by Ross and colleagues (1991) and others, particularly in patients under the age of 45 years (Elkins et al., 1992; Matsuki et al., 1988a). This procedure transfers the pulmonic valve and root to the aortic annulus and replaces the pulmonic valve and root with a pulmonary root homograft. In children, the pulmonary autograft has shown some capacity for growth and has had 93% freedom from reoperation at 5.6 years (Elkins et al., 1992) and 85% freedom from reoperation at 20 years (Ross et al., 1991).

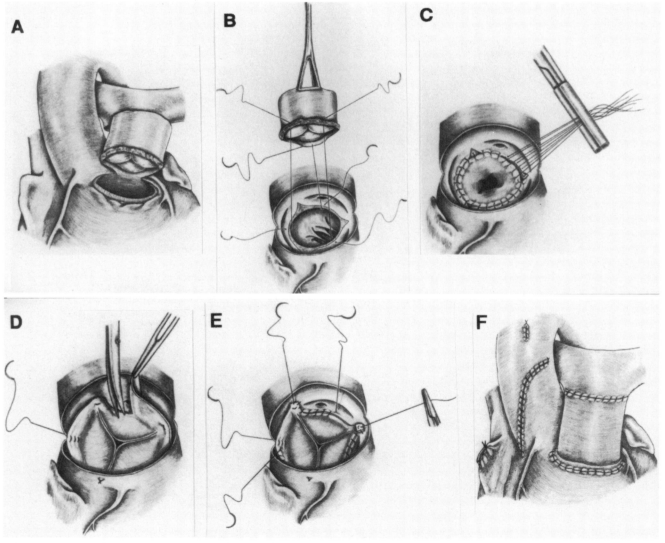

**FIGURE 52–15.** Technique of aortic valve replacement with a pulmonary autograft. *A,* Harvest of the pulmonary trunk and valve. *B,* Proximal suture line begun at the midpoint of each sinus of Valsalva. *C,* Interrupted proximal suture line with the autograft inverted. Completion with the free-hand technique. *D,* Anchoring of each commissure and scalloping of sinuses to expose coronary ostia. *E,* Incorporation of noncoronary sinus into aortotomy closure. The distal suture line runs below the coronary ostia. *F,* Closure of aortotomy and reconstruction of pulmonary outflow tract with cryopreserved pulmonary homograft.

■ **Table 52–4.** TYPICAL TRANSVALVULAR GRADIENTS AND VALVE ORIFICE AREAS IN SMALLER VALVE SIZES

| Valve | 19 mm | | 21 mm | |
|---|---|---|---|---|
| | Mean Gradient (mm Hg) | Area (cm²) | Mean Gradient (mm Hg) | Area (cm²) |
| Hancock modified orifice porcine valve (Khan et al., 1990) | 17 | 0.9 | 15 | 1.1 |
| Carpentier-Edwards porcine valve (Khan et al., 1990) | 32 | 0.8 | 22 | 0.9 |
| Carpentier-Edwards pericardial valve (Cosgrove et al., 1985) | 23 | 1.1 | 20 | 1.4 |
| Ionescu-Shiley pericardial valve (Ionescu and Tandon, 1978) | 8 | 1.1 | 8 | 1.4 |
| Björk-Shiley valve (Björk et al., 1973; Schaff et al., 1981) | 16 peak | 1.06 | 25 peak | 1.3 |
| Starr-Edwards 1260 valve (Pyle et al., 1978) | — | — | 29 | 1.0 |
| St. Jude Medical valve (Wortham et al., 1981) | 17 peak | 1.2 | 6 | 1.4 |
| Medtronic-Hall (Tatineni et al., 1989) | — | — | — | 1.5 |
| Björk-Shiley monostrut valve (Björk and Lindblom, 1985) | 11 | — | 9 | 1.4 |
| CarboMedics valve (Ihlen et al., 1992) | 17 | 1.1 | 12 | 1.5 |

After the aortotomy is performed and the aortic valve excised, the pulmonary valve autograft is then excised up to the pulmonary artery bifurcation, with care taken to not injure septal coronaries (Ross, 1991) (Fig. 52–15A–C). The pulmonary valve autograft shoulder is then oriented with the anterior convexity toward the patient's right so that the pulmonic sinuses accurately overly the aortic valve sinuses. After the valve is inverted, the proximal anastomosis is performed using interrupted 4-0 Prolene sutures. The valve is then everted, and the commissures are secured with individual sutures. The pulmonic sinuses are scalloped for the coronary ostia, and the distal anastomosis is performed using continuous 4-0 Prolene suture, with each suture tied over pledgets at the commissures (Fig. 52–15D–F). The aortotomy is closed, and a pulmonary homograft is sewn distally and proximally into the pulmonic outflow tract with running 4-0 Prolene. Alternatively, the pulmonary autograft may be completed as an aortic root replacement in a manner similar to aortic root replacement with an aortic homograft (Fig. 52–15G–J).

**Starr-Edwards Valve.** Of the valves currently available, the Starr-Edwards model 1200/1260 ball cage prosthesis has the longest performance record, having been available in essentially unmodified form since 1965 in 21-mm to 31-mm sizes. The durability of this prosthesis has been excellent, with no structural dysfunction observed in over 1100 patients followed up to 20 years (Cobanoglu et al., 1988; Miller et al.,

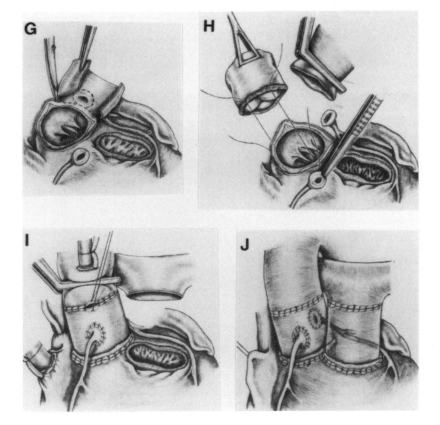

FIGURE 52–15 *Continued* Completion as a root replacement. *G*, Trimming the aortic root to split the distance between the coronary ostia and the valve annulus. *H*, Root alignment to allow coronary reimplantation as buttons. *I*, Completion of proximal and distal anastomoses. *J*, Reconstruction of pulmonary outflow tract with cryopreserved pulmonary homograft. (*A–F*, Modified from Randolph, J. D., Toal, K., Stelzer, P., and Elkins, R. C.: Aortic valve and left ventricular outflow tract replacement using allograft and autograft valves: A preliminary report. Reprinted with permission from the Society of Thoracic Surgeons [The Annals of Thoracic Surgery, 1989, Vol. 48, pp. 345–349]; *G–J*, Modified from Stelzer, P.: Pulmonary autograft replacement of the aortic valve. *In* Emery, R. W., and Arom, K. V. [eds]: The Aortic Valve. Philadelphia, Hanley & Belfus, Inc., 1991.)

1984). Freedom from explanation in mixed series of aortic and mitral valves varied from 92% at 20 years (Cobanoglu et al., 1988) to 90% at 10 years (Miller et al., 1984). The incidence of thrombosis is low at 0.1% per patient-year (Swanson and Starr, 1989). Potential disadvantages of the Starr-Edwards valve include significant transvalvular gradients in sizes less than 23 mm (see Table 52–4), and the high profile makes the valve unsuitable for narrow aortic roots.

**Björk-Shiley Valve.** The standard Björk-Shiley valve is a tilting disk that first became available in 1969. After problems with strut fracture in the 60-degree convexoconcave and 70-degree convexoconcave models, all Björk-Shiley valves were withdrawn from the market in 1986. At most, estimated rates of strut fracture are 0.47 and 1.3% per patient-year for the 60-degree and 70-degree aortic valve models, respectively, in the 29- to 33-mm sizes only. Although valve replacement is indicated for any instance of strut fracture, prophylactic valve replacement is generally not warranted except in certain batches of the 70-degree convexoconcave valve released only in Europe (Birkmeyer et al., 1992). Flemma and co-workers (1988) reported no structural deterioration in 785 patients followed up to 15 years with standard Björk-Shiley valves, but valve thrombosis was observed at a rate of 0.36% per patient-year.

**St. Jude Valve.** The St. Jude bileaflet valve is constructed of pyrolytic carbon and has been in use since 1977. The St. Jude valve is available in 19-mm to 31-mm sizes with either a standard sewing cuff or an expanded sewing cuff. A newer HP model available in the 17-mm to 21-mm sizes is designed to sit in a supra-annular position and provide slightly larger effective orifice areas. The St. Jude valve provides superior hemodynamics in small sizes (see Table 52–4) and excellent durability of 100% freedom from structural deterioration at 10 years (Arom et al., 1989; Czer et al., 1990). Nonstructural dysfunction has been primarily related to leaflet entrapment, and thrombosis is rare (0.1% per patient-year) (Swanson and Starr, 1989). These prostheses have the advantages of being low profile and excellent flow characteristics (see Table 52–4), making the St. Jude valve a desirable mechanical device in annular sizes less than 23 mm.

**Medtronic-Hall Valve.** The Medtronic-Hall valve is a pyrolytic carbon and metal tilting disk prosthesis first implanted in 1977 and now available in 20-mm to 31-mm sizes. This valve has excellent flow characteristics (see Table 52–4), and freedom from prosthetic dysfunction has been 100% at 10 years (Nitter-Hauge et al., 1989). Like other tilting disk valves, the Medtronic-Hall valve may have a slightly higher incidence of prosthetic thrombosis than do the bileaflet valves (Fig. 52–16).

**Björk-Shiley Monostrut Valve.** The Björk-Shiley monostrut valve became available in 1982 with a pyrolytic carbon tilting disk in metal housing. This valve is available in 17-mm to 33-mm sizes, has excellent flow characteristics (see Table 52–4), and has demonstrated 100% freedom from prosthetic dysfunction at 7 years (Aris et al., 1992).

**Omniscience Valve.** The Omniscience valve with a pyrolytic carbon tilting disk in metal housing became available in 1978 in 19-mm to 31-mm sizes. Freedom from structural dysfunction has been 100% at 9 years (Kazui et al., 1991).

**CarboMedics Valve.** The CarboMedics valve is a pyrolytic carbon bileaflet valve that became available in 1986 in 19-mm to 27-mm sizes. This valve has excellent flow characteristics (see Table 52–4), and freedom from prosthetic dysfunction has been 100% at 5 years (CarboMedics, 1993).

## Coronary Artery Bypass Grafting

The indication for coronary artery bypass grafting concurrent with aortic valve replacement is significant stenosis of a graftable coronary artery supplying a significant amount of viable myocardium. The additional operative risk of combining coronary bypass grafting with aortic valve replacement is small yet probably real (Lytle et al., 1988, 1989). On the other hand, failure to perform coronary bypass grafting may increase operatic mortality owing to perioperative myocardial infarction (Miller et al., 1979) and may contribute to 5 to 20% of late deaths after aortic valve replacement in patients with significant coronary disease (Lund et al., 1990a; Mullaney et al., 1987).

Saphenous vein has been the conduit most frequently used for coronary bypass grafting concurrent

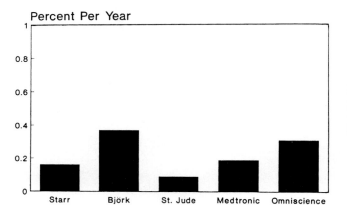

FIGURE 52–16. Pooled rates of valve thrombosis (% per patient-year) for selected mechanical valves. (From Swanson, J. S., and Starr, A.: The ball valve experience over three decades. Reprinted with permission from the Society of Thoracic Surgeons [The Annals of Thoracic Surgery, 1989, Vol. 48, pp. S51–S52].)

with aortic valve replacement, owing to the short harvest time for saphenous vein, the ability to administer cardioplegia down the saphenous vein, and the technical difficulties of performing subsequent redo aortic valve replacement in the presence of patent mammary grafts. However, increasing consideration should be given to use of internal mammary arteries in patients felt to have a life expectancy of more than 10 to 15 years and in whom the valvular prosthesis is expected to last 15 years.

Although many techniques may be used to perform concurrent aortic valve replacement and coronary artery bypass grafting, most surgeons will perform the distal coronary anastomoses first. After initial cardiac arrest, subsequent doses of cardioplegia may be administered through the coronary sinus, down the vein grafts, or by cannulation of the coronary ostia with the aorta open. Aortic valve replacement is then performed in the standard manner, the aortic cross-clamp is released, and the proximal anastomoses are performed after restoration of sinus rhythm and evacuation of intracardiac air.

## Replacement of the Ascending Aorta

The presence of dissection or aneurysm of the ascending aorta is the primary indication for ascending aortic replacement at the time of aortic valve operation. A more controversial indication for grafting the ascending aorta may be extensive ascending aortic atherosclerosis likely to produce atheroembolism. Details of replacing the ascending aorta are described further in Chapter 33, Section IV.

## Narrow Aortic Root

Adult patients with a small aortic root less than 21 mm may often be managed by selection of a prosthesis that provides an acceptable mild degree of residual aortic stenosis, particularly in small and inactive patients (Foster et al., 1986; Kallis et al., 1992). Narrowing of the supravalvular aorta can be relieved by closing the aortotomy with a gusset of pericardium or Dacron material if the aortic annulus itself is of adequate size (Hopkins, 1989; Piehler et al., 1983). In those patients where a satisfactory aortic valve orifice area cannot be obtained by any available prosthesis, the aortic root may be enlarged by one of several techniques. In certain patients, a larger prosthetic valve may be seated at an oblique angle by placing the noncoronary cusp suture ring in the supra-annular position (Olin et al., 1983). Using the technique of Nicks and associates (1970), the aortotomy may be extended through the mid-noncoronary sinus down onto the anterior leaflet of the mitral valve. An elliptical patch of Dacron or expanded *polytetrafluoroethylene* material is then sewn into place onto the mitral valve leaflet using continuous 4-0 Prolene suture, and the aortic valve is secured in the aortic root now enlarged by 2 to 4 mm (Fig. 52–17).

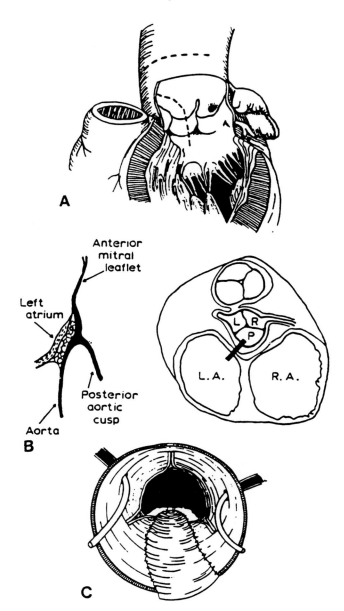

**FIGURE 52–17.** Aortic root enlargement by the technique of Nicks. *A,* The incision. *B,* Anatomic section of the aortic root through noncoronary sinus of Valsalva *(left panel).* Origins of the aortic and mitral valves as seen by the surgeon from above *(right panel).* (L.A. = left atrium; R.A. = right atrium; L = left; R = right; P = posterior. *C,* Final patch. *(A–C,* From Nicks, R., Cartmill, T., and Bernstein, L.: Hypoplasia of the aortic root: The problem of aortic valve replacement. Thorax, 24:339, 1970.)

Alternatively, more extensive patch enlargement of the aortic root by 3 to 5 mm is possible by extending the incision into the left noncoronary commissure and onto the left atrium (Manouguian and Seybold-Epting, 1979; Rittenhouse et al., 1979) (Fig. 52–18). Placement of an aortic homograft "miniroot" (Glazier et al., 1991; Hopkins, 1989) often allows significant enlargement of a narrowed aortic root using the incision of either Nicks or Manouguian. Finally, in unusual patients where the subvalvular left ventricular outflow tract is also narrowed, the aortotomy may be

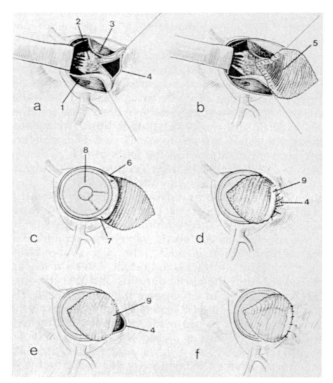

**FIGURE 52–18.** Aortic root enlargement by the technique of Manouguian. (1 = Left aortic leaflet; 2 = anterior mitral leaflet; 3 = noncoronary aortic leaflet; 4 = left atrial wall; 5 = patch; 6–7 = enlargement of the aortic valve ring; 8 = aortic valve prosthesis; 9 = sewing ring of the prosthesis.) *a*, The incision. *b*, Initial suture of patch. *c*, Implantation of prosthesis. *d*, Suture of left atrium and patch to sewing ring with same suture for small atriotomies. *e* and *f*, Separate closure of larger left atriotomy following larger posterior enlargements. (*a–f*, From Manouguian, S., and Seybold-Epting, W.: Patch enlargement of the aortic valve by extending the aortic incision into the anterior mitral leaflet. J. Thorac. Cardiovasc. Surg., *78*:402, 1979.)

extended anteriorly through the right coronary cusp onto the right ventricular outflow tract. Separate ventricular septal and right ventricular outflow tract patches of Dacron are placed obtaining roughly 3 to 5 mm increase in aortic valve size (Konno et al., 1975). In rare patients, a valve conduit has been placed between the left ventricular apex and the descending thoracic or abdominal aorta (Norman et al., 1980).

## Redo Aortic Valve Replacement

In redo aortic valve replacement, consideration should be given to cannulation of the femoral artery, particularly if extensive aortic disease is present. Usual precautions are taken to avoid injuring cardiac structures on entering the chest, and generally no more mediastinal dissection should be performed than is necessary. In the rare event that the ascending aorta is adherent to the sternum, an alternative technique would be to institute femoral venous-to-femoral arterial cardiopulmonary bypass and cool to 20° C. The median sternotomy may then be safely performed and circulatory arrest instituted if hemorrhage

from the aorta occurs on entering the chest (Bojar et al., 1988).

Aortic valve repair rather than replacement may be feasible if the underlying valve pathology is valve thrombosis or sterile perivalvular leakage. Otherwise, the prosthetic valve should be excised and replaced. If the previous valve was stented, the old sewing ring should ideally be excised, but leaving residual sewing ring is preferable to excessive débridement of the aortic annulus. If the previous valve was a free-hand aortic homograft, these prostheses can almost always be removed in their entirety by careful dissection. The conduct of the operation is otherwise as with first-time aortic valve replacement.

## Aortic Valve Endocarditis

The indications for aortic valve operation during active endocarditis include persistent sepsis, heart failure due to significant regurgitation, aortic root abscess, and occasionally, recurrent embolism due to endocarditis. Although aortic valve repair for endocarditis has been attempted, results have generally been less satisfactory than in mitral valve endocarditis (Dreyfus et al., 1990). Therefore, patients undergoing operation for endocarditis generally require aortic valve replacement. All patients with aortic valve endocarditis require appropriate antibiotic therapy whether or not the aortic valve is replaced (Love, 1991), and most patients with native aortic valve endocarditis respond to antibiotic therapy without operation (Kaye, 1973). Once endocarditis has been eradicated medically, aortic valve operation may still be indicated for aortic insufficiency. Because of difficulty eradicating infection with antibiotics alone, aortic valve operation is more likely to be needed in prosthetic valve endocarditis, fungal endocarditis, and staphylococcal endocarditis (Ivert et al., 1984; Richardson et al., 1978; Utley et al., 1975). Operation for acute endocarditis should generally be performed on a relatively urgent basis once any of these criteria are met, to avoid rapid hemodynamic deterioration, and operation during active endocarditis does not appear to carry significantly increased risk of subsequent endocarditis.

Operation for aortic valve endocarditis is conducted as in standard aortic valve replacement except that great care should be taken to remove all infected material along with the aortic valve. Small aortic annular abscesses may be closed primarily with pledgeted mattress sutures either separate from the valve sewing ring or incorporated into the valve sewing ring anastomosis. Large annular abscesses may be closed using a Dacron patch after careful débridement (Jault et al., 1993). However, in the presence of extensive annular abscesses, consideration should be given to use of a homograft root replacement owing to the technical ease of obtaining a secure closure (Hopkins, 1989). A more radical approach is supracoronary translocation of the prosthetic aortic valve and aortocoronary bypass (Jault et al., 1993). Survival 5 years after repair of prosthetic endocarditis with ring abscess is 50 to 70% (Jault et al., 1993).

## Combined Aortic and Mitral Valve Replacement

Combined aortic and mitral valve replacement is indicated for significant disease of both aortic and mitral valves, or for significant disease of one valve and mild to moderate disease of the other valve likely to require intervention before reoperation on the more severely diseased valve. Cardiopulmonary bypass is initiated as described previously, using bicaval cannulation. The aorta is cross-clamped, cardioplegia administered, and the left ventricle vented simply by opening the left atrium. With the heart arrested, an aortotomy is performed and the aortic valve is excised and sized. If a free-hand aortic homograft is used, the aortic valve should be replaced first. Otherwise, the left atrium is opened fully and the mitral valve replacement is completed, leaving a Foley catheter across the mitral valve as a left ventricular vent. Left atrial retractors are removed, and the aortic valve replacement is completed with closure of the aortotomy and removal of the aortic cross-clamp. The left ventricular vent is removed, and the left atriotomy is repaired during rewarming once air has been adequately evacuated from the heart and left ventricular distention is not occurring. Caution should be used in elevating the left ventricular apex to aspirate air, because this could contribute to atrioventricular disruption posteriorly, and air may be adequately removed without this maneuver. Transesophageal echocardiography may be of benefit in evaluating left ventricular wall motion, presence of intracardiac air, and function of the aortic mitral and tricuspid valves (de Bruijn et al., 1987).

## Aortic Valve Repair

Aortic valve repair for aortic stenosis was one of the first open heart operations performed (Kirklin and Mankin, 1960). In the child with aortic stenosis, aortic valve repair (primarily commissurotomy) continues to have a clear role as a palliative procedure until the patient grows larger. In the adult, aortic valve repair for aortic stenosis involves both aortic valve commissurotomy and débridement of the aortic valve calcium deposits (King et al., 1986). For the latter, ultrasonic débridement has been used extensively in several institutions (Craver, 1990). Duran (1988) reported acceptable results repairing mixed rheumatic aortic stenosis and regurgitation by commissurotomy, unfolding free cusp edges, commissural annuloplasty, and supra-aortic crest enlargement with 78% freedom from reoperation at 13 years; yet few centers have been able to duplicate these results. In general, aortic valve repair for aortic stenosis in the adult has a high incidence of early recurrent stenosis or progression to aortic regurgitation (Craver, 1990). The current role

for aortic valve repair in the adult with aortic stenosis is very limited.

Patients with chronic aortic regurgitation may have several underlying valvular pathologies potentially amenable to aortic valve repair. Blunt or penetrating trauma may result in leaflet laceration amenable to direct valve suture or patch using fine 5-0 polyester suture. Patients with certain forms of aortic regurgitation owing to leaflet prolapse (generally in bicuspid valves) have undergone successful aortic valve repair with resection or plication of the redundant leaflet as well as an aortic annuloplasty (Cosgrove et al., 1991; Frater, 1986). Similarly, prolapse of one leaflet has been repaired by securing excessive leaflet at the commissure (Cohn, 1983). Although results in selected patients have been good with these procedures, long-term results await further data (Cosgrove et al., 1991; Duran, 1988). Resuspension of the aortic valve for aortic regurgitation secondary to acute aortic dissection has proved to be quite successful in both short-term and long-term results, with a relatively low incidence of requiring further aortic valve surgery in the absence of underlying aortic valvular disease (Fann et al., 1991). Repair may be accomplished by transmural 3-0 Prolene pledgeted mattress sutures at each of the three commissures (Wolfe, 1980), or by placing the proximal aortic anastomosis low just above the aortic annulus and coronary ostia, thereby resuspending the aortic valve with the proximal anastomosis suture line (Miller, 1991).

## Operation for Hypertrophic Cardiomyopathy

The most widely applied operation for correction for hypertrophic cardiomyopathy with left ventricular outflow obstruction is the septal myotomy-myectomy as described by Morrow and colleagues (1975). With a transaortic approach, a tunnel of septal tissue is excised (Fig. 52–19). Some authors have used a finger placed in the right ventricle to help prevent excessive septal thinning and secondary ventricular septal defect. Others have used a combined transventricular and transaortic approach to achieve similar results. The results of septal myectomy have been excellent, with 70% of patients having significant symptomatic relief up to 25 years postoperatively, although no studies have found any conclusive survival benefit from operation (Maron et al., 1987b). Septal myotomy-myectomy for hypertrophic cardiomyopathy carries an operative mortality rate of 5 to 8%, with complications such as ventricular septal defect, complete heart block, and aortic or mitral valve damage occurring in 8% of patients (Morrow et al., 1975). Intraoperative transesophageal echocardiography can be quite helpful in assessing the adequacy of the result.

Mitral valve replacement has also been applied extensively to relieve left ventricular outflow tract obstruction in patients with hypertrophic cardiomyopathy, with excellent results (Cooley et al., 1973;

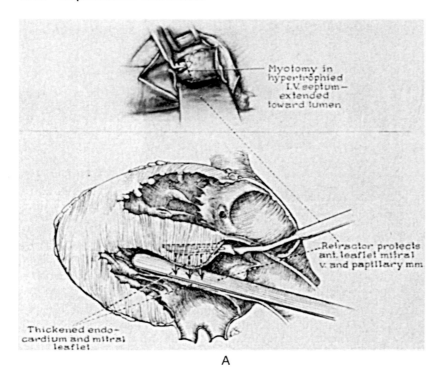

A

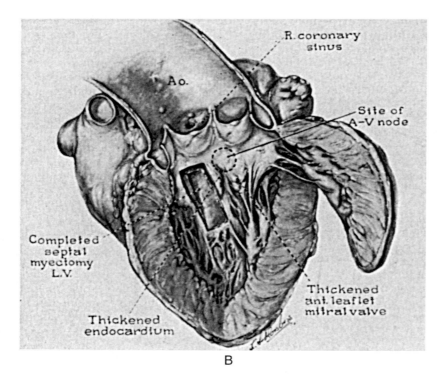

B

FIGURE 52–19. Technique of myotomy-myectomy for idiopathic hypertrophic subaortic stenosis. *A*, A flat ribbon retractor is used to displace and protect the anterior mitral leaflet and papillary muscle. A knife blade is passed into the muscular septum just below the base of the right coronary leaflet of the aortic valve at a point 2 to 3 mm to the right of the intercoronary commissure. After a second incision has been made parallel and approximately 1 cm to the right of the first incision, the bar of muscle between the two myotomies is excised. *B*, Resected area of the septum is shown with its relationship to the aortic valve, the area of the conduction system, and the anterior leaflet of the mitral valve. (*A* and *B*, From Morrow, A. G., Reitz, B. A., Epstein, S. E., et al.: Operative treatment in hypertrophic subaortic stenosis: Techniques and results of pre- and postoperative assessment in 83 patients. Circulation, *52*:88, 1975. By permission of the American Heart Association, Inc.)

McIntosh et al., 1989). Mitral valve replacement may be preferable to septal myotomy-myectomy in patients with a previous myectomy, a thin septum (<18 mm) in the area of usual resection, atypical septal morphology, or significant mitral regurgitation. The conduct of the operation does not differ from standard mitral valve replacement except that the anterior mitral valve leaflet should always be excised.

## Postoperative Care

All patients with aortic valve operation require careful control of postoperative hypertension, generally using an intravenous nitroprusside drip. Postoperative hypertension can be especially common in patients with preoperative aortic stenosis and left ventricular hypertrophy, now successfully relieved by aortic valve replacement. Because aortic valve patients may have impaired left ventricular diastolic compliance owing to left ventricular hypertrophy or dilatation, patients may require left ventricular filling pressures higher than normal to maintain forward cardiac output. Similarly, these patients may be especially susceptible to the loss of the atrial systole during atrial fibrillation. Because of the possibility of transient or permanent atrioventricular conduction disturbance, patients are not routinely digitalized until atrioventricular conduction has been established postoperatively.

Patients with bioprostheses may be placed on aspirin beginning on the first postoperative day. According to standard practice and manufacturer's recommendations, most patients with bioprosthetic aortic valves are placed on warfarin for 6 to 8 weeks (Carpentier et al., 1982), yet more recent data suggest that patients with aortic bioprostheses may be placed on aspirin alone without increased risk of thromboembolism or the risks of anticoagulant-related hemorrhage (Louagie et al., 1992). Patients with mechanical prostheses requiring anticoagulation are begun on warfarin between the second and the fourth postoperative days. Ultimate prothrombin ratios of 1.3 to 1.5 times control (INR 2.0 to 2.5) may be adequate for patients with isolated aortic valve replacement with modern valves (DiSesa et al., 1989; Saour et al., 1990). Whether low-dose warfarin in conjunction with antiplatelet therapy may minimize thromboembolism and hemorrhage in aortic valve patients remains to be determined (Edmunds, 1987). Although aortic valve replacement with a mechanical prosthesis is generally an indication for long-term anticoagulation, most mechanical aortic valves can be managed with aspirin alone with thromboembolism increased to roughly 8% per patient-year (Czer et al., 1985).

Temporary ventricular and atrial pacing wires are discontinued on the fifth postoperative day, and telemetry monitoring is continued through the fifth postoperative day because of the relatively high frequency of serious ventricular and atrial arrhythmias in patients with aortic valve disease. In all patients with repaired, replaced, or abnormal valves, endocarditis prophylaxis is indicated for procedures potentially associated with bacteremia, including dental procedures, urologic manipulation, or manipulation of the gastrointestinal tract (Table 52–5).

## RESULTS OF SURGICAL THERAPY

### Operative Mortality

The in-hospital or 30-day mortality for isolated aortic valve replacement in large recent series has varied from 2 to 5% (Lytle et al., 1989). Mortality is increased to 6 to 15% by a prior median sternotomy (Lytle et al.,

■ **Table 52–5.** CURRENT RECOMMENDATIONS FOR INFECTIOUS ENDOCARDITIS PROPHYLAXIS

**Standard Regimen**

| | |
|---|---|
| For dental procedures; upper respiratory tract surgery; minor GI and GU tract procedures | Amoxicillin 3.0 g PO 1 hr before, then 1.5 g 6 hr later |

**Special Regimens**

| | |
|---|---|
| Oral regimen for penicillin-allergic patients (oral and respiratory tract only) | Erythromycin 1.0 g PO 1–2 hr before, then 0.5 g 5 hr later |
| Parenteral regimen for high-risk patients; also for GI and GU tract procedures | Ampicillin 2.0 g IM or IV plus gentamicin 1.5 mg/kg IM or IV 0.5 hr before |
| Parenteral regimen for penicillin-allergic patients | Vancomycin 1.0 g IV slowly over 1 hr before; add gentamicin 1.5 mg/kg IM or IV if GI or GU tract involved |
| Cardiac surgery including implantation of prosthetic valves | Cefazolin 2 g IV at induction of anesthesia, repeated 8 and 16 hr later or Vancomycin 1.0 g IV slowly over 1 hr at induction then 0.5 g IV 8 and 16 hr later |

From Durack, D. T.: Prophylaxis of infective endocarditis. In Mandell, G. L., and Bennet, J. E. (eds): Principles and Practice of Infectious Diseases. 3rd ed. Douglas, R. G., Jr., Churchill Livingstone, New York, 1990.
*Key:* GI = gastrointestinal; GU = genitourinary; PO = by mouth; IM = intramuscularly; IV = intravenously

1986), increased to 6% by the addition of concurrent coronary bypass grafting (Lytle et al., 1988), and increased to 10% by the addition of mitral valve replacement. Mortality for patients over the age of 80 years with aortic stenosis has been 9% (Levinson et al., 1989). Other significant predictors of increased mortality in a series of 1689 primary isolated aortic valve replacements were increased age, decreased left ventricular function, poor preoperative functional status, renal insufficiency, and atrial fibrillation (Lytle et al., 1989). The most common causes of operative mortality were cardiac failure or infarction in 58% of deaths, hemorrhage in 11%, infection in 7%, arrhythmia in 5%, and stroke in 4% (Lytle et al., 1989).

### In-Hospital Complications

The most common serious complications after aortic valve operation include stroke in 1 to 2%, mediastinal bleeding requiring reoperation in 5 to 11%, wound infection in 1 to 2%, heart block requiring a permanent pacemaker in less than 1%, renal failure requiring dialysis in 0.7%, prolonged ventilation in 3%, and perioperative myocardial infarction in 2% (Lytle et al., 1989). These risks are similar for all aortic valve operations. Strokes may be embolic or related to atherosclerosis, and strokes are best avoided by meticulous removal of air and potential embolic debris from the heart. The somewhat higher incidence of bleeding after aortic valve replacement relative to coronary bypass grafting suggests that meticulous hemostasis at the aortotomy and in previously operated fields is indicated.

## Late Complications

The most frequent late complications from aortic replacement are thromboembolism and anticoagulant-related hemorrhage. The incidence of each of these is related to the valve prosthesis implanted, patient age, the presence of atrial fibrillation, and the degree of anticoagulation employed. For most bioprosthetic valves, incidence of thromboembolism is roughly 0.2 to 1.3% per patient-year for isolated aortic valve replacement (see Table 52–3). For mechanical aortic valves, the rate of thromboembolism increases to 1.5 to 2.0% per patient-year (see Table 52–3). The rate of anticoagulant-related hemorrhage is 0.3% for bioprostheses (Jamieson et al., 1990) and 2 to 3% per patient-year for mechanical valves requiring warfarin anticoagulation (Edmunds, 1987). Whether anticoagulant-related hemorrhage is more likely in elderly patients remains controversial.

Endocarditis is another late complication occurring after aortic valve operation with an incidence of roughly 0.5 to 1.0% per patient-year after the first 6 months (Lytle et al., 1989). Most data currently available suggest that the type of aortic prosthesis has little effect on the incidence of prosthetic endocarditis (Hammermeister et al., 1993). The type of prosthesis does affect the incidence of aortic root abscess in patients developing prosthetic endocarditis, with the incidence of aortic root abscess being 65% for infected mechanical valves, 36% for porcine valves, and 20% for unstented homografts (Miller, 1990).

Clinically significant hemolysis is unusual, and hemolysis is generally related to perivalvular leak and occasionally results from prosthetic dysfunction or small mechanical valve sizes (Dale and Myhre, 1978; Björk et al., 1974). The incidence of perivalvular leak is 0.2 to 0.5% and is associated with infection in a significant number of cases (Bortolotti et al., 1991; Czer et al., 1990; Jamieson et al., 1988). Although some perivalvular leaks may be present at the time of operation, sterile perivalvular leak may occur weeks or even years after valve replacement. Risk factors for perivalvular leak may include endocarditis, prior operation, and large valve size.

Prosthetic dysfunction is an important late complication after aortic valve replacement, especially for biologic prostheses. Risk factors for prosthetic dysfunction may include the valve model, patient age, and valve size (Glower et al., 1994). Additional risk factors for aortic allografts include greater donor age, and valve preparation technique (Barratt-Boyes et al., 1987; Kirklin and Barratt-Boyes, 1993). False aneurysm or aortic dissection at the aortotomy site are extremely rare and probably related to aortic tissue characteristics and technical details of aortic closure. Symptomatic postoperative aortic stenosis may occur with stented mechanical or biologic valves of 21-mm size or less when the effective valve orifice area is inadequate for the cardiac output at rest or exercise (Schaff et al., 1981).

## Long-Term Survival

Long-term survival after aortic valve replacement is decreased by many factors including older patient age, impaired left ventricular function, coronary artery disease, renal insufficiency, and other co-morbidity (Lytle et al., 1989). Typical survival 10 years after aortic valve replacement is 60 to 70% (Lund et al., 1990b; Lytle et al., 1989) with primary causes of death including cardiac failure or sudden death in 42 to 83% (Lund et al., 1990b; Lytle et al., 1989), and hemorrhage (4%), infection (5%), thromboembolism (6%), and other noncardiac causes in the remainder (Lund et al., 1990b).

## Symptomatic Relief

Most patients with aortic valve replacement for aortic valve disease notice fairly immediate improvement in preoperative symptoms. This improvement persists long-term, with 96% of patients being New York Heart Association functional Class I or II 6 years after operation (Cohn et al., 1989). In many patients, especially those with normal preoperative left ventricular function or with mildly depressed ejection fraction owing to aortic stenosis, exercise capacity postoperatively may be relatively normal.

## SELECTED BIBLIOGRAPHY

Hammermeister, K. E., Sethi, G. K., Henderson, W. G., et al.: Veterans Affairs Cooperative Study: A comparison of outcomes in men 11 years after heart-valve replacement with a mechanical valve or bioprosthesis. N. Engl. J. Med., 328:1289, 1993.

Eleven-year follow-up data from the Veterans Affairs Cooperative Study of 575 patients revealed no differences in patient survival, total valve-related complications, or thromboembolism between mechanical or bioprosthetic valves. Mechanical valves had a higher incidence of bleeding complications, whereas bioprostheses were more likely to develop structural failure.

Edmunds, L. H. Jr.: Thrombotic and bleeding complications of prosthetic heart valves. Ann. Thorac. Surg., 44:430, 1987.

An excellent review of the literature regarding anticoagulation and thromboembolism after valve replacement. Discussions include anticoagulation regimens, comparison of valve prostheses, risk factors for hemorrhage or thromboembolism, and the pharmacology of anticoagulation and antiplatelet therapy.

Emery, R. W., and Arom, K. V. (eds): The Aortic Valve. Philadelphia, Hanley & Belfus, 1991.

This is a current and authoritative text regarding the pathophysiology, diagnosis, and treatment of aortic valve disease. Chapters regarding operative technique are well illustrated, including the use of homografts, autografts, and aortic root enlargement.

Hopkins, R. A. (ed): Cardiac Reconstructions with Homograft Valves. New York, Springer-Verlag, 1989.

This thorough and well-illustrated treatise discusses the use of homograft tissues in reconstruction of the aortic and pulmonic outflow tracts. The history and biology of homografts, techniques of homograft banking, and surgical techniques applying homografts are thoroughly reviewed.

Lytle, B. W., Cosgrove, P. M., Taylor, P. C., et al.: Primary isolated aortic valve replacement. Early and late results. J. Thorac. Cardiovasc. Surg., 97:675, 1989.

Analysis of the Cleveland Clinic experience with 1689 patients found that age, renal dysfunction, functional class, atrial fibrillation, and no use of cardioplegia were predictors of in-hospital mortality. Age, left ventricular dysfunction, coronary disease, and renal dysfunction impaired long-term survival. A detailed retrospective comparison of outcome using biologic versus mechanical prostheses is also provided.

# BIBLIOGRAPHY

Aris, A., Padro, J. M., Camara, M. L., et al.: The Monostrut Björk-Shiley valve: Seven years' experience. J. Thorac. Cardiovasc. Surg., 103:1074, 1992.

Arom, K. V., Nicoloff, D. M., Kersten, T. E., et al.: Ten years' experience with the St. Jude medical valve prosthesis. Ann. Thorac. Surg., 47:831, 1989.

Bache, R. J.: Effects of hypertrophy on the coronary circulation. Prog. Cardiovasc. Dis., 31:403, 1988.

Bahnson, H. T., Spencer, F. C., Busse, E. F. G., and Davis, F. W., Jr.: Cusp replacement in coronary artery perfusion in open operations on the aortic valve. Ann. Surg., 152:494, 1960.

Bailey, C. P., Ramirez, H. P., and Larselere, H. B.: Surgical treatment of aortic stenosis. J.A.M.A., 150:1647, 1952.

Barratt-Boyes, B. G., Ko, P. H., and Jaffe, W. M.: The zero-pressure fixed Medtronic intact porcine valve: Clinical results over a 6-year period, including serial echocardiographic assessment. J. Card. Surg., 6(Suppl.):562, 1991.

Barratt-Boyes, B. G., Roche, A. H. G., Subramanyan, R., et al.: Long-term follow-up of patients with the antibiotic-sterilized aortic homograft valve inserted freehand in the aortic position. Circulation, 75:768, 1987.

Binet, J. P., Duran, C. G., Carpentier, A., and Langlois, J.: Heterologous aortic valve transplantation. Lancet, 2:1275, 1965.

Birkmeyer, J. D., Marrin, C. A. S., and O'Connor, G. T.: Should patients with Björk-Shiley valves undergo prophylactic replacement? Lancet, 340:520, 1992.

Björk, V. O., Henze, A., and Holmgren, A.: Five years' experience with the Björk-Shiley tilting disc valve in isolated aortic valvular disease. J. Thorac. Cardiovasc. Surg., 68:393, 1974.

Björk, V. O., Henze, A., Holmgren, A., and Szamosi, A.: Evaluation of the 21-mm Björk-Shiley tilting disc valve in patients with narrow aortic roots. Scand. J. Thorac. Cardiovasc. Surg., 7:203, 1973.

Björk, V. O., and Lindblom, D.: The monostrut Björk-Shiley heart valve. J. Am. Coll. Cardiol., 6:1142, 1985.

Bojar, R. M., Payne, D. D., Sheffield, A. B., et al.: Successful repair of postoperative ascending aortic mycotic false aneurysms using circulatory arrest. Ann. Thorac. Surg., 46:182, 1988.

Bonow, R. O., Borer, J. S., Rosing, D. R., et al.: Preoperative exercise capacity in symptomatic patients with aortic regurgitation as a predictor of postoperative left ventricular function and long-term prognosis. Circulation, 62:1280, 1980.

Bonow, R. O., Dodd, J. T., Maron, B. J., et al.: Long-term serial changes in left ventricular function and reversal of ventricular dilatation after valve replacement for chronic aortic regurgitation. Circulation, 78:1108, 1988.

Bonow, R. O., Rosing, D. R., McIntosh, C. L., et al.: The natural history of asymptomatic patients with aortic regurgitation and normal left ventricular function. Circulation, 68:509, 1983.

Borer, J. S., Herrold, E. M., Hochreiter, C., et al.: Natural history of left ventricular performance at rest and during exercise after aortic valve replacement for aortic regurgitation. Circulation, 84:III-133, 1991.

Borkon, A. M., Soule, L. M., Baughman, K. L., et al.: Aortic valve selection in the elderly patient. Ann. Thorac. Surg., 46:270, 1988.

Bortolotti, U., Milano, A., Testolin, L., et al.: Influence of type of prosthesis on late results after combined mitral-aortic valve replacement. Ann. Thorac. Surg., 52:84, 1991.

CarboMedics: Summary of clinical investigation. Clin. Rep., 5:1, 1993.

Carpentier, A., Deloche, A., Relland, J., et al.: Six-year follow-up of glutaraldehyde-preserved heterografts. J. Thorac. Cardiovasc. Surg., 68:771, 1974.

Carpentier, A., Dubost, C., Lane, E., et al.: Continuing improvements in valvular bioprostheses. J. Thorac. Cardiovasc. Surg., 83:27, 1982.

Carroll, J. D., Carroll, E. P., Feldman, T., et al.: Sex-associated differences in left ventricular function in aortic stenosis of the elderly. Circulation, 86:1099, 1992.

Cartwright, R. S., Giacobine, J. W., Ratan, R. S., et al.: Combined aortic and mitral valve replacement. J. Thorac. Cardiovasc. Surg., 45:35, 1963.

Cobanoglu, A., Fessler, C. L., Guvendik, L., et al.: Aortic valve replacement with the Starr-Edwards prosthesis: A comparison of the first and second decades of follow-up. Ann. Thorac. Surg., 45:248, 1988.

Cohn, L. H. (ed.): Modern Technics in Surgery/Cardiac Thoracic Surgery. Mt. Kisco, NY: Futura, 1983.

Cohn, L. H., Allred, E. N., DiSesa, V. J., et al.: Early and late risk of aortic valve replacement: A 12-year concomitant comparison of the porcine bioprosthetic and tilting disc prosthetic aortic valves. J. Thorac. Cardiovasc. Surg., 88:695, 1984.

Cohn, L. H., Collins, J. J., DiSesa, V. J., et al.: Fifteen-year experience with 1678 Hancock porcine bioprosthetic heart valve replacements. Ann. Thorac. Surg., 210:435, 1989.

Cohn, L. H., Couper, G. S., Aranki, S. F., et al.: The long-term follow-up of the Hancock modified orifice porcine bioprosthetic valve. J. Card. Surg., 6(Suppl. 4):557, 1991.

Cooley, D. A., Leachman, R. D., and Wukasch, D. C.: Diffuse muscular subaortic stenosis. Am. J. Cardiol., 31:1, 1973.

Cosgrove, D. M., Lytle, B. W., and Williams, G. W.: Hemodynamic performance of the Carpentier-Edwards pericardial valve in the aortic position. Circulation, 72:II-146, 1985.

Cosgrove, D. M., Rosencranz, E. R., Hendren, W. G., et al.: Valvuloplasty for aortic insufficiency. J. Thorac. Cardiovasc. Surg., 102:571, 1991.

Craver, J. M.: Aortic valve débridement by ultrasonic surgical aspirator: A word of caution. Ann. Thorac. Surg., 49:746, 1990.

Czer, L. S. C., Chaux, A., Matloff, J. M., et al.: Ten-year experience with the St. Jude Medical valve for primary valve replacement. J. Thorac. Cardiovasc. Surg., 100:44, 1990.

Czer, L. S. C., Matloff, J., Chaux, A., et al.: A 6-year experience with the St. Jude Medical valve: Hemodynamic performance, surgical results, biocompatibility, and follow-up. J. Am. Coll. Cardiol., 6:904, 1985.

Dale, J., and Myhre, E.: Intravascular hemolysis in the late course of aortic valve replacement: Relation to valve type, size, and function. Am. Heart J., 96:24, 1978.

Daly, R. C., Orszulak, T. A., Schaff, H. V., et al.: Long-term results of aortic valve replacement with nonviable homografts. Circulation, 84:III-81, 1991.

Davidson, C. J., Harrison, J. K., Leithe, M. E., et al.: Failure of balloon aortic valvuloplasty to result in sustained clinical improvement in patients with depressed left ventricular function. Am. J. Cardiol., 65:72, 1990.

de Bruijn, N. P., Clements, F. M., and Kisslo, J. A.: Intraoperative transesophageal color-flow mapping: Initial experience. Anesth. Analg., 66:386, 1987.

DiSesa, V. J., Collins, J. J., and Cohn, L. H.: Hematological complications with the St. Jude valve and reduced-dose Coumadin. Ann. Thorac. Surg., 48:280, 1989.

Dreyfus, G., Serraf, A., Jebara, V. A., et al.: Valve repair in acute endocarditis. Ann. Thorac. Surg., 49:706, 1990.

Duran, C. G.: Reconstructive techniques for rheumatic valve disease. J. Cardiac. Surg., 3:23, 1988.

Edmunds, L. H., Jr.: Thrombotic and bleeding complications of prosthetic heart valves. Ann. Thorac. Surg., 44:430, 1987.

Elkins, R. C., Santangelo, K., Randolph, J. D., et al.: Pulmonary autograft replacement in children. The ideal solution? Ann. Surg., 216:363, 1992.

Ellis, F. H., Jr., and Kirklin, J. W.: Aortic stenosis. Surg. Clin. North Am., 35:1029, 1955.

Fananapazir, L., Cannon, R. O., Tripodi, D., and Panza, J. A.: Impact of dual-chamber permanent pacing in patients with obstructive hypertrophic cardiomyopathy with symptoms refractory to verapamil and β-adrenergic blocker therapy. Circulation, 85:2149, 1992.

Fann, J. I., Glower, D. D., Miller, D. C., et al.: Preservation of aortic valve in type A aortic dissection complicated by aortic regurgitation. J. Thorac. Cardiovasc. Surg., 102:62, 1991.

Fenoglio, J., Jr., McAllister, H. A., Jr., DeCastro, C. M., et al.: Congenital bicuspid aortic valve after age 20. Am. J. Cardiol., 39:164, 1977.

Flemma, R. J., Mullen, D. C., Kleinman, L. H., et al.: Survival and event-free analysis of 785 patients with Björk-Shiley spherical-disc valves at 10 to 16 years. Ann. Thorac. Surg., 45:258, 1988.

Florenzano, F., and Glantz, S. A.: Left ventricular mechanical adaptation to chronic aortic regurgitation in intact dogs. Am. J. Physiol., 252:H969, 1987.

Folts, J. D., and Rowe, G. G.: Coronary and hemodynamic effects of temporary and acute aortic insufficiency in intact anesthetized dogs. Circ. Res., 35:238, 1974.

Foster, A. H., Tracy, C. M., Greenberg, G. J., et al.: Valve replacement in narrow aortic roots: Serial hemodynamics and long-term clinical outcome. Ann. Thorac. Surg., 42:506, 1986.

Frater, R. W. M.: Aortic valve insufficiency due to aortic dilation: Correction by sinus rim adjustment. Circulation, 47:I-136, 1986.

Frater, R. W. M., Salomon, N. W., Rainer, W. G., et al.: The Carpentier-Edwards pericardial aortic valve: Intermediate results. Ann. Thorac. Surg., 53:764, 1992.

Gibbon, J. H.: Application of a mechanical heart and lung apparatus to cardiac surgery. Minn. Med., 37:171, 1954.

Glazier, J. J., Verwilghen, J., Donaldson, R. M., and Ross, D. N.: Treatment of complicated prosthetic aortic valve endocarditis with annular abscess formation by homograft aortic root replacement. J. Am. Coll. Cardiol., 17:1177, 1991.

Glower, D. D., Murrah, R. L., Olsen, C. O., et al.: Mechanical correlates of the third heart sound. J. Am. Coll. Cardiol., 19:450, 1992.

Glower, D. D., White, W. D., Hatton, A. C., et al.: Determinants of reoperation after 960 valve replacements with Carpentier-Edwards prostheses. J. Thorac. Cardiovasc. Surg., 107:381, 1994.

Gonzales-Lavin, L., Gonzales-Lavin, J., Chi, S., et al.: The pericardial valve in the aortic position ten years later. J. Thorac. Cardiovasc. Surg., 101:75, 1991.

Gorlin, R., and Gorlin, S. G.: Hydraulic formula for calculation of the area of the stenotic mitral valve, other valves, and central circulatory shunts. Am. Heart J., 41:1, 1951.

Grossman, W., Jones, D., and McLaurin, L. P.: Wall stress and patterns of hypertrophy in the human left ventricle. J. Clin. Invest., 56:56, 1975.

Gula, S. S., Pomerance, A., Bennet, M., and Yacoub, M. H.: Homograft replacement of aortic valve and ascending aorta in a patient with nonspecific giant cell arteritis. Br. Heart J., 39:581, 1977.

Hammermeister, K. E., Sethi, G. K., Henderson, W. G., et al.: A comparison of outcomes in men 11 years after heart-valve replacement with a mechanical valve or bioprosthesis. N. Engl. J. Med., 328:1289, 1993.

Harken, D. E., Soroff, H. S., Taylor, W. J., et al.: Partial and complete prostheses in aortic insufficiency. J. Thorac. Cardiovasc. Surg., 40:744, 1960.

Harpole, D. H., and Jones, R. H.: Serial assessment of ventricular performance after valve replacement for aortic stenosis. J. Thorac. Cardiovasc. Surg., 99:645, 1990.

Hegglin, R., Scheu, H., and Rothlin, M.: Aortic insufficiency. Circulation, 37, 38:V-77, 1968.

Hejtmancik, J. F., Brink, P. A., Towbin, J., et al.: Localization of gene for familial hypertrophic cardiomyopathy to chromosome 14q1 in a diverse US population. Circulation, 83:1592, 1991.

Hopkins, R. A.: Cardiac Reconstructions with Allograft Valves. New York: Springer-Verlag, 1989.

Hufnagel, C. A., and Harvey, W. P.: The surgical correction of aortic regurgitation: Preliminary report. Bull. Georgetown U. Med. Ctr., 6:60, 1953.

Hwang, M. H., Hammermeister, K. E., Oprian, C., et al.: Preoperative identification of patients likely to have left ventricular dysfunction after aortic valve replacement. Circulation, 80:I-65, 1989.

Ihlen, H., Molstad, P., Simonsen, S., et al.: Hemodynamic evaluation of the CarboMedics prosthetic heart valve in the aortic position: Comparison of noninvasive and invasive techniques. Am. Heart J., 123:151, 1992.

Ionescu, M. I., Pakrashi, B. C., Holden, M. P., et al.: Results of aortic valve replacement with frame-supported fascia lata and pericardial grafts. J. Thorac. Cardiovasc. Surg., 64:340, 1972.

Ionescu, M. I., and Tandon, A. P.: Long-term clinical and hemodynamic evaluation of the Ionescu-Shiley pericardial xenograft heart valve. Thoraxchir., 26:250, 1978.

Ivert, T. S. A., Dismukes, W. E., Cobbs, G. C., et al.: Prosthetic valve endocarditis. Circulation, 69:223, 1984.

Jaffe, W. M., Barratt-Boyes, B. G., Sadri, A., et al.: Early follow-up of patients with the Medtronic intact porcine valve: A new cardiac bioprosthesis. J. Thorac. Cardiovasc. Surg., 98:942, 1989.

Jamieson, W. R. E., Allen, P., Miyagishima, R. T., et al.: The Carpentier-Edwards standard porcine bioprosthesis. J. Thorac. Cardiovasc. Surg., 99:543, 1990.

Jamieson, W. R. E., Munro, A. I., Miyagishima, R. T., et al.: The Carpentier-Edwards supra-annular porcine bioprosthesis: A new generation tissue valve with excellent intermediate clinical performance. J. Thorac. Cardiovasc. Surg., 96:652, 1988.

Jamieson, W. R. E., Tyers, G. F. O., Miyagishima, R. T., et al.: Carpentier-Edwards porcine bioprostheses: Comparison of standard and supra-annular prostheses at 7 years. Circulation, 84:III-145, 1991.

Jault, F., Ganjbakhch, I., Chastre, J. C., et al.: Prosthetic valve endocarditis with ring abscess: Surgical management and long-term results. J. Thorac. Cardiovasc. Surg., 105:1106, 1993.

Johnson, A. M.: Aortic stenosis, sudden death, and the left ventricular baroreceptors. Br. Heart J., 33:1, 1971.

Kallis, P., Sneddon, J. F., Simpson, I. A., Fung, A., et al.: Clinical and hemodynamic evaluation of the 19-mm Carpentier-Edwards supra-annular aortic valve. Ann. Thorac. Surg., 54:1182, 1992.

Kass, D. A., Maughan, W. L., Guo, Z. M., et al.: Comparative influence of load versus inotropic states on indexes of ventricular contractility: Experimental and theoretical analysis based on pressure-volume relationships. Circulation, 76:1422, 1987.

Kawasuji, M., Hetzer, R., Oelert, H., et al.: Aortic valve replacement and ascending aorta replacement in ankylosing spondylitis: Report of three surgical cases and a review of the literature. Thorac. Cardiovasc. Surg., 30:310, 1982.

Kaye, D.: Changes in the spectrum, diagnosis, and management of bacterial and fungal endocarditis. Med. Clin. North Am., 57:941, 1973.

Kazui, T., Yamada, O., Yamagishi, M., et al.: Aortic valve replacement with omniscience and omnicarbon valves. Ann. Thorac. Surg., 52:236, 1991.

Khan, S. S., Mitchell, R. S., Derby, G. C., et al.: Differences in Hancock and Carpentier-Edwards porcine xenograft aortic valve hemodynamics: Effect of valve size. Circulation, 82:IV-117, 1990.

King, R. M., Pluth, J. R., Giuliani, E. R., and Piehler, J. M.: Mechanical decalcification of the aortic valve. Ann. Thorac. Surg., 42:269, 1986.

Kirklin, J. W., and Barratt-Boyes, B. G.: Cardiac Surgery. 2nd ed. New York, Churchill Livingstone, 1993.

Kirklin, J. W., and Mankin, H. T.: Open operation in the treatment of calcific aortic stenosis. Circulation, 21:578, 1960.

Klues, H. G., Maron, B. J., Dollar, A. L., and Roberts, W. C.: Diversity of structural mitral valve alterations in hypertrophic cardiomyopathy. Circulation, 85:1651, 1992.

Konno, S., Imai, Y., Iida, Y., et al.: New method for prosthetic valve replacement in congenital aortic stenosis associated with hypoplasia of the aortic valve ring. J. Thorac. Cardiovasc. Surg., 70:909, 1975.

Lakier, J. B., Copans, H., Rosman, H. S., et al.: Idiopathic degeneration of the aortic valve: A common cause of isolated aortic regurgitation. J. Am. Coll. Cardiol., 5:347, 1985.

Levinson, J. R., Akins, C. W., Buckley, M. J., et al.: Octogenarians with aortic stenosis. Outcome after aortic valve replacement. Circulation, 80:I-49, 1989.

Lieberman, E. B., Bashore, T. M., Hermiller, J. B., et al.: Balloon aortic valvuloplasty in the elderly: The final chapter? Circulation, (in press).

Lillehei, C. W., Barnard, C. N., Long, D. M., et al.: Aortic valve reconstruction and replacement by total valve prostheses. In Merendino, K. A. (ed): Prosthetic Heart Valves for Cardiac Surgery. Springfield, IL, Charles C. Thomas, 1961, p. 527.

Louagie, Y., Noirhomme, P., Aranguis, E., et al.: Use of the Carpentier-Edwards porcine bioprosthesis: Assessment of a patient selection policy. J. Thorac. Cardiovasc. Surg., 104:1013, 1992.

Love, K.: Infective endocarditis of the aortic valve. In Emery, R. W., and Arom, K. V, (eds): The Aortic Valve. Philadelphia, Hanley & Belfus, 1991.

Lund, O., Neilson, T. T., Pilegaard, H. K., et al.: The influence of coronary artery disease and bypass grafting on early and late survival after valve replacement for aortic stenosis. J. Thorac. Cardiovasc. Surg., 100:327, 1990a.

Lund, O., Pilegaard, H. K., Magnussen, K., et al.: Long-term prosthesis-related and sudden cardiac-related complications after valve replacement for aortic stenosis. Ann. Thorac. Surg., 50:396, 1990b.

Lytle, B. W., Cosgrove, D. M., Gill, C. C., et al.: Aortic valve replacement combined with myocardial revascularization. Late results and determinants of risk for 471 in-hospital survivors. J. Thorac. Cardiovasc. Surg., 95:402, 1988.

Lytle, B. W., Cosgrove, D. M., Taylor, P. C., et al.: Primary isolated aortic valve replacement: Early and late results. J. Thorac. Cardiovasc. Surg., 97:675, 1989.

Lytle, B. W., Cosgrove, D. M., Taylor, P. C., et al.: Reoperations for valve surgery: Perioperative mortality and determinants of risk for 1000 patients, 1958–1984. Ann. Thorac. Surg., 42:632, 1986.

Manouguian, S., and Seybold-Epting, W.: Patch enlargement of the aortic valve ring by extending the aortic incision into the anterior mitral leaflet: New operative technique. J. Thorac. Cardiovasc. Surg., 78:402, 1979.

Maron, B. J., Bonow, R. O., Cannon, R. O., et al.: Hypertrophic cardiomyopathy: Interrelations of clinical manifestations, pathophysiology, and therapy. Part I. N. Engl. J. Med., 316:780, 1987a.

Maron, B. J., Bonow, R. O., Cannon, R. O., et al.: Hypertrophic cardiomyopathy: Interrelations of clinical manifestations, pathophysiology, and therapy. Part II. N. Engl. J. Med., 316:780, 1987b.

Maron, B. J., and Fananapazir, L.: Sudden cardiac death in hypertrophic cardiomyopathy. Circulation, 85:I-57, 1992.

Maron, B. J., Ferrans, V. J., and Roberts, W. C.: Myocardial ultrastructure in patients with chronic aortic valve disease. Am. J. Cardiol., 35:725, 1975.

Masters, R. G., Pipe, A. L., Bedard, J. P., et al.: Long-term clinical results with the Ionescu-Shiley pericardial xenograft. J. Thorac. Cardiovasc. Surg., 101:81, 1991.

Matsuki, A., Okita, Y., Almieda, R. S., et al.: Two decades' experience with aortic valve replacement with pulmonary autograft. J. Thorac. Cardiovasc. Surg., 95:705, 1988a.

Matsuki, O., Robles, A., Gibbs, S., et al.: Long-term performance of 555 aortic homografts in the aortic position. Ann. Thorac. Surg., 46:187, 1988b.

McGoon, D. C.: Prosthetic reconstruction of the aortic valve. Staff Meet. Mayo Clin., 36:88, 1961.

McIntosh, C. L., Greenberg, G. J., Maron, B. J., et al.: Clinical and hemodynamic results after mitral valve replacement in patients with obstructive hypertrophic cardiomyopathy. Ann. Thorac. Surg., 47:236, 1989.

McKenna, W. J.: Arrhythmia and prognosis in hypertrophic cardiomyopathy. Eur. Heart J., 4:225, 1983.

McKenna, W. J., Harris, L., and Rowland, E.: Amiodarone for long-term management of patients with hypertrophic cardiomyopathy. Am. J. Cardiol., 54:802, 1984.

Miller, D. C.: Predictors of outcome in patients with prosthetic valve endocarditis (PVE) and potential advantages of homograft aortic root replacement for prosthetic ascending aortic valve–graft infections. J. Cardiac Surg., 5:53, 1990.

Miller, D. C.: Surgical management of acute aortic dissection: New data. Semin. Thorac. Cardiovasc. Surg., 3:225, 1991.

Miller, D. C., Oyer, P. E., Mitchell, R. S., et al.: Performance characteristics of the Starr-Edwards model 1260 aortic valve prosthesis beyond ten years. J. Thorac. Cardiovasc. Surg., 88:193, 1984.

Miller, D. C., Stinson, E. B., Oyer, P. E., et al.: Surgical implications and results of combined aortic valve replacement and myocardial revascularization. Am. J. Cardiol., 43:494, 1979.

Monrad, E. S., Hess, O. M., Murakami, T., et al.: Time course of regression of left ventricular hypertrophy after aortic valve replacement. Circulation, 77:1345, 1988.

Morrow, A. G., Reitz, B. A., Epstein, S. E., et al.: Operative treatment in hypertrophic subaortic stenosis: Techniques and the results of pre- and postoperative assessment in 83 patients. Circulation, 52:88, 1975.

Morrow, A. G., Roberts, W. C., and Ross, J., Jr.: Obstruction to left ventricular outflow. Ann. Intern. Med., 69:1255, 1968.

Mullaney, C. J., Elveback, L. R., Frye, R. L., et al.: Coronary artery disease and its management: Influence on survival in patients undergoing aortic valve replacement. J. Am. Coll. Cardiol., 10:66, 1987.

Muller, W. H., Jr., Littlefield, J. B., and Dammann, J. F.: Subcoronary prosthetic replacement of the aortic valve. In Merendino, K. A. (ed): Prosthetic Heart Valves for Cardiac Surgery. Springfield, IL, Charles C. Thomas, 1961, p. 493.

Murray, G.: Homologous aortic valve segment transplant as surgical treatment for aortic and mitral insufficiency. Angiology, 7:466, 1956.

Nicks, R., Cartmill, T., and Bernstein, L.: Hypoplasia of the aortic root. Thorax, 25:339, 1970.

Nitter-Hauge, S., and Abdelnoor, M.: Ten-year experience with the Medtronic Hall valvular prosthesis. A study of 1104 patients. Circulation, 80:I-43, 1989.

Norman, J. C., Nihill, M. R., and Cooley, D. A.: Valved apico-aortic composite conduits for left ventricular outflow tract obstruction. Am. J. Cardiol., 45:1265, 1980.

O'Brien, M. F., Stafford, E. G., Gardner, M. A., et al.: A comparison of aortic valve replacement with viable cryopreserved and fresh allograft valves, with a note on chromosomal studies. J. Thorac. Cardiovasc. Surg., 94:812, 1987.

Okita, Y., Franciosi, G., Matsuki, O., et al.: Early and late results of aortic root replacement with antibiotic-sterilized aortic homograft. J. Thorac. Cardiovasc. Surg., 95:696, 1988.

Olin, C. L., Bomfim, V., Halvazulis, V., et al.: Optimal insertion technique for the Bjork-Shiley valve in the narrow aortic ostium. Ann. Thorac. Surg., 36:567, 1983.

Ovil, Y., Wahi, R., Liu, P., et al.: Aortic valvuloplasty for traumatic aortic insufficiency: A two-year follow-up. Ann. Thorac. Surg., 49:43, 1990.

Perier, P., Mihaileanu, S., Fabiani, J. N., et al.: Long-term evaluation of the Carpentier-Edwards pericardial valve in the aortic position. J. Card. Surg., 6:589, 1991.

Piehler, J. M., Danielson, G. K., Pluth, J. R., et al.: Enlargement of the aortic root or annulus with autogenous pericardial patch during aortic valve replacement. J. Thorac. Cardiovasc. Surg., 86:350, 1983.

Pyle, R. B., Mayer, J. E., Jr., Lindsay, W. G., et al.: Hemodynamic evaluation of Lillehei-Kaster and Starr-Edwards prostheses. Ann. Thorac. Surg., 26:336, 1978.

Richardson, J. V., Karp, R. B., Kirklin, J. W., and Dismukes, W. E.: Treatment of infective endocarditis: A 20-year comparative analysis. Circulation, 58:589, 1978.

Rittenhouse, E. A., Sauvage, L. R., Stamm, S. J., et al.: Radical enlargement of the aortic root and outflow tract to allow valve replacement. Ann. Thorac. Surg., 27:367, 1979.

Roberts, W. C., and Honig, H. S.: The spectrum of cardiovascular disease in the Marfan syndrome: A clinicomorphologic study of 18 necropsy patients and comparison of 151 previously reported necropsy patients. Am. Heart J., 104:115, 1982.

Roger, V. L., Tajik, A. J., Bailey, K. R., et al.: Progression of aortic stenosis in adults: New appraisal using Doppler echocardiography. Am. Heart J., 119:331, 1990.

Ross, D. N.: Homograft replacement of the aortic valve. Lancet, 2:487, 1962.

Ross, D. N.: Replacement of aortic and mitral valve with a pulmonary autograft. Lancet, 2:956, 1967.

Ross, D. N.: Replacement of the aortic valve with a pulmonary autograft: The "switch" operation. Ann. Thorac. Surg., 52:1346, 1991.

Ross, D. N., Jackson, M., and Davies, J.: Pulmonary autograft aortic valve replacement: Long-term results. J. Card. Surg., 6:529, 1991.

Ross, D. N., Martelli, V., and Wain, W. H.: Allograft and autograft valves used for aortic valve replacement. In Ionescu M. I. (ed): Tissue Heart Valves. London, Butterworths, 1979.

Ross, J., Jr., and Braunwald E.: Aortic stenosis. Circulation, 38:V-61, 1968.

Saour, J. N., Sieck, J. O., Mamo, L. A. R., and Gallus, A. S.: Trial of different intensities of anticoagulation in patients with prosthetic heart valves. N. Engl. J. Med., 322:428, 1990.

Schaff, H. V., Borkon, A. M., Hughes, C., et al.: Clinical and hemodynamic evaluation of the 19-mm Björk-Shiley aortic valve prosthesis. Ann. Thorac. Surg., 32:50, 1981.

Sellers, R. D., Levy, M. J., Amplatz, K., and Lillehei, C. W.: Left retrograde cardioangiography in acquired cardiac disease: Technic, indications, and interpretations in 700 cases. Am. J. Cardiol., 14:437, 1964.

Senning, A.: Fascia lata replacement of aortic valves. J. Thorac. Cardiovasc. Surg., 54:465, 1967.

Smedira, N. G., Ports, T. A., Merrick, S. H., and Rankin, J. S.: Balloon aortic valvuloplasty as a bridge to aortic valve replacement in critically ill patients. Ann. Thorac. Surg., 55:914, 1993.

Smithy, H. G., and Parker, E. F.: Experimental aortic valvulotomy: A preliminary report. Surg. Gynecol. Obstet., 34:625, 1947.

Smucker, M. L., Manning, S. B., Stuckey, T. D., et al.: Preoperative left ventricular wall stress, ejection fraction, and aortic valve gradient as prognostic indicators in aortic valve stenosis. Cathet. Cardiovasc. Diagn., 17:133, 1989.

Spagnuolo, M., Kloth, H., Taranta, A., et al.: Natural history of rheumatic aortic regurgitation: Criteria predictive of congestive heart failure and angina in young patients. Circulation, 44:368, 1971.

Starling, M. R., Kirsch, M. M., Montgomery, D. G., and Gross, M. D.: Mechanisms for left ventricular systolic dysfunction in aortic regurgitation: Importance for predicting the functional response to aortic valve replacement. J. Am. Coll. Cardiol., 17:887, 1991.

Starr, A., Edwards, M. L., McCord, C. W., and Griswold, H. E.: Aortic replacement: Clinical experience with a semirigid ball-valve prosthesis. Circulation, 27:779, 1963.

Starr, A., Edwards, M., McCord, C. W., et al.: Multiple-valve replacement. Circulation, 29:30, 1964.

Swanson, J. S., and Starr, A.: The ball valve experience over three decades. Ann. Thorac. Surg., 48:S51, 1989.

Tatineni, S., Barner, H. B., Pearson, A. C., et al.: Rest and exercise evaluation of St. Jude Medical and Medtronic Hall prostheses: Influence of primary lesion, valvular type, valvular size, and left ventricle function. Circulation, 80:I-16, 1989.

Teare, R. D.: Asymmetrical hypertrophy of the heart in young adults. Br. Heart J., 20:1, 1958.

Tuffier, T.: Etude experimentale sur la chirurgie des valves de coeur. Bull. Acad. Med. Paris, 71:293, 1914.

Tuna, I. C., Orszulak, T. A., Schaff, H. V., and Danielson, G. K.: Results of homograft aortic valve replacement for active endocarditis. Ann. Thorac. Surg., 49:619, 1990.

Utley, J. R., Mills, J., and Roe, B. B.: The role of valve replacement in the treatment of fungal endocarditis. J. Thorac. Cardiovasc. Surg., 69:255, 1975.

Williams, M. A.: Tissue valves in young patients—A recipe for disaster. J. Card. Surg., 6:620, 1991.

Wolfe, W. G.: Acute ascending aortic dissection. Ann. Surg., 192:658, 1980.

Wortham, D. C., Tri, T. B., and Bowen, T. E.: Hemodynamic evaluation of the St. Jude Medical valve prosthesis in the small aortic annulus. J. Thorac. Cardiovasc. Surg., 81:615, 1981.

Wynne, J., and Braunwald, E.: The cardiomyopathies and myocarditides. In Braunwald, E. (ed): Heart Disease: A Textbook of Cardiovascular Medicine. Philadelphia, W. B. Saunders, 1988, p. 1410.

# 53

## Cardiac Pacemakers and Implantable Cardioverter-Defibrillators

James E. Lowe and J. Marcus Wharton

Although studies in electrical stimulation of the heart started in the eighteenth century, it has been only relatively recently that cardiac pacemakers and defibrillators have become widely available for clinical use. Technologic advances in the past three decades have allowed the advent and steady improvement in implantable devices for control of bradyarrhythmias and tachyarrhythmias. It is now estimated that over 1 million persons living in the United States have pacemakers and that the implantation rate is approximately 130,000 per year. Estimated worldwide rates are 400,000 per year. By 1992, over 30,000 implantable cardioverter defibrillators had been implanted worldwide. As implantable arrhythmia control devices are continually improved and as new indications are discovered, the rate of implantations should increase further. The development and application of future pacemakers and antiarrhythmia devices require an interdisciplinary interface among cardiovascular surgeons, cardiologists, basic electrophysiologists, and biomedical engineers in an era of continued cost containment and expense justification.

## HISTORICAL ASPECTS

Cardiac electrostimulation began in the mid-eighteenth century with the use of currents from the Leyden jar or voltaic pile to stimulate cardiac nerves and cardiac muscle in animals and to attempt resuscitation of intact dead animals (Schechter, 1971). Electrostimulation was suggested for human resuscitation in a number of communications to the Royal Humane Society of London by Squires, Henley, and Fothergill between 1774 and 1784 (Registers of the Royal Humane Society of London, 1774–1784; Schechter, 1971). However, Aldini, in 1774, was the first to use intermittent precordial electrical stimulation to successfully revive a child who had fallen downstairs (Aldini, 1819). These reports may have led Hunter (1776) to recommend that electrostimulation be attempted as a last resort in the resuscitation of drowning victims. Nysten (1802), using the body of a recently executed convict, demonstrated that the heart lost its ability to be electrically reactivated first in the left ventricle, then in the right ventricle, then in the left atrium, and then in the right atrium. Later in the nineteenth century, Walshe (1862) and Duchenne (1872) advocated electrostimulation for cardiac standstill. During this same period, Althaus (1864) and Steiner (1871) reported successful resuscitation of cardiac arrest victims by electrical currents applied through transthoracic needles.

Von Ziemssen (1882) reported a 42-year-old woman, Catharina Serafin, who had a huge defect of the anterior left chest wall after resection of an enchondroma. The heart was covered only by a thin layer of skin and was visible and palpable (Fig. 53–1). Von Ziemssen noted that application of electrodes to the heart produced rhythmic stimulation only if the rate of stimulation was greater than the spontaneous heart rate. Slower stimulation rates produced erratic and occasionally slower heart rates. He also noted while placing the electrodes that the most sensitive area for stimulation was in the region of the atrioventricular (AV) groove. This observation was made more than a decade before His (1893) and Kent (1893) described the location of the AV node and the bundle of His.

Albildgaard (1775) demonstrated that a small shock applied to a chicken would cause it to fall lifeless and that a stronger shock applied across the chest would resuscitate the animal. This may be the first report of electrical induction of ventricular fibrillation and electrical defibrillation. The first description of electrical defibrillation in humans was reported by Kite (1788), who observed that transchest electrical discharge successfully resuscitated a 3-year-old child (Stilling, 1976).

Prevost and Battelli (1899) showed that electrical currents could cause ventricular fibrillation that often could be reversed by another powerful discharge of alternating or direct current. Robinovitch (1907–1909), in a series of reports, confirmed this work and designed the first portable electrical resuscitative apparatus for ambulances. MacWilliam, in many publications beginning in 1899 and extending until World War I, further elucidated the pathophysiology of ventricular fibrillation and described deterioration of cardiac pump function by both tachyarrhythmias and bradyarrhythmias (Schechter, 1972).

These early experimental and clinical experiences did not lead to immediate clinical trials of cardiac pacing or electrical defibrillation. Schechter suggested that this initial apathy may have been due to the

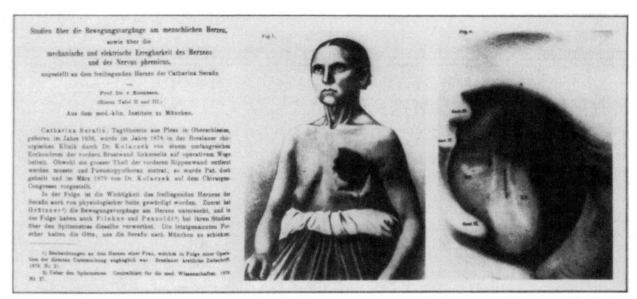

**FIGURE 53–1.** Hugo von Ziemssen's manuscript describing Catharina Serafin. Frau Serafin had a large defect in the left anterior chest wall after resection of an enchondroma. As shown in the second panel, the heart was covered only by skin, thus allowing von Ziemssen the opportunity to electrically stimulate various parts of the human heart. (From Schechter, D. C.: Exploring the origins of electrical cardiac stimulation. VII World Symposium on Cardiac Pacing, Vienna, Austria, May 1983. Minneapolis, Medtronic, Inc., 1983. Reprinted with permission of Medtronic, Inc.)

medical profession's interest in other techniques of cardiac reanimation, including pharmacologic injections, blood transfusions, electrolyte infusions, and cardiac massage (Schechter, 1971, 1972). The efforts of Kouwenhoven and colleagues (1932) and Beck and associates (1947) helped electrical defibrillation become widely applied clinically. Delayed communications and unnoticed publications were also an obstacle to progress in the development of cardiac pacing (Samet and El-Sherif, 1980). Studies in Europe by Marmorstein (1927) using both transvenous and transthoracic electrodes to pace the right atrium, right ventricle, and left ventricle in dogs were essentially unnoticed in the United States. This is evident from the reports of Bigelow and colleagues (1950), who independently described similar studies using transvenous electrodes to pace the right atrium of dogs. If these investigators had advanced electrodes into the right ventricle, which was done by Marmorstein, a clinical method to treat complete heart block might have been developed earlier. Similarly, the contributions of Gould, who designed a pulse generator and transthoracic pacing needle electrode and successfully resuscitated a patient, went unnoticed in the United States. This work was presented in Australia but was not published except for mention of it later by Hyman (1932). However, a report by Mond and associates (1982) suggests that Gould did not exist and that the Australians actually responsible for the development of the first impulse generator were Lidwill and Booth.

## Developments Leading to the Modern Pacemaker

Hyman (1932) developed a machine for controlled repetitive electrostimulation of the heart and called this device "the artificial cardiac pacemaker" (Fig. 53–2). This device was used successfully in a number of animal experiments. By using a transthoracic needle electrode, the artificial cardiac pacemaker was subsequently used to resuscitate for brief intervals several patients with complete heart block and syncope. Unfortunately, these reports were never published because Hyman was subjected to abusive correspondence and even lawsuits from those who regarded his attempts at resuscitation by pacing as tampering with "Divine Providence" (Schechter, 1983).

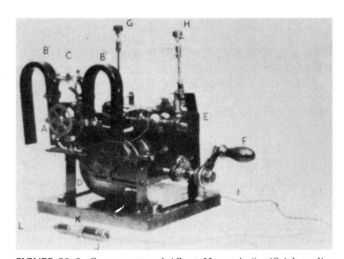

**FIGURE 53–2.** Components of Albert Hyman's "artificial cardiac pacemaker." Regular-spaced, repeated stimuli were delivered through a needle passed across the intact chest wall into the right atrium. (From Schechter, D. C.: Exploring the origins of electrical cardiac stimulation. VII World Symposium on Cardiac Pacing, Vienna, Austria, May 1983. Minneapolis, Medtronic, Inc., 1983. Reprinted with permission of Medtronic, Inc.)

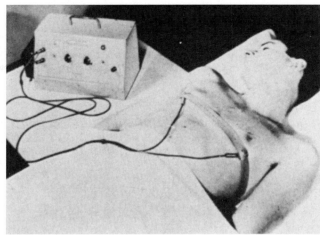

FIGURE 53–3. Zoll's successful pacing technique using external metal electrodes applied to the anterior chest wall. Zoll's contributions convinced the medical profession as well as the general public that cardiac pacing was both feasible and lifesaving. (From Schechter, D. C.: Exploring the origins of electrical cardiac stimulation. VII World Symposium on Cardiac Pacing, Vienna, Austria, May 1983. Minneapolis, Medtronic, Inc., 1983. Reprinted with permission of Medtronic, Inc.)

Zoll (1952) first described successful pacing through external metal electrodes applied to the anterior chest wall in two patients (Fig. 53–3). The initial impulse generator was a Grass stimulator. This noninvasive technique was easy to apply and was much better accepted than the invasive techniques of Hyman or Bigelow and Callaghan. Zoll's continued work and many publications convinced the medical profession as well as the general public that cardiac pacing was both feasible and lifesaving. Disadvantages of the external pacing technique included skin burns when inadequate electrode jelly was applied, painful chest wall muscle contractions, and inability to pace in thick-chested or emphysematous patients.

The new field of cardiac operations provided a major impetus in pacemaker development, because complete heart block was sometimes created during operations such as pulmonic commissurotomy and closure of ventricular septal defect (VSD). Brockman and colleagues (1958) used a wire electrode to successfully pace the heart of an infant who developed complete heart block after closure of a VSD. Although this patient died, pacing was effective and uninterrupted for 10 hours. Intramyocardial electrodes placed at the time of operation or introduced percutaneously through a needle were popularized in 1957 by the researchers at the University of Minneapolis (Allen and Lillehei, 1957; Gott et al., 1960; Lillehei et al., 1960, 1964; Thevenet et al., 1958; Weirich and Roe, 1961; Weirich et al., 1957, 1958a, 1958b). The electrodes were insulated silver-plated copper wires with exposed tips. These intramyocardial electrodes were connected to a self-contained external pacemaker containing transistors and a mercury battery. The disadvantages of this technique included lead dislodgment and steadily rising pacing thresholds of the myocardial wire electrode.

In August of 1958, Furman and Schwedel used a right ventricular endocardial wire electrode connected to an external generator to successfully pace for 96 hours a 76-year-old patient with complete heart block (Furman and Robinson 1959; Furman et al., 1961; Schwedel et al., 1960) (Fig. 53–4). This experience

showed that prolonged cardiac pacing with low voltages could be accomplished with an endocardial right ventricular electrode connected to an external pacemaker. Other important and independent developments in the field of cardiac electrostimulation also occurred during this period. Elmquist and Senning (1960) first implanted a rechargeable pacemaker in an epigastric pocket connected to electrodes that passed subcutaneously to the heart. Glenn and associates (1959) developed a method of cardiac pacing that

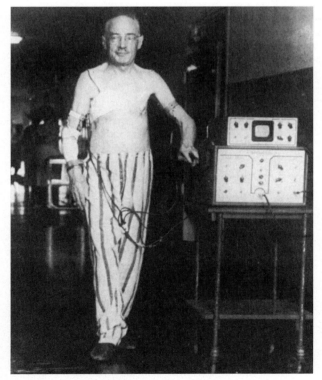

FIGURE 53–4. The feasibility of prolonged cardiac pacing using a right ventricular endocardial wire electrode connected to an external generator was demonstrated by Furman in 1958. Successful pacing was maintained for 96 days. The unipolar catheter attached to the external impulse generator allowed the patient to ambulate. (Courtesy of Dr. Seymour Furman.)

used radiofrequency transmission. This method required an external pulse generator but had the advantage of leaving the skin intact.

Chardack and colleagues (1960) developed a transistorized, self-contained implantable pacemaker connected to modified Hunter-Roth epicardial electrodes (Hunter et al., 1959). This was the first implantable permanent pacemaker with the pacing lead attached to the heart by thoracotomy (Fig. 53–5). Other completely implantable units developed by Zoll and colleagues (1961) and by Kantrowitz and associates (1962) followed. The technique for inserting a permanent transvenous bipolar pacemaker lead was developed in the United States by Parsonnet and colleagues (1962) and in Sweden by Ekestrom and associates (1962). In the most common method of pacing, the permanent impulse generator is now implanted near the site where the lead enters the cephalic or subclavian vein.

These initial implantable permanent pacemakers were fixed-rate asynchronous devices that delivered the impulse independently of the underlying cardiac rate. Noncompetitive demand pacing of the ventricles was later introduced by Leatham and associates (1956) and by Nicks and co-workers (1962) using external pacemakers. A brief period of asystole (1 to 2 seconds) triggered the onset of pacing, but deactivation of pacing required manual intervention. The use of implantable demand pacemakers that initiated pacing automatically in response to a single R-R interval prolongation with suppression on return of rhythm to a baseline R-R rate was first reported by Lemberg and associates (1965). Extensive clinical trials showing the efficacy of demand pacing were later reported by Goetz and associates (1966), Parsonnet and colleagues (1966), and Furman and co-workers (1967).

During the late 1960s, increased numbers of patients with sinus bradycardia and intact conduction were recognized. R wave–inhibited and synchronous pulse generators began to be applied to the atrium, and eventually dual-chamber pacemakers were designed to provide AV sequential pacing in patients with sinus bradycardia and heart block (Berkovits et al., 1969; Smyth et al., 1971). During the 1960s, new and improved pacemaker power sources were developed. Mercury-zinc batteries were used initially and usually lasted for less than 2 years. The mass of these cells accounted for two-thirds to three-quarters of the volume and even more of the weight of the pacemaker. Although various new power sources were

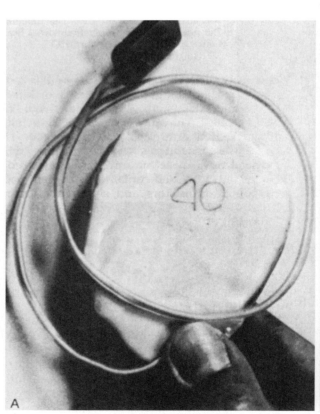 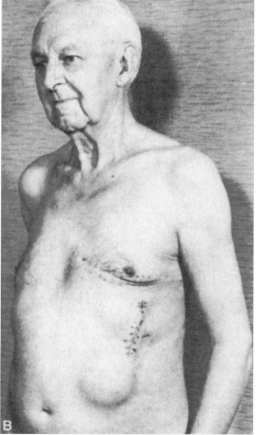

FIGURE 53–5. *A*, The first totally implantable pacemaker developed in 1960 by Chardack, Gage, and Greatbach. The pacemaker was connected to modified Hunter-Roth epicardial electrodes. *B*, The first patient to receive a Chardack, Gage, Greatbach totally implantable pacemaker. (*A* and *B*, From Schechter, D. C.: Exploring the origins of electrical cardiac stimulation. VII World Symposium on Cardiac Pacing, Vienna, Austria, May, 1983. Minneapolis, Medtronic, Inc., 1983. Reprinted with permission of Medtronic, Inc.)

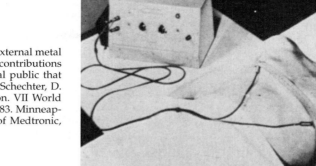

**FIGURE 53–3.** Zoll's successful pacing technique using external metal electrodes applied to the anterior chest wall. Zoll's contributions convinced the medical profession as well as the general public that cardiac pacing was both feasible and lifesaving. (From Schechter, D. C.: Exploring the origins of electrical cardiac stimulation. VII World Symposium on Cardiac Pacing, Vienna, Austria, May 1983. Minneapolis, Medtronic, Inc., 1983. Reprinted with permission of Medtronic, Inc.)

Zoll (1952) first described successful pacing through external metal electrodes applied to the anterior chest wall in two patients (Fig. 53–3). The initial impulse generator was a Grass stimulator. This noninvasive technique was easy to apply and was much better accepted than the invasive techniques of Hyman or Bigelow and Callaghan. Zoll's continued work and many publications convinced the medical profession as well as the general public that cardiac pacing was both feasible and lifesaving. Disadvantages of the external pacing technique included skin burns when inadequate electrode jelly was applied, painful chest wall muscle contractions, and inability to pace in thick-chested or emphysematous patients.

The new field of cardiac operations provided a major impetus in pacemaker development, because complete heart block was sometimes created during operations such as pulmonic commissurotomy and closure of ventricular septal defect (VSD). Brockman and colleagues (1958) used a wire electrode to successfully pace the heart of an infant who developed complete heart block after closure of a VSD. Although this patient died, pacing was effective and uninterrupted for 10 hours. Intramyocardial electrodes placed at the time of operation or introduced percutaneously through a needle were popularized in 1957 by the researchers at the University of Minneapolis (Allen and Lillehei, 1957; Gott et al., 1960; Lillehei et al., 1960, 1964; Thevenet et al., 1958; Weirich and Roe, 1961; Weirich et al., 1957, 1958a, 1958b). The electrodes were insulated silver-plated copper wires with exposed tips. These intramyocardial electrodes were connected to a self-contained external pacemaker containing transistors and a mercury battery. The disadvantages of this technique included lead dislodgment and steadily rising pacing thresholds of the myocardial wire electrode.

In August of 1958, Furman and Schwedel used a right ventricular endocardial wire electrode connected to an external generator to successfully pace for 96 hours a 76-year-old patient with complete heart block (Furman and Robinson 1959; Furman et al., 1961; Schwedel et al., 1960) (Fig. 53–4). This experience

showed that prolonged cardiac pacing with low voltages could be accomplished with an endocardial right ventricular electrode connected to an external pacemaker. Other important and independent developments in the field of cardiac electrostimulation also occurred during this period. Elmquist and Senning (1960) first implanted a rechargeable pacemaker in an epigastric pocket connected to electrodes that passed subcutaneously to the heart. Glenn and associates (1959) developed a method of cardiac pacing that

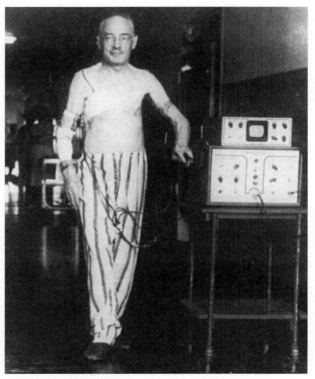

**FIGURE 53–4.** The feasibility of prolonged cardiac pacing using a right ventricular endocardial wire electrode connected to an external generator was demonstrated by Furman in 1958. Successful pacing was maintained for 96 days. The unipolar catheter attached to the external impulse generator allowed the patient to ambulate. (Courtesy of Dr. Seymour Furman.)

used radiofrequency transmission. This method required an external pulse generator but had the advantage of leaving the skin intact.

Chardack and colleagues (1960) developed a transistorized, self-contained implantable pacemaker connected to modified Hunter-Roth epicardial electrodes (Hunter et al., 1959). This was the first implantable permanent pacemaker with the pacing lead attached to the heart by thoracotomy (Fig. 53–5). Other completely implantable units developed by Zoll and colleagues (1961) and by Kantrowitz and associates (1962) followed. The technique for inserting a permanent transvenous bipolar pacemaker lead was developed in the United States by Parsonnet and colleagues (1962) and in Sweden by Ekestrom and associates (1962). In the most common method of pacing, the permanent impulse generator is now implanted near the site where the lead enters the cephalic or subclavian vein.

These initial implantable permanent pacemakers were fixed-rate asynchronous devices that delivered the impulse independently of the underlying cardiac rate. Noncompetitive demand pacing of the ventricles was later introduced by Leatham and associates (1956) and by Nicks and co-workers (1962) using external pacemakers. A brief period of asystole (1 to 2 seconds) triggered the onset of pacing, but deactivation of pacing required manual intervention. The use of implantable demand pacemakers that initiated pacing automatically in response to a single R-R interval prolongation with suppression on return of rhythm to a baseline R-R rate was first reported by Lemberg and associates (1965). Extensive clinical trials showing the efficacy of demand pacing were later reported by Goetz and associates (1966), Parsonnet and colleagues (1966), and Furman and co-workers (1967).

During the late 1960s, increased numbers of patients with sinus bradycardia and intact conduction were recognized. R wave–inhibited and synchronous pulse generators began to be applied to the atrium, and eventually dual-chamber pacemakers were designed to provide AV sequential pacing in patients with sinus bradycardia and heart block (Berkovits et al., 1969; Smyth et al., 1971). During the 1960s, new and improved pacemaker power sources were developed. Mercury-zinc batteries were used initially and usually lasted for less than 2 years. The mass of these cells accounted for two-thirds to three-quarters of the volume and even more of the weight of the pacemaker. Although various new power sources were

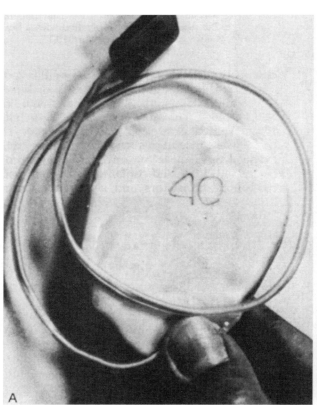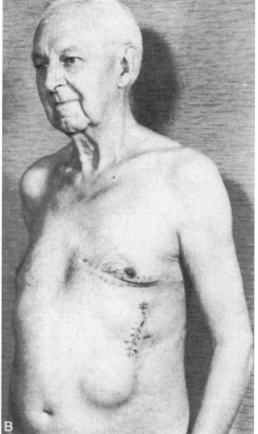

FIGURE 53–5. A, The first totally implantable pacemaker developed in 1960 by Chardack, Gage, and Greatbach. The pacemaker was connected to modified Hunter-Roth epicardial electrodes. B, The first patient to receive a Chardack, Gage, Greatbach totally implantable pacemaker. (A and B, From Schechter, D. C.: Exploring the origins of electrical cardiac stimulation. VII World Symposium on Cardiac Pacing, Vienna, Austria, May, 1983. Minneapolis, Medtronic, Inc., 1983. Reprinted with permission of Medtronic, Inc.)

tested, the lithium-iodine battery was soon recognized to be the best power source. In general, it is thought that the modern lithium-iodine battery may last for as long as 10 to 12 years. Nuclear-powered plutonium pacemakers are thought to last for a minimum of 10 to more than 20 years. However, cost and environmental restrictions have essentially eliminated their use in the United States.

## NORMAL CARDIAC CONDUCTION SYSTEM

### Impulse Formation

In the resting state, the myocardial cell maintains an electrical gradient or voltage potential across its cell membrane known as the *resting membrane potential.* The cell membrane is a semipermeable barrier through which ions can pass with various degrees of ease. In addition to the passive diffusion of ions along chemical or electrical gradients, active transport processes or "pumps" move ions against these gradients. The resting potential is the result of transmembrane differences in the concentrations of various ions, mainly sodium and potassium. The intracellular potassium concentration is much higher than that in the extracellular fluid. The opposite is true for sodium ions. The cell membrane is more permeable to potassium than to sodium, and potassium ions tend to pass outward through the cell membrane down the concentration gradient. This outward flow of positively charged ions causes a voltage gradient across the cell membrane. Because the flux of potassium ions is greater, potassium is the chief determinant of the voltage gradient at equilibrium. This equilibrium potential can be approximated by Nernst's equation, which relates the transmembrane potential to the ratio of extracellular and intracellular potassium concentrations:

$$V = \frac{RT}{F} \ln \frac{[K^+]_o}{[K^+]_i}$$

where R is the universal gas constant, T is the absolute temperature, and F is the Faraday constant. The cell membrane is a biologic system subject to variation, and the relationship between transmembrane potential and potassium levels becomes nonlinear at extremes of intra- or extracellular potassium concentrations. Changes in membrane permeability to other ions such as sodium at these extremes may also make their contribution to transmembrane potential more significant.

At equilibrium, when there is no net change in ion concentrations across the cell membrane, the equilibrium or resting potential is constant. For myocardial cells, the equilibrium potential is approximately −90 mV. *Depolarization* refers to a change in membrane potential to a less negative value (toward zero). When cell membranes are depolarized to a particular critical value, the threshold potential, a chain reaction of

events is triggered, resulting in complete, rapid depolarization followed by repolarization. When these events are recorded from a microelectrode placed inside the cell, an action potential is obtained (Fig. 53–6A). The phases of the action potential are the result of various transmembrane ionic currents, and rapid inward flux of sodium is mainly responsible for the rapid upstroke (phase 0) of the action potential recorded from myocardial cells and Purkinje fibers.

Certain cells, notably those in the sinoatrial (SA) node, display the property of automaticity. Automaticity refers to the spontaneous phase IV depolarization noted in recordings from these cells (Fig. 53–6B). The resting membrane potential of these cells is considerably lower (less negative) than that in myocardial cells and Purkinje fibers, and phase 0 is slower. The depolarization of these cells depends on slow channel currents, thought to be carried by calcium as well as sodium ions. The transmembrane potential in cells displaying automaticity does not remain constant in phase IV, but undergoes spontaneous depolarization until the threshold potential is reached and

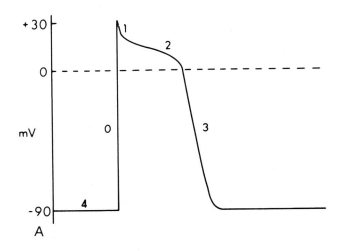

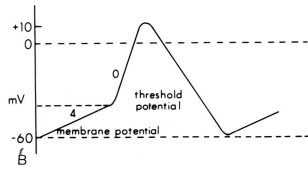

**FIGURE 53–6.** *A,* An action potential typical of a Purkinje fiber or ventricular myocardial cell. The resting membrane potential is −90 mV, and there is no spontaneous phase 4 depolarization. The upstroke (phase 0) is rapid. *B,* An action potential recorded from a cell displaying automaticity such as found in the sinoatrial (SA) and atrioventricular (AV) nodes. Spontaneous phase IV depolarization is present. The resting membrane potential is lower (−60 mV), and the upstroke is slower.

an action potential is generated. A wave of depolarizing current then passes from one cell to another throughout the myocardium. Automaticity is normally a property of cells in the SA node and, to a lesser extent, cells of the AV node. Under abnormal conditions, Purkinje fibers and myocardial cells may also develop automaticity.

Myocardial cells can also be depolarized by means of artificially applied electrical stimuli. The stimulus must have sufficient strength to bring a critical number of cells up to the threshold potential, which creates a propagated impulse. When an activation wavefront is initiated by an artificial stimulus, it propagates throughout the myocardium. This unique property of myocardial cells forms the basis for artificial cardiac pacing.

## Functional Anatomy of the Conduction System

The SA node is a group of specialized cells located subepicardially at the lateral junction of the superior vena cava with the right atrium, although some anatomic variation may occur with extension of the node anteriorly across the caval-atrial junction. The SA node extends for several centimeters along the crista terminalis to the mid-high posterolateral right atrium. The SA node is especially vulnerable to surgical trauma because of its location. Three types of cells can be found in the human SA node, in addition to supporting elements of fibrocytes, nerves, and vessels (Lowe et al., 1988). Pacemaker or polygonal cells are polyhedral and contain prominent nuclei and sparse numbers of contractile elements. These cells are believed to be the site of impulse formation in the SA node, although electrophysiologic confirmation in humans is lacking. Transitional cells are found surrounding pacemaker cells and interposed between nodal cells and atrial myocardium. These cells have some features of both nodal cells and myocardial cells, with larger numbers of contractile elements. Atrial myocardial cells with prominent longitudinally oriented myofibrils may also be found in SA node tissue.

The AV node is located subendocardially in the triangle of Koch, an anatomic region on the medial wall of the right atrium formed by the tendon of Todaro, the eustachian valve of the coronary sinus, and the tricuspid annulus. The AV node is composed of a transitional zone and a compact zone. Transitional cells gradually merge into the compact zone that rests along the most inferior portion of the interatrial septum. Three distinct inputs of transitional cells into the AV node have been identified—posterior, right septal, and left septal inputs (Meijler and Janse, 1988).

There are probably three preferential pathways of interatrial conduction between the SA node and the AV node (James, 1963). The posterior internodal pathway, which is the crista terminalis, extends from the SA node to merge with the posterior input to the AV node in the region of the coronary sinus ostium. The middle and anterior preferential interatrial pathways extend from the SA node across the posterior and anterior interatrial septum to provide the right septal input to the AV node. Although the orientation of atrial muscle fibers appears to produce preferential pathways of conduction, evidence for functionally distinct conduction pathways across the atrium from the SA node is lacking in humans.

The compact AV nodal cells can be identified along the length of Koch's triangle with the greatest proportion anteriorly (Meijler and Janse, 1988). From the annular side of the small compact AV nodal cells, large, linear Purkinje cells gradually emerge and coalesce to form the penetrating His bundle within the central fibrous body. The His bundle courses a short distance along the crest of the muscular interventricular septum below the membranous septum to branch into the right and left bundle branches. The right bundle branch is a discrete fascicle that runs along the endocardial surface of the right ventricular septum to the moderator band where initial branches to the apical septum exit. The right bundle then provides a dense network of Purkinje fibers across the right ventricular endocardium. The left bundle branch is occasionally a discrete fascicle of approximately a centimeter in length, but more usually there is no discrete left bundle. Instead, a complex, interdigitating network of left-sided Purkinje fascicles fan out from the bifurcation at the distal His bundle to run across the left ventricular endocardium (Massing and James, 1976). Although electrocardiographic patterns of left anterior and left posterior fascicle conduction block have been defined and have clinical utility, discrete left anterior and posterior fascicle cannot be identified anatomically in most patients.

Decremental conduction is a characteristic feature of conduction through the AV node. This refers to the normal slowing of conduction that occurs as the rate of impulse transmission to the AV node increases. In the absence of changes in autonomic tone, as the atrial rate increases, the AV nodal conduction time likewise increases to the point that physiologic block (Wenckebach's or Mobitz I second-degree AV block) occurs. This usually occurs at rates of 150 to 170 beats per minute. However, conduction through the AV node depends heavily on autonomic tone. Withdrawal of vagal tone due to exercise or administration of atropine results in accelerated AV conduction, whereas increased vagal tone results in slower AV conduction or transient AV block. Increased sympathetic tone likewise improves conduction through the AV node. Thus, during exercise or stress, autonomic changes improve AV nodal conduction concomitantly with increases in heart rate, allowing maintenance of AV conduction.

The delay in conduction that occurs in the AV node is responsible for the majority of the P-R interval of the standard electrocardiogram (ECG) as well as the AH interval of the bundle of His recording. Normal conduction times across the AV node are between 60 and 120 msec, whereas conduction from the SA node to AV node is 30 to 40 msec and from the His bundle to ventricle 35 to 45 msec.

Conduction of impulses may proceed retrogradely from ventricle to atrium across the AV node. Retrograde conduction has been estimated to be intact in two-thirds of normal humans (Akhtar, 1981). Retrograde VA block often occurs in or below the bundle of His, compared with antegrade conduction block that normally occurs in the AV node.

## INDICATIONS FOR PACEMAKER THERAPY

Artificial pacing has clearly prolonged and improved the lives of thousands of patients with symptomatic bradyarrhythmias. The recognition of this impact on patient care has steadily increased pacemaker implantations worldwide. In the United States, approximately 360 pacemakers are inserted annually per million population, and this has been increasing at a rate of about 19 implants per million per year (Bernstein and Parsonnet, 1992). Analysis of trends since 1975 indicates an increasing awareness of the benefits of pacing in patients with sinus node dysfunction. Implantation of a pacemaker for sinus node dysfunction accounted for 23% of primary implants in 1975 and 48% by 1989. Atrioventricular node and His-Purkinje conduction disturbances were indications for pacing in 45% of patients in 1989, drug-induced bradycardia in 4%, and tachyarrhythmias in 2% (Bernstein and Parsonnet, 1992). Furthermore, there has been an increasing dependence on dual-chamber pacing in a number of clinical conditions as the multiple benefits of this pacing modality are demonstrated. It is estimated that over 30% of pacemakers implanted today are dual-chamber devices, and this percentage is anticipated to increase further in the next decade (Bernstein and Parsonnet, 1992). In addition, the availability of various sensors to increase the pacemaker rate during periods of physiologic stress has improved exercise capabilities in patients receiving pacemakers. Single-chamber, rate-responsive devices now account for another third of all pacemakers implanted (Bernstein and Parsonnet, 1992). As pacemaker technology continues to improve, new indications for pacemakers are identified, and the percentage of the elderly in the population increases, it is anticipated that the need for permanent pacemakers will continue to increase.

Although there is still some controversy regarding indications for temporary and permanent cardiac pacing as well as the type of pacing system chosen, most physicians would agree with the following guidelines.

### Indications for Temporary Pacing

Three major factors that help to determine the indications for temporary pacing include (1) symptoms such as dizziness, near syncope, frank syncope, hypotension, and heart failure; (2) ventricular rate; and (3) clinical circumstances, which include the patient's underlying heart disease and the direct cause of the dysrhythmia being evaluated for temporary pacing. In general, ventricular rates less than 40 beats per minute produce symptoms and require temporary pacing. Acute bradyarrhythmias require temporary pacing more often than chronic arrhythmias. This appears to be particularly important in dealing with acute bradyarrhythmias associated with recent myocardial infarction. Indications for temporary pacing are shown in Table 53–1.

**Symptomatic, Second-Degree, and Complete AV Block.** Wenckebach (Mobitz Type I) second-degree AV block rarely requires temporary pacing unless the patient is symptomatic, which may occur if there is predominantly 2:1 AV conduction or even higher grades of conduction block. Because Wenckebach block is typically due to increased vagal tone, atropine or other means to decrease vagal tone may be helpful in those symptomatic patients and obviate the need for temporary pacing. However, if the precipitating cause is expected to last hours to days, temporary pacing is a safer and more reliable therapy than repeated dosing with atropine. Asymptomatic Mobitz Type II second-degree block probably does not require temporary pacing if a permanent pacemaker can be implanted promptly, given the relatively low risk in most situations for progression to complete heart block over the short term (although the long-term risk is high). However, Mobitz Type II second-degree AV block in acute situations such as during a myocardial infarction should prompt temporary pacemaker implantation, given the much higher acute risk for progressing to higher grades of conduction disturbance. In high-grade (i.e., transient periods of 3:1 or greater ratios of AV conduction) and complete heart block, symptoms and the ventricular rate are the determining factors for insertion of a temporary pacemaker. Generally, temporary pacing is indicated in this group of patients who have symptoms that include dizziness, syncope, near syncope, hypotension, or congestive heart failure. In addition, patients who develop high-grade or complete heart block in clini-

---

■ **Table 53–1.** INDICATIONS FOR TEMPORARY PACING

Symptomatic second-degree and complete AV block
Symptomatic bradyarrhythmias after acute myocardial infarction
New bifascicular or trifascicular block after acute myocardial infarction
Sick sinus syndrome (selected patients before permanent pacemaker insertion)
Symptomatic drug-induced bradyarrhythmias
Drug-resistant tachyarrhythmias (selected patients)
Carotid sinus syncope (selected patients)
Before permanent pacemaker implantation in selected patients
Therapeutic trial in patients with medically refractory low cardiac output
After cardiac surgery
Ventricular tachycardia (torsades de pointes) associated with long Q-T interval or bradycardia

*Key:* AV = atrioventricular.

cally unstable situations should undergo temporary pacemaker placement even if the heart block is well tolerated. Infranodal advanced or complete AV block frequently requires permanent pacing. Temporary pacing may be indicated before implantation of a permanent pacemaker, depending on the patient's ventricular rate and on the presence or absence of symptoms.

**Symptomatic Bradyarrhythmias After Acute Myocardial Infarction.** Acute diaphragmatic myocardial infarction often leads to bradyarrhythmias that are usually transient and seldom require artificial pacing. However, when the ventricular rate is significantly slow (less than 40 beats per minute), or when the bradyarrhythmia becomes refractory to pharmacologic agents such as atropine and isoproterenol, or if symptoms develop, temporary pacing is indicated. In the setting of inferior myocardial infarction with heart block and a right ventricular infarct syndrome, temporary AV sequential pacing is necessary to provide maximum hemodynamic benefit. Although less common, AV block due to anterior myocardial infarction usually represents infranodal block. Given the frequent instability of escape rhythms in this situation, all patients should receive a temporary pacemaker, even if they are asymptomatic. These patients may also benefit from permanent pacing, even if the heart block resolves.

**New Bifascicular or Trifascicular Block After Acute Myocardial Infarction.** In general, prophylactic temporary pacing should be considered in patients with acute bifascicular block or trifascicular block after acute myocardial infarction. Controversy still exists as to whether temporary pacing is sufficiently useful in the setting of new left bundle branch block and anterior myocardial infarction to justify its use. Isolated right bundle branch block, left anterior fascicular block, or left posterior fascicular block are not indications for prophylactic pacing during acute infarction. In addition, prophylactic temporary pacing is usually not indicated in patients with acute infarction and pre-existing bundle-branch blocks, including old bifascicular or trifascicular block. Most of the studies analyzing the need for prophylactic pacing for conduction disturbances during acute myocardial infarction occurred before the era of widespread use of acute thrombolytic therapy. Whether successful reperfusion significantly alters the risk for developing complete heart block in patients with new bifascicular or trifascicular block and acute infarction is not known, and prophylactic temporary pacing is still recommended.

**Sick Sinus Syndrome.** Patients with advanced sick sinus syndrome often require permanent pacing. Many develop bradyarrhythmias as well as tachyarrhythmias and require a combination of pacemaker therapy and antiarrhythmic drug therapy. Temporary cardiac pacing is occasionally necessary before permanent pacemaker implantation in those patients who are symptomatic and have near syncope or syncope. In most of these patients, temporary pacing can be accomplished with conventional ventricular demand pacing. However, in those who require the atrial component to cardiac filling, temporary atrial pacing or dual-chamber pacing may be required.

**Symptomatic Digitalis-Induced Bradyarrhythmias.** Temporary cardiac pacing is indicated in symptomatic patients with marked bradyarrhythmia due to digitalis toxicity. Digitalis-induced bradyarrhythmias include sinus bradycardia, sinus arrest, second-degree AV block, and advanced or complete AV block.

**Drug-Resistant Tachyarrhythmias.** When tachyarrhythmias, particularly ventricular tachycardia, become refractory to antiarrhythmic drug therapy, artificial overdrive pacing (80 to 120 beats per minute) is occasionally effective. Various modes of temporary pacing can be attempted, but atrial or coronary sinus pacing is usually ideal, particularly in patients in whom the atrial contribution to cardiac output is essential. However, given the difficulties in maintaining stable atrial pacing and frequently associated impaired AV nodal conduction, temporary ventricular or AV sequential pacing is often necessary.

**Carotid Sinus Syncope.** Permanent pacemaker implantation is indicated in patients with carotid sinus syncope or near syncope resulting from bradycardia. Syncope due to hypotension (vasodepressor syncope) does not respond to pacing. In some patients, hypersensitive carotid sinus reactions may be greatly exaggerated by drugs such as digitalis, methyldopa, and propranolol. Temporary pacing is occasionally indicated in this group while the offending drug is withdrawn.

**Before Permanent Pacemaker Implantation.** Most patients requiring permanent pacemaker implantation do not require a preoperative temporary pacemaker. However, temporary pacing is essential before permanent implantation in patients with acute arrhythmias, especially after acute myocardial infarction or in symptomatic patients with complete AV block.

**Therapeutic Trial for Congestive Heart Failure, Cardiogenic Shock, and Cerebral or Renal Insufficiency.** It is becoming increasingly apparent that some patients with intractable congestive heart failure, cardiogenic shock, and cerebral or renal hypoperfusion may be improved by an increased heart rate. Generally, atrial pacing is chosen because the atrial contribution to cardiac output appears to be essential in patients with low perfusion states. Therefore, temporary pacing should be considered as a therapy in this difficult subgroup of patients. In patients who respond, permanent pacemaker implantation may be considered for long-term therapy.

**After Cardiac Surgery.** Temporary atrial or AV sequential pacing through temporary epicardial electrodes may decrease the need for inotropic support in the perioperative period. Transient conduction disturbances are often encountered in the immediate perioperative period, and temporary epicardial pacing is essential. An additional advantage is that atrial dysrhythmias that occur perioperatively can be diagnosed more accurately through recording of electrograms from these temporary wires, and overdrive pacing can often be used to convert perioperative atrial flutter and occasionally atrial fibrillation (Waldo and MacLean, 1980). Most cardiac surgeons routinely attach temporary atrial and ventricular pacing wires after major cardiac surgical procedures.

## Indications for Permanent Pacing

Implantation of a permanent pacemaker commits the patient to a lifetime with an implantable device with its associated costs, inconveniences, and potential complications. Therefore, the decision to implant a permanent pacemaker must consider both the benefits and the risks and complications associated with its use. Fortunately, pacemaker and lead technology and implantation techniques have been so greatly improved that the acute and long-term risk associated with permanent pacemakers is small. Nonetheless, the decision to implant a permanent pacemaker needs to be made with the aim of improving the patient's quality of life and longevity.

Because controversy exists about appropriate indications for implantation of a permanent pacemaker, guidelines have been written by a task force of the American College of Cardiology and American Heart Association (Committee of Pacemaker Implantation, 1991). Indications for permanent pacemaker implantation have been grouped in this report into three classifications:

*Class I:* Conditions for which there is general agreement that a permanent pacemaker should be implanted.

*Class II:* Conditions for which permanent pacemakers are frequently used but in which there may be a divergence of opinion with respect to the necessity of their implantation.

*Class III:* Conditions in which there is general agreement that permanent pacemaker implantation is not indicated.

Thus, Class I and II indications are those in which the patient definitely or probably benefits from implantation of a permanent pacemaker, whereas in Class III indications, there is no or minimal potential benefit to the patient. The ACC/AHA guidelines for implantation of permanent pacemakers in different clinical situations are listed in Table 53–2.

### Acquired AV Block in Adults

Before permanent pacemakers were available, 50% of patients with complete heart block died within 1 year (Friedberg et al., 1964; Johansson, 1969). The most common cause of acquired complete heart block is sclerodegenerative disease of the cardiac skeleton and AV conduction system. Other causes of complete heart block include ischemic heart disease, cardiomyopathic processes, Chagas' disease, and traumatic injury. Permanent pacemaker implantation is indicated in any patient with symptomatic complete, high-grade, or second-degree AV block. Symptoms include congestive heart failure, altered mental status,

or other end-organ failure, particularly if it can be shown that temporary pacing improves the symptom. Permanent pacing is usually recommended for surgically induced complete heart block that persists more than 1 week after the operation. Symptomatic complete or high-grade AV block in the setting of atrial fibrillation or other atrial tachyarrhythmias is also an indication unless the AV block is due to digitalis or other drugs and these drugs are not necessary for the patients' management. In patients with second-degree AV block, symptoms should be shown to be related to the episodes of AV block. Patients with asymptomatic Mobitz Type II are frequently considered to benefit from permanent pacing given the high risk for development of complete heart block in these patients (Dhingra et al., 1974). Patients with Wenckebach (Mobitz Type I) second-degree AV block shown to be due to block in or below the His bundle during electrophysiologic testing are also candidates for permanent pacing, because their risk for developing complete heart block is similar to that of patients with classic Mobitz Type II second-degree AV block. Patients with Wenckebach second-degree AV block due to intra- or infra-Hisian Wenckebach conduction patterns usually have associated bundle-branch block. Wenckebach second-degree AV block with a narrow QRS complex is almost always due to AV nodal block, and three-fourths of the cases associated with bundle-branch block are also due to AV nodal block and thus are not indications for permanent pacemaker implantation (Peuch et al., 1976).

### AV Block After Myocardial Infarction

Unlike those for acquired AV block in other conditions, indications for permanent pacemaker implantation in the setting of recent myocardial infarction do not necessarily require the presence of symptoms. Patients with persistent complete or high-grade AV block after myocardial infarction, whether associated with symptoms or not, should be permanently paced given their poor prognosis. In addition, patients with transient complete heart block during acute myocardial infarction who have persistent bundle-branch block have been shown in some studies to have a high risk of late complete heart block and thus should be permanently paced (Domenghetti and Perret, 1980; Hindman et al., 1978). Because alternating bundle-branch blocks have high rates of progression to complete heart block, they also should be permanently paced, even if episodes of transient complete or high-grade AV block have not been documented (Wu et al., 1976).

### Chronic Bifascicular and Trifascicular Block

Bifascicular and trifascicular block suggest extensive damage to the His bundle and bundle branches. Although the overall risk for progression to permanent or symptomatic complete heart block is low, certain patients with bi- and trifascicular blocks are at considerably higher risks. Patients with bi- or tri-

■ **Table 53–2.** INDICATIONS FOR PERMANENT PACING (GUIDELINES OF THE AMERICAN COLLEGE OF CARDIOLOGY/ AMERICAN HEART ASSOCIATION TASK FORCE)

**Indications for Permanent Pacing in Acquired AV Block in Adults**
**Class I**
  A. Complete heart block, permanent or intermittent, at any anatomic level, associated with any one of the following complications:
   1. Symptomatic bradycardia. In the presence of complete heart block, symptoms must be presumed to be due to the heart block unless proved otherwise
   2. Congestive heart failure
   3. Ectopic rhythms and other medical conditions that require drugs that suppress the automaticity of escape pacemakers and cause symptomatic bradycardia
   4. Documented periods of asystole ≥ 3.0 seconds or any escape rate < 40 beats/min in symptom-free patients
   5. Confusional states that clear with temporary pacing
   6. Post–AV-junction ablation, myotonic dystrophy
  B. Second-degree AV block, permanent or intermittent, regardless of the type or the site of block, with symptomatic bradycardia
  C. Atrial fibrillation, atrial flutter, or rare cases of supraventricular tachycardia with complete heart block or advanced AV block, bradycardia, and any of the conditions described under Class IA. The bradycardia must be unrelated to digitalis or drugs known to impair AV conduction

**Class II**
  A. Asymptomatic complete heart block, permanent or intermittent, at any anatomic site, with ventricular rates of 40 beats/min or faster
  B. Asymptomatic type II second-degree AV block, permanent or intermittent
  C. Asymptomatic type I second-degree AV block at intra-His or infra-His levels

**Class III**
  A. First-degree AV block (see section IV on bifascicular and trifascicular block)
  B. Asymptomatic type I second-degree AV block at the supra-His (AV node) level

**Indications for Permanent Pacing After Myocardial Infarction**
**Class I**
  A. Persistent advanced second-degree AV block or complete heart block after acute myocardial infarction with block in the His-Purkinje system (bilateral bundle-branch block)
  B. Patients with transient advanced AV block and associated bundle-branch block

**Class II**
  A. Patients with persistent advanced block in the AV node

**Class III**
  A. Transient AV conduction disturbances in the absence of intraventricular conduction defects
  B. Transient AV block in the presence of isolated left anterior hemiblock
  C. Acquired left anterior hemiblock in the absence of AV block
  D. Patients with persistent first-degree AV block in the presence of bundle-branch block not demonstrated previously

fascicular block with intermittent complete heart block, high-grade AV block, or Mobitz Type II second-degree AV block represent such a high-risk group, and should undergo permanent pacemaker implantation. Because syncope is the usual symptom associated with transient complete or high-grade AV block, patients with syncope and bi- or trifascicular block should undergo electrophysiologic testing to determine if infra-Hisian block can be induced by pacing, in which case a pacemaker should be implanted. It has also been suggested that even asymptomatic patients with a markedly prolonged infranodal conduction time (HV interval > 100 msec) should undergo prophylactic permanent pacing given their high risk for progression to complete heart block (Scheinmann et al., 1983). Even in the absence of pacing-induced infra-Hisian block or a markedly prolonged HV interval, patients with syncope and bi- or trifascicular block in whom a cause for syncope cannot be identified with extensive testing should receive a permanent pacemaker given the high probability that their syncope was secondary to a high-grade though transient conduction disturbance and their potential increased risk of death from a bradyarrhythmia. Although patients with bi- and trifascicular disease have a relatively high mortality rate, this is largely due to the underlying heart disease that caused the conduc-

tion disorder, not to the development of complete heart block. Thus, routine implantation of pacemakers in asymptomatic patients with bi- and trifascicular block is not indicated (McAnulty et al., 1982).

### Sinus Node Dysfunction

Patients with sinus node dysfunction may develop a number of arrhythmias, such as inappropriate sinus bradycardia, chronotropic incompetence, SA exit block, and sinus arrest. This group of rhythm disorders typically occurs in older patients with or without underlying heart disease and is collectively known as the "sick sinus syndrome." In addition, many patients with sick sinus syndrome have associated atrial tachyarrhythmias, particularly atrial fibrillation. This association of atrial tachyarrhythmias in patients with the sick sinus syndrome is called the tachycardia-bradycardia (or tachy-brady) syndrome. Patients with symptomatic bradycardia not due to reversible cause are candidates for permanent pacing. In addition, patients with the tachycardia-bradycardia syndrome frequently require digitalis, other AV nodal blocking agents, or antiarrhythmic drugs to control atrial tachyarrhythmias, which cause an exaggerated suppression of sinus node function. If these drugs are not avoidable in this situation, then permanent pacing

■ **Table 53–2.** INDICATIONS FOR PERMANENT PACING (GUIDELINES OF THE AMERICAN COLLEGE OF CARDIOLOGY/ AMERICAN HEART ASSOCIATION TASK FORCE) *(Continued)*

**Indications for Permanent Pacing in Bifascicular and Trifascicular Block**
**Class I**
  A. Bifascicular block with intermittent complete heart block associated with symptomatic bradycardia (as defined)
  B. Bifascicular or trifascicular block with intermittent type II second-degree AV block without symptoms attributable to the heart block

**Class II**
  A. Bifascicular or trifascicular block with syncope that is not proved to be due to complete heart block, but other possible causes for syncope are not identifiable
  B. Markedly prolonged HV (> 100 ms)
  C. Pacing-induced infra-His block

**Class III**
  A. Fascicular block without AV block or symptoms
  B. Fascicular block with first-degree AV block without symptoms

**Indications for Permanent Pacing in Sinus Node Dysfunction**
**Class I**
  A. Sinus node dysfunction with documented symptomatic bradycardia; in some patients this will occur as a consequence of long-term (essential) drug therapy of a type and dose for which there are no acceptable alternatives

**Class II**
  A. Sinus node dysfuncton, occurring spontaneously or as a result of necessary drug therapy, with heart rates < 40 beats/min when a clear association between significant symptoms consistent with bradycardia and the actual presence of bradycardia has not been documented

**Class III**
  A. Sinus node dysfunction in asymptomatic patients, including those in whom substantial sinus bradycardia (heart rate < 40 beats/min) is a consequence of long-term drug treatment
  B. Sinus node dysfunction in patients in whom symptoms suggestive of bradycardia are clearly documented not to be associated with a slow heart rate

**Indications for Permanent Pacing in Hypersensitive Carotid Sinus and Neurovascular Syndromes**
**Class I**
  A. Recurrent syncope associated with clear, spontaneous events provoked by carotid sinus stimulation; minimal carotid sinus pressure induces asystole of > 3 seconds' duration in the absence of any medication that depresses the sinus node or AV conduction

**Class II**
  A. Recurrent syncope without clear, provocative events and with a hypersensitive cardioinhibitory response
  B. Syncope with associated bradycardia reproduced by a head-up tilt with or without isoproterenol or other forms of provocative maneuvers and in which a temporary pacemaker and a second provocative test can establish the likely benefits of a permanent pacemaker

**Class III**
  A. A hyperactive cardioinhibitory response to carotid sinus stimulation in the absence of symptoms
  B. Vague symptoms, such as dizziness, lightheadedness, or both, with a hyperactive cardioinhibitory response to carotid sinus stimulation
  C. Recurrent syncope, light-headedness, or dizziness in the absence of a cardioinhibitory response

---

will be needed to protect against drug-induced bradycardia. Some patients with intermittent symptoms suggestive of bradycardia and documented bradycardias with rates less than 40 beats per minute but in whom the symptoms have not been documented to occur with bradycardia may be candidates for permanent pacing. However, a concerted effort should be made to confirm the presence of bradycardia with symptoms.

### Neurovascular Syndromes

Several neurovascular syndromes cause exaggerated parasympathetic tone with resultant sinus bradycardia, asystole, and transient high-grade AV block (cardioinhibitory effect). In addition, reflex withdrawal of sympathetic tone may further exacerbate the bradyarrhythmias and also produce profound vasodilatation (vasodepressor effect), sometimes without significant bradyarrhythmias. The most common of these syndromes is the carotid sinus hypersensitiv-

ity syndrome when it is associated with a significant cardioinhibitory response and syncope. In these patients, mild carotid sinus massage will cause significant asystole (> 3 seconds) (Morley and Sutton, 1984). Some individuals, however, may have a hypersensitive response to carotid sinus massage and remain asymptomatic. For this reason, it is useful to document significant bradyarrhythmia during a spontaneous episode of syncope or near syncope in patients suspected of having carotid sinus hypersensitivity syndrome. However, in some patients with recurrent syncope, clear documentation of bradycardia during a spontaneous episode is not possible, although demonstration of a hypersensitive response to carotid massage suggests the diagnosis. The most common neurovascular syndrome is the neurally mediated syncope syndrome, which results from an exaggerated Bezold-Jarisch reflex induced when relative hypovolemia and increased sympathetic tone create left ventricular chamber obliteration during systole. Some patients may have palliation of symptoms with permanent pacing to alleviate the bradycardia component of the Bezold-Jarisch reflex if pacing demonstrates improvement in symptoms during provocative tilt table testing (Fitzpatrick et al., 1989).

### Tachyarrhythmias

Permanent pacing can be useful in some cases of medically refractory supraventricular and ventricular tachycardia if pacing the atria or ventricles, respectively, at tolerated rates above the intrinsic heart rate will prevent arrhythmia recurrence (overdrive suppression). However, a prolonged period of overdrive suppression using a temporary pacemaker should be tried before implanting a permanent pacemaker to demonstrate the efficacy of this approach. Patients with syndromes and torsades de pointes can be effectively treated with overdrive pacing if reversible causes are not found (Eldar et al., 1992). Permanent pacemakers have been designed to detect and terminate with pacing both supraventricular and ventricular tachycardias. With the advent of highly effective catheter ablation techniques for treatment of paroxysmal supraventricular tachycardias, the use of pacemakers for overdrive suppression or termination of supraventricular tachycardias is rarely needed. Pacemakers that only pace terminate ventricular tachycardia can accelerate the tachycardia to a poorly tolerated ventricular tachycardia or fibrillation. These have been incorporated as part of implantable defibrillators to administer high-energy shocks if pacing causes degeneration of an initially hemodynamically stable arrhythmia.

### Intractable Congestive Heart Failure and Cerebral or Renal Insufficiency Benefited by Temporary Pacing

As described earlier, patients with refractory congestive heart failure and decreased perfusion causing cerebral or renal insufficiency may be improved occasionally by increasing heart rate with temporary pacing. If temporary pacing has proved to be effective under these conditions and long-term therapy is indicated, permanent pacing should be considered. Most of these patients require atrial contraction to improve cardiac output. Therefore, dual-chamber atrial synchronous pacing is usually indicated in this subgroup. Recent studies have suggested that AV sequential pacing with relatively short AV intervals may improve left ventricular function in patients with dilated cardiomyopathies without overt bradycardia (Hochleitner et al., 1990, 1992), but further evaluation of this phenomenon is needed before this indication can be recommended. Patients with hypertrophic obstructive cardiomyopathy are also favorably influenced by ventricular pacing, presumably because of the asyneresis induced by pacing the ventricular apex that partially alleviates outflow tract obstruction (Fanapazir et al., 1992).

## IMPULSE GENERATOR

An implantable cardiac pacemaker consists of an impulse generator, lead wire, and electrode (Fig. 53–7). The impulse generator contains a power source or battery, hybrid circuits, and a lead connector (Fig.

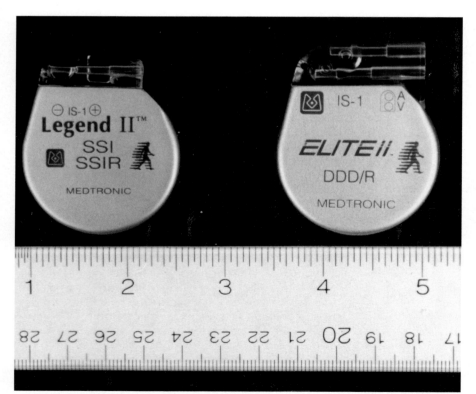

**FIGURE 53–7.** Modern single- *(left)* and dual- *(right)* chamber rate-responsive pacemaker generators. Note the small size and the header for connecting one or two leads, respectively. (Courtesy of Medtronic, Inc.)

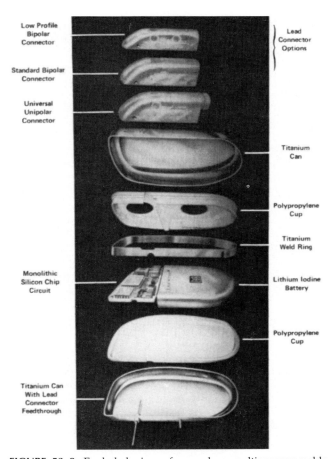

**FIGURE 53–8.** Exploded view of a modern multiprogrammable impulse generator. Various lead connectors are available to accept a variety of epicardial and transvenous leads. The battery and pacemaker electronics are enclosed in a titanium metal case. Hybrid circuit technology allows all components of the circuit, including semiconductors, resistors, and capacitors, to be diffused into a substrate to produce what is called a *monolithic silicon chip.* As shown, the major advantage of the silicon chip circuit is its extremely small size. This technology, combined with the improved lithium power source, has allowed modern multiprogrammable pacemakers to be much smaller, lighter, and more reliable than earlier pacemakers. (Courtesy of Paul Craven, Joe Hitselberger, and Gene Boone, Medtronic, Inc.)

53–8). All of these components are kept in a hermetically sealed metal container. The size and weight of the impulse generator depend on the size of the battery and the number of electronic components. Impulse generators are usually kept in rectangular or oval packages with rounded edges and weigh between 20 and 50 g.

## Power Sources

The power source used in a totally implantable pacemaker may be biologic, rechargeable, nuclear, or chemical. Biologic power sources convert mechanical or chemical energy of the body into electrical energy using piezoelectric crystals, biogalvanic cells, or bio-fuel cells (Armour et al., 1966; Cywinski et al., 1978; Myers et al., 1964). Theoretically, these power sources

can be renewed potentially for the patient's lifetime, but they have not been developed to a point at which they are clinically practical. In 1973, a highly reliable, hermetically sealed, nickel-cadmium rechargeable pacemaker was developed at Johns Hopkins University and introduced commercially by Pacesetter, Inc. (Fischell et al., 1975). The useful battery life of such a rechargeable pacemaker has been calculated to be 70 to 80 years. Rechargeable pacemakers, although reliable, are not used, primarily because of the necessity for weekly recharging. Nuclear-powered impulse generators have been implanted in more than 3,000 patients worldwide. Their longevity is predicted to be longer than 20 years; however, nuclear generators are no longer used because of cost, the improved longevity of newer chemical power sources, legislative restrictions, and concerns about the risk of chronic low-level radiation exposure. Chemical power sources continue to be the primary component of power cells in implantable pacemakers.

The modern power cell or battery is composed of an anode, a cathode, and an electrolyte. The power cell is generally named for the materials used in the anode and cathode—for example, lithium-iodine. Current solid-state cells have a dry, crystalline electrolyte between the anode and cathode. Electric current is produced by ionization of the anode, resulting in the migration of positively charged metallic ions through the electrolyte toward the cathode. Electrons are left behind on the anode, which becomes negatively charged relative to the cathode. When the anode and cathode are connected by a conductive pathway, a flow of electrons passes from the anode to the cathode. The higher the resistance in the conductor, the slower the flow of electrons and the longer the power cell will last. In the modern lithium-iodine power cell, the migrating or positively charged ions are lithium, which combines with iodine from the cathode to form a lithium-iodide electrolyte barrier. Most currently available lithium-powered pacemakers contain a single power cell, unlike the original mercury-zinc generators, which were powered by multiple-cell batteries.

Lithium power cells are available in five chemical types: lithium-iodine (polyvinyl pyridine), lithium-lead sulfide, lithium-silver chromate, lithium-copper sulfide, and lithium-thionyl chloride (Tyers and Brownlee, 1981). All of these lithium power sources have been extremely reliable and durable when compared with the earlier mercury-zinc systems. Most current pacemaker implants worldwide contain a solid-state lithium-iodine cell, which appears to be the power source of choice. Overall, pulse generator performance based on the type of power source is shown in Figure 53–9. The results with rechargeable impulse generators are essentially parallel to those of the nuclear power sources. The power source longevity of lithium pacemakers is estimated to be 10 to 12 years. However, battery longevity is determined by a number of factors, including percentage of time the generator is pacing, requirements for single- or dual-chamber pacing, lead impedance, programmed volt-

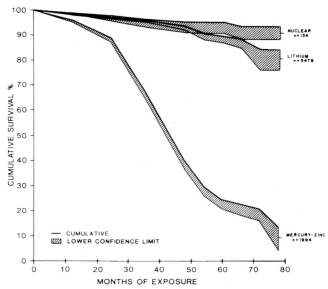

FIGURE 53–9. Impulse generator performance based on the type of power source. (From Bilitch, M., Hauser, R. G., Goldman, B. S., et al.: Performance of cardiac pacemaker pulse generators. PACE, 4:254, 1981.)

age and pulse width, and power drainage from monitoring, sensor, and special function circuits. Because of wound, lead-electrode, and functional problems relating to pacing and sensing, it appears that fewer than about 10% of patients have required reoperation 4 to 5 years after implantation of a lithium-powered pacemaker (Gross et al., 1992). Therefore, it is unwise to suggest to a patient that the life of the pacemaker is governed only by the predicted life expectancy of the power cell. Even modern lithium-powered pacemakers have been associated with a small incidence of random failure (Welti, 1981).

## Pacemaker Electronics

The first implantable pacemakers contained individual or discrete components including resistors, capacitors, diodes, transistors, reed switches, and wire coils for induction. These individual components were mounted on or between printed circuit boards. A major advance in pacemaker electronics has been the development of "hybrid" circuits. Hybrid technology allows all components of the circuit including semiconductors, resistors, and capacitors to be diffused into a substrate to produce a monolithic silicon chip (Fig. 53–10). The major advantage of the single-chip circuit is its small size. Customized digital, silicon, large-scale integrated circuits are used in almost all multiprogrammable pacemakers and may include as many as 40,000 transistors on a 4-mm² wafer. This technology combined with the improved lithium power source has allowed modern multiprogrammable pacemakers to be much smaller, lighter, and more reliable than earlier, simpler pacemakers. The lithium-powered pacemaker containing a custom integrated

circuit design is exceptionally reliable and capable of providing both multiprogrammable and physiologic pacing functions and extensive monitoring capabilities. Future pacemakers will most likely use low current drain, custom microcomputers consisting of a central processing unit, a memory unit, and an input-output circuit (Barold and Mugica, 1982). Pacemakers containing microcomputers are now capable of monitoring various physiologic changes to control in on-line manner pacemaker function. Physiologic changes that can be monitored include cardiac output requirements as determined by online measurement of temperature, Q-T interval, oxygen saturation, right ventricular pressure change, depolarization gradient, body motion, and respiratory rate. Moreover, microcomputer-based pacemakers can automatically select an appropriate pacing technique for the control of various dysrhythmias. Future pacemakers will be able to automatically detect loss of capture due to threshold changes and adjust their output accordingly.

## Hermetic Seal

The electronics and power source of the first totally implantable pacemakers were protected by epoxy resins and silicone rubber (Tyers and Brownlee, 1981). Gradually, however, moisture gained access to the interior of the pacemaker, causing short circuits, sudden cessation of pacing, battery explosion, pacemaker runaway, and occasionally even ventricular fibrillation (Tyers and Brownlee, 1976). Fluid infiltration problems were responsible for the massive recalls that

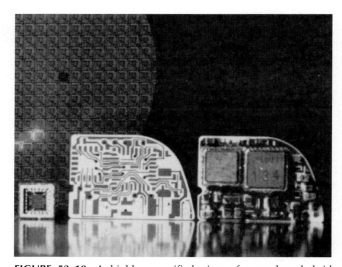

FIGURE 53–10. A highly magnified view of a modern hybrid circuit. Hybrid technology allows all components of the circuit, including semiconductors, resistors, and capacitors, to be diffused into a substrate to produce what is called a *monolithic silicon chip*. The obvious advantage of the single-chip circuit is its small size. Such hybrid circuits are used in almost all multiprogrammable pacemakers and may include as many as 40,000 transistors on a 4-mm² wafer. Such a hybrid circuit is exceptionally reliable and capable of providing both multiprogrammable and physiologic pacing functions. However, its capacity for monitoring and data processing is limited, and it may be replaced in the future by single-chip microcomputers.

eventually terminated the use of mercury-zinc, epoxy-enclosed pacemakers (Tyers and Brownlee, 1976).

The modern pacemaker is hermetically enclosed, rendering it airtight and fluid tight. Pacemaker manufacturers determine the quality of the hermetic seal in terms of a leak rate for an inert gas under standard conditions (Tyers and Brownlee, 1981). For example, an acceptable helium leak rate of $10^{-8}$ ml/sec at one atmosphere involves the passage of less than 0.01 ml of helium per 24 hours. Permeability to fluid is many orders of magnitude lower. Hermetic seal is now achieved by encasing the power source and electronics in a sealed metal container, which usually requires laser welding. The materials chosen for enclosure have included stainless steel, Haynes' alloy, and titanium. Most modern pacemakers are enclosed in titanium.

## Lead Connector

Impressive advances have been made in leads and electrodes and in pacemaker power sources and circuitry. As described by Tyers (1981), the ideal pacemaker connector should be tangential to reduce electrode stress, universal to accept all available leads without adapters, simple, and short-circuit proof. A standard coaxial bipolar connector that has been developed is an industry standard that eliminates incompatibilities between various leads and pacemakers. This universal lead connector is referred to as the VS-1 (voluntary standard) and is a 3.2-mm-diameter connector designed to fit potentially all bipolar pacemakers (Calfee and Saulson, 1986) as well as to reduce the size of the connector itself (see Fig. 53–8).

## LEAD–ELECTRODE SYSTEM

A pacemaker lead is an insulated wire used to connect the pacemaker impulse generator to the heart. The electrode is the uninsulated, electrically active metal tip that is in contact with the myocardium (see Fig. 53–7). The lead-electrode system in a demand pacemaker has two equally important functions: It conducts the electric stimulus from the impulse generator to the myocardium and transmits an endocardial electrogram from the heart to the pacemaker. In unipolar systems, only the cathode is in the heart and the indifferent electrode, or anode, which is a part of the metallic pacemaker case, is in soft tissue. In a bipolar system, a double wire runs from the pacemaker to the heart and the two electrodes are separated by approximately 1 cm within the heart. The lead wire is most often a continuous helical coil that is resistant to fracture caused by repeated flexion.

In the past, the lead was most commonly insulated with silicone rubber. Polyurethane insulation has been introduced because of its greater elasticity and tensile strength, which allows lead diameter to be reduced. Furthermore, polyurethane has a smoother surface, which improves handling characteristics during

multilead placement. However, several models of bipolar polyurethane leads have been shown to increase the risk of compression fracture of the polyurethane coating, causing early lead failure (Hayes et al., 1992). Similarly constructed bipolar silicone rubber leads have been much less likely to demonstrate insulation breaks. This argues strongly for the continued use of silicone rubber insulation, at least for bipolar leads. Newer polymers of polyurethane with greater compression strength are now being used on some polyurethane leads, but whether these newer polymers will prevent the increased risk of insulation fracture awaits long-term follow-up in a large number of patients.

The uninsulated electrically active metal tip of the lead in contact with the myocardium is the electrode. This exposed tip is usually made of platinum, iridium, nickel alloys, or activated carbon. Platinum-iridium electrodes are now the most common and may be either porous or solid. Steroid-eluding lead tips improve chronic sensing and pacing function by decreasing scar formation at the tip as it heals into place (Wish et al., 1990). Recent studies have suggested that porous-tipped, steroid-eluding suture-on epicardial leads also have improved chronic sensing and pacing thresholds in pediatric patients (Johns et al., 1991).

Two general types of lead-electrode systems exist. The most common are the systems passed transvenously to embed within the subendocardium of the right atrium or right ventricle or both. The second group are those placed transthoracically; they are directly attached to the myocardium of any chamber. These leads have been referred to as epicardial leads, but this term is a misnomer because they are actually embedded within the myocardium and not just within the epicardium. Transthoracic leads are used primarily in small infants and children, after repeated failure of the transvenous approach, and sometimes when the chest is already open, such as after cardiac surgical procedures. Generally, transvenous lead-electrode systems are preferred because of their improved chronic thresholds and decreased incidence of lead fracture.

Transvenous lead systems are referred to as active or passive. Passive leads have a small flanged expansion just proximal to the exposed distal electrode or have short, flexible tines (Fig. 53–11A). These tined leads are designed to catch beneath trabeculas and reduce the incidence of dislodgment, which should be less than 1% (Furman et al., 1981). Currently used active fixation leads contain sharpened screws that may be remotely activated and retracted (Fig. 53–11B). Active fixation leads are used in the ventricular location when the right ventricle is smooth-walled, when there is significant tricuspid regurgitation, or when a site other than the right ventricular apex is needed. Active fixation of the atrial lead is typically performed in the setting of a markedly dilated right atrium or in patients who have undergone prior cardiopulmonary bypass with resultant trauma to the right appendage. Passive leads designed primarily for placement in the atrial appendage by the transvenous route differ from

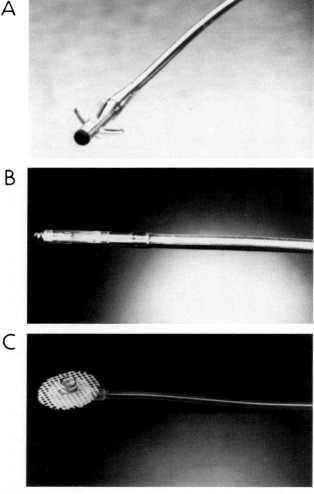

**FIGURE 53–11.** Examples of *(A)* a passive-fixation (tined) bipolar endocardial pacing lead, *(B)* an active-fixation (retractable helical screw) bipolar endocardial lead, and *(C)* a screw-in epicardial pacing lead. *(A–C,* Courtesy of Medtronic, Inc.)

plantation) (Mond, 1991). With the advent of programmable polarity of both sensing and pacing functions, the use of bipolar leads allows programming of either unipolar or bipolar functions, whereas unipolar pacing leads restrict options to unipolar modes only. Although personal preferences vary, the increased benefits of bipolar pacing leads make them preferable to unipolar leads in most cases.

To a certain extent, decreasing electrode tip size results in lower thresholds, both at the time of implant as well as chronically because of higher current density. However, better sensing function is directly related to electrode area and is adversely affected by small electrode size (Hughes et al., 1976). Therefore, a compromise between pacing and sensing efficiency is required. Typical electrode surface areas for pacing are between 8 and 10 mm$^2$. The effective surface area for sensing is increased many times through the use of microporous electrodes. These porous-tip electrodes improve sensing for a given electrode size because the interstices increase the sensing area without increasing overall electrode size and subsequent stimulation energy requirements (Lagergren and Johansson, 1963) (see Fig. 53–11$A$). Techniques such as platinization of the electrode or use of activated carbon result in lower stimulation thresholds by reducing polarizing currents at the electrode surface.

## OPERATIVE TECHNIQUES AND EVALUATION OF PACEMAKER FUNCTION

### Operative Techniques

Implantation of a permanent impulse generator and lead-electrode system should be done in a fluoroscopic unit or a cardiac catheterization laboratory under sterile conditions. Various impulse generators and lead electrodes as well as a pacing system analyzer should be readily available. Most commonly, the pacemaker lead-electrode is passed transvenously under local anesthesia to become embedded within the subendocardium of the right atrium or right ventricle. Transthoracic leads are used primarily in small infants and children, after repeated failure of the transvenous approach, and sometimes after cardiac procedures when a permanent pacemaker is indicated. In general, for elective permanent pacemakers, transvenous leads are preferred because of their improved chronic sensing and pacing thresholds and decreased incidence of lead fracture.

Preoperatively, patients receive a therapeutic dose of an antistaphylococcal antibiotic based on the proven beneficial effects of prophylactic antibiotic administration in general and thoracic surgical procedures. Antibiotics are discontinued 24 hours postoperatively. Regardless of the planned approach for implantation, the entire anterior chest from the chin to the umbilicus should be prepared and draped as a sterile field. This wide field of preparation allows conversion from one transvenous approach to another

ventricular leads in that when the stylet is withdrawn they assume a J shape, which allows them to be positioned well up into the atrial appendage (see Fig. 53–7).

As mentioned earlier, pacing lead systems are either bipolar or unipolar. Possible advantages of unipolar lead systems include smaller lead diameter with an attendant slight decreased risk of right ventricular perforation, increased stimulus artifact size, allowing easier identification of pacemaker function, and more simple connection. Earlier concerns about better sensing and pacing function have been eliminated by improvements in bipolar lead design (Mond, 1991). Advantages of bipolar pacing leads include reduced risk of skeletal muscle stimulation, lower susceptibility of electromagnetic interference, elimination of pacemaker inhibition by skeletal muscle myopotential sensing, decreased risk of cross-talk between atrial and ventricular stimuli, and greater range of location for placement of the pulse generator without concern for skeletal muscle stimulation (e.g., submuscular im-

and permits a limited anterior thoracotomy without interruption of the procedure.

Based on the work of Lagergren and Johansson (1963) in Sweden and by Furman and Schwedel (1959) and Chardack and colleagues (1965) in the United States, the transvenous approach under local anesthesia is now used in more than 90% of patients requiring pacemakers. The venous anatomy of the anterior chest wall is particularly well suited for implantation of pacing leads (Fig. 53–12). Generally, the pacemaker pocket is placed over the anterior side of the chest beneath the junction of the inner and middle thirds of the clavicle on the patient's nondominant side. The cephalic or subclavian veins are the preferred venous approaches for lead introduction. Implantation through the external or internal jugular veins requires a separate neck incision, and the lead must be tunneled over or under the clavicle to reach the pacemaker pocket and generator. Passing the lead over the clavicle predisposes to skin erosion and lead fracture; tunneling beneath the clavicle increases the risk of hemorrhage due to vascular injury.

An oblique incision on the anterior chest wall inferior to the deltopectoral groove provides excellent exposure to the cephalic vein and also allows introducer cannulation of the subclavian vein (Fig. 53–13).

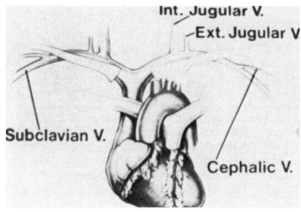

FIGURE 53–12. Anatomy for preferred venous approaches. Any vein in the neck, chest, or shoulder may be used for a permanent transvenous lead, but it is preferable to expose the vein through the same incision used for making the pocket. In order of preference, acceptable veins are as follows: (1) Cephalic vein, a tributary of the subclavian vein. It lies in the deltopectoral groove and is usually big enough to admit a lead up to No. 7 or 8 French. In 10% of patients, it is quite delicate and may not be usable. It is occasionally absent. (2) Subclavian vein or tributary. If the cephalic vein cannot be used, it is always possible to expose another tributary of the subclavian or the subclavian vein itself through the same incision by freeing the pectoralis major from its lateral origin from the inferior surface of the clavicle. The subclavian vein is now commonly used as the primary choice for lead insertion with introducer techniques. (3) External jugular vein. This is usually the most prominent visible vein in the neck, although it may be absent in 10% of patients. Because of the necessity of tunneling the electrode over or under the clavicle, with an increased incidence of fracture and erosion, this is a poor choice for permanent pacing. (4) Internal jugular vein. This is also a poor choice, unless purulent infections exist at every other potential site or an unusually large electrode is required as for an implantable defibrillator. (From Parsonnet, V.: Implantation of Transvenous Pacemakers. Tarpon Springs, FL, Tampa Tracings, 1972.)

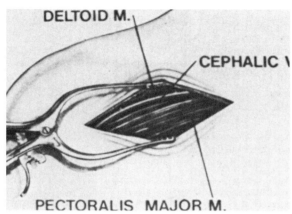

FIGURE 53–13. Cephalic vein approach. After the incision is made below the clavicle, the deltopectoral groove is identified. The cephalic vein is usually found with ease in the fat pad that fills the groove. Division of a few fibers of the pectoralis major from the clavicle will allow dissection of the vein proximally, and if gentle traction is applied, the angle of entrance of the cephalic vein into the subclavian vein can be made more oblique. Passage of the electrode toward the heart rather than into the axilla is thus facilitated. (From Parsonnet, V.: Implantation of Transvenous Pacemaker. Tarpon Springs, FL, Tampa Tracings, 1972.)

The pacemaker pocket should be as far medial as is comfortable for the patient to minimize pectoral stimulation. It should be made only slightly larger than the impulse generator so that migration laterally, which tends to follow the curvature of the chest wall, is minimized. Small arterial and venous bleeders are ligated or electrocoagulated to avoid postoperative hematoma formation. The pacemaker generator pocket should be just superficial to the pectoralis major in thick-chested individuals or beneath the premuscular fascia or muscle itself in thin-chested patients.

Several techniques have evolved for cannulating the venous system for insertion of permanent pacing leads. With the cephalic vein approach, the lead is directly inserted into the small incision made in the vein (Figs. 53–13 and 53–14). There are two subclavian vein approaches. In the commonly performed intrathoracic approach, the subclavian vein is cannulated with a thin wall introducer needle underneath the middle portion of the clavicle within the thoracic cavity (Fig. 53–15). Care should be taken to approach the subclavian vein as laterally as possible, because more medial subclavian vein approaches are more apt to create lead compression between the first rib and clavicle and soft tissue entrapment in the subclavius muscle, which may cause lead fracture (Jacobs et al., 1993; Magney et al., 1993). Recently, an extrathoracic approach for subclavian vein cannulation has been described (Byrd, 1992). In this approach, the subclavian vein is cannulated with the thin wall needle as it crosses the first rib before entering the thoracic catheter underneath the clavicle (Fig. 53–16). The vein is located in this position by maneuvering the thin wall needle posteriorly along the first rib until the vein is punctured. The extrathoracic approach may be better than the intrathoracic approach because of

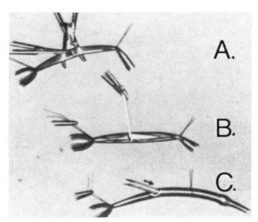

**FIGURE 53–14.** Small-vein introduction technique. If the vein is large, an electrode can be inserted simply by any standard method. When the vein is small, gentle handling and care permit insertion of an electrode that at first may seem to be much larger than the vein. The vein is ligated distally, a loose, nonabsorbable suture is placed proximally, and a transverse incision is made one-third of the way across the anterior wall of the vessel (A). A plastic inserter (present in the lead packages from many manufacturers) is carefully slipped into the opening (B). With upward traction on the inserter, which is concave on its inferior surface, the electrode can be passed underneath the inserter, which is not withdrawn until the tip of the electrode has passed medially a centimeter or so. As the electrode is advanced, the proximal ligature is loosened and then tightened to prevent bleeding. Countertraction on the distal ligature is maintained to assist passage into the subclavian vein (C). Traction on the distal ligature is easily maintained by pulling it over the self-retaining retractor shown in Figure 53–13 and by placing a straight hemostat across it, with the tip of the hemostat underneath the ratchet of the retractor. (A–C, From Parsonnet, V.: Implantation of Transvenous Pacemakers. Tarpon Springs, FL, Tampa Tracings, 1972.)

the decreased risk of pneumothorax and avoidance of lead fracture due to compression between the first rib and clavicle seen with the more medial intrathoracic approach (Byrd, 1992).

After the subclavian vein is cannulated, a guidewire is initially placed into the venous system through the thin wall needle (see Fig. 53–15). A lead introducer sheath is then advanced over the guidewire into the venous system to the superior vena cava. The guidewire and dilator to the sheath are removed, and the pacing lead is advanced through the sheath to the level of the right atrium. The sheath can then be peeled away from the lead to remove it from the body while leaving the pacing lead in the vein. The flexible pacing lead is made more steerable by use of an internal stylet to give the lead some rigidity. Once the lead is in the right atrium, the standard straight stylet is exchanged for one with a J tip, which allows the lead to be passed across the tricuspid valve (Fig. 53–17). The lead is then advanced across the pulmonic valve to confirm that the right ventricle has been cannulated, not the coronary sinus. The lead is then withdrawn into the cavity of the right ventricle, and the curved stylet is replaced with a straight one. The lead is then gradually withdrawn until the electrode falls and points toward the apex of the right ventricle. The stylet is then withdrawn a few millimeters and the lead is gently maneuvered to

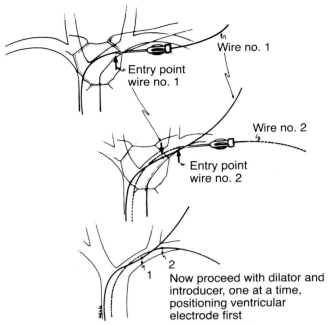

**FIGURE 53–15.** Two–entry-point dual-lead introducer technique. Method for inserting separate guidewires, introducers, and sheaths with a small distance between the electrode entrance sites. (From Parsonnet V., Werres R., Atherley, T., et al.: Transvenous insertion of double set of permanent electrodes: Atraumatic technique for atrial synchronous and atrial ventricular sequential pacemakers. J. A. M. A., 243:62–64, 1980. Copyright 1980, American Medical Association.)

lodge the pacing and sensing electrode beneath right ventricular trabeculae (see Fig. 53–17). If a dual-chamber procedure is planned, ventricular lead placement is accomplished first, followed by placement of an atrial J lead, which is designed to lodge in the right atrial appendage. If stable positioning of an atrial J

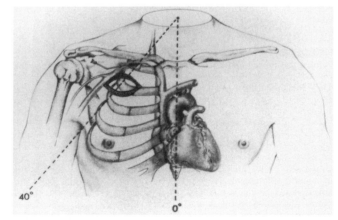

**FIGURE 53–16.** Extrathoracic approach to subclavian vein cannulation. The thin-walled introducer needle is shown inserted into the subclavian vein outside of the thoracic cavity as the vein crosses over the first rib. The introducer needle is initially advanced to the anterior portion of the first rib and then advanced more posteriorly by a series of partial insertions and withdrawals along the body of the first rib until the subclavian vein is cannulated. (From Byrd, C. L.: Safer introducer technique for pacemaker lead implantation. PACE, 15:262–267, 1992.)

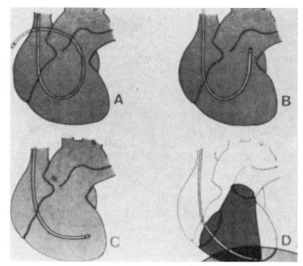

FIGURE 53–17. Right ventricular lead positioning technique. If the catheter is advanced into the pulmonary artery (A), which is easily confirmed by seeing the tip in the lung fields, there can be no question that, on slow withdrawal of the electrode tip (B), it will fall into the ventricle (C), assuming the absence of ventricular septal defects. D, The *shaded area* reflects the approximate shape of the right ventricle. Note that the apex is far lateral and that the electrode usually lies below the dome of the left diaphragm as seen fluoroscopically. (A–D, From Parsonnet, V.: Implantation of Transvenous Pacemakers. Tarpon Springs, FL, Tampa Tracings, 1972.)

lead cannot be accomplished, an endocardial screw-in lead is placed into the wall of the right atrium. After transvenous positioning and testing of thresholds, the lead is anchored at the fascial or venous exit site to prevent dislodgment by tying a suture around the movable sewing ring provided on the pacing lead.

Tying directly onto the pacing lead will frequently result in fracture of the lead's insulation and subsequent lead malfunction. The wound is irrigated with a diluted bacitracin-saline solution. The pacing lead is then connected to the impulse generator, which is positioned in its pocket, and the wound is closed in layers by absorbable suture.

Permanent transthoracic leads can be placed through either a small left anterior thoracotomy or subxiphoid mediastinotomy. Generally, sutureless screw-in or hook leads are used and tunneled beneath the costal margin to the pacemaker pocket, which is created over the left upper quadrant of the abdomen well above the belt line or occasionally placed retroperitoneally in either lower quadrant in small infants (Fig. 53–18). The electrode is placed by opening the pericardium and by identifying a fat-free area on the anterior or lateral aspect of the left ventricle. The electrode should not be placed too close to the apex of the heart because of its thinness and because increased motion in this area may cause electrode dislodgment or lead fracture. In addition, the electrode should not be placed in myocardium adjacent to the pericardial course of the phrenic nerve, which could cause diaphragmatic pacing.

## Evaluation of Pacemaker Function

A thorough evaluation of pacing threshold energy requirements, atrial and ventricular sensing thresholds, and impulse generator parameters should be done at the time of initial pacemaker implantation as well as the time of replacement. A pacing system analyzer simulates the function of the pacemaker's output and sensing circuits and is also capable of

FIGURE 53–18. Chest film of a 36-hour-old infant born with congenital complete heart block. A fishhook lead electrode (Medtronic, Inc., model 4951) was embedded over the lateral aspect of the left ventricle. The lead was then tunneled beneath the musculature of the anterior abdominal wall down to the left lower quadrant. A left lower-quadrant incision was made, and the anterior abdominal wall musculature was split. The peritoneum was identified and swept down and medially to create a retroperitoneal pacemaker pocket. The lead was connected to a Pacesetter Programalith III unipolar impulse generator. Most children who require pacemakers do not require a retroperitoneal pocket because of the small size of current impulse generators. However, in an extremely small infant, it is occasionally necessary to place the impulse generator in a retroperitoneal position.

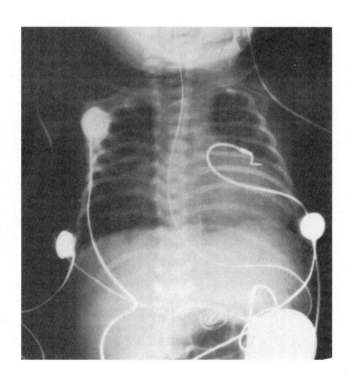

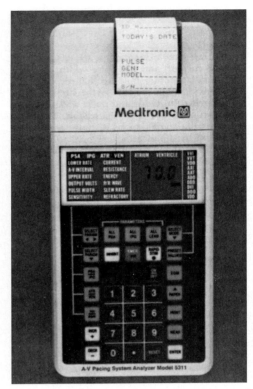

**FIGURE 53–19.** A pacing system analyzer (PSA) simulates the function of the pacemaker's output and sensing circuits and can evaluate the integrity of the impulse generator itself. A thorough evaluation of pacing threshold energy requirements, atrial and ventricular endocardial electrograms, and impulse generator parameters should be performed at the time of initial pacemaker implantation as well as at the time of generator or lead electrode replacement.

evaluating the integrity of the impulse generator itself (Fig. 53–19). The pacemaker's energy output and sensing circuits communicate with the myocardium through the implanted lead at the electrode-myocardial interface. The pacemaker generator delivers an electrical impulse, which passes through its output circuit into the lead, to the electrode-myocardial interface, and back through body tissue to an indifferent electrode. This system is a simple series electrical circuit described by Ohm's law (resistance = voltage/current). The factors determining resistance are summarized in Figure 53–20.

The electrical pulse discharged by the impulse generator's output circuit is designed to initiate cardiac depolarization. The pacing threshold of the electrode-myocardial interface can be expressed in terms of energy, current, or voltage. The electrical energy discharged by the impulse generator is defined as follows: energy = voltage × current × time. This electrical energy has both an amplitude (voltage or current) and a time component (pulse width or duration). The lowest voltage or current that is delivered to the heart at a given pulse width and that produces cardiac depolarization is referred to as the stimulation threshold. A strength-duration curve (Fig. 53–21) is a graphic plot that shows the stimulation threshold for each pulse width. Any amplitude pulse width combination on or above the strength-duration curve is sufficient to initiate cardiac depolarization. As shown in Figure 53–21, the amplitude component approaches an infinite value at very short pulse widths, such as less than 0.1 msec, and it approaches a minimal value at long pulse widths, such as greater than 1.5 msec. As can be seen from the strength-duration curve, at a short pulse width, the stimulation threshold may exceed the output of the pacemaker and produce loss of pacing. Conversely, excessively long pulse widths do not lower the pacing threshold and waste energy. In right ventricular implants using currently available transvenous electrodes, a pulse width of at least 0.5 msec is usually used acutely to obtain a voltage threshold of less than or equal to 1 V. Generally, an acute threshold greater than 1 V is unsatisfactory. Atrial pacing thresholds are usually comparable with ventricular thresholds but may be slightly higher. Atrial thresholds greater than 1.5 V are unsatisfactory. In general, a low acute threshold provides a substantial safety margin because acute thresholds generally rise to higher values during the first several weeks and then decline slightly to their chronic levels secondary to maturation of the electrode-myocardial interface.

In addition to measuring pulse amplitude (voltage

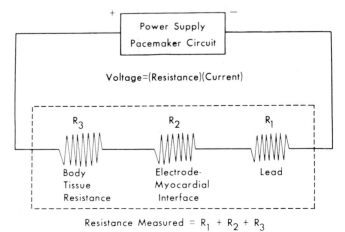

**FIGURE 53–20.** Simple series circuit. A simple series circuit is an accurate model for the standard pacemaker-body circuit. The electrical properties of this circuit are expressed by Ohm's law: $V = R \times I$. The resistance of the lead ($R_1$), the electrode-myocardial interface ($R_2$), and the body tissue acting as the return pathway back to the pacemaker's indifferent electrode ($R_3$) are series resistances that add up to the total resistance of the circuit (i.e., total resistance of the circuit = $R_1 + R_2 + R_3$). This is the resistance measured across the circuit by a PSA device. (From Byrd, C.: *In* Samet, P., and El-Sherif, N. [eds]: Cardiac Pacing. 2nd ed. New York, Grune & Stratton, 1980, p. 229.)

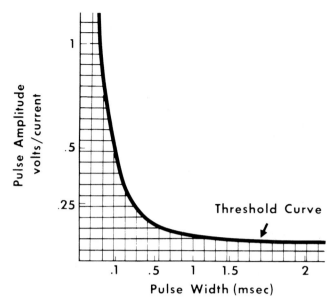

**FIGURE 53–21.** Strength-duration curve. A strength-duration curve demonstrates the relationship between the pulse amplitude (volts and current) and the pulse width. Each point on the curve is the stimulation threshold for that respective pulse amplitude and pulse width. The area above the strength-duration curve represents the pulse amplitude and pulse width combinations that will stimulate an endocardial depolarization. The area below the curve represents the combinations of pulse amplitude and pulse width insufficient to stimulate a depolarization. (From Byrd, C.: *In* Samet, P., and El-Sherif, N. [eds]: Cardiac Pacing. 2nd ed. New York, Grune & Stratton, 1980.)

and current) and pulse width, resistance is also determined. As described by Ohm's law, resistance is calculated by dividing voltage by current. Resistance calculations are made at a voltage near that of the pacemaker's output. The calculated resistance at 5 V should range from 300 to 800 ohms. Low resistances result in higher currents and are unsatisfactory for pacing. An unsatisfactorily low resistance can develop secondary to location of the electrode in the ventricular chamber or because of a separate competing electrical pathway (parallel circuit) (Fig. 53–22). If a competing pathway exists, current flows through a stimulating and nonstimulating pathway. The current

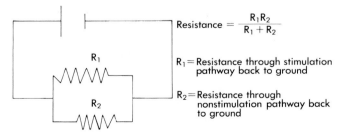

$$\text{Resistance} = \frac{R_1 R_2}{R_1 + R_2}$$

$R_1$ = Resistance through stimulation pathway back to ground

$R_2$ = Resistance through nonstimulation pathway back to ground

**FIGURE 53–22.** Parallel circuit. A stimulating and a nonstimulating circuit represent two separate pathways back through the body tissue to the indifferent electrode. Parallel circuits may occur in bipolar lead implants, epicardial lead implants, and with current leaks from a damaged lead system. (From Byrd, C.: *In* Samet, P., and El-Sherif, N. [eds]: Cardiac Pacing. 2nd ed. New York, Grune & Stratton, 1980, p. 229.)

flow through the nonstimulating pathway lowers the resistance and represents wasted energy. This phenomenon can be seen with poorly positioned endocardial electrodes, as well as with epicardial electrodes. Very low acute resistances are unsatisfactory because current is wasted and battery life is shortened, which creates a potential for exit block or an increased incidence of muscle stimulation due to increased current. Conversely, excessively high resistances (> 800 ohms) increase battery life but decrease the current delivered to the heart for both constant-voltage and constant-current pacemakers. For example, current flow from a 5-V battery through a resistance greater than 1000 ohms is reduced below 5 mA, which is an inadequate safety margin to compensate for eventual chronic threshold elevation.

In addition to measuring stimulation thresholds and resistance, the sensing circuit of the pacemaker must be evaluated. The sensing circuit monitors spontaneous myocardial depolarizations. The voltage change at the electrode caused by cardiac depolarization (P wave or R wave) is transmitted via the lead to the sensing circuit of the impulse generator. The sensing circuit is designed to detect electrical signals above a particular amplitude within the frequency range of endocardial electrograms. Measurements of amplitude and frequency are essential to ensure proper operation of the sensing circuit. As shown in Figure 53–23, an endocardial waveform has both an amplitude and a frequency component. The frequency component of the endocardial signal is approximated by the slew rate for the measured portion of the waveform. The slew rate represents the maximum rate of change in electrogram amplitude with respect to time and is expressed as millivolts per millisecond (or more simply, volts per second). As shown in Figure 53–23, the amplitude of the atrial or ventricular electrogram is measured in millivolts. As this waveform passes through the sensing circuit of the pacemaker, both the amplitude and the slew rate (rate of amplitude rise or frequency) must be acceptable for the signal to be detected. In general, ventricular endocardial electrograms should be at least 6 mV, and atrial endocardial electrograms greater than 2.0 mV in amplitude can be detected and provide a safety margin over time. A slew rate of 0.5 or greater is sufficient for detection of both types of signal. Although these values of electrogram amplitude and slew rate represent acceptable minimum values, every effort should be made at the time of lead placement to maximize these parameters to ensure appropriate chronic setting.

A pacing system analyzer that is capable of simulating the function of a given pacemaker's output and sensing circuits is provided by each pacemaker manufacturer. In addition, the pacing system analyzer is used to evaluate the pacemaker's rate, interval, pulse width, voltage, current, sensitivity, refractory period, and AV interval in dual-chamber devices. After complete testing of threshold energy requirements, atrial and ventricular endocardial signals, and pacemaker parameters, high-voltage settings are used to detect

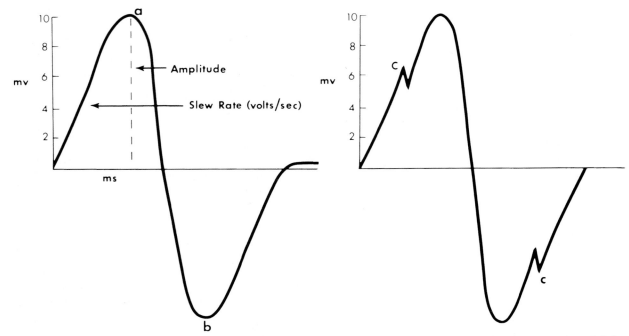

**FIGURE 53–23.** Endocardial waveform analysis. An endocardial waveform, as demonstrated on an electrogram, consists of deflections above and below the baseline. The pacemaker sensing circuit evaluates these deflections by rapidly determining the slew rate (rate of change of the amplitude with respect to time) and amplitude of that deflection. The amplitude is defined by a sensing circuit as the maximal uninterrupted excursion of the wave deflection at a constant slew rate (point a and point b). A change in the slew rate for a deflection such as a notch (point c) on the wave will be interpreted as a point of maximal excursion (the amplitude or peak for that deflection). Modern sensing circuits can determine not only the peak deflections (points a, b, and c) from the baseline but the peak-to-peak deflections across the baseline (point a to point b). The sensing circuit samples only a small portion of the waveform to determine the slew rate and amplitude. The slew rate obtained from a peak deflection above and below the baseline or a peak-to-peak analysis can be extrapolated into a frequency measurement, assuming the entire waveform has that slew rate. (From Byrd, C.: *In* Samet, P., and El-Sherif, N. [eds]: Cardiac Pacing. 2nd ed. New York, Grune & Stratton, 1980, p. 229.)

diaphragmatic or phrenic nerve stimulation, which require lead repositioning. The patient is then asked to do deep-breathing and coughing exercises to attempt to produce electrode dislodgment before securing the pacemaker leads and implanting the generator.

## PHYSIOLOGY OF PACING

### Pacing Modes

Perhaps the most dramatic example of the advancement in pacemaker technology is the various ways in which the heart can be paced. The way in which an impulse generator functions is referred to as the pacing mode. An accurate description of pacing mode must convey not only the chamber of the heart that is being paced, but also the chamber sensed by the pacemaker and the manner in which the pacemaker responds to sensed activity. Simple descriptive terms such as *ventricular-demand pacemaker* sufficed well for single-chamber devices but have become more awkward as the complexity of pacemakers increases. Devices that pace and sense both atrial and ventricular activity are now frequently implanted. To meet the need for a uniform method of describing pacemaker function, the Intersociety Commission for Heart Disease Resources (ICHD) recommended a five-letter code that succinctly and accurately described various pacing modes (Parsonnet et al., 1981). This code was updated in 1987 to accommodate newer pacemakers (Bernstein et al., 1987) (Table 53–3).

The ICHD code uses the letters A and V for atrium and ventricle. The letter D stands for "dual," indicating both chambers, or when indicating a mode of response, more than one mode. The two traditional response modes to sensed activity, either inhibition or triggering, are indicated by I and T. When no function or response is possible, the letter O is used. In the three-letter code system, the first letter designates the chamber(s) paced, the second letter the chamber(s) sensed, and the third letter the mode of response of the pacemaker to sensed activity. Thus, a pacemaker that paces only the ventricle senses ventricular activity when intrinsic beats are present, and it responds to the sensed activity by inhibiting its output (the well-known ventricular-demand pacemaker); this is designated VVI in the ICHD code. An asynchronous ventricular pacemaker that does not sense but that paces at a constant rate regardless of intrinsic cardiac rhythm would be designated VOO (the ventricle is paced, neither chamber is sensed, and there is therefore no response mode to sensed events). In the case

■ **Table 53–3.** NBG (NASPE/BPEG) GENERIC PACEMAKER CODE

| Position/Category | I Chamber(s) Paced | II Chamber(s) Sensed | III Response to Sensing | IV Programmability, Rate Modulation | V Antitachyarrhythmia Function(s) |
|---|---|---|---|---|---|
| | O = None | O = None | O = None | O = None | O = None |
| | V = Ventricle | V = Ventricle | T = Triggers pacing | P = Simple programmable | P = Pacing (antitachy-arrhythmia) |
| Letter Codes | A = Atrium | A = Atrium | I = Inhibits pacing | M = Multiprogrammable | S = Shock |
| | D = Dual (A + V) | D = Dual (A + V) | D = Dual (T + I) | C = Communicating (telemetry) | D = Dual (P + S) |
| | | | | R = Rate modulation | |

*NOTE:* Positions I through III are used exclusively for antibradyarrhythmia pacing.
　　　Manufacturers may use "S" in positions I and II to indicate single chamber (A or V).
　　　A minimum of four positions is required to describe a pacemaker.

Adapted from Bernstein, A. D., Camm, A. J., Fletcher, R. D., et al.: The NASPE/BPEG Generic Pacemaker Code for antibradyarrhythmia and adaptive-rate pacing and antitachyarrhythmia devices. PACE, *10*:794, 1987.
*Key*: NASPE = North American Society of Pacing and Electrophysiology; BPEG = British Pacing and Electrophysiology Groups.

of the standard AV sequential pacemaker in which both the atrium and ventricle are paced but only ventricular activity is sensed, the designation is DVI.

The five-letter code has a tremendous advantage in describing not only a certain pacemaker, but also various possible modes of function incorporated into a single programmable pacemaker. The magnet mode of a pacemaker may also be described. This is the test mode in which a pacemaker functions when the internal reed switch is closed by the external application of a strong magnet. Thus, a VVI pacemaker generally functions in the VOO (asynchronous) mode when an external magnet is applied. Likewise, a sophisticated DDD pacemaker, discussed later, may be programmed to function in one of many modes, including DVI, VVI, AAI, AOO, VDD, and many more.

Fourth and fifth letters of the ICHD code are used to denote programmability and antitachycardia capabilities, respectively (see Table 53–3). In this system, the letter P in the fourth position indicates the ability to program one or two parameters, and the letter M represents multiprogrammability. However, because all modern pacemakers have multiple programmable features, the M is usually omitted. The letter R in the fourth position is used to designate a rate-modulated pacemaker (e.g., VVI-R); an O in the fourth position indicates a nonprogrammable pacemaker. In the fifth position, various antitachycardia functions may be indicated, including P for pacing, S for shock, and D (for both pacing and shock). These modes are discussed later in detail.

Multiple pacing modes are potentially feasible, although only seven modes have real significance in clinical practice. Of these, two (VVI and DDD) have comprised the majority of pacing applications (Table 53–4).

**VVI Pacing.** Single-chamber ventricular pacing has been the main type of cardiac pacing but is being replaced by more physiologic pacing modes. This mode, often referred to as ventricular-demand pacing, is the simplest of the pacing modes that is routinely used. As the ICHD code states, the pacemaker senses intrinsic ventricular activity and is inhibited when

this activity exceeds the standby or escape rate of the pacemaker. When the intrinsic ventricular rate falls below the escape rate of the pulse generator, the pacemaker begins to function at its programmed rate. The escape rate and the automatic rate (pacing rate) may be identical or may be different if hysteresis is programmed into the pacemaker.

Potential disadvantages of VVI pacing are the lack of AV synchrony and the inability to increase heart rate with physiologic stress. Loss of coordinated contraction of the atria and ventricles may cause unpleasant symptoms due to atrial contraction against a closed tricuspid valve and may produce symptoms of low cardiac output referred to as the pacemaker syndrome. The magnet mode for VVI pacemakers (VOO) allows the function of the pacemaker to be observed even when an intrinsic rhythm is present that would otherwise inhibit pacemaker function.

Asynchronous ventricular pacing was used clinically before units capable of inhibition were available. Because of the potential dangers of asynchronous pacemaker function, with paced beats falling in the T wave of preceding spontaneous beats and inducing ventricular arrhythmias, VOO pacing is now relegated to the rare situation in which oversensing produces inappropriate inhibition that cannot be corrected by reprogramming.

**AAI Pacing.** Atrial pacing is potentially of great benefit in patients with intact AV conduction and sinus bradycardia, as in the sick sinus syndrome.

■ **Table 53–4.** COMMONLY USED PACING MODES

| ICHD Code | Description |
|---|---|
| VVI | Ventricular demand |
| VOO | Ventricular asynchronous |
| AAI | Atrial demand |
| AOO | Atrial asynchronous |
| DVI | AV sequential fixed rate |
| VDD | Atrial synchronous |
| DDD | AV "universal" |
| VVI-R | Ventricular rate modulated |

*Key*: ICHD = Intersociety Commission for Heart Disease.

Until recently, atrial pacing was not used extensively because of technical problems related to stability of endocardial atrial leads. In addition to achieving stable pacing, the atrial electrode must be able to sense an adequate atrial electrogram to avoid asynchronous atrial pacing, which can induce atrial fibrillation. Advances in electrode technology have resulted in preformed J-shaped atrial tined leads that may be placed in position in the atrial appendage and active fixation leads that can be screwed into the atrial endocardium in other locations. These leads are capable of providing reliable atrial pacing in most patients.

**Single-Chamber Rate-Modulated Pacing.** Single-chamber rate-modulated pacing (VVI-R or AAI-R) has become an important and frequently used pacing mode with the commercial availability of pacemakers using various sensors to regulate the pacing rate. In rate-modulated pacing, the pacing rate is determined by a physiologic parameter, other than atrial rate, that is measured by a special sensor in the pacemaker or pacing lead. During exertion, the required increase in cardiac output is obtained mostly by the increase in heart rate, although increased venous filling and maintenance of AV synchrony are also important contributors. The most commonly used physiologic parameters used in rate-modulated pacemakers at present are body motion and minute ventilation. Other parameters that are less commonly used or under evaluation include QT interval, venous blood temperature, mixed venous oxygen saturation, contractility, stroke volume, pH, and the paced depolarization gradient. Although the commonly used body motion sensors increase heart rate (and thus cardiac output) with exercise, the newer physiologic sensors can theoretically respond to a wider variety of physiologic states. However, whether more physiologic sensors improve the quality of life of patients compared with body motion sensors remains controversial. One particular problem with some special sensors is that they require specialized pacing leads to detect the physiologic parameter, such as an oxygen or pH detector on the distal portion of the lead. Whether such specialized leads will be more prone to premature lead or sensor failure remains to be determined.

Patients who have chronic or intermittent atrial fibrillation and in whom atrial synchronous pacing is impossible may be able to maintain normal heart rate responses to exercise through the use of ventricular-rate–modulated pacing. In patients with normal AV conduction and sinus bradycardia that does not respond to exercise, rate-modulated atrial pacing may be indicated.

**DVI Pacing.** Dual-chamber pacing provides an important improvement over simple ventricular pacing in patients in whom optimal cardiac function depends on the atrial contribution to cardiac output. Before the development of atrial synchronous pacing, AV sequential pacing was the only modality available.

In this mode, both the atrium and the ventricle are paced, with an artificial AV delay programmed between the atrial and ventricular impulses. In other respects, these devices function similarly to VVI pace-makers. Only ventricular activity is sensed, thus atrial stimulation is asynchronous if the spontaneous atrial rate exceeds the paced rate. DVI pacemakers may be of two varieties: committed or noncommitted. Committed systems are those in which the ventricular output must be delivered when the atrial pulse has occurred. In these systems, a QRS appearing in the AV interval will not inhibit ventricular output, and the ventricular pulse will fall in the QRS or ST segment (Fig. 53–24). The advantage of the committed system is that false inhibition of the ventricular output due to cross-talk from the atrial channel cannot inappropriately fail to pace. In noncommitted systems, ventricular activity occurring in the AV interval inhibits the ventricular output. Cross-talk from the atrial channel is prevented by means of a blanking period of approximately 20 to 30 msec after atrial output during which the ventricular sensing circuits are closed. Some systems have used a compromise between these two modes in which sensed ventricular activity after the atrial output results in a paced beat with a shortened AV interval, thus providing protection from failure to pace and diminishing the chance that the paced beat will fall in the vulnerable period, causing an arrhythmia.

**VDD Pacing.** One of the primary limitations of

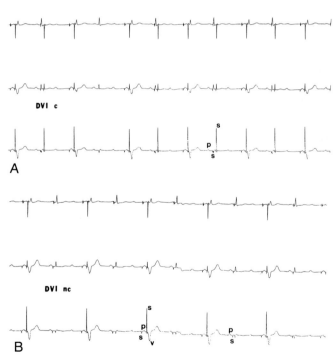

**FIGURE 53–24.** *A,* Simultaneous three-channel rhythm strip showing a normally functioning DVI pacemaker in the committed mode. Even though a normally conducted QRS occurs in the AV interval (second, sixth, eighth, and tenth complexes), a ventricular pacing output occurs after the QRS. Note that there is no atrial sensing in the DVI mode. The pacemaker is completely inhibited only when a QRS occurs sufficiently early to inhibit both atrial and ventricular outputs (fourth complex). *B,* A normally functioning noncommitted DVI pacemaker. P waves are not sensed in the DVI mode (second, fourth, sixth, eighth, and tenth complexes) and atrial pacing artifacts occur in the P-R interval. Conducted QRS complexes that follow these P waves inhibit the ventricular output.

DVI pacing is its fixed rate and the need for pacing at a rate faster than the patient's intrinsic sinus rate if the benefits of AV synchrony are to be maintained. Atrial synchronous pacing allows the ventricle to be paced after sensed atrial activity (Fig. 53–25). This method has the advantage of preserving AV synchrony and allowing the ventricular rate to vary as the sinus rate varies. VDD pacing is differentiated from an earlier form of atrial synchronous pacing (VAT) in which the ventricle was paced synchronously with atrial activity, but without sensing in the ventricle.

Older VDD pacemakers required both an atrial and a ventricular lead and had no advantage over DDD units. However, recent advancements in lead technology have allowed the development of a single-lead VDD pacemaker (Antonioli et al., 1993). A single lead is placed into the right ventricle for pacing and sensing. However, unlike traditional pacing leads, the lead also has a sensing electrode located several centimeters proximal to the ventricular leads in the right atrial chamber. This proximal electrode can sense atrial activity remotely, although the lack of contact with atrial myocardium precludes atrial pacing. Single-lead VDD pacemakers allow many of the advantages of two-lead DDD units but obviate the difficulties of pacing an atrial lead. However, because a VDD pacemaker cannot pace the atrium when the atrial rate decreases below the programmed lower rate limit, VVI pacing results, with its potential disadvantages. Furthermore, failure to sense the atrium will result in ventricular pacing at the lower rate despite the faster atrial activity.

**DDD and DDD-R Pacing.** "Universal" or DDD pacing increasingly has been shown to have many benefits over other pacing modalities, including the ability to track the intrinsic sinus rate, pace the atrium and ventricle, maintain atrioventricular synchrony, and avoid the pacemaker syndrome. Recognition of these benefits has steadily increased the use of DDD pacemakers in the last decade (Bernstein and Parsonnet, 1992). Recent studies have suggested that the overall impact on the quality of life in patients with pacemakers may be greater than previously recognized (Sulke et al., 1992). Thus, DDD pacing is the preferred pacing modality in most patients unless chronic or frequent atrial tachyarrhythmias are present or the anticipated frequency of pacing is expected to be minimal. If chronotropic incompetence is present intrinsically or if drugs suppressing sinus node automaticity must be, or are anticipated to be, used, then a rate-modulated dual chamber pacemaker (DDD-R) should be selected.

The primary difference between early DDD pacemakers and VDD pacemakers was the ability to pace the atrium at the lower rate limit. Thus, instead of VVI pacing at the low rate, AV synchrony was maintained by DVI pacing. DDD pacemakers can be programmed to almost every pacing mode conceivable in addition to DDD, including AAI, VVI, DVI, and VOO. Thus, another benefit of DDD pacemakers is flexibility in programmable options. With newer DDD-R pacemakers, rate-modulated options for each available pacing mode are available (e.g., AAI and AAI-R or VVI and VVI-R). Such flexibility in programmable options allows the greatest freedom to change pacing function as the patient's condition changes over time.

With atrial rates above the lower limit of the DDD pacemaker, the atrial output is inhibited and the pacemaker tracks atrial activity and responds with ventricular pacing after the programmed AV delay if intrinsic ventricular activation is not detected prior to completion of the AV interval. The ability of the pacemaker to track intrinsic atrial activity provides a range of rates between the lower and upper programmed rate limits. Dual-chamber pacemakers (both VDD and DDD) have a programmable upper rate limit or an atrial rate beyond which the pacemaker does not continue to track atrial activity. This is a programmable function that can be set according to the patient's needs and to avoid excessive paced rates in the event of rapid atrial arrhythmias.

Two responses to rapid atrial rates can be seen, and these depend on how the pacemaker is programmed. If atrial activity exceeds the programmed upper rate limit before encountering programmed refractoriness of the pacemaker to sense atrial activity, the pacemaker maintains a fixed upper ventricular rate. This produces an apparent Wenckebach sequence with gradual lengthening of the AV intervals before an atrial beat occurs in the atrial refractory period of the pacemaker and creates a "nonconducted" atrial beat (Fig. 53–26). The total atrial refractory period (TARP) is the sum of two programmed intervals: the AV interval and the postventricular atrial refractory pe-

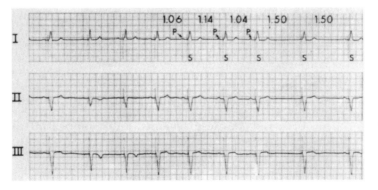

**FIGURE 53–25.** A normally functioning VDD pacemaker. Spontaneous atrial activity is sensed and followed by paced ventricular beats, resulting in slight variation in cycle length. When the atrial activity falls below the lower rate limit of the pacemaker, in this case a rate of 40 beats per minute (R-R interval of 1.5 second), ventricular pacing results. In the case of a DDD device, DVI pacing as seen in Figure 53–24 would be present at the lower rate.

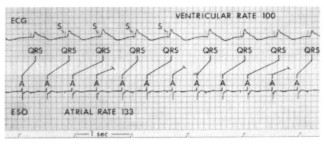

**FIGURE 53–26.** An atrial synchronous pacemaker functioning at the upper rate limit. The atrial rate is 133 beats per minute, and the upper rate limit of the pacemaker has been programmed to 100 beats per minute. The interval between sensed atrial activity recorded from an esophageal lead and the pacing stimulus progressively lengthens until a P wave cannot be "tracked," which results in a dropped beat.

■ **Table 53–5.** COMMONLY PROGRAMMABLE FUNCTIONS OF A MULTIPROGRAMMABLE PULSE GENERATOR

| | |
|---|---|
| Mode | Hysteresis |
| Rate | Polarity |
| Pulse width | AV interval* |
| Output | Upper rate limit* |
| Sensitivity | Lower rate limit* |
| Refractory period | |

*Dual-chamber devices only.

riod (PVARP). The PVARP is the interval after a paced or sensed ventricular event during which the pacemaker does not respond to sensed atrial complexes. For Wenckebach behavior to occur, the TARP must be less than the upper rate interval (i.e., 60,000 msec-min$^{-1}$/upper rate min$^{-1}$ = upper rate interval [msec]). In other words, atrial rates exceeding the upper rate limit will not encounter refractoriness of the pacemaker to sense atrial activity. When the upper rate interval is programmed to a value less than TARP and the atrial rate is faster than that allowed by the TARP, then alternating P waves fall during the pacemaker's period of atrial refractoriness and the pacemaker will track only every other P wave (the 2:1 block point). Thus, in programming VDD and DDD pacemakers, TARP should be programmed at less than the upper rate interval. Injudicious programming of the atrial refractory period may cause an abrupt conversion to 2:1 conduction by the pacemaker at or near the upper rate limit, and the patient will have an abrupt and frequently symptomatic decrease in heart rate.

## Programmability

Programmability is defined as the ability to permanently and noninvasively change one or more of the operating characteristics of an implanted pacemaker. The advantages of modifying pacemaker function after implantation have been apparent for a long time. Early devices were made with the capability of changing rate by inserting a transcutaneous needle that turned a potentiometer in the pacemaker. Noninvasive programming was made possible originally through the use of an external magnet that activated a switch inside the pacemaker and changed its rate in incremental steps.

Almost all pacemakers implanted now have multiple programmable functions. The use of programmability in terms of avoiding reoperation for pacing system malfunction and in improving the patient's tolerance of the pacemaker has been documented (Billhardt et al., 1982). No indications exist for the implantation of nonprogrammable pacemakers. Sim-

ple programmability usually includes the ability to change rate, pulse width, mode (usually from inhibited to asynchronous), and refractory period. The ability to change many parameters is called multiprogrammability (Table 53–5). The various programmable functions found on current devices are discussed in detail later in this section.

To effect programming of an implanted pacemaker, a signal must be sent from a programmer to the pacemaker (Fig. 53–27). In practical terms, a programmer must be placed relatively close to the pacemaker to transmit coded information to the pacemaker that is specific for the change desired. The pacemaker must be able to reject inappropriate signals from the environment or from other programmers that could potentially cause unwanted changes in pacemaker function. The pacemaker may respond by returning a signal to the programmer, indicating acceptance of the programming instructions.

Programming features that are desirable include the ability of the programmer to interrogate the pacemaker and to retrieve three kinds of information: the programmed settings of the pacemaker—that is, what the pacemaker is supposed to be doing; measured data from the pacemaker that indicate what the pacemaker is actually doing, what kind of sensed electrograms the pacemaker is receiving, lead impedance, and the battery status; and an increasing variety of

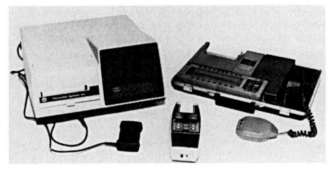

**FIGURE 53–27.** Three programmers currently in use, showing the range of complexity and size. *A,* The programmer for Pacesetter Systems, Inc., models 281, 283, and 285 pacemakers. The programming head is placed over the pacemakers for programming or interrogation. *B,* A portable hand-held programmer that can perform many of the same functions as the larger unit on the left. The programming head is incorporated into the device itself. *C,* The Medtronic model 9710 programmer with printer and programming head. This device is compatible with all programmable Medtronic pulse generators.

stored monitoring data, such as the percentage of time spent at various heart rates and the percentage of paced or sensed beats.

Most pacemakers now use radiofrequency signals to transmit coded information to and from the pacemaker. The functions that can be programmed in a given pacemaker vary considerably depending on the manufacturer and model. Obviously, the functions subject to programmability depend a great deal on the type of pacemaker (e.g., VVI, DDD-R). The most important functions for programmability are generally considered to be rate, pulse width, pulse amplitude, and sensitivity. Most of the potentially correctable problems encountered with implanted pacemakers can be managed by using these functions. Other functions that can be programmed in various models include refractory period, mode, and hysteresis. In dual-chamber pacemakers, the AV interval, upper and lower rate limits, and the mode of response to upper rate limit may be programmed. In sophisticated units, the pacemaker may actually be programmed off, blanking periods on atrial and ventricular channels can be changed, polarity can be programmed from bipolar to unipolar, and the pacemaker can even be programmed to respond or not respond to an external magnet.

**Rate Programmability.** The ability to change the rate of an implanted pacemaker is the single most useful programmable function. In patients with chronic cardiac disease, cardiac output may be highly rate dependent. The ability to increase rate allows the individual patient's heart rate to be changed to accommodate temporary changes in physical condition (e.g., cardiac procedures, heart failure, angina pectoris). Some patients develop an unpleasant sensation during pacemaker function or may actually have adverse hemodynamic effects from ventricular pacing. These situations may be remedied by lowering the pacing rate to allow more time in sinus rhythm. The ability to change rate also allows one pacemaker model to be used in all patient age groups, obviating the need for different models for use in pediatric patients who may require higher rates. In most pacemakers, rate can be programmed in steps from 40 to 150 pulses per minute. In rate-responsive pacemakers, the upper sensor drive rate can often be programmed even higher (150 to 180 pulses per minute). In some rate-responsive DDD units, the upper rate limit for tracking intrinsic atrial activity can be programmed to different values than the upper rate drive by the sensor.

**Output Programmability.** The output of the pacemaker in terms of total pacing energy is a function of both voltage and pulse width. The energy consumed varies by the square of the voltage but linearly with pulse width; thus, when possible, it is preferable to adjust pulse width rather than amplitude for changes in stimulation threshold. Standard lithium-iodine batteries have an output of approximately 2.5 V. The nominal voltage output of most pacemakers is 5 V, achieved by the use of a voltage multiplier circuit. The ability to program the voltage output down to

the lower value may help greatly in prolonging the battery life when chronic lead thresholds permit a lower stimulation energy. In addition, some models have the capability of increasing voltage output to the 7- to 10-V range, thus accommodating unusually high pacing thresholds although substantially shortening the longevity of the impulse generator.

Pulse width programmability also allows the output of the pacemaker to be lowered to prolong battery life. Lowering pulse width below 0.3 msec is not generally recommended, because very high stimulation voltages may be required. Unfortunately, as evident from the strength-duration curve, increasing the pulse width beyond approximately 1 msec does little to lower the stimulation threshold; thus, raising pulse width in situations of high threshold has often little value (see Fig. 53–21).

**Sensitivity Programmability.** The sensitivity setting of the pacemaker determines the amplitude of the patient's intrinsic cardiac activity required for proper sensing to occur. A balance must be reached between settings that are oversensitive and may allow inhibition by extraneous signals such as myopotentials or T waves, and settings that are too insensitive and thus fail to sense intrinsic electrograms. Most pacemakers have a ventricular R-wave sensitivity ranging from 1.25 to 8 mV (the lower value representing the highest sensitivity). In the atrium, sensitivity values of 0.5 to 4.0 mV are usual. Whether a given electrogram is sensed by a pacemaker depends not only on the actual amplitude of the electrogram, but also on the slew rate, or change in voltage per time (dV/dt). Thus, the programmed sensitivities do not necessarily guarantee adequate sensing of an electrogram based on its peak-to-peak amplitude. The ability to program sensitivity frequently corrects sensing problems that might otherwise require lead repositioning. Failure to sense premature ventricular contractions (PVCs) is a common example of a situation in which failure to sense may develop, despite proper sensing of sinus beats.

**Refractory Period Programmability.** The refractory period of the pacemaker is the interval after a sensed or paced event during which the pacemaker does not respond to sensed electrical activity. This feature prevents inappropriate inhibition of the pacemaker due to artifacts from the stimulus and prevents sensing of other waveforms of the ECG such as the T wave. When electrodes are implanted in the atrium for AAI pacing, the refractory period should be extended to prevent sensing of farfield R waves. The PVARP of DDD pacemakers should be programmed so that retrograde atrial activation generated by PVCs falls within the PVARP. If the retrograde atrial activation is sensed and triggers the pacemaker to pace the ventricle, retrograde atrial activation may again occur and the process continue to repeat itself to generate a pacemaker-mediated tachycardia (endless loop tachycardia). Dual-chamber pacemakers frequently have a programmable or fixed PVARP extension in which the PVARP is automatically prolonged when two consecutive ventricular events occur without an intervening atrial event, such as occurs with PVCs.

**Hysteresis.** Hysteresis is a feature that has more theoretical appeal than practical applicability. Hysteresis is usually expressed in terms of the number of pulses per minute below the programmed rate required to initiate pacing. Thus, the escape interval is longer than the automatic or pacing interval. A pacemaker programmed to pace at a rate of 60 pulses per minute with a hysteresis rate of 40 pulses per minute would remain inhibited until a sensed rate of 40 pulses per minute was present, at which time the pacemaker would begin to pace at a rate of 60 pulses per minute. The theoretical advantage of this function is that the patient is allowed to remain in sinus rhythm at intermediate rates between 40 and 60 beats per minute, but when pacing is required, the heart rate is maintained at the faster rate. A problem often encountered with hysteresis is that the patient's intrinsic rate must exceed the automatic rate to inhibit the pacemaker again. For patients who tend to maintain slow rates, hysteresis works well on the front end of the loop, but when pacing is initiated, patients may be unable to elevate their heart rate sufficiently to once again inhibit the pacemaker.

## Physiologic Pacing

*Physiologic pacing* is a term used to describe pacing modes that attempt to duplicate normally conducted sinus rhythm (Sutton et al., 1980; Wirtzfield et al., 1987). This concept assumes an understanding of the physiologic relationships between the conduction of the cardiac impulse and the hemodynamic events it initiates and implies that duplication of this physiology can be achieved with an artificial pacemaker. At best, current artificial pacemakers are only crude substitutes for normal sinus rhythm; therefore, the term *physiologic pacing* must be considered to be an oversimplification. Physiologic pacing has also been recognized as synonymous with dual-chamber pacing, although this is not necessarily true.

It has been well established that AV synchrony—that is, the contraction of the atria and the ventricles with normal sequence and timing—provides some margin of improved cardiac output when compared with ventricular pacing alone at comparable rates (Kappenberger et al., 1982; Ogawa et al., 1978; Sutton et al., 1980, 1983; Wirtzfield et al., 1987). Appropriately timed atrial contraction has been shown to increase cardiac output by as much as 25% (Kappenberger et al., 1982; Reiter and Hindman, 1982; Samet et al., 1965). This difference may be even greater during exercise or in certain pathologic states (Narahara and Blettel, 1983; Rickards and Donaldson, 1983; Shapland et al., 1983). The deleterious effects of AV dissociation due to ventricular pacing vary greatly from one patient to another and depend on the heart's ability to compensate for a fixed rate, the presence of retrograde VA conduction, and the patient's overall level of activity.

The ability to increase heart rate to meet increased metabolic demand is also an important feature of normal cardiac conduction. Cardiac output is related directly to heart rate and stroke volume, and when cardiac disease impairs the ability to increase stroke volume, increased heart rate is the only mechanism remaining to increase cardiac output. Therefore, a physiologic pacing system has two aspects: the maintenance of AV synchrony and the preservation of rate variation. AV synchrony is maintained by atrial pacing in the presence of intact AV conduction or dual-chamber pacing in the presence of heart block. Preservation of rate variation is achieved by pacemakers that either track sinus rhythm or imitate normal rate variation using sensors to artificially modulate heart rate.

The pacing modes that offer some preservation of normal physiologic function include AAI-R, DVI, VVI-R, DDD, and DDD-R. AAI-R pacing has the advantages of maintaining normal AV conduction, requiring only one electrode, and offering rate variation. It is used in patients with chronic sinus bradycardia with intact AV conduction. DVI obviates the concern for AV conduction but has the limitation of fixed rate (no atrial tracking) and has been replaced by DDD and DDD-R pacing. In patients with chronic atrial fibrillation, VVI-R pacemakers allow more physiologic increases in heart rate with stress. DDD pacing offers both rate variation and AV synchrony, and is the optimal form of pacing when sinus node function is normal. DDD-R pacing is preferable when sinus node dysfunction is present or medications blunting sinus node function are necessary. Because DDD-R pacemakers can be programmed to the DDD mode, it can be argued that all candidates for DDD pacemakers should receive a DDD-R unit so that the rate response option is available for use in the future should it be required.

The acute benefits of AV sequential or atrial synchronous pacing compared with ventricular pacing have been well documented (Reiter and Hindman, 1982). Numerous studies have also substantiated a sustained hemodynamic benefit of physiologic pacing modalities compared with fixed-rate ventricular pacing. Improvement in acute and chronic exercise capacity, symptoms (dyspnea and fatigue), and even survival have been attributed to rate-modulated and dual-chamber atrial synchronous pacing when compared with simple ventricular pacing (Alpert et al., 1986; Faerestrand and Ohm, 1985; Kappenberger et al., 1982; Kristensson et al., 1985; Kruse and Ryder, 1981; Kruse et al., 1982; Levy et al., 1979; Perrins et al., 1983; Rickards and Donaldson, 1983; Sutton et al., 1983; Videen et al., 1986; Wirtzfield et al., 1987; Yee et al., 1984).

The AV interval is an important programmable feature of DDD and DDD-R pacemakers. The optimal AV interval must be defined in relationship to the pacing rate, because AV conduction shortens with increasing heart rate under physiologic stresses. Thus, a shorter AV interval may be needed during exercise than at rest. Many modern DDD pacemakers have a function called rate-adaptive AV delay, in which the AV interval is shortened as the intrinsic or sensor-driven rate increases. Besides potential hemodynamic benefits, the shortening of the AV delay allows higher programmable upper rate limits by decreasing the total atrial refractory period (see earlier). Recent studies have suggested that optimal programming of the AV interval allows optimal timing between left atrial and left ventricular contraction rather than between right atrial and right ventricular contraction (Wish et al., 1987). In the setting of prolonged intra-atrial conduction, relatively normal programmed AV intervals (e.g., 150 msec) may not allow sufficient time for left atrial activation before left ventricular activation and may cause left-sided atrioventricular dyssynchrony with its potential adverse hemodynamic sequelae. Other investigators have seen improvement in hemodynamic parameters in patients with severe cardiomyopathies when programmed to short AV intervals, presumably due to prolonged intraventricular conduction (Hochleitner et al., 1990, 1992). Optimal selection of an AV interval in any patient may depend on monitoring blood pressure during dual chamber pacing at a number of AV intervals and choosing the interval associated with the best hemodynamic response. A final consideration of the AV interval is that the latency from the atrial stimulus to the onset of atrial systole creates a longer AV interval during atrial pacing than occurs when ventricular pacing follows a sensed atrial event. Newer pacemakers have the feature of different programmable AV intervals for sensed and paced events to adjust for this problem.

It might be held that patients with normal cardiac function and potentially high levels of normal activity should benefit the most from physiologic pacing systems, whereas patients with limited exercise capacity should benefit the least. However, the former patients are probably best able to compensate for a fixed-rate ventricular pacing system through an increase in stroke volume, whereas patients with cardiac disease may depend completely on an increase in heart rate to increase their cardiac output.

An aspect of pacing that may also have significance in terms of physiologic pacing is the pacing site. Normal ventricular contraction is related to the sequence of myocardial depolarization. Ventricular dyssynergy is present during artificial ventricular pacing. This may cause an increase in myocardial oxygen consumption, inefficient ventricular emptying, and abnormal mitral valve function. The deleterious effects of artificial ventricular stimulation may depend on pacing site and are present even when AV synchrony is maintained with dual-chamber pacing. Thus, in patients with intact AV conduction and sinus bradycardia, atrial pacing can be expected to be superior to both VVI and DDD pacing.

## Indications for Pacing Modes

**AAI Pacing.** Atrial fixed-rate pacing may be indicated in patients with resting sinus bradycardia and intact AV conduction. Patients with the sick sinus syndrome may be included in this category; however, the potential effects of antiarrhythmic drugs on AV conduction must be considered before an atrial pacing system is implanted. Likewise, the intermittent occurrence of atrial fibrillation would render this pacing mode ineffective. AAI-R (rate-modulated) pacing is indicated when a normal increase in sinus rate with exercise is absent.

Technical problems with atrial lead stability have been mainly overcome with the use of tined J leads, as well as the availability of endocardial screw-in leads. These active fixation leads make atrial pacing possible in patients who have had cardiac procedures with cannulation of the right atrial appendage. Screw-in leads may also be useful in other patients in whom a stable pacing site cannot be found in the atrial appendage. Atrial pacing from the coronary sinus has also been an effective method.

**VVI Pacing.** VVI pacing is indicated for patients with chronic atrial fibrillation and symptomatic bradycardia and for patients with infrequent and intermittent symptoms who have sinus rhythm. VVI pacemakers should not be implanted in patients with sick sinus syndrome and frequent pacing requirements because of the increased risk of atrial fibrillation, embolic events, and heart failure in addition to the pacemaker syndrome. VVI pacing systems should not be implanted in patients who would benefit from dual-chamber units because of unfamiliarity with these units or difficulties with atrial lead placement. VVI-R pacing is indicated when dual-chamber pacing is not possible because of atrial arrhythmias and when normal chronotropic response to exercise is not present.

**DDD Pacing.** Over the past decade, there has been an increasing use of dual-chambered pacemakers, for several reasons. First, dual-chamber pacing maintains normal AV synchrony with its hemodynamic benefits. Patients with compromised cardiac systolic function or diastolic dysfunction are particularly likely to benefit from maintaining AV synchrony. Second, overt pacemaker syndrome occurs relatively frequently in patients with ventricular pacing and intact VA conduction (Figure 53–28). Patients with the pacemaker syndrome classically present with fatigue, lightheaded spells, decreased exercise capacity, dyspnea, headaches, pulsations in the abdomen or neck, chest pain, syncope, and other frequently vague symptoms. It may be difficult to prove a causal relationship between nonspecific symptoms such as fatigue or decreased exercise capacity and the presence of ventricular pacing, although careful monitoring and correlation of symptoms with periods of ventricular pacing can be helpful. However, VA conduction and thus symptoms may be intermittent during ventricular pacing. It has been demonstrated that many patients who do not report symptoms of pacemaker syndrome feel substantially better when their pacemaker is upgraded to a dual-chamber device (Sulke et al., 1992). Thus, many patients with single-chamber ventricular pacemaker actually have a subclinical

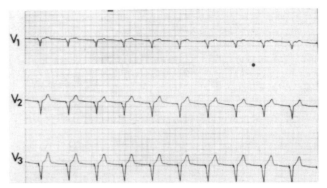

**FIGURE 53–28.** VVI pacing at a rate of 60 beats per minute with retrograde conduction. A retrograde P wave can be seen in the ST segment of each paced beat. This patient had symptoms of low cardiac output due to pacemaker syndrome.

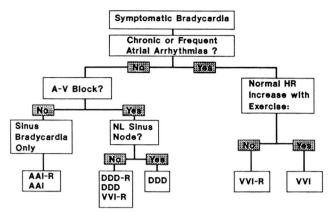

**FIGURE 53–29.** Algorithm for choosing pacing mode. Patients with frequent atrial arrhythmias are generally not considered to be candidates for dual-chamber systems, but may do well with a rate-modulated pacemaker if their heart rate does not increase with exercise. Patients with an insufficient heart rate response to exercise and AV conduction abnormalities are candidates for the newer DDD-R pacemakers. Atrial pacing alone should be used only when AV conduction is known to be reliably intact.

pacemaker syndrome that is not manifested unless dual-chamber pacing is initiated.

Another benefit of DDD pacing is that it decreases the risk of atrial fibrillation in selected patients. Several large studies have demonstrated that VVI pacing in the sick sinus syndrome is associated with a several-fold increase risk of development of atrial fibrillation, strokes, peripheral emboli, heart failure, and possibly death, compared with dual-chamber (or atrial) pacing (Sutton and Kenny, 1986; Lamas et al., 1992; Rosenqvist 1988). The increased risk of these events with VVI pacing may be due to the adverse hemodynamic effects of this pacing modality. In addition to maintaining AV synchrony, DDD pacing (or AAI pacing with intact AV conduction) prevents atrial bradycardia, which may allow the escape of atrial arrhythmias. Finally, between 20 and 50% of patients with sick sinus syndrome or heart block have some evidence of chronotropic incompetence, and thus these patients would best be treated with a DDD-R device in order to maximize exercise capacity. Furthermore, DDD-R pacemakers, because of their wide range of programmable options, can be programmed to VVI-R should refractory atrial fibrillation or atrial lead malfunction occur.

For these reasons, DDD or DDD-R pacemakers are the preferable options for most patients with symptomatic bradycardias and an underlying sinus rhythm. The numerous benefits that have been well documented in the patients with sick sinus syndrome appear to extend to the patients with heart block as well. Dual-chamber pacing is also the preferable mode of pacing in patients with carotid sinus hypersensitivity and neurally mediated syncope, given the greater attenuation of hypotension if a vasodepressor component is present (Fitzpatrick et al., 1989; Morley and Sutton, 1984).

An algorithm for choosing pacing modes based on the presence of atrial arrhythmias and AV conduction is shown in Figure 53–29.

## COMPLICATIONS

As summarized in Table 53–6, pacemaker complications can be divided into four categories: immediate

surgical complications, wound problems, delayed complications, and pacemaker malfunctions. Fortunately, all are relatively uncommon, making pacemaker insertion an exceptionally safe procedure when done by experienced surgeons.

## Immediate Surgical Complications

As described earlier, perhaps the safest way of inserting a permanent transvenous lead-electrode system is via the cephalic vein. The risk of pneumothorax, vascular injury, air embolism, and air entrapment within the pacing pocket are increased when the subclavian vein access route is chosen. Air entrapment within the pacemaker pocket secondary to either pneumothorax with subcutaneous emphysema or secondary to air entrapped during pacemaker pocket

■ **Table 53–6.** PACEMAKER COMPLICATIONS

| *Immediate Surgical Complications* | *Delayed Complications* |
|---|---|
| Pneumothorax | Venous thrombosis |
| Vascular injury | Pulmonary embolism |
| Air embolism | Twiddler's syndrome |
| Cardiac perforation | Constrictive pericarditis |
| Tamponade | Tricuspid insufficiency |
| Lead-electrode dislodgment | Pacemaker syndrome |
| Neural injury—phrenic, recurrent laryngeal | *Pacemaker Malfunctions* |
| Air entrapment in pocket | Radiation damage |
| *Wound Problems* | Runaway pacemaker |
| Hematoma | Pacemaker-induced ventricular fibrillation |
| Infection | Irregular pacing |
| Skin erosion | Failure of sensing |
| Migration of impulse generator | Failure of capture |
| Skeletal muscle stimulation | Electrode fracture |
| | Knotting of lead |
| | Inhibition of pacemaker by skeletal myopotentials |
| | Electromagnetic interference |

closure can cause pacemaker failure in unipolar systems secondary to insulation of the unipolar anodal plate (indifferent electrode) from the subcutaneous tissues (Hearne and Maloney, 1982; Kreis et al., 1979; Lasala et al., 1979). Neural injury to both the phrenic and recurrent laryngeal nerves has been reported when the lead-electrode system is introduced through the internal jugular vein (Dieter et al., 1981). Regardless of the venous access route chosen, cardiac perforation can occur but fortunately rarely leads to hemopericardium and tamponade (Irwin et al., 1987) (Fig. 53–30). A final complication is immediate electrode dislodgment. The risk of this complication can be reduced by doing provocative maneuvers such as coughing and deep breathing at the time of initial implantation. Transvenous electrode dislodgment problems have not been significantly increased in patients with congenitally corrected transposition of the great vessels, although this would have been expected because of the decreased trabeculation of the embryologic left ventricle, which is where the pacing lead lies (Estes et al., 1983).

## Wound Problems

Perhaps the most common wound problem associated with permanent pacemaker implantation is a hematoma. Obviously, this complication can be prevented by strict attention to hemostasis at the time of implantation. In patients who require impulse generator change, the pacemaker pocket should be débrided of excess pseudocapsule to prevent the formation of a sterile seroma. Fortunately, wound infection is a rare problem prevented by meticulous operative technique and the appropriate use of prophylactic antibiotics. In general, when infection occurs, the entire pacing system including the impulse generator and lead-electrode system should be removed, the patient should be treated with appropriate intravenous antibiotics, and a temporary pacemaker should be used for an interim period. When infection has completely cleared, a new pacemaker system is implanted through another access site. Skin erosion by either the impulse generator or lead can be prevented by proper positioning of pacemaker hardware deep within the subcutaneous tissues or beneath the fascia of the pectoralis major muscle. Unipolar impulse generators can cause muscle stimulation if placed immediately adjacent to skeletal muscle. However, bipolar impulse generators can be placed either in the subcutaneous tissue or beneath muscle. Migration of the impulse generator most commonly occurs in infraclavicular pacemaker pockets. Migration tends to follow the curvature of the chest wall, and the impulse generator

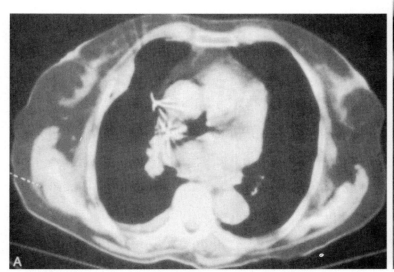
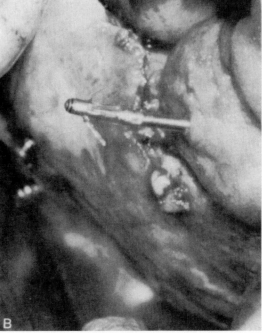

**FIGURE 53–30.** Transvenous atrial lead perforation. An 80-year-old woman was referred to Duke University Medical Center several months after implantation of a DDD pacemaker system. The patient initially had done well but was referred for evaluation of a recent syncopal episode. During evaluation, she was noted to have hiccups that coincided with atrial pacing. An ECG demonstrated atrial pacing without atrial capture. The admission chest film showed a new right pleural effusion and suggested displacement of the atrial lead outside of the cardiac silhouette. A repeat echocardiogram could not show the position of the atrial lead, but a chest computed tomographic scan (A) clearly showed that the atrial lead perforated the atrium. A pneumomediastinum was also noted. The patient was taken to the operating room and underwent a right anterior thoracotomy (B) for removal of the lead and atrial repair under direct visualization. An atrial epicardial lead was placed and tunneled across the chest subcutaneously to the chronic left pectoral pacemaker pocket, where the ventricular endocardial lead was still attached. The patient recovered uneventfully. This case demonstrates that unlike ventricular perforations, which often seal with retraction of the pacing wire, the thin-walled atrium may not seal and indeed, as in this case, may require surgical repair. (A and B, From Irwin, J. M., Greer, G. S., Lowe, J. E., et al.: Atrial lead perforation: A case report. PACE, 10:1378, 1987.)

tends to migrate laterally. This can be prevented by creating an anteromedial pocket sufficiently large to contain the impulse generator and lead. In susceptible individuals, the impulse generator can be further secured to the chest wall to prevent migration.

## Delayed Complications

Unusual delayed complications associated with transvenous pacemakers include thrombosis of the superior vena cava with resultant superior vena caval syndrome, axillary vein thrombosis with upper-extremity edema, cerebral venous sinus thrombosis, and right atrial and right ventricular thrombosis (Bradof et al., 1982; Branson, 1978; Cholankeril et al., 1982; Fritz et al., 1983; Girard et al., 1980; Gundersen et al., 1982; Kinney et al., 1979; Krug and Zerbe, 1980; Mitrovic et al., 1983; Nicolosi et al., 1980; Pauletti et al., 1979; Youngson et al., 1980). Pulmonary thromboembolism has also been recognized as a rare but lethal complication that occurs most often in patients with low cardiac output and underlying right atrial or right ventricular thrombi (Kinney et al., 1979). Constrictive pericarditis has been reported in patients who have received both transvenous and transthoracic electrodes (Foster, 1982; Schwartz et al., 1979). Tricuspid insufficiency is rare, usually asymptomatic, and is secondary to either lead placement or lead removal (Gibson et al., 1980; Ong et al., 1981). Electrode dislodgment and lead fracture can be caused by unconscious or habitual "twiddling" of the impulse generator (Fig. 53–31). Twiddler's syndrome has been reported most commonly in patients with transvenous pacing systems but has also been reported in those with transmediastinal pacing systems (Rodan et al., 1978). An uncommon late complication is an allergic reaction to the pacemaker, usually to the titanium components. This can be confirmed by skin testing to various pacemaker components. However, many cases of pacemaker allergic reactions are actually smoldering pocket infections with nonvirulent bacteria and should be treated as outlined earlier (Peters et al., 1984).

## Pacemaker Malfunctions

Most pacemaker system malfunctions are due to abnormalities of the pacing lead or lead-tissue interface. Primary pacemaker generator malfunction is uncommon, because biomedical engineering improvements have produced exceptionally durable and reliable permanent pacemakers. The possibility of pacemaker generator and lead malfunction and failure emphasizes the need for appropriate long-term follow-up. Pacemaker system malfunction may cause failure to capture the myocardium, over- or under-sensing, alterations in the preset pacing rate (either acceleration or slowing), and various combinations of these events. These abnormalities may be either persistent or intermittent, the latter presenting a diagnostic challenge to confirm if it occurs infrequently.

When patients present with presumed pacemaker malfunction, they should be extensively monitored to detect periods of inappropriate pacemaker function. A chest film sometimes helps detect lead fracture or displacement (Fig. 53–32). However, the most useful information usually comes from a careful and methodical interrogation of the pacemaker to assess whether the pacemaker is sensing or pacing appropriately. Intermittent lead malfunction can sometimes be manifested by stressing the lead with direct compression of the lead at the clavicle or by having the patient raise the arms over the head. Usually detailed evaluation of the patient will uncover the nature of the pacemaker malfunction.

Failure of the pacemaker to capture the myocar-

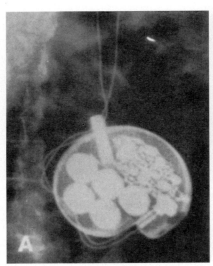 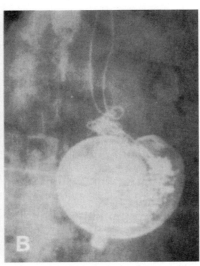 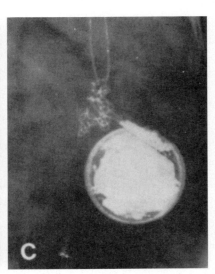

**FIGURE 53–31.** Abdominal films. *A,* Film 1 year after initial implant shows normal relationship between the wires and the impulse generator. *B,* Film 2 years later shows rotation of impulse generator 180 degrees and twisting of wires close to the generator. *C,* 6 months after implantation of a new impulse generator, additional twisting is evident. (*A–C,* From Rodan, B. A., Lowe, J. E., and Chen, J. T. T.: Abdominal twiddler's syndrome. Am. J. Roentgenol., *131*:1084, 1978. Copyright © 1978 by Williams & Wilkins Company.)

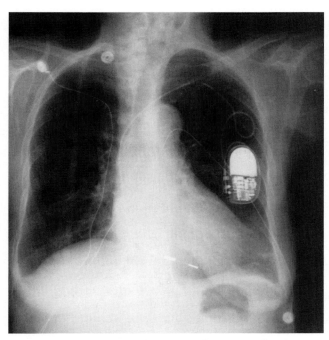

**FIGURE 53-32.** Chest film of a patient who presented with pacing and sensing malfunction. Note the fracture of the outer coil of the pacing lead at the junction of the clavicle. Lead fracture probably occurred at this location because of compression between the clavicle and the first rib.

dium may be persistent or intermittent. Pacing failure may be due to a number of factors, but most commonly these are lead problems such as displacement, perforation, fracture, disruption of insulation, and poor generator-lead connection. An increased stimulation threshold may also cause failure to capture. The increase in stimulation threshold may simply be related to the increase in pacing requirements seen in new leads as they heal into place, or it may be due to other factors such as acute inferior myocardial infarction, hyperkalemia, hypokalemia, or drug effect or toxicity (especially with antiarrhythmic drugs such as amiodarone or flecainide). Measurement of telemetered lead impedance may help define the cause of pacing failure. If the lead impedance is high (> 1000 ohms), a lead discontinuity is present such as is seen in a lead fracture. If the impedance is low (< 300 ohms) an insulation break is probably present. A normal lead impedance suggests a stimulation threshold problem; however, the lead impedance may also be normal in the setting of intermittent fractures or insulation disruption. If none of these factors are present, the impulse generator itself may be malfunctioning.

Inappropriate sensing by the pacemaker may result from either under- or oversensing of electrical signals. The most common cause of failure to sense appropriate signals is poor initial positioning of the lead electrode or lead dislodgment. Disruption of insulation around the lead elements, electrolyte disturbances, drug effects, and primary pacemaker malfunction may also cause undersensing. Oversensing refers to the detection of electrical signals that were not meant to be detected by the pacemaker. Such

signals could be generated by the T wave, by electrical noise from motion at a lead fracture or other source, by myopotentials generated by the pectoral muscles (with unipolar pacemakers), or by far-field, high-voltage sources such as electrocautery. Most modern pacemakers can record intracardiac electrograms or event markers, which permits direct documentation of under- and oversensing.

Sudden accelerations in the paced rate may be due to several factors. With DDD pacemakers, the most common cause is the development of an atrial tachyarrhythmia which is tracked by the pacemaker to produce ventricular pacing near the upper rate limit. Application of the magnet typically places the pacemaker in the asynchronous pacing mode and allows detection or termination of the underlying atrial arrhythmia. Recording intracardiac atrial electrograms or event markers also allows the diagnosis to be made. Rate-responsive pacemakers may have erratic fluxes in rate if the sensor is programmed too sensitively; this can be corrected by reprogramming. Motion sensors respond to vibration to cause accelerations in paced rate, as exemplified by very rapid paced rates in patients with activity sensor–driven pacemakers transported by helicopters. Acutely, this can be corrected by magnet applications, to deactivate sensor activity or by eliminating the source of vibration.

Pacemaker-mediated tachycardia (PMT) occurs in the setting of intact ventriculoatrial (VA) conduction. Typically, premature ventricular contractions may be conducted retrogradely through the AV conduction system and cause retrograde activation of the atrium. If this retrograde atrial activation occurs after completion of the PVARP, the atrial event is sensed by the DDD pacemaker and evokes a paced ventricular event that may cause further VA conduction. If each ventricularly paced event produces retrograde atrial activation sensed by the pacemaker, PMT (or endless loop tachycardia) will be generated. Because PMT is caused by sensing of retrograde atrial activation, placement of the pacemaker in the asynchronous mode by application of the magnet or programming will terminate the tachycardia. Another alternative is to reprogram the PVARP to a larger value so that retrograde atrial activation occurs during the refractory period of the pacemaker and cannot be sensed to continue tachycardia. Prevention of further episodes of PMT can be achieved by prolonging the PVARP or using PVARP extension. Some newer pacemakers have programmable options to terminate possible PMT episodes, such as dropping ventricular paced events intermittently when the pacemaker reaches maximum atrial tracking rates. Occasionally, drugs that block AV nodal conduction must be used to prevent retrograde atrial activation after premature ventricular contractions.

Primary pacemaker malfunction may abruptly accelerate the pacing rate, called "runaway pacemaker," creating pacemaker-induced ventricular tachycardia. Fortunately, runaway pacemaker is rarely encountered with modern pacemaker generators. Runaway pacemaker is a medical emergency that should be treated by immediate replacement of the malfunctioning pacemaker. Persistent slowing of the pacemaker rate below the programmed lower rate may be an indication that the pacemaker's battery is nearly depleted. Knowledge of the pacing rates that suggest generator end of life is important for recognition of this problem. Electrical interference, such as with electrocautery during surgical procedures, may alter the paced rate in some pacemakers (the "noise reversion mode"). Oversensing the T wave can also result in apparent slowing of the paced rate.

## Environmental Interactions

Electrocautery may have a number of adverse effects on pacemaker function, depending on the amplitude of the radiofrequency current used and its proximity to the pacing lead and pacemaker generator. In general, unipolar pacemakers are more apt to be affected by electrocautery, given their increased sensitivity to detect noncardiac electrical events. If the pacemaker senses electrocautery potentials of sufficient amplitude, this may inhibit the pacing output. Atrial sensing of electrocautery in DDD pacemakers may result is rapid pacing of the ventricles. Electrocautery can also cause pacemaker reprogramming, fall back to noise reversion mode, permanent pacemaker generator damage, and permanent or temporary pacing or sensing abnormalities by damaging the myocardium adjacent to the lead electrodes. Patients with pacemakers who are scheduled for surgical procedures in which electrocautery is used should probably be programmed to asynchronous modes to avoid inhibition or oversensing, or they should have the magnet placed over the pacemaker to obtain asynchronous pacing during periods of electrocautery.

## PACEMAKER FOLLOW-UP

An organized follow-up program for pacemaker patients should be provided by every clinic engaged in implanting permanent pacemakers. An adequate follow-up program must do more than merely document normal or abnormal function of a pacemaker, and the purpose of pacemaker follow-up is not just to detect pacemaker failure. Instead, a comprehensive program should provide preimplant and postimplant teaching, continued reassurance for the patient and family, transtelephonic monitoring of both the pacemaker and the patient's spontaneous rhythm, office or clinic visits when necessary, and assistance when admission to the hospital is required for complications, for routine battery changes, or for reasons not related to the pacemaker directly.

A properly designed follow-up program should not only provide support for the patient with a pacemaker, but should also be capable of providing important information concerning the patient's pacemaker for the physicians who are involved in care.

The functions of the pacemaker follow-up program may be summarized as involving the education of both the patient and physician, documentation of normal and abnormal pacemaker function, detection of complications (surgical and related to pacemaker function), facilitation of efficient medical care for the patient with the pacemaker, and storage of critical data regarding the pacemaker and electrodes for each patient in an organized system so that it is available to any physician who takes care of the patient. Commercial services can provide transtelephonic ECG tracings and monitor pacemaker function, but these services cannot substitute for a program that involves the medical personnel involved in pacemaker implantation and patient follow-up.

Although commonly thought to involve primarily transtelephonic ECG recording, pacemaker follow-up should be an integrated system of postimplant teaching, clinic visits, and telephone transmissions. The purposes of teaching the patient when the pacemaker is implanted are to allay the patient's and family's concerns about the pacemaker, to inform the patient about the normal function of the pacemaker, and to teach the patient how to use the telephone transmission equipment. A schedule of call-in times should be arranged before discharge, and the use of the transmitter should be practiced with the personnel who will receive the calls. Baseline recordings should be made of the ECG with and without magnet and an overpenetrated chest film obtained to document lead position.

The patient should be observed as an outpatient at 6 weeks after implantation, at which time a noninvasive assessment of pacing threshold should be made. This assessment is done in different ways, depending on the model and manufacturer of the pacemaker. Pulse generator output can be decreased in a stepwise manner by shortening pulse width in some generators and by lowering output voltage in others. By observing the point at which capture is lost, an estimation of the chronic pacing threshold can be obtained and the pacemaker's output programmed down to lower levels to prolong battery life. A margin of safety of at least 3:1 over the capture threshold should be maintained. Because pacing thresholds may rise during the first few weeks after implantation, decreasing pacing output, either by reprogramming pulse width or voltage, should not be done earlier than 4 to 6 weeks after implantation.

The return visit also provides an opportunity to examine carefully the surgical site for signs of excessive skin tension, inflammation, or improper wound healing.

Telephone transmissions should begin immediately after discharge and are done weekly for the first 4 weeks to document proper function. Subsequent telephone transmissions should be made regularly, but at longer intervals. In most patients, transmissions are probably not required more frequently than every 2 to 3 months in the absence of symptoms. At the time of the telephone transmission, recordings should be made of the spontaneous rhythm, and then with the application of the external magnet. Readings of pulse width and AV interval (for dual-chamber devices) can also be obtained. These data are recorded in the follow-up files so that proper pacemaker function can be documented and future malfunctions ascertained.

The response of a pacemaker to application of the magnet varies with the manufacturer and model number, and the appropriate magnet response of each patient's pacemaker should be noted in the records. Application of the magnet usually converts the pacemaker to an asynchronous functional mode, typically VOO for a VVI pacemaker and DOO for a DDD pacemaker, although this rule has exceptions. The pacing rate with application of the magnet usually relays information about battery status, with predefined decreases in rate indicating either approaching or imminent battery depletion. Some pacemakers demonstrate an increase in the pulse width above the programmed value as the battery approaches its end of life. When rate changes or pulse width increases suggest approaching battery depletion, transtelephonic follow-up should be increased in frequency to at least once a month to monitor for the occurrence of an elective replacement indicator. Magnet application also allows assessment of the pacing function of the pacemaker during asynchronous pacing, even if the intrinsic rhythm is more rapid. Some pacemakers perform threshold tests during application of the magnet. The most commonly encountered method is the threshold margin test, in which three pulses are generated at a relatively rapid rate by the pacemaker on application of the magnet, with the last of the three pulses being 25% of the programmed pulse width. If the third pulse does not capture the appropriate chamber and the previous pulses do, the safety margin for capture is too small and pacing outputs need to be programmed to higher values. Some pacemakers are placed in the vario mode with magnet application, during which the rate is accelerated slightly for 16 beats and the voltage output is decreased by 1/15 between each beat. By calculating the number of complexes that capture the paced chamber, one can ascertain the relative safety margin for pacing.

Finally, records of any reprogramming should be maintained in the follow-up files so that changes in pacemaker function that appear on routine tracings can be properly interpreted.

## FUTURE TRENDS

Future trends in cardiac pacing will undoubtedly continue to follow the advances in technology that have characterized the field during the last 10 years. Improvements in lead-electrode technology can be expected to produce smaller leads and improved electrodes with lower chronic pacing thresholds, and therefore lower energy requirements and longer battery life. The ability to pace with less energy output may permit the use of smaller batteries, and thus smaller pulse generators.

The proliferation of programmable pacemakers has required pacemaker centers to stock an increasingly large number of different manufacturers' programmers. At present, there is no compatibility between the various programmers. Unfortunately, it is unlikely that a device will be devised to program all existing pacemakers. In the future, it would seem to be in the best interests of efficiency and cost reduction to work toward a universal system for pacemaker programmability.

Finally, continued advances in physiologic pacing devices can also be expected. Among these advances will be pacemakers that respond to various physiologic parameters and allow changes in heart rate that correspond with the patient's physiologic needs (Wirtzfeld et al., 1987).

With further technologic advances in the field of physiologic pacing, improved ways of determining which patients will benefit from these devices will be necessary. This can be accomplished only through clinical databases located at centers that implant and closely monitor large numbers of patients with pacemakers.

## ANTITACHYCARDIA PACING

The 1980s saw rapid developments in the application of pacing technology to the treatment of supraventricular and ventricular tachycardia, which culminated in implantable pacemakers designed specifically to treat these arrhythmias. These antitachycardia pacemakers were needed because pharmacologic therapy so often was ineffective in controlling arrhythmia recurrence. Although atrial antitachycardia pacemakers were very effective in terminating episodes of paroxysmal supraventricular tachycardia due to various mechanisms (e.g., AV nodal re-entrant tachycardia, AV reciprocating tachycardia, atrial tachycardia, and atrial flutter), the concomitant development of curative and highly effective technique of transcatheter radiofrequency current ablation has virtually eliminated the need for atrial antitachycardia devices. Although catheter ablation techniques have not been as successful in the treatment of ventricular tachycardia in the setting of structural heart disease, the occurrence of pacing-induced acceleration of ventricular tachycardia to a more rapid and poorly tolerated ventricular tachycardia or to ventricular fibrillation necessitated the application of antitachycardia pacing only in conjunction with backup defibrillation capabilities. Third-generation automatic implantable cardioverter-defibrillators now provide both antitachycardia pacing and low-energy synchronized cardioversion and high-energy defibrillation should the ventricular tachycardia be accelerated to a more malignant arrhythmia (see later).

Antitachycardia pacing techniques are most effective in terminating re-entrant arrhythmias. Tachycardias due to abnormal automaticity are not terminated by pacing, although arrhythmias due to triggered automaticity can be so terminated.

Several pacing techniques have been used to prevent or terminate arrhythmias. Commonly used techniques include overdrive pacing and various forms of burst pacing. Overdrive pacing (pacing at rates slower than the tachycardia but faster than the baseline intrinsic rhythm) often is used temporarily to suppress atrial and ventricular arrhythmias. Permanent overdrive pacing in the treatment of tachyarrhythmias is used when relative bradycardia allows the "escape" of an atrial or ventricular tachyarrhythmia. A standard antibradycardia pacemaker is used for this purpose. This technique is most commonly employed in the treatment of patients with the long QT syndrome and torsades de pointes (Eldar et al., 1992). Occasionally, overdrive pacing can be shown to suppress tachycardia in conjunction with antiarrhythmic medications in patients with bradycardia-related monomorphic ventricular tachycardia or atrial tachyarrhythmias. In all of these examples, however, it is important to document the suppression of tachycardia with overdrive pacing using a temporary pacemaker prior to implantation of a permanent device.

*Burst pacing* is defined as pacing during tachycardia at a rate faster than the rate of the tachycardia (generally more than 30 beats per minute faster) (Fig. 53–33). Burst pacing is the pacing modality most commonly used to terminate re-entrant arrhythmias using an antitachycardia device (Fisher et al., 1982). After detection of a tachyarrhythmia, the device will automatically deliver a burst of pacing pulses at a programmed rate and will reiterate the process or else progress to more aggressive burst pacing protocols, depending on how the device is programmed. Antitachycardia pacemakers can be programmed to deliver bursts in several ways. The rate and number of beats of a burst can be fixed and repeated several times, or the rate or number of beats in the burst can be increased by a fixed amount after each successive attempt. The pacing rate can also be accelerated during each burst (ramp pacing). The coupling interval between the last sensed tachycardia beat and the first beat of the burst can also be programmed, as can the

number of paced beats in a burst. By adjusting these various parameters, the most appropriate burst pacing technique can be chosen for the patient. Obviously, determining the best pacing algorithm for an individual patient requires extensive electrophysiologic testing (1) before implantation of the device to determine if antitachycardia pacing is an appropriate therapeutic modality for the patient and (2) after implantation of the device to optimally program the antitachycardia functions. Fortunately, most pacemakers also can deliver programmed stimulation as directed by the pacemaker programmer (so-called noninvasive programmed stimulation). This programmed stimulation function allows repeated induction of the tachycardia in most patients without having to insert temporary pacing catheters, and thus greatly facilitates testing of the antitachycardia device after its implantation. Antitachycardia pacemakers also can manage bradycardias that occur after termination of tachycardia or that allow escape of the tachyarrhythmia.

The major limitation of the widespread use of antitachycardia pacemakers in the treatment of ventricular tachycardia has been the potential for arrhythmia acceleration or fibrillation. For this reason, ventricular tachycardia that can be terminated by burst pacing is best treated with an implantable cardioverter-defibrillator with antitachycardia pacing capabilities.

## IMPLANTABLE CARDIOVERTER–DEFIBRILLATORS

Sudden cardiac death due to ventricular tachyarrhythmias is the major cause of death in the United States, accounting for approximately 400,000 lives per year. In patients with ventricular tachycardia or fibrillation, antiarrhythmic drugs can be identified to control the arrhythmia in only 20 to 50% of patients if electrophysiologic studies are used to guide therapy (ESVEM, 1993; Mitchell et al., 1987; Waller et al., 1987; Wilber et al., 1988). In patients whose arrhythmia cannot be controlled with antiarrhythmic drugs, the risk of sudden cardiac death and recurrent ventricular tachycardia remains high. A small number of these patients may be candidates for surgical ablation of their arrhythmogenic focus. However, for most patients who are refractory to medical therapy, surgical ablation is not an option, and an *implantable cardioverter-defibrillator* (ICD) is the optimal form of therapy.

Mirowski designed the first ICD in the late 1960s and demonstrated that ICDs were effective in terminating ventricular fibrillation in animals with electrically induced ventricular fibrillation (Mirowski et al., 1978). In 1980, the first ICDs were implanted in humans with medically refractory ventricular tachyarrhythmias and were shown to effectively prevent sudden death and to decrease mortality in this high-risk group of patients. As the general safety and efficacy of ICDs were demonstrated, their use has greatly expanded: Over 30,000 have been implanted. Retrospective analyses have demonstrated that ICDs effec-

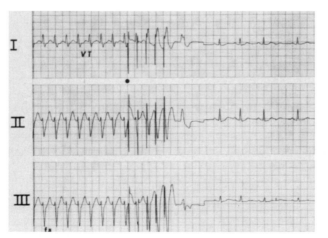

**FIGURE 53–33.** Termination of ventricular tachycardia with a manually activated radiofrequency pacemaker. A short burst of pacing stimuli results in interruption of the tachycardia. Extensive preimplantation testing was done to show safety and efficacy.

tively reduce sudden cardiac death (Fogoros et al., 1990; Fromer et al., 1992; Newman et al., 1992; Tchou et al., 1988) (Fig. 53–34). Most retrospective studies suggest that ICDs are superior to pharmacologic therapy (Akhtar et al., 1992). Prospective trials are assessing the efficacy of ICDs in medical therapy, especially with amiodarone.

## Mechanism of Cardioversion and Defibrillation

Modern ICDs provide three antiarrhythmic functions: antitachycardia pacing, cardioversion, and defibrillation. As discussed earlier, antitachycardia pacing terminates an arrhythmia by causing refractoriness within the re-entrant circuit. Cardioversion refers to the delivery of relatively low-energy shocks (usually 0.1 to 5.0 J) to terminate ventricular tachycardia. The low-energy shock must be synchronized to the QRS complex of the tachycardia to avoid precipitation of ventricular fibrillation by delivering a low-energy shock on the T wave. Low-energy synchronized shocks presumably cardiovert by depolarizing excitable segments within the re-entrant circuit to prevent further re-entry. The energy required for successful cardioversion depends on the proximity of the shock electrode to the re-entrant circuit, the presence of excitable elements within the re-entrant circuit, and the ability of the shock to depolarize these excitable elements. Besides terminating ventricular tachycardia, synchronized cardioversion shocks can also accelerate ventricular tachycardia or cause it to degenerate into polymorphic ventricular tachycardia or fibrillation. Acceleration of ventricular tachycardia or precipitation of ventricular fibrillation presumably occurs by changing the re-entrant circuit to a more unstable one or by stimulating myocardium that exists within or outside the circuit, which is in its vulnerable period when most of the myocardium is being activated (i.e., during the QRS complex). Because of the risk of acceleration or degeneration of ventricular tachycardia by low-energy cardioversion shocks, defibrillation backup is necessary in implantable cardioversion devices.

During ventricular fibrillation, multiple re-entrant wavefronts chaotically activate the ventricles. Unlike ventricular tachycardia, in which there is a single fixed re-entrant circuit and thus a constant QRS morphology, ventricular fibrillation is generated by multiple wavelets that are continually shifting direction and colliding with one another. Thus, a consistent QRS pattern is not generated during ventricular fibrillation. The only reliable means of terminating ventricular fibrillation is with a high-energy electrical shock.

Three hypotheses attempt to explain electrical defibrillation (Wharton et al., 1991). The total extinction hypothesis proposes that successful defibrillation shocks depolarize all excitable gaps between the multiple re-entrant wavelets on the ventricles (Wiggers, 1940). Thus, further re-entry is not possible, and ventricular fibrillation is terminated. However, the frequent observation that ventricular fibrillation appears to continue for a few beats before terminating after a successful shock cannot be readily explained by this hypothesis. The critical mass hypothesis is a modification of the total extinction hypothesis. It suggests that a critical amount of myocardium, typically assumed to be about 75% of the ventricles, must be depolarized for defibrillation to occur (Zipes et al., 1975). Although wavelets of fibrillation can continue in areas not directly depolarized by the shock, there is insufficient excitable myocardium after the shock for ventricular fibrillation to be maintained, and the residual wavefronts would gradually die out.

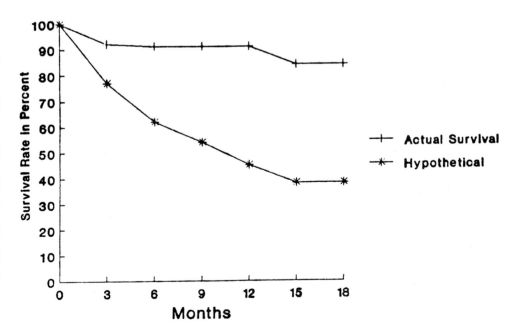

FIGURE 53–34. Actuarial survival with a third-generation implantable cardioverter-defibrillator (ICD) in patients with medically refractory ventricular tachyarrhythmias. The actual survival probability is compared with a theoretical survival rate, which is based on the delivery of a high-energy defibrillation shocks. It is presumed that if a defibrillation energy shock was needed, death would have ensued if the ICD were not present. Episodes of antitachycardia pacing for termination of ventricular tachycardia were not included in this analysis. (From Fromer, M., et al.: Efficacy of automatic multimodal device therapy for ventricular tachyarrhythmias as delivered by a new implantable pacing cardioverter-defibrillator. Circulation, 86:363–374, 1992. Reproduced with permission. Copyright 1992 American Heart Association.)

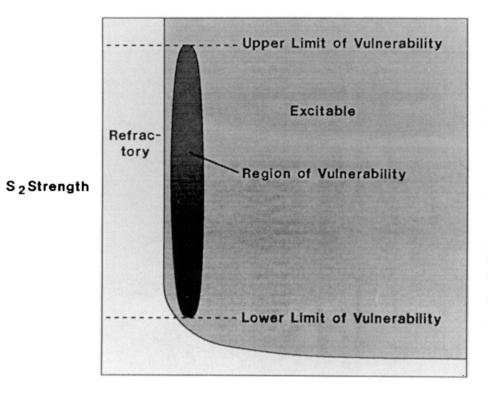

**FIGURE 53–35.** Diagram of the region of vulnerability to shocks delivered during the relatively refractory period of the ventricles. The abscissa indicates the coupling interval between the shock ($S_2$) and the preceding paced beat ($S_1$). The ordinate indicates increasing strength of the shock. At short coupling intervals or low shock strength, the ventricles are not activated by the shock (labeled "Refractory"). At longer coupling intervals and at higher shock strengths, the myocardium is excitable. A region of vulnerability exists at coupling intervals slightly longer than where refractoriness begins. As noted in the diagram, there exists a lower and upper limit of shock strength that will induce ventricular fibrillation when delivered in the vulnerable period.

Most recent studies suggest a third hypothesis, known as the upper limit of vulnerability hypothesis. When a shock of sufficient amplitude is delivered during sinus rhythm near the peak of the T wave, ventricular fibrillation can be induced. The period during the T wave in which a sufficiently strong shock can induce fibrillation is known as the vulnerable period (Fig. 53–35). The lowest-strength shock that can induce ventricular fibrillation defines the lower limit of vulnerability, or the ventricular fibrillation threshold. Less well appreciated is that there exists

an upper limit to the shock strength that will induce ventricular fibrillation if the shocks are delivered to defibrillation electrodes. Thus, shocks with an energy level exceeding this upper limit of vulnerability will not induce fibrillation no matter when the shock is delivered in the vulnerable zone. Several investigators have shown that the shock strength at the defibrillation threshold is closely related to that of the upper limit of vulnerability (Chen et al., 1986; Fabiato et al., 1967; Lesigne et al., 1976; Wharton et al., 1990). The upper limit of vulnerability appears to best define the

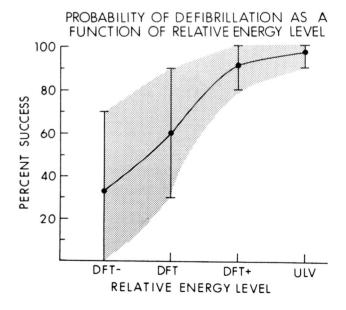

**FIGURE 53–36.** Probability of successful defibrillation curve from pooled animal data. Shock strengths are expressed in relative terms as the energy determined from a single defibrillation threshold (DFT) determination, the upper limit of vulnerability (ULV) energy, an energy halfway between the DFT and the ULV (DFT+), and an equal energy decrement less than DFT (DFT−). Shocks of each strength were delivered on ten attempts at defibrillation to generate the probability of success. As can be seen, the probability of successful defibrillation can be best described by a sigmoidal dose-response relation, illustrated in this figure as a mean *(line)* and a range *(stippled area)*. The energy at the ULV was effective more than 95% of the time. (From Wharton, J. M., Richard, V. J., Murray, C. E., et al.: Electrophysiologic effects of monophasic and biphasic stimuli in normal and infarcted dogs. PACE, *13*:1158–1172, 1990.)

lowest strength shocks with the greatest probability of successful defibrillation when given repetitively (Wharton et al., 1990) (Fig. 53–36). However, shocks with a strength of the defibrillation threshold, defined as the lowest energy shock that successfully defibrillated at least once, are effective on average for only 60% of attempts. Finally, interventions that decrease the defibrillation threshold also decrease the upper limit of vulnerability. Thus, the upper limit of vulnerability appears to be closely linked to successful defibrillation.

The upper limit of vulnerability hypothesis states that successful shocks halt fibrillation not only by depolarizing all excitable gaps but, more importantly, by not reinducing ventricular fibrillation. Because the multiple re-entrant wavelets during fibrillation create multiple sites in the vulnerable period at any point in time, shocks of insufficient strength could reinduce fibrillation by stimulating during the vulnerable period at one or more sites on the ventricles (Chen et al., 1986, 1990). Shocks with a strength exceeding the upper limit of vulnerability would not reinduce fibrillation. It has been demonstrated that a minimum voltage gradient (which is related to current density) of approximately 6 V/cm has to be generated over all of the ventricles for successful defibrillation, regardless of the electrode configuration used (Wharton et al., 1991). This voltage gradient is much higher than that needed for stimulation of excitable myocardium and is required over all of the ventricles. Both of these observations are contrary to predictions of the total extinction or critical mass hypotheses and further support the upper limit of vulnerability hypothesis.

From a practical standpoint, the lowest energy for defibrillation is obtained by electrode configurations that distribute current most uniformly over the ventricles (Fig. 53–37). Thus, defibrillation electrodes should be placed such that the greatest amount of myocardium is interposed as evenly as possible between the electrodes. Defibrillation electrodes placed asymmetrically to one side require higher energy to defibrillate because more current must be given in order to raise regions remote from the shock electrodes to a certain threshold current density.

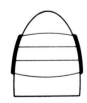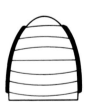

**FIGURE 53–37.** Current distribution across the ventricles based on relative defibrillation patch location and size. The diagram illustrates the ventricles with patches placed on the right and left epicardial surfaces. *Current lines* connecting patches represent relative distribution of current. The most uniform distribution of current (and thus the lowest defibrillation threshold) is achieved with large patches evenly spaced across the heart *(leftmost drawing).* Smaller patches or asymmetric patch location result in less uniformity of current distribution and probably higher defibrillation thresholds.

## Indications

As mentioned earlier, ICDs are probably the preferred treatment option for most patients with medically refractory ventricular tachycardia and fibrillation. Given the poor prognosis in these patients and their high risk for recurrent ventricular tachycardia and sudden cardiac death, ICDs provide the greatest and most reliable degree of protection. In addition, some patients with ventricular tachycardia or fibrillation have no inducible arrhythmia during electrophysiologic testing or insufficient ventricular ectopy during Holter monitoring to guide antiarrhythmic drug therapy. Because empiric antiarrhythmic drug therapy may increase rather than decrease their risk of recurrent sudden death and ventricular tachycardia, these patients are probably best treated with ICDs (Committee of Pacemaker Implantation, 1991).

Patients being considered for ICD therapy must be carefully evaluated before implantation. Reversible or transient etiologies of ventricular tachyarrhythmia should be excluded, such as acute myocardial infarction or severe ischemia, electrolyte disturbances, and drug toxicity. Given the pain generated by high-energy shocks, the frequency of the ventricular tachycardia must be controlled medically before the defibrillator is implanted. An ICD is not a therapeutic option for patients with incessant or frequent episodes of ventricular tachycardia. In addition, supraventricular tachyarrhythmias must also be controlled, or else the rapid ventricular rates during the supraventricular tachycardia will precipitate unnecessary ICD shocks. Given the discomfort and cost of defibrillators, an ICD is probably not the best option for patients with a limited short-term prognosis due to end-stage cardiac or pulmonary disease, metastatic cancer, or other similar processes. Before receiving an ICD, the patient needs to be extensively evaluated by electrophysiologic testing so that the rate, hemodynamic stability, and susceptibility to termination by pacing techniques of the ventricular tachyarrhythmia can be established. This allows the selection of the most appropriate ICD for the individual patient and the optimal programming of the device. Further, the patient needs to be evaluated for the presence of underlying coronary artery disease or other cardiac disorders, not only to establish the process causing the patient's arrhythmia, but also to guide the surgical procedure, because concomitant coronary artery revascularization or other procedures may be needed in addition to placement of the ICD.

Before implantation of an ICD, patients and their families must be counseled about the impact, both good and bad, of ICDs on their lifestyle. Most patients who receive ICDs are able to return to their previous employment and lead active lives (Kalbfleisch et al., 1989). However, although ICDs effectively treat ventricular tachycardia, some patients tolerate shocks poorly and develop marked anxiety and depression (Fricchione et al., 1989; Keren et al., 1991). The development of ICDs with antitachycardia pacing has decreased the frequency with which most patients receive shocks, and thus patients may be more likely to accept this form of therapy. It is important to advise patients that their license to drive an automobile may be revoked for 6 to 12 months or longer in some states after they receive an ICD, because this restriction may affect the patient's decision about using this form of therapy. Because driving restrictions vary from state to state, implanting physicians should know the regulations applicable to their patient population (Strickberger et al., 1991). Adequate preparation of patients and their families before implantation of the ICD greatly facilitates their acceptance of and adaptation to this form of therapy afterward.

## ICD Generator and Leads

ICDs are composed of three parts: the ICD generator, the shocking electrodes, and the sensing electrode (Fig. 53–38). The sensing circuit in the ICD generator constantly monitors the ventricular rate and other

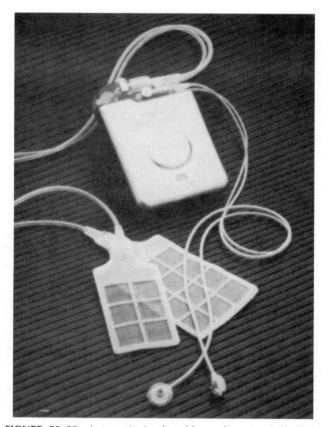

**FIGURE 53–38.** Automatic implantable cardioverter-defibrillator (AICD). Through a median sternotomy, epicardial sensing electrodes are attached at the level of the anterior aspect of the interventricular septum. Plaque electrodes are sutured onto the right ventricle (RV) and lateral aspect of the left ventricle (LV). The defibrillating shock is delivered from the smaller RV plaque, and the large LV plaque serves as a grounding electrode. After implantation of the sensing electrodes and defibrillating electrodes, all leads are tunneled beneath the xiphoid to a left upper-quadrant pocket, where they are attached to the AICD generator.

features of the cardiac rhythm through the sensing electrode. If ventricular tachycardia or fibrillation is detected, electrical therapy is delivered through the shocking electrodes. The first generation of ICD generators were relatively simple devices that were designed to recognize a rapid heart rate and deliver a high-energy (30-J) shock. The initial ICDs had no programmable features. The heart rate that had to be exceeded for shock delivery was preset by the manufacturer and could not be changed if the patient's arrhythmia slowed, as could occur after changes in antiarrhythmic drug therapy. In addition, the early ICDs delivered only a 30-J shock appropriate for defibrillation; low-energy synchronized cardioversion was not possible, nor was antitachycardia or antibradycardia pacing. The early ICD generators had no monitoring capabilities to allow determination of how often and for what arrhythmia therapy had been delivered. Lastly, the only reliable ICDs had to be connected to epicardial shocking electrodes to achieve reliable defibrillation.

ICD technology has improved greatly in recent years. The second generation of ICDs had the addition of low-energy synchronized cardioversion shocks, which could be used to treat less painfully well-tolerated ventricular tachycardia. In addition, the second-generation devices had some programmable features, such as the rate cutoff for detection of tachycardia. The present third-generation devices provide a complex array of programmable features. Besides high-energy defibrillation shocks and low-energy synchronized cardioversion shocks, third-generation devices have extensive, programmable antitachycardia pacing functions. In many patients with hemodynamically stable monomorphic ventricular tachycardia, rapid ventricular burst pacing may terminate tachycardia, circumventing the need for painful cardioversion shocks (Fromer et al., 1992; Porterfield et al., 1993). The device can be programmed for various means of delivering burst pacing, the specific means in any patient being determined with extensive electrophysiologic testing to ensure the efficacy and safety of the antitachycardia pacing algorithm used. The ICD can be programmed to deliver increasingly progressive antitachycardia pacing protocols and subsequent cardioversion or defibrillation shocks if antitachycardia pacing is not successful or if ventricular tachycardia is accelerated or deteriorates into ventricular fibrillation. In addition, up to three tiers of therapy can be delivered, one for slower ventricular tachycardia, one for faster tachycardia, and one for ventricular fibrillation or very rapid ventricular tachycardia. The options of tiered therapy allow prescription of different therapies for patients with several tachyarrhythmias. The number of attempts with antitachycardia pacing is also programmable. If after the prescribed number of attempts antitachycardia pacing has not been successful, cardioversion or defibrillation shocks will be tried as programmed.

Third-generation ICDs also have enhanced tachycardia detection functions. A problem with early ICDs was that simple rate criteria for detection of tachycardia did not discriminate between ventricular tachycardia and supraventricular tachycardias, such as atrial fibrillation, atrial flutter, and even sinus tachycardia above the programmed upper rate cutoff. Some first- and second-generation ICDs had a function called *probability density function* (PDF), which attempted to separate supraventricular tachycardias from ventricular tachycardia. PDF determined the percentage of the duty cycle detected on the shock electrode configuration at which the electrical signal was significantly above baseline. If this percentage was beyond a certain limit, implying a wide QRS complex tachycardia such as ventricular tachycardia, then PDF criteria would be met and the shock delivered. PDF did not gain wide acceptance as a means to separate supraventricular from ventricular tachycardia because of obvious problems encountered with relatively narrow QRS morphologies of ventricular tachycardia or supraventricular tachycardias with bundle-branch block patterns. Third-generation ICDs have programmable detection enhancements that include suddenness of onset of the arrhythmia, stability of rate, sustained rate duration, and morphologic criteria. Because ventricular tachycardia usually occurs prematurely in the cardiac cycle, sudden-onset criteria require a certain percentage of shortening of the first complex of a tachycardia meeting the programmed rate criteria. This helps distinguish ventricular tachycardia from rhythms with gradual onset, such as sinus tachycardia. Rate stability criteria require a certain level of regularity of rate to help distinguish ventricular tachycardia from irregular arrhythmias, such as atrial fibrillation. Finally, sustained-rate duration criteria allow separation of the arrhythmia from nonsustained variants. Early ICDs were committed devices—that is, once arrhythmia detection criteria had been met, therapy would be delivered even if the arrhythmia spontaneously terminated. Thus, shocks would be delivered even for nonsustained episodes of ventricular tachycardia. Third-generation ICDs are either fixed or programmable noncommitted devices because they have "relook" capabilities that reassess whether detection criteria are met before delivering therapy. If tachycardia is still detected, therapy is delivered; if not, therapy is aborted.

In addition to extensive antitachycardia pacing and detection functions, third-generation ICDs also have programmable antibradycardia ventricular pacing capabilities. This allows fixed rate pacing to correct postshock or spontaneous bradycardia. In ICD patients who require continuous pacing for bradycardia, it is now preferable to implant a permanent pacemaker in addition to the third-generation ICD, because continuous pacing from the latter will prematurely deplete the battery. Extreme caution is needed in combining pacemakers with ICDs, given the potential for adverse interactions (Epstein et al., 1989). In particular, unipolar pacemakers or pacemakers with programmable polarity should not be used. Unipolar pacing can produce double counting by the ICD due to detection of the pacing stimulus and evoked QRS, so that antitachycardia therapy is delivered for paced

rhythm. In pacemakers with programmable polarity, ICD shock delivery can reprogram the pacemaker from bipolar pacing to unipolar pacing. Thus, only dedicated bipolar pacemakers should be implanted in patients with ICDs. Care must also be taken to ensure that pacing during ventricular fibrillation (from failure to sense the low-amplitude ventricular signal during fibrillation) is not detected by the sensing circuit of the ICD, because this may inhibit ICD therapy delivery. Given the potential for adverse interactions, it is best to avoid pacemakers in patients with ICDs if possible.

Newer ICDs also monitor delivery of therapies, storing the information for subsequent telemetry during follow-up of the patient (Marchlinski et al., 1993). The stored information typically includes the time and type of each therapy delivery and information about the cycle length or the recorded intracardiac electrograms at the time of therapy. Such information allows precise monitoring of the appropriateness of programmed therapies for the patient. Moreover, newer generations of ICDs can be programmed to deliver programmed electrical stimulation noninvasively, allowing testing of ICD function without placement of temporary catheters.

The early ICDs required placement of two epicardial patches or an intravascular right atrial spring-coil electrode and left ventricular epicardial patch. Thus, implantation of ICDs required an open chest procedure. Given the poor left ventricular function and other co-morbid processes usually seen in the group of patients with medically refractory ventricular tachyarrhythmias, the operative mortality rate was relatively high (2 to 4%), and the procedure precluded use of ICDs in sicker patients (Horowitz, 1992). Recent development of electrode arrays using right-sided intravascular leads with or without leads in the coronary sinus or a subcutaneous or submuscular patch along the left lateral chest have allowed most implantable defibrillators to be implanted without open chest procedures—the so-called nonthoracotomy systems (Bardy et. al., 1992; Block et al., 1992; McGowan et al., 1991) (Fig. 53–39). Another development that has allowed implantation of nonthoracotomy ICDs is the use of biphasic shock waveforms. Most ICDs use monophasic shock waveforms in which the current path is in the same direction throughout the shock. Biphasic shock waveforms, in which the current direction is switched to the opposite direction part way through the shock, decrease the energy required for defibrillation, compared with monophasic waveforms, in most patients (Bardy et al., 1989; Fain et al., 1989). ICDs with biphasic shock capabilities connected to nonthoracotomy lead configurations can be implanted successfully in most patients, obviating the need for an open chest procedure with its morbidity and mortality. The operative mortality rate associated with new nonthoracotomy systems is less than 1%, and hospital stays have been dramatically decreased (Bardy et al., 1992; Block et al., 1992; McGowan et al., 1991).

Present ICDs are relatively large devices with rela-

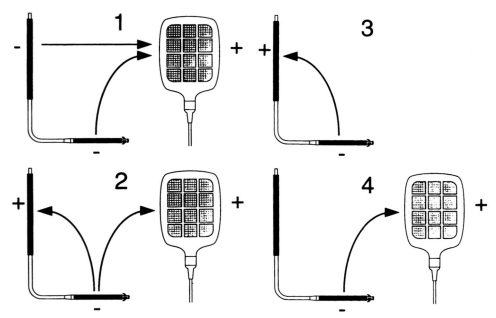

**FIGURE 53–39.** Various possible lead configurations using an intravascular lead with or without a subcutaneous patch. The intravascular lead (Endotak, CPI, St. Paul, MN) has a coiled defibrillation electrode at its distal end, which is situated in the right ventricular apex, and more proximally, which is usually located in the high right atrium. A lead-alone system can be used (configuration 3) with the distal electrode as cathode ($-$) and the proximal electrode as anode ($+$), or the patch can be utilized in conjunction with the lead (configurations 1, 2, and 4). The most commonly used are configurations 2 and 3. (From McGowan R., Maloney, J., Wilkoff, B., et al.: Automatic implantable cardioverter-defibrillator implantation without thoracotomy using an endocardial and submuscular patch system. J. Am. Coll. Cardiol., 17:415–521, 1991. Reprinted with permission from the American College of Cardiology [Journal of the American College of Cardiology, 1991, Vol. 17, pp. 415–521].)

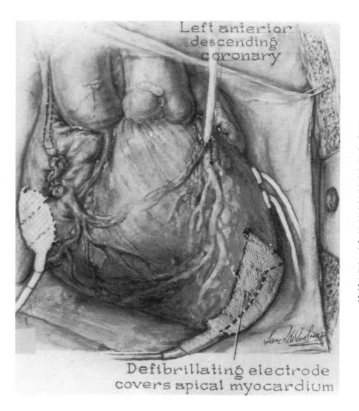

**FIGURE 53–40.** Defibrillation patches placed via a midline sternotomy on the lateral left ventricle (large patch) and the lateral right atrium (small patch). Instead of the small right atrial patch, an intravascular spring coil electrode *(dashed outline)* could have been placed in the high right atrium from a subclavian vein approach. Epicardial screw-in sensing electrodes are attached to the high lateral left ventricle. Alternatively, an endocardial pacing lead could have been placed into the right ventricle via the subclavian vein for rate sensing. An advantage of the midline sternotomy approach is the ability to perform concomitant procedures, such as the revascularization of the left anterior descending coronary artery. (From Watkins, L., Jr., Guarnieri, T., and Taylor, E., Jr.: The surgical approaches to ICD implantation. *In* Naccarelli, G. V., and Veltri, E. P. [eds]: Implantable Cardioverter-Defibrillators. Boston, Blackwell Scientific, 1993, pp. 86–101. Reprinted by permission of Blackwell Scientific Publications, Inc.)

tively short life spans (approximately 3 years). Most of the size of ICDs encompasses the capacitors, which allow 30 J of energy output and lithium batteries for charging the capacitors. Ongoing developments in capacitor technology will create smaller generators with potentially greater longevity. ICDs small enough for pectoral implantation are presently under clinical evaluation.

## Implantation Technique

The shock electrode configuration used and the necessity for other cardiac procedures determines the surgical approach to the patient. If epicardial patches are used, access can be obtained by midline sternotomy, left-sided thoracotomy, subxiphoid, and subcostal approaches (Figs. 53–40, 53–41, and 53–42). When concomitant cardiac procedures are not indicated, a subxiphoid or subcostal approach has the advantage of smaller surgical incisions; however, visibility and access to the heart are limited. Midline sternotomy offers the greatest range of patch placements as well as safety and is preferred in many centers. In addition, it is the preferred approach when concomitant surgery such as coronary artery revascularization is required. A left-sided thoracotomy may be used in patients with prior sternotomies, but access to the right side of the heart may be difficult. Because epicardial patches should be placed on opposite sides of

the heart to enclose as much of the myocardial mass as possible, left-sided thoracotomies may not allow adequate defibrillation thresholds to be obtained (Tedder et al., 1993).

Epicardial shocking patches may be sewn directly onto the myocardium or attached to the inside or outside of the pericardium. Care must be taken to ensure that the patches do not buckle or crinkle during their application to the heart or pericardium and during closure of the chest, because this buckling will decrease the effective surface area of the lead and potentially elevate the defibrillation threshold. Extrapericardial attachment is advantageous in that it does not violate the pericardial space, which could hamper any subsequent cardiac procedures, but it is technically more difficult. Typical epicardial lead locations include lateral right atrial–lateral left ventricular or anterior right ventricular–posterior left ventricular configurations. Anterior left ventricular–posterior left ventricular lead configurations should be avoided if possible, because defibrillation thresholds may be too high (Tedder et al., 1993). In general, a lead configuration should incorporate as much of the right and left ventricular mass between the patches as possible in order to obtain the lowest defibrillation thresholds. Defibrillation thresholds also decrease with increasing surface area of the lead system used, so the surface area of the lead should be as large as possible (Troup et al., 1985). However, if epicardial patch size is too large so that edges are not roughly equidistant, cur-

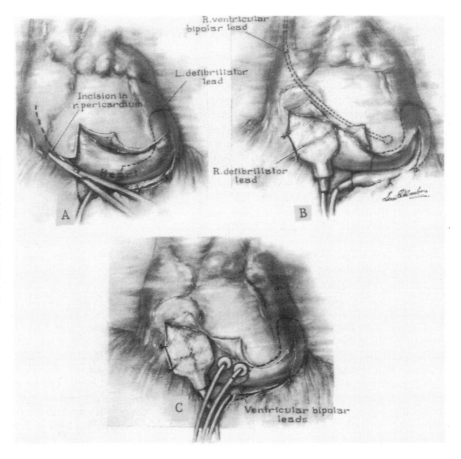

FIGURE 53–41. Subxiphoid approach to placement of an ICD. Through a subxiphoid incision, the dissection is carried down to the pericardial sac, which is incised (A) to allow placement of two epicardial patches, either with an endocardial rate sensing lead (B) or epicardial rate sensing leads (C). (From Watkins, L., Jr., Guarnieri, T., and Taylor, E., Jr.: The surgical approaches to ICD implantation. In Naccarelli, G. V., and Veltri, E. P. [eds]: Implantable Cardioverter-Defibrillators. Boston, Blackwell Scientific, 1993, pp. 86–101. Reprinted by permission of Blackwell Scientific Publications, Inc.)

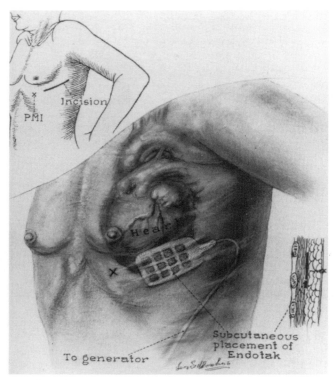

**FIGURE 53–42.** Location of the left lateral thoracic subcutaneous patch to be used with a right-sided intracardiac defibrillation lead for a nonthoracotomy approach. (From Watkins, L., Jr., Guarnieri, T., and Taylor, E., Jr.: The surgical approaches to ICD implantation. *In* Naccarelli, G. V., and Veltri, E. P. [eds]: Implantable Cardioverter-Defibrillators. Boston, Blackwell Scientific, 1993, pp. 86–101. Reprinted by permission of Blackwell Scientific Publications, Inc.)

rent shunting can occur where the edges of the two patches are too close. Different sizes of epicardial patches are available and should be selected for the individual patient to optimize surface area while maintaining appropriate interelectrode distance.

Nonthoracotomy defibrillation lead systems use intravascular shock electrodes. These electrodes may have a distal and proximal coil electrode for delivering the electrical shock. With this design, the distal shocking electrode is located in the right ventricle when the lead is positioned in the right ventricular apex, similar to a typical ventricular pacing lead. The proximal shocking electrode is located roughly at the right atrial–superior vena cava junction. Defibrillation can use the lead only or may be between the lead and a subcutaneous or submuscular patch placed along the left lateral or posterior thorax (see Fig. 53–42). A defibrillation lead system using one shocking electrode placed into the right ventricular apex and another in the coronary sinus is also effective and presently under evaluation (Yee et al., 1992). Defibrillation with up to 30 J appears to be safe using these leads in the coronary sinus.

Rate-sensing leads may be composed of either two epicardial screw-in electrodes or an endocardial bipolar lead placed in the right ventricle via the subclavian vein and tunneled to the ICD generator, which, because of its size, must be placed in a subcutaneous or subrectus abdominal wall site. Endocardial sensing electrodes are preferred to epicardial leads, given the improved sensing and pacing characteristics and better long-term survival of endocardial leads. The abdominal pocket should be fashioned carefully to allow sufficient overlying tissue to prevent subsequent erosion. A subrectus pocket probably provides the greatest degree of protection from this complication. The pocket should also be fashioned so that the ICD generator does not rub against the costal margin. Because healing tends to retract the ICD toward the costal margin, the margin of distance from the costal margin should be sufficient. As mentioned earlier, ICDs small enough for subcutaneous or submuscular pectoral implantation are now being evaluated and should further simplify the implantation procedure.

During implantation of an ICD, it is critically important to ensure that supplemental means of defibrillation are available and functional *before* the procedure starts. Supplemental defibrillation means are needed in case the external defibrillator used for ICD testing fails or in case ventricular tachycardia or fibrillation occurs before the defibrillator is implanted. For open chest procedures, a stand-alone defibrillator with external and internal paddles is often sufficient. If a subxyphoid or subcostal implantation route is used, large adhesive cutaneous defibrillation pads should be placed before the patient is prepped and draped. External defibrillation pads should also be used during placement of nonthoracotomy systems.

## Intraoperative Testing

A critical component of ICD implantation is intraoperative testing of each component of the device to ensure appropriate postoperative function. Three components need to be tested. First, the rate-sensing leads must be tested to determine if the ventricular electrogram is of sufficient magnitude. The minimum acceptable electrogram amplitude is 6 mV, and a value greater than 10 mV is preferable. This aspect of electrogram testing is important, because the ventricular electrogram becomes much smaller in ventricular fibrillation than it is in sinus rhythm. Thus, a sufficiently large electrogram in sinus rhythm is required to ensure an adequate electrogram during ventricular fibrillation; otherwise, failure to detect ventricular fibrillation and deliver therapy may occur.

The second component of the ICD system that must be tested intraoperatively is the defibrillation electrode system. After placement of epicardial patches or the nonthoracotomy lead system, the leads are connected to an external cardioverter-defibrillator that mimics the function of the device to be implanted. Using an external source to induce ventricular fibrillation, the external device is used to deliver defibrillation shocks at various shock strengths. Using a systematic protocol that involves repeated inductions of fibrillation and shock delivery, one determines the lowest shock strength that successfully defibrillates (called the *defibrillation threshold,* or DFT). The defibrillation threshold should be *at least* 10 J less than the maximum output of the ICD to be implanted (typically 30 to 35 J) (Marchlinski et al., 1988). The safety margin is needed to ensure that defibrillation occurs despite a change in clinical status of the patient.

Although this method of testing defines a defibrillation "threshold," in actuality an absolute threshold does not exist (Rattes et al., 1987). That is, the DFT does not represent a point above which all shocks are always successful. Rather, the probability of successful defibrillation of different-strength shocks is best defined by a sigmoidal dose-response curve (see Fig. 53–36). As shock strength is increased, the probability of successful defibrillation progressively increases. Usual means of determining the DFT used intraoperatively typically define a shock strength that is successful approximately 60% of the time. If two out of two sequential attempts are successful at a given energy, the probability of success at that energy approaches 80%. Maintenance of an adequate safety margin above the DFT for the defibrillation shocks also ensures that the delivered shock is nearly 100% effective. Obviously, the lower the DFT that can be obtained intraoperatively, the greater the available safety margin.

High DFTs (> 25 J) occur in approximately 5% of patients using epicardial patch electrode configurations and monophasic waveforms (Epstein et al., 1992). The most common causes of increased DFTs with epicardial patch systems are inadequate surface area of the defibrillation electrodes and inadequate placement of the patches to incorporate both ventricles within the interelectrode axis. As previously mentioned, electrode configurations that do not incorporate both ventricles have the highest DFT (Tedder et al., 1993). Other correctable causes for elevated DFTs include poor contact of the electrode with the myocardium, crinkling of the patches, too much fluid in the pericardial sac, or close apposition of the edges of the patches to allow current shunting, and shunting of current away from the patient through poorly grounded monitoring equipment. Patient-related factors include ischemia, antiarrhythmic drug use, hypothermia, and increased myocardial mass. Cardiopulmonary bypass does not appear to affect the DFTs (Klein et al., 1986). Identification and correction of these problems usually decrease the DFT to an acceptable range (< 25 J). Typically, the left ventricular shock electrode is the cathode and the right ventricular or right atrial electrode is the anode. Reversing this polarity will occasionally help decrease the DFT (O'Neill et al., 1991). More recently, use of ICDs with biphasic waveforms has greatly decreased the frequency of high DFT using epicardial patch systems (Bardy et al., 1989; Fain et al., 1989). With nonthoracotomy lead systems, similar factors can decrease the efficacy of defibrillation. Relatively small degrees of lead dislodgment may significantly affect the DFT and may be corrected by lead repositioning. Options for increasing defibrillation lead surface area include the placement of subcutaneous or submuscular patches along the left lateral thorax. As mentioned earlier, the use of biphasic waveforms has greatly decreased the frequency of elevated DFTs, precluding the use of the nonthoracotomy system.

The third component of the ICD system that must be tested intraoperatively is the ICD to be implanted connected to the defibrillation lead system. This tests the integrity of the final system as a unit and the appropriate function of the ICD generator. Minimally, the ICD should be tested to see if ventricular fibrillation is appropriately sensed and terminated. Intraoperative assessment of antitachycardia pacing and low-energy cardioversion for termination of ventricular tachycardia can also be tested, but this is more conveniently tested postoperatively in the electrophysiology laboratory. Antibradycardia functions, if available in the device, should also be tested. Finally, the ICD is programmed to the desired parameters. The ICD should be programmed off until the surgical implantation is completed and reactivated before the patient leaves the operating suite or else in the recovery room. The ICD is deactivated to prevent inadvertent shock delivery due to sensing of electrocautery or motion artifact during lead connection.

## Postoperative Management

Several specific management problems arise postoperatively in the patient with ICD. Probably the most common is the occurrence of atrial fibrillation with a ventricular rate that triggers the ICD to shock inappropriately. This problem is handled best by programming the ICD to a rate above that encountered in atrial fibrillation if this would not exclude recognition of the patient's ventricular tachyarrhythmia. More commonly, the ICD must be temporarily programmed off until pharmacologic slowing of the ventricular rate can be obtained. Older model ICDs could be programmed off by holding a doughnut-shaped magnet over the header end of the ICD. With an activated device, beeping tones synchronous with ventricular sensing will be emitted for several seconds (indicating that the device was activated) before a continuous beeping tone is emitted indicating deactivated status.

Some recent models cannot be altered by magnet application or may be programmed to be activated or deactivated by magnet application. Information regarding how the patient's ICD can be deactivated needs to be charted to ensure prompt care of the patient if repetitive discharges for atrial arrhythmias occur. However, if the patient's ICD is programmed off, the patient must be closely monitored so that therapy for recurrent ventricular tachycardia can be administered if necessary. The agents used to control atrial fibrillation may also slow the rate of spontaneous ventricular tachycardia below the programmed rate cutoff. This issue can be addressed at the time of postoperative testing. Careful reporting of the functional status of the patient's ICD must be maintained so that the device is not left deactivated after the patient's course is stabilized. Another problem that can be encountered in patients with ICDs is that frequent recurrent episodes of ventricular tachycardia can cause repetitive ICD shocks. Administering antiarrhythmic drugs, controlling ischemia and heart failure, and limiting the use of adrenergic agonists are potential means of controlling the repetitive episodes of ventricular tachycardia. Both the problems of recurrent atrial and ventricular tachyarrhythmias are seen much less frequently in the era of nonthoracotomy lead system. As with any prosthetic device, postoperative infections should be treated aggressively to prevent infection of the ICD system.

Before discharge from the hospital, the patient should undergo testing of the function of the ICD. The device should be tested for appropriate recognition and termination of ventricular fibrillation and, if applicable, ventricular tachycardia. In addition, the low-energy cardioversion thresholds for each of the patient's ventricular tachycardia morphologies can be obtained and antitachycardia pacing algorithms tested. Detailed postoperative testing thus allows optimal programming of the patient's ICD. With optimal management and programming, the frequency of painful high-energy shocks has significantly decreased in most patients, improving their acceptance of this form of therapy.

### ICD Follow-Up

Routine follow-up of ICD patients includes clinic visits every 2 to 3 months, at which time a detailed cardiac history and physical examination are obtained, and the device is interrogated and reprogrammed as clinically indicated. In addition, the capacitors should be reformed, because this improves the function and longevity of the ICD. A chemical reaction occurs between the capacitor plate and the dielectric between the plates; application of a charge across the capacitor reverses this chemical reaction to restore, or reform, the capacitor. Some recent ICD models automatically reform the capacitors periodically. During follow-up, careful attention should also be focused on the patient's other clinical problems, such as ischemia or heart failure. Exacerbation of ischemia or heart failure may increase the frequency of ventricular arrhythmias and shock delivery.

After any change in antiarrhythmic drug therapy, whether for ventricular or for supraventricular arrhythmias, the ICD should be retested to ensure that it continues to function appropriately at the programmed settings. Frequently, changes in antiarrhythmic drug therapy decrease the rate of ventricular tachycardia, potentially below the rate cutoff for recognition of tachycardia. In addition, some antiarrhythmic drugs increase the defibrillation threshold, although typically the change is relatively small. Amiodarone, flecainide, and propafenone may have the greatest effect on increasing the defibrillation threshold, whereas quinidine, procainamide, disopyramide, and mexiletine may have modest or inconsistent ef-

fects (Gremillion and Echt, 1993). Sotalol appears to have a minimal effect. Despite these generalizations, the effect of any drug on tachycardia rate or defibrillation threshold is unpredictable, so ICD function should be re-evaluated carefully after any change in the antiarrhythmic drug regimen.

Careful records should be maintained on each patient with an ICD. Changes in programmed values, details of therapy delivery, and the battery status should be recorded. The battery status of older models of ICDs was followed by measuring the charge time. Once the charge time exceeded a predetermined value, the ICD had to be replaced promptly so that therapy could be continued. Newer models still display charge times, but they also label the battery status to indicate when an *elective replacement indicator* (ERI) is present. In addition, some newer models can be programmed to deliver a series of beeping tones at regular intervals once an ERI has been reached. Transtelephonic evaluation of ICDs is now possible but not yet widely used (Porterfield et al., 1991).

### Future

In a little more than a decade, ICDs have dramatically changed the approach to management of patients with ventricular tachycardia and fibrillation. ICD technology has evolved rapidly given the need and success of this form of therapy. Improvements in nonthoracotomy lead systems and downsizing of the ICD generator size will continue over the next few years so that pectoral implants will be feasible for most patients. ICDs with both ventricular and dual-chamber pacing capabilities that do not prematurely deplete ICD generator lifespan are being designed. Limited-capability ICDs placed prophylactically in patients who have not had, but are at high risk for, ventricular tachyarrhythmias may also become feasible.

### SELECTED BIBLIOGRAPHY

Committee on Pacemaker Implantation: Guidelines for implantation of cardiac pacemakers and antiarrhythmia devices. J. Am. Coll. Cardiol., 18:1–13, 1991.

These are the most recent published guidelines for implantation of permanent pacemakers, antiachycardia pacemakers, and implantable cardioverter-defibrillators, as established by a joint committee of the American Heart Association and the American College of Cardiology. These guidelines provide practical information on acceptable and unacceptable indications for pacemaker and defibrillator implantation, and they provide useful clinical background information supporting the indications. This should be read in detail by anyone prescribing or implanting pacemakers or defibrillators.

Barold, S. S. (ed): Modern Cardiac Pacing. Mt. Kisco, NY, Futura, 1985.

This is a comprehensive reference concerning detailed discussions of all aspects of cardiac pacing. The text includes well-written chapters that provide technical information on pacemakers and pacing leads, and it serves as a valuable resource on pacemaker technology. Also included are excellent discussions on practical aspects of cardiac pacing including indications, troubleshooting, pacemaker timing cycles, implantation techniques, and the like. This text provides more in-depth information for the reader interested in understanding the intricacies of cardiac pacemakers.

Benditt, D. G. (ed): Rate-Adaptive Pacing. Boston, Blackwell Scientific, 1993.

The area of rate-adaptive pacing is rapidly changing. This text reviews in detail the specifics of the hemodynamic and clinical benefits of rate-adaptive pacing and discusses advances in rate-adaptive pacing technology. There are excellent chapters reviewing each of the sensors presently being evaluated for use in rate-adaptive pacemakers.

Naccarelli, G. V., and Veltri, E. P. (eds): Implantable Cardioverter-Defibrillators. Boston, Blackwell Scientific, 1993.

This well-written, multiauthored text concerns technical and clinical aspects of the implantable cardioverter-defibrillators. It provides practical information for individuals involved in the care of patients with implantable cardioverter-defibrillators. The preoperative evaluation, intraoperative testing, and postoperative management of patients with defibrillators are discussed.

Schechter, D. C.: Exploring the Origins of Electrical Cardiac Stimulation. Minneapolis, Medtronics, Inc., 1983.

This monograph contains selected works of Schechter on the history of electrotherapy. Areas covered in detail include the origins of electrotherapy, the background of clinical cardiac electrostimulation, and early observations on the pathophysiology of ventricular fibrillation. This special volume is exceptionally well illustrated and referenced and represents an outstanding source for those interested in the fascinating history of cardiac pacing.

## BIBLIOGRAPHY

Akhtar, M.: Retrograde conduction in man. PACE, 4:548, 1981.
Akhtar, M., Avitall, B., Jazayeri, M., et al.: Role of implantable cardioverter defibrillator therapy in the management of high-risk patients. Circulation, 85(Suppl. I):131–139, 1992.
Aldini, G.: General Views on the Application of Galvanism to Medical Purposes. London, J. Callow, 1819.
Allen, P., and Lillehei, C. W.: Use of induced cardiac arrest in open heart surgery: Results in seventy patients. Minn. Med., 40:672, 1957.
Alpert, M. A., Curtis, J. J., San Felippo, J. F., et al.: Comparative survival after permanent ventricular and dual chamber pacing for patients with chronic high degree atrioventricular block with and without pre-existent congestive heart failure. J. Am. Coll. Cardiol., 7:925, 1986.
Althaus, J.: Report of the committee appointed by the Royal Medical and Chirurgical Society to inquire into the uses and the physiological, therapeutical and toxic effects of chloroform. Med. Chir. Trans., 47:416, 1864.
Antonioli, G. E., Anscani, L., Barbieri, D., et al.: Single-lead VDD pacing. In Barold, S. S., and Mugica, J. (eds): New Perspectives in Cardiac Pacing 3. Mt. Kisco, NY, Futura, 1993, pp. 359–381.
Armour, J. A., Roy, O. Z., Firor, W. B., et al.: A battery-less biological cardiovascular pacemaker. Surg. Forum, 17:164, 1966.
Bardy, G. H., Ivey, T. D., Allen, M. D., et al.: A prospective randomized evaluation of biphasic versus monophasic waveform pulses on defibrillation efficacy in humans. J. Am. Coll. Cardiol., 14:728–733, 1989.
Bardy, G. H., Troutman, C., Poole, J. E., et al.: Clinical experience with a tiered-therapy, multiprogrammable antiarrhythmia device. Circulation, 85:1689–1698, 1992.
Barold, S. S., and Mugica, J.: Advances in technology and clinical applications. In Barold, S. S. (ed): The Third Decade of Cardiac Pacing. Mt. Kisco, NY, Futura, 1982.
Beck, C. S., Pritchard, W. H., and Feil, H. S.: Ventricular fibrillation of long duration abolished by electric shock. J. A. M. A., 135:985, 1947.
Berkovits, B. V., Castellanos, A., Jr., and Lemberg, L.: Bifocal demand pacing. Circulation, 39:44, 1969.
Bernstein, A. D., Camm, A. J., Fletcher, R. D., et al.: The NASPE/BPEG generic pacemaker code for antibradyarrhythmia and adaptive-rate pacing and antitachyarrhythmia devices. PACE, 10:794, 1987.
Bernstein, A. D., and Parsonnet, V.: Survey of cardiac pacing in the United States in 1989. Am. J. Cardiol., 69:331–338, 1992.
Bigelow, W. G., Callaghan, J. C., and Hopps, J. A.: General hypothermia for experimental intracardiac surgery. The use of electrophrenic respirations, an artificial pacemaker for cardiac standstill, and radio-frequency rewarming in general hypothermia. Ann. Surg., 132:531, 1950.
Billhardt, R. A., Rosenbush, S. W., and Hauser, R. G.: Successful

management of pacing system malfunctions without surgery: The role of programmable pulse generators. PACE, 5:675, 1982.
Block, M., Hammel, D., and Isbruch, F.: Results and realistic expectations with transvenous lead systems. PACE, 15(Part III):665–670, 1992.
Bradof, J., Sands, M. J., and Lakin, P. C.: Symptomatic venous thrombosis of the upper extremity complicating permanent transvenous pacing: Reversal with streptokinase infusion. Am. Heart J., 104:1112, 1982.
Branson, J. A.: Radiology of cardiac pacemakers and their complications with three cases of superior vena caval obstruction. Australas. Radiol., 22:125, 1978.
Brockman, S. K., Webb, R. C., Jr., and Bahnson, H. T.: Monopolar ventricular stimulation for the control of acute surgically produced heart block. Surgery, 44:910, 1958.
Byrd, C. L.: Safe introducer technique for pacemaker lead implantation. PACE, 15:262–267, 1992.
Calfee, R. V., and Saulson, S. H.: A voluntary standard for 3.2 mm unipolar and bipolar pacemaker leads and connectors. PACE, 9:1181, 1986.
Chardack, W. M., Gage, A. A., Federico, A. J., et al.: Five years' clinical experience with an implantable pacemaker: An appraisal. Surgery, 58:915, 1965.
Chardack, W. M., Gage, A. A., and Greatbatch, W.: A transistorized self-contained, implantable pacemaker for the long-term correction of heart block. Surgery, 48:643, 1960.
Chen, P.-S., Shibata, N., Dixon, E. G., et al.: Activation during ventricular defibrillation in open-chest dogs. J. Clin. Invest., 77:810–823, 1986.
Chen, P.-S., Shibata, N., Dixon, E. G., et al.: Comparison of the defibrillation threshold and the upper limit of ventricular vulnerability. Circulation, 73:1022–1028, 1986.
Chen, P.-S., Wolf, P. D., Melnick, S. D., et al.: Comparison of activation during ventricular fibrillation and following unsuccessful defibrillation shocks in open-chest dogs. Circ. Res., 66:1544–1560, 1990.
Cholankeril, J. V., Joshi, R. R., and Ketyer, S.: Benign superior vena cava syndrome caused by transvenous cardiac pacemaker. Cardiovasc. Intervent. Radiol., 5:40, 1982.
Cywinski, J. K., Hahn, A. W., Nichols, M. F., et al.: Performance of implanted biogalvanic pacemakers. PACE, 1:117, 1978.
Dhingra, R. C., Denes, P., Wu, D., et al.: The significance of second degree atrioventricular block and bundle branch block: Observations regarding site and type of block. Circulation, 49:638, 1974.
Dieter, R. A., Jr., Asselmeier, G. H., Hamouda, F., et al.: Neural complications of transvenous pacemaker implantation: Hoarseness and diaphragmatic paralysis: Case reports. Milit. Med., 146:647, 1981.
Domenighetti, G., and Perret, C.: Intraventricular conduction disturbances in acute myocardial infarction: Short- and long-term prognosis. Eur. J. Cardiol., 11:51, 1980.
Driscol, T. E., Ratnoff, O. D., and Nygaard, O. F.: The remarkable Dr. Abildgaard and countershock. Ann. Intern. Med., 83:878–882, 1975.
Duchenne de Boulogne: De L'Electrisation Localisée et son Application à la Pathologie et à la Therapeutique. Paris, Baillière, 1872.
Ekestrom, S., Johansson, L., and Lagergren, H.: Behandling av Adams-Stokes syndrom med en intracardiell pacemaker elektrod. Opusc. Med., 7:1, 1962.
Eldar, M., Griffin, J. C., Van Hare, G. F., et al.: Combined use of beta-adrenergic blocking agents and long-term cardiac pacing for patients with the long QT syndrome. J. Am. Coll. Cardiol., 20:830–837, 1992.
Elmquist, R., and Senning, A.: Implantable pacemaker for the heart. In Smyth, C. N. (ed): Medical Electronics. Proceedings of the Second International Conference on Medical Electronics. Paris, June, 1959; London, Iliffe & Sons, 1960.
Epstein, A. E., Ellenbogen, K. A., Kirk, K. A., et al.: Clinical characteristics and outcome of patients with high defibrillation thresholds. Circulation, 86:1206–1216, 1992.
Epstein, A. E., Kay, G. N., Plumb, V. J., et al.: Combined automatic implantable cardioverter-defibrillator and pacemaker systems: Implantation techniques and follow-up. J. Am. Coll. Cardiol., 13:121–131, 1989.

Estes, N. A. M., III, Salem, D. N., Isner, J. M., and Gamble, W. J.: Permanent pacemaker therapy in corrected transposition of the great arteries: Analysis of site of lead placement in 40 patients. Am. J. Cardiol., 52:1091, 1983.

ESVEM Investigators: Determinants of predicted efficacy of antiarrhythmic drugs in the electrophysiologic study versus electrocardiographic monitoring trial. Circulation, 87:323–329, 1993.

Fabiato, A., Coumel, P., Gourgon, R., and Saumont, R.: Le seuil de response synchrone des fibres myocardiques. Application à la comparaison expérimentale de l'efficacité des différentes formes de chocs electriques de défibrillation. Arch. Mal. Coeur, 60:527–544, 1967.

Faerestrand, S., and Ohm, O-J.: A time-related study of the hemodynamic benefit of atrioventricular synchronous pacing evaluated by Doppler echocardiography. PACE, 8:838, 1985.

Fain, E. S., Sweeney, M. B., and Franz, M. R.: Improved internal defibrillation efficacy with a biphasic waveform. Am. Heart J., 117:358–364, 1989.

Fananapazir, L., Cannon, R. O., Tripodi, D., and Panza, J. A.: Impact of dual-chamber permanent pacing in patients with obstructive hypertrophic cardiomyopathy with symptoms refractory to verapamil and β-adrenergic blocker therapy. Circulation, 85:2149–2161, 1992.

Fischell, R. E., Lewis, K. B., Schulman, J. H., et al.: A long-lived, reliable, rechargeable cardiac pacemaker. In Schaldach, M. (ed): Advances in Pacemaker Technology. New York, Springer-Verlag, 1975, p. 357.

Fisher, J. D., Kim, S. G., Furman, S., and Matos, J. A.: Role of implantable pacemakers in control of recurrent ventricular tachycardia. Am. J. Cardiol., 49:194, 1982.

Fitzpatrick, A., and Sutton, R.: Tilting towards a diagnosis in recurrent unexplained syncope. Lancet, March 25, 658–660, 1989.

Fogoros, R. N., Elson, J. J., Bonnet, C. A., et al.: Efficacy of the automatic implantable cardioverter-defibrillator in prolonging survival in patients with severe underlying cardiac disease. J. Am. Coll. Cardiol., 16:381–386, 1990.

Foster, C. J.: Constrictive pericarditis complicating an endocardial pacemaker. Br. Heart J., 47:497, 1982.

Fricchione, G. L., Olson, L. C., and Vlay, S. C.: Psychiatric syndromes in patients with the automatic internal cardioverter defibrillator: Anxiety, psychological dependence, abuse, and withdrawal. Am. Heart J., 117:1411–1414, 1989.

Friedberg, C. K., Donoso, E., and Stein, W. G.: Nonsurgical acquired heart block. Ann. N. Y. Acad. Sci., 111:835, 1964.

Fromer, M., Brachmann, J., Block, M., et al.: Efficacy of automatic multimodal device therapy for ventricular tachyarrhythmias as delivered by a new implantable pacing cardioverter-defibrillator. Circulation, 86:363–374, 1992.

Fritz, T., Richeson, J. F., Fitzpatrick, P., and Wilson, G.: Venous obstruction: A potential complication of transvenous pacemaker electrodes. Chest, 83:534, 1983.

Furman, S., Escher, D. J. W., Solomon, N., et al.: Electrocardiographic manifestation of standby pacing. J. Thorac. Cardiovasc. Surg., 54:723, 1967.

Furman, S., Pannizzo, F., and Campo, I.: Comparison of active and passive leads for endocardial pacing. II. PACE, 4:78, 1981.

Furman, S., and Robinson, G.: Stimulation of the ventricular endocardial surface in control of complete heart block. Ann. Surg., 150:841, 1959.

Furman, S., and Schwedel, J. B.: An intracardiac pacemaker for Stokes-Adams seizures. N. Engl. J. Med., 261:943, 1959.

Furman, S., Schwedel, J. B., Robinson, G., and Hurwitt, E. S.: Use of an intracardiac pacemaker in the control of heart block. Surgery, 49:98, 1961.

Gibson, T. C., Davidson, R. C., and DeSilvey, D. L.: Presumptive tricuspid valve malfunction induced by a pacemaker lead: A case report and review of the literature. PACE, 3:88, 1980.

Girard, D. E., Reuler, J. B., Mayer, B. S., et al.: Cerebral venous sinus thrombosis due to indwelling transvenous pacemaker catheter. Arch. Neurol., 37:113, 1980.

Glenn, W. W. L., Mauro, A., Longo, E., et al.: Remote stimulation of the heart by radiofrequency transmission: Clinical application to a patient with Stokes-Adams syndrome. N. Engl. J. Med., 261:948, 1959.

Goetz, R. H., Dormandy, J. A., and Berkovits, B.: Pacing on demand

in the treatment of atrioventricular conduction disturbances of the heart. Lancet, 2:599, 1966.

Gott, V. L., Sellers, R., and Lillehei, C. W.: The development of an epicardial-endocardial electrode for permanent placement in Stokes-Adams disease. Surg. Forum, 11:250, 1960.

Gremillion, S. T., and Echt, D. S.: Drug-device interactions. In Naccarelli, G. V., and Veltri, E. P. (eds): Implantable Cardioverter-Defibrillators. Boston, Blackwell Scientific, 1993, pp. 185–204.

Gross, J. N., Moser, S., Benedek, Z. M., et al.: DDD pacing mode survival in patients with a dual-chamber pacemaker. J. Am. Coll. Cardiol., 19:1536–1541, 1992.

Gundersen, T., Abrahamsen, A. M., and Jorgensen, I.: Thrombosis of superior vena cava as a complication of transvenous pacemaker treatment. Acta Med. Scand., 212:85, 1982.

Hayes, D. L., Graham, K. J., Irwin, M., et al.: A multicenter experience with a bipolar tined polyurethane ventricular lead. PACE, 15:1033–1039, 1992.

Hearne, S. F., and Maloney, J. D.: Pacemaker system failure secondary to air entrapment within the pulse generator pocket: A complication of subclavian venipuncture for lead placement. Chest, 82:651, 1982.

Hindman, M. C., Wagner, G. S., Jo Ro, M., et al.: The clinical significance of bundle branch block complicating acute myocardial infarction. II: Indications for temporary and permanent pacemaker insertion. Circulation, 58:689, 1978.

His, W.: Die Thatigkeit des embryonalen Herzens und deren Bedeutung fur die tehre von der Herzbewegung beim Erwachsenen. In Curschmaun, H. (ed): Arbeiten aus der Medicinschen Klinik zu Leipzig. Leipzig, Vogel, 1893.

Hochleitner, M., Hortnagl, H., Hortnagl, H., et al.: Long-term efficacy of physiologic dual-chamber pacing in the treatment of end-stage idiopathic dilated cardiomyopathy. Am. J. Cardiol., 70:1320–1325, 1992.

Hochleitner, M., Hortnagl, H., Ng, C.-K., et al.: Usefulness of physiologic dual-chamber pacing in drug-resistant idiopathic dilated cardiomyopathy. Am. J. Cardiol., 66:198–202, 1990.

Horowitz, L. N.: The automatic implantable cardioverter defibrillator: Review of clinical results, 1980–1990. PACE, 15:604–609, 1992.

Hughes, H. C., Jr., Brownlee, R. R., and Tyers, G. F.: Failure of demand pacing with small surface area electrodes. Circulation, 54:128, 1976.

Hunter, J.: Proposals for recovery of people apparently drowned. Philos. Trans. R. Soc. Lond., 66:412, 1776.

Hunter, S. W., Roth, N. A., Bernardez, D., et al.: A bipolar myocardial electrode for complete heart block. Lancet, 70:506, 1959.

Hyman, A. S.: Resuscitation of the stopped heart by intracardial therapy. II: Experimental use of an artificial pacemaker. Arch. Intern. Med., 50:283, 1932.

Irwin, J. M., Greer, G. S., Lowe, J. E., et al.: Atrial lead perforation: A case report. PACE, 10:1378, 1987.

Jacobs, D. M., Fink, A. S., Miller, R. P., et al.: Anatomical and morphological evaluation of pacemaker lead compression. PACE, 16:434–444, 1993.

James, T. N.: The connecting pathways between the sinus node and A-V node and between the right and left atrium in the human heart. Am. Heart J., 66:498–508, 1963.

Johansson, B. W.: Longevity in complete heart block. Ann. N. Y. Acad. Sci., 167:1031, 1969.

Johns, J. A., Fish, F. A., Burger, J. D., et al.: Steroid-eluting epicardial leads in pediatric patients: Encouraging early results [Abstract]. PACE, 14:633, 1991.

Kalbfleisch, K. R., Lehmann, M. H., Steinman, R. T., et al.: Reemployment following implantation of the automatic cardioverter defibrillator. Am. J. Cardiol., 64:199–202, 1989.

Kantrowitz, A., Cohen, R., Raillard, H., et al.: The treatment of complete heart block with an implanted, controllable pacemaker. Surg. Gynecol. Obstet., 115:415, 1962.

Kappenberger, L., Gloor, H. O., Babotai, I., et al.: Hemodynamic effects of atrial synchronization in acute and long-term ventricular pacing. PACE, 5:639, 1982.

Kent, A. F. S.: Researches on the structure and function of the mammalian heart. J. Physiol. (Lond.), 14:233, 1893.

Keren, R., Aarons, D., and Veltri, E. P.: Anxiety and depression in patients with life-threatening ventricular arrhythmias: Impact of the implantable cardioverter-defibrillator. PACE, 14:181–187, 1991.

Kinney, E. L., Allen, R. P., Weidner, W. A., et al.: Recurrent pulmonary emboli secondary to right atrial thrombus around a permanent pacing catheter: A case report and review of the literature. PACE, 2:196, 1979.

Klein, G. J., Jones, D. L., Sharma, A. D., et al.: Influence of cardiopulmonary bypass on internal cardiac defibrillation. Am. J. Cardiol., 57:1194–1195, 1986.

Kouwenhoven, W. G., Hooker, D. R., and Langworthy, O. R.: Current flowing through the heart under conditions of electric shock. Am. J. Physiol., 100:344, 1932.

Kreis, D. J., Jr., Licalzi, L., and Shaw, R. K.: Air entrapment as a cause of transient cardiac pacemaker malfunction. PACE, 2:641, 1979.

Kristensson, B. E., Arnmon, K., Smedgard, P., and Ryden, L.: Physiological versus single-rate ventricular pacing: A double-blind cross-over study. PACE, 8:73, 1985.

Krug, H., and Zerbe, F.: Major venous thrombosis: A complication of transvenous pacemaker electrodes. Br. Heart J., 44:158, 1980.

Kruse, I., Arnman, K., Conradson, T. B., and Ryden, L.: A comparison of the acute and long-term hemodynamic effects of ventricular inhibited and atrial synchronous ventricular inhibited pacing. Circulation, 65:846, 1982.

Kruse, I. B., and Ryder, L.: Comparison of physical work capacity and systolic time intervals with ventricular inhibited and atrial synchronous ventricular inhibited pacing. Br. Heart J., 46:129, 1981.

Lagergren, H., and Johansson, L.: Intracardiac stimulation for complete heart block. Acta Chir. Scand., 125:562, 1963.

Lamas, G. A., Estes, N. M., Schneller, S., and Flaker, G. C.: Does dual chamber or atrial pacing prevent atrial fibrillation? The need for a randomized controlled trial. PACE, 15:1109–1113, 1992.

Lasala, A. F., Fieldman, A., Diana, D. J., and Humphrey, C. B.: Gas pocket causing pacemaker malfunction. PACE, 2:183, 1979.

Leatham, A., Cook, P., and Davies, J. G.: External electric stimulator for treatment of ventricular standstill. Lancet, 2:1185, 1956.

Lemberg, L., Castellanos, A., Jr., and Berkovits, B.: Pacing on demand in AV block. J. A. M. A., 191:12, 1965.

Lesigne, C., Levy, B., Saumont, R., et al.: An energy-time analysis of ventricular fibrillation and defibrillation thresholds with internal electrodes. Med. Biol. Eng., 14:617–622, 1976.

Levy, S., Gerard, R., Jausseran, J. M., et al.: Long-term results of permanent atrioventricular sequential demand pacing. PACE, 2:175, 1979.

Lillehei, C. W., Gott, V. L., Hodges, P. C., Jr., et al.: Transistor pacemaker for treatment of complete atrioventricular dissociation. J. A. M. A., 172:2007, 1960.

Lillehei, C. W., Levy, M. J., Bonnabeau, M. D., Jr., et al.: The use of a myocardial electrode and pacemaker in the management of acute postoperative and postinfarction complete heart block. Surgery, 56:463, 1964.

Lowe, J. E., Hartwich, T., Takla, M. W., and Schaper, J.: Ultrastructure of electrophysiologically identified human sinoatrial nodes. Basic Res. Cardiol. 83:401, 1988.

Magney, J. E., Flynn, D. M., Parsons, J. A., et al.: Anatomical mechanisms explaining damage to pacemaker leads, defibrillator leads, and failure of central venous catheters adjacent to the sternoclavicular joint. PACE, 16:445–457, 1993.

Marchlinski, F. E., Flores, B., Miller, J. M., et al.: Relation of the intraoperative defibrillation threshold to successful postoperative defibrillation with an automatic implantable cardioverter defibrillator. Am. J. Cardiol., 62:393–398, 1988.

Marchlinski, F. E., Gottlieb, C. D., Sarter, B., et al.: ICD data storage: Value in arrhythmia management. PACE, 16:527–533, 1993.

Marmorstein, M.: Contribution à l'étude des excitations électriques localisées sur le coeur en rapport avec la topographie de l'innervation du coeur chez le chien. J. Physiol. (Paris), 25:617, 1927.

Massing, G. K., and James, T. N.: Anatomical configuration of the His bundle and bundle branches in the human heart. Circulation, 53:609–621, 1976.

McAnulty, J. H., Rahimtoola, S. H., Murphy, E., et al.: Natural history of "high-risk" bundle-branch block. N. Engl. J. Med., 307:137–143, 1982.

McGowan, R., Maloney, J., Wilkoff, B., et al.: Automatic implantable cardioverter-defibrillator implantation without thoracotomy using an endocardial and submuscular patch system. J. Am. Coll. Cardiol., 17:415–521, 1991.

Meijler, F. L., and Janse, M. J.: Morphology and electrophysiology of the mammalian atrioventricular node. Physiol. Rev., 68:608–647, 1988.

Mirowski, M., Mower, M. M., Langer, A., et al.: A chronically implanted system for automatic defibrillation in active conscious dogs. Circulation, 58:90–94, 1978.

Mitchell, L. B., Duff, H. J., Manyari, D. E., and Wyse, D. G.: A randomized clinical trial of the noninvasive and invasive approaches to drug therapy of ventricular tachycardia. N. Engl. J. Med., 317:1681–1687, 1987.

Mitrovic, V., Thormann, J., Schlepper, M., and Neuss, H.: Thrombotic complications with pacemakers. Int. J. Cardiol., 2:363, 1983.

Mond, H. G., Sloman, J. G., and Edwards, R. H.: The first pacemaker. PACE, 5:278, 1982.

Mond, H. G.: Unipolar versus bipolar pacing-poles apart. PACE, 14:1411–1424, 1991.

Morley, C. A., and Sutton, R.: Carotid sinus syncope. Int. J. Cardiol., 6:287–293, 1984.

Myers, G. H., Parsonnet, V., Zucker, I. R., et al.: Biologically-energized cardiac pacemakers. Am. J. Med. Electron., 3:233, 1964.

Narahara, K. A., and Blettel, M. L.: Effects of rate on left ventricular volumes and ejection fraction during chronic ventricular pacing. Circulation, 67:323, 1983.

Newman, D., Sauve, M. J., Herre, J., et al.: Survival after implantation of the cardioverter defibrillator. Am. J. Cardiol., 69:899–903, 1992.

Nicks, R., Stening, G. F., and Hulme, E. C.: Some observations on the surgical treatment of heart block in degenerative heart disease. Med. J. Aust., 49:857, 1962.

Nicolosi, G. L., Charmet, P. A., and Zanuttini, D.: Large right atrial thrombosis: Rare complication during permanent transvenous endocardial pacing. Br. Heart J., 43:199, 1980.

Nysten, P. H.: Expériences sur le Coeur et les Autres Parties d'un Homme Décapité le 14 Brumaire, Au XI. Paris, Levkault, 1802.

Ogawa, S., Dreifus, L. S., Shenoy, P. N., et al.: Hemodynamic consequences of atrioventricular and ventriculoatrial pacing. PACE, 1:8, 1978.

O'Neill, P. G., Boahene, K. A., Lawrie, G. M., et al.: The automatic implantable cardioverter-defibrillator: Effect of patch polarity on defibrillation threshold. J. Am. Coll. Cardiol., 17:707–711, 1991.

Ong, L. S., Barold, S. S., Craver, W. L., et al.: Partial avulsion of the tricuspid valve by tined pacing electrode. Am. Heart J., 102:798, 1981.

Parsonnet, V., Bernstein, A. D., and Galasso, D.: Cardiac pacing practices in the United States in 1985. Am. J. Cardiol., 62:71–77, 1988.

Parsonnet, V., Furman, S., and Smyth, N. P.: A revised code for pacemaker identification. PACE, 4:400, 1981.

Parsonnet, V., Zucker, I. R., Gilbert, L., et al.: An intracardiac bipolar electrode for interim treatment of complete heart block. Am. J. Cardiol., 10:261, 1962.

Parsonnet, V., Zucker, I. R., Gilbert, L., et al.: Clinical use of an implantable standby pacemaker. J. A. M. A., 196:784, 1966.

Pauletti, M., Pingitore, R., and Contini, C.: Superior vena cava stenosis at site of intersection of two pacing electrodes. Br. Heart J., 42:487, 1979.

Perrins, E. J., Morley, C. A., Chen, S. L., and Sutton, R.: Randomized controlled trial of physiological and ventricular pacing. Br. Heart J., 50:112, 1983.

Peters, M. S., Schroeter, A. L., van Hale, H. M., and Broadbent, J. C.: Pacemaker contact sensitivity. Contact Dermatitis, 11:214–218, 1984.

Peuch, P., Grolleau, R., and Guimond, C.: Incidence of different types of A-V block and their localization by His bundle recordings. In Wellens, H. J. J., Lie, K. I., Janse, M. J. (eds): The Conduction System of the Heart. Lieden, H. E. Stenfert Kroese, 1976, pp. 467–484.

Porterfield, J. G., Porterfield, L. M., Bray, L., and Sugalski, J., Jr.: A prospective study utilizing a transtelephonic electrocardiographic transmission program to manage patients in the first several months post-ICD implant. PACE, 14(Part II):308–311, 1991.

Porterfield, J. G., Porterfield, L. M., Smith, B. A., et al.: Conversion rates of induced versus spontaneous ventricular tachycardia by a third generation cardioverter defibrillator. PACE, 16:170–173, 1993.

Prevost, J. L., and Battelli, F.: La mort par les courant électriques. Courant alternatif à bas voltage. J. Physiol. (Paris), 1:399, 1899.

Rattes, M. F., Jones, D. L., Sharma, A. D., and Klein, G. J.: Defibrillation threshold: A simple and quantitative estimate of the ability to defibrillate. PACE, 10:70–77, 1987.

Registers of the Royal Humane Society of London. London, Nichols and Sons, 1774–1784.

Reiter, M. J., and Hindman, M. C.: Hemodynamic effects of acute atrioventricular sequential pacing in patients with left ventricular dysfunction. Am. J. Cardiol., 49:687, 1982.

Rickards, A. F., and Donaldson, R. M.: Rate responsive pacing. Clin. Prog. Pacing Electrophysiol., 1:12, 1983.

Robinovitch, L. G.: Triple interrupter of direct currents for resuscitation: Portable model for ambulance service. J. Ment. Pathol., 8:195, 1907–1909.

Rodan, B. A., Lowe, J. E., and Chen, J. T. T.: Abdominal twiddler's syndrome. Am. J. Roentgenol., 131:1084, 1978.

Rosenqvist, M., Brandt, J., and Schuller, H.: Long-term pacing in sinus node disease: Effects of stimulation mode on cardiovascular morbidity and mortality. Am. Heart J., 116:16–22, 1988.

Samet, P., Bernstein, W. H., Nathan, D. A., and Lopez, A.: Atrial contribution to cardiac output in complete heart block. Am. J. Cardiol., 16:1, 1965.

Samet, P., and El-Sherif, N.: Cardiac Pacing. 2nd ed. New York, Grune & Stratton, 1980, pp. 631–643.

Schechter, D. C.: Background of clinical cardiac electrostimulation. I: Responsiveness of quiescent, bare heart to electricity. N. Y. State J. Med., 71:2575, 1971.

Schechter, D. C.: Background of clinical cardiac electrostimulation. IV: Early studies on the feasibility of accelerating heart rate by means of electricity. N. Y. State J. Med., 72:395, 1972.

Schechter, D. C.: Early experience with resuscitation by means of electricity. Surgery, 69:360, 1971.

Schechter, D. C.: Exploring the origins of electrical cardiac stimulation. Minneapolis, Medtronic, 1983, p. 91.

Scheinmann, M. M., Peters, R. W., Morady, F., et al.: Electrophysiologic studies in patients with bundle branch block. PACE, 6:1157, 1983.

Schwartz, D. J., Thanavaro, S., Kleiger, R. E., et al.: Epicardial pacemaker complicated by cardiac tamponade and constrictive pericarditis. Chest, 76:226, 1979.

Schwedel, J. B., Furman, S., and Escher, D. J. W.: Use of an intracardiac pacemaker in the treatment of Stokes-Adams seizures. Prog. Cardiovasc. Dis., 3:170, 1960.

Shapland, J. E., MacCarter, D., Tockman, B., and Knudson, M.: Physiologic benefits of rate responsiveness. PACE, 6:329, 1983.

Smyth, N. P. D., Basu, A. P., Bacos, J. M., et al.: Permanent transvenous synchronous cardiac pacing. Chest, 59:493, 1971.

Steiner, F.: Ueber die Electropunctur des Herzens als Wiederbelebungsmittel in der Choroformsyncope zugleich eine Studie uber Stichwunden des Herzens. Arch. Klin. Chir., 12:741, 1871.

Stillings, D.: The first defibrillation? Medical Instrumentation, 10:168, 1976.

Strickberger, S. A., Cantillon, C. O., and Friedman, P. L.: When should patients with lethal ventricular arrhythmia resume driving? Ann. Intern. Med., 115:560–563, 1991.

Sulke, N., Dritsas, A., Bostock, J., et al.: "Subclinical" pacemaker syndrome: A randomized study of symptom free patients with ventricular demand (VVI) pacemakers upgraded to dual chamber devices. Br. Heart J., 67:57–64, 1992.

Sutton, R., and Kenny, R.-A.: The natural history of sick sinus syndrome. PACE, 9:1110–1114, 1986.

Sutton, R., Morley, C., Chan, S. L., and Perrins, J.: Physiological benefits of atrial syncrony in paced patients. PACE, 6:327, 1983.

Sutton, R., Perrins, J., and Citron, P.: Physiological cardiac pacing. PACE, 3:207, 1980.

Sutton, R., Perrins, E. J., Morley, C., and Chen, S. L.: Sustained improvement in exercise tolerance following physiological cardiac pacing. Eur. Heart J., 4:781, 1983.

Tchou, P. J., Kadri, N., Anderson, J., et al.: Automatic implantable cardioverter defibrillators and survival of patients with left ventricular dysfunction and malignant ventricular arrhythmias. Ann. Intern. Med., 109:529–534, 1988.

Tedder, M., Wharton, J. M., Anstadt, M. P., et al.: Optimal defibrillation patch configuration includes the right heart and left ventricle. Am. J. Cardiol., 71:349–350, 1985.

Thevenet, A., Hodges, P. C., and Lillehei, C. W.: The use of a myocardial electrode inserted percutaneously for control of complete atrioventricular block by an artificial pacemaker. Dis. Chest, 34:621, 1958.

Troup, P. J., Chapman, P. D., Olinger, G. N., and Kleinman, L. H.: The implanted defibrillator: Relation of defibrillating lead configuration and clinical variables to defibrillation thresholds. J. Am. Coll. Cardiol., 6:1315–1321, 1985.

Tyers, G. F., and Brownlee, R. R.: The non-hermetically sealed pacemaker myth, or, Navy-Ribicoff 22,000—FDA-Weinberger. J. Thorac. Cardiovasc. Surg., 71:253, 1976.

Tyers, G. F. O., and Brownlee, R. R.: Power pulse generators, electrodes and longevity. Prog. Cardiovasc. Dis., 23:421, 1981.

Videen, J. S., Huang, S. K., Bazgan, I. D., et al.: Hemodynamic comparison of ventricular pacing, atrioventricular sequential pacing, and atrial synchronous ventricular pacing using radionuclide ventriculography. Am. J. Cardiol., 57:1305, 1986.

Waldo, A. L., and MacLean, W. A. H.: Diagnosis and treatment of cardiac arrhythmias following open heart surgery: Emphasis on the use of atrial and ventricular epicardial wire electrodes. Mt. Kisco, NY, Futura, 1980, p. 115.

Waller, T. J., Kay, H. R., Spielman, S. R., et al.: Reduction in sudden death and total mortality by antiarrhythmic therapy evaluated by electrophysiologic drug testing: Criteria of efficacy in patients with sustained ventricular tachyarrhythmia. J. Am. Coll. Cardiol., 10:83–89, 1987.

Walshe, W. H.: A Practical Treatise on the Diseases of the Heart and Great Vessels Including the Principles of Physical Diagnosis. Philadelphia, Blanchard & Lee, 1862.

Watkins, L., Jr., Guarnieri, T., Taylor, E., Jr.: The surgical approaches to ICD implantation. In Naccarelli, G. V., and Veltri, E. P. (eds): Implantable Cardioverter-Defibrillators. Boston, Blackwell Scientific, 1993, pp. 86–101.

Weirich, W. L., Gott, V. L., and Lillehei, C. W.: The treatment of complete heart block by the combined use of myocardial electrode and an artificial pacemaker. Surg. Forum, 8:360, 1957.

Weirich, W. L., Paneth, M., Gott, V. L., and Lillehei, C. W.: Control of complete heart block by use of an artificial pacemaker and a myocardial electrode. Circ. Res., 6:410, 1958a.

Weirich, W. L., Paneth, M., Gott, V. L., and Lillehei, C. W.: The treatment of complete heart block by the use of an artificial pacemaker and a myocardial electrode. Am. J. Cardiol., 2:250, 1958b.

Weirich, W. L., and Roe, B. B.: The role of pacemakers in the management of surgically induced complete heart block. Am. J. Surg., 102:293, 1961.

Welti, J. J.: Premature lithium batteries depletion. PACE, 4:349, 1981.

Wharton, J. M., Richard, V. J., Murry, C. E., et al.: Electrophysiological effects of monophasic and biphasic stimuli in normal and infarcted dogs. PACE, 13:1158–1172, 1990.

Wharton, J. M., Smith, W. M., Wolf, P. D., and Ideker, R. E.: Mechanisms of electrical defibrillation. In Luderitz, B., and Saksena, S. (eds): Interventional Electrophysiology in the Management of Cardiac Arrhythmias. Mt. Kisco, NY, Futura, 1991, pp. 361–376.

Wharton, J. M., Wolf, P. D., Smith, W. M., et al.: Cardiac potential and potential gradient fields generated by single, combined, and sequential shocks during ventricular defibrillation. Circulation, 85:1510–1523, 1992.

Wiggers, C. J.: The physiologic basis for cardiac resuscitation from ventricular fibrillation—Method for serial defibrillation. Am. Heart. J., 20:413–421, 1940.

Wilber, D. J., Garan, H., Finkelstein, D., et al.: Out-of-hospital cardiac arrest. N. Engl. J. Med., 318:19–24, 1988.

Wirtzfield, A., Schmidt, G., Himmler, F. C., and Stangl, K.: Physiologic pacing: Present status and future developments. PACE, *10*:41, 1987.

Wish, M., Fletcher, R. D., Gottdiener, J. S., and Cohen, A. I.: Importance of left atrial timing in the programming of dual-chamber pacemakers. Am. J. Cardiol., *60*:566–571, 1987.

Wish, M., Swartz, J., and Cohen, A.: Steroid-tipped leads versus porous platinum permanent pacemaker leads: A controlled study. PACE, *13*:1887–1890, 1990.

Wu, D., Denes, P., Dhingra, R. C., et al.: Electrophysiological and clinical observations in patients with alternating bundle branch block. Circulation, *53*:456–464, 1976.

Yee, R., Benditt, D. G., Kostuk, W. J., et al.: Comparative functional effects of chronic ventricular demand and atrial synchronous ventricular inhibited pacing. PACE, *7*:23, 1984.

Yee, R., Klein, G. J., Leitch, J. W., et al.: A permanent transvenous lead system for an implantable pacemaker cardioverter-defibrillator. Circulation, *85*:196–204, 1992.

Youngson, G. G., McKenzie, F. N., and Nichol, P. M.: Superior vena cava syndrome: Case report. A complication of permanent transvenous endocardial cardiac pacing requiring surgical correction. Am. Heart J., *99*:503, 1980.

Ziemssen, H. von: Studien uber die Bewegungsvorgange am menschlichen Herzen, sowie uber die mechanische und elektrische Erregbarkeit des Herzens und des Nervus phrenicus, angestellt an dem freiliegenden Herzen der Catharina Serafin. Dtsch. Arch. Klin. Med., *30*:270, 1882.

Zipes, D. P., Fischer, J., King, R. M., et al.: Termination of ventricular fibrillation in dogs by depolarizing a critical amount of myocardium. Am. J. Cardiol., *36*:37–44, 1975.

Zoll, P. M.: Resuscitation of the heart in ventricular standstill by external electric stimulation. N. Engl. J. Med., *247*:768, 1952.

Zoll, P. M., Frank, H. A., Zarsky, L. R. N., et al.: Long-term electric stimulation of the heart for Stokes-Adams disease. Ann. Surg., *154*:330, 1961.

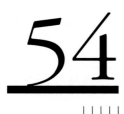

# 54 The Coronary Circulation
## ■ I Physiology of Coronary Blood Flow, Myocardial Function, and Intraoperative Myocardial Protection

J. Scott Rankin and David C. Sabiston, Jr.

A detailed knowledge of normal and pathologic physiology of the heart is of primary importance to the practice of cardiac surgery. Many patients come to the operating room with pre-existing myocardial ischemia or hypertrophy, and most cardiac operations superimpose further transient physiologic impairment. Unlike other organs, the heart must resume adequate function immediately after the procedure, so prevention of intraoperative myocardial injury and subsequent optimization of cardiac performance are critical to the survival of the patient. This section summarizes the normal and pathologic physiology of the heart, briefly reviews the general topic of intraoperative myocardial preservation, and describes practical myocardial protection techniques that have been useful in cardiac surgical practice.

## NORMAL PHYSIOLOGY

Coronary blood flow delivers oxygen and metabolic substrates to the myocardium and removes carbon dioxide and metabolic byproducts via transcapillary exchange. The function of the heart is to transfer metabolic energy in the form of oxygen and substrates into mechanical energy in the form of circulatory pressure and flow. Therefore, the cardiac ventricles and their fundamental units, the sarcomeres, can be viewed physiologically as chemomechanical energy transducers. Normal coronary blood flow approximates 0.7 to 0.9 ml/g of myocardium per minute and delivers 0.1 ml of oxygen per gram per minute to the heart, which is a high rate of energy use compared with the rest of the body. The extraction of oxygen in the coronary bed is very high, averaging 75% under normal conditions and increasing to nearly 100% during stress (Berne and Rubio, 1979).

Coronary artery blood flow occurs primarily during diastole because myocardial contraction increases intramyocardial vascular resistance during systole (Sabiston and Gregg, 1957) (Fig. 54–1). Normally, mean coronary resistance is 3 to 6 times the totally vasodilated value, and because of the high baseline oxygen extraction, increasing oxygen delivery during stress is provided primarily by vasodilatation. Assuming adequate perfusion pressure, total and regional myocardial blood flow under normal conditions is determined by autoregulation of regional arteriolar resistance modulated by local metabolic demand.

According to the most accepted theory, the fundamental unit of muscular contraction is the myosin cross-bridge (Squire, 1981). With electrical depolarization of the myocardial cell membrane, ionized calcium fluxes into the cytoplasm from *sarcoplasmic reticulum* (SR) stores, causing the myosin molecule to hydrolyze *adenosine triphospate* (ATP) into adenosine diphosphate and inorganic phosphate. When ATP is split, a considerable amount of chemical energy is released from the ATP molecule and transferred into a conformational change in the myosin cross-bridge. This chemomechanical alteration in the cross-bridge produces sliding of myosin filaments relative to actin and shortening of the sarcomere. Over the physiologic range of sarcomere lengths (1.6 to 2.0 μm), the surface area of available cross-bridge interactions, and thus the metabolic energy transferred into mechanical energy during sarcomere contraction, is linearly proportional to end-diastolic sarcomere length (Fig. 54–2). This length dependency of cross-bridge interaction at the sarcomere level constitutes the fundamental basis of the Frank-Starling relationship. As final steps in the process, calcium is removed from the cytosol by active transport of the SR, and ATP is regenerated at the mitochondrial level by aerobic metabolism of oxygen and substrates.

In many ways, the intact cardiac ventricles function as an integrated sum of their component sarcomeres. Mechanical energy production, in the form of external stroke work, is a direct linear function of end-diastolic volume (Fig. 54–3) and is not influenced significantly by physiologic changes in afterload (Glower et al., 1985). Therefore, short-term alterations in myocardial inotropism (defined as load-independent intrinsic myocardial performance) can be assessed by the slope of the stroke work/end-diastolic volume (SW/EDV) relationship. This fundamental Frank-Starling prop-

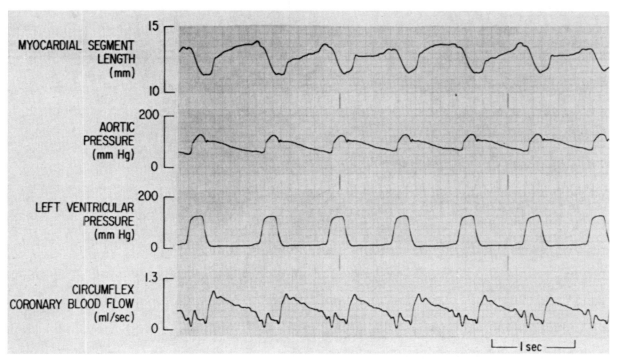

**FIGURE 54–1.** Coronary blood flow and myocardial functional characteristics observed under normal conditions in the conscious dog. Myocardial segment length was measured with pulse transit ultrasonic dimension transducers, pressures were obtained with high-fidelity micromanometers, and coronary blood flow was assessed with an implanted electromagnetic flow transducer.

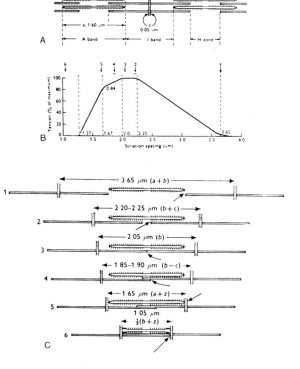

**FIGURE 54–2.** The alteration of tension actively generated by the contractile apparatus as a function of sarcomere length *(B)* and its interpretation in terms of the changing overlap of the thick and thin filaments (*A* and *C*). (*A–C*, From Gordon, A. M., Huxley, A. F., and Julian, F. J.: The variation in isometric tension with sarcomere length in vertebrate muscle fibres. J. Physiol. [London], *184*:170, 1966.)

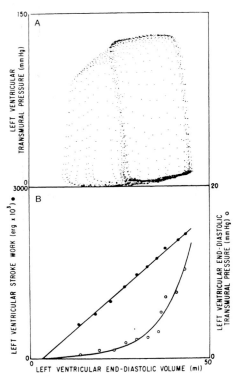

**FIGURE 54–3.** *A,* Dynamic left ventricular pressure-volume loops obtained in the conscious dog during vena caval occlusion with data digitized at 200 Hz. *B,* Stroke work–end-diastolic volume and diastolic pressure-volume curves.

erty of the heart probably directly reflects sarcomere and myosin cross-bridge dynamics.

Energetically, cardiac metabolic activity over time can be assessed by myocardial oxygen consumption ($MVO_2$). Each milliliter of oxygen utilized by the heart provides 2.02 joules of energy to the contractile apparatus via aerobic metabolic pathways and ATP. Thus, oxygen consumption can be used to quantify myocardial energy use. *Myocardial energy expenditure* has two components: external energy, which is stroke work or the integral of the ventricular pressure (P) volume (V) loop; and internal energy, which is the thermodynamic cost of maintaining systolic ventricular pressure at a given volume. Internal energy expenditure is estimated as the product of ventricular mean ejection pressure ($P_{ME}$) and end-diastolic volume ($V_{ED}$) and constitutes the sole mechanical energy production during isovolumic contraction. Thus, total mechanical energy expenditure (TME) for each cardiac cycle can be calculated as follows:

$$TME = \int PdV + P_{ME} \cdot V_{ED}$$

Because 1 mm Hg ml is equivalent to $1.333 \times 10^{-4}$ joules, TME expenditure can be compared with metabolic energy use ($MVO_2$) to obtain a linear measure of metabolic-to-mechanical energy transfer efficiency (Elbeery et al., in press; Feneley et al., 1987) (Fig. 54–4).

## PATHOPHYSIOLOGY

The pathophysiology of coronary blood flow is complex. Reduction in myocardial oxygen supply during ischemia or increasing oxygen demand during hemodynamic stress produces regulatory coronary vasodilatation. With decreasing arteriolar resistance, impedance to coronary blood flow is shifted proximally in the coronary circuit, and diastolic intramyocardial pressure becomes a relatively more important determinant of mean myocardial perfusion. In the presence of adequate arterial pressure and low diastolic cavitary pressure, the modest transmural gradient of diastolic intramyocardial force has little effect on regional myocardial perfusion through the dilated vascular bed. However, in this situation, transmural flow becomes pressure-dependent, and if perfusion pressure decreases or diastolic intracavitary pressure increases, coronary blood flow may be redistributed away from the subendocardium, where intramural compressive forces are the highest. This redistribution of flow can cause subendocardial ischemia, even in the presence of normal coronary arteries (Buckberg et al., 1972), and, together with an inherent subendocardial metabolic vulnerability (Lowe et al., 1983), contributes to subendocardial myocardial infarction.

When an atherosclerotic plaque in a proximal coronary artery decreases the cross-sectional area by 75% or more, the resistance to flow caused by the plaque becomes significant (Sabiston, 1974). The dominant point of coronary vascular impedance moves even more proximal, and the critical stenosis can limit myocardial perfusion to a fixed value. Although flow may be adequate at rest, exercise or other factors that increase myocardial oxygen demand can induce relative ischemia, a fall in coronary pressure distal to the stenosis, and redistribution of blood flow away from the subendocardium. This appears to be the mechanism of exercise-induced angina pectoris and associated myocardial dysfunction. Superimposed on the phenomenon, coronary vasospasm or unstable thrombotic plaques can compound the obstructive physiology.

Because of high metabolic demand and tight coupling between energy use and expenditure, acute coronary occlusion immediately decreases myocardial performance (Fig. 54–5). Work function of the ischemic segment ceases, and myocardial necrosis begins in the subendocardium after about 15 to 20 minutes. Reperfusion in the first hours after occlusion can create partial functional recovery, but after approximately 4 to 6 hours, infarction becomes irreversible. There are exceptions, however, including infarcted arteries with minor persistent antegrade flow and those with well-established collaterals.

Even with a totally reversible injury produced by a 15-minute coronary occlusion, dysfunction can be prolonged, and 24 to 48 hours can be required for full recovery (Fig. 54–6). Ischemic myocardial dysfunction is characterized by a diminished slope of the stroke work (end-diastolic segment length relationship) together with a rightward shifting of the X-intercept ($l_o$)

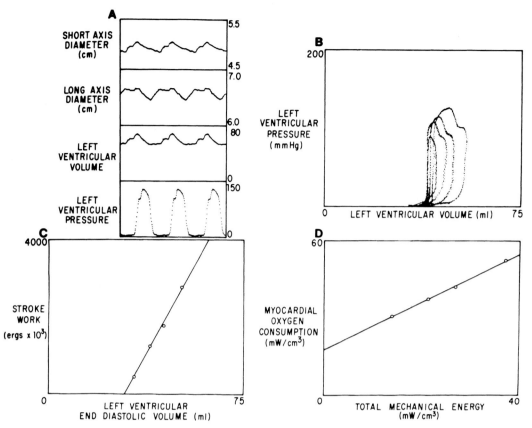

**FIGURE 54–4.** Hemodynamic variables obtained from an isolated heart. *A,* Digitized raw pressure, dimension, and derived left ventricular volume data. *B,* Digitized pressure-volume loops at four different preloads. *C,* Representative stroke work–end-diastolic volume relationship. *D,* Representative myocardial energy transfer relationship. Note that the slope of this relationship approximates unity with a finite y-axis intercept.

that has been called *diastolic creep.* With reperfusion, the slope recovers rapidly, but ($l_o$) remains stretched, diminishing work capacity at any given end-diastolic length (Fig. 54–7). Recovery of systolic function occurs slowly and is associated with a reversal of the ischemic-induced creep (Glower et al., 1987). Pressure afterloading or a second ischemic event during early reperfusion can produce prolonged dysfunction and delay ultimate recovery.

The functional and energetic changes accompanying all forms of myocardial failure (whether induced by coronary or valvular heart disease) appear exactly the same as those observed in transient ischemia. The X-intercept of the SW/EDV relationship shifts rightward, the slope falls, and the linear $MVO_2$/TME curve shifts downward in a parallel fashion (Figs. 54–8 and 54–9). This finding suggests that all forms of myocardial dysfunction may have the same functional and metabolic/energetic characteristics. Perhaps some sort of *low-grade ischemic injury* is common to each. Certainly, each form of global dysfunction could have abnormalities in diastolic coronary perfusion pressure or diastolic perfusion time. The corollary is that the cellular/molecular basis of myocardial dysfunction may also be similar among the various etiologies. Studies implicating SR abnormalities (Bentivegna et al., 1991; Limbruno et al., 1989),

together with the finding of excitation-contraction coupling problems (downward shift in Y-intercept of the $MVO_2$/TME curve in Fig. 54–9) in both ischemic and valvular disorders, suggest that SR dysfunction may be a common factor in these various settings (Koutlas et al., 1990; Lilly et al., 1990; Lucke et al., 1990, 1991).

It is clear now that atherosclerotic plaque rupture and acute coronary thrombosis constitute the dominant mechanism of myocardial infarction. At an ultrastructural level, acute postocclusion systolic dysfunction and diastolic creep can be correlated with myofilament relaxation, increased Z band separation, and widening of I bands (Fig. 54–10). Thus, ischemic myocardial dysfunction seems to represent some degree of disengagement of actin-myosin filaments and possibly some fundamental abnormality in crossbridge performance. With persistent ischemia, ultrastructural changes become more prominent, and distinct irreversible alterations are evident by 30 to 40 minutes. The cell nucleus exhibits peripherally aggregated chromatin and numerous swollen perinuclear mitochondria (Fig. 54–11). Some mitochondria contain amorphous matrix densities, and the Z bands bisect the I bands of the myofibrils. After 60 minutes of ischemia, glycogen becomes virtually absent, and the myofibrils are stretched even further (Fig. 54–12). Mi-

*Text continued on page 1822*

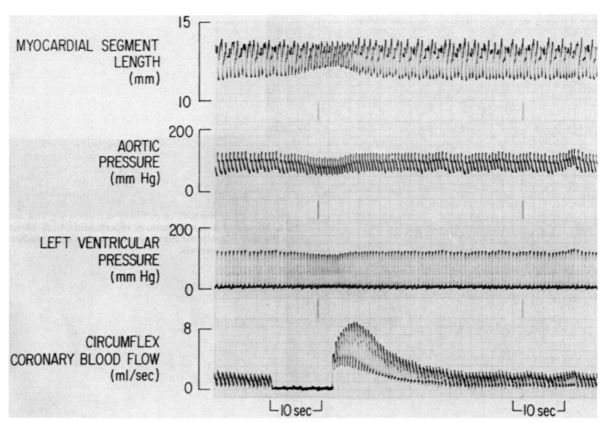

**FIGURE 54–5.** Myocardial dimension, pressure, and blood flow data obtained during a 12-second coronary occlusion in the conscious dog. Note that myocardial shortening begins to diminish rapidly after coronary occlusion and that vasodilatation associated with postischemic reactive hyperemia increases coronary blood flow by several times.

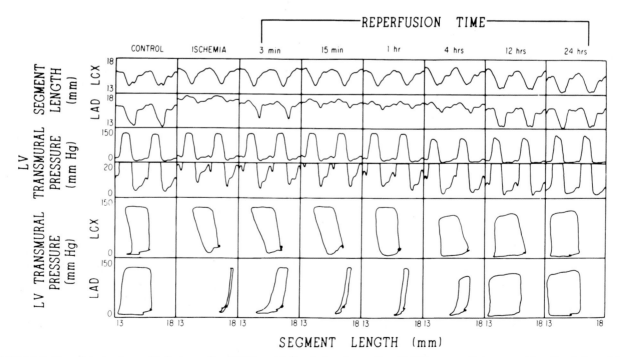

**FIGURE 54–6.** Raw data tracings of left circumflex (LCX) and left anterior descending (LAD) myocardial segment lengths, left ventricular transmural pressure, and pressure-length work loops in the control state, during 15 minutes of LAD occlusion, and after 3 minutes, 15 minutes, 1 hour, 4 hours, 12 hours, and 24 hours of LAD reperfusion. (From Glower, D. D., Spratt, J. A., Kabas, J. S., et al.: Quantification of regional myocardial function after acute ischemic injury: Application of preload recruitable stroke work. Am. J. Physiol., 255:H85, 1988.)

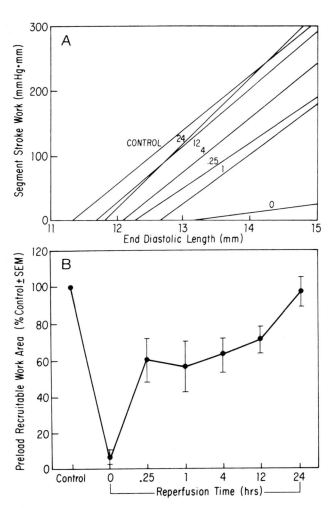

**FIGURE 54–7.** Segment stroke work–end-diastolic segment length relationships for a representative dog under control conditions, after 15 minutes of coronary occlusion (0), and after 0.25, 1, 4, 12, and 24 hours of coronary reperfusion (A). B, Mean values for area beneath the curve observed in eight studies over the same intervals.

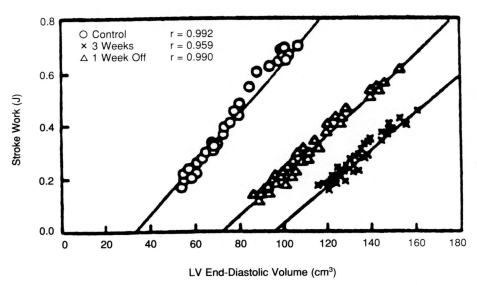

**FIGURE 54–8.** Left ventricular stroke work–end-diastolic volume relationships obtained in a conscious dog in the control state, after 3 weeks of pacing tachycardia–induced heart failure, and after 1 week of discontinuing pacing. Notice the rightward shift in the x-axis intercept (diastolic creep) associated with ventricular dilatation and the recovery of creep after cessation of pacing.

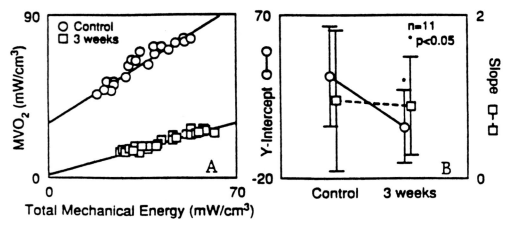

**FIGURE 54–9.** Corresponding energy transfer data in conscious dogs with pacing-induced heart failure. Myocardial dysfunction was associated primarily with a downward shift in the y-axis intercept, characteristic of excitation-contraction abnormalities or SR malfunction.

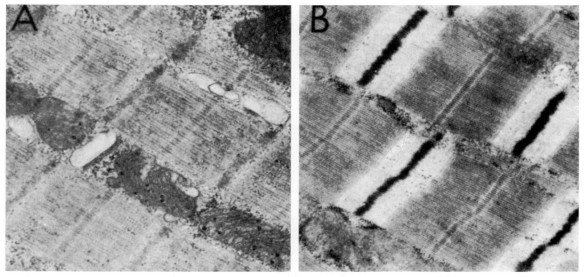

**FIGURE 54–10.** Typical electron micrographs of nonischemic *(A)* and ischemic *(B)* myocardium after 15 minutes of coronary occlusion. Note that ischemic tissue displays myofilament relaxation with increased Z band separation and widening of I bands. *(A and B,* From Glower, D. D., Schaper, J., Kabas, J. S., et al.: Relation between reversal of diastolic creep and recovery of systolic function after ischemic myocardial injury in conscious dogs. Circ. Res., *60*:850, 1987.)

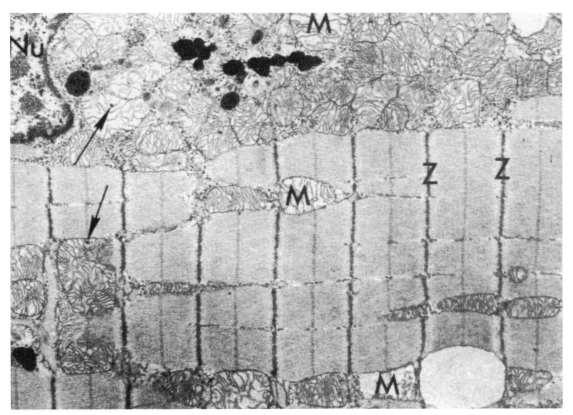

**FIGURE 54–11.** Electron micrograph of myocardial ultrastructure after 40 minutes of ischemia, showing irreversible injury. This portion of a myocardial cell illustrates a nucleus (Nu) with peripherally aggregated chromatin and numerous swollen perinuclear mitochondria (M). Some mitochondria contain tiny amorphous matrix densities. The Z bands (Z) bisect the I bands of the myofibrils. The dark bodies in the perinuclear zone are pigment granules (lysosomes, lipofuscin) and are structurally intact. (Osmium fixation; magnification × 31,000.) (From Jennings, R. B., and Ganote, C. E.: Structural changes in myocardium during acute ischemia. Circ. Res., *34, 35*[Suppl. 3]:156, 1974.)

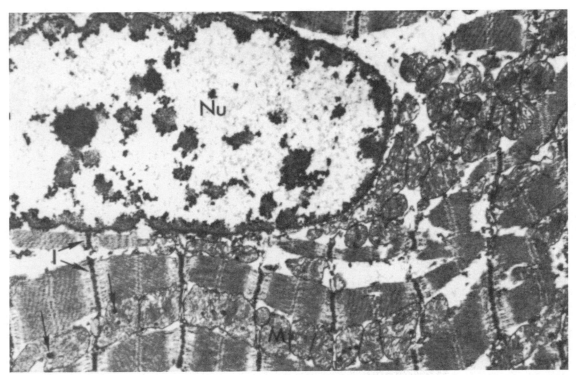

**FIGURE 54–12.** Myocardial ultrastructure after 60 minutes of ischemia, with irreversible injury. Note the margination of the chromatin in the nucleus (Nu). The myofibrils are relaxed and have prominent I bands (I); an N band is also present in the I bands. The mitochondria (M) are swollen and contain amorphous matrix densities at the *arrows*. Little or no glycogen is expected at this time, but this tissue cannot be used to illustrate this fact because the fixative extracts glycogen during processing. (Osmium fixation with uranyl acetate in block; magnification × 16,628.) (From Jennings, R. B., and Ganote, C. E.: Structural changes in myocardium during acute ischemia. Circ. Res., *34, 35*[Suppl. 3]:156, 1974.)

tochondrial and sarcolemmal abnormalities progress to total myofibrillar disruption and distortion of Z lines. When irreversibly injured myocardium is reperfused, explosive cellular swelling, deposition of calcium phosphate, and intense contracture are observed, which progress to cell rupture and death. Healing of infarcted myocardium is characterized by resorption of necrotic tissue, wall thinning, and replacement of infarcted myofibrils by fibrous tissue (Jennings and Ganote, 1974).

## PRINCIPLES OF INTRAOPERATIVE MYOCARDIAL PROTECTION

### Minimizing Operative Injury

Most cardiac operations require arrest of the heart and interruption of coronary blood flow; thus, a precise technical procedure can be performed in a quiet, bloodless field. The historical development of surgical cardioplegia is reviewed in the fifth edition of this book (Rankin and Sabiston, 1990). At present, everyone would agree that the period of induced operative ischemia should be kept as short as possible by appropriate planning of the procedure. Even with the most advanced methods of myocardial protection, ischemic tissue injury progresses exponentially with time, thus emphasizing the importance of an expeditiously per-

formed operation. With modern surgical technique, however, even the most complicated intracardiac procedures can be accomplished within 90 to 150 minutes, a period of ischemia that is well tolerated with appropriate preservation methods. Care should be taken during the operation to minimize retraction of cardiac structures, because direct damage to the heart may negate even the best method of myocardial protection.

During cardiopulmonary bypass, close attention should be given to maintaining adequate coronary perfusion pressure and ensuring satisfactory transmural blood flow distribution. Ventricular distention can limit subendocardial flow and should be prevented by appropriate perfusion techniques. Direct cardiac venting is rarely used at present. Ventricular fibrillation creates continuous myocardial wall stress, which, together with increased oxygen demand, predisposes the heart to subendocardial injury; therefore, periods of ventricular fibrillation should be avoided or minimized. Finally, there is no substitute for a well-performed operation. Good myocardial protection combined with complete correction of the physiologic defect will produce optimal operative results.

### Hypothermia

Hypothermia remains the most important technique of myocardial preservation during ischemia.

The protective effects of hypothermia are related to reduction in cardiac cellular metabolism, which diminishes energy and ATP consumption during ischemia and reduces the toxic products of metabolism such as carbon dioxide and hydrogen ions. As illustrated in Figure 54–13, oxygen consumption at 10° C in the chemically arrested, nonworking heart is less than 5% of the normal value (Chitwood et al., 1979), permitting safe ischemic arrest for prolonged periods without permanent injury.

Initial rapid induction of myocardial hypothermia is best accomplished by infusion of cold cardioplegic solution into the aortic root after aortic clamping. In current practice, 1.2 l of hypercooled 4° C crystalloid solution are infused over 3 to 4 minutes to achieve a measured myocardial temperature below 10° C. Such extreme levels of hypothermia appear to have additive protective effects (Karck et al., 1992), and are readily achievable clinically. Occasionally, with markedly hypertrophied ventricles or in the presence of a highly developed noncoronary collateral circulation, more cardioplegic solution is required to produce the desired myocardial hypothermia. Recirculation and hypercooling of the cardioplegic solution between infusions is accomplished with a commercially available cannula system (DLP, Walker, MI), a roller pump, and a heat exchanger immersed in an alcohol-ice mixture. Cardioplegic solution is periodically reinfused at 4° C to help maintain hypothermia.

Myocardial hypothermia also is maintained using combinations of other techniques. *External topical cooling* is one important method. It is readily accomplished by a continuous infusion of 4° C saline at 50 to 100 ml/min over the heart and into the pericardial cavity (Shumway et al., 1959). Excess fluid is removed by a suction catheter in the inferior aspect of the incision. Endocardial right ventricular cooling can be facilitated by continuous *intracavitary infusion* of cold saline directly into the heart, as in mitral valve replacement through an indwelling right atrial catheter (Rosenfeldt and Watson, 1979; Hearse et al., 1981; Daily et al., 1987).

Along with bronchial blood flow and noncoronary collateral circulation, return of the systemic perfusate to the heart is the major source of rewarming during hypothermic arrest (Rosenfeldt and Watson, 1979). Therefore, an additional technique, *low-flow systemic hypothermia*, is highly important in minimizing rewarming during the period of aortic occlusion (Grover et al., 1981). In current practice, systemic perfusate temperature is lowered to 24° C and systemic pump flow to 50 to 67% of calculated values during the cardioplegia period, and rewarming is begun 5 to 10 minutes before release of the aortic clamp. Lowering systemic blood flow not only reduces noncoronary collateral flow but assists in maintaining cardiac decompression with single venous cannulation. The importance of systemic hypothermia should not be underestimated; clinical experience suggests that it is a major factor in myocardial protection.

## Cardioplegic Additives

Rapid metabolic arrest of the heart can be achieved with a number of chemical components. Perhaps the most widely used at present is potassium (Gay and Ebert, 1973). High extracellular potassium reduces the transmembrane potassium gradient, depolarizes the cell, and eliminates the energy cost of maintaining membrane ionic pumps. The concentration of potassium is critical, with 15 to 20 mM/l achieving optimal results in most studies (Hearse et al., 1981).

Magnesium is a major intracellular cation contained primarily within mitochondria and myofibrils. On the cell membrane, magnesium competes for calcium receptor sites and delays calcium influx into the cell. It is an important component of high-energy phosphate molecules and a co-factor for cellular enzyme systems. When used to induce arrest, magnesium seems to inhibit excitation-contraction coupling, although it is not a very good arresting agent because of its slow onset of action. Absence of magnesium during ischemia or reperfusion can impair synthesis of ATP. Therefore, magnesium can be useful in cardioplegic solutions.

Calcium is an essential component of actin-myosin interaction and fundamentally contributes to the regulation of myocardial contraction. Calcium also is required for maintenance of membrane integrity and numerous intracellular functions. Because intracellular calcium deposition plays a significant role in is-

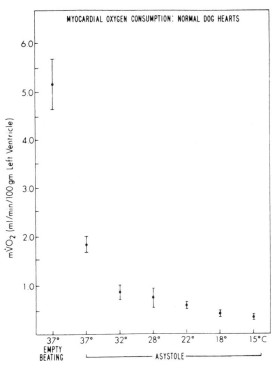

**FIGURE 54–13.** Effects of hypothermia on myocardial oxygen consumption in the potassium-arrested dog heart. (From Chitwood, W. R., Sink, J. D., Hill, R. C., et al.: The effects of hypothermia on myocardial oxygen consumption and transmural coronary blood flow in the potassium-arrested heart. Ann. Surg., *190*:106, 1979.)

chemic and reperfusion injury (Shen and Jennings, 1972), extracellular calcium should be regulated carefully during cardioplegic arrest. Reduction in calcium can diminish the cellular influx associated with ischemic injury and improve functional recovery (Hearse et al., 1981). Minute quantities of calcium, however, are essential for maintenance of cellular integrity, so maintaining a minimum concentration of calcium is useful.

The availability of calcium during the ischemic period can be diminished in a number of ways. First, in crystalloid solutions, the concentration of calcium can be reduced to the range of 0.5 to 1.0 mM/l, which has been beneficial in numerous studies (Hearse et al., 1981). When blood cardioplegia is used, calcium in the blood can be chelated with small amounts of citrate (Follette et al., 1978a). Cellular calcium influx can also be limited by cardioplegia additives such as magnesium and procaine.

## Buffering

Maintenance of appropriate myocardial pH is important for repletion of ATP and for sustaining low levels of cellular function. Hydrogen ions are produced continuously during the ischemic period, so that a stable source of buffering is required. In most cardioplegic formulations, pH is carefully controlled by the addition of specific buffering systems. The choice of cardioplegic buffers varies, but most clinically tested solutions use bicarbonate, phosphate, or tris(hydroxymethyl)aminomethane (TRIS) as the major buffering component. Lactate should be avoided because of its poor buffering capacity and because lactate inhibits anaerobic metabolism independent of pH (Hearse et al., 1981).

Available information suggests that cellular function during hypothermia is best maintained with a slightly alkaline pH (Becker et al., 1981; Rahn et al., 1975). Normally, when blood is cooled, pH increases approximately 0.15 per 10° C of hypothermia. Thus, at temperatures below 20° C, cellular pH in excess of 7.7 may be necessary. This concept is further substantiated by the observation that the pH of poikilothermic animals increases to about 7.8 with hypothermia. Recovery of myocardial function has been better when a pH of 7.6 to 7.8 was maintained (Follette et al., 1981), and most investigators currently recommend appropriate composition and buffering of cardioplegic solutions to maintain pH in the alkaline range of normal.

## Osmolarity

Cellular swelling and myocardial edema consistently accompany ischemic injury (Leaf, 1970). The primary mechanisms responsible seem to be altered cellular energetics and permeability related to the ischemic state (MacKnight and Leaf, 1977). Thus, one important aspect of minimizing water gain is the efficacy of myocardial protection; less edema occurs in well-protected hearts. The osmolarity of the perfusate also influences myocardial edema, and hearts perfused with hypotonic solutions rapidly gain water (Foglia et al., 1979). Conversely, hyperosmotic formulations in excess of 400 mOsm/kg of $H_2O$ produce myocardial dehydration and impair functional recovery. Although the direct influence of minor degrees of cellular edema on ultimate functional recovery is unclear, most authors would recommend slightly hyperosmolar cardioplegic solutions. Oncotic agents such as albumin or mannitol also can be used to prevent myocardial edema and can contribute to functional preservation.

## Oxygen Delivery/Blood Cardioplegia

The use of blood as the vehicle for cardioplegic arrest was popularized by Buckberg and associates (Follette et al., 1978a, 1978b). Blood is diluted to a hematocrit of 20% with cardioplegic solution, such that the final potassium concentration is 25 to 30 mM/l. The solution is oxygenated, cooled, and delivered through standard cannulas. Initially, 500 to 750 ml are administered at 16 to 20° C, and then 250 ml are reinfused every 20 minutes. Before the aortic clamp is released, 500 to 750 ml of blood cardioplegic solution at 37° C are infused to warm and reoxygenate the heart while arrest is maintained (Follette et al., 1981).

When so used, blood cardioplegia has several potential advantages. Blood is the most physiologic of all solutions. The heart is arrested while being oxygenated, so that ATP is not depleted before asystole. Reinfusion of oxygenated blood provides a source of oxygen for continued metabolism and ATP repletion during the period of hypothermic arrest. Although little oxygen is released from hemoglobin during hypothermia, enough is probably dissolved in the plasma to sustain metabolism when reinfusion is performed every 20 minutes. Reinfusing the solution maintains myocardial hypothermia, washes out waste products, and provides metabolic substrate. Hyperkalemia maintains chemical arrest with its inherently lower metabolic requirements. Formulation of the blood from the oxygenator is simple, and hemodilution usually is not significant. The buffering and oncotic characteristics of blood are excellent. Trace metals, co-factors, hormones, or other undefined but important constituents are provided. Finally, reperfusion with alkalotic, hyperkalemic, hypocalcemic blood is facilitated with this system, which minimizes fibrillation and reperfusion injury and provides a source of oxygen during the initial rewarming period (Follette et al., 1981).

Clinical experience with blood cardioplegia has been very positive. Follette and associates (1978b) reduced the perioperative myocardial infarction rate from 6.4% with intermittent ischemia to 1.3% with blood cardioplegia, and operative mortality also diminished. Similar results have been reported by Cunningham and associates (1979), who also noted good preservation of myocardial ultrastructure and ATP. These authors indicated that the "safe" aortic clamping time was extended beyond 2 hours with this technique, and Barner and colleagues (1981) confirmed these findings. Blood cardioplegia may offer distinct advantages in certain clinical situations. The disadvantage, as compared with hypercooled crystalloid methods, is that myocardial hypothermia in the range of 8 to 10° C usually is not achievable with blood cardioplegia, so some of the protective effects of hypothermia are lost.

## Retrograde Cold Blood Cardioplegia/Warm Blood Cardioplegia

Retrograde delivery of cold cardioplegia solution to the myocardium via coronary sinus perfusion has been evaluated for some time (Fabiani et al., 1986; Guiraundon et al., 1986; Menasché and Piwnica, 1987; Schaper et al., 1985). In its current form, cold blood cardioplegia usually is employed and is delivered through commercially available coronary sinus catheters (DLP, Walker, MI) at high flows and low pressures. Frequently, cardiac arrest is induced with antegrade cold blood cardioplegia and maintained with retrograde reinfusion. Potential advantages of this approach include better regional cardioplegia solution delivery in highly obstructed coronary beds, improved protection in reoperative situations with obstructed atherosclerotic vein grafts (Rosengart et al., 1993), and technical simplification in aortic valve procedures. Many surgeons use this method routinely (Bhayana et al., 1989; Loop et al., 1992). Disadvantages include the potential for coronary sinus injury (Onitsuka et al., 1990), inadequate right ventricular hypothermia (Hoshino, 1989), and inadequate capillary nutrient perfusion (Gates et al., 1993). Nevertheless, antegrade/retrograde cold blood cardioplegia is a well-established technique that provides excellent intraoperative myocardial protection. A modification of blood cardioplegia, continuous retrograde warm blood cardioplegia (Salerno et al., 1991), has been studied widely in animals and humans. Although this topic is still evolving, current enthusiasm for continuous retrograde warm blood cardioplegia is waning because of inferior myocardial protection (Ko et al., 1993; VanCamp et al., in press), reduced clarity in the operative field (Lajos et al., 1993), and a greater potential for neurologic injury with normothermic perfusion (Martin et al., 1994).

## A PRACTICAL CRYSTALLOID CARDIOPLEGIA SYSTEM

Although the methods of myocardial protection are numerous and probably vary somewhat among all surgeons, a simple technique that we have used since the early 1980s is described in this section. The method is a variant of the St. Thomas' Hospital tech-

nique and has produced excellent results in wide-ranging clinical practice.

Aortic arch cannulation is employed, using the metal-tip Sarns cannula (Sarns, Ann Arbor, MI). For most coronary bypass and aortic valve procedures, single venous cannulation is accomplished through the right atrial appendage, and direct cardiac venting is avoided. Cardiopulmonary bypass is initiated at 32° C, distal coronary grafting sites are visualized, and internal mammary artery flow is measured. As the DLP cardioplegia cannula is inserted into the distal ascending aorta, pump inflow temperature is reduced transiently to 16° C to precool the myocardium. A silicone rubber catheter is passed into the posterior pericardium via the transverse sinus and connected to a cold saline infusion system. A metal coil submerged in an alcohol-ice mixture acts as a heat exchanger to maximally cool the pericardial saline lavage, which is begun at 100 ml/min. A suction catheter at the inferior aspect of the incision collects the pericardial lavage and returns it to a cell-saver to scavenge any shed blood. A myocardial temperature probe is placed to the right of the left anterior descending artery into the interventricular septum. When the myocardial temperature falls below 24° C, the aorta is cross-clamped, and 1200 ml of cold crystalloid cardioplegia (Table 54–1) is infused via the DLP cannula over 4 to 5 minutes. Myocardial precool-

■ **Table 54–1.** CONGENITAL VARIATIONS OF THE CORONARY ARTERIES IN 224 PATIENTS

| Congenital Variations | No. of Cases |
|---|---|
| *Major Coronary Anomalies (75 Cases)* | |
| Coronary "arteriovenous" fistula* | 31 |
| Anomalous origin from the pulmonary artery | 44 |
| Left coronary artery | 39 |
| Right coronary artery | 4 |
| Both coronary arteries | 1 |
| *Minor Coronary Variations (63 Cases)* | |
| High takeoff | 2 |
| Multiple ostia | 6 |
| Anomalous circumflex artery origin | 14 |
| Anomalous anterior descending artery origin | 11 |
| Absent proximal ostium/single ostium in other aortic sinus | 10 |
| Absent proximal ostium/multiple ostia in other aortic sinus | 10 |
| Hypoplastic proximal coronary artery | 5 |
| Congenital proximal stenosis | 2 |
| Congenital distal stenosis | 1 |
| Coronary artery from the posterior aortic sinus | 1 |
| Ventricular origin of an accessory coronary artery | 1 |
| *Secondary Coronary Anomalies (86 Cases)* | |
| Secondary coronary "arteriovenous" fistula | 3 |
| Variations in transposition of the great vessels | 65 |
| Variations in truncus arteriosus | 6 |
| Variations in tetralogy of Fallot | 4 |
| Ectasia or coronary arteries in supravalvular aortic stenosis | 5 |
| Mural coronary artery | 3 |

Adapted from Ogden, J. A.: Congenital anomalies of the coronary arteries. Am. J. Cardiol., 25:474, 1970.
*This category does not include cases of adult anomalous origin of the right or left coronary artery from the pulmonary artery.

ing with the bypass circuit allows better and more uniform myocardial cooling for a given volume of cardioplegia solution. Reduction in myocardial temperature below 10° C is achieved routinely. If myocardial cooling is inadequate, additional volumes of cardioplegia solution are infused to attain the desired hypothermia. Coincident with aortic clamping, systemic perfusate temperature is returned to 24° C, and flow is reduced to 1.0 to 1.5 l/min/m², producing a systemic arterial pressure of approximately 40 mm Hg. A side arm on the cardioplegia cannula is used for aortic venting during aortic clamping. The cardiac procedure is performed, and additional 200- to 500-ml volumes of cardioplegia solution are infused every 30 to 45 minutes to maintain myocardial temperature below 15° C. Five to 10 minutes before aortic unclamping, full rewarming is begun, and lidocaine (200 mg) is administered into the oxygenator to diminish reperfusion arrhythmias. After aortic unclamping, additional procedures such as proximal aorto-vein graft anastomoses are performed, and cardiopulmonary bypass is discontinued after a bladder temperature of 35° C is achieved.

For mitral valve procedures or for unusual cases in which long periods of arrest are required in the presence of preoperative ventricular impairment, individual caval cannulation is used with occluding types. A side arm from the pericardial lavage system is inserted into the right atrium adjacent to one of the venous cannulas, and the purse-string is left loose to allow uninhibited egress of the endocardial saline lavage. Experimental and clinical evidence suggests that the right atrium and ventricle are particularly prone to rewarming (Chen et al., 1991), and the additional hypothermia provided by this method can significantly enhance myocardial protection for procedures requiring over 90 minutes of cardiac arrest (Velardi et al., 1989). Thus, endocardial cold saline lavage is used primarily in complex mitral valve-coronary or multiple valve operations, and the simplified method is used for most coronary bypass and aortic valve procedures, with or without coronary bypass. This simple approach to crystalloid cardioplegia has been assessed clinically in both coronary and valve procedures and has preserved myocardial functional integrity extremely well (Harpole et al., 1989; Rankin and Sabiston, 1990; Rankin et al., 1985).

Current myocardial protection techniques have been developed to the point that postoperative myocardial dysfunction should no longer be a major problem in cardiac surgery. Whichever method one chooses to employ, the incidence of cardiac dysfunction after coronary or valve procedures should now be extremely low. Although techniques will undoubtedly be refined in future years, current excellent results in cardiac surgery are significantly attributable to advances in myocardial protection over the past two decades.

## SELECTED BIBLIOGRAPHY

Berne, R. M., and Rubio, R.: Coronary circulation. In Handbook of Physiology. Vol. I. Bethesda, MD, American Physiology Society, 1979, pp. 873–952.

This comprehensive review of the physiology of coronary blood flow is by two outstanding authorities.

Follette, D. M., Fey, K., Mulder, D., et al.: Advantages of intermittent blood cardioplegia over intermittent ischemia during prolonged hypothermic aortic clamping. Circulation, 58(Suppl. 1):200, 1978.

This is the original work on blood cardioplegia on which clinical application has been based.

Gay, W. A., and Ebert, P. A.: Functional, metabolic and morphologic effects of potassium-induced cardioplegia. Surgery, 74:284, 1973.

This paper was responsible for reintroducing potassium cardioplegia into clinical practice. The work is not only a major contribution but also a model of simplicity and innovation.

Hearse, D. J., Braimbridge, M. V., and Jynge, P.: Protection of the Ischemic Myocardium: Cardioplegia. New York, Raven Press, 1981.

This is a definitive work on myocardial preservation, with emphasis on both basic science and practical surgical technique.

Sabiston, D. C., Jr.: The coronary circulation. The William F. Rienhoff, Jr. Lecture. Johns Hopkins Med. J., 134:314, 1974.

This is a review of the anatomy, physiology, and pathologic aspects of the coronary circulation. The data presented are based on experimental and clinical findings in normal and pathologic conditions.

## BIBLIOGRAPHY

Barner, H. B., Kaiser, G. C., Codd, J. E., et al.: Clinical experience with cold blood as the vehicle for hypothermic potassium cardioplegia. Ann. Thorac. Surg., 29:224, 1981.
Becker, H., Vinten-Johansen, J., Buckberg, G. D., et al.: Myocardial damage caused by keeping pH 7.40 during systemic deep hypothermia. J. Thorac. Cardiovasc. Surg., 81:810, 1981.
Bentivegna, L. A., Ablin, W. A., Kihara, Y., Morgan, J. P.: Altered calcium handling in left ventricular pressure-overload hypertrophy as detected with aequorin in the isolated, perfused ferret heart. Circ. Res., 69:1538–1545, 1991.
Berne, R. M., and Rubio, R.: Coronary circulation. In Handbook of Physiology. Vol. I. Bethesda, MD, American Physiological Society, 1979, pp. 873–952.
Bhayana, J. N., Kalmbach, T., Booth, F. V., et al.: Combined antegrade/retrograde cardioplegia for myocardial protection: A clinical trail. J. Thorac. Cardiovasc. Surg., 98(5 Part 2):956–960, 1989.
Buckberg, G. D., Fixler, D. D., Archie, J. D., and Hoffman, J. I. E.: Experimental subendocardial ischemia in dogs with normal coronary arteries. Circ. Res., 30:67, 1972.
Chen, Y. F., Lin, Y. F., and Wu, S. F.: Inconsistent effectiveness of myocardial preservation among cardiac chambers during hyopthermic cardioplegia. J. Thorac. Cardiovasc. Surg., 102(5):684–687, 1991.
Chitwood, W. R., Sink, J. D., Hill, R. C., et al.: The effects of hypothermia on myocardial oxygen consumption and transmural coronary blood flow in the potassium-arrested heart. Ann. Surg., 190:106, 1979.
Cunningham, J. N., Jr., Adams, P. X., Knopp, E. A., et al.: Preservation of ATP, ultrastructure, and ventricular function after aortic crossclamping and reperfusion: Clinical use of blood potassium cardioplegia. J. Thorac. Cardiovasc. Surg., 78:708, 1979.
Daily, P. O., Pfeffer, T. A., Wisniewski, J. B., et al.: Clinical comparisons of methods of myocardial protection. J. Thorac. Cardiovasc. Surg., 93:324, 1987.
Elbeery, J. R., Lucke, J. C., Feneley, M. P., et al.: The mechanical determinants of myocardial oxygen consumption in the conscious dog. Am. J. Physiol. (in press).
Fabiani, J., Deloche, A., Swanson, J., and Carpentier, A.: Retrograde cardioplegia through the right atrium. Ann. Thorac. Surg., 41:101, 1986.
Feneley, M. P., Maier, G. W., Gayor, J. W., et al.: Comparison of elastic and non-elastic predictive models of myocardial oxygen consumption in conscious dogs. Circulation, 76(Suppl. 4):543, 1987.
Foglia, R. P., Steed, D. L., Follette, D. M., et al.: Iatrogenic myocar-

dial edema with potassium cardioplegia. J. Thorac. Cardiovasc. Surg., 78:217, 1979.

Follette, D. M., Fey, K., Mulder, D., et al.: Advantages of blood cardioplegia over continuous coronary perfusion or intermittent ischemia: Experimental and clinical study. J. Thorac. Cardiovasc. Surg., 76:604, 1978a.

Follette, D. M., Fey, K., Buckberg, G. D., et al.: Reducing postischemic damage by temporary modification of reperfusate calcium, potassium, pH, and osmolarity. J. Thorac. Cardiovasc. Surg., 82:221, 1981.

Follette, D. M., Steed, D. L., Foglia, R., et al.: Advantages of intermittent blood cardioplegia over intermittent ischemia during prolonged hypothermic aortic clamping. Circulation, 58(Suppl. 1):200, 1978b.

Gates, R. N., Laks, H., Drinkwater, D. C., et al.: Gross and microvascular distribution of retrograde cardioplegia in explanted human hearts. Ann. Thorac. Surg., 56:410, 1993.

Gay, W. A., and Ebert, P. A.: Functional, metabolic and morphologic effects of potassium-induced cardioplegia. Surgery, 74:284, 1973.

Glower, D. D., Schaper, J., Kabas, J. S., et al.: Relation between reversal of diastolic creep and recovery of systolic function after ischemic myocardial injury in conscious dogs. Circ. Res., 60:850, 1987.

Glower, D. D., Spratt, J. A., Snow, N. D., et al.: Linearity of the Frank-Starling relationship in the intact heart: The concept of preload recruitable stroke work. Circulation, 71:994, 1985.

Grover, F. L., Fewel, J. G., Ghidoni, J. J., and Trinkle, J. K.: Does lower systemic temperature enhance cardioplegic myocardial protection? J. Thorac. Cardiovasc. Surg., 81:11, 1981.

Guiraudon, G. M., Campbell, C. S., Mclellan, D. G., et al.: Retrograde coronary sinus versus aortic root perfusion with cold cardioplegia: Randomized study levels of cardiac enzymes in 40 patients. Circulation, 74(Suppl 3):105, 1986.

Harpole, D. H., Wolfe, W. G., Rankin J. S., et al.: Assessment of left ventricular functional preservation during isolated cardiac valvular operation. Circulation, 80:III-1, 1989.

Hearse, D. J., Braimbridge, M. V., and Jynge, P.: Protection of the Ischemic Myocardium: Cardioplegia. New York, Raven Press, 1981.

Hoshino, R.: Right ventricular function in retrograde cardioplegia for myocardial protection—An experimental study. J. Jpn. Assoc. Thorac. Surg., 37(7):1287–1296, 1989.

Jennings, R. B., and Ganote, C. E.: Structural changes in myocardium during acute ischemia. Circ. Res., 34, 35(Suppl. 3):156, 1974.

Karck, M., Vivi, A., Tassini, M., et al.: Optimal level of hypothermia for prolonged myocardial protection assessed by 31P nuclear magnetic resonance. Ann. Thorac. Surg. 54(2):345–351, 1992.

Ko, W., Zelano, J., Isom, O. W., and Krieger, K. H.: The effects of warm versus cold blood cardioplegia on endothelial function, myocardial function, and energetics. Circulation, 88(5 Pt 2):359–365, 1993.

Koutlas, T. C., Lucke, J. C., Gall, S. A., et al.: Effects of blood cardioplegia reperfusion on recovery of ventricular function after global myocardial ischemia. Surg. Forum, 41:230–233, 1990.

Lajos, T. Z., Espersen, C. C., Lajos, P. S., et al.: Comparison of cold versus warm cardioplegia: Crystalloid antegrade or retrograde blood? Circulation, 88(5 Pt 2):344–349, 1993.

Leaf, A.: Regulation of intracellular fluid volume and disease. Am. J. Med., 49:291, 1970.

Lilly, R. E., Lucke, J. C., Livesey, S. A., et al.: Effects of chronic left ventricular failure on myocardial energetics in the conscious dog. Circulation, 82(Suppl 3):566, 1990.

Limbruno, U., Zucchi, R., Ronca-Testoni, S., et al.: Sarcoplasmic reticulum function in the stunned myocardium. J. Mol. Cell. Cardiol., 21:1063–1072, 1989.

Loop, F. D., Higgins, T. L., Panda, R., et al.: Myocardial protection during cardiac operations. Decreased morbidity and lower cost with blood cardioplegia and coronary sinus perfusion. J. Thorac. Cardiovasc. Surg., 104(3):608–618, 1992.

Lowe, J. E., Cummings, R. G., Adams, D. H., and Hull-Ryde, E. A.: Evidence that ischemic cell death begins in the subendocardium independent of variations in collateral flow or wall tension. Circulation, 28(68):190, 1983.

Lucke, J. C., Elbeery, J. R., Koutlas, T. C., et al.: Metabolic to mechanical energy transfer after regional and global myocardial ischemia. J. Am. Coll. Cardiol., 17:44A, 1991.

Lucke, J. C., Koutlas, T. C., Gall, S. A., et al.: Effects of global ischemia on metabolic to mechanical energetic transfer characteristics of the left ventricle. Surg. Forum, 41:254–257, 1990.

MacKnight, A., and Leaf, A.: Regulation of cellular volume. Physiol. Rev., 57:510, 1977.

Martin, T. D., Craver, J. M., Gott, J. P., et al.: A prospective randomized trial of retrograde warm blood cardioplegia: Myocardial benefit and neurologic threat. Ann. Thorac. Surg., 57:298, 1994.

Menasché, P., and Piwnica, A.: Retrograde cardioplegia through the coronary sinus. Ann. Thorac. Surg., 44:214, 1987.

Onitsuka, T., Yonezawa, T., Kuwabara, M., et al.: A case of coronary sinus rupture following retrograde coronary perfusion for myocardial protection. Jpn. J. Thorac. Surg., 43(7):562–564, 1990.

Rahn, H., Reeves, R. B., and Howell, B. J.: Hydrogen ion regulation, temperature and evolution. Am. Rev. Respir. Dis., 112:165, 1975.

Rankin, J. S., Newman, G. E., Muhlbaier, L. H., et al.: The effects of coronary revascularization on left ventricular function in ischemic heart disease. J. Thorac. Cardiovasc. Surg., 90:818, 1985.

Rankin, J. S., and Sabiston, D. C., Jr.: Physiology of coronary blood flow, myocardial function, and intraoperative myocardial protection. In Sabiston, D. C., Jr., and Spencer, F. C. (eds): Gibbon's Surgery of the Chest. 5th ed. Philadelphia, W. B. Saunders, 1990.

Rosenfeldt, F. L., and Watson, D. A.: Interference with local myocardial cooling by heat gain during aortic cross-clamping. Ann. Thorac. Surg., 27:13, 1979.

Rosengart, T. K., Krieger, K., Lang, S. J., et al.: Reoperative coronary artery bypass surgery. Improved preservation of myocardial function with retrograde cardioplegia. Circulation, 88(5 Part 2):330–335, 1993.

Sabiston, D. C., Jr.: The coronary circulation. The William F. Rienhoff, Jr. Lecture. Johns Hopkins Med. J., 134:314, 1974.

Sabiston, D. C., Jr., and Gregg, D. E.: Effect of cardiac contraction on coronary blood flow. Circulation, 15:14, 1957.

Salerno, T. A., Houck, J. P., Barrozo, C. A., et al.: Retrograde continuous warm blood cardioplegia: A new concept in myocardial protection. Ann. Thorac. Surg., 51(2):245–247, 1991.

Schaper, J., Walter, P., Scheld, H., and Hehrlein, F.: The effects of retrograde perfusion of cardioplegic solution in cardiac operations. J. Thorac. Cardiovasc. Surg., 90:882, 1985.

Shen, A. C., and Jennings, R. B.: Myocardial calcium and magnesium in acute ischemic injury. Am. J. Pathol., 67:417, 1972.

Shumway, N. E., Lower, R. R., and Stofer, R. C.: Selective hypothermia of the heart in anoxic cardiac arrest. Surg. Gynecol. Obstet., 109:750, 1959.

Squire, J.: The Structural Basis of Muscular Contraction. New York, Plenum Press, 1981.

VanCamp, J. R., Brunsting, L. A., Childs, K. F., and Bollig, S. F.: Functional recovery after acute ischemia: Warm continuous retrograde versus cold intermittent antegrade cardioplegia. Ann. Thorac. Surg. (in press).

Velardi, A. R., Widner, S. J., Cilley, J. H., Jr., et al.: Right ventricular myocardial protection through intracavitary cooling in cardiac operations. J. Thorac. Cardiovasc. Surg., 98(6):1077–1082, 1989.

# 54

# ■ II Congenital Malformations of the Coronary Circulation

James E. Lowe and David C. Sabiston, Jr.

Congenital coronary arterial malformations have long been recognized, but the frequency of these reports in the literature has increased greatly since Sones introduced selective coronary arteriography in 1959 (Sones and Shirey, 1960). In a review of 224 patients with coronary malformations, Ogden (1970) proposed three basic classifications: major anomalies, in which there is an abnormal communication between an artery and a cardiac chamber or abnormal origin of a major coronary artery from the pulmonary artery; minor anomalies, in which there is variation of the origin of the vessels from the aorta but the distal circulation is normal; and secondary anomalies, in which the coronary arterial variation probably represents a circulatory response of the primary intracardiac pathologic defect. The distribution of coronary artery anomalies in these 224 patients is shown in Table 54–1.

Major anomalies that are amenable to surgical correction include congenital coronary fistulas, anomalous origin of either the left or the right coronary artery from the pulmonary artery, congenital aneurysms of the coronary arteries, and congenital membranous obstruction of the ostium of the left main coronary artery. Minor anomalies, in which there is variation in the origin of the coronary arteries from the aorta with normal distal circulation, and secondary anomalies, associated with congenital heart defects such as transposition of the great vessels, truncus arteriosus, and tetralogy of Fallot, seldom require surgical intervention. This section describes the clinical manifestations, evaluation, and surgical management of patients with major coronary anomalies, including congenital coronary artery fistulas, congenital origin of either the left or the right coronary artery from the pulmonary artery, congenital coronary artery aneurysms, and membranous obstruction of the ostium of the left main coronary artery.

The authors' experience, supported by that of others, indicates that most patients with major congenital coronary arterial malformations should be considered candidates for surgical correction. In most cases, the natural history of these lesions is not associated with a normal life expectancy, with the possible exception of patients with congenital origin of the right coronary artery from the pulmonary artery. Because these malformations can be corrected safely and long-term results are gratifying, surgical intervention should be strongly recommended when a precise diagnosis has been established.

## CORONARY ARTERY FISTULAS

Since Krause first described a coronary artery fistula in 1865, over 400 additional patients with this malformation have been reported in the literature. Increasing numbers of patients with this anomaly are being recognized each year because of the widespread use of cardiac catheterization and selective coronary arteriography in the evaluation of various cardiac problems.

Coronary artery fistulas are characterized by normal origin of the coronary artery from the aorta with a fistulous communication with the atria or ventricles or with the pulmonary artery, coronary sinus, or superior vena cava. These fistulas represent the most common of the congenital coronary malformations. Coronary artery fistulas are found in 1 of every 50,000 patients with congenital heart disease and in 1 of every 500 patients who have coronary arteriography (Wenger, 1978). The right coronary artery is involved most frequently, and the abnormal communication most often is to the right ventricle, followed in incidence by drainage into the right atrium and pulmonary artery. Left coronary artery fistulas are less common but may drain into the right ventricle, right atrium, or coronary sinus. On rare occasion, right or left coronary artery fistulas may communicate with the left ventricle (Podolsky et al., 1991) (Fig. 54–14). The size of the fistulous communication may vary widely, but it generally becomes larger with time.

### Clinical Manifestations

It is commonly believed that most patients with coronary artery fistulas are asymptomatic. However, the authors' experience with 36 patients, supported by a review of 258 other patients reported in the literature, shows that 55% are symptomatic at the time of presentation (Lowe et al., 1981; Lowe and Sabiston, 1982). Because the underlying pathophysiology is essentially that of a left-to-right cardiac shunt, it follows that the most common manifestation is congestive heart failure (CHF). Another common

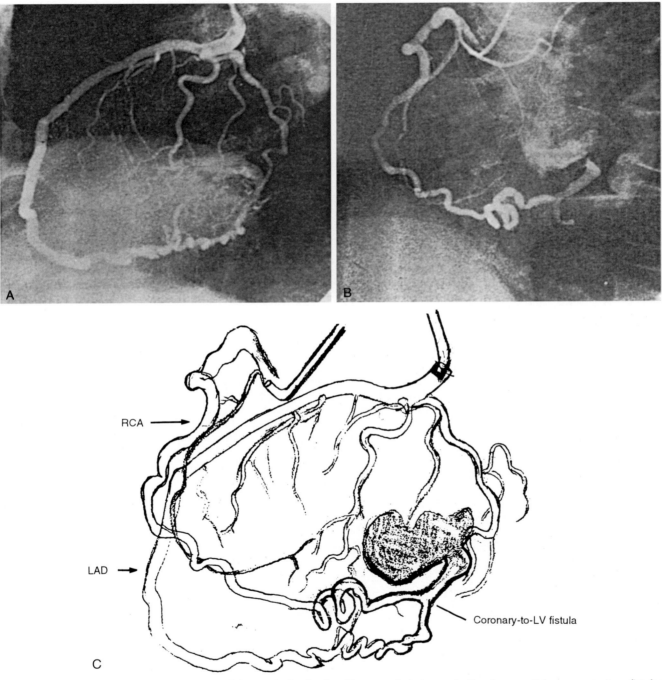

**FIGURE 54–14.** *A*, Bilateral coronary artery to left ventricular fistulas. The overwhelming majority of congenital coronary artery fistulas involve the right coronary artery and the abnormal communication most often is to the right ventricle, right atrium, or pulmonary artery. Left coronary artery fistulas are uncommon, but when they occur, they usually drain into the right ventricle, right atrium, or coronary sinus. This is the first case report of a patient with both left and right coronary artery fistulas emptying into the left ventricle. The patient was a 64-year-old man who was admitted to the hospital for evaluation of chest pain. Selective coronary arteriography of the left anterior descending coronary artery shows a fistulous tract entering into the posterior aspect of the left ventricle. *B*, A lateral view of the right coronary angiogram reveals that the right coronary artery also empties into a fistulous tract communicating with the left ventricle. *C*, Schematic drawing of the coronary anatomy with both left and right coronary artery fistulas draining into the left ventricle (LV). (RCA = right coronary artery; LAD = left anterior descending coronary artery.) (*A–C*, From Podolsky, L., Ledley, G. S., Goldstein, J., et al.: Bilateral coronary artery to left ventricular fistulas. Cathet. Cardiovasc. Diagn., 24:271, 1991. Copyright © 1991 by John Wiley & Sons. Reprinted by permission of John Wiley & Sons, Inc.)

■ **Table 54–2.** MAJOR PRESENTING CLINICAL MANIFESTATIONS OF CORONARY ARTERY FISTULAS WHEN PRESENT AS SOLE CARDIAC ANOMALY

| Manifestation | No. of Cases | Percentage of Total |
|---|---|---|
| Asymptomatic murmur | 67 | 45 |
| Dyspnea on exertion; fatigue | 34 | 22 |
| Congestive heart failure | 21 | 14 |
| Angina or nonspecific chest pain | 10 | 7 |
| Bacterial endocarditis | 9 | 6 |
| Frequent upper respiratory infections | 9 | 6 |
| Total | 150 | |

From Daniel, T. M., Graham, T. P., and Sabiston, D. C., Jr.: Coronary artery-right ventricular fistula with congestive heart failure. Surgical correction in the neonatal period. Surgery, 67:985, 1970.

symptom is angina pectoris, secondary to a steal of coronary arterial flow through the fistulous communication. Bacterial endocarditis, anemia, and glomerulonephritis in the same patient have been reported (Sabiston et al., 1963). Infants and children with this lesion may fail to thrive. Less commonly, patients present with acute myocardial infarction, aneurysm formation with subsequent rupture or embolization, or symptoms secondary to pulmonary hypertension.

The major presenting features of coronary artery fistulas are shown in Table 54–2 (Daniel et al., 1970). The age of onset of CHF in 21 patients who had this feature in a group of 150 studied is shown in Figure 54–15. In addition, the age of onset of dyspnea on exertion, the appearance of bacterial endocarditis, and the age of onset of angina pectoris in this series are shown in Figures 54–16 to 54–18.

CHF may actually appear quite early; the chest

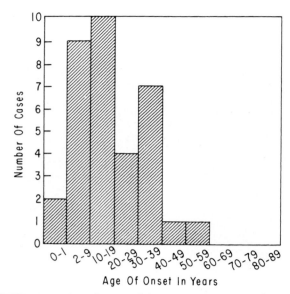

**FIGURE 54–16.** Age of onset of dyspnea on exertion or fatigue in patients with isolated coronary artery fistula. (From Daniel, T. M., Graham, T. P., and Sabiston, D. C. Jr.: Coronary artery-right ventricular fistula with congestive heart failure: Surgical correction in the neonatal period: Surgery, 67:985, 1970.)

films and arteriogram of a 1-month-old infant with this complication are shown in Figures 54–19 and 54–20. The infant was managed by closing the communication between the anterior descending coronary artery and the right ventricle, with complete cure. The postoperative aortogram is shown in Figure 54–21B (Daniel et al., 1970).

In patients who are asymptomatic, the diagnosis is usually made after coronary angiography is performed to evaluate asymptomatic murmurs, mild car-

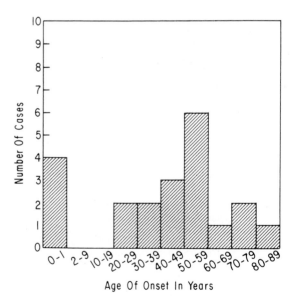

**FIGURE 54–15.** Age of onset of congestive heart failure in patients with an isolated coronary artery fistula. (From Daniel, T. M., Graham, T. P., and Sabiston, D. C., Jr.: Coronary artery-right ventricular fistula with congestive heart failure: Surgical correction in the neonatal period. Surgery, 67:985, 1970.)

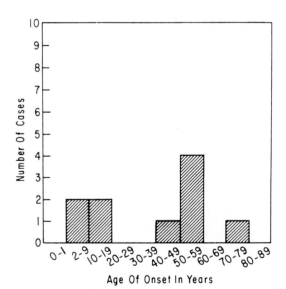

**FIGURE 54–17.** Age of onset of angina or chest pain in patients with an isolated coronary artery fistula. (From Daniel, T. M., Graham, T. P., and Sabiston, D. C., Jr.: Coronary artery-right ventricular fistula with congestive heart failure: Surgical correction in the neonatal period. Surgery, 67:985, 1970.)

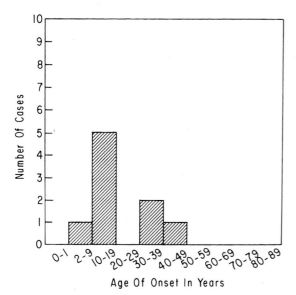

FIGURE 54–18. Age of onset of bacterial endocarditis in patients with an isolated coronary artery fistula. (From Daniel, T. M., Graham, T. P., and Sabiston, D. C., Jr.: Coronary artery-right ventricular fistula with congestive heart failure: Surgical correction in the neonatal period. Surgery, 67:985, 1970.)

■ Table 54–3. CONGENITAL CORONARY ARTERY FISTULAS–INVOLVED CORONARY ARTERY IN 286 PATIENTS

| Involved Artery | % |
| --- | --- |
| Right coronary artery | 56 |
| Left coronary artery | 36 |
| Both right and left coronary arteries | 5 |
| Single coronary artery | 3 |

From Lowe, J. E., Oldham, H. N., Jr., and Sabiston, D. C., Jr.: Surgical management of congenital coronary artery fistulas. Ann. Surg., 194:371, 1981.

drain into the left atrium or left ventricle (Podolsky et al., 1991) (see Fig. 54–14).

## Evaluation

The successful surgical management of patients with congenital coronary artery fistulas depends on a thorough preoperative evaluation that precisely defines the anatomy and pathophysiology of the anomaly. Although echocardiography (Barton et al., 1986; Pickoff et al., 1982; Reeder et al., 1980) and computed chest tomography (Slater et al., 1984) have been used to noninvasively identify coronary fistulas, the precise diagnosis requires arteriographic demonstration of the involved coronary artery, the recipient cardiac chamber, and the exact site of communication. The clinical manifestations and the radiographic and electrocardiographic findings do not exclude other lesions such as patent ductus arteriosus, sinus of Valsalva fistulas, or a ventricular septal defect with aortic insufficiency. In patients with a large fistula, injection of contrast medium into the aortic root may clearly delineate the lesion. In patients with a smaller fistula or fistulous communications from both coronary arteries, selective coronary arteriography is preferable and may be essential to establish the diagnosis.

Almost all patients with a major coronary artery fistula should be considered candidates for surgical correction. In most cases, the natural history of these lesions is not associated with a normal life expectancy because of the eventual development of CHF, angina, myocardial infarction, subacute bacterial endocarditis, aneurysm formation with rupture or embolization, or pulmonary hypertension. Spontaneous closure of a coronary fistula is rare, and only three documented

diomegaly discovered on routine chest film, or persistent electrocardiographic abnormalities.

The main clinical manifestation of coronary artery fistulas is a continuous murmur over the site of the abnormal communication. This murmur may closely resemble that of a patent ductus arteriosus, and in fact, the first patient on whom closure was performed was operated on by Björk and Crafoord in 1947 for a presumed patent ductus. Because a patent ductus was not found, the pericardium was opened, and a coronary artery fistula draining into the pulmonary artery was identified and obliterated. The differential diagnosis of coronary artery fistulas, in addition to patent ductus arteriosus, includes congenital aortic-pulmonary fistulas, sinus of Valsalva fistulas, ventricular septal defect with aortic insufficiency, pulmonary arteriovenous malformations, and fistulas of systemic vessels such as the subclavian and internal mammary arteries connecting to veins of the chest wall or to the lung.

### Involved Coronary Artery and Site of Fistulous Communication

The right coronary artery is most often involved in the development of a congenital coronary artery fistula (56%) (Table 54–3) and most commonly communicates with a chamber of the right side of the heart (Table 54–4). The fistula usually involves the right ventricle (39%), followed closely in incidence by drainage into the right atrium (33%), including the coronary sinus and superior vena cava, or the pulmonary artery (20%). Left coronary artery fistulas are less common but usually drain into the right ventricle or right atrium. Rarely, coronary artery fistulas may

■ Table 54–4. CONGENITAL CORONARY ARTERY FISTULAS—SITE OF FISTULOUS COMMUNICATION IN 286 PATIENTS

| Site of Fistulous Communication | % |
| --- | --- |
| Right ventricle | 39 |
| Right atrium (coronary sinus, superior vena cava) | 33 |
| Pulmonary artery | 20 |
| Left atrium | 6 |
| Left ventricle | 2 |

From Lowe, J. E., Oldham, H. N., Jr., and Sabiston, D. C., Jr.: Surgical management of congenital coronary artery fistulas. Ann. Surg., 194:371, 1981.

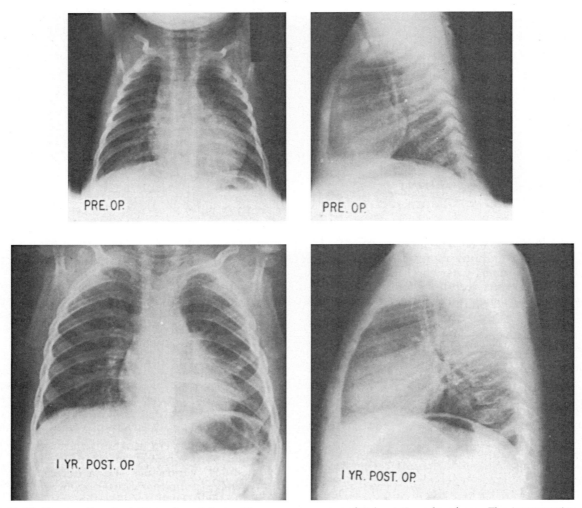

**FIGURE 54–19.** Preoperative chest films of an infant with a coronary artery fistula at 5 weeks of age. The interpretation included biventricular enlargement, left atrial enlargement, and increased pulmonary vasculature. Chest films 1 year after operation show decrease in cardiomegaly. (From Daniel, T. M., Graham, T. P., and Sabiston, D. C., Jr.: Coronary artery-right ventricular fistula with congestive heart failure: Surgical correction in the neonatal period. Surgery, *67*:985, 1970.)

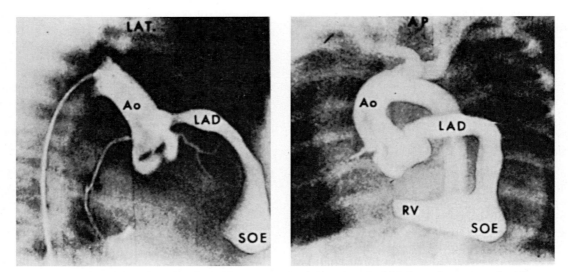

**FIGURE 54–20.** Ascending aortogram (lateral and anteroposterior views) in a 6-week-old infant who presented with severe congestive heart failure. The aortogram shows a left coronary artery-right ventricular fistula. (Ao = aorta; LAD = left anterior descending coronary artery; SOE = site of entry of the fistula into the right ventricle; RV = incompletely opacified right ventricle.) (From Daniel, T. M., Graham, T. P., and Sabiston, D. C., Jr.: Coronary artery-right ventricular fistula with congestive heart failure: Surgical correction in the neonatal period. Surgery, *67*:985, 1970.)

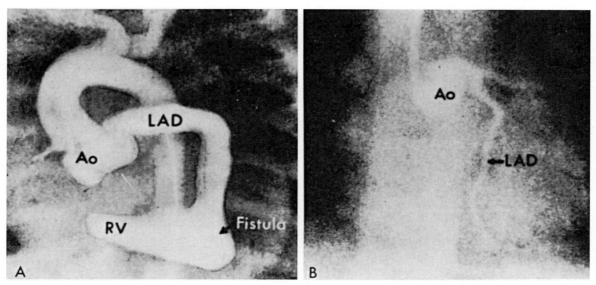

FIGURE 54–21. *A*, Preoperative aortogram of patient in Figure 54–20. (LAD = left anterior descending coronary artery; Ao = aorta; RV = right ventricle.) *B*, Repeat aortogram 1 year after successful surgical obliteration of the fistula. The left anterior descending coronary artery has returned to normal size. (*A* and *B*, From Daniel, T. M., Graham, T. P., and Sabiston, D. C., Jr.: Coronary artery-right ventricular fistula with congestive heart failure: Surgical correction in the neonatal period. Surgery, *67*:985, 1970.)

cases have been reported (Griffiths et al., 1983; Hacket and Hallidie-Smith, 1984; Mahoney et al., 1982). The ideal time for elective surgical closure is before the development of symptoms and major pathologic changes in the heart, the coronary arteries, and the pulmonary circulation. As shown by Liberthson and associates (1979), most patients with congenital coronary artery fistulas develop both symptoms and fistula-related complications with increased age and are subject to increased morbidity and mortality when surgery is performed later in life.

## Surgical Management

Because patients with coronary artery fistulas have had a precise and detailed angiographic examination showing the involved coronary artery, the recipient cardiac chamber, and the exact site of communication, the need for cardiopulmonary bypass can often be anticipated preoperatively. Patients with a single communication that is easily dissected usually do not require bypass for suture obliteration. However, in patients with multiple communications or large, tortuous, draining channels, the fistula is best obliterated by opening the recipient cardiac chamber with the patient on bypass to completely close all fistulous tracts. Finally, if fistula obliteration in any way jeopardizes distal coronary arterial flow, a saphenous vein or internal mammary bypass graft should be placed with the patient under cardioplegic arrest.

After a median sternotomy or anterior thoracotomy is performed and a pericardial cradle is created, the fistulous communication is dissected and obliterated by using multiple transfixion sutures of nonabsorbable material. If a cardiac chamber or the main pulmonary artery must be opened to close larger or multiple fistulous tracts, the patient is placed on cardiopulmonary bypass (Figs. 54–22 to 54–24). An arterial perfusion cannula is placed in the ascending aorta, and venous return cannulas are placed in the superior and inferior venae cavae. Tapes are placed around both the inferior and the superior venae cavae. If the right atrium, right ventricle, or pulmonary artery is opened, the tapes are drawn tightly around the venous cannulas to prevent venous return to the right side of the heart except for coronary sinus flow. The heart is then fibrillated, and the recipient cardiac chamber is opened. If the fistulous communication is with the left side of the heart and obliteration requires opening the left atrium or left ventricle or if bypass grafting is planned, the aorta is cross-clamped and the heart arrested using cardioplegia and topical hypothermia. After operative correction, intraoperative shunt curves or transesophageal echocardiography is obtained to be certain that there is no residual left-to-right shunt.

Thirty-six patients with congenital coronary artery fistulas have been evaluated at the Duke University Medical Center. These patients were between 6 weeks and 76 years of age, with a mean of 32 years and equal distribution between males and females. Half of the patients came to surgical attention because of symptoms such as CHF, angina, or failure to thrive. The remainder were asymptomatic and came to operation after evaluation of asymptomatic heart murmurs or cardiomegaly found on a routine chest film. Twenty-nine of these patients have had operative repair. All procedures were performed through a median sternotomy, and 14 (48%) patients had suture obliteration of the fistula without bypass. Seven (24%) patients had cardiopulmonary bypass to open the recipient cardiac chamber and successfully occlude multiple draining fistulous tracts. Two (7%) patients

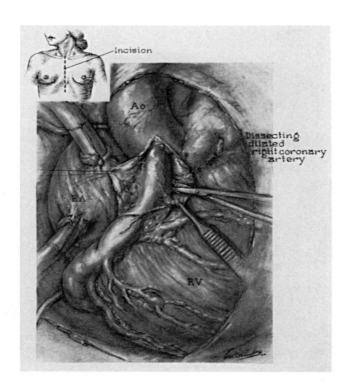

**FIGURE 54–22.** Right coronary-right atrial congenital coronary fistula as seen at operation in a 76-year-old woman who presented with severe congestive heart failure. Through a median sternotomy, the patient was placed on cardiopulmonary bypass with separate venous return cannulas placed in the superior and inferior venae cavae. (From Lowe, J. E., and Sabiston, D. C., Jr.: Congenital coronary malformations. *In* Cohn, L. [ed]: Modern Technics in Surgery: Cardiac-Thoracic Surgery. Mt. Kisco, NY, Futura, 1981.)

**FIGURE 54–23.** Tapes are secured around the superior (SVC) and inferior (IVC) venae cavae to eliminate venous return to the right atrium. The heart is then fibrillated and the right atrium is opened. The large fistulous opening is identified and closed by using interrupted nonabsorbable piedgeted sutures (*A*). (Ao = aorta.) The site of entry into the right coronary fistula is shown in *B*. (*A* and *B*, From Lowe, J. E., and Sabiston, D. C., Jr.: Congenital coronary malformations. *In* Cohn, L. [ed]: Modern Technics in Surgery: Cardiac-Thoracic Surgery. Mt., Kisco, NY, Futura, 1981.)

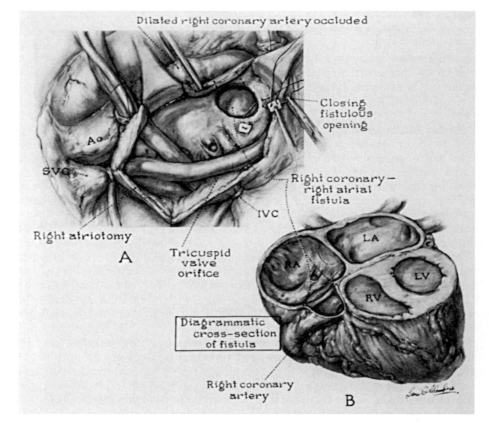

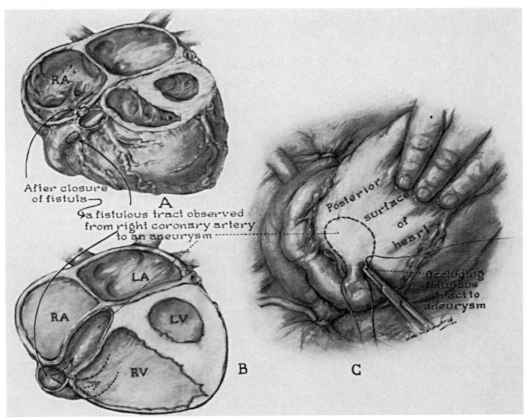

**FIGURE 54–24.** After closure of the site of entry into the right atrium, a second fistulous tract was found entering an aneurysm over the posterior surface of the heart (*A* and *B*). This fistulous tract was closed by using multiple transfixion sutures (*C*). (*A–C*, From Lowe, J. E., and Sabiston, D. C., Jr.: Congenital coronary malformations. *In* Cohn, L. [ed]: Modern Technics in Surgery: Cardiac-Thoracic Surgery. Mt. Kisco, NY, Futura, 1981.)

had saphenous vein bypass grafting after fistula obliteration in order to reconstitute distal coronary flow. The mean time of follow-up for these 29 patients has been 10 years. There were no operative deaths, and all patients are well and have no evidence of recurrent fistula formation, although 1 patient with a complex fistula of the circumflex coronary artery to the right ventricle has a small residual shunt (Lowe and Sabiston, 1982). Urrutia-S and co-workers (1983) reported similar surgical results in 56 patients at the Texas Heart Institute with an overall survival of 98.3%. The update of the Texas Heart experience by Fernandes and colleagues (1992) further documents excellent long-term results in 93 patients.

## CONGENITAL ORIGIN OF THE LEFT CORONARY ARTERY FROM THE PULMONARY ARTERY

Abbott (1908) first described a left coronary artery originating from the pulmonary artery. Abrikossoff (1911) reported a 5-month-old infant who died of CHF and was found to have an aneurysm of the left ventricle at postmortem examination. Photomicrographs of the ventricle revealed infarction, including areas of calcification. Bland and associates (1933) de-

scribed the electrocardiographic changes in an infant with this malformation and showed for the first time that a diagnosis could be established during life.

It is generally recognized that the prognosis for most patients with origin of the left coronary artery from the pulmonary artery is poor. It has been estimated that 95% of patients with this anomaly die within the first year of life unless surgical therapy is undertaken (Keith, 1959).

The pathophysiology of this malformation was poorly understood for many years, but evidence in the past has now made this aspect relatively straightforward. Numerous studies of postmortem specimens clearly reveal the presence of many collaterals that originate from the right coronary artery and connect to the left coronary artery. If the right coronary artery is injected in postmortem specimens, branches of the left coronary artery fill easily and in significant amounts (Case et al., 1958). It has also been observed at the time of operation that occlusion of the left coronary artery at its anomalous origin from the pulmonary artery causes an increase in pressure within the artery, suggesting that flow originates from the right coronary artery by collaterals (Sabiston et al., 1960a, 1960b). Of additional significance is the fact that blood withdrawn from the left coronary artery at operation has been fully saturated with oxygen.

Collectively, these findings are sound evidence that the direction of blood flow is from the right coronary artery by collaterals into the left coronary artery and then into the pulmonary artery. The resultant symptoms and clinical manifestations are secondary to left ventricular myocardial ischemia, which results either from inadequate collateral flow from the right coronary artery to the left coronary artery or from a steal of adequate collateral flow into the low-pressure pulmonary arterial system.

## Clinical Manifestations

The clinical manifestations of origin of the left coronary artery from the pulmonary artery become apparent in infancy in most patients. The infant usually appears to be normal at birth because the pulmonary arterial pressure at this age is elevated and allows perfusion of the left coronary artery from the pulmonary artery. Nevertheless, symptoms may be present at birth, especially if there are associated cardiac malformations. Symptoms are most likely to occur during the first few months of life, as left ventricular ischemia becomes more pronounced. When symptoms appear, the course is usually one of progressive deterioration. Unless operative therapy is undertaken, progressively worsening left ventricular dysfunction occurs, usually leading to death in infancy. Although most patients with this malformation develop symptoms in infancy (95%), a rare patient will survive to adult life with few, if any, symptoms (Abbott, 1927). In a collected review, Harthorne and co-workers (1966) reported 28 adults with this condition, and Moodie and colleagues (1983) studied 10 adult patients with this malformation and provided long-term follow-up after surgical correction. Purut and Sabiston (1991) described the oldest patient with this malformation, a 61-year-old female who underwent successful surgical repair.

### Symptoms

It was originally believed that symptoms resulted from poorly oxygenated blood from the pulmonary artery flowing into the left coronary arterial system. As described earlier, however, various studies have shown that blood flow is actually from the right coronary artery via collaterals into the left coronary artery and subsequently into the pulmonary artery. Symptoms derive either from poor collateral flow from the right coronary artery or secondary to a steal phenomenon of blood passing through well-developed collaterals into the left coronary arterial system with drainage into the pulmonary artery. Because of the low pressures in the pulmonary artery, blood flow is selectively shunted into the pulmonary system instead of perfusing left ventricular myocardium.

Two of the earliest and most characteristic symptoms are tachypnea and dyspnea. Coughing, wheezing, and cyanosis usually follow. One interesting finding that may be present has been called the "an-gina of feeding," in which the infant shows evidence of pain during and immediately after feeding. As CHF worsens, cyanosis and pallor become apparent.

### Physical Examination

The characteristic findings on physical examination include a rapid respiratory rate, tachycardia, and cardiac enlargement. A murmur is not usually present early in life, and congenital origin of the left coronary artery from the pulmonary artery is one of the few malformations that in infancy can cause CHF without a murmur. In older infants and children, mitral regurgitation develops secondarily either to left ventricular dilatation (Burchell and Brown, 1962) or to chronic ischemia or infarction, which causes papillary muscle dysfunction. Buist, in 1991, reported a 6-month-old male who presented with physical signs and chest film findings suggestive of a foreign body in the tracheobronchial tree. However, the patient subsequently was found to have extrinsic compression of the left main bronchus by a markedly enlarged left atrium. Anomalous origin of the left coronary artery from the pulmonary artery was found at cardiac catheterization, and the patient was cured by operation.

The liver is usually enlarged, and the spleen is palpable in a smaller number of patients. Occasionally, patients first present with signs of cardiovascular collapse and shock similar to those manifested by adults with sudden coronary artery occlusion.

## Evaluation

### Chest Film

The chest film shows cardiomegaly, especially involving the left ventricle. Evidence of CHF may be present as well. Aneurysmal dilatation may result from marked thinning of the left ventricular wall. In many cases, the left border of the heart extends to the lateral rib margin. As a result of left ventricular failure, the pulmonary vascular markings are usually exaggerated.

### Electrocardiography

Considerable emphasis has been placed on the changes that occur in the electrocardiogram leading to the establishment of a diagnosis. Bland and associates (1933) first described myocardial ischemia on the electrocardiogram of an infant with this condition. Based on this work, congenital origin of the left coronary artery from the pulmonary artery has also been called *Bland-White-Garland syndrome*. Generally, it is possible to make a relatively firm diagnosis on the basis of electrocardiographic changes. Tachycardia is almost always present. The T waves are characteristically inverted in the standard limb leads, and slight ST-segment elevation may be noted in lead I. The T waves in the precordial leads, especially $V_5$ and $V_6$, are usually inverted, and deep Q waves are frequently present. The body surface potential distribution has also been helpful in diagnosis and in providing evidence of improved coronary blood flow after operative therapy (Flaherty et al., 1967).

## Noninvasive Techniques

Noninvasive tests to diagnose anomalous origin of the left coronary artery from the pulmonary artery include two-dimensional echocardiography (Fisher et al., 1981), thallium scans (Finley et al., 1978), pulsed-wave Doppler echocardiography (King et al., 1985), and most recently, magnetic resonance imaging (Duoard et al., 1988). So far, too few patients have been reported to determine whether these techniques can eliminate the need for preoperative cardiac catheterization. However, available results suggest that noninvasive studies can be used to accurately assess and monitor postoperative patients (Fyfe et al., 1987).

## Angiocardiography

The right side of the heart is usually normal. The pulmonary vasculature may show slight engorgement and enlargement. The most striking feature is enlargement of the left atrium and particularly of the left ventricle. The wall of the left ventricle may be quite thin, especially the anterolateral aspect near the apex. A true ventricular aneurysm with paradoxical pulsations may be present, and mitral insufficiency is relatively common. Contrast medium passing into the aorta demonstrates a single right coronary artery, although selective coronary arteriography is more reliable for precise demonstration of this feature.

## Aortography

Injection of contrast medium into a catheter passed into the proximal aorta (or, when possible, directly into the right coronary ostium) shows the classic findings. Contrast medium enters the right coronary artery as it originates from the aorta and passes through dilated collaterals that communicate with the left coronary artery. The contrast material can then be followed into the left circumflex and anterior descending coronary arteries, where it converges to enter the left main coronary artery, with ultimate drainage into the pulmonary artery. This finding is impressive and conclusive, and large amounts of radiopaque contrast medium can be seen flowing freely into the pulmonary artery. Thus, retrograde flow of blood in the left coronary artery can be shown convincingly in such a study, and this finding establishes an objective diagnosis (Fig. 54–25).

## Cardiac Catheterization

Cardiac catheterization also helps establish the diagnosis. The right ventricular and pulmonary artery pressures may be elevated. Moreover, injection of contrast medium usually shows a left-to-right shunt at the pulmonary artery level. Although the oxygen sat-

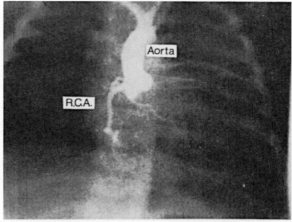
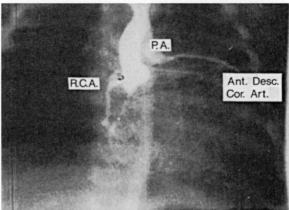
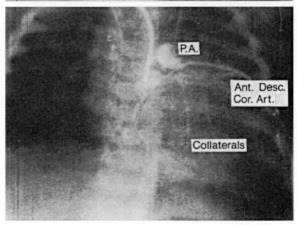

FIGURE 54–25. Several cine frames taken from a series illustrating coronary arterial filling during aortography. A, Filling of the right coronary artery (RCA) as it arises normally from the aorta. Note that its size is slightly greater than normal. B, Filling of the branches of the left coronary artery through collaterals from the right coronary artery, (PA = pulmonary artery.) C, Filling of the pulmonary artery by retrograde flow from the left coronary artery. (A–C, From Sabiston, D. C., Jr., and Orme, S. K.: Congenital origin of the left coronary artery from the pulmonary artery. J. Cardiovasc. Surg., 9:543, 1968.)

uration may sometimes show a significant increase from the right ventricle to the pulmonary artery, this increase is not always present, even when it can be shown that the left coronary artery arises from the pulmonary artery.

The ejection fraction in patients with anomalous origin of the left coronary artery was measured by Menke and associates (1972) in eight preoperative patients, in whom it ranged from 0.13 to 0.72. Among those who died, the ejection fraction was less then 0.36, but in the survivors it was more then 0.55. Similar finds were reported by Vouhé and colleagues (1992) in 31 patients who underwent preoperative determination of left ventricular shortening fraction measured by echocardiography. There was a 31% operative mortality rate among patients with a left ventricular shortening fraction of less than 0.20 versus no deaths among patients with a left ventricular shortening fraction of 0.20 or more ($p = .03$).

### Pathology

The major pathologic features of this condition are apparent at the time of operation. The left ventricle is greatly dilated and the wall is thin. The left coronary artery is larger than normal, and numerous collateral vessels connect the right and left coronary arteries and these are usually tortuous and thin-walled. The right coronary artery arises in its normal position and is also enlarged. Its branches tend to be more tortuous than usual as they emit various collateral vessels. With time, and especially in adults, the right coronary artery may become quite large and increasingly tortuous. Similarly, the left coronary artery may also become quite enlarged, up to 10 mm or more in diameter at its origin. The left coronary artery arises from the left or posterior cusp of the pulmonary artery. The branches and course of the anterior descending and circumflex branches are usually otherwise normal. On section, the left ventricle may be very thin and in area is totally replaced by scar tissue (Fig. 54–26). Various degrees of subendocardial fibroelastosis may be present. Calcification is often present in the fibrotic portion of the left ventricle. Infarction of the ventricle may involve a papillary muscle, producing mitral insufficiency. If the left ventricle is dilated, the mitral ring may be sufficiently enlarged to prevent normal coaptation of the valve leaflets, also causing mitral insufficiency.

## Surgical Management

The main objective in surgical correction of origin of the left coronary artery from the pulmonary artery is to establish adequate blood flow in the left coronary artery and its branches. Historically, several surgical procedures were advocated to accomplish this: Mustard's left common carotid artery anastomosis to the left coronary artery (1962), Potts' aortopulmonary anastomosis (1955), the pulmonary artery banding of Case and associates (1958), and the technique of pericardial poudrage and de-epicardialization (Paulson and Robbins, 1955). However, disappointing results with these procedures led to their abandonment.

In the modern era, two basic approaches are used in the surgical treatment of this malformation: simple

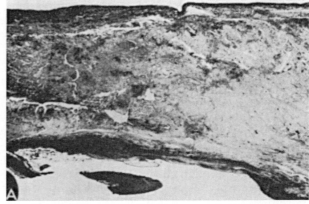
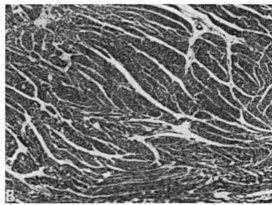

**FIGURE 54–26.** *A,* Histologic section of full thickness of left ventricle. Note that the left ventricular wall is almost totally replaced with scar tissue. The section represents the full thickness of the ventricle and is magnified 12 times, showing the extreme thinness of the left ventricle. *B,* Histologic section of right ventricular myocardium in the same patient showing normal cardiac muscle. (*A* and *B,* From Sabiston, D. C., Jr., and Orme, S. K.: Congenital origin of the left coronary artery from the pulmonary artery. J. Cardiovasc. Surg., *9:*543, 1968.)

ligation at the site of origin of the anomalous left coronary artery and the establishment of a two–coronary artery system.

Simple ligation at the site of origin from the pulmonary artery is an effective treatment if enough collaterals from the right coronary artery exist to supply the left coronary system adequately (Fig. 54–27A). Ligation prevents the "coronary steal" into the pulmonary artery, increases the coronary artery pressure, and improves myocardial blood flow (Sabiston and Orme, 1968). Long-term follow-up of patients undergoing this procedure has demonstrated the beneficial effects of simple ligature with relief of symptoms and decrease in heart size (De Salazar et al., 1990; Shrivistava et al., 1978).

Simple ligation alone, however, has led to high mortality because the number of intercoronary collaterals varies and simple ligature is unable to produce immediate and sufficient improvement in left ventricular myocardial perfusion in all patients (Backer et al., 1992; Hurwitz et al., 1989; Wilson et al., 1977). Survivors of this procedure are left with a single coronary artery system, which is theoretically less

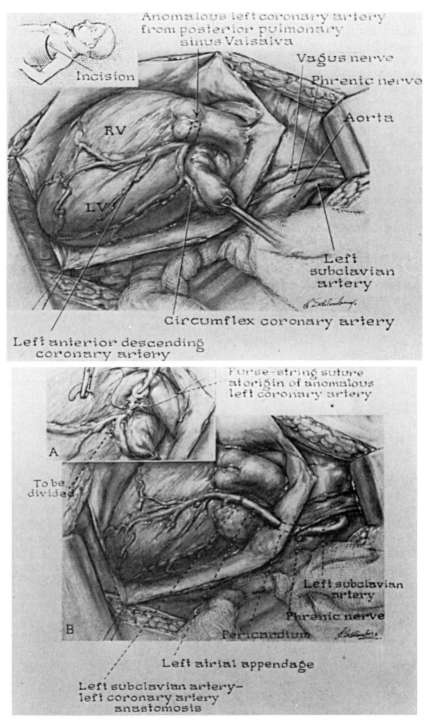

**FIGURE 54–27.** *A,* Congenital origin of the left coronary artery from the pulmonary artery. Through a left anterior third interspace thoracotomy, the left coronary artery is occluded at its site of origin with suture ligatures and is then divided. *B,* The left subclavian artery is then anastomosed to the left coronary artery in end-to-end fashion by using interrupted 7-0 nonabsorbable sutures. (*A* and *B,* From Lowe, J. E., and Sabiston, D. C., Jr.: Congenital coronary malformations. *In* Cohn, L. [ed]: Modern Technics in Surgery: Cardiac-Thoracic Surgery. Mt. Kisco, NY, Futura, 1981.)

physiologic and at greater risk of atherosclerosis (Roberts and Loube, 1947). Also, the incidence of sudden death is higher in patients who had undergone simple ligation than in those who had a two-coronary artery system established (Backer et al., 1992; Wilson et al., 1977). Poorer performance on treadmill exercise testing (McNamara and Elsaid, 1973) and higher late mortality (not due to sudden death) (Bunton et al., 1987) have also been reported in patients with simple ligature or nonfunctioning grafts (ligature equivalent) compared with those with two–coronary artery systems. Therefore, simple ligature should be reserved for only those critically ill patients in whom it may be lifesaving (Kirklin and Barratt-Boyes, 1986; Vouhé et al., 1987) and creation of a two–coronary artery system can be accomplished later in life (Cooley et al., 1966).

Surgical reestablishment of a two–coronary artery system is the treatment of choice for anomalous left coronary artery arising from the pulmonary artery (Arciniegas et al., 1980; Backer et al., 1992; Elsaid et al., 1973; Hurwitz et al., 1989; Kesler et al., 1989; Smith et al., 1989; Tkebuchava et al., 1992; Vigneswaran et al., 1989; Vouhé et al., 1987, 1992). The surgical alternatives include left subclavian-left coronary artery anastomosis (Kesler et al., 1989; Meyer et al., 1968; Pinsky et al., 1973; Stephenson et al., 1981) (see Fig. 54–27B) or connection of the left coronary artery to the aorta. The latter can be performed by direct implantation (Backer et al., 1992; Grace et al., 1977; Hurwitz et al., 1989; Neches et al., 1974; Vouhé et al., 1992) (Fig. 54–28), autologous artery (Laborde et al., 1981; Neches et al., 1974; Pirk et al., 1993) (Figs. 54–29 and 54–30), venous bypass grafting (Elsaid et al., 1973; Kesler et al., 1989), or intrapulmonary tunneling (Figs. 54–31 and 54–32). This transpulmonary aorta-left coronary artery continuity has been accomplished by using a flap of anterior pulmonary wall (Sese and Imoto, 1992; Takeuchi et al., 1979), autologous pericardium (Hamilton et al., 1979), a free segment of left subclavian artery (Arciniegas et al., 1980), or polytetrafluoroethylene (PTFE; Gore-Tex) (Bunton et al., 1987) to connect a side-to-side aortopulmonary window to the left coronary ostium within the lumen of the pulmonary artery.

In older children and adults, a two–-coronary artery system can be reconstructed using a saphenous vein graft (Wilson et al., 1977) or internal mammary bypass grafting (Fig. 54–33). These methods are technically difficult in infants and small children. Moreover, graft

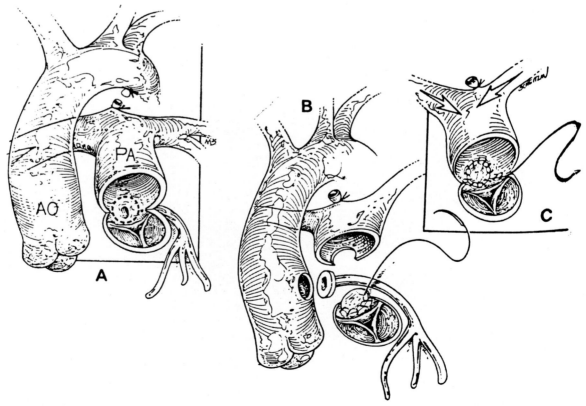

**FIGURE 54–28.** Direct aortic reimplantation of anomalous origin of the left coronary artery from the pulmonary artery (PA) is becoming the procedure of choice by many surgeons for both infants and adults. *A,* Excision of the anomalous origin of the left coronary ostium from the pulmonary artery. (Ao = aorta.) *B,* Aortic reimplantation of the coronary ostium to the aorta using an 8-0 absorbable continuous suture. Mobilization of the pulmonary bifurcation and division of the ligamentum arteriosum allow end-to-end reconstruction of the pulmonary artery in most patients. However, when compression of the reimplanted left coronary artery is apparent, a patch of autologous pericardium is used to close the defect created in the pulmonary wall. *C,* Reconstruction of the pulmonary artery. (*A–C,* From Vouhé, P. R., Tamisier, D., Sidi, D., et al.: Anomalous left coronary artery from the pulmonary artery: Results of isolated aortic reimplantation. Reprinted by permission. From the Society of Thoracic Surgeons [The Annals of Thoracic Surgery, 1992, Vol. 54, pp. 621–627].)

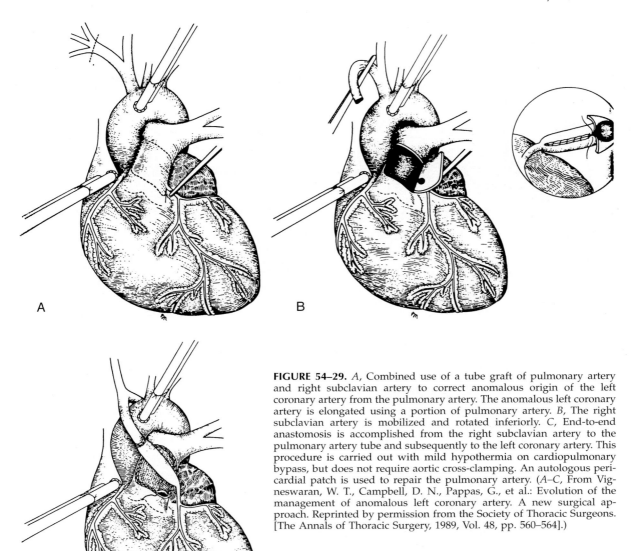

**FIGURE 54–29.** *A,* Combined use of a tube graft of pulmonary artery and right subclavian artery to correct anomalous origin of the left coronary artery from the pulmonary artery. The anomalous left coronary artery is elongated using a portion of pulmonary artery. *B,* The right subclavian artery is mobilized and rotated inferiorly. *C,* End-to-end anastomosis is accomplished from the right subclavian artery to the pulmonary artery tube and subsequently to the left coronary artery. This procedure is carried out with mild hypothermia on cardiopulmonary bypass, but does not require aortic cross-clamping. An autologous pericardial patch is used to repair the pulmonary artery. (*A–C,* From Vigneswaran, W. T., Campbell, D. N., Pappas, G., et al.: Evolution of the management of anomalous left coronary artery. A new surgical approach. Reprinted by permission from the Society of Thoracic Surgeons. [The Annals of Thoracic Surgery, 1989, Vol. 48, pp. 560–564].)

occlusion in infants is a problem (Arciniegas et al., 1980; McNamara and Elsaid, 1973). Given the inability of a graft to grow with the child, bypass grafting with veins is considered an unsatisfactory method of reconstruction of a two–coronary vessel circulation in infants (Grace et al., 1977).

Direct implantation of the anomalous left coronary artery into the root of the aorta is a method of establishing a two–coronary vessel circulation by recreating the normal anatomy. Excellent patency rates of 100% have been reported in patients who survived direct aortic reimplantation (Backer et al., 1992; Laborde et al., 1981; Tkebuchava et al., 1992; Vouhe et al., 1992). Technical difficulties in mobilizing adequate length may also preclude the use of this technique. Moreover, reimplantation alters both the shape of the left coronary orifice and the angle it subtends with

the aorta (Smith et al., 1989). The clinical significance of these changes awaits further follow-up of survivors and detailed study of coronary blood flow and ventricular function in these infants.

The technique of subclavian-left coronary anastomosis (see Fig. 54–27*B*) was first described by Apley and co-workers in 1951; Meyer and colleagues first performed this successfully in 1968. This procedure can be performed through a left thoracotomy without cardiopulmonary bypass or with cardiopulmonary bypass through a median sternotomy or bilateral anterior thoracotomies with transverse sternotomy. Excellent results have been reported using this procedure (Kesler et al., 1989; Stephenson et al., 1981). Technical advantages over other revascularizing techniques include the avoidance of aortic cross-clamping (which may increase the ongoing ischemic injury of

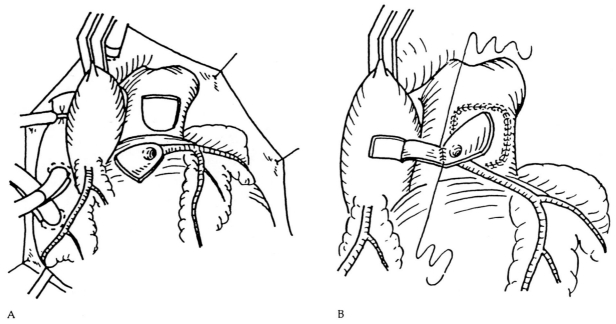

A                                                        B

**FIGURE 54–30.** Creation of a two–coronary artery system in the treatment of anomalous origin of the left coronary artery from the pulmonary artery using a new elongation technique. *A,* With the patient under cardiopulmonary bypass with moderate hypothermia, the aorta is cross-clamped. The pulmonary trunk was incised, and the orifice of the left coronary artery was identified. The anomalous left coronary artery was excised with a wide and long cuff of pulmonary artery. The defect in the pulmonary artery is closed with an autologous pericardial patch. *B,* The aorta is then incised to make a swinging-door-shaped flap. The cuff of the left coronary artery was then sutured onto the aortic flap with a continuous 6-0 polydioxanone suture. (*A* and *B,* From Sese, A., and Imoto, Y.: New technique in the transfer of an anomalously originated left coronary artery to the aorta. Reprinted with permission from the Society of Thoracic Surgeons [The Annals of Thoracic Surgery, 1992, Vol. 53, pp. 527–529].)

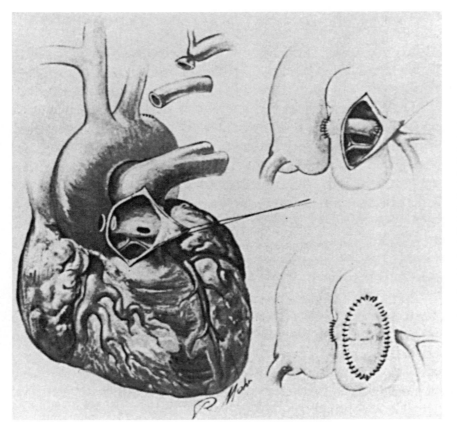

**FIGURE 54–31.** Transpulmonary arterial aortocoronary bypass grafting is performed with a free segment of the left subclavian artery (LSCA). A 4-mm aortopulmonary window is constructed and the LSCA segment is sutured within the pulmonary artery to the aortopulmonary anastomosis and around the ostium of the anomalous left coronary artery. A pericardial angioplasty prevents luminal compromise of the pulmonary artery containing the transpulmonary arterial bypass graft. (Reproduced with permission from Arciniegas, E. A., Farooki, Z. Q., Haimi, M., and Green, E. W.: Management of anomalous left coronary artery from the pulmonary artery. Circulation, *62* [Suppl. I]:180, 1980. Copyright 1980 American Heart Association.)

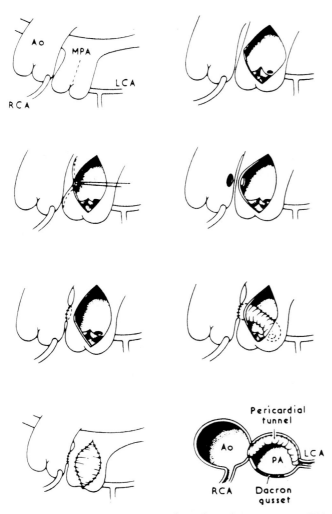

**FIGURE 54–32.** An opening is made in the pulmonary artery (PA) and an aortopulmonary window is created. A pericardial tunnel is then constructed and connects the aortopulmonary window within the pulmonary artery to the anomalous origin of the left main coronary artery (LCA) from the pulmonary artery. The defect in the anterior pulmonary arterial wall is repaired using a Dacron patch. (Ao = aorta; RCA = right coronary artery; MPA = main pulmonary artery.) (From Hamilton, D. E., Ghosh, P. K., and Donnelly, R. J.: An operation for anomalous origin of left coronary artery. Br. Heart J., *41*:121, 1979.)

flap to direct blood from a created aortopulmonary window into the anomalous left coronary artery ostium. As noted previously, modifications have been made to this technique. Preliminary experience has shown this method to be technically applicable to infants and small children (as well as adults) with favorable improvements in clinical status and left ventricular function (Bunton et al., 1987). Operative complications include aortic valve incompetence secondary to valve damage during creation of the aortopulmonary window and pulmonic stenosis as a result of pulmonary arteriotomy or the intrapulmonary conduit. Long-term patency and survival have shown this to be a simple and effective means of establishing a two–coronary artery system. Transpulmonary arterial bypass is now considered by some to be the procedure of choice in infants because it has low mortality and good patency rates (Arciniegas et al., 1980; Bunton et al., 1987).

The best form of surgical treatment for this disorder is unknown. Clearly, the establishment of a two–coronary vessel circulation is superior to simple ligation. Simple ligation should be reserved for neonates whose critical illness precludes a lengthy cardiac bypass procedure. The Meyer operation is an excellent alternative because it can be performed without bypass. In older children and adults, a two–coronary artery system can be reconstructed by using saphenous vein or internal mammary artery bypass grafting. In young children, infants, and neonates, the

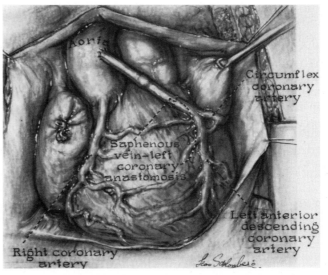

**FIGURE 54–33.** Congenital origin of the left coronary from the pulmonary artery can also be managed by division of the left coronary artery at its site of origin and reconstruction of a two-coronary artery system using a saphenous vein graft. Through a median sternotomy, and with a patient on cardiopulmonary bypass, the saphenous vein graft is attached to the ascending aorta using a partial occluding clamp. The left coronary artery is then divided at its site of origin from the pulmonary artery. The saphenous vein graft is anastomosed in end-to-end manner to the left coronary artery using interrupted 7-0 nonabsorbable sutures. (From Lowe, J. E., and Sabiston, D. C., Jr.: Surgical correction of congenital malformations of the coronary circulation. Reprinted by permission from the Southern Medical Journal *75*:1508, 1982.)

the myocardium) and the avoidance of direct surgical procedures involving the pulmonary artery that may lead to late stenosis. Among infants, however, graft occlusion can be a problem and occlusion rates as high as 50% have been reported (Pinsky et al., 1973). The tendency for the left subclavian artery to kink as it arises from the left aortic arch predisposes it to late graft occlusion. However, this technique may have a role in the establishment of a two–coronary artery system in critically ill infants because it can be performed without cardiopulmonary bypass or aortic occlusion (Kesler et al., 1989).

In 1979, Takeuchi and associates described a technique that involved the creation of a transpulmonary artery aortocoronary bypass in which the anterior wall of the pulmonary artery was used as a tunnel surgical alternatives include direct implantation of the anomalous coronary artery into the aorta, intrapulmonary conduits, and left subclavian-left coronary artery anastomosis. Bypass grafting with venous autograft or prosthetic graft is not a satisfactory option in this age group because of technical difficulty and poor graft patency. Direct aortic reimplantation or intrapulmonary artery conduits are increasingly being used with good results and are becoming the procedures of choice in all age groups.

## Results

The authors have evaluated 40 patients with anomalous origin of the left coronary artery from the pulmonary artery, and 30 have been surgically treated. Twenty-two had severe CHF. Six had angina and 2 infants came to attention because of failure to thrive. The remaining 10 patients were evaluated for murmurs of uncertain cause, cardiomegaly on physical examination, or chest films or unexplained dyspnea. All 10 patients not operated on died within several hours to several months after diagnosis. Of the 30 patients undergoing repair, 17 had simple ligation at the origin of the left coronary artery from the pulmonary artery, with 6 operative deaths (35%) and 1 additional death 4 months postoperatively. Seven patients had ligation of the left coronary artery followed by saphenous vein or left internal mammary artery grafting. There were no operative deaths and all 7 have been well 4 to 14 years after operation. Five of 7 grafts were clotted on repeat angiography performed 4 months to 2 years postoperatively. One patient treated with ligation of the left coronary artery from its origin had left subclavian-left coronary artery anastomosis at 14 months of age. This patient, at age 13 years, is a gymnast. Two patients underwent a pulmonary artery tunnel procedure and 1 died 1 hour postoperatively. Early in the authors' experience, 2 patients were treated with de-epicardialization and are long-term survivors. One early patient had pulmonary-aortic anastomosis and died shortly after operation, and 1 died during thoracotomy before a planned simple ligation. Among the 30 patients, there were 9 operative deaths with overall operative mortality of 30%. Because of the 95 to 100% mortality in those treated nonoperatively, surgical treatment is always recommended following diagnosis.

## ORIGIN OF THE RIGHT CORONARY ARTERY FROM THE PULMONARY ARTERY

Brooks in 1886 originally described this rare malformation in two cadavers studied in the anatomic dissection laboratory at the University of Dublin. Both lesions occurred in adults, neither of whom had evidence of heart disease. Brooks noted dilated collaterals from the left coronary artery feeding the right coronary artery and correctly postulated, based on this observation, that flow in the right coronary artery might actually be retrograde into the pulmonary artery.

## Clinical Manifestations

The clinical manifestations of this condition are usually minimal or absent. In 17 cases collected from the literature (reviewed by Tingelstad et al., 1972), the abnormal artery was discovered in individuals whose ages ranged from 17 to 90 years. The malformation was thought to have been associated with death in only 2 cases. One of these was a 17-year-old female who died suddenly. Autopsy showed complete occlusion of the left coronary artery by thrombus with evidence of left ventricular infarction. The only other death occurred in a 55-year-old woman who presented with angina and CHF. In 3 additional patients, the anomaly was found in association with other congenital malformations.

Even though origin of the right coronary artery from the pulmonary artery is a rare anomaly with a benign natural history in most patients, it can cause myocardial ischemia, infarction, CHF, and myocardial fibrosis (Coe et al., 1982; Ross et al., 1987; Saenz et al., 1986; Vairo et al., 1992). Because it can be safely corrected when diagnosed, operative management is indicated.

## Evaluation

In the rare patient with this condition who comes to medical attention, the diagnosis is established by aortography and selective coronary arteriography. The left coronary artery is found to be dilated, and large intercoronary collaterals feed the right coronary artery. As Brooks correctly suggested, flow in the right coronary artery is retrograde, emptying into the pulmonary artery. In contrast with patients who have the more frequently occurring malformation of origin of the left coronary artery from the pulmonary artery, there are usually no electrocardiographic or radiographic abnormalities. The diagnosis is therefore established only in those who have selective coronary arteriography. Two-dimensional echocardiography has been used to diagnose this malformation, which was confirmed later by coronary arteriography (Saenz et al., 1986; Worsham et al., 1985).

## Surgical Management and Results

Tingelstad and colleagues (1972) reported a fascinating case of a 12-year-old boy who was asymptomatic but had a to-and-fro systolic and diastolic murmur along the left sternal border in the third intercostal space. The chest film showed slight cardiac enlargement and normal pulmonary vasculature. Mild left ventricular hypertrophy was shown by a scalar electrocardiogram. An aortogram revealed a dilated left coronary artery arising normally from the left sinus of Valsalva of the aorta and the right coronary artery was filled through tortuous intercoronary anastomoses from the left coronary artery and drained into the main pulmonary artery. At operation, a narrow rim of tissue from the pulmonary artery was removed with the origin of the right coronary artery and this was successfully reimplanted into the ascending aorta. This represents the ideal form of surgical management and has also been performed successfully by others (Bregman et al., 1976; Coe et al., 1982; van Meura-van Woezik et al., 1984; Vairo et al., 1992). Other alternatives include simple ligation at the site of anomalous origin with or without saphenous vein bypass grafting (Rowe and Young, 1960).

## ORIGIN OF BOTH CORONARY ARTERIES FROM THE PULMONARY ARTERY

Twenty-five infants in whom both coronary arteries arose from the pulmonary artery have been reported. These patients have been reviewed in detail by Heifetz and associates (1986). The survival time ranged from 9 hours to 7 years. The patient who lived to age 7 years was able to do so because of severe pulmonary hypertension secondary to a ventricular septal defect and congenital mitral stenosis (Feldt et al., 1965). The pressure in the pulmonary artery was sufficient to force blood into the myocardial capillary bed and the child lived for an amazingly long time. This malformation has been diagnosed by cardiac catheterization, and surgical repair has been attempted (Goldblatt et al., 1984; Keeton et al., 1983; Ogasawara et al., 1985).

## ANEURYSMS OF THE CORONARY ARTERIES

In 1812, Bougon first reported an aneurysm of the coronary arteries (cited by Packard and Wechsler, 1929). These lesions have been reported from infancy to adult life (Crocker et al., 1957). Congenital aneurysms of the coronary arteries are rare, constituting only 15% of coronary artery aneurysms in the 89 patients reported by Daoud and co-workers (1963). Other causes of aneurysms of the coronary arteries include atherosclerosis, mycosis, syphilis, rheumatic heart disease, and mucocutaneous lymph node syndrome (Kawasaki's disease).

These lesions most often are asymptomatic until complications occur, including thrombosis or embolization with subsequent myocardial ischemia or infarction or actual rupture of the aneurysm. Wei and Wang (1986) reported a 26-year-old woman who presented with a 3-month history of cough, shortness of breath, and vomiting. The patient was found to have a giant congenital right coronary aneurysm measuring 15 cm in diameter. The aneurysm was excised and the symptoms resolved completely. An intramural coronary aneurysm has also been reported, which produced reversed flow during systole owing to bulging of the thin-walled chamber into the left ventricular cavity. The narrow neck of the aneurysm was closed successfully at operation. An example of a congenital coronary artery aneurysm involving the left circumflex vessel is shown in Figure 54–34A. In this patient, a mural thrombus occurred in the aneurysm; it embolized and produced acute myocardial infarction (Fig. 54–34B). The aneurysm was resected and a saphenous vein autograft was inserted (Ebert et al., 1971) (Fig. 54–34C). Surgical management of a coronary artery aneurysm is indicated if the aneurysm is symptomatic, especially if there is evidence of emboli arising from the aneurysm, producing myocardial ischemia in the distal coronary bed.

## MEMBRANOUS OBSTRUCTION OF THE OSTIUM OF THE LEFT MAIN CORONARY ARTERY

Hypoplasia or atresia of the coronary arteries in infancy and childhood has been reported and usually causes severe impairment of ventricular function and sudden death. Congenital atresia of the left main coronary artery has been reported in 9 patients, all of whom presented with signs and symptoms of myocardial ischemia or CHF, or both. Histopathologic studies in these patients showed that the left main coronary artery had been replaced by fibromuscular tissue and that the left coronary ostium was absent. These conditions are not surgically correctable. However, three patients have been reported with membranous obstruction at the ostium of the left main coronary artery, associated with a normal distal coronary artery. The first patient was a 6-month-old infant who died following myocardial infarction; the diagnosis was established at the time of autopsy (Verney et al., 1969). Josa and colleagues (1981) reported two cases diagnosed at the time of operation. One patient, a 2-year-old child being operated on for congenital aortic stenosis, was found to have a membrane markedly obstructing the ostium of the left main coronary artery. The second patient was an 8-year-old boy with Type I truncus arteriosus who also had membranous obstruction of the ostium of the left main coronary artery at operation. Both patients showed evidence of myocardial ischemia preoperatively, and after the membrane was excised at operation, the symptoms were totally relieved. Grossly, the membranous structure appeared to be continuous with the aortic intima, and histologic studies revealed that its structure was similar to that of normal aortic root media. These two examples indicate the importance of careful evaluation of the origin and distribution of the coronary arteries in patients with congenital heart disease, especially when the signs and symptoms of ischemia and heart failure are disproportionate to the congenital lesion being evaluated (Josa et al., 1981).

Lea and associates (1986) reported a patient with congenital ostial stenosis of the right coronary artery that was successfully repaired by vein patch angioplasty.

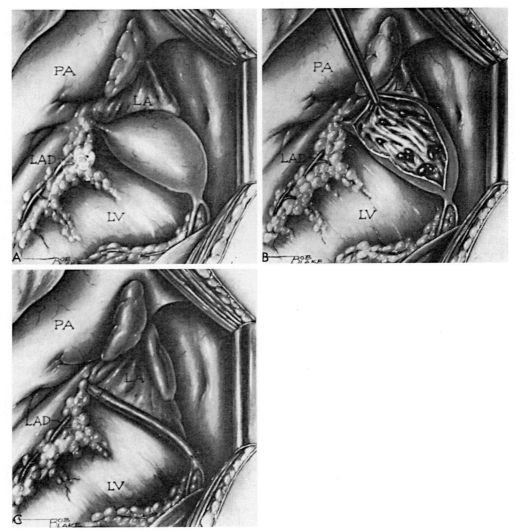

**FIGURE 54–34.** *A,* Congenital aneurysm of the left circumflex coronary artery as seen at operation in a 31-year-old woman who presented with an acute myocardial infarction with subsequent disabling angina. (PA = pulmonary artery; LAD = left anterior descending coronary artery; LV = left ventricle; LA = left atrium.) *B,* Numerous small fresh thrombi are shown adherent to the rough, irregular surface of the aneurysm. The proximal opening into the aneurysm was a discrete, mildly dilated vessel of good quality and normal-appearing intima. The distal branches of the circumflex coronary artery are of normal size. *C,* The entire aneurysm was excised, and an interposition graft of saphenous vein was placed. There was only minimal discrepancy in the size of the saphenous vein graft and the ends of the circumflex coronary artery. A continuous 7-0 nonabsorbable suture was used at each anastomosis. (From Ebert, P. A., Peter, R. H., Gunnells, J. C., and Sabiston, D. C., Jr.: Resecting and grafting of coronary artery aneurysms. Circulation, *43*:593, 1971. By permission of the American Heart Association, Inc.)

## SELECTED BIBLIOGRAPHY

Abrikossoff, A.: Aneurysma des linken Herzventrikels mit abnormer Abgangsstelle der linken Koronararterie von der Pulmonalis bei einem funfmonatlichen Kinde. Virchows Arch. (Pathol. Anat.), *203*:413, 1911.

The classic description of anomalous origin of the left coronary artery from the pulmonary artery is made in this historic paper. Both the gross and the microscopic illustrations are excellent. The author describes in detail the clinical manifestations and postmortem findings.

Ebert, P. A., Peter, R. H., Gunnells, J. C., and Sabiston, D. C., Jr.: Resecting and grafting of coronary artery aneurysm. Circulation, *43*:593, 1971.

This paper describes an aneurysm of the circumflex coronary artery containing a thrombus that later embolized and produced myocardial infarction. The problem, clinical manifestations, and management are discussed.

Feldt, R. H., Ongley, P. A., and Titus, J. L.: Total coronary arterial circulation from pulmonary artery with survival to age seven: Report of a case. Mayo Clin. Proc., *40*:539, 1965.

This paper presents the amazing report of a child who survived to 7 years of age with a coronary circulation arising solely from the pulmonary artery. This case report is clearly a fascinating one and is an example of the marked compensatory power of the coronary circulation.

Heifetz, S. A., Robinowitz, M., Mueller, K. H., and Virmani, R.: Total anomalous origin of the coronary arteries from the pulmonary artery. Pediatr. Cardiol., *7*:11, 1986.

Four patients with total anomalous origin of the coronary arteries from the pulmonary artery are presented and compared with 21 previously reported patients. Of the 19 patients in whom a clinical history was available, 16 were symptomatic before 3 days of age. All patients died, 60% before 2 weeks of age. Longer survival was associated with additional cardiovascular malformations that resulted in pulmonary hypertension or increased oxygen saturation, or both. Cardiomegaly was present in 56% of patients, and most had myocardial fibrosis or infarction. Surgical correction had been attempted in 2 patients, but both attempts failed secondary to severe preexistent myocardial injury.

Lea, J. W., IV, Page, D. L., and Hammon, J. W., Jr.: Congenital ostial stenosis of the right coronary artery repaired by vein patch angioplasty. J. Thorac. Cardiovasc. Surg., 92:796, 1986.

This is the first report of a patient with congenital ostial stenosis of the right coronary artery in which successful repair was accomplished by saphenous vein patch angioplasty. A biopsy from the region of stenosis revealed markedly thickened intima containing well-oriented fibrous tissue, whereas the media contained smooth muscle cells in mild disarray separated focally by mucoid material. There was no evidence of atheromatous involvement.

Lowe, J. E., Oldham, H. N., Jr., and Sabiston, D. C., Jr.: Surgical management of congenital coronary artery fistulas. Ann. Surg., 194:371, 1981.

This article reports the clinical manifestations of 28 patients with congenital coronary artery fistulas seen at one institution and summarizes the results of surgical management in 22 patients. An additional 258 patients reported earlier are also reviewed. The natural history and pathophysiology of coronary fistulas are discussed, and the reason for early surgical intervention is presented.

Sabiston, D. C., Jr., and Orme, S. K.: Congenital origin of the left coronary artery from the pulmonary artery. J. Cardiovasc. Surg., 9:543, 1968.

In this report, 23 patients with origin of the left coronary artery from the pulmonary artery are described. The youngest patient was 1 day old and the oldest patient was 31 years old. The natural history, clinical findings, laboratory data, and ultimate course are presented.

Stephenson, L. W., Edmunds, L. H., Jr., Friedman, S., et al.: Subclavian-left coronary artery anastomosis (Meyer operation) for anomalous origin of the left coronary artery from the pulmonary artery. Circulation, 64(Suppl. II):130, 1981.

Six patients, ages 2 to 76 months, had subclavian-to-coronary artery anastomosis for anomalous origin of the left coronary artery from the pulmonary artery. Five of the six patients had congestive heart failure and ongoing ischemia. All six had cardiomegaly, and preoperative left ventricular ejection fractions averaged $0.46 \pm 0.171$. Five patients survived operation and were alive at 8 to 92 months after operation, and four of the five anastomoses were patent at postoperative cardiac catheterization. None of the surviving patients has required cardiac medications, and all of them are symptom-free at follow-up. In addition to subclavian-left coronary anastomosis, multiple other surgical options, including intrapulmonary shunts, are discussed in detail.

Vouhé, P. R., Tamisier, D., Sidi, D., et al.: Anomalous left coronary artery from the pulmonary artery: Results of isolated aortic reimplantation. Ann. Thorac. Surg., 54:621, 1992.

The authors report 31 consecutive children with anomalous origin of the left coronary artery from the pulmonary artery who underwent direct aortic reimplantation of the anomalous artery. There were 5 deaths (16%), 3 in the hospital and 2 within 3 months postoperatively. The severity of preoperative left ventricular dysfunction was the only incremental risk factor for mortality: 31% among patients with a left ventricular shortening fraction of less than 0.20, versus 0% among patients with a left ventricular shortening fraction of 0.20 or more ($p = .03$). There were no late deaths up to 6 years following operation, and the overall survival rate was 84%. Extensive follow-up was carried out in 23 survivors having a follow-up of longer than 12 months. Ninety-six per cent were free of symptoms. Left ventricular function returned to normal in all patients and moderate to severe mitral regurgitation decreased to minimal or no regurgitation in the majority of patients (5 of 7). Most importantly, the reimplanted anomalous left coronary artery was patent in all patients. The authors feel strongly that direct aortic reimplantation is the operation of choice for this anomaly and that intrapulmonary tunnel repair may be indicated in only a very few patients in whom coronary arterial transfer appears to be impossible. In addition, the authors believe that the mitral valve should not be repaired or replaced at the initial operation because mitral regurgitation almost always decreases after successful revascularization.

Wei, J., and Wang, D.: A giant congenital aneurysm of the right coronary artery. Ann. Thorac. Surg., 41:322, 1986.

The authors report a 26-year-old patient who presented with shortness of breath and a chronic cough. A chest film showed a huge mass on the right ventricular border, and the patient was admitted with a tentative diagnosis of mediastinal tumor. Coronary arteriography showed a giant coronary aneurysm arising from the right coronary artery. At the time of operation, the aneurysm measured 15 cm in diameter. The aneurysm was resected, and histologic examination of the aneurysmal wall showed no evidence of atheromatous change. The patient recovered, and symptoms resolved completely.

# BIBLIOGRAPHY

Abbott, M. E.: Congenital cardiac disease. In Osler, W. (ed.): Modern Medicine. Vol. 4. Philadelphia, Lea & Febiger, 1908.

Abbott, M. E.: Congenital cardiac disease. In Osler, W. (ed.): Modern Medicine. 3rd ed. Philadelphia, Lea & Febiger, 1927.

Abrikossoff, A.: Aneurysma des linken Herzventrikels mit abnormer Abgangsstelle der linken Koronararterie von der Pulmonalis bei einem funfmonatlichen Kinde. Virchows Arch. (Pathol. Anat.), 203:413, 1911.

Apley, J., Horton, R. E., and Wilson, M. G.: The possible role of surgery in the treatment of anomalous left coronary artery. Thorax, 12:28, 1951.

Arciniegas, E. A., Farooki, Z. Q., Haimi, M., and Green, E. W.: Management of anomalous left coronary artery from the pulmonary artery. Circulation, 62(Suppl. I):168, 1980.

Backer, C. L., Stout, M. J., Zales, V. R., et al.: Anomalous origin of the left coronary artery. J. Thorac. Cardiovasc. Surg., 103:1049, 1992.

Barton, C. W., Snider, A. R., and Rosenthal, A.: Two-dimensional and Doppler echocardiographic features of left circumflex coronary artery-to-right ventricle fistula: Case report and literature review. Pediatr. Cardiol., 7:167, 1986.

Björk, G., and Crafoord, C.: Arteriovenous aneurysm on the pulmonary artery stimulating patent ductus arteriosus botalli. Thorax, 2:65, 1947.

Bland, E. F., White, P. D., and Garland, J.: Congenital anomalies of coronary arteries: Report of an unusual case associated with cardiac hypertrophy. Am. Heart J., 8:787, 1933.

Bougon: Bibl. Med., 37:183, 1812. Cited by Packard, M., and Wechsler, H. F.: Aneurysm of the coronary arteries. Arch. Intern. Med., 43:1, 1929.

Bregman, D., Brennan, J., Singer, A., et al.: Anomalous origin of the right coronary artery from the pulmonary artery. J. Thorac. Cardiovasc. Surg., 72:626, 1976.

Brooks, H. St. J.: Two cases of an abnormal coronary artery of the heart arising from the pulmonary. J. Anat. Physiol., 20:26, 1886.

Buist, R. J.: An unusual cause of obstructive emphysema. Anesthesia, 46:283, 1991.

Bunton, R., Jonas, R. A., Lang, P., et al.: Anomalous origin of left coronary artery from pulmonary artery: Ligation versus establishment of a two–coronary artery system. J. Thorac. Cardiovasc. Surg., 93:103, 1987.

Burchell, H. B., and Brown, A. L., Jr.: Anomalous origin of the coronary artery from the pulmonary artery masquerading as mitral insufficiency. Am. Heart J., 63:388, 1962.

Case, R. B., Morrow, A. G., Stainsby, W., and Nestor, J. O.: Anomalous origin of the left coronary artery: The physiologic defect and suggested surgical treatment. Circulation, 17:1062, 1958.

Coe, J. Y., Radley-Smith, R., and Yacoub, M.: Clinical and hemodynamic significance of anomalous origin of the right coronary artery from the pulmonary artery. Thorac. Cardiovasc. Surg., 30:84, 1982.

Cooley, D. A., Hallman, G. L., and Bloodwell, R. D.: Definitive surgical treatment of anomalous origin of left coronary artery from pulmonary artery: Indications and results. J. Thorac. Cardiovasc. Surg., 52:798, 1966.

Crocker, D. W., Sobin, S., and Thomas, W. C.: Aneurysms of the coronary arteries. Report of three cases in infants and review of the literature. Am. J. Pathol., 33:819, 1957.

Daniel, T. M., Graham, T. P., and Sabiston, D. C., Jr.: Coronary artery-right ventricular fistula with congestive heart failure: Surgical correction in the neonatal period. Surgery, 67:985, 1970.

Daoud, A. S., Pankin, D., Tulgan, H., and Florentin, R. A.: Aneurysms of the coronary artery. Am. J. Cardiol., 11:228, 1963.

De Salazar, A. O., Juanena, C., Aramendi, J. I., et al.: Anomalous origin of the left coronary artery from the pulmonary artery. Surgical alternatives depending on the age of the patient. J. Cardiovasc. Surg., 31:801, 1990.

Duoard, H., Barat, J. L., Laurent, F., et al.: Magnetic resonance imaging of an anomalous origin of the left coronary artery from the pulmonary artery. Eur. Heart J., 9:1356, 1988.

Ebert, P. A., Peter, R. H., Gunnells, J. C., and Sabiston, D. C., Jr.: Resecting and grafting of coronary artery aneurysm. Circulation, 43:593, 1971.

Elsaid, G. M., Ruzyllo, W., Williams, W. L., et al.: Early and later results of saphenous vein graft for anomalous origin of left coronary artery from pulmonary artery. Circulation, 48(Suppl.):382, 1973.

Feldt, R. H., Ongley, P. A., and Titus, J. L.: Total coronary arterial circulation from pulmonary artery with survival to age seven: Report of a case. Mayo Clin. Proc., 40:539, 1965.

Fernandes, E. D., Kadivar, H., Hallman, G. L., et al.: Congenital malformation of the coronary arteries: The Texas Heart Institute experience. Ann. Thorac. Surg., 54:732, 1992.

Finley, J. P., Holman-Giles, R., Gilday, D. L., et al.: Thallium-201 myocardial imaging in anomalous left coronary artery arising from the pulmonary artery: Applications before and after medical and surgical treatment. Am. J. Cardiol., 42:675, 1978.

Fisher, E. A., Sepehri, B., Lendrum, B., et al.: Two-dimensional echocardiographic visualization of the left coronary artery in anomalous origin of the left coronary artery from the pulmonary artery. Circulation, 63:698, 1981.

Flaherty, J. T., Spach, M. S., Boineau, J. P., et al.: Cardiac potentials on body surface of infants with anomalous left coronary artery (myocardial infarction). Circulation, 36:345, 1967.

Fyfe, D. A., Sade, R. M., Gillette, P. C., and Kline, C. H.: Pre- and postoperative Doppler echocardiographic evaluation of anomalous left coronary artery arising from the pulmonary artery. J. Ultrasound Med., 6:101, 1987.

Goldblatt, E., Adams, A. P. S., Ross, I. K., et al.: Single-trunk anomalous origin of both coronary arteries from the pulmonary artery. J. Thorac. Cardiovasc. Surg., 87:59, 1984.

Grace, R. R., Angelini, P., and Cooley, D. A.: Aortic implantation of anomalous left coronary artery arising from pulmonary artery. J. Cardiol., 39:608, 1977.

Griffiths, S. P., Ellis, K., Hordof, A. J., et al.: Spontaneous complete closure of a congenital coronary artery fistula. J. Am. Coll. Cardiol., 2:1169, 1983.

Hacket, D., and Hallidie-Smith, K. A.: Spontaneous closure of coronary artery fistula. Br. Heart J., 52:477, 1984.

Hamilton, D. E., Ghosh, P. K., and Donnelly, R. J.: An operation for anomalous origin of left coronary artery. Br. Heart J., 41:121, 1979.

Harthorne, J. W., Scannell, J. G., and Dinsmore, R. E.: Anomalous origin of the left coronary artery: Remediable cause of sudden death in adults. N. Engl. J. Med., 275:660, 1966.

Heifetz, S. A., Robinowitz, M., Mueller, K. H., and Virmani, R.: Total anomalous origin of the coronary arteries from the pulmonary artery. Pediatr. Cardiol., 7:11, 1986.

Hurwitz, R. A., Caldwell, R. L., Girod, D. A., et al.: Clinical and hemodynamic course of infants and children with anomalous left coronary artery. Am. Heart J., 118:1176, 1989.

Josa, M., Danielson, G. K., Weidman, W. H., and Edwards, W. D.: Congenital ostial membrane of left main coronary artery. J. Thorac. Cardiovasc. Surg., 81:338, 1981.

Keeton, B. R., Keenan, D. J. M., and Monro, J. L.: Anomalous origin of both coronary arteries from the pulmonary trunk. Br. Heart J., 49:397, 1983.

Keith, J. D.: The anomalous origin of the left coronary artery from the pulmonary artery. Br. Heart J., 21:149, 1959.

Kesler, K. A., Pennington, G., Nouri, S., et al.: Left subclavian-left coronary artery anastomosis for anomalous origin of the left coronary artery: Long-term follow-up. J. Thorac. Cardiovasc. Surg., 98:25, 1989.

King, D. H., Danford, D. A., Huhta, J. C., and Gutgesell, H. P.: Noninvasive detection of anomalous origin of the left main coronary artery from the main pulmonary trunk by pulsed Doppler echocardiography. Am. J. Cardiol., 55:608, 1985.

Kirklin, J. W., and Barratt-Boyes, B. A.: Congenital anomalies of the coronary arteries. In Kirklin, J. W., and Barratt-Boyes, B. A. (eds): Cardiac Surgery. New York, John Wiley & Sons, 1986, p. 945.

Laborde, F., Marchand, M., Leca, F., et al.: Surgical treatment of anomalous origin of the left coronary artery in infancy and childhood: Early and late results in 20 consecutive cases. J. Thorac. Cardiovasc. Surg., 82:423, 1981.

Lea, J. W., IV, Page, D. L., and Hammon, J. W., Jr.: Congenital ostial stenosis of the right coronary artery repaired by vein patch angioplasty. J. Thorac. Cardiovasc. Surg., 92:796, 1986.

Liberthson, R. R., Sagar, K., Behocoben, J. P., et al.: Congenital coronary arteriovenous fistula. Circulation, 59:849, 1979.

Lowe, J. E., and Sabiston, D. C., Jr.: Surgical correction of congenital malformations of the coronary circulation. South. Med. J., 75:1508, 1982.

Lowe, J. E., Oldham, H. N., Jr., and Sabiston, D. C., Jr.: Surgical management of congenital coronary artery fistulas. Ann. Surg., 194:371, 1981.

Mahoney, L. T., Schieken, R. M., and Lauer, R. M.: Spontaneous closure of a coronary artery fistula in childhood. Pediatr. Cardiol., 2:311, 1982.

McNamara, D. G., and Elsaid, G.: Treatment of anomalous origin of the left coronary artery from the pulmonary artery. Eur. J. Cardiol., 1:497, 1973.

Menke, J. A., Shaher, R. M., and Wolff, G. S.: Ejection fraction in anomalous origin of the left coronary artery from the pulmonary artery. Am. Heart J., 84:325, 1972.

Meyer, W., Stefanik, G., Stiles, Q. R., et al.: A method of definitive surgical treatment of anomalous origin of left coronary artery. J. Thorac. Cardiovasc. Surg., 56:104, 1968.

Moodie, D. S., Fyfe, D., Gill, C. C., et al.: Anomalous origin of the left coronary artery from the pulmonary artery (Bland-White-Garland syndrome) in adult patients: Long-term follow-up after surgery. Am. Heart J., 26:597, 1985.

Mustard, W. T.: Anomalies of the coronary artery. In Benson, C. D., Mustard, W. T., Ravitch, M. M., et al. (eds): Pediatric Surgery. Vol. 1. Chicago, Year Book Medical, 1962, p. 433.

Neches, W. H., Mathews, R. A., Pack, S. C., et al.: Anomalous origin of the left coronary artery from the pulmonary artery. Circulation, 50:582, 1974.

Ogasawara, K., Aizawa, T., Fijii, J., et al.: A case with fistulas from both coronary arteries and the left bronchial artery to the pulmonary artery. Jpn. Heart J., 26:597, 1985.

Ogden, J. A.: Congenital anomalies of the coronary arteries. Am. J. Cardiol., 25:474, 1970.

Paulson, R. M., and Robbins, S. G.: A surgical treatment proposed for either endocardial fibroelastosis or anomalous left coronary artery. Pediatrics, 16:147, 1955.

Pickoff, A. S., Wolff, G. S., Bennett, V. L., et al.: Pulsed Doppler echocardiographic detection of coronary artery to right ventricle fistula. Pediatr. Cardiol., 2:145, 1982.

Pinsky, W. W., Fagan, L. R., Kraeger, R. R., et al.: Anomalous left coronary artery. J. Thorac. Cardiovasc. Surg., 65:810, 1973.

Pirk, J., Fabian, J., and Kovac, J.: Reconstructing an anomalous left coronary artery origin using the internal iliac artery. Ann. Thorac. Surg., 56:1163, 1993.

Podolsky, L., Ledley, G. S., Goldstein, J., et al.: Bilateral coronary artery to left ventricular fistulas. Cathet. Cardiovasc. Diagn., 24:271, 1991.

Potts, quoted by Kittle, C. F., Diehl, A. M., and Heilbrake, A.: Anomalous left coronary artery arising from the pulmonary artery. J. Pediatr., 47:198, 1955.

Purut, C. M., and Sabiston, D. C., Jr.: Origin of the left coronary artery from the pulmonary artery in older adults. J. Thorac. Cardiovasc. Surg., 102:566, 1991.

Reeder, G. S., Tajik, A. J., and Smith, H. C.: Visualization of coronary artery fistula by two-dimensional echocardiography. Mayo Clin. Proc., 55:185, 1980.

Roberts, J. T., and Loube, S. D.: Congenital single coronary artery in man. Am. Heart J., 34:100, 1947.

Ross, T. C., Latham, R. D., and Craig, W. E.: Anomalous origin of the right coronary artery from the main pulmonary artery: Incidental finding in a case of dilated cardiomyopathy. South. Med. J., 80:783, 1987.

Rowe, G. G., and Young, W. P.: Anomalous origin of the coronary arteries with special reference to surgical treatment. J. Thorac. Cardiovasc. Surg., 39:777, 1960.

Sabiston, D. C., Jr., and Orme, S. K.: Congenital origin of the left coronary artery from the pulmonary artery. J. Cardiovasc. Surg., 9:543, 1968.

Sabiston, D. C., Jr., Neill, C. A., and Taussig, H. B.: The direction of blood flow in anomalous left coronary artery arising from the pulmonary artery. Circulation, 22:591, 1960a.

Sabiston, D. C., Jr., Pelargonio, S., and Taussig, H. B.: Myocardial infarction in infancy: The surgical management of a complication of congenital origin of the left coronary artery from the pulmonary artery. J. Thorac. Cardiovasc. Surg., 40:321, 1960b.

Sabiston, D. C., Jr., Ross, R. S., Criley, J. M., et al.: Surgical management of congenital lesions of the coronary circulation. Ann. Surg., 157:908, 1963.

Saenz, C. B., Taylor, J. L., Soto, B., et al.: Acute myocardial infarction in a patient with anomalous right coronary artery. Am. Heart J., 112:1092, l986.

Sese, A., and Imoto, Y.: New technique in the transfer of an anomalously originated left coronary artery to the aorta. Ann. Thorac. Surg., 53:527, 1992.

Shrivistava, S., Castañeda, A. R., and Moller, J. H.: Anomalous left coronary artery from pulmonary trunk. Long-term follow-up after ligation. J. Thorac. Cardiovasc. Surg., 76:130, 1978.

Slater, J., Lighty, G. W., Jr., Winer, H. E., et al.: Doppler echocardiography and computed tomography in diagnosis of left coronary arteriovenous fistula. J. Am. Coll. Cardiol., 4:1290, 1984.

Smith, A., Arnold, R., Anderson, R. H., et al.: Anomalous origin of the left coronary artery from the pulmonary trunk: Anatomic findings in relation to pathophysiology and surgical repair. J. Thorac. Cardiovasc. Surg., 98:16, 1989.

Sones, F. M., and Shirey, E. K.: Collateral arterial channels in living human with coronary artery disease. Circulation, 22:815, 1960.

Stephenson, L. W., Edmunds, L. H., Jr., Friedman, S., et al.: Subclavian-left coronary artery anastomosis (Meyer operation) for anomalous origin of the left coronary artery from the pulmonary artery. Circulation, 64(Suppl. II):130, 1981.

Takeuchi, S., Imamura, H., Katsumoto, K., et al.: New surgical method for repair of anomalous left coronary artery from pulmonary artery. J. Thorac. Cardiovasc. Surg., 78:7, 1979.

Tingelstad, J. B., Lower, R. R., and Eldredge, W. J.: Anomalous origin of the right coronary artery from the main pulmonary artery. Am. J. Cardiol., 30:670, 1972.

Tkebuchava, T., Carrel, T., von Segesser, L., et al.: Repair of anoma-

lous origin of the left coronary artery from the pulmonary artery without early and late mortality in 9 patients. J. Cardiovasc. Surg. (Torino), 33:479, 1992.

Urrutia-S, C. O., Falaschi, G., Ott, D. A., and Cooley, D. A.: Surgical management of 56 patients with congenital coronary artery fistulas. Ann. Thorac. Surg., 35:300, 1983.

Vairo, U., Marino, B., De Simone, G., and Marcelletti, C.: Early congestive heart failure due to origin of the right coronary artery from the pulmonary artery. Chest, 102:1610, 1992.

van Meura-van Woezik, H., Serruys, P. W., Reiber, J. H. C., et al.: Coronary artery changes 3 years after reimplantation of an anomalous right coronary artery. Eur. Heart J., 5:175, 1984.

Verney, R. N., Monnet, P., Arnaud, P., et al.: Infarctus du myocarde chez un nourrisson de cinq mois—Ostium coronaire gauche punctiforme. Ann. Pedaiatr. (Paris), 16:260, 1969.

Vigneswaran, W. T., Campbell, D. N., Pappas, G., et al.: Evolution of the management of anomalous left coronary artery: A new surgical approach. Ann. Thorac. Surg., 48:560, 1989.

Vouhé, P. R., Baillot-Vernant, F., Trinquet, F., et al.: Anomalous left coronary artery from pulmonary artery in infants: Which operation? When? J. Thorac. Cardiovasc. Surg., 94:192, 1987.

Vouhé, P. R., Tamisier, D., Sidi, D., et al.: Anomalous left coronary artery from the pulmonary artery: Results of isolated aortic reimplantation. Ann. Thorac. Surg., 54:621, 1992.

Wei, J., and Wang, D.: A giant congenital aneurysm of the right coronary artery. Ann. Thorac. Surg., 41:322, 1986.

Wenger, N. K.: Rare causes of coronary heart disease. In Hurst, J. W. (ed): The Heart. New York, McGraw-Hill, 1978.

Wilson, C. L., Dlabal, P. W., Holeyfield, R. W., et al.: Anomalous origin of left coronary artery from pulmonary artery: Case report and review of literature concerning teenagers and adults. J. Thorac. Cardiovasc. Surg., 73:887, 1977.

Worsham, C., Sanders, S. P., and Burger, B. M.: Origin of the right coronary artery from the pulmonary trunk: Diagnosis by two-dimensional echocardiography. Am. J. Cardiol., 55:232, 1985.

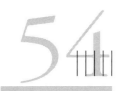

# ■ III Pathology of Coronary Atherosclerosis

William C. Roberts

Atherosclerotic *coronary artery disease* (CAD) is the most common cause of death in the Western world. One American dies every minute of atherosclerotic CAD. In the United States alone, 5.5 to 7.5 million individuals have symptomatic myocardial ischemia because of atherosclerotic CAD. The cause of atherosclerosis is now clear: The evidence is overwhelming that atherosclerosis is a cholesterol problem. The higher the blood total cholesterol level (especially the low-density lipoprotein level), the greater is the risk for developing symptomatic CAD, fatal CAD, and atherosclerotic plaques. Lowering the blood total cholesterol level decreases the chances of development of symptomatic or fatal CAD, and the possibility increases that some atherosclerotic plaques will actually regress.

Although the coronary arteries have been examined

visually at necropsy for more than 100 years, only recently has the extent of the atherosclerotic process in the coronary arteries in patients with symptomatic or fatal CAD become appreciated. This chapter concerns the status of the major epicardial coronary arteries in patients with fatal atherosclerotic CAD.

## AMOUNTS OF CORONARY ARTERIAL LUMINAL NARROWING

The amounts of coronary arterial narrowing observed at necropsy in patients with *unstable angina pectoris* (UAP), *acute myocardial infarction* (AMI), and *sudden coronary death* (SCD) are generally enormous (Roberts, 1989b). As shown in Table 54–5 from a study of 80 patients at necropsy with these three coronary

■ **Table 54–5.** NUMBER OF MAJOR (RIGHT, LEFT MAIN, LEFT ANTERIOR DESCENDING, AND LEFT CIRCUMFLEX) CORONARY ARTERIES NARROWED MORE THAN 75% IN CROSS-SECTIONAL AREA BY ATHEROSCLEROTIC PLAQUE IN FATAL CORONARY ARTERY DISEASE

| Coronary Event | Patients (n) | Mean Age (Yrs) | Number of Four Arteries/Patient Narrowed More Than 75% in Cross-Sectional Area by Plaque | | | | |
| | | | 4 | 3 | 2 | 1 | Mean |
| --- | --- | --- | --- | --- | --- | --- | --- |
| Sudden coronary death | 31 | 47 | 3 | 20 | 6 | 2 | 2.8 |
| Acute myocardial infarction | 27 | 59 | 3 | 14 | 10 | 0 | 2.7 |
| Unstable angina pectoris | 22 | 48 | 10 | 8 | 3 | 1 | 3.2 |
| Totals | 80 | 51 | 16 (20%) | 42 (52%) | 19 (24%) | 3 (4%) | 2.9 |
| Controls | 40 | 52 | 0 (0) | 5 (5%) | 12 (13%) | 21 (23%) | 0.7 |

events (SCD in 31, AMI in 27, and UAP in 22), an average of 2.9 of the four major (right, left main, left anterior descending, and left circumflex) coronary arteries were severely narrowed (more than a 75% decrease in cross-sectional area) at some point, and no significant differences were observed among the three coronary subsets. The patients with UAP had a much higher frequency of severe narrowing of the left main coronary artery (10 of 22 patients [45%]), compared with those with AMI (3 of 27 patients [11%]) and SCD (3 of 31 patients [10%]).

A more sophisticated approach to determining degrees of luminal narrowing is to examine the entire lengths of the four major epicardial coronary arteries. One technique involves incising each of the four major coronary arteries transversely at 5-mm intervals and then preparing a histologic section from each 5-mm segment. Normally, the total length of the four major arteries is about 27 cm (right = 10 cm; left main = 1 cm; left anterior descending = 10 cm, and left circumflex = 6 cm), and thus about 55 five-mm segments are available for examination from each heart. Studies using this approach in the patients with UAP, AMI, and SCD are summarized in Table 54–6. Of the 4016 five-mm segments studied in the 80 patients, 38% were narrowed 76 to 100% in cross-sectional area by plaque alone (controls = 3%); 34% were narrowed 51 to 75% (controls = 3%); 34% were narrowed 51 to 75% (controls = 22%); 20% were narrowed 26 to 50% (controls = 44%); and only 7% were narrowed 25% or less (controls = 31%). Similar degrees of narrowing by plaque alone at all four

categories of narrowing were observed in the patients with AMI and SCD; the patients with UAP had significantly more severe coronary narrowing than did the other two groups.

Thus, in general, patients with fatal UAP have more extensive severe narrowing by plaque alone of the four major epicardial coronary arteries than do patients with either AMI or SCD. And the patients with UAP, compared with the other two groups, have a significantly higher frequency of severe narrowing of the left main coronary artery.

The information derived at necropsy quantitating the severity and extent of atherosclerosis in the four major epicardial coronary arteries in fatal CAD is potentially useful clinically in two areas: in interpreting degrees of coronary narrowing by angiography during life and in deciding which of the major coronary arteries needs a conduit at the time of *coronary artery bypass grafting* (CABG) (Fig. 54–35).

Without coronary angiography, neither CABG nor angioplasty would be performed. The only way during life to obtain information on the status of the epicardial coronary arteries is through angiography; therefore, this procedure revolutionized diagnosis of CAD just as aortocoronary bypass grafting revolutionized therapy of CAD. However, angiography—as good as it is—has certain deficiencies. An angiogram is a luminogram, and a narrowed segment is compared with a less narrowed segment that is assumed to be normal. The angiogram does not delineate the internal elastic membrane of the artery, so the artery's true lumen is still uncertain.

■ **Table 54–6.** AMOUNTS OF CROSS-SECTIONAL AREA NARROWING OF EACH 5-MM SEGMENT OF THE FOUR MAJOR (RIGHT, LEFT MAIN, LEFT ANTERIOR DESCENDING, AND LEFT CIRCUMFLEX) EPICARDIAL CORONARY ARTERIES BY ATHEROSCLEROTIC PLAQUES IN SUBJECTS WITH FATAL CORONARY ARTERY DISEASE

| Subgroup | Patients (n) | Mean Age (Yrs) | Number of 5-mm Segments | Percentage of Segments Narrowed | | | | |
| | | | | 0–25% | 25–50% | 51–75% | 76–100% | Mean Score |
| --- | --- | --- | --- | --- | --- | --- | --- | --- |
| Sudden coronary death | 31 | 47 | 1564 | 7 | 23 | 34 | 36 | 2.98 |
| Acute myocardial infarction | 27 | 59 | 1403 | 5 | 23 | 38 | 34 | 3.01 |
| Unstable angina pectoris | 22 | 48 | 1049 | 11 | 12 | 29 | 48 | 3.12 |
| Totals | 80 | 51 | 4016 | 7 | 20 | 34 | 38 | 3.02 |
| Controls | 40 | 52 | 1849 | 31 | 44 | 22 | 3 | 1.97 |

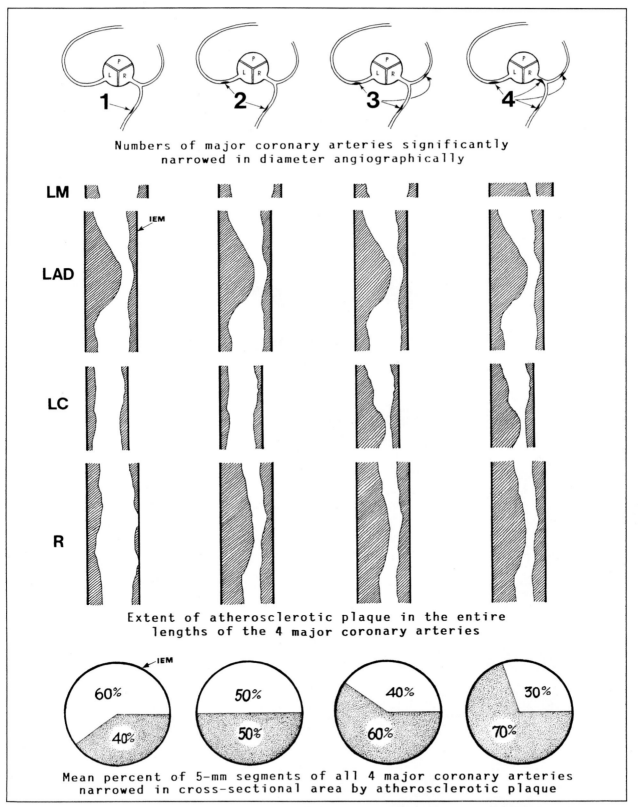

**FIGURE 54–35.** *Top,* The numbers of major coronary arteries severely narrowed in diameter by angiogram. *Middle,* The average amount of atherosclerotic plaque in the left main (LM), left anterior descending (LAD), left circumflex (LC), and right (R) coronary arteries in their full lengths according to the numbers of coronary arteries significantly narrowed by angiogram. *Bottom,* The average amount of cross-sectional area narrowing by atherosclerotic plaque in each 5-mm segment of the four major epicardial coronary arteries. (Reproduced with permission from Roberts, W. C.: Coronary "lesion," coronary "disease," "single-vessel disease," "two-vessel disease": Word and phrase misnomers providing false impressions of the extent of coronary atherosclerosis in symptomatic myocardial ischemia. Am. J. Cardiol., 66:121, 1990.)

The aforementioned coronary quantitative studies demonstrated in fatal CAD that 93% of the 5-mm segments of the four major epicardial coronary arteries were narrowed more than 25% in cross-sectional area by atherosclerotic plaque. Thus, only 7% of the 5-mm segments approached normal and almost none was normal. Thus, at least in fatal CAD and probably also in live patients with symptomatic myocardial ischemia, it is infrequent that an angiographically severely narrowed segment of a coronary artery can be compared with a segment of coronary artery that is actually normal. In other words, in patients with symptomatic myocardial ischemia, the coronary angiogram measures degrees of narrowing by comparing severely narrowed segments with segments that are less narrowed but by no means normal (Fig. 54–36). Accordingly, coronary angiograms in patients with symptomatic myocardial ischemia usually underestimate the degrees of luminal narrowing (Arnett et al., 1979; Isner et al., 1981). This fact is well appreciated by most cardiac surgeons, but is less well appreciated by cardiologists.

The unit of measuring degrees of narrowing by angiography differs from the unit of measurement at necropsy. In anatomic studies, the unit is usually *cross-sectional area* narrowing. The unit of angiography is *diameter* narrowing. Generally, a 75% cross-sectional area narrowing is equivalent to a 50% diameter reduction, and therefore, a 50% or more diameter narrowing during life generally has been considered the cut-off point between clinically significant and clinically insignificant coronary narrowing (see Fig. 54–36).

The second potential use of the information derived

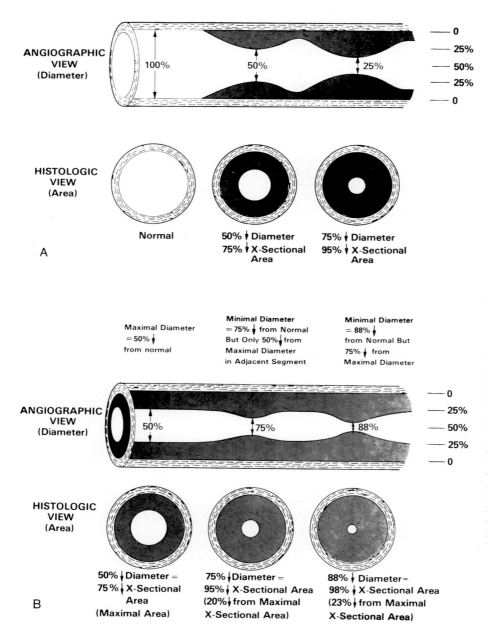

**FIGURE 54–36.** The relationship between longitudinal narrowing (diameter reduction) as seen by coronary angiography and cross-sectional area narrowing as seen by histologic examination of a coronary artery. A coronary arterial segment with a 50% diameter narrowing has a 75% reduction in cross-sectional area. A 75% reduction in diameter corresponds to a 95% reduction in cross-sectional area. The theoretical situation by which a narrowing is compared with an adjacent perfectly normal segment of artery is shown (*A*) and the usual real situation is shown (*B*). The least-narrowed segment below has a 50% reduction in diameter (75% loss of cross-sectional area) and a central, round residual lumen. Because the angiogram is a luminogram and the width of the original arterial lumen is unknown, the least narrowed segment is often presumed to be normal. The width of more narrowed segments is compared with that of the least narrowed segments. If the least narrowed segment is 50% narrowed, what appears to be a 50% narrowing in an adjacent segment is really a 75% diameter narrowing (95% reduction in cross-sectional area); what appears to be a 75% narrowing in an adjacent segment is really an 88% diameter narrowing (98% reduction in cross-sectional area). (From Arnett, E. N., Isner, J. M., Redwood, D. R., et al.: Coronary artery narrowing in coronary heart disease: Comparison of cineangiographic and necropsy findings. Ann. Intern. Med., *91*:350, 1979.)

from the detailed CAD studies at necropsy is the appreciation that the atherosclerotic process in patients with symptomatic myocardial ischemia is usually diffuse and severe and, therefore, that more rather than fewer aortocoronary conduits provide a higher frequency of relief or improvement in symptomatic myocardial ischemia, of improvement of exercise testing, and of prolonging life. Among patients surviving for fewer than 30 days or at later periods after aortocoronary bypass operations, the amount of severe narrowing in the *nonbypassed native* coronary arteries is usually similar to that in the *bypassed native* coronary arteries. From study at necropsy of 102 patients dying either early (60 days or less) or late (2.5 to 108 months [mean, 35 months]) after bypass operations (Waller and Roberts, 1980), it was found that the bypassed and nonbypassed native coronary arteries had similar degrees of severe luminal narrowing by atherosclerotic plaques. Specifically, in 213 (94%) of the 226 bypassed native arteries and in 73 (91%) of 80 nonbypassed native arteries, the lumens were narrowed more than 75% in cross-sectional area by atherosclerotic plaque. The reason why the native arteries were not bypassed was not that they were too small or severely narrowed distally, but that by angiogram the lumens were judged not sufficiently narrowed to warrant the insertion of a conduit. Thus, if two of the major coronary arteries are severely narrowed by angiography and the third major artery is "insignificantly" narrowed and if a bypass operation is to be performed, the insertion of a conduit in all three major coronary arteries could be reasonably considered. There is, of course, potential danger in inserting a conduit in an artery that is insignificantly narrowed; nevertheless, it may be more advantageous to err on the side of too many conduits than too few. At necropsy, three-vessel disease is more frequent than two-vessel disease, and when only two of the three major arteries at necropsy are narrowed more than 75% in cross-sectional area, the third one is usually narrowed at least 51–75% in cross-sectional area. Thus, an appreciation of the diffuse nature of coronary atherosclerosis in fatal CAD and probably also in symptomatic myocardial ischemia encourages the use of more rather than fewer conduits at CABG operations.

## COMPOSITION OF ATHEROSCLEROTIC PLAQUES IN FATAL CAD

Kragel and associates (1989, 1990) studied at necropsy atherosclerotic plaque composition in the four major (right, left main, left anterior descending, and left circumflex) coronary arteries in 15 patients who died of consequences of AMI, in 12 patients with SCD without associated AMI, and in 10 patients with isolated UAP with pain at rest. The coronary arteries were sectioned at 5-mm intervals, and a Movat-stained section of each segment of artery was prepared and analyzed using a computerized morphometric system. Among the three subsets of coronary

patients, there were no differences in plaque composition among any of the four major epicardial coronary arteries. Within all three groups, the major component of plaque was a combination of dense acellular and cellular fibrous tissue, with much smaller portions of plaque being composed of pultaceous debris, calcium, foam cells with and without inflammatory cells, and foam cells alone (Table 54–7). Within all three groups, plaque morphology varied as a function of cross-sectional area narrowing of the segments. In all three groups, the amount of dense, relatively acellular fibrous tissue, calcified tissue, and pultaceous debris (amorphous debris containing cholesterol clefts, presumably rich in extracellular lipid) increased in a linear manner with increasing degrees of cross-sectional area narrowing of the segments, and the amount of cellular fibrous tissue decreased. Multiluminal channels were most frequent in the subgroup with UAP. The studies by Kragel and associates (1989, 1990) were the first to analyze quantitatively the composition of coronary arterial plaques in the various subsets of coronary patients.

## EFFECTS OF PERCUTANEOUS TRANSLUMINAL CORONARY ANGIOPLASTY ON ATHEROSCLEROTIC PLAQUES AND RELATION OF PLAQUE COMPOSITION AND ARTERIAL SIZE TO OUTCOME

To delineate their relation to outcome of *percutaneous transluminal coronary angioplasty* (PTCA), the atherosclerotic plaque composition and coronary artery size in 82 five-mm segments at 28 PTCA sites were determined by Potkin and Roberts (1988) in 26 patients having PTCA. The 26 patients were subdivided into three groups according to the degree of angiographic patency at the end of the PTCA procedure and to the duration of survival after PTCA (30 days

■ **Table 54–7.** MEAN COMPOSITION OF CORONARY ARTERIAL ATHEROSCLEROTIC PLAQUES IN THE FOUR MAJOR EPICARDIAL CORONARY ARTERIES

| Components of Plaque | Mean Percent of Plaque Containing Various Components in the Four Major Coronary Arteries (1438 segments) | | |
|---|---|---|---|
| | *Unstable Angina Pectoris (n = 10)* | *Acute Myocardial Infarction (n = 15)* | *Sudden Coronary Death (n = 12)* |
| Dense fibrous tissue | 35 | 46 | 29 |
| Loose fibrous tissue | 1 | 3 | 3 |
| Cellular fibrous tissue | 52 | 32 | 50 |
| Calcium | 4 | 4 | 8 |
| Pultaceous debris | 4 | 8 | 4 |
| Foam cells | 0 | 1 | 0 |
| Foam cells and lymphocytes | 3 | 4 | 6 |
| Inflammatory infiltrates without significant number of foam cells | 1 | 2 | 1 |

or less versus more than 30 days): early success (13 patients, 16 PTCA sites, and 16 five-mm segments) and late success (9 patients, 8 PTCA sites, and 17 five-mm segments). The mean percentage of plaque composed of fibrous tissue among the three groups was $80 \pm 18\%$, $71 \pm 23\%$, and $82 \pm 16\%$; the mean percentage of plaque composed of lipid was $17 \pm 16\%$, $21 \pm 24\%$, and $16 \pm 15\%$; and of calcium was $3 \pm 4\%$, $8 \pm 10\%$, and $2 \pm 3\%$. The mean coronary arterial internal diameter was $3.3 \pm 0.6$, $3.9 \pm 1.2$, and $3.2 \pm 0.7$ mm. Plaque tear was present in 1 or more histologic sections in 25 of the 26 patients. Plaque tear extending from intima into media with dissection was observed only in the early and late success groups. Hemorrhage into plaque was present in 16 (80%) of 20 PTCA sites in the two early groups and in 3 (37%) of 8 sites in the late group. Occlusive thrombus (5 of 16, 1 of 4, and 1 of 8) and plaque debris (7 of 16, 1 of 4, and 2 of 8) in residual lumens were insignificantly different among the three groups and their 82 five-mm segments. Plaques that had more than 25% lipid content had an increased frequency of hemorrhage into plaque, occlusive thrombus, and plaque debris in residual lumens. These findings suggest that coronary arterial size and plaque composition are strong determinants of PTCA outcome. The ideal coronary arterial atherosclerotic narrowing for both technically and clinically successful PTCA appears to be a small (less than 3.3 mm in interval diameter) artery in which the plaque contains relatively little calcium and lipid.

## MORPHOLOGIC FINDINGS IN SAPHENOUS VEINS USED AS CABG CONDUITS

Saphenous veins, when used as aortocoronary conduits, undergo changes in their intimal, medial, and adventitial layers. The predominant late intimal change is a proliferation of fibrous tissue, a finding observed within 2 months after CABG. Other late changes in saphenous vein grafts include deposits of lipid, thrombus, and rarely, aneurysm formation. Most published studies describing changes in saphenous veins used as bypass conduits have involved few necropsy patients, involved only operatively excised specimens, or involved cases with relatively short intervals from CABG to death or reoperation. Kalan and Roberts (1990) studied at necropsy the hearts and grafts of 53 patients who lived longer than 1 year after CABG. They examined 123 saphenous vein grafts and 1865 five-mm segments of the grafts in the 53 patients, some of whom died of consequences of myocardial ischemia and some of whom died of noncardiac conditions.

The 53 patients died from 13 to 53 months (mean, 58 months) after a single aortocoronary bypass operation. Of the 53 patients, 32 (60%) died of a cardiac cause, and of their 72 saphenous vein aortocoronary conduits, 36 (49%) were narrowed at some point more than 75% in cross-sectional area by atherosclerotic plaque. The remaining 21 patients (40%) died of a

noncardiac cause, and of their 50 saphenous vein conduits, 10 (20%) were narrowed at some point more than 75% in cross-sectional area by plaque. Thus, the noncardiac mode of death in a large percentage of the patients suggests that the bypass operation prolonged life to a degree sufficient for another condition to develop. The 123 saphenous vein conduits were divided into 5-mm segments, and a histologic section was prepared from each. Of the 1104 five-mm segments in the 32 patients dying as a consequence of symptomatic myocardial ischemia, 291 (26%) were narrowed more than 75% in cross-sectional area by plaque; in contrast, of the 761 five-mm segments of veins in the 21 patients with a noncardiac mode of death, 86 (11%) were narrowed more than 75% by plaque. Of the total 1865 five-mm segments of vein, only 395 (21%) were narrowed 25% or less in cross-sectional area by plaque. Thus, in patients dying late after CABG, the atherosclerotic process continues in all segments of the saphenous veins used as aortocoronary conduits. Therapy after the operation must be directed toward prevention of progression of the atherosclerosis in the "new" coronary "arteries."

In the 1990 study by Kalan and Roberts, the amount of luminal narrowing in the saphenous veins used as aortocoronary conduits was significantly greater in those patients who died of a cardiac cause than in those who died of a noncardiac cause. Additionally, the percentage of vein conduits and the percentage of 5-mm segments of the vein conduits totally occluded or nearly so (more than 95% in cross-sectional area) were significantly greater in the patients dying of a cardiac cause than in those dying of a noncardiac cause (22 [30%] of 73 veins versus 7 [14%] of 50 veins, and 152 [14%] of 1104 segments versus 57 [27%] of 213 segments).

The interval from CABG to death did not correlate with either the percentage of vein conduits or the percentage of 5-mm segments of vein conduit narrowed more than 75% in cross-sectional area by plaque. The percentage of venous conduits narrowed severely (more than 75%) was similar in the 18 conduits (7 patients) in place from 13 to 24 months and in the 9 conduits (5 patients) in place for longer than 10 years. Moreover, the percentage of 5-mm segments of saphenous vein conduit severely narrowed was similar in the 35 patients surviving up to 5 years compared with the 18 patients surviving more than 5 years (268 [19%] of 1387 segments versus 113 [24%] of 478 segments).

Why some saphenous vein conduits became severely narrowed or occluded or nearly so and others did not may be related more to the status of the native coronary artery containing the graft than to the graft itself. Of the 123 native coronary arteries containing a saphenous vein conduit, 49 (40%) of the arteries distal to the anastomotic site were narrowed more than 75% in cross-sectional area by plaque, and the anastomosed saphenous vein was severely narrowed in 33 (67%) of them. In contrast, of the 74 native coronary arteries narrowed less than 75% distal to the anastomotic site, the attached saphenous vein was severely narrowed in only 14 (19%). Thus, the amount of narrowing in the native coronary artery distal to the anastomotic site plays a major determining role in the fate of the attached saphenous vein.

The composition of the plaques in the saphenous venous conduits is similar to that in the native coronary arteries (Mautner et al., 1993). Fibrous tissue or fibromuscular tissue was the dominant component of the plaques in the saphenous vein conduits, just as it is the dominant component of plaques in the native coronary arteries in patients with fatal CAD without CABG. Lipid was present in plaques in saphenous veins in much smaller amounts than was fibrous tissue. Intracellular lipid was found in a saphenous vein as early as 14 months after CABG, and it did not increase in either frequency or amount as the interval from bypass to death increased. Extracellular lipid was first seen at 26 months after bypass, and it did not appear to increase thereafter as the interval from bypass increased. Hemorrhage into plaque, which occurred almost entirely into extracellular lipid deposits (containing cholesterol clefts within pultaceous debris), was first seen at 32 months after bypass. Intraluminal thrombus was found in saphenous veins in 14 patients (26%) and was first observed at 32 months. Thrombus was always superimposed on underlying lipid plaque. Calcific deposits were found in saphenous vein conduits in 11 patients (21%), they were first noted at 34 months after bypass, and they did increase in frequency with time.

The frequency of the various modes of death among the patients dying late after CABG is a bit different from that of patients with symptomatic myocardial ischemia without CABG. Of the 53 coronary bypass patients studied, only 32 (60%) died of a cardiac cause, and therefore 21 (40%) died of a noncardiac cause. Among patients with symptomatic myocardial ischemia who did not have CABG, approximately 95% died of a cardiac cause, and therefore only about 5% died of a noncardiac cause. The fact that 40% of the bypass patients studied died of a noncardiac cause supports the view that the bypass operation prolongs life long enough in many patients for various fatal noncardiac conditions to develop. Of the 53 bypass patients studied by Kalan and Roberts (1990), 10 (19%) died of cancer, a percentage far higher than in patients with symptomatic myocardial ischemia not having coronary surgery.

The Kalan and Roberts study (1990) reemphasizes that CABG is useful but that it does not deter progression of the underlying atherosclerotic process. In a slight way, the bypass operation might even accelerate the atherosclerotic process because in about 25% of persons having coronary bypass the serum total

cholesterol increases and the body weight increases substantially during the first year after operation. Because lowering the serum (or plasma) total cholesterol level (and specifically the low-density lipoprotein cholesterol) causes some portion of atherosclerotic plaques to regress and the chances of a fatal or nonfatal subsequent atherosclerotic event to decrease, a strong case can be advanced for combined simultaneous initiation of both low-fat, low-cholesterol diet therapy and lipid-lowering drug therapy as soon as is reasonably feasible after a CABG operation (Roberts, 1989a).

## BIBLIOGRAPHY

Arnett, E. N., Isner, J. M., Redwood, D. R., et al.: Coronary artery narrowing in coronary heart disease: Comparison of cineangiographic and necropsy findings. Ann. Intern. Med., 91:350, 1979.
Isner, J. M., Kishel, J., Kent, K. M., et al.:Accuracy of angiographic determination of left main coronary arterial narrowing: Angiographic-histologic correlative analysis in 28 patients. Circulation, 63:1056, 1981.
Kalan, J. M., and Roberts, W. C.: Morphologic findings in saphenous veins used as coronary arterial bypass conduits for longer than 1 year: Necropsy analysis of 53 patients, 123 saphenous veins, and 1865 five-millimeter segments of veins. Am. Heart J., 119:1164, 1990.
Kragel, A. H., Reddy, S. G., Wittes, J. T., and Roberts, W. C.: Morphologic analysis of the composition of atherosclerotic plaques in the four major epicardial coronary arteries in acute myocardial infarction and in sudden coronary death. Circulation, 80:1747, 1989.
Kragel, A. H., Reddy, S. G., Wittes, J. T., and Roberts, W. C.: Morphometric analysis of the composition of coronary arterial plaques in isolated unstable angina pectoris with pain at rest. Am. J. Cardiol. 66:893, 1990.
Mautner, S. L., Lin, F., Mautner, G. C., and Roberts, W. C.: Comparison in women versus men of composition of atherosclerotic plaques in native coronary arteries and in saphenous veins used as aortocoronary conduits. J. Am. Coll. Cardiol., 21:1312, 1993.
Mautner, S. L., Mautner, G. C., Hunsberger, S. A., and Roberts, W. C.: Comparison of composition of atherosclerotic plaques in saphenous veins used as aortocoronary bypass conduits with plaques in native coronary arteries in the same men. Am. J. Cardiol., 70:1380, 1992.
Potkin, B. N., and Roberts, W. C.: Effects of percutaneous transluminal coronary angioplasty on atherosclerotic plaques and relation of plaque composition and arterial size to outcome. Am. J. Cardiol., 62:41, 1988.
Roberts, W. C.: Lipid-lowering therapy after an atherosclerotic event. Am. J. Cardiol., 64:693, 1989a.
Roberts, W. C.: Qualitative and quantitative comparison of amounts of narrowing by atherosclerotic plaques in the major epicardial coronary arteries at necropsy in sudden death, transmural acute myocardial infarction, transmural healed myocardial infarction and unstable angina pectoris. Am. J. Cardiol., 64:324, 1989b.
Waller, B. F., and Roberts, W. C.: Amount of narrowing by atherosclerotic plaque in 44 nonbypassed and 52 bypassed major epicardial coronary arteries in 32 necropsy patients who died within 1 month of aortocoronary bypass grafting. Am. J. Cardiol., 46:956, 1980.

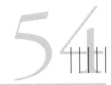

## ■ IV   Coronary Arteriography

Charles J. Davidson, J. Kevin Harrison, and Thomas M. Bashore

## HISTORICAL ASPECTS

Forssmann (1929) is credited with having performed the first human cardiac catheterization. While receiving training as a surgeon in Eberswalde, Germany, he used fluoroscopic guidance to advance a catheter through his own left antecubital vein into the right atrium. In attempting to develop a technique for direct delivery of drugs into the heart, he catheterized himself on several occasions. However, after intense criticism, he eventually abandoned this pursuit and became a urologist. Zimmerman and co-workers (1950) did the first left-sided heart catheterization. This technique was further facilitated by Seldinger (1953) who developed the percutaneous technique for catheter introduction. Early attempts to visualize the coronary arteries in humans were accomplished with nonselective injection of radiopaque contrast media into the ascending aorta (Radner, 1945). In 1958, Sones and colleagues did the first selective injection of contrast media into the coronary arteries (Sones et al., 1959). Several percutaneous transfemoral coronary arteriographic techniques were developed by Ricketts and Abrams (1962), Amplatz and associates (1967), and Judkins (1967), but the femoral technique introduced by Judkins and the brachial technique pioneered by Sones and colleagues are the most widely used today. Each method has its own set of advantages and disadvantages—for example, the brachial technique is useful particularly in patients with severe peripheral vascular disease involving the abdominal aorta and the iliac and femoral arteries, but is generally performed via cutdown of the brachial artery. The femoral approach offers the advantage of not requiring arteriotomy and arterial repair. It can therefore be done several times in the same patient, is more quickly performed, and demands less technical skill to do the procedure in its entirety.

Gruentzig and co-workers (1977, 1979) developed *percutaneous transluminal coronary angioplasty* (PTCA). While working in Zurich, and later at Emory University, Gruentzig introduced an intra-arterial therapeutic technique that has revolutionized the approach to patients with coronary artery disease (CAD). His innovation opened a new era in the interventional approach to coronary artery stenoses and has enabled other percutaneous modalities for treatment of CAD such as atherectomy, laser, and stenting techniques.

## ANATOMY

Physicians performing coronary arteriography as well as cardiac surgeons require a clear understanding of the normal coronary artery anatomy and its common anomalies. In most patients, two separate ostia arise from the ascending aorta to supply the left and right main coronary arteries. Variations of the usual pattern are discussed under "Coronary Artery Anomalies," later in this chapter.

### Normal Arterial Anatomy (Fig. 54–37)

#### Left Main Coronary Artery

The left main coronary artery (LMCA) arises from the left posterior coronary sinus. It courses laterally between the posterior portion of the pulmonary artery and the anterior portion of the left atrial appendage. After a distance of less than 1 mm to as much as 30 mm, it bifurcates into two major branches, the left anterior descending (LAD) and left circumflex arteries. A trifurcation often occurs when the ramus intermedius originates between the anterior descending and the circumflex arteries. It may be difficult angiographically to distinguish the third branch from a proximal diagonal branch of the LAD or marginal branch of the circumflex artery. Infrequently, the LMCA is absent, and the LAD and circumflex arteries arise from common or separate ostia. In these cases, selective arteriography of the LAD and circumflex arteries is performed to visualize the left coronary artery (LCA).

#### Left Anterior Descending Artery

The LAD courses behind the pulmonary trunk into the anterior interventricular sulcus, extending to and often around the left ventricular apex. The LAD provides major branches that penetrate the interventricular septum and left ventricular free wall. A variable number of small right ventricular branches may also arise proximally and distally from the LAD. A large proximal branch may course toward similar branches of the right conus artery to form the circle of Vieussens.

Many septal perforating branches provide arterial

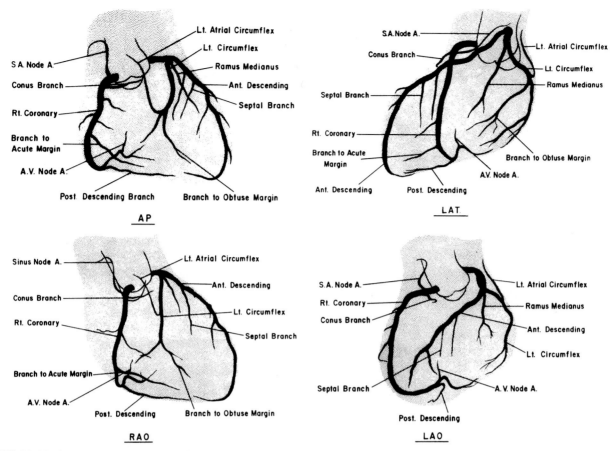

**FIGURE 54–37.** Anatomic representation of the coronary arteries in four projections: anteroposterior (AP), lateral (LAT), right anterior oblique (RAO), and left anterior oblique (LAO). (From Abrams, H. L., and Adams, D. F.: The coronary arteriogram: Structural and functional aspects. N. Engl. J. Med., *281*:1276, 1969.)

supply to the anterior two-thirds and apical portions of the interventricular septum; these are the characteristic landmarks of the anterior descending artery. The first and usually largest septal perforator supplies the base of the septal myocardium. Septal perforators tend to become progressively smaller toward the left ventricular apex.

### Diagonal Branches

As the LAD courses along the interventricular sulcus, several branches arise diagonally over the left ventricular surface. The diagonal (anterolateral) branches arise, as their name implies, diagonally over the left ventricular surface. Two to six diagonal branches may be present, parallel to each other. Generally, the largest diagonal arteries originate from the proximal portion of the LAD and become progressively smaller distally. If a ramus intermedius artery is present, these diagonal branches may be less prominent because the intermediate artery supplies this area of myocardium. Occasionally, diagonal branches may be the source of septal perforating arteries.

### Left Circumflex Artery

The left circumflex artery originates from the LMCA at an acute angle or occasionally from a sepa-

rate ostium of the left coronary sinus. It courses posteriorly under the left atrial appendage along the left atrioventricular (AV) groove. Its termination is highly dependent on the length of the right coronary artery (RCA); in most cases, it terminates at the acute left margin of the heart. From the obtuse margin of the heart, one to four marginal branches of various dimensions emerge from the main circumflex artery. These obtuse marginal arteries course along the lateral aspect of the left ventricle and are named by the order of emergence from the main body of the circumflex artery. Branches arising most distally are often referred to as posterolateral branches from the circumflex artery and course toward the apex perpendicular to the AV groove.

In approximately 10% of patients, the circumflex artery extends to the interventricular groove and beyond the crux of the heart. In these cases, it supplies the posterior descending and, frequently, AV nodal arteries as it courses along the posterior interventricular sulcus. This pattern of circulation is called *left dominant* or *predominant* (Fig. 54–38).

A large left atrial branch arises proximally from the left circumflex artery in 30 to 40% of patients. It courses superiorly along the left atrium, posterior to the aorta, continuing to the anterior interatrial sulcus.

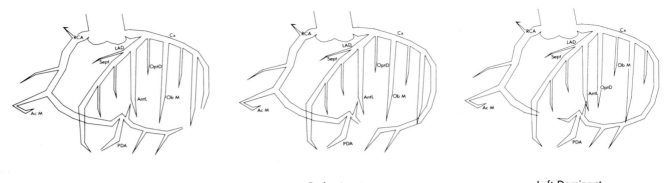

Right Dominant          Codominant          Left Dominant

**FIGURE 54–38.** Diagrams of the coronary artery tree demonstrating right and left dominance and co-dominance based on the variation in blood supply to the posterior diaphragmatic surface of the heart. (RCA = right coronary artery; LAD = left anterior descending coronary artery; Cx = circumflex artery; PDA = posterior descending artery; Ac M = acute marginal artery; AntL = anterolateral [diagonal] arteries; OptD = optional diagonal artery; Op M = obtuse marginal arteries; Sept = septal perforator artery.)

Besides being an important source of blood supply to the left atrium and providing collateral flow to the RCA, it initiates the sinus node artery in slightly less than 50% of human hearts.

### Right Coronary Artery

The RCA emerges from its ostium in the right coronary sinus. Lying deep in epicardial fat, it courses anteriorly along the right AV sulcus between the right atrium and the right ventricle. The extent of the RCA is usually related inversely to the length of the circumflex artery. In approximately 90% of patients, it courses in the AV sulcus to the posterior interventricular sulcus. Therefore, it has a C shape in left anterior oblique (LAO) projection. If any vessels arise after the posterior descending origin, the system is referred to as *right dominant.*

The conus artery may originate as a separate ostium anterior to the RCA or as the most proximal branch of the RCA. It is an important collateral artery

source to the LAD distribution. The conus artery courses across the anterior surface of the right ventricle near the pulmonic valve and terminates in the anterior interventricular sulcus.

The sinus node artery arises from the proximal RCA in about half of patients studied. It takes a course posteriorly along the right atrium, traveling in an almost opposite direction as the conus artery. While supplying small branches to both atria and the interatrial septum, the sinus node artery terminates as it encircles the superior vena cava. Many small atrial branches arise from the RCA, but they usually have little significance as sources for collateral circulation to the left ventricle (see "Collateral Circulation," later in this chapter).

Other prominent branches of the RCA include the acute marginal artery and anterior (or right) ventricular branches. The acute marginal artery courses along the right aspect of the heart and may occasionally supply all or a portion of the posterior descending artery (PDA). In a left dominant circulation, the acute

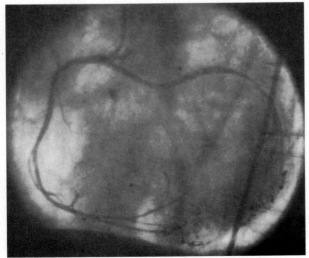
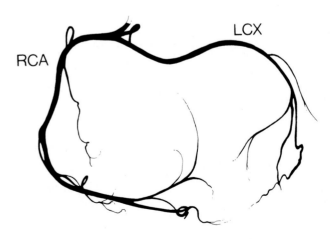

**FIGURE 54–39.** Coronary arteriogram and diagram of the most common anomaly, which is in the left circumflex coronary artery (LCX) arising from the right sinus of Valsalva and coursing between the aorta and the main pulmonary artery. (RCA = right coronary artery.)

■ **Table 54–8.** ANOMALIES OF THE CORONARY ARTERIES

**Minor Anomalies**
Circumflex artery from the right coronary artery (RCA) or right sinus of Valsalva
Left anterior descending artery from RCA or right sinus of Valsalva
Left main coronary artery (LMCA) from the right sinus of Valsalva
RCA from the left sinus of Valsalva
RCA from the posterior (noncoronary) sinus of Valsalva
Single coronary artery
Multiple coronary ostia

**Major Anomalies**
Coronary artery fistula
Anomalous origin of the LMCA or RCA from the pulmonary artery
Coronary artery atresia
Coronary artery hypoplasia
Congenital coronary artery aneurysms
Congenital coronary artery stenosis

marginal artery may represent the last prominent branch of the RCA.

In most cases, the RCA bifurcates into the PDA and posterior left ventricular branches (posterolateral arteries to the left ventricle). The PDA courses toward the apex through the interventricular groove. The actual length of the PDA is related inversely to the extent of the LAD. Several small anterior branches are usually present. These branches arise from the PDA and perforate the interventricular septum supplying the lower one-third of the septum. These septal perforating arteries may help angiographically to distinguish between the PDA and the larger left ventricular branches. Posterolaterals to the left ventricular branches are a continuation of the RCA beyond the origin of the PDA.

The AV node artery arises from the RCA in approximately 90% of patients. The location of the AV node artery is related to whether the RCA or left circumflex artery crosses the posterior interventricular groove (crux). In 90%, the RCA extends beyond the crux and supplies the PDA and the left ventricular branches (right dominant). In 10% of patients, the left circumflex crosses the crux and supplies branches to the right ventricle (left dominant). Occasionally, PDAs arise from both the RCA and the left circumflex artery and produce a balanced, mixed, or co-dominant circulation (see Fig. 54–38). Angiographically, if the RCA terminates in the PDA with no further branches to the left ventricle, the anatomy is considered to be *co-dominant.*

## Coronary Artery Anomalies

With widespread use of coronary arteriography, a knowledge of coronary artery anomalies is essential to avoid potential misdiagnoses or complications. Two reviews of 4250 and 3750 patients having diagnostic cardiac catheterization indicate that the incidence of anomalies is approximately 1% (Chaitman et al., 1976; Engel et al., 1975). These congenital abnor-

malities may or may not be clinically significant. Insignificant anomalies are due primarily to an abnormal origin from the aorta or unusual distribution of the coronary arteries. Hemodynamically significant anomalies such as coronary fistulas or the origin of a coronary artery from the pulmonary artery may cause abnormalities of coronary perfusion. Table 54–8 lists coronary artery anomalies.

The most common congenital variation encountered by the angiographer is the origin of the circumflex artery from the RCA or the right coronary sinus (Figs. 54–39 and 54–40). This malformation occurs in approximately 0.5% of patients (Chaitman et al., 1976; Engel et al., 1975). Typically, this anomalous circumflex artery takes a posterior course behind the great vessels to reach the left AV groove. This anomaly may be associated with transposition of the great vessels (Ogden, 1970) and is generally considered to be benign.

Anomalous origin of the anterior descending artery from the right sinus of Valsalva is similar in several respects to the origin of LMCA from the right sinus of Valsalva. The anterior descending artery may arise

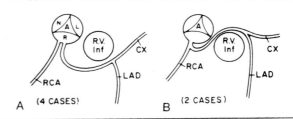

● ABERRANT ORIGIN OF THE LAD and LEFT CX (6 CASES)

A  (4 CASES)          B  (2 CASES)

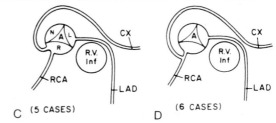

● ABERRANT ORIGIN OF THE LEFT CX (11 CASES)

C  (5 CASES)          D  (6 CASES)

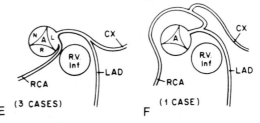

● ABERRANT RCA  (4 CASES)

E  (3 CASES)          F  (1 CASE)

**FIGURE 54–40.** Schematic representation of aberrant coronary artery patterns. (A = aorta; R.V. Inf = right ventricular infundibulum; R = right sinus of Valsalva; L = left sinus of Valsalva; N = noncoronary sinus; CX = circumflex artery; LAD = left anterior descending coronary artery.) *Numbers in parentheses* indicate the frequency of the aberrant pattern in this series of 21 cases. (From Leberthson, R. R., Dinsmore, R. E., Bharad, S., et al.: Aberrant coronary artery origin from the aorta. Circulation, *50*:774, 1974. By permission of the American Heart Association, Inc.)

from a separate ostium in the right sinus of Valsalva or directly from the RCA (see Fig. 54–40). Initially, it courses similarly to the conus artery. It then extends across the anterior aspect of the right ventricular infundibulum to reach the anterior interventricular sulcus. This is the most common coronary artery anomaly associated with tetralogy of Fallot and has been reported to occur in 2% of these patients (McManus et al., 1982; Meng et al., 1965). Because inadvertent transection of this anomalous anterior descending artery has been reported to occur during repair of tetralogy of Fallot, preoperative coronary arteriography has been recommended (McManus et al., 1982) for these patients. Compared with the LMCA from the right sinus of Valsalva, origin of the anterior descending artery from the RCA or right sinus of Valsalva is generally considered to be benign.

Origin of the LMCA and the RCA from the right sinus of Valsalva is a rare anomaly that has been associated with sudden death in young adults. The LMCA may take one of three courses. Most commonly, it originates anterior to the RCA and courses between the pulmonary artery and the aorta, and then bifurcates into the anterior descending and circumflex arteries (see Fig. 54–40). More rarely, the LMCA may pass either anterior to the right ventricular outflow tract or posterior to the aorta. Leberthson and colleagues (1974) postulated that sudden death may result from acute occlusion of this aberrant LMCA. Because cardiac output rises during exercise, the LMCA could become compressed between the dilated aorta and the pulmonary artery or stretched between them, with subsequent occlusion of the sharply angulated proximal segment of the vessel.

Anomalous origin of the RCA from the left sinus of Valsalva has been reported to be present in 0.17% (Engel et al., 1975) and 0.16% (Chaitman et al., 1976) of patients having routine cardiac catheterization (Fig. 54–41). In this anatomic variation, the RCA courses between the ascending aorta and the pulmonary ar-

tery to reach the right AV sulcus. Roberts and associates (1982) reported that, in 10 patients with this anomaly, the ostium of the RCA was slit-like. They postulated that coronary blood flow might be altered when the aorta dilated and further compressed the RCA during exercise.

The origin of both coronary arteries from a single ostium has been reported to occur in from 0.04% (Sharbaugh and White, 1974) to 0.1% (Douglas et al., 1985) of the population. Single RCAs and LMCAs are present in about equal numbers (Sharbaugh and White, 1974). An example of a single RCA is shown in Figure 54–42. As described earlier for other coronary artery anomalies, the clinical features of this anomaly depend on the luminal diameter of the orifice and the degree of compression or angulation of the artery as it courses through or around the great vessels. Myocardial infarction, angina pectoris, congestive heart failure, or sudden death have been reported before the age of 40 years in as many as 15% of patients with a single coronary artery (Douglas et al., 1985).

The most common hemodynamically significant coronary anomaly is a precapillary fistula that connects a major coronary artery directly with a cardiac chamber, coronary sinus, superior vena cava, or pulmonary artery (Levin et al., 1978). Although a physiologic left-to-right shunt is present, except in rare cases in which termination is in a left-sided heart chamber, approximately 50% of patients have catheterization for an asymptomatic continuous murmur (Oldham et al., 1971). However, others may develop congestive heart failure, endocarditis (endarteritis), myocardial ischemia owing to a steal phenomenon, or rupture of an aneurysmal fistula (Oldham et al., 1971). Levin and colleagues (1978) reviewed 363 reported cases of coronary artery fistulas and noted that 50% arose from the RCA, 42% arose from the LMCA, and 5% arose from both coronary arteries. Drainage occurred most commonly into the right ventricle (41%), fol-

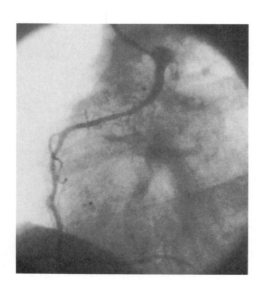

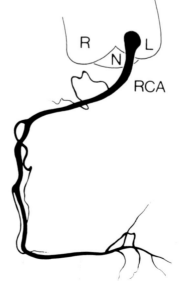

**FIGURE 54–41.** Anomalous origin of the right coronary artery (RCA) from the left sinus of Valsalva (L) (LAO view). (R = right sinus of Valsalva; N = noncoronary sinus.)

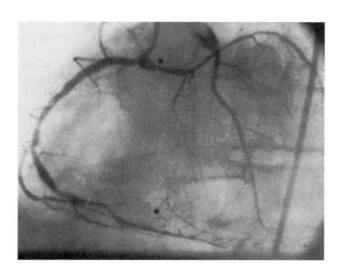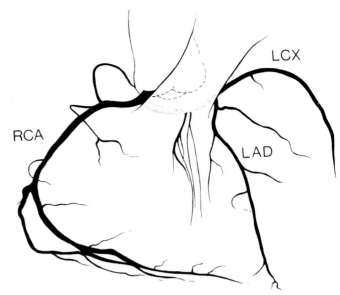

**FIGURE 54–42.** Coronary arteriogram and diagram of the LAO view showing a single right coronary ostium initiative, right and left main coronary arteries. Note that the course of the left main coronary artery is between the pulmonary artery and the aorta (AP view). (LAD = left anterior descending coronary artery; LCX = left circumflex coronary artery; RCA = right coronary artery.)

lowed by the right atrium (26%), pulmonary artery (16%), coronary sinus (7%), left atrium (5%), left ventricle (3%), and superior vena cava (1%). An example of an RCA-to-right atrial fistula is shown in Figure 54–43. Angiography provides the definitive diagnosis, although oximetry may help to estimate the size of the shunt (but the degree of the shunt is frequently too small for accurate assessment). The originating coronary artery is usually dilated and tortuous and often resembles saccular aneurysms. In approximately 3% of patients with coronary artery fistulas, the contralateral coronary artery is absent.

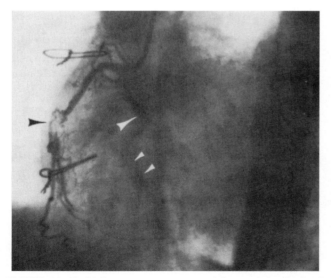

**FIGURE 54–43.** Right coronary artery to right atrial fistula (LAO view) *(single, large, white arrowhead)*. Note the area of contrast dye pooling in the right atrium *(double white arrowheads)*. Incidental severe stenosis of the right coronary artery *(black arrowhead)* is shown.

The four types of anomalous origin of the coronary arteries from the pulmonary trunk are origins of the LMCA, the RCA, both arteries, or an accessory coronary artery. In approximately 90% of patients with this anomaly, the LMCA arises from the pulmonary artery (Ogden, 1970). Angina-like symptoms of dyspnea, tachypnea, pallor, and restlessness often begin soon after birth as pulmonary artery pressures decline, leading to a coronary artery steal and inadequate perfusion of the myocardium. Myocardial infarction, papillary muscle dysfunction with mitral insufficiency, and sudden death are common. Aortography reveals a large RCA, an absent LMCA, and delayed appearance of collateral vessels from the RCA that opacify the LAD and left circumflex arteries. When an extensive collateral circulation is present, contrast appears in the pulmonary artery and outlines the left-to-right shunt.

Congenital coronary artery stenosis occurs most commonly in conjunction with other congenital lesions, such as calcific coronary sclerosis, supravalvular aortic stenosis, homocystinuria, Friedreich's ataxia, Hurler's syndrome, and rubella syndrome (Levin et al., 1978). Congenital coronary artery aneurysm is a rare lesion because most aneurysms occur secondary to conditions such as atherosclerosis, inflammatory processes, or a coronary fistula. These aneurysms are caused presumably by structural weakness in the arterial wall and often are difficult to distinguish from acquired coronary artery aneurysms.

## Coronary Venous Anatomy

Gensini and co-workers (1965) explored the anatomy of the coronary circulation with coronary venography in living humans. Specially designed balloon-tip catheters were used. Satisfactory balloon inflation and occlusion were determined by a characteristic change from the atrial waveform of the nonoccluded coronary sinus to ventricular complexes of occluded coronary venous pressure.

The normal anatomy of coronary veins can be represented diagramatically by two large triangles with apices on either side of the apex of the heart and hinged at their bases by the great cardiac vein and the coronary sinus (Fig. 54–44). The first triangle is larger and medially located. The sides of the triangle are formed by the anterior and posterior interventricular veins. The second triangle is smaller and is located on the free wall of the left ventricle. Its sides are formed by the left diagonal and obtuse marginal veins.

This entire system drains approximately 85% of coronary blood flow, including the interventricular septum, left ventricular free wall, and part of the right ventricle. The remaining 15% is drained by the anterior cardiac veins and thebesian channels.

A small left atrial vein of great anatomic significance is the oblique vein of Marshall. It courses diagonally on the posterior surface of the left atrium and is directed medially and caudally. The great cardiac vein becomes the coronary sinus at the point at which the vein of Marshall drains into it.

Hutchins and associates (1986) investigated the interrelationships between the intramural arteries and the intramural veins by angiography, serial sectioning, and graphic microconstruction. They showed that epicardial vessels begin to divide within the epicardium and that muscle fibers are oriented in the same direction as the interstitial space. An unconventional pattern of branching exists: The vein begins as a large vessel that divides and then rejoins its branches, forming a large vessel. The arteriole intertwines between veins.

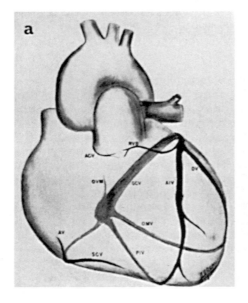
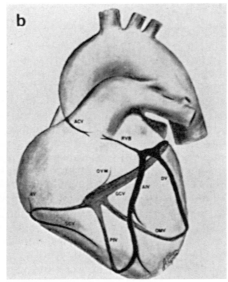
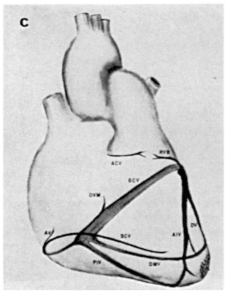
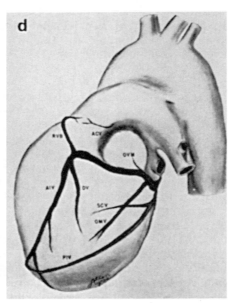

FIGURE 54–44. Four projections of the human coronary venous anatomy. *a*, AP view; *b*, LAO; *c*, RAO; *d*, Left LAT. Black vessels are anteriorly located; gray are posteriorly located. (GCV = great cardiac vein; AIV = anterior interventricular vein; OMV = obtuse marginal vein; DV = diagonal vein; PIV = posterior interventricular vein [middle cardiac vein]; OVM = oblique vein of Marshall; SCV = small cardiac vein [right marginal vein]; ACV = anterior cardiac vein.) (*a–d*, From Gensini, G. G., DiGiorgi, S., Coskun, O., et al.: Anatomy of the coronary circulation in living man: Coronary venography. Circulation, *31*:778, 1965. By permission of the American Heart Association, Inc.)

Penetrating arteries lie in the interstitial spaces and are related closely to accompanying veins. The interstitial veins partially surround and are indented by branch arteries. A second system of veins lies within the muscle fascicles between interstitial spaces and is not related to arteries. The isolated veins have collateral connections with interstitial veins and join them in the subepicardium. Therefore, there are twice as many veins as arteries. The auxiliary venous system not adjacent to the artery could be an alternative route for increased blood flow, preventing rapid washout of metabolic end-products during ischemia (Hutchins et al., 1986).

## PATHOANATOMIC CORRELATES

### Interpretation of CAD

In the angiographic evaluation of CAD, it is imperative to define the degree of stenosis that constitutes either prognostic or hemodynamic significance. Generally, the severity of stenosis is assessed by visually comparing the percentage diameter reduction relative to an adjacent "normal" segment. Although angiographically normal, most reference segments have varying degrees of atherosclerosis. Thus, angiography often underestimates the true severity of CAD, including LMCA disease. Intracoronary ultrasound has demonstrated that the degree of plaque mass is similar in angiographically normal and abnormal LMCAs in patients undergoing interventional therapy (Hermiller et al., 1993a). The inability of silhouette angiography to assess a true normal segment means that the severity of CAD can be underestimated. Although a 50% narrowing in diameter has been considered to be clinically significant, the American Heart Association Committee Report (1975) has recommended that an 80% decrease in luminal diameter should be considered to be a significant lesion. This recommendation is based on data obtained at the time of operation indicating that this degree of stenosis was necessary to measure a pressure gradient. It has further been shown that a 50% decrease in diameter represents a small reduction in peak coronary artery flow, whereas a 70% stenosis results in a severe reduction in peak flow (McMahon et al., 1979; Peterson et al., 1983). Exercise-induced ischemia has been documented by first-pass radionuclide angiography in patients with 75% stenosis determined by cardiac catheterization, and 40 mm Hg pressure gradients allowed discrimination of patients with and without exercise ischemia (American Heart Association Committee Report, 1975). Length of stenosis, although not generally measured, has been shown to limit coronary flow when greater than 10 mm (Feldman et al., 1978).

Studies of coronary flow reserve measured by Doppler flowmeters have shown the inadequacy of measurement of percentage diameter narrowing alone (Gould et al., 1986; Kirkeeide et al., 1986; White et al., 1984). Consideration of all dimensions may be necessary to adequately evaluate the physiologic significance of a lesion. These dimensions of a lesion include percentage diameter stenosis, absolute minimal cross-sectional area, absolute stenosis diameter, and minimal stenosis luminal area. The entry and exit angles entering and leaving the lesion also affect lesion resistance. Thus, consideration of all parameters of lesion length, absolute diameter, and percentage narrowing may be necessary to correctly predict the functional severity of stenosis, at least as defined by coronary flow reserve (Gould et al., 1986; Kirkeeide et al., 1986).

Despite the fact that prognostic information based on the number of diseased vessels can be obtained by qualitative interpretation, it must be appreciated that visual interpretation has multiple sources of error. Various studies have documented the wide interobserver and intraobserver variation that exists when cineangiograms are visually evaluated. DeRouen and co-workers (1977) reported that, when 11 experienced angiographers interpreted 10 angiograms, disagreement regarding the number of vessels with greater than 70% stenosis occurred in one-third of the cases. The Coronary Artery Surgery Study (CASS) (Kennedy et al., 1982) found that in the PDA one observer did not identify a lesion in 28.5% of patients, and another reader identified a lesion of greater than 50%. A second area in which interobserver variation was large was in the LMCA; whereas one angiographer interpreted a lesion of greater than 50%, a second reader failed to identify the same lesion 15.7% of the time. The scattergram results of the CASS study describing interobserver and intraobserver variation in the proximal LAD are shown in Figure 54–45.

Similarly, a poor correlation exists between visually assessed coronary arteriograms and corresponding postmortem coronary artery specimens. In general, coronary arteriography tends to understimate the severity of most lesions. The presence of diffuse atherosclerosis in patients with clinically symptomatic disease (Blankenhorn and Curry, 1982) or dilatation of the nearby normal vessel as a result of aging or poststenotic enlargement may make definition of a normal segment difficult. Intravascular ultrasound studies have further highlighted the limitation of silhouette angiograms to adequately assess the true luminal narrowings that are present (Hermiller et al., 1993b). Also, owing to adaptive enlargement of coronary arteries in the early stages of atherosclerosis, the reference segment may actually dilate and overcompensate when stenosis of less than 30% is present (Glagov et al., 1987; Hermiller et al., 1993b). The agreement between angiography and pathology is improved when either minimal lesions or severe lesions are present; variation increases when the stenosis is from 51 to 75%. Minimal lumen area may be a better predictor of the physiologic significance of a coronary lesion than the calculated percentage of stenosis (Harrison et al., 1984).

The first attempts to quantitate coronary artery stenosis used calipers. Electronic calipers are available that can be used to measure reference and lesion segment dimensions; methods using handheld cali-

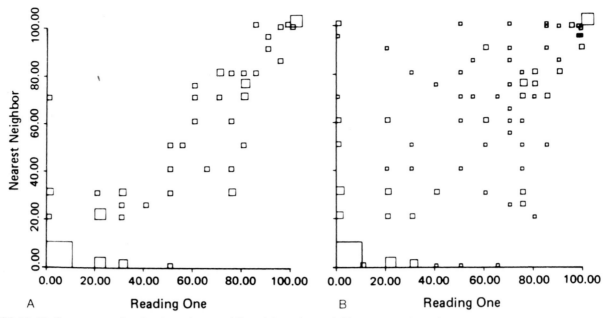

**FIGURE 54–45.** Scattergram showing intraobserver (A) and interobserver (B) variation. Data from visually interpreted stenosis of the proximal LAD in the Coronary Artery Stenosis Study (CASS) registry. The size of each square represents the number of each observation. (A and B, From Kennedy, J. W., Fisher, L. D., and Killip, T.: Coronary angiography quality control in CASS study. In Bond, M. A., Insull, W., and Glagov, S. [eds]: Clinical Diagnosis of Atherosclerosis: Quantitative Methods of Evaluation. New York, Springer-Verlag 1982, pp. 475–491.)

pers are widely employed owing to simplicity of use and low cost. Absolute dimensions can be calibrated using the coronary catheter or a grid and percentage diameter stenosis.

However, comparison of caliper of cine film with a computed quantitative coronary angiographic system showed that reproducibility was significantly superior with quantitative coronary angiography (r = 0.95 vs. r = 0.63) (Kalbfleisch et al., 1990), yet overall correlation of the two techniques was good (r = 0.72). These authors conclude that calipers are not adequate substitutes for quantitative coronary angiography because overestimation of noncritical stenosis and underestimation of severe stenosis can occur. There is also question whether calipers offer any real advantage over visual techniques. Despite these known limitations, caliper techniques are being employed in several large clinical trials evaluating bypass surgery and PTCA including the Bypass Angioplasty Revascularization Investigation (BARI).

Computed edge-detection algorithms have been applied to digitally acquired image data or to standard cine film that has been digitized. Some of these techniques of analysis are labor-intensive and time-consuming and may require two orthogonal views of the lesion. There are several validated computed quantitative coronary arteriographic methods for evaluating stenosis severity. These methods use automated edge-detection algorithms that can be applied to either digitized 35-mm cine film or directly acquired digital images. Examples of these commercially available systems are ARTREK, developed by LeFree and colleagues (1986), Duke University Quantitative/Qualitative Evaluation System (DUQUES) (Cusma et al.,

1990; Hermiller et al., 1992), and Cardiovascular Angiographic Analysis System (CAAS) (Reiber et al., 1984).

Quantitative coronary arteriography may be divided into film digitization, image calibration, and contour detection. For digitization, the cine film is placed on a cinevideo converter and projected onto a high-resolution camera. For calibration and estimation of absolute dimensions of coronary artery diameters, the diagnostic or guiding catheter can be used for scaling. The operator then selects a region of interest that contains the proximal and distal ends of the calibration catheter or lesion. Linear density profiles are then sampled along the vessel length, and the centerline is derived. A weighted average of the first and second derivative function is used to define the edge points of the vessel. The edges are then smoothed by discarding outliers, and individual points are connected using an automated algorithm. Using the known diameter of the catheter as a calibration factor expressed in millimeters per pixel, the absolute coronary dimensions can be defined. This automated algorithm can be used to detect the edges of digitized cineangiograms or digitally subtracted images (Fig. 54–46). Measurements done on digital subtraction angiograms have compared favorably with pathologic data of vessels fixed in barium gelatin and contrast injections into perfused hearts (Skelton et al., 1987).

The interobserver and intraobserver variability for percentage diameter stenosis are approximately ±3.0% and for minimal lesion diameter 0.10 to 0.18 mm (Hermiller et al., 1992; Mancini et al., 1987). Mancini and colleagues (1987) have shown anatomic and

physiologic validation in vivo of a fully automated edge-detection algorithm by performing digital coronary arteriograms and cineangiograms on dogs with intraluminal stenosis created by plastic cylinders. An excellent correlation was found between known and measured minimal diameter stenosis (r = 0.87 to 0.98). Interobserver and intraobserver analyses were highly reproducible (r = 0.9 to 0.97). Furthermore, measures of percentage diameter stenosis, percentage area stenosis (geometric and videodensitometric), and

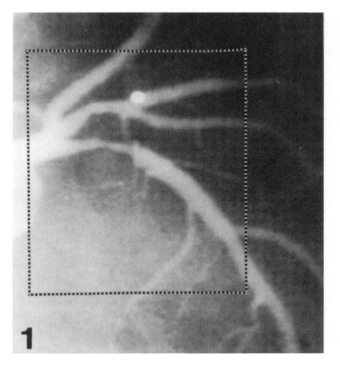

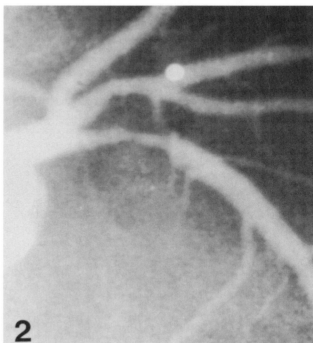

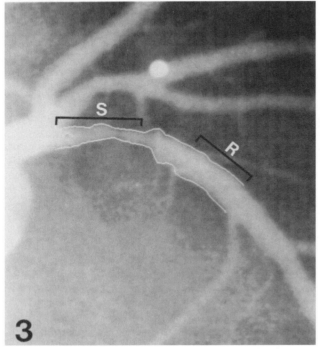

| | Reference segment (mm) | Stenotic segment (mm) |
|---|---|---|
| Max | 3.79 | 2.46 |
| Min | 3.35 | 1.33 |
| Mean | 3.60 | 1.79 |
| Length | 4.71 | 9.60 |
| **% diameter stenosis** | | **63.17%** |
| **% area stenosis** | | **86.44%** |

calibration 0.0900

**FIGURE 54–46.** Quantitative coronary angiography evaluating stenosis in the proximal LAD. *1,* Digitized angiogram of the proximal left coronary system viewed in the anterior-posterior cranial projection. The left main in this case trifurcates into the circumflex artery, a large ramus intermedius, and the LAD. A diffuse stenosis exists at the origin of the LAD. *2,* Magnified image of the proximal LAD stenosis. *3,* Computer-generated edge-detection algorithm employed to define the vessel edges in the stenotic area (S) and in the LAD reference area (R), distal to the stenosis. *4,* Quantitative data resulting from this analysis defining absolute vessel diameter in the stenosis and reference segments, lesion length, and percent diameter and area stenosis.

absolute minimal cross-sectional diameter (geometric and videodensitometric) all significantly correlated with coronary blood flow measured by electromagnetic flow probes.

Videodensitometry has been used to quantitate artery diameter and percentage stenosis. This method analyzes the optical density of selected cross-sections of the artery. Abrupt changes identify the borders of the arteriographic lumen. This concept forms the basis of the edge-detection algorithms used for quantitative coronary arteriography described previously. With videodensitometric techniques, the optical density of an arterial segment can be expressed as a function of the volume of contrast media within the lumen of the artery, and represents the volume of the segment. The optical density profile can thus provide an estimate of the cross-sectional area of the artery. Three-dimensional information can therefore be derived from two-dimensional images. Normal segment optical density can then be compared with the area of greatest vessel narrowing, and a percentage area reduction can be determined (Laufer and Buda, 1985).

The motivation for developing videodensitometric techniques has been to avoid the need for geometric assumptions characteristic of the previously described quantitative coronary arteriographic techniques. In comparison, measurements of videodensitometry data of either cineangiograms or digital images theoretically yield measurements of cross-sectional area and vessel thickness for any shape of lesion. Nichols and associates (1984) have validated that relative cross-sectional area determinations from digitized cine-film correlate well with phantoms and postmortem specimens.

Videodensitometry has been difficult to validate in vivo. Interobserver and intraobserver variability immediately after PTCA is significantly less precise than geometric methods, and correlation with geometric methods is poor. The use of videodensitometric methods is still limited because the linearity of the relationship between the video signal and the thickness of the contrast-filled vasculature often deviates from the ideal situation. Contrast streaming, variation in film processing, and fluctuations in light source during projection or variable digital acquisition are potential sources of error with this technique. Other limitations include x-ray scatter and veiling glare within the image intensifier.

## LIMITATIONS OF QUANTITATIVE ANGIOGRAPHY

Despite the improved reliability and reproducibility of quantitative coronary angiography, several limitations can have an impact on accurate measurements. Cardiac motion, pincushion distortion, veiling glare, quantum mottling, and spherical observation can affect the angiographic analysis (Hermiller et al., 1992). Additionally, successful quantitative coronary angiography depends on obtaining the proper angiographic view. Although two orthogonal views have been advocated as the optimal method for defining asymmetric geometric lesion contour, this is obtainable in only about 50% of patients. Therefore, the "worst view" analysis has become clinically acceptable because it differs only slightly from the average of two orthogonal views (Lesperance et al., 1989).

Inaccurate calibration of the angiographic catheter as a scaling device can lead to an error in calibration of absolute luminal dimensions. Particularly problematic are smaller diagnostic catheters (Nos. 5 or 6 French sizes) (Fortin et al., 1991). When it is possible to use them, larger diagnostic catheters (No. 7 French) or guide catheters (Nos. 8 to 10 French) are superior and introduce less error into the calibration. This problem, however, is only apparent when absolute dimensions are determined and does not apply to relative percentage diameter stenosis, which is the more widely clinically applied terminology.

Along with radiographic and angiographic parameters, biologic factors affect vasomotor tone. Thus, intracoronary vasodilators (e.g., nitroglycerin) should be administered before angiography to improve reproducibility. Angiography's ability to predict functional significance of the stenosis is discussed under "Coronary Blood Flow Determinations in the Cardiac Catheterization Laboratory," later in this chapter.

## LESION MORPHOLOGY

Quantitation and imaging of coronary artery atherosclerosis ideally should be concerned with four related, yet distinguishable, anatomic manifestations of lesion: extent, severity, lesion composition, and complication (Glagov and Zarins, 1982) (Fig. 54–47). Extent of disease refers to the mass of atherosclerotic intimal tissue in an artery or arterial segment. The location of narrowing should be defined as precisely as possible because diffuse disease may be distributed in various patterns. Severity of disease is a measure of the degree to which atherosclerosis has narrowed the lumen of the artery and compromised flow. This may be quantitated by measuring absolute diameter and length of each stenosis with respect to the number of stenoses in an artery. In most cases, severity is expressed as percentage stenosis by comparing nearby "normal" segments with disease segments.

The composition of the lesion involves the nature, consistency, and distribution of the stenosis. It evaluates the cellular and matrix constituents of lesions. Stenosis can be dense, hard, and calcific or soft and semisolid. A complicated lesion entails fragmentation, ulceration, plaque hemorrhage, or thrombosis of the lesion.

Minor irregularities of the arterial wall are an early manifestation of atherosclerosis. This intimal plaque formation can be seen in many patients older than 45 years. These plaques occur irregularly along the vessel but are more evident on proximal segments.

Atheroma and vessel calcification are frequently associated. Calcification may be visible during fluoroscopy before injection of contrast, and tends to be

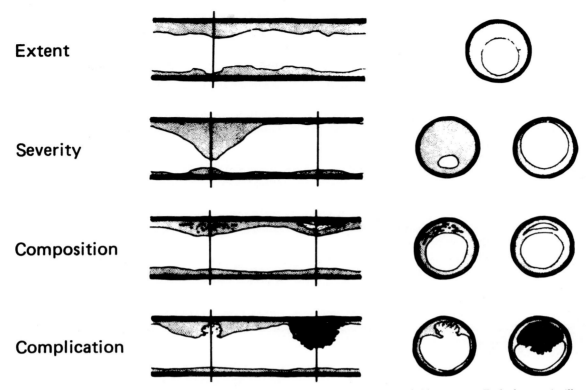

Extent

Severity

Composition

Complication

**FIGURE 54–47.** Schematic representation of atherosclerotic lesions demonstrating quantifiable aspects. Each feature is illustrated in longitudinal (*left*) and transverse (*right*) cross-section. *Vertical lines* indicate the level of transverse cross-section. *Shaded areas* are intimal lesions. See the text for a description of the extent, severity, composition, and complication. (From Glagov, S., and Zarins, C. K.: Quantitative atherosclerosis: Problems of definition. *In* Bond, M. G., Insull, W., and Glagov, S. [eds]: Clinical Diagnosis of Atherosclerosis: Quantitative Methods of Evaluation. New York, Springer-Verlag, 1982, pp. 11–35.)

most extensive proximally. Calcium within the coronary arteries is associated with significant disease in 50 to 75% of patients, although the stenosis may not be at the site of calcification (Bartel et al., 1974; Hamby et al., 1974).

An angiographic lesion-specific characterization has been described by an American College of Cardiology/American Heart Association (ACC/AHA) Task Force (Ryan et al., 1988). These lesion descriptors were designed to help stratify potential success rates with PTCA. They have been slightly modified and validated as clinically useful determinants of procedural outcomes with PTCA (Ellis et al., 1990). Type A lesions are discrete, concentric, and nonangulated (less than 45 degrees), have smooth contours and little or no calcification, are less than totally occlusive, and are nonostial. They have no major branch involvement and no thrombus present. Type B lesions are subclassified into Types B1 and B2. Type B2 indicates that more than one B characteristic is present. Type B lesions are characterized by the presence of any of the following: irregular contours, moderate to heavy calcium, totally occluded vessels less than 3 months old, ostial, bifurcation, some thrombus present, tubular (10 to 20 mm in length), eccentric, or moderately tortuous proximal to segment. Type C lesions have the least favorable outcome with PTCA. Lesion morphology of Type C lesions include diffuseness (greater than 2 cm), excessive tortuosity of proximal segment,

extremely angulated segments (more than 90 degrees), total occlusion greater than 3 months old, or degenerated vein grafts with friable lesions. Although with newer devices and increased operator experience, PTCA success rates for these lesion types have improved, it remains a clinically useful grading system for identifying lesions likely to benefit from PTCA. However, interobserver and intraobserver assessment for qualitative characteristics is variable, as is visual assessment of luminal dimensions (Ellis et al., 1990).

To assess the degree of coronary perfusion with cineangiography, the Thrombosis in Myocardial Infarction (TIMI) study group suggested standard criteria that have been used in thrombolytic studies (Sheehan et al., 1987). TIMI flow can be employed in the setting of acute myocardial infarction or in any lesion in which antegrade flow is impaired.

TIMI Grade 0 flow involves no perfusion; no contrast flows through the stenosis. TIMI Grade 1 flow (penetration with minimal perfusion) occurs when a small amount of contrast flows through a stenosis, but does not completely opacify the distal artery. TIMI Grade 2 flow (partial perfusion) is contrast flow through the stenotic area with slow but eventual opacification of the terminal artery segment. Contrast enters the terminal segment more slowly than the more proximal segments and neighboring vessels. Grade 3 flow (complete reperfusion) is normal flow in which contrast enters and clears a stenotic segment with equal promptness. Successful reperfusion after thrombolytics has generally been considered to be TIMI Grade 2 or 3 flow. However, more recent data have suggested that TIMI Grade 3 flow predicts significantly better outcomes than lesser grades of flow (Anderson et al., 1993).

In reality, the actual extent of disease or the composition of lesions cannot be well defined by coronary arteriography. The irregularities and stenoses visualized may represent ulcerations or thrombi or alternatively complex lesions that override one another. Even detection of thrombus depends on the size and type of thrombus. Although small thrombi may be difficult to discern, organizing thrombi may conform to the atherosclerotic lesions and be difficult to distinguish from underlying plaque. Large and fresh thrombi extending from the wall into the lumen and those associated with disintegration of plaque often can be detected when multiple views are obtained. Intracoronary ultrasound as well as angioscopy provides much more detailed assessments of coronary artery morphology and should be used as adjuncts to angiography for detailed morphologic examination of coronary arteries.

## CORONARY BLOOD FLOW DETERMINATIONS IN THE CARDIAC CATHETERIZATION LABORATORY

Four methods are generally used to measure human coronary blood flow in the cardiac catheterization laboratory: thermodilution, digital subtraction angiography, electromagnetic flowmeters, and Doppler velocity probes. Although most current methods measure relative changes in coronary blood flow, useful information regarding the physiologic significance of stenosis (Wilson et al., 1987), cardiac hypertrophy (Marcus, 1983), and pharmacologic interventions (Klocke et al., 1987) can be obtained from these measurements.

Ganz and co-workers (1971) introduced thermodilution methods for measuring coronary sinus flow in humans. This inexpensive, widely available technique is the most frequently applied method for measuring global coronary blood flow in humans (Marcus et al., 1987). By injecting iced saline solution in the distal end of the catheter placed in the coronary sinus and measuring the temperature change from a proximal thermistor, the rate of change in temperature can be used to define coronary flow. The frequency response of this system is sufficient to measure flow changes that occur in 2 to 3 seconds and are greater than 30% (Ganz et al., 1971). This technique suffers from several serious limitations, however (Marcus et al., 1987). Although the method has been validated in vitro with the thermodilution catheter attached to the coronary sinus (Ganz et al., 1971), weaker correlations have been shown when the thermodilution catheter is allowed to move within the coronary sinus (Mathey et al., 1978). Meanwhile, no studies have clearly demon-

strated the accuracy of this method in patients with severe CAD or myocardial infarction. Other fundamental limitations include the facts that rapid changes in flow cannot be assessed because of the slow time constant of the technique, right atrial and ventricular perfusion cannot be evaluated because the venous drainage is not via the coronary sinus, and regional function and specifically transmural coronary flow cannot be assessed.

To use digital subtraction angiography to measure coronary flow, contrast medium is power-injected into a coronary artery at a rate of quantity sufficient to completely replace blood within the artery. It is assumed that the contrast bolus is undiluted until the peak concentration has been imaged distally in the arterial segment. Regional flow reserve can be calculated in a number of ways, including the use of downstream appearance time and maximal contrast concentration before and during reactive hyperemia (Klocke, 1987). The assumption is that transit time within a region is inversely proportional to coronary blood flow in that region. This is true if the volume of distribution is constant. The technique is limited by a slow time constant and the inability to measure absolute flow. This method of evaluation of coronary flow reserve has been validated in dogs by comparing digital flow ratio estimate with electromagnetic flow ratio measurements (Cusma et al., 1987; Hodgson et al., 1985). In humans, flow reserve has been shown to be abnormal in stenosed arteries and bypass grafts and after coronary angioplasty (Vogel, 1985). Further validation in humans is necessary.

The electromagnetic flowmeter is based on Faraday's induction law, which states that a conductor moving in an electric field produces current. A major advantage of electromagnetic flowmeters is the high-frequency response (Marcus, 1983). Although these flowmeters have been used to measure aortic blood flow velocity in humans (Klinke et al., 1980), they have not developed to the point at which they are useful for measuring coronary blood flow at catheterization, partly because most methods require placement directly around the coronary artery. Electromagnetic flowmeters are occasionally still used intraoperatively to evaluate flow in aortocoronary bypass grafts.

The Doppler flowmeter is based on the principle of the Doppler effect and is the most widely applied technique for measuring coronary flow in humans. High-frequency sound waves are reflected from moving red blood cells and undergo a shift in sound frequency that is proportional to the velocity of the blood flow. In pulsed-wave Doppler methods, a single piezoelectric crystal can both transmit and receive high-frequency sound waves. These methods have been applied successfully in humans by using tiny crystals fixed to the tip of catheters.

Recent developments in technology have further miniaturized steerable Doppler guidewires to 0.014 inch in diameter. Therefore, flow can be assessed distal and proximal to a stenosis. The Doppler guidewire measures phasic flow velocity patterns and tracks linearly with flow rates in small straight coronary arteries (Doucette et al., 1992). It has been advocated for use to determine the severity of intermediate stenosis (40 to 60%) and to evaluate whether normal blood flow has been restored after PTCA. Validation studies compared Doppler flow probes with labeled microspheres (Wangler et al., 1981) and electromagnetic flow probes (Marcus et al., 1981). The use of this technique in 200 patients in the cardiac catheterization laboratory has been reported (Wilson and White, 1987). It permits repeated sampling at high frequency, thus allowing measurements after physiologic or pharmacologic interventions. With the use of smaller Doppler catheters, selective coronary artery flow velocity can be measured. By noting the increase in flow velocity following a strong coronary vasodilator, such as papaverine, the catheters can define the coronary flow reserve. *Coronary flow reserve* (CFR) provides an index of the functional significance of coronary lesions that obviates some of the ambiguity of anatomic description (Wilson et al., 1987).

Animal data indicate that stenosis greater than 50% is associated with a reduction in absolute flow reserve. It has been suggested that *stenosis flow reserve* (SFR) is a more reliable method of functional severity (Dehmer et al., 1988). For a fixed arterial dimension and stenosis geometry, directly measured arterial CFR can be 0, if no aortic perfusion is present, or may change with other physiologic conditions. Thus, CFR can be broken into its component parts of SFR, i.e., the flow reserve of the proximal arterial stenosis, and *myocardial perfusion reserve* (MPR), i.e., the flow reserve of the distal vascular bed. SFR is defined by geometric quantitative coronary dimensions using standard physiologic conditions. MPR is directly or indirectly measured and is affected by geometric as well as physiologic variables. The equation relating pressure change across a lesion and flow is:

$$\Delta P = Pa - Pc = A(Q/Qrest) + B(Q/Qrest)^2$$

where $\Delta P$ is the translesional gradient, Pc is distal coronary pressure, Pa is aortic pressure, Q and Qrest are flow and rest flow and A and B are related to lesion geometry. A and B are defined by lesion length, minimal cross-sectional area of the lesion and reference segment, and blood viscosity.

The limitation of the current Doppler probe method is that only changes in flow velocity, rather than absolute velocity or flow, are measurable. Furthermore, there is concern that changes in luminal diameter and arterial cross-sectional area during interventions are not reflected in measurements of flow velocity, thus potentially causing underestimation of the true volume flow (Klocke, 1987).

## COLLATERAL CIRCULATION

Coronary collaterals provide an alternative blood supply to a major artery that has become obstructed. In humans, the collaterals represent an initially un-used pathway that can be recruited when the original vessel is unable to provide adequate flow. Collateral vessels may arise de novo or alternatively be preexisting, with dilatation and expansion in response to severe obstruction. Collaterals are classified as *intercoronary* if they connect branches of different arteries. *Intercoronary collaterals* are present in individuals with fixed CAD, and have been visualized acutely during angiography when coronary artery spasm occurs (Maseri et al., 1978). Intracoronary collaterals have been divided into two subtypes, secondary and tertiary. Secondary connections link branches of the same coronary artery, are found in 50 to 60% of normal hearts, and form one-third of the normal heart's collateral network (Cohen, 1985). Tertiary collaterals join proximal and distal segments of the same branch, and are observed only in patients with occlusive CAD (Cohen, 1985).

Levin (1974) examined 200 coronary arteriograms and left ventriculograms of patients with significant coronary disease and found that collateral circulation was usually visualized when the degree of stenosis exceeded 90% diameter narrowing. The major patterns of these collateral routes to the coronary arteries are shown in Figures 54–48 to 54–50. In patients with severe narrowing of the RCA, the most common collateral source involves the LAD via septal branches to the posterior descending branch of the RCA or distal left circumflex to the distal RCA (Fig. 54–48). Individuals with severe or complete obstruction of the LAD most commonly show intercoronary collaterals via the acute marginal branch of the RCA and intracoronary collaterals via proximal septal branches (Fig. 54–49). In circumflex artery occlusion, intracoronary collaterals are frequently observed. These collaterals include the left atrial circumflex branch to the distal circumflex artery and the proximal obtuse marginal branch to a more distal obtuse marginal artery (Fig. 54–50). Finally, in patients with adequate collaterals manifested by good distal runoff, regional left ventricular function is often preserved.

## CORONARY SPASM

Coronary artery spasm when detected by angiography can be clinically benign catheter-induced spasm, spontaneous spasm occurring in patients with variant (Prinzmetal's) angina, or provocatively induced spasm in patients with variant angina. When no vasodilating agents have been administered before catheterization, coronary artery spasm has occurred in 1 to 3% of patients (Chahine et al., 1975; Linhart, 1974). In most cases, spasm is mechanically induced by the catheter tip and is especially frequent when the RCA is cannulated. It is presumably due to local irritation, rarely produces symptoms, and usually responds to removal of the catheter and administration of nitroglycerin. A repeat angiogram should be performed after administration of nitroglycerin if associated coronary spasm is suspected.

Coronary artery spasm may also occur spontane-

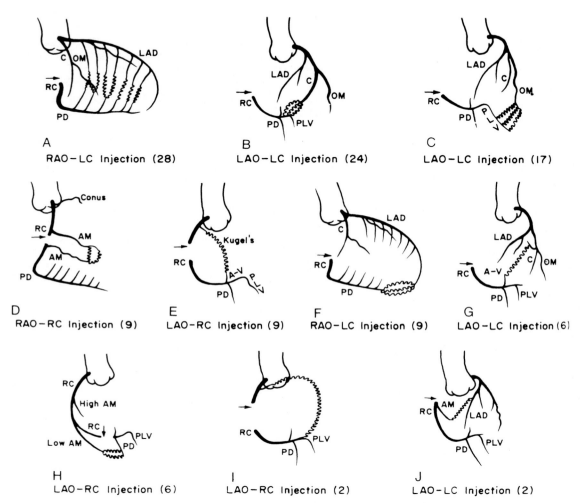

**FIGURE 54–48.** *A–J,* Coronary collateral pathways observed in patients with right coronary artery obstruction (*arrow*). (RAO = right anterior oblique projection; LAO = left anterior oblique projection; LC = left coronary artery; RC = right coronary artery; AM = acute marginal branch of the right coronary artery; PD = posterior descending branch of the right coronary artery; PLV = posterior left ventricular branch of the right coronary artery; A-V = atrioventricular node artery; LAD = left anterior descending artery; C = circumflex artery; OM = obtuse marginal branch of circumflex artery.) *Numbers in parentheses* signify the frequency of a particular collateral pathway in this series. (*A–J,* From Levin, D. C.: Pathways and functional significance of the coronary collateral circulation. Circulation, *50*:831, 1973. By permission of the American Heart Association, Inc.)

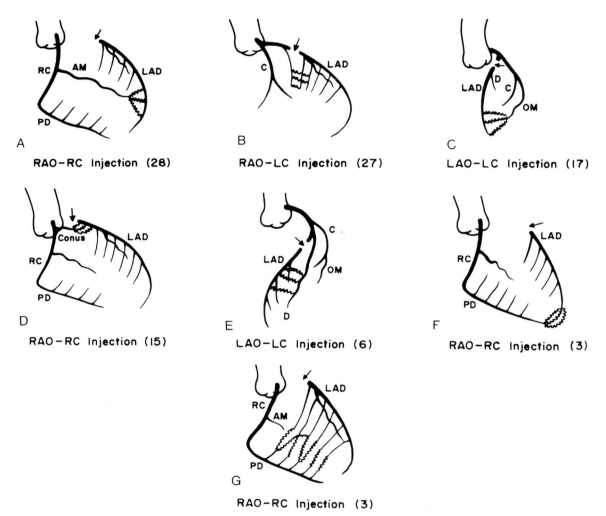

**FIGURE 54–49.** *A–G,* Collateral pathways observed with left anterior descending artery obstruction (*arrow*). (RAO = right anterior oblique projection; LAO = left anterior oblique projection; RC = right coronary artery; LC = left coronary artery; Am = acute marginal branch of the right coronary artery; C = circumflex artery; D = diagonal [anterolateral] branch of the left anterior descending artery; LAD = left anterior descending artery; OM = obtuse marginal branch of circumflex artery; PD = posterior descending branch of the right coronary artery.) (*A–G,* From Levin, D. C.: Pathways and functional significance of the coronary collateral circulation. Circulation, *50*:831, 1973. By permission of the American Heart Association, Inc.)

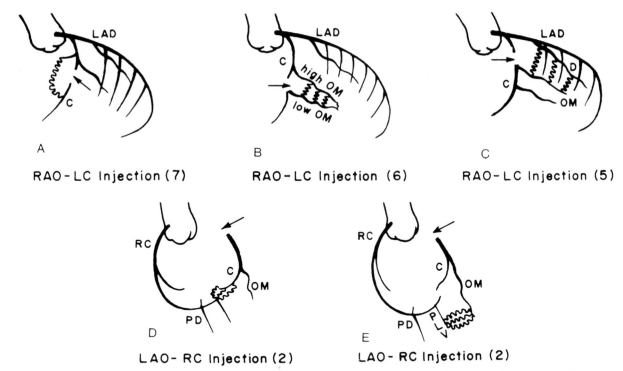

**FIGURE 54–50.** *A–E,* Collateral pathways observed in circumflex artery obstruction (*arrow*). (RAO = right anterior oblique projection; LAO = left anterior oblique projection; RC = right coronary artery; LC = left coronary artery; AM = acute marginal branch of the right coronary artery; C = circumflex artery; D = diagonal [anterolateral] branch of the left anterior descending artery; LAD = left anterior descending artery; OM = obtuse marginal branch of the circumflex artery; PD = posterior descending branch of the right coronary artery; PLV = posterior left ventricular branch of the right coronary artery.) (*A–E,* From Levin, D. C.: Pathways and functional significance of the coronary collateral circulation. Circulation, *50:*831, 1973. By permission of the American Heart Association, Inc.)

ously in angiographically normal coronary arteries, producing transient ST segment elevation and angina. When it occurs, spasm is most frequently noted in the section of the coronary artery with atheromatous involvement (MacAlpin, 1980). It is often irregular and eccentric and may involve long segments of single or multiple arteries. Even in patients with known Prinzmetal's angina, spontaneous spasm occurs only in a minority of patients during coronary angiography (Maseri et al., 1978). Therefore, provocative testing to precipitate spasm during arteriography can be used in patients who have symptoms that suggest variant angina and in whom insignificant stenosis of a major coronary artery is seen. Provocative testing should generally not be used if significant stenoses are evident on the initial coronary angiogram or if there is well-documented electrocardiographic evidence of transluminal ischemia.

The most commonly used provocative test for coronary artery spasm is intravenous administration of ergonovine maleate (Harding et al., 1992; Heupler et al., 1978; Waters et al., 1983), which is an alpha-adrenergic, and serotonin receptor agonists in epicardial coronary vessels. Spasm can often be induced in patients with known variant angina and has been reported to occur in approximately 5% of patients with atypical anginal symptoms (Bertrand et al., 1982). Other agents that have been used include intravenous methacholine, epinephrine, propranolol, tris-

buffer, or the use of the cold pressor test (placing the hands in iced saline solution). Intracoronary injection of acetylcholine has been reported to be a useful, safe, and reliable method to document multivessel coronary spasm in patients with variant angina (Okumura et al., 1988). The patient should be withdrawn from nitrates and calcium antagonists before provocative testing.

For ergonovine testing, progressive incremental doses of 0.05 mg, 0.1 mg, and then 0.15 mg are administered intravenously at 3- to 5-minute intervals. Because severe spasm can occur instantly, intracoronary nitroglycerin (usual dose 300 to 500 μg) should be made available for use. The patient should be asked about the presence of symptoms, and multilead electrocardiography should be performed before and during the procedure. Even in the absence of symptoms or electrocardiographic changes, repeat arteriography of the LCA and RCA should be done. Traditionally, a positive response is identified if focal vasospasm exceeding 70% diameter narrowing is associated with typical anginal symptoms or electrocardiographic ST segment changes. However, based on the previous discussion of the role of lesion length, diffuse spasm might also be considered to be flow-limiting. An example of intense spasm of the RCA after administration of ergonovine maleate in a patient with variant angina is shown in Figure 54–51.

The utility of ergonovine treating for coronary artery spasm was assessed in 3447 patients at Duke University (Harding et al., 1992). Patients with angiographically insignificant disease or no CAD without Prinzmetal's variant angina were evaluated. Overall, 4% had positive tests and complications occurred in 0.03%. Independent predictors of spasm were the amount of visible fixed CAD on the angiogram or a history of smoking.

## MYOCARDIAL BRIDGES

The major coronary arteries pass primarily along the epicardial surface of the heart. Segments of the epicardial artery occasionally course below the surface into the myocardium. The myocardial fibers thus form a bridge over the involved arterial segment. Myocardial bridging is shown angiographically by systolic compression of the intramyocardial arterial segment that reverts to a normal caliber during diastole. It is most often observed in the middle segment of the LAD. Systolic compression is angiographically apparent in 1.6 to 5% of patients studied (Bertrand et al., 1982; Huepler et al., 1978; MacAlpin, 1980; Waters et al., 1983). Myocardial bridges are more frequently discovered during autopsy than during cardiac catheterization. The incidence is higher in men and in patients with hypertrophic cardiomyopathy. In the latter disease, bridging of septal vessels is particularly prominent.

Rare reports have suggested that myocardial bridges cause ischemia and resultant angina (Ishimori et al., 1977; Kramer et al., 1982), myocardial infarction (Dander et al., 1980), and sudden death (Angelini et al., 1983; Morales et al., 1980). Although these data are inconclusive, it appears that in some patients bridging may alter coronary flow sufficiently to produce symptoms of ischemia. In one report (Hill et al., 1981), the persistence of luminal narrowing in early diastole

appeared to blunt the normal early influx of coronary perfusion observed at this time; loss of early diastolic filling may therefore contribute to reduced coronary flow. There appears to be a decreased incidence of atherosclerotic changes at the level of intramural coronary arteries. In 1100 consecutive patients with CAD studied with angiography, no luminal defects were noted in diastole at the level of systolic narrowing (Angelini et al., 1983).

## TECHNIQUES

Before cardiac catheterization, the procedure and potential complications should be explained to the patient and a written informed consent should be obtained. The patient is generally fasting and is often premedicated with antihistamines such as diphenhydramine, 25 to 50 mg intravenously. Sedatives including intravenous or oral benzodiazepines may help before the procedure. An intravenous line should be established before the catheterization. The patient is brought to the catheterization laboratory and prepared and draped in a sterile manner.

Electrocardiographic monitoring and recording should be visible to the angiographer and the catheterization team. Systemic blood pressure should be monitored through the intra-arterial catheter and displayed on the same screen as the electrocardiogram (see Chapter 31, part I, for further details). Judkins' technique (1967), because of its relative ease, speed, reliability, and slightly lower complication rate (Davis et al., 1979), has become the most widely used method of coronary arteriography in the United States.

The type of contrast media used during cardiac catheterization can affect the incidence of complications. When compared with ionic contrast agents, nonionic contrast agents have reduced the incidence of adverse cardiovascular events such as bradycardia,

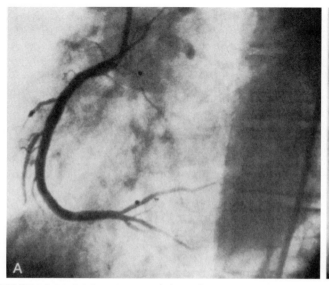
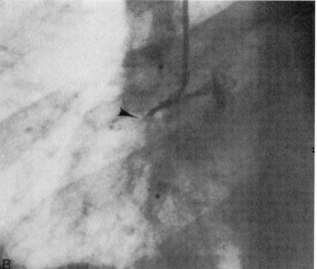

**FIGURE 54–51.** LAO projection of the right coronary artery before (*A*) and after (*B*) intravenous ergonovine injection. Note the severe spasm resulting in total occlusion of the coronary (*arrowhead*).

ventricular fibrillation, hypotension, electrocardiographic changes, and depressed left ventricular function. Cardiovascular events were evaluated in 8517 patients undergoing diagnostic cardiac catheterization (Davidson et al., 1990). Death occurred in 2 patients (0.02%), prolonged chest pain in 29 (0.3%), ventricular tachycardia or fibrillation in 5 (0.06%), and profound bradycardia in 15 (1.8%). Stroke occurred in 5 (0.06%) and transient ischemic attacks in 2 (0.02%). Thrombotic complications occurred in 15 (0.18%). These data indicate that nonionic contrast can reduce the incidence of cardiovascular events compared with ionic contrast and at no increased risk for thrombotic events. Contrast-induced nephropathy, defined as a rise in creatinine equal to or greater than 0.5 mg/dl, occurs in 6% of patients (Davidson et al., 1989). Patients with elevated baseline serum creatinine appear to be at increased risk. The risk appears to be directly related to the severity of baseline renal insufficiency.

## Percutaneous Femoral Technique—Judkins' Technique

The preformed catheters used for Judkins' technique are shown in Figure 54–52. These catheters are made of polyurethane and polyethylene, and contain either steel braid or nylon in the wall of the catheter shaft to allow better torque control. The catheters are designed with a single end hole for contrast injection and a tapered blunt tip to reduce intimal trauma. Although the original catheters were usually No. 8 French, Nos. 5, 6, and 7 French of a standard 100-cm length are currently available for use. The Nos. 5, 6, and 7 French catheters are the most commonly used for adult coronary arteriography. All catheters have a primary, secondary, and tertiary curve. The Judkins left and right coronary catheters are available in four

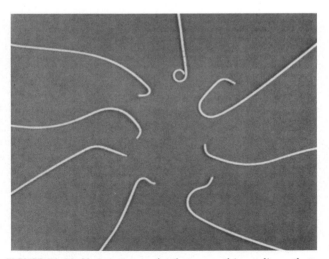

**FIGURE 54–52.** Various types of catheters used in cardiac catheterization with the percutaneous femoral technique. Beginning clockwise from 12 o'clock, the pigtail catheter, the left and right Judkins catheters, the left and right Amplatz catheters, a multipurpose catheter, a bypass graft catheter, and an internal mammary artery catheter.

sizes and are commonly referred to as JL3.5, JL4, JL5, JL6 (left) and JR3.5, JR4, JR6 (right). The numbers describe the length in centimeters of the secondary arm of the catheters. The JL4 catheter is most commonly used in patients with normal-sized aortic roots, whereas the JL5 and JL6 catheters are used in patients with progressively elongated or dilated aortic roots. The secondary bend constitutes the major difference in the left and right coronary catheters. The secondary bend of the left coronary catheter approaches 180 degrees, whereas the right coronary bend is approximately 30 degrees.

After local anesthesia with 1% lidocaine (Xylocaine), percutaneous entry of the femoral artery is achieved by puncturing the vessel 1 to 3 cm below the inguinal ligament. The ligament, which can be palpated as it courses from the anterior superior iliac spine to the superior pubic ramus, should be the landmark used, rather than the inguinal crease, which is often misleading. A transverse skin incision is made over the femoral artery with a scalpel. A No. 18-gauge thin-wall needle is inserted at a 30- to 45-degree angle into the femoral artery, and a 0.035-inch J-tip Teflon-coated guidewire is advanced into the needle. The wire should pass freely up the aorta. Fluoroscopy should be used to reveal the cause of any resistance to advancement. While pressure is firmly applied over the femoral artery, the needle is removed and a dilator equal in size to the catheters to be used is introduced. Alternatively, an arterial sheath of equal size to the coronary catheter can be placed in the femoral artery. With the guidewire within the aorta, the coronary catheter is passed over the wire to the ascending aorta. After the guidewire is removed, 3 to 4 ml of blood is aspirated from the catheter, which is then flushed with heparinized saline solution. The catheter is attached to the catheter-syringe manifold assembly, which allows pressure monitoring as well as contrast injection. Patients should receive systemic heparinization (3000 to 5000 units) after arterial access is achieved.

The left coronary catheter is initially advanced near but not into the orifice of the LMCA using fluoroscopic guidance in the left anterior oblique (LAO) projection. A flush injection of contrast is made to visualize the left main ostium before entry of the catheter. After this and each subsequent injection, arterial pressure should be noted first before selective angiography. If damping (decrease in catheter tip pressure) or ventricularization (normal systolic pressure but low diastolic pressure) occurs, it may indicate a significant stenosis of the LMCA, perhaps that the catheter tip has created total or almost total obstruction of the vessel. Alternatively, it suggests an adverse position of the catheter end hole against the wall of the artery. In either situation, the catheter should be removed immediately from the ostium. The angiographer should reevaluate the possibility of high-grade proximal coronary stenosis with further flush injections of the artery in multiple views. If ostial stenosis is present, additional injections must be made quickly, followed by immediate withdrawal of the catheter. Lengthy injections in this situation may cause prolonged ischemia or dissection of the artery.

After arteriography of the LMCA is performed in multiple views with satisfactory visualization of any abnormalities (see "Angiographic Views," later in this chapter), the left coronary catheter is withdrawn to the level of the diaphragm. The guidewire is reintroduced, and the left coronary catheter is replaced with the Judkins right catheter. The catheter is advanced to the ascending aorta approximately 3 cm above the right sinus of Valsalva, and the patient is imaged in the LAO position. The Judkins left catheter almost automatically seeks out the left coronary ostium, but the right catheter may require considerable manipulation. The right coronary catheter tip is slowly rotated clockwise (anteriorly) and steadily withdrawn until it enters the orifice of the artery. The withdrawal is necessary because the catheter tends to descend within the aortic root as it is torqued clockwise.

Unlike in the LMCA, damping and ventricularization of the RCA are commonly due to catheter tip–induced spasm. Other potential causes include a small caliber of the ostia, superselective cannulation of the conus artery, or severe proximal stenosis. The cause can usually be determined by nonselective test injections or administration of nitroglycerin. Once again, cautious injections with rapid catheter withdrawal should be accomplished to avoid unnecessary ischemic complications.

Selective injection of aortocoronary bypass grafts via the percutaneous femoral approach can be accomplished with a right Judkins catheter, a right Amplatz catheter, or specifically designed graft catheters. To engage posterior or medial grafts, a specifically designed Judkins bypass catheter, which is similar to a right coronary catheter but modified so the tip has a smooth downward terminal curve, may be used (see Fig. 54–52). Injection of these grafts with contrast media often causes patients various degrees of pain in the extremities.

After coronary arteriography has been performed, the catheters are removed and firm pressure is applied to the femoral area for 10 to 15 minutes, either by hand or by a mechanical clamp. The patient should be instructed to lie in bed for several hours, usually 4 to 6 hours, with the leg remaining straight to prevent formation of hematoma.

The main advantage of Judkins' technique is the speed and ease of selective catheterization. However, these attributes should not preclude gaining extensive operator experience to ensure quality studies with an acceptable degree of safety. The main disadvantage of this technique is that its use in patients with iliofemoral atherosclerotic disease may prevent retrograde passage of catheters through areas of extreme narrowing or tortuosity.

## Brachial Artery Technique

Sones and colleagues (1959) introduced the first technique for selective coronary artery angiography via a brachial artery cutdown. Sones' technique is still popular in many centers. The Sones catheter is available in a thin-walled woven Dacron or polyurethane design. It is 100 cm long and No. 7 or 8 French in diameter, tapering to No. 5.5 French at the tip. It has an end hole and two to four side holes near the catheter tip. After direct exposure of the brachial artery (usually the right brachial artery), an arteriotomy is made. The catheter is connected to a manifold and is advanced through the subclavian artery and innominate artery to the ascending aorta under fluoroscopic and pressure control. If a tortuous innominate or subclavian artery is encountered, a guidewire may be useful. The patient may attempt maneuvers such as shrugging the shoulders, turning the head to the left, or taking a deep breath in these situations. Pressure monitoring and safety precautions are the same as those with Judkins' technique.

With the catheter in the central aorta, systemic heparinization is administered. In Sones' technique, the same catheter is used for both right and left coronary injections. After a flush injection of the LMCA, selective left and right coronary arteriography may be performed. With the patient in the LAO projection, the catheter is advanced to the left sinus of Valsalva and a J loop is made. The catheter is then advanced and withdrawn until the left ostium is engaged.

To cannulate the RCA, the catheter is withdrawn from the LMCA while a gentle loop is maintained and clockwise rotation is applied. Damping owing to spasm, selective catheterization of the conus artery, or wedging within a stenosis may also occur with Sones' technique.

When the catheter is removed from the brachial artery, proximal and distal bleeding are permitted to flush potential small thrombi. A small probe may be placed gently into the distal artery if distal flow is inadequate. A Fogarty thrombectomy catheter may be used for this purpose. The arteriotomy site is usually closed with a purse-string suture. After the skin is closed, a light pressure dressing is placed over the area.

Disadvantages of Sones' technique are that it is more difficult to master and that the LMCA may be extremely difficult to cannulate. Furthermore, catheter seating may be less stable than with Judkins' technique, and biplane ventriculography or aortography may be difficult because the patient is being studied from the arm. Left internal mammary grafts may require the use of a left brachial approach. Advantages of Sones' technique are that the entire procedure, including bypass grafts, may be performed with one catheter, and the technique is especially useful in patients with severe iliofemoral vascular disease. Patients who are receiving oral anticoagulation with prolonged prothrombin times may benefit from this approach. In addition, patients can ambulate soon after the procedure.

A modification of Sones' technique is the percutaneous brachial technique with preformed Judkins catheters. This technique uses the Seldinger method of percutaneous brachial artery entry. A No. 5 or 6

French sheath is placed into the brachial artery, and 5000 units of heparin are infused into the side port. A guidewire is then advanced to the ascending aorta under fluoroscopic control. No. 5 or 6 French Judkins left, right, and pigtail catheters are passed over the guidewire for routine arteriography and ventriculography. The guidewire may be necessary occasionally to direct the left coronary catheter into the left sinus of Valsalva and the ostium of the LMCA. The main advantage of the percutaneous brachial technique is that it avoids a brachial artery cutdown and repair.

## Angiographic Views

To visualize coronary arteries adequately, it is necessary to identify the LMCA and RCA in multiple projections. Because of considerable overlap, tortuosity, and branching of vessels, additional views may be required to assess atherosclerotic lesions. As discussed under "Pathoanatomic Correlates," earlier in this chapter, eccentric lesions require orthogonal views to quantify the severity of stenosis.

Early angiographic studies of the heart depend on transverse views. Therefore, only different degrees of LAO and right anterior oblique (RAO) views were performed. As expected, these limited views were often inadequate to assess the severity of the lesion with eccentricity, and branching obscured visualization.

Several reports in the 1970s documented the use of cranial and caudal angulation of the x-ray beam (Aldridge, 1984; Aldridge et al., 1975; Arani et al., 1975; Sos and Baltaxe, 1977). These sagittal plane views have allowed improved evaluation of foreshortened and partially obscured vessels (Fig. 54–53). In particular, it has been well documented that stenosis of the origin of the PDA and the distal LMCA may be difficult to quantify reliably, even when multiple views are available (Kennedy et al., 1982).

X-ray systems now in routine use are able to provide any combination of transverse angulation with cranial or caudal angulation. The proposed and generally accepted terminology (Aldridge et al., 1975; Sos and Baltaxe, 1977) for angiographic views is based on how one views the arteries from the image intensifier. Thus, in the LAO cranial view, one visualizes the coronary arteries as if looking over the patient's left shoulder. Likewise, in the RAO caudal view, coronary arteries are viewed as if looking from the inferior aspect of the right thorax.

The LMCA with its major branches may require as many as six views to assess the anatomy adequately. RAO, LAO, LAO cranial, RAO cranial, RAO caudal, and LAO caudal are the standard projections used. The LMCA typically is best viewed in a shallow LAO and RAO projection, with the artery just off the spine. However, in many cases, additional injections with cranial and caudal angulation are necessary.

The LAD should be seen at the minimum in the LAO and RAO projections. The addition of cranial angulation to these views may facilitate identification of lesions, especially those in the proximal LAD, the septal perforators, and the diagonal (anterolateral) branches (Figs. 54–54 and 54–55; see also Fig. 54–53). The left circumflex coronary artery is best evaluated in the LAO caudal, RAO caudal, and LAO projections (Fig. 54–56; see also Fig. 54–53). The LAO caudal view (spider view) allows evaluation of the LMCA, proximal LAD, and proximal circumflex artery, including the optional diagonal artery. In a left dominant circulation, the PDA from the circumflex artery is best visualized in the LAO and LAO cranial projections. A RAO caudal projection aids in separation and visualization of the marginal branches. Although all views may not be necessary in all patients, the angiographer should individualize the examination to obtain the maximal amount of information with the least number of injections. Occasionally, complex overlap of proximal LMCA vessels can be better defined by rolling the camera during the view.

The RCA is usually viewed in shallow RAO and LAO projections (Figs. 54–57 and 55–58). However, when the PDA or the origin of the RCA is obscured, an LAO cranial or a steep RAO view may be useful to overcome foreshortening. Cranial angulation of the LAO view helps to visualize the bifurcation of the RCA into the PDA and the distal left ventricular branches.

## UNUSUAL CORONARY ANATOMY

Coronary artery aneurysms and ectasia are usually caused by atherosclerotic infiltration of the media of the artery, although congenital aneurysms may also occur (Fujita et al., 1983). Other less common causes include periarteritis, syphilis, trauma, rheumatic fever, bacterial endocarditis, and Kawasaki's disease. Coronary aneurysms are present angiographically or at autopsy in as many as 1.5% of patients (Glickel et al., 1978). Aneurysms have been classified as being *diffuse* or *localized* (Kalke and Edwards, 1968). *Diffuse aneurysms* are generally considered to be congenital, whereas *localized aneurysms* can be caused by atherosclerosis or inflammatory disease. They are frequently encountered when arteriovenous fistulas are present. The diagnosis of coronary artery aneurysms and ectasia can best be made by coronary arteriography (Figs. 54–59 and 54–60). Multiple views should be obtained to exclude the presence of coexisting atherosclerotic disease.

Angiographically, a fresh or organized coronary artery thrombus appears as an eccentric filling defect that usually extends from the arterial wall into the lumen. It may be difficult to distinguish in vivo from fixed atherosclerotic stenosis and, in many cases, are attached to an atherosclerotic plaque. Coronary artery thrombus appears to be a frequent occurrence in patients with acute myocardial infarction or unstable angina. However, coronary artery emboli are separate from the intima of the artery and may have a tail-like appearance. Coronary artery embolism may result from endocarditis, mural thrombi secondary to valvu-

*Text continued on page 1881*

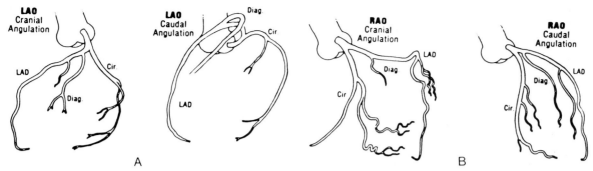

**FIGURE 54–53.** Diagrammatic representation of the left coronary artery when visualized with cranial and caudal angulation of the x-ray beam. (LAD = left anterior descending artery; Cir. = circumflex artery; Diag. = diagonal artery.) (*A* and *B*, From Sos, T. A., and Baltaxe, H. A.: Cranial and caudal angulation for coronary angiography revisited. Circulation, *56*:119, 1977. By permission of the American Heart Association, Inc.)

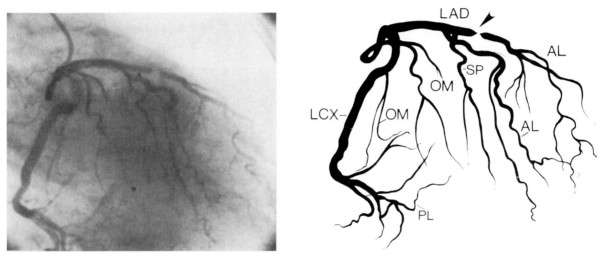

**FIGURE 54–54.** Coronary arteriogram and diagram in RAO projection of severe stenosis (*arrowhead*) of the mid left anterior descending coronary artery (LAD). (AL = anterolateral [diagonal] artery; LCX = left circumflex coronary artery; OM = obtuse marginal branch of circumflex artery; SP = septal perforator; PL = posterolateral artery.)

**FIGURE 54–55.** Coronary arteriogram and diagram of LAO cranial view of left anterior descending artery (LAD) stenosis (*arrowhead*) described in Figure 54–54. (AL = anterolateral [diagonal] artery; LCX = left circumflex coronary artery; LM = left main coronary artery; OM = obtuse marginal branch of circumflex artery; PL = posterolateral artery.)

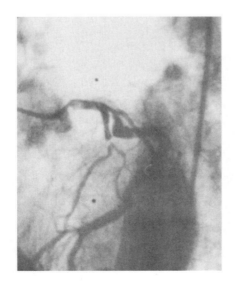

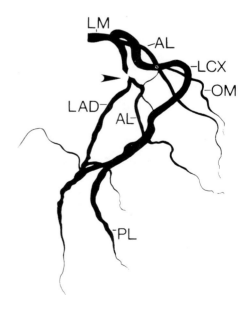

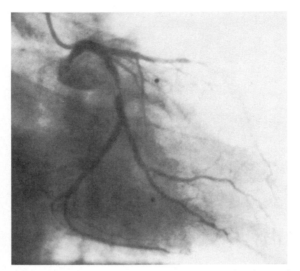
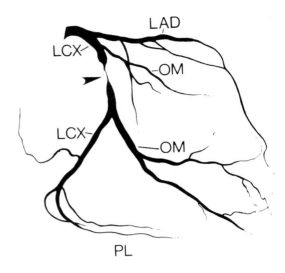

**FIGURE 54–56.** RAO caudal view of mid left circumflex lesion (*arrowhead*). (LAD = left anterior descending coronary artery; LCX = left circumflex coronary artery; OM = obtuse marginal branch of circumflex artery; PL = posterolateral artery.)

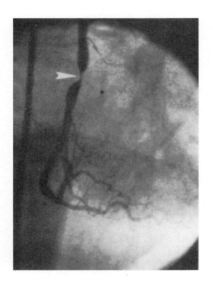
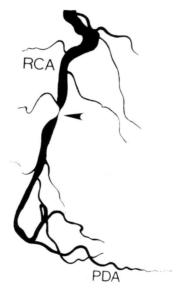

**FIGURE 54–57.** RAO view of mid right coronary artery obstruction (*arrowheads*). (RCA = right coronary artery; PDA = posterior descending artery.)

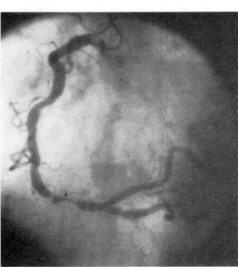
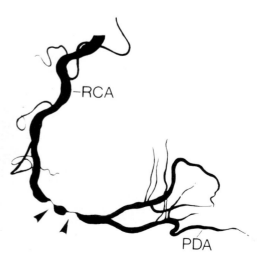

**FIGURE 54–58.** Shallow LAO view of multiple right coronary artery stenosis (*arrowheads*). (RCA = right coronary artery; PDA = posterior descending artery.)

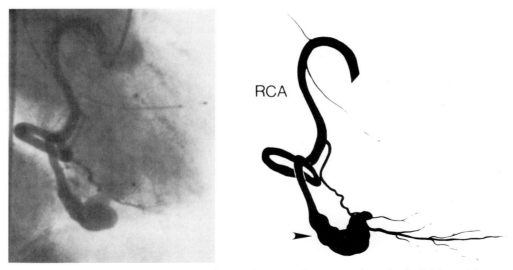

**FIGURE 54–59.** RAO view of right coronary artery (RCA) showing large distal aneurysm (*arrowhead*). (RCA = right coronary artery.)

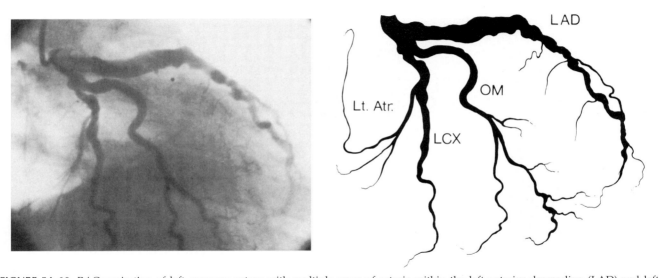

**FIGURE 54–60.** RAO projection of left coronary artery with multiple areas of ectasia within the left anterior descending (LAD) and left circumflex (LCX) arteries. (OM = obtuse marginal branch of circumflex artery; Lt. Atr. = left atrial branch.)

**FIGURE 54–61.** RAO projection of the right coronary with intracoronary thrombus present at the site of severe stenosis (*arrowhead*). Thrombus occurred as a complication of routine coronary arteriography.

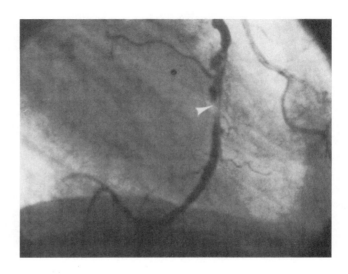

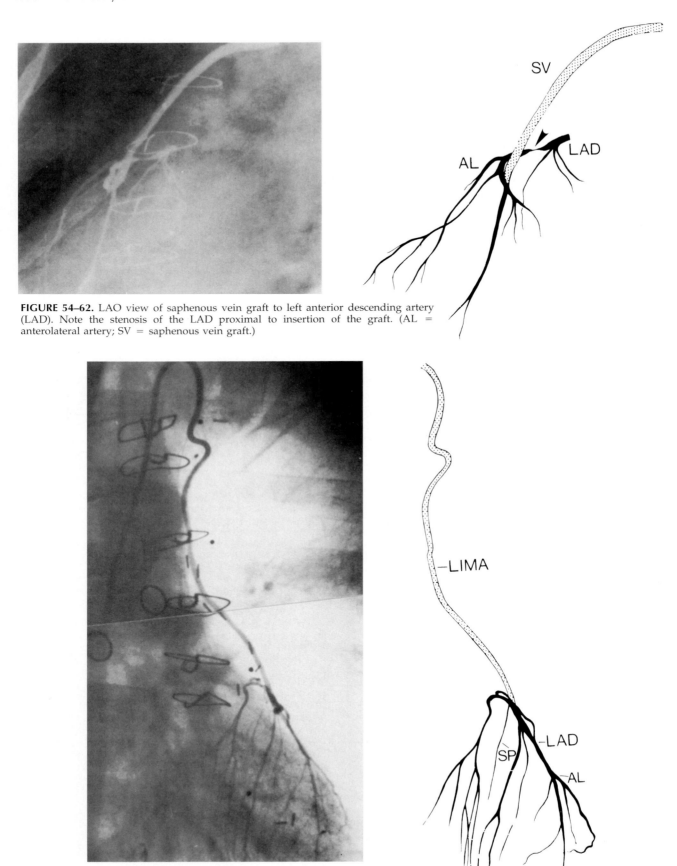

**FIGURE 54–62.** LAO view of saphenous vein graft to left anterior descending artery (LAD). Note the stenosis of the LAD proximal to insertion of the graft. (AL = anterolateral artery; SV = saphenous vein graft.)

**FIGURE 54–63.** RAO view of left internal mammary artery (LIMA) graft to left anterior descending (LAD) artery. (AL = anterolateral artery; SP = septal perforator.)

lar disease or cardiomyopathy, or intracardiac tumors (particularly myxoma). Iatrogenic coronary occlusion due to embolism is a well-recognized complication of coronary arteriography (Fig. 54–61).

## CORONARY ARTERY BYPASS GRAFTS
(Figs. 54–62 and 54–63)

Coronary artery bypass grafts should appear smooth and equal to or larger in size than the native coronary artery. Stenosis may occur at the proximal anastomosis, in the body of the graft, or at distal anastomosis. In aortocoronary bypass grafts, stenosis of the origin is best viewed in multiple orthogonal projections because of the potential eccentricity of the lesion. Total occlusion of the graft appears as a dimple or stump arising from the aortic root during selective angiography. If total stenosis occurs anywhere within the graft, the graft usually occludes back to the aortic anastomosis. Although aortography may assist in localizing unmarked grafts, an inability to visualize graft patency by this method should not be taken as conclusive evidence of graft occlusion. Selective angiography is necessary to fully evaluate the patency of a graft.

Mid-graft or distal-graft stenosis may appear as either smooth intimal proliferation or a typical atherosclerotic plaque. To avoid confusion, the significance of a lesion within an aortocoronary bypass graft should probably be interpreted in relation to the diameter of the normal native artery rather than the "normal" part of the saphenous vein.

## SELECTED BIBLIOGRAPHY

Chaitman, B. R., Lesperance, J., Saltiel, J., and Bourassa, M. G.: Clinical, angiographic, and hemodynamic findings in patients with anomalous origin of the coronary arteries. Circulation, 53:122, 1976.

This study describes the clinical and angiographic features of 31 patients with an anomalous origin of the coronary arteries. The course of aberrant circumflex artery, left coronary artery, and right coronary artery is described. The relationship between each anomaly and its clinical significance is reviewed. In addition, coronary blood flow during exercise and myocardial metabolism during pacing are assessed in 5 patients with aberrant left coronary arteries. It is concluded that aberrant left coronary artery origin from the right sinus of Valsalva can cause significant myocardial ischemia and infarction.

Ellis, S. G., Vandormael, M. G., Cowley, M. J., et al.: Coronary morphologic and clinical determinants of procedural outcome with angioplasty for multivessel coronary disease. Implications for patient selection. Circulation, 82:1193, 1990.

This important study assesses the likelihood of procedural success after percutaneous transluminal coronary angioplasty (PTCA) based on coronary morphology, lesion severity, and clinical determinants. Three hundred fifty consecutive patients and 1100 stenoses were evaluated. The authors demonstrate that a modified American College of Cardiology/ American Heart Association (ACC/AHA) task force classification of morphology can determine success rates and complications after PTCA. Type A stenosis had a 92% success rate and a 2% complication rate compared with a 61% success rate and a 21% complication rate with Type C lesions. Types B1 and B2 were intermediate in success and complications. The stenosis characteristics of chronic total occlusion, high-grade (80 to 99% diameter) stenosis, stenosis on a bend greater than 60 degrees, and excessive tortuosity are particularly high-risk. These data indicate that risk stratification for PTCA can be elucidated from morphologic and quantitative characteristics of the baseline cineangiogram.

Harding, M. B., Leithe, M. E., Mark, D. B., et al.: Ergonovine maleate testing during cardiac catheterization: A 10-year perspective in 3447 patients without significant coronary artery disease or Prinzmetal's variant angina. J. Am. Coll. Cardiol., 20:107, 1992.

This study analyzed the utility of ergonovine testing for coronary artery spasm in 3447 patients with angiographically insignificant (less than or equal to 50% visual diameter stenosis) or no coronary artery disease. No patient had clinical evidence of Prinzmetal's variant angina. There was a 4% incidence of positive ergonovine test results, which was defined as spasm causing greater than or equal to 75% focal narrowing. Complications occurred in 11 patients (0.03%), with myocardial infarction in 4 and ventricular tachycardia or fibrillation in 7.

To identify the major predictors of a positive ergonovine test result, the 3447 patients were separated into two groups, a training sample and a test sample. In the training sample, two independent predictors of spasm were found in the multivariate analysis: the amount of visible coronary artery disease on the cineangiogram ($p < .0001$) and a smoking history ($p = .001$). To demonstrate the utility of the model in the validation sample, a risk score was developed that assigned 1 point for a stenosis less than or equal to 50% and 1 point for a history of smoking. With a score of 0, 1% of patients had a positive ergonovine test, with a score of 1, 3% were positive; and with a score of 2, 10% were positive. The logistic regression model allowed identification of 400 patients in the validation sample who had a 10% positive test rate compared with 2% in the remaining patients.

These data should be useful for clinicians who use provocative testing to reserve ergonovine testing for the subset of patients most likely to have abnormal findings.

Hermiller, J. B., Cusma, J. T., Spero, L. A., et al.: Quantitative and qualitative coronary angiographic analysis: Review of methods, utility, and limitations. Cathet. Cardiovasc. Diagn., 25:131, 1992.

This review article describes various methods of quantitative coronary artery analysis currently in use both commercially and institutionally. Caliper, computer-derived geometric techniques, and video densitometry are described. The utility and pitfalls of quantitative coronary arteriography are elucidated.

The second part of the review concentrates on morphologic evaluation of coronary artery disease utilizing contrast angiography. The authors demonstrate that the qualitative morphologic characteristics are at least equally as important as quantitative measures in determining lesion stability and prognosis.

Levin, D. C.: Pathways and functional significance of the coronary collateral circulation. Circulation, 50:831, 1974.

This classic article reports the results of 200 coronary arteriograms and left ventriculograms in patients with significant coronary artery disease. The diagrams of collateral circulation outline the pathways observed in left anterior descending, left circumflex, and right coronary artery obstruction. These diagrams are reproduced in this chapter.

The author examines the role of collateral circulation in preserving myocardial function and concludes that regional wall motion is preserved in the presence of adequate collateral circulation.

Mancini, G. B. J., Simon, S. B., McGillem, M. J., et al.: Automated quantitative coronary arteriography: Morphologic and physiologic validation in vivo of a rapid digital angiographic method. Circulation, 75:452, 1987.

This study assesses for the first time the performance in vivo of the fully automatic rapid coronary quantitation program. Dogs were instrumented with high-fidelity micromanometer catheters, electromagnetic flow, and plastic cylinders to create intraluminal stenoses of the left anterior descending and circumflex arteries. Interobserver and intraobserver variation was low, and the correlation between known and measured luminal diameter was high. The measures of percentage diameter stenosis, percentage area stenosis (geometric and video densitometric), and absolute minimal cross-sectional area (geometric and video densitometric) all were correlated with independent measures of coronary flow reserve. Therefore, this report provides direct anatomic and physiologic validation of a quantitative method of analysis for digital angiograms and cineangiograms.

Marcus, M. L., Wilson, R. F., and White, C. W.: Methods of measurement of myocardial blood flow in patients: A critical review. Circulation, 76:245, 1987.

This article critically reviews the currently available methods of studying coronary flow in humans and provides insight into newer methods under investigation and development. The methods discussed include thermodilution, gas clearance, densitometry, electromagnetic, and Doppler flow probes, positron-emission tomography, ultra-fast computed tomography, contrast echocardiography, and magnetic resonance imaging. The article discusses the relative merits and limitations of each technique and strongly recommends more widespread use of Doppler catheters. An extensive list of current references is provided.

Wilson, R. F., Marcus, M. L., and White, C. W.: Prediction of the physiologic significance of coronary artery lesions by quantitative lesion geometry in patients with limited coronary artery disease. Circulation, 75:723, 1987.

This study examines the relationship between coronary flow reserve measured by Doppler coronary catheter and luminal stenosis of individual lesions in patients with discrete coronary artery stenoses. The authors show that, in patients with limited coronary atherosclerosis, precise angiographic measurements by quantitative angiography correlated closely with a physiologic measurement of coronary obstruction. Lesions in major coronary arteries with less than a 70% area stenosis or minimal cross-sectional area greater than 2.5 mm$^2$ did not functionally impair coronary blood flow or result in significant translesional pressure gradient.

The physiologic conclusions emerging from this study are: (1) Coronary stenosis of more than 90% luminal area stenosis was associated with a wide range of coronary flow reserve. (2) Lesions of less than a 70% area stenosis or greater than 2.5 mm$^2$ cross-sectional area usually do not result in myocardial ischemia. This is not always the case because coronary lesions are known to be dynamic. Lesions may not result in functional obstruction when vasodilatory agents are used. (3) There is usually only modest reduction in coronary blood flow reserve in lesions with 70 to 80% area obstruction.

# BIBLIOGRAPHY

Aldridge, H. E.: A decade or more of cranial and caudal angled projections in coronary arteriography—Another look. Cathet. Cardiovasc. Diagn., 10:539, 1984.

Aldridge, H. E., McLoughlin, M. J., and Taylor, L. W.: Improved diagnosis in coronary cinearteriography with routine use of 110-degree oblique views and cranial and caudal angulations: Comparison with standard oblique views in 100 patients. Am. J. Cardiol., 36:568, 1975.

American Heart Association Committee Report: A reporting system on patients evaluated for coronary artery disease. Circulation, 51:7, 1975.

Amplatz, K., Formonek G., Stranger, P., and Wilson, W.: Mechanics of selective coronary artery catheterization via the femoral approach. Radiology, 89:1040, 1967.

Anderson, J. L., Karagounis, L. A., and Becker, L. C.: TIMI perfusion grade 3, but not grade 2, results in improved outcome after thrombolysis for myocardial infarction. Circulation, 87:1829, 1993.

Angelini, P., Trivellato, M., Donis, J., and Leachman, R. D.: Myocardial bridges: A review. Prog. Cardiovasc. Dis., 26:75, 1983.

Arani, D. T., Bunnel, I. L., and Greene, D. G.: Lordotic right posterior oblique projection of the left coronary artery: A special view for special anatomy. Circulation, 52:504, 1975.

Bartel, A. G., Chen, J. T., Peter, R. H., et al.: The significance of coronary artery calcification detected by fluoroscopy. Circulation, 49:1247, 1974.

Bertrand, M. E., La Blanche, J. M., Tilmant, P. Y., et al.: Frequency of provoked coronary arterial spasm in 1089 consecutive patients undergoing coronary arteriography. Circulation, 65:1299, 1982.

Blankenhorn, D. H., and Curry, P. J.: The accuracy of arteriography and ultrasound imaging for atherosclerotic measurement. Arch. Pathol. Lab. Med., 106:483, 1982.

Chahine, R. A., Raizner, A. E., Ishimon, T., et al.: The incidence and clinical implications of coronary artery spasms. Circulation, 52:972, 1975.

Chaitman, B. R., Lesperance, J., Saltiel, J., and Bourassa, M. G.: Clinical, angiographic, and hemodynamic findings in patients with anomalous origin of the coronary arteries. Circulation, 53:122, 1976.

Cohen, M. V.: Morphologic considerations of the coronary collateral circulation in man. In Cohen, M. V. (ed): Coronary Collaterals: Clinical and Experimental Observation. Mount Kisco, NY, Futura Publishing, 1985, pp. 1–91.

Cusma, J. T., Spero, L. A., Hanemann, J. D., et al.: A multi-user environment for the display and processing of digital cardiac angiographic images. Proc. SPIE, 310:1233, 1990.

Cusma, J. T., Toggart, E. J., Folts, J. D., et al.: Digital subtraction

angiographic imaging of coronary flow reserve. Circulation, 75:461, 1987.

Dander, B., Rossi, L., Nidasio, G. P., et al.: Myocardial bridges and ischemic heart disease. Eur. Heart J., 1:239, 1980.

Davidson, C. J., Hlatky, M., Morris, G. G., et al.: Cardiovascular and renal toxicity of a nonionic radiographic contrast agent after cardiac catheterization. Ann. Intern. Med., 110:119, 1989.

Davidson, C. J., Mark, D. B., Pieper, K. S., et al.: Thrombotic and cardiovascular complications related to nonionic contrast media during cardiac catheterization. Analysis of 8517 patients. Am. J. Cardiol., 65:1481, 1990.

Davis, K., Kennedy, J. W., Kemp, H. G., et al.: Complications of coronary arteriography. Circulation, 59:1105, 1979.

Dehmer, L., Gould, K. L., and Kirkeeide, R.: Assessing stenosis severity, coronary flow reserve, collateral function, quantitative coronary arteriography, position imaging, and digital subtraction angiography. A review and analysis. Prog. Cardiovasc. Dis., 30:307, 1988.

DeRouen, T. A., Murray, J. A., and Owen, W.: Variability in the analysis of coronary arteriograms. Circulation, 55:324, 1977.

Doucette, J. W., Corl, P. D., Payne, H. M., et al.: Validation of a Doppler guidewire for intravascular measurement of coronary artery flow velocity. Circulation, 85:1899, 1992.

Douglas, J. S., Franch, R. H., and King, S. B.: Coronary artery anomalies. In King, S. B., and Douglas, J. S. (eds): Coronary Arteriography and Angioplasty. New York, McGraw-Hill, 1985, pp. 33–85.

Ellis, S. G., Vandormael, M. G., Cowley, M. J., et al.: Coronary morphologic and clinical determinants of procedural outcome with angioplasty for multivessel coronary disease. Circulation, 82:1516, 1990.

Engel, H. J., Torres, C., and Page, H. L.: Major variations in anatomical origin of the coronary arteries. Cathet. Cardiovasc. Diagn., 1:157, 1975.

Feldman, R. L., Nichols, W. W., Pepine, C. J., and Cond, C. R.: Hemodynamic significance of the length of the coronary arterial narrowing. Am. J. Cardiol., 41:865, 1978.

Forssmann, W.: The catheterization of the right side of the heart. Klin. Wochenschr., 8:2085, 1929.

Fortin, D. F., Spero, L. A., Cusma, J. T., et al.: Pitfalls in the determination of absolute dimensions using angiographic catheters as calibration devices in quantitative angiography. Am. J. Cardiol., 68:1176, 1991.

Fujita, S., Murakami, E., Takekoshi, N., et al.: Congenital coronary arterial aneurysm without arteriovenous fistula resulting in myocardial infarction. Jpn. Circ. J., 47:363, 1983.

Ganz, W., Tamura, K., Marcus, H. S., et al.: Measurement of coronary sinus blood flow by continuous thermodilution in man. Circulation, 44:181, 1971.

Gensini, G. G., DiGiorgi, S., Coskun, O., et al.: Anatomy of the coronary circulation in living man: Coronary venography. Circulation, 31:778, 1965.

Glagov, S., Weisenberg, E., Zarines, C. K., et al.: Compensatory enlargement of human atherosclerotic coronary arteries. N. Engl. J. Med., 316:1371, 1987.

Glagov, S., and Zarins, C. V.: Quantitative atherosclerosis: Problems of definition. In Bond, M. A., Insull, W., Glagov, S., et al. (eds): Clinical Diagnosis of Atherosclerosis: Quantitative Methods of Evaluation. New York, Springer-Verlag, 1982.

Glickel, S. Z., Maggs, P. R., and Ellis, F. H.: Coronary artery aneurysm. Ann. Thorac. Surg., 25:372, 1978.

Gould, K. L., Goldstein, R. A., Mullani, N. A., et al.: Noninvasive assessment of coronary stenoses by myocardial perfusion imaging during pharmacologic coronary vasodilatation. VII: Clinical feasibility of positron cardiac imaging without a cyclotron using generator produced rubidium-82. J. Am. Coll. Cardiol., 7:775, 1986.

Gruentzig, A. R., Myler, R. K., Hanna, E. S., et al.: Coronary transluminal angioplasty [Abstract]. Circulation, 56:III-84, 1977.

Gruentzig, A. R., Senning, A., and Siegenthaler, W. E.: Nonoperative dilation of coronary artery stenoses: Percutaneous transluminal coronary angioplasty. N. Engl. J. Med., 301:61, 1979.

Hamby, R. I., Tabrah, R., Wisoff, B. G., and Hartenstein, M. L.: Coronary artery calcification: Clinical implications and angiographic correlates. Am. Heart J., 87:565, 1974.

Harding, M. B., Leithe, M. E., Mark, D. B., et al.: Ergonovine maleate testing during cardiac catheterization: A 10-year perspective in 3447 patients without significant coronary artery disease or Prinzmetal's variant angina. J. Am. Coll. Cardiol., 20:107, 1992.

Harrison, D. G., White, C. W., and Hiratzka, L. F.: The value of cross-sectional area determined by quantitative coronary arteriography in assessing the physiologic significance of proximal left anterior stenosis. Circulation, 69:1111, 1984.

Hermiller, J. B., Buller, C. E., Tenaglia, A. N., et al.: Unrecognized left main coronary artery disease in patients undergoing interventional procedures. Am. J. Cardiol., 71:173, 1993a.

Hermiller, J. B., Cusma, J., Spero, L., et al.: Quantitative and qualitative coronary angiographic analysis: Review of methods, utility and limitations. Cathet. Cardiovasc. Diagn., 25:110, 1992.

Hermiller, J. B., Tenaglia, A. N., Kisslo, K. B., et al.: In vivo validation of compensatory enlargement of atherosclerotic coronary arteries. Am. J. Cardiol., 71:665, 1993b.

Heupler, F. A., Proudfit, W. L., Razavi, M., et al.: Ergonovine maleate: Provocative test for coronary artery spasm. Am. J. Cardiol., 41:631, 1978.

Hill, R., Chitwood, W. R., Bashore, T. M., et al.: Coronary flow and regional function before and after supra-arterial myotomy for myocardial bridging. Ann. Thorac. Surg., 31:176, 1981.

Hodgson, J. M., LeGrand, V., Bates, E. R., et al.: Validation in dogs of a rapid digital angiographic technique to measure relative coronary blood flow during routine cardiac catheterization. Am. J. Cardiol., 55:188, 1985.

Hutchins, G. M., Moore, G. W., and Hatton, E. V.: Arterial-venous relationships in the human left ventricular myocardium: Anatomic basis for countercurrent regulation of blood flow. Circulation, 74:1195, 1986.

Ishimori, T., Raizner, A. E., Chahine, R. A., et al.: Myocardial bridges in man: Clinical correlation and angiographic accentuations with nitroglycerin. Cathet. Cardiovasc. Diagn., 3:59, 1977.

Judkins, M. P.: Selective coronary arteriography. I: A percutaneous transfemoral technique. Radiology, 89:815, 1967.

Kalbfleisch, S. J., McGillem, M. J., Pinto, I. M. F., et al.: Comparison of automated quantitative coronary angiography with caliper measurements of percent diameter stenosis. Am. J. Cardiol., 65:1181, 1990.

Kalke, B., and Edwards, J. E.: Localized aneurysms of the coronary arteries. Angiology, 19:460, 1968.

Kennedy, J. W., Fisher, L. D., and Killip, T.: Coronary angiography quality control in CASS study. In Bond, M. G., Insull, W., Glagov, S., et al. (eds): Clinical Diagnosis of Atherosclerosis: Quantitative Methods of Evaluation. New York, Springer-Verlag, 1982, pp. 475–491.

Kirkeeide, R. L., Gould, K. L., and Parsel, L.: Assessment of coronary stenoses by myocardial perfusion imaging during pharmacologic coronary vasodilatation. VII: Validation of coronary flow reserve as a single integrated functional measure of stenosis severity reflecting all its geometric dimensions. J. Am. Coll. Cardiol., 7:103, 1986.

Klinke, W. P., Christie, L. G., Nichols, W. W., et al.: Use of catheter-tip velocity-pressure transducer to evaluate left ventricular function in man: Effects of intravenous propranolol. Circulation, 61:946, 1980.

Klocke, F. J.: Measurement of coronary flow reserve: Defining pathophysiology versus making decisions about patient care. Circulation, 76:1183, 1987.

Klocke, F. J., Ellis, A. K., and Canty, J. M., Jr.: Interpretation of changes in coronary flow that accompany pharmacologic interventions. Circulation, 75(Suppl. V):34, 1987.

Kramer, J. R., Kitazume, H., Proudfit, W. L., and Sones, F. M.: Clinical significance of isolated coronary bridges: Benign and frequent condition involving the left anterior descending artery. Am. Heart J., 103:283, 1982.

Laufer, N., and Buda, A.: Quantitative coronary arteriography. In Buda, A. J., and Delp, E. J. (eds): Digital Cardiac Imaging. Boston, Martinus Nijhoff, 1985, pp. 119–139.

Leberthson, R. R., Dinsmore, R. E., Bharak, S., et al.: Aberrant coronary artery origin from the aorta: Diagnosis and clinical significance. Circulation, 50:774, 1974.

LeFree, M. T., Simon, S. B., Mancini, G. B. J., and Vogel, R. A.: Digital radiographic assessment of coronary artery diameter and video densitometric cross-sectional area. Proc. SPIE, 626:334, 1986.

Lesperance, J., Hudson, G., White, C., et al.: Comparison by quantitative angiographic assessment of coronary stenosis of one view showing the severest narrowing with two orthogonal views. Am. J. Cardiol., 64:462, 1989.

Levin, D. C.: Pathways and functional significance of the coronary collateral circulation. Circulation, 50:831, 1974.

Levin, D. C., Fellows, K. E., and Abrams, H. L.: Hemodynamically significant primary anomalies of the coronary arteries. Circulation, 58:25, 1978.

Linhart, J. W.: Prinzmetal variant of angina pectoris. J. A. M. A., 228:342, 1974.

MacAlpin, R. N.: Relation of coronary artery spasm to sites of organic stenosis. Am. J. Cardiol., 46:143, 1980.

Mancini, G. B. J., Simon, S. B., McGillem, M. J., et al.: Automated quantitative coronary arteriography: Morphologic and physiologic validation in vivo of a rapid digital angiographic method. Circulation, 75:452, 1987.

Marcus, M. L.: Effects of cardiac hypertrophy on the coronary circulation. In Marcus, M. L. (ed): The Coronary Circulation in Health and Disease. New York, McGraw-Hill, 1983, p. 285.

Marcus, M. L., Wilson, R. F., and White, C. W.: Methods of measurement of myocardial blood flow in patients: A critical review. Circulation, 76:245, 1987.

Marcus, M., Wright, C., Doty, D., et al.: Measurement of coronary velocity and reactive hyperemia in the coronary circulation in humans. Circ. Res., 49:877, 1981.

Maseri, A., Severi, S., deNes, M., et al.: "Variant" angina: One aspect of a continuous spectrum of vasospastic myocardial ischemia: Pathogenetic mechanisms, estimated incidence, and clinical and coronary arteriographic findings in 138 patients. Am. J. Cardiol., 42:1019, 1978.

Mathey, D. G., Chatterjee, K., Tyberg, J. V., et al.: Coronary sinus reflux: A source of error in the measurement of thermodilution coronary sinus flow. Circulation, 57:778, 1978.

McMahon, M. M., Brown, G. B., Cuckingnon, R., et al.: Quantitative coronary angiography: Measurement of the critical stenosis in patients with unstable angina and single-vessel disease without collaterals. Circulation, 60:106, 1979.

McManus, B. M., Waller, B. F., Jones, M., et al.: The case for preoperative coronary angiography in patients with tetralogy of Fallot and the complex congenital heart disease. Am. Heart J., 103:451, 1982.

Meng, C. C., Eckner, F. A., and Lev, M.: Coronary artery distribution in tetralogy of Fallot. Arch. Surg., 90:363, 1965.

Morales, A. R., Romanell, R., and Boucek, R. J.: The mural left anterior descending coronary artery, strenuous exercise and sudden death. Circulation, 62:230, 1980.

Nichols, A. B., Gabrieli, C. F., Fenoglio, J. J., and Esser, P. D.: Quantification of relative coronary arteriosis stenosis by cinevideodensitometric analysis of coronary arteriograms. Circulation, 69:512, 1984.

Ogden, J. A.: Congenital anomalies of the coronary arteries. Am. J. Cardiol., 25:474, 1970.

Okumura, K., Yasue, H., Horio, Y., et al.: Multivessel coronary spasm in patients with variant angina: A study with intracoronary injection of acetylcholine. Circulation, 77:535, 1988.

Oldham, H. N., Ebert, P. A., Young, W. G., and Sabiston, D. C., Jr.: Surgical management of congenital coronary artery fistula. Ann. Thorac. Surg., 12:503, 1971.

Peterson, R. J., King, S. B., Farjam, W. A., et al.: Relationship of coronary artery stenosis and gradient to exercise-induced ischemia. J. Am. Coll. Cardiol., 1:673, 1983.

Radner, S.: Attempt at roentgenologic visualization of coronary blood vessels in man. Acta Radiol., 26:492, 1945.

Reiber, J., Kooijman, C., Slager, C., et al.: Coronary artery dimensions from cineangiograms: Methodology and validation of a computer-assisted analysis procedure. I. E. E. E. Trans. Med. Imag., M12:131, 1984.

Ricketts, J. H., and Abrams, H. L.: Percutaneous selective coronary arteriography. J. A. M. A., 181:620, 1962.

Roberts, W. C., Siegel, R. J., and Zipes, D. P.: Origin of the right coronary artery from the left sinus of Valsalva and its functional consequences: Analysis of 10 necropsy patients. Am. J. Cardiol., 49:863, 1982.

Ryan, T. S., Faxon, D. P., Gunnar, R. M., et al.: Guidelines for percutaneous transluminal coronary angioplasty. J. Am. Coll. Cardiol., 12:529, 1988.

Seldinger, S. I.: Catheter replacement of the needle in percutaneous arteriography: A new technique. Acta Radiol., 39:368, 1953.

Sharbaugh, A. H., and White, R. S.: Single coronary artery: Analysis of the anatomic variation, clinical importance, and report of five cases. J. A. M. A., 230:243, 1974.

Sheehan, F., Braunwald, E., Canner, P., et al.: The effect of intravenous thrombolytic therapy on left ventricular function. Circulation, 75:815, 1987.

Skelton, T. N., Kisslo, K. B., Mikat, E. M., and Bashore, T. M.: Accuracy of digital angiography for quantitation of normal coronary luminal segments in excised, perfused hearts. Am. J. Cardiol., 59:1261, 1987.

Sones, F. M., Jr., Shivey, E. K., Proudfit, W. L., and Westcott, R. N.: Cinecoronary arteriography [Abstract]. Circulation, 20:773, 1959.

Sos, T. A., and Baltaxe, H. A.: Cranial and caudal angulation for coronary arteriography revisited. Circulation, 56:119, 1977.

Vogel, R. A.: Digital radiographic assessment of coronary flow reserve. In Buda, A. J., and Delp, E. J. (eds): Digital Cardiac Imaging. Boston, Martinus Nijhoff, 1985, pp. 106–118.

Wangler, R. D., Peters, K. G., Laughlin, D. E., et al.: A method for continuously assessing coronary velocity in the rat. Am. J. Physiol., 10:H816, 1981.

Waters, D. D., Szlachic, J., and Bonan, R.: Comparative sensitivity of exercise, cold pressor, and ergonovine testing in provoking attacks of variant angina in patients with active disease. Circulation, 67:310, 1983.

White, C. W., Wright, C. B., Doty, D. B., et al.: Does visual interpretation of the coronary arteriogram predict the physiologic importance of a coronary stenosis? N. Engl. J. Med., 310:819, 1984.

Wilson, R. F., Marcus, M. L., and White, C. W.: Prediction of the physiologic significance of coronary artery lesions by quantitative lesion geometry in patients with limited coronary artery disease. Circulation, 75:723, 1987.

Wilson, R. F., and White, C. W.: Measurement of maximal coronary flow reserve: A technique for assessing the physiologic significance of coronary arterial lesions in humans. Herz, 12:163, 1987.

Zimmerman, H. A., Scott, R. W., and Becker, N. O.: Catheterization of the left side of the heart in man. Circulation, 1:357, 1950.

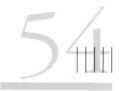

# ■ V Surgical Management of Coronary Artery Disease

## 1 Bypass Grafting for Coronary Artery Disease

Frank C. Spencer, Aubrey C. Galloway, and Stephen B. Colvin

## HISTORICAL ASPECTS

Bypass grafting for coronary artery disease was developed between 1967 and 1968 at three major centers in the United States: the Cleveland Clinic; the University of Wisconsin in Milwaukee; and New York University.

The principal credit belongs to the pioneering efforts of Favaloro, Effler, and associates at the Cleveland Clinic, although Sabiston performed the *first* human saphenous vein-coronary artery bypass graft at Johns Hopkins in 1962 (Favaloro, 1992; Naif, 1990; Sabiston, 1974). Johnson in Milwaukee also deserves considerable credit for his early contributions (1969). Investigation of coronary artery disease had been a major effort at his institution for several years. The development of coronary angiography by F. Mason Sones around 1959 was the landmark achievement that permitted precise definition of the anatomic obstruction and laid the foundation for bypass surgery. The first operations in Cleveland used the saphenous vein to bypass segments of the right coronary artery, first demonstrating its impressive short-term patency. Johnson quickly perceived the significance of this

technique and extended the procedure to the left coronary artery. Within 2 years, 1969, Johnson reported to the American Surgical Association on his successful operations on the left coronary artery in 301 patients, with a mortality rate of 12% (Johnson et al., 1969). The magnitude of this achievement is illustrated by the fact that before 1967, the mortality rate of operative procedures on the left coronary artery exceeded 50% and had been almost abandoned. Johnson's report firmly launched the modern era of coronary bypass grafting, which has since grown exponentially. Over 300,000 bypass operations have been done annually for the past few years in the United States.

At New York University (NYU), the concept of anastomosis of the internal mammary artery to the left anterior descending artery using a dissecting microscope was developed by Green and Tice in 1968 (Green et al., 1970). Spencer and associates, in 1964, had previously demonstrated in the laboratory both the feasibility and the durability of this type of anastomosis.

In 1967 in Russia, Kolessov did an end-to-end anastomosis between the mammary artery and the coronary artery on a beating heart; the next year, he did a similar end-to-side anastomosis on another patient.

He was chairman of the department of surgery at the first Leningrad Medical Institute between 1953 and 1976. During this time, he performed bypass procedures in 132 patients, performing most of these on a beating heart. His work for many years was largely unknown in the United States, but in 1988 his contributions were well summarized by Olearchyk (1988).

In the three decades before 1967, numerous indirect procedures to increase coronary blood flow were evaluated. Almost all were designed to enhance the growth of collateral circulation to the myocardium. Some were ingenious, others bizarre; all have been discarded. The only procedure that offered some durable benefit was the Vineberg procedure of implanting the internal mammary artery into the ischemic myocardium. Surprisingly enough, the artery remained patent in most patients, but because the magnitude of flow through the implanted artery remained disappointingly small in most of them, it has been virtually abandoned.

In the 1970s, bypass grafting was widely adopted as the operation became simpler and safer. The introduction of potassium cardioplegia greatly facilitated both the performance and safety of the procedure. Large randomized studies were done, as discussed in detail by Frye and co-workers (1987). The three major studies were the Veterans Administration Study, the European Cooperative Study (European Coronary Surgery Study Group, 1980, 1982), and the Coronary Artery Surgery Study (CASS) of about 25,000 patients with coronary disease undergoing catheterization between 1974 and 1979 (CASS Principal Investigators and Their Associates, 1983).

Several major changes occurred in the 1980s. The 1983 report by Campeau and colleagues from the Montreal Heart Institute, which assessed angiographic findings in 82 patients 10 years after bypass, was a sobering milestone. Previously, 5-year postoperative studies had shown good patency rates and minimal atherosclerosis in bypass venous grafts. However, between 5 and 10 years following operation, significant atherosclerosis developed in a high percentage of vein grafts such that, at 10 years after operation, 40% of vein grafts were closed, another 30% had significant atherosclerosis, and only 30% remained satisfactory.

By contrast, Campeau's studies found that internal mammary grafts remained patent without degenerative changes in more than 90% of patients, a number of whom showed significant enlargement of the artery, which apparently dilated in response to increased "demand" in the distal coronary tree. This important report quickly led to frequent, worldwide use of the mammary artery. Previously, as late as 1981, the internal mammary was used in less than 15% of bypass operations. Additional techniques that were soon developed included the use of bilateral mammary grafts or sequential mammary grafts (Lytle et al., 1986; Rankin et al., 1986).

Loop and associates (1986) subsequently reported in 1986 that, 10 years following operation, longevity was much better in patients in whom the internal mammary had been used, as compared with those in whom only saphenous veins had been used.

Another major development was the evolution of angioplasty, first done by Gruentzig and colleagues in 1977 and subsequently applied worldwide with increasing frequency. Angioplasty is now performed in hundreds of thousands of patients each year, and it seems to be the initial procedure of choice for most patients with single- or double-vessel disease.

Also significant was the introduction of effective thrombolytic therapy, initially streptokinase and urokinase but subsequently *tissue plasminogen activator* (TPA). TPA first was approved for clinical use in late 1987. Topol and associates summarized events with this remarkable therapy in December 1988, describing results in 708 patients from the Thrombosis in Angioplasty and Myocardial Infarction (TAMI) studies.

Administration of TPA in the first few hours after onset of coronary thrombosis reopened the obstructed artery in about 75% of patients. Some restoration of ventricular function occurred when therapy was initiated within 1 to 4 hours after coronary occlusion began. With thrombolytic therapy, the mortality rate for acute myocardial infarction decreases from 11 to 12% to under 8%.

Progress in preventing progressive coronary atherosclerosis, however, has been slow. The most encouraging results have been with therapy to lower the blood cholesterol level and to modify dietary lipid intake. These developments are well described by Dunn and Morris in the fifth edition of this book (1990). In the 1980s, the National Institutes of Health (NIH) convened two major conferences, a Consensus Development Conference on lowering blood cholesterol in 1984 and a National Cholesterol Education Program (NCEP) in 1985. Available data indicate an increased risk for coronary artery disease with any elevation of blood cholesterol above 200 mg/dl, with the risk rising markedly with cholesterol levels above 240 mg/dl. The American Heart Association currently recommends a Step I diet that basically consists of limiting cholesterol intake to less than 300 mg a day, total fat calories to less than 30% of daily intake, and saturated fat to less than 10%. If satisfactory decrease in blood elevated cholesterol does not occur within 3 months, a Step II diet is recommended, with a daily cholesterol intake less than 200 mg and saturated fat less than 7% of total calories. A registered dietitian is often needed to develop this therapy.

If diet therapy is ineffective, drug therapy is begun. The development of lovostatin, which inhibits cholesterol biosynthesis, has made drug therapy far more effective for lowering cholesterol levels below 200 mg/dl. The usual dose varies from 20 mg a day to 40 mg twice a day.

## FREQUENCY AND EPIDEMIOLOGY

Coronary atherosclerosis apparently is the most common serious disease in the Caucasian male throughout the world. In the United States, it causes more than 600,000 deaths annually. Worldwide epidemiologic studies (Stamler, 1978) found that the United States had the second highest frequency of coronary disease in the world, exceeded only by Finland. Japan had the lowest frequency.

The disease is seldom found in populations in which the average cholesterol concentration is below 200 mg/100 ml. In Japan, the average cholesterol level is approximately 160 mg/100 ml. The disease is more common in men in the first five decades of life, with a male/female ratio of about 4:1. A report from the Bureau of Vital Statistics for 1976 described 644,000 deaths (360,000 men, 280,000 women); only 34,000 deaths occurred in women under 65 years of age.

The frequency of deaths from coronary disease increases 2 to 4 times with each decade of life. For example, in 1976, the death rate for men between 45 and 54 years of age was 281 per 100,000, compared with 66 per 100,000 for men between 35 and 44 years of age. Between 55 and 65 years of age, the number of deaths rose to 756. This striking increase with age probably indicates the progressive growth of coronary atherosclerosis as well as the inability of collateral circulation to compensate for the progressive obstruction.

For unclear reasons, there was a 21% decrease in mortality from major cardiovascular disease in the United States between 1958 and 1976. This was analyzed in detail at a 2-day conference at the NIH in 1978, because the reduction had not occurred in most countries over the world (U.S. Department of Health, Education, and Welfare, 1979).

Further reduction in the mortality from coronary artery disease can be anticipated with the widespread emphasis in the last decade on decreasing blood cholesterol levels and lipid intake. This national effort was highlighted by the NCEP initiated by the National Heart, Lung, and Blood Institute in 1985. By June 1993, the average cholesterol was found to have decreased to near 200 mg/dl (Sempos et al., 1993).

## ETIOLOGY

Coronary atherosclerosis is a disorder of lipid metabolism of unknown origin. The three major theories are the response to injury, the lipogenic hypothesis, and the monoclonal hypothesis. These theories are discussed in detail by Dunn and Morris in Chapter 54 of the fifth edition of this book (1990).

Several risk factors clearly have been long recognized as increasing the frequency of coronary disease. The major ones include cigarette smoking, hypertension, hypercholesterolemia, diabetes, and severe obesity. Additional risk factors include increasing age, male sex, and the family history. Lack of physical exercise or "stress" are plausible factors but they lack scientific proof (Froelicher et al., 1985).

Among the different risk factors, tobacco smoking clearly has a very strong adverse effect, for the death rate in smokers is about 3 times greater than in non-smokers. Hypertension is another strong risk factor. Numerous studies have found an association between high blood cholesterol levels and an increased frequency of coronary disease. Apparently, any cholesterol level above 200 mg/dl is associated with an increased risk, especially with levels above 240 mg/dl.

## PATHOLOGY

Coronary atherosclerosis is a segmental disease that occurs primarily in the proximal portion of the three major coronary arteries within 5 cm of their origin from the aorta. Fortunately, part of the distal arterial segment is usually patent.

As described in Chapter 54 of the fifth edition of this book, Roberts (1990) did detailed studies of 516 major coronary arteries in 129 patients dying from coronary disease and compared these with 160 arteries from 40 control patients, most of whom had died from leukemia. Histologic segments were taken for each 5-mm segment of artery, for a total of 6461 5-mm segments for comparison with 1849 segments from the 40 control patients. He found that in the patients with coronary disease, 92% of the over 6000 5-mm segments were narrowed at least 25% by an atherosclerotic plaque and so concluded that coronary atherosclerosis is a diffuse process, the severity of which is easily underestimated by the arteriogram. The standard terminology is *single-*, *double-*, or *triple-*vessel disease, designating the number of major coronary arteries involved. Most patients with severe disease have triple-vessel involvement. A common pattern is stenosis or occlusion of the proximal right coronary, the anterior descending, and the circumflex artery. However, the distal right coronary artery is usually patent near the bifurcation into the posterior descending and atrioventricular groove branches. The anterior descending is usually patent in its middle or distal third; one or more marginal branches usually remain patent. This fortunate segmental variation in severity of disease is the basis for bypass grafting. In their 1978 monograph, Ochsner and Mills described six different pathologic variations encountered in more than 1000 patients.

It is well established that a 50% decrease in the diameter of a coronary artery, corresponding to a 75% reduction in cross-sectional area, is required to decrease coronary blood flow a moderate amount. A reduction in diameter of two-thirds corresponds to a reduction in cross-sectional area of about 90%, representing severe stenosis. There is considerable debate among different surgical groups about whether or not vessels with only 50% reduction in diameter should be bypassed, because previous studies have shown that insertion of a bypass graft often accelerates atherosclerosis, with subsequent occlusion of the proximal vessel.

The decrease in coronary blood flow from the atherosclerotic obstructions usually first shows symptoms of myocardial ischemia, "angina," during physical activities that increase cardiac oxygen demand, such as exercise, eating, or intense emotion. Such episodes usually subside without permanent structural injury, either spontaneously or with vasodilator therapy (nitroglycerine).

Myocardial infarction results when severe ischemia develops acutely, often associated with thrombosis of a major artery. The precipitating event apparently is rupture or "fissuring" of an atherosclerotic plaque with resulting deposition of platelets and occlusion of the lumen from a blood clot. A curious observation is that large infarctions often develop from thrombosis of major arteries that previously had minimal atherosclerotic narrowing, perhaps because patients with more severe stenosis had better coronary collateral circulation to the zone of ischemia.

A more subtle form of muscle dysfunction and necrosis results from silent ischemia, a serious condition that can lead to progressive myocardial fibrosis without clinical symptoms. It is somewhat analogous to the gradual trophic changes that evolve in the feet from progressive atherosclerosis in the femoral and popliteal arteries. Detection and early treatment of patients with significant silent ischemia remain an important goal in future therapy to prevent extensive destruction of left ventricular muscle, with an ejection fraction near 20%.

The two dominant factors that determine prognosis are the number of vessels involved (single-, double-, or triple-vessel disease) and the function of the left ventricle. The left ventricle's ability to maintain normal function through collateral circulation, despite an increase in coronary atherosclerotic obstruction, is apparently an individual variation that unfortunately has been influenced little by therapy. Coronary collaterals develop in a goal-directed manner toward the ischemic zone of myocardium but often develop too slowly to be of clinical significance. In some patients, however, the collaterals can grow enough to protect the underlying myocardium despite total proximal coronary occlusion.

Left ventricular function is customarily expressed as ejection fraction, measured either by cineangiography or by radionuclide scanning. An ejection fraction between 60 and 75% is considered normal. A mild-to-moderate depression of ventricular function is represented by an ejection fraction of 40 to 60%; those below 40% represent moderate depression, and below 30% severe depression.

Symptoms of congestive heart failure appear with increasing frequency with an ejection fraction below 30% and are common with an ejection fraction below 20%. Effective bypass surgery that relieves all major obstructions is usually associated with an increase in ejection fraction of at least 10% if viable myocardium is significant, apparently because blood flow is restored to viable but nonfunctioning ischemic muscle.

Chronic hypoxia also impairs diastolic function of the left ventricle, manifested by a rise in left ventricular end-diastolic pressure above the normal upper limit of 12 mm Hg. With moderate left ventricular injury, the end-diastolic pressure rises to the range of 12 to 20 mm Hg; levels of 20 to 30 mm Hg are present with severe cardiac dysfunction.

The influence of ventricular function on prognosis is striking. For patients with triple-vessel disease and normal ventricular function, the 5-year survival rate is well above 90%. However, with increasing severity of ventricular dysfunction, there is a sharp decrease in the 5-year survival rate to 40% in patients with severely decreased cardiac function.

## Clinical Considerations

Progressive myocardial ischemia can cause one of three serious events: angina pectoris, myocardial infarction, or sudden death. Angina is the most frequent symptom, stemming from activities that increase myocardial oxygen demand. Unfortunately, myocardial infarction or sudden death may occur without any preceding symptoms.

*Angina* typically appears when myocardial oxygen consumption is increased from exercise, eating, or emotional stress. It subsides with rest or with treatment to increase coronary vasodilatation, such as sublingual nitroglycerin. In about 80% of patients angina is "typical," described as a constricting, vise-like sensation over the precordium. In at least 15 to 20% of cases, however, angina is "atypical" and can mimic a wide variety of diseases, the most common of which are esophagitis, hiatal hernia, cholecystitis, bursitis, or even dental disorders. Because angina is a symptom arising from ischemic metabolism, it is analogous to claudication, appearing with exercise but subsiding with rest.

Unfortunately, a significant number of patients, probably 10 to 20%, do not have angina despite continuing myocardial ischemia. Such silent ischemia has been recognized with increasing frequency, primarily by 24-hour monitoring with an electrocardiogram.

*Unstable angina* is an important clinical syndrome that is intermediate between classic angina and myocardial infarction. The precordial discomfort persists despite nitroglycerin therapy, but there are no signs of myocardial necrosis. The syndrome probably comes from acutely decreased regional myocardial flow produced by rupture of an atherosclerotic plaque with subsequent thrombosis. If the ischemia resolves, recovery ensues without permanent injury. If it does not, myocardial infarction or death may occur. Unstable angina is thus an acute medical emergency, treated by urgent hospitalization and intensive medical therapy with intravenous heparin, intravenous nitroglycerin, and beta-adrenergic blockers to decrease myocardial oxygen demand.

*Myocardial infarction* is the most common serious life-threatening complication. Over one million myocardial infarctions occur in the United States annually. With current therapy, the mortality rate has steadily decreased to below 8 to 10%.

Infarction usually results from acute thrombosis of the diseased coronary artery, probably from disruption of an atherosclerotic plaque with subsequent thrombosis. As mentioned earlier, especially large infarctions may occur in the distribution of arteries that were only minimally narrowed from an atherosclerotic plaque but that suddenly thrombose. The significance of the infarction depends on how much the myocardium is injured.

*Sudden death,* defined as occurring within 1 hour after the onset of symptoms (Holmes and Davis, 1986), is the most common form of death from coronary disease. The risk varies with the extent of disease and the degree of impairment of ventricular function, ranging from as low as 2% to as high as 10%. Over 400,000 deaths occur each year in the United States, many before a patient arrives at a hospital. Death is caused by either acute infarction or arrhythmia, usually ventricular fibrillation, at times occurring from ischemia without transmural infarction.

It is extremely important, therefore, for a wide range of people to be familiar with techniques of cardiopulmonary resuscitation, as was dramatically emphasized by Cobb and associates (1980), who described experiences in Seattle with 10 years of cardiac resuscitation outside the hospital. Over 300 patients were resuscitated each year by trained laypersons outside the hospital. Although most patients had coronary disease, more than one-half of the patients resuscitated did not have any signs of transmural myocardial necrosis.

How long attempts at resuscitation should be continued in such circumstances is an important ethical, legal, and economic question. In this regard, the report by Murphy and Murray in 1989 is of particular interest. They studied outcome following resuscitation for 503 cardiac arrests in patients over 70 years of age. Two hundred forty-four of these occurred outside the hospital. A heartbeat was restored in 112 patients, but only a few survived without incapacitating neurologic injury. The most significant finding was that most effective resuscitations required massage for less than 5 minutes, which probably distinguishes those with fibrillation from those with significant myocardial injury.

In a small percentage of patients, congestive heart failure develops from extensive destruction of ventricular muscle from multiple infarctions. Some patients have a clinical history of multiple infarctions. In others, the clinical history is both puzzling and ominous, because significant events are absent. Apparently, extensive destruction of myocardium had "silently" advanced from progressive ischemia. Recognizing and treating such patients before extensive destruction occurs remains a major frontier in cardiology.

Chronic congestive failure has an ominous outlook. Although modern treatment with afterload reduction and diuresis is often effective, such patients often die within 1 to 2 years. Some are candidates for cardiac transplantation. Bypass grafting is of value in such patients only if there are significant areas of ischemic but viable myocardium.

## LABORATORY EVALUATION

Coronary artery disease produces no abnormalities on physical examination until infarction supervenes.

Therefore, the diagnosis of coronary disease depends on eliciting a history of angina or previous infarctions. Unless angina is present, coronary disease can be detected only by laboratory studies.

The chest film shows a heart of normal size unless previous infarctions have produced cardiac dilatation. The electrocardiogram is normal at rest in about 70% of patients. The simplest and most widely used study is the exercise electrocardiogram, the "stress test," which detects electrocardiographic signs of ischemia during graded amounts of exercise. Because silent ischemia is common, an annual stress test should be seriously considered in all patients with known coronary disease, regardless of whether the symptoms are present.

More complex studies include radionuclide angiography to measure myocardial contractility (gated blood pool scan), expressing contractility as "ejection fraction"; myocardial perfusion can also be evaluated with radioactive thallium. The ejection fraction normally increases with exercise from the normal range of 50 to 70% to above 75 to 80%. With significant coronary disease, however, the ejection fraction falls with exercise, a significant abnormality. Exercise stress testing, with echocardiography, can detect inducible abnormalities in left ventricular wall movement.

## Coronary Arteriography

Cineangiography, including coronary arteriography and ventriculography, is the crucial diagnostic study. Arteriography outlines the location and severity of the atherosclerotic disease; ventriculography measures ventricular function and permits calculation of ejection fraction, approximately indicating the degree to which the growth of collateral circulation has compensated for the atherosclerotic obstruction. Moderate stenosis is present with a diameter reduction of 50%, equivalent to 75% reduction in cross-sectional area. Severe stenosis is present with a reduction in diameter of more than 70%, which corresponds to a reduction in cross-sectional area of at least 90%.

Regional ventricular contraction usually is evaluated from the right anterior oblique view in the cineangiogram. The left ventricular outline is divided into five segments: anterobasal, anterolateral, apical, diaphragmatic, and posterobasal. The motion of each segment is judged as normal, hypokinetic, akinetic, dyskinetic. A myocardial numeric score is commonly used, from No. 1 for normal function to No. 6 for dyskinesia or paradoxic contraction; with five segments, a normal myocardial score is 5, whereas the worst score is 30. Impaired myocardial contractility is often described as "left ventricular scores greater than 10."

Although cineangiography is the best method for evaluating coronary disease, it has significant limitations. Unwarranted conclusions are often made. First, the angiogram usually underestimates the severity of the disease. Stenosed or obstructed vessels are compared with those that are not visibly stenosed. However, as Roberts' (1990) extensive pathologic findings have shown, the atherosclerotic process is diffuse, usually involving over half of the coronary vessels. Intracoronary ultrasonography has produced similar insights.

A second common error is concluding that vessels are "too small" for bypass. Coronary arteries distal to an obstruction may appear small for different reasons, either from inadequate amounts of dye entering through collateral vessels or from lack of distention of the vessel wall from normal perfusion pressure. However, surgical experience has demonstrated that in more than 95% of patients, a coronary artery over 1 mm in internal diameter can be found distal to the area of obstruction, so that bypass grafting can be effectively performed.

When an angiogram is performed on patients for recurrent symptoms after a previous bypass operation, some of the previously inserted grafts are often found occluded. For unclear reasons, the vessels beyond the occluded grafts are often not opacified at the time of repeat angiography but may be found patent at operation.

Another frequent error is concluding that regional myocardial contractility is irreversibly injured (dyskinetic or akinetic) and that bypass to this area of myocardium is therefore futile. Usually at operation, these akinetic areas are found to contain large areas of viable myocardial tissue rather than simple avascular scar. Recovery of some function in such segments has been demonstrated to occur weeks or even months following bypass (Kirklin and Barratt-Boyes, 1993; Sabiston and Spencer, 1990).

## TREATMENT: MEDICAL, ANGIOPLASTY, OR BYPASS?

### Medical Therapy

The importance of lifelong medical therapy should be strongly emphasized to each patient with coronary disease. Coronary bypass can effectively correct existing myocardial ischemia, but the underlying disease, coronary atherosclerosis, is incurable by present knowledge and will progress at a variable rate. A simple analogy is to compare coronary disease with diabetes. Both are biochemical disorders of unknown origin that can be treated effectively in most patients but at present are incurable.

Details of medical therapy are beyond the scope of this textbook. Only basic essentials are described here. The most important three measures are complete cessation of cigarette smoking, control of hypertension, and dietary modification to lower the blood cholesterol below 200 mg/dl and sharply decrease the type and quantity of lipids in the diet. As described earlier, guidelines for daily lipid intake are well described by the American Heart Association. The moderate Step I diet limits cholesterol intake to 300 mg a day, total fat calories to less than 30% of total intake, and saturated fats to less than 10%. The Step II diet includes a cholesterol intake less than 200 mg per day and saturated fat intake less than 7% of total calories.

If dietary measures are inadequate, drug therapy can be undertaken to lower blood cholesterol below 200 mg/dl. Lovostatin therapy has made this process far simpler than in the past.

Weight reduction and physical exercise are plausible goals, although their precise benefit is difficult to measure. For patients with angina, drug therapy includes aspirin, nitrates, beta-adrenergic blockers, and calcium channel blockers.

The effectiveness of medical therapy in slowing and stopping progressive coronary atherosclerosis is probably unpredictable for any given patient and can be determined only by periodic evaluation. Some studies have demonstrated that coronary atheroma regresses after strict modification of diet in combination with exercise programs.

### Angioplasty

This procedure was developed by Gruentzig in Switzerland in 1978 and quickly spread worldwide. Although indications and contraindications are still evolving, over 300,000 angioplasties were performed in 1992 in the United States alone. The number of angioplasties and coronary artery bypass procedures in the state of New York has been roughly equal over the past several years, ranging from 12,000 to 16,000 yearly for each procedure.

Angioplasty usually has been employed in patients with single- or double-vessel disease. In general, stenotic lesions judged suitable for dilatation can be treated successfully in approximately 90%; "success" is defined as a reduction in the severity of the stenosis to less than 50% of the diameter of the artery.

Both mortality and morbidity with angioplasty vary with the severity of the disease treated and the experience of the interventional cardiologist. The mortality rate is usually near 1%; myocardial infarction occurs in 3 to 4% of patients. A small percentage of patients require emergency bypass, discussed later. At New York University, less than 1% of 500 patients treated required emergency bypass.

When angioplasty is successful, angina is relieved. However, the stenosis can recur in 25 to 30% of patients within 6 to 12 months. Some of these patients receive repeat angioplasty; others require bypass operation.

Long-term results after angioplasty will not be available for some years. The key question is the status of the area of atherosclerotic stenosis 5 or more years later. Most theories of coronary atherosclerosis accept the concept of injury to the vessel wall, especially the intima, with subsequent permeation of the vessel wall by lipids from the bloodstream. "Angioplasty" is actually a misnomer, because the pneumatic dilatation clearly disrupts the atherosclerotic plaque, with resulting intramural hemorrhage. It is remarkable that complications such as thrombosis or distal embolization are infrequent. Whether this procedure, which is traumatic to the vessel wall, can permanently retard the growth of an atherosclerotic plaque is a key biologic question.

Newer procedures, now FDA-approved, include coronary atherectomy and, more recently, rotational atherectomy and stents (Gianturco-Roubin stent). Unfortunately, any procedure that removes the intimal lining of a small artery, exposing the media to lipids and growth factors in the bloodstream, inevitably is associated with progressive cicatricial stenosis and occlusion over 2 to 3 years. This process was demonstrated in the 1960s with extensive endarterectomy of the femoral and popliteal arteries. These procedures all have been abandoned because of the inevitable contraction and occlusion even in vessels as large as the popliteal artery, 4 to 5 mm. It is possible that coronary arteries following atherectomy will behave similarly. Certainly, newer data are encouraging about the molecular blockage of local growth factor and lipid uptake in the injured vessel wall after atherectomy or angioplasty and may lead to improved long-term results.

A major question is the choice of therapy for an individual patient. To address this issue, large randomized trials comparing angioplasty and bypass have been instituted; two large ones are the RITA trial in England and the Bypass Angioplasty Revascularization Investigation (BARI) trial in the United States.

The early results with the RITA trial were published in 1993. Sixteen centers participated, and over 3 years nearly 28,000 patients underwent coronary angiography. Among these, 17,000 (70%) were referred for bypass, 25% were referred for percutaneous transluminal coronary angioplasty (PTCA), and 4.8% (about 1000 patients) were chosen for randomization. Those chosen for randomization had comparable clinical characteristics. After an average of 2.5 years follow-up in the 1011 patients randomized, 34 deaths had occurred, a nearly equal number of each treatment group. Hence, the early frequency of infarction or death was similar in the two groups. However, a significant number of patients treated initially with angioplasty required a second revascularization procedure. Among those treated by angioplasty, single-vessel disease was present in 45%, double-vessel disease in 43%, and triple-vessel disease in 12%. Among the PTCA patients requiring further revascularization, 19% underwent bypass, whereas 18% underwent further PTCA. Long-term results remain to be reported. Results of the BARI trial are not yet available.

Angioplasty is best done in a hospital, with immediate access to an operating room, because emergency operation may be required in a small percentage of patients. Even though operation is performed quickly, there is still a significant mortality rate of 2 to 4% and a perioperative infarction rate of 40 to 50%. Greene and associates (1991) describe experiences with over 1200 angioplasties, 60 of which required emergency bypass grafting, a frequency near 5%. Among the 60 patients, 7 had signs of an infarction before angioplasty and were excluded from the study. Twenty-

seven of the remaining 53 (51%) had a perioperative infarction; the mortality rate was 4%.

This report is typical of those from most centers describing experiences with emergency bypass for failed angioplasty. Hence, the data are very clear that both mortality and morbidity are greatly increased if emergency bypass has to be done after an unsuccessful angioplasty.

## Coronary Artery Bypass

Leape and co-workers reported in 1993 a study by the Rand Corporation of the appropriateness of coronary artery bypass surgery in New York State in 1990. A sample of 1338 operations were reviewed. Operations were performed for chronic stable angina in 43% of patients, unstable angina in 22%, and post-infarction angina in 28%. Seventy-six per cent of patients either had three-vessel disease or left-sided main disease. Ninety-one per cent of operations were considered appropriate, 7% uncertain, and only 2.4% inappropriate.

### For Left-Sided Main Disease

There is widespread agreement that significant disease in the left main coronary, narrowing the diameter more than 50%, requires prompt surgery even though the patient is completely asymptomatic. Stenosis of this severity is found in 5 to 10% of patients at catheterization. At NYU, operation is performed as soon as possible after the diagnosis has been established at catheterization. These patients are placed on intravenously administered heparin, and monitored in the hospital, and operation is performed promptly.

### For Stable Angina of Varying Severity

There is general agreement that patients with severe angina who do not respond to drug therapy should undergo surgery electively. Therapeutic choices arise with patients with extensive disease but minimal or no angina. As discussed earlier, if single- or double-vessel disease is present, angioplasty is commonly performed as the initial procedure if the anatomy of the stenotic area is favorable. The short-term results have been good. What to do with the patient with few symptoms, triple-vessel disease, and good ventricular function was evaluated with the CASS study in the 1970s, which included over 25,000 patients studied by angiography and subsequently followed for at least 5 years until 1983. Disease was considered significant if the vessel diameter was narrowed more than 70% or more than 50% in the left main coronary artery. Left ventricular function was evaluated with the left ventricular score rating described earlier, based on segmental contraction of different ventricular segments. In the patients with good ventricular function treated with medical therapy, the 4-year survival rate was 97% for the control group, the patients without coronary disease. It was 95% for those with single-vessel disease, 93% with double-vessel disease, and 82% with triple-vessel disease, reflecting the strong influence of extent of disease on survival. However, during the 4-year study period 20%, 30%, and 45% of patients, respectively, "crossed over" for surgical therapy because of increasing angina.

The CASS studies indicated that patients with minimal symptoms and single- or double-vessel disease did not do better with operation than with medical therapy. At present, most such patients are treated by angioplasty, often when the diagnosis is established. Thus, many published angioplasty results are not comparable with the surgical results, because bypass is usually performed in patients with more severe disease.

The findings in patients with triple-vessel disease and normal ventricular function were of particular interest. If symptoms did not change, there was no benefit with surgical therapy over medical therapy. However, that nearly 40% of patients originally randomized to medical therapy developed increasing angina during the 5 years of observation and crossed over to surgical therapy reflects the relentless progression of the atherosclerotic process.

In patients with triple-vessel disease and impaired ventricular function (ejection fraction below 50%), bypass operation should be performed regardless of symptoms. Such loss of ventricular function indicates that growth of collateral circulation has not compensated adequately for the progressive decrease in coronary flow from the atherosclerotic process. Symptoms should seldom be used as the sole guide for operation: The patient with few symptoms is at greater risk from loss of ventricular function, because there is little warning that the disease is progressively destroying functioning myocardium. In the CASS study, 7 years following operation, survival in the surgical group was nearly 88% but only 65% in the medical group (Passamani et al., 1985).

The benefit of bypass in patients with a severe depression of ejection fraction to the range of 15 to 20% depends partly on the degree of improvement in ventricular function following bypass, which, in turn, probably reflects how much of the preoperative decrease in ejection fraction was due to irreversible scar instead of reversible ischemia. Diagnostic studies, such as stress thallium scans or positron emission tomography (PET), can assess myocardial viability but have not totally resolved this question. Preoperative severe angina clearly indicates viable, but ischemic, muscle.

A separate benefit from revascularization, more difficult to demonstrate, is preventing future additional loss of ventricular function. The virulence of the native atherosclerotic process is already evident from the preoperative severe loss in ventricular function. Obviously, a future similar loss would be incompatible with life. Hence, there may be some long-term benefit with effective revascularization, even if the ventricular function does not improve. The degree of survival benefit depends, to some extent, on the ability to control the significant ventricular arrhythmias that commonly cause death in these patients.

In 1993, Milano and associates reported experiences with bypass in 118 patients with an ejection fraction of 25% or less treated over a period of 10 years at Duke University. Many of the patients were acutely ill; over 50% presented with an acute event such as pulmonary edema, myocardial infarction, or unstable angina. Over 80% had Class IV angina. The operative mortality rate was 11%. The one-year survival rate was 77%, the estimated 5-year survival rate 58%. The estimated 5-year survival rate in a comparable medically treated group was only 38%. Nevertheless, the average improvement in ejection fraction was small, only about 5%.

Twenty reports from other groups, describing experiences with bypass in patients with a severe reduction in ejection fraction, were tabulated in this report, six of which had occurred in the previous decade. Seven studies of medical therapy alone were also tabulated. With medical therapy alone, the late mortality rate was high, ranging from 38% at 2 years in one report to 96% at 5 years in another.

At NYU, virtually all such patients undergo operation, even though cardiac failure with some pulmonary hypertension is present. With current techniques of myocardial preservation, the operative mortality rate is no greater than 3 to 4%.

Dramatic results have been obtained in a few patients who were initially seen as a "second opinion" after they had been placed on a waiting list for cardiac transplantation at another institution. In other patients undergoing operation with chronic congestive failure, angina has been relieved, but congestive failure has improved little.

### For Unstable Angina

As described earlier, this condition is a semiemergency that requires immediate hospitalization in a coronary care unit. The condition evolves when blood flow to a segment of myocardium has been seriously jeopardized but necrosis has not yet occurred. This sudden decrease in regional blood flow probably results from rupture of an atherosclerotic plaque with subsequent thrombosis.

The mainstay of therapy is intravenous heparin and nitroglycerin in varying amounts. Other elements of medical therapy include beta-adrenergic blockers and calcium channel blockers. If angina persists despite intensive medical therapy, an intra-aortic balloon is almost always effective.

Once the patient's condition has stabilized, coronary arteriography should be done to see if either angioplasty or bypass is indicated. In New York State in 1990, 22% of bypass operations were done for unstable angina (Leape et al., 1993).

### For Acute Infarction

The availability of effective thrombolytic agents, especially tissue plasminogen activator, has greatly decreased the indications for urgent bypass. As reported by Berg and colleagues, in 1984, bypass can be safely and effectively done soon after the onset of acute infarction. Thrombolytic therapy, however, is simpler and safer.

Thrombolytic therapy or immediate angioplasty is clearly more logical because irreversible myocardial necrosis may develop within as quickly as 30 to 60 minutes following occlusion of a major coronary artery. Subsequent evolution of the infarction, however, is complicated, with reperfusion from adjacent collateral circulation as well as edema formation from the inflammatory reaction to the infarction. This process may continue for several hours. Thrombolytic therapy has been particularly beneficial if initiated within 4 hours after onset—the sooner the better. Data also indicate, however, that restoration of vessel patency has some value even when thrombolytic therapy is started after several hours. If thrombolytic therapy is not available, for some unusual reason, immediate bypass can be performed with an operative risk no greater than 3 to 4%. Some studies have suggested that emergency angiography and angioplasty may yield initial results that are as good as those with thrombolysis and may be followed by fewer complications. However, most centers reserve emergency angioplasty for patients in shock or for those who have persistent or recurrent pain after thrombolysis.

Cardiogenic shock following myocardial infarction is the most severe complication seen in surviving patients, with a mortality rate well above 50%. Thrombolytic therapy, per se, has been of limited benefit, probably because of the time required for lysis of the clot. Initial treatment should begin with insertion of an intra-aortic balloon, although this is seldom adequate. Immediate catheterization should then be performed to determine whether angioplasty or immediate bypass is indicated.

Allen and associates in Los Angeles (1986) have presented experimental data that muscle ischemia for over 4 hours can be salvaged if the initial reperfusion is "modified" with a low-calcium mixture and other agents to avoid permanent intracellular permeation of calcium.

Allen and associates reported experiences from UCLA in 1989 with emergency bypass for cardiogenic shock following myocardial infarction in 80 patients treated over 6 years using Buckberg's techniques of reperfusion. Patients underwent surgery an average of 3.4 days after onset of infarction, usually for failure of medical therapy. Special techniques of reperfusion were used, including warm induction with glutamate aspartate and warm terminal cardioplegia.

Impressive cardiac results were reported: The left ventricular power failure was reversed in about 94% of patients. Three deaths occurred in 45 patients undergoing surgery within 18 hours, a mortality rate of 7%, whereas 11 deaths occurred in 35 patients undergoing surgery after 18 hours, a mortality rate of 31%. A large number of late deaths occurred from end-stage cardiac disease over the next 1 to 2 years, for a total mortality rate in the series near 44%.

The data indicated that the earlier operations produced excellent results, but operations undertaken even after 2 to 3 days were not futile. Similar data from other institutions are meager.

Guyton and colleagues in 1987 reported experiences with 17 emergency bypass procedures for cardiogenic shock, with two operative deaths and a 3-year survival rate near 90%. Ten of the 17 patients were treated with a balloon pump beforehand. Rapid revascularization was the key, with the first distal anastomosis completed in less than 5 hours in all but 1 of the 17 patients. Crystalloid cardioplegia was used. No attempt was made to modify the reperfusate.

Kirklin and Barratt-Boyes have stated that at least 50% of patients with cardiogenic shock can be saved with emergency coronary bypass. They advise using a different form of myocardial protection, possibly including "cold cardioplegia, controlled aortic root reperfusion, and warm cardioplegia induction" (Kirklin and Barratt-Boyes, 1993).

In 1993, Beyersdorf in Germany described experiences with 163 patients undergoing urgent operation for acute coronary occlusion, most cases of which developed after failed angioplasty. These experiences occurred over 15 years, during which time four different methods of cardioplegia were employed. The best results were obtained among the 37 patients treated between 1989 and 1992, in whom a controlled reperfusion of the type recommended by Buckberg was employed. There were only 2 deaths among the 37 patients.

### For Postinfarction Angina

Abundant data show that with current techniques of myocardial preservation, a patient recovering from a myocardial infarction can undergo surgery promptly at any time. Mortality among patients undergoing surgery in the first few days after infarction differs little from that of patients undergoing surgery within 3 to 4 weeks. Therefore, if angina continues after infarction or recurs, bypass should be undertaken promptly. Such patients often have a critical stenosis in one or more large coronary arteries that jeopardizes flow to viable but ischemic myocardium. With current techniques of preservation, the operative mortality rate is seldom greater than 2 to 3%.

## CONTRAINDICATIONS TO OPERATION

At NYU, the only cardiac contraindication to bypass is severe chronic congestive failure and pulmonary hypertension, manifested by a right atrial pressure above 15 mm Hg and hepatomegaly. Cardiac transplantation should be considered in appropriate patients.

Virtually no other contraindications to operation exist. The angiogram's unreliability in predicting that vessels are too small or too diseased for bypass has already been discussed. We have found that segmental revascularization into multiple diseased arteries is almost always feasible and is highly effective. Although endarterectomy is infrequently performed at NYU, Johnson, Brenowitz, and colleagues in Milwaukee have published extensive experiences with radical triple endarterectomy in patients with severe disease. In 1988, Brenowitz and associates reported 144 consecutive patients in all of whom extensive endarterectomy was performed in all three major coronary arteries, the anterior descending, the circumflex, and right coronary arteries. An average of five grafts were inserted in each patient. The operative mortality rate was 10%. One hundred two patients were evaluated 30 months following operation. Twelve late deaths had occurred. The five-year actuarial overall survival rate was 71% for the entire group, and 87% for 106 low-risk patients.

Advanced age is clearly not a contraindication. At NYU, less attention is given to the chronologic age of the patient than to the "physiologic age." A useful prognostic guide in the elderly is the muscle mass, because a history of substantial weight loss with associated weakness in the previous year has an unfavorable prognosis. Patients in their mid- or late eighties with intact mental status frequently undergo surgery; occasionally, bypass is effective in vigorous patients early in their tenth decade.

Several reports indicate a higher mortality and morbidity rate in such patients but excellent results in surviving patients. Weintraub's 1991 report from Emory University describes the influence of age in a series of over 13,000 patients undergoing coronary bypass. One hundred forty-six were over 80 years of age. The death rate in this group was about 8%. The frequency of stroke also rose from 1.9% in the sixth decade to 3.4% in the seventh and 4.1% in the eighth.

Mullany and colleagues reported experiences at the Mayo Clinic in 1990 with bypass operations in 156 patients over 80 years of age. The overall mortality rate was 10% and only 4% in patients without disease in other organs. The estimated 5-year survival rate for hospital survivors was 80%.

In 1991, Tsai and associates reported experiences with 157 patients with a mean age of 82 years over a period of 9 years. The mortality rate was 7%, the stroke rate 4%. The 5-year actuarial survival rate was estimated to be 62%.

## OPERATIVE TECHNIQUE

The two major considerations with coronary bypass are complete revascularization, grafting all major arteries with stenoses that narrow the diameter more than 50 to 70%, and prevention of myocardial infarction.

### Preoperative Therapy

Platelet inhibitor therapy is routinely used, modified from the original report by Chesebro and Fuster in 1982 (Chesebro et al., 1984). Dipyridamole is started 24 to 48 hours before operation, usually 75 mg 4 times a day until a few hours before operation. A few hours after operation, aspirin, 325 mg, is given by nasogastric tube or by rectal suppository. Aspirin is then continued with a single daily dose of 325 mg for at least 1 year. Dipyridamole usually is given for only a short time after operation, because randomized studies have not found additional long-term benefit beyond that provided by aspirin alone.

Cardiac medications, especially beta-adrenergic blockers and calcium channel blockers, are continued in decreased doses until the operation. Preferably, propranolol should be decreased to less than 160 mg a day; otherwise, inotropic agents may be needed for 1 to 2 days after the operation.

With unstable angina, intravenous nitroglycerin is invaluable, sometimes in large amounts, as much as 100 to 200 μg/minute or more. These patients are fully heparinized if rest angina or extremely "tight lesions" are present. The heparin is continued until the patient arrives in the operating room. With hypertensive patients, afterload can be reduced by nitroprusside infusion. If angina persists despite other measures, an intra-aortic balloon pump can be inserted preoperatively. This is a valuable form of therapy, although it has seldom been necessary with the management scheme noted earlier.

## Stroke Considerations

This is the major cause of serious morbidity following bypass surgery. Virtually all studies have reported an increasing frequency of stroke with age. Guyton, studying over 13,000 patients, reported a frequency of stroke in the fifth decade of life of only 1%, but over 4% in the eighth decade. Obvious calcification of the ascending and transverse aortic arch is a particularly serious risk factor for stroke. Available data strongly suggest, but do not prove, that the main source of stroke is atherosclerotic debris in the aortic arch not associated flow restrictive disease in the carotid and vertebral vessels.

Wareing and associates, in 1992, reported studies with intraoperative ultrasonography of the ascending aorta in 500 patients over 50 years of age. Sixty-eight patients, 13% of the total, with an average age of 72, had significant atheromatous disease. Several variations of the standard operative technique were employed. No strokes occurred in this group, although 1% of the patients in the overall group suffered a stroke.

In 1992, Blauth and co-workers described studies of the frequency of atheroembolism at autopsy in 221 patients who died after cardiac surgery. Atheroemboli were identified in 22% of the group. There was remarkably high correlation of atheroemboli found at autopsy with severe atherosclerosis in the ascending aorta. Atheroemboli were found in 37% of patients with ascending aortic atherosclerosis, but only in 2% of 98 patients without significant aortic disease.

This subject has been studied at NYU in some detail for over a decade. The data indicate, but do not prove, that with current techniques the major cause of stroke following bypass is atheroembolism from the aorta. A particularly important event occurred with the development of transesophageal echocardiography, which detects significant aortic arch atherosclerosis that could not be found by palpation or other methods. This was developed at NYU by both the department of cardiology and the department of anesthesiology (Katz et al., 1992; Tunick and Kronzon, 1993). It has been of such great value in older patients that it is used in most cardiac operations, both to evaluate cardiac function and to detect aortic arch disease.

Ribakove and co-workers from NYU in 1992 reported findings in 97 patients over 65 years of age studied with perioperative transesophageal echocardiography. Ten of the 97 had protruding mobile atheroma, the type associated with the highest frequency of perioperative stroke. Such atheromas appear as wavy fronds of atherosclerotic debris that protrude into the lumen and oscillate with the flow of blood. Findings on echocardiography were compared with findings on palpation. On palpation, 78% were considered normal, 13% had moderate disease, and 8% had severe disease. Virtually no correlation existed between the abnormal findings on palpation and the mobile atheroma detected on echocardiography.

Four intraoperative strokes occurred, a frequency of 4%. Significantly, the aorta in all four patients was considered normal on palpation in the operating room.

Three of the four strokes occurred in patients with the mobile protruding atheroma. The 10 patients with this most severe abnormality were treated as follows: Four had aortic arch débridement performed during a short period of hypothermic circulatory arrest; all recovered uneventfully. The other six patients were treated with more standard operative approaches, varying the site of arterial cannulation; three of the four strokes in the entire series occurred in this group of six patients.

The current approach preferred by the senior author is to perform transesophageal echocardiography in all patients over 70 years of age, so that the operative technique can be modified accordingly. The ascending aorta is also often studied with a hand-held echocardiographic probe. If mobile protruding atheromas are seen, distal cannulation with an aortic "arch cannula" and aortic endarterectomy are performed. The technique is described in subsequent paragraphs.

## ANESTHETIC CONSIDERATIONS

The importance of a precise anesthetic technique can scarcely be overemphasized. In the early 1970s, we were astonished to find in a cooperative study among several institutions that more than 20 to 25% of patients had enzymatic changes of myocardial necrosis before bypass was started. Changes in anesthetic technique greatly decreased this frequency. Na-

tional recognition of the particular importance of the anesthetic technique of course led to the subspecialty of cardiac anesthesiology.

At NYU, a Swan-Ganz catheter is inserted routinely after anesthesia is induced. This permits precise monitoring of pulmonary capillary wedge pressure as well as cardiac output. Particular attention is given to at least four measurements before bypass: blood pressure and pulse, electrocardiogram for signs of ischemia or arrhythmia, pulmonary wedge pressure, and cardiac output. Serious abnormalities can be readily corrected by the anesthesiologist by appropriate adjustment in drug therapy or intravenous fluids. Both intravenous nitroglycerin and intravenous diltiazem have been extremely helpful in controlling myocardial ischemia before bypass. This technique is especially crucial in patients with severe angina, which indicates ongoing myocardial ischemia before operation, because control of ischemia before bypass improves results after revascularization.

## MYOCARDIAL PRESERVATION

Hypothermic potassium cardioplegia with cold blood, described in a later paragraph, has been used routinely since 1979. The technique evolved from joint investigations between the NYU Cardiac Laboratories and those of Buckberg at UCLA. An alternative approach used at Duke University with crystalloid cardioplegia is described in part I of Chapter 54. For short periods of aortic occlusion, results reported with the two techniques are similar, but with longer periods of occlusion or with serious pre-existing myocardial ischemia, blood cardioplegia is strongly preferred.

At operation, arterial cannulation is done with a standard technique except in patients over 70 years of age or in those with atherosclerosis in the aortic arch. In such patients, a special aortic arch cannula is inserted and carefully placed so the tip of the cannula is beyond the orifice of the left carotid artery, near the ostium of the left subclavian. The concept of a special aortic arch cannula was initially reported by Culliford from NYU in 1986. Placing the cannula tip distally prevents the sandblast effect of the jet of arterial blood emerging from the cannula striking an atherosclerotic plaque and dislodging fragments, which can subsequently embolize into the innominate or left carotid artery. Venous cannulation may be done with two caval cannulas (preferred by the senior author) or by a single large two-stage cannula placed in the inferior vena cava and right atrium (preferred by most of the NYU faculty). The membrane oxygenator is employed. A crystalloid prime is used, maintaining a hematocrit above 20% and an oncotic pressure above 9 to 10 mm Hg after cardiopulmonary bypass is initiated. Perfusion rates are usually 2 to 2.5 $l/m^2$ at a temperature of 30° C, maintaining a perfusion pressure near 60 mm Hg. The left ventricle may be vented, most often with a catheter inserted through the right pulmonary vein.

## Aortic Arch Endarterectomy During Circulatory Arrest

A special problem exists if transesophageal echocardiography reveals the presence of mobile atherosclerotic fronds in the transverse aortic arch. These fronds evolve from ulceration of atherosclerotic intimal plaques with subsequent mobile fragments of intima at the edges of the ulceration. These were found in about 10% of the 97 elderly patients reported by Ribakove and Katz and their colleagues (1992) and were associated with the highest frequency of perioperative stroke. This type of abnormality, an ulcerated protuberant plaque, is the most severe form of aortic arch atherosclerosis and is associated with the highest risk of embolization, because the atherosclerotic fragments are fragile and easily dislodged with the slightest manipulation.

The preferred approach is as follows: The transverse aortic arch is exposed by dissection in the mediastinum, so that an aortic arch cannula can be inserted distal to the left carotid artery, with the tip placed near or just beyond the left subclavian. The location of the cannula tip often can be seen on the transesophageal echocardiogram. Bypass is then begun, and the temperature is lowered over 20 to 25 minutes to a tympanic membrane temperature of 15 to 17° C. (Tympanic membrane temperature is routinely monitored.) The head is lowered and packed in ice, and steroids are given. As cooling progresses, ventricular fibrillation occurs. At this time, the right atrium is opened and a coronary sinus catheter inserted. When the tympanic membrane temperature reaches 17° C, which requires 20 to 30 minutes of perfusion, the pump flow rate is decreased to about 500 ml/min, and the aortic arch is incised 5 to 7 cm with a longitudinal incision. Coronary sinus cardioplegia is started at this time, infusing 500 to 1000 ml to facilitate myocardial preservation. The mobile atherosclerotic fragments are removed easily by a combination of suction, gentle abrasion by twirling a sponge in the aortic lumen, and direct excision of loose intimal flaps with rongeurs. A formal endarterectomy is not attempted; the goal is to simply remove any loose debris that could embolize during perfusion. The area is then copiously lavaged with cold saline solution. Visualization of the aortic arch and the ostia of the three great vessels is usually excellent. Rarely, atherosclerotic ulcers are found at the orifice of either the innominate or left carotid artery, obviously constituting a serious hazard for stroke.

Following arch débridement, the pump flow rate is gradually increased as the aortotomy is sutured, displacing air from the lumen as the suture line is completed. Perfusion is restarted at a normal rate and the temperature raised to 30° C. The ascending aorta is clamped, and additional cardioplegia is infused through the coronary sinus. The time needed for aortic arch débridement varies with the severity of the disease, ranging from 4 to 5 minutes to longer than 30 minutes in one patient.

In the past 2 years, during which over 800 coronary bypass operations were performed, aortic arch exploration during circulatory arrest was performed in 10 patients. No ulceration of the intima was found in three patients, so the aortotomy was simply closed, requiring circulatory arrest for 3 to 6 minutes. In seven others, multiple ulcerated atheroma were debrided, as described earlier. Nine of the 10 patients recovered uneventfully. One died from massive multiple strokes with an unusual clinical course suggesting retrograde embolization from extensive atheromatous disease in the *descending* thoracic aorta.

Atherosclerotic disease in the ascending aorta, as described by Kouchoukos (Wareing et al., 1992), can be assessed both by palpation and with a sterile hand-held echocardiographic probe on the operative field. A variation of the circulatory arrest technique is used in these patients. The patient is cooled to less than 20° C by the methods described. The pump is then stopped and the ascending aorta opened near the innominate artery to permit inspection of the lumen, both to choose the site for application of the aortic clamp and to detect any ulceration in the ascending aorta. It is crucial that the aortic clamp is not placed across an area of ulceration. This requires only 3 to 5 minutes of circulatory arrest. Subsequently, the bypass grafts may be attached to the aorta while the aortic clamp is in place, obviating any risk of atherosclerotic embolism.

## Cardioplegia

Since the previous edition of this book, coronary sinus cardioplegia has become a valuable method of cardioplegia and has been widely adopted at NYU. This technique has been used either exclusively or in combination with antegrade cardioplegia through the ascending aorta.

In patients with normal ventricular function, *antegrade cardioplegia* is simpler and is usually employed. After clamping of the ascending aorta, the heart is arrested by infusing a cold blood cardioplegic solution (6° C), with a potassium concentration of 25 to 30 mEq/l, into the aortic root at a rate sufficient to develop an aortic root pressure near 70 mm Hg. The infusion rate is usually over 200 ml/min. The amount infused is greater than that described in reports from many institutions, at 15 to 20 ml/kg, 1000 to 1500 ml of blood. After the first injection, the potassium concentration is decreased to about 8 to 10 mEq/l. Regional myocardial temperatures are measured routinely with a thermistor, usually infusing sufficient cardioplegia to lower even the warmest area, the most ischemic, below 15° C.

Topical hypothermia is routinely employed, usually by intermittently flooding the operative field with cold electrolyte solution or by constant pericardial infusion of cold electrolyte solution, which is removed by continuous sump suction—a modification of Shumway's original technique. Care is taken to be certain the right side of the heart is empty and wrinkled, so that reflux of blood from the vena cava does not occur. Temperature is checked frequently to make sure that all areas of the myocardium remain below 15° C.

Cold blood cardioplegia is reinfused for 1 to 2 minutes after each distal anastomosis, or every 20 to 30 minutes. If distal anastomoses are done first, blood is often perfused during periods of reinjection through the vein grafts as these are constructed.

Opinions differ about the importance of hypothermia. Our strong preference at NYU is to keep the myocardial temperature at 15° C or lower.

The *coronary sinus technique* of administering cardioplegia is frequently used, either alone or in combination with antegrade aortic injections. The technique is used especially in patients with a significant decrease in ventricular function, which in turn manifests poor collateral circulation. It is also used routinely with acute ischemia, where maldistribution may occur with antegrade injection. Contrary to most reports, an open technique is often employed, using separate venous cannulas in the venae cavae that are snared. The right atrium is opened with a short incision, and the coronary sinus catheter is inserted under direct vision and secured with a purse-string suture after the balloon has been inflated. Alternatively, closed administration using a transatrial coronary sinus catheter has been highly effective. Cold blood cardioplegia is infused at a rate that maintains a coronary sinus pressure between 25 and 40 mm Hg, usually a rate of 100 to 200 ml/min. Coronary sinus pressures above 40 mm Hg are avoided, because significant myocardial edema may develop. The amount given is similar to that given by the antegrade technique, 15 to 20 ml/kg.

The NYU methods of myocardial preservation are extremely effective. With these techniques, periods of aortic occlusion for as long as 2 to 3 hours are easily tolerated; a few patients with exceedingly complex conditions have been clamped for 3 to 4 hours with no subsequent detectable myocardial injury.

## Technique of Graft Procurement

The left internal mammary is used in most bypass operations. The mammary artery is mobilized from the chest wall with a narrow (1 to 2 cm) strip of soft tissue from the sixth interspace inferiorly to the first interspace superiorly. During mobilization of the mammary pedicle, care is taken to minimize injury from the electric cautery, which in turn can significantly decrease blood flow to the sternum. This is especially important when bilateral mammary grafts are done in older patients or in those with diabetes. Experimental studies reported from our laboratories by Parish and associates in 1992 found a significant decrease in blood flow to the sternum, depending on the width of the pedicle harvested. The decrease in blood flow was least if the mammary vessels were skeletonized by making a very narrow pedicle. All techniques of internal mammary mobilization decreased sternal blood flow to less than 30% of control

values, but blood flow with a skeletonized pedicle was about twice as large as that in a standard pedicle. A more detailed discussion of use of the internal mammary artery is given by Rankin in a later part of this chapter.

After the internal mammary pedicle has been mobilized, the artery is divided and the free flow noted. A small cannula is then inserted, and 2 to 3 ml of papaverine (1 mg/ml) is gently injected, after which the artery is occluded with a hemaclip and put aside. The pulsatile arterial pressure over the next 10 to 15 minutes will gently dilate the papaverine-filled artery.

At the time of grafting of the internal mammary to the anterior descending, the adequacy of free flow is again confirmed. Confirming adequate flow is most important, because disasters can occur from anastomosing a mammary artery with an inadequate flow to a large anterior descending. Proximal obstruction to flow in the mammary artery can occur from injury or from atherosclerotic stenosis in the subclavian artery. If flow appears inadequate, a vein graft is obtained and used. In 1989, Jones and colleagues reported grim experiences over 2 years with five patients in whom flow through the internal mammary artery seemed inadequate. Three of the five died; another required cardiac transplantation.

Appropriate segments of saphenous vein larger than 3.5 mm are removed from the lower extremity. Large veins, over 6 mm, are avoided if possible, although there is little correlation between the size of the vein used and subsequent results. The veins are distended with heparinized electrolyte solution (plasmalyte). High-pressure distention (> 100 to 150 mm Hg) is avoided, because it can cause endothelial injury with resultant premature intimal hyperplasia. Veins with significant disease, manifested by scarring and thickening, are avoided.

If the greater saphenous veins are not satisfactory, the lesser saphenous veins are used. These are usually obtained by flexion of the knee and appropriate rotation of the lower extremity. An alternate approach, simple but awkward, is to have the foot held upward by an assistant while the vein is removed.

If neither the internal mammary arteries nor the greater or lesser saphenous veins are available, the last choice is to use veins from the arm, either the cephalic or basilic, whichever is more satisfactory. These have been used regularly at New York University for many years in such instances, and most commonly have been needed in the unfortunate patient who has had extensive ligation and stripping of all veins in both lower extremities. The arm veins are thin, usually requiring the use of 8-0 proline for the anastomoses. Short-term results are excellent. Long-term results from NYU are not available, but major complications have not been observed. The limited data published by others about long-term results with arm veins describe a high frequency of late degeneration and occlusion, probably because of the thin vein wall.

In 1990, Wijnberg and associates, in Holland, reported angiographic findings in 28 patients in whom

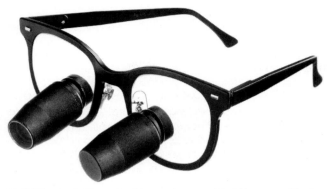

**FIGURE 54–64.** Binocular loupes that provide 3.5× magnification for coronary bypass surgery (Designs for Vision, Inc., 760 Koehler Avenue, Ronkonkoma, NY 11779).

44 arm vein grafts were performed. The average follow-up was 4.6 years. Angiography found 47% of the arm veins patent, compared to 77% of leg vein grafts.

Earlier, in 1984, both Stoney and associates and Prieto and co-workers separately reported their experiences. Stoney reviewed experiences with 59 patients over 9 years. Angiograms in 28 patients with 56 grafts found a 57% patency rate at about 2 years following operation, but among the 32 patent grafts, 7 had a localized stenosis. Prieto and associates described short-term results in 13 patients with a total of 24 grafts. At repeat catheterization in less than 9 months, 9 out of the 10 were patent, but studies after a year found that only 5 of 8 veins were patent, 2 of which had gross abnormalities.

The incisions in the lower extremity are closed with absorbable vicryl sutures. We prefer figure-of-eight sutures rather than continuous sutures, which were used for years. The continuous suture can create significant fat necrosis if large bites are taken, which in turn can cause serious morbidity. The leg incisions may be closed after the veins are removed, or closure may be deferred until after bypass following neutralization of heparin with protamine.

## CORONARY GRAFTING TECHNIQUE

The technique of distal anastomosis must be precise to construct a smooth anastomosis with no disruption of the intimal surface. Binocular loupes that magnify to 4 times normal are used regularly (Fig. 54–64). These were developed at NYU in 1971 (Spencer, 1971) and quickly adopted throughout the world.

A short arteriotomy (6 to 8 mm) is made beyond the site of obstruction, after which the lumen is gently probed with a calibrated metal probe, usually 1.5 to 2 mm, to confirm patency of the distal vessel. The venous-arterial anastomosis is then constructed end-to-side with a continuous suture of 7-0 prolene, usually with suture "bites" about 1 mm deep and 1 mm apart (Fig. 54–65). The mammary-coronary anastomosis is performed with continuous 8-0 Prolene (Fig. 54–66). Before the sutures are tied, blood is injected

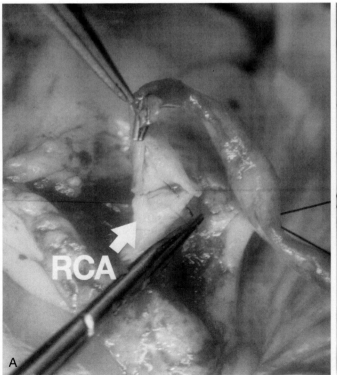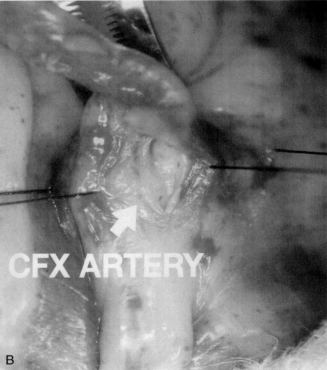

**FIGURE 54–65.** Operative photograph of saphenous vein used for coronary artery bypass. *A,* Coronary anastomosis. (RCA = right coronary artery.) *B,* Coronary anastomosis of the circumflex (CFX) artery.

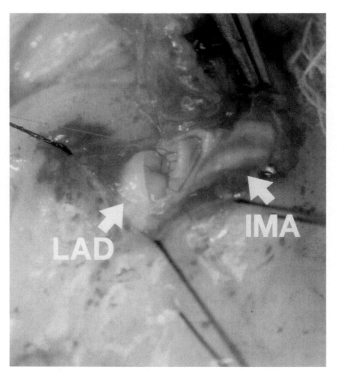

**FIGURE 54–66.** Intraoperative photograph of left internal mammary artery (IMA)/left anterior descending (LAD) anastomosis.

down the vein graft to displace any air. Additional cardioplegic solution is injected for 1 to 2 minutes to perfuse the region of myocardium grafted.

The aortic anastomosis is a standard one, placing the grafts either to the left or to the right of the midline. A small tangential clamp is applied to the anterior surface of the aorta, after which a small button of aorta is then constructed with a continuous 6-0 Prolene suture.

The aortic anastomoses may be constructed before the aorta is clamped, or else the distal anastomoses may be constructed initially and the proximal vessels attached while the aorta is cross-clamped or later with the heart beating. The former method is simpler and preferable for most patients. If there are signs of significant myocardial ischemia, however, it is preferable to establish bypass promptly and decompress the ventricle.

A variant technique is to attach the grafts while the aorta is clamped. This should surely be done if atherosclerotic disease is present in the ascending aorta, in order to avoid atherosclerotic embolization. Attaching the proximal anastomoses with the aorta clamped has the advantage of immediate reperfusion of the heart following unclamping, but it has the disadvantage of a longer period of aortic occlusion.

Sequential anastomoses are commonly used, although not nearly as often as those described by Kirklin and Barratt-Boyes (1993). The most common sequential anastomosis is to the left anterior descending and diagonal arteries. It is unusual to do more than four or five distal anastomoses. A more radical

approach, described by Kirklin, is to graft all vessels 1.5 mm in diameter or larger that are narrowed more than 50%. With multiple sequential anastomoses, as many as 8 to 10 anastomoses have been done in a few patients (Kirklin and Barratt-Boyes, 1993, Table 7–11, p. 317).

Endarterectomy is seldom performed because it is preferable to graft beyond the distal obstruction into segmental zones. The experiences of Johnson and Brenowitz in Milwaukee (1988) are followed with particular interest, but serious doubt remains concerning long-term patency (after 1 to 3 years) in endarterectomized vessels because of progressive cicatricial contraction of fibrous tissue. This phenomenon led to abandonment long ago of endarterectomy in the popliteal arteries, which are much larger than the coronary arteries. When endarterectomy is necessary, the microvascular technique, with a small arteriotomy, is used.

Following bypass, graft flow rates are measured routinely with a Doppler flowmeter, usually finding peak flows in the range of 70 to 100 ml/minute. The flow rates, of course, vary with the size of the distal vessel grafted and the arterial pressure.

Before the operative incision is closed, soft tissues are approximated in the superior mediastinum to cover the grafts, leaving the pericardium open inferiorly. Pacemaker wires are routinely left in the right ventricle and right atrium for control of postoperative arrhythmias. A small plastic catheter for monitoring left atrial pressure is often left in the right superior pulmonary vein. A Swan-Ganz catheter in the pulmonary artery is used routinely.

## BILATERAL MAMMARY GRAFTS

The feasibility of bilateral mammary grafts has been well established over the past decade. There is little increase in morbidity except in older diabetic patients, in whom risk of sternal infection is increased sharply to at least 3 to 4%.

Free grafts of the mammary artery have been used sporadically. Loop and associates in (1986a) reported experiences with 156 patients treated over 15 years. Not enough data are available to determine whether long-term results with a free graft are comparable with those with a conventional pedicle graft (Mills et al., 1993). This is an important question, because the remarkable durability of the pedicled left internal mammary graft may be due to inherent properties in the mammary artery or to leaving the mammary artery as a pedicle with an intact innervation and lymphatic and venous drainage. The apparently equally good results with "skeletonized" mammary arteries suggest that the lymphatic and venous drainage is not a crucial factor. Denervation of the mammary artery, however, may be a significant factor, especially influencing the remarkable ability of the pedicled internal mammary artery to enlarge over 5 to 10 years following operation.

In 1990, Fiore and co-workers reported a retrospective comparison of 100 patients who underwent placement of double mammary grafts with 100 matched patients who underwent placement of only a single mammary graft. They concluded that the data indicated substantial benefit from the use of double mammary grafts. However, Kirklin and Barratt-Boyes (1993) stated that Fiore's report included a number of untraced patients. These were subsequently located and the analysis was repeated, after which no difference in long-term survival was found between patients with a double mammary graft and those with a single mammary graft.

Galbut and colleagues, in 1990, reported experiences of over 1000 patients with bilateral mammary grafts treated over 17 years. Eighty-two have been followed over 10 years. Among the 959 survivors, nonfatal myocardial infarction occurred at a rate of about 1% per patient year. Overall 10-year survival was about 80%. Among the 82 late deaths, 34 were cardiac-related, 27 were not, and 21 were unknown.

## OTHER ARTERIAL CONDUITS

Most work in the past few years has been with the right gastroepiploic artery as an arterial conduit. Fewer data are available from use of the inferior epigastric artery, the radial artery, or the subscapular artery.

### Right Gastroepiploic Artery

Anatomic studies have found that the gastroepiploic is at least 1.5 mm or larger in more than 95% of patients. The artery is very susceptible to spasm, so intraluminal papaverine is usually needed to counteract the spasm resulting from mobilization and manipulation. Pym, in Canada, was the first to systematically use the gastroepiploic artery, beginning in 1984. In 1987, three separate reports appeared from different parts of the world—Pym in Canada, Suma in Japan, and Carter in Australia. In 1993, Suma reported cumulative experiences with 200 patients over 5 years, using the artery as a pedicle graft in 182 patients and as a free graft in 18. Postoperative angiography in 152 patients in the first few months after operation found a patency rate of 95%. Angiography was performed in 40 patients an average of 2 years after operation, again finding a patency rate near 95%.

Mills, discussing Suma's 1993 paper, stated that he had used the gastroepiploic in about 150 patients but had abandoned use of the artery as a free graft because of the frequency of spasm. These data, however, clearly indicate that the initial durability and patency of the gastroepiploic is well established. Long-term results are as yet unknown.

### Inferior Epigastric Artery

Mills and Everson in 1991 reported experiences with 18 patients with inferior epigastric artery grafts.

The technique of obtaining the inferior epigastric graft is well illustrated in the publication. The grafts measured from 11 to 17 cm in length, with a distal internal diameter of 1.0 to 2.5 mm. Follow-up, however, was only 1 year to 18 months. Only three patients underwent postoperative angiography in the first several days after operation, which found all vessels widely patent.

In 1991, Milgalter from UCLA reported experiences with 28 patients. A preoperative duplex scan was found useful in determining the diameter of the vessel and deciding which vessel was best for harvesting as a graft. No differences in size were found between the right and left inferior epigastric arteries. Distal diameter ranged between 2 and 3 mm. The usable length of artery was near 11 cm. Short-term results were satisfactory, but no postoperative angiograms had been performed.

In 1992, Buche from Belgium reported experiences with 73 patients undergoing surgery over 3 years. Postoperative angiograms in 61 patients found that 63 of 65 distal anastomoses were patent. Angiograms in 19 patients more than 6 months after operation found that 17 of 19 grafts were patent.

### Radial Artery

Use of the radial artery was proposed by Carpentier in 1977, but abandoning the graft was recommended 2 years later because the rate of significant stenosis or occlusion was 35%. The use of radial artery grafting was revived by Acar and Carpentier in 1992. This reinvestigation was prompted after it was found that several patients who had undergone radial artery grafting in the early 1970s still had excellent patent grafts 15 to 18 years later. The 1992 report discussed experiences with 104 patients since 1989. No ischemia of the hand was observed. On the assumption that denervation of the artery could be responsible for the previous poor results, diltiazem was started intraoperatively and continued after discharge. Angiography in the first 50 patients performed within 2 weeks of operation found 100% patency in 56 grafts. Late angiograms were performed about 9 months later in 27 patients, finding a patency rate of 93%. The dosage of diltiazem was 1 $\mu g/kg/min$. Postoperatively it was given orally, 250 mg/day.

An en-bloc dissection was used to minimize spasm, leaving the artery in a pedicle of soft tissue. After division, the artery was dilated with blood and papaverine. An Allen test and Doppler studies were routinely performed beforehand.

### Subscapular Artery

In 1992, Mills and co-workers (1993) reported use of the subscapular artery via a left-sided thoracotomy in three patients, having previously noted its usefulness in conjunction with muscle flaps. All three patients were in desperate circumstances, requiring reoperations and having no available conduits. The subscapular was connected to marginal branches of the circumflex coronary system. There were good results over a short-term follow-up of 6 to 21 months.

## POSTOPERATIVE CARE

The principal considerations in the first 12 to 24 hours after operation are blood pressure, adequacy of ventilation, postoperative bleeding, cardiac output, and arrhythmias. Ventilation is usually done through an endotracheal tube until the patient awakes, usually within a few hours, but varying with the anesthetic agent used. Once the patient is awake, extubation is done. The blood gas tensions are periodically monitored. Significant ventilatory problems are uncommon.

In the recovery room, the arterial pressure, electrocardiogram, and left atrial pressure (or pulmonary artery pressure) are usually displayed continuously. The basic goal is to maintain a systolic blood pressure of 100 to 120 mm Hg with a cardiac index above 2.5 l/min/m². Hypertension and increased peripheral vascular resistance can be treated by low-dose intravenous infusion of sodium nitroprusside. Nitroglycerin is given to prevent coronary spasm, and intravenous diltiazem likewise has proved helpful for coronary spasm and for hypertension and tachycardia. Low doses of beta-adrenergic blockers also are occasionally necessary. Blood volume is adjusted by infusion of appropriate fluids, depending on both blood loss and the degree of vasoconstriction or vasodilatation. Left atrial pressure is usually maintained between 8 and 12 mm Hg.

If an adequate cardiac output is not present despite an adequate left atrial pressure and a peripheral vascular resistance of 1000 to 1200 dynes, inotropic agents are given. These are usually either dobutamine (5 to 15 µg/kg/min) or amrinone (5 to 10 µg/kg/min). Epinephrine is used as a second-line agent. With the myocardial preservation technique previously described, a significant sustained depression of cardiac output after an uncomplicated bypass is uncommon.

Significant postoperative bleeding is unusual. The usual blood loss is about 300 to 750 ml in the first 24 hours. Shed blood is collected sterilely and reinfused. With intraoperative cell-saving techniques and postoperative reinfusion of shed blood, many patients do not require exogenous blood transfusion.

However, if significant bleeding from a coagulopathy requires multiple transfusions, particular attention is given to replacing all blood components on a "1 for 1" basis, rather than simply infusing packed red cells. For example, if 500 ml of blood drains from a chest tube, replacement requires four separate ingredients: packed cells, fresh frozen plasma, platelets, and cryoprecipitate. With significant bleeding from a major coagulopathy, this requires considerable "book-keeping" to be certain that all four components are properly replaced. If coagulopathy is significant, coagulation tests are done and appropriate therapy is undertaken.

The unusual patient with a blood loss of more than 1000 to 1500 ml is returned to the operating room for exploration, regardless of the hemodynamic status. This approach not only excludes a discrete site of surgical bleeding but also removes intrapericardial clots that could cause tamponade.

A patient with a low cardiac output who does not respond to infusion of fluids or inotropic agents is usually promptly returned to the operating room. The four most common causes are thrombosis of a bypass graft, tamponade, edematous myocardium compressed within the pericardium, and diffuse myocardial injury.

Three of these four can be treated by appropriate surgical maneuvers. Severe myocardial depression is an uncommon cause, because it is usually diagnosed previously in the operating room. Sustained low-output syndrome can be treated by insertion of an intraaortic balloon pump. However, a balloon pump is almost never inserted empirically in the recovery room because of the difficulty of excluding the other three possible causes of depressed cardiac function.

Atrial arrhythmias are common, and usually are treated by overdrive pacing. Atrial fibrillation may require intravenous digoxin or beta-adrenergic blockers for rate control, intravenous procainamide, or electrical cardioversion. Electrical pacing may also be necessary for transient bradycardia for 24 to 48 hours. Ventricular arrhythmias are treated with intravenous lidocaine or procainamide.

A small perioperative infarction probably occurs in 2 to 4% of patients, though precise data are not available. This is usually diagnosed from the appearance of Q waves on the electrocardiogram. Myocardial enzymes (CPK-MB isoenzyme) are measured regularly, although the precise significance of various levels remains uncertain. Hemodynamic instability suggesting a major infarction is rare with present methods of myocardial preservation.

With modern techniques, most patients recover uneventfully and are discharged from the hospital within 5 to 10 days following operation.

## EARLY RESULTS

### Operative Mortality and Morbidity

The operative mortality rate in the past few years has risen to the range of 2 to 3%, probably because good-risk patients are more frequently treated by angioplasty, whereas patients with more complicated conditions are referred for coronary bypass.

The crude mortality, expected mortality, and risk-adjusted mortality rates at NYU Medical Center and in New York State are shown in Table 54–9 for a period of 4 years, 1989 through 1992. At NYU, the crude mortality rate ranged between 2 and 4.38%, whereas the risk-adjusted mortality rate decreased

■ **Table 54–9.** OPERATIVE MORTALITY RATES (CRUDE, EXPECTED, RISK–ADJUSTED) FOLLOWING ISOLATED CABG AT NYU AND IN NEW YORK STATE 1989–1992

| Year | NYU Medical Center | | | | New York State | | | |
|---|---|---|---|---|---|---|---|---|
| | No. of Patients | Crude (%) | Expected (%) | Risk-Adjusted (%) | No. of Patients | Crude (%) | Expected (%) | Risk-Adjusted (%) |
| 1989 | 745 | 3.22 | 4.26 | 2.52 | 12,269 | 3.52 | 2.68 | 4.25 |
| 1990 | 694 | 3.60 | 4.09 | 2.75 | 13,946 | 3.14 | 3.26 | 3.11 |
| 1991 | 707 | 4.38 | 5.38 | 2.51 | 14,944 | 3.08 | 3.66 | 2.72 |
| 1992 | 636 | 2.04 | 4.13 | 1.38 | 16,028 | 2.78 | — | — |

*Key*: CABG = coronary artery bypass graft; NYU = New York University.

from 2.8 to 1.4%. During this time, 600 to 700 coronary bypass operations were done annually.

In New York State, between 12,000 and 16,000 operations were performed yearly. Crude mortality rates varied from 2.8 to 3.5%, whereas the risk-adjusted mortality rates varied from 2.7 to 4.3%.

In the 1990 analysis of the New York State mortality by Leape, the overall mortality rate was 2% in the patients studied, ranging from a low of 0.5% for operations for chronic stable angina to 15% for complications of PTCA or angiography, and 30% for cardiogenic shock following myocardial infarction. Seven per cent of patients had at least one major cardiac complication (perioperative infarction, 2.3%; cardiac arrest, 2.9%; arrhythmias requiring defibrillation, 1.7%; permanent pacemaker, 1%). Two per cent had a stroke. Sternal wound infections occurred in 2%, acute renal failure in 1%.

The 1993 textbook by Kirklin and Barratt-Boyes mathematically analyzes the importance of several classic risk factors (Kirklin and Barratt-Boyes, 1993). The most serious ones are advanced age, decrease in ejection fraction, and incomplete revascularization. Both diabetes and hypertension are also significant risk factors. Nonuse of the internal mammary artery has become a clear risk factor, especially apparent between 5 and 10 years following operation.

At NYU, a tertiary university center, a firm, longstanding policy has been to accept virtually all patients for operation if a problem is correctable, no matter how gravely ill the patient. A significant number of patients undergo surgery who have been considered "inoperable," usually because of depressed ventricular function or diffuse distal coronary disease. With present techniques of myocardial preservation, the operative mortality rate even in these very seriously ill patients is gratifyingly low, less than 5%. For 1992, the expected mortality rate for the 636 patients undergoing bypass at NYU was 4.13%, but the risk-adjusted mortality was only 1.38% (Table 54–9).

## Significant Operative Complications

The four most serious operative complications are stroke, myocardial infarction, renal failure, and wound infection. A large myocardial infarction, as discussed in the preceding paragraphs, is uncommon

with present techniques of myocardial preservation. Electrocardiographic signs of a small perioperative infarction of minimal hemodynamic significance occur in a small percentage of patients.

A stroke is the most disabling complication, fortunately decreasing in frequency in recent years to a range between 1 and 2% at NYU (Table 54–10). As discussed earlier, this low frequency may be related to the method of surgically assessing the diseased aorta as well as to liberal use of perioperative transesophageal echocardiography. As noted above, the techniques used for patients with known atherosclerotic disease in the aortic arch include a special aortic arch cannula as well as operative débridement during circulatory arrest for severe cases. The preliminary experiences with this technique were reported by Culliford and associates from this institution in 1986.

Blossom and co-workers reported in 1992 a retrospective analysis of 46 strokes that occurred after more than 3400 bypass operations, a frequency of 1.3%. Sixteen of the 46 were considered intraoperative. The other 30 patients became symptomatic between 1 and 7 days following operation. About one-half of these were considered to have had an embolic event, whereas the others seemed to have had cerebral hypoperfusion. The mortality rate was 35%, with a high percentage of disability in the surviving patients.

Concomitant procedures for co-existing carotid and coronary disease are rarely done and are reserved for the unusual patient with acute symptoms from both coronary and carotid disease. We no longer believe that asymptomatic carotid disease, even though hemodynamically significant, is a significant cause of perioperative stroke. Usually with severe disease in both carotid and coronary systems, the most symptomatic disease is treated first, followed within a few

■ **Table 54–10.** FREQUENCY OF STROKE FOLLOWING ISOLATED CABG AT NYU 1989–1992

| Year | No. of Patients | No. of Strokes | Incidence of Stroke |
|---|---|---|---|
| 1989 | 745 | 14 | 1.88% |
| 1990 | 694 | 12 | 1.73% |
| 1991 | 707 | 11 | 1.56% |
| 1992 | 636 | 13 | 2.04% |

days by treatment of the other disease. The low frequency of stroke in recent years is consistent with the theory that perioperative strokes arise primarily from atheroma in the aortic arch, not from the carotid arteries.

Experiences with a combined approach of carotid endarterectomy and coronary bypass at the same operation in 127 patients were reported by Rizzo from the Brigham and Women's Hospital over 13 years (Rizzo et al., 1992). The results were unimpressive, because there were seven deaths and seven strokes, a mortality rate of 5.5% and a similar stroke rate.

Significant *sternal infection* fortunately has become rare, less than 1%. Particular emphasis is given to minimal use of the cautery, minimal use of bone wax, and appropriate use of intravenous antibiotics and topical antibiotic irrigation. Meticulous attention to operative technique is probably the most important factor of all.

Sternal infection occurs more often in older diabetic patients, especially with bilateral mammary grafts. When bilateral mammary grafts are done, particular attention is given to preparation of a narrow mammary pedicle, with minimal use of the cautery. Both of these methods minimize devascularization of the sternum.

Loop in 1990 reviewed experiences with 72 sternal infections that occurred in a group of 6500 patients undergoing coronary artery bypass grafting over a period of 3 years, a frequency of 1%. A detailed analysis found that bilateral internal mammary grafting in a diabetic patients had a 5-fold increase in the risk of sternal infection. By contrast, a repeat sternotomy for a second bypass had no increased risk of infection (Loop et al., 1990).

Fortunately, significant renal failure is rare. It occurs more frequently in older patients with pre-existing renal disease, especially when undergoing surgery in urgent circumstances soon after catheterization. Peritoneal dialysis is used as necessary and is continued until the patient is hemodynamically stable enough to permit hemodialysis. Most patients recover after a short period of dialysis as long as postoperative cardiac function remains good.

## Relief of Angina

Immediate relief of angina has long been recognized as the most dramatic feature of coronary bypass surgery, because angina is completely relieved in most patients with complete revascularization. This dramatic response was responsible for the rapid rise in the frequency of coronary bypass grafting after its introduction in 1967 to 1968.

## Neuropsychiatric Abnormalities

Several studies in recent years have documented a significant frequency of transient neuropsychiatric abnormalities following coronary bypass, usually in the absence of gross neurologic deficits. The two principal causes are perfusion emboli from the pump oxygenator and inadequate cerebral blood flow. Unanswered questions are whether these are less common with a membrane oxygenator than a bubble oxygenator, the value of an arterial in-line filter, and the value of pulsatile blood flow in maintaining better cerebral perfusion. Significant permanent neurologic abnormalities have not been noted among the vast majority of patients treated at NYU, and, when present, these have been thought to be embolic in origin.

An excellent prospective study by Townes and colleagues in 1989 evaluated 90 patients, 65 of whom underwent coronary bypass and 25 of whom underwent intracardiac operations. These were compared with 47 nonsurgical control subjects. Extensive neuropsychologic tests were done before operation, before hospital discharge, and about 7 months later. The operations were performed by four different surgeons, a bubble oxygenator was used, and blood pressure was maintained intraoperatively, when necessary, with phenylephrine. An arterial line filter was not used. Neuropsychologic abnormalities were frequently found soon after operation, but 7 months later these had disappeared in all but about 11% of patients. In most patients, there were no difficulties with problem-solving, memory, motor speed, sensory perceptual functions, visual motor abilities, expressive language, or concentration. A good number of patients improved in performance, compared with the control group, presumably from improvement in cardiac function and overall well-being. The 11% with residual abnormalities were, in general, older than the other patients. There were no gross neurologic defects. Surprisingly, the abnormalities occurred with equal frequency among the coronary patients and those undergoing intracardiac operations.

A less extensive study was reported by Sellman and associates from the Karolinska Institute in Stockholm in 1991. Sixty-six patients younger than 70 years were studied before and 1 week following bypass grafting. Twenty were randomized to a bubble oxygenator without an arterial line filter; 22 had a filter, whereas 24 had a membrane oxygenator without a filter. No gross neurologic abnormalities occurred in any group. However, some abnormalities developed in about 20% of patients in whom a bubble oxygenator was used, regardless of whether a filter was present. Only 8% of patients in whom a membrane oxygenator was used developed an abnormality, although the authors state that the numbers were not large enough to be statistically significant.

Henz and colleagues in Germany in 1990 reported an evaluation of 22 patients undergoing bypass grafting, 14 of whom had nonpulsatile flow, 8 of whom had pulsatile flow. Transient neurologic abnormalities developed in both groups with equal frequency, implying that pulsatile flow, per se, did not correct the problem. Obviously, numbers were small.

Blauth and co-workers, in London, reported in 1988 and 1990 interesting studies with fluorescein angiography of the retina during cardiopulmonary bypass.

Tiny microvascular particles causing transitory or permanent occlusion were seen. Sixty-four patients were studied before bypass, shortly before bypass was terminated, and about 30 minutes following bypass. Neuropsychiatric studies were also done before operation and about a week later in approximately 20 patients. The retinal abnormalities occurred in 100% of those on the bubble oxygenator, in about 56% of those on the membrane oxygenator. It was felt that the abnormalities were due to emboli that subsequently fragmented; whether these were microaggregates of fibrin or gaseous emboli was uncertain.

Their clinical significance was unclear. Only one patient had slight visual changes. The neuropsychiatric studies showed little correlation with the presence of emboli: About two-thirds of the patients had no change when studied about 9 days after operation. The 35% that had at least one abnormality showed little correlation with the number of emboli seen.

## CONVALESCENCE

Convalescence is uneventful in most patients. Some fatigue is common for at least 2 to 3 weeks. Within a month after operation, most patients have regained much of their preoperative physical stamina. Full recovery, however, does not occur for 2 to 3 months in most patients, including both physical stamina and intellectual capacity. In some patients, one of the last functions to return is the capacity for concentration and concept formation. Moderate sedentary activity, such as walking, travel, or driving a car, is permitted after a month, but strenuous physical exercise is avoided for 2 to 3 months.

If ventricular function was normal before operation, patients can anticipate a normal exercise capacity within 3 months of complete revascularization with virtually no limit on physical activity. This ability to return to a normal lifestyle is one of the major attractions of bypass operations. Generally, a stress test is recommended before beginning a vigorous exercise schedule.

Postoperative improvement in ventricular function can be anticipated in many patients with decreased ejection fraction beforehand, probably reflecting improved flow to "stunned" or "hibernating" myocardium. The degree of improvement in ejection fraction averages about 5 to 10%, for example, rising from 30% to 35 to 40%. In some patients, improvement in hypokinetic and dyskinetic segments may continue for several months after operation as the chronically ischemic myocardium recovers.

Return to light work is permitted within a month after operation, if desired. Patients are allowed to choose their work schedule thereafter, but return to normal working capacity should not be expected for about 3 months.

Lifelong dietary therapy is strongly recommended. This was discussed previously and is also discussed by Guyton in Chapter 54, Part VI. It is most important for the patient to understand that he has a permanent biochemical lipid defect, not unlike diabetes, the severity of which can be greatly lessened by modification of the lipid intake in the diet. Tight control of other risk factors is essential for optimal long-term results.

A regular exercise program of moderate intensity is usually recommended. The benefits are plausible, although not proved (Froelicher et al., 1985). For most patients, enrollment in a cardiac rehabilitation program is reasonable if not too inconvenient or expensive. Alternatively, the patient can arrange this herself. However, exercise in patients with depressed left ventricular function should be closely monitored with the electrocardiogram to prevent hazardous or even lethal arrhythmias.

## LONG-TERM RESULTS

### Patency of Vein Grafts

With appropriate technique combined with antiplatelet therapy, a patency rate of 93 to 95% can be expected 1 month following operation, decreasing only slightly in subsequent months to a patency rate of near 90% 1 year after operation (Bourassa, 1991).

Intimal *hyperplasia* probably develops uniformly in all vein grafts in the first few months after operation, representing a histologic response of the vein to arterial pressure; it stops after 12 to 18 months. This process, which Barratt-Boyes called a "remodeling," continues until, after several months, the diameter of the vein has decreased to more closely resemble that of the distal coronary artery (Kirklin and Barratt-Boyes, 1993). This decrease in diameter is probably beneficial, because the velocity of blood flow in the graft is increased to near that in the coronary artery. If unusually large veins are used, however, the decrease in diameter does not occur to that extent.

A localized *anastomotic stenosis* may be found on angiography in a small percentage of patients. This is perhaps due to surgical technique, probably from excessive traction on the suture tearing the intima with subsequent localized accumulation of blood in the vessel wall. Injury of the endothelial lining of the grafted vessel is another possible explanation. If the stenosis is severe, the likelihood of progression to complete occlusion within the next few months or years is high. Angioplasty has been successful in such patients.

A separate phenomenon is the development of *localized stenoses in the vein graft*, which at times are severe. These appear too early to be due to atherosclerosis. Probably these result from localized trauma to the wall of the vein during surgical handling or to overdistention with endothelial sloughing, which leads to progressive fibrosis and stenosis.

*Atherosclerosis* rarely is identified within the first 3 years after operation, but the frequency progressively increases between 3 and 7 years after operation. Bourassa and colleagues (1986) stated that their studies found atherosclerosis in at least 17% of vein grafts within 7 years after operation, a third of which narrowed the lumen more than 50%. The progression of atherosclerosis is subsequently rapid, however, so that by 10 years after operation, 46% of grafts show significant atherosclerosis, over two-thirds of which constrict the lumen more than 50%.

In 1991, Fitzgibbon and associates reported long-term angiographic studies in a large series of patients with findings similar to those reported by Bourassa and associates in 1986 (Fitzgibbon et al., 1991). In 222 patients, 741 vein grafts were studied periodically at 1 year and an average of 9.6 years after operation; most were also examined 5 years after operation.

The frequency of graft occlusion rose from 13% at 1 year to 20% at 5 years and 41% at 10 years. Abnormalities interpreted as due to atherosclerosis were present in 38% of grafts at 5 years, and 75% at 10 years. The atherosclerotic lesions in general tended to gradually progress to complete occlusion. Thus, in a group of 590 grafts free of disease 1 year following operation, at 10 years after operation, 41% of grafts were occluded; 75% of those that were patent were diseased.

Aspirin was routinely given to all patients throughout the series. Unfortunately, avoiding gross technical errors did not prevent later atherosclerosis, for a significant percentage of grafts that appeared normal at 1 year were found significantly diseased or occluded at the 5-year study.

The combination of fibrous stenoses and progressive atherosclerosis decreases patency from near 80% 5 years after operation to about 40% at 10 years. Of the remaining patent grafts, at least 75% have significant atherosclerotic narrowing.

Preventing or retarding the development of atherosclerosis in vein grafts remains a major challenge. It is hoped that intensive lipid therapy, reducing both the lipid intake as well as lowering blood cholesterol below 200 mg/dl, will be beneficial. To date, unfortunately, only a few reports have been able to demonstrate much benefit. The importance of intense lipid therapy in all patients following operation cannot be overemphasized, however. The role of local growth factors in this process is also currently under investigation. Unfortunately, the normal appearance of a vein graft 5 years following operation has not guaranteed that atherosclerosis would not develop in the next 5 years. An unanswered question is whether the 25 to 30% of vein grafts functioning well at 10 years will remain so indefinitely, or whether all vein grafts will subsequently become atherosclerotic and occlude. This is an important surgical consideration, because some centers recommend the routine removal of all vein grafts more than 5 to 7 years old at the time of repeat operation.

Lytle and colleagues in 1985 reported that 5 to 12 years after operation (average 7 years), 36% of vein grafts were occluded, 18% were stenotic, and 45% appeared satisfactory.

## Progression of Atherosclerosis

Serial angiograms following operation uniformly demonstrate a variable progression of native athero-sclerosis in both grafted and ungrafted arteries. The most severe progression occurs in severe stenoses proximal to the site of anastomosis in a grafted vessel. This is probably a flow phenomenon, because flow through the bypass graft greatly reduces flow through the stenotic vessel proximally.

The progression of atherosclerosis in other vessels is variable but usually continuous. As stated previously, the ability to slow or stop progression of atherosclerosis in native vessels is a major future challenge for effective lipid therapy. The postoperative patient provides an ideal model for evaluating lipid programs, because the rate of progression of disease before and after operation can be well documented. We have seen several patients 7 to 10 years following operation whose angiograms showed little progression of native atherosclerosis, although these observations are of no statistical value. The patients almost invariably had voluntarily adopted an unusually strenuous low-fat diet, virtually becoming vegetarians.

## Recurrence of Angina

Angina recurs in 10 to 15% of patients within 5 years after operation and in about 40% within 10 years. Interestingly enough, return of angina is not an ominous event, for the longevity of patients with recurrent angina is nearly as good as that of asymptomatic patients (Kirklin and Barratt-Boyes, 1993). Recurrence of angina almost always indicates either occlusion of a previous functioning graft or the development of additional disease in the native coronary circulation. Hence, recurrence of significant angina is a strong indication for a repeat coronary angiogram, because stenotic lesions may be treated effectively by angioplasty or repeat operation. Reoperative coronary bypass is now a common procedure, with an operative risk little greater than with elective bypass. Lytle reported experiences with 1500 repeat operations in 1987 (Lytle et al., 1987). Repeat coronary operations are discussed separately by Loop in Part III of Chapter 54.

## Freedom from Myocardial Infarction

Myocardial infarction is uncommon after coronary bypass. About 96% of patients are free of infarction 5 years after operation, about 64% at 15 years.

## Sudden Death

Fortunately, sudden death is rare following coronary bypass, probably one of the most important benefits. According to Kirklin, 97% of patients were free of sudden death at 10 years (Kirklin and Barratt-Boyes, 1993). A major risk factor for late sudden death is low ejection fraction. Patients with a normal preoperative ejection fraction have only about a 4% chance of sudden death within 15 years, compared with those with an ejection fraction of 25%, who have a 15% risk.

## Arrhythmias

Unfortunately, only a few significant preoperative arrhythmias improve following coronary bypass. Arrhythmias primarily result from scar from previous myocardial infarctions; an uncommon cause is ischemic but viable muscle that can be revascularized. This is reflected in the previously cited data from Kirklin (Kirklin and Barratt-Boyes, 1993). These data showed a very small risk of sudden death over a period of 15 years following operation in patients with normal ventricular function, but the frequency rose to 15% in those with a low preoperative ejection fraction.

When coronary bypass is performed in patients with poor ventricular function, which is a high percentage of patients, the presence of significant ventricular arrhythmias should be carefully determined postoperatively. Electrocardiographic monitoring with a 24-hour Holter monitor should be done. In patients with significant arrhythmias refractory to standard drug therapy, further studies should be done, usually electrophysiologic studies. From these, a decision about appropriate medications or even implantation of a permanent defibrillator can be considered. The surgical management of cardiac arrhythmias is considered in more detail in Chapter 55 by Cox.

## LONGEVITY

In the first 1100 patients undergoing surgery at NYU between 1968 and 1975, the 5-year survival rate, including operative deaths, was 88%. Only 49 cardiac deaths occurred after the patients were discharged from the hospital, an average mortality rate of 1.5% per year for the next 5 years. This was almost identical to a matched population group of similar age and sex distribution.

The beneficial effect of complete revascularization with bypass grafting is demonstrated by noting that 5-year survival is similar after bypass for single-, double-, or triple-vessel disease, whereas there is a major difference in mortality for patients treated medically with single-, double-, or triple-vessel disease. In general, of patients treated medically, about 88% of patients survive 5 years after operation, 75% at 10 years, and 60% at 15 years.

Three large randomized trials have been completed in the past several years: the CASS Randomized Trial, the European Randomized Trial, and the VA Randomized Trial. In these three studies, the 5- and 10-year survival rates were 95 and 82% for the CASS, 91 and 77% for the European study, and 83 and 64% for the VA study. These differences probably reflect a difference in risk factors in the patients before operation. Kirklin and Barratt-Boyes described an overall

5-year survival rate of 92%, decreasing to 81% at 10 years and 57% at 15 years (1993, Fig. 7–14).

Hence, data from several sources agree with the 1978 report from NYU that the risk of death following bypass with reasonably good ventricular function is similar to that of the normal population for the first 5 years (Isom et al., 1978).

After 5 years, there is a gradual increase in the risk of death, reflecting both progression of the native atherosclerotic process and progressive occlusion of the venous grafts. Loop and associates (1986b) first demonstrated the important difference in 10-year survival between patients in whom an internal mammary was used and in those who had only vein grafts. A significant benefit in longevity from double mammary grafting has not been conclusively demonstrated, but this may well require 10 to 15 years of follow-up after comparable operations. The benefits of single mammary grafting did not become evident until 5 to 10 years after operation.

A significant decrease in ejection fraction before operation is a significant risk factor for late death, possibly because the decrease in ejection fraction reflects the inability of the individual patient's collateral circulation to compensate for the rapid progression of the native atherosclerotic process. Kirklin and Barratt-Boyes (1993) compared late survival between patients who had ejection fractions of 60 and 30%. Five years after operation, survival rates were 96 and 90%, at 10 years 86 and 69%, and at 15 years 61 and 34%, respectively.

In 1993, Rahimtoola and colleagues published long-term survival studies of a group of over 7500 patients undergoing bypass over 20 years (1969 to 1988). The 5-, 10-, 15-, and 20-year survival rates were 88, 73, 53, and 38%, respectively. A comparison of four cohorts undergoing surgery at 5-year intervals showed that the results in the first 5 years (1969 to 1973) were not as good as those in subsequent ones; in the last 15 years, the three cohorts had similar results. The 1977 to 1988 cohort had 10- and 15-year survival rates of 74 and 55%, respectively.

The influence of ventricular function on survival was clearly shown. Patients with a "normal" left ventricular function had 10- and 15-year survival rates of 82 and 64%, respectively, compared with 64 and 37%, respectively, for those with impaired ventricular function. Fifteen years following operation, about 33% of patients had undergone reoperation; about 26% had suffered myocardial infarction.

Hence, complete revascularization greatly decreases the risk of cardiac death for at least 5 years. Subsequently, there is a gradual increased risk of cardiac death from graft closure, as well as from progression of native atherosclerosis. In the future, increased use of arterial grafts may decrease the former hazard. Effective lipid dietary therapy and control of the molecular aspects of atherosclerosis may decrease the latter.

## SELECTED BIBLIOGRAPHY

Baumann, F. G., Catinella, F. P., Cunningham, J. N., Jr., and Spencer, F. C.: Vein contraction and smooth muscle cell extensions as causes of endothelial damage during graft preparation. Ann. Surg., *194*:199, 1981.

A striking phenomenon with removal of a saphenous vein is the development of spasm. This concentric contraction of the vessel, with contraction of the internal elastic membrane, may rupture the endothelial lining with exposure of the underlying vessel wall to elements in the blood. Thus, the graft is no longer a tube completely lined with endothelium and is more susceptible to thrombosis. This paper demonstrates with electron microscopy the mechanism of this phenomenon. It can be minimized by the use of papaverine at the time of removal of the saphenous vein.

Bounos, E. P., Mark, D. B., Pollock, B. G., et al.: Surgical survival benefits for coronary disease patients with left ventricular dysfunction. Circulation, *78*(Suppl. I):151, 1988.

In a group of 710 patients with an ejection fraction of less than 40%, 301 patients were treated surgically. Three-year surgical survival was 86% compared with a medical survival of only 68%. The greatest surgical benefits occurred in the patients with the most severe left ventricular dysfunction, contradicting the common opinion that patients with severe impairment of ventricular function benefit little from bypass.

CASS Principal Investigators and Their Associates: Coronary Artery Surgery Study (CASS): A randomized trial of coronary artery bypass surgery: Survival data. Circulation, *68*:939, 1983.

This important report was one of the first from the extensive CASS of patients between 1975 and 1979, including almost 25,000 patients. This report discussed 780 patients with stable coronary disease with good ventricular function. During a period of 5 years, the longevity was very good in both medical and surgical groups (almost 93%). Thus, there was no benefit from performance of elective bypass.

An important point, however, is that these conclusions were valid only for patients whose angina did not increase in severity. In patients with triple-vessel disease, more than 7% of the patients each year developed symptoms and were treated with a bypass operation; thus within 5 years, 38% had had a bypass, emphasizing the importance of continued periodic evaluation.

Catinella, F. P., Cunningham, J. N., Jr., Srungaram, R. K., et al.: Cold blood should not be used for vein preparation prior to coronary bypass grafting. J. Thorac. Cardiovasc. Surg., *82*:904, 1981.

There is an increasing amount of data that indicate that the method of handling the saphenous vein at the time of coronary bypass grafting is crucial and determines both early and long-term patency and possibly also the susceptibility of the vein to atherosclerosis. This paper indicates that cold blood is actually harmful. The cold causes a contraction of the vein with disruption of the endothelium, and the platelets in the blood then accumulate and initiate a thrombotic reaction. Moderately cold plasmanate is superior.

Chesebro, J. H., Clements, I. P., Fuster, V., et al.: A platelet-inhibitor-drug trial in coronary-artery bypass operations: Benefit of perioperative dipyridamole and aspirin therapy on early postoperative vein graft patency. N. Engl. J. Med., *307*:73, 1982.

This important report was the first to show the significant influence of preoperative antiplatelet therapy on patency rate of vein grafts following operation. With some modifications, this therapeutic regimen has now been widely adopted throughout the United States.

Cobb, L. A., Werner, J. A., and Trobaugh, G. B.: Sudden cardiac death. I: A decade's experience with out-of-hospital resuscitation. Mod. Concepts Cardiovasc. Dis., *49*:31, 1980.

This remarkable paper from Seattle summarizing several years' experience with resuscitation of patients who develop cardiac arrest outside the hospital should be studied in detail. The data are especially significant because of the 600,000 deaths that occur annually in the United States, approximately two-thirds occur outside the hospital. The data are remarkable in that only one-fifth of the patients resuscitated had a transmural infarction, and more than half had no signs of myocardial necrosis whatsoever. About 75% of the patients had triple-vessel disease, indicating that the event causing ventricular fibrillation was an arrhythmia, not an infarction. The implications for prompt cardiopulmonary resuscitation, as well as for the long-term monitoring for malignant arrhythmias, are clear.

European Coronary Surgery Study Group: Prospective randomised study of coronary artery bypass surgery in stable angina pectoris: Second interim report. Lancet, *2*:491, 1980.

The most important question with coronary bypass grafting is its influence on longevity. This randomized study is probably the best of its kind in the world. It was the first to conclusively show a significant difference in 5-year survival in patients with triple-vessel disease and good ventricular

function. Patients with triple-vessel disease had a 5-year survival rate of 95% after operation and one of 85% after medical therapy.

Fitzgibbon, G. M., Leach, A. J., Kafka, H. P., et al.: Coronary bypass graft fate: Long-term angiographic study. J. Am. Coll. Cardiol., *17*:1075, 1991.

In 222 patients, 741 venous coronary bypass grafts were studied angiographically at 1 year and later (mean 9.6 years). The grafts were graded for patency and for significant atherosclerotic disease. Absence of early disease had little prognostic significance for late patency. Graft occlusion rates were 8% at 1 year, 20% at 5 years, 41% at 10 years, and 45% at 11.5 years. Only 17% of the original grafts were healthy at late follow-up. This study documents the progression of graft atherosclerosis, which severely limits the long-term utility of saphenous vein grafts.

Froelicher, V., Jensen, D., Sullivan, M.: A randomized trial of the effects of exercise training after coronary artery bypass surgery. Arch. Intern. Med., *145*:689, 1985.

This carefully designed study randomized 53 patients after bypass surgery to determine the influence of a specific exercise program in the year after bypass. Although about one-third of the patients had signs or symptoms of residual ischemia after revascularization, little benefit from the exercise program could be shown.

Galbut, D. L., Traad, E. A., Dorman, M. J., et al.: Seventeen-year experience with bilateral internal mammary artery grafts. Ann. Thorac. Surg., *49*:195, 1990.

This study reviews 1087 patients who received bilateral internal mammary artery grafts, with supplemental vein grafts, between 1972 and 1988. The hospital mortality rate was 2.7%. Follow-up was completed on 1058 hospital survivors. The actuarial survival rate for patients discharged from the hospital was 80% at 10 years and 60% at 15 years. Over 90% of the patients were asymptomatic at the time of follow-up. This in-depth longitudinal analysis demonstrates that bilateral IMA grafting has a low operative risk and yields excellent long-term functional results and survival.

Isom, O. W., Spencer, F. C., Glassman, E., et al.: Does coronary bypass increase longevity? J. Thorac. Cardiovasc. Surg., *75*:28, 1978.

This paper reports experiences at New York University with the first 1174 patients operated on between 1968 and 1975. The overall operative mortality rate was 5%. In the subsequent 5 years, an additional 7% of the patients died, an 88% 5-year survival rate. This actuarial survival curve parallels that of a matched population of similar age and sex, and thus, this was one of the first papers to show the strong likelihood that bypass grafting greatly increased longevity.

Loop, F. D., Cosgrove, D. M., Lytle, B. W., et al.: An eleven year evolution of coronary arterial surgery (1967–1978). Ann. Surg., *190*:444, 1979.

This paper summarizes much of the extensive experience at the Cleveland Clinic for a period of several years. Graft patency rates for four different groups, each studied around 20 months after operation, ranged from 77 to 87%. The 5-year survival rate for these four groups ranged from 89 to 92%.

Loop, F. D., Lytle, B. W., Cosgrove, D. M., et al.: Influence of internal mammary artery grafts on 10 year survival and other cardiac events. N. Engl. J. Med., *314*:1, 1986.

This important paper was one of the first to show the significant influence of internal mammary artery grafting on longevity 10 years after operation. This influence is not apparent 5 years after operation but appears later on as significant disease develops in vein grafts. Another reason for the difference may be that the internal mammary artery often enlarges. The studies presented in the paper included more than 2300 patients with an internal mammary graft, 855 of whom had postoperative catheterization. Patency of the internal mammary 10 years after operation was 96%. Catheterization studies also found that patency rate was similar both 1 year and 10 years after operation, which indicates the absence of a significant frequency of late occlusion.

Lytle, D. W., Cosgrove, D. M. K., et al.: Perioperative risk of bilateral internal mammary artery grafting: Analysis of 500 cases 1971 to 1984. Circulation, *71*(Suppl. 3):37, 1986.

This significant report clearly showed that bilateral internal mammary artery grafting could be done with little increase in mortality or morbidity. During the year preceding this report, 25% of all patients having bypass had bilateral mammary grafts.

Milano, C. A., White, W. D., Smith, R., et al.: Coronary artery bypass in patients with severely depressed ventricular function. Ann. Thorac. Surg., *56*:487, 1993.

This study reviews 118 consecutive patients with an ejection fraction of

25% or less who underwent coronary bypass grafting at Duke University Medical Center between 1981 and 1991. The operative mortality rate was 11%. Ventricular arrhythmias requiring treatment were found in 27% of patients postoperatively. One-year and 5–year survival rates were 77% and 58%, respectively. Survivors improved in the resting ejection fraction and were significantly improved symptomatically, with less angina and congestive heart failure. These data suggest that patients with coronary artery disease and severely depressed ejection fraction benefit significantly from coronary artery bypass grafting.

Mock, M. B., Fisher, L. D., Holmes, D. R., Jr., et al.: Comparison of effects of medical and surgical therapy on survival in severe angina pectoris and two-vessel coronary artery disease with and without left ventricular dysfunction: A Coronary Artery Surgery Study Registry Study. Am. J. Cardiol., 61:1198, 1988.

In a group of about 2000 patients in the CASS with double-vessel disease, 1317 were treated with bypass grafting. A definite benefit from surgical intervention was shown in the patients who either had severe left-ventricular dysfunction or severe angina, with one or two proximal stenoses. Six-year survival was 78% in the surgical group and 49% in the medical group.

Murphy, D. J., Murray, A. M., Robinson, B. E., and Campion, E. W.: Outcomes of cardiopulmonary resuscitation in the elderly. Ann. Intern. Med., 111:199, 1989.

This study assessed the results of cardiopulmonary resuscitation in 503 consecutive patients over 70 years of age. Twenty-two per cent survived initially, but only 3.8% were discharged from the hospital. Risk factors for poor outcome were unwitnessed cardiac arrest, terminal arrhythmias such as asystole or electromechanical dissociation, and a cardiopulmonary resuscitation time of more than 15 minutes. Fewer than 1% of patients in these high-risk groups ultimately survive. Patients undergoing cardiopulmonary resuscitation for ventricular arrhythmias with a witnessed arrest had a much greater chance of survival. The study concludes that cardiopulmonary resuscitation for unwitnessed or out-of-hospital cardiac arrest in elderly patients is seldom successful.

Passamani, E., Davis, K. B., Gillespie, M. J., et al.: A randomized trial of coronary artery bypass surgery: Survival of patients with a low ejection fraction. N. Engl. J. Med., 312:1665, 1985.

This study evaluated by randomization the influence of operation on 780 patients with an ejection fraction between 0.34 and 0.5. Seven years later, there was a significant benefit from operation in those with triple-vessel disease. Of the surgical group 88% were alive compared with 65% of the medical group.

Ribakove, G. H., Katz, E. S., Galloway, A. C., et al.: Surgical implications of transesophageal echocardiography to grade the atheromatous aortic arch. Ann. Thorac. Surg., 53:758, 1992.

This study uses intraoperative transesophageal echocardiography to assess atheromatous disease in the aortic arch in 97 high-risk patients undergoing open heart surgery. The mean age was 73 years. Atheromatous disease in the aortic arch was graded according to mobility and protrusion into the lumen. The study found that clinical evaluation of the aorta did not always correlate with echocardiographic grade, yet the incidence of stroke correlates significantly with the echocardiographic assessment of atheromatous grade. Four patients had perioperative strokes, three of whom were found to have grade V lesions on TEE. Four of 10 Grade V TEE patients were treated with hypothermic circulatory arrest and aortic arch débridement, and none suffered strokes. The other six were treated with standard techniques, and three suffered strokes. These results suggest that patients with mobile atheromatous disease in the aortic arch are at high risk for embolic strokes that are not predicted by routine intraoperative clinical evaluation. Selective use of circulatory arrest in the presence of TEE detects mobile arch atheromas and may reduce the risk of intraoperative stroke.

Spencer, F. C.: The internal mammary artery: The ideal coronary bypass graft? [Editorial]. N. Engl. J. Med., 314:50, 1986.

This editorial summarized the sequence of events that led to the performance of the first successful internal mammary artery bypass graft in people in the United States by Green and Tice at New York University in 1968. More than a decade later, after 1980, internal mammary grafts were used in less than 15% of bypass operations done in the United States, but after the demonstration of the serious deterioration of vein grafts between 5 and 10 years after operation, internal mammary artery grafting was widely accepted as indicated in almost all patients having bypass.

Topol, E. J., Califf, R. M., George, B. S., et al.: Insights derived from the thrombolysis and angioplasty in myocardial infarction (TAMI) trials. J. Am. Coll. Cardiol., 12:24-A, 1988.

This report describes experiences with the first three TAMI studies in 708 patients. In general, thrombolysis therapy reopened the thrombosed vessel in almost 80% of patients. With patent vessels, immediate angioplasty had

no advantage over deferred angioplasty. If vessels remained occluded, however, angioplasty was successful in more than 50%. Morbidity was significant, however, because 14 patients developed a stroke, five of which were from intracranial hemorrhage. Bleeding was significant; approximately 30% of the patients required transfusion of at least two units of blood.

Weiner, D. A., Ryan, T. A., McCabe, C. H., et al.: Comparison of coronary artery bypass surgery and medical therapy in patients with exercise-induced silent myocardial ischemia: A report from the coronary artery surgery study (CASS) registry. J. Am. Coll. Cardiol., 12:595, 1988.

Six hundred ninety-two patients were studied, 268 of whom underwent surgical therapy. Definite benefit from operation was found in the group with triple-vessel disease and impaired ventricular function, because the 7-year survival was 90% in the surgical group and only 37% in the medical group.

## BIBLIOGRAPHY

Acar, C., Deloche, A., Guermonprez, J. L., et al.: Revival of the radial artery for coronary bypass grafting. Ann. Thorac. Surg., 54:652–660, 1992.
Allen, B. S., Okamoto, F., Buckberg, G. D., et al.: Immediate functional recovery after six hours of regional ischemia by careful control of conditions of reperfusion and composition of reperfusate. J. Thorac. Cardiovasc. Surg., 92:621–635, 1986.
Allen, B. S., Rosenkranz, E., Buckberg, G. D., et al.: Studies on prolonged acute regional ischemia. VI. Myocardial infarction with left ventricular power failure: A medical/surgical emergency requiring urgent revascularization with maximal protection of remote muscle. J. Thorac. Cardiovasc. Surg., 98:691–703, 1989.
Berg, R., Jr., Selinger, S. L., Leonard, J. L., et al.: Acute evolving myocardial infarction. A surgical emergency. J. Thorac. Cardiovasc. Surg., 88:902–906, 1984.
Beyersdorf, F., Mitrev, Z., Sarai, K., et al.: Changing patterns of patients undergoing emergency surgical revascularization for acute coronary occlusion. Importance of myocardial protection techniques. J. Thorac. Cardiovasc. Surg., 106:137–148, 1993.
Blauth, C. I., Arnold, J. V., Schulenberg, W. E., et al.: Cerebral microembolism during cardiopulmonary bypass: Retinal microvascular studies in vivo with fluorescein angiography. J. Thorac. Cardiovasc. Surg., 95:668–676, 1988.
Blauth, C. I., Cosgrove, D. M., Lytle, B. W., et al.: Atheroembolism from the ascending aorta: An emerging problem in cardiac surgery. J. Thorac. Cardiovasc. Surg., 103:1104–1112, 1992.
Blauth, C. I., Smith, P. L., Arnold, J. V., et al.: Influence of oxygenator type on the prevalence and extent of microembolic retinal ischemia during cardiopulmonary bypass. Assessment by digital image analysis. J. Thorac. Cardiovasc. Surg., 99:61–69, 1990.
Blossom, G. B., Fietsam, R., Jr., Bassett, J. S., et al.: Characteristics of cerebrovascular accidents after coronary artery bypass grafting. Am. Surg., 58:584–589, 1992.
Bourassa, M. G.: Fate of venous grafts: The past, the present and the future [Editorial]. J. Am. Coll. Cardiol., 17:1081–1083, 1991.
Bourassa, M. G., Campeau, L., Lespérance, J., et al.: Atherosclerosis after coronary artery bypass surgery: Results of recent studies and recommendations regarding prevention. Cardiology, 73:259, 1986.
Brenowitz, J. B., Kayser, K. L., and Johnson, W. D.: Results of coronary artery endarterectomy and reconstruction. J. Thorac. Cardiovasc. Surg., 95:1, 1988.
Buche, J., Schoevaerdts, J. C., Louagie, Y., et al.: Use of the inferior epigastric artery for coronary bypass. J. Thorac. Cardiovasc. Surg., 103:665–670, 1992.
Campeau, L., Grondin, C. M., and Bourassa, M. G.: Atherosclerosis and late closure of aortocoronary saphenous vein grafts: Sequential angiographic studies at 2 weeks, 1 year, 5 to 7 years, and 10 to 12 years after surgery. Circulation, 68(Suppl. II):1–7, 1983.
Carter, M. J.: The use of the right gastroepiploic artery in coronary artery bypass grafting. Aust. N. Z. J. Surg., 57:317–321, 1987.
CASS Principal Investigators and Their Associates: Coronary artery surgery study (CASS): A randomized trial of coronary artery bypass surgery: Survival data. Circulation, 68:939, 1983.

Chesebro, J. H., Fuster, V., Elveback, L. R., et al.: Effect of dipyridamole and aspirin on late vein graft patency after coronary bypass operations. N. Engl. J. Med., *310*:209, 1984.

Cobb, L. A., Werner, J. A., and Trobaugh, G. B.: Sudden cardiac death. I: A decade's experience with out-of-hospital resuscitation. Mod. Concepts Cardiovasc. Dis., *49*:31, 1980.

Culliford, A. T., Colvin, S. B., Rohrer, K., et al.: The atherosclerotic ascending aorta and transverse arch: A new technique to prevent cerebral injury during bypass: Experiences with 13 patients. Ann. Thorac. Surg., *41*:27, 1986.

Dunn, F. L. and Morris, P. B.: Dietary and pharmacologic management of atherosclerosis. *In* Sabiston, D. C., Jr., and Spencer F. C. (eds): Surgery of the Chest. 5th ed. Philadelphia, W. B. Saunders, 1990.

European Coronary Surgery Study Group: Prospective randomised study of coronary artery bypass surgery in stable angina pectoris. Second interim report. Lancet, 2:491, 1980.

European Coronary Surgery Study Group: Long-term results of prospective randomised study of coronary artery bypass surgery in stable angina pectoris. Lancet, 2:1173, 1982.

Favaloro, R. G.: The Challenging Dream of Heart Surgery. Cleveland, Cleveland Clinic Foundation, 1992.

Fiore, A. C., Naunheim, K. S., McBride, L. R., et al.: Results of internal thoracic artery grafting over 15 years: Single verses double grafts. Ann. Thorac. Surg., *49*:2102–2109, 1990.

Fitzgibbon, G. M., Leach, A. J., Kafka, H. P., and Keon, W. J.: Coronary bypass graft fate: Long-term angiographic study. J. Am. Coll. Cardiol., *17*:1075–1080, 1991.

Froelicher, V., Jensen, D., and Sullivan, M.: A randomized trial of the effects of exercise training after coronary artery bypass surgery. Arch. Intern. Med., *145*:689, 1985.

Frye, R. L., Fisher, L., Schaff, H. V., et al.: Randomized trial in coronary artery bypass surgery. Prog. Cardiovasc. Dis., *30*:1, 1987.

Galbut, D. L., Traad, E. A., Gentsch, T. O., et al.: Seventeen-year experience with bilateral internal mammary artery grafts. Ann. Thorac. Surg., *49*:195–201, 1990.

Green, G. E., Spencer, F. C., Tice, D. A., and Stertzer, S. H.: Arterial and venous microsurgical bypass grafts for coronary artery disease. J. Thorac. Cardiovasc. Surg., *60*:491, 1970.

Greene, M. A., Gray, L. A., Jr., Slater, D., et al.: Emergency aortocoronary bypass after failed angioplasty. Ann. Thorac. Surg., *51*:194–199, 1991.

Gruentzig, A., Myler, A., Hanna, E. S., and Turina, M.: Transluminal angioplasty of coronary artery stenosis [Abstract]. Circulation, *56*(Part 21):84, 1977.

Guyton, R. A., Arcidi, R. M., Jr., Langford, D. A., et al.: Emergency coronary bypass for cardiogenic shock. Circulation, *76*(Suppl. V):22, 1987.

Henz, T., Stephan, H., and Sonntag, H.: Cerebral dysfunction following extracorporeal circulation for aortocoronary bypass surgery: No differences in neurophychological outcome after pulsatile versus nonpulsatile flow. J. Thorac. Cardiovasc. Surg., *38*:65–68, 1990.

Holmes, D. R., and Davis, K. B.: The effect of medical and surgical treatment on subsequent sudden cardiac death in patients with coronary artery disease: A report from the coronary artery surgery study. Circulation, *73*:1254, 1986.

Isom, O. W., Spencer, F. C., Glassman, E., et al.: Does coronary bypass increase longevity? J. Thorac. Cardiovasc. Surg., *75*:28, 1978.

Johnson, W. D., Flemma, R. J., Lepley, D., Jr., and Ellison, E. H.: Extended treatment of severe coronary artery disease: A total surgical approach. Ann. Surg., *170*:460, 1969.

Jones, E. L., Lattouf, O. M., and Weintraum, W. S.: Catastrophic consequences of internal mammary artery hypoperfusion. J. Thorac. Cardiovasc. Surg., *98*:902–907, 1989.

Katz, E. S., Tunick, P. A., Ribakove, G., et al.: Protruding aortic atheromas predict stroke in elderly patients undergoing cardiopulmonary bypass: Experience with intraoperative transesophageal echocardiography. J. Am. Coll. Cardiol., *20*(1):70–77, 1992.

Kirklin, J. W., and Barratt-Boyes, B. G.: Cardiac Surgery. New York, John Wiley & Sons, 1986.

Kirklin, J. W., and Barratt-Boyes, B. G.: Cardiac Surgery: Morphology, Diagnostic Criteria, Natural History, Techniques, Results, and Indications. 2nd ed. New York, Churchill Livingstone, 1993.

Leape, L. L., Hilborne, L. H., Park, R. E., et al.: The appropriateness of use of coronary artery bypass graft surgery in New York State. J. A. M. A., *269*:753–760, 1993.

Loop, F. D., Lytle, B. W., Cosgrove, D. M., et al.: Free (aortocoronary) internal mammary artery graft. Late results. J. Thorac. Cardiovasc. Surg., *92*:827–831, 1986a.

Loop, F. D., Lytle, B., Cosgrove, D. M., et al.: Influence of internal mammary artery grafts on 10 year survival and other cardiac events. N. Engl. J. Med., *314*:1, 1986b.

Loop, F. D., Lytle, B. W., Cosgrove, D. M., et al.: Sternal wound complications artery bypass grafting: Early and late mortality, morbidity, and cost of care. Ann. Thorac. Surg., *49*:179–187, 1990.

Lytle, B. W., Cosgrove, D. M., Loop, F. D., et al.: Perioperative risk of bilateral internal mammary artery grafting: Analysis of 500 cases 1971 to 1984. Circulation, *74*(Suppl. 3):37, 1986.

Lytle, B. W., Loop, F. D., Cosgrove, D. M., et al.: Long-term (5–12 years) serial studies of internal mammary artery and saphenous vein coronary bypass grafts. J. Thorac. Cardiovasc. Surg., *89*:248–258, 1985.

Lytle, B. W., Loop, F. D., Cosgrove, D. M., et al.: Fifteen hundred coronary reoperations. Results and determinants of early and late survival. J. Thorac. Cardiovasc. Surg., *93*:847–859, 1987.

Milano, C. A., White, W. D., Smith, L. R., et al.: Coronary artery bypass in patients with severely depressed ventricular function. Ann. Thorac. Surg., *56*:487–493, 1993.

Milgalter, E., Laks, H., Elami, A., et al.: Preoperative duplex scan assessment of the inferior epigastric artery as a coronary bypass conduit. Ann. Thorac. Surg., *52*:567–568, 1991.

Mills, N. L., and Everson, C. T.: Technique for use of the inferior epigastric artery as a coronary bypass graft. Ann. Thorac. Surg., *51*:208–214, 1991.

Mills, N. L., Dupin, C. L., Everson, C. T., and Leger, C. L.: The subscapular artery: An alternative conduit for coronary bypass. J. Card. Surg., *8*:66–71, 1993.

Mock, M. B., Ringqvist, I., Fisher, L. D., et al.: Survival of medically treated patients in the Coronary Artery Surgery Study (CASS) Registry. Circulation, *66*:562, 1982.

Mullany, C. J., Darling, G. E., Pluth, J. R., et al.: Early and late results after isolated coronary artery bypass surgery in 159 patients aged 80 years and older. Circulation, *82*(Suppl. IV):229–236, 1990.

Murphy, D. J., and Murray, A. M.: Outcomes of cardiopulmonary resuscitation in the elderly. Ann. Intern. Med., *111*:199–205, 1989.

Naef, A. P.: The story of thoracic surgery. Toronto, Hogrefe and Huber, 1990.

Ochsner, J. L., Mills, N. L., and Béthea, M. C.: Operative technique of myocardial revascularization. World J. Surg., 2:767, 1978.

Olearchyk, A. S.: Coronary revascularization: Past, present and future. JUMANA (J. Ukr. Med. Assoc. North Am.), *35*:3, 1988.

Parish, M. A., Asai, T., Grossi, E. A., et al.: The effects of different techniques of internal mammary artery harvesting on sternal blood flow. J. Thorac. Cardiovasc. Surg., *104*:1303–1307, 1992.

Passamani, E., Davis, K. B., Gillespie, M. J., et al.: A randomized trial of coronary artery bypass surgery: Survival of patients with a low ejection fraction. N. Engl. J. Med., *312*:1665, 1985.

Prieto, I., Basile, F., and Abdulnour, E.: Upper extremity vein graft for aortocoronary bypass. Ann. Thorac. Surg., *37*:221, 1984.

Pym, J., Brown, P. M., Charrette, E. J., et al.: Gastroepiploic-coronary anastomosis. A viable alternative bypass graft. J. Thorac. Cardiovasc. Surg., *94*:256–259, 1987.

Rahimtoola, S., Fessler, C. L., Grunkemeier, G. L., and Starr, A.: Survival 15 to 20 years after coronary artery bypass for angina. J. Am. Coll. Cardiol., *21*:151–157, 1993.

Read, R. C., Murphy, M. L., Hultgren, H. N., and Takaro, T.: Survival of men treated for chronic stable angina pectoris: A cooperative randomized study. J. Thorac. Cardiovasc. Surg., *75*:1, 1978.

Ribakove, G. H., Galloway, A. C., Kronzon, I., et al.: Surgical implications of transesophageal echocardiography to grade the atheromatous aortic arch. Ann. Thorac. Surg., *53*:758–763, 1992.

Ribakove, G. H., Katz, E. S., Galloway, A. C., et al.: Surgical implications of transesophageal echocardiography to grade the atheromatous aostic arch. Ann Thorac. Surg., 53:758, 1992.

RITA Trial Participants: Coronary angioplasty versus coronary artery bypass surgery: The randomised intervention treatment of angina (RITA) trial. Lancet, 341:573–580, 1993.

Rizzo, R. J., Whittemore, A. D., Couper, G. S., et al.: Combined carotid and coronary revascularization: The preferred approach to the severe vasculopath. Ann. Thorac. Surg., 54:1099, 1992.

Roberts, W. C.: Diffuse extent of coronary atherosclerosis in fatal coronary artery disease. Am. J. Cardiol., 65:2F–6F, 1990.

Sabiston, D. C., Jr.: The coronary circulation. William F. Rienhoff, Jr. lecture. Johns Hopkins Med. J., 134:314, 1974.

Sabiston, D. C., Jr., and Spencer, F. C.: Surgery of the Chest. 5th ed. Philadelphia, W. B. Saunders, 1990.

Sellman, N., Ivert, T., Wahlgreen, N. G., et al.: Early neurological and electroencephalographic changes after coronary artery surgery in low-risk patients younger than 70 years. J. Thorac. Cardiovasc. Surg., 39:76–80, 1991.

Sempos, C. T., Cleeman, J. I., Carroll, N. D., et al.: Prevalence of high blood cholesterol among US adults. An update based on guidelines from the second report of the national cholesterol education program adult treatment panel. J. A. M. A., 269:3009–3014, 1993.

Spencer, F. C.: Binocular loupes (microtelescopes) for coronary artery surgery. J. Thorac. Cardiovasc. Surg., 62:163, 1971.

Spencer, F. C.: The internal mammary artery: The ideal coronary bypass graft? [Editorial]. N. Engl. J. Med., 314:50–51, 1986.

Stamler, J.: Dietary and serum lipids in the multifactorial etiology of atherosclerosis. Arch. Surg., 113:21, 1978.

Stoney, W. S., Alford, W. C., Jr., Thomas, C. S., Jr., et al.: The fate of arm veins used for aorto-coronary bypass grafts. J. Thorac. Cardiovasc. Surg., 88:522–526, 1984.

Suma, H., Fukumoto, H., and Takeuchi, A.: Coronary artery bypass grafting by utilizing in situ right gastroepiploic artery: Basic study and clinical application. Ann. Thorac. Surg., 44:394–397, 1987.

Suma, H., Wanibuchi, Y., Terada, Y., et al.: The right gastroepiploic artery graft: Clinical and angiographic midterm results in 200 patients. J. Thorac. Cardiovasc. Surg., 105:615–623, 1993.

Topol, E. J., Califf, R. M., George, B. S., et al.: Insights derived from the thrombolysis and angioplasty in myocardial infarction (TAMI) trials. J. Am. Coll. Cardiol., 12:24A, 1988.

Townes, B. D., Bashein, G., Hornbein, T. F., et al.: Neurobehavioral outcomes in operations. A prospective controlled study. J. Thorac. Cardiovasc. Surg., 98:774–782, 1989.

Tsai, T. P., Nessim, S., Kass, R. M., et al.: Morbidity and mortality after coronary artery bypass in octogenarians. Ann. Thorac. Surg., 51:983–986, 1991.

Tunick, P. A., and Kronzon, I.: Protruding atheromas in the thoracic aorta: A newly recognized source of cerebral and systemic embolization. Echocardiography, 10(4):419–428, 1993.

Uppal, R., Mills, N. L., Wechsler, A. S., Smith, P. K: 1985: Left thoracotomy for reoperative coronary artery bypass procedures: 1993 update. Ann. Thorac. Surg., 55:1275–1276, 1993.

U. S. Department of Health, Education and Welfare: Proceedings of the Conference on the Decline in Coronary Heart Disease Mortality. NIH Publication 79–1610. Washington, D.C., U. S. Government Printing Office, May 1979.

Wareing, T. H., Kouchoukos, N. T., et al.: Management of the severely atherosclerotic ascending aorta during cardiac operation. J. Thorac. Cardiovasc. Surg., 103:453–462, 1992.

Weintraub, W. S., Craver, J. M., Cohen, C. L., et al.: Influence of age on results of coronary artery surgery. Circulation, 84(Suppl. III):226–235, 1991.

Wijnberg, D. S., Boeve, W. J., van der Heide, J. N. H., et al.: Patency of arm vein grafts used in aorto-coronary bypass surgery. Eur. J. Cardiothorac. Surg., 4:510–513, 1990.

# 2  Utilization of Autologous Arterial Grafts for Coronary Artery Bypass

J. Scott Rankin and James J. Morris

Over a quarter of a century after its general clinical introduction, coronary artery bypass is well established as one of the most effective operations in history. In 1991, over 400,000 coronary revascularizations were performed in the United States alone, and the procedure has been definitively shown to improve long-term survival and well-being in virtually all categories of coronary artery disease (Califf et al., 1989; Muhlbaier et al., 1992). Perhaps even more interesting is the fact that operative techniques are still evolving rapidly, and clinical results continue to improve, despite worsening of average patient characteristics (Jones et al., 1991; Pryor et al., 1987).

The most significant operative modification in recent years is the general acceptance of routine *internal mammary artery* (IMA) grafting. This trend was initiated in the early 1980s through several new insights. First, it became clear that long-term patency of IMA grafts was superior to that of venous conduits. Second, several studies observed improved clinical re-

sults in patients undergoing IMA operations. Third, multiple new methods emerged to expand the general applicability of arterial grafting to most anatomic situations, including early data documenting the efficacy of *gastroepiploic artery* (GEA) grafts (Suma et al., 1993).

Few would question that this trend has improved the clinical outlook of surgically treated patients. However, several controversies remain, such as the extent to which arterial grafts should be employed. It is now generally agreed that a single left IMA graft is the minimal acceptable procedure in routine practice. However, some authors suggest that multiple IMA or all arterial graft procedures should be performed more frequently and that clinical results will be further enhanced by this policy. The purpose of this section is to review the development and current understanding of autologous arterial grafts as conduits for coronary revascularization, to provide a detailed description of standardized operative techniques, and to assess recent clinical results of arterial grafting procedures with specific reference to the indications for multiple arterial conduit operations.

## HISTORICAL DEVELOPMENT

As with most aspects of cardiovascular surgery, arterial bypass of the coronary circulation was first performed experimentally by Alexis Carrel (Carrel, 1910). A free graft of carotid artery was interposed between the descending thoracic aorta and the left coronary artery in the dog using vascular anastomotic techniques, but the animal died of ventricular fibrillation. Although limitations in circulatory support precluded success at that time, Carrel clearly understood the clinical implications of such a procedure. As early as the 1940s, Murray experimented with coronary suture anastomosis (Murray, 1940) and in 1954 reported successful coronary bypass in dogs using both in situ subclavian and free carotid arteries (Murray et al., 1954). Two papers describing experimental IMA to coronary bypass were published in 1956 (Absolon et al., 1956; Thal et al., 1956), and a succession of animal studies followed (Baker and Grindley, 1959; Ballinger et al., 1964; Hall et al., 1961; Julian et al., 1957; Mamiya et al., 1961; Moore and Riberi, 1958).

In pioneering experiments published in 1964, Spencer and co-workers combined microsurgical anastomotic techniques with cardiopulmonary bypass and hypothermic cardiac arrest in dogs to achieve a controlled operative field and excellent long-term patency of IMA-coronary grafts (Spencer et al., 1964). In 1967, Kolessov from the Soviet Union reported six clinical cases of IMA bypass performed without coronary angiography or cardiopulmonary bypass (Kolessov, 1967). However, Green and associates should be credited with initiating the first modern clinical series of left IMA grafts to the left anterior descending (LAD) in 1968 with documented excellent postoperative patency (Green et al., 1968, 1970). Loop (Loop et al., 1973, 1986) and Barner (1973) later advocated the use of free IMA conduits; subsequently, bilateral and sequential IMA techniques were described (Barner et al., 1985; Galbut et al., 1985; Harjola et al., 1984; Kabbani et al., 1983; Kamath et al., 1985; Lytle et al., 1983; McBride and Barner, 1983; Orszulak et al., 1986; Schimert et al., 1975; Tector et al., 1986).

With the overwhelming rise in popularity of saphenous vein grafts in the early 1970s, the more complicated and technically demanding IMA bypass never emerged as a routine procedure, with a few notable exceptions (Barner et al., 1982; Hutchinson et al., 1974; Loop et al., 1977; Tector et al., 1976). However, increasing knowledge of limitations in long-term vein graft patency (Bourassa et al., 1986), together with several studies demonstrating excellent IMA performance, dramatically changed the situation. By 1983, it became clear that IMA grafts should be used routinely, and this concept has been largely accepted by the medical community. More recently, GEA grafts have become routine clinical practice (Lytle et al., 1989; Mills et al., 1989b; Suma et al., 1991, 1993), and newer types of arterial conduits, such as the *inferior epigastric artery* (IEA) and the radial artery, are being evaluated (Acar et al., 1992; Barner et al., 1991; Buche et al., 1992; Milgalter et al., 1992).

## GRAFT PATENCY

The long-term patency of IMA grafts in the coronary position has been firmly established to be superior to that of venous conduits (Barner et al., 1982; Geha and Baue, 1979; Grondin et al., 1984; Jones et al., 1980; Lytle et al., 1985; Okies et al., 1984; Siegel and Loop, 1976; Singh et al., 1983; Tector et al., 1976, 1983). In most studies, early IMA patency rates approximated 95%; more important, 10-year functional patency rates approached 90%, compared with 25 to 50% for vein grafts. The propensity for saphenous veins to develop late postoperative graft atherosclerosis was largely responsible for this difference, whereas IMAs remained relatively free of disease. Although most long-term patency studies were performed in patients with recurrent symptoms or in highly selected subgroups, the observed superiority of IMA grafts was so significant and consistent that the principle of better IMA patency appears to be correct. More recent studies have confirmed early patency rates in excess of 95% for more complex forms of IMA grafting, including right IMA grafts, sequential IMAs, and free IMA grafting (Rankin et al., 1986).

Patency characteristics of other forms of arterial grafts are less well defined. The best studied at present is the GEA, which has been used primarily to bypass the right coronary system as an in situ pedicle graft. In Suma's study, the angiographic patency rate in 152 grafts at 2 months was 95% and in 40 grafts, studied at 2 years, was also 95% (Suma et al., 1993). Clinical symptomatic status and scintigraphic perfusion were correspondingly enhanced. Although late studies will be important, early data are good enough to justify the GEA for routine clinical use.

Insufficient data are available on the long-term patency of IEA grafts, but early studies are encouraging. Of course, IEA conduits are always used as free grafts from the aorta, and because of short length and inadequate late patency data, the IEA has been used primarily to graft proximal, less important coronary arteries. Available studies suggest that the early patency rate will exceed 90% (Barner et al., 1991; Buche et al., 1992), but more data are needed. Nevertheless, one can be justified at present in using the IEA in limited-conduit situations (Louagie et al., 1992). As more patency data accrue, the IEA may become more generally applicable. Finally, a reassessment of free radial artery grafts suggests that intraoperative and postoperative administration of diltiazem may prevent the postoperative spasm that has characterized previous studies of this conduit (Acar et al., 1992). Although it may be prudent to defer use of the radial artery until more data are available, the excellent technical characteristics of this graft make it an attractive potential alternative if this observation can be confirmed.

The biologic explanation for superior arterial graft performance is not entirely clear. An arterial graft more closely approximates the diameter of the coronary artery; for an equivalent flow volume, blood velocity is greater than for vein grafts, which may reduce stasis. Similarly, vascular turbulence may be lower because transitional differences in graft to coronary geometry are negligible and because arterial grafts have no varicosities or valves. The elastic and collagen support of the arterial wall is suited to arterial pressures that may be injurious to vein graft structure (Barbour and Roberts, 1984; Kalan and Roberts, 1987).

The incidence of atherosclerosis in the native IMA is low (Kay et al., 1976; Singh, 1983), and, perhaps most important, the IMA is a living graft (Singh et al., 1986). Thin-walled visceral arteries, such as the IMA, have few vasa vasorum in the arterial wall and receive the majority of their nutrition from luminal diffusion (Landymore and Chapman, 1987). Thus, the biologic processes of the vessel remain intact after grafting, even when used as a free graft (Loop et al., 1986). A list of potentially vital vascular mechanisms includes intact vasomotor activity, the capacity to enlarge with increasing flow demands, and an intact endothelium, producing prostacyclin compounds, nitric oxide, fibrinolysins, or as yet undefined substances (Buikema et al., 1992; Chaikhouni et al., 1986; Dobrin, 1984; Pearson et al., 1992; Singh et al., 1986; von Son et al., 1990; Werner et al., 1990). Each of these factors, individually or in combination, may contribute to the excellent long-term patency of arterial conduits.

## INDICATIONS FOR ARTERIAL BYPASS GRAFTING

In early series, a common indication for employing arterial grafts was the absence of suitable saphenous veins. Arterial conduits have been demonstrated for some time to be superior to other alternatives, such as cephalic veins (Prieto et al., 1984), venous allografts (Gelbfish et al., 1986), cryopreserved bovine IMAs (Mitchell et al., 1993), cryopreserved vein grafts (Laub et al., 1992), and synthetic materials (Sapsford et al., 1981). As long-term patency data became available and the use of arterial grafts increased, several other considerations became apparent. Young adults with coronary artery disease, almost by definition, have an accelerated atherogenic diathesis and are especially prone to early vein graft failure. In the Cleveland Clinic study (Lytle et al., 1984), which examined patients undergoing coronary bypass at age 35 years or younger, 4-year vein graft patency was only 56%, as compared with 93% for IMAs. Persistent smoking, hyperlipemia, diabetes, and a family history of coronary artery disease all negatively influenced long-term survival. Thus, it is increasingly apparent that arterial grafts should be used maximally in younger

patients, both because vein grafts are more susceptible to early failure and because a longer-term result is desired. This trend has led to increasing application of all-arterial conduit operations in this population, especially in the presence of refractory hyperlipidemia (Lemma et al., 1991; Ramstrom et al., 1990; Suma et al., 1989; Takahashi et al., 1992). Young patients may be one group in which a late (10 to 20 years) prognosis is improved by multiple arterial grafts (Cosgrove et al., in press).

Diabetes mellitus is a significant risk factor influencing the late results of coronary revascularization. Perioperative mortality and complications such as sternal infections and strokes are significantly more frequent in diabetics, but diabetes and reduced long-term survival also are independently associated (Morris et al., 1991; Salomon et al., 1983). After 5 to 10 years, the survival of diabetic patients is 15 to 20% lower than that of nondiabetics, and the quality of survival is significantly worse, despite similarities in other baseline characteristics. This suboptimal prognosis is at least partially due to accelerated atherosclerosis, both in native vessels and in vein grafts. Use of arterial grafts, which enhances long-term patency, has been shown to improve prognosis in diabetics (Morris et al., 1991), and at least a single IMA should be standard policy for coronary revascularization among this population.

In patients undergoing reoperation for vein graft failure, every effort should be made to employ arterial conduits (Galbut et al., 1991; Lytle et al., 1987). Because these patients already have experienced a negative result with venous grafts, reutilization of primarily venous material appears illogical. IMA grafts have reduced the subsequent need for reoperation (Cosgrove et al., 1986), so that employing arterial conduits in reoperative cases may significantly lessen the likelihood of eventual third or fourth procedures.

Difficult anatomic situations, such as limited graft material, poor-quality saphenous veins in the elderly, small coronary vessels in females, or diffusely diseased but important coronary arteries, may meet with better patency and overall clinical success with arterial grafts (Louagie et al., 1992; Olearchyk and Magovern, 1986). In patients with severe ascending aortic calcification, or in Type I aortic dissections with associated coronary disease, proximal vein graft anastomoses often are precluded. Arterial grafts expand the versatility with which each of these difficult problems can be managed (Peigh et al., 1991; Suma et al., 1989).

As most surgeons have become increasingly comfortable with arterial grafting, unstable angina, reoperations, severe left ventricular dysfunction, and advanced age no longer contraindicate the use of IMA, although ensuring adequate graft function in critical situations is crucial (Azariades et al., 1990; Galbut et al., 1991; Gardner et al., 1990; Rankin et al., 1985, 1986; Wareing et al., 1990). Acute evolving myocardial infarction requiring emergency surgical revascularization also is not a uniform contraindication to IMA grafting, and up to 90% of patients in some series have had arterial grafts (Morris et al., 1990). If a perfusion balloon catheter has been placed, the operation can be approached in a stable manner, and arterial grafts can be constructed. A single IMA graft can be employed even without a perfusion catheter if the patient is otherwise stable, because IMA dissection adds only an extra 10 to 15 minutes to the ischemic period. With extreme hemodynamic compromise, however, more rapid revascularization with saphenous vein grafts can be prudent. Finally, children requiring coronary bypass for Kawasaki's disease appear especially prone to late vein graft occlusion; IMA conduits function better in these patients and even enlarge with time in proportion to the child's growth (Hirose et al., 1986; Kawachi et al., 1991; Kitamura et al., 1987).

Arterial conduits are rarely inferior to vein grafts in achieving better patency and improved long-term results. For this reason, at least one arterial graft, usually the left IMA to the LAD, is attempted in virtually every patient undergoing coronary revascularization. Practically, a small percentage of IMAs have inadequate flow capacity and length, but at least one arterial graft can be constructed in over 95% of patients (Morris et al., 1990; Rankin et al., 1986). For multiple IMA or all arterial graft operations, the additional clinical benefits of performing a second or third arterial conduit need to be considered. Patients with inadequate venous conduit are clearly candidates, as are younger patients or those with ascending aortic disease, as described above. However, further long-term analysis of early risks versus long-term benefits will be required to establish fully the propriety of routine multiple arterial grafting procedures in other subsets of the coronary disease population. In general, a trend toward moderation in the use of multiple arterial procedures has characterized the past 5 years. This topic is discussed in more detail in later sections.

## PITFALLS OF MAMMARY GRAFTING

Several problems peculiar to IMA grafting deserve special emphasis. The most important is operative recognition of the "inadequate mammary graft." Use of an IMA with inadequate flow for bypass of a critically jeopardized and important coronary artery may cause perioperative myocardial infarction and circulatory failure. If an IMA graft is suspected to be inadequate at the conclusion of cardiopulmonary bypass, the preferred approach is to rearrest the heart and to construct a distal vein graft to the coronary artery in question. It should be emphasized, however, that routine operative testing of IMA grafts, including quantitative flow capacity measurement, virtually eliminates this problem (Jones et al., 1989; Rankin et al., 1986).

Causes for inadequate IMA grafts include intimal flaps or wall dissection secondary to operative injury, arterial spasm, unrecognized subclavian artery stenosis, anomalous arterial origins, intrinsic atherosclerotic obstruction, and occlusion of the subclavian artery by the intra-aortic balloon pump. Significantly,

each of these problems can be identified by routine IMA flow capacity testing and thereby can be avoided. IMA occlusion by an intimal flap or spasm usually reflects operative trauma and can be prevented by more gentle handling of the IMA pedicle during chest wall dissection. The incidence of IMA injury diminishes with operator experience, but injury can occur even in the most experienced hands. Thus, routine flow testing should be an integral part of IMA procedures.

With either subclavian stenosis or intrinsic atherosclerotic disease, the IMA can still be used as a free graft if segments are sufficiently long. Subclavian stenosis developing late postoperatively can lead to the "coronary steal syndrome," which is readily managed with subclavian bypass or balloon angioplasty. Finally, if the IMA is not properly positioned, it can be tented up and become obstructed by expansion of the upper lobe of the lung. Strict attention to suturing the IMA in a lateral mediastinal position, parallel to the phrenic nerve and medial to the upper lobe of the lung, will prevent this complication.

## OPERATIVE TECHNIQUE

As the sternotomy is performed, intravenous heparin is administered, so that blood shed during IMA dissection may be returned to the oxygenator. With exposure provided by a Favaloro retractor, the IMA is transected at the level of the xyphoid, and the distal branch is controlled with a metal clip. Early transection of the IMA helps identify the vessel and prevents the forceful retraction and damage that can occur when the vessel is left as a sling. Narrow mammary pedicles are dissected from the chest wall, primarily using low-energy electrocautery and working toward the apex of the chest. Excessive cauterization of the chest wall and intercostal nerves is avoided to lessen the incidence of a chronic chest wall dysesthesia syndrome. Care is taken to retract the mammary artery gently and to divide the small branches at some distance from the main IMA. In the superior aspect of the dissection, the IMA pedicle is left attached medially to the thymus to prevent phrenic nerve injury, but the graft is dissected completely from the chest wall anteriorly and laterally to the level of the subclavian vein. All proximal branches are divided to prevent competitive flow. Above the level of the inferior thymus, sharp dissection and metallic clips are employed rather than electrocautery to prevent electrical injury to the phrenic or recurrent laryngeal nerves, both of which can lie close to the IMA at the apex. After topical infiltration of papaverine solution by forceful spraying with a 25-gauge needle, the pedicle is wrapped with a papaverine-soaked sponge and placed in the pleural space while cardiopulmonary bypass is instituted.

As systemic cooling is begun, the locations of the distal coronary anastomoses are identified, the thymic fat pads are excised, and the pericardial edges are divided laterally with scissors to within 2 cm of the phrenic nerves. Proximal dissection of the IMA pedicles and the lateral pericardial incisions allows the grafts to lie along the lateral mediastinum, adjacent to the phrenic nerve and medial to the lung. This course provides the shortest distance to the heart, prevents stretching of the graft by lung inflation, and may lessen the likelihood of IMA injury if reoperation is required (Baillot et al., 1985). The distance to the coronary anastomotic site is measured, allowing a gentle curve of the pedicle without tension. If extra IMA length is needed, the mammary vein and medial thymic attachments are divided, again using sharp technique. Occasionally, the endothoracic fascia and adjacent pedicle tissue are incised transversely at multiple levels to attain extra length (Cosgrove and Loop, 1985). After determining the necessary graft length and finalizing the anastomotic plan, the mammary artery is marked at the appropriate level with methylene blue.

The IMA pedicle then is transected a few millimeters beyond the planned anastomotic site, and free flow from the papaverine-dilated IMA is measured on cardiopulmonary bypass by allowing the artery to bleed into a 50-ml syringe for 20 to 30 seconds. IMA flow ranges from 50 to 250 ml/min at a mean arterial pressure of 60 mm Hg and can be used to estimate the "flow capacity" of the graft. A flow rate of 50 ml/min is acceptable for small coronary vessels, but flows approaching 100 ml/min or greater are required for large LAD arteries or sequential grafts. Some authors prefer intraluminal distension of the IMA with a papaverine solution (Mills et al., 1989a), which improves acute flow, but intimal damage from luminal instrumentation with metallic dilators should be avoided. If a free IMA graft is planned, flow is still measured in situ before disconnecting the graft to assure adequate function. If a question of free IMA adequacy remains, the proximal aortic anastomosis can be performed first, and flow can be measured in the eventual anatomic position. To a certain extent, the flow rate is evaluated relative to the coronary vessel being grafted; a small IMA with a flow of 50 ml/min would be acceptable for a woman with a small LAD but inadequate for larger coronary arteries. If measured flow seems marginal, the IMA is discarded or used to graft a secondary vessel, such as a diagonal. With satisfactory harvesting techniques and papaverine infiltration, however, IMA performance should be adequate for the primary vessel in approximately 95% of patients.

After cardioplegic arrest, a 3- to 4-mm coronary arteriotomy is performed, and the IMA pedicle is transected cleanly at the predetermined level. The interior of the IMA orifice is inspected, and if a small branch that may cause bleeding is visualized, the artery is transected again proximal to the branch. For large, thick-walled, or calcified coronary arteries such as the proximal LAD or RCA, a small ellipse is removed from the arterial wall. After turning the mammary pedicle 180 degrees so that the pleura lies away from the epicardium, the IMA is beveled on its undersurface for 2 to 3 mm. Care is taken not to strip the

pedicle tissue from around the artery or to touch the arterial wall with instruments.

The pedicle is grasped by the assistant (Fig. 54–67), and the suture line is begun on the side opposite the surgeon, with 7-0 or 8-0 polypropylene suture and an 8- to 12-suture running technique. After the heel sutures are placed, the anastomosis is tightened and the toe sutures are completed. The most important IMA (usually to the LAD) is constructed as the last graft, the clamp on the IMA is released, and the suture is tied as flow is established into the coronary artery. The myocardium should warm rapidly, become pink, and begin contracting within 30 seconds. When this does not occur, an anastomotic error or other problem must be considered and the suture line possibly revised. Other factors to be considered include unsuspected distal coronary occlusive disease or inadequate IMA performance relative to flow requirements.

If such a problem is suspected, the coronary artery is explored more carefully with calibrated probes, and then a different grafting site is chosen or a vein graft inserted. Having the myocardium of the grafted region begin beating with flow through only the most

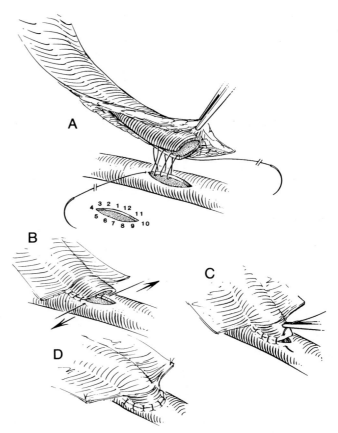

**FIGURE 54–67.** Technique of end-to-side internal mammary artery (IMA)–coronary anastomosis. A–D, Stitches 1–6 are placed with the IMA elevated off the coronary artery. The assistant grasps the pedicle with a forceps in the right hand and controls the suture loops with a forceps in the left hand. After stitch 6, the suture line is tightened, and the remaining toe sutures are placed. For smaller coronary arteries, the IMA is bevelled less, and 10 stitches (omitting 3 and 5) or 8 stitches (omitting 3, 5, 9, and 11) are employed. See text for details.

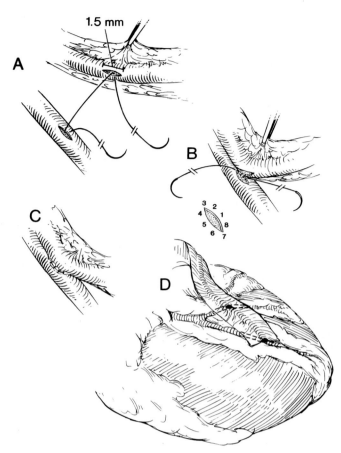

**FIGURE 54–68.** *A–D,* Technique for sequential IMA-coronary grafting. See text for details.

important IMA is an *absolute final requirement* that prevents the disastrous consequences of constructing an inadequate bypass to a critical vessel such as the LAD (Rankin et al., 1986).

Sequential IMA grafting (Fig. 54–68) is most often employed with the diagonal-LAD combination but is satisfactory for multiple vessels in the circumflex or right systems as well. A good-sized IMA with a mea-

sured flow exceeding 100 ml/min is required for sequential grafting, as is ample pedicle length to reach the distal vessel without tension. After both coronary arteries are opened and the suitability for sequential grafting is determined, the distance from the proximal to the distal IMA anastomotic site is defined as the intercoronary distance plus 1 cm. To perform the side-to-side anastomosis, the underside (chest wall side) of the IMA is carefully freed of adventitia and opened with a microsurgical knife.

With microsurgical scissors, short (1.5 to 2.0 mm) longitudinal arteriotomies are performed in both the IMA and the coronary artery; each opening tends to stretch during the anastomosis. An eight-suture running technique is employed with 8-0 polypropylene suture, beginning on the side opposite the surgeon and proceeding counterclockwise. The distal anastomosis of the pedicle is then completed in an end-to-side manner, and the graft is opened. A parallel technique is used for diagonal-LAD combinations, but for circumflex sequentials, both proximal and distal anastomoses are turned 90 degrees. The pedicle is sutured carefully to the epicardium proximally and distally to prevent torsion or kinking around the anastomotic sites. As the final step before cardiopulmonary bypass is discontinued, the IMA pedicles, the anastomoses, and especially the tips of the pedicles are inspected for bleeding, and any obvious branches are clipped. When the lungs are first inflated, care is taken to position the IMA pedicles medial to the upper lobes.

Three general types of IMA grafts are performed. Using the *in situ left IMA* (LIMA) (Fig. 54–69), single or as many as three sequential anastomoses can be constructed to the LAD or circumflex systems. Most sequential grafts have two distal anastomoses, and for a rare triple sequential, one would require good coronary vessels and a very good IMA with high flow. The *in situ right IMA* (RIMA) (Fig. 54–70) is anastomosed as a simple graft to the LAD, to the right (RCA) or posterior descending (PD) coronary arteries and, less commonly, to the high circumflex marginal artery (CMA) over the top of the pulmonary

## In Situ Left Mammary Grafting

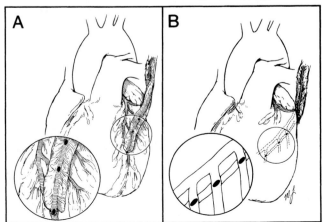

**FIGURE 54–69.** *A* and *B,* Methods of in situ left IMA grafting.

## In Situ Right Mammary Grafting

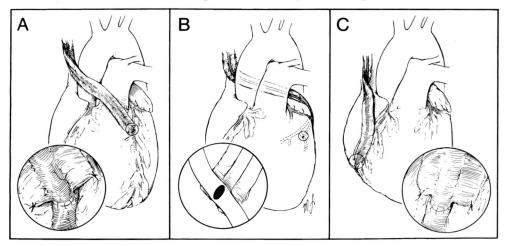

**FIGURE 54–70.** *A–C,* Techniques of in situ right IMA grafting.

artery. With adequate mobilization of the RIMA pedicle, the PD can be reached in most patients. Occasionally, a pledget-supported traction suture between the right atrioventricular groove and right lateral aorta is required to maintain a RIMA-PD graft without tension as the right atrium expands with filling. If the RIMA is grafted to the LAD, the thymus is mobilized as a pedicle and used to cover the RIMA as it crosses the midline at the conclusion of the procedure. This maneuver lessens the chance of RIMA injury if repeat sternotomy is required. *Free IMA* grafts (Fig. 54–71) with either simple or sequential distal anastomoses can be constructed to all three coronary systems. The proximal aortic anastomosis of free IMA grafts is accomplished using a method similar to that of vein grafts (Fig. 54–72), except that 7-0 polypropylene suture is employed and only a 2.5- to 3.0-mm circular aortotomy is performed. Obviously, a soft, nondiseased aorta is desirable for this delicate anastomosis. Representative arteriographic appearances of the various types of IMA grafts are illustrated in Figure 54–

73. RIMA grafts to the CMA via the transverse sinus (Puig et al., 1984) have been discontinued because of their propensity for retroaortic compression (Rankin et al., 1986).

The right GEA is harvested by extending the median sternotomy incision into the upper abdominal midline. The artery is identified along the greater curvature of the stomach and divided 10 to 15 cm to the left of the pylorus. With metallic chips used to control branches, the GEA is dissected as a pedicle from the greater curvature of the stomach to its origin. The artery is then soaked in papaverine, and after initiation of cardiopulmonary bypass, graft flow capacity is tested, similar to the IMA. After the grafting site on the right coronary artery system is selected, a hole is made in the central aspect of the diaphragm, and the GEA pedicle is brought anterior to the left hepatic lobe near the right coronary artery. Under cardioplegic arrest, the GEA is anastomosed to the coronary, using a technique similar to that for the IMA (see Fig. 54–67). The pedicle is sutured to the

## Free Mammary Grafting

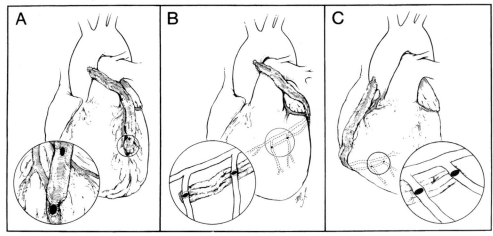

**FIGURE 54–71.** *A–C,* Methods of free IMA grafting.

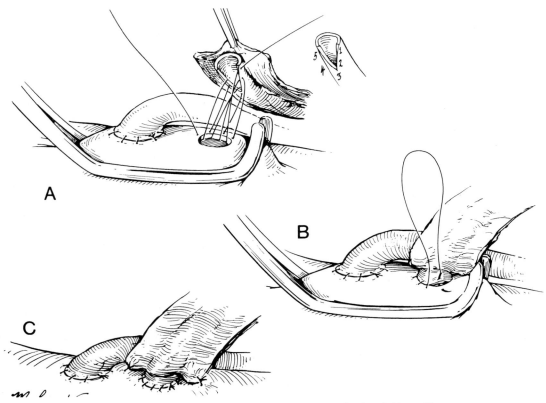

**FIGURE 54–72.** *A–C,* Proximal aortic anastomosis for free IMA grafting.

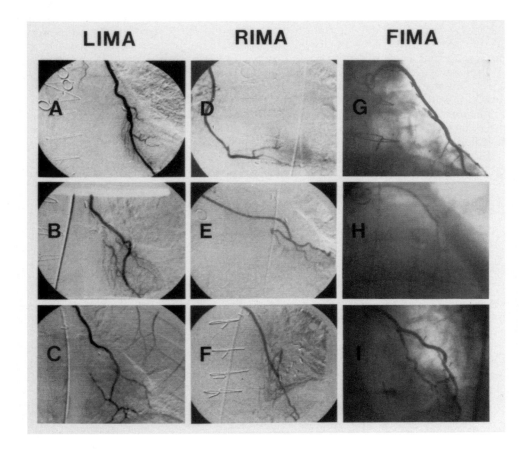

**FIGURE 54–73.** Radiographic images of IMA grafts. *A–F,* Images obtained with digital subtraction angiography. *G* and *I,* Frames from standard selective arteriograms; *H,* An unsubtracted digital arteriogram. *A,* Simple left IMA (LIMA) to LAD. *B,* Sequential LIMA to diagonal/LAD. *C,* Sequential LIMA to the first and second circumflex marginal arteries. *D,* Right IMA (RIMA) to RCA. *E,* RIMA to circumflex marginal artery. *F,* RIMA to LAD. *G,* Free IMA (FIMA) to LAD. *H,* FIMA to circumflex marginal artery. *I,* Sequential FIMA to the first and second circumflex marginal arteries.

epicardium and diaphragm to prevent torsion; the final position is illustrated in Figure 54–74. The comfort in using this graft increases proportionally with user experience. The incidence of abdominal and other complications has been quite low (Suma et al., 1993), and the GEA is now established as a routine alternative for arterial grafting.

The IEA is harvested from the rectus sheath through lower abdominal midline or paramedian incisions. The artery is fragile and requires careful technique during dissection. One or both IEAs are removed from their origins to the level of the umbilicus, although usually only the proximal 6- to 8-cm segment is large enough to use. Often the vessels appear small, but if they are anastomosed to the aorta before cardioplegic arrest, their flow capacity can be tested and usually is quite good. Proximal and distal anastomoses are performed similarly to free IMA grafts (see Figs. 54–71 and 54–72). The potential for wound breakdown or other complications with bilateral IMA and IEA harvesting would seem significant but has actually been low in practice (Barner et al., 1991). If long-term patency of the IEA can be confirmed, it could become a routine conduit.

Three factors are considered in choosing the coronary arteries to be grafted with arterial conduits. First, the size and flows of the IMAs or GEA must be matched to the coronaries, as described above. Second, an arterial graft may be used to revascularize the vessels with the largest regions of normally functioning myocardium. This concept, in practice, translates into using a LIMA for the LAD in most patients. If the anterior wall is infarcted, however, a vein graft may be selected for the LAD, and the RIMA and LIMA pedicles, for example, can be used for the viable RCA and CMA regions. Thus, arterial grafts are performed not to the best vessels but to the best myocardium. In fact, the IMAs often are chosen for small or diffusely diseased coronary arteries if the regional myocardium is judged to be important for the long-term maintenance of ventricular function. Clearly, IMA grafts maintain better long-term patency to such vessels than do veins. One example of this problem is the diffusely diseased or segmented LAD. If a good-sized LIMA is available with high flow, up to three sequential anastomoses can be performed along the LAD, ending the mammary artery at the apex. With a smaller LIMA, the mammary artery usually is used to graft the distal LAD, and a vein is chosen for the intermediate segment. Sequential IMA grafting, with its excellent patency, is a more favorable approach than extensive endarterectomy for LAD revascularization in this setting.

The third factor to be considered is technical feasibility. For example, an optional diagonal artery that courses lateral on the anterior wall is more difficult to sequence to the LAD than a more medial diagonal. In this situation, the lay of the LIMA graft is better if a vein graft is constructed to the lateral optional diagonal, and a simple LIMA to the LAD. Similarly, LIMA or RIMA grafts used for the right or circumflex coronary system must be long enough to reach the distal vessel with adequate flow capacity. Because of length constraints, the right GEA graft is most commonly used as a pedicle to the right coronary system in proximity to the diaphragmatic surface of the heart. Although the GEA can be used for other coronary vessels, this is usually not feasible. Finally, free IEA grafts tend to be short and are used primarily for proximal and less important branches of right, circumflex, or diagonal systems. Using an IEA for grafting the LAD is avoided, because long-term patency data are not yet available. It should be emphasized that with bilateral IMA dissection, liberal use of free and sequential IMA grafts, and application of GEA and IEA conduits, at least two and frequently all three coronary systems can be revascularized with arterial grafts in patients requiring such an approach.

## THERAPEUTIC RESULTS

### Operative Mortality and Morbidity

Complex arterial grafting procedures are more technically demanding and usually require more operative time than saphenous vein bypasses. Therefore, operations involving multiple IMAs may increase complications, morbidity, and mortality. However, experienced surgeons can liberally apply complex arterial grafting methods without an excessive increase in operative morbidity or mortality (Azariades et al.,

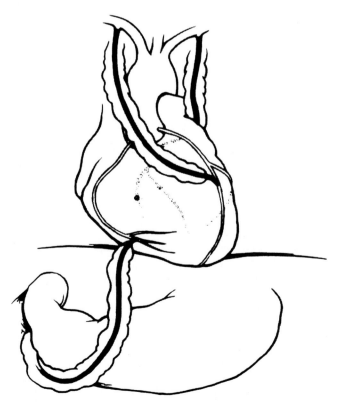

**FIGURE 54–74.** Technique of using the gastroepiploic artery (GEA) for a bypass graft to the right coronary system. See text for details.

1990; Barner et al., 1985; Cosgrove et al., 1985; Galbut et al., 1985; Gardner et al., 1990; Jones et al., 1986, 1987; Lytle et al., 1983; Rankin et al., 1986; Russo et al., 1986; Sauvage et al., 1986; Suma et al., 1991, 1993; Tector et al., 1986; Wareing et al., 1990). In many series, multiple arterial grafting in elective cases has been associated with less than a 1% hospital mortality rate. Urgent or emergency IMA procedures performed for unstable angina, postinfarction angina, or acute evolving myocardial infarction are associated with a hospital mortality rate of 3 to 5%, which compares favorably with vein graft operations (Rankin et al., 1984, 1986). In emergency cases when immediate adequacy of revascularization is critical, however, careful IMA flow testing and graft selection are especially important.

Patient morbidity may be influenced by mammary grafting. Early reoperation rates for bleeding may be slightly higher, and postoperative blood loss may be greater because of more extensive IMA and chest wall dissection (Cosgrove et al., 1988). Blood conservation techniques, including autotransfusion (Cosgrove et al., 1985), are useful after IMA procedures to minimize transfusion requirements. With contemporary blood conservation, exogenous blood transfusion can be avoided in over 90% of patients (Ovrum et al., 1991). Contemporary perioperative myocardial infarction rates for IMA grafting are quite low and should now approximate 2%; in fact, enhanced IMA patency may have a role in achieving low infarction rates.

A higher incidence of postoperative respiratory insufficiency has been observed with bilateral IMA grafting, but it may have been caused by electrocautery injury to both phrenic nerves. This complication usually can be avoided with proper operative technique. IMA harvesting *does* detrimentally influence postoperative pulmonary function (Berrizbeitia et al., 1989; Shapiro et al., 1990; Vargas et al., 1992); however, these effects usually are transient and produce little clinical disability. Use of IMA grafts in patients with ascending aortic atherosclerosis may reduce the incidence of cerebral embolization and stroke.

The relationship between bilateral IMA dissection and postoperative sternotomy infection has been controversial (Cosgrove et al., 1988; Green et al., 1993; Grmoljez and Barner, 1978; Grossi et al., 1991; Hazelrigg et al., 1989; Morris et al., 1990; Nkongho et al., 1984). Many studies of multiple mammary grafting have reported a low incidence of sternal infections, and others suggest that bilateral sternal devascularization predisposes to mediastinitis, especially in diabetics. In most contemporary analyses, however, the incidence of deep sternal infections with bilateral IMA grafting is quite low, suggesting that bilateral IMAs can be used liberally without excessively increasing morbidity. Most would suggest, however, that obese patients with diabetes should usually undergo only a single IMA, because this group is most at risk for sternal infection. With current management methods, including aggressive application of pectoralis and rectus muscle flaps, a sternal infection

should rarely cause mortality, and morbidity also should be low (Cheung et al., 1985; Prevosti et al., 1989).

## Long-Term Survival

Several studies have examined the influence of IMA procedures on long-term patient survival. Loop and associates (Loop et al., 1986b) assessed 10-year survival and cardiac events in 5931 patients undergoing coronary revascularization for non–left main coronary disease in the 1970s. Sixty per cent of the total underwent only vein graft operations, and in 40% an IMA graft was performed additionally. Differences between the groups were significant, reflecting operative selection biases: IMA patients less often had left ventricular dysfunction, multivessel disease, severe angina, advanced age, and incomplete revascularization. In addition, IMA procedures became more frequent in the later years of the study. After attempts to adjust for differences in baseline risk factors using the Cox proportional hazards model, improved survival was observed with IMA grafting in most anatomic subsets (Fig. 54–75) and in patients with ventricular dysfunction (Fig. 54–76). Moreover, IMA grafting significantly reduced the incidence of subsequent reoperation (Fig. 54–77) as well as nonfatal cardiac events (Cosgrove et al., 1986).

Similar findings were published about 748 patients followed for 15 years postoperatively (Cameron et al., 1986). Survival appeared to be improved in patients receiving IMA grafts, the incidence of reoperation was less in the IMA patients, and event-free survival also was enhanced. As in the Loop study, however, selection biases for IMA grafting produced significant differences in baseline characteristics: IMA patients less often had ventricular impairment, left main disease, or incomplete revascularization. After adjustment for these baseline differences using the Cox model, the long-term clinical benefits of IMA grafting still appeared significant.

Moreover, operative mortality and complications were equivalent between groups, except that perioperative infarction was less common in IMA patients. Thus, routine use of a single IMA graft seems to improve long-term survival and quality of life in all subsets of coronary disease patients. Similar results recently have been presented from multiple sources, and the propriety of routine *single IMA grafting* is now established (Acinapura et al., 1989; Cameron et al., 1988; Morris et al., 1990, 1991; Proudfit et al., 1990).

The clinical effects of *multiple arterial grafts* on long-term clinical outcome are less well understood. In one study (Morris et al., 1990), 1063 patients underwent coronary revascularization over 3 years, 420 by a surgeon favoring single IMA use (Group I) and 643 by a surgeon in the same practice who maximized arterial grafts (Group II). No differences were noted in the incidence of preoperative risk factors between groups (Table 54–11), and the series were concurrent. Variables reflecting operative technique, including clamp

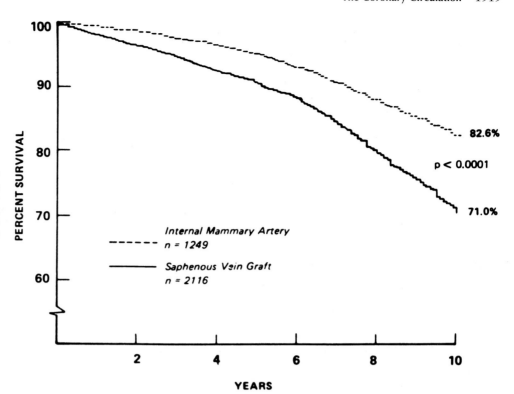

**FIGURE 54–75.** Unadjusted raw survival data for patients with three-vessel disease who were selected for coronary grafting with and without IMA utilization in the Cleveland Clinic series. See text for details.

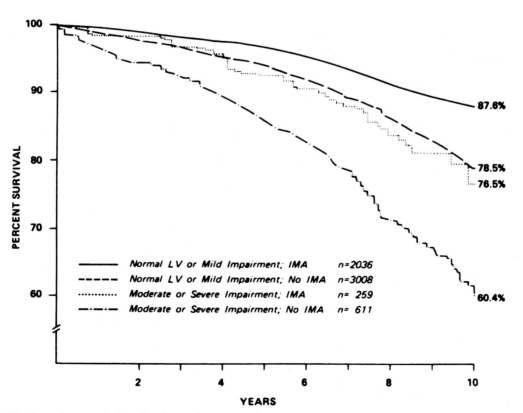

**FIGURE 54–76.** Unadjusted survival data for four subgroups undergoing coronary revascularization with and without IMA in the Cleveland Clinic series. See text for details.

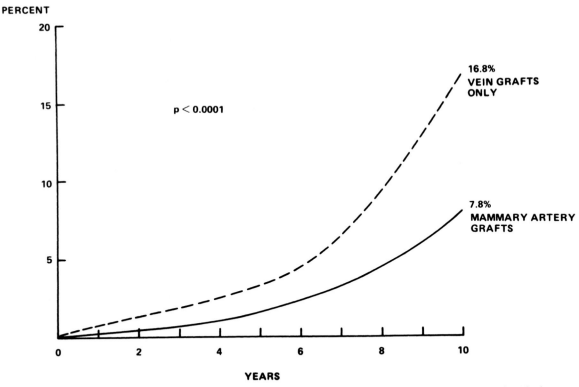

PERCENT

**FIGURE 54–77.** Reoperation rates versus postoperative years for patients receiving vein grafts only, as compared with those receiving at least one IMA graft.

time per graft, bypass time per graft, and number of grafts per patient, were similar. The distribution of single versus multiple IMA grafts between groups reflected the differing operative philosophies (see Table 54–11). For example, 74% of patients in Group I with multivessel or left main disease received a single IMA and adjunctive vein grafts, whereas 71% of patients with multivessel or left main disease in Group II had multiple arterial grafts with proportionally less use of saphenous vein.

Overall 30-day survival rates and the incidence of sternal infections did not differ between the groups (see Table 54–11). Moreover, using the Cox proportional hazards model and taking into account all relevant preoperative variables, researchers found that long-term survival over 7 postoperative years was not statistically or clinically different between the groups (Fig. 54–78), whether assessed as single IMA versus multiple IMA policy (*panel A*) or all patients receiving single or multiple IMA grafts (*panel B*). Moreover, patient age had no effect to a follow-up of 7 years (Fig. 54–79). Thus, it is possible that most of the clinical benefit of arterial grafting is provided by a single IMA, and further use is associated, on average, with diminishing clinical returns. Alternatively, many of the potential clinical advantages of multiple arterial grafting might be expected in later years, so 7 years of follow-up may be inadequate to test the hypothesis.

In this regard, a more recent study from the Cleveland Clinic suggests that the benefits of multiple

arterial grafting will be significant but will occur primarily in younger patients and potentially in the follow-up period beyond 8 to 10 years (Cosgrove et al., in press). Thus, a consensus is developing that routine multiple arterial grafting is appropriate in younger patients in an effort to improve results into the second postoperative decade. We currently prefer the procedure illustrated in Figure 54–74 for most multiple arterial operations in young patients. In the remainder of the population, however, multiple IMA grafting is reserved for specific indications, as defined earlier.

Finally, one would be remiss to omit discussion of therapy for the underlying atherosclerotic process. Patients and referring physicians should be encouraged to modify long-term risk factors and aggressively manage persistent hyperlipidemias after coronary bypass grafting. Normalization of lipids significantly improves late prognosis of surgical patients (Blankenhorn et al., 1987) and reduces cardiac events and reoperation rates. The combination of *surgical bypass* of established coronary obstructions using arterial grafts, long-term *risk factor modification,* and effective *medical management of underlying hyperlipidemias* is the most effective and highly documented therapeutic approach available today for this most prevalent disease of modern society.

## CONCLUSION

The development of IMA to coronary artery bypass, and especially the routine application of this proce-

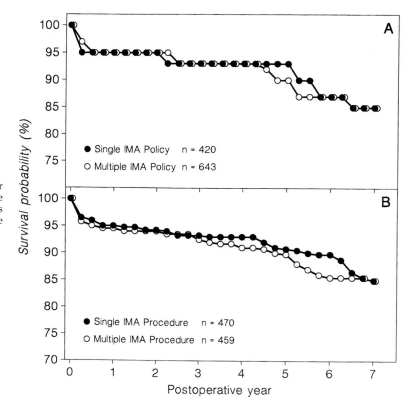

FIGURE 54–78. Seven-year survival data grouped for patients managed with a single IMA versus a multiple IMA policy (*A*) and grouped according to all patients receiving a single IMA versus multiple IMA (*B*). See text for details.

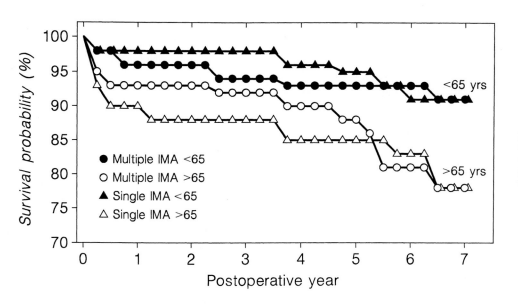

FIGURE 54–79. Seven-year survival data for patients managed with single versus multiple IMA policies, subgrouped according to age. See text for details.

■ **Table 54–11.** SINGLE VERSUS MULTIPLE IMA COMPARISON

| | Group I | Group II |
|---|---|---|
| | *Preoperative Risk Factors* | |
| No. of patients | 420 | 643 |
| MVD/LMD | 89% | 91% |
| Elective | 53% | 52% |
| USA/PIA | 41% | 43% |
| AEMI | 6% | 5% |
| > 65 years old | 33% | 34% |
| Mean EF | 0.5 ± 0.10 | 0.49 ± 0.11 |
| EF < 0.4 | 26% | 26% |
| Age | 60 ± 10 years | 60 ± 10 years |
| ***All Patients*** | *Operative Variables (%)* | |
| No IMA | 16 | 3 |
| Single IMA | 73 | 30 |
| Multiple IMA | 11 | 67 |
| Any IMA | 84 | 97 |
| ***Single-Vessel Disease*** | | |
| IMA Used | 90 | 97 |
| ***MVD/LMD*** | | |
| No IMA | 14 | 3 |
| Single IMA | 74 | 26 |
| Multiple IMA | 12 | 71 |
| ***Subgroups*** | *30-Day Survival Probability (%)* | |
| Overall | 96 | 98 |
| Elective | 98 | 99 |
| USA/PIA* | 93 | 97 |
| Age ≥ 65 | 92 | 97 |
| Age < 65 | 98 | 99 |
| EF ≥ 0.4 | 96 | 99 |
| EF < 0.4 | 96 | 96 |
| Nondiabetic | 97 | 98 |
| Diabetic | 91 | 97 |
| ***Sternal Infection*** | 2.1% | 1.0% |

From Morris, J. J., Smith, L. R., Glower, D. D., et al.: Clinical evaluation of single versus multiple mammary artery bypass. Circulation, 82(Suppl. 5):218–223, 1990.

*Key*: AEMI = acute evolving myocardial infarction; EF = ejection fraction; IMA = internal mammary artery; LMD = left main disease; MVD = multivessel disease; PIA = postinfarction angina*; Reop. = repeat coronary bypass; USA = unstable angina.*

*As defined narrowly (Rankin, J. S., Newton, J. R., Califf, R. M., et al.: Clinical characteristics and current management of medically refractory unstable angina. Ann. Surg., 200:457, 1984).

dure to the general coronary disease population, constitutes one of the major advances in cardiac surgery. At present, most coronary revascularizations probably should include at least one IMA graft, and multiple IMA procedures should be employed for specific indications. Alternative arterial conduits, such as the GEA and IEA, are being used more frequently. It is now well established that long-term patient survival and well-being are enhanced with routine arterial grafting, but more follow-up time, together with careful analysis of graft patency and clinical outcome variables, will continue to improve the understanding of this topic.

## BIBLIOGRAPHY

Absolon, K. B., Aust, J. B., Varco, R. L., and Lillehei, C. W.: Surgical treatment of occlusive coronary artery disease by endarterectomy or anastomotic replacement. Surg. Gynecol. Obstet., 103:180, 1956.

Acar, C., Jebara, V. A., Portoghese, M., et al.: Revival of the radial artery for coronary artery bypass grafting. Ann. Thorac. Surg., 54(4):652–659, 1992.

Acinapura, A. J., Rose, D. M., Jacobwitz, I. J., et al.: Internal mammary artery bypass grafting: Influence on recurrent angina and survival in 2,100 patients. Ann. Thorac. Surg., 48(2):186–191, 1989.

Azariades, M., Fessler, C. L., Floten, H. S., and Starr, A.: Five-year results of coronary bypass grafting for patients older than 70 years: Role of internal mammary artery. Ann. Thorac. Surg., 50(6):940–945, 1990.

Baillot, R. G., Loop, F. D., Cosgrove, D. M., and Lytle, B. W.: Reoperation after previous grafting with the internal mammary artery: Technique and early results. Ann. Thorac. Surg., 40:271, 1985.

Baker, N. H., and Grindlay, J. H.: Technic of experimental systemic-to coronary-artery anastomosis. Staff Meetings of the Mayo Clinic, 34:497, 1959.

Ballinger, W. F., Padula, R. T., Fishman, N. H., and Camishion, R. C.: Operations upon coronary arteries: Evaluation of absorbable intraluminal gelatin tubes, sutures, and tissue adhesive. J. Thorac. Cardiovasc. Surg., 48:790, 1964.

Barbour, D. J., and Roberts, W. C.: Additional evidence for relative resistance to atherosclerosis of the internal mammary artery compared to saphenous vein when used to increase myocardial blood supply. Am. J. Cardiol., 56:488, 1984.

Barner, H. B.: The internal mammary artery as a free graft. J. Thorac. Cardiovasc. Surg., 66:219, 1973.

Barner, H. B., Naunheim, K. S., Fiore, A. C., et al.: Use of the inferior epigastric artery as a free graft for myocardial revascularization. Ann. Thorac. Surg., 52:429–437, 1991.

Barner, H. B., Standeven, J. W., and Reese, J.: Twelve-year experience with internal mammary artery for coronary artery bypass. J. Thorac. Cardiovasc. Surg., 90:668, 1985.

Barner, H. B., Swartz, M. T., Mudd, J. G., and Tyras, D. H.: Late patency of the internal mammary artery as a coronary bypass conduit. Ann. Thorac. Surg., 34:408, 1982.

Berrizbeitia, L. D., Tessler, S., Jacobwitz, I. J., et al.: Effect of sternotomy and coronary bypass surgery on postoperative pulmonary mechanics. Comparison of internal mammary and saphenous vein bypass grafts. Chest, 96(4):873–876, 1989.

Blankenhorn, D. H., Nessim, S. A., Johnson, R. L., et al.: Beneficial effects of combined colestipol-niacin therapy on coronary atherosclerosis and coronary venous bypass grafting. J. A. M. A., 257:3233, 1987.

Bourassa, M. G., Campeau, L., Lesperance, J., and Solymoss, B. C.: Atherosclerosis after coronary artery bypass surgery: Results of recent studies and recommendations regarding prevention. Cardiology, 73:259, 1986.

Buche, M., Schoevaerdts, J. C., Louagie, Y., et al.: Use of the inferior epigastric artery for coronary bypass. J. Thorac. Cardiovasc. Surg., 103(4):665–670, 1992.

Buikema, H., Grandjean, J. G., van den Broek, S., et al.: Differences in vasomotor control between human gastroepiploic and left internal mammary artery. Circulation, 86(Suppl. 5):205–209, 1992.

Califf, R. M., Harrell, F. E., Lee, K. L., et al.: The evolution of medical and surgical therapy for coronary artery disease: A 15-year perspective. J. A. M. A., 261:2077–2086, 1989.

Cameron, A., Davis, K. B., Green, G. E., et al.: Clinical implications of internal mammary artery bypass grafts: The Coronary Artery Surgery Study experience. Circulation, 77:815, 1988.

Cameron, A., Kemp, H. G., and Green, G. E.: Bypass surgery with the internal mammary artery graft: 15 year follow-up. Circulation, 74(Suppl. III):30, 1986.

Carrel, A.: On the experimental surgery of the thoracic aorta and the heart. Ann. Surg., 52:83, 1910.

Chaikhouni, A., Crawford, F. A., Kochel, P. J., et al.: Human internal mammary artery produces more prostacyclin than saphenous vein. J. Thorac. Cardiovasc. Surg., 92:88, 1986.

Cheung, E. H., Craver, J. M., Jones, E. L., et al.: Mediastinitis after cardiac valve operations. J. Thorac. Cardiovasc. Surg., 90:517, 1985.

Cosgrove, D. M., Amiot, D. M., and Meserko, J. J.: An improved technique for autotransfusion of shed mediastinal blood. Ann. Thorac. Surg., 40:519, 1985.

Cosgrove, D. M., and Loop, F. D.: Techniques to maximize mammary artery length. Ann. Thorac. Surg., 40:78, 1985.

Cosgrove, D. M., Loop, F. D., Lytle, B. W., et al.: Predictors of reoperation after myocardial revascularization. J. Thorac. Cardiovasc. Surg., 92:811, 1986.

Cosgrove, D. M., Lytle, B. W., Hill, A. C., et al.: Are two internal thoracic arteries better than one? J. Thorac. Cardiovasc. Surg. (in press).

Cosgrove, D. M., Lytle, B. W., Loop, F. D., et al.: Does bilateral internal mammary artery grafting increase surgical risk? J. Thorac. Cardiovasc. Surg., 95:850, 1988.

Dobrin, P. B.: Mechanical behavior of vascular smooth muscle in cylindrical segments of arteries in vitro. Ann. Biomed. Engineering, 12:497, 1984.

Galbut, D. L., Traad, E. A., Dorman, M. J., et al.: Bilateral internal mammary artery grafts in reoperative and primary coronary bypass surgery. Ann. Thorac. Surg., 52(1):20–27, 1991.

Galbut, D. L., Traad, E. A., Dorman, M. J., et al.: Twelve-year experience with bilateral internal mammary artery grafts. Ann. Thorac. Surg., 40:264, 1985.

Gardner, T. J., Greene, P. S., Rykiel, M. F., et al.: Routine use of the left internal mammary artery graft in the elderly. Ann. Thorac. Surg., 49(2):188–193, 1990.

Geha, A. S., and Baue, A. E.: Early and late results of coronary revascularization with saphenous vein and internal mammary artery grafts. Am. J. Surg., 137:456, 1979.

Gelbfish, J., Jacobowitz, I. J., Rose, D. M., et al.: Cryopreserved homologous saphenous vein: Early and late patency in coronary artery bypass surgical procedures. Ann. Thorac. Surg., 42:70, 1986.

Green, G. E., Stertzer, S. H., Gordon, R. B., and Tice, D. A.: Anastomosis of the internal mammary artery to the distal left anterior descending coronary artery. Circulation, 41, 42(Suppl. II):79, 1970.

Green, G. E., Stertzer, S. H., and Reppert, E. H.: Coronary arterial bypass grafts. Ann. Thorac. Surg., 5:443, 1968.

Green, G. E., Swistel, D. G., Castro, J., et al.: Sternal blood flow during mobilization of the internal thoracic arteries. Ann. Thorac. Surg., 55(4):967–970, 1993.

Grmoljez, P. F., and Barner, H. B.: Bilateral internal mammary artery mobilization and sternal healing. Angiology, 29:272, 1978.

Grondin, C. M., Campeau, L., Lesperance, J., et al.: Comparison of late changes in internal mammary artery and saphenous vein grafts in two consecutive series of patients 10 years after operation. Circulation, 70(Suppl. I):208, 1984.

Grossi, E. A., Esposito, R., Harris, L. J., et al.: Sternal wound infections and use of internal mammary artery grafts. J. Thorac. Cardiovasc. Surg., 102(3):342–346, 1991.

Hall, R. J., Khouri, E. M., and Gregg, D. E.: Coronary-internal mammary artery anastomosis in dogs. Surgery, 50:560, 1961.

Harjola, P. T., Frick, M. H., Harjula, A., et al.: Sequential internal mammary artery (IMA) grafts in coronary artery bypass surgery. J. Thorac. Cardiovasc. Surg., 32:288, 1984.

Hazelrigg, S. R., Wellons, H. A., Jr., Schneider, J. A., and Kolm, P.: Wound complications after median sternotomy: Relationship to internal mammary grafting. J. Thorac. Cardiovasc. Surg., 98(6):1096–1099, 1989.

Hirose, H., Kawashima, Y., Nakano, S., et al.: Long-term results in surgical treatment of children 4 years old or younger with coronary involvement due to Kawasaki disease. Circulation, 74(Suppl I):77, 1986.

Hutchinson, J. E., III, Green, G. E., Mekhjian, H. A., and Kemp, H. G.: Coronary bypass grafting in 376 consecutive patients, with three operative deaths. J. Thorac. Cardiovasc. Surg., 67:7, 1974.

Jones, E. L., Lattouf, O., Lutz, J. F., and King, S. B.: Important anatomical and physiological considerations in performance of complex mammary-coronary artery operations. Ann. Thorac. Surg., 43:469, 1987.

Jones, E. L., Lattouf, O. M., and Weintraub, W. S.: Catastrophic consequences of internal mammary artery hypoperfusion. J. Thorac. Cardiovasc. Surg., 98(5 Part 2):902–907, 1989.

Jones, E. L., Lutz, J. F., King, S. B., et al.: Extended use of the internal mammary artery graft: Important anatomic and physiologic considerations. Circulation, 74(Suppl. III):42, 1986.

Jones, E. L., Weintraub, W. S., Craver, J. M., et al.: Coronary bypass surgery: Is the operation different today? J. Thorac. Cardiovasc. Surg., 101(1):108–115, 1991.

Jones, J. W., Oschner, J. L., Mills, N. L., and Hughes, L.: Clinical comparison with saphenous vein and internal mammary artery as a coronary graft. J. Thorac. Cardiovasc. Surg., 80:334, 1980.

Julian, O. C., Lopez-Belio, M., Moorehead, D., and Lima, A.: Direct surgical procedures of the coronary arteries: Experimental studies. J. Thorac. Surg., 34:654, 1957.

Kabbani, S. S., Hanna, E. S., Bashour, T. T., et al.: Sequential internal mammary-coronary artery bypass. J. Thorac. Cardiovasc. Surg., 86:697, 1983.

Kalan, J. M., and Roberts, W. C.: Comparison of morphologic changes and luminal sizes of saphenous vein and internal mammary artery after simultaneous implantation for coronary arterial bypass grafting. Am. J. Cardiol., 60:193, 1987.

Kamath, M. L., Matysik, L. S., Schmidt, D. H., and Smith, L. L.: Sequential internal mammary artery grafts. J. Thorac. Cardiovasc. Surg., 89:163, 1985.

Kawachi, K., Kitamura, S., Seki, T., et al.: Hemodynamics and coronary blood flow during exercise after coronary artery bypass grafting with internal mammary arteries in children with Kawasaki disease. Circulation, 84(2):618–624, 1991.

Kay, H. R., Korns, M. E., Flemma, R. J., et al.: Atherosclerosis of the internal mammary artery. Ann. Thorac. Surg., 21:504, 1976.

Kitamura, S., Kawachi, K., Morita, R., et al.: Excellent patency and growth capacity of internal mammary artery (IMA) grafts in pediatric coronary artery bypass surgery: New evidence of a "live conduit." Circulation, 76(Suppl. IV):1395, 1987.

Kolessov, V. I.: Mammary artery-coronary artery anastomosis as method of treatment for angina pectoris. J. Thorac. Cardiovasc. Surg., 54:535, 1967.

Landymore, R. W., and Chapman, D. M.: Anatomical studies to support the expanded use of the internal mammary artery graft for myocardial revascularization. Ann. Thorac. Surg., 44:4, 1987.

Laub, G. W., Muralidharan, S., Clancy, R., et al.: Cryopreserved allograft veins as alternative coronary artery bypass conduits: Early phase results. Ann. Thorac. Surg., 54(5):826–831, 1992.

Lemma, M., Vanelli, P., Bozzi, G., and Santoli, C.: Myocardial revascularization with arterial grafts alone: Our experience. Giornale Italiano di Cardiologia, 21(10):1057–1063, 1991.

Loop, F. D., Irarrazaval, M. J., Bredee, J. J., et al.: Internal mammary artery graft for ischemic heart disease: Effects of revascularization on clinical status and survival. Am. J. Cardiol., 39:516, 1977.

Loop, F. D., Lytle, B. W., Cosgrove, D. M., et al.: Free (aorto-coronary) internal mammary artery graft: Late results. J. Thorac. Cardiovasc. Surg., 92:827, 1986a.

Loop, F. D., Lytle, B. W., Cosgrove, D. M., et al.: Influence of the internal mammary artery graft on 10-year survival and other cardiac events. N. Engl. J. Med., 314:1, 1986b.

Loop, F. D., Spampinato, N., Cheanvechai, C., and Effler, D. B.: The free internal mammary artery bypass graft. Ann. Thorac. Surg., 15:50, 1973.

Louagie, Y. A., Buche, M., Schroder, E., and Schoevaerdts, J. C.: Coronary bypass with both internal mammary and inferior epigastric arteries. Ann. Thorac. Surg., 53(6):1117–1119, 1992.

Lytle, B. W., Cosgrove, D. M., Ratliff, N. B., and Loop, F. D.: Coronary artery bypass grafting with the right gastrepiploic artery. J. Thorac. Cardiovasc. Surg., 97(6):826–831, 1989.

Lytle, B. W., Cosgrove, D. M., Saltus, G. L., et al.: Multivessel coronary revascularization without saphenous vein: Long-term results of bilateral internal mammary artery grafting. Ann. Thorac. Surg., 36:540, 1983.

Lytle, B. W., Kramer, J. R., Golding, L. R., et al.: Young adults with coronary atherosclerosis: 10 year results of surgical myocardial revascularization. J. Am. Coll. Cardiol., 4:445, 1984.

Lytle, B. W., Loop, F. D., Cosgrove, D. M., et al.: Fifteen hundred coronary reoperations. J. Thorac. Cardiovasc. Surg., 93:847, 1987.

Lytle, B. W., Loop, F. D., Cosgrove, D. M., et al.: Long-term (5 to 12 years) serial studies of internal mammary artery and saphenous vein coronary bypass grafts. J. Thorac. Cardiovasc. Surg., 89:248, 1985.

Mamiya, R. T., Cooper, T., Willman, V. L., et al.: Distal relocation of the origin of the left coronary artery by subclavian left coronary anastomosis. Surg. Gynecol. Obstet., 113:599, 1961.

McBride, L. R., and Barner, H. B.: The left internal mammary artery as a sequential graft to the left anterior descending system. J. Thorac. Cardiovasc. Surg., 86:703, 1983.

Milgalter, E., Pearl, J. M., Laks, H., et al.: The inferior epigastric arteries as coronary bypass conduits: Size preoperative duplex scan assessment of suitability, and early clinical experience. J. Thorac. Cardiovasc. Surg., 103(3):463–465, 1992.

Mills, N. L., and Bringaze, W. L., III: Preparation of the internal mammary artery graft: Which is the best method? J. Thorac. Cardiovasc. Surg., 98(1):73–77, 1989a.

Mills, N. L., and Everson, C. T.: Right gastroepiploic artery: A third arterial conduit for coronary artery bypass. Ann. Thorac. Surg., 47(5):706–711, 1989b.

Mitchell, I. M., Essop, A. R., Scott, P. J., et al.: Bovine internal mammary artery as a conduit for coronary revascularization: Long-term results. Ann. Thorac. Surg., 55(1):120–122, 1993.

Moore, T. C., and Riberi, A.: Maintenance of coronary circulation during systemic-to-coronary artery anastomosis. Surgery, 43:245, 1958.

Morris, J. J., Smith, L. R., Glower, D. D., et al.: Clinical evaluation of single versus multiple mammary artery bypass. Circulation, 82(Suppl. 5):214–223, 1990.

Morris, J. J., Smith, L. R., Jones, R. H., et al.: Influence of diabetes and mammary artery grafting on survival after coronary bypass. Circulation, 84(Suppl. 5):275–284, 1991.

Muhlbaier, L. H., Pryor, D. B., Rankin, J. S., et al.: Observational comparison of event-free survival with medical and surgical therapy in patients with coronary artery disease: 20 years of follow up. Circulation, 86(Suppl. 5):198–204, 1992.

Murray, G.: Heparin in surgical treatment of blood vessels. Arch. Surg., 40:307, 1940.

Murray, G., Porcheron, R., Hilario, J., and Roschlau, W.: Anastomosis of a systemic artery to the coronary. Can. Med. Assoc. J., 71:594, 1954.

Nkongho, A., Luber, J. M., Bell-Thompson, J., and Green, G. E.: Sternotomy infection after harvesting of the internal mammary artery. J. Thorac. Cardiovasc. Surg., 88:788, 1984.

Okies, J. E., Page, U. S., Bigelow, J. C., et al.: The left internal mammary artery: The graft of choice. Circulation, 70(Suppl. I):213, 1984.

Olearchyk, A. S., and Magovern, G. J.: Internal mammary artery grafting. J. Thorac. Cardiovasc. Surg., 92:1082, 1986.

Orszulak, T. A., Schaff, H. V., Chesebro, J. H., and Holmes, D. R., Jr.: Initial experience with sequential internal mammary artery bypass grafts to the left anterior descending and diagonal coronary arteries. Mayo Clin. Proc., 61:3, 1986.

Ovrum, E., Holen, E. A., Abdelnoor, M., and Oystese, R.: Conventional blood conservation techniques in 500 consecutive coronary artery bypass operations. Ann. Thorac. Surg., 52(3):500–505, 1991.

Pearson, P. J., Evora, P. R., and Schaff, H. V.: Bioassay of EDRF from internal mammary arteries: Implications for early and late bypass graft patency. Ann. Thorac. Surg., 54(6):1078–1084, 1992.

Peigh, P. S., DiSesa, V. J., Collins, J. J., Jr., and Cohn, L. H.: Coronary bypass grafting with totally calcified or acutely dissected ascending aorta. Ann. Thorac. Surg., 51(1):102–104, 1991.

Prevosti, L. G., Subramainian, V. A., Rothaus, K. O., and Dineen, P.: A comparison of the open and closed methods in the initial treatment of sternal wound infections. J. Cardiovasc. Surg., 30(5):757–763, 1989.

Proudfit, W. L., Kramer, J. R., Goormastic, M., and Loop, F. D.: Ten-year survival of patients with mild angina or myocardial infarction without angina: A comparison of medical and surgical treatment. Am. Heart J., 119(4):942–948, 1990.

Pryor, D. B., Harrell, F. E., Rankin, J. S., et al.: The changing survival benefits of coronary revascularization over time. Circulation, 76(Suppl. V):13, 1987.

Puig, L. B., Neto, L. F., Rati, M., et al.: A technique of anastomosis of the right internal mammary artery to the circumflex artery and its branches. Ann. Thorac. Surg., 38:533, 1984.

Ramstrom, J., Henze, A., Thuren, J., and Nystrom, S. O.: Myocardial revascularization with three native in situ arteries: Gastroepiploic and bilateral internal mammary artery grafting. Scand. J. Thorac. Cardiovasc. Surg., 24(3):177–180, 1990.

Rankin, J. S., Newman, G. E., Bashore, T. M., et al.: Clinical and angiographic assessment of complex mammary artery bypass grafting. J. Thorac. Cardiovasc. Surg., 95:832, 1986.

Rankin, J. S., Newton, J. R., Califf, R. M., et al.: Clinical characteristics and current management of medically refractory unstable angina. Ann. Surg., 200:457, 1984.

Rankin, J. S., Newman, G. E., Muhlbaier, L. H., et al.: The effects of coronary revascularization on left ventricular function in ischemic heart disease. J. Thorac. Cardiovasc. Surg., 90:818, 1985.

Russo, P., Orszulak, T. A., Schaff, H. V., and Holmes, D. R.: Use of internal mammary artery grafts for multiple coronary artery bypasses. Circulation, 74(Suppl. III):48, 1986.

Salomon, N. W., Page, U. S., Okies, J. E., et al.: Diabetes mellitus and coronary artery bypass. J. Thorac. Cardiovasc. Surg., 85:264, 1983.

Sapsford, R. N., Oakley, G. D., and Talbot, S.: Early and late patency of expanded polytetrafluoroethylene vascular grafts in aorta-coronary bypass. J. Thorac. Cardiovasc. Surg., 81:860, 1981.

Sauvage, L. R., Wu, H. D., Kowalsky, T. E., et al.: Healing basis and surgical techniques for complete revascularization of the left ventricle using only the internal mammary arteries. Ann. Thorac. Surg., 42:449, 1986.

Schimert, G., Vidne, B. A., and Lee, A. B.: Free internal mammary artery graft: An improved technique. Ann. Thorac. Surg., 19:474, 1975.

Shapiro, N., Zabatino, S. M., Ahmed, S., et al.: Determinants of pulmonary function in patients undergoing coronary bypass operations. Ann. Thorac. Surg., 50(2):268–273, 1990.

Siegel, W., and Loop, F. D.: Comparison of internal mammary artery and saphenous vein bypass grafts for myocardial revascularization. Circulation, 54:III-1, 1976.

Sims, F. H.: A comparison of coronary and internal mammary arteries and implications of the results in the etiology of arteriosclerosis. Am. Heart J., 105:560, 1983.

Singh, R. N.: Atherosclerosis and the internal mammary arteries. Cardiovasc. Intervent. Radiol., 6:72, 1983.

Singh, R. N., Beg, R. A., and Kay, E. B.: Physiological adaptability: The secret of success of the internal mammary artery grafts. Ann. Thorac. Surg., 41:247, 1986.

Singh, R. N., Sosa, J. A., and Green, G. E.: Long-term fate of the internal mammary artery and saphenous vein grafts. J. Thorac. Cardiovasc. Surg., 86:359, 1983.

Spencer, F. C., Eiseman, B., Yong, N. K., and Prachuabmoh, K.: Experimental coronary arterial surgery with hypothermia and cardiopulmonary bypass. Circulation (Cardiovascular Surgery Supplement), 29:140, 1964.

Suma, H.: Coronary artery bypass grafting in patients with calcified ascending aorta: Aortic no-touch technique. Ann. Thorac. Surg., 48(5):728–730, 1989.

Suma, H., Takeuchi, A., and Hirota, Y.: Myocardial revascularization with combined arterial grafts utilizing the internal mammary and the gastroepiploic arteries. Ann. Thorac. Surg., 47(5):712–715, 1989.

Suma, H., Wanibuchi, Y., Furuta, S., and Takeuchi, A.: Does use of gastroepiploic artery graft increase surgical risk? J. Thorac. Cardiovasc. Surg., 101(1):121–125, 1991.

Suma, H., Wanibuchi, Y., Terada, Y., et al.: The right gastroepiploic artery graft: Clinical and angiographic midterm results in 200 patients. J. Thorac. Cardiovasc. Surg., 105(4):615–622, 1993.

Takahashi, T., Nakano, S., Kaneko, M., et al.: Coronary bypass using arterial grafts in homozygous familial hypercholesterolemia. Ann. Thorac. Surg., 53(3):510–512, 1992.

Tector, A. J., Davis, L., Gabriel, R., et al.: Experience with internal mammary artery grafts in 298 patients. Ann. Thorac. Surg., 22:515, 1976.

Tector, A. J., Schmahl, T. M., and Canino, V. R.: Expanding the use of the internal mammary artery to improve patency in coronary artery bypass grafting. J. Thorac. Cardiovasc. Surg., 91:9, 1986.

Tector, A. J., Schmahl, T. M., and Canino, V. R.: The internal mammary artery graft: The best choice for bypass of the diseased left anterior descending coronary artery. Circulation, 68(Suppl. II):214, 1983.

Thal, A., Perry, J. F., Miller, F. A., and Wangensteen, O. H.: Direct suture anastomosis of the coronary arteries in the dog. Surgery, 40:1023, 1956.

Vargas, F. S., Cukier, A., Terra-Filho, M., et al.: Relationship between pleural changes after myocardial revascularization and pulmonary mechanics. Chest, 102(5):1333–1336, 1992.

von Son, J. A., Smedts, F., Vincent, J. G., et al.: Comparative anatomic studies of various arterial conduits for myocardial revascularization. J. Thorac. Cardiovasc. Surg., 99(4):703–707, 1990.

Wareing, T. H., Saffitz, J. E., and Kouchoukos, N. T.: Use of single internal mammary artery grafts in older patients. Circulation, 82(Suppl. 5):224–228, 1990.

Werner, G. S., Wiegand, V., and Kreuzer, H.: Effect of acetylcholine on arterial and venous grafts and coronary arteries in patients with coronary artery disease. Eur. Heart J., 11(2):127–137, 1990.

# 3 Repeat Coronary Artery Bypass Grafting for Myocardial Ischemia

Floyd D. Loop

As the number of coronary artery bypass patients has increased, reoperations have become commonplace. Some 42,000 isolated coronary artery reoperations were performed in 1993, and this number is estimated to rise to 54,000 in 1995. Certain factors influence the occurrence and timing of reoperative coronary artery procedures. The *single* greatest determinant of reoperation is the use of vein bypass conduits at the first operation (Cosgrove et al., 1986). Other determining factors include one- or two-vessel coronary atherosclerosis, incomplete revascularization, good ventricular performance, and young age at first operation.

As a result of randomized trials and observational studies, the indications for primary and reoperative coronary artery surgery have been refined since the late 1960s. Angina continues to be the principal reason for initial and subsequent coronary artery operations. However, arteriographic findings and the perception of myocardial jeopardy frequently underlie recommendations for primary operation (Alderman et al., 1982). Today, earlier surgical consideration is given to patients with persistent pain or discomfort, which, despite a good medical program, interferes with the patient's life-style. Symptoms should correlate with objective evidence of ischemia, and with few exceptions, most surgical candidates and almost all reoperation patients have multivessel coronary atherosclerosis. Patients with severe proximal stenoses in all major coronary vessels, demonstrated by exercise testing or with scintigraphic proof of ischemia, should be considered for bypass grafting. Particular attention should be given to patients with high-grade lesions in the proximal anterior descending coronary artery. Subtotal obstruction above the first diagonal, and especially at or above the first septal, perforator is recognized as prognostically dangerous and more likely to cause fatal myocardial infarction than vessel involvement at any other site (Klein et al., 1986; Schuster et al., 1981). Among patients with multivessel disease, severe left ventricular dysfunction (defined as an ejection fraction of less than 0.35) is best treated surgically (Passamani et al., 1985).

As selection criteria have evolved, so too has the operation. In the late 1970s, myocardial protection progressed from systemic hypothermia to the use of cold potassium cardioplegia. This advance reduced mortality and morbidity and allowed the performance of more grafts per patient. The luxuries of time and a dry, motionless field accelerated the trend toward arterial bypass grafting and provided greater safety when coronary artery surgery was combined with other cardiac reconstructive procedures.

A coronary artery bypass procedure is performed for a degenerative disease and, like many other operations, does not provide a cure. The clinical result depends on the anatomic result, which tends to deteriorate over time. After the first postoperative year, a 5% or greater rate of angina recurrence may accrue annually and is almost always related to bypass graft closure, progressive atherosclerosis in ungrafted vessels, or less frequently, development of lesions beyond the distal graft sites. Later on, mainly after the fifth to seventh postoperative year, vein graft atherosclerosis becomes the dominant reason for graft closure. These events weigh heavily on the incidence of reoperation, which increases with time.

## INCIDENCE OF REOPERATION

Incidence estimates for coronary artery reoperation encompass experience in coronary bypass surgery during the 1970s (Loop et al., 1983). Five years after the initial operation, the rate of reoperation is low, at about 3% (Cosgrove et al., 1986; Foster et al., 1984). Early reoperations were attributed to technical problems that caused graft stenosis or closure (Culliford et al., 1979). The cumulative rate of reoperation escalated to 12 and 17% at 10 and 12 years, respectively, and 30% at 15 years after the first operation (Fig. 54–80). This incidence may be altered by demographics, type of conduits used in the first operation, and use of new therapies, notably coronary artery balloon angioplasty, which affects the initial surgical case mix and thus may influence the incidence of reoperations. Prototypic variations in catheter interventions (e.g., atherectomy devices, stents, and laser ablation) may further postpone operation and reduce reoperation rates, but their impact now is only speculative.

One factor that definitely modifies the probability of reoperation is the choice of conduits used during the first operation. Sustained patency of the internal thoracic artery graft has decreased the incidence of coronary artery reoperation (Cameron et al., 1986; Loop et al., 1986). A single thoracic arterial graft anastomosed to the anterior descending coronary artery solely or combined with aortocoronary vein grafts to other major coronary vessels reduces the rate of reoperation by half during the first decade after primary operation.

The question that remains is whether multiple internal thoracic artery grafts provide additional benefit. Some authors have not found long-term benefit from bilateral internal thoracic artery grafting (Johnson et al., 1989; Kirklin et al., 1989). It is more difficult to show the additive effect of multiple thoracic artery grafts because the first graft is almost invariably grafted to the anterior descending artery, and this vessel influences survival more than any other coronary artery except the left main. The survival advantage may accrue to younger patients with two internal thoracic artery grafts (Cosgrove et al., in press). For patients less than 60 years of age, survival, reoperation-free survival, and freedom from cardiac events

were significantly improved for those who received bilateral internal thoracic artery grafts compared with cohorts who received one thoracic artery graft and vein grafts only. For older patients, this was not true. Late patency of the internal thoracic (mammary) arterial graft is significantly greater than that of a vein graft bypass to the anterior descending coronary artery. Internal thoracic artery graft patency up to 12 years is consistently greater than 90% in all years surveyed (Loop et al., 1986), whereas vein graft patency declines to approximately 60% at 10 years (Campeau et al., 1984; Lytle et al., 1985).

Of late patent grafts, approximately half show evidence of luminal irregularity connoting vein graft atherosclerosis (Reeves et al., 1991). In the Cleveland Clinic experience, late stenosis in an anterior descending vein graft has been identified as an incremental risk factor associated with decreased survival, reoperation-free survival, and event-free survival (Lytle et al., 1992). Late vein graft stenoses, particularly involving the left anterior descending coronary artery, are more dangerous than early vein graft stenoses or early anterior descending coronary artery stenoses, and they predict a high rate of death and cardiac events. Thus, an anterior descending *vein graft* narrowing years after the original operation should be considered an indication for reoperation, even when associated with mild symptoms. The comparative effect of anterior descending coronary artery atherosclerosis and vein graft atherosclerosis on survival is shown in Figure 54–81. New or progressive lesions beyond distal graft anastomoses appear significantly less frequently than progressive proximal lesions (Bourassa et al., 1978).

In vein grafts, fibrinolysis is greater, lipolysis is slower, and prostacyclin production is diminished in comparison with internal thoracic artery grafts (Grondin, 1986). The internal thoracic artery may differ from the radial and gastroepiploic arteries in that it may have a more impermeable internal elastic mem-

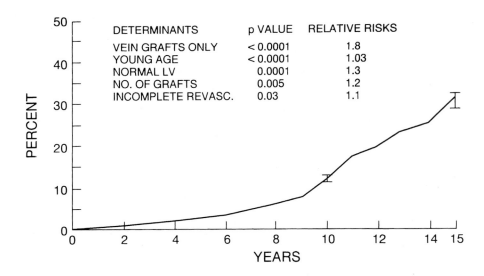

FIGURE 54–80. The incidence of coronary artery reoperation among patients who were first operated on at the Cleveland Clinic from 1971 through 1978. At 5 years postoperatively, 3% were reoperated on. Thereafter, the incidence rose progressively and even accelerated further after the tenth postoperative year. Thirty per cent of the surviving complement underwent reoperation by year 15. The significant determinants of reoperation are listed. The single greatest predictor of reoperation was the use of vein grafts only during the initial surgery. (LV = left ventricle.)

| DETERMINANTS | p VALUE | RELATIVE RISKS |
|---|---|---|
| VEIN GRAFTS ONLY | < 0.0001 | 1.8 |
| YOUNG AGE | < 0.0001 | 1.03 |
| NORMAL LV | 0.0001 | 1.3 |
| NO. OF GRAFTS | 0.005 | 1.2 |
| INCOMPLETE REVASC. | 0.03 | 1.1 |

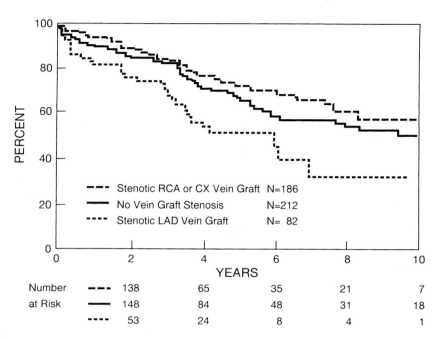

**FIGURE 54–81.** Patients who develop late anterior descending coronary artery vein graft stenosis (50–99%) experience worse survival after late cardiac catheterization (mean, 5 years) than either patients with native vessel anterior descending coronary artery stenosis or a control group with no angiographic evidence of vein graft stenoses. Patients with late stenotic vein grafts had survival of 70% and 50% 2 and 5 years after the *late* catheterization compared with 97% and 80% survival for patients with native anterior descending stenoses. (RCA = right coronary artery; CX = circumflex artery; LAD = left anterior descending artery.) (Data from Lytle, B. W., Loop, F. D., Taylor, P. C., et al.: Vein graft disease: The clinical impact of stenoses in saphenous vein bypass grafts to coronary arteries. J. Thorac. Cardiovasc. Surg., *103*:831–840, 1992.)

brane, which may limit smooth muscle cell migration (Sims, 1987). Endothelium-derived relaxing factor released from endothelial cells causes vascular smooth muscle relaxation, increasing blood flow and reducing platelet aggregation and adhesion. Although the relative immunity to late atherosclerosis is not fully explained by these metabolic findings, they do reveal differences between artery and vein bypass conduits.

Graft thrombosis may occur within 3 to 6 months after bypass surgery and is usually attributed to technical error, poor distal runoff, or vein graft damage (Shark and Kass, 1981). Serial angiograms showed that of vein grafts found to be stenotic 1 year postoperatively, 60% progressed to complete occlusion by the time of the second postoperative angiogram, a mean of 7 years later (Lytle et al., 1985). Early intimal fibroplasia is more stable than vein graft atherosclerosis. Atherosclerotic narrowing in the vein graft is usually encountered after the fifth postoperative year and frequently progresses rapidly to complete occlusion, suggesting that even early vein graft atherosclerosis has an unstable history and a poor prognosis for continued graft patency. Vein grafts that were patent at the first postoperative arteriogram but stenotic or occluded at the second postoperative arteriogram were associated with lengthening interval between arteriograms, diabetes, and hyperlipidemia; and these patients had significantly more cardiac events than patients without progressive graft disease.

Thrombosis superimposed on a ruptured atheromatous plaque may cause acute late thrombotic graft occlusion (Walts et al., 1982). Thrombosis usually occurs at the site of a preexisting atherosclerotic plaque that severely compromises the lumen (Qiao et al., 1991). This is in contrast to native vessel plaques that may rupture at the site of relatively mild lesions. Therefore, thrombolytic therapy for old vein grafts is unlikely to restore patency.

## INDICATIONS FOR REOPERATION

Clinical indications for coronary artery reoperation and primary operation are identical. The difference is that the magnitude of risk is higher, and therefore the selection process is more conservative for reoperation. Because of the higher risk involved, the cautious practice of recommending reoperation for only very symptomatic patients is probably justifiable. However, the patient's functional disability seems to carry more weight than pathoanatomy in decision making. Age, clinical characteristics, and interval between operations are depicted in Figure 54–82.

Angiographic indications for reoperation are more complex than for primary operation and have been categorized into three groups: graft closure (or dysfunction), progressive atherosclerosis, and a combination of both graft disease and progressive native ves-

| | 1967-78 | 1979-81 | 1982-84 | 1985-87 |
|---|---|---|---|---|
| Women | 9% | 13% | 15% | 12% |
| Mean age at reoperation | 52.3 | 56.3 | 58.2 | 60.9 |
| Severe angina NYHA III or IV | 73% | 71% | 67% | 64% |
| Diabetes on insulin | 14% | 15% | 17% | 23% |
| Current hypertension | 27% | 33% | 33% | 35% |
| Peripheral vascular disease | 7% | 12% | 12% | 14% |
| Cigarette use | 28% | 21% | 21% | 24% |
| Interval between surgeries in months | 50 | 72 | 84 | 101 |

**FIGURE 54–82.** The characteristics of 2509 consecutive patients who underwent reoperation are shown. They are categorized into surgical periods. Note that mean age at reoperation has steadily increased and the interval between surgeries has more than doubled in 20 years. (NYHA = New York Heart Association.) (Data from Loop, F. D., Lytle, B. W., Cosgrove, D. M., et al.: Reoperation for coronary atherosclerosis. Changing practice in 2509 consecutive patients. Ann. Surg., *212*:378–386, 1990.)

sel disease. In the author's group's most recent experience, graft closure occurring alone or combined with progressive native vessel coronary atherosclerosis accounted for 85% of the angiographic reasons for reoperative surgery (Loop et al., 1990). Early graft failure caused by technical errors from conduit twisting, kinks, short grafts producing "tenting" of the distal anastomosis, or vein grafts traumatized by high distention pressures during preparation or long storage in saline solution is encountered less frequently today. Graft construction to small vessels with poor arterial runoff is also performed less frequently. The finding of graft closure mainly applies to aortocoronary saphenous vein grafts. As greater reoperation experience has been compiled, late vein graft obstruction has become the predominant angiographic reason for reoperation.

Age at the first operation, gender, and the artery bypassed do not predict graft closure, but risk factors associated with atherosclerosis in native vessels, notably hypercholesterolemia, may affect atherosclerosis in aortocoronary vein bypass grafts (Barboriak et al., 1978; Neitzel et al., 1986). Mechanical trauma in vein graft preparation and elevated serum lipid levels are strongly implicated in degeneration of vein bypass conduits. Increased endothelial permeability of vein grafts allows migration of neutrophils and monocytes into subintimal layers of the vein graft. Vein graft atherosclerosis is frequently associated with an inflammatory reaction that invades the media and may extend through the adventitia. Atherosclerotic graft lesions are characterized by foam cells, cholesterol clefts, and calcium deposits. They are unstable, prone to rupture and hemorrhage, and thus may cause thrombosis and graft occlusion (Cox et al., 1991).

The interval between operations is increasing: Most reoperations occur between the fifth and tenth years (the mean is now close to the tenth year), although reoperations beyond the tenth year are increasing in frequency. Therefore, candidates for reoperation are often 10 years older than they were before the first operation, and they show an increased prevalence of diabetes, more diffuse atherosclerosis (often in more than one arterial system), and significantly more left main coronary artery stenosis. During this sometimes lengthy interval between operations, most patients have had additional cardiac events that may further increase operative risk. One-third of patients in the Cleveland Clinic series showed perceptible deterioration in left ventricular performance during the intervening years. Despite this deterioration, myocardial infarctions that occur in patients who have had previous bypass operations tend to be smaller than the myocardial infarctions in patients who have not had bypass operations (Crean et al., 1985). Coronary artery procedures may offer protection by bypassing the major vessels so that only minor vessels are involved in a subsequent myocardial infarction.

Advanced age is not a contraindication to either first or subsequent coronary artery procedures, but chronologic age cannot be dismissed as a risk factor. An accurate assessment of physiologic age is im-

portant and includes prior activity, mental attitude including an understanding of the potential risks and benefits, and co-morbidity (Loop et al., 1988). Concomitant diseases may include hypertension, diabetes, pulmonary disease, peripheral vascular atherosclerosis, and cancer, none of which contraindicates operation but which must be evaluated in the appraisal of the whole patient. Some patients reach a point in their aging process at which additional higher-risk, expensive surgical therapy is not warranted because there is a meager potential for effective rehabilitation.

The candidate for reoperation may be referred for *percutaneous transluminal coronary angioplasty* (PTCA). Percutaneous interventions may be recommended for early or late graft stenosis or dilatation of previously ungrafted vessels. Early results are good for discrete native vessel lesions and distal anastomotic narrowing. Stenoses of distal anastomoses are generally recognized and treated at an early stage; however, the success rate of less than 50% for dilatation of aortic anastomoses and dilatation of lesions in the graft body is significantly lower than the success rate for native vessel dilatation (Douglas, 1994). PTCA for intimal hyperplasia frequently leads to restenosis from fibrocellular proliferation. Dilatation of stenoses in the body of vein grafts implanted for over 3 years has a high risk of embolization, and long lesions in either vein grafts or native vessels have a high recurrence rate after dilatations. The relationship between graft age and recurring stenosis is significant; e.g., for grafts implanted for less than 36 months, stenosis recurred in 42%, compared with 83% for grafts implanted for more than 36 months (Platko et al., 1989). In contrast, PTCA of internal thoracic artery graft distal anastomoses has a high success rate, and improvement is sustained (Dimas et al., 1991). Overall, PTCA in patients who have had coronary artery surgery is moderately successful for relief of angina, but less than that achieved in patients undergoing PTCA without bypass surgery and similar to that of PTCA for multivessel disease (Reed et al., 1989).

Patients should be advised of different risks and outcomes that depend on the age of their vein grafts (Loop and Whitlow, 1990). The longer the interval between surgery and angioplasty, the greater the risk (Weintraub et al., 1990). An emergency reoperation is hazardous when the patient is acutely ischemic. If the patient with failed PTCA is stable and without ischemia, risk is the same as for elective reoperation. Few reports have addressed urgent or emergency reoperation after failed angioplasty, but there is a lower incidence of arterial graft usage in that setting. As in primary emergency revascularization, not only is risk elevated but the probability of perioperative myocardial infarction is also high (Golding et al., 1986). Although results of emergency operation are improving (Ferguson et al., 1988), the patient having an emergency reoperation represents one of the most demanding challenges of myocardial protection. The composition of the reperfusate, dispersion of cardioplegia, and decompression of the left ventricle determine regional wall recovery.

## PREOPERATIVE ASSESSMENT

Because the profile of the candidate for reoperation is changing, the surgeon must pay particular attention to risk among the increased numbers of patients who are women, 70 years or older, patients with left main stenosis 50% or greater, those with patent atherosclerotic vein grafts, and patients with abnormal left ventricular function. In-hospital risk may be estimated from clinical and angiographic studies. A stratified clinical risk index may be applied. In developing a prospectively validated clinical scoring system, Cleveland Clinic investigators (Higgins et al., 1992) found that the most influential risk factors were emergency surgery, elevated serum creatinine, reoperation, and combined cardiac surgical procedures. Advanced age and left ventricular dysfunction were additive. The clinical severity score predicts mortality and morbidity with reasonable specificity and sensitivity based on clinical information. These models must be refined over time as the population and the operation change. The current model tends to overpredict morbidity in higher-risk patients. Nevertheless, a clinical severity score enables the surgical team to estimate risk and to better advise the patient about the potential dangers of reoperative surgery.

The reoperation experience of the institution and its surgeons' results serve as a background for preoperative discussion. Patients should understand that risk assessment is only an educated estimate. Factors that influence the outcome include the type and number of previous operations, current stability, status and location of old grafts, and coronary pathoanatomy. Gender is a risk factor that relates to body size and coronary vessel diameter. The risk of coronary artery reoperation is about two to three times that of the first operation (Fig. 54–83).

Patients and their families should be informed that major morbidity is generally higher with reoperation, specifically perioperative myocardial infarction, respiratory complications, and bleeding that requires exploration. However, stroke, wound, renal, and gastrointestinal complications occur with about the same frequency as in the first operation. Obviously, morbidity differs among institutions, but it behooves surgeons to be aware of their personal experience in these more complicated coronary artery bypass operations.

Risk assessment is aided by a thorough review of the patient's history. What were the indications for the first operation, and are they different for the second operation? What procedure was done initially? It may make a difference technically if the patient previously had Beck's talc poudrage, Vineberg's implant, or coronary endarterectomy. Whenever possible, original hospital records and the original operative note should be surveyed for information on co-morbidity, technical problems, or perioperative complications. The surgeon should ask patients if they have copies of missing or inaccessible records (Bahn and Annest, 1986).

The patient's physical appearance is important, not only as part of a standard physical examination but also for information that could affect surgical technique. Persons with small body surface area (less than 1.7 m²) are less likely to require more blood and blood products. Women with previous mastectomy may have had chest wall irradiation, which could affect

| Mortality and Morbidity | Primary* (n=16.996) | | Reoperation (n=2509) | | p value |
|---|---|---|---|---|---|
| | (n) | (%) | (n) | (%) | |
| Operative mortality | 240 | 1.4 | 80 | 3.2 | <.0001 |
| Perioperative myocardial infarction | 415 | 2.4 | 148 | 5.9 | <.0001 |
| Bleeding | 891 | 5.2 | 155 | 6.2 | <.0001 |
| Respiratory insufficiency | 377 | 2.2 | 98 | 3.9 | <.0001 |
| Neurologic deficit | 294 | 1.7 | 46 | 1.8 | NS |
| Wound complication | 302 | 1.7 | 41 | 1.6 | NS |

**\*First 1000 causes annually from 1971 to 1987.**

FIGURE 54–83. Mortality and morbidity are shown for primary coronary artery surgery and compared with a consecutive reoperation series. Operative mortality, myocardial infarction, bleeding, and respiratory insufficiency occurred in significantly more patients in the reoperation series; however, neurologic deficit and wound complications were virtually the same in primary and reoperation cases. (Data from Loop, F. D., Lytle, B. W., Cosgrove, D. M., et al.: Reoperation for coronary atherosclerosis. Changing practice in 2509 consecutive patients. Ann. Surg., 212:378–386, 1990.)

wound healing and may preclude internal thoracic artery use. Mediastinal radiation may have caused atherosclerosis of the ascending aorta. In the author's group's experience, previous mediastinitis does not necessarily affect reentry or adhesion formation; however, when the sternum has been destroyed by osteomyelitis, removed and replaced with a muscle flap, reentry presents a problem that must be solved on an individual basis or may not be amenable to midline reentry. The responsible surgeon should be cognizant of peripheral vascular disease and previous arterial reconstruction, both of which could affect femoral cannulation and intra-aortic balloon insertion.

A carotid bruit requires further investigation to confirm or disprove significant internal carotid disease. When internal carotid narrowing is present in a neurologically asymptomatic patient, unless subtotal, the coronary artery reoperation generally takes precedence; however, the patient should be informed of the findings of carotid disease and the plan for follow-up. A history of neurologic problems in a patient with documented carotid disease may require a strategy that takes into account the severity and bilaterality of the lesion, current cardiac symptoms, coronary pathoanatomy, and magnitude of the planned cardiac reoperation. When the condition is stable, carotid endarterectomy may be staged first. In patients with dangerous coexisting carotid and coronary disease, simultaneous operation may be required, but the additional potential for stroke should be conveyed to the patient.

The preoperative lateral chest film may reveal proximity of the cardiac structures and the overlying sternum, and a posteroanterior view may show the location of a viable internal thoracic artery graft that could modify the plan of reentry. Preoperative evaluation should include questions about unusual bleeding events related to surgery, medication history (including aspirin or other antiplatelet drugs), an assessment of liver function, a family history of bleeding problems and easy bruisability, and laboratory tests of hematocrit, hemoglobin, and platelet count (Goodnough et al., 1990). Some have recommended prothrombin time and partial thromboplastin time studies to assess coagulation factor activity preoperatively. If a patient is thrombocytopenic, the possibility of heparin-induced thrombocytopenia should be considered.

Reoperation transfusion requirements depend on the patient's age, gender, and initial circulating red blood cell volume, as well as number of previous reoperations. Autologous blood is still underutilized. Predeposit of blood for autologous use should be encouraged for patients who are in stable condition without serious co-morbidity or anemia that contraindicates blood donation. Factors that may preclude autologous blood donation include idiopathic hypertrophic subaortic stenosis, aortic stenosis, congenital cyanotic heart disease, unstable angina, congestive heart failure, malignant cardiac arrhythmias, atrioventricular block, and severe left main coronary disease. Designated blood transfusion may be no safer than banked blood and may increase the risk of graft-

versus-host disease. All red cell and platelet transfusions from blood relatives must now be irradiated. Routine coagulation tests have not been found to be helpful in predicting postoperative bleeding. Discontinuation of aspirin and other antiplatelet drugs 10 or more days (Ferraris et al., 1988) and anticoagulants 2 to 3 days preoperatively is indicated.

A thorough review of the most recent cine coronary arteriogram may reveal vein graft atherosclerosis, especially when the vein graft was placed more than 5 years previously. The course of mild vein graft atherosclerosis is not known, but severe atherosclerotic vein graft narrowing may progress rapidly to closure (Fig. 54–84). It is not unusual to find complete occlusion of a vein graft that was patent but severely narrowed on the most recent pre-reoperative film. The ramifications of patent atherosclerotic vein grafts should be communicated to the patient because of their potential source of morbidity, even mortality, in the reoperation. Atherosclerotic emboli may lodge in the microcirculatory system and cause myocardial infarction.

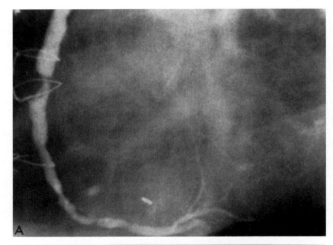

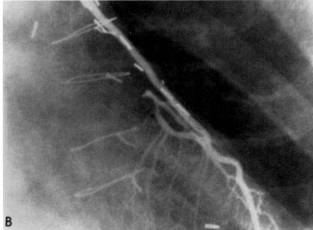

**FIGURE 54–84.** Diffuse atherosclerosis of vein grafts occurs with increased frequency after the fifth postoperative year. *A,* Diffuse atherosclerosis in a 7-year-old vein bypass graft to the right coronary artery. *B,* A normal-appearing internal thoracic artery graft to the left anterior descending coronary artery in the same patient.

Should a graft that looks normal 5 or more years after the first operation be replaced when another vein graft is atherosclerotic in the same patient? The answer is probably yes. The decision is also made easier if the old but normal-appearing vein graft perfuses the anterior descending artery and could be replaced with an internal thoracic artery graft. This is more of a dilemma 5 years or so after the first operation but less of an issue 7 to 10 years after the operation, when most vein grafts show atherosclerosis. The decision to replace old vein grafts depends on the pathoanatomic findings, the extent of regional perfusion of that graft, the status of the myocardium in that region, and the patient's overall risk profile. If severe narrowing is apparent on the pre-reoperative angiogram, the grafts should be replaced. Minimal atherosclerosis in vein grafts as shown by arteriography generally proves to be more diffuse when examined after the graft is removed. Angiographic studies tend to underestimate the severity of atherosclerotic degeneration, and because of the propensity of atherosclerotic disease in grafts to progress unpredictably, some surgeons recommend routine replacement of all saphenous vein grafts at the time of reoperation if done 5 or more years after the initial procedure (Marshall et al., 1986). The decision to replace a vein graft with an internal thoracic artery graft depends on the size of the vein and regional perfusion. If the old vein graft carries a high flow, replacement with an internal thoracic graft may cause a hypoperfusion syndrome (Navia et al., 1994). Each case must be considered individually.

As experience with reoperation has become greater, problems with heparin and protamine have been recognized. Protamine sensitivity is discussed under "Reoperation Techniques" later in this chapter. A syndrome termed *heparin-induced platelet activation* has already been described (Kappa et al., 1987). Although the condition is rare, these patients have been exposed previously to heparin, usually continuous heparin therapy over days, and have had severe thrombocytopenia or thrombosis. The platelet count may be normal preoperatively. However, when a low platelet count exists preoperatively (less than 50,000/mm$^3$ or there is history of thromboembolism during previous heparin administration, the surgeon should recognize that the condition may exist. Heparin-induced platelet activation is characterized by platelet aggregation and C-serotonin release. When reexposed to heparin, the patient could experience thrombocytopenia, intravascular thrombosis, arterial emboli, and hemorrhage. Surveillance of the platelet count does not prevent thrombosis (King and Kelton, 1984). Aspirin may prevent platelet aggregation in vitro, but it has not been consistently efficacious in vivo. A stable analog of prostacyclin appears to stimulate adenylcyclase and to elevate intracellular levels of cyclic adenosine monophosphate. Starting prostacyclin analog as an infusion preoperatively and continuing it throughout the operation until the administration of protamine has led to a successful outcome (Addonizio et al., 1987).

Finally, the preoperative arteriogram should be reviewed again immediately before the reoperation. A clear strategy for reentry, cannulation, and grafting should be formulated. Reoperation that is based on a plan for preventing complications is the best method to avoid them.

## REOPERATION TECHNIQUES

In recent years the author's group has been able to increase the number of grafts per patient, but reoperation patients receive fewer grafts because of diffuse coronary atherosclerosis, new transmural scars, and the fact that some original grafts remain open and functioning well. The internal thoracic graft is a good investment in any coronary artery operation, and arterial graft usage is increasing in reoperations. Interestingly, left ventricular function before reoperation is frequently better preserved in patients who had internal thoracic artery grafting initially (Coltharp et al., 1991). In the author's group's most recent experience, patent internal thoracic artery grafts were damaged during reoperation in 3.5% of cases. The use of arterial grafts at the first procedure does not appear to increase the risk of reoperation (Lytle et al., 1993).

### Induction of Anesthesia

In the immediate preoperative period, premedication protocols are essentially the same as in patients having a primary operation, and they depend on age and clinical stability. Packed red blood cells should be available when the patient arrives in the operating room. Most anesthesiologists insert two large-bore peripheral intravenous catheters, one of which may be a pulmonary artery catheter. Although thermodilution pulmonary artery catheters are used inconsistently in primary coronary operations, most anesthesiologists and surgeons believe that the greater risk of hemodynamic instability with repeat operation requires serial recording of filling pressures and cardiac output (Camann et al., 1987). An alternative method is placement of a pulmonary artery thermistor and a left atrial line postoperatively.

The principle of anesthesia for patients undergoing reoperation is to select anesthetic agents and techniques that will ensure hemodynamic stability, prevent or minimize cardiac ischemia, and protect vital organ function. There is a trend toward monitoring the brachial artery in lieu of the radial artery for greater accuracy. Some anesthesiologists prefer to insert a catheter in the arm opposite the side of internal thoracic artery dissection to avoid subclavian artery or arm compression by the sternal retractor. Femoral artery monitoring is avoided because of the potential for femoral cannulation and the possibility of the need for an intra-aortic balloon pump postoperatively. Calcium-channel blockers and beta-blockers may cause a lower heart rate preoperatively. Calcium-channel blockers may cause arterial vasodilatation, and these patients may experience hypotension, especially if they are dehydrated.

Electrocardiographic monitoring of two leads is standard, and most anesthesia teams have the option to display eight leads. Potent opioid anesthetics (fentanyl and sufentanil) provide improved hemodynamic stability during induction compared with benzodiazepines, inhalational anesthetics, or barbiturates. The new muscle relaxants (such as doxacurium, vecuronium, pipecuronium) are advantageous for further hemodynamic stability. Since inhalation agents may affect ventricular function in reoperations, lower concentrations of inhalation agents may be appropriate. Halothane, enflurane, and isoflurane all produce dose-related myocardial depression.

The author's group uses pulmonary artery catheters for all reoperations; they allow measurement of cardiac output, calculation of cardiac index, and comparison of right and left ventricular function. Transesophageal echocardiography may also provide valuable information about ischemia and the status of ventricular and valvular function. The prevalence of left ventricular dysfunction may limit the level of hemodilution in these reoperation patients. In patients with severe left ventricular dysfunction, cardiac output may be insufficient to compensate for decreased systemic vascular resistance. In these cases, experimental studies indicate that hematocrit levels should not be less than 28 to 30% (Estafanous et al., 1990).

## Reentry and Cannulation

The objective is to avoid complications during reentry and cannulation. It may be wise to expose the femoral vessels in patients who show dense adherence of cardiac structures to the sternum, in patients undergoing a second or more reoperation, in patients who have a patent right internal thoracic artery crossing the midline or a vein graft adhering to the sternotomy, in patients who have received mediastinal irradiation, in patients with aneurysms of the ascending aorta or aortic arch, and in some elderly patients, especially those who have long-standing mitral or tricuspid valve dysfunction or fragile, osteoporotic sternums. In these selected cases, the surgeon should consider cannulating the femoral artery and vein before reopening the sternum. Cardiopulmonary bypass could then be initiated through the femoral artery, which would provide some support if catastrophic bleeding occurred. In cannulating the femoral vein, a long cannula is advanced into the vena cava or right atrium. A second venous cannula may be placed through the right atrium after the sternotomy.

A number of safeguards may prevent bleeding associated with reentry (Loop, 1984): (1) appreciate beforehand that a high-risk situation exists; (2) in the most hazardous circumstance, cannulate the femoral vessels before opening the sternum; (3) use a nitrogen-powered oscillating saw at low power and first divide the outer sternal table only; (4) simultaneously retract the sternum upward with rakes (Fig. 54–85) and request that the anesthesiologist deflate the lungs; (5) avoid probing retrosternally, which may cause penetration of a thin right ventricle; (6) when the sternum is divided, mobilize each side 2 to 4 cm before inserting a retractor; (7) mobilize the innominate vein; (8) if hemorrhage occurs, temporarily approximate the sternum with rakes, initiate femoral arterial venous bypass, and collect mediastinal blood in the cardiotomy reservoir. Core cooling should be immediately initiated, and after hypothermic arrest, the sternal tables should be mobilized before inserting the retractor and visualizing the defect. Large rents may require a patch to alleviate tension on the suture line.

Some surgeons (Burlingame et al., 1988; Uppal et al., 1993) advocate a left thoracotomy for reoperative coronary bypass. The technique limits versatility in grafting and should be considered only in unusual cases, such as patients prone to catastrophic hemorrhage, or unique emergency situations. It requires femoral artery and left atrial or pulmonary artery cannulation. Proximal anastomoses are performed on the descending aorta or subclavian artery, and the site should be marked for future catheterization. In the rare case of reoperation in the presence of a tracheostoma, a bilateral thoracotomy approach separates the stoma from the operative field (Marshall et al., 1988).

Various synthetic and bioprosthetic membranes

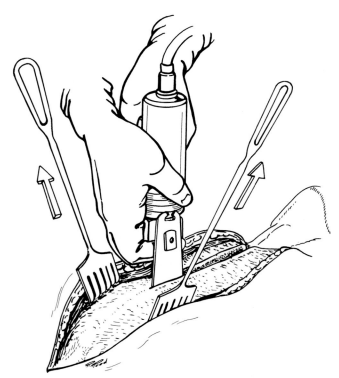

**FIGURE 54–85.** Sternotomy is accomplished with a nitrogen-powered oscillating saw. The anesthesiologist deflates the lungs while an assistant simultaneously pulls outward with rakes fastened to subcutaneous tissue. The objective of these maneuvers is to move the sternum away from the underlying mediastinal structures.

have been used to reduce pericardial and mediastinal adhesions. None has worked consistently, and they may be detrimental in the midst of infection. The effect on future adhesions of pericardial closure after cardiac surgery is unpredictable. Closure of the pericardium may or may not decrease the extent of adhesions. Instead of bioprosthetic or plastic material, the safest material is the patient's own pericardial or mediastinal tissue approximated in the midline after the first operation.

After sternal reentry, the next maneuver is to expose the right atrium and aorta. A plane around the right atrium is entered by dividing adhesions between the right ventricular margin and the diaphragm. One should use sharp dissection instead of blunt, which might tear the myocardium or thin atrial wall. When the aorta is exposed, heparin is administered. Many surgeons prefer to give heparin prior to procuring the lower extremity veins. Gentle technique in vein procurement, avoidance of vein distention, and storage of the specimen in dilute papaverine reduces endothelial sloughing. Consensus has not been reached regarding the optimal storage medium, but only a short period of storage is recommended to reduce endothelial damage. If the internal thoracic arteries and greater saphenous veins do not supply adequate conduits, the next choice is the lesser saphenous veins. Arm veins and synthetic conduits provide lower patency rates. The gastroepiploic artery holds promise, but its versatility as an in situ conduit is limited. The patency of free gastroepiploic arteries as coronary artery bypass grafts is too preliminary to recommend for routine use.

Appropriate heparin dosage cannot always be predicted, yet activated clotting time should be maintained at 480 seconds or higher. A consistently reliable and practical method for anticipating the extremes of heparin responsiveness has not been identified (Gravlee et al., 1987). In most reoperation cases, the aorta is cannulated for arterial perfusion and a two-stage right atrial cannula extending into the inferior vena cava is inserted for venous drainage. In patients who have poor left ventricular function or who require reoperative coronary bypass combined with other cardiac operations, the surgeon may use two caval cannulas, caval tourniquets, and a left atrial or left atrioventricular vent. This full cannulation results in lower septal temperature and consistent decompression.

## Myocardial Protection

Cardioplegic solution is delivered antegrade into the aortic root and retrograde into the coronary sinus. A double-lumen retrograde catheter is inserted through a right atrial purse-string suture and advanced into the coronary sinus. Retrograde perfusion improves the distribution of cardioplegia (Weisel et al., 1983), which is beneficial for patients who have diffuse coronary atherosclerosis, poor left ventricular function, open internal thoracic artery grafts, patent

atherosclerotic vein grafts, or total obstruction of the anterior descending and other coronary arteries.

In recent years, surgeons have advocated normothermic perfusion and continuous warm retrograde cardioplegia (Lichtenstein et al., 1991). This technique is fraught with frequent hyperkalemia and metabolic alkalosis, poor visibility for coronary surgery, maldistribution and inadequate arrest, systemic vasodilatation possibly due to inactivation of the complement system, increased degranulation of neutrophils and increased histamine release, and a theoretical risk of cerebral complications (Martin et al., 1994).

The many cardioplegic techniques probably all provide satisfactory protection for stable patients with normal left ventricular function who undergo primary coronary artery bypass grafting. The differences between techniques arise when patients are unstable preoperatively or have reoperations in the face of severe diffuse coronary atherosclerosis, patent internal thoracic artery grafts, or poor left ventricular performance (Barner, 1991).

Based on the author's group's experience in reoperation, core cooling is recommended, followed by aortic cross-clamping and cardioplegia delivery *before* mobilizing the left ventricle. In cardiac reoperations, blood cardioplegia appears advantageous over crystalloid cardioplegia (Loop et al., 1992). Antegrade/retrograde blood cardioplegia reduces morbidity, specifically perioperative myocardial infarction, wound complications, and overall length of stay in reoperation patients. Despite longer cross-clamp time for patients who received blood cardioplegia, this method of myocardial protection resulted in significantly less morbidity. In the author's group's experience, crystalloid cardioplegia patients were 1.7 times more likely to have a morbid event. Use of blood cardioplegia has also reduced the time required in the intensive care unit and the overall length of stay; consequently, hospital costs are lower. The greatest measure of cost saving is the absence of complications.

Ascending aortic atherosclerosis is a potential source of stroke. Suspected atherosclerosis of the aorta may be further evaluated by intraoperative echocardiography (Blauth et al., 1992; Mills and Everson, 1991). Aortic atheroemboli are related to advanced age, peripheral vascular disease, left main coronary artery narrowing, and a long history of cigarette smoking. The findings of aortic atherosclerosis may contraindicate aortic cross-clamping. Freeing a cold, flaccid heart is technically easier than mobilizing a beating heart, and is less traumatic. In cases of patent, atherosclerotic vein grafts, dissection begins inferiorly and is extended down along the diaphragmatic surface of the left ventricular wall between the heart and the diaphragm (Fig. 54-86). First, the dissection proceeds inferiorly to gain a plane between the inferior and left ventricular wall and the diaphragm. The surgeon then gently sweeps the right hand around the posterolateral surface and up anteriorly under the fused pleuropericardial resection, which may then be opened widely toward the left ventricular apex. The pericar-

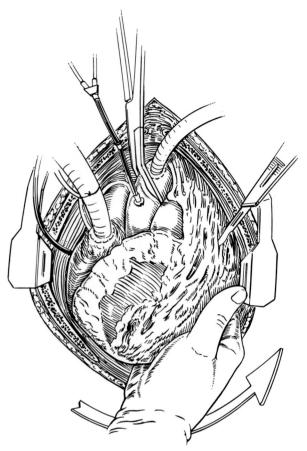

**FIGURE 54–86.** After cannulation and institution of cardiopulmonary bypass and cardioplegia, dissection begins inferiorly to mobilize the cold, flaccid heart. When the surgeon frees the posterolateral surface of the left ventricle, the pleural-pericardial reflection may be opened anteriorly to gain access to the pericardial space.

dium may be dissected back sharply to expose the anterior descending coronary artery (Fig. 54–87).

The regrafting sequence is important, and priorities should be established. Totally occluded atherosclerotic vein grafts are rarely a source of embolization, but atheroembolism from patent atherosclerotic vein grafts is a real threat (Grondin et al., 1984; Keon et al., 1982). Even mild atherosclerosis in vein grafts constitutes a hazard for embolization. Rather than base the decision for replacement on angiographic studies, which underestimate the extent of atherosclerotic involvement of these grafts, some surgeons have recommended replacing all veins more than 5 years old because almost all vein grafts explanted before that time show evidence of atherosclerosis. Reoperation mortality and incidence of myocardial infarction have been reduced by minimal graft handling, prompt division of old grafts before repeated cardioplegic infusion, and performance of all anastomoses (distal and proximal) under one period of cross-clamping.

In the author's group's experience, the first dose of cardioplegic solution may be given via the aortic root and down the old vein graft if it is patent and has

not been manipulated. Subsequent doses are administered after the patent vein grafts are divided (Fig. 54–88). Cardioplegia is delivered at 15- to 20-minute intervals throughout the reoperation. The cardioplegic solution may be administered into the new graft through a side-arm cannula, or the graft may be connected to the aorta and the root reperfused. Proximal anastomoses may be performed at the site of an old graft aortic anastomosis (Fig. 54–89). In patients having reoperation, it is technically easier to construct aortic anastomoses with the aorta fully clamped. After regrafting of arteries perfused by open atherosclerotic vein grafts, attention is turned to other vessels.

In reoperation patients who have a patent internal thoracic artery graft to the anterior descending artery, the procedure is essentially the same except that during mobilization of the left side of the heart, the arterial conduit must be identified so that a small bulldog clamp may be temporarily applied to it (Baillot et al, 1985) (Fig. 54–90). This maneuver is necessary so that continued flow through the thoracic artery does not rewarm the myocardium or wash out the effect of cardioplegia. After this maneuver, additional cardioplegia cools the area supplied by the patent thoracic artery. If thoracic artery perfusion of

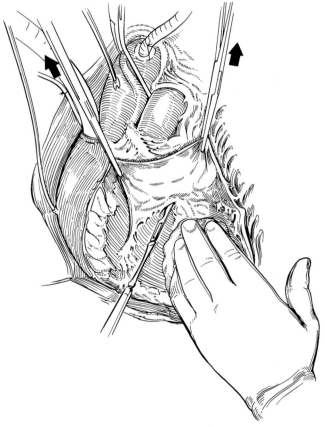

**FIGURE 54–87.** The most anterior leaf of pericardium is grasped and, with gentle countertraction, a flap of adherent pericardium is raised by sharp dissection to expose the anterior descending coronary artery.

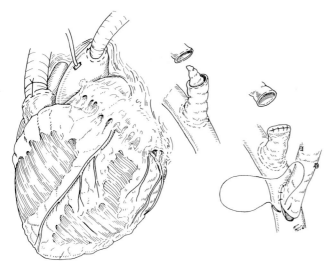

FIGURE 54–88. An atherosclerotic vein graft is divided distally near the old anastomosis. Cardioplegic solution is given retrograde through the coronary sinus to flush out remaining debris. A new distal anastomosis is performed, and the stump of the old graft is oversewn.

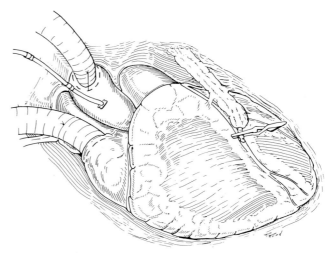

FIGURE 54–90. The patent internal thoracic artery graft has been located and is clamped temporarily to stop blood flow to the anterior descending distribution. Failure to temporarily occlude the internal thoracic artery graft usually produces continued myocardial metabolic activity and less than optimal myocardial protection in that region.

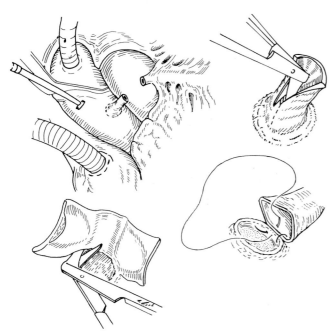

FIGURE 54–89. The new proximal anastomosis frequently may be centered at the site of the previous vein graft aortic anastomosis. In cases of multiple grafting, this maneuver conserves space on the aorta.

the coronary bed is allowed during the operation, protection may be less than optimal because of persistent electrical activity in that region. The internal thoracic artery may even be reused when stenosis has developed immediately beyond the distal anastomosis or the old arterial graft may be removed and reapplied to other vessels, either still as an in situ graft or detached from the subclavian and connected as a free aortocoronary graft (Noyez and Lacquet, 1993).

## Blood Transfusion

Reoperation patients require blood transfusion more than those undergoing primary operations, because of the presence of bleeding adhesions and the generally longer period of cardiopulmonary bypass. Nevertheless, blood conservation has reduced the use of banked blood or blood products from 8 units in the earliest reoperation experience to approximately 2 units today. The risks of blood transfusion include infection, stimulation of antibodies, graft-versus-host disease, and hemolytic transfusion reactions. Hepatitis C virus is the most frequent cause of hepatitis transmitted by blood transfusion. However, the rate of infection with hepatitis C has decreased more than 90%, to 0.03% (Donahue et al., 1992).

Blood conservation should be practiced throughout the operation (Cosgrove et al., 1979; Thurer and Hauer, 1982; Utley et al., 1981). The following methods may be used to reduce transfusion requirements in all cardiac operations: (1) Secure hemostasis throughout the procedure; persistent oozing requires greater use of cardiotomy suction with attendant hemolysis. (2) Restrict total crystalloid infusion to minimize dilutional anemia. (3) Use a regionally heparinized blood processing system to collect intraoperative blood shed before heparinization and after administration of protamine; these cells are washed, concentrated, and transfused at the end of the procedure. (4) Allow normovolemic anemia (25 to 30% hematocrit), depending on preoperative left ventricular function. (5) Control arterial pressure. (6) Transfuse all oxygenator contents at the conclusion of the procedure.

(7) Transfuse shed mediastinal and pleural cavity blood postoperatively. This blood may be collected in the cardiotomy reservoir and transfused without washing or concentration (Cosgrove et al., 1985).

Transfusion requirements vary widely among institutions (Goodnough et al., 1992). Older patients, patients with small blood volume, and patients with preoperative anemia generally require more blood and blood products. Some transfusion practices are questionable, however, and include platelet transfusions in patients who have not received aspirin in the 7 days prior to surgery, plasma transfusion in the absence of multiple blood transfusions, and underutilization of autologous blood. Anemia is tolerated better in younger patients with good left ventricular function and no complications. Some physicians transfuse blood automatically when the hemoglobin/hematocrit falls below 10/30 prior to hospital discharge. A better practice is to individualize based on the patient's appearance, physical progress, and age.

## Hemostasis and Closure

When the aorta is unclamped, cardiopulmonary bypass perfusion is continued until the patient is normothermic and cardiac activity has fully recovered. During this interval of support, hemostasis is obtained, and when indicated, temporary pacemaker wires and additional monitor lines are applied. Anastomoses should be inspected and management should be discussed with the anesthesiologist while the patient is on pump support. After decannulation, anastomotic or other bleeding that requires control by lifting or retraction of the heart may have devastating consequences.

Protamine administration requires careful monitoring. The cardiovascular effects of protamine are those of vasodilatation and negative inotropism. Three types of adverse responses have been identified: hypotensive, anaphylactoid, and catastrophic pulmonary vasoconstriction (Gupta et al., 1989; Horrow, 1988). Patients who have neutral protamine Hagedorn (NPH) insulin-dependent diabetes and those with allergies to fish (commercial protamine is prepared from the sperm of salmon) should have protamine administered cautiously (Stewart et al., 1984). These patients are susceptible to protamine reactions that simulate anaphylaxis. Anyone who has previously received protamine is suspect, although major adverse reactions among nondiabetic patients are rare. The NPH insulin-dependent diabetic patient may have had a long exposure to protamine and thus may have an allergic reaction when rechallenged with a large dose. The use of alternate routes for protamine delivery is conjectural. The safest approach is to administer a test dose, and if no signs of allergy are noted, protamine is given slowly to neutralize heparin.

After protamine is delivered and clot formation is established, hemostatic agents may be useful. Raw sites, especially over the anterior right ventricle, may be managed effectively by a cellulose gauze. Anastomotic oozing may be controlled by fibrin glue applied as a topical hemostatic agent (Borst et al., 1982; Matthew et al., 1990). This sealant is best used after heparin has been neutralized by protamine.

Aprotinin appears effective in reducing bleeding, overall blood loss, and transfusion requirements, but there is also evidence that it may increase the risk of vein graft thrombosis (Cosgrove et al., 1992). Improved hemostasis with aprotinin is attributed to preserved adhesive capacity of platelets, not increased platelet aggregation (van Oeveren et al., 1990). Further reports indicate that aprotinin may be more detrimental in elderly patients who undergo deep hypothermia during thoracic or thoracoabdominal aortic reconstruction, because of the increased risk of renal failure, myocardial infarction, and death (Sundt et al., 1993).

An organized, methodical cleanup phase should be accomplished expeditiously; random cauterization and purposeless movement should be minimized. Pleural chest tubes are best inserted at the time of pleural entry. If the pleura has been entered earlier, extensive lysis of adhesions should be avoided owing to their vascularity. Dense pleural adhesions may bar entry, and in those cases, drainage by mediastinal tubes only is prudent. A heavy No. 6 stainless-steel wire ensures tight sternal approximation and generally prevents dehiscence even if respiratory complications ensue. Interrupted sutures are recommended for fascial and subcutaneous closure, and interrupted monofilament or braided plastic is preferable for skin closure in diabetic patients, obese patients, patients with bilateral internal thoracic artery grafting, and patients with previous mastectomy (Loop et al., 1990). The author's group recommends rescrubbing before sternal closure because microscopic glove perforation occurs frequently and the incidence is related to the duration of surgery.

## Immediate Postoperative Care

In the early phase of postoperative management, attention to afterload reduction, judicious volume replacement, and maintenance of normal hemodynamic parameters help to ensure a favorable outcome. Hypotension secondary to vasodilatation should be treated carefully with controlled doses of vasopressors until the systemic vascular resistance is normalized. Injudicious blood or crystalloid infusion may be harmful and will increase lung water, possibly causing prolonged postoperative ventilation. Antiplatelet drugs are indicated whenever possible to enhance vein graft patency (Chesebro et al., 1982). However, giving aspirin *preoperatively* increases bleeding complications and offers no additional benefit in early vein graft patency (Goldman, 1991). Aspirin does not seem to affect internal thoracic artery patency.

## CLINICAL RESULTS

Despite evidence of a worsening clinical profile of patients with reoperation, early results are improving.

After coronary bypass surgery began in 1967, several years elapsed before publication of the first reports of reoperation. Adam and colleagues (1972) and Johnson and associates (1972) reported an operative mortality rate of approximately 10% and higher morbidity in patients requiring second procedures. Higher risk in coronary artery reoperation was attributed to greater extent of coronary atherosclerosis, interim left ventricular damage, accidents during reentry, technical difficulty caused by adhesions, and longer pump oxygenator time. In the mid-1970s, other reports confirmed that reoperation was more hazardous, but early relief of angina approached that achieved after the first operation (Benedict et al., 1974; Londe and Sugg, 1974; Macmanus et al., 1975; Skow et al., 1973; Stiles et al., 1976; Thomas et al., 1976; Winkle et al., 1975).

The author's group has reviewed a 20-year experience in coronary artery reoperations, from 1967 to 1987 (Loop et al., 1990). In these 2 decades, hospital mortality ranged from 2 to 5%. The internal thoracic artery graft was used in reoperations in 67% of patients. Perioperative Q-wave myocardial infarction was reduced from 8 to 4%. Logistic regression analysis of a number of clinical, angiographic, and operative variables predictive of hospital death found that older age, three-vessel disease, left main coronary artery narrowing greater than or equal to 50%, current cigarette smoking, no internal thoracic arterial graft at the first operation, severe angina, and poor left ventricular function all increased operative risk.

In addition to left main coronary artery disease, open but stenotic grafts are believed by some investigators (Schaff et al., 1983) to pose a higher surgical risk because graft injury or manipulation leading to embolism of atherosclerotic material could compromise myocardial blood supply. Any manipulation, external or internal, may disrupt the fragile debris and cause an embolic myocardial infarction (Case Records of Massachusetts General Hospital, 1987). In the hospital, most deaths after coronary artery reoperation are related to myocardial dysfunction; in the author's group's experience, 82% of early deaths were from cardiac causes (Lytle et al., 1987). Major morbidity in reoperation series has been due to perioperative myocardial infarction (47%), stroke (1 to 2%), reoperation for bleeding (4 to 5%), respiratory distress (2 to 3%), wound complication (1%), and renal failure (less than 1%) (Foster et al., 1984; Loop et al., 1990).

Freedom from angina after the initial coronary artery operation must be judged as the base line to compare results after reoperation. In one study, the freedom from angina after primary revascularization was 95%, 83%, and 63% at 1, 5, and 10 years after initial surgery (Sergeant et al., 1991). The incidence of late angina is increased by hyperlipidemia and hypertension; the severity of preoperative symptoms and return of angina were more frequent in women. However, the freedom from sudden death was 97% at 10 years.

After reoperation, relief of angina is less than after the first operation (Cameron et al., 1988; Loop et al., 1983; Schaff et al., 1983), mainly because of high recurrence of angina in the first year postoperatively. Rather than studying freedom from angina per se, which is approximately 50% at 10 years after reoperation (Lytle et al., 1987), angina should be included in an assessment of cardiac events. Cardiac events are analyzed in terms of event-free survival, and the end points depend on which cardiac events are included in the follow-up. Schaff and co-workers (1983) calculated that angina-free survival was 40% at 3 years, 28% at 5 years, and 26% at 7 years. Freedom from New York Heart Association Class III or IV angina was 73% at 3 years and 63% at 5 to 7 years. Thus, a relatively high proportion of patients having reoperation had mild angina 5 years postoperatively, but severe angina was less common. In one report, a low serum cholesterol level was the best correlate of an improved symptomatic response after the first operation (Lamas et al., 1986). However, after a reoperation, the principal correlate of a better symptomatic response was normal or almost normal ventricular ejection fraction before reoperation.

Information about reoperation graft patency is scarce because few patients who have one or more coronary reoperations will be restudied by postoperative angiography unless they have recurrent symptoms of angina that substantially affect life-style. The records of 256 patients were assessed from a reoperation series of 1500 patients who had angiography after reoperation (Lytle et al., 1987). Patency of both vein and internal thoracic artery grafts was almost the same as that reported after the first operation: 70% for vein grafts and 91% for internal thoracic artery grafts at an average of 4 years postoperatively.

## SURVIVAL

Longevity after coronary reoperation must be considered as a continuum of survival that began with the first coronary operation. These patients were operated on initially for angina in most cases, but they tended to be a decade or more younger than the average surgical candidate today. Furthermore, these patients, who were operated on originally in the 1970s, tended to have less extensive coronary atherosclerosis, had normal left ventricular function, or had incomplete revascularization (i.e., not all significantly narrowed major coronary arteries received bypass grafts). This profile is different today. The average age of surgical patients has increased; 75% or more have three-vessel disease, and half have impaired left ventricular performance. Complete revascularization is achieved in 90% or more, and one or both internal thoracic artery grafts are used more liberally.

The point is that both the patient and the operation have changed since the early 1980s, and these changes affect both the incidence and the outcome of reoperations. In this continuum, the patient has survived the first operation and later on, mainly after the fifth postoperative year, has a cardiac event that initiates reevaluation and sometimes a reoperation. These reoperation patients have shown 5-year and 10-year actuarial survival rates of 90 and 75%, respectively (Fig. 54–91). The survival rate is more impressive if one takes into account that longevity began with the first operation. From an analysis of 2509 consecutive reoperation patients, advanced age, hypertension, and abnormal left ventricular function are found to adversely affect late survival (Loop et al., 1990; Lytle et al., 1987). The angiographic indication for reoperation (i.e., graft closure, progressive atherosclerosis, or a combination of these two indications) did not affect survival. Data on subsets indicate a 3-year survival of 85% for patients 70 years or older and a 5-year survival of 82% for patients with severely impaired left ventricular function. Preliminary data indicate that a new internal thoracic artery graft to the anterior descending coronary artery favorably influences intermediate-term survival after reoperation (Lytle et al., 1994). Patency, freedom from coronary events, and survival are extended (Galbut et al., 1991).

In the Cleveland Clinic report of patients who underwent angiography 5 or more years after the original operation, surgery for late anterior descending vein graft stenosis resulted in significant improvement in survival over medical treatment (Lytle et al., 1993) (Fig. 54–92). The 2- to 4-year survival after late catheterization was 84 and 74% respectively, versus 76 and 53% for the medically treated group. This improvement applied also to patients with mild symptoms. Patients with totally obstructed grafts to the anterior descending artery also had improved survival with early reoperative surgery. Interestingly, patients with a patent internal thoracic artery graft to the anterior descending artery were at lower risk with medical treatment, and early reoperation did not appear to improve their survival.

Results of two or more coronary artery reoperations indicate higher mortality for each successive reoperation. For hospital survivors, however, the outlook was reasonably good, with 87% alive 5 years later (Breno-

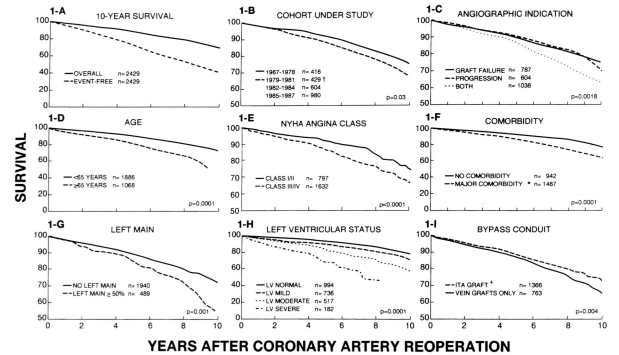

YEARS AFTER CORONARY ARTERY REOPERATION

†1979–81, 1982–84, 1985–87 curves are superimposed
*Diabetes, hypertension, peripheral vascular disease, or cigarette smoking
+Internal thoracic artery (ITA) graft used at either first or second operation

**FIGURE 54–91.** *1–A,* Ten-year actuarial survival and event-free survival rates are shown after reoperation for 2429 hospital survivors, 69.3% and 41.2%, respectively. *1–B,* The earliest group, 1967–1978, enjoyed a significantly higher 10-year survival rate (74.5%) than the first three cohorts, whose curves are virtually superimposed and reach 67.4% at 10 years. *1–C,* Analysis of longevity by angiographic indication shows that patients reoperated on for graft failure or progressive atherosclerosis had a better ($p = .0018$) 10-year survival rate than patients who experienced both progression and graft failure, 75.5% and 70.4% versus 63.4%. *1–D,* Patients younger than 65 years before reoperation had a significantly better 10-year survival rate (72.0%) than their older counterparts (50.8%) ($p = .0001$). *1–E,* Survival rate by NYHA angina functional class shows Classes I and II achieved 69.1% and III and IV, 63.5% ($p < .0001$). *1–F,* Co-morbidity was defined as diabetes, hypertension, peripheral vascular disease, and cigarette smoking. Those with no co-morbidity had a 10-year survival rate (77.1%) significantly greater than those with one or all co-morbid conditions (63.7%) ($p = .0001$). *1–G,* The presence or absence of left main coronary artery narrowing ≥ 50% significantly influenced 10-year survival rate, 71.9% versus 55.2% ($p = .001$). *1–H,* Left ventricular performance before operation, stratified subjectively, demonstrated a wide range of 10-year survival rates: normal function, 77.4%; mild impairment, 70.3%; moderate dysfunction, 56.4%; and severe impairment, 45.1%. The survival difference between normal and poor performance is significant ($p = .0001$). *1–I,* The performance of an internal thoracic artery graft at either the first or the second operation affected long-term survival rate (72.6%) compared with vein grafts at both operations (65.5%) ($p = .004$). (*1–A* to *1–I,* From Loop, F. D., Lytle, B. W., Cosgrove, D. M., et al.: Reoperation for coronary atherosclerosis: Changing practice in 2509 consecutive patients. Ann. Surg., 212:378–386, 1990.)

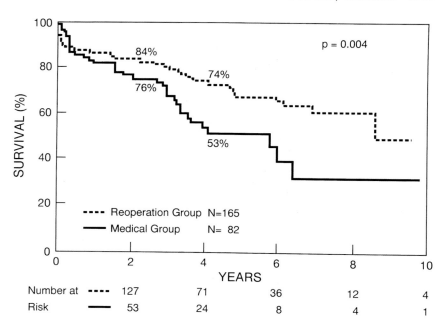

**FIGURE 54–92.** Actuarial survival comparisons for patients with late severe anterior descending coronary artery vein graft stenosis treated surgically and medically. The zero point in time is 5 or more years after the first operation. Subsequent years listed on the horizontal axis are years after postoperative catheterization. Patients undergoing reoperation had significantly improved survival compared with their medical counterparts. (From Lytle, B. W., Loop, F. D., Taylor, P. C., et al.: The effect of coronary reoperation on the survival of patient with stenoses in saphenous vein bypass grafts to coronary arteries. J. Thorac. Cardiovasc. Surg., *105*:605–614, 1993.)

witz et al., 1988). Few reports on reoperation in women are available, but the in-hospital death rate may not be higher overall than that generally encountered in the first operation (Kahn et al., 1993).

## LONG-TERM CARE

The surgeon should advise the patient who smokes to stop smoking completely (Hermanson et al., 1988), eat a low-fat diet, monitor serum lipid levels (Landymore, 1991), keep diabetes (Hoogwerf, 1992) and hypertension under good control (Campeau et al., 1984), maintain ideal weight, and exercise with progress monitored through a cardiovascular rehabilitation program (Hedback et al., 1990; Juneau et al., 1991). Modification of Type A behavior remains controversial (Rose and Robbins, 1992), but some type of stress management is important for many patients (Swenson and Abbey, 1992). Reduction of serum lipids is an attainable goal for most patients (Agren et al., 1989; Nessim et al., 1983). Although bypass surgery has no effect on the underlying cause of the disease, secondary prevention that modifies risk factors may reduce recurrent coronary heart disease and death (Murray and Beller, 1983; Siegel et al., 1988). Dietary recommendations should be individualized to the specific lipoprotein abnormality and ideal body weight (Lavie et al., 1988). A registered dietitian with a particular interest in coronary heart disease may provide the patient with advice and encouragement (Brown et al., 1990).

Patients who do not respond to dietary efforts and who have lipoprotein abnormalities are candidates for drug therapy (Blankenhorn et al., 1987). Most of the lipid-lowering drugs are expensive and may have major side effects. The 3-hydroxy-3-methylglutaryl coenzyme A reductase inhibitors, such as lovastatin,

are the most promising of these agents, but the long-term efficacy and safety of these drugs is not yet proved. Although regression of the complicated plaque has been considered a rare event, the advent of new lipid-lowering agents may slow the progression of disease and may even make regression of coronary atherosclerosis a reality (Brown et al., 1990; Sheperd and Packard, 1988).

The Cholesterol-Lowering Atherosclerosis Study found that therapeutic reduction of total plasma and low density lipoprotein cholesterol was associated with a reduction in percentage of new vein bypass graft lesions (Blankenhorn et al., 1987). These and other clinical trials were done in middle-aged men, so the extrapolation to women and elderly persons may not apply. Optimal weight and exercise in keeping with norms for age and previous activity are part of any rehabilitation plan (Blackburn, 1992). A recent study showed a beneficial effect of regular physical exercise and a low-fat diet on progression of coronary lesions (Schuler et al., 1992a, 1992b). Eight to 12 weeks of exercise training provide reconditioning for return to normal activities and help establish the concept of regular exercise (Pashkow, 1993), but 3 months of supervised exercise training are recommended for patients who desire to do strenuous exercise such as jogging, tennis, and handball (Thompson, 1988). This advice applies particularly to reoperation patients who are at higher risk because of more diffuse coronary atherosclerosis and abnormal left ventricular function (Pashkow, 1991).

Because platelet function inhibition appears to improve vein graft patency up to 1 year after coronary bypass surgery (Chesebro et al, 1984), aspirin/dipyridamole or aspirin alone is prescribed for at least 1 year for patients who tolerate salicylates and have not had peptic ulcer disease or blood dyscrasia and are not receiving anticoagulants (Fuster and Chesebro, 1986). No clinical studies currently address the effect of antiplatelet agents on the development of vein graft atherosclerosis, although data in animals suggest that such therapy may reduce vein graft atherogenesis (Boerboom et al., 1990; Landymore et al., 1991). There is no reason to believe that new vein grafts are any more immune to atherosclerosis than the first ones. Exercise electrocardiographic testing with some type of noninvasive imaging can be used to assess residual ischemia when clinically indicated or on a periodic basis in those with suspected silent ischemia (Dubach et al., 1989). Ten years after the first or subsequent coronary bypass operation, another coronary arteriogram is advisable, even if no cardiac events have occurred.

## BIBLIOGRAPHY

Adam, M., Geisler G. F., Lambert, C. J., and Mitchel, B. F., Jr.: Reoperation following clinical failure of aorta-to-coronary artery bypass vein grafts. Ann. Thorac. Surg., 14:272, 1972.

Addonizio, V. P., Jr., Fisher, C. A., Kappa, J. R., and Ellison, N.: Prevention of heparin-induced thrombocytopenia during open heart surgery with Illoprost (ZK 36374). Surgery, 102:796, 1987.

Agren, B., Olin, C., Castentors, J., and Nilsson-Ehle, P.: Improvements of the lipoprotein profile after coronary bypass surgery: Additional effects of an exercise training program. Eur. Heart J., 10:451, 1989.

Alderman, E. L., Fisher, L., Maynard, C., et al.: Determinants of coronary surgery in a consecutive patient series from geographically dispersed medical centers: The Coronary Artery Surgery Study. Circulation, 66(Suppl. I):6, 1982.

American Association of Blood Banks: Standards for Blood Banks and Transfusion Services. 15th ed. Bethesda, MD, American Association of Blood Banks, 1993.

Bahn, C. H., and Annest, L. S.: Reoperation without medical records: Avoidable? J. Thorac. Cardiovasc. Surg., 91:139, 1986.

Baillot, R. G., Loop, F. D., Cosgrove, D. M., and Lytle, B. W.: Reoperation after previous grafting with the internal mammary artery: Technique and early results. Ann. Thorac. Surg., 40:271, 1985.

Barboriak, J. J., Barboriak, D. P., Anderson, A. J., et al.: Risk factors in patients undergoing a second aorta-coronary bypass procedure. J. Thorac. Cardiovasc. Surg., 76:111, 1978.

Barner, H.: Blood cardioplegia: A review and comparison with crystalloid cardioplegia. Ann. Thorac. Surg., 52:1354, 1991.

Benedict, J. S., Buhl, T. L., and Henney, R. P.: Re-revascularization of the ischemic myocardium. Arch. Surg., 108:40, 1974.

Blackburn, G. G.: Exercise prescription development and supervision: Perspectives on the formulation of exercise prescriptions. In Pashkow, F., and Dafoe, W. (eds): Clinical Cardiac Rehabilitation: A Cardiologist's Guide. Baltimore, Williams & Wilkins, 1992, pp. 3–24.

Blankenhorn, D. H., Nessim, S. A., Johnson, R. L., et al.: Beneficial effects of combined colestipol-niacin therapy on coronary atherosclerosis and coronary venous bypass grafts. J.A.M.A., 257:3233, 1987.

Blauth, C. L., Cosgrove, D. M., Webb, B. W., et al.: Atheroembolism from the ascending aorta. J. Thorac. Cardiovasc. Surg., 103:1104, 1992.

Boerboom, L. E., Olinger, G. N., Liu, T. Z., et al.: Histologic, morphometric, and biochemical evolution of vein bypass grafts in a nonhuman primate model. III. Long-term changes and their modification by platelet inhibition with aspirin and dipyridamole. J. Thorac. Cardiovasc. Surg., 99:426, 1990.

Borst, H. G., Haverich, A., Walterbusch, G., and Maatz, W.: Fibrin adhesive: An important hemostatic adjunct in cardiovascular operations. J. Thorac. Cardiovasc. Surg., 84:548, 1982.

Bourassa, M. G., Lesperance, J., Corbara, F., et al.: Progression of obstructive coronary artery disease 5 to 7 years after aortocoronary bypass surgery. Circulation, 58(Suppl. I):100, 1978.

Brenowitz, J. B., Johnson, W. D., Kayser, K. L., et al.: Coronary

artery bypass grafting for the third time or more: Results of 150 consecutive cases. Circulation, 78:(Suppl. I):166, 1988.

Brown, G., Albers, J. J., Fisher, L. D., et al.: Regression of coronary artery disease as a result of intensive lipid-lowering therapy in men with high levels of apolipoprotein B. N. Engl. J. Med., 323:1289, 1990.

Burlingame, M. W., Bonchek, L. L., and Vazales, B. E.: Left thoracotomy for reoperative coronary bypass. J. Thorac. Cardiovasc. Surg., 95:508, 1988.

Camann, W. R., Wojtowicz, S. R., and Mark, J. B.: Reoperation for coronary artery bypass grafting: Anesthetic challenge. J. Card. Anes., 1:458, 1987.

Cameron, A., Kemp, H. G., Jr., and Green, G. E.: Bypass surgery with the internal mammary artery graft: 15-year follow-up. Circulation, 74(Suppl. III):30, 1988.

Cameron, A., Kemp, H. G., Jr., and Green, G. E.: Reoperation for coronary artery disease: 10 years of clinical follow-up. Circulation, 78(Suppl. I):158, 1988.

Campeau, L., Enjalbert, M., Lesperance, J., et al.: The relation of risk factors to the development of atherosclerosis in saphenous-vein bypass grafts and the progression of disease in the native circulation: A study 10 years after aorto-coronary bypass surgery. N. Engl. J. Med., 311:1329, 1984.

Case Records of the Massachusetts General Hospital: Case 6–1987. N. Engl. J. Med., 316:321, 1987.

Chesebro, J. H., Clements, I. P., Fuster, V., et al.: A platelet inhibitor-drug trial in coronary-artery bypass operations: Benefit of perioperative dipyridamole and aspirin therapy on early postoperative vein-graft patency. N. Engl. J. Med., 307:73, 1982.

Chesebro, J. H., Fuster, V., Elveback, L. R., et al.: Effect of dipyridamole and aspirin on late vein-graft patency after coronary bypass operations. N. Engl. J. Med., 310:209, 1984.

Coltharp, W. H., Decker, M. D., Lea, J. W., et al.: Internal mammary artery graft at reoperation: Risks, benefits and methods and preservation. Ann. Thorac. Surg., 52:225, 1991.

Cosgrove, D. M., Amiot, D. M., and Meserko, J. J.: An improved technique of autotransfusion of shed mediastinal blood. Ann. Thorac. Surg., 40:519, 1985.

Cosgrove, D. M., Heric, B., Lytle, B. W., et al.: Aprotinin therapy for reoperative myocardial revascularization: A placebo-controlled study. Ann. Thorac. Surg., 54:1031, 1992.

Cosgrove, D. M., Loop, F. D., Lytle, B. W., et al.: Predictors of reoperation after myocardial revascularization. J. Thorac. Cardiovasc. Surg., 92:811, 1986.

Cosgrove, D. M., Lytle, B. W., Hill, A. C., et al.: Are two internal thoracic arteries better than one? J. Thorac. Cardiovasc. Surg. (in press).

Cosgrove, D. M., Thurer, R. L., Lytle, B. W., et al.: Blood conservation during myocardial revascularization. Ann. Thorac. Surg., 28:184, 1979.

Cox, J. L., Chiasson, D. A., and Gotlieb, A. I.: Stranger in a strange land: The pathogenesis of saphenous vein graft stenosis with emphasis on structural and functional differences between veins and arteries. Prog. Cardiovasc. Dis., 34:45, 1991.

Crean, P. A., Waters, D. D., Bosch, X., et al.: Angiographic findings after myocardial infarction in patients with previous bypass surgery: Explanations for smaller infarcts in this group compared with control patients. Circulation, 71:693, 1985.

Culliford, A. T., Girdwood, R. W., Isom, O. W., et al.: Angina following myocardial revascularization: Does time of recurrence predict etiology and influence results of operation? J. Thorac. Cardiovasc. Surg., 77:899, 1979.

Dimas, A. P., Arora, R. R., Whitlow, P. L., et al.: Percutaneous transluminal angioplasty involving internal mammary artery grafts. Am. Heart J., 122:423, 1991.

Donahue, J. G., Munoz, A., Ness, P. M., et al.: The declining risk of post-transfusion hepatitis C virus infection. N. Engl. J. Med., 327:369, 1992.

Douglas, J. S.: Percutaneous intervention in patients with prior coronary bypass surgery. In Topol, E. J. (ed): Textbook of Interventional Cardiology, 2nd ed. Philadelphia, W. B. Saunders, 1994.

Dubach, P., Froelicher, V., Klein, J., and Detrano, R.: Use of the exercise test to predict prognosis after coronary artery bypass graft. Am. J. Cardiol., 63:530, 1989.

Estafanous, F. G., Smith, C. E., Selim, W. M., and Tarazi, R. C.: Cardiovascular effects of acute normovolemic hemodilution in rats with disopyramide-induced myocardial depression. Basic Res. Cardiol., 85:227, 1990.

Ferguson, T. B., Jr., Muhlbaier, L. H., Salai, D. L., and Wechsler, A. S.: Coronary bypass grafting after failed elective and failed emergent percutaneous angioplasty. J. Thorac. Cardiovasc. Surg., 95:761, 1988.

Ferraris, V. A., Ferraris, S. P., Lough, F. C., and Berry, W. R.: Preoperative aspirin ingestion increases operative blood loss after coronary artery bypass grafting. Ann. Thorac. Surg., 45:71, 1988.

Foster, E. D., Fisher, L. D., Kaiser, G. C., and Myers, W. O.: Comparison of operative mortality and morbidity for initial and repeat coronary artery bypass grafting: The Coronary Artery Surgery Study (CASS) Registry experience. Ann. Thorac. Surg., 38:563, 1984.

Fuster, V., and Chesebro, J. H.: Role of platelets and platelet inhibitors in aortocoronary artery vein-graft disease. Circulation, 73:227, 1986.

Galbut, D. L., Traad, E. A., Dorman, M. J., et al.: Bilateral internal mammary artery grafts in reoperative and primary coronary bypass surgery. Ann. Thorac. Surg., 52:20, 1991.

Golding, L. A. R., Loop, F. D., Hollman, J. L., et al.: Early results of emergency surgery following coronary angioplasty. Circulation, 74(Suppl. III):26, 1986.

Goldman, S., Copeland, J., Moritz, T., et al.: Starting aspirin therapy after operation: Effects on early graft patency. Circulation, 84:520, 1991.

Goodnough, L. T., Johnston, M. F., Ramsey, G., et al.: Guidelines for transfusion support in patients undergoing coronary artery bypass grafting. Ann. Thorac. Surg., 50:675, 1990.

Goodnough, L. T., Johnston, M. F. M., Toy, P. T. C. Y.: The variability of transfusion practice in coronary artery bypass surgery. J.A.M.A., 265:86, 1992.

Gravlee, G. P., Brauer, S. D., Roy, R. C., et al.: Predicting the pharmacodynamics of heparin. A clinical evaluation of the Hepcon System 4. J. Card. Anes., 1:379, 1987.

Grondin, C. M.: Graft disease in patients with coronary bypass grafting [Editorial]. J. Thorac. Cardiovasc. Surg., 92:323, 1986.

Grondin, C. M., Pomar, J. L., Hebert, Y., et al.: Reoperation in patients with patent atherosclerotic coronary vein grafts: A different approach to a different disease. J. Thorac. Cardiovasc. Surg., 87:379, 1984.

Gupta, S. K., Veith, F. J., Ascer, E., et al.: Anaphylactoid reactions to protamine: An often lethal complication in insulin-dependent diabetic patients undergoing vascular surgery. J. Vasc. Surg., 9:342, 1989.

Hedback, B. E., Perk, J., Engvall, J., and Areskog, N. H.: Cardiac rehabilitation after coronary artery bypass grafting: Effects on exercise performance and risk factors. Arch. Phys. Med. Rehabil., 71:1069, 1990.

Hermanson, B., Omenn, G. S., Kronmal, R. A., et al.: Beneficial six-year outcome of smoking cessation in older men and women with coronary artery disease: Results from the CASS Registry. N. Engl. J. Med., 319:1365, 1988.

Higgins, T. L., Estafanous, F. G., Loop, F. D., et al.: Stratification of morbidity and mortality outcome by preoperative risk factors in coronary artery bypass patients: A clinical severity score. J.A.M.A., 267:2344, 1992.

Hoogwerf, B. J.: Cardiac rehabilitation in the diabetic patient. In Pashkow, F., and Dafoe, W. (eds), Clinical Cardiac Rehabilitation: A Cardiologist's Guide. Baltimore, Williams & Wilkins, 1992, pp. 169–177.

Horrow, J. C.: Protamine allergy. J. Card. Anes., 2:225, 1988.

Johnson, W. D., Brenowitz, J. B., and Kayser, K. L.: Factors influencing long-term (10-year to 15-year) survivial after a successful coronary artery bypass operation. Ann. Thorac. Surg., 48:19, 1989.

Johnson, W. D., Hoffman, J. F., Jr., Flemma, R. J., and Tector, A. J.: Secondary surgical procedure for myocardial revascularization. J. Thorac. Cardiovasc. Surg., 64:523, 1972.

Juneau, M., Geneau, S., Marchand, C., and Brosseau, R.: Cardiac rehabilitation after coronary bypass surgery. Cardiovasc. Clin., 21:25, 1991.

Kahn, S. S., Nessim, S., Gray, R., et al.: Outcome of coronary bypass reoperation in women. J. Am. Coll. Cardiol., 21(Suppl. A):132A, 1993.

Kappa, J. R., Horn, M. K., III, Fisher, C. A., et al.: Efficacy of iloprost (ZK36374) versus aspirin in preventing heparin-induced platelet activation during cardiac operations. J. Thorac. Cardiovasc. Surg., 94:405, 1987.

Keon, W. J., Heggtveit, H. A., and Leduc, J.: Perioperative myocardial infarction caused by atheroembolism. J. Thorac. Cardiovasc. Surg., 84:849, 1982.

King, D. J., and Kelton, J. G.: Heparin-associated thrombocytopenia. Ann. Intern. Med., 100:535, 1984.

Kirklin, J. W., Naftel, D. C., Blackstone, E. H., and Pohost, G. M.: Summary of a consensus concerning death and ischemic events after coronary artery bypass grafting. Circulation, 79(Suppl. I):81, 1989.

Klein, L. W., Weintraub, W. D., Agarwal, J. B., et al.: Prognostic significance of severe narrowing of the proximal portion of the left anterior descending coronary artery. Am. J. Cardiol., 58:42, 1986.

Lamas, G. A., Mudge, G. H., Jr., Collins, J. J., Jr., et al.: Clinical response to coronary artery reoperations. J. Am. Coll. Cardiol., 8:274, 1986.

Landymore, R. W.: Inaccuracy of serum lipid measurements after open heart operations. Can. J. Cardiol., 7:24, 1991.

Landymore, R. W., MacAulay, M. A., and Fris, J.: Effect of aspirin on intimal hyperplasia and cholesterol uptake in experimental bypass grafts. Can. J. Cardiol., 7:87, 1991.

Lavie, C. J., Gau, G. T., Squires, R. W., and Kottke, B. A.: Management of lipids in primary and secondary prevention of cardiovascular diseases. Mayo Clin. Proc., 63:512, 1988.

Lichtenstein, S. V., Ashe, K. A., El Dalati, H., et al.: Warm heart surgery. J. Thorac. Cardiovasc. Surg., 101:269, 1991.

Londe, S., and Sugg, W. L.: The challenge of reoperation in cardiac surgery. Ann. Thorac. Surg., 17:157, 1974.

Loop, F. D.: Catastrophic hemorrhage during sternal reentry. Ann. Thorac. Surg., 37:271, 1984.

Loop, F. D., Higgins, T. L., Panda, R., et al.: Myocardial protection during cardiac operations. J. Thorac. Cardiovasc. Surg., 104:608, 1992.

Loop, F. D., Lytle, B. W., Cosgrove, D. M., et al.: Coronary artery bypass graft surgery in the elderly: Indications and outcome. Cleve. Clin. J. Med., 55:23, 1988.

Loop, F. D., Lytle, B. W., Gill, C. C., et al., Trends in selection and results of coronary artery reoperations. Ann. Thorac. Surg., 36:380, 1983.

Loop, F. D., Lytle, B. W., Cosgrove, D. M., et al.: Influence of the internal mammary artery graft on 10-year survival and other cardiac events. N. Engl. J. Med., 314:1, 1986.

Loop, F. D., Lytle, B. W., Cosgrove, D. M., et al.: Reoperation for coronary atherosclerosis: Changing practice in 2509 consecutive patients. Ann. Surg., 212:378, 1990.

Loop F. D., and Whitlow, R. L.: Coronary angioplasty in patients with previous bypass surgery. J. Am. Coll. Cardiol., 16:1348, 1990.

Lytle, B. W., Loop, F. D., Cosgrove, D. M., et al.: Long-term (5 to 12 years) serial studies of internal mammary artery and saphenous vein coronary bypass grafts. J. Thorac. Cardiovasc. Surg., 89:248, 1985.

Lytle, B. W., Loop, F. D., Cosgrove, D. M., et al.: Fifteen hundred coronary reoperations: Results and determinants of early and late survival. J. Thorac. Cardiovasc. Surg., 93:847, 1987.

Lytle, B. W., Loop, F. D., Taylor, P. C., et al.: The effect of coronary reoperation on the survival of patients with stenoses in saphenous vein bypass grafts to coronary arteries. J. Thorac. Cardiovasc. Surg., 105:605, 1993.

Lytle, B. W., Loop, F. D., Taylor, P. C., et al.: Vein graft disease: The clinical impact of stenoses in saphenous vein bypass grafts to coronary arteries. J. Thorac. Cardiovasc. Surg., 103:831, 1992.

Lytle, B. W., McElroy, D., McCarthy, P., et al.: The influence of arterial coronary bypass grafts on the mortality of coronary reoperations. J. Thorac. Cardiovasc. Surg., 107:675, 1994.

Macmanus, O., Okies, J. E., Phillips, S. J., and Starr, A.: Surgical considerations in patients undergoing repeat median sternotomy. J. Thorac. Cardiovasc. Surg., 69:138, 1975.

Marshall, W. G., Meng, R. L., and Ehrenhaft, J. L.: Coronary artery bypass grafting in patients with a tracheostoma: Use of a bilateral thoracotomy incision. Ann. Thorac. Surg., 46:465, 1988.

Marshall, W. G., Saffitz, J., and Kouchoukos, N. T.: Management during reoperation of aortocoronary saphenous vein grafts with minimal atherosclerosis by angiography. Ann. Thorac. Surg., 42:163, 1986.

Martin, T. D., Craver, J. M., Gott, J. P., et al.: Prospective, randomized trial of retrograde warm blood cardioplegia: Myocardial benefit and neurologic threat. Ann. Thorac. Surg., 57:298, 1994.

Matthew, T. L., Spotnitz, W. D., Kron, I. L., et al.: Four years' experience with fibrin sealant in thoracic and cardiovascular surgery. Ann. Thorac. Surg., 50:40, 1990.

Mills, N. L., and Everson, C. T.: Atherosclerosis of the ascending aorta and coronary artery bypass. J. Thorac. Cardiovasc. Surg., 102:546, 1991.

Murray, G. C., and Beller, G. A.: Cardiac rehabilitation following coronary artery bypass surgery. Am. Heart J., 105:1009, 1983.

Navia, D., Cosgrove, D. M., Lytle, B. W., et al.: Is the internal thoracic artery the conduit of choice to replace a stenotic vein graft? Ann. Thorac. Surg., 57:40, 1994.

Neitzel, G. F., Barboriak, J. J., Pintar, K., and Qureshi, I.: Atherosclerosis in aortocoronary bypass grafts: Morphologic study and risk factor analysis 6 to 12 years after surgery. Arteriosclerosis, 6:594, 1986.

Nessim, S. A., Chin, H. P., Alaupovic, P., and Blankenhorn, D. H.: Combined therapy of niacin, colestipol, and fat-controlled diet in men with coronary bypass. Effect on blood lipids and apolipoproteins. Arteriosclerosis, 3:568, 1983.

Noyez, L., and Lacquet, L. K.: Recycling of the internal mammary artery in coronary reoperation. Ann. Thorac. Surg., 55:597, 1993.

Pashkow, F. J.: Issues in contemporary cardiac rehabilitation: A historical perspective. J. Am. Coll. Cardiol., 21:822, 1993.

Pashkow, F. J.: Rehabilitation strategies for the complex cardiac patient. Cleve. Clin. J. Med., 58:70, 1991.

Passamani, E., Davis, K. B., Gillespie, M. G. J., and Killip, T.: A randomized trial of coronary artery bypass surgery: Survival of patients with a low ejection fraction. N. Engl. J. Med., 313:1665, 1985.

Platko, W. P., Hollman, J., Whitlow, P. L., and Franco, I.: Percutaneous transluminal angioplasty of saphenous vein graft stenosis: Long-term follow-up. J. Am. Coll. Cardiol., 14:1645, 1989.

Qiao, J. H., Walts, A. E., and Fishbein, M. C.: The severity of atherosclerosis at sites of plaque rupture with occlusive thrombosis in saphenous vein coronary artery bypass grafts. Am. Heart J., 122:955, 1991.

Reed, D. C., Beller, G. A., Nygaard, T. W., et al.: The clinical efficacy and scintigraphic evaluation of post-coronary bypass patients undergoing percutaneous transluminal coronary angioplasty for recurrent angina pectoris. Am. Heart J., 117:60, 1989.

Reeves, F., Bonan, R., Cote, G., et al.: Long-term angiographic follow-up after angioplasty of venous coronary bypass grafts. Am. Heart J., 122:620, 1991.

Rose, M., and Robbins, B.: Psychosocial recovery issues and strategies in cardiac rehabilitation. In Pashkow, F., and Dafoe, W. (eds): Clinical Cardiac Rehabilitation: A Cardiologist's Guide. Baltimore, Williams and Wilkins, 1992, pp. 248–262.

Schaff, H. V., Orszulak, T. A., Gersh, B. J., et al.: The morbidity and mortality of reoperation for coronary artery disease and analysis of late results with use of actuarial estimate of event free interval. J. Thorac. Cardiovasc. Surg., 85:508, 1983.

Schuler, G., Hambrecht, R., Schlierf, G., et al.: Myocardial perfusion and regression of coronary artery disease in patients on a regimen of intensive physical exercise and low-fat diet. J. Am. Coll. Cardiol., 19:34, 1992.

Schuler, G., Hambrecht, R., Schlierf, G., et al.: Regular physical exercise and low-fat diet: Effects on progression of coronary artery disease. Circulation, 86:1, 1992b.

Schuster, E. H., Griffith, L. S., and Bulkley, B. H.: Preponderance of acute proximal left anterior descending coronary arterial lesions in fatal myocardial infarction: A clinicopathologic study. Am. J. Cardiol., 47:1189, 1981.

Sergeant, P., Lesaffre, E., Flameng, W., et al.: The return of clinically evident ischemia after coronary artery bypass grafting. Eur. J. Cardiothorac. Surg., 5:446, 1991.

Shark, W. M., and Kass, R. M.: Repeat myocardial revascularization in coronary disease therapy: Consideration of primary bypass failures and success of second graft surgery. Am. Heart. J., 102:303, 1981.

Sheperd, J., and Packard, C. J.: Regression of coronary atherosclerosis: Is it possible? Br. Heart J., 59:149, 1988.

Siegel, D., Grady, D., Browner, W. S., and Hulley, S. B.: Risk factor modification after myocardial infarction. Ann. Intern. Med., 109:213, 1988.

Sims, F. H.: The internal mammary artery as a bypass graft? Ann. Thorac. Surg., 44:2, 1987.

Skow, J. R., Carey, J. S., Plested, W. G., and Mulder, D. G.: Saphenous vein bypass as a secondary cardiac procedure. Arch. Surg., 107:34, 1973.

Stewart, W. J., McSweeney, S. M., Kellett, M. A., et al.: Increased risk of severe protamine reactions in NPH insulin-dependent diabetics undergoing cardiac catheterization. Circulation, 70:788, 1984.

Stiles, O. R., Lindesmith, G. G., Tucker, B. L., et al.: Experience with fifty repeat procedures for myocardial revascularization. J. Thorac. Cardiovasc. Surg., 72:849, 1976.

Sundt, T. M., Kouchoukos, N. T., Saffitz, J. E., et al.: Renal dysfunction and intravascular coagulation with aprotinin and hypothermic circulatory arrest. Ann. Thorac. Surg., 55:1418, 1993.

Swenson, R., and Abbey, S.: Management of depression and anxiety disorders in the cardiac patient. In Pashkow, F., and Dafoe, W. (eds): Clinical Cardiac Rehabilitation: A Cardiologist's Guide. Baltimore, Williams & Wilkins, 1992, pp. 263–288.

Thomas, C. S., Jr., Alford, W. C., Jr., Burrus, G. R., et al.: Results of reoperation for failed aortocoronary bypass grafts. Arch. Surg., 111:1210, 1976.

Thompson, P. D.: The benefits and risks of exercise training in patients with chronic coronary artery disease. J.A.M.A., 259:1537, 1988.

Thurer, R. L., and Hauer, J. L.: Autotransfusion and blood conservation. Curr. Probl. Surg., 19:97, 1982.

Uppal, R., Mills, N. L., Wechsler, A. S., and Smith, P.: Left thoracotomy for reoperative coronary artery bypass procedures. Ann. Thorac. Surg., 55:275, 1993.

Utley, J. R., Moores, W. Y., and Stephens, D. B.: Blood conservation techniques. Ann. Thorac. Surg., 40:11, 1981.

van Oeveren, W., Harder, M. P., Roozendaal, K. J., et al.: Aprotinin protects platelets against the initial effect of cardiopulmonary bypass. J. Thorac. Cardiovasc. Surg., 99:788, 1990.

Walts, A. E., Fishbein, M. C., Sustaita, H., and Matloff, J. M.: Ruptured atheromatous plaques in saphenous vein coronary artery bypass grafts: A mechanism of acute, thrombotic, late graft occlusion. Circulation, 65:197, 1982.

Weintraub, W. S., Cohen, C. L., Curling, P. E., et al.: Results of coronary surgery after failed elective coronary angioplasty in patients with prior coronary surgery. J. Am. Coll. Cardiol., 16:1341, 1990.

Weisel, R. D., Hoy, F. B. Y., Baird, R. J., et al.: Improved myocardial protection during a prolonged cross-clamp period. Ann. Thorac. Surg., 36:664, 1983.

Winkle, R. A., Alderman, E. L., Shumway, N. E., and Harrison, D. C.: Results of reoperation for unsuccessful coronary artery bypass surgery. Circulation, 51, 52 (Suppl. 1):61, 1975.

# 4 Left Ventricular Aneurysm

Michael A. Grosso and Alden H. Harken

## HISTORICAL ASPECTS

In 1955, Bailey (Likoff and Bailey, 1955) developed a surgical approach for the repair of left ventricular aneurysm without cardiopulmonary bypass. Through a left-sided thoracotomy, a large clamp was applied to the bulging, beating aneurysm, and the adjacent ventricle was plicated. Interestingly, in 1937, Sauerbruch was probably the first to operate on a patient with a cardiac aneurysm (Sauerbruch and O'Shaughnessy, 1937). Before surgery, he diagnosed a mediastinal tumor, but at the time of operation, he found a mass that contained blood. The mass was opened and found to communicate with the right ventricle. Sauerbruch placed two fingers into the communication to control the bleeding and ligated the neck of the sac as he withdrew his fingers. In 1944, Beck concluded that Sauerbruch had operated on a false aneurysm of the right ventricle. In the same year, Beck treated a ventricular aneurysm by buttressing it with strips of fascia lata.

Early reports of cardiac aneurysms were confounded by failure to distinguish generalized cardiomegaly from aneurysm formation. Sternberg (1914) catalogued descriptions of cardiac enlargement by Baillow in 1538 and Lancisius in 1740. Schlichter and colleagues (1954) attribute the first reports of ventricular aneurysm to Dominicus Gusmanus Galeati (Galeati, 1757) and John Hunter (1757). Hunter's description specifically identified aneurysmal thinning of the left ventricular apex "lined with a thrombus just the shape of the pouch in which it lay." In 1816, Cruveilhier first recognized that a ventricular aneurysm was myocardial fibrosis, but the pathogenesis of this fibrosis was unclear (Rokitansky, 1844). Toward the end of the nineteenth century, several cases of left ventricular aneurysm were convincingly suspected ante mortem (Voelcker, 1902), and Cohnheim and Shulthess-Rechberg traced the etiology of ventricular aneurysm to myocardial infarction. By 1914, Sternberg recognized the clinical sequence of angina preceding myocardial infarction leading to ventricular aneurysm. He correctly diagnosed ventricular aneurysm based on the pathogenic concept of coronary artery occlusion and even predicted the feasibility of radiologic confirmation.

In the early part of this century, x-rays greatly facilitated diagnosis, and Sezary and Alibert first visualized an aneurysm in 1922. Ten years later, mural calcification was noted radiologically. Subsequently, paradoxic systolic ventricular motion was appreciated fluoroscopically (Schwedel et al., 1950), and Dolly and co-workers demonstrated a ventricular aneurysm by angiography in 1951.

The development of cardiopulmonary bypass permitted Cooley and associates (1958) to establish the open heart technique of aneurysmectomy. By 1973, Loop and associates had established indications and provided surgical rehabilitation for a large group of patients with left ventricular aneurysms. Refinements by Jatene, Dor, Fontan, and Cooley in the surgical reconstruction of the left ventricular defect created by aneurysmectomy continue to spark debate and will be discussed in this chapter.

## PATHOLOGY: CLASSIFICATION

The continuum from a true left ventricular aneurysm through left ventricular dyskinesia and akinesia to normally contractile ventricle remains a controversial spectrum. Most authors agree, however, that a left ventricular aneurysm is a well-defined transmural scar that is thin, contains fibrous tissue with little or no contractile muscle, and during systole, displays a characteristic paradoxic bulging (Fig. 54–93). Cardiac aneurysms may therefore be classified by both their location and their type (Cabin and Roberts, 1980).

**Location.** Following an acute transmural myocardial infarction, approximately 10 to 15% of patients develop a true left ventricular aneurysm. Most (approximately 85%) involve the left ventricular anterolateral wall and apex (Nagle and Williams, 1974). Only 5 to 10% involve the posterobasal portion of the left ventricle. Interestingly, most anterolateral aneurysms are "true aneurysms," whereas over one-half of posterobasal aneurysms are "false" aneurysms.

**Type.** A true aneurysm is a full-thickness, well-delineated outpouching of all layers (endocardium, myocardium, and epicardium) of the ventricle (Fig. 54–94). The walls are thin, fibrotic, and often calcified. Harding and associates (1989) isolated human myocytes from both developing and chronic ventricular aneurysms. The sarcomere length in the myocytes from a developing aneurysm was significantly higher than that of cells from chronic aneurysms. These developing aneurysm cells did not contract even in the presence of high calcium concentrations. Electron microscopy confirmed the presence of elongated sarcomeres. These overstretched cells may account for the weakness of the wall of developing aneurysms and be a cause of enlargement or even rupture. A true aneurysm has a wide mouth or base. Approximately one-half contain mural thrombus (Rao, 1974). True aneurysms rarely rupture. A false or pseudoaneurysm develops following a postinfarction ventricular rupture. Patients survive ventricular rupture only when

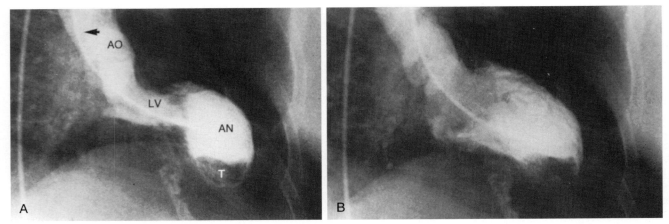

**FIGURE 54–93.** Contrast ventriculography with catheter (*arrow*) injection of dye into the left ventricle (LV). *A,* Large anteroapical left ventricular aneurysm (AN). Mural thrombus (T) is seen within the aneurysm. (AO = aorta.) *B,* During diastole, noninfarcted left ventricular segments relax, while the aneurysm remains unchanged. (*A* and *B,* From Patel, R., and Shenoy, M. M.: Left ventricular aneurysm. Reprinted, by permission of the New England Journal of Medicine, *329:*246, 1993.)

it is contained by dense localized adhesions to the pericardium, typically produced by prior postinfarction pericardial inflammation (Dressler's syndrome). This contained ventricular disruption (false aneurysm) usually has a narrow base that, following re-endothelialization, communicates freely with the ventricular cavity. With time, false aneurysms do enlarge and tend to lethally rupture even into adherent pericardial scar (Vlodaver, 1975).

Aneurysms of both the right and the left atrium have also been described (Galeati, 1757). Atrial false aneurysms following valvuloplasty have been reported (Fojo-Echevarria et al., 1955). Right ventricular aneurysms occur and also tend to be ischemic in origin (Stansel et al., 1963). Iatrogenic "patch" pseudoaneurysms are a late complication of surgical repair (Sarkar and Fagan, 1991). Congenital ventricular aneurysms and cardiac diverticula have been described

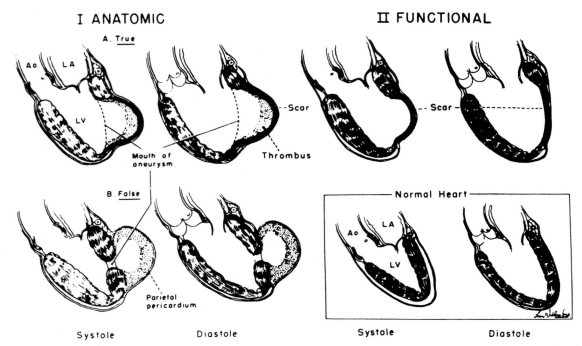

**FIGURE 54–94.** Anatomic aneurysms protrude during both systole and diastole. The true aneurysm consists of all layers of the heart wall (endocardium, myocardium, and epicardium) along with a wide mouth or base. The false aneurysm wall consists of parietal pericardium and has a narrow base. Functional aneurysms protrude during systole but not diastole and represent ventricular dyskinesia. *Inset,* Normal heart in systole and in diastole. (Adapted from Cabin, H. S., and W. C.: True left ventricular aneurysm and healed myocardial infarction: Clinical and necropsy observations including quantification of degrees of coronary artery narrowing. Am. J. Cardiol., *46:*754, 1980.)

(Arnold, 1894) and are associated with hypoplasia of the aorta (Grossi et al., 1991). Pseudoaneurysms of both the right (Stansel et al., 1963) and the left ventricle (Lyons and Perkins, 1958) can occur secondary to trauma. Mycotic aneurysms secondary to bacterial endocarditis (Schlichter et al., 1954) have also been described. Rare combinations of pseudoaneurysms arising from true aneurysms have also been identified and repaired (St. Cyr and Fullerton, 1992).

## PATHOPHYSIOLOGY

Chronic ventricular aneurysms must be distinguished from transient functional aneurysm formation, which is the regional left ventricular dyskinesia and dilatation following acute myocardial infarction (Eaton et al., 1979). Acute regional left ventricular dilatation is functionally equivalent to a chronic ventricular aneurysm (Cabin and Roberts, 1980). Meizlish and associates (1984) obtained radionuclide angiocardiograms of 51 patients immediately after acute anterior myocardial infarction. Functional "aneurysms" developed in 18 of the patients within 48 hours. Progressive imbalance of oxygen supply and demand leads to an ultimate failure of blood supply, with consequent myocardial infarction. Three aspects of this pathologic process lead directly to the three clinical stigmata associated with left ventricular aneurysm.

**Left Ventricular Dysfunction and Congestive Failure.** First, as a thin layer of necrotic muscle and fibrous tissue replaces the contracting myocardium, paradoxic systolic motion "steals" left ventricular stroke volume, thus decreasing cardiac output (Alpert and Braunwald, 1980; Swan et al., 1972). A strong predictor of aneurysm formation is the presence of total occlusion of the proximal *left anterior descending* artery (LAD) without collateral vessels on angiogra-

phy (Shen et al., 1992). By LaPlace's law, wall tension increases as the ventricle dilates; thus, factors conspire to promote even further global or regional ventricular dilatation. Progressive ventricular dysfunction eventually results in congestive heart failure.

**Mural Thrombus and Systemic Emboli.** Second, transmural or subendocardial infarction transforms the glimmering, smooth, metabolically active endocardium into a microscopically rough surface that encourages thrombus formation (Sater et al., 1988) (Figs. 54–93 and 54–95). Endothelial injury promotes release of thromboxanes, which vigorously induce platelet aggregation (Didisheim and Foster, 1978). Evidence for platelet involvement is provided by elevations of circulating platelet factor four (PF-4), which is a marker of platelet activation. Although conformational changes in the left ventricle may produce relative stasis that contributes to thrombus formation (Rosenthal and Braunwald, 1980), aneurysm formation is not essential to the development of endocardial clot (Cabin and Roberts, 1980). Although ventricular thrombus may mature, laminate, and remain in situ, this process is the basis for emboli.

**Ventricular Tachyarrhythmias.** Third, the thin wall of a left ventricular aneurysm and the adjacent jeopardized border are composed of a mixture of fibrous tissue, necrotic muscle, and viable myocardium (Schlichter et al., 1954) (Fig. 54–96). The electrophysiologic properties of conduction and refractoriness in these disparate tissues are logically different (Grosso et al., 1983; Harken, 1993). The conditions for re-entrant ventricular arrhythmias are satisfied when two or more electrically heterogeneous pathways (with respect to conduction and refractoriness) are connected proximally and distally (Rosenthal and Braunwald, 1980; Wellens, 1975). An impulse must travel in only one direction along one of these pathways (unidirectional block). When this impulse arrives at the distal connection, it may return along

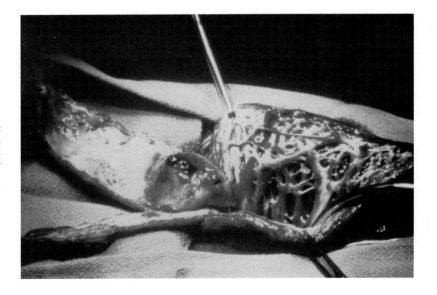

**FIGURE 54–95.** Intraoperative photograph of a left ventricular aneurysm opened to show a mural thrombus. Note also the junction of the thin-walled fibrous aneurysmal wall and the muscular trabeculations of viable ventricular endocardium.

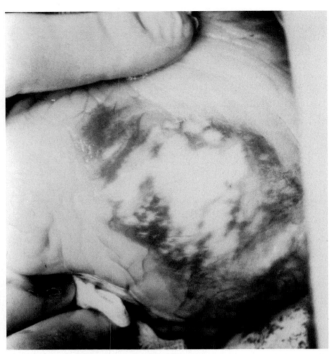

**FIGURE 54–96.** Intraoperative photograph of a heterogeneous post-infarction myocardial scar that predisposes to re-entrant arrhythmias.

the originally blocked pathway. If conduction of this impulse is sufficiently slow to permit repolarization of the origin, the impulse may re-enter the circuit (Fig. 54–97). Normal hearts contain a network of interarterial anastomotic collateral channels that are 50 to 100 μ in diameter. In patients with coronary occlusive disease, these coronary collaterals become extensive (Gorlin, 1976). Subsequent myocardial infarction with multiple zones of pericollateral salvage produces a heterogeneously injured zone that predisposes to re-entrant arrhythmias (Harken, 1993). Levett and colleagues (1991) evaluated alterations in adrenergic receptor density in patients with postinfarction left ventricular aneurysms. Resected specimens revealed up-regulation of beta-receptors in the perianeurysm tissue. This study suggests that aneurysm formation can alter adrenergic receptor density, which may also predispose to arrhythmogenesis.

## NATURAL HISTORY OF LEFT VENTRICULAR ANEURYSM

The decrease in left ventricular function associated with myocardial infarction is related to the volume of muscle damage (Pfeffer et al., 1979). Because of the virtual absence of oxygen reserve, contractility decreases significantly 4 to 6 seconds after cessation of blood flow (Harden et al., 1979). In the normothermic working heart, some cells are irreversibly damaged after 20 minutes of ischemia (Mitchell et al., 1993). With continued ischemia, four sequential contraction abnormalities result (Forrester et al., 1976): *dyssynchrony*, dissociation of electrical and mechanical events in the same muscle region; *hypokinesia*, decreased muscle shortening; *akinesia*, absence of muscle shortening; and *paradoxic motion*, systolic muscle bulging. By 6 to 8 hours, edema and neutrophil infiltration increase left ventricular wall stiffness (decreased compliance), which transiently improves function by decreasing paradoxic systolic wall motion (Vokonas et al., 1976). As pump function deteriorates, cardiac output, stroke volume, blood pressure, and contractility are decreased (Pfeffer et al., 1979).

Left ventricular aneurysm formation after myocardial infarction has been associated with elongation of infarcted tissue in response to wall stress. In an elegant experimental study, Connelly and associates (1991) came to three conclusions: First, that an increase in afterload is more likely to lead to aneurysm development than an increase in preload. Second, acutely ischemic tissue is most vulnerable to systemic hypertension (afterload). And third, that for a given wall stress, *healed* scar tissue is as susceptible to irreversible elongation (aneurysm formation) as is acutely infarcted tissue. This study suggests that acute and long-term medical control of afterload in patients following myocardial infarctions may be beneficial in preventing aneurysm formation.

The relationship among congestive heart failure, angiographic evidence of regional left ventricular dysfunction, and poor prognosis (regardless of medical or surgical therapy) is well established (Cohn and Braunwald, 1980). Indeed, of the myriad risk factors currently related to prognosis in ischemic heart disease, left ventricular function is unquestionably the dominant variable. Epidemiologic studies have classi-

**FIGURE 54–97.** Schema of the mechanism of ventricular tachycardia associated with coronary artery disease. *Left,* A portion of the left ventricle is shown with normal muscle shown in *oblique lines* and ischemically damaged muscle in the *stippled area.* Islands of dead tissue are represented by the *empty spaces* enclosed with the ischemic area. An electrocardiogram and an electrogram from this area that represent the border of an infarct at the left ventricular aneurysm (LV-An) is shown alongside each of the panels. *A,* During sinus rhythm, the cardiac impulse enters the ischemically injured area and conducts slowly but cannot exit because the surrounding area is refractory. The slow conduction is shown by a fractionated electrogram in the LV-An recording. *B,* During ventricular pacing (V₁), a premature ventricular stimulus (V₂) is delivered that results in marked slowing of impulse propagation through this damaged area. This is associated with more marked fractionation of the electrogram in the LV-An. *C,* A slightly more premature impulse is introduced during ventricular pacing, and conduction of the impulse is slow enough to allow recovery of the surrounding tissue. Re-entry occurs, resulting in ventricular tachycardia. Note that the fractionated electrogram in the LV-An extends through diastole, becoming continuous before and between complexes of the tachycardia.

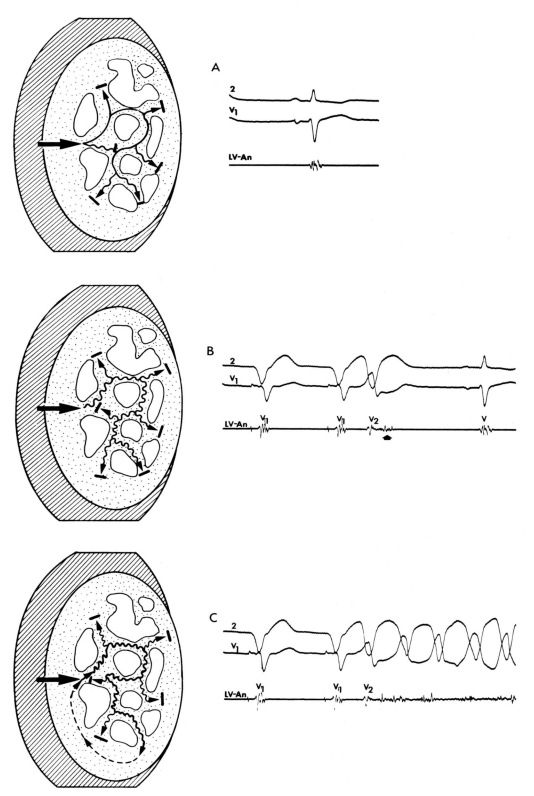

**FIGURE 54–97** *See legend on opposite page*

cally presented a bleak outlook for patients with left ventricular aneurysm. Natural history studies are no longer ethically permissible. It is therefore necessary to examine old studies, when medical therapy was arguably different. In a group of 102 patients with pathologically proven aneurysms, only 27% survived for 3 years, and 12% survived for 5 years (Schlichter et al., 1954). Schattenberg and co-workers (1970) found a 76% mortality rate within 39 months in a similar group of patients. Proudfit (1979) followed 74 patients with angiographically proven left ventricular aneurysms and observed a 5-year survival rate of 47% and a 10-year survival rate of 18%. Some studies (Puglielli et al., 1991) have suggested that the prognostic implication of the presence of a left ventricular aneurysm can be stratified solely on the basis of left ventricular ejection fraction. At 36 months, the overall mortality rate was 34%; however, in those patients with an ejection fraction less than 50%, the mortality rate was nearly doubled. Management of refractory congestive heart failure remains a perplexing medical problem (Patel and Shenoy, 1993). Similarly, surgical results of aneurysmectomy depend almost entirely on the quantity of residual contracting ventricle (Brooks et al., 1991; Cox, 1989; Kim et al., 1992). In fact, in a population-based cohort study, Benediktsson and colleagues (1991) concluded that the reduced survival of patients with chronic left ventricular aneurysm compared with control subjects with akinetic scar was accounted for by the more extensive myocardial damage and not by the presence of aneurysm per se.

In the classic study (that can never ethically be repeated) by Bruschke and colleagues (1973), 490 patients were angiographically identified as having significant coronary artery disease and then treated medically, with a follow-up of 5 to 9 years. Again, survival depended primarily on the extent of coronary disease and left ventricular function. In the years since publication of this report, medical therapy has improved immeasurably. No one is willing to accept these statistics as the currently achievable medical standard. For ethical, moral, perhaps legal, and certainly practical reasons, however, it will not be possible to improve on this study. Patients are necessarily culled out for surgery following angiographic documentation of left main coronary artery disease (Murphy et al., 1977) or triple-vessel disease (European Coronary Surgery Study Group, 1979) even with regional ventricular dysfunction.

Prolongation of life as an isolated indication for surgery in patients with left ventricular aneurysm remains controversial. Use of programmed stimulation (electrophysiologic study) and signal-averaged electrocardiogram (ECG) may help those patients at significant risk for sudden death and hence serve as indications for intervention. Simonson and associates (1991) found that the filtered QRS duration on the signal-averaged ECG was an independent predictor of inducible ventricular arrhythmias (high-risk group for sudden death) in patients with ventricular aneurysm (Harken, 1993). In symptomatic patients with medically intractable ventricular failure, angina,

thromboemboli, and ventricular arrhythmias, the role of surgery is now well established.

## MOLECULAR BIOLOGY OF VENTRICULAR REMODELING

Molecular biology is based on the belief that signals external to a cell can be perceived at the cell surface and transduced internally to influence nuclear regulation. Following sublethal stress, cardiac myocytes exhibit a spectrum of functional and metabolic responses ranging from preconditioning to hibernating to stunning to infarction (Mitchell et al., 1993). Indeed, the inflammation produced by local cardiac cell death (myocardial infarction) may be the stimulus for adjacent regional hyperdynamic function through a nitric oxide–mediated mechanism (Finkel et al., 1992). Alterations in steady-state messenger RNA (mRNA) levels typically reflect functional modifications in their protein products. The stressed or failing heart appears to compensate by reverting to a fetal program of "immediate early response" genes (Brown et al., 1990). DNA encoding atrial natriuretic peptide (characteristic of fetal myocardium) is expressed in abundance in failing human heart, whereas the structural genes encoding beta-myosin heavy chain and cytoskeletal beta-actin are unchanged (Feldman et al., 1991). For the foreseeable future, surgeons will have access to coronary arterial vessels during revascularization procedures and to the donor heart during transplantation in a manner simply unapproachable in other disciplines. It behooves us to therapeutically regulate protective gene expression by distinct cell surface signaling pathways (Bading et al., 1993), provoke protective myocardial preconditioning (Banerjee et al., 1993), or transfect resilient genes into diseased endothelial or myocardial cells (Friedman, 1989) while we have the heart in our hands.

## SURGICAL INDICATIONS

**Left Ventricular Dysfunction and Angina.** Ultimately, myocardial ischemia results when oxygen demand exceeds supply, and wall-motion abnormalities are seen universally in patients following clinical infarction (Wynne et al., 1977). The peri-ischemic "border zone" may contract weakly, whereas a compensatory increase in the force of contraction has been described in surrounding nonischemic muscle (Mitchell et al., 1993). Braunwald and Sobel (1980) have identified the increase in wall tension associated with left ventricular dilatation as one of the primary determinants of myocardial oxygen consumption, and Harken and colleagues (1981), using a high-precision fluorophotographic technique, have demonstrated the exquisite sensitivity of the peri-ischemic border zone (thus infarct volume) to alterations in oxygen demand. According to LaPlace's law, wall tension (force/cm) is the product of intraventricular pressure and ventricular radius. With an increase in either global or regional left ventricular dimensions, there is an obligatory increase in wall tension and a concurrent augmentation in muscle oxygen demand. Clinically, the largest cross-sectional wall tension at the equator of the ventricle is presented as circumferential wall stress (Mirsky, 1979) (dynes/cm² × 103):

LaPlace's law:

$$\text{Tension} = \text{pressure} \times \text{radius}$$

Mirsky's modification:

$$CWS = (P \times Y) (1 - Y^2/2X^2 - H/2Y + H^2/8 \times 2)/H$$

where H is wall thickness, P is left ventricular pressure (dynes/cm²), and X and Y are the horizontal and vertical axes (in centimeters) of the ventricle. Circumferential wall stress, and thus myocardial oxygen consumption, is a function of left ventricular dimensions. The rationale for surgical aneurysmectomy in congestive heart failure is firmly based on the principle that a smaller ventricular chamber will pump more efficiently while consuming less oxygen. Savage and co-workers (1992), in an experimental study of anteroapical left ventricular aneurysm, found that plication of an aneurysm produced a shorter, more spherical ventricle with reduced end-systolic wall stress in the perianeurysm border zone as well as in remote areas of myocardium. Monsieur LaPlace assists the surgeon.

**Thromboemboli.** Endocardial thrombosis frequently accompanies myocardial infarction (Sater et al., 1988). Mural thrombus is identified at autopsy (Schlichter et al., 1954) or operation (Rao et al., 1974) in approximately half of the patients with a left ventricular aneurysm. In about half of these patients, systemic emboli are found (Schlichter et al., 1954). In fact, 10% of all clinically evident thromboembolic strokes are due to left ventricular aneurysm mural thrombus (Arnow, 1991). Many emboli are "silent" or not evident clinically. In a study of 500 patients, Davies and colleagues (1976), however, found that half of the emboli identified at autopsy were cerebral. Not all intraventricular clotting is clinically obvious (see Figs. 54–93 and 54–95). The use of indium-111 labeled platelet scintigraphy is reportedly capable of identifying active left ventricular mural thrombi (Tsuda et al., 1989), although our personal experience has been disappointing. When thrombus is apparent (in the absence of an embolic event), this constitutes a relative indication for surgery.

**Tachyarrhythmias.** The common denominator of both left ventricular aneurysm and ventricular irritability is myocardial ischemia. One does not necessitate the other, but they frequently co-exist. When a rhythm originates in the ventricle, the pattern of ventricular activation is aberrant (wide QRS complex). The mechanism of premature ventricular contractions or ventricular tachycardia is enhanced automaticity, re-entry, or both (Harken, 1993). Automatic ventricular rhythms due to local myocardial irritability are common in the perioperative and peri-infarction periods. These rhythms are exacerbated by hypokalemia,

catecholamines, or digitalis. As mentioned, a re-entrant rhythm (see Fig. 54–97) may occur when two or more electrically heterogeneous (with respect to conduction and refractoriness) pathways are connected proximally and distally. An impulse must travel in only one direction along one of these pathways (unidirectional block). When this impulse arrives at the distal connection, it may return by the initially blocked pathway. If conduction of the impulse is sufficiently slow to allow the originally blocked site to recover excitability, the impulse may re-enter the circuit (see Figs. 54–96 and 54–97). A re-entrant arrhythmia may be induced by a technique of specially timed paced beats called programmed stimulation. This technique permits pharmacologic testing and eventual mapping of re-entrant rhythms such as ventricular tachycardia. Automatic arrhythmias cannot be induced and therefore cannot be tested or mapped. Surgery has proven to be a viable therapeutic option for re-entrant ventricular tachycardia (Cox, 1989; Grosso and Harken, 1991). Currently, there is no evidence to support a surgical approach to automatic ventricular tachycardia and no reason to operate for isolated premature ventricular contractions. Each year, one-third of a million Americans die suddenly. The popularity of educating civilians in cardiopulmonary resuscitation and emergency medical systems has increased the salvage in this epidemic (Brooks et al., 1991). Patients who survived episodes of recurrent ventricular tachycardia or sudden death are subjected to pharmacologic testing during programmed induction of their arrhythmias (Hassapoyannes et al., 1991). In addition, those patients without clinical ventricular tachycardia or who have not died suddenly, but in whom an abnormal signal averaged ECG has been identified and who are at significant risk for sudden death, should also undergo electrophysiologic study (Harken, 1993; Kulakowski et al., 1991). If the rhythm cannot be suppressed with high-dose antiarrhythmic agents, these patients are considered candidates for surgical excision of the re-entrant circuit.

**Ventricular Rupture.** Although ventricular rupture occurs in 10% of patients dying of acute myocardial infarction (Bjorck et al., 1960), late rupture of a matured (true, not false) aneurysm almost never occurs (Vlodaver et al., 1975). The incidence of cardiac rupture is high only during the acute phase of infarct evolution. During this phase, the pathophysiologic and technical risks associated with surgical intervention are high. The avoidance of possible ventricular rupture for acute and certainly for chronic left ventricular aneurysms in the setting of acute myocardial infarction therefore does not routinely constitute an indication for surgery.

## DIAGNOSIS

### Physical Examination

A ventricular aneurysm may be suspected from the history and physical examination. A patient who has suffered a transmural anterior myocardial infarction who presents with congestive heart failure, embolic events, or sustained ventricular arrhythmias should raise suspicion for the presence of an aneurysm. Physical signs, such as a forceful cardiac impulse concurrent with a weak peripheral pulse or a late systolic bulge, indicate left ventricular aneurysm (Schlichter et al., 1954). Libman (1932) emphasized that a distinct pulsation independent of the apical impulse and associated with a gallop rhythm and a dull first heart sound was pathognomonic of an aneurysm.

## Contrast Ventriculography

Regional contractility can be localized by superimposing the angiographic outlines of end-diastole and end-systole (Herman et al., 1967). There is a spectrum of ventricular function from normal to grossly paradoxic motion and/or discrete aneurysm. Akinesia exists when parts of the diastolic and systolic ventriculographic silhouettes share a common line. Dyskinesia is present when the end-systolic silhouette protrudes outside the end-diastolic outline. Persistence of this protrusion throughout the cardiac cycle defines the presence of an aneurysm (see Figs. 54–93 and 54–94). Often the aneurysm wall may be calcified. Mural thrombus within the aneurysm may also be detected (see Figs. 54–93 and 54–95).

Ventriculography also allows the surgeon to assess regional "contractile reserve" and the quantity of residual functioning myocardium (see Fig. 54–93). Akinesis of the ventricular septum is a poor prognostic sign. In contrast, an acceptable outcome can be expected, even in the presence of a large aneurysm, if residual contractile function is good (Ba'Albaki and Clements, 1989).

## Echocardiography

Echocardiography provides a precise, noninvasive, and almost universally available assessment of intracardiac structures. M-mode, two-dimensional, transthoracic echocardiography, transesophageal echocardiography, and color-flow or pulsed Doppler ultrasonography have all been used to diagnose left ventricular aneurysms (Catherwood et al., 1980). M-mode echocardiography may reveal an echo-free space suggesting aneurysm. A pericardial effusion, pleural effusion, or pericardial cyst, however, can mimic these findings. Two-dimensional echocardiography can also identify the presence of ventricular aneurysms. Two-dimensional echo may reveal a narrow or wide "mouth" or base and differentiating true from false aneurysm. In addition, the functional characteristics of the residual myocardium can best be assessed by two-dimensional echocardiography, thus providing important prognostic information (Visser et al., 1985). Unusual variations, such as aneurysms arising from the mitral valve apparatus, can be well-delineated by two-dimensional echocardiography

(Lawson et al., 1991). In addition, two-dimensional echocardiography may be more sensitive than contrast ventriculography in identifying the presence of thrombus within the left ventricular aneurysm (Asinger et al., 1981). The availability of color Doppler can augment the echocardiographic diagnosis of both true and false left ventricular aneurysms. Demonstration of flow into a color Doppler two-dimensional echocardiographic free space clearly establishes the diagnosis (Alam et al., 1989). The recent availability of *transesophageal echocardiography* (TEE) has greatly enhanced our diagnostic ability. It is particularly useful in identifying posterior left ventricular pseudoaneurysms. Burns and co-workers (1992) described two patients in whom TEE identified posterior pseudoaneurysms that had been undiagnosed by other modalities. In addition, the intraoperative repair of these lesions was aided by TEE. Repair of these pseudoaneurysms, which were located close to the posteromedial papillary muscle, was successfully accomplished without compromising function of the mitral valve, as evidenced by intraoperative TEE. These authors (Burns et al., 1992) emphasize the utility of TEE in both the diagnosis and the management of ventricular aneurysms.

## Nuclear Imaging

**Radionuclide Cineangiography.** This modality (gated blood-pool scan) is a safe, simple, and noninvasive method for evaluating the presence of a left ventricular aneurysm. In a study by Friedman and Cantor (1979), the radionuclide scintigram correctly identified all of 54 apical and anteroapical aneurysms and one inferior aneurysm. Conversely, scintigraphy did not detect one of six anterior aneurysms and two of three posterobasal aneurysms; in addition, there were two false-positive scans. Overall, the accuracy of scintigraphy in detecting a left ventricular aneurysm is 96%. The posterobasal region (in contrast to TEE) is a relative "blind" spot. Valette and associates (1990), however, combined Fourier analysis with gated blood-pool scans and improved the detection rate (sensitivity) to 100%.

**Magnetic Resonance Imaging (MRI).** Flowing blood in the cardiovascular system spatially dissociates the MRI signal, so there is substantial natural contrast between blood and cardiac chambers (Higgins, 1986). Iga and colleagues (1992) reported that MRI can supplement echocardiographic diagnosis of left ventricular aneurysm by providing detailed anatomic delineation of the left ventricular apex and posterobasilar segments. Improved detection of left ventricular thrombus has also been described (Lalisang et al., 1990). The radionuclide scan also offers additional information not available with other noninvasive modalities, such as ejection fraction and regional contractility (Sharaf el-Deane et al., 1989). In fact, in a multivariate analysis of preoperative variables, systolic dyskinesia (paradoxic left ventricular wall motion), as defined best by radionuclide ventriculography, was found to be the only independent predictor of a favorable surgical outcome (Mangschau, 1989). Thallium-201 scintigraphy also can be used to detect left ventricular aneurysms with good sensitivity and specificity (Mangschau, 1989). It also provides additional information regarding the presence or absence of ischemia in the myocardium remote from the aneurysm.

## TECHNIQUE OF ANEURYSMECTOMY

All preoperative medications are continued until operation (Fullerton and Harken, 1990). The standard approach for left ventricular aneurysm repair is a median sternotomy. The aorta is cannulated; a single venous cannula is sufficient unless an associated ventricular septal defect is suspected. A postinfarction left ventricular aneurysm often presents with dense pericardial adhesions (secondary to Dressler's syndrome). Premature placement of the sternal retractor can cause a catastrophic right ventricular tear. Cardiopulmonary bypass decompresses the heart and may facilitate "take down" of the adhesions. With the initiation of cardiopulmonary bypass, the patient is cooled until the heart fibrillates. The aorta is then cross-clamped to prevent left ventricular distention. With proper decompression, the aneurysmal zone should collapse, while viable left ventricle remains firm. A linear incision is made in the collapsed aneurysm while cold, blood-potassium cardioplegic solution is infused retrograde into the coronary sinus.

Retrograde cardioplegia delivery prevents aortic root air from embolizing into the coronary circulation. If coronary bypass or valve replacement is to be done concurrently, the ventricular aneurysm is always opened first. This optimizes ventricular decompression.

The entire ventricle is then inspected for mural thrombus (see Figs. 54–93 and 54–95). Thrombus should be removed, and the underlying endocardium should be cleaned with a sponge. The ventricular cavity is irrigated with iced saline solution to cool the myocardium and to remove any residual thrombotic debris. Concurrent coronary artery bypass grafting or valvular procedures are done at this time in a cold, flaccid, decompressed heart. The temptation of resecting the aneurysm too early should be avoided. The fibrotic aneurysmal edges may be grasped with clamps (damaged) and subsequently resected without weakening the heart.

If the indication for operation is recurrent sustained ventricular tachycardia, the left ventricular endocardium should be mapped when the aneurysm is opened (Harken, 1993; Harken et al., 1980a). After the area of earliest activation (tachycardia origin) is located, this endocardial zone is peeled back beyond the aneurysmal edge into grossly viable myocardium (Horowitz et al., 1980). (Fig. 54–98). Again, at this point, concomitant coronary bypass or valve replacement is done. The aneurysmectomy and ventricular repair may then be approached via one of three techniques: linear repair, plication/patch repair, or patch "endoaneurysmorrhaphy."

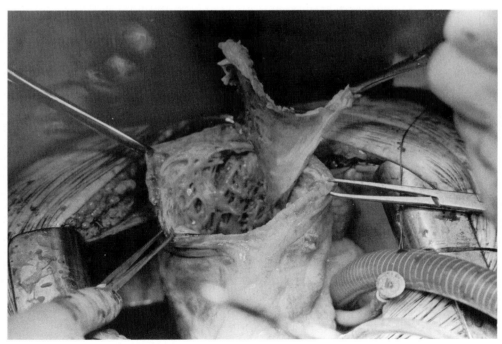

**FIGURE 54–98.** Intraoperative photograph. The left ventricular aneurysm has been opened, and the earliest site of ventricular activation (origin of the tachyarrhythmias) has been identified within the endocardium. The endocardial resection (peel) is near completion. (From Harken, A. H., Horowitz, L. N., and Josephson, M. E.: The surgical treatment of ventricular tachycardia. Ann. Thorac. Surg., *30:*499, 1980.)

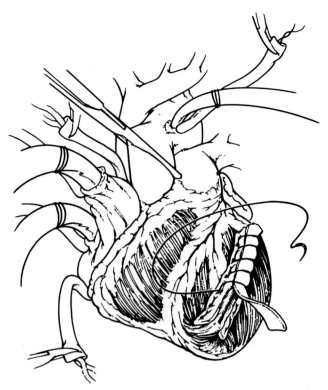

**FIGURE 54–99.** Linear closure technique. The aneurysmectomy defect is closed by reapproximating the fibrous rims of the aneurysm in a horizontal mattress fashion over felt buttresses. (Adapted from Cooley, D. A.: Ventricular endoaneurysmorrhaphy: A simplified repair for extensive postinfarction aneurysm. J. Card. Surg., 4:200, 1989.)

**Linear Repair.** In 1958, Cooley and co-workers (1958) reported the first definitive repair of left ventricular aneurysm using cardiopulmonary bypass. The aneurysm edge is trimmed, leaving 1 cm of fibrous rim. The aneurysm is closed with 0 monofilament sutures in a horizontal mattress manner over long felt buttresses. Felt strips that are 1 cm wide facilitate closure. Separate sutures are initiated at either end, brought to the middle, and tied. Before this row is tied, the ventricle is filled with blood by inflating the lungs. The atrial appendage should be inserted. A second row of 0 monofilament sutures is placed in an over-and-over technique at both ends and tied over a felt buttress in the middle (Fig. 54–99). Closed in this manner, the ventriculotomy will never bleed. Seemingly minor traction on the felt buttresses, however, can tear the heart at the lateral junction between the ventricle and the suture line. Repair of this complication requires recooling and decompression of the heart. Sutures placed (even with pledgets) into a firm beating ventricle are prone to tear. Before removing the cross-clamp, we reperfuse the myocardium with hypocalcemic (0.25 mg/dl), hyperkalemic (9 mEq/l), normothermic blood cardioplegic solution for 2 minutes to minimize reperfusion injury (Brown et al., 1988).

**Plication/Patch.** Jatene (1985) believed that closing a left ventricular aneurysmectomy incision linearly distorted the ventricle, impairing left ventricular function. He introduced a repair that attempted a geometric reconstruction of the left ventricle using a prosthetic patch (Fig. 54–100). The aneurysm is incised linearly while the patient is on normothermic cardiopulmonary bypass with the heart beating. This allows palpation of contracting, viable myocardium and determines the extent of the aneurysm resection. The aneurysmal orifice is then plicated to reduce its size and return the ventricle to a more spherical configuration. The plication is performed by placing purse-string sutures around the aneurysmal orifice at the junction between normal muscle and fibrotic scar. The orifice should be closed to a size that estimates the

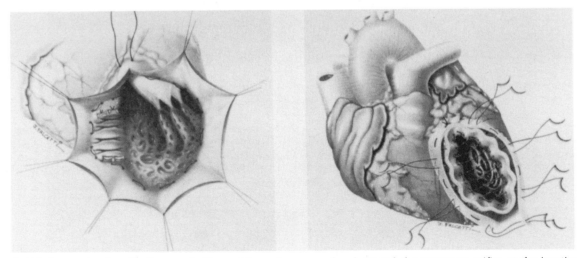

**FIGURE 54–100.** Jatene circular plication repair. Purse-string sutures are placed around the aneurysm orifice at the junction between normal muscle and fibrotic scar. Following plication, the defect is closed with horizontal mattress sutures over felt buttresses as in the linear repair. If the defect is too large for plication, a Dacron patch is secured to the junction of endocardial muscle and scar tissue (Dor modification). (Adapted from Sosa, E., Jatene, A., Kaeriyama, J. V., et al.: Recurrent ventricular tachycardia associated with postinfarction aneurysm. Results of left ventricular reconstruction. J. Thorac. Cardiovasc. Surg., *103*[5]:855, 1992.)

size of the original infarcted area. The remaining defect is then closed with horizontal mattress sutures tied over Teflon buttresses in a manner similar to the linear repair technique. A Dacron patch is used to close the aneurysmal orifice if direct closure will produce excessive ventricular cavity distortion. The patch may be backed with pericardium on the endocardial surface to prevent thrombus formation. The patch is anchored between Teflon buttresses placed through the fibrous border of the aneurysm. Dor and associates (1989) described a similar technique using a pericardium-lined Dacron buttressed patch secured at the junction of viable endocardial muscle and scarred tissue. The margins of the cut ventricle are then oversewn with circular suture to control bleeding. This variation has been called "endoventricular circular plasty."

**Patch "Endoaneurysmorrhaphy."** As mentioned, Cooley and associates (1958) performed the first definitive repair of left ventricular aneurysm and used the linear closure technique for the next 31 years. Since then, however, Cooley has used an intracavitary repair technique that he calls "ventricular endoaneurysmorrhaphy" (Cooley et al., 1992). A Dacron patch (usually 2 × 4 cm) is tailored to conform to the baseline left ventricular volume (Fig. 54–101).

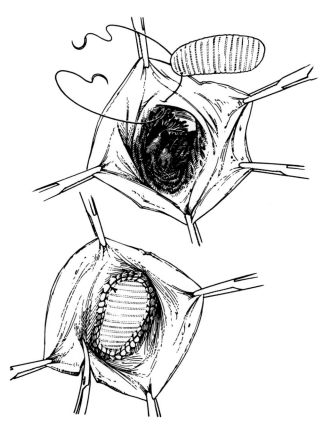

FIGURE 54–101. Cooley endoaneurysmorrhaphy. A Dacron patch is anchored to the myocardium at the transition zone between scarred and normal myocardium. The ventriculotomy is closed directly with a continuous double row of sutures without buttresses. (Adapted from Cooley, D. A.: Ventricular endoaneurysmorrhaphy: A simplified repair for extensive postinfarction aneurysm. J. Card. Surg., 4:200, 1989.)

The patch is then anchored to the myocardium at the visible transition zone between scarred and normal myocardium with 3-0 polypropylene continuous suture. The ventriculotomy is then closed with a continuous double row of sutures. Felt buttresses are not necessary because the ventriculotomy closure is not exposed to intracavitary pressure. By avoiding epicardial buttresses, this technique optimizes access to left anterior descending artery bypass (if the vessel is patent).

## SURGICAL RESULTS

A surgical procedure is indicated when the documented results and prognosis are better than those of the natural history of the disease. Global left ventricular dysfunction is an ominous prognostic risk factor. Left ventricular aneurysm has been dissociated from global ventricular dysfunction as an independent and grave prognostic indicator (Meizlish et al., 1984). The 1-year mortality rate of patients with a left ventricular aneurysm after an anterior myocardial infarction was 61%. Patients who develop a detectable aneurysm within 48 hours of myocardial infarction had an 80% mortality rate. Surgical results are superior to those of available medical therapy. The current operative mortality rate is approximately 5 to 10%. One- and 5-year survival rates following surgery approximate 85 and 65% respectively (Harken et al., 1980a; Tebbe and Kreuzer, 1989). Magovern and colleagues (1989) retrospectively reviewed the 10-year experience with surgical therapy for ventricular aneurysms. Medical therapy has produced 30 to 45% 5-year survival rates. Magovern's reported survival rates after operation were 79% at 5 years and 67% at 10 years. Oxelbark and co-workers (1992) reported 20 survivors of 22 patients who underwent resection of left ventricular aneurysm in the face of a preoperative ejection fraction less than 20%. This survival advantage was present even in patients who did *not* undergo concomitant coronary artery bypass grafting. The only prospective comparison between medical and surgical therapy was obtained by the Coronary Artery Surgery Study (CASS) (Faxon et al., 1982). The 4-year survival rates of the medically and surgically treated groups did not differ significantly. However, survival in the medically treated group was rated at 71%, a marked deviation (and improvement) from all other reported medical treatment data. Tebbe and Kreuzer (1989) compiled the available literature to amass an amazing 5528 patients treated for ventricular aneurysms. Surgical therapy was clearly advantageous (Fig. 54–102). Louagie and associates (1989) identified a group of patients (good contractile segment ejection fraction and myocardial score) whose 5-year survival rate was 93% despite a preoperative ejection fraction of 30% or less. In addition, for patients in whom aneurysmectomy is undertaken for control of ventricular arrhythmias (15% of all surgically treated patients), the benefit of surgical therapy is clear-cut. Medical therapy (when successful) yields a 1-year survival rate of 30 to 50% (Kastor et al., 1981). With surgical aneurysmec-

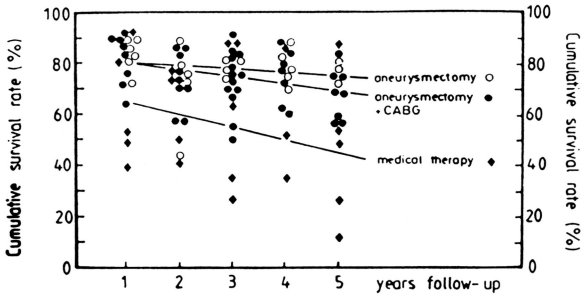

**FIGURE 54–102.** Cumulative survival in left ventricular aneurysmectomy with and without coronary artery bypass graft (CABG) in over 5500 patients. (Adapted from Tebbe, J., and Kreuzer, H.: Pros and cons of surgery of the left ventricular aneurysm—A review. Reprinted with permission from Journal of Thoracic and Cardiovascular Surgery, 37:3, 1989, Thieme Medical Publishers, Inc.)

tomy and endocardial resection, 80% of patients are expected to survive for the first year (Harken, 1993; Harken et al., 1980b; Kastor et al., 1981; Martin et al., 1982).

Multivariate analysis has identified the following predictors of early postoperative mortality: operation within 30 days of myocardial infarction, advanced age, operative intervention for congestive heart failure or arrhythmia, and preoperative cardiogenic shock (Baciewicz et al., 1991; Cooper et al., 1990; Svennevig et al., 1989). Intra- and postoperative mortality predictors were excision of an akinetic rather than a dyskinetic scar and the need for intra-aortic balloon support (Cooper et al., 1990; Magovern et al., 1989). Interestingly, late mortality and length of survival were not predicted by any preoperative variable (Magovern et al., 1989).

Symptomatic relief occurs in only 20 to 40% of patients treated medically for left ventricular aneurysm (Magovern et al., 1989). In contrast, surgery offers relief of angina in 90% of patients and improvement in New York Heart Association (NYHA) class in 85% of patients (Mills et al., 1993). This correlates with numerous studies documenting improvement in postoperative ejection fraction (Louagie et al., 1989; Oxelbark et al., 1992).

Whether a specific repair technique significantly alters surgical outcome remains to be convincingly demonstrated. Each technique has its proponents. The linear repair, in use since 1958, remains the standard for comparison. Cooley has used this technique in over 4000 patients with gratifying results. We have demonstrated objective (pre- and postoperative ventriculography) improvement in left ventricular function using the linear repair (Martin et al., 1982). Mickleborough and colleagues (1992) report a 7% operative mortality rate in 54 patients undergoing aneurysmec-

tomy and linear repair. Similarly, Magovern and colleagues (1989) report a 9.6% operative mortality rate in 197 patients treated with the linear repair and a 5-year survival rate of 85%, with 85% of patients exhibiting improvement in their preoperative NYHA class.

Using the circular plication and patch repair, Jatene (1985) and Sosa and associates (1992) have reported a significant decrease in operative and late mortality rates (4.3% and 3.5%, respectively) in 508 patients. Besa (1992) also reports a low operative mortality rate (3.9%) and an excellent survival rate (90% at 3 years) using Jatene's technique. Dor (1989) described results with his "endoventricular circular plasty" technique in 152 patients. The operative mortality rate was 9%; global ejection fraction improved from a mean preoperative level of 36 to 52% postoperatively. A recent update from the same group (DiDonato et al., 1992) revealed an operative mortality rate of 4.8% along with an improvement in ventricular hemodynamics and ejection fraction. Fontan (1990), using Dor's technique, also has experienced excellent results (operative mortality rate of 8%, 79% of postoperative patients in NYHA Class 1).

As mentioned, Cooley introduced the concept of linear repair. Recently, however, he described six patients who underwent repair of very large aneurysms. In this group, he felt there was insufficient normal myocardium to allow a linear repair (Cooley, 1989). The closure technique was dubbed "ventricular endoaneurysmorrhaphy" and was modeled after the technique introduced by Matas (1888) more than a century ago for arterial aneurysm repair. All six patients survived the operation; one patient's ejection fraction improved from 19% preoperatively to 55% following surgery. In 1992, Cooley reported the results with this technique in 136 patients (Cooley et al., 1992). One hundred patients (Group I) had not sustained a recent myocardial infarction (within 30 days of operation), nor had they undergone previous cardiac surgery. Thirty-six patients (Group II) had sustained an acute myocardial infarction or had undergone previous cardiac surgery. The operative mortality rate in Group I was 4%; the 1-year survival rate was 85%. The operative mortality rate in Group II was 31%. In both groups, functional class and ejection fraction improved significantly. Mills and colleagues (1993) adopted Cooley's technique in 22 consecutive aneurysm repairs. The operative mortality rate was a low 3.3%. Few studies have directly compared the repair techniques. Kesler and co-workers (1992) compared linear closure with circular/patch repair in 66 patients. Clinical outcome and two-dimensional echocardiography data were not different between the two groups. A larger study reviewing the outcome of 336 patients has been reported by Komeda and associates (1992). Again, the technique of repair was not an independent predictor of mortality. However, when patients with poor left ventricular function were analyzed separately, the operative mortality rate was reduced from 12.5 to 6.5% when the "geometric" (nonlinear) technique was employed.

Should these high-risk patients be candidates for heart transplantation rather than "experimental" repairs? Several studies have addressed this issue. Mangschau and colleagues (1989) analyzed data from 26 patients with left ventricular aneurysm and severe congestive heart failure. Fourteen patients underwent aneurysm resection, and 12 were accepted for heart transplantation. Mortality and overall outcome were similar among the two groups. In addition, in the United States alone, more than 2000 patients await heart transplantation. Approximately one-third will die before a donor organ becomes available (Alexander et al., 1991). Therefore, the lack of donor organs seems to justify our current aggressive surgical approach to ventricular aneurysm, even in high-risk patients.

It is difficult to draw firm conclusions or recommendations from the above studies. Even the definition of an aneurysm remains elusive; additionally, most studies do not consistently describe aneurysm size, aneurysm location, aneurysm function (akinetic vs. dyskinetic), contractile state of the noninfarcted myocardium, complete versus incomplete operative revascularization, and the presence or absence of arrhythmias, mural thrombus, or valvular dysfunction. Many, if not all, of these variables may have a more significant impact on outcome than the type of repair used in surgical aneurysmectomy. Suffice it to say, surgical therapy for ventricular aneurysms remains the most attractive treatment option in most patients. Additional debate will fuel further investigations.

## SELECTED BIBLIOGRAPHY

Boineau, J. P., and Cox, J. L.: Slow ventricular activation in acute myocardial infarction: A source of re-entrant premature ventricular contractions. Circulation, 48:702, 1973.

This study was the first to suggest that a heterogeneous pattern of myocar-

dial ischemia (see Fig. 54–96) led to zones of slow conduction that predisposed to re-entrant ventricular arrhythmias. Automatic and re-entrant arrhythmias are explained and related to fragmentation of intramyocardial potentials.

Harken, H. A.: Surgical treatment of cardiac arrhythmias. Sci. Am., 269:68–74, 1993.

This is a comprehensible description of the microelectroanatomy of re-entrant ventricular arrhythmias. The concept that slow conduction, rapid refractoriness, and ischemic heterogeneity conspire to promote re-entry is graphically presented. The signal averaged surface electrocardiogram is depicted as a method of assessing arrhythmogenic potential in ventricular aneurysmal tissue.

Harken, A. H., Horowitz, L. N., and Josephson, M. E.: Comparison of standard aneurysmectomy and aneurysmectomy with directed endocardial resection for the treatment of recurrent sustained ventricular tachycardia. J. Thorac. Cardiovasc. Surg., 80:527, 1980.

This is the only comparative study that relates standard aneurysmectomy to electrophysiologically directed endocardial excision plus aneurysmectomy in patients with recurrent ventricular tachycardia.

Kesler, K. A., Fiore, A. C., Naunheim, K. S., et al.: Anterior wall left ventricular aneurysm repair: A comparison of linear versus circular closure. J. Thorac. Cardiovasc. Surg., 103:841–848, 1992.

Forty patients surviving closure of an anterior left ventricular aneurysm by standard linear repair are compared with 22 patients surviving repair by the circular closure technique. At a mean follow-up interval of 3 years, no differences were noted in anginal class, New York Heart Association functional classification, or survival. Long-axis left ventricular systolic diameter and short-axis systolic and diastolic areas were determined by echocardiography. No differences in the linear versus circular closure techniques were appreciated.

Martin, J. L., Untereker, W. J., Harken, A. H., et al.: Aneurysmectomy and endocardial resection for ventricular tachycardia: Favorable hemodynamic and antiarrhythmic results in patients with global left ventricular dysfunction. Am. Heart J., 103:960, 1982.

This is still the largest series of patients undergoing left ventricular aneurysmectomy who have all been studied both pre- and postoperatively with contrast ventriculography. Sixty-two patients were catheterized before and after aneurysmectomy. Ejection fraction increased from $28 \pm 8\%$ to $39 \pm 10\%$ ($p < 0.001$), and left ventricular end-diastolic pressure decreased from $17 \pm 8$ to $14 \pm 5$ mm Hg ($p < .005$). Objectively, aneurysmectomy improves left ventricular function.

Meizlish, J. L., Berger, H. J., Plankey, M., et al.: Functional left ventricular aneurysm formation after acute anterior transmural myocardial infarction. N. Engl. J. Med., 311:1001, 1984.

The incidence, natural history, and prognostic implications of an anterior transmural myocardial infarction are critically examined. The authors obtained serial radionuclide angiocardiograms of patients after an anterior myocardial infarction. Patients with and without aneurysms had comparable depression of left ventricular function (31% vs. 27% ejection fraction). The 1-year mortality rates were very different (61% vs. 9%).

Mills, N. L., Everson, C. T., Hockmuth, D. R.: Technical advances in the treatment of left ventricular aneurysm. Ann. Thorac. Surg., 55:792, 1993.

A thoughtful inquiry by a superb surgical group examines whether a prosthetic patch aneurysmorrhaphy can redirect normal muscle bundles to their normal orientation with improved functional results over standard linear aneurysmectomy. The authors conclude that patch aneurysmorrhaphy is the preferred surgical approach in patients with large aneurysms.

Schlichter, J., Hellerstein, H. K., and Katz, L. N.: Aneurysm of the heart: A correlative study of 102 proved cases. Medicine, 33:43, 1954.

This natural history study will never be repeated. It is a classic clinicopathologic correlation of 102 confirmed cases of left ventricular aneurysm treated nonoperatively. The history, diagnosis, pathology, and prognosis are reviewed in detail. The authors indicate that three-quarters of patients were dead in 3 years and that there was a 12% 5-year survival rate. This study is still the classic example of the natural history of medically treated left ventricular aneurysm.

## BIBLIOGRAPHY

Alam, M., Rosman, H. S., Lewis, J. W., and Brymen, J. F.: Color Doppler features of left ventricular pseudoaneurysm. Chest, 95(1):231, 1989.

Alexander, J. W., and Vaughn, W. K.: The use of "marginal" donors for organ transplantation. The influence of donor age on outcome. Transplantation, *51*:135, 1991.

Alpert, J. S., and Braunwald, E.: Pathological and clinical manifestations of acute myocardial infarction. *In* Braunwald, E. (ed): Heart Disease: A Textbook of Cardiovascular Medicine. Philadelphia, W. B. Saunders, 1980, p. 1309.

Arnold, J.: Ueber angeborene divertikel des herzens. Virchows Arch. (Pathol. Anat.), *137*:318, 1894.

Arnow, W. S.: Etiology and pathogenesis of thromboembolism. Herz, *16*(6):395, 1991.

Asinger, R. W., Mitchell, F. L., Sharma, B., and Hodges, M.: Observations on detecting left ventricular thrombus with two-dimensional echocardiography: Emphasis on avoidance of false positive diagnoses. Am. J. Cardiol., *47*:145, 1981.

Ba'Albaki, H. A., and Clements, S. D., Jr.: Left ventricular aneurysm: A review. Clin. Cardiol., *12*:5, 1989.

Baciewicz, P. A., Weintraub, W. S., Jones, E. L. et al.: Late follow-up after repair of left ventricular aneurysm and associated coronary bypass grafting. Am. J. Cardiol., *68*:193, 1991.

Bading, H., Ginty, D. D., and Greenberg, M. E.: Regulation of gene expression in hippocampal neurons by distinct calcium signalling pathways. Science, *260*:181–188, 1993.

Banerjee, A., Locke-Winter, C. R., Rogers, K. B., et al.: Preconditioning against myocardial dysfunction after ischemia reperfusion by an alpha-1 adrenergic mechanism. Circ. Res., *73*:656–670, 1993.

Benediktsson, R., Eyjolfsson, O., and Thorgeirsson, G.: Natural history of chronic left ventricular aneurysm: A population based cohort study. J. Clin. Epidemiol., *44*(11):1131, 1991.

Besa, G.: Left ventricular aneurysmectomy: Technical evolution and results. Ital. Cardiol., *22*:331, 1992.

Bjorck, G., Morgensen, L., Nyquist, O., et al.: Studies of myocardial rupture with cardiac tamponade in acute myocardial infarction. Concours Med., *82*:2637, 1960.

Braunwald, E., and Sobel, B. E.: Coronary blood flow and myocardial ischemia. *In* Braunwald, E. (ed): Heart Disease: A Textbook of Cardiovascular Medicine. Philadelphia, W. B. Saunders, 1980, p. 1279.

Brooks, R., McGovern, B. A., Garan, H., and Ruskin, J. N.: Current treatment of patients surviving out-of-hospital cardiac arrest. J. A. M. A., *265*:762–768, 1991.

Brown, J. M., Grosso, M. A., Whitman, G. J. R., et al.: Cardiac oxidase systems mediate oxygen metabolite reperfusion injury. Surgery, *104*:266, 1988.

Brown, J. M., Harken, A., and Sharefkin, J. B.: Recombinant DNA and surgery. Ann. Surg., *212*:178–186, 1990.

Bruschke, A. V. G., Proudfit, W. F., and Sones, F. M.: Progressive study of 490 consecutive nonsurgical cases of coronary disease followed 5 to 9 years. II: Ventriculographic and other correlations. Circulation, *47*:1154, 1973.

Burns, C. A., Pauisen, W., Arrowood, J. A., et al.: Improved identification of posterior left ventricular pseudoaneurysms by transesophageal echocardiography. Am. Heart J., *124*(3):796, 1992.

Cabin, H. S., and Roberts, W. C.: True left ventricular aneurysm and healed myocardial infarction: Clinical and necropsy observations including quantification of degrees of coronary artery narrowing. Am. J. Cardiol., *46*:754, 1980.

Catherwood, E., Mintz, G. S., Kotler, M. N., et al.: Two dimensional echocardiographic recognition of left ventricular pseudoaneurysm. Circulation, *62*:294, 1980.

Cohn, P. F., and Braunwald, E.: Chronic coronary artery disease. *In* Braunwald, E. (ed): Heart Disease: A Textbook of Cardiovascular Medicine. Philadelphia, W. B. Saunders, 1980, p. 1387.

Connelly, C. M., McLaughlin, R. J., Vogel, W. M., and Apstein, C. S.: Reversible and irreversible elongation of ischemic, infarcted, and healed myocardium in response to increases in preload and afterload. Circulation, *84*(1):387, 1991.

Cooley, D. A.: Ventricular endoaneurysmorrhaphy: A simplified repair for extensive postinfarction aneurysm. J. Card. Surg., *4*:200, 1989.

Cooley, D. A., Collins, H. A., Morris, G. C., and Chapman, D. W.: Ventricular aneurysm after myocardial infarction. Surgical excision with use of temporary cardiopulmonary bypass. J. A. M. A., *167*:557, 1958.

Cooley, D. A., Frazier, D. H., Duncan, J. M., et al.: Intracavitary repair of ventricular aneurysm and regional dyskinesia. Ann. Surg., *215*:417, 1992.

Cooper, G. S., Burton, R. W., Birjiniuk, V., et al.: Relative risks of left ventricular aneurysmectomy in patients with akinetic scars versus true dyskinetic aneurysms. Circulation, *82*(Suppl. 5):248, 1990.

Cox, J. L.: Ventricular tachycardia surgery: A review of the first decade and a suggested contemporary approach. Semin. Thorac. Cardiovasc. Surg., *1*:83–87, 1989.

Davies, M. J., Woolf, N., and Robertson, W. B.: Pathology of acute myocardial infarction with particular reference to occlusive coronary thrombi. Br. Heart J., *38*:659, 1976.

Didisheim, P., and Foster, V.: Actions and clinical status of platelet suppressive agents. Semin. Hematol., *15*:55, 1978.

DiDonato, M., Barletta, G., Mailoa, M., et al.: Early hemodynamic results of left ventricular reconstructive surgery for anterior wall left ventricular aneurysm. Am. J. Cardiol., *69*:886, 1992.

Dolly, C. H., Dotter, C. T., and Steinberg, H.: Ventricular aneurysm in a 29-year-old man studied angiocardiographically. Am. Heart J., *42*:894, 1951.

Dor, V., Soab, M., Coste, P., et al.: Left ventricular aneurysm: A new surgical approach. J. Thorac. Cardiovasc. Surg., *37*:11, 1989.

Eaton, L. W., Weiss, J. L., Bulkley, B. H., et al.: Regional cardiac dilatation after acute myocardial infarction: Recognition by two dimensional echocardiography. N. Engl. J. Med., *300*:57, 1979.

European Coronary Surgery Study Group: Coronary artery bypass surgery in stable angina pectoris: Survival at two years. Lancet, *1*:889, 1979.

Faxon, D. P., Ryan, T. J., Davis, K. B., et al.: Prognostic significance of angiographically documented left ventricular aneurysm from the coronary artery surgery study (CASS). Am. J. Cardiol., *50*:157, 1982.

Feldman, A. M., Ray, P. E., Silan, C. M., et al.: Selective gene expression in failing human hearts. Circulation, *83*:1866–1872, 1991.

Finkel, M. S., Oddis, C. V., Jacob, T. D., et al.: Inotropic effects of cytokines in the heart mediated by nitric oxide. Science, *257*:387–389, 1992.

Fojo-Echevarria, P., Muniz-Sotolongo, J. C., and Aixala, R.: Aneurysma de la autioula izquierda cumo sequela de comisurotomia. Revista Cubana de Cardiologia, *16*:377, 1955.

Fontan, F.: Transplantation of knowledge. J. Thorac. Cardiovasc. Surg., *99*:387, 1990.

Forrester, J. S., Wyatt, H. L., Oaluz, P. L., et al.: Functional significance of regional ischemic contraction abnormalities. Circulation, *54*:64, 1976.

Friedman, M. L., and Canter, R. E.: Reliability of gated heart scintigrams for detection of left ventricular aneurysms. J. Nucl. Med., *20*:720, 1979.

Friedman, T.: Progress toward human gene therapy. Science, *244*:1275, 1989.

Fullerton, D., and Harken, A. H.: Preoperative cardiac assessment. *In* Wilmore, D., Brennan, M., Harken, A. H., et al. (eds): Care of the Surgical Patient. New York, Scientific American, 1989.

Galeati, D. G.: DeBononiensi scientiarum et atrium instituto atque academia commentarii. DeMorbis Duobus, *4*:25, 1757.

Gorlin, R.: Coronary collaterals. *In* Gorlin, R. (ed): Coronary Artery Disease. Philadelphia, W. B. Saunders, 1976, p. 59.

Grossi, E. A., Colvin, S. B., Galloway, A. C., et al.: Repair of posterior left ventricular aneurysm in a six-year-old boy. Ann. Thorac. Surg., *51*:484, 1991.

Grosso, M. A., and Harken, A. H.: Antiarrhythmic surgery. Curr. Opin. Cardiol., *6*:66–71, 1991.

Grosso, M. A., Simson, M. B., Kobayashi, K., et al.: Myocardial ischemic pattern determines predisposition to ventricular arrhythmias. Surgical Forum, *34*:239, 1983.

Harden, W. R., Barlow, C. H., Simson, M. J., and Harken, A. H.: Temporal relation between the onset of cell anoxia and ischemic contractible failure. Am. J. Cardiol., *44*:741, 1979.

Harding, S. E., Vescovo, G., Jones, S. M., et al.: Morphological and functional characteristics of myocytes isolated from human left ventricular aneurysms. J. Pathol., *159*(3):191, 1989.

Harken, A. H.: Surgical treatment of cardiac arrhythmias. Sci. Am., *269*(1):68–74, 1993.

Harken, A. H., Horowitz, L. N., and Josephson, M. E.: Comparison of standard aneurysmectomy and aneurysmectomy with directed endocardial resection for the treatment of recurrent sustained ventricular tachycardia. J. Thorac. Surg., 80:527, 1980a.

Harken, A. H., Horowitz, L. N., and Josephson, M. E.: The surgical treatment of ventricular tachycardia. Ann. Thorac. Surg., 30:499, 1980b.

Harken, A. H., Simson, M. B., Wetstein, L. W., et al.: Early ischemia following complete coronary ligation in the rabbit, dog, pig and monkey. Am. J. Physiol., 241:202, 1981.

Hassapoyannes, C. A., Hornung, C. A., Berbin, M. C., and Flowers, N. C.: Effect of left ventricular aneurysm on risk of sudden and nonsudden cardiac death. Am. J. Cardiol., 67(6):454, 1991.

Herman, M. V., Heinle, R. A., Klein, M. D., and Gorlin, R.: Localized disorders in myocardial contraction: Asynergy and its role in congestive heart failure. N. Engl. J. Med., 277:222, 1967.

Higgins, C. B.: Overview of magnetic resonance of the heart. Am. J. Roentgenol., 146:907, 1986.

Horowitz, L. N., Harken, A. H., Kastor, J. A., and Josephson, M. E.: Ventricular resection guided by epicardial and endocardial mapping for the treatment of recurrent ventricular tachycardia. N. Engl. J. Med., 302:589, 1980.

Hunter, J.: An account of the dissection of morbid bodys. A manuscript copy in the Library of the Royal College of Surgeons, No. 32, 1757, pp. 30–32.

Iga, K., Matsuo, M., Tsuji, A., et al.: Usefulness of magnetic resonance imaging (MRI) in evaluation of left ventricular apical aneurysm [English abstract]. Kokyu-To-Junkan, 40(6):593, 1992.

Jatene, A. D.: Left ventricular aneurysmectomy: Resection or reconstruction. J. Thorac. Cardiovasc. Surg., 89:321, 1985.

Kastor, J. A., Horowitz, L. N., Harken, A. H., and Josephson, M. E.: Clinical electrophysiology of ventricular tachycardia. N. Engl. J. Med., 304:1004, 1981.

Kesler, K. A., Fiore, A. C., Neunheim, K. S., et al.: Anterior wall left ventricular aneurysm repair: A comparison of linear versus circular closure. J. Thorac. Cardiovasc. Surg., 103:841, 1992.

Kim, S. G., Fisher, J. D., Chove, C. W., et al.: Influence of left ventricular function on outcome of patients treated with implantable defibrillators. Circulation, 85:1304–1310, 1992.

Komeda, M., David, T. E., Malik, A., et al.: Operative risks and long-term results of operation for left ventricular aneurysm. Ann. Thorac. Surg., 53:22, 1992.

Kulakowski, P., Dluzniewski, M., Budoj, A., and Ceremuzynski, L.: Relationship between signal-averaged electrocardiography and dangerous ventricular arrhythmias in patients with left ventricular aneurysm after myocardial infarction. Eur. Heart J., 12(11):1170, 1991.

Lalisang, R. R., Baur, L. H., VanderWall, E. E., et al.: Left ventricular aneurysmectomy after myocardial infarction following detection of left ventricular thrombus by magnetic resonance imaging. Magn. Reson. Imaging, 8(5):661, 1990.

Lawson, C. S., Venn, G. E., and Webb-Peploe, M. M.: Thrombus within a submitral left ventricular aneurysm: Diagnosis on cross sectional echocardiography. Br. Heart J., 66(2):179, 1991.

Levett, J. M., McGrath, L. B., and Bianchi, J. M.: Beta receptor derangement in postinfarction left ventricular perianeurysm tissue. Clin. Cardiol., 14(11):909–912, 1991.

Libman, E.: Affections of the coronary arteries. Interst. Postgrad. Med. Assoc. North Am., 2:405, 1932.

Likoff, W., and Bailey, C. P.: Ventriculoplasty: Excision of myocardial aneurysm. J. A. M. A., 158:915, 1955.

Louagie, Y., Alouini, T., Lesperance, J., and Pelletier, L. C.: Left ventricular aneurysm complicated by congestive heart failure: An analysis of long-term results and risk factors of surgical treatment. J. Cardiovasc. Surg. (Torino), 30:648, 1989.

Lyons, C., and Perkins, R.: Resection of a left ventricular aneurysm secondary to a cardiac stab wound. Ann. Surg., 147:256, 1958.

Magovern, G. J., Sakert, T., Simpson, K., et al.: Surgical therapy for left ventricular aneurysms. A ten-year experience. Circulation, 79(6 pt 2):1102, 1989.

Mangschau, A.: Akinetic versus dyskinetic left ventricular aneurysms diagnosed by gated scintigraphy: Difference in surgical outcome. Ann. Thorac. Surg., 47(5):746, 1989.

Mangschau, A., Geiran, O., Forfang, K., et al.: Left ventricular

aneurysm and severe cardiac dysfunction: Heart transplantation or aneurysm surgery? J. Heart Transplant., 8:486, 1989.

Martin, J. L., Untereker, W. J., Harken, A. H., et al.: Aneurysmectomy and endocardial resection for ventricular tachycardia: Favorable hemodynamic and antiarrhythmic results in patients with global left ventricular dysfunction. Am. Heart J., 103:960, 1982.

Matas, R.: Traumatic aneurysm of the left brachial artery. Med. New, 43:462, 1888.

Meizlish, J. L., Berger, H. J., Plankey, M., et al.: Functional left ventricular aneurysm formation after acute anterior transmural myocardial infarction. N. Engl. J. Med., 311:1001, 1984.

Mickleborough, L. L., Mizuno, S., Downer, E., and Gray, C. C.: Late results of operation for ventricular tachycardia. Ann. Thorac. Surg., 54:832, 1992.

Mills, N. L., Everson, C. T., and Hockmuth, D. R.: Technical advances in the treatment of left ventricular aneurysm. Ann. Thorac. Surg., 55:792, 1993.

Mirsky, I.: Elastic properties of the myocardium: A quantitative approach with physiological and clinical applications. In Berne, L. M. (ed): Handbook of Physiology. Vol. 1: The Heart. Bethesda, MD, American Physiological Society, 1979, p. 501.

Mitchell, M. B., Winter, C. A., Banerjee, A., and Harken, A. H.: The relationship between ischemia-reperfusion injury, myocardial "stunning" and cardiac preconditioning. Surg. Gynecol. Obstet., 177:97, 1993.

Murphy, M. L., Hultgren, H. N., Detre, K., et al.: Treatment of chronic stable angina. N. Engl. J. Med., 297:621, 1977.

Nagle, R. E., and Williams, D. O.: Natural history of ventricular aneurysm without surgical treatment. Br. Heart J., 36:1037, 1974.

Oxelbark, S., Mannting, F., Morgan, M. G., and Henze, A.: Left ventricular aneurysmectomy in patients with poor left ventricular function. Scand. J. Thorac. Cardiovasc. Surg., 26:47, 1992.

Patel, R., and Shenoy, M. M.: Left ventricular aneurysm. N. Engl. J. Med., 329:246, 1993.

Pfeffer, M. A., Pfeffer, J. M., Fishbein, M. C., et al.: Myocardial infarct size and ventricular function in rats. Circ. Res., 44:503, 1979.

Proudfit, W. L.: Personal communication. Cited in Grondin, P., Kretz, J. G., Bical, O., et al.: Natural history of saccular aneurysms of the left ventricle. J. Thorac. Cardiovasc. Surg., 77:57, 1979.

Puglielli, L., Incalz, R. A., Capparello, O., and Carbonin, P.: Verification of the prognostic significance of often a first myocardial infarct. Cardiologia, 36(7):557, 1991.

Rao, G., Zikria, E. A., and Miller, W. H.: Experience with sixty consecutive ventricular aneurysm resections. Circulation, 49(Suppl. 2):149, 1974.

Rokitansky, C.: Handbuch der Pathologischen Anatomie. Vol. II. Vienna, Braumuller and Seidel, 1844, p. 449.

Rosenthal, D. S., and Braunwald, E.: Hematologic oncologic disorders and heart disease. In Braunwald, E. (ed): Heart Disease: A Textbook of Cardiovascular Medicine. Philadelphia, W. B. Saunders, 1980, p. 1771.

St. Cyr, J. A., and Fullerton, D. A.: Successful repair of a pseudoaneurysm originating from a true left ventricular aneurysm. Am. Heart J., 124:1381, 1992.

Sarkar, P. K., and Fagan, A. M.: Ventriculo-pulmonary fistula. Case report, literature review and possible surgical approach to the infected LV suture line. Eur. J. Cardiothorac. Surg., 5(9):503, 1991.

Sater, P. T., Perlmutter, R. A., Rosenfeld, L. E., et al.: Electrophysiologic effects of thrombolytic therapy in patients with a transmural anterior infarction complicated by left ventricular aneurysm formation. J. Am. Coll. Cardiol., 12(1):19–24, 1988.

Sauerbruch, F., and O'Shaughnessy, L.: Thoracic Surgery. Baltimore, William Wood & Company, 1937, p. 245.

Savage, E. B., Downing, S. W., Ratcliffe, M. B., et al.: Repair of left ventricular aneurysm. Changes in ventricular mechanics, hemodynamics, and oxygen consumption. J. Thorac. Cardiovasc. Surg., 104(3):752, 1992.

Schattenberg, T. T., Giuliana, E. R., Campion, B. C., and Danielson, G. K., Jr.: Postinfarction ventricular aneurysm. Mayo Clin. Proc., 45:13, 1970.

Schlichter, J., Hellerstein, H., and Katz, L. N.: Aneurysm of the heart: A correlative study of 102 proved cases. Medicine, 33:43, 1954.

Schwedel, J. B., Samet, P., and Mednick, H.: Electrokymographic studies of abnormal left ventricular pulsations. Am. Heart J., 40:410, 1950.

Sharaf el-Deane, M. S., Logan, K. W., Parker, B. M., and Holmes, R. A.: Aneurysmectomy prognosticators by equilibrium multigated cardiac blood pool scintigraphy. Am. J. Physiol. Imag., 4(4):124, 1989.

Shen, W. F., Tribouilloy, C., Mirode, A., et al.: Left ventricular aneurysm and prognosis in patients with first acute transmural anterior myocardial infarction and isolated left anterior descending artery disease. Eur. Heart J., 13(1):39, 1992.

Simonson, J. S., Gang, E. S., Diamond, G. A., et al.: Selection of patients for programmed ventricular stimulation: A clinical decision making model based on multivariate analysis of clinical variables. J. Am. Coll. Cardiol., 20(2):317, 1991.

Sosa, E., Jontene, A., Kaeriyama, J. V., et al.: Recurrent ventricular tachycardia associated with postinfarction aneurysm. Results of left ventricular reconstruction. J. Thorac. Cardiovasc. Surg., 103(5):855, 1992.

Stansel, J. C., Jr., Julian, O. C., and Dye, W. S.: Right ventricular aneurysm. J. Thorac. Cardiovasc. Surg., 46:66, 1963.

Sternberg, M.: Das chronische partielle herzaneurysma. Vienna and Leipzig, Franz Deuticke, 1914.

Svennevig, J. L., Semb, G., Fjeld, N. B., et al.: Surgical treatment of left ventricular aneurysm. Analysis of risk factors, morbidity and mortality in 205 cases. Scand. J. Thorac. Cardiovasc. Surg., 23:229, 1989.

Swan, H. J. C., Forrester, J. S., Diamond, G., et al.: Hemodynamic spectrum of myocardial infarction and cardiogenic shock. Circulation, 45:1097, 1972.

Tebbe, J., and Kreuzer, H.: Pros and cons of surgery of the left ventricular aneurysm—A review. J. Thorac. Cardiovasc. Surg., 37:3, 1989.

Tsuda, T., Kubota, M., Akiba, H., et al.: Availability of [111]In–labeled platelet scintigraphy in patients with postinfarction left ventricular aneurysm. Ann. Nucl. Med., 3(1):15, 1989.

Valette, H. B., Bourguignon, M. H., Merlet, P., et al.: Improved detection of left ventricular aneurysm with multi-harmonic fourier analysis. J. Nucl. Med., 31:1306, 1990.

Vlodaver, Z., Coe, J. L., and Edwards, J. E.: True and false left ventricular aneurysms: propensity for the latter to rupture. Circulation, 51:576, 1975.

Voelcker, A. F.: Aneurysms of the heart. Trans. Pathol. Soc. (Lond.), 53:409, 1902.

Vokonas, P. S., Pirzada, F. A., Hood, W. B., Jr.: Experimental myocardial infarction. XII: Dynamic changes in segmental mechanical behavior of infarcted and non-infarcted myocardium. Am. J. Cardiol., 37:853, 1976.

Wynne, J., Birnholz, J., Fineberg, H., and Alpert, J. S.: Assessment of regional left ventricular wall motion in acute myocardial infarction by two-dimensional echocardiography. Circulation, 56(Suppl. 2):152, 1977.

# 5  Postinfarction Rupture of the Papillary Muscles and Ischemic Mitral Insufficiency

Kevin P. Landolfo

The left atrioventricular valve was first compared in morphology to the bishop's miter by Vesalius. The name was subsequently adapted from the Latin *mitra*, meaning cap, and the Greek *mitra*, meaning headdress. Of the conditions affecting the mitral valve, few are as challenging to the cardiac surgeon as the problem of ischemic mitral insufficiency, the moderate to severe incompetence precipitated by an acute myocardial infarction. Acute mitral insufficiency in the setting of myocardial infarction was identified at post mortem as early as 1935 at Johns Hopkins Hospital (Stevenson and Turner, 1935), and subsequently described clinically in 1948 (Davidson). Successful mitral valve replacement for papillary muscle rupture was first performed at the Massachusetts General Hospital by Austin in 1965. This was followed in 1967 by the first combined mitral valve replacement and coronary bypass procedure for ischemic mitral insufficiency (Spencer et al., 1967).

The concept of papillary muscle dysfunction without frank rupture was introduced by Burch in 1963. This abnormality, also termed *papillary-annular dysfunction*, has been recognized increasingly as treatment strategies for ischemic mitral insufficiency have developed (Kay et al., 1986).

In patients with coronary artery disease, the complication of moderate or severe mitral insufficiency is demonstrated in approximately 3% of patients undergoing coronary angiography (Hickey et al., 1988; Rankin et al., 1989). However, with only half of these patients referred for surgical consideration in most centers, this represents less than 10% of patients who undergo mitral valve procedures (Hendren et al., 1991; Hickey et al., 1988). The combination of coronary bypass grafting with mitral valve procedures is associated with a perioperative mortality ranging from 3 to 53%. The highest mortality rates are seen in patients with ischemic mitral insufficiency (Connolly et al., 1986), and therefore, careful consideration must be given to patients referred with this problem.

## ANATOMIC CONSIDERATIONS

A thorough knowledge of the anatomy and morphology of the normal mitral valve is crucial to both the understanding of pathophysiologic consequences and the application of reconstructive principles in the operating room. Specific abnormalities of the valve and supporting structures are often detected by direct visual inspection at the time of surgery.

The functional apparatus of the mitral valve has six components (Perloff and Roberts, 1972; Roberts and Perloff, 1972):

1. Posterior left atrial wall
2. Left ventricular wall
3. Annulus
4. Chordae tendineae
5. Valve leaflets
6. Papillary muscles

The precise mode of closure of the normal mitral valve is not completely understood, although each of these components plays a significant role in normal valve function. Ventricular systole is initiated with contraction of the papillary muscles, and the resulting vertical forces cause apposition of the anterior and posterior leaflets (Cheng, 1969; Rushmer et al., 1956). During contraction, the free edges of the leaflets coapt along a significant portion of their atrial surfaces. The mitral annulus is a dynamic component of valvular function, and during ventricular contraction the annular circumference is significantly reduced (Brolin, 1967; Davis and Kinmoth, 1963). Under normal circumstances, the vertical axis of the left ventricle shortens during systole, and as this occurs, concomitant contraction of the papillary muscles and the contiguous left ventricular wall provides a counterbalancing force, exerted through the chordae tendineae, to prevent prolapse of the leaflets into the left atrium (Perloff and Roberts, 1972).

The papillary muscles and corresponding left ventricular wall from which they originate are the muscular components of the mitral apparatus. These muscles vary in size and configuration, although both arise from the caudal one-third of the posterior free wall of the left ventricle and are oriented along the long axis of the heart (Fishbein, 1989). The papillary muscles make up part of the subendocardium, and the vascular supply to the muscular heads is determined in part by their configuration. The shape of the papillary muscles has been categorized into three morphologic types: finger-like, tethered, and mixed (Ranganathan and Burch, 1969). The papillary muscles of the tethered and mixed configurations have subendocardial anastomosis in their attachment areas, whereas those of the finger-like type are perfused by a single central artery and are therefore at greater risk of ischemia. The normal function of the papillary muscles is also closely related to regional left ventricular wall motion. Akinetic or dyskinetic wall motion in the region of the papillary muscle origin may lead to significant valvular insufficiency (van Rijk-Zwikker).

The anterolateral papillary muscle, the larger of the two muscles, arises as a single head at the level of the obtuse margin of the heart. The arterial supply to this structure is derived from the circumflex coronary artery, with contributions from diagonal branches of the anterior descending artery (Perloff and Roberts, 1972).

The posteromedial papillary muscle arises from the ventricle along the septal border and forms two or

three columns, with a single arterial supply determined by the vascular dominance of the coronary circulation. The right coronary artery supplies the muscle in right-dominant hearts, and the circumflex artery supplies patients with left-dominant circulations (Perloff and Roberts, 1972).

Ischemic coronary artery disease may affect the normal function of any of the components of the mitral valve apparatus but isolated or combined abnormalities of the papillary muscles, the mitral annulus, or the left ventricular wall are most frequently observed. The severity of the mitral insufficiency is often graded on a scale from 1 to 4, based on observational ventriculography.

## CLINICAL PRESENTATION

Approximately 1.5 million people in the United States annually suffer an acute myocardial infarction (American Heart Association, 1987). The postinfarction development of ischemic mitral insufficiency in these patients presents as a continuum of disease that relates in part to the mechanism of the valvular abnormality. The anatomic cause should be determined in each patient before operative intervention is considered. These abnormalities may be classified as shown in Table 54–12 and are based on echocardiographic findings or direct visual inspection of the valve and surrounding structures (David, 1994).

**Transient Mitral Insufficiency.** This abnormality occurs with varying frequency in patients with ischemic coronary artery disease, but its mechanism is poorly understood. A transient myocardial ischemic episode causes intermittent regional wall dyskinesis at the site of the papillary muscle origin or failure of leaflet coaptation owing to papillary muscle displacement (David, 1994; Fehrenbacher et al., 1991). Patients may present with moderate to severe mitral insufficiency and recurrent episodes of pulmonary edema (LeFeuvre et al., 1992).

**Fixed Mitral Insufficiency.** Fixed mitral insufficiency may also occur following myocardial in-

■ **Table 54–12.** CAUSES OF MITRAL REGURGITATION IN ISCHEMIC HEART DISEASE

Leaflet(s) prolapse
1. Transient ischemia
2. Papillary muscle rupture
   Papillary muscle trunk
   Papillary muscle head
   Chordal avulsion
3. Papillary muscle elongation

Lack of coaptation of leaflets*
1. Transient ischemia
2. Annular dilatation
3. Dyskinetic/akinetic wall with apical displacement of papillary muscle and leaflets
4. Distortion of papillary muscles

From David, T. E.: Techniques and results of mitral valve repair for ischemic mitral regurgitation. J. Card. Surg., 9(Suppl.):274, 1994.
*Caused by apical displacement of the papillary muscle.

farction. In a series reported from Duke University, 55 patients were collected from 1981 to 1987 with 3+ to 4+ ischemic mitral insufficiency (graded on a scale from 1 to 4). Valvular abnormalities were categorized into those with papillary muscle rupture (partial or complete), those with papillary muscle dysfunction, and those with extensive left ventricular infarction or aneurysm associated with generalized annular dilatation (Rankin et al., 1988). This allowed for classification of patients with ischemic mitral insufficiency on a clinical and anatomic basis.

**Papillary Muscle Rupture.** A papillary muscle rupture is the least common mechanical complication following an acute myocardial infarction (Vlodaver and Edwards, 1977). In the series from Duke, this abnormality accounted for only 16% of the patients undergoing surgery. However, as many as 0.4 to 5% of all deaths following myocardial infarction are related to papillary muscle rupture, which reflects the severity of the problem when it does occur (Wei et al., 1979).

The clinical and pathologic features have been described in a series of 22 patients with ruptured papillary muscles. Two-thirds of the patients were men in the sixth decade of life. The location of the myocardial infarction was inferior in 90%, and the papillary muscle rupture occurred within 2 to 7 days of the acute event in virtually all patients. Most patients (81%) presented in shock or with symptomatic congestive heart failure following papillary muscle rupture. The myocardial infarction was relatively localized in most patients, suggesting that shear forces from maintained ventricular wall motion may have caused the papillary muscle rupture.

The common pathology found in these patients is demonstrated in Figure 54–103. The posteromedial papillary muscle was involved most frequently (73% of patients). Rupture of only one muscular head, as opposed to complete papillary muscle avulsion, was seen in 75% of patients (Barbour and Roberts, 1986).

Associated coronary artery disease is common. The right coronary artery, as the only vascular supply to the posteromedial papillary muscle, is involved as single-vessel disease, or in combination with circumflex artery disease in the majority of patients (Kishon et al., 1992).

**Papillary Muscle Dysfunction.** In the Duke University series, posterior papillary muscle dysfunction, also known as papillary-annular dysfunction, accounted for 56% of the patients undergoing valve surgery, and was the most common variety of ischemic mitral insufficiency observed. The pathophysiologic abnormalities include significant posterior annular dilatation, papillary muscle elongation, and loss

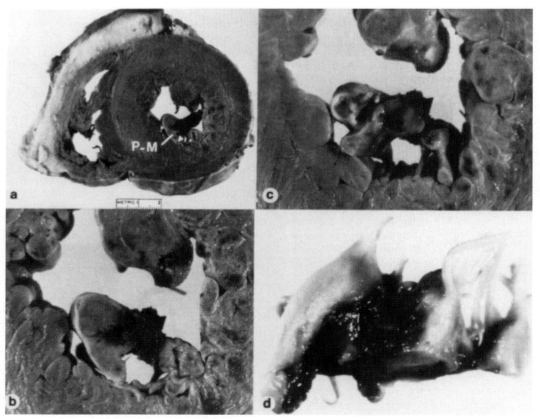

**FIGURE 54–103.** *a–c,* Transverse section of the cardiac ventricles showing acute infarction and incomplete rupture of the posteromedial (P-M) papillary muscle. *d,* The avulsed papillary muscle head with attached chordae tendineae. (*a–d,* From Barbour, D. J., and Roberts, W. C.: Rupture of a left ventricular papillary muscle during acute myocardial infarction: Analysis of 22 necropsy patients. Reprinted with permission from the American College of Cardiology [Journal of the American College of Cardiology, 1986, Vol. 8, pp. 558–565].)

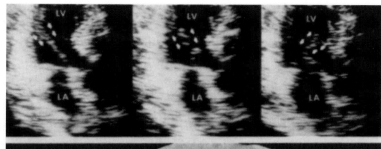

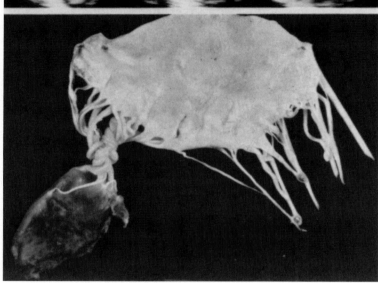

**FIGURE 54–104.** *Top,* Two-dimensional echocardiographic pictures from apical position of ruptured posteromedial papillary muscle. Note freely mobile head of papillary muscle (*arrows*) attached to mitral valve chordae. (LA = left atrium; LV = left ventricle.) *Bottom,* Surgical specimen of ruptured papillary muscle and excised mitral valve from the same patient. (From Nishimura, R. A., Schaff, H. V., Gersh, B. J., et al.: Early repair of mechanical complication after acute myocardial infarction. J. A. M. A., *256:*47–50, 1986. Copyright 1986, American Medical Association.)

of papillary muscle shortening with resultant insufficiency (Godley et al., 1981; Mittal et al., 1971). Other reports have questioned the role of posterior annular dilatation in this condition, emphasizing instead the concomitant elongation and fibrosis of the papillary muscle coupled with fibrosis and regional wall motion abnormality beneath the muscle bundles. In this case, mitral insufficiency results from restricted leaflet motion (Hendren et al., 1992; Tsakiris et al., 1970). These patients frequently presented several months following myocardial infarction, and elective surgical intervention was performed in half of these patients. Most patients sustained inferior myocardial infarctions with resultant posterior wall motion abnormalities.

**Generalized Annular Dilatation.** This was seen in 27% of the patients and was associated with severe left ventricular dysfunction. A history of multiple previous myocardial infarctions had caused left ventricular dilatation and diminished ejection fraction. Many patients presented with progressive congestive heart failure owing to poor myocardial reserve rather than valvular dysfunction.

## DIAGNOSIS

Detection of associated mitral insufficiency in the setting of myocardial ischemia is in part determined by the diagnostic method used. A clinical diagnosis can be made from the presence of a V-wave in the

pulmonary wedge pressure tracing obtained from a pulmonary artery catheter, and an accompanying systolic murmur. The rate of transient mitral insufficiency detected by auscultation has varied from 17% in a series of 1653 patients (Maisel et al., 1986) to as high as 55% (Heikkila, 1967). However, auscultatory findings alone are relatively insensitive; an audible murmur may be absent in as many as 50% of patients who have moderate or severe mitral insufficiency demonstrated angiographically (Tcheng et al., 1992). Angiographic evaluation allows quantitation and accurate detection of mitral insufficiency as well as precise delineation of the coronary anatomy. Specific information regarding the valve apparatus and associated pathology may be difficult to obtain from angiographic studies alone.

Echocardiographic evaluation is useful both preoperatively for diagnosis and intraoperatively in patients undergoing surgical exploration. Echocardiography may also obviate the need for right-side heart catherization and cine ventriculography in critically ill patients (Harrison et al., 1989). Transthoracic two-dimensional echocardiography with color-flow Doppler can quantitate the degree of mitral insufficiency and characterize the nature of the valve abnormality. The distinction between papillary muscle dysfunction, in which the papillary muscle may appear hypokinetic, and papillary muscle rupture is clear, as shown in Figure 54–104 (Erbel et al., 1981; Izumi et al., 1985; Prachar et al., 1990). Color-flow Doppler imaging also allows differentiation of acquired ventricular septal defects from acute mitral insufficiency complicating myocardial infarction (Harrison et al., 1989; Kishon et al., 1993).

The demonstration of increased resolution of left atrium and mitral valve apparatus with transesophageal echocardiography has expanded as use of this technique has become more widespread (Patel et al., 1989; Sakai et al., 1991; Stoddard et al., 1990). Transesophageal echocardiography has proved highly accurate even in cases where transthoracic examination failed to demonstrate a significant abnormality (Kishon et al., 1993) (Fig. 54–105).

## SURGICAL TREATMENT

The surgical management of patients with ischemic mitral insufficiency poses a difficult challenge for the thoracic surgeon. Although this relatively uncommon problem occurs in only 3% of patients with coronary artery disease, published mortality rates have ranged from 9 to 53% and the patients affected are quite diverse. The elderly patient referred from the coronary care unit with papillary muscle rupture in cardiogenic shock and progressive organ damage is clearly not analogous to a patient presenting with moderate to severe mitral insufficiency several months following myocardial infarction. Risk stratification of these patients using baseline prognostic indicators is necessary so that management strategies can be developed for similar patients and compared among institutions with a large patient experience (Rankin et al., 1989).

Additionally, the anatomic cause of ischemic mitral valve dysfunction, as well as the classification of these abnormalities, remains controversial. This is important because valve reconstructive techniques, which correct specific anatomic disturbances of the valve apparatus, are increasingly being employed. Despite these limitations, basic principles in the approach to patients with ischemic mitral insufficiency can be applied and modified based on the individual surgeon's experience and ability.

Several studies support the premise that mitral insufficiency, in patients with coronary artery disease, is a predictor of decreased survival, and this correlation extends to the severity of the valvular insufficiency determined angiographically (Rankin et al., 1989; Tcheng et al., 1992) (Fig. 54–106). Therefore, even mild degrees of ischemic mitral insufficiency must be thor-

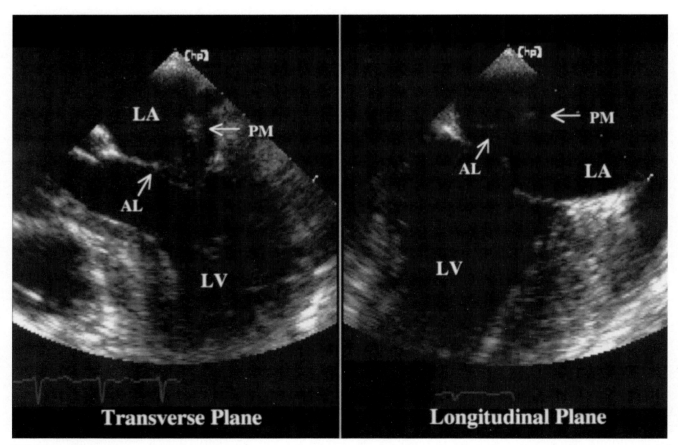

**FIGURE 54–105.** Transesophageal echocardiography was performed preoperatively in a patient in cardiogenic shock following a myocardial infarction. This study revealed a flail anterior leaflet of the mitral valve and, although less common, a ruptured anterolateral papillary muscle. The patient underwent successful mitral valve replacement following this diagnosis. (LA = left atrium; LV = left ventricle; AL = anterior leaflet of the mitral valve; PM = disrupted papillary muscle.)

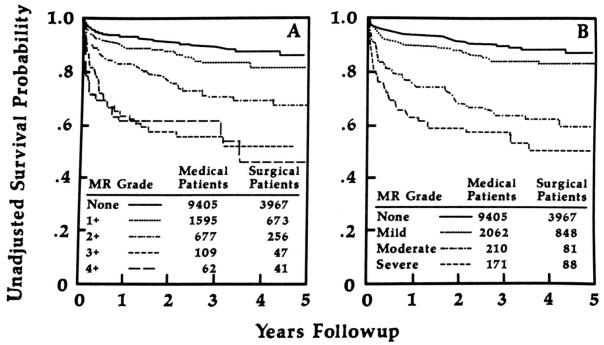

**FIGURE 54–106.** Unadjusted survival characteristics of all patients ($n = 11,849$) with significant coronary artery disease diagnosed at catheterization from 1981 to 1987, stratified according to associated mitral regurgitation (MR) Grades 1+ to 4+ (A) and Mild to Severe (B). (A and B, From Rankin, J. S., Livesay, S. A., Smith, L. R., et al.: Trends in the surgical treatment of ischemic mitral regurgitation: Effects of mitral valve repair on hospital mortality. Semin. Thorac. Cardiovasc. Surg., 1:149, 1989.)

oughly evaluated in patients with coronary artery disease. Surgical decisions are based on the degree and anatomic nature of the valvular dysfunction, as well as specific patient factors.

## Transient Mitral Insufficiency

This abnormality should be suspected in patients with a normal valve apparatus and transient episodes of moderate to severe mitral insufficiency and coexistent coronary artery lesions. The aim of therapy in these patients is complete myocardial revascularization. This may be achieved with either angioplasty or coronary bypass grafting, which ameliorates the valvular dysfunction in most patients (Heuser et al., 1987; LeFeuvre et al., 1992; Rankin et al., 1989). Resolution of valvular dysfunction should be confirmed by Doppler echocardiography following angioplasty or in the operating room following revascularization. Volume loading can be performed to raise the left atrial pressure to 12 to 15 mm Hg; if significant mitral insufficiency occurs, it can be corrected surgically by annuloplasty or valve replacement (David, 1994; Rankin et al., 1989).

The surgical treatment of lesser degrees (1+ to 2+) of ischemic mitral insufficiency remains controversial. Some argue for an aggressive approach to this problem because of the impact of mitral insufficiency on survival and the published results of mitral valve repair that demonstrate a low perioperative mortality

in patients who undergo concomitant coronary artery bypass grafting (Hendren et al., 1991; Rankin et al., 1989).

However, others suggest a more conservative approach to lesser degrees of ischemic mitral insufficiency and recommend myocardial revascularization alone (Connolly et al., 1986). In a study by Arcidi and colleagues (1988), 58 patients with moderate ischemic mitral insufficiency (3+ on a scale of 1 to 4) were managed with coronary bypass alone. The patients presented with symptoms of significant angina (Class III or greater in 90%) but not congestive heart failure. Although most of the patients had ischemic mitral insufficiency (75%) identified as the cause of their valvular lesion, 15 patients had mitral insufficiency from other causes. The operative mortality was low at 3.4%, although 50% of patients required inotropic support in the immediate postoperative period. The 5-year survival rate in this group of patients was 77%, comparing favorably with other reports in which the mitral insufficiency was corrected surgically.

On balance, although mitral insufficiency does have prognostic significance, treatment of mild (1+ to 2+), asymptomatic ischemic mitral insufficiency should consist of complete myocardial revascularization, with intraoperative transesophageal echocardiographic assessment to confirm the severity of the valvular dysfunction. The value of surgical correction of persisting mitral insufficiency in this setting is as yet unproved. However, moderate to severe ischemic mitral insufficiency in patients with associated congestive heart failure symptoms warrants surgical consideration.

## Fixed Mitral Insufficiency

### Papillary Muscle Rupture

Patients with rupture of the papillary muscles are subject to a high operative mortality because of the acuity of presentation. The rupture is usually partial, and in most patients it involves the posteromedial papillary muscle. Some patients may be well compensated on medical management, but most present in cardiogenic shock within the first week following myocardial infarction, and often require intraaortic balloon pump support. If a complete rupture is left untreated, it is almost uniformly fatal, with 70% mortality in the first 24 hours (Saunders et al., 1957; Wei et al., 1979).

Although the optimal timing for surgical intervention is not known, correction before the onset of severe pulmonary edema and organ dysfunction is recommended (Cohn, 1992; Kishon et al., 1992; Tepe and Edmunds, 1985). The preoperative assessment should include delineation of coronary anatomy even in critically ill patients. In a Mayo Clinic study (Kishon et al., 1992) involving 22 patients with acute papillary muscle rupture, 50% had associated coronary artery disease remote from the right coronary artery that, when bypassed, was associated with improved survival. In these critically ill patients with complete papillary muscle rupture, the appropriate treatment is mitral valve replacement, with preservation of at least the posterior leaflet chordal attachments and papillary muscle whenever possible, and concomitant coronary bypass grafting (Cohn, 1992; Kishon et al., 1992; Tepe and Edmunds, 1985). In the group of patients from the Mayo Clinic, the perioperative mortality was 27% and the estimated 7-year survival rate for discharged patients was 67%.

The importance of chordal papillary integrity for the preservation of ventricular function is now well established (David et al., 1983; David and Ho, 1986; Harpole et al., 1990; Pitarys et al., 1990). Attempts to preserve the mitral valve apparatus have led to a resurgence in valvular reconstructive techniques. Recognized advantages of mitral valve repair over prosthetic replacement include better preservation of ventricular function, reduced valve-related complications, decreased anticoagulation requirements, savings in cost, lower operative mortality, and improved long-term survival (Cohn et al., 1988; Galloway et al., 1988; Goldman et al., 1987; Hendren et al., 1991; King and Pluth, 1986; Weintraub et al., 1986). In complete ruptures of the papillary muscle, the presence of necrotic and friable tissue makes successful repair less feasible (Cohn, 1992; Loisance et al., 1990). However, reparative techniques have been described using a strip of Teflon felt as a sling to support the papillary muscle and allow replantation as illustrated in Figure 54–107.

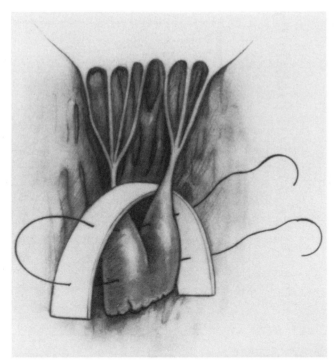

**FIGURE 54–107.** Reimplantation of a ruptured papillary muscle with the sling pledget method. (From Rankin, J. S., Livesay, S. A., Smith, L. R., et al.: Trends in the surgical treatment of ischemic mitral regurgitation: Effects of mitral valve repair on hospital mortality. Semin. Thorac. Cardiovasc. Surg., 1:149, 1989.)

Rupture of a single papillary muscle head may also be amenable to repair techniques. A unique transventricular approach has been used to repair the mitral valve (Fig. 54–108), including papillary muscle rupture. The authors conclude that for patients with papillary muscle rupture and preserved left ventricular function, this approach may damage viable myocardium, and therefore they advocate repair through the standard transatrial approach (Rankin et al., 1988).

### Papillary Muscle Dysfunction

The surgical approach to patients with papillary muscle dysfunction has been altered most with the resurgence of mitral valve repair techniques. A unique method used at Duke University has been to approach the mitral valve transventricularly in the presence of a transmural infarction or aneurysm, as shown in Figure 54–109. A longitudinal posterior ventriculotomy to the left of the posterior descending artery was performed. The incision is then continued to within 1 cm of the base of the heart, exposing both the valve and the subvalvular apparatus. An annuloplasty suture is then placed deep to the posteromedial commissure, as shown in Figure 54–109A, to correct posterior annular dilatation. The elongated posteromedial papillary muscle heads are then individually displaced apically, as shown in Figure 54–109B. Associated abnormalities can also be repaired using this approach, including specific chordal short-

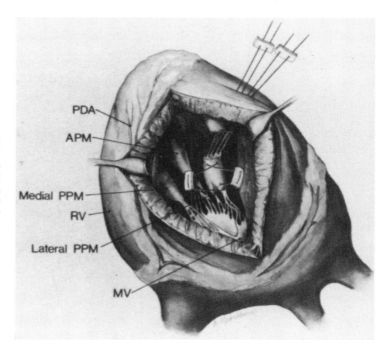

**FIGURE 54–108.** Reimplantation of a ruptured lateral head of the posterior papillary muscle (PPM) complex. (PDA = posterior descending coronary artery; APM = anterior papillary muscles; RV = right ventricle; MV = mitral valve.) See text for details. (From Rankin, J. S., Feneley, M. P., Hickey, M., et al.: A clinical comparison of mitral valve repair versus valve replacement in ischemic mitral regurgitation. J. Thorac. Cardiovasc. Surg., 95:165, 1988.)

ening (Carpentier, 1983), as well as annuloplasty of the anterior commissure (Fig. 54–110).

Intraoperative echocardiography should be used to characterize the mitral valve repair following completion in the same way it is used to define the valvular abnormality. Significant mitral insufficiency following repair should not be tolerated, and reexploration for a second repair or conversion to valve replacement is a possibility in any patient (Cohn et al., 1988; Hendren et al., 1991). As the long-term durability of mitral valve repair is increasingly reported and extensive experience with this technique is acquired, the per-

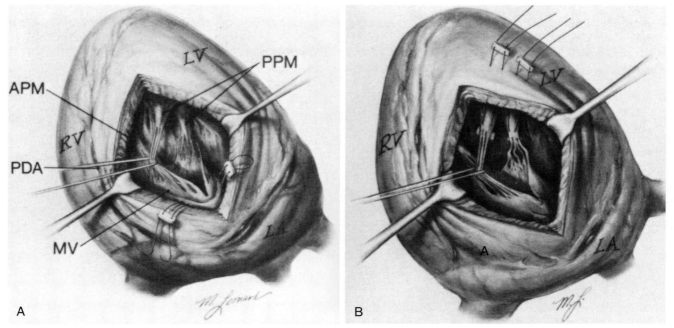

**FIGURE 54–109.** *A,* Initial steps of transventricular mitral valve (MV) reconstruction, The apex of the heart is lifted superiorly, and the ventriculotomy is performed to the left of the posterior descending coronary artery (PDA) through the posterior infarct. The posterior annuloplasty suture is illustrated, as are the posterior (PPM) and anterior (APM) papillary muscles. The ventriculotomy is shown larger for illustrative purposes. See text for details. (RV = right ventricle; LV = left ventricle; LA = left atrium.) *B,* The annuloplasty suture has been tied, and pledget-supported mattress sutures have been placed to shorten the PPM. (*A* and *B,* From Rankin, J. S., Feneley, M. P., Hickey, M., et al.: A clinical comparison of mitral valve repair versus valve replacement in ischemic mitral regurgitation. J. Thorac. Cardiovasc. Surg., 95:165, 1988.)

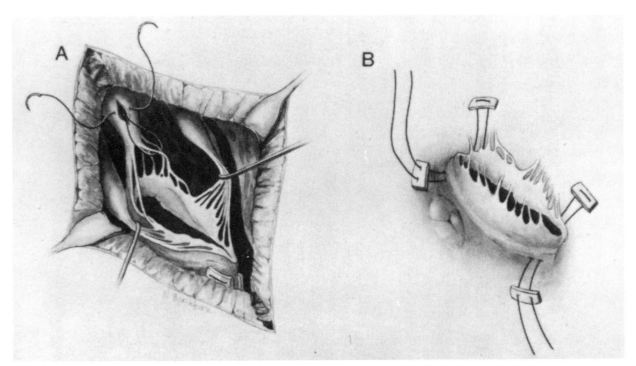

**FIGURE 54–110.** A Carpentier chordal shortening procedure, as performed transventricularly for elongated anterior chordae to the central posterior leaflet (*A*), and a transventricular bilateral commissural annuloplasty (*B*). (*A* and *B*, From Rankin, J. S., Feneley, M. P., Hickey, M., et al.: A clinical comparison of mitral valve repair versus valve replacement in ischemic mitral regurgitation. J. Thorac. Cardiovasc. Surg., *95*:165, 1988.)

centage of patients for whom mitral valve repair is applied will increase.

These repairs were performed following the distal coronary anastomosis where required. The ventriculotomy was then closed using Teflon felt strips. The mitral valve repair was carried out transventricularly in 18 patients, with a hospital mortality rate of 26%; in a similar group having mitral valve replacement, mortality was 53%. This comparison suggests that mitral valve repair has a survival advantage over replacement. The authors conclude that the transventricular approach is safe and effective and should be considered in the presence of a significant wall motion defect and transmural infarction.

A similar experience with valve repair has been described for patients with ischemic mitral insufficiency at the Cleveland Clinic (Hendren et al., 1991). In a series of 84 patients, 65 (77%) had mitral valve repair performed through the left atrial approach. Most of the patients (83%) presented with chronic mitral insufficiency. Various established techniques (Carpentier, 1983) were used to correct the valvular insufficiency, including leaflet resection (3), chordal shortening (15), papillary muscle reimplantation (10), and papillary muscle shortening (3). Annuloplasty (63) was performed in almost all patients. The mean degree of residual mitral insufficiency was minimal (0.6+ as a mean). Two patients had to be reexplored postoperatively for failed repair. Excellent results were achieved, and the hospital mortality rate was low, at 9.2%. Improved hospital mortality and long-term survival were seen in patients who presented with chronic ischemic mitral insufficiency and underwent valve repair, compared with valve replacement. In this series, 80% of patients with ischemic mitral insufficiency underwent successful valve repair. Follow-up to 3 years demonstrated an overall survival of 63% for all patients undergoing mitral valvuloplasty for ischemic dysfunction.

### Generalized Annular Dilatation

This group of patients did poorly regardless of surgical treatment. All patients with generalized dilatation and anterior aneurysm in the Duke University series died in the postoperative period, regardless of whether they underwent valve repair or replacement. Further, poor outcomes among these patients have been described by others (Najafi et al., 1975; Pinson et al., 1984). A suggested management approach to these patients is referral to assess suitability for cardiac transplantation (Rankin et al., 1988).

### CONCLUSION

Ischemic mitral insufficiency, a relatively uncommon problem, is significant because of a high operative mortality. Mitral insufficiency of any degree caused by coronary artery disease is associated with a poorer long-term survival. Patients with moderate to severe dysfunction should be evaluated for surgical correction. The increasing use of mitral valve repair, especially in patients who present with chronic valvular dysfunction, necessitates precise anatomic determination of the valvular pathology before surgical intervention. Mitral valve repair continues to demonstrate a lower hospital mortality and a more favorable long-term outcome than valve replacement in many patients with ischemic mitral insufficiency.

## SELECTED BIBLIOGRAPHY

Barbour, D. J., and Roberts, W. C.: Rupture of a left ventricular papillary muscle during acute myocardial infarction: Analysis of 22 necropsy patients. J. Am. Coll. Cardiol., 8:558, 1986.

This is a careful review of the postmortem findings in a group of 22 patients following papillary muscle rupture in the setting of an acute myocardial infarction. The patient characteristics and pathologic data present a clear picture of this entity.

Hendren, W. G., Nemec, J. J., Lytle, B. W., et al.: Mitral valve repair for ischemic mitral insufficiency. Ann. Thorac. Surg., 52:1246, 1991.

This is an extensive review of a study from the Cleveland Clinic over a 5-year period that included 1292 patients with mitral valve abnormalities. From this group, 84 patients with ischemic mitral insufficiency who underwent valve repair are presented. The study compares valve replacement with valve repair and contains an extensive review of the literature. This paper contains compelling data regarding the effectiveness of mitral valve repair from a group with extensive experience with this problem.

Kishon, Y., Oh, J. K., Schaff, H. V., et al.: Mitral valve operation in postinfarction rupture of a papillary muscle: Immediate results and long-term follow-up of 22 patients. Mayo Clin. Proc., 67:1023, 1992.

This is a review from the Mayo Clinic of 22 patients managed with papillary muscle rupture collected over a 31-year period. The demographic and clinical features are clearly represented. The management principles are clearly stated and prognostic indicators stated. The series presents good results and excellent follow-up in this group of patients with papillary muscle rupture.

Rankin, J. S., Feneley, M. P., Hickey, M., et al.: A clinical comparison of mitral valve repair versus valve replacement in ischemic mitral regurgitation. J. Thorac. Cardiovasc. Surg., 95:165, 1988.

This is the first of two significant papers from the same authors outlining the features and surgical management of patients with ischemic mitral insufficiency. A novel surgical approach to the mitral valve apparatus via ventriculotomy is presented. A classification of valvular abnormalities in patients with ischemic valve dysfunction is also presented. The outcomes of patients undergoing valve repair are compared with those of patients treated with valve replacement. Significant reduction in hospital mortality was demonstrated in patients whose valvular dysfunction was managed by valve repair as opposed to replacement.

Rankin, J. S., Livesay, S. A., Smith, L. R., et al.: Trends in the surgical treatment of ischemic mitral regurgitation: Effects of mitral valve repair on hospital mortality. Semin. Thorac. Cardiovasc. Surg., 1:149, 1989.

This paper is an overview of the current treatment strategies for patients with ischemic mitral insufficiency. The prognostic significance of mitral insufficiency is demonstrated and a detailed analysis of mitral valve repair techniques is outlined.

Roberts, W. C., and Perloff, J. K.: A clinicopathologic survey of the conditions causing the mitral valve to function abnormally. Ann. Intern. Med., 77:939, 1972.

This report is an in-depth discussion of the anatomy, pathology, and pathophysiology of a variety of mitral valve abnormalities. A thorough discussion of all aspects of the mitral valve apparatus is provided. The anatomic descriptions of specific mitral valve abnormalities form the basis for attempted corrective surgery.

## BIBLIOGRAPHY

American Heart Association: 1987 Heart Facts. Dallas, American Heart Association National Center, 1987.
Arcidi, J. M., Hebeler, R. F., Craver, J. M., et al.: Treatment of moderate mitral regurgitation and coronary disease by coronary bypass alone. J. Thorac. Cardiovasc. Surg., 95:951, 1988.
Austin, W. E., Sanders, C. A., Auerill, J. H., and Friedlich, A. L.: Ruptured papillary muscle: Report of a case with successful mitral valve replacement. Circulation, 32:597, 1965.
Barbour, D. J., and Roberts, W. C.: Rupture of a left ventricular papillary muscle during acute myocardial infarction: Analysis of 22 necropsy patients. J. Am. Coll. Cardiol., 8:558, 1986.
Brolin, I.: The mitral orifice. Acta Radiol. [Diagn.] (Stockh.), 6:273, 1967.
Burch, G. E., Depasquale, N. P., and Philips, J. H.: Clinical manifestations of papillary muscle dysfunction. Arch. Intern. Med., 112:158, 1963.
Carpentier, A.: Cardiac valve surgery—The "French correction." J. Thorac. Cardiovasc. Surg., 86:323, 1983.
Cheng, T.: Some new observations on the syndrome of papillary muscle dysfunction. Am. J. Med., 47:924, 1969.
Cohn, L. H.: Surgical treatment of postinfarction rupture of a papillary muscle. Mayo Clin. Proc., 67:1109, 1992.
Cohn, L. H.: Surgery for mitral regurgitation. J.A.M.A., 260:2883, 1988.
Cohn, L. H., Kowalker, W., Bhatia, S., et al.: Comparative morbidity of mitral valve repair versus replacement for mitral regurgitation with and without coronary artery disease. Ann. Thorac. Surg., 45:284, 1988.
Connolly, M. W., Gelbfish, J. S., Jacobowitz, I. J., et al.: Surgical results for mitral regurgitation from coronary artery disease. J. Thorac. Cardiovasc. Surg., 91:379, 1986.
David, T. E.: Techniques and results of mitral valve repair for ischemic mitral regurgitation. J. Card. Surg., 9(Suppl.):274, 1994.
David, T. E., and Ho, W. C.: The effect of preservation of chordae tendineae on mitral valve replacement for post infarction mitral regurgitation. Circulation, 74(Suppl. I):II-16, 1986.
David, T. E., Uden, D. E., and Strauss, H. D.: The importance of the mitral apparatus in left ventricular function after correction of mitral regurgitation. Circulation, 68(Suppl. II):II-76, 1983.
Davidson, S.: Spontaneous rupture of a papillary muscle of the heart: A report of three cases and a review of the literature. Mt. Sinai J. Med., 14:941, 1948.
Davis, P. K. B., and Kinmouth, J. B.: The movements of the annulus of the mitral valve. J. Cardiovasc. Surg. (Torino), 4:427, 1963.
Erbel, R., Schweizer, P., Bardos, P., and Meyer, J.: Two-dimensional echocardiographic diagnosis of papillary muscle rupture. Chest, 79:595, 1981.
Fehrenbacher, G., Schmidt, D. H., and Bommer, W. J.: Evaluation of transient mitral regurgitation in coronary artery disease. Am. J. Cardiol., 68:868, 1991.
Fishbein, M. C.: Mitral insufficiency in coronary artery disease. Semin. Thorac. Cardiovasc. Surg., 1:129, 1989.
Galloway, A. C., Colvin, S. B., Baumann, F. G., et al.: Current concepts of mitral valve reconstruction for mitral insufficiency. Circulation, 78:1087, 1988.
Godley, R. W., Wann, L. S., Rogers, E. W., et al.: Incomplete mitral leaflet closure in patients with papillary muscle dysfunction. Circulation, 63:565, 1981.
Goldman, M. E., Mora, F., Guarino, T., et al.: Mitral valvuloplasty is superior to valve replacement for preservation of left ventricular function: An operative two-dimensional echocardiographic study. J. Am. Coll. Cardiol., 10:568, 1987.
Harpole, D. H., Jr., Rankin, J. S., Wolfe, W. G., et al.: Effects of standard mitral valve replacement on left ventricular function. Ann. Thorac. Surg., 49:866, 1990.
Harrison, M. R., MacPhail, B., Gurley, J. C., et al.: Usefulness of color Doppler flow imaging to distinguish ventricular septal defect from acute mitral regurgitation complicating acute myocardial infarction. Am. J. Cardiol., 64:697, 1989.
Heikkila, J.: Mitral incompetence complicating acute myocardial infarction. Br. Heart. J., 29:162, 1967.
Hendren, W. G., Nemec, J. J., Lytle, B. W., et al.: Mitral valve repair for ischemic mitral insufficiency. Ann. Thorac. Surg., 52:1246, 1991.
Heuser, R. R., Maddoux, G. L., Goss, J. E., et al.: Coronary angioplasty for acute mitral regurgitation due to myocardial infarction. Ann. Intern. Med., 107:852, 1987.
Hickey, M. St. J., Smith, L., Muhlbaier, L. H., et al.: Current prognosis of ischemic mitral regurgitation. Implications for future management. Circulation, 78(Suppl. I):I-51, 1988.

Izumi, S., Miyatake, K., Beppu, S., et al.: Mechanism of mitral regurgitation in patients with myocardial infarction: A study using real-time two-dimensional Doppler flow imaging and echocardiography. Circulation, 76:777, 1987.

Kay, E. L., Kay, J. H., Zubiate, P., et al.: Mitral valve repair for mitral regurgitation secondary to coronary artery disease. Circulation, 74(Suppl. I):88, 1986.

King, R. M., and Pluth, J. R.: Concomitant mitral valve repair or replacement and coronary revascularization. J. Card. Surg., 1:233, 1986.

Kishon, Y., Iqbal, A., Oh, J. K., et al.: Evolution of echocardiographic modalities in detection of postmyocardial infarction ventricular septal defect and papillary muscle rupture: Study of 62 patients. Am. Heart J., 126:667, 1993.

Kishon, Y., Oh, J. K., Schaff, H. V., et al.: Mitral valve operation in postinfarction rupture of a papillary muscle: Immediate results and long-term follow-up of 22 patients. Mayo Clin. Proc., 67:1023, 1992.

LeFeuvre, C., Metzger, J. P., Lachurie, M. L., et al.: Treatment of severe mitral regurgitation caused by papillary muscle dysfunction: Indications for coronary angioplasty. Am. Heart J., 123:860, 1992.

Loisance, D. Y., Deleuze, P., Hillion, M. L., and Cachera, J. P.: Are there indications for reconstructive surgery in severe mitral regurgitation after acute myocardial infarction? Eur. J. Cardiothorac. Surg., 4:394, 1990.

Maisel, A. S., Gilpen, E. D., Klein, L., et al.: The murmur of papillary muscle dysfunction in acute myocardial dysfunction: Clinical features and prognostic implications. Am. Heart J., 112:705, 1986.

Mittal, A. K., Langston, M., Jr., Cohn, K. E., et al.: Combined papillary muscle and left ventricular wall dysfunction as a cause of mitral regurgitation. Circulation, 44:174, 1971.

Najafi, H., Javid, H., Hunter, J. A., et al.: Mitral insufficiency secondary to coronary heart disease. Ann. Thorac. Surg., 20:529, 1975.

Patel, A. M., Miller, F. A., Jr., Khandheria, B. K., et al.: Role of transesophageal echocardiography in the diagnosis of papillary muscle rupture secondary to myocardial infarction. Am. Heart J., 118:1330, 1989.

Perloff, J. K., and Roberts, W. C.: Functional anatomy of mitral regurgitation. Circulation, 46:227, 1972.

Pinson, C. W., Cobanoglu, A., Metzdorff, M. T., et al.: Late surgical results for ischemic mitral regurgitation. J. Thorac. Cardiovasc. Surg., 88:663, 1984.

Pitarys, C. J., Forman, M. B., Panayiotou, H., and Hansen, D. E.: Long-term effects of excision of the mitral apparatus on global and regional ventricular function in humans. J. Am. Coll. Cardiol., 15:557, 1990.

Prachar, H., Dittel, M., and Enenkel, W.: Acute mitral regurgitation due to short periods of ischemia during percutaneous transluminal coronary angioplasty: An angiographic study. Int. J. Cardiol., 29:185, 1990.

Ranganathan, N., and Burch, G. E.: Gross morphology and arterial supply of the papillary muscles of the left ventricle of man. Am. Heart J., 77:506, 1969.

Rankin, J. S., Feneley, M. P., Hickey, M., et al.: A clinical comparison of mitral valve repair versus valve replacement in ischemic mitral regurgitation. J. Thorac. Cardiovasc. Surg., 95:165, 1988.

Rankin, J. S., Livesay, S. A., Smith, L. R., et al.: Trends in the surgical treatment of ischemic mitral regurgitation: Effects of mitral valve repair on hospital mortality. Semin. Thorac. Cardiovasc. Surg., 1:149, 1989.

Roberts, W. C., and Perloff, J. K.: A clinicopathologic survey of the conditions causing the mitral valve to function abnormally. Ann. Intern. Med., 77:939, 1972.

Rushmer, R. F., Finlayson, B. L., and Nash, A. A.: Movements of the mitral valve. Circ. Res., 4:337, 1956.

Sakai, K., Nakamura, K., and Hosoda, S.: Transesophageal echocardiographic findings of papillary muscle rupture. Am. J. Cardiol., 68:561, 1991.

Saunders, R. J., Neuberger, K. T., and Ravin, A.: Rupture of papillary muscles: Occurrence of rupture of the posterior muscle in posterior myocardial infarction. Dis. Chest, 31:316, 1957.

Spencer, F. C., Reppert, E. H., and Stertzer, S. H.: Surgical treatment of mitral insufficiency secondary to coronary artery disease. Arch. Surg., 95:853, 1967.

Stevenson, R. R., and Turner, W. J.: Rupture of a papillary muscle in the heart as a sudden cause of death. Bull. Johns Hopkins Hosp., 57:235, 1935.

Stoddard, M. F., Keedy, D. L., and Kupersmith, J.: Transesophageal echocardiographic diagnosis of papillary muscle rupture complicating acute myocardial infarction. Am. Heart J., 120:690, 1990.

Tcheng, J. E., Jackman, J. D., Nelson, C. L., et al.: Outcome of patients sustaining acute ischemic mitral regurgitation during myocardial infarction. Ann. Intern. Med., 117:18, 1992.

Tepe, N. A., and Edmunds, L. H., Jr.: Operation for acute postinfarction mitral insufficiency and cardiogenic shock. J. Thorac. Cardiovasc. Surg., 89:525, 1985.

Tsakiris, A. G., Rastell, G. C., Amorim, D., et al.: Effect of experimental papillary muscle dysfunction on mitral valve closure in intact anaesthetized dogs. Mayo Clin. Proc., 45:275, 1970.

van Rijk-Zwikker, G. L., Delemarre, B. J., and Huysmans, H. A.: Mitral valve anatomy and morphology: Relevance to mitral valve replacement and valve reconstruction J. Card. Surg., 9(Suppl.):255, 1994.

Vlodaver, Z., and Edwards, J. E.: Rupture of the ventricular septum or papillary muscle complicating myocardial infarction. Circulation, 55:815, 1977.

Wei, J. Y., Hutchins, E. M., and Bulkley, B. H.: Papillary muscle rupture in fatal acute myocardial infarction: A potentially treatable form of cardiogenic shock. Ann. Intern. Med., 90:149, 1979.

Weintraub, R. M., Wei, J. Y., and Thurer, R. L.: Surgical repair of remediable postinfarction cardiogenic shock in the elderly. J. Am. Geriatr. Soc., 34:389, 1986.

# *6  Postinfarction Ventricular Septal Defect*

J. Scott Rankin

Rupture of the interventricular septum following myocardial infarction is uncommon and is associated with an extremely poor prognosis. Without surgical management, most patients die of severe congestive heart failure within hours to days, and less than 20% survive 2 months. Thus, expeditious diagnosis and almost uniform operative intervention should be the standard of therapy.

Septal rupture most commonly occurs within 1 to 4 days of infarction and involves the anterior septum (*left anterior descending* [LAD] infarct) in approximately 60% of cases and the posterior septum (right coronary infarct) in the remainder. Anterior defects are more commonly simple and located toward the apex. Posterior defects are frequently complex, with multiple septal tracts or aneurysms, and are often

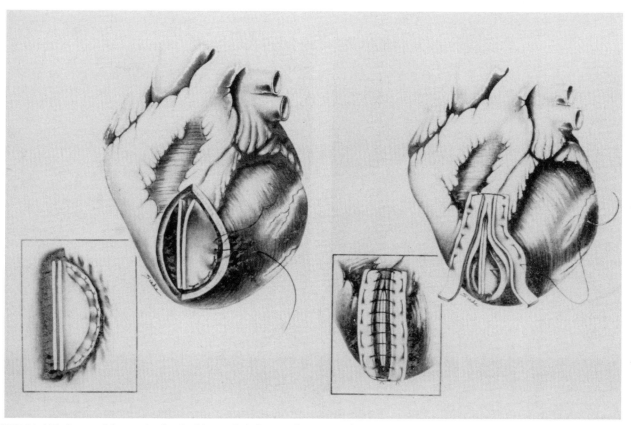

**FIGURE 54–111.** Sequential steps in the double-patch technique for repair of anterior postinfarction ventricular septal defect. See text for details. (Modified from Ochsner, J. L., and Mills, N. L.: Coronary Artery Surgery. Philadelphia, Lea & Febiger, 1978.)

**FIGURE 54–112.** Survival characteristics of 100 patients undergoing repair of postinfarction ventricular septal defect to a mean follow-up of 4 years. *Vertical bars* represent plus or minus one standard error for each calculation. *Numbers above bars* refer to number of surviving patients for each period. (From Skillington, P. D., Davies, H. R., Luff, A. J., et al.: Surgical treatment for infarct-related ventricular septal defects. J. Thorac. Cardiovasc. Surg., *99*:798–808, 1990.)

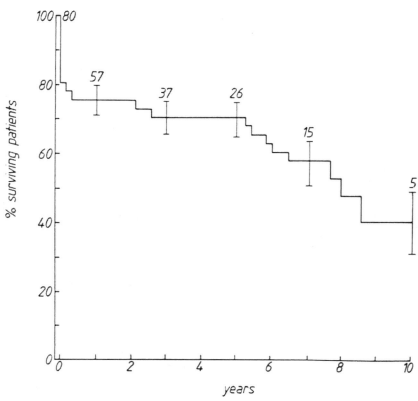

1970    The Coronary Circulation

located toward the base, near or even involving the A-V valve ring (Mann and Roberts, 1988).

Posterior defects also are associated with large right ventricular infarctions if the right coronary occlusion is proximal, whereas anterior defects usually have more left ventricular necrosis, especially if the LAD occlusion is proximal. Both lesions are associated with an acute left-to-right shunt, producing pulmonary overcirculation, pulmonary edema, and acute failure of the volume-overloaded right ventricle. The combination of acute volume overload and right ventricular infarction can have ominous consequences in patients with posterior defects (Anderson et al., 1989; Cummings et al., 1989).

The condition should be suspected in a patient recovering from myocardial infarction in whom cardiogenic shock or congestive heart failure suddenly develops. A harsh holosystolic murmur usually is present along the left sternal border, and many patients demonstrate a palpable thrill. Currently, the diagnosis can be made quickly in the CCU setting with transthoracic Doppler echocardiography and, if necessary, confirmed with transesophageal echocardiography (Fortin et al., 1991; Harrison et al., 1989). Cardiac catheterization should be performed immediately to document coronary anatomy, and efforts should be directed to minimize dye load and contrast nephropathy.

In most patients, an *intra-aortic balloon pump* (IABP) should be placed at the conclusion of catheterization. Even if the patient seems hemodynamically stable, IABP support helps maintain myocardial and multiorgan perfusion during transport to the operating room and induction of anesthesia. Postinfarction *ventricular septal defect* (VSD) is a true surgical emergency, and immediate intervention should be the rule (Daggett, 1990; Daggett et al., 1982; Gaudiani et al., 1981). Delay can be associated with pulmonary and multiorgan deterioration, as well as worsening right ventricular injury due to the acute volume overload.

Surgical repair of postinfarction VSD was first accomplished by Cooley in a relatively stable patient, several weeks after infarction (Cooley et al., 1957). An approach through a longitudinal right ventriculotomy was used, as employed in congenital VSD at the time. Subsequently, it was demonstrated that the right ventricle was less injured when the defect was approached through the infarct, and transventricular repair became the standard approach (Stinson et al., 1969).

Currently, the surgical procedure is performed with transesophageal echocardiographic monitoring before and after bypass. When the pericardium is opened, the right ventricle usually appears dilated and hypocontractile. Cardiopulmonary bypass is instituted with bicaval cannulation, although a single right atrial cannula can be used for simple anterior defects. When caval cannulation is used, endocardial right ventricular cold saline lavage is employed to assist with right ventricular preservation (Dailey et al., 1987; Rankin and Sabiston, 1995). This is especially important in

right coronary infarcts, in which extensive preoperative right ventricular injury may be present.

After cardioplegic arrest, an incision is made in the area of infarction, and good exposure to the interiors of both the left and right ventricles is obtained. A portion of the necrotic edge of the defect is resected, and a double-patch technique is used for repair (Fig. 54–111). For posterior defects, an identical procedure is performed with the apex elevated and the incision in the posterior interventricular groove. Although other methods have been advocated by various authors, the double-patch technique remains applicable to virtually all cases. This approach is simple and expeditious, and it has been associated with a negligible incidence of persistent or recurrent VSD.

Coronary bypass grafts are constructed routinely to all diseased vessels, including the right coronary artery in cases of right ventricular infarction (Angelini et al., 1989). A minimal degree of right ventricular functional recovery can make the difference between patient survival and demise and is extremely important for proximal right coronary occlusions. If the LAD requires grafting in posterior VSD, the left internal mammary artery is usually employed.

Obtaining optimal surgical results in postinfarction VSD requires multidisciplinary teamwork among primary care physicians, cardiologists, anesthesiologists, and surgeons. Early recognition and diagnosis of the problem, together with adequate hemodynamic support (IABP in most cases) during coronary angiography, minimizes preoperative patient injury. Recent advances in cardiac anesthetic techniques, surgical approaches, and postoperative care have made postoperative survival routine. The operative mortality rate now should approximate 20% (Fig. 54–112), even though most patients present with some degree of cardiogenic shock and multiorgan failure (Skillington et al., 1990). Long-term results after repair have been shown to be better if concomitant complete coronary revascularization is performed (Muehrcke et al., 1992). Risk factors for mortality include the preoperative presence of cardiogenic shock (especially if prolonged), severe multiorgan failure, posterior as compared with anterior defects (Moore et al., 1986), and advanced age (Skillington et al., 1990). Most patients should be considered operative candidates unless multiorgan failure is advanced. Surgical results have improved dramatically in recent years, and this trend is likely to continue as methods of diagnosis and treatment become more standardized.

## BIBLIOGRAPHY

Anderson, D. R., Adams, S., Bhat, A., and Pepper, J. R.: Post-infarction ventricular septal defect: The importance of site of infarction and cardiogenic shock on outcome. Eur. J. Cardiothorac. Surg., 3(6):554–557, 1989.
Angelini, G. D., Penny, W. J., Ruttley, M. S., et al.: Post-infarction ventricular septal defect: The importance of right ventricular coronary perfusion in determining surgical outcome. Eur. J. Cardiothorac. Surg., 3(2):156–161, 1989.
Cooley, D. A., Belmonte, B. A., Zels, L. B., and Schnur, S.: Surgical repair of ruptured interventricular septum following acute myocardial infarction. Surgery, 41:930–937, 1957.

Cummings, R. G., Califf, R., Jones, R. N., et al.: Correlates of survival in patients with postinfarction ventricular septal defect. Ann. Thorac. Surg., 47(6):824–830, 1989.

Daggett, W. M.: Postinfarction ventricular septal defect repair: Retrospective thoughts and historical perspectives. Ann. Thorac. Surg., 50(6):1006–1009, 1990.

Daggett, W. M., Buckley, M. J., Akins, C. W., et al.: Improved results of surgical management of postinfarction ventricular septal rupture. Ann. Surg., 196:269–277, 1982.

Daily, P. O., Pfeffer, T. A., Wisniewski, J. B., et al.: Clinical comparisons of methods of myocardial protection. J. Thorac. Cardiovasc. Surg., 93:324, 1987.

Fortin, D. F., Sheikh, K. H., and Kisslo, J.: The utility of echocardiography in the diagnostic strategy of postinfarction ventricular septal rupture: A comparison of two-dimensional echocardiography versus Doppler color flow imaging. Am. Heart J., 121 (1 Pt 1):25–32, 1991.

Gaudiani, V. A., Miller, D. C., Stinson, E. B., et al.: Postinfarction ventricular septal defect: An argument for early operation. Surgery, 89:48–55, 1981.

Harrison, M. R., MacPhail, B., Gurley, J. C., et al.: Usefulness of color Doppler flow imaging to distinguish ventricular septal defect from acute mitral regurgitation complicating acute myocardial infarction. Am. J. Cardiol., 64(12):697–701, 1989.

Mann, J. M., and Roberts, W. C.: Acquired ventricular septal defect during acute myocardial infarction: Analysis of 38 unoperated necropsy patients and comparison with 50 unoperated necropsy patients without rupture. Am. J. Cardiol., 62(1):8–19, 1988.

Moore, C. A., Nygaard, T. W., Kaiser, D. L., et al.: Postinfarction ventricular septal rupture: The importance of location of infarction and right ventricular function in determining survival. Circulation, 74:45–55, 1986.

Muehrcke, D. D., Daggett, W. M., Buckley, M. J., et al.: Effect of coronary bypass grafting on long-term survival after postinfarction ventricular septal defect repair. Ann. Thorac. Surg., 54:876–883, 1992.

Rankin, J. S., and Sabiston, D. C., Jr.: Physiology of coronary blood flow, myocardial function, and intraoperative myocardial protection. In Sabiston, D. C., Jr., and Spencer, F. C. (eds): Gibbon's Surgery of the Chest. 6th ed. Philadelphia: W. B. Saunders, 1995.

Skillington, P. D., Davies, R. H., Luff, A. J., et al.: Surgical treatment for infarct-related ventricular septal defects. J. Thorac. Cardiovasc. Surg., 99:798–808, 1990.

Stinson, E. B., Becker, J., and Shumway, N. E.: Successful repair of postinfarction ventricular septal defect and bi-ventricular aneurysm. J. Thorac. Cardiovasc. Surg., 58:20, 1969.

# 7  Prinzmetal's Variant Angina and Other Syndromes Associated with Coronary Artery Spasm

James E. Lowe

In 1768, William Heberden described chest pain associated with effort, eating, or anxiety. He called this pain angina pectoris from the Greek word *anchein,* meaning "to choke." Subsequently, it was shown that the pain of angina pectoris is associated with myocardial ischemia, although the neurophysiology of how this pain is perceived is still unknown.

Since Heberden's original description of angina pectoris, several anginal syndromes have been described that have different clinical implications. Until relatively recently, it was thought that the pathophysiology in these syndromes was related to various degrees of subtotal or totally obstructive atherosclerotic coronary artery disease and that clinically identifiable subgroups of patients had similar degrees of obstruction at certain anatomic sites that caused similar degrees of myocardial ischemic dysfunction.

Although Osler (1910) postulated that coronary vasospasm was a cause of angina pectoris, most pathologists and clinicians at the time, including Herrick (1912), thought that atherosclerotic obstruction alone was responsible for both angina and myocardial infarction. In 1959, Prinzmetal and associates reported 32 patients with a different type of anginal syndrome that could not be explained solely by the degree of atherosclerotic coronary artery disease thought to be present. Prinzmetal suggested that transient coronary artery spasm was occurring in this subgroup. Subsequently, coronary artery spasm was documented in many other patients and was associated with various clinical presentations, which are discussed in this chapter.

Coronary arterial spasm is a sudden increase in coronary vascular tone with localized or diffuse vasoconstriction. The degree of vasoconstriction is an abnormal vascular phenomenon and should be distinguished from normal coronary vasomotor changes. Although spasm is most often identified in large extramural coronary arteries, there is evidence that it may also occur in small resistance arterioles. Recognition of patients with coronary artery spasm and selection of appropriate therapeutic interventions are two problems that challenge both cardiologists and cardiovascular surgeons.

## CLASSIFICATION OF ANGINAL SYNDROMES

Since Heberden's original description of angina pectoris, it has been shown that there are various subgroups of patients with different types of angina, which must be identified because they have different clinical courses. *Stable angina* is the pain syndrome described by Heberden and is associated with effort, anxiety, or eating. Although the frequency of attacks can increase over time, this type of angina is usually predictable and stable over long periods. *Unstable angina* is a rapidly progressing pain syndrome that often causes myocardial infarction unless it is relieved by medical therapy, PTCA, or coronary artery bypass grafting. *Variant angina* is a distinctly different pain syndrome caused by coronary artery spasm, which can occur in normal coronary arteries or, more commonly, in coronary arteries with atherosclerotic lesions. Unlike stable and unstable angina, variant angina is usually not brought on by effort, eating, or anxiety. *Atypical angina* is a vague term that has various meanings. To some physicians, it represents chest pain secondary to coronary artery disease (with or without concomitant spasm) with a different kind of pain pattern—for example, pain that radiates into the right side of the chest or right arm; others use the term to refer to chest pain that may not even be related to coronary disease. Finally, angina occurs in patients with congenital coronary arterial malformations such as coronary artery fistulas or anomalous origin of the left coronary artery from the pulmonary artery. In these patients, angina results not from atherosclerotic disease or spasm but from a "steal" of normal coronary flow into the recipient cardiac chamber.

Each of these anginal syndromes is referred to by various names. Stable angina is called typical angina, classic angina, or Heberden's angina. Stable angina is also known as effort angina because of its association with exercise, eating, or anxiety, and Maseri and associates (1978a) called it secondary angina because it is secondary to fixed obstructive atherosclerotic coronary artery disease. Unstable angina is also known as preinfarction or crescendo angina because of its rapid progression. Stenosis of the left main coronary artery is one anatomic cause of this type of pain, and its clinical recognition is important because survival can be improved by coronary artery bypass grafting. Variant angina is also known as Prinzmetal's angina, vasospastic angina, and angina decubitus, because it usually occurs at rest, and Maseri and associates (1978a) called it primary angina because it is caused by spasm of the coronary arteries and is not secondary to atherosclerotic disease alone. For clarification, the terminology used to describe these various anginal syndromes is summarized in Table 54–13.

## PRINZMETAL'S VARIANT ANGINA

Stable angina, or classic Heberden's angina, is a distinct syndrome with two major clinical manifestations. First, the pain occurs when more work is demanded of the heart and the pain is relieved by rest or administration of nitroglycerin. Second, the electrocardiogram during an episode of pain often shows ST-segment depression in certain leads without reciprocal elevation. Prinzmetal and associates (1959) reported 32 patients, 20 of whom were personally observed, with a different anginal syndrome. They described this syndrome as "a variant form of angina

■ **Table 54–13.** ANGINAL SYNDROMES

**Stable Angina**

Heberden's angina
Classic angina
Typical angina
Effort angina
Secondary angina

**Unstable Angina**

Preinfarction angina
Crescendo angina

**Variant Angina**

Prinzmetal's angina
Vasospastic angina
Angina decubitus
Primary angina

**Atypical Angina**

**Angina Secondary to a Steal Phenomenon**

(Congenital coronary fistulas and anomalous origin of the left coronary artery from the pulmonary artery)

pectoris." Prinzmetal noted that this form of angina appeared to occur at rest or during ordinary activity and was not brought on by exercise, eating, or emotional stress. The pain was in the same location as classic angina, although the duration was usually longer and the pain was more severe. Attacks often occurred at the same time each day or night, and the waxing and waning of the pain were of equal duration. Nitroglycerin promptly relieved the pain of variant angina but, unlike the situation in classic angina, the electrocardiogram often showed ST-segment elevation similar to that in patients with acute myocardial infarction (Fig. 54–113). The ST-segment elevations usually were related to the distribution of one

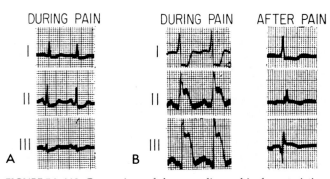

**FIGURE 54–113.** Comparison of electrocardiographic characteristics of classic angina pectoris and the variant form. *A,* Classic angina pectoris: ST segments show depression without reciprocal ST elevation. Electrocardiogram obtained after exercise. *B,* Variant form of angina pectoris: During spontaneous pain, ST segments show elevation in leads II and III with reciprocal ST depression in lead I. Immediately after pain, the electrocardiogram returns to normal or to prepain pattern. (*A* and *B,* From Prinzmetal, M., Kennamer, R., Merliss, R., et al.: Angina pectoris. I: A variant form of angina pectoris. Am. J. Med., 27:375, 1959.)

large coronary artery. Testing of these patients showed that exercise could cause ST-segment depression but did not cause pain unless the patient also had angina secondary to fixed obstructive disease. Dysrhythmias were common during the pain of variant angina, and transient Q waves were occasionally observed. Prinzmetal observed that infarction occurred in some patients weeks or months later in areas of previous ST-segment elevation. Finally, Prinzmetal noted that the pain of variant angina was often relieved by myocardial infarction, whereas the pain of stable angina often increased after myocardial infarction. These observations are still the classic clinical criteria for establishing a diagnosis of variant angina.

Prinzmetal also noted that "it is not uncommon for both the variant and classic forms of angina pectoris to occur together in the same patient." This clinically significant observation is discussed in detail later. It has been well documented that coronary artery spasm is most common in patients with concomitant atherosclerotic coronary artery disease, but a number of patients have variant angina and coronary arteries that appear to be normal on arteriography. This subgroup of patients with "normal coronary arteries" and variant angina have been described as patients with a "variant of the variant" anginal syndrome of Prinzmetal (Cheng et al., 1973; Guazzi et al., 1976).

Finally, in his classic manuscript, Prinzmetal postulated that "temporary increased tonus of a large coronary artery is suggested as the cause of pain in the variant form of angina." Arteriographic evidence of coronary artery spasm during an attack of Prinzmetal's variant angina was shown by Oliva and associates in 1973 (Fig. 54–114).

Since Prinzmetal's initial observations and the demonstration of coronary artery spasm in patients with variant angina by Oliva and associates, various other syndromes have been recognized in which coronary artery spasm causes the clinical manifestations or at least contributes to the clinical course of events. These syndromes are discussed later.

## Diagnosis and Incidence

It is accepted that coronary artery spasm may occur in both normal and diseased coronary arteries, but, until the late 1970s, spasm was considered a rare phenomenon. The clinical significance of coronary artery spasm has been under-rated by some because of its rarity during selective coronary arteriography (0.26 to 0.93%) and the frequent absence of associated symptoms when spasm is documented (Demany et al., 1968; Lavine et al., 1973; O'Reilly et al., 1970). Chahine and associates (1975) reviewed 274 consecutive coronary angiograms obtained during a 1-year period and documented eight cases of spasm (3%). This incidence, which was higher than that reported earlier, was attributed to a systematic prospective search for the phenomenon and avoidance of vasodilators and premedication before arteriography. Although many cases of arteriographically demon-strated spasm are related to catheter-tip irritation, Chahine suggested that catheter-induced spasm may occur only in patients with a predisposition to spasm. Spasm often is not specifically looked for because most patients with spasm also have fixed obstructive coronary lesions, which are thought to explain their symptoms.

Clinically, it is often difficult to obtain an electrocardiogram during an episode of spontaneous chest pain because attacks may be infrequent and often occur during sleep. Numerous provocation tests have been studied such as ergonovine infusion. Ergonovine is an ergot alkaloid and smooth muscle constrictor. Conti and associates (1979), Oliva (1979), and Waters and associates (1986) observed that ergonovine produces spasm in nearly all patients with Prinzmetal's angina and has diagnostic value if carefully administered during cardiac catheterization. However, deaths after ergonovine administration have been reported, and this test is not universally accepted (Buxton et al., 1980). Yasue and associates (1986) reported that intracoronary injection of acetylcholine can provoke coronary spasm in susceptible arteries and may be safer than ergonovine infusion.

Most recently, inducement of transient systemic alkalosis (arterial pH > 7.65) by a combination of hyperventilation and infusion of an alkaline solution has been used as a provocative test for coronary spasm. Weber and associates (1988) used this technique in 237 patients with infrequent angina at rest. Infusion of alkaline solution followed by hyperventilation increased arterial pH above the 7.65 value necessary for diagnostic significance in 196 (83%) patients. Twenty-four patients (12%) had significant ST-segment changes. Chest pain and ECG changes were reversed within 5 minutes in all patients by intravenous nitroglycerin. Coronary arteriography was performed in 36 patients with a negative response, and 33 (92%) had normal arteriograms and a negative response to ergonovine infusion. This technique appears to be a safe and specific diagnostic procedure that may gain increased use in the future to identify patients with coronary spasm.

When spasm is looked for, the incidence appears to increase dramatically. Maseri and associates (1978b) reported that the incidence of variant angina in their experience increased from 2% to more than 10% of patients admitted for evaluation of anginal pain when systematic measures were used for its detection. These authors proposed that variant angina is only one manifestation of coronary artery spasm and that spasm contributes to practically all phases of ischemic heart disease.

Although the true incidence of variant angina is unknown, coronary artery spasm may be more common than was previously assumed and may contribute to the clinical manifestations of various syndromes besides variant angina.

## Natural History

Myocardial infarction and death from infarction or ventricular arrhythmias are common in patients with

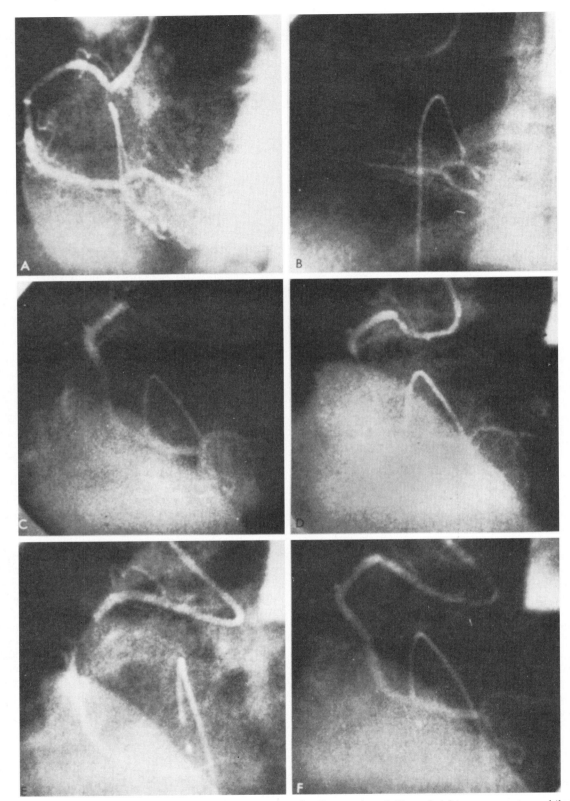

**FIGURE 54–114.** Documentation of coronary spasm during episodes of variant angina. *A,* Normal right coronary artery while the patient was pain-free, without electrocardiographic changes. *B,* During a spontaneous attack of angina, with electrocardiographic changes and spasm of a long segment of the midportion of the right coronary artery. *C,* During an injection while the patient was pain-free, showing a normal vessel (spasm could not be induced by the catheter or the contrast medium). *D,* Spasm of a long segment extending into the distal right coronary artery and posterior descending artery during the next attack of pain. *E,* During a subsequent but separate attack of angina, when a segmental area of spasm is noted. *F,* Within 2 minutes the angina subsided, and the vessel appeared normal.

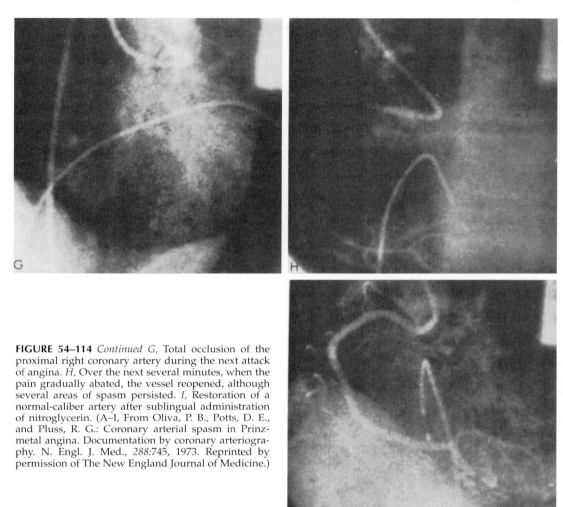

FIGURE 54–114 *Continued G,* Total occlusion of the proximal right coronary artery during the next attack of angina. *H,* Over the next several minutes, when the pain gradually abated, the vessel reopened, although several areas of spasm persisted. *I,* Restoration of a normal-caliber artery after sublingual administration of nitroglycerin. (A–I, From Oliva, P. B., Potts, D. E., and Pluss, R. G.: Coronary arterial spasm in Prinzmetal angina. Documentation by coronary arteriography. N. Engl. J. Med., *288:*745, 1973. Reprinted by permission of The New England Journal of Medicine.)

documented but untreated variant angina. Bentivoglio and associates (1974) viewed 90 patients reported between 1959 and 1972 for whom long-term follow-up data were available. As pointed out by Raizner and Chahine (1980), this group of patients is most representative of the natural history of variant angina because, in 1972, the pathophysiology of the syndrome was not fully appreciated, and appropriate therapy was not in widespread use. Of these 90 patients, 22 (24%) developed acute myocardial infarction within several months after the onset of variant angina, and 13 patients (14%) died suddenly. Catastrophic events, therefore, occurred in 38% of the group, usually soon after onset of symptoms. Stenson and associates (1975) observed that variant angina first seen after acute myocardial infarction has an even higher mortality rate (33%). Although the incidence of myocardial infarction and death in patients with variant angina has decreased with more aggressive medical therapy, patients with Prinzmetal's angina should be considered a high-risk subgroup of patients with ischemic heart disease. Infarction or death of patients with variant angina usually occurs soon after symptoms or electrocardiographic changes. In survivors, long phases of complete remission are common (Cipriano et al., 1981; Madias, 1986; Rothman and Khan, 1991; Severi et al., 1980).

Approximately half of the patients with variant angina experience spontaneous remission, which most commonly occurs in the first 6 to 12 months after the onset of symptoms (Rothman and Khan, 1991). As a rule, patients with variant angina and concomitant significant coronary artery disease are at greater risk than the less common group of patients with variant angina and normal coronary arteries (Madias, 1986; Rothman and Khan, 1991; Selzer et al., 1976).

## OTHER SYNDROMES ASSOCIATED WITH CORONARY ARTERY SPASM

In addition to Prinzmetal's variant angina, coronary artery spasm may contribute to the clinical manifestations observed in various ischemic heart disease syndromes (Table 54–14).

■ **Table 54–14.** SYNDROMES ASSOCIATED WITH CORONARY ARTERY SPASM

---

Prinzmetal's angina
"Silent" variant angina
Partial coronary artery spasm mimicking stable angina
Stable angina and coronary artery spasm
Preinfarction angina
Acute myocardial infarction
Sudden death
Nitrate withdrawal
Perioperative arrest after myocardial revascularization
Other vasospastic disorders
    Raynaud's phenomenon
    Migraine headaches
    Peripheral venous spasm

---

**"Silent" Variant Angina.** Since Prinzmetal's original description of variant angina in 1959, a number of patients have been reported who have ST-segment elevation and documented coronary artery spasm without chest pain (Bodenheimer et al., 1974; Gorfinkel et al., 1973; Guazzi et al., 1970; Lasser and de la Paz, 1973; Maseri, 1987; Prohkov et al., 1974). Clinically, these patients are difficult to identify, because their symptoms are often vague and not directly referable to the heart or they present with a catastrophic event such as acute myocardial infarction or life-threatening arrhythmia. This subgroup of patients with variant angina were said to have "silent" variant angina (Prohkov et al., 1974) because they have all of the hallmarks of Prinzmetal's angina with the important exception that there is no accompanying chest pain.

**Partial Spasm Mimicking Stable Angina.** ST-segment elevation, chest pain, and documented coronary artery spasm are the classic clinical criteria for a diagnosis of Prinzmetal's angina. Maseri and associates (1975) reported two patients, and Chahine and associates (1975) reported a third patient with documented partial coronary artery spasm who had pain both at rest and with exercise. Compared with Prinzmetal's angina, the episodes of pain were associated with ST-segment depression that mimicked the usual electrocardiographic findings in classic angina secondary to fixed obstructive atherosclerotic coronary disease. Because most patients with coronary artery spasm have concomitant atherosclerotic disease, the importance of spasm in explaining a patient's clinical course is perhaps often overlooked.

**Coronary Artery Spasm and Stable Angina.** Numerous patients with variant angina at rest have classic effort-induced angina with characteristic ST-segment depression in the same leads that demonstrated ST-segment elevation at rest (Maseri et al., 1977). Advances in the medical treatment of coronary artery spasm make identification of these patients important so that appropriate treatment can be instituted to maximize control of the most important contributor to the chest pain syndrome. As discussed later, beta-blockers can exacerbate spasm in some patients and may be contraindicated in patients with both fixed obstructive disease and vasospastic disease in which spasm is the predominant feature.

**Coronary Artery Spasm Causing Preinfarction Angina.** Patients with Prinzmetal's angina can develop a worsening pain syndrome and can have subsequent myocardial infarction. Distinct from this group are patients with long-standing stable angina or with recent onset of angina who have definite severe atherosclerotic coronary disease and later develop an accelerating pain syndrome that leads to infarction unless medical or surgical therapy is given. Several patients who have stable, fixed obstructive disease, by serial coronary angiograms, progress to preinfarction angina. Linhart and associates (1972) and Bolooki and associates (1972) reported patients with atherosclerotic coronary artery disease and preinfarction angina who had ST-segment elevation with episodes of pain without evidence of subsequent myocardial infarction. These findings suggest that the addition of spasm to long-standing fixed obstructive disease caused preinfarction angina. The patients in both reports were managed successfully by coronary artery bypass grafting. These observations do not implicate spasm in all cases of preinfarction angina but suggest that in some patients, the addition of spasm to fixed obstructive disease can explain the transition from stable to unstable or preinfarction angina.

**Coronary Artery Spasm Causing Acute Myocardial Infarction.** It is well documented that coronary artery spasm can cause acute myocardial infarction in patients with variant angina and normal coronary arteries (Johnson and Detwiler, 1977; King et al., 1973) as well as in patients without antecedent signs or symptoms of variant angina who have atherosclerotically diseased vessels (Oliva and Breckinridge, 1977). In a study reported by Oliva and Breckinridge in 1977, 15 patients who presented with acute myocardial infarction underwent coronary arteriography within 6 hours after the onset of infarction. Coronary angiograms were obtained before and after administration of nitroglycerin. Six of the patients (40%) had coronary artery spasm superimposed on a high-grade atherosclerotic lesion. The involved coronary artery remained patent after the initial relief of spasm in two patients who were maintained on sublingual nitrates and heparin. The authors concluded that their results show the occurrence of spasm in significant numbers of patients with acute myocardial infarction, but do not establish the importance of spasm in the pathophysiology of acute myocardial infarction, or whether relief of spasm has a beneficial or harmful effect on myocardium rendered ischemic for a prolonged period before reperfusion. This important study emphasizes the need for further investigations of the role of spasm in patients with acute myocardial infarction because of the possible therapeutic implications.

There are conflicting recent reports regarding the possible role of coronary spasm in the subsequent development of atherosclerotic coronary obstruction. Nobuyoshi and associates (1991) performed serial coronary arteriograms with concomitant ergonovine infusion and found a strong association between areas of spasm and subsequent development of fixed obstructive disease. However, Kaski and associates (1992) found that stenosis progression was not frequently observed at spastic sites despite the recurrence of focal coronary spasm over long periods.

**Coronary Artery Spasm After Acute Myocardial Infarction.** Stenson and associates (1975) identified an interesting group of 9 patients of a total of 57 patients who presented with acute myocardial infarction during a 1-year period. These 9 patients (16%) had episodes of angina more than 24 hours after initial infarction associated with transient ST-segment elevation. Seven of these patients (78%) had a second myocardial infarction within 2 weeks to 4½ months after their first infarction. Three of the 9 patients died after reinfarction, an overall mortality rate of 33%. All of these patients had severe atherosclerotic coronary artery disease in addition to clinical evidence for coronary artery spasm. None had symptoms of variant angina before their first infarction. Thus, spasm became manifest in these patients after infarction and appears to have greatly increased subsequent morbidity and mortality.

**Coronary Artery Spasm Causing Sudden Death.** Many patients who die suddenly have normal coronary arteries at postmortem examination. Presumably, they died of an arrhythmia of uncertain etiology or died secondary to vasospasm and severe ischemia or vasospasm that initiated an arrhythmia. Cheng and associates (1973) described four patients with variant angina and normal coronary arteries at the time of catheterization. Because Prinzmetal originally postulated that spasm was most likely to be associated with atherosclerotic lesions, Cheng suggested that spasm in normal coronary arteries was a variant of Prinzmetal's angina and coined the term "a variant of the variant" angina to describe the condition. When one of these patients, a 60-year-old man with angina associated with ST-segment elevation, underwent coronary arteriography, no atherosclerotic disease was revealed. The patient later developed ventricular fibrillation and died. Postmortem examination confirmed that he had completely normal coronary arteries and strongly implicated coronary artery spasm as the cause of sudden death.

In further support of coronary artery spasm as the underlying mechanism in certain cases of sudden death are numerous reports of ventricular fibrillation in patients with documented coronary artery spasm (Fellows et al., 1987; Myerburg et al., 1992). Prohkov and associates (1974) reported a patient who presented with ventricular fibrillation. The patient was successfully resuscitated, and coronary arteriography showed total spasm of the right coronary artery, which resolved after sublingual administration of nitroglycerin. Because the patient's coronary arteries were free of atherosclerotic lesions and before ventricular fibrillation the patient had no symptoms of angina, the authors described this as "silent" variant angina and suggested that coronary artery spasm should be considered a cause of sudden death syn-

drome. Cipriano and associates (1981) reported the clinical course of 25 patients with coronary artery spasm documented by arteriography. Ventricular tachycardia occurred in 7 patients (28%) and led to death in 1 patient. Four of the 7 patients had absent or minimal atherosclerotic coronary disease, and 3 had severe atherosclerotic disease in addition to spasm. Waters and associates (1982) reported that myocardial infarction can occur in the absence of severe fixed lesions and despite apparent clinical improvement with administration of calcium channel blockers. MacAlpin (1993) reviewed 81 patients with variant angina to determine which clinical features were associated with the greatest risk of angina-linked cardiac arrest (13 patients) or sudden unexpected death (9 patients). The risk of occurrence of one of these events was tripled by the presence of either a history of angina-linked syncope or a serious arrhythmia complicating attacks of coronary spasm. Unexpectedly, the risk was increased 1.5-fold in patients with absence of concomitant high-grade fixed coronary obstruction. Collectively, these reports show that spasm in both normal and diseased coronary arteries can produce life-threatening arrhythmias and the sudden death syndrome.

**Coronary Artery Spasm and the Nitrate Withdrawal Syndrome.** Lange and associates (1972) described clinical, angiographic, and hemodynamic findings for nine patients who presented with nonatheromatous ischemic heart disease induced by chronic industrial exposure to nitroglycerin and subsequent withdrawal. This group accounted for almost 5% of a group of 200 workers who had similar exposure. Five of these patients had coronary arteriography, which showed reversible spasm with no atherosclerotic coronary artery disease. Two patients died suddenly, most likely secondary to reflex coronary artery spasm after nitrate withdrawal. The authors suggested that long-term exposure to nitroglycerin produced chronic vasodilatation, which evoked a homeostatic vasoconstrictive response that in turn produced severe spasm and ischemia after nitrate withdrawal.

**Coronary Artery Spasm Causing Perioperative Arrest.** Pichard and associates (1980) reported a patient who had both angina at rest and effort-induced angina. Before the angina became worse, the patient had an 8-year history of stable angina. Exercise testing showed ST-segment elevation in lead AVL and leads $V_2$ to $V_4$ in addition to a short run of ventricular tachycardia. Cardiac catheterization showed 70% obstruction of the right coronary artery in its proximal third, with 90% obstruction in the left anterior descending artery proximal to the first septal perforator and 50% obstruction at the origin of a posterolateral circumflex branch. The left main coronary artery was normal, and the ejection fraction was 90%. Because of his severe obstructive disease and increased angina, the patient had uncomplicated internal mammary-to–left anterior descending coronary artery grafting and saphenous vein bypass grafting to the right coronary and posterolateral circumflex coronary arteries. He was easily separated from cardiopulmonary bypass in normal sinus rhythm and showed evidence of good left ventricular contractility. However, as the chest was being closed, the patient developed rapid atrial fibrillation followed by ventricular arrhythmias and hypotension. He required multiple countershocks and reinstitution of cardiopulmonary bypass support.

The patient was eventually stabilized and again weaned from bypass uneventfully and moved to the intensive care unit. Two hours later, he again became hypotensive, with increased left atrial pressures and associated ST-segment elevations on monitor leads. These changes progressed to rapid atrial fibrillation and recurrent ventricular tachycardia, which degenerated to ventricular fibrillation refractory to external countershock and intravenous lidocaine and procainamide. The chest was reopened; there was no evidence of tamponade, and all three grafts were patent. With the patient was stabilized again and the chest was closed, only to be reopened again 40 minutes later for resuscitation because of another episode of refractory ventricular fibrillation. The patient remained refractory to all resuscitative agents until papaverine (1 mg) was injected into each graft and nitrol paste (2%) was applied to the skin, after which he had successful cardioversion. An intra-aortic balloon pump was inserted, and the patient subsequently recovered uneventfully. Serial postoperative electrocardiograms showed no evidence of postoperative myocardial infarction. Thirteen days postoperatively, repeat cardiac catheterization showed that all three grafts were patent. The native coronary circulation and ejection fraction were unchanged from findings before operation. When the internal mammary artery graft was injected with contrast medium, the patient developed ST-segment elevation without chest pain or arrhythmias. Repeat internal mammary artery visualization showed severe, diffuse spasm of the entire left anterior descending coronary artery, which resolved after administration of nitroglycerin. The patient was subsequently maintained on nitroglycerin and aspirin without further problems and returned to work 6 weeks after operation.

Retrospectively, it appears that this patient had fixed obstructive disease and manifested spasm when his angina increased. Spasm persisted perioperatively and produced the course of clinical events reported. Based on these observations, the authors suggest that coronary artery spasm be considered strongly in the differential diagnosis of perioperative hemodynamic deterioration in patients after coronary artery bypass graft surgery, especially in the presence of ST-segment elevation or intractable ventricular arrhythmias. Buxton and associates (1981) reported six patients who had similar problems immediately after myocardial revascularization.

Perioperative spasm also can involve arterial conduits used for revascularization, such as the internal mammary artery (Gurley et al., 1990; He, 1993; Zaiac et al., 1990) and the gastroepiploic artery (Mills and Everson, 1989; Suma, 1990), as well as saphenous vein grafts (Blanche and Chaux, 1988). These reports suggest that coronary artery spasm and conduit

spasm after coronary artery bypass grafting may be more than a rare phenomenon. Lemmer and Kirsh (1988) reviewed in detail published reports of postoperative coronary spasm and identified important predisposing factors, which are discussed later.

**Coronary Artery Spasm Associated with Other Vasospastic Disorders.** There is some evidence, although not conclusive, that coronary artery spasm is more common in patients with other vasospastic diseases such as Raynaud's phenomenon, progressive systemic sclerosis, peripheral venous spasm, and migraine headaches. Robertson and Oates (1978) described three patients with both variant angina and Raynaud's phenomenon. One patient had continuous electrocardiographic monitoring for 26 days, and 569 episodes of ST-segment elevation occurred without chest pain ("silent" variant angina). None of these patients had chest pain simultaneous with attacks of Raynaud's phenomenon, and although a cool environment could trigger signs of Raynaud's phenomenon, it was unrelated to episodes of variant angina. Spasm in normal coronary arteries that causes myocardial infarction and sudden death has been associated with progressive systemic sclerosis in patients who previously had Raynaud's phenomenon (Bulkley et al., 1978). Miller and associates (1981) studied 62 patients with variant angina and noted a statistically increased incidence of both Raynaud's phenomenon and migraine headaches, compared with patients who had atherosclerotic coronary disease without signs or symptoms of variant angina. This study did not show that the prevalence of Raynaud's phenomenon in women with variant angina was statistically higher than that in men with variant angina, although Raynaud's phenomenon is 5 times more common in women than in men (Coffman and Cohen, 1981).

Dagenais and associates (1970) described a 15-year-old female with tetralogy of Fallot with severe peripheral venous spasm observed during cardiac catheterization. In association with venous spasm, the patient developed simultaneous chest pain and ST-segment elevation, which resolved at the same time that the venous spasm resolved.

Because Raynaud's phenomenon, migraine headaches, and peripheral venous spasm sometimes appear to be triggered by emotional stress, some suggested that investigations into the etiology of variant angina include the possibility of a central neurogenic trigger mechanism (Coffman and Cohen, 1981).

## PATHOPHYSIOLOGY OF CORONARY ARTERY SPASM

Spasm can occur in both normal and atherosclerotically diseased coronary arteries, and it is an important component in various ischemic heart disease syndromes other than Prinzmetal's variant angina. Furthermore, spasm can completely or partially occlude a coronary artery, involve one or more vessels, and be diffuse or segmental (Conti et al., 1979). Cannon and Epstein (1988) described patients with angiographically normal coronary arteries who had increased sensitivity to vasoconstrictor stimuli only within coronary arterioles. They called this syndrome "microvascular angina" and found that symptoms were improved by calcium antagonists. Despite the wealth of clinical information about Prinzmetal's angina and the apparently ubiquitous nature of spasm in other coronary syndromes, little is known about the exact pathogenesis of coronary spasm.

Two general areas of investigation appear promising: one involves the study of neurogenic mechanisms, and the other involves humoral and metabolic factors that affect vascular smooth muscle tone. A number of clinical studies and studies of animals can be cited to show that either of these possibilities is important in the pathogenesis of coronary spasm. It may eventually be shown that both mechanisms are interrelated or that either can be important in specific groups of patients with spasm.

## Neurogenic Mechanisms

Considerable evidence suggests that neurogenic stimulation that originates centrally or via the autonomic nervous system is important in the etiology of coronary artery spasm.

**Central Nervous System.** As discussed earlier, there may be an increased incidence of variant angina in patients with generalized vasospastic disorders such as Raynaud's phenomenon, progressive systemic sclerosis, peripheral venous spasm, and migraine headaches. Because these disorders can be triggered by emotional stress, it has been suggested that variant angina may also be initiated by perceived stress (Coffman and Cohen, 1981). Melville and associates (1969) showed that severe coronary constriction can result from electrical stimulation of the central nervous system in monkeys. Also, reports have described patients with subarachnoid hemorrhage who had transient and repeated episodes of ST-segment elevation with reciprocal ST-segment depression, presumably secondary to coronary artery spasm (Goldman et al., 1975; Toyama et al., 1979; Yuki et al., 1991). However, Cipriano and associates (1979) showed that ergonovine can cause coronary artery spasm in susceptible, totally denervated, transplanted human hearts, which suggests that the final trigger mechanism is within intramyocardial autonomic receptors or that a humoral trigger mechanism is of primary importance.

**Autonomic Nervous System**

*Sympathetic Influences.* A network of autonomic nerve fibers that supply coronary arteries is demonstrated by electron microscopic and histochemical studies. Both parasympathetic and sympathetic components of the autonomic nervous system have been implicated in coronary artery spasm.

Sympathetic nerves in large numbers connect with the smooth muscle cells of coronary arteries. Beta-adrenergic stimulation produces coronary arterial dilatation by both direct and indirect mechanisms. Stimulation of smooth muscle beta$_2$-receptors directly dilates coronary arteries. Stimulation of beta$_1$-recep-

tors creates metabolically mediated dilatation due to an increase in heart rate and contractility. Alpha-sympathetic receptor stimulation causes coronary arterial constriction. The balance between alpha and beta$_1$-beta$_2$ sympathetic discharge is thought to account for a component of normal coronary arteriolar resistance or "tone." Kelley and Feigl (1978) showed in dogs that alpha-receptor–induced coronary constriction can be produced by pretreatment with propranolol to block beta-vasodilatory sympathetic responses, followed by intracoronary injection of norepinephrine and simultaneous electrical stimulation of the left stellate ganglion. The increase in large vessel resistance was approximately 60% of the total observed for the entire coronary bed, which suggests that sympathetically mediated coronary vasoconstriction affects distal small vessels, not just large epicardial vessels.

Ricci and associates (1979) showed that coronary artery spasm in eight patients was rapidly reversed by intravenous administration of the alpha-adrenergic blocker phentolamine. In four additional patients with recurrent episodes of coronary spasm, oral administration of the alpha-adrenergic blocker phenoxybenzamine prevented symptoms of spasm during 1 year of follow-up. Also, some patients with vasospastic angina have had attacks triggered by exposure to a cold environment, and it has been suggested that the stress of cold exposure activates alpha-sympathetic discharge that causes coronary artery spasm. To test this hypothesis, Mudge and associates (1976) exposed susceptible patients to cold after intravenous administration of the alpha-adrenergic blocker phentolamine. The results showed that coronary vasoconstriction could be prevented in this group by pretreatment with phentolamine.

It has not been possible to document increased alpha-sympathetic tone in patients susceptible to spasm. Robertson and associates (1979) found normal levels of urinary and plasma catecholamines and metabolite levels of catecholamines in three patients with coronary artery spasm. They obtained blood samples from two patients at the onset and termination of spontaneous episodes of ST-segment elevation and found no significant changes in catecholamine levels. There was no evidence for a generalized increase in sympathetic discharge in patients during episodes of coronary artery spasm. These data, however, do not exclude the possibility that alpha-beta$_1$, beta$_2$ sympathetic imbalance is operative in patients with coronary artery spasm.

*Parasympathetic Influences.* Compared with the dense network of sympathetic fibers that supply coronary arteries, parasympathetic fibers are found in much smaller numbers in the heart (Hillis and Braunwald, 1978). There is evidence that increased activity of the parasympathetic system can trigger spasm. The fact that patients with variant angina usually have attacks of coronary artery spasm at rest supports this theory, because parasympathetic activity is maximal at rest and is suppressed during exercise.

Both sympathetic and parasympathetic fibers are found in parasympathetic vagal ganglia that innervate the heart. Stimulation of the vagus (para-sympathetic) nerve or intracoronary injection of its neurotransmitter, acetylcholine, creates coronary vasodilatation (Berne et al., 1965; Blesa and Ross, 1970; Blumenthal et al., 1968; Feigl, 1969; Hackett et al., 1972; Levy and Zieske, 1969). However, besides causing direct vasodilatation, acetylcholine appears to release norepinephrine from postganglionic sympathetic nerve endings in the heart (Blumenthal, 1968; Burn, 1967; Cabrera et al., 1966; Dempsey and Cooper, 1969; Levy, 1971). Normally, coronary blood flow is regulated primarily by metabolic requirements of the heart (an increase in myocardial oxygen consumption causes coronary vasodilatation), and neurogenic control is less important. Excess parasympathetic activity decreases heart rate, blood pressure, and myocardial contractility, all of which reduce myocardial oxygen consumption and thus eliminate metabolic factors that normally control coronary vascular tone.

Yasue and associates (1974) and Endo and associates (1976) postulated that increased parasympathetic activity stimulates alpha-sympathetic nerves in parasympathetic ganglia, which can cause severe coronary artery spasm under resting conditions. Yasue and associates (1974), in a study of 10 patients with Prinzmetal's angina, found that administration of the parasympathomimetic drug methacholine could induce spasm, and that the parasympathetic blocker atropine could prevent attacks of spasm. Epinephrine provoked attacks of spasm in some patients if resting parasympathetic tone appeared to be increased but had little effect if resting parasympathetic tone was normal. Administration of the beta-adrenergic blocker propranolol could not prevent attacks, but administration of the alpha-adrenergic blocker phenoxybenzamine could prevent spasm. The authors concluded that parasympathetic activity may be excessive in patients who are prone to coronary artery spasm, that increased parasympathetic activity selectively stimulates alpha-sympathetic fibers in parasympathetic ganglia, and that alpha-adrenergic stimulation is the final common pathway to coronary artery spasm. This work is supported by the observation that attacks of variant angina usually occur in patients at rest when baseline parasympathetic tone is increased. Further support for this theory was provided by Nowlin and associates (1965) and Murao and associates (1972), who reported that attacks of variant angina in susceptible individuals are associated with the rapid eye movement (REM) period of sleep. REM sleep is triggered by acetylcholine, which indicates increased parasympathetic activity, and is suppressed by atropine, which blocks acetylcholine release. Yasue and associates (1986) reported that intracoronary injection of acetylcholine produced coronary spasm in patients with variant angina.

Recently, power spectral analysis of heart rate variability has been used as a noninvasive means to determine the level of autonomic nervous activity. The power spectrum has two main components: a low-frequency component (0.04 to 0.12 Hz), which is an index of sympathetic activity with vagal modulation,

and a high-frequency component (0.22 to 0.32 Hz), which is a specific index of parasympathetic activity. Yoshio and associates (1993) used Holter monitoring and spectral analysis of heart rate variability to assess the role of the autonomic nervous system in the development of nocturnal angina in seven patients with nocturnal variant angina. Parasympathetic activity increased 10 minutes before attacks of spasm, whereas sympathetic activity with vagal modulation increased 5 minutes before attacks.

The studies described suggest that parasympathetic-sympathetic imbalance in the autonomic nervous system of patients with coronary artery spasm may be an important trigger mechanism (Fig. 54–115). Whether higher-level central nervous system input is related to this imbalance is unknown. The only evidence against neurogenic mechanisms is the fact that denervated hearts susceptible to spasm can still be provoked to show coronary artery spasm by administration of agents such as ergonovine (Clark et al., 1977). However, ergonovine appears to work by stimulation of alpha-receptors in coronary arteries; thus, this evidence does not disprove the theories that postulate that the final pathway in the initiation of coronary artery spasm involves alpha-receptor activity in coronary arteries.

## Humoral-Metabolic Mechanisms

**Platelet-Prostaglandin–Vessel Wall Interactions.** The role of prostaglandins in initiating and mediating various physiologic responses is under intense investigation. It has been suggested that platelet-prostaglandin and coronary vessel wall interactions are important in the pathophysiology of myocardial is-

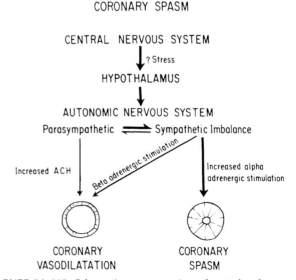

**FIGURE 54–115.** Schematic representation of postulated parasympathetic-sympathetic imbalances leading to increased alpha-sympathetic activity and coronary spasm. *Heavy arrows* indicate direction of the imbalance.

chemia. It is generally accepted that platelet aggregation on atherosclerotic plaques can initiate thrombosis, and there is evidence that platelets also may be involved in the initiation of coronary artery spasm.

Platelets release thromboxane $A_2$ as they aggregate. Thromboxane $A_2$ is a powerful endogenous vasoconstrictor as well as a stimulator for further platelet aggregation. Within vessel walls a prostaglandin, prostacyclin ($PGI_2$), is normally synthesized, which has biologic actions that directly oppose those of thromboxane $A_2$. Specifically, $PGI_2$ causes vasodilatation and inhibits platelet aggregation (Bunting et al., 1976; Dusting et al., 1978). It has been suggested that the balance between $PGI_2$ release and thromboxane release contributes to normal coronary vascular tone and the stimulation or inhibition of platelet aggregation (Boullin et al., 1979; Dusting et al., 1978; Moncada et al., 1977). This balance may be disrupted in coronary artery disease. Studies in both humans and animals showed that atherosclerotic coronary arteries have a decreased ability to synthesize prostacyclin (D'Angelo et al., 1978; Dembinska-Kiec et al., 1977). Furthermore, platelets from patients who survive acute myocardial infarction synthesize increased quantities of thromboxane $A_2$ (Szczeklik et al., 1978). These studies suggest that in coronary artery disease, an imbalance between prostacyclin release and thromboxane release favors vasoconstriction and platelet aggregation. Increased thromboxane release can cause vasoconstriction but has not been proved to cause coronary artery spasm. However, Lewy and associates (1979) and Tada and associates (1981) reported increased levels of thromboxane $B_2$, the major metabolite of thromboxane $A_2$, in patients with Prinzmetal's angina. Whether thromboxane release initiated spasm or was secondary to spasm and platelet aggregation is unknown.

Synthesis of both thromboxane and prostacyclin begins with arachidonic acid, a free fatty acid. The metabolism of arachidonic acid and the possible relationship between platelets, prostaglandins, and vessel walls in initiating coronary artery spasm are shown schematically in Figure 54–116.

As described earlier, variant angina frequently occurs during the REM phase of sleep or very early in the morning, which is a period of transition from parasympathetic to sympathetic predominance. Acetylcholine induces dilatation of the aorta and other arteries via muscarinic receptors of medial smooth muscle cells. Once endothelial cells are injured or denuded, arteries cannot be dilated even by acetylcholine because of reduced nitric oxide production (Sakurai, 1991). Therefore, injury or loss of endothelial cells may play a major role in the pathogenesis of coronary spasm. This hypothesis fits well with the clinical observation that most patients with coronary spasm are usually beyond middle age, and many of them have various degrees of coronary atherosclerotic changes that may affect endothelial cell function even without coronary luminal obstruction (Sakurai, 1991). Shirai and associates (1993) found that the serum level of apolipoprotein A-I in patients with vasospastic an-

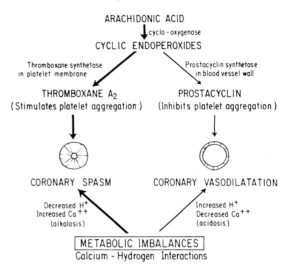

FIGURE 54–116. Schematic representation of humoral-metabolic imbalances that have been postulated to initiate coronary spasm. *Heavy arrows* indicate direction of the imbalance. (Adapted from Conti, C. R., Pepine, C., and Curry, R. C.: Coronary artery spasm: An important mechanism in the pathophysiology of ischemic heart disease. Curr. Probl. Cardiol., 4:1, 1979. Reproduced with permission.)

gina was significantly lower in patients without vasospasm. Thus, apolipoprotein A-I may play a role in preventing early endothelial injury and subsequent vasospastic angina.

**Hydrogen, Calcium, and Magnesium Ion Imbalances.** Contraction of vascular smooth muscle depends on the presence of calcium ions, which are necessary for the activation of myofibrillar ATPase (Bohr, 1973; Fleckenstein et al., 1976). Physiologically, hydrogen ions exert a potent calcium antagonist action by competition with calcium ions for transport across cell membranes as well as for binding sites at the myofibrillar level (Fleckenstein et al., 1976). Vasoconstriction can occur if calcium ion concentration increases or hydrogen ion concentration decreases. Vasodilatation is produced by decreased transmembrane calcium flux or increased hydrogen ion concentration. Yasue and associates (1978) gave nine patients with documented Prinzmetal's angina an infusion of 100 ml of TRIS buffer over 5 minutes, followed by hyperventilation for a second 5-minute period. Arterial pH increased from normal values to 7.65 with this protocol, and eight of the nine patients developed ST-segment elevation. With the onset of alkalosis and ST-segment elevation, simultaneous coronary angiograms revealed spasm. The patients were then pretreated with the calcium blocker diltiazem, and the experimental protocol was repeated. After pretreatment with diltiazem, alkalosis did not induce attacks of Prinzmetal's angina. Because hydrogen ion production decreases at rest, particularly during sleep, when metabolism slows, and the respiratory rate often increases during REM sleep, alkalosis may result. Prinzmetal's angina is more likely to occur at rest and during periods of REM sleep, and the authors suggest that hydrogen ion/calcium ion imbalances may trigger coronary artery spasm (see Fig. 54–116).

An interesting study by Goto and associates (1990) suggests that magnesium deficiency is present in many patients with variant angina. The mean serum magnesium concentrations in patients with variant angina were no different from those of control patients without coronary spasm. Magnesium retention, however, after an intravenous load of magnesium was 60 ± 5% in patients with variant angina, compared with 36 ± 3% ($p < 0.001$) in control patients. After treatment with calcium channel blockers, the 24-hour magnesium retention decreased significantly from 60 ± 6% to 34 ± 7% ($p < 0.01$). These data suggest that intracellular magnesium deficiency is present in many patients with variant angina, and that this deficiency is corrected by treatment with calcium antagonists.

## MANAGEMENT OF PATIENTS WITH CORONARY ARTERY SPASM

Coronary artery spasm appears to be an important component in various syndromes other than Prinzmetal's angina, and appropriate therapy must be carefully individualized. Most patients with coronary artery spasm also have atheromatous disease, and it is important to try to identify the relative contribution of each of these processes so that treatment can be successful. A rational approach to therapy must also take into account that over time, the clinical manifestations of ischemia may at one point be secondary to spasm and later be due to increased atherosclerotic with concomitant spasm. Appropriate therapy, therefore, involves both medical and surgical interventions (Table 54–15).

■ **Table 54–15.** THERAPY FOR CORONARY ARTERY SPASM

**Medical Therapy**

Calcium antagonists (nifedipine, verapamil, diltiazem, perhexiline maleate)
Nitrates
Nonsteroidal anti-inflammatory agents (aspirin, indomethacin, dipyridamole, sulfinpyrazone, ibuprofen)
Alpha-adrenergic blockers (phentolamine, phenoxybenzamine)
Beta-adrenergic blockers (selected patients with atherosclerotic disease and spasm)

**Surgical Therapy (Selected Patients Only)**

Coronary artery bypass grafting
Cardiac denervation

## Medical Therapy

Nitroglycerin often effectively terminates acute attacks of coronary artery spasm and should be given at the onset of symptoms. Maintenance therapy is directed toward preventing recurrent attacks of spasm by the addition of long-acting nitrates. Patients should be warned about the possible provocation of spasm by drugs such as Cafergot, an ergot alkaloid used to treat migraine headaches, and by environmental influences such as sudden exposure to cold. Some patients have developed coronary spasm after alcohol ingestion (Takizawa et al., 1984), alcohol withdrawal (Pijls and van der Werf, 1988), cigarette smoking (Caralis et al., 1992), emotional stress (Schiffer et al., 1980), extradural anesthesia (Krantz et al., 1980), biliary colic (Antonelli and Rosenfeld, 1987), hyperventilation (Hisano et al., 1984), aspirin ingestion (Miwa et al., 1983), naproxen ingestion (Cistero et al., 1992), calcium injection (Bouglanger et al., 1984), phenylephrine eyedrop administration (Alder et al., 1981), cytotoxic chemotherapy (Kleiman et al., 1987; Shachor et al., 1985), and cocaine ingestion (Ascher et al., 1988). These reports show the importance of a careful history in identifying possible "trigger events" in individual patients with variant angina. Many of the above "trigger events" are allergic reactions mediated by histamine release, which can cause coronary spasm, and this subgroup of patients has been referred to as having "allergic angina" (Kounis and Zavras, 1991).

Most patients with coronary artery spasm have concomitant atheromatous disease, and beta-adrenergic blockers have been tried with various success rates. Evidence summarized by Conti and associates (1979) suggests that beta-blockers are "effective, occasionally useful, ineffective or possibly harmful" in patients with attacks of coronary artery spasm. Theoretically, beta-blockade can initiate spasm by allowing alpha-adrenergic sympathetic activity to predominate, with subsequent vasoconstriction. However, in patients with ischemia due to fixed obstructive disease as well as intermittent spasm, beta-blockers such as propranolol may be an important adjunct to medical therapy. Therapy with beta-blockers should be initiated slowly and under careful supervision. Patients have been reported who have variant angina that does not respond to calcium channel blocking drugs but does respond to combined calcium channel and beta-blocking drugs (Bourmayan et al., 1983).

Isolated reports show that alpha-adrenergic receptor blocking agents prevent coronary artery spasm. Mudge and associates (1976) showed that administration of the alpha-adrenergic blocker phentolamine can block reflex coronary constriction caused by exposure to cold. Tzivoni and associates (1983) reported beneficial effects with the selective alpha$_1$-blocker prazosin, whereas Winniford and associates (1983) found that prazosin treatment produced no improvement in symptoms or decrease in episodes of spasm identified by Holter monitoring. To date, no large clinical trials have investigated the efficacy of various alpha-block-

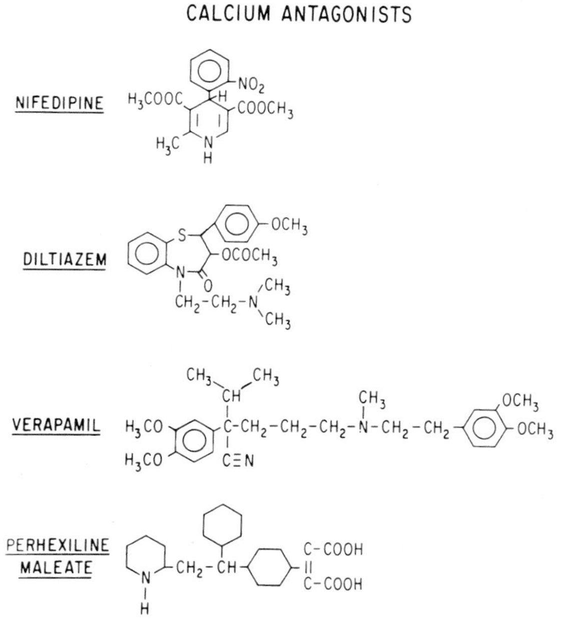

## CALCIUM ANTAGONISTS

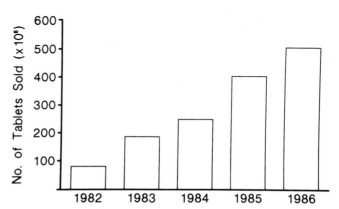

NIFEDIPINE

DILTIAZEM

VERAPAMIL

PERHEXILINE MALEATE

**FIGURE 54–117.** Structural formulas of the commonly used calcium antagonists.

ers. Because the final pathogenesis of spasm may well involve alpha-adrenergic receptors, alpha-blockers may deserve further clinical investigation in refractory patients.

Humoral theories suggest that platelet-vessel wall interactions are important in the pathogenesis of spasm, and drugs such as aspirin, indomethacin, sulfinpyrazone, dipyridamole, and ibuprofen are being investigated. These drugs are nonsteroidal anti-inflammatory agents that appear to inhibit platelet aggregation and prevent release of the potent vasoconstrictor thromboxane $A_2$ from platelet membranes. However, in some patients, coronary spasm has been induced by anti-inflammatory agents such as aspirin. Coronary arteries synthesize $PGI_2$, which causes vasodilatation, and aspirin suppresses the synthesis of prostaglandins by blocking cyclo-oxygenase. Therefore, it is postulated that in certain patients, aspirin therapy can cause vasoconstriction and coronary spasm (Miwa et al., 1983).

At present, the most effective treatment of Prinzmetal's angina and other syndromes that involve coronary artery spasm is the addition of calcium antagonists (Fig. 54–117). These agents are powerful vasodilators, and numerous clinical studies indicate impressive results in prevention of coronary artery spasm. Nitroglycerin causes vasodilatation by blocking calcium influx into smooth-muscle cells of large epicardial coronary arteries, and adenosine preferentially dilates smaller intramyocardial coronary branches, also by blockade of calcium influx (Harder et al., 1979). Calcium antagonists, including nifedipine, verapamil, diltiazem, and perhexiline maleate, appear to dilate both large epicardial and small intramural coronary arteries. It is thought that the primary beneficial effect of these agents is via their vasodila-

tory actions, but diltiazem and verapamil are also potent inhibitors of platelet aggregation (Shinjo et al., 1978).

Increasing numbers of patients are being treated with calcium blockers, and many reports have shown impressive efficacy. Endo and associates (1975) reported 35 patients with variant angina (16 with spasm and atherosclerotic disease and 19 with spasm in normal coronary arteries). Twenty-six patients were treated medically, with one death and persistence of symptoms in most patients. Addition of nifedipine to the treatment regimen of the remaining 25 patients completely relieved symptoms in each case. Antman and associates (1980) studied 127 patients with coronary spasm and found that nifedipine (40 to 160 mg/day) significantly decreased mean weekly anginal attacks from 16 to 2 ($p < .001$). Encouraging results have been reported for verapamil (Johnson et al., 1981; Severi et al., 1979), diltiazem (Feldman et al., 1979; Pepine et al., 1981; Rosenthal et al., 1980; Schroeder et al., 1982), and perhexiline maleate (Conti et al., 1979; Raabe, 1979). Kimura and Kishida (1981) found that the efficacy rates of nifedipine, diltiazem, and verapamil were 94%, 90.8%, and 85.7%, respectively, in 286 patients with variant angina. Glazier and associates (1988) have noted a dramatic decrease in the number of in-hospital patients with coronary spasm since the widespread use of calcium channel blockers began in the mid-1980s (Fig. 54–118). In addition, since the practice of using calcium channel blockers in all patients undergoing PTCA became widespread, the incidence of spasms complicating PTCA has decreased from greater than 4 to 1% (Detre et al., 1987). Rutitzky and associates (1982) reported that amiodarone is effective in the prevention of coronary spasm. However, amiodarone has many toxic side effects and should be used only in patients refractory to calcium channel antagonists. In most of these reports, calcium antagonists have proved most

**FIGURE 54–118.** The use of calcium channel blocking agents in the United States from 1982 to 1986 (data from Pharmaceutical Services reports). The widespread use of calcium channel blockers has dramatically affected survival and has decreased myocardial infarction in patients with variant angina. (From Glazier, J. J., Faxon, D. P., Melidossian, C., and Ryan, T. J.: The changing face of coronary artery spasm: A decade of experience. Am. Heart J., 116:572–576, 1988.)

■ **Table 54–16.** RESULTS OF MEDICAL TREATMENT OF PRINZMETAL'S ANGINA

| No. of Patients | Atheromatous Coronary Disease | | Asymptomatic or Improved (%) | Same or Worse (%) | Myocardial Infarction (%) | Died (%) |
|---|---|---|---|---|---|---|
| | None (%) | One or More Arteries Involved (%) | | | | |
| 275 | 22 | 78 | 47 | 47 | 23 | 6 |

Adapted from Raizner, A. E., and Chahine, R. A.: The treatment of Prinzmetal's variant angina with coronary bypass surgery. *In* Hurst, J. W. (ed): Update II: The Heart—Bypass Surgery for Obstructive Coronary Disease. Chap. 9. New York, McGraw-Hill, 1980.

efficacious when used with long-acting nitrates. The addition of calcium channel blockers to the medical therapy of coronary artery spasm has been a major contribution that has decreased subsequent morbidity and mortality (Scholl et al., 1988; Yasue et al., 1988).

## Surgical Therapy

Coronary artery bypass grafting effectively relieves angina in patients with obstructive coronary artery disease. Life is prolonged in specific subgroups such as those with left main coronary artery disease or severe three-vessel disease with impaired left ventricular function. Furthermore, numerous large series show that these benefits can be achieved with very low operative morbidity and mortality. Surgical intervention in the management of patients with coronary artery spasm is a more complex issue.

Since the initial report by Silverman and Flamm in 1971 of two patients with coronary disease and variant angina treated by bypass grafting, numerous small series have been reported with various results. Conti and associates (1979) and Raizner and Chahine (1980) reviewed the results of coronary artery bypass grafting in patients with variant angina with both normal and atherosclerotically diseased coronary arteries. As shown in Tables 54–16 to 54–19, these reviews have shown that:

1. Coronary artery bypass grafting is generally contraindicated in patients with variant angina who do not have concomitant significant atherosclerotic disease.

2. Coronary artery bypass grafting may be an important adjunct to the medical treatment of patients with variant angina and concomitant atherosclerotic disease.

Addition of calcium channel blockers to the medical treatment of variant angina may control spasm so effectively that patients with concomitant atherosclerotic disease may have bypass grafting with morbidity and mortality rates that approach those achieved in patients with obstructive disease alone (Schick et al., 1982). At present, the effect of calcium antagonist therapy on the selection of patients for bypass grafting is an unsettled issue. In general, patients with variant angina and normal coronary arteries should be treated medically, and those with significant obstructive disease and variant angina should be considered for operation only if they are refractory to medical therapy or, more ideally, if medical therapy is successful in relieving spasm but the patient remains symptomatic secondary to significant obstructive disease.

In addition to coronary bypass grafting, various other procedures have been used to prevent coronary spasm. Bertrand and associates (1981a) used extensive cardiac denervation (plexectomy) followed by coronary bypass grafting in 30 patients, with two operative deaths (6.7%). Twenty-eight patients on no medical therapy were followed for an average of 23 months, and only two patients had recurrent attacks of angina. Similar results were reported by Betriu and associates (1983) and DiPaolo and associates (1985). Cardiac denervation was also accomplished by autotransplantation (Bertrand et al., 1981b; Clark et al., 1977) with mixed results. Sussman and associates (1981) placed bypass grafts distal to areas of focal spasm followed by proximal ligation of the native coronary. Both patients were asymptomatic without anginal medication at 24 and 66 months. The authors recommend this approach only in patients who are completely refractory to calcium antagonists.

■ **Table 54–17.** RESULTS OF CORONARY BYPASS GRAFTING IN PATIENTS WITH PRINZMETAL'S ANGINA AND ATHEROSCLEROTIC CORONARY ARTERY DISEASE

| No. of Patients | Asymptomatic or Improved (%) | Same or Worse (%) | Myocardial Infarction (%) | Died (%) |
|---|---|---|---|---|
| 90 | 73 | 19 | 12 | 8 |

Adapted from Raizner, A. E., and Chahine, R. A.: The treatment of Prinzmetal's variant angina with coronary bypass surgery. *In* Hurst, J. W. (ed): Update II: The Heart—Bypass Surgery for Obstructive Coronary Disease. Chap. 9. New York, McGraw-Hill, 1980.

■ **Table 54–18.** RESULTS OF MEDICAL THERAPY IN PATIENTS WITH PRINZMETAL'S ANGINA AND "NORMAL" CORONARY ARTERIES

| No. of Patients | Asymptomatic or Improved (%) | Same or Worse (%) | Myocardial Infarction (%) | Died (%) |
|---|---|---|---|---|
| 41 | 66 | 27 | 7 | 7 |

Adapted from Raizner, A. E., and Chahine, R. A.: The treatment of Prinzmetal's variant angina with coronary bypass surgery. *In* Hurst, J. W. (ed): Update II: The Heart—Bypass Surgery for Obstructive Coronary Disease. Chap. 9. New York, McGraw-Hill, 1980.

■ **Table 54–19.** RESULTS OF CORONARY ARTERY BYPASS GRAFTING IN PATIENTS WITH PRINZMETAL'S ANGINA AND "NORMAL" CORONARY ARTERIES

| No. of Patients | Asymptomatic or Improved (%) | Same or Worse (%) | Myocardial Infarction (5) | Died (%) |
|---|---|---|---|---|
| 8 | 50 | 25 | 13 | 25 |

Adapted from Raizner, A. E., and Chahine, R. A.: The treatment of Prinzmetal's variant angina with coronary bypass surgery. *In* Hurst, J. W. (ed): Update II: The Heart—Bypass Surgery for Obstructive Coronary Disease. Chap. 9. New York, McGraw-Hill, 1980.

## Management of Coronary Artery Spasm After Coronary Artery Bypass Grafting

Although the importance of spasm in patients with atherosclerotic coronary artery disease and angina is becoming more apparent, its role is often overlooked, and spasm may first be recognized in the perioperative period. A dramatic example is the case report of Pichard and associates (1980), cited earlier. This report and that of six additional patients described by Buxton and associates (1981) show that coronary artery spasm after coronary artery bypass grafting can cause cardiac arrest. Several cardiovascular surgeons have had similar unreported experiences, and this phenomenon may be frequent enough to require further investigation. As suggested by Pichard and associates (1980), coronary artery spasm should be suspected perioperatively in the patient who has myocardial revascularization and displays ventricular arrhyth-

■ **Table 54–20.** MANAGEMENT OF EARLY POST–CORONARY ARTERY BYPASS CORONARY ARTERY SPASM

| Situation | Management Plan |
|---|---|
| Preoperative | 1. Identify patients at risk<br>2. Maintain oral calcium channel antagonists until time of operation |
| Intraoperative | 1. Inject intragraft nitroglycerin (0.2-mg increments)<br>2. Administer sublingual nifedipine (10-mg increments) or intravenous verapamil (2.5- to 5.0-mg increments)<br>3. Avoid vasoconstricting agents |
| Postoperative<br>*Patient stable* | 1. Perform cardiac catheterization<br>2. If spasm present, inject nitroglycerin (0.2-mg increments) directly into coronary artery or vein graft |
| *Patient unstable* | 1. Quickly exclude other causes of deterioration<br>2. Administer sublingual nifedipine or intravenous verapamil<br>3. If patient is severely hypotensive or arrested, perform emergency sternotomy for open cardiac massage and direct injection into vein grafts |

Reprinted with permission from The Society of Thoracic Surgeons (The Annals of Thoracic Surgery, Vol. 46, 1988, p. 108).

mias or hemodynamic instability associated with ST-segment elevation. Prompt therapy with coronary vasodilators may be life-saving.

An excellent review of coronary spasm after coronary surgery was published by Lemmer and Kirsh

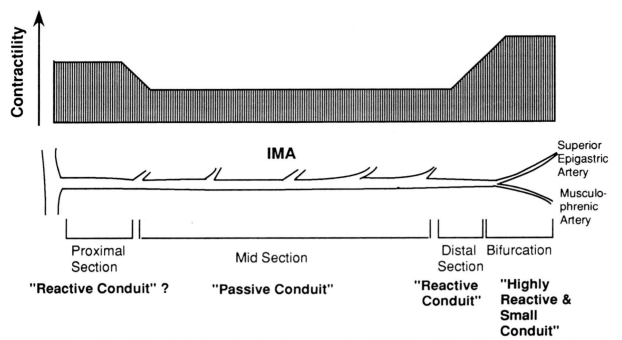

**FIGURE 54–119.** Contractility at different sites along the internal mammary artery (IMA). The middle section of the IMA is a large "passive conduit," whereas the distal section is a pharmacologically reactive conduit. The contractility increases toward the distal end of the IMA. The bifurcation is highly reactive and susceptible to spasm. (From He, G.-W.: Contractility of the human internal mammary artery at the distal section increases toward the end: Emphasis on not using the end of the internal mammary artery for grafting. J. Thorac. Cardiovasc. Surg., *106*:406–411, 1993.)

(1988). The authors found that perioperative angina at rest was an important factor in the development of postoperative native coronary spasm. Also, in 79% of patients with postoperative spasm, inferior electrocardiographic changes indicated right coronary artery involvement. The right coronary artery was angiographically free of significant obstruction and was not grafted at the time of operation. Infusion of catecholamines, especially dopamine, induced postoperative spasm. The authors emphasized that reluctance to use vasodilating agents must be overcome, even if hypotension is present, when evidence of postoperative coronary spasm is apparent. The management of perioperative coronary spasm is shown in Table 54–20.

The widespread use of the internal mammary artery for coronary artery bypass has led to many case reports of perioperative mammary artery spasm (Sarabu et al., 1987). Recent experimental studies of human internal mammary artery segments by He (1993) have convincingly shown that the distal end is highly susceptible to spasm and should be removed before bypass grafting whenever possible (Fig. 54–119).

Conti and associates (1979) and Raizner and Chahine (1980) reviewed in detail the results of medical and surgical therapy for variant angina. As shown in Tables 54–16 and 54–17, there is only a slight difference in mortality between patients with variant angina and coronary artery disease treated medically and patients treated by coronary artery bypass grafting. These groups are not directly comparable, however; as shown in Table 54–16, 22% of medically treated patients had no significant atherosclerotic coronary disease. However, symptoms appear to decrease in patients with variant angina and coronary disease who underwent successful coronary artery bypass grafting (73% asymptomatic or improved, compared with 47% asymptomatic or improved with medical therapy).

Tables 54–18 and 54–19 compare medical and surgical results in the treatment of variant angina in patients without significant coronary artery disease. These data show that coronary artery bypass grafting is contraindicated in this subgroup of patients and that medical therapy, although not ideal, is superior. If spasm can be controlled effectively by calcium antagonists, selection of patients who would benefit from coronary artery bypass grafting or possible cardiac denervation procedures may become more objective. It is hoped that these agents also will decrease the incidence of perioperative myocardial infarction as well as operative mortality secondary to the persistence of spasm.

## SELECTED BIBLIOGRAPHY

Cannon, R. O., and Epstein, S. E.: "Microvascular angina" as a cause of chest pain with angiographically normal coronary arteries. Am. J. Cardiol., 61:1338, 1988.

It has long been recognized that coronary vasospasm can occur in large epicardial coronary arteries. This clinical investigation is the first to show that some patients can develop angina secondary to an increased sensitivity to vasoconstrictor stimuli of small coronary arterioles. The authors called this vasospastic disorder microvascular angina, and they suggested that it is caused by a basic derangement of cellular calcium regulation, because this group of patients responded favorably to calcium antagonist agents.

He, G. W.: Contractility of the human internal mammary artery at the distal section increases toward the end. J. Thorac. Cardiovasc. Surg., 106:406–411, 1993.

The distal section of the internal mammary artery was collected from patients undergoing aortocoronary bypass grafting and studied in organ baths. Maximal contraction forces were determined using various vasoconstrictor agents. It was found that the contractility of the distal section of the internal mammary artery is inversely correlated to the diameter; that is, the smaller the diameter, the greater the tendency for spasm to develop. These in vitro experimental data suggest that trimming off the distal end of the internal mammary artery as much as possible may be the best way to prevent internal mammary artery graft spasm.

Kimura, E., and Kishida, H.: Treatment of variant angina with drugs: A survey of 11 cardiology institutes in Japan. Circulation, 63:844, 1981.

This clinical study summarizes data from 11 cardiology institutes in Japan to determine the effectiveness of various calcium antagonists in variant angina. There were 286 patients available for comparison. The efficacy rates of nifedipine, diltiazem, and verapamil were 94%, 90.8%, and 85.7%, respectively. Regardless of the presence or absence of organic coronary lesions, the agents were effective in 92.3% of patients with normal or almost normal coronary arteries and in 82.6% of patients with stenosis of more than 50% of the luminal diameter.

Lemmer, J. H., and Kirsh, M. M.: Coronary artery spasm following coronary artery surgery. Ann. Thorac. Surg., 46:108, 1988.

This is an excellent review of perioperative coronary artery spasm after myocardial revascularization procedures. The literature on perioperative coronary spasm is reviewed, and methods of prevention, diagnosis, and treatment are discussed in detail. Preoperative angina at rest appears to be an important factor in patients who have postoperative coronary spasm. Anatomically, the presence of a relatively normal, dominant right coronary artery may also indicate risk for early postoperative spasm. Acute hypotension is often the first sign of coronary artery spasm, and conventional treatment methods may increase the vasospastic reaction. Peripheral intravenous nitroglycerin effusion has often been unsuccessful. Intragraft or intracoronary nitroglycerin injection or administration of calcium channel-blocking drugs, or both, has effectively reversed the coronary artery spasm and ventricular dysfunction. The authors emphasize that reluctance to use vasodilating agents must be overcome, even if one is confronted with hypotension, when evidence for postoperative spasm is present.

MacAlpin, R. N.: Cardiac arrest and sudden unexpected death in variant angina: Complications of coronary spasm that can occur in the absence of severe organic coronary stenosis. Am. Heart J., 125:1011, 1993.

The clinical course of 81 patients with variant angina was reviewed to determine which clinical features were associated with the greatest risk of angina-linked cardiac arrest (13 patients) or sudden unexpected death (9 patients). The presence of either a history of angina-linked syncope or documentation of serious arrhythmia complicating vasospastic anginal attacks tripled the likelihood of potentially fatal events. An unexpected finding was that the risk was increased 1.5-fold by the absence of high-grade coronary obstructing lesions. These clinical data show that cardiac arrest and sudden death are important risks of variant angina that can occur without the presence of severe obstructing coronary artery disease.

Maseri, A.: Role of coronary artery spasm in symptomatic and silent myocardial ischemia. J. Am. Coll. Cardiol., 9:249, 1987.

A detailed discussion of the diagnosis, treatment, and pathophysiology of vasospastic angina is presented. Maseri and associates have contributed greatly to our understanding of the clinical manifestations of coronary artery spasm and have accumulated convincing evidence that spasm may contribute to practically all aspects of ischemic heart disease.

Prinzmetal, M., Kennamer, R., Merliss, R., et al.: Angina pectoris. I: A variant form of variant pectoris. Am. J. Med., 27:375, 1959.

This classic article describes the clinical manifestations of 32 patients with a different kind of anginal syndrome referred to as variant angina. Unlike typical angina, variant angina is not associated with effort, eating, or anxiety. Prinzmetal correctly postulated that "temporary increased tonus of a large coronary artery" occurred in these patients during episodes of chest pain. The clinical manifestations of variant angina, initially described by Prinzmetal, are still the criteria for establishing a diagnosis of vasospastic angina. Variant angina is commonly referred to as Prinzmetal's angina in recognition of this major contribution.

Raizner, A. E., and Chahine, R. A.: The treatment of Prinzmetal's variant angina with coronary bypass surgery. *In* Hurst, J. W. (ed): Update II: The Heart—Bypass Surgery for Obstructive Coronary Disease. New York, McGraw-Hill, 1980.

*This review summarizes the results of medical and surgical therapy for Prinzmetal's angina. The evidence presented indicates that patients with spasm and insignificant coronary artery disease are best treated medically, and that some patients with spasm and significant atherosclerotic coronary disease are candidates for myocardial revascularization.*

Yasue, H., Takizawa, A., Nagao, M., et al.: Long-term prognosis for patients with variant angina and influential factors. Circulation, 78:1–9, 1988.

*Two-hundred forty-five patients with documented variant angina were followed for an average of 80.5 months. Survival at 1, 3, 5, and 10 years was 98%, 97%, 97%, and 93%, respectively. Survival without myocardial infarction at 1, 3, 5, and 10 years was 86%, 85%, 83%, and 81%, respectively. Multivariate analysis using the Cox proportional hazards model showed that intake of calcium antagonist, extent and severity of coronary artery disease, and ST-segment elevation in both the anterior and inferior leads were independent predictors of survival without myocardial infarction. These results show that the long-term prognosis for patients with variant angina is improved by the aggressive use of calcium antagonist.*

# BIBLIOGRAPHY

Alder, A. G., McElwain, G. E., and Martin, J. H.: Coronary artery spasm induced by phenylephrine eyedrops. Arch. Intern. Med., 141:1384, 1981.

Antman, E., Muller, J., Goldberg, S., et al.: Nifedipine therapy for coronary artery spasm. N. Engl. J. Med., 302:1269, 1980.

Antonelli, D., and Rosenfeld, T.: Variant angina induced by biliary colic. Br. Heart. J., 58:417, 1987.

Ascher, E. K., Stauffer, J. E., and Gaasch, W. H.: Coronary artery spasm, cardiac arrest, transient electrocardiographic Q waves and stunned myocardium in cocaine-associated acute myocardial infarction. Am. J. Cardiol., 61:939, 1988.

Bentivoglio, L. G., Ablaza, S. G. G., and Greenberg, L. F.: Bypass surgery for Prinzmetal angina. Arch. Intern. Med., 134:313, 1974.

Berne, R. M., Degust, H., and Levy, M. N.: Influence of the cardiac nerves on coronary resistance. Am. J. Physiol., 208:763, 1965.

Bertrand, M. E., Lablanche, J. M., and Tilmant, P. Y.: Treatment of Prinzmetal's variant angina. Am. J. Cardiol., 47:174, 1981a.

Bertrand, M. E., Lablanche, J. M., Tilmant, P. Y., et al.: Complete denervation of the heart (autotransplantation) for treatment of severe, refractory coronary spasm. Am. J. Cardiol., 47:1375, 1981b.

Betriu, A., Pomar, J. L., Bourassa, M. G., and Grondin, C. M.: Influence of partial sympathetic denervation on the results of myocardial revascularization in variant angina. Am. J. Cardiol., 51:661, 1983.

Blanche, C., and Chaux, A.: Spasm in mammary artery grafts. Ann. Thorac. Surg., 45:586, 1988.

Blesa, M. I., and Ross, G.: Cholinergic mechanism on the heart and coronary circulation. Br. J. Pharmacol., 39:93, 1970.

Blumenthal, M. R., Wang, H. H., Markee, S., and Wang, S. G.: Effects of acetylcholine on the heart. Physiology, 214:1280, 1968.

Bodenheimer, M., Lipski, J., Donoso, E., and Dack, S.: Prinzmetal's variant angina: A clinical and electrocardiographic study. Am. Heart J., 87:304, 1974.

Bohr, D. F.: Vascular smooth-muscle updates. Circ. Res., 32:665, 1973.

Bolooki, H., Vargas, A., Gharamani, A., et al.: Aortocoronary bypass graft for preinfarction angina. Chest, 61:312, 1972.

Boulanger, M., Maille, J., Pelletier, G. B., and Michalk, S.: Vasospastic angina after calcium injection. Anesth. Analg., 63:1124, 1984.

Boullin, D., Bunting, S., Blasp, W., et al.: Responses of human and baboon arteries to prostaglandin endoperoxides and biologically generated and synthetic prostacyclin: Their relevance to cerebral arterial spasm in man. Br. J. Clin. Pharmacol., 7:139, 1979.

Bourmayan, C., Artigou, J. Y., Barrillon, A. G., et al.: Prinzmetal's variant angina unresponsive to calcium channel-blocking drugs but responsive to combined calcium channel- and beta-blocking drugs. Am. J. Cardiol., 51:1792, 1983.

Bulkley, B., Klacsmann, P., and Hutchins, G.: Angina pectoris, myocardial infarction, and sudden death with normal coronary arteries: A clinicopathologic study of 9 patients with progressive systemic sclerosis. Am. Heart J., 95:563, 1978.

Bunting, S., Gryglewski, R., Moncada, S., and Vane, J.: Arterial walls generate from prostaglandin endoperoxides a substance (prostaglandin X) which relaxes strips of mesenteric and coeliac arteries and inhibits platelet aggregation. Prostaglandins, 12:897, 1976.

Burn, J. H.: Release of noradrenaline from the sympathetic postganglionic fiber. Br. Med. J., 2:197, 1967.

Buxton, A. E., Goldberg, S., Harken, A., et al.: Coronary artery spasm immediately after myocardial revascularization: Recognition and management. N. Engl. J. Med., 304:1249, 1981.

Buxton, A. E., Goldberg, S., and Hirshfield, J. W.: Refractory ergonovine-induced coronary vasospasm: Importance of intracoronary nitroglycerin. Am. J. Cardiol., 46:329, 1980.

Cabrera, R., Cohen, A., Middleton, S., et al.: The immediate source of noradrenaline released in the heart by acetylcholine. Br. J. Pharmacol., 27:46, 1966.

Cannon, R. O., and Epstein, S. E.: "Microvascular angina" as a cause of chest pain with angiographically normal coronary arteries. Am. J. Cardiol., 61:1338, 1988.

Caralis, D. G., Deligonul, U., Kern, M. J., and Cohen, J. D.: Smoking is a risk factor for coronary spasm in young women. Circulation, 85:905–909, 1992.

Chahine, R., Raizner, A., Ishimori, T., et al.: The incidence and clinical implications of coronary artery spasm. Circulation, 52:972, 1975.

Cheng, T. O., Bashour, T., Kelser, G. A., et al.: Variant angina of Prinzmetal with normal coronary arteriograms. A variant of the variant. Circulation, 47:476, 1973.

Cipriano, P., Guthaner, D., Orlick, A., et al.: The effects of ergonovine maleate on coronary arterial size. Circulation, 59:82, 1979.

Cipriano, P., Koch, F., Rosenthal, S. J., and Schroeder, J. S.: Clinical course of patients following the demonstration of coronary artery spasm by angiography. Am. Heart J., 101:127, 1981.

Cistero, A., Urias, S., Guindo, J., et al.: Coronary artery spasm and acute myocardial infarction in naproxen-associated anaphylactic reaction. Allergy, 47:576–578, 1992.

Clark, D. A., Quint, R. A., Mitchell, R. L., and Angell, W. W.: Coronary artery spasm. Medical management, surgical denervation, and autotransplantation. J. Thorac. Cardiovasc. Surg., 73:332, 1977.

Coffman, J. D., and Cohen, R. A.: Vasospasm—Ubiquitous? N. Engl. J. Med., 304:780, 1981.

Conti, C. R., Pepine, C. J., and Curry, R. C.: Coronary artery spasm: An important mechanism in the pathophysiology of ischemic heart disease. Curr. Probl. Cardiol., 4:1, 1979.

Dagenais, G., Gundel, W., and Conti, C.: Peripheral venospasm associated with signs of transient myocardial ischemia. Am. Heart J., 80:544, 1970.

D'Angelo, V., Ville, S., Mysliwiec, M., et al.: Defective fibrinolytic and prostacyclin-like activity in human atheromatous plaques. Thromb. Haemost., 39:535, 1978.

Demany, M., Tambe, A., and Zimmerman, H.: Coronary arterial spasm. Dis. Chest., 53:714, 1968.

Dembinska-Kiec, A., Gryglewski, T., Zmuda, A., and Gryglewski, R. J.: The generation of prostacyclin by arteries and by the coronary vascular bed is reduced in experimental atherosclerosis in rabbits. Prostaglandins, 14:1025, 1977.

Dempsey, P. J., and Cooper, T.: Ventricular cholinergic receptor systems: Interaction with adrenergic systems. J. Pharmacol. Exp. Ther., 167:282, 1969.

Detre, K., Costigan, T., Kelsey, S., et al.: PTCA in 1985; NHLBI PTCA Registry. J. Am. Coll. Cardiol., 9:9a, 1987.

DiPaolo, C., Kerin, N. Z., Rubenfire, M., and Levine, F.: Surgical treatment of medically refractory variant angina pectoris: Segmental coronary resection with aortocoronary bypass and plexectomy. Am. J. Cardiol., 56:792, 1985.

Dusting, G., Chapple, D., Hughes, R., et al.: Prostacyclin ($PG_2$) induced coronary vasodilatation in anaesthetized dogs. Cardiovasc. Res., 12:720, 1978.

Endo, M., Hirosawa, K., Kaneko, N., et al.: Prinzmetal's variant angina: Coronary arteriogram and left ventriculogram during angina attack induced by methacholine. N. Engl. J. Med., 294:252, 1976.

Endo, M., Kanda, I., Hosoda, S., et al.: Prinzmetal's variant form of angina pectoris. Circulation, 52:33, 1975.

Faxon, D. P., Melidossian, C., and Ryan, T. J.: The changing face of coronary artery spasm: A decade of experience. Am. Heart J., 116:572–576, 1988.

Feigl, E. O.: Parasympathetic control of coronary blood flow in dogs. Circ. Res., 25:509, 1969.

Feldman, R. L., Pepine, C. J., Whittle, J., and Conti, C. R.: Short and long-term responses to diltiazem in patients with variant angina. Am. J. Cardiol., 49:554, 1982.

Fellows, C. L., Weaver, W. D., and Greene, H. L.: Cardiac arrest associated with coronary artery spasm. Am. J. Cardiol., 60:1397–1399, 1987.

Fleckenstein, A., Nakayama, K., Fleckenstein-Grun, G., and Byon, Y. K.: Interactions of hydrogen ions, calcium antagonistic drugs and cardiac glycosides with excitation-contraction coupling of vascular smooth-muscle. In Beta, E. (ed): Ionic Actions on Vascular Smooth Muscle. Berlin, Springer-Verlag, 1976, p. 117.

Goldman, M., Rogers, E., and Rogers, M.: Subarachnoid hemorrhage: Association with unusual electrocardiographic changes. J. A. M. A., 234:957, 1975.

Gorfinkel, H. J., Inglesby, T. V., Lansing, A. M., and Goodin, R. R.: ST-segment elevation, transient left-posterior hemiblock, and recurrent ventricular arrhythmias unassociated with pain: A variant of Prinzmetal's anginal syndrome. Ann. Intern. Med., 79:795, 1973.

Goto, K., Yasue, H., Okumura, K., et al.: Magnesium deficiency detected by intravenous loading test in variant angina pectoris. Am. J. Cardiol., 65:709–712, 1990.

Guazzi, M., Fiorentini, C., Polese, A., and Magrini, F.: Continuous electrocardiographic recording in Prinzmetal's variant angina pectoris: A report of four cases. Br. Heart J., 32:611, 1970.

Guazzi, M., Olivari, M., Polese, A., et al.: Repetitive myocardial ischemia of Prinzmetal type without angina pectoris. Am. J. Cardiol., 37:923, 1976.

Gurley, J. C., Booth, D. C., and DeMaria, A. N.: Circulatory collapse following coronary bypass surgery: Multivessel and graft spasm reversed in the catheterization laboratory by intracoronary papaverine. Am. Heart J., 119:1194–1195, 1990.

Hackett, J. G., Abboud, F. M., Mark, A. L., et al.: Coronary vascular responses to stimulation of chemoreceptors and baroreceptors: Evidence for reflex activation of vagal cholinergic innervation. Circ. Res., 31:8, 1972.

Harder, D., Belardinello, L., Sperelakis, N., et al.: Differential effects of adenosine and nitroglycerin on the action potentials of large and small coronary arteries. Circ. Res., 44:176, 1979.

He, G. W.: Contractility of the human internal mammary artery at the distal section increases toward the end: Emphasis on not using the end of the internal mammary artery for grafting. J. Thorac. Cardiovasc. Surg., 106:406–411, 1993.

Heberden, W.: Some account of a disorder of the breast. Medical Transactions of the Royal College of Physicians of London, 2:59, 1772.

Herrick, J. B.: Clinical features of sudden obstruction of the coronary arteries. J. A. M. A., 59:2015, 1912.

Hillis, L., and Braunwald, E.: Coronary artery spasm. N. Engl. J. Med., 299:695, 1978.

Hisano, K., Matsuguchi, T., Oatsubo, H., et al.: Hyperventilation induced variant angina. Am. Heart. J., 108:423, 1984.

Johnson, A. D., and Detwiler, J. H.: Coronary spasm, variant angina, and recurrent myocardial infarctions. Circulation, 55:947, 1977.

Johnson, S. M., Mauritson, D. R., Willerson, J. T., and Hillis, L. D.: Comparison of verapamil and nifedipine in the treatment of variant angina pectoris: Preliminary observations in 10 patients. Am. J. Cardiol., 47:1295, 1981.

Kaski, J. C., Tousoulis, D., McFadden, E., et al.: Variant angina pectoris: Role of coronary spasm in the development of fixed coronary obstructions. Circulation, 85:619–626, 1992.

Kelley, K., and Feigl, E.: Segmental alpha-receptor mediated vasoconstriction in the canine coronary circulation. Circ. Res., 43:908, 1978.

Kimura, E., and Kishida, H.: Treatment of variant angina with drugs: A survey of 11 cardiology institutes in Japan. Circulation, 63:844, 1981.

King, S., Mansour, K., Hatcher, C., et al.: Coronary artery spasm producing Prinzmetal's angina in myocardial infarction in the absence of coronary atherosclerosis. Ann. Thorac. Surg., 16:337, 1973.

Kleiman, N. S., Lehane, D. E., Geyer, C. E., Jr., et al.: Prinzmetal's angina during 5-fluorouracil chemotherapy. Am. J. Med., 82:566, 1987.

Kounis, N. G., and Zavras, G. M.: Histamine-induced coronary artery spasm: The concept of allergic angina. BJCP, 45:121–128, 1991.

Krantz, E. M., Viljoen, J. F., and Gilbert, M. S.: Prinzmetal's variant angina during extradural anaesthesia. Br. J. Anaesth., 52:945, 1980.

Lange, R., Reid, M., Tresch, D., et al.: Nonatheromatous ischemic heart disease following withdrawal from chronic industrial nitroglycerin exposure. Circulation, 46:666, 1972.

Lasser, R. T., and de la Paz, N. D.: Repetitive transient myocardial ischemia, Prinzmetal type, without angina pectoris, presenting with Stokes-Adams attacks. Chest, 64:350, 1973.

Lavine, P., Kimbiris, D., and Linhart, J.: Coronary artery spasm during selective coronary arteriography: A review of 8 years experience [Abstract]. Circulation, 49(Suppl. 4):89, 1973.

Lemmer, J. H., Jr., and Kirsh, M. M.: Coronary artery spasm following coronary artery surgery. Ann. Thorac. Surg., 46:108, 1988.

Levy, M. N.: Sympathetic-parasympathetic interactions in the heart. Circ. Res., 29:437, 1971.

Levy, M. N., and Zieske, H.: Comparison of the cardiac effects of vagus nerve stimulation and of acetylcholine infusions. Am. J. Physiol., 216:890, 1969.

Lewy, R., Smith, J., Silver, M., et al.: Detection of thromboxane B2 in the peripheral blood of patients with Prinzmetal's angina. Prostaglandins Med., 2:243, 1979.

Linhart, J. W., Beller, B. M., and Talley, R. C.: Preinfarction angina: Clinical, hemodynamic and angiographic evaluation. Chest, 61:312, 1972.

MacAlpin, R. N.: Cardiac arrest and sudden unexpected death in variant angina: Complications of coronary spasm that can occur in the absence of severe organic coronary stenosis. Am. Heart J., 125:1011–1917, 1993.

Madias, J. E.: The long-term outcome of patients who suffered and survived an acute myocardial infarction in the midst of recurrent attacks of variant angina. Clin. Cardiol., 9:277, 1986.

Maseri, A.: Role of coronary artery spasm in symptomatic and silent myocardial ischemia. J. Am. Coll. Cardiol., 9:249, 1987.

Maseri, A., Klassen, G. A., and Lesch, M. (eds): Primary and Secondary Angina Pectoris. New York, Grune & Stratton, 1978a.

Maseri, A., L'Abbate, A., Pesola, A., et al.: Coronary vasospasm in angina pectoris. Lancet, 1:713, 1977.

Maseri, A., Mimmo, R., Chierchia, S., et al.: Coronary spasm as a cause of acute myocardial ischemia in man. Chest, 68:625, 1975.

Maseri, A., Severi, S., Nes, M. D., et al.: "Variant" angina: One aspect of a continuous spectrum of vasospastic myocardial ischemia. Am. J. Cardiol., 42:1019, 1978b.

Melville, K., Garvey, H., Shister, E., et al.: Central nervous system stimulation and cardiac ischemic changes in monkeys. Ann. N. Y. Acad. Sci., 156:241, 1969.

Miller, D., Waters, D. D., Warnica, W., et al.: Is variant angina the coronary manifestation of a generalized vasospastic disorder? N. Engl. J. Med., 304:763, 1981.

Mills, N. L., and Everson, C. T.: Right gastroepiploic artery: A third arterial conduit for coronary artery bypass. Ann. Thorac. Surg., 47:706–711, 1989.

Miwa, K., Kambara, H., and Kawai, C.: Effect of aspirin in large doses on attacks of variant angina. Am. Heart J., 105:351, 1983.

Moncada, S., Higgs, E., and Vane, J.: Human arterial and venous tissues generate prostacyclin (prostaglandin X), a potent inhibitor of platelet aggregation. Lancet, 1:18, 1977.

Mudge, G., Grossman, W., Miles, R., et al.: Reflex increase in coronary vascular resistance in patients with ischemic heart disease. N. Engl. J. Med., 295:1333, 1976.

Murao, S., Harumi, K., Katayama, S., et al.: All-night polygraphic studies of nocturnal angina pectoris. Jpn. Heart J., 13:295, 1972.

Myerburg, R. J., Kessler, K. M., Mallon, S. M., et al.: Life threatening ventricular arrhythmias in patients with silent myocardial ischemia due to coronary artery spasm. N. Engl. J. Med., 326:1451–1455, 1992.

Nobuyoshi, M., Tanaka, M., Nosaka, H., et al.: Progression of coronary atherosclerosis: Is coronary spasm related to progression? J. Am. Coll. Cardiol., 18:904–910, 1991.

Nowlin, J. B., Troyer, W. G., Collens, W. S., et al.: The association of nocturnal angina pectoris with dreaming. Ann. Intern. Med., 63:1040, 1965.

Oliva, P. B.: Coronary artery spasm: An important mechanism in the pathophysiology of ischemic heart disease [Editorial Comment]. Curr. Probl. Cardiol., 4:1, 1979.

Oliva, P. B., and Breckinridge, J.: Arteriographic evidence of coronary arterial spasm in acute myocardial infarction. Circulation, 56:366, 1977.

Oliva, P. B., Potts, D. E., and Pluss, R. G.: Coronary peripheral spasm in Prinzmetal angina. Documentation by coronary arteriography. N. Engl. J. Med., 288:745, 1973.

O'Reilly, R., Spellberg, R., and King, T.: Recognition of proximal right coronary artery spasm during coronary arteriography. Radiology, 95:305, 1970.

Osler, W.: The Lumleian lectures on angina pectoris. Lancet, 1:699, 1910.

Pepine, C. J., Feldman, R. L., Whittle, J., et al.: Effect of diltiazem in patients with variant angina: A randomized double blind trial. Am. Heart J., 101:719, 1981.

Pichard, A. D., Ambrose, J., Mindrich, B., et al.: Coronary artery spasm and perioperative cardiac arrest. J. Thorac. Cardiovasc. Surg., 80:249, 1980.

Pijls, N. H. J., and van der Werf, T.: Prinzmetal's angina associated with alcohol withdrawal. Cardiology, 75:226–229, 1988.

Prinzmetal, M., Kennamer, R., Merliss, R., et al.: Angina pectoris. I: A variant form of angina pectoris. Am. J. Med., 27:375, 1959.

Prohkov, V. K., Mookherjee, S., Schiess, W., and Obeid, A. L.: Variant anginal syndrome, coronary artery spasm and ventricular fibrillation in absence of chest pain. Ann. Intern. Med., 81:858, 1974.

Raabe, D.: Treatment of variant angina pectoris with perhexiline maleate. Chest, 75:152, 1979.

Raizner, A. E., and Chahine, R. A.: The treatment of Prinzmetal's variant angina with coronary bypass surgery. In Hurst, J. W. (ed): Update II: The Heart—Bypass Surgery for Obstructive Coronary Disease. New York, McGraw-Hill, 1980.

Ricci, D., Orlick, A., Cipriano, P., et al.: Altered adrenergic activity in coronary arterial spasm. Insight into mechanism based on study of coronary hemodynamics and the electrocardiogram. Am. J. Cardiol., 43:1073, 1979.

Robertson, D., and Oates, J.: Variant angina and Raynaud's phenomenon [Letter]. Lancet, 1:452, 1978.

Robertson, D., Robertson, R., Nies, A., et al.: Variant angina pectoris: Investigation of indexes of sympathetic nervous system functioning. Am. J. Cardiol., 43:1080, 1979.

Rosenthal, S. J., Ginsburg, R., Lamb, I. H., et al.: Efficacy of diltiazem for control of symptoms of coronary arterial spasm. Am. J. Cardiol., 46:1027, 1980.

Rothman, M. T., and Kahn, B.: Coronary artery spasm. BJCP, 45:129–134, 1991.

Rutitzky, B., Girotti, A. L., and Rosenbaum, M. B.: Efficacy of chronic amiodarone therapy in patients with variant angina pectoris and inhibition of ergonovine coronary constriction. Am. Heart J., 103:38, 1982.

Sakurai, I.: Coronary artery spasm and vascular biology: Cholinergic constriction. Acta Pathol. Jpn., 41:865–873, 1991.

Sarabu, M. R., McClung, J. A., Fass, A., and Reed, G. E.: Early postoperative spasm in left internal mammary artery bypass graft. Ann. Thorac. Surg., 44:199–200, 1987.

Schick, E. C., Davis, Z., Lavery, R. M., et al.: Surgical therapy for Prinzmetal's variant angina. Ann. Thorac. Surg., 33:359, 1982.

Schiffer, F., Hartley, H., Schulman, C. L., and Abelmann, W. H.: Evidence for emotionally induced coronary arterial spasm in patients with angina pectoris. Br. Heart J., 44:62, 1980.

Scholl, J.-M., Veau, P., Benacerraf, A., et al.: Long-term prognosis of medically treated patients with vasospastic angina and no fixed significant coronary atherosclerosis. Am. Heart J., 115:559–564, 1988.

Schroeder, J. S., Feldman, R. L., Giles, T. D., et al.: Multiclinic

controlled trial of diltiazem for Prinzmetal's angina. Am. J. Med., 72:227, 1982.

Selzer, A., Langston, M., Ruggeroli, C., and Cohn, K.: Clinical syndrome of variant angina with normal coronary arteriogram. N. Engl. J. Med., 295:1343, 1976.

Severi, S., Davies, G., Maseri, A., et al.: Long-term prognosis of "variant" angina with medical treatment. Am. J. Cardiol., 46:226, 1980.

Shachor, J., Beker, B., Geffen, Y., and Bruderman, I.: Acute ECG changes during cyclophosphamide infusion in a patient with bronchogenic carcinoma. Cancer, 69:734, 1985.

Shinjo, A., Sasaki, Y., Inamasu, M., and Morita, T.: In vivo effects of the coronary vasodilator diltiazem on human and rabbit platelets. Thromb. Res., 13:941, 1978.

Shirai, K., Nii, T., Imamura, M., et al.: Low serum apolipoprotein A-I level in patients with vasospastic angina. Am. Heart J., 125:320, 1993.

Silverman, M., and Flamm, M.: Angina pectoris. Anatomic findings and prognostic implications. Ann. Intern. Med., 75:339, 1971.

Stenson, R. E., Flamm, M. D., Zaret, B. L., and McGowan, R. L.: Transient ST-segment elevation with postmyocardial infarction angina: Prognostic significance. Am. Heart J., 89:449, 1975.

Suma, H.: Spasm of the gastroepiploic artery graft [Letter]. Ann. Thorac. Surg., 49:168–169, 1990.

Sussman, E. J., Goldberg, S., Poll, D. S., et al.: Surgical therapy of variant angina associated with nonobstructive coronary disease. Ann. Intern. Med., 94:771, 1981.

Szczeklik, A., Gryglewski, R. J., Musial, J., et al.: Thromboxane generation and platelet aggregation in survivors of myocardial infarction. Thromb. Haemost., 40:66, 1978.

Tada, M., Kuzuya, T., Inoue, M., et al.: Elevation of thromboxane $B_2$ levels in patients with classic and variant angina pectoris. Circulation, 64:1107, 1981.

Takizawa, A., Yasue, H., Omote, S., et al.: Variant angina induced by alcohol ingestion. Am. Heart J., 107:25, 1984.

Toyama, Y., Tanaka, H., Nuruki, K., and Shirao, T.: Prinzmetal's variant angina associated with subarachnoid hemorrhage: A case report. Angiology, 30:211, 1979.

Tzivoni, D., Keren, A., Benhorin, J., et al.: Prazosin therapy for refractory variant angina. Am. Heart J., 105:262, 1983.

Waters, D. D., Crean, P. A., Roy, D., and Theroux, P.: Problems related to the detection of myocardial ischemia. Can. J. Cardiol., (Suppl. A):173A, 1986.

Waters, D. D., Szlachcic, J., Miller, D., and Theroux, P.: Clinical characteristics of patients with variant angina complicated by myocardial infarction or death within 1 month. Am. J. Cardiol., 49:658, 1982.

Weber, S., Cabanes, L., Simon, J.-C., et al.: Systemic alkalosis as a provocative test for coronary artery spasm in patients with infrequent resting chest pain. Am. Heart J., 115:54–59, 1988.

Winniford, M. D., Filipchuk, N., and Hillis, L. D.: Alpha-adrenergic blockade for variant angina: A long-term, double-blind, randomized trial. Circulation, 67:1185, 1983.

Yasue, H., Horio, Y., Nakamura, N., et al.: Induction of coronary spasm by acetylcholine in patients with variant angina: Possible role of the parasympathetic nervous system in the pathogenesis of coronary spasm. Circulation, 74:955, 1986.

Yasue, H., Nagao, M., Omote, S., et al.: Coronary arterial spasm and Prinzmetal's variant form of angina induced by hyperventilation and TRIS-buffer infusion. Circulation, 58:56, 1978.

Yasue, H., Takizawa, A., Nagao, M., et al.: Long-term prognosis for patients with variant angina and influential factors. Circulation, 78:1–9, 1988.

Yasue, H., Touyama, M., Shimamoto, M., et al.: Role of autonomic nervous system in the pathogenesis of Prinzmetal's variant form of angina. Circulation, 50:534, 1974.

Yoshio, H., Shimizu, M., Sugihara, N., et al.: Assessment of autonomic nervous activity by heart rate spectral analysis in patients with variant angina. Am. Heart J., 125:324, 1993.

Yuki, K., Kodama, Y., Onda, J., et al.: Coronary vasospasm following subarachnoid hemorrhage as a cause of stunned myocardium. J. Neurosurgery, 75:308–311, 1991.

Zaiac, M., Renzulli, A., and Hilton, C. J.: Coronary artery spasm following coronary artery bypass grafting: Treatment with intracoronary ISDN followed by systemic intravenous Nifedipine infusion. Eur. J. Cardiothorac. Surg., 4:109–111, 1990.

# 8  Kawasaki's Disease

Thomas A. D'Amico

Kawasaki's disease is a multisystemic disorder of undetermined etiology that is an important cause of cardiovascular disease in children. Described by Kawasaki in 1967, the acute illness is characterized by fever, conjunctivitis, cervical lymphadenopathy, and vasculitic changes. Although the syndrome usually is indolent and self-limiting, in its advanced stage it is characterized by coronary aneurysms, peripheral aneurysms, mitral valve insufficiency, and left ventricular dysfunction.

Kawasaki's disease predominantly affects infants and children, the highest incidence being at 12 to 16 months. The overall incidence in children younger than 5 years is 1.1 per 100,000 population, equivalent to the incidence of acute rheumatic fever (Rauch, 1987). Although various causative agents have been proposed, the etiology of Kawasaki's disease is still unclear. The pathophysiology has been well described, but the infrequent progression to severe cardiovascular manifestations is not well understood. Increased awareness of the potential severity of Kawasaki's disease has contributed to more prompt diagnosis and earlier institution of therapy. Current management consists of antiplatelet and anti-inflammatory agents; surgical intervention is reserved for patients with advanced disease. An ideal treatment that ameliorates the early inflammatory symptoms, arrests the vasculitic progression, and prevents the formation of coronary aneurysms has not yet been discovered.

## CLINICAL MANIFESTATIONS

### Symptoms

Kawasaki's original description of the clinical features of the syndrome has been consistently supported by others. The diagnostic criteria, including the principal symptoms and associated findings, are shown in Table 54–21 (Hicks and Melish, 1986). The diagnosis of Kawasaki's disease is secured by the presence of five of the six major criteria. The presentation of this syndrome is acute, and the symptoms evolve during a period of a few days, a stereotypical clinical pattern that leads to certain diagnosis. However, various reports of atypical presentations suggest that a high index of suspicion is required to prevent delayed diagnosis and late recognition of cardiovascular complications.

The principal presenting symptom is fever, which usually has an abrupt onset, may be prolonged or intermittent, and does not respond to antibiotics. The fever lasts from 7 to 14 days but may persist in more severe cases. The fever is often accompanied by congested conjunctivae, bilateral and sterile. After the appearance of conjunctivitis, several changes in the lips and oral cavity occur. Commonly, there is a reddening of the lips, which may then become dry and fissured. The tongue may appear prominently, with protuberant papillae ("strawberry tongue"), or there may be only diffuse reddening of the oropharyngeal mucosa (Rowley et al., 1988).

By the third day of the illness, a polymorphous macular erythematous rash appears. The rash begins with reddening of the palms and soles; individual lesions may coalesce as the rash progresses proximally to spread over the trunk, usually over 48 hours. As the rash resolves, secondary changes in digits appear. A unique desquamation begins at the junction of the nails and the skin on the tips of the digits. In approximately 50% of patients, nonpurulent cervical lymphadenopathy develops (Bligard, 1987).

### Physical Examination

The principal physical findings are easily recognized. Elicitation of the more subtle physical findings early in the course of Kawasaki's disease may facili-

■ **Table 54–21.** SYMPTOMS AND ASSOCIATED FINDINGS OF KAWASAKI'S DISEASE

**Principal Symptoms (Five Needed for Diagnosis)**

1. Fever
2. Conjunctivitis
3. Changes in the mouth and oral cavity
   Dry, fissured, or reddened lips
   Prominent reddened tongue
   Diffuse reddening of the oral mucosa
4. Changes of the extremities
   Reddening of the palms or soles
   Indurative edema of the hands or feet
   Desquamation
5. Polymorphous truncal rash
6. Cervical adenopathy

**Associated Findings**

Arthralgia
Arthritis
Aseptic meningitis
Diarrhea
Hydrops of the gall bladder
Jaundice
Myocarditis
Pericarditis
Proteinuria
Urethritis

tate the prompt diagnosis of its numerous complications.

The cardiac examination should be performed twice daily to ensure detection of cardiovascular abnormalities. Examination of the heart may reveal tachycardia, distant heart sounds, or a gallop, suggestive of myocarditis or congestive failure; a holosystolic murmur signifies mitral valve insufficiency. Palpation of the peripheral arteries, especially in the axillary and inguinal regions, may reveal an aneurysm (Fig. 54–120). Palpation of the abdomen may show congestive hepatomegaly, or right upper-quadrant tenderness, secondary to hydrops of the gallbladder (Nehme and Mikhail, 1983). Although infrequent, the presence of peritoneal signs suggests vascular compromise in the mesenteric arteries (Mercer and Carpenter, 1981). Auscultation of the abdomen may reveal the bruit of an aneurysm of the renal, celiac, mesenteric, or iliac arteries. Neurologic examination may show meningeal signs, irritability, stupor, or coma, secondary to aseptic meningitis. Examination of the neck often yields prominent cervical lymphadenopathy, an early finding that precedes other classic findings. It has been suggested that lymph node biopsy should be performed to ascertain the diagnosis of Kawasaki's disease and thereby institute therapy earlier (Giesker et al., 1982).

## Laboratory Studies

Leukocytosis is invariably present and is often accompanied by a leftward shift in the differential. Anemia and thrombocytosis may be present. Other findings include an increase in interleukin-6, interleukin-8, tumor necrosis factor alpha (Lin et al., 1992), erythrocyte sedimentation rate (ESR), C-reactive protein, Factor VII concentration, and fibrinogen level, as well as low antithrombin III level (Rowley et al., 1988).

The electrocardiographic findings are abnormal in 70% of patients. The most common findings are sinus tachycardia, prolonged PQ and QR intervals, second-degree atrioventricular block, decreased voltage, ST-segment changes, and T wave changes (Daniels et al., 1987).

Admission radiographic studies often yield abnormal results. Chest films may reveal cardiomegaly or pleural effusion. Echocardiograms yield positive results in 45% of patients, providing early objective evidence of cardiovascular dysfunction (Chung et al., 1988).

## ETIOLOGY

Kawasaki's disease is the predominant cause of acquired heart disease in children in the United States (Rowley and Shulman, 1987). Despite the prevalence of the disorder, investigations of the etiology have been inconclusive; the pathogenesis of Kawasaki's disease has not yet been discovered. Many clinical aspects of the syndrome suggest a communicable causative factor. The acute presentation of fever, rash, conjunctivitis, and lymphadenopathy in children suggests an infectious disease. That the disease affects children exclusively and spares adults suggests a mechanism of acquired immunity. Epidemiologic evidence supports the theory of an infectious etiology. In addition to the geographic areas where it appears

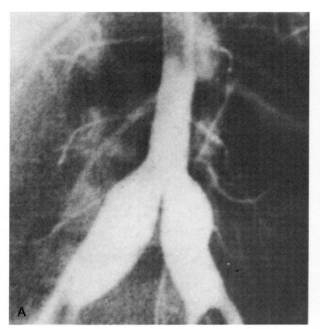 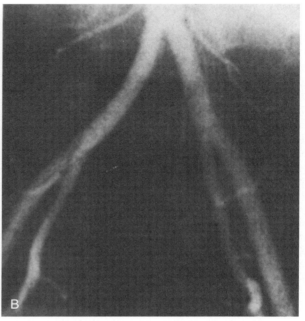

**FIGURE 54–120.** *A,* Aortogram in an infant with Kawasaki's disease demonstrates bilateral iliac artery aneurysms. *B,* After regression of the aneurysms 1 year later, the arteries appear radiographically normal. (*A* and *B,* From Chung, K. J., Fulton, D. R., Lapp, R., et al.: One-year follow-up of cardiac and coronary artery disease in infants and children with Kawasaki disease. Am. Heart J., *115:*1263, 1988.)

to be endemic, such as Japan, seasonal epidemic outbreaks are common.

The search for a single etiologic agent has been unsuccessful. Possibilities include rickettsiae, spirochetes, *Propionibacterium, Borrelia, Pseudomonas,* Epstein-Barr virus, and superantigens, all without confirmation (Leung, 1993). The lack of evidence for person-to-person transmissibility has made it difficult to isolate a single causative factor. Variable immunity or low communicability could explain this phenomenon.

Investigation of peripheral lymphocytes isolated from the blood during the acute stage of Kawasaki's disease has shown increased helper T-lymphocyte activity and decreased suppressor T-lymphocyte activity, which suggests a retroviral component in the etiology of Kawasaki's disease (Shulman and Rowley, 1986). In contrast to the human immunodeficiency virus I, the helper-to-suppressor T-lymphocyte ratio is increased, which is compatible with a suppressor T-lymphocytic virus (Rauch, 1987). That Kawasaki's disease is recurrent in 3% of patients suggests a cell-associated agent that persistently infects lymphocytes (Marchette et al., 1987). Reverse transcriptase, which synthesizes DNA from a template of RNA, is the hallmark of retroviral activity. Analysis of supernatants from cultures of lymphocytes from patients with Kawasaki's disease showed significantly increased reverse transcriptase activity compared with controls. Although this finding has been confirmed by multiple laboratories, there has been no conclusive evidence of a specific viral agent, because cell lines and culture conditions have not been discovered, and there is no serologic evidence of a specific antiviral antibody (Burns et al., 1986; Shulman et al., 1987).

## NATURAL HISTORY

The pathologic basis of Kawasaki's disease is the progression of a nonspecific vasculitis that involves the microvasculature of the aorta and its major branches, manifested by endarteritis of the vasa vasorum of the coronary, brachiocephalic, celiac, renal, and iliofemoral systems. As the inflammatory process of the intima and adventitia progresses, aneurysms form in these vessels and cause stenosis, thromboembolism, ischemia, rupture, or healing.

There are three clinical stages of Kawasaki's disease (Hicks and Melish, 1986). The acute phase lasts approximately 10 days, during which fever and the development of the characteristic rash predominate. The subacute phase ensues, during which the cardiac complications commonly occur. The convalescent phase is defined as the period during which the ESR remains elevated. Although the course of Kawasaki's disease is typically acute, with resolution of symptoms and complications, it may recur with vasculitic symptoms or with sudden death (Feild et al., 1987).

A spectrum of cardiovascular manifestations may occur in Kawasaki's disease, usually self-limited (Crowley, 1984). Myocarditis is present in as many as 50% of patients (Takahashi, 1989). One study, in which endomyocardial biopsies were taken during cardiac catheterization for coronary arteriography, showed inflammatory changes in each of 201 patients (Kato et al., 1979). In the acute phase, myocarditis may cause exercise intolerance, congestive heart failure, or death.

Mitral regurgitation occurs in only 5% of patients with Kawasaki's disease; however, in patients with coronary aneurysms, the incidence is 25% (Kitamura et al., 1980). Ischemia to the papillary muscles secondary to coronary artery involvement is responsible for most cases, although diffuse myocarditis and annular dilatation may also contribute (Takao et al., 1987).

Myocardial infarction, a rare complication of Kawasaki's disease, may occur after diffuse ischemia or a thromboembolic event. Myocardial ischemia is due to profound fibrotic changes or is secondary to multiple stenotic lesions. The presence of collateral circulation usually preserves ventricular function, despite multiple stenotic lesions; however, left ventricular hypertrophy associated with diffuse hypokinesia sometimes develops.

The most serious complication of Kawasaki's disease is the formation of coronary artery aneurysms, which has an incidence of 10 to 40% (Akagi et al., 1992; Kato et al., 1986). Coronary artery aneurysms are responsible for at least 85% of the mortality associated with Kawasaki's disease. The mortality among boys with Kawasaki's disease is twice that among healthy boys, and most deaths occur within 2 months of the diagnosis (Nakamura et al., 1992). A spectrum of coronary artery involvement is associated with Kawasaki's disease. Echocardiographic studies have demonstrated that coronary arterial wall changes occur in all patients, which progress to dilatation in half and to true aneurysms in over one-quarter of patients (Kamiya and Suzuki, 1987). The aneurysms may be asymptomatic, or may not become symptomatic until years later, whereas other aneurysms present initially with myocardial infarction, cardiogenic shock, or sudden death (Kato, 1987).

Serial angiographic studies have shown "resolution" of aneurysms that are discovered as early as the second week; several studies have demonstrated resolution of 50% of coronary aneurysms 1 year after initial presentation (Chung et al., 1988; Kato et al., 1982). Pathologic analysis has shown that angiographic resolution may be caused by intimal proliferation rather than by healing, which leaves these arteries at further risk for stenosis and thromboembolism (Nakano et al., 1986). The risk of chronic coronary involvement and development of premature atherosclerosis is uncertain (Bierman and Gersony, 1987). The sequelae of coronary artery disease from childhood Kawasaki's disease may be manifested as early-onset coronary disease in adults (Kato et al., 1992).

Coronary artery aneurysms follow inflammatory changes in the intima and adventitia, caused by perivasculitis of the major coronary arteries. As in atherosclerotic coronary artery disease, the lesions occur most commonly at the bifurcation of the *left anterior descending* (LAD) and circumflex vessels (found in 74% of patients with coronary aneurysms) and at the origin of the *right coronary artery* (RCA) (48%) (Nakanishi et al., 1985). Most patients have multiple aneurysms, but only aneurysms that reach 4 mm in diameter are considered clinically significant (Fujiwara et al., 1987). Within the aneurysm, turbulence and stagnation produce platelet aggregation and thrombosis. Advanced thrombosis causes critical stenoses in the coronary arteries, the most common indication for surgical intervention. Thromboembolic phenomena are also common and may produce acute myocardial infarction.

Cardiac fatalities occur in less than 1% of patients with Kawasaki's disease (Melish, 1987). Patients with aneurysms larger than 8 mm have the worst prognosis, and this group constitutes nearly all the late deaths from Kawasaki's disease.

The diagnosis of Kawasaki's disease should be accompanied routinely by echocardiography, which has demonstrated a sensitivity of greater than 90% in detecting coronary aneurysms (Daniels et al., 1987). However, echocardiography is not effective in detecting stenotic lesions. Early detection and treatment of coronary lesions are necessary to reduce the mortality of Kawasaki's disease. To ensure prompt institution of therapy, the severity of the disease in a particular patient must be evaluated at a stage before most aneurysms can be detected by echocardiography. Thus, many clinicians have developed a scoring system, using risk factors, to anticipate major cardiac complications (Ichida et al., 1987; Nakano et al., 1986). The accepted risk factors for the development of coronary aneurysms are listed in Table 54–22.

Selective coronary angiography is reserved for patients with complications of known coronary aneurysms (Fig. 54–121). Analysis of these data has shown groups of patients who are most likely to develop aneurysms and who require serial coronary echocardiograms, selective coronary angiography, and surgical intervention (Koren et al., 1986; Nakano et al., 1985). The indications for cardiac catheterization are shown in Table 54–23.

## TREATMENT

The mortality rate of Kawasaki's disease before 1976 was 1 to 2%. Since 1976, the mortality rate has decreased to approximately 0.5%, owing to earlier diagnosis and the evolution of effective therapy, including surgical intervention (Suma et al., 1982). Early diagnosis and recognition of the appearance of cardio-

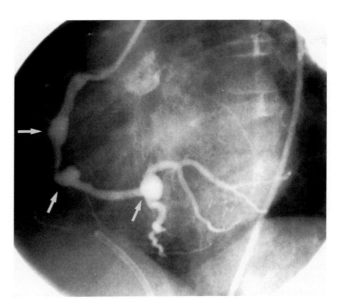

**FIGURE 54–121.** Coronary arteriogram demonstrating three aneurysms of the right coronary artery in a 10-year-old boy with Kawasaki's disease.

vascular complications are critical in the successful management of patients with Kawasaki's disease, because death may occur in the first week of the illness.

## Aspirin

When Kawasaki's disease is diagnosed, children are given a regimen of aspirin, 100 mg/kg/day, which is continued until defervescence. Thereafter, they are maintained on aspirin, 10 mg/kg/day, for 8 weeks or until the ESR is normal. In children who develop aneurysms, low-dosage (3 to 5 mg/kg/day) aspirin therapy may be continued indefinitely (Gersony, 1992); the risk of associated salicylate complications, including Reye's syndrome, is low. The goal of aspirin therapy is to ameliorate symptoms and to prevent the thrombotic and embolic complications of Kawasaki's disease. Aspirin does not decrease the risk of developing coronary aneurysms, nor does it prevent the obstruction of giant aneurysms (Ichida et al., 1987).

## Immune Globulin

Treatment with intravenous immune globulin has been shown to decrease the duration of fever (Furu-

■ **Table 54–22.** RISK FACTORS FOR THE DEVELOPMENT OF CORONARY ANEURYSMS IN KAWASAKI'S DISEASE

Male sex
Age under 1 year
Duration of fever greater than 16 days
White blood cell count greater than 30
Erythrocyte sedimentation rate greater than 100
Elevated C-reactive protein
Thrombocytosis

■ **Table 54–23.** INDICATIONS FOR CARDIAC CATHETERIZATION IN KAWASAKI'S DISEASE

Severe symptoms at onset
Symptoms of ischemic heart disease
Symptoms of congestive heart failure
Mitral regurgitation
Coronary calcifications evident on chest films
Persistent coronary aneurysms

sho et al., 1984), to decrease the prevalence of cardio-vascular complications (Nagashima, 1987), and to prevent the progression to giant coronary aneurysms (Rowley and Shulman, 1988). A cooperative study compared aspirin therapy alone for 14 days with the combination of intravenous immune globulin (400 mg/kg/day for 5 days) and aspirin for 14 days. A decreased incidence of cardiovascular complications at 14 days (8% vs. 23.1%) and at 49 days (3.8% vs. 17.7%) was reported in the group treated with both aspirin and immune globulin (Newburger et al., 1986). Further studies have demonstrated that 200 mg/kg/day of intravenous immune globulin is equally effective (Furusho et al., 1987). Moreover, immune globulin therapy improves cardiac function in patients with wall-motion abnormalities secondary to myocarditis (Newburger et al., 1989). Proposed mechanisms to explain the efficacy of intravenous immune globulin therapy include competition for endothelial cell receptors, negative feedback on the B cell lymphocyte system, and direct neutralization of a viral agent (Leung et al., 1987).

## Surgical Management

Advanced cardiovascular complications require surgical intervention. The first use of *coronary artery bypass grafting* (CABG) for obstructive coronary aneurysms in Kawasaki's disease was reported in 1976 by Kitamura and colleagues (1976). The procedure involved a 4-year-old boy with coronary aneurysms that obstructed the LAD and the RCA, diagnosed 10 months after presentation with Kawasaki's disease. General problems with CABG became apparent with experience, however. Further use of homologous and autologous *saphenous vein grafts* (SVGs) showed frequent early occlusion. In many patients, the distal coronary arteries appeared to be too small to accept vein grafts. Also, autogenous SVGs are not available in some children. The potential for SVGs to grow as the heart grows and the thoracic cavity expands is unknown.

Alternative grafts have been used in place of autogenous SVGs. Mains and associates (1983) have successfully used the right subclavian artery bypass to the LAD, and Kitamura and associates (1985) described the first use of the *internal mammary artery* (IMA) to treat patients with Kawasaki's disease. In a study by Hirose and associates (1986), the early patency rate of IMA grafts was 100%, and the overall early patency rate with both IMA and SVG was 83%. In that study, the late patency rate of the IMA was 50%, compared with 38% for the SVG. A study by Kitamura and colleagues (1988) showed 100% early and late patency (more than 1 year) of the IMA, compared with 90% early patency and 50% late patency of the SVG. In children younger than 8 years of age, patency of the SVG was 65%, compared with 87% in children older than 8 years. The use of the IMA provides greater patency and the potential for growth, both elongation and dilatation. The operative

■ **Table 54–24.** CRITERIA FOR CORONARY ARTERY BYPASS GRAFTING IN KAWASAKI'S DISEASE

Progressive coronary lesions
No distal coronary aneurysms or stenoses
Localized aneurysm with significant stenosis in the left main coronary artery
Significant stenosis in two coronary arteries
Progressive stenosis in the left anterior descending coronary artery
Presence of left ventricular aneurysm

indications for coronary bypass grafting are shown in Table 54–24 (Suzuki et al., 1985).

## SUMMARY

Kawasaki's disease is a fascinating disorder with many cardiovascular manifestations. Aspects of this disease yet to be explained include etiology, selectivity for children, and ability to progress to severe stages in view of its usually benign and self-limited nature.

## BIBLIOGRAPHY

Akagi, T., Rose, V., Benson, L. N., et al.: Outcome of coronary artery aneurysms after Kawasaki disease. J. Pediatr., 121:689, 1992.
Bierman, F. Z., and Gersony, W. M.: Kawasaki disease: Clinical perspective. J. Pediatr., 111:789, 1987.
Bligard, C. A.: Kawasaki disease and its diagnosis. Pediatr. Dermatol., 4:75, 1987.
Burns, J. C., Wiggins, J. W., Jr., Toews, W. H., et al.: Clinical spectrum of Kawasaki disease in infants younger than 6 months of age. J. Pediatr., 109:759, 1986.
Chung, K. J., Fulton, D. R., Lapp, R., et al.: One-year follow-up of cardiac and coronary artery disease in infants and children with Kawasaki disease. Am. Heart. J., 115:1263, 1988.
Crowley, D. C.: Cardiovascular complications of mucocutaneous lymph node syndrome. Pediatr. Clin. North Am., 31:1321, 1984.
Daniels, S. R., Specker, B., Capannari, T. E., et al.: Correlates of coronary artery aneurysm formation in patients with Kawasaki disease. Am. J. Dis. Child., 141:205, 1987.
Feild, C., Brady, S., and Lowe, B.: Relapsing Kawasaki's disease. Int. J. Cardiol., 15:241, 1987.
Fujiwara, T., Fujiwara, H., and Hamashima, Y.: Frequency and size of coronary arterial aneurysm at necropsy in Kawasaki disease. Am. J. Cardiol., 59:808, 1987.
Furusho, K., Kamiya, T., Nakano, H., et al.: High-dose intravenous gammaglobulin for Kawasaki disease. Lancet, 2:1055, 1984.
Furusho, K., Kamiya, T., Nakano, H., et al.: Japanese gamma globulin trials for Kawasaki disease. Prog. Clin. Biol. Res., 250:425, 1987.
Gersony, W. M.: Long-term issues in Kawasaki disease. J. Pediatr., 121:731, 1992.
Giesker, D. W., Pastuszak, W. T., Forouhar, F. A., et al.: Lymph node biopsy for early diagnosis in Kawasaki disease. Am. J. Surg. Pathol., 6:493, 1982.
Hicks, R. V., and Melish, M. E.: Kawasaki syndrome. Pediatr. Clin. North Am., 33:1151, 1986.
Hirose, H., Kawashima, Y., Nakano, S., et al.: Long-term results in surgical treatment of children 4 years old or younger with coronary involvement due to Kawasaki disease. Circulation, 74(Suppl. I):77, 1986.
Ichida, F., Fatica, N. S., Engle, M. A., et al.: Coronary artery involvement in Kawasaki syndrome in Manhattan, New York: Risk factors and role of aspirin. Pediatrics, 80:828, 1987.
Kamiya, T., and Suzuki, A.: Ischemic heart disease in Kawasaki disease. Prog. Clin. Biol. Res., 250:347, 1987.

Kato, H.: Cardiovascular involvement in Kawasaki disease. Prog. Clin. Biol. Res., 250:277, 1987.

Kato, H., Ichinose, E., and Kawasaki, T.: Myocardial infarction in Kawasaki disease: Clinical analysis in 195 cases. J. Pediatr., 108:923, 1986.

Kato, H., Ichinose, E., Yoshioka, F., et al.: Fate of coronary aneurysms in Kawasaki disease: Serial coronary angiography and long-term follow-up study. Am. J. Cardiol., 49:1758, 1982.

Kato, H., Koike, S., Tanaka, C., et al.: Coronary heart disease in children with Kawasaki disease. Jpn. Circ. J., 43:469, 1979.

Kato, H., Inoue, O., and Kawasaki, T.: Adult coronary artery disease probably due to childhood Kawasaki disease. Lancet, 340:1127, 1992.

Kawasaki, T.: Acute febrile mucocutaneous syndrome with lymphoid involvement with specific desquamation of the fingers and toes in children. Jpn. J. Allerg., 16:178, 1967.

Kitamura, S., Kawashima, Y., Fujita, T., et al.: Aortocoronary bypass grafting in a child with coronary artery obstruction due to mucocutaneous lymph node syndrome. Circulation, 53:1035, 1976.

Kitamura, S., Kawashima, Y., Kawachi, K., et al.: Severe mitral regurgitation due to coronary arteritis of mucocutaneous lymph node syndrome. A new surgical entity. J. Thorac. Cardiovasc. Surg., 80:629, 1980.

Kitamura, S., Kawachi, K., Oyama, C., et al.: Severe Kawasaki heart disease treated with an internal mammary graft in pediatric patients. A first successful report. J. Thorac. Cardiovasc. Surg., 89:860, 1985.

Kitamura, S., Seki, S., Kawachi, K., et al.: Excellent patency and growth potential of internal mammary artery grafts in pediatric coronary artery bypass surgery. New evidence for a "live" conduit. Circulation, 78(Suppl. I):129, 1988.

Koren, G., Lavi, S., Rose, V., et al.: Kawasaki disease: Review of risk factors for coronary artery aneurysms. J. Pediatr., 108:388, 1986.

Leung, D. Y. M.: Kawasaki disease. Curr. Opin. Rheum., 5:41, 1993.

Leung, D. Y., Burns, J. D., Newburger, J. W., et al.: Reversal of lymphocyte activation in vivo in the Kawasaki syndrome by intravenous gammaglobulin. J. Clin. Invest., 79:468, 1987.

Lin, C. Y., Lin, C. C., Hwang, B.: Serial changes of serum interleukin-6, interleukin-8, and tumor necrosis factor alpha among patients with Kawasaki disease. J. Pediatr., 121:924, 1992.

Mains, C., Wiggins, J., Groves, G., et al.: Surgical therapy for a complication of Kawasaki's disease. Ann. Thorac. Surg., 35:197, 1983.

Marchette, N. J., Ho, D., Kihara, S., et al.: Search for retrovirus etiology of Kawasaki syndrome. Prog. Clin. Biol. Res., 250:131, 1987.

Melish, M. E.: Kawasaki syndrome: A 1986 perspective. Rheum. Dis. Clin. North Am., 13:7, 1987.

Mercer, S., and Carpenter, B.: Surgical complications of Kawasaki disease. J. Pediatr. Surg., 16:444, 1981.

Nagashima, M., Matasushima, M., Matsuoka, H., et al.: High-dose gammaglobulin therapy for Kawasaki disease. J. Pediatr., 110:710, 1987.

Nakamura, Y., Yanagawa, H., and Kawasaki, T.: Mortality among children with Kawasaki disease in Japan. N. Engl. J. Med., 326:1246, 1992.

Nakanishi, T., Takao, A., Nakazawa, M., et al.: Mucocutaneous lymph node syndrome: Clinical and angiographic features of coronary obstructive disease. Am. J. Cardiol., 55:662, 1985.

Nakano, H., Ueda, K., Saito, A., et al.: Repeated quantitative angiograms in coronary arterial aneurysms in Kawasaki disease. Am. J. Cardiol., 56:846, 1985.

Nakano, H., Ueda, K., Saito, A., et al.: Scoring method for identifying patients with Kawasaki disease at high risk of coronary artery aneurysms. Am. J. Cardiol., 58:739, 1986.

Nehme, A. E., and Mikhail, R. A.: Kawasaki syndrome. An abdominal crisis. Am. Surg., 49:275, 1983.

Newburger, J. W., Sanders, S. P., Burns, J. C., et al.: Left ventricular contractility in Kawasaki syndrome. Effect of intravenous gamma-globulin. Circulation, 79:1237, 1989.

Newburger, J. W., Takahashi, M., Burns, J. C., et al.: The treatment of Kawasaki syndrome with intravenous gamma globulin. N. Engl. J. Med., 315:341, 1986.

Rauch, A. M.: Kawasaki syndrome: Review of new epidemiologic and laboratory developments. Pediatr. Infect. Dis. J., 6:1016, 1987.

Rowley, A. H., and Shulman, S. T.: The search for the etiology of Kawasaki disease. Pediatr. Infect. Dis. J., 6:506, 1987.

Rowley, A. H., and Shulman, S. T.: What is the status of intravenous gamma-globulin for Kawasaki syndrome in the United States and Canada? Pediatr. Infect. Dis. J., 7:463, 1988.

Rowley, A. H., Gonzalez-Crussi, F., and Shulman, S. T.: Kawasaki syndrome. Rev. Infect. Dis., 10:1, 1988.

Shulman, S. T., and Rowley, A. H.: Does Kawasaki disease have a retroviral etiology? Lancet, 2:545, 1986.

Shulman, S. T., Rowley, A. H., Fresco, R., et al.: The etiology of Kawasaki disease: Retrovirus? Prog. Clin. Biol. Res., 250:117, 1987.

Suma, K., Takeuchi, Y., Shiroma, K., et al.: Early and late postoperative studies in coronary arterial lesions resulting from Kawasaki's disease in children. J. Thorac. Cardiovasc. Surg., 84:224, 1982.

Suzuki, A., Kamiya, T., Ono, Y., et al.: Indication of aortocoronary bypass for coronary arterial obstruction due to Kawasaki disease. Heart-Vessels, 1:94, 1985.

Takahashi, M.: Myocarditis in Kawasaki syndrome. Circulation, 79:1398, 1989.

Takao, A., Niwa, K., Kondo, C., et al.: Mitral regurgitation in Kawasaki disease. Prog. Clin. Biol. Res., 250:311, 1987.

# 9  Assisted Circulation

Mark P. Anstadt and James E. Lowe

## HISTORICAL ASPECTS

Cardiogenic shock is a preterminal condition that complicates most cardiac disease states. As recently as the early 1970s, patients experiencing cardiogenic shock, even for a few hours, were expected to perish, hence the term *irreversible shock* (Burton, 1972). This concept originated before clinically feasible methods of assisted circulation became available. Assist devices now offer a completely new therapeutic alternative for patients in cardiogenic shock. Circulatory support devices can reverse the physiology of shock by restoring normal hemodynamics. The relatively safe methods that have been developed to assist the circulation represent phenomenal progress in both medicine and engineering and have broadened the therapeutic approach to cardiovascular disease. Whereas previous therapies merely prolonged an "irreversible" state of shock, assist devices can provide a unique opportunity for myocardial recovery.

Most influential in the development of modern assist devices was the introduction (Dennis et al., 1951) and successful application (Gibbon, 1954) of the pump-oxygenator. Initial success with *cardiopulmonary bypass* (CPB) marks the cornerstone in the field of assisted circulation. CPB remains the most common means for assisting the circulation. Although primarily known for its use during cardiac operations, CPB circuits are also employed for life support in other settings. In the 1950s, investigators (Connolly et al., 1958; Stuckey et al., 1957) used CPB to support the failing heart. Their success, however, was limited by the absence of appropriate patient selection criteria and insufficient means for achieving left ventricular unloading.

Other breakthroughs led to new approaches for assisting the circulation. Improved myocardial perfusion was described by the Kantrowitz brothers (1953), who experimentally delayed the arrival of systolic pressure to the coronary circulation by an interposed rubber conduit. This phenomenon, termed *diastolic augmentation*, was further exploited in compressing the aorta during diastole using a surgically transferred hemidiaphragm (Kantrowitz and McKinnon, 1959). Harken (1958) later postulated that aspiration of arterial blood during systole and reinfusion during diastole could diminish cardiac work without compromising perfusion. A device developed by Clauss and associates (1961) subsequently achieved "diastolic counterpulsation" by withdrawing and infusing blood via two femoral artery cannulas.

The most practical means of achieving diastolic augmentation was reported by Clauss and colleagues (1962) and Moulopoulos and co-workers (1962), who worked in independent laboratories. Both teams of investigators demonstrated that balloons positioned in the central aorta could augment diastolic pressure if inflated and deflated synchronous to the cardiac cycle. This simple yet ingenious method of intravascular volume displacement has evolved into the modern *intra-aortic balloon pump* (IABP) (Fig. 54–122).

Other important advancements in the field of circulatory support have addressed the interaction of blood with artificial surfaces. Innovative designs have reduced stasis within blood pumps, decreasing the incidence of thrombus formation. Furthermore, materials have been developed that cause less procoagulate activation. Heparin bonding of biomaterials can significantly decrease the necessary level of systemic anticoagulation (Lazzara et al., 1993). Another approach employs textured surfaces to stimulate blood elements to form an adherent neointima (Graham et al., 1990). This biologic coating serves as a thromboresistant barrier between the bloodstream and the blood pump's artificial surfaces. These innovations may reduce the bleeding and thromboembolic events that remain major complications of mechanical circulatory support.

Two techniques have been developed that avoid blood contact altogether. Described in the 1960s,

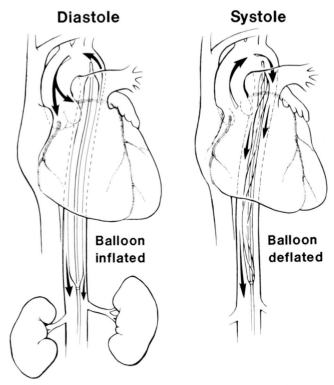

**FIGURE 54–122.** Schematic representation of a properly positioned intra-aortic balloon pump. Arrows indicate direction of blood volume displacement. During diastole, balloon inflation displaces blood, which augments coronary perfusion pressure. During systole, balloon deflation reduces resistance to forward flow. (From Anstadt, M. P.: Acquired cardiac conditions: Cardiac assist devices and the artificial heart. *In* Sabiston, D. C., and Lyerly, H. K. [eds]: *Sabiston Essentials of Surgery.* 2nd ed. Philadelphia, W. B. Saunders, 1994.)

both approaches physically massage the heart. One method, *dynamic cardiomyoplasty* (DCM), was first described by Kantrowitz (1960). With this technique, skeletal muscle is surgically wrapped around the heart and electrically stimulated to compress the cardiac chambers. The concept of muscle transformation (Salmons and Sreter, 1967), combined with subsequent developments in skeletal muscle stimulation (Drinkwater et al., 1980), may provide a role for cardiomyoplasty in the treatment of end-stage cardiac failure. A different approach for prolonged circulatory support, *direct mechanical ventricular actuation* (DMVA), was described by Anstadt and associates (1965). This method uses a "heart-cup," with a pneumatically regulated inner diaphragm for direct cardiac massage. DMVA has shown efficacy for prolonged circulatory support in humans (Lowe et al., 1991). To date, only DMVA and DCM can definitively circumvent the complications inherent to blood contact.

## PHYSIOLOGIC CONSIDERATIONS

Cardiogenic shock can result from either myocardial pump failure or peripheral vascular collapse. The underlying problem requiring circulatory support is most commonly pump failure secondary to myocardial ischemia, cardiomyopathy, or valvular disease. Conditions such as septicemia, intoxication, and metabolic disorders can lead to shock through a profound decrease in peripheral vascular resistance independent of cardiac failure. The use of assist devices in these latter settings is usually not indicated.

Assist devices typically are employed temporarily, with two primary therapeutic goals. First, they improve systemic blood flow and arterial pressure to achieve adequate organ perfusion. The preservation of vital organ function is essential to the ultimate success of any assist device. Second, these devices improve hemodynamics, thus reducing cardiac work and interrupting progressive myocardial injury. Reversing the pathophysiologic consequences of heart disease can effect myocardial recovery.

Normal myocardial function is possible only if the heart's right and left ventricles operate uniformly, as two pumps in series. The left ventricle most commonly requires assistance when significant cardiac decompensation occurs. For this reason, most cardiovascular compensatory mechanisms have been characterized for the *left ventricle* (LV) and the systemic circulation. However, these principles can also be applied to the *right ventricle* (RV) and pulmonary circulation. Because the RV and LV function in series, their outputs must be balanced with each other and, simultaneously, respond to a wide range of physiologic demands. These conditions are satisfied by the Frank-Starling law of the heart. Normally, each ventricle operates within a relatively narrow range of *end-diastolic volumes* (EDVS) or preloads. Changes in preload occur with fluctuations in venous return and are accommodated by variations in ventricular geometry. The degree of ventricular distention, in turn, alters the alignment of actin and myosin filaments, thereby modulating myocardial contractility. In this manner, the Frank-Starling relationship accounts for most normal changes in cardiac output and accounts for maintaining balanced flow between the right and the left ventricles.

The Frank-Starling relationship is best illustrated by ventricular pressure-volume curves. *Starling curves* (Fig. 54–123) depict changes in myocardial performance that result from physiologic alterations in preload and contractility. Load-dependent adjustments in performance help maintain ventricular output within an optimal range. When this mechanism is not sufficient to meet increased physiologic demands, other factors (e.g., increased heart rate, endogenous catecholamines) can independently influence the heart's contractile state and shift the Starling curve upward. On the other hand, myocardial ischemia depresses cardiac function, causing a downward shift in the Starling curve. Consequentially, the ischemic heart contracts less vigorously for any given EDV and is less responsive to further increases in preload.

In the setting of myocardial ischemia, increased EDV may initially compensate for decreased contractility. However, these salutary effects become less ade-

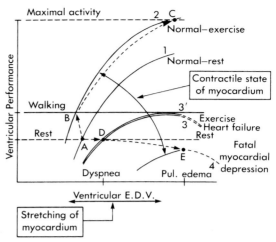

**FIGURE 54–123.** Starling's left ventricular function curves representing normal left ventricular function at rest and exercise (*upper curves* represent increased ventricular end-diastolic volume [E.D.V.]). Depressed left ventricular function may result from myocardial ischemia or infarction (*lower curves* show varying degrees of myocardial dysfunction). Progressive myocardial dysfunction may eventually lead to fatal myocardial depression. (From Braunwald, E., Ross, J., Jr., and Sonnenblick, E. H.: Control of cardiac performance and cardiac output: A synthesis. *In* Mechanisms of Contraction of the Normal and Failing Heart, edited by Braunwald, E., Ross, J., and Sonnenblick, E. H. Boston, Little Brown, 1968. Published by Little, Brown and Company.)

quate as cardiac pathology worsens. If LV distention continues to progress, the optimal wall tension for actin and myosin interactions is surpassed, further impairing contractile function. Reduced ventricular compliance is exhibited by disproportionate elevations in end-diastolic pressure with further increases in preload. Continued cardiac injury eventually eliminates the compensatory response as the heart dilates.

The deleterious effects of ventricular distension are based on the law of Laplace:

$$T = P \times R/h$$

where T = ventricular wall tension, P = intraventricular pressure, R = intracavitary radius, and h = ventricular wall thickness. Ventricular dilatation increases wall tension, creating an even greater demand for effective ventricular contraction. The cycle then set in motion places increasing stress on an already compromised heart. Cardiac output further declines, exacerbating the ischemic process that initiated these events.

The physiologic response to low cardiac output is mediated largely by the sympathetic nervous system. However, these acclimations often place increased demands on the failing heart. Endogenous catecholamines directly stimulate the heart to contract more vigorously and also increase peripheral vascular resistance. It has long been known that increases in afterload (pressure work) are significantly more costly in terms of myocardial oxygen consumption than increases in cardiac output (volume work) (Sarnoff et al., 1958) (Fig. 54–124). Other factors such as heart

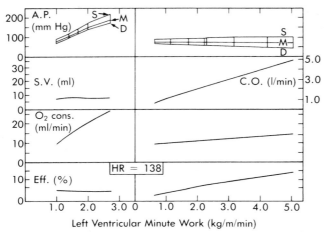

**FIGURE 54–124.** Relationship of myocardial oxygen consumption (demand) relative to increases in mean aortic pressure (A.P.) (pressure work—*left panel*) with constant cardiac output (C.O.) compared with increases in C.O. (volume work—*right panel*) with constant mean A.P. (left ventricular afterload). Pressure work is much more costly in terms of myocardial oxygen demand than volume work. Therapeutic interventions to relieve progressive myocardial ischemia should attempt to reduce left ventricular afterload. (From Sarnoff, S. J., Braunwald, E., Welch, G. H., et al.: Hemodynamic determinants of oxygen consumption of the heart with special reference to the tension-time index. Am. J. Physiol., *192*:148, 1958.)

rate and temperature affect myocardial oxygen demand, but to a lesser degree. Therefore, the primary hemodynamic determinants of myocardial oxygen consumption are best delineated by the *time-tension*

index (TTI) (Fig. 54–125). In contrast, the *diastolic pressure time index* (DPTI) represents the driving force for coronary blood flow, and measures myocardial oxygen delivery. The balance between myocardial oxygen supply and demand, or the DPTI:TTI ratio, is the *endocardial viability ratio* because of the endocardium's marked susceptibility to ischemia.

Optimal medical management of severe left ventricular power failure should be directed toward improving the unfavorable balance between myocardial oxygen supply and demand. Beta-blocking agents decrease myocardial oxygen demand, but may decrease ventricular performance, further compromising end-organ perfusion (Pierce et al., 1993). Patients in cardiogenic shock generally require high doses of inotropic agents to maintain organ perfusion by increasing myocardial contractility (Loisance et al., 1993). These agents cause a concomitant increase in myocardial oxygen consumption and frequently exacerbate myocardial ischemia. Afterload-reducing agents repress these negative effects by reducing ventricular work, but caution must be exercised to avoid jeopardizing coronary perfusion. No pharmacologic therapy is ideal, and ideally, correction of the underlying pathology should be accomplished before the onset of cardiogenic shock. Advances in interventional cardiology using thrombolytic agents and angioplasty have significantly improved the ability to acutely revascularize ischemic myocardium (Ghitis et al., 1991; Lee et al., 1988). If these measures fail to adequately restore hemodynamics, mechanical circulatory support should be considered.

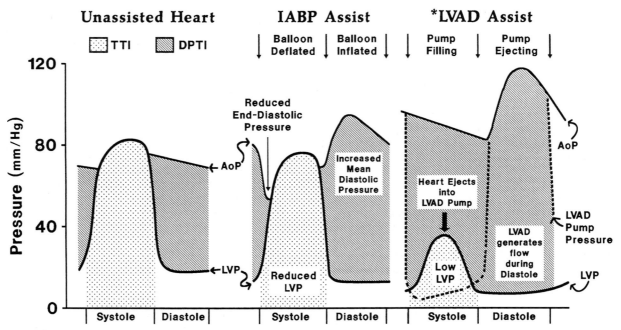

**FIGURE 54–125.** Hemodynamic determinants of myocardial oxygen demand (time tension index [TTI]) and delivery (diastolic pressure time index [DPTI]) are illustrated for the unassisted heart, and during intra-aortic balloon pump (IABP) and left ventricular assist device (LVAD) therapies. (AoP = aortic pressure; LVP = left ventricular pressure; asterisk = hemodynamic alterations representative for synchronized, LVAD counterpulsation.) (From Anstadt, M. P.: Acquired cardiac conditions: Cardiac assist devices and the artificial heart. *In* Sabiston, D. C., and Lyerly, H. K. [eds]: Sabiston Essentials of Surgery. 2nd ed. Philadelphia, W. B. Saunders, 1994.)

## THE INTRA-AORTIC BALLOON PUMP

When circulatory support is necessary, the IABP is generally considered the most appropriate initial therapy. This device assists the failing heart by decreasing afterload and increasing coronary perfusion pressure. Furthermore, IABP insertion requires minimal technical skill and can be accomplished at the bedside.

The IABP is not a true blood pump, but it improves the balance between myocardial oxygen supply and demand by displacing intravascular volume (see Fig. 54–122). The device's balloon occupies (inflation) and vacates (deflation) space within the central aorta during diastole and systole, respectively. Two favorable hemodynamic changes result (Bregman, 1976; Hanloser et al., 1966) (see Fig. 54–124). First, mean diastolic blood pressure increases owing to aortic volume displacement during balloon inflation. Second, afterload is reduced by the sudden vacancy of aortic volume caused by balloon deflation just before ventricular emptying. *Diastolic augmentation*, the term adopted to describe these hemodynamic alterations, highlights the increase in coronary perfusion pressure that can alleviate myocardial ischemia (Cox et al., 1975; Maroko et al., 1972). However, it should be emphasized that afterload reduction is the IABP's most beneficial effect on the failing heart (Buckley et al., 1970; Rose et al., 1979).

The myocardium has a better opportunity for recovery when provided afterload reduction combined with augmented diastolic pressure (Bregman, 1976; Corday et al., 1970). In addition, afterload reduction lowers the resistance to forward flow, which enhances ventricular emptying, so that cardiac output is increased. Reductions in EDV further reduce myocardial oxygen demand by lowering ventricular wall tension. The resulting improvements in myocardial function allow further increases in cardiac output and end-organ perfusion. Thus, the IABP can reverse the ongoing deterioration that characterizes medically refractory cardiogenic shock (Scheidt et al., 1973).

## Indications and Results

In general, most patients suffering cardiogenic shock who do not adequately respond to maximal pharmacologic measures are considered potentialcandidates for IABP support (Tables 54–25 and 54–26). However, the appropriate regimen of pharmacologic therapy before initiating IABP support remains controversial. Some argue that earlier institution of IABP therapy may decrease the risk of further end-organ damage that frequently complicates the prolonged use of high-dose inotropic agents. These unresolved issues, along with the fact that some therapeutic indications remain controversial, explain the apparent variations in IABP use among reporting institutions, (Naunheim et al., 1992) (Table 54–27). This discussion reviews the current indications for use of the

■ **Table 54–25.** GENERAL CRITERIA FOR IABP SUPPORT FOLLOWING CARDIAC SURGERY

Inability to separate from CPB despite multiple interventions after 30 minutes
Inadequate hemodynamics despite maximal inotropic support including:
  Persistent hypotension (systolic blood pressure <70 mm Hg)
  Low cardiac index (<2.0 l/min/m$^2$)
  Elevated left atrial pressure (>20 mm Hg)
  High peripheral vascular resistance (>2500 dynes/sec/cm$^{-5}$)
Requirement of inotropic agents at deleterious levels
Persistent malignant ventricular arrhythmias

*Key:* IABP = intra-aortic balloon pump; CPB = cardiopulmonary bypass.

IABP along with the reported outcome for these applications.

### Cardiogenic Shock Secondary to Acute Myocardial Infarction

It has been well established that patients suffering acute *myocardial infarction* (MI) who meet hemodynamic criteria for cardiogenic shock (mean arterial pressure less than 60 mm Hg or systolic pressure less than 90 mm Hg, pulmonary capillary wedge pressure greater than 18 to 20 mm Hg, cardiac index less than 1.8 to 2.0 l/m$^2$/min, and urine output less than 20 ml/hr) experience a mortality of 100% when there is no improvement with medical therapy (Scheidt et al., 1970). When the IABP first became clinically available, it was used most commonly for treating patients who experienced medically refractory shock secondary to MI (Weber and Janicki, 1974). In more than 75% of such patients, IABP support can produce significant hemodynamic improvement (Dunkman et al., 1972; Levine and Austen, 1983). However, survival for this group of patients has remained consistently low (less than 20%) except in those whose underlying pathology can be corrected (Allen et al., 1989; Bolooki, 1989; Bolooki et al., 1976). When IABP therapy leads to revascularization or repair of other underlying pathology, prognosis can be significantly improved (Bolooki, 1985; Pennington et al., 1983). Therefore, the IABP's role has changed significantly; today's approach is to use the IABP as an adjunct for other

■ **Table 54–26.** INDICATIONS FOR IABP SUPPORT

Postcardiotomy cardiogenic shock (most commonly, inability to separate from CPB)
Cardiogenic shock secondary to myocardial infarction in addition to:
  Postinfarction ventricular septal defect
  Postinfarction papillary muscle rupture with mitral regurgitation
Myocardial ischemia refractory to medical therapy including:
  Unstable angina
  Refractory ventricular tachyarrhythmias
Postoperative cardiogenic shock
Preoperative prophylaxis (less common)
Failed coronary angioplasty with myocardial ischemia (preoperative)

*Key:* IABP = intra-aortic balloon pump; CPB = cardiopulmonary bypass.

■ **Table 54–27.** MODERN SURVIVAL RESULTS FOR POSTCARDIOTOMY IABP

| Series | n | Frequency of IABP Insertion | | Thirty-day Mortality (%) | Two-year Survival (%) |
| --- | --- | --- | --- | --- | --- |
| | | *No* | % | | |
| Washington University | 6877 | 432 | 6.3 | 34 | 56 |
| Duke University | 3297 | 90 | 3.0 | 40 | 42 |
| T.H.I.–B.C.M. | 2813 | 322 | 11.4 | 48 | — |
| St. Louis University | 6856 | 473 | 6.9 | 42 | 49 |

From Naunheim, K. S., Swartz, M. T., Pennington, D. G., et al.: Intra-aortic balloon pumping in patients requiring cardiac operations. J. Thorac. Cardiovasc. Surg., *104*:1654, 1992.
*Key:* IABP = intra-aortic balloon pump; T.H.I.–B.C.M. = Texas Heart Institute and Baylor College of Medicine.

interventions. Approximately two-thirds of patients who receive IABP therapy in this manner are found to have operable coronary anatomy. Thrombolysis or coronary angioplasty can acutely reestablish perfusion in a number of patients and the decision for surgery can be made later (Ghitis et al., 1991; Lee et al., 1988). In other situations, the IABP provides a period of hemodynamic stabilization before emergent surgical revascularization. Survival following these strategies has been improved to approximately 50% in those patients amenable to definitive therapy (McEnany et al., 1978; Naunheim et al., 1992; Pierri et al., 1980) versus the nearly uniform mortality among those with uncorrectable disease.

The IABP's ability to improve outcome in the setting of cardiogenic shock secondary to acute MI stems from the current approach to acute cardiac ischemia. It is now well established that timely reperfusion can salvage ischemic myocardium at risk of infarction (Reimer et al., 1977) and improve survival following MI (Moritz and Wolner, 1993). The IABP provides critical, temporizing support that stabilizes the patient for further evaluation and reperfusion therapy when appropriate. Successful reperfusion is in turn associated with improved survival. Selection of the appropriate reperfusion technique is determined by the patient's condition, coronary anatomy, and the availability of treatment options. However, the most efficacious method for revascularization will remain somewhat controversial until long-term patency rates and patient outcome are assessed adequately.

### Mechanical Complications of Acute MI

Treatment options are relatively limited when support is required for an acutely ruptured ventricular septum or papillary muscle. Ischemic *ventricular septal defect* (VSD) or *mitral valve regurgitation* (MR) demand early surgical intervention to avoid an otherwise exceedingly high mortality. Both MR and VSD result from tissue necrosis (Mallory et al., 1939; Sanders et al., 1957; Wei et al., 1979) and can complicate MI by days to 1 or 2 weeks. The IABP can provide emergent, preoperative support when these complications occur (Heitmiller et al., 1986), whereas pharmacologic agents may be counterproductive.

In the case of VSD, vasoconstrictors further accentuate left-to-right shunting, and afterload-reducing agents can further jeopardize coronary perfusion. The IABP is an ideal therapy because it decreases left-to-right shunting by lowering peak systolic pressures while augmenting diastolic pressures, which, in turn, enhance myocardial perfusion (Gold et al., 1973). The IABP therefore provides a critical period of hemodynamic stabilization, which prepares the patient for surgery while minimizing risks of further cardiac or other end-organ damage. The mortality rates for VSD following acute MI have thereby been reduced from more than 80% with no surgical intervention (Oyamada and Queen, 1961; Sanders et al., 1956) to approximately 25% with successful VSD repair (Dagget et al., 1982; Gaudiani et al., 1981).

The successful treatment of MR following acute MI has also been improved with use of the IABP. This catastrophic event responds poorly to medical therapy. Inotropic agents that are used to restore contractility cause increases in afterload and myocardial oxygen consumption that can exacerbate both mitral insufficiency and cardiac ischemia. As in the therapy of VSD, the IABP can reduce the mechanical impairment of MR by reducing afterload while augmenting coronary blood flow through elevations in diastolic perfusion pressure (Mueller et al., 1972). Unfortunately, the surgical mortality for the treatment of this condition is nearly 50% and is probably related to the extent of underlying cardiac dysfunction (DiSesa et al., 1982; Magovern et al., 1985; Radford et al., 1979; Tepe and Edmunds, 1985). Although discouraging, these results represent a significant improvement of the more than 90% overall mortality rate without surgical therapy (DeBusk and Harrison, 1969; DePasquale and Burch, 1971; Morrow et al., 1968; Sanders et al., 1957; Wei et al., 1979). There is some evidence that mitral repair as opposed to replacement may lead to better results in the treatment of MR (Connolly et al., 1986). Regardless of the choice of operative repair, the IABP is a valuable adjunct for the treatment of ischemic MR or VSD.

### Postcardiotomy Cardiogenic Shock

Since the early 1970s, the largest subpopulation of IABP recipients has been those who undergo cardiac surgery and either cannot separate from CPB or experience cardiac failure during the early postoperative period. In the United States, postoperative IABP support is used in 2 to 12% of adult cardiac operations (Baldwin et al., 1993; Creswell et al., 1992; Di Lello et al., 1988; Golding et al., 1980; Naunheim et al., 1992; Pennington et al., 1983), which accounts for 30 to 50% of all IABP applications (Bolooki, 1985).

Most patients who receive postcardiotomy IABP support can be weaned, with 30-day and 2-year survival ranging from 52 to 65% and 42 to 56%, respectively (see Table 54–27). Long-term survival differs little from that of patients with similar LV function who do not require IABP support (Davies et al., 1980; Golding et al., 1980), corroborating clinical reviews that identify ventricular function as the most influential prognostic factor for the postcardiotomy patient (Force et al., 1990; Lytle et al., 1987; Myers et al., 1989). Ventricular function, and therefore patient outcome, can be jeopardized when IABP therapy is not instituted expeditiously (Anstadt et al., 1992; Bolooki et al., 1976; Norman et al., 1977).

Predicting the need for IABP support has been difficult, if not impossible. Univariate, preoperative factors (i.e., LV function, congestive heart failure, emergent operation) can estimate the likelihood for poor outcome following cardiac surgery (Adler et al., 1986; Brahos et al., 1985; Chaitman et al., 1990; Edwards et al., 1990; Freed et al., 1988; Miller et al., 1983; Sergeant et al., 1986). However, the need for postcardiotomy support can only be objectively determined when weaning from CPB. Most commonly, postcardiotomy low-output syndromes result from preexisting myocardial dysfunction, inadequate intraoperative myocardial protection, or perioperative MI. Technical errors and prolonged CPB times can also be important contributing factors. In most patients, the IABP can successfully reverse hemodynamic deterioration, but mortality rates still approach 50% (Bolooki, 1985; Di Lello et al., 1988; Gottlieb et al., 1984; Naunheim et al., 1992; Pennington et al., 1983; Wasfie et al., 1988) (see Table 54–27).

Hemodynamic criteria can help identify patients who need IABP support following cardiac surgery (see Table 54–25). Patients who cannot maintain peak systolic pressures of more than 90 mm Hg, pulmonary capillary wedge pressures of less than 18 to 20 mm Hg, or cardiac indices of more than 1.8 to 2.0 l/min/m² despite appropriate therapeutic measures (volume replacement, correction of acid/base imbalances, inotropic support, afterload reduction, and temporary pacing) should receive an IABP without further delay (Norman et al., 1977). These standards can be confounded by pharmacologic regimens and the trial periods used to assess each therapy. Universal protocols that would dictate these critical decisions do not yet exist.

Only clinical trials can objectively determine the optimal therapeutic regimens prior to IABP insertion. Until then, miscalculations can subject patients to excessive doses of inotropic agents or unnecessary IABP support, which are both attended by significant risks. Some investigators have shown that delaying IABP therapy can increase mortality; "delay," however, requires further definition (Anstadt et al., 1992; Bolooki et al., 1976; Golding et al., 1980; Parascandola et al., 1988; Pierce et al., 1993). Timing becomes more ambiguous when IABP therapy manifests marginal results and ventricular assist device (VAD) therapy is considered.

## MI Refractory to Medical Therapy

The IABP's ability to enhance myocardial recovery has led to other applications. One example is the treatment of medically refractory (unstable) angina. In general, unstable angina before surgical revascularization is associated with a poor prognosis (Fischl et al., 1973; Fulton et al., 1974; Gazes et al., 1973; Schuster and Bulkley, 1981). This condition can occur in two groups of patients. One group has no evidence of MI, termed *preinfarction unstable angina*, and the other is in convalescence from infarction, termed *postinfarction unstable angina*. IABP before revascularization may benefit patients in either group (Bardet et al., 1977; Gold et al., 1976; Harris et al., 1980; Levine et al., 1978). Clearly, IABP support benefits those patients whose condition before revascularization is complicated by hemodynamic instability.

## IABP as an Adjunct to Coronary Angioplasty

*Percutaneous transluminal coronary angioplasty* (PTCA) is now a common treatment for coronary artery disease. Major complications occur in 3 to 8% of PTCA procedures and usually derive from occlusion or dissection of the treated coronary artery (Abdelmeguid and Ellis, 1994). A significant number of these complications cause hemodynamic instability, and the IABP plays an important role in stabilizing these patients before surgical revascularization. Other IABP applications are being evaluated in the cardiac catheterization suite, such as "prophylactic" IABP-assisted PTCA in patients determined to be at high risk for these procedures. However, until criteria have been established that identify those patients who benefit from IABP-assisted angioplasty, such applications should be considered investigational.

## Bridge-to-Cardiac Transplantation

The first successful bridge-to-cardiac transplantation using an IABP was reported by Reemstma and colleagues (1978), before cardiac transplantation was popularized. Subsequent use of cyclosporine led to the acceptance of heart transplantation as a standard therapy in select patients (Hunt and Schroeder, 1994). Cardiac transplants have since reached a plateau because donor availability has been limited (Kaye, 1992; McManus et al., 1993). The combination of fewer organ donors and broader criteria for recipients has left a growing number of patients awaiting cardiac replacement. Because there is no therapeutic alternative to heart transplantation, mechanical devices are the only life-sustaining alternative for patients who deteriorate hemodynamically prior to transplantation. The IABP is generally considered the initial therapy of choice for patients with hemodynamic instability who are awaiting transplantation (Dembitsky et al., 1992; Hardesty et al., 1986; Marks et al., 1992; Reedy et al., 1992). Criteria established for postcardiotomy patients help determine the need for mechanical support (see Table 54–25). The IABP provides sufficient stabilization in more than 50% of patients (Birovljev et al., 1992; Marks et al., 1992; Oaks et al., 1989; O'Connell et al., 1988; Pifarre et al., 1992; Reedy et al., 1992). However, questions still exist regarding the acceptable level of pharmacologic support both before and after inserting an IABP. Even more controversial is the inclination to use VADs as a first-line therapy instead of the IABP (Hetzer et al., 1992).

Patients awaiting cardiac transplantation exhibit distinguishing features that affect these therapeutic algorithms (Dembitsky et al., 1992; Hetzer et al., 1992; Loisance et al., 1993; Pennington et al., 1993). The response to inotropic agents may be blunted in end-stage cardiac failure, particularly when these agents have already been required for extended periods. Physiologic changes that accompany these chronic disease states may make end-organs more tolerant of deleterious hemodynamic conditions. Although each of these factors should be taken into account, the clinician's primary concern is the preservation of end-organ function (Pierce et al., 1993). The IABP can improve organ perfusion, but adds risk of other complications that can preclude transplantation (Copeland et al., 1985; Pifarre et al., 1992; Reedy et al., 1992). This dilemma requires careful consideration; patients awaiting transplantation on mechanical support are subject to the same strict selection criteria as those not requiring such measures.

### Other Indications

The IABP has been applied less frequently in other conditions associated with MI or myocardial dysfunction. One example is the treatment of medically refractory ventricular arrhythmias (Bolooki, 1985; Bregman, 1976; Mundth et al., 1975; Willerson et al., 1975). The IABP can often abate ischemically induced ventricular arrhythmias by augmenting perfusion to the ischemic zone. Patients who respond should be evaluated promptly for revascularization. The IABP has also been used to treated septic shock, with modest results (Berger et al., 1973; McEneny et al., 1978; O'Rouke, 1977), as well as patients with inoperable coronary artery disease who develop MI during general surgical procedures (Grotz and Yeston, 1989).

Although there appears to be an ever-expanding potential for the IABP, a few conditions represent contraindications to its implementation. Both aortic aneurysm and acute aortic dissection should discourage IABP insertion. Finally, *aortic insufficiency* (AI) is considered a contraindication to IABP support, because diastolic augmentation generally aggravates regurgitation. However, when hemodynamic instability is associated with less severe forms of AI, the benefits of afterload reduction may outweigh the relatively moderate increases in valvular insufficiency (Yellin et al., 1973).

### Balloon Use and Complications

Use of the IABP is relatively easy. First, the common femoral artery is accessed by surgical exposure or percutaneous techniques (Bolooki, 1985; Bregman, 1976). Approaching the femoral artery midway between the inguinal ligament and the origin of the profunda femoris artery is ideal. More proximal cannulation risks bleeding that is difficult to control, and entry near the profunda femoris can jeopardize arterial patency. Percutaneous catheters of graduated size are passed over a guidewire until the balloon can be accommodated. The balloon's tip is advanced just below the origin of the left subclavian artery, with its proximal portion above the renal arteries (see Fig. 54–122). Deviations above or below this location may cause aortic arch trauma or renal artery occlusion, respectively.

Balloon insertion is not possible in 5 to 10% of patients because of severe aortoiliac or femoral disease (Bahn et al., 1979; Beckman et al., 1977; McEnany et al., 1978). One alternative during surgery is to introduce the balloon via a small Dacron graft sewn to the ascending aorta (Bolooki, 1984). The graft is exteriorized at sternotomy closure, which facilitates nonoperative removal. Other insertion sites can be used, but they are more technically difficult and may lead to significant complications. In all cases, fluoroscopic guidance or a postinsertion chest radiograph is necessary to confirm proper IABP positioning.

Proper insertion can minimize the reported 9 to 36% incidence of leg ischemia, the most common complication during IABP support (Alderman et al., 1987; Alpert et al., 1976; Hauser et al., 1982; Kantrowitz et al., 1986). Serial evaluations of the lower extremities following balloon insertion are important to identify ischemic complications early and avoid limb loss. Significant ischemia requires balloon withdrawal and exploration of the femoral artery with a Fogarty catheter to remove clots. Another balloon can then be placed in the contralateral extremity. An alternative for patients unable to tolerate balloon withdrawal is to employ a femoral-femoral crossover graft to reestablish flow to the ischemic leg.

Less common complications of IABP support include infection and bleeding. Anticoagulation reduces the incidence of thrombosis and embolic sequelae, but increases the risk of bleeding. Associated hematoma formation at the balloon insertion site provides an ideal media for wound infections. Fortunately, when infections occur, they usually remain localized and can be effectively treated without further sequelae. The incidence of infectious complications (1 to 3%), increases with the use of percutaneous insertion, and may be as high as 30% in obese and diabetic patients (Martin et al., 1983). Therefore, prophylactic antibiotics have been recommended during IABP support (Goldman et al., 1982). Proper balloon positioning reduces the incidence of other complications. Incorrect balloon positioning may cause inadequate counterpulsation or occlusion of major aortic branches (Pennington et al., 1983; Weber and Janicki, 1974). Furthermore, improperly situated balloons increase the risk for balloon rupture. Balloon rupture is a serious complication, and it may occur significantly more often than reported (Alvarez et al., 1992).

After proper placement, balloon pumping must be carefully synchronized with the cardiac cycle (Bregman, 1976; Corday et al., 1970). Inflation should coincide with the dicrotic notch and be maintained through diastole. Balloon deflation just before the aortic valve opens optimizes afterload reduction (see Fig. 54–123). If balloon inflation is too prolonged, the heart may experience periods of increased afterload, which would be counterproductive. On the other hand, early balloon deflation will diminish the desired hemodynamic effect and may cause counterproductive periods of decreased or even retrograde diastolic coronary flow (Corday et al., 1970; Weber and Janicki, 1974).

Aberrant cardiac rhythms and rapid heart rates are common clinical conditions that unfavorably alter the IABP's efficacy (Kantrowitz et al., 1992; Weber and Janicki, 1974). Arrhythmias can be so severe that synchronous support is not possible, in which case, a fixed rate independent of the heart's rhythm can be used. Tachycardia presents yet another problem because the IABP can fill and empty only at a limited rate. Although heart rates up to 140/minute can generally be followed with smaller balloon sizes, rates that exceed 100/minute often limit effective augmentation to every other beat (1 to 2 mode). Unfortunately, reducing the frequency of augmentation not only reduces effectiveness but also abruptly increases afterload with each unassisted cardiac cycle, which may be detrimental.

IABP support is continued until cardiac recovery permits reduction or discontinuation of inotropic agents. Weaning can be accomplished by one of two methods. The most common technique is *rate weaning*, in which the frequency of augmentation (1 : 2, 1 : 3, etc.) is gradually decreased. However, sudden increases in afterload that accompany each unassisted cardiac cycle may hinder myocardial recovery. An alternative technique, *volume weaning*, gradually reduces balloon inflation volume. When cardiac function is deemed adequate, the IABP is temporarily turned off or "fluttered," and the patient's hemodynamic stability is assessed before the balloon is withdrawn.

A comment should be made regarding IABP development: The efficacy of diastolic augmentation is directly related to the volume displacement (Weber and Janicki, 1974). The latest developments in percutaneous balloons allow rapid insertion and diversify the IABP's clinical utility (Kantrowitz et al., 1992). However, the small size of percutaneous balloons further limits their effectiveness. Balloon responsiveness may also be restricted because of the relatively slender catheters being used for gas delivery. Finally, reports indicate that percutaneous insertion techniques may

increase the incidence of complications during IABP support (Collier et al., 1986). These trends deserve careful evaluation to determine if IABP performance is being significantly sacrificed.

## VENTRICULAR ASSIST DEVICES

The IABP can benefit only the marginally impaired LV. *Ventricular assist devices* (VADs) provide more effective support of the severely impaired ventricle. Unlike the IABP, VADs are true pumps that temporarily substitute for the *left* (LVAD), *right* (RVAD), or *both* ventricles (BVAD). The complexity and expense of VADs is reflected by their technically demanding installation, and their use frequently causes significant morbidity and mortality (Hill et al., 1993; Miller et al., 1990; Moritz and Wolner, 1993; Pae et al., 1992; Pierce et al., 1993). For these reasons, VAD use requires both surgical skill and careful clinical judgment (Pennington et al., 1993).

Vascular access is similar for most VAD systems (Hahn et al., 1993a; Lick et al., 1993; Magovern et al., 1993; Pennington and Swartz, 1990). LVADs are most commonly used owing to the predominance of LV failure. In these circumstances, an inlet cannula is positioned in the left atrium or LV and a return cannula in the ascending aorta (Figs. 54–126A and B). Biventricular support requires that an additional set

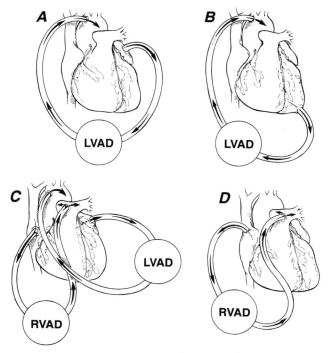

FIGURE 54–126. Four common configurations for ventricular devices. Left ventricular assist devices (LVADs) usually employ an inlet cannula placed in either the left atrium (*A*) or the left ventricular apex (*B*) and an outlet cannula in the ascending aorta. Right ventricular assist devices (RVADs) have an inlet and outlet cannula positioned in the right atrium and the pulmonary artery, respectively (*D*). Biventricular support entails a combination of an RVAD and an LVAD (*C*).

of inlet and outlet cannulas be placed in the right atrium and pulmonary artery (Fig. 54–126C). These latter cannulation sites are also employed during isolated right ventricular support (Fig. 54–126D).

It is important to underscore that all forms of cardiac failure affect both the LV and the RV to some degree. Inotropic agents and volume loading are often sufficient for RV dysfunction, but LV failure requires mechanical support on a more frequent basis. Nevertheless, RV function must always be carefully assessed during LVAD support; significant right ventricular failure that remains unrecognized is associated with a high mortality.

During severe left ventricular failure, LVADs can reinstate normal flow, improving arterial pressures and organ perfusion. The LV benefits from decreased end-diastolic pressure as blood is diverted to the filling VAD. The decrease in LV preload reduces myocardial wall tension, which in turn attenuates oxygen demand. Reductions in left atrial pressure also relieve pulmonary congestion. As pulmonary arterial pressures decline, there is less resistance to RV emptying. Consequently, the pulmonary edema and RV dysfunction that result from LV failure are usually reversed by an LVAD.

Optimal reductions in cardiac work are achieved when a pulsatile VAD provides synchronous counterpulsation (Axelrod et al., 1987; Laas et al., 1981) (see Fig. 54–125). In this situation, the heart ejects directly into the filling VAD. The VAD, in turn, pumps during cardiac diastole. TTI is thereby markedly reduced owing to the low resistance offered by the LVAD pump. DPTI is also optimized by the augmented diastolic pressures of LVAD counterpulsation. Unfortunately, synchronous LVAD support has proved difficult to achieve in most clinical settings owing to technical problems with device timing. Most pulsatile systems are instead operated in a nonsynchronous, "fill-to-empty" mode (Farrar and Hill, 1993; Pennington et al., 1988). Sensors detect when the pump is full and signal VAD emptying. As a result, the pump is more completely "washed" during each cycle, which reduces blood stagnation and the likelihood of thrombus formation within the pump.

A broad assortment of blood pumps can support the failing heart (Rowles et al., 1993). Although a detailed description of each device is another subject in itself, certain properties that differentiate VADs from one another provide a basis for selecting a device. One such feature is the generation of either pulsatile or nonpulsatile flow.

Nonpulsatile VADs generally are easier to use and less expensive (Dembitsky et al., 1993; Hill et al., 1992; Magovern, 1993; Pennington et al., 1984; Phillips, 1986). These systems employ either roller or, more commonly, centrifugal pumps (Fig. 54–127), as do conventional CPB circuits. Use of such devices has curtailed exhaustive regulatory restraints, and thus has kept costs relatively low and availability of the pumps widespread. Centrifugal pumps are the most frequently used nonpulsatile VADs. The three centrifugal VADs available for clinical use are manufactured

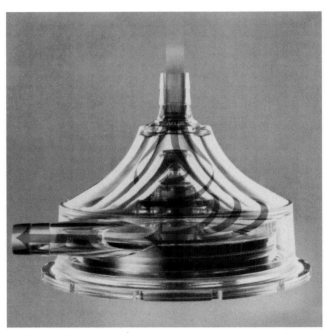

**FIGURE 54–127.** A Medtronic Biomedicus assist device (Eden Prairie, MN), the most frequently used centrifugal pump. The inlet and outlet ports are in the central and the outer aspects of the pump housing, respectively. A rotating cone located within the housing creates a vortex, which causes blood to flow as indicated by the arrows. Centrifugal pumps generate nonpulsatile flow and are the most common form of assist device in use. (Courtesy of Medtronic Biomedicus.)

by Medtronic Biomedicus (Eden Prairie, MN), Sarns 3M Health Care (Ann Arbor, MI), and St. Jude Medical (Chelmsford, MA). Each device generates flow by vortexing blood with rotating cones or impellers. The vortex creates a central area of low pressure where blood enters the pump housing. Blood then exits the housing's outer perimeter, where maximal pressures are developed. The housing and impeller designs of each available pump have different theoretical advantages. Of these systems, the Biomedicus is the most widely used. However, Food and Drug Administration (FDA) regulations may be implemented to restrict use of all centrifugal pumps to 6 hours or less. If these are enforced, new approval processes will be required to permit the flexible use nonpulsatile VADs have previously enjoyed.

Unlike nonpulsatile pumps, which generate continuous flow, pulsatile VADs oscillate flow in a manner that more closely mimics the normal hemodynamic state (Champsaur et al., 1990; Portner, 1993; Sato et al., 1993; Takano et al., 1993). Generally, pulsatile VADs propel blood with motorized pusher plates (Fig. 54–128) or hydraulically actuated, flexible sacs (Fig. 54–129). Although relatively complex, pulsatile VADs are more reliable and less likely to cause embolic or hemolytic complications than are nonpulsatile VADs. Clinical experience has not yet demonstrated a significant difference in patient outcome following hours to days of support with either pulsatile or nonpulsatile systems (Miller et al., 1990; Pae et al.,

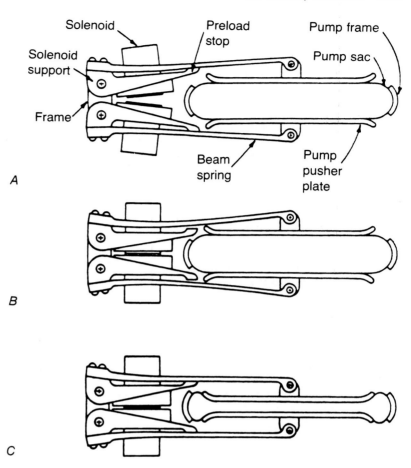

**FIGURE 54–128.** *A,* The Novacor left ventricular assist device (Baxter Healthcare, Oakland, CA). Pusher plates are regulated by a solenoid to compress (*C*) and dilate (*B*) a pump sac. In this manner, the device generates pulsatile flow. The pump is implanted. (*A–C,* From Bernhard, W. F., Warren, C., Howell, N. A., et al.: Ventricular assist devices for left and right heart support: Clinical and experimental considerations. *In* Kapoor, A. S., and Laks, H. [eds]: Cardiomyopathies and Heart-Lung Transplantation. New York, McGraw-Hill, 1991. Reproduced with permission.)

1992). Yet, despite technically difficult installation, pulsatile VADs do appear to offer a better opportunity for either long-term (Farrar and Hill, 1993; Hahn et al., 1993b), or even permanent circulatory support (Portner et al., 1993). For these reasons, pulsatile VADs are presently being developed for long-term or permanently implantable support, whereas most nonpulsatile VADs have remained extracorporeal and are intended for short-term use.

Numerous extracorporeal pulsatile VADs are cur-

rently available for temporary circulatory support (Hahn et al., 1993a; Takano et al., 1993). These pneumatic pumps are tethered to external-drive systems, which can limit patient mobility. The Pierce-Donachy Ventricular Assist Device (Thoratec Laboratories, Berkeley, CA) uses a smooth, sac-like pump contained within a rigid housing (Pennington et al., 1988). The flexible pouches are pneumatically regulated to pump blood (see Fig. 54–129). A fill-to-empty mode reduces the thromboembolic complications that have been as-

**FIGURE 54–129.** A Pierce-Donachy ventricular assist device (Thoratec Laboratories, Berkeley, CA). The flexible sac within the pump's rigid housing is pneumatically regulated to generate pulsatile blood flow. Blood flows (arrows) only in one direction because of valves positioned in the inlet and outlet of the pump housing. This pneumatic pump is the most common type of pulsatile ventricular assist device in use. (From Pennington, G. D., and Swartz, M. T.: Assisted circulation and artificial hearts: *In* Greenfield, L. J. [ed]: Surgery: Scientific Principles and Practice. Philadelphia, J. B. Lippincott, 1993.)

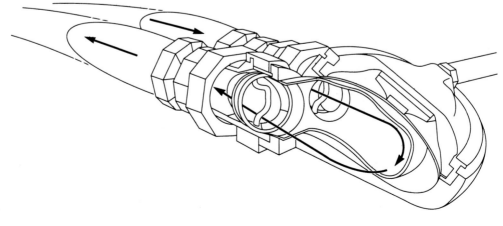

sociated with incomplete pump ejection. Heparin is still administered during VAD support unless bleeding is a problem. The Pierce-Donachy device has been used clinically more than any other pulsatile VAD (Farrar and Hill, 1993), but is not yet FDA approved.

One extracorporeal pulsatile VAD (ABIOMED, Danvers, MA) has been granted FDA approval for market in the United States (Champsaur et al., 1990). Distinctive features of this system include a dual-chambered blood pump and trileaflet polyurethane valves (Fig. 54–130). The upper chamber serves as an "artificial atrium" allowing continuous, uninterrupted gravity-filling, which may reduce the risk of hemolysis associated with vacuum-assisted filling. The lower chamber represents an "artificial ventricle" that ejects in a fill-to-empty mode. Polyurethane valves contribute to the device's affordability, compared with VADs, which require commercially available valves. Like other extracorporeal VADs, the ABIOMED is somewhat cumbersome, restricting patient mobility.

The problems surrounding patient mobility can be improved dramatically with implantable VADs (Port-

ner et al., 1993). First-generation systems are still tethered to external drive consoles. However, "wearable" power sources that are carried as lightweight backpacks are now being investigated. Currently, two wearable VADs are being evaluated in clinical trials: the Novacor LVAD (Baxter Healthcare, Oakland, CA) and the HeartMate LVAD (Thermo Cardiosystems, Woburn, MA). The Novacor system (Fig. 54–131; see also Fig. 54–128) has clearly demonstrated the most significant progress toward a totally implantable VAD (Portner, 1993). On the other hand, textured biomaterials used to construct the blood-contacting components of the HeartMate system (Fig. 54–132) may alter the requirement for long-term systemic anticoagulation (Poirier, 1993). A combination of these technologic achievements may be achieved in future, state-of-the-art devices.

Totally implantable VADs represent the most sophisticated development goal in the field of circulatory support (see Fig. 54–131). Planned systems eliminate percutaneous lines and use transformers for inductive power transmission across the skin. The

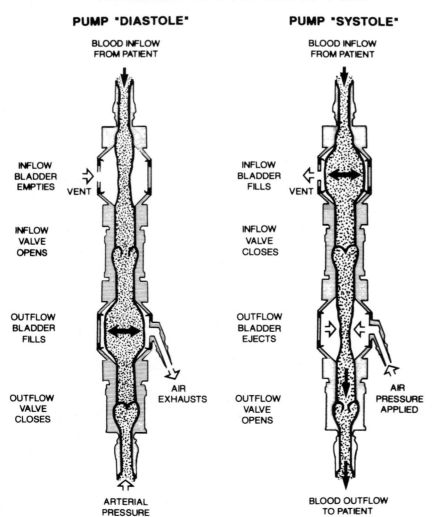

**ABIOMED BVS 5000 BLOOD PUMP**

PUMP "DIASTOLE"

PUMP "SYSTOLE"

BLOOD INFLOW FROM PATIENT

BLOOD INFLOW FROM PATIENT

INFLOW BLADDER EMPTIES        VENT

INFLOW BLADDER FILLS        VENT

INFLOW VALVE OPENS

INFLOW VALVE CLOSES

OUTFLOW BLADDER FILLS

OUTFLOW BLADDER EJECTS

OUTFLOW VALVE CLOSES

AIR EXHAUSTS

OUTFLOW VALVE OPENS

AIR PRESSURE APPLIED

ARTERIAL PRESSURE

BLOOD OUTFLOW TO PATIENT

**FIGURE 54–130.** The ABIOMED assist device (Danvers, MA). This dual-chambered blood pump has trileaflet polyurethane valves, which reduces the cost compared with other commercially available valves. The upper chamber allows continuous, uninterrupted gravity-filling, which may reduce the risk of hemolysis associated with vacuum-assisted filling. The ABIOMED is the only pulsatile assist device commercially available in the United States. (Courtesy of ABIOMED, Inc., Danvers, MA.)

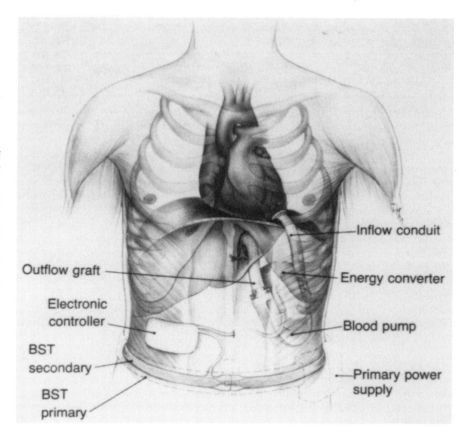

**FIGURE 54–131.** Anatomic placement of the Novacor left ventricular assist device (Baxter Healthcare, Oakland, CA). The Novacor is the only totally implantable system currently under clinical investigation in the United States. (From Bernard, W. F., Warren, C., et al.: Ventricular assist devices for left and right heart support: Clinical and experimental considerations. *In* Kapoor, A. S., and Laks, H. [eds]: Cardiomyopathies and Heart-Lung Transplantation. New York, McGraw-Hill, 1991. Reproduced with permission.)

systems should reduce infection rates and permit patient ambulation, which becomes more important as support durations increase (Hahn et al., 1993a; Hill et al., 1993).

## Indications and Results

Strictly speaking, VADs should be instituted only after fluid replacement, inotropic agents, and IABP

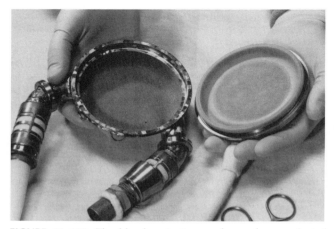

**FIGURE 54–132.** The blood-contacting surfaces of an explanted Thermo-Cardiosystems left ventricular assist device (Thermo-Cardiosystems, Woburn, MA). This pulsatile assist device employs a specially textured biomaterial that promotes fibrin deposition and formation of a "pseudoendothelium" and reduces the required level of systemic anticoagulation. (Courtesy of Thermo-Cardiosystems, Inc., Woburn, MA.)

support prove inadequate. However, experience has shown that high-dose inotropic agents and delays that result from assessing alternative therapies are detrimental. Therefore, the pharmacologic regimens and need for IABP support remain controversial prerequisites for instituting a VAD. Some institutions have developed protocols to address these issues. Generally, the hemodynamic criteria for instituting an IABP are combined with clinical indicators of end-organ compromise to predict the need for VAD support (Pennington et al., 1993; Pennington and Swartz, 1990).

After VAD support is initiated, hemodynamic parameters are reassessed. Preload should be increased to optimize VAD filling. These maneuvers sometimes unmask RV failure during LV support. An LVAD reduces left atrial pressure while augmenting systemic flow and venous return. Excessive central venous pressure may indicate that significant RV dysfunction cannot accommodate increases in venous return. If this condition persists despite pharmacologic therapy, biventricular support should be instituted without hesitation. Less commonly, initial hemodynamics may indicate predominant RV failure, in which case a RVAD in combination with inotropic agents or an IABP may be sufficient.

The largest group of VAD recipients comprises patients who cannot separate from CPB or deteriorate in the intensive care unit shortly after cardiac surgery (Magovern et al., 1993; Pae, 1993; Pae et al., 1992; Pennington and Swartz, 1990). Although the IABP usually provides sufficient support, approximately 1 to 2% of all patients undergoing cardiac operations require more aggressive therapy. VADs can improve hemodynamics by providing partial or nearly complete circulatory support. Unfortunately, less than 50% of patients who require VADs for postcardiotomy cardiogenic shock wean from these devices (Table 54–28). Furthermore, of those patients who are successfully weaned, roughly half die before leaving the hospital. Both the critical status of these patients and the complications of VAD support contribute to poor outcome. However, those patients who wean from VAD support and survive generally enjoy a good quality of life (Pae, 1993; Pennington et al., 1988).

Patient outcome is best when VAD support is brief, partly because cardiac dysfunction is limited and exposure to device-related complications is reduced. Therefore, assessment of cardiac recovery should begin early by briefly turning the VAD off. As cardiac function improves, VAD flows are gradually decreased. As with IABP therapy, inotropic agents should be reduced before VAD support is discontinued. In patients who successfully separate from VAD support, 2 to 4 days of assisted circulation is usually required for adequate myocardial recovery (Pae et al., 1992; Pennington et al., 1988). Patients who require more than 1 to 2 weeks of support are presumed to have irreversible myocardial damage and should be considered for cardiac transplantation.

Bridge-to-transplant is the second most common ⁻ation for VAD support (Farrar and Hill, 1993; ⁻ et al., 1990; Pae, 1993). Recipients must meet the same selection criteria as other patients considered for cardiac transplantation (Kaye, 1992). One criterion, frequently difficult to assess during VAD support, requires that *pulmonary vascular resistance* be no greater than 6 to 8 Woods units. Therefore, careful clinical judgment must be exercised when estimating the pulmonary vascular resistance in the bridge-to-transplant setting. Increased pulmonary vascular resistance incrementally correlates with right ventricular failure and poor outcome in cardiac transplant recipients (Kirklin et al., 1988).

Selection criteria and transplant therapy combine to give this group of VAD recipients the best prognosis overall (Birovljev et al., 1992; Farrar and Hill, 1993; Hetzer et al., 1992; Miller et al., 1990; Pifarre et al., 1992; Reedy et al., 1992) (Table 54–28). Two-thirds are successfully transplanted, with subsequent survival

rates similar to those patients not requiring VADs. One distinct problem during bridge-to-transplant support is the potentially long wait for a donor heart. Therefore, patients expected to have long waiting periods (e.g., large body habitus, O-negative blood, or high panel reactive antibody test) may be best served by totally implantable devices.

Unlike bridge-to-transplant, postcardiotomy VAD support introduces clinical predicaments that appear difficult to resolve (Pae et al., 1992; Pennington et al., 1988, 1993). The limitations of hemodynamic criteria for evaluating cardiac function are shadowed by obstacles surrounding assessment of other end-organs. Patients should not be considered for VAD support if they meet one of any exclusion criteria, including chronic renal failure, severe peripheral vascular disease, symptomatic cerebral vascular disease, cancer, chronic liver disease, blood dyscrasias, significant chronic obstructive pulmonary disease, or severe infection. Time constraints can hinder recognition of these conditions, and interpretation of their severity is often subjective. An expedient, objective assessment of end-organ function is generally not possible. Clearly, patients without underlying pathology do better than those with end-organ dysfunction. Nevertheless, procrastination while evaluating a potential VAD candidate increases the risk for poor patient outcome (Anstadt et al., 1992; Parascandola et al., 1988; Pierce et al., 1993). Unavoidably, patients both too ill or lacking genuine need will occasionally receive VAD support. These misadventures contribute to the high costs and complication rates associated with postcardiotomy VAD support.

## Complications of VAD Use

Although VAD technology in itself is expensive (Hahn et al., 1993b), installation and subsequent patient care are even more costly. Because VADs are not routinely used, specially trained teams are generally employed for installation and postoperative care (Shinn et al., 1993). Following implantation, complications frequently cause significant morbidity and mortality (Table 54–29). The underlying culprit for most major complications is blood contact (Copeland et al., 1993; Gristina, 1987; Pifarre, 1993; Termuhlen et al., 1989). Bleeding occurs frequently and demands reop-

■ **Table 54–28.** OUTCOME FOLLOWING VAD SUPPORT

| | Postcardiotomy Support | | | Bridge-to-Transplant | | |
|---|---|---|---|---|---|---|
| | *Patient #* | *Weaned* | *Discharged* | *Patient #* | *Transplanted* | *Discharged* |
| LVAD | 587 | 299 (51%) | 161 (27%) | 166 | 119 (72%) | 107 (64%) |
| RVAD | 160 | 63 (39%) | 39 (24%) | 5 | 2 (40%) | 0 (0%) |
| BVAD | 476 | 190 (40%) | 102 (21%) | 189 | 116 (61%) | 76 (40%) |
| Total | 1223 | 552 (45%) | 302 (25%) | 360 | 237 (66%) | 183 (51%) |

Data from the Clinical Registry of Mechanical Ventricular Assist Pumps and Artificial Hearts, the International Society for Heart Transplantation, and the American Society for Artificial Internal Organs, 1993; Courtesy of Walter E. Pae, M.D.
*Key:* VAD = ventricular assist device; LVAD = left ventricular assist device; RVAD = right ventricular assist device; BVAD = both ventricular assist devices.

■ **Table 54–29.** COMPLICATIONS FOLLOWING VAD SUPPORT

| | Postcardiotomy | | Bridge-to-Transplant | |
|---|---|---|---|---|
| Complications | *All Patients* (*n = 1223*) | *Discharged* (*n = 302*) | *All Patients* (*n = 551*) | *Discharged* (*n = 249*) |
| Bleeding/DIC | 50% | 40% | 38% | 25% |
| BV failure/low c.o. | 36% | 18% | 13% | 5% |
| Renal failure | 31% | 16% | 20% | 8% |
| Infection | 13% | 17% | 23% | 18% |
| Thrombus/emboli | 11% | 10% | 17% | 15% |
| Neurologic | 11% | 8% | 8% | 3% |
| Hemolysis | 6% | 6% | 9% | 6% |
| Technical problems | 4% | 2% | 5% | 5% |

Data from the Clinical Registry of Mechanical Ventricular Assist Pumps and Artificial Hearts, the International Society for Heart Transplantation, and the American Society for Artificial Internal Organs, 1993; courtesy of Walter E. Pae, M.D.

*Key:* VAD = ventricular assist device; DIC = disseminated intravascular coagulation; BV = biventricular; c.o. = cardiac output.

eration in nearly half of all VAD recipients. These complications would be reduced if VADs did not generally require CPB for insertion. The incidence of bleeding does appear to decrease with clinical experience, explained by meticulous surgical technique, adequate reversal of heparin, and use of thrombostatic agents such as fibrin glue.

Once hemostasis is achieved, anticoagulants must be instituted to prevent thrombus formation (Copeland et al., 1993; Montoya et al., 1993). Thromboembolic events are thereby reduced, but not without increasing the risk for bleeding. The level of anticoagulation often has a direct impact on the patient's clinical course. Simple systems such as roller and centrifugal pumps generally require continuous heparin administration. More sophisticated pulsatile devices only require dextran until oral regimens of warfarin and antiplatelet therapy can be started. In any case, aggressive anticoagulation regimens are frequently employed in an attempt to further reduce potential thromboembolic events.

Innovative biomaterials may curtail some problems associated with blood contact. Artificial surfaces activate platelets and leukocytes, as well as the complement, coagulation-kinin, and fibrinolytic systems (Pifarre, 1993; Sharma and Szycher, 1991; Termuhlen et al., 1989). Heparin bonding localizes thrombin inactivation at the artificial surface (Breillat and Hsu, 1993; Lazzara et al., 1993; Magovern et al., 1993). This methodology reduces systemic anticoagulant requirements, but demands maintenance of endogenous antithrombin III, which complexes with heparin to inhibit coagulation. Furthermore, heparin does not suppress the inflammatory response and platelet activation that persists at the blood-contacting surface. Specially textured biomaterials may help solve this problem (Graham et al., 1990). One such material is employed in a pulsatile VAD (Thermocardiosystems, Woburn, MA). The surface's unique features promotes fibrin deposition and formation of a "pseudoendothelium." This biologic shield reduces the need for anticoagulation, but its tendency to loosen or embolize has not yet been clearly defined (Copeland et al., 1993; Frazier, 1993; Poirer, 1993). These new technologies may help

reduce the frequent bleeding and thromboembolic complications associated with VAD support.

The interactions between blood and biomaterials may have other derogatory effects that remain to be identified (Pifarre, 1993; Sharma and Szycher, 1991). In particular, the immunologic consequences of blood-to-artificial surface contact are poorly understood. Biomaterial-centered infections are considered one of the main barriers to the success of totally implantable devices (Gristina, 1987). Even temporary VAD support is associated with a 10 to 25% incidence of infectious complications (Hill et al., 1993; Pae et al., 1992). These complications are most concerning when bridge-to-cardiac transplantation is the indication for VAD insertion. Infections are a significant cause of morbidity and mortality in the postcardiac transplant setting (Kaye, 1992). Patients who require mechanical support before transplant have significantly more infections than those not requiring such therapy (Pifarre et al., 1992). Permanently implantable devices may reduce infectious complications by eliminating percutaneous drive lines. However, blood contact in itself may increase the risk of infection (Gristina, 1987), which is a subject of some controversy (Termuhlen et al., 1989).

Advances in biomaterials, however, will not be fully realized unless paralleled by improved patient selection criteria. Perioperative assessment of end-organ function is essential to the success of VAD therapy. The associated morbidity and mortality of organ dysfunction is surpassed only by bleeding; for example, renal failure during VAD support has been identified as an independent predictor of poor outcome and is nearly always fatal when requiring hemodialysis. The assessment of renal function is limited by the brief time one has to determine the need for an assist device. However, devices that are instituted easily may decrease the period of hemodynamic instability. Measures that reduce the period of hypoperfusion should minimize the risk of organ failure. To better expedite mechanical support, some advocate use of less complex (e.g., nonpulsatile) devices before embarking on the technically demanding installation of most pulsatile VADs.

## OTHER APPROACHES TO ASSIST THE CIRCULATION

Three methods of circulatory support that are currently gaining increased attention deserve mention. One device, the Hemopump (Johnson & Johnson Interventional Systems, Rancho Cordova, CA), is based on rotating turbopump technology (Flameng, 1991) (Fig. 54–133). Connected to an external motor by a rotating flexible drive shaft, the device rotates rapidly within a cylindrical housing and generates nonpulsatile flow. The Hemopump can be positioned across the aortic valve without a major surgical procedure so that its inlet rests within the LV and its outlet in the ascending aorta. The pump can provide effective circulatory support while actively decompressing the LV.

Clinical trials using the Hemopump began in 1988 (Magovern et al., 1993). Early problems involved a high failed insertion rate (23%) and fractures of the flexible drive shaft (9%). A No. 14 French pump, which provides flow up to 2.5 l/min, was developed to reduce previous insertion difficulties. The original device provides flows of more than 4 l/min and is now intended for aortic placement via sternotomy. The Hemopump is being evaluated for aorta-coronary bypass grafting without use of a membrane oxygenator. As with other VADs, the hemopump requires anticoagulation to prevent thrombus formation.

Two methods require no anticoagulation because they function outside the bloodstream. One, *dynamic cardiomyoplasty* (DCM), uses transformed, fatigue-resistant *latissimus dorsi* (LD) muscle to assist the failing heart (Fig. 54–134). The LD is wrapped around the heart and stimulated in synchrony with cardiac systole. The technique was conceived as a mode of assisting cardiac contraction, but it may also reduce myocardial stress by prohibiting excessive distention during diastole. Clinical trials using DCM have identified three limiting factors: The procedure required to position the LD has a high surgical risk in severely ill patients; postoperatively, patients must survive for several weeks of LD conditioning before effective support begins; and DCM provides only limited support, which may be inadequate for many patients with severe refractory congestive heart failure or who experience frequent malignant arrhythmias.

Despite these potential obstacles, clinical experience since DCM's first application in 1985 has increased (Moreira et al., 1993). Results demonstrated that DCM can significantly improve the functional status in some patients who suffer from chronic, end-stage heart disease. However, prospective trials are needed to determine whether this method will favorably affect survival. The efficacy of DCM may be improved by better patient selection, improved surgical technique, development of muscle conditioning protocols that provide improved assist, and use of implantable

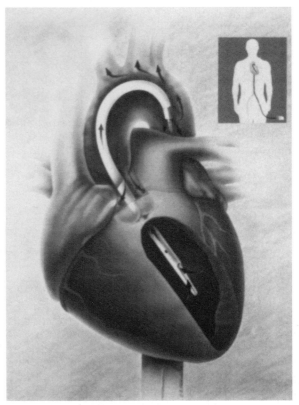
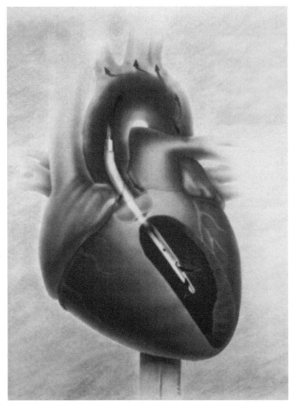

**FIGURE 54–133.** The Hemopump assist device (Johnson and Johnson, Interventional Systems, Rancho Cordova, CA). This axial flow pump unloads the left ventricle (LV) as blood is pumped from within the LV into the proximal aorta. The pump can be placed percutaneously via a femoral artery access site or directly into the aorta via a sternotomy. (Courtesy of Johnson & Johnson Interventional Systems, Rancho Cordova, CA.)

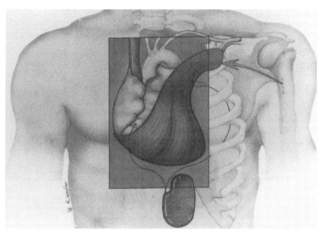

FIGURE 54–134. The use of dynamic cardiomyoplasty (DCM) to assist the heart. DCM uses transformed, fatigue-resistant latissimus dorsi muscle, which is wrapped around the heart and stimulated in synchrony with the cardiac cycle. The method avoids blood contact but requires a fairly extensive operation and can only partially assist the heart. (From Moreira, L. F. P., Stolf, N. A. G., and Janene, A. D.: Hemodynamic benefits of cardiomyoplasty in clinical and experimental myocardial dysfunction. *In* Chiu, R. C. J., and Bourgeois, I. M. [eds]: Transformed Muscle for Cardiac Assist and Repair, New York, Futura Publishing, 1990.)

defibrillators and antiarrhythmic pacemakers for adjunctive therapy.

*Direct mechanical ventricular actuation* (DMVA) is the only other non-blood-contacting method in clinical use. Unlike cardiomyoplasty, DMVA can provide total circulatory support and can be instituted in a matter of minutes. DMVA employs a "heart cup" (Fig. 54–135) that is vacuum-attached to the heart. A pneumatically regulated diaphragm within the cup compresses and dilates the ventricles. Early clinical experience with DMVA was very encouraging when it was first used for resuscitative circulatory support. Skinner and co-workers (1968) and Baue and associates (1968) demonstrated that DMVA could provide hemodynamic stabilization more rapidly than is possible by any other means. Postcardiotomy support for up to 36 hours revealed no adverse effects on saphenous vein grafts. In 1971, one patient was discharged from the hospital after 3 days of DMVA was used to support her failing heart (Lambert, 1992).

Initially, DMVA was overshadowed by noninvasive resuscitation techniques (closed-chest cardiopulmonary resuscitation), and the evolution of other VAD technology. However, the poor outcome of cardiac arrest victims and unresolved obstacles of blood contact has renewed interest in DMVA. DMVA has now been used successfully as a bridge-to-cardiac transplantation (Lowe et al., 1991). More recently, a patient suffering cardiac arrest secondary to an acute viral myocarditis was supported for over 1 week; she recovered and is well today with no evidence of cardiac dysfunction. DMVA's limitations for long-term support remain to be determined. However, the device's greatest potential appears to be its ability for providing rapid, life-saving, resuscitative support (Anstadt et al., 1991a, 1991b, 1993).

## RESUSCITATIVE CIRCULATORY SUPPORT

John Gibbon (1954) began work on the heart-lung machine to resuscitate moribund patients suffering from massive pulmonary embolus. However, the early applications of CPB for resuscitative support were discouraging because of poor patient selection. Kouwenhoven and colleagues (1960) subsequently described application of an alternating current defibrillator to patients receiving closed-chest *cardiopulmonary resuscitation* (CPR). It was Kouwenhoven's rather anecdotal experience that led to closed-chest CPR's becoming the accepted therapy for cardiac arrest.

The outcome following cardiac arrest remains discouragingly low. Although closed-chest compressions can sustain life, the potential to definitively treat cardiac arrest is extremely short-lived. The low-flow states that characterize closed-chest CPR create an increasing oxygen debt. If perfusion is not readily restored, organ dysfunction and eventual death are inevitable. The vital organ with the least tolerance to ischemia is the brain, so cerebral resuscitation is the predominant challenge when treating cardiac arrest. Furthermore, the return of neurologic function following resuscitation from cardiac arrest is the most important predictor of outcome.

It is paradoxical that 30 to 50% of the patients for

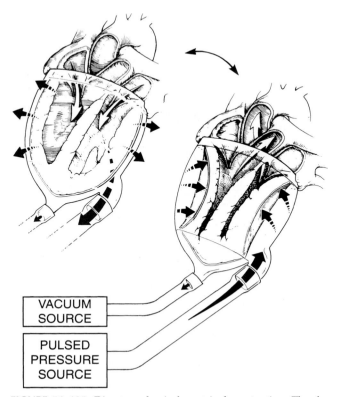

VACUUM SOURCE

PULSED PRESSURE SOURCE

FIGURE 54–135. Direct mechanical ventricular actuation. The device pneumatically actuates the ventricles into systolic and diastolic configurations, providing total circulatory support without contacting the blood. The device can be rapidly applied via a left anterior thoracotomy for emergent resuscitative circulatory support.

■ **Table 54–30.** OUTCOME FOLLOWING CPB RESUSCITATION IN WITNESSED CARDIAC ARREST

| Time from Arrest to Bypass | Patient # | Outcome | | |
|---|---|---|---|---|
| | | Alive > 30 Days | Alive < 30 Days | Unsuccessful Resuscitation |
| <15 min | 51 | 29% | 16% | 55% |
| 15–30 min | 55 | 29% | 7% | 64% |
| 30–45 min | 28 | 7% | 7% | 86% |
| 45–60 min | 26 | 19% | 8% | 73% |
| >60 min | 34 | 9% | 6% | 85% |

Data from National Cardiopulmonary Registry for Emergent Applications, 1993; courtesy of Jonathan G. Hill, M.D.
*Key:* CBC = cardiopulmonary bypass.

whom sophisticated *circulatory* support devices are being developed will die annually because effective devices for *resuscitative* support are not yet available (McManus et al., 1993). This only represents a small fraction of the half million deaths occurring annually from cardiac arrest in the United States alone. To address these problems, a variety of portable CPB systems have been developed for percutaneous application (Dembitsky et al., 1993; Hill et al., 1992; Moritz and Wolner, 1993).

Because no other alternatives are currently available, the use of CPB for resuscitating patients in refractory cardiac arrest has gradually increased. To date, more than 200 patients have been reported to a national volunteer registry. Twenty-one per cent of these patients were successfully resuscitated and experienced short-term survival. However, the 10 to 20 minutes required to institute percutaneous systems can decrease the probability of survival during cardiac arrest (Table 54–30). Once CPB has been initiated, flow restrictions of the percutaneous cannulas and blood contact of the membrane oxygenator create further limitations.

Alternatively, mechanical (DMVA) and manual methods of cardiac massage may create better opportunities for successful resuscitation. Magovern (1993) noted that the incidence of neurologic injury was lower when manual cardiac massage was used instead of percutaneous bypass during the transport of patients in cardiac arrest to the operating room. These findings may be explained by the suboptimal characteristics of nonpulsatile flow during CPB. Pulsatile flow generated during DMVA has improved cerebral oxygen consumption, the distribution of cerebral flow (Anstadt et al., 1993), and neurologic outcome (Anstadt et al., 1993) when compared with nonpulsatile flow following experimental cardiac arrest.

## SUMMARY

A growing assortment of devices is becoming available to support the circulation. Clearly, the IABP remains the mainstay of therapy if cardiac failure does not adequately respond to standard medical management. When the IABP proves insufficient, VADs provide additional life-saving potential, but are associated with significant morbidity and mortality. The

primary goal of these devices is to allow recovery of the patient's cardiac function or bridge to other therapies, such as revascularization, valvular repair, or cardiac transplantation.

The field of mechanical circulatory support can only reach its greatest potential through organized, prospective clinical trials. Otherwise, controversies that surround patient selection and therapeutic strategies will continue to overshadow these technologic marvels with unfavorable connotations. The ideal biomaterial remains to be discovered; that is probably the most critical goal that needs to be met for permanently implantable devices to reach fruition. Furthermore, effective methods of resuscitative circulatory support need to be examined and made more readily available. This latter endeavor could improve the outlook of cardiac arrest victims and afford select patients a critical link to other existing technologies.

## SELECTED BIBLIOGRAPHY

Anstadt, M. P., Anstadt, G. L., and Lowe, J. E.: Direct mechanical ventricular actuation: A review. Resuscitation, 21:7, 1991.

*Direct mechanical ventricular actuation* (DMVA) provides total circulatory support without blood contact and can be rapidly applied for resuscitation through a small anterior thoracotomy. This manuscript summarizes clinical and laboratory data published before 1991. Studies that examined DMVA for prolonged support during ventricular fibrillation, resuscitation, organ preservation, and profound hypothermia are discussed. Comparisons are made between DMVA and other relevant therapies including standard methods of cardiopulmonary resuscitation and cardiopulmonary bypass (CPB).

Chiu, R. C. J., and Bourgeois, I. M. (eds.): Transformed Muscle for Cardiac Assist and Repair. Mount Kisco, NY, Futura Publishing, 1990.

Transformed skeletal muscle may be a feasible means for achieving partial biomechanical cardiac assist. This text reviews the basic science of fatigue-resistant, transformed skeletal muscle. The authors describe laboratory and clinical experiences with dynamic cardiomyoplasty that address both the benefits and the limitations of this method when used for a number of disease states. Hybrid devices that incorporate skeletal muscle to power mechanical blood pumps are also discussed.

Flameng, W. (ed): Temporary Cardiac Assist with an Axial Pump System. Darmstadt, Steinkopff Verlag, 1991.

The axial flow pump is a very unique method for assisting the heart. This book reviews developmental studies that led to the only currently available device that uses this principle, the Hemopump (Johnson & Johnson Interventional Systems). A review of the laboratory and clinical applications of this investigational device is provided.

Kay, P. H. (ed): Techniques in Extracorporeal Circulation. Oxford, Butterworth-Heinemann, 1992.

CPB is the method of assisted circulation from which all other blood pumps have evolved. The institution of most assist devices requires application of CPB. Furthermore, modified CPB systems are commonly used to assist the failing heart, particularly in the resuscitation setting. This text reviews historical, physiologic, and biomechanical aspects of CPB and the membrane oxygenator. Advances in rheology and material science are discussed as they relate to potential complications associated with CPB. The use of other related methods of circulatory support is also discussed in this text.

Pifarre, R. (ed): Anticoagulation, Hemostasis, and Blood Preservation in Cardiovascular Surgery. Philadelphia, Hanley & Belfus, 1993.

The morbidity and mortality associated with mechanical circulatory support is frequently related to hemostasis. This text reviews the pharmacology and biologic aspects of anticoagulation. Complications of blood contact as well as the various anticoagulants are discussed. The indications and mechanism of action for a host of therapeutic strategies are presented. The complex interactions of blood formed elements and hemostatic systems during cardiovascular procedures are central to this text. The potential for future biomaterials and pharmacologic agents to reduce complications of blood contact also is covered.

Rowles, J. R., Mortimer, B. J., and Olsen, D. B.: Ventricular assist and total artificial heart devices for clinical use in 1993. ASAIO J., 39:840, 1993.

Several circulatory support devices currently are being developed for clinical use. This manuscript reviews those blood pumps that have been used in the United States. Emphasis is placed on the description of each device, including relevant specifications and methods of implantation. The recommended indications and brief discussion of clinical results are also included. Each of the described devices is accompanied with well-selected photographs.

Sarnoff, S. J., Braunwald, E., Welch, G. H., Jr., et al.: Hemodynamic determinants of oxygen consumption of the heart with special reference to the tension-time index. Am. J. Physiol., 192:148, 1958.

The hemodynamic determinants of myocardial oxygen consumption are central to the potential effectiveness of circulatory support devices. This historical article describes experimental results used to identify which hemodynamic parameters have the greatest influence on myocardial oxygen consumption. The tension-time index, described as the area beneath the systolic pressure curve, was determined to have the greatest impact on myocardial oxygen consumption and efficiency. A clear understanding of these principles is important for determining which methods of ventricular support are most likely to result in myocardial recovery.

Sharma, C. P., and Szycher, M. (ed): Blood Compatible Materials and Devices. Lancaster, PA, Technomic Publishing, 1991.

Widely varying of biomaterials have been evaluated for use in the fabrication of ventricular assist devices. This text provides an in-depth review of these resources. The properties that characterize the texture, physical strength, and durability of materials are discussed in detail. Various methods used to assess the biologic response of materials are defined. The use and assessment of materials for specific applications, including blood pumps, heart valves, vascular grafts, and pacing leads, are discussed under separate chapters.

Unger, F. (ed): Assisted Circulation 4. Berlin, Heidelberg, Germany, Springer-Verlag, 1995.

This text offers a comprehensive review of mechanical circulatory support devices. Historic and developmental aspects of nearly all forms of assisted circulation are covered. Devices in various stages of development are discussed in terms of bioengineering and laboratory tests. Clinical experiences are generally furnished by individuals with international reputation. This is an excellent overall review of the field of assisted circulation.

## BIBLIOGRAPHY

Abdelmeguid, A. E., and Ellis, S. G.: Complications of percutaneous transluminal coronary angioplasty. In Vlietstra, R. E., and Holmes, D. R., Jr. (eds): Coronary Balloon Angioplasty. Cambridge, MA, Blackwell Scientific, 1994, pp. 399–451.
Adler, D. S., Goldman, L., O'Neil, A., et al.: Long-term survival of more than 2000 patients after coronary artery bypass grafting. Am. J. Cardiol., 58:195, 1986.
Alderman, J. D., Gabliani, G. I., McCabe, C. H., et al.: Incidence and management of leg ischemia with percutaneous wire guided intraortic balloon catheters. J. Am. Coll. Cardiol., 9:524, 1987.
Allen, B. S., Rosenkranz, E., Buckberg, G. D., et al.: Studies on prolonged acute regional ischemia. IV. Myocardial infarction with left ventricular power failure: A medical surgical emer-
gency requiring urgent revascularization with maximal protection of remote muscle. J. Thorac. Cardiovasc. Surg., 98:691, 1989.
Alpert, J., Bhaktan, E. K., Gielchinsky, I., et al.: Vascular complications in intraaortic balloon pumping. Arch. Surg., 111:1190, 1976.
Alvarez, J. M., Brady, P. W., and McWilson, R.: Intra-aortic balloon rupture. An increasing trend? ASAIO J., 38:862, 1992.
Anstadt, G. L., Blakemore, W. S., and Baue, A. E.: A new instrument for prolonged mechanical massage [Abstract]. Circulation, 31(Suppl. 2):43, 1965.
Anstadt, M. P., Anstadt, G. L., and Lowe, J. E.: Direct mechanical ventricular actuation: A review. Resuscitation, 21:7, 1991a.
Anstadt, M. P., Stonnington, M. J., Tedder, M., et al.: Pulsatile reperfusion after cardiac arrest improves neurologic outcome. Ann. Surg., 214:478, 1991b.
Anstadt, M. P., Tedder, M., Hegde, S. S., et al.: Intraoperative timing may provide criteria for use of post-cardiotomy ventricular assist devices. ASAIO J., 38:M147, 1992.
Anstadt, M. P., Tedder, M., Hegde, S. S., et al.: Pulsatile versus nonpulsatile reperfusion improves cerebral blood flow after cardiac arrest. Ann. Thorac. Surg., 56:453, 1993.
Axelrod, H. I., Galloway, A. C., Murphy, M. M. S., et al.: Percutaneous cardiopulmonary bypass with a synchronous pulsatile pump combines effective unloading with ease of application. J. Thorac. Cardiovasc. Surg., 93:358, 1987.
Bahn, C. H., Bitikainen, K. J., Anderson, C. L., et al.: Vascular evaluation for balloon pumping. Ann. Thorac. Surg., 27:475, 1979.
Baldwin, R. T., Slogoff, S., Noon, G. P., et al.: A model to predict survival at time of postcardiotomy intra-aortic balloon pump insertion. Ann. Thorac. Surg., 55:908, 1993.
Bardet, J., Rigaud, M., Kahn, J. C., et al.: Treatment of postmyocardial infarction angina by intra-aortic balloon pumping and emergency revascularization. J. Thorac. Cardiovasc. Surg., 74:299, 1977.
Baue, A. E., Tragus, E. T., Anstadt, G. L., and Blakemore, W. S.: Mechanical ventricular assistance in man. Circulation, 37(Suppl. 2):33, 1968.
Beckman, C. B., Geha, A. S., Hammond, G. L., et al.: Results and complications of intra-aortic balloon counterpulsation. Ann. Thorac. Surg., 24:550, 1977.
Berger, R. L., Saini, V. K., Long, W., et al.: The use of diastolic augmentation with the intra-aortic balloon pump in human septic shock with associated coronary artery disease. Surgery, 74:601, 1973.
Birovljev, S., Radovancevic, B., Burnett, C. M., et al.: Heart transplantation after mechanical circulatory support: Four years' experience. J. Heart Lung Transplant., 11:240, 1992.
Bolooki, H.: Current status of circulatory support with an intra-aortic balloon pump. Cardiol. Clin., 3:123, 1985.
Bolooki, H.: Emergency cardiac procedures in patients in cardiogenic shock due to complications of coronary artery disease. Circulation, 79(Suppl. 1):137, 1989.
Bolooki, H.: Methods of insertion of intraaortic balloon catheter. In Bolooki, H. (ed): Clinical application of intra-aortic balloon pump. New York, Futura Publishing, 1984, p. 103.
Bolooki, H., Williams, W., Thurer, R. J., et al.: Clinical and hemodynamic criteria for use of intra-aortic balloon pump in patients requiring cardiac surgery. J. Thorac. Surg., 72:756, 1976.
Brahos, G. J., Baker, N. H., Ewy, H. G., et al.: Aortocoronary bypass following unsuccessful PTCA: Experience in 100 consecutive patients. Ann. Thorac. Surg., 40:7, 1985.
Bregman, D.: Mechanical support of the failing heart. In Ravitch, M. M. (ed): Current Problems in Surgery. Chicago, Year Book Medical, 1976.
Breillatt, J., and Hsu, L. C.: Antithrombotic biomaterials for cardiovascular surgery. In Pifarre, R. (ed): Anticoagulation, Hemostasis, and Blood Preservation in Cardiovascular Surgery. Philadelphia, Hanley & Belfus, 1993, pp. 353–362.
Buckley, M. J., Leinbach, R. C., Kaston, J. A., et al.: Hemodynamic evaluation of intra-aortic balloon pumping in man. Circulation, 46(Suppl. 2):130, 1970.
Burton, A. C. (ed): Physiology and Biophysiology of the Circulation. Chicago, Year Book Medical, 1972, pp. 72, 207.

Chaitman, B. R., Ryan, T. J., Kronmal, R.A., et al.: Coronary Artery Surgery Study (CASS): Comparability of 10-year survival in randomized and randomizable patients. J. Am. Coll. Cardiol., 16:1071, 1990.

Champsaur, G., Ninet, J., Vigneron, M., et al.: Use of the Abiomed BVS System 5000 as a bridge to cardiac transplantation. J. Thorac. Cardiovasc. Surg., 100:122, 1990.

Clauss, R. H., Birtwell, W. C., Albertal, G., et al.: Assisted circulation. I. The arterial counterpulsator. J. Thorac. Cardiovasc. Surg., 41:447, 1961.

Clauss, R. H., Misser, P., Reed, G. E., and Tice, D.: Assisted circulation by counterpulsation with an intra-aortic balloon. Methods and effects. In Digest, 15th Annual Conference on Engineering in Medicine and Biology. Vol. 4. Chicago, Northwestern University, 1962, p. 44.

Collier, P. E., Liebler, G. A., Park, S. B., et al.: Is percutaneous insertion of the intra-aortic balloon pump through the femoral artery the safest technique? J. Vasc. Surg., 3:629, 1986.

Connolly, J. E., Bacaner, M. B., Bruns, E. L., et al.: Mechanical support of the circulation in acute heart failure. Surgery, 44:225, 1958.

Connolly, M. W., Gelbfish, J. S., Jacobowitz, I. J., et al.: Surgical results for mitral regurgitation from coronary artery disease. J. Thorac. Cardiovasc. Surg., 91:379, 1986.

Copeland, J. G., Emery, R. W., Levinson, M. M., et al.: The role of mechanical support and transplantation in treatment of patients with end-stage cardiomyopathy. Circulation, 72:7, 1985.

Copeland, J. G., III, Frazier, O. H., McBride, L. R., et al.: Anticoagulation. Ann. Thorac. Surg., 55:213, 1993.

Corday, E., Swan, J. C., Lang, T. W., et al.: Physiologic principles in the application of circulatory assist for the failing heart. Am. J. Cardiol., 26:595, 1970.

Cox, J. L., Pass, H. I., Anderson, R. N., et al.: Augmentation of coronary collateral blood flow in acute myocardial infarction. Surg. Forum, 26:238, 1975.

Creswell, L. L., Rosenbloon, M., Cox, J. L., et al.: Intra-aortic balloon counterpulsation: Patterns of usage and outcome in cardiac surgery patients. Ann. Thorac. Surg., 54:11, 1992.

Daggett, W. M., Buckley, W. J., Akins, C. W., et al.: Improved results of surgical management of postinfarction ventricular septal rupture. Ann. Surg., 196:269, 1982.

Davies, R., Laks, H., Berger, H., et al.: Follow-up radionuclide assessment of left ventricular function and perfusion in patients requiring intra-aortic balloon pump to wean from cardiopulmonary bypass. Am. J. Cardiol., 45:488, 1980.

DeBusk, R. F., and Harrison, D. C.: The clinical spectrum of papillary-muscle disease. N. Engl. J. Med., 281:1458, 1969.

Dembitsky, W. P., Moore, C. H., Holman, W. L., et al.: Successful mechanical circulatory support for noncoronary shock. J. Heart Lung Transplant., 11:129, 1992.

Dembitsky, W. P., Moreno-Cabral, R. J., Adamson, R. M., and Daily, P. O.: Emergency resuscitation using portable extracorporeal membrane oxygenation. Ann. Thorac. Surg., 55:304, 1993.

Dennis, C., Spreng, D. S., Nelson, G. E., et al.: Development of a pump-oxygenator to replace the heart and lungs: An apparatus applicable to human patients and an application to one case. Ann. Surg., 134:709, 1951.

DePasquale, N. P., and Burch, G. E.: Papillary muscle dysfunction in coronary (ischemic) heart disease. Annu. Rev. Med., 22:327, 1971.

Di Lello, F., Mullen, D. C., Flemma, R. J., et al.: Results of intra-aortic balloon pumping after cardiac surgery: Experience with the Percor balloon catheter. Ann. Thorac. Surg., 46:442, 1988.

DiSesa, V. J., Cohn, L. H., Collins, J. J., Jr., et al.: Determinants of operative survival following combined mitral valve replacement and coronary revascularization. Ann. Thorac. Surg., 34:482, 1982.

Drinkwater, D. C., Chiu, R. C. J., Modry, D., et al.: Cardiac assist and myocardial repair with synchronously stimulated skeletal muscle. Surg. Forum, 31:271, 1980.

Dunkman, W. B., Leinbach, R. C., Buckley, M. J., et al.: Clinical and hemodynamic results of intra-aortic balloon pumping for cardiogenic shock. Circulation, 46:465, 1972.

Edwards, F. H., Bellamy, R. F., Burge, J. R., et al.: True emergency coronary artery bypass surgery. Ann. Thorac. Surg., 49:603, 1990.

Farrar, D. J., and Hill, J. D.: Univentricular and biventricular Thoratec VAD support as a bridge to transplantation. Ann. Thorac. Surg., 55:276, 1993.

Fischl, S. J., Herman, M. J., and Gorlin, R.: The intermediate coronary syndrome. Clinical, angiographic and therapeutic aspects. N. Engl. J. Med., 288:1193, 1973.

Flameng, W. (ed): Temporary Cardiac Assist with an Axial Pump System. Darmstadt, Steinkopff Verlag, 1991.

Force, T., Hibberd, P., Weeks, G., et al.: Perioperative myocardial infarction after coronary artery bypass surgery. Clinical significance and approach to risk stratification. Circulation, 82:903, 1990.

Frazier, O. H.: Chronic left ventricular support with a vented electric assist device. Ann. Thorac. Surg., 55:273, 1993.

Freed, P. S., Wasfie, T., Zado, B., and Kantrowitz, A: Intra-aortic balloon pumping for prolonged circulatory support. Am. J. Cardiol., 61:554, 1988.

Fulton, M., Lutz, W., Donald, K. W., et al.: Natural history of unstable angina. Lancet, 1:860, 1974.

Gaudiani, V. A., Miller, D. C., Stinson, E. B., et al.: Postinfarction ventricular septal defect: An argument for early operation. Surgery, 89:48, 1981.

Gazes, P. C., Mobley, E. M., Jr., Farais, H. M., Jr., et al.: Preinfarction (unstable) angina—A prospective study. Ten-year follow-up. Prognostic significance of electrocardiographic changes. Circulation, 48:331, 1973.

Ghitis, A., Flaker, G. C., Meinhardt, S., et al.: Early angioplasty in patients with acute myocardial infarction complicated by hypotension. Am. Heart J., 122:380, 1991.

Gibbon, J. H., Jr.: Application of a mechanical heart and lung apparatus to cardiac surgery. Minn. Med., 37:171, 1954.

Gold, H. K., Leinbach, R. C., Buckley, M. J., et al.: Refractory angina pectoris: Follow-up after intra-aortic balloon pumping and surgery. Circulation, 54(Suppl. III):III–41, 1976.

Gold, H. K., Leinbach, R. C., Sanders, C. A., et al.: Intra-aortic balloon pumping for ventricular septal defect on mitral regurgitation complicating acute myocardial infarction. Circulation, 47:1191, 1973.

Golding, L. A. R., Loop, F. D., Peter, M., et al.: Late survival following use of intra-aortic balloon pump in revascularization operations. Ann. Thorac. Surg., 30:48, 1980.

Goldman, B. S., Hill, T. J., Rosenthal, G. A., et al.: Complications associated with the use of the intra-aortic balloon pump. Can. J. Surg., 25:153, 1982.

Gottlieb, S. O., Brinker, J. A., Borkon, A. M., et al.: Identification of patients at high risk for complications of intra-aortic balloon counterpulsation: A multivariate risk factor analysis. Am. J. Cardiol., 53:1135, 1984.

Graham, T. R., Dasse, K. A., Coumbe, A., et al.: Neo-intimal development on textured biomaterial surfaces during clinical use of an implantable left ventricular assist device. Eur. J. Cardiothorac. Surg., 4:182, 1990.

Gristina, A. G.: Biomaterial-centered infection: Microbial adhesion versus tissue integration. Science, 237:1588, 1987.

Grotz, R. L., and Yeston, N. S.: Intra-aortic balloon counterpulsation in high-risk cardiac patients undergoing noncardiac surgery. Surgery, 106:1, 1989.

Hahn, C. J., Holman, W. L., Copeland, J. G., III, and Champsaur, G.: External pulsatile circulatory support. Ann. Thorac. Surg., 55:257, 1993a.

Hahn, C. J., Pierce, W. S., Olsen, D. B., et al.: Long-term biventricular assist. Ann. Thorac. Surg., 55:227, 1993b.

Hanloser, P. B., Gallow, E., and Schenk, W. G.: Hemodynamics of counterpulsation. J. Thorac. Cardiovasc. Surg., 51:366, 1966.

Hardesty, R. L., Griffith, B. P., Trento, A., et al.: Mortally ill patients and excellent survival following cardiac transplantation. Ann. Thorac. Surg., 41:126, 1986.

Harken, D. E.: Presented at the International College of Cardiology Meeting, Brussels, 1958.

Harris, P. L., Woollard, K., Bartoli, A., et al.: The management of impending myocardial infarction using coronary bypass grafting and an intra-aortic balloon pump. J. Cardiovasc. Surg., 21:405, 1980.

Hauser, A. M., Gordon, S., Gangadharen, V., et al.: Percutaneous intra-aortic balloon counterpulsation. Clinical effectiveness and hazards. Chest, 82:442, 1982.

Heitmiller, R., Jacobs, M. L., and Dagget, W. M.: Surgical management of postinfarction ventricular septal rupture. Ann. Thorac. Surg., 41:683, 1986.

Hetzer, R., Hennig, E., Schiessler, A., et al.: Mechanical circulatory support and heart transplantation. J. Heart Lung Transplant., 11:S175, 1992.

Hill, J. D., Griffith, B. P., Meli, M., and Didisheim, P.: Infections—Prophylaxis and treatment. Ann. Thorac. Surg., 55:217, 1993.

Hill, J. G., Bruhn, P. S., Cohen, S. E., et al.: Emergent applications of cardiopulmonary support: A multi-institutional experience. Ann. Thorac. Surg., 54:699, 1992.

Hunt, S. A., and Schroeder, J. S.: Cardiac transplantation. In Hurst, J. W. (ed): Current Therapy in Cardiovascular Disease. St. Louis, Mosby–Year Book, 1994, p. 285–291.

Kantrowitz, A.: Functioning ectogenous muscle used experimentally as an auxiliary ventricle. Trans. Am. Soc. Artif. Intern. Organs, 6:305, 1960.

Kantrowitz, A., Cardona, R. R., and Freed, P. S.: Percutaneous intra-aortic balloon counterpulsation. Crit. Care Clin., 8:819, 1992.

Kantrowitz, A., and Kantrowitz, A.: Experimental augmentation of coronary flow by retardation of arterial pressure pulse. Surgery, 34:678, 1953.

Kantrowitz, A., and McKinnon, W. M. P.: The experimental use of the diaphragm as an auxiliary myocardium. Surg. Forum, 9:265, 1959.

Kantrowitz, A., Wasfie, T., Freed, P. S., et al.: Intra-aortic balloon pumping 1967 through 1982: Analysis of complications in 733 patients. Am. J. Cardiol., 57:976, 1986.

Kaye, M. P.: The registry of the international society for heart and lung transplantation: Ninth official report—1992. J. Heart Lung Transplant., 11:599, 1992.

Kirklin, J. K., Naftel, D. C., Kirklin, J. W., et al.: Pulmonary vascular resistance and the risk of heart transplantation. J. Heart Transplant., 7:331, 1988.

Kouwenhoven, W. B., Jude, J. R., and Knickerbocker, G. G.: Closed chest cardiac massage. J.A.M.A., 173:1064, 1960.

Laas, J., Campbell, C. D., Takanashi, Y., et al.: Critical analysis of intra-aortic balloon counterpulsation and transapical left ventricular bypass in the sufficient and insufficient circulation. Thorac. Cardiovasc. Surg., 29:17, 1981.

Lambert, C. J.: Clinical experience with direct mechanical ventricular actuation at Baylor University, Dallas. Personal communication, 1992.

Lazzara, R. R., Magovern, J. A., Benckart, D. H., et al.: Extracorporeal membrane oxygenation for adult post-cardiotomy cardiogenic shock using a heparin-bonded system. ASAIO J., 39:M444, 1993.

Lee, L., Bates, E. R., Pitt, B., et al.: Percutaneous transluminal angioplasty improves survival in acute myocardial infarction complicated by cardiogenic shock. Circulation, 78:1345, 1988.

Levine, F. H., and Austen, W. G.: Intra-aortic balloon assistance. In Glenn, W. W. L. (ed): Thoracic and Cardiovascular Surgery. 4th ed. Norwalk, CT, Appleton-Century-Crofts, 1983, p. 1157.

Levine, F. H., Gold, H. K., Leinbach, R. C., et al.: Management of acute myocardial ischemia with intra-aortic balloon pumping and surgery. Circulation, 58(Suppl. I):I–69, 1978.

Lick, S., Copeland, J. G., III, Smith, R. G., et al.: Use of the symbion biventricular assist device in bridging to transplantation. Ann. Thorac. Surg., 55:283, 1993.

Loisance, D. Y., Deleuze, P. H., Houel, R., et al.: Pharmacological bridge to cardiac transplantation: Current limitations. Ann. Thorac. Surg., 55:310, 1993.

Lowe, J. E., Anstadt, M. P., Van Trigt, P., et al.: First successful bridge to cardiac transplantation using direct mechanical ventricular actuation. Ann. Thorac. Surg., 52:1237, 1991.

Lytle, B. W., Loop, F. D., Cosgrove, D. M., et al.: Fifteen hundred coronary reoperations. Results and determinants of early and late survival. J. Thorac. Cardiovasc. Surg., 93:847, 1987.

Magovern, G. J., Jr.: The biopump and postoperative circulatory support. Ann. Thorac. Surg., 55:245, 1993.

Magovern, G. J., Jr., Wampler, R. W., Joyce L. D., and Wareing, T. H.: Nonpulsatile circulatory support: Techniques of insertion. Ann. Thorac. Surg., 55:266, 1993.

Magovern, J. A., Pennock, J. L., Campbell, D. B., et al.: Risks of

mitral valve replacement and mitral valve replacement with coronary artery bypass. Ann. Thorac. Surg., 39:346, 1985.

Mallory, G. K., White, P. D., and Salcedo-Salgar, J.: The speed of healing of myocardial infarction. Am. Heart J., 18:647, 1939.

Marks, J. D., Karwande, S. V., Richenbacher, W. E., et al.: Perioperative mechanical circulatory support for transplantation. J. Heart Lung Transplant., 11:117, 1992.

Maroko, P. R., Bernstein, E. F., Libby, P., et al.: Effects of intra-aortic balloon counterpulsation on the severity of myocardial ischemic injury following acute coronary occlusion. Circulation, 45:1150, 1972.

Martin, R. S., Moncure, A. C., Buckley, M. J., et al.: Complications of percutaneous intra-aortic balloon insertion. J. Thorac. Cardiovasc. Surg., 85:186, 1983.

McEnany, M. T., Kay, H. R., Buckley, M. J., et al.: Clinical experience with intra-aortic balloon pump support in 728 patients. Circulation, 58(Suppl. I):I–24, 1978.

McManus, R. P., O'Hair, D. P., Beitzinger, J. M., et al.: Patients who die awaiting heart transplantation. J. Heart Lung Transplant., 12:159, 1993.

Miller, C. A., Pae, W. E., Jr., and Pierce, W. S.: Combined registry for the clinical use of mechanical ventricular assist pumps and the total artificial heart in conjunction with heart transplantation: Fourth official report—1989. J. Heart Transplant., 9:453, 1990.

Miller, D. C., Stinson, E. B., Oyer, P. E., et al.: Discriminant analysis of the changing risks of coronary artery operations: 1971–1979. J. Thorac. Cardiovasc. Surg., 85:197, 1983.

Montoya, A., Lonchyna, V. A., and Moreno, N.: Anticoagulation for ventricular assist device. In Pifarre, R. (ed): Anticoagulation, Hemostasis, and Blood Preservation in Cardiovascular Surgery. Philadelphia, Hanley & Belfus, 1993, pp. 265–270.

Moreira, L. F. P., Bocchi, E. A., Stolf, N. A. G., et al.: Current expectations in dynamic cardiomyoplasty. Ann. Thorac. Surg., 55:299, 1993.

Moritz, A., and Wolner, E.: Circulatory support with shock due to acute myocardial infarction. Ann. Thorac. Surg., 55:238, 1993.

Morrow, A. G., Cohen, L. S., Roberts, W. C., et al.: Severe mitral regurgitation following acute myocardial infarction and rupture of papillary muscle. Circulation, 37(Suppl. II):II–124, 1968.

Moulopoulos, S. D., Topaz, S., and Kolff, W. J.: Diastolic balloon pumping (with carbon dioxide) in the aorta: Mechanical assistance to the failing circulation. Am. Heart J., 63:669, 1962.

Mueller, H., Aynes, S. M., Gianelli, S., Jr., et al.: Cardiac performance and metabolism in shock due to acute myocardial infarction in man: Response to catecholamines and mechanical cardiac assist. Trans. N. Y. Acad. Sci., 34:309, 1972.

Mundth, E. D., Buckley, M. J., Daggett, W. M., et al.: Intra-aortic balloon pump assistance and early surgery in cardiogenic shock. Integrated medical-surgical care in acute coronary artery disease. Adv. Cardiol., 15:159, 1975.

Myers, W. O., Schaff, H. V., Gersh, B. J., et al.: Improved survival of surgically treated patients with triple-vessel coronary artery disease and severe angina pectoris. A report from the Coronary Artery Surgery Study (CASS) registry. J. Thorac. Cardiovasc. Surg., 97:487, 1989.

Naunheim, K. S., Swartz, M. T., Pennington, D. G., et al.: Intra-aortic balloon pumping in patients requiring cardiac operations. J. Thorac. Cardiovasc. Surg., 104:1654, 1992.

Norman, J. C., Cooley, D. A., Igo, S. R., et al.: Prognostic indices for survival during postcardiotomy intra-aortic balloon pumping. J. Thorac. Cardiovasc. Surg., 74:709, 1977.

Oaks, T. E., Wisnan, C. B., Pae, W. E., et al.: Results of mechanical assistance before heart transplantation. J. Heart Transplant., 8:113, 1989.

O'Connell, J. B., Renlund, D. G., Robinson, J. A., et al.: Effect of preoperative hemodynamic support on survival after cardiac transplantation. Circulation, 78(Suppl. III):III–78, 1988.

O'Rouke, M. F.: Arterial counterpulsation in the management of ischemic heart disease. Aust. N. Z. J. Surg., 47:1, 1977.

Oyamada, A., and Queen, F. B.: Spontaneous rupture of the interventricular septum following acute myocardial infarction with some clinicopathologic observations on survival in five cases. Presented at the First Pan-Pacific Pathology Congress, Tripler, U.S. Army Hospital, Honolulu, Hawaii, October 12, 1961.

Pae, W. E., Jr.: Ventricular assist devices and total artificial hearts: A combined registry experience. Ann. Thorac. Surg., 55:295, 1993.

Pae, W. E., Jr., Miller, C. A., Matthews, Y., and Pierce, W. S.: Ventricular assist devices for postcardiotomy cardiogenic shock. A combined registry experience. J. Thorac. Cardiovasc. Surg., 104:541, 1992.

Parascandola, S. A., Pae, W. E., Davis, P. K., et al.: Determinants of survival in patients with ventricular assist devices. ASAIO Trans., 34:222, 1988.

Pennington, D. G., Farrar, D. J., Loisance, D., et al.: Panel selection. Ann. Thorac. Surg., 55:206, 1993.

Pennington, D. G., Kanger, K. R., McBride, L. R., et al.: Seven years' experience with the Pierce-Donachy ventricular assist device. J. Thorac. Cardiovasc. Surg., 96:901, 1988.

Pennington, D. G., Merjavy, J. P., Codd, J. E., et al.: Extracorporeal membrane oxygenation for patients with cardiogenic shock. Circulation, 70(Suppl.):130, 1984.

Pennington, D. G., and Swartz, M. T.: Current status of temporary circulatory support. In Karp, R. B. (ed): Advances in Cardiac Surgery. Vol. 1. Chicago, Year Book Medical, 1990, pp. 177–198.

Pennington, D. G., Swartz, M. T., Codd, J. E., et al.: Intra-aortic balloon pumping in cardiac surgical patients: A nine-year experience. Ann. Thorac. Surg., 36:125, 1983.

Phillips, S. J.: Percutaneous cardiopulmonary bypass and innovations in clinical counterpulsation. Crit. Care Clin., 2:297, 1986.

Pierce, W. S., Hershon, J. J., Kormos, R. L., et al.: Management of secondary organ dysfunction. Ann. Thorac. Surg., 55:222, 1993.

Pierri, M. K., Zema, M., Kligfield, P., et al.: Exercise tolerance in late survivors of balloon pumping and surgery for cardiogenic shock. Circulation, 62(Suppl. I):I–138, 1980.

Pifarre, R. (ed): Anticoagulation, Hemostasis, and Blood Preservation in Cardiovascular Surgery. Philadelphia, Hanley & Belfus, 1993.

Pifarre, R., Sullivan, H., Montoya, A., et al.: Comparison of results after heart transplantation: Mechanically supported versus nonsupported patients. J. Heart Lung Transplant., 11:235, 1992.

Poirier, V. L.: The quest for a solution we must continue. We must push forward. The 16th Hastings lecture. ASAIO J., 39:856, 1993.

Portner, P. M.: A totally implantable heart assist system: The Novacor program. In Akutsu, T., and Koyanagi, H. (eds): Artificial Heart 4. Heidelberg, Springer-Verlag, 1993.

Portner, P. M., Baumgartner, W. A., Cabrol, C., et al.: Internal pulsatile circulatory support. Ann. Thorac. Surg., 55:261, 1993.

Radford, M. J., Johnson, R. A., Buckley, M. J., et al.: Survival following mitral valve replacement for mitral regurgitation due to coronary artery disease. Circulation, 60(Suppl. II):II–39, 1979.

Reedy, J. E., Pennington, D. G., Miller, L. W., et al.: Status I heart transplant patients: Conventional versus ventricular assist device support. J. Heart Lung Transplant., 11:246, 1992.

Reemstma, K., Drusin, R., Edie, R., et al.: Cardiac transplantation for patients requiring mechanical circulatory support. N. Engl. J. Med., 298:670, 1978.

Reimer, K. A., Lowe, J. E., and Rasmussen, M. M.: The wavefront phenomenon of ischemic cell death. Circulation, 56:786, 1977.

Rose, E. A., Marrin, C. A. S., Bregman, D., et al.: Left ventricular mechanics of counterpulsation and left heart bypass, individually and in combination. J. Thorac. Cardiovasc. Surg., 77:127, 1979.

Rowles, J. R., Mortimer, B. J., and Olsen, D. B.: Ventricular assist and total artificial heart devices for clinical use in 1993. ASAIO J., 39:840, 1993.

Salmons, S., and Sreter, F. A.: Significance of impulse activity in the transformation of skeletal muscle type. Nature, 263:30, 1967.

Sanders, R. J., Kern, W. H., and Blount, S. G.: Perforation of the interventricular septum complicating myocardial infarction. Am. Heart J., 51:736, 1956.

Sanders, R. J., Neubuerger, K. T., and Ravin, A.: Rupture of papillary muscles. Occurrence of rupture of the posterior muscle and posterior myocardial infarction. Dis. Chest, 31:316, 1957.

Sarnoff, S. J., Braunwald, E., Welch, G. H., Jr., et al.: Hemodynamic determinants of oxygen consumption of the heart with special reference to the tension-time index. Am. J. Physiol., 192:148, 1958.

Sato, N., Mohri, H., Fujimasa, I., et al.: Multivariate analysis of risk factors for thrombus formation in University of Tokyo ventricular assist device. J. Thorac. Cardiovasc. Surg., 106:520, 1993.

Scheidt, S., Ascheim, R., and Killip, T.: Shock after acute myocardial infarction: A clinical and hemodynamic profile. Am. J. Cardiol., 26:556, 1970.

Scheidt, S., Wilner, G., Mueller, H., et al.: Intra-aortic balloon counterpulsation in cardiogenic shock: Report of a cooperative clinical trial. N. Engl. J. Med., 288:979, 1973.

Schuster, E. H., and Bulkley, B. H.: Early postinfarction angina. N. Engl. J. Med., 305:1101, 1981.

Sergeant, P., Wouters, L., Dekeyser, L., et al.: Is the outcome of coronary artery bypass graft surgery predictable in patients with severe ventricular function impairment? J. Cardiovasc. Surg. (Torino), 27:618, 1986.

Sharma, C. P., and Szycher, M. (eds): Blood compatible materials and devices. Lancaster, PA, Technomic Publishing, 1991.

Shinn, J. A., Abou-Awdi, N., Ley, S. J., et al.: Nursing care of the patient on mechanical circulatory support. Ann. Thorac. Surg., 55:288, 1993.

Skinner, D. B., Schechter, E., Hood, R. H., et al.: Mechanical ventricular assistance in human beings. Ann. Thorac. Surg., 5:131, 1968.

Stuckey, J. H., Newman, M. M., Dennis, C., et al.: The use of the heart-lung machine in selected cases of acute myocardial infarction. Surg. Forum, 8:342, 1957.

Takano, H., Nakatani, T., and Taenaka, Y.: Clinical experience with ventricular assist systems in Japan. Ann. Thorac. Surg., 55:250, 1993.

Tepe, N. A., and Edmunds, L. H., Jr.: Operation for acute postinfarction mitral insufficiency and cardiogenic shock. J. Thorac. Cardiovasc. Surg., 89:525, 1985.

Termuhlen, D. F., Pennington, D. G., Roodman, S. T., et al.: T cells in ventricular assist device patients. Circulation, 80(Suppl. III):III–174, 1989.

Wasfie, T., Freed, P. S., Rubenfire, M., et al.: Risks associated with intra-aortic balloon pumping in patients with and without diabetes mellitus. Am. J. Cardiol., 61:558, 1988.

Weber, K. T., and Janicki, J. S.: Intraaortic balloon counterpulsation. Ann. Thorac. Surg., 17:602, 1974.

Wei, J. Y., Hutchins, G. M., and Bulkley, B. M.: Papillary muscle rupture and fatal acute myocardial infarction. Ann. Intern. Med., 90:149, 1979.

Willerson, J. T., Curry, G. C., Watson, J. T., et al.: Intra-aortic balloon counterpulsation in patients with cardiogenic shock, medically refractory left ventricular failure and/or recurrent ventricular tachycardias. Am. J. Med., 58:183, 1975.

Yellin, E., Levy, L., and Bregman, D.: Hemodynamic effects of intraaortic balloon pumping in dogs with aortic incompetence. Trans. Am. Soc. Artif. Intern. Organs, 19:389, 1973.

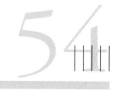

# ■ VI Dietary and Pharmacologic Management of Atherosclerosis

## John R. Guyton

Accumulating experience from epidemiology, research trials, and clinical practice indicates that it is possible to prevent atherosclerotic disease with a high expectation of success and also to achieve regression of established disease in many, if not most, patients. Since the 1960s, a 40% decline in overall cardiovascular mortality has occurred in the United States (Sytkowski et al., 1990). This decline may be attributed to a number of factors: lower plasma cholesterol, improved treatment of hypertension, reduced smoking rates, intensive care for acute ischemia, or intervention by bypass surgery and angioplasty. Most recently, it has become clear that established coronary heart disease can regress with lipid-lowering treatment and that the anatomic improvement is accompanied by symptomatic clinical benefit and marked reduction of risk for thrombotic events (Brown et al., 1993; Ornish et al., 1990). Aggressive medical regimens for atherosclerosis regression are difficult to implement, however, and the simpler regimens for prevention remain underused among the population. Thus, atherosclerotic vascular disease, which currently accounts for approximately one-third of all deaths in the United States, is likely to remain a dominant clinical concern for decades to come.

This chapter primarily describes effective preventive and regressive therapy of atherosclerosis. To set the stage, lesion pathology and arterial wall biology are discussed. Because lipid-oriented therapy is so important, basic aspects of lipids and lipoproteins are described. A guide to practical decision making in atherosclerosis treatment is the last and largest section of the chapter.

## ATHEROSCLEROSIS

### Vascular Biology

Endothelial cells are flat cells arranged like paving stones to form a continuous, tightly sealed monolayer on the luminal surface. Their primary function is to act as a permeability barrier, preventing exudation of plasma into arterial tissue, but they have important effects on blood clotting, inflammation, and arterial muscle tone as well. The influence on blood clotting is weighted toward antithrombotic effects. Endothelium synthesizes prostacyclin and nitric oxide, which in-

hibit platelet aggregation. The endothelial cell surface provides molecular mechanisms for the activation of antithrombin III, protein C, and tissue plasminogen activator. However, endothelial cells can also promote clotting via synthesis of tissue factor and Factor VIII/ von Willebrand's factor (Nachman, 1992). Inflammatory stimuli cause the expression of endothelium-leukocyte adhesion molecules, such as vascular cell adhesion molecule-1, E-selectin, and others. When stimulated by certain chemical mediators or by increased blood flow, endothelial cells secrete increased amounts of nitric oxide, which relaxes underlying smooth muscle and thus dilates the artery (Ross, 1993).

The cell that provides shape, bulk, and strength to the arterial wall is the vascular smooth muscle cell. Collagen, elastin, and proteoglycans in the tunica media are synthesized by smooth muscle cells. In small animals and in small arteries of large animals (e.g., pig or human), smooth muscle resides entirely in the tunica media, or middle coat of the artery. Beginning at birth in larger arteries, and especially in such arteries as the coronaries, which encounter longitudinal as well as radial pulsatile stretching, smooth muscle cells migrate into the subendothelial zone of the tunica intima. The thickened intima formed postnatally by migrating smooth muscle cells in large arteries is the locus for atherosclerosis development.

Studies of vascular smooth muscle in vivo demonstrate that tensile stress is an important regulator of growth and fibrous protein synthesis (Guyton, 1987). Hypertension causes thickening of the arterial media and intima. Arterial injury can cause exuberant smooth muscle cell proliferation, apparently mediated by basic fibroblast growth factor (Reidy, 1992). In atherosclerosis, smooth muscle growth and migration may be stimulated partly by *platelet-derived growth factor* (PDGF). Macrophages in arterial lesions synthesize PDGF B-chain, and smooth muscle cells themselves make PDGF A-chain. In late stages of atherosclerosis, platelets adhering to sites of intimal ulceration or endothelial denudation can provide PDGF as well. The most important cytokine for stimulation of collagen synthesis may be transforming growth factor–beta (Ross, 1993).

The entry of monocytes into the arterial wall and their transformation into macrophages may be early events in atherogenesis (Fig. 54–136). In addition to

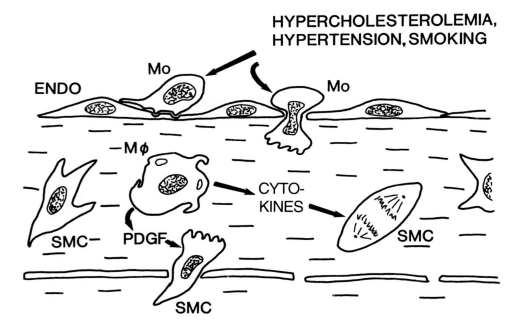

FIGURE 54–136. Role of monocyte-macrophages in atherogenesis. Monocytes (Mo) adhere to endothelium (ENDO) and enter the arterial intima in large numbers under conditions of hypercholesterolemia, hypertension, or smoking. After entering the intima, monocytes change gene expression and become macrophages (Mø). Platelet-derived growth factor (PDGF), which actually can be made by many cells besides platelets, is secreted by macrophages and can induce migration of smooth muscle cells (SMC). This and other cytokines from macrophages may cause SMC proliferation.

producing cytokines that affect smooth muscle cells, macrophages take up modified lipoproteins avidly, forming foam cells. Macrophages also undergo mitosis and cell division in atherosclerotic lesions (Ross, 1993).

## Lesion Development

Fatty streaks are early atherosclerotic lesions that first appear normally in teenagers in the coronaries and the aorta. These lesions are flat and small, do not disrupt the endothelial lining, and have no clinical consequence in themselves. Histologically, fatty streaks usually consist of lipid-filled macrophages with lesser numbers of lipid-bearing smooth muscle cells. Feeding of cholesterol to animals causes within a few weeks the adherence of large numbers of circulating monocytes to the arterial endothelium. Adherence and subsequent transmigration of monocytes are mediated by several distinct sets of cellular adhesion molecules expressed on the surface of both endothelial cells and monocytes. The monocytes squeeze through interendothelial junctions to enter the arterial intima, where they activate a program of gene expression leading to their development into macrophages.

Beginning at about age 20 years, especially in males, raised lesions appear in the proximal coronaries and in the iliac arteries. Progression of raised atherosclerosis extends from the iliac arteries proximally into the abdominal and later the thoracic aorta, and distally toward the femorals. In addition, the carotid bulb and many branch points of larger arteries become involved. The raised character of the lesions is due to proliferation of smooth muscle cells and macrophages and to elaboration of large amounts of fibrous tissue, especially collagen. Raised lesions with an intact intimal surface are called *fibrous plaques*. Most raised lesions possess a lipid-rich, hypocellular or acellular core region. Recently, a putative core region has been described in early, flat aortic lesions that resemble fatty streaks (Guyton and Klemp, 1993). This finding is compatible with the hypothesis that most fibrous plaques are derived from preexisting fatty streaks (Fig. 54–137).

Under certain circumstances, fibrous plaques may develop with little or no accompanying lipid deposition. The concentric intimal thickening that develops in coronary arteries of transplanted hearts, often to a severe degree, appears to be immunologically mediated and largely independent of lipid deposition. The extent to which ordinary fibrous plaques in native arteries can develop without lipid is uncertain.

As the fibrous plaque enlarges and begins to impinge on the arterial lumen, a compensatory enlargement of the entire artery occurs. This is probably due to physiologic regulation of arterial lumen diameter in response to blood velocity and shear rate. However, the compensatory enlargement eventually fails, perhaps when the collagenous lesion extends circumferentially almost all the way around the artery, leaving little normal wall to respond to blood flow (Glagov et al., 1987).

The most hazardous component of the atherosclerotic lesion is the core region, which expands and erodes the fibrous cap of the lesion with time. When the fibrous cap finally ruptures, blood dissects rapidly into the core, and the thrombogenic contents of the core erupt into the vessel lumen, causing partial or complete thrombosis of the artery within one to a few minutes. This final process appears to be inhibitable by aspirin (Fuster et al., 1990).

## LIPOPROTEIN METABOLISM

### Lipids

A high content of carbon and hydrogen makes all lipid molecules hydrophobic, so that lipids tend to

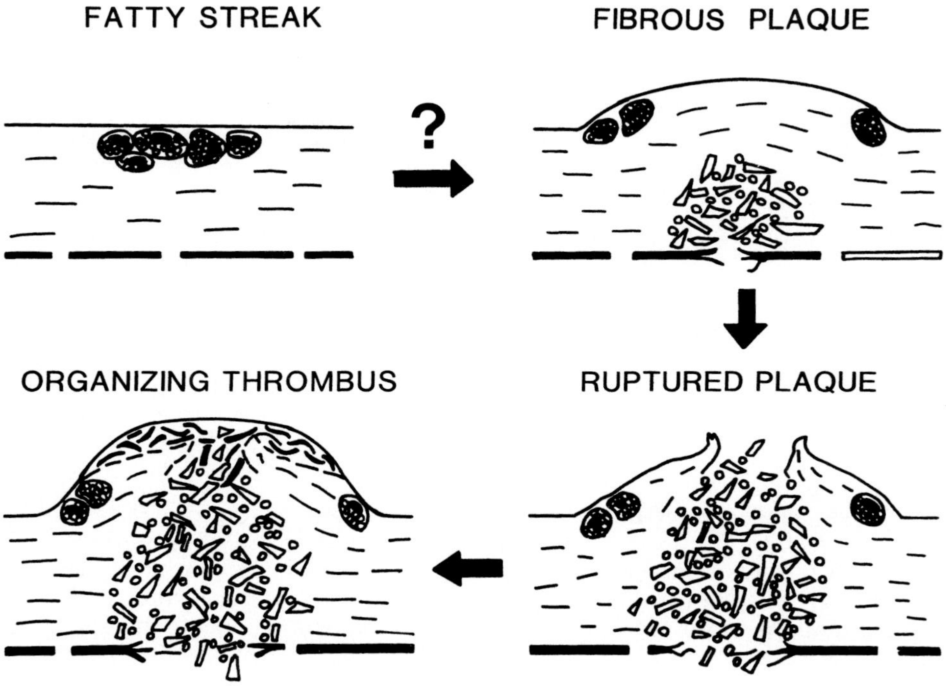

## FATTY STREAK

## FIBROUS PLAQUE

## ORGANIZING THROMBUS

## RUPTURED PLAQUE

FIGURE 54–137. Lesion development. The fatty streak is a flat lesion composed of foam cells. Fibrous plaques are raised lesions that usually, but not always, contain a cholesterol-rich, acellular core. Rupture of a fibrous plaque occurs after the expanding core weakens the support of the endothelial surface to the breaking point. The luminal thrombus resulting from plaque rupture is organized by ingrowth and proliferation of smooth muscle cells, leading to rapid, episodic growth of advanced lesions. (From Guyton, J. R.: Lipid metabolism and atherogenesis. *In* Garson, A., Jr., Bricker, J. T., and McNamara, D. G. [eds]: The Science and Practice of Pediatric Cardiology. Philadelphia, Lea & Febiger, 1990.)

associate with other lipids in an aqueous environment, forming membranes, oily droplets, and micelles. Phospholipids are the broad, diverse class of phosphorus-containing lipids that form cell membranes and perform many other essential biologic functions. Phospholipids are not a target for antiatherosclerotic therapies at present.

Cholesterol is an essential component of most cell membranes. Fatty acids are the principal fuel used by muscle and most other body tissues. These lipids also serve as hormone precursors—steroids from cholesterol, prostaglandins and leukotrienes from arachidonic acid—but lipid-lowering treatment generally produces no adverse endocrine effects.

Cholesteryl ester and triglyceride are lipid esters that provide efficient storage or transport of the corresponding active molecules, cholesterol and fatty acids. These lipid esters are so hydrophobic that they practically cannot enter or move across cell membranes. A recurring theme in lipoprotein metabolism is either formation or hydrolysis of lipid esters, accompanying the movement of cholesterol or fatty acids in and out of cells.

### Lipoproteins and Apolipoproteins

Human plasma lipoproteins transport triglyceride and cholesterol/cholesteryl ester in plasma. They are spherical particles ranging from 100 to 1 million lipid molecules combined with one or more protein molecules. The oily core of the lipoprotein is composed of triglyceride and cholesteryl ester. Based on which of these species predominates in the oily core, lipoproteins can be classified as triglyceride-rich or cholesterol-rich. Phospholipids, free (unesterified) cholesterol, and protein are found in a surface layer. Lipoprotein classes are listed in Table 54–31.

The protein components, termed *apolipoproteins*, bear specific binding sites for lipoprotein receptors or for enzymes involved in lipoprotein metabolism and thus target the lipoproteins for tissue uptake or lipid delivery (Table 54–32). All normal human lipoproteins contain either *apolipoprotein A-I* (apoA-I) or *apolipoprotein B* (apoB), or in the case of chylomicrons, both. Thus apoA-I and apoB appear to determine lipoprotein formation and structure as well as metabolic targeting. *High density lipoproteins* (HDLs) characteristically contain apoA-I, and all lipoproteins of larger size and lower density contain apoB.

### Lipoprotein Pathways

Chylomicrons are intestinally derived triglyceride-rich lipoproteins of very large size, which appear transiently for several hours after the ingestion of fat in the diet. Chylomicrons are secreted into intestinal lymph and enter the bloodstream via the thoracic duct. From there, chylomicrons travel to peripheral capillaries, where they encounter an enzyme, lipoprotein lipase, that hydrolyzes triglyceride ester bonds to deliver free fatty acids to the tissues. Following lipoprotein lipase action, the chylomicron remnant is released and circulates back to the liver, where it is taken up very rapidly by a process that depends partly on apolipoprotein E present on the lipoprotein surface.

The metabolic pathways of apoB-containing lipoproteins originating in the liver are shown in Figure

■ **Table 54–31.** PLASMA LIPOPROTEINS

| Lipoprotein | Density (g/ml) | Diameter (nm) | Molecular Weight (kilodaltons) | Electrophoretic Mobility | Most Abundant Chemical Constituents |
|---|---|---|---|---|---|
| Chylomicrons* | <0.93 | 75–1200 | ~400,000 | Origin | Triglyceride |
| VLDL | 0.93–1.006 | 30–80 | 10,000–80,000 | Prebeta | Triglyceride |
| IDL* | 1.006–1.019 | 25–35 | 5000–10,000 | Slow prebeta | Cholesteryl ester, triglyceride |
| LDL | 1.019–1.063 | 18–25 | 2300 | Beta | Cholesteryl ester |
| Lp[a]* | 1.050–1.125 | 24–26 | 3000–5000 | Slow prebeta | Cholesteryl ester |
| HDL₂ | 1.063–1.125 | 9–12 | ~360 | Alpha | Protein, phospholipid, cholesteryl ester |
| HDL₃ | 1.125–1.210 | 5–9 | ~175 | Alpha | Protein, phospholipid, cholesteryl ester |

Data from Gotto et al., 1986; Havel et al., 1980; Morrisett et al., 1987; Smith et al., 1983.

*Key:* IDL = intermediate density lipoprotein; LDL = low density lipoprotein; VLDL = very low density lipoprotein; Lp[a] = lipoprotein [a]; HDL₂, HDL₃ = HDL subfractions.

*These lipoproteins usually are not major components in fasting plasma. Chylomicrons normally circulate only postprandially. IDL are formed continuously from VLDL but are rapidly cleared or metabolized to LDL. Lp[a] is a minor lipoprotein in most individuals, but some persons have substantial plasma Lp[a] concentrations on a genetic basis.

54–138. A single molecule of apoB is incorporated into *very low density lipoprotein* (VLDL) before secretion from the liver, and this apoB molecule remains with the lipoprotein throughout all of its subsequent transformations, until the entire lipoprotein is taken up and degraded by a cell. VLDLs, which are triglyceride-rich, encounter lipoprotein lipase and deliver fatty acids to tissues in exactly the same manner as chylomicrons. As shown in Figure 54–138, some of the VLDL remnants (also known as *intermediate density lipoproteins* [IDLs]) are processed within the hepatic microcirculation to become *low density lipoproteins* (LDLs), the major cholesterol-carrying particles in plasma. Physiologic removal of LDLs from plasma depends on the presence of LDL receptor molecules found on the surface of hepatocytes and peripheral cells.

## Triglyceride Metabolism

The level of triglycerides in plasma depends on the balance of entry, in the form of VLDLs and chylomicrons, and exit via the action of lipoprotein lipase. Deficiency of lipoprotein lipase action can be due to partial or complete genetic defects in the enzyme itself or in its cofactor, apoC-II, or to suppression by diabetes mellitus or ethanol abuse. Any of these factors can raise plasma triglyceride levels greatly. The most important regulator of VLDL production is body fat. Intracellular lipase activity in adipose tissue releases fatty acids, which circulate as plasma free fatty acids to the liver. The liver re-esterifies the fatty acids, making triglyceride for secretion in VLDL. Thus, excess body fat stimulates a fatty acid-triglyceride cycle with concomitant excess production of VLDLs. Improved caloric balance—i.e., reduced dietary calories or increased caloric expenditure with exercise—is the only way to reduce body fat and eliminate this stimulus to high plasma triglycerides. A lesser, but sometimes important, stimulus to high plasma triglycerides is a high percentage of carbohydrates in the diet.

## Cholesterol Metabolism

Between 30 and 60% of dietary cholesterol is absorbed and reaches the liver largely via chylomicron remnants. A more important source of cholesterol, however, is synthesis in the liver from acetyl coenzyme A (acetyl CoA). A rate-limiting step in synthesis is catalyzed by *3-hydroxy-3-methylglutaryl CoA reductase*, which is potently inhibited by the "statin" category of cholesterol-lowering drugs. The liver is also the site of exit for most of the cholesterol leaving the body's metabolic pools. Cholesterol cannot be bro-

■ **Table 54–32.** MAJOR APOLIPOPROTEINS

| Apolipoprotein | Molecular Weight (kilodaltons) | Distribution | Function |
|---|---|---|---|
| A-I | 28,000 | HDL, chylomicrons | Structural role in HDL; activates lecithin-cholesterol acyltransferase |
| A-II | 17,000 | HDL, chylomicrons | Structural role in HDL |
| B-48 | 264,000 | Chylomicrons | Structural role in intestine-derived lipoproteins |
| B-100 | 550,000 | LDL, IDL, VLDL, chylomicrons | Structural role; ligand for LDL receptor binding |
| C-II | 9100 | VLDL, IDL, HDL, chylomicrons | Activates lipoprotein lipase |
| C-III | 8750 | VLDL, IDL, HDL, chylomicrons | Inhibits hepatic uptake of lipoproteins |
| E | 34,000 | IDL, VLDL, chylomicrons, HDL | Ligand for LDL receptor binding of IDL; promotes hepatic uptake of chylomicron remnants |
| [a] | 400,000–700,000 | Lp[a], chylomicrons | Unknown |

Data from Havel et al., 1980; Morrisett et al., 1987; Smith et al., 1983.

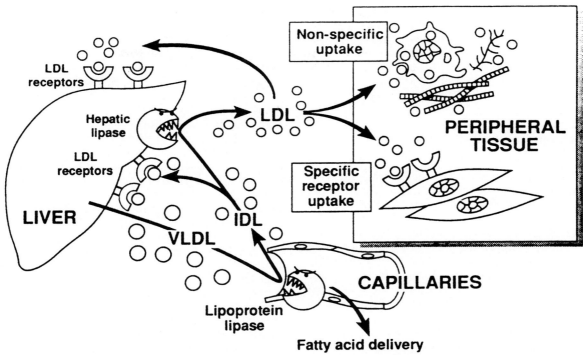

**FIGURE 54–138.** Pathways of apoB-containing lipoproteins derived from the liver. Triglyceride-rich very low density lipoproteins (VLDL) encounter lipoprotein lipase, which hydrolyzes triglyceride, resulting in smaller intermediate density lipoproteins (IDL), also called *VLDL remnants*. Some IDLs are taken up by the liver, and some are converted to low density lipoprotein (LDL) by hepatic lipase. There are three fates for LDL: (1) uptake in the liver, (2) uptake in peripheral cells via specific receptors, and (3) nonspecific disposition in tissues via uptake in macrophages or adherence to collagen, elastin, or proteoglycans. (Reproduced with permission. ©Medical Education Slides for the American Heart Association/Bristol-Myers Squibb Lipid Disorders Training Centers, 1990. Copyright American Heart Association.)

ken down by mammalian cells to simple metabolic end-products such as carbon dioxide. The liver converts cholesterol into bile acids; biliary secretion of these and of cholesterol itself account for the bulk of cholesterol removal from the body. More than 95% of bile acids ordinarily are reabsorbed in the terminal ileum (Grundy, 1978). The use of nonabsorbable resins (cholestyramine, colestipol), which bind bile acids in the gut, can lead to far greater net excretion and effectively reduce body cholesterol via bile acid conversion. This strategy is particularly effective when combined with agents that block a compensatory increase in cholesterol synthesis.

The liver plays a major role in the production of plasma LDL via secretion of VLDL and via processing of VLDL remnants to LDL. The liver also expresses cellular LDL receptors that mediate the removal of a large percentage of LDL particles exiting the plasma compartment. This is the reason that liver transplantation can reverse the extreme hypercholesterolemia that occurs in patients with homozygous deficiency of LDL receptors.

When a person has a heterozygous deficiency of functional LDL receptors, a relatively common, highly atherogenic condition occurring in 1 of 500 persons worldwide, plasma LDL levels are approximately twice normal (Goldstein and Brown, 1989). Recently, a similar condition, familial defective apoB, has been described, in which the receptor binding site on apoB is genetically dysfunctional (Innerarity et al., 1990).

The most common genetic hyperlipidemia that leads to coronary artery disease is neither of these, however, but is a less well understood, probably multifactorial or polygenic condition characterized by oversecretion of VLDLs. Among different members of a single family or even in a single individual at different times, either LDLs (plasma cholesterol) or VLDLs (plasma triglycerides), or both, may be elevated (Goldstein et al., 1973).

Peripheral cells derive essentially all of their cholesterol by endocytic uptake of LDLs via LDL receptors. Macrophages and other cells, which clear proteinaceous debris from body tissue, express other receptors able to bind chemically altered, oxidized, or aggregated LDLs. One of these latter receptors, the "scavenger" or "acetyl-LDL" receptor, has been cloned and studied in detail (Krieger et al., 1993).

Reverse cholesterol transport—i.e., movement of cholesterol from peripheral tissues back to the liver—is complex and incompletely understood. There is no clear, direct measurement that quantifies reverse cholesterol transport. HDL and apoA-I are clearly involved in the uptake of unesterified cholesterol from tissues and in the conversion of cholesterol to cholesteryl ester to facilitate reverse transport in lipoproteins. However, one cannot assume that reverse cholesterol transport is simply proportional to HDL cholesterol or apoA-I levels. Probucol and vegetarian diets both reduce HDL cholesterol levels, yet the former can reduce cholesterol-laden tendon xanthomas and the latter can largely prevent coronary disease (Yamamoto et al., 1986). Nevertheless, generally speaking, HDL cholesterol levels (including both subfractions $HDL_2$ and $HDL_3$) do correlate with coronary protection and with antiatherosclerotic efficacy of medical maneuvers (Levy et al., 1984).

## Role of Lipoproteins in Atherogenesis

The concentration of LDLs in the arterial intima is approximately equal to plasma LDL concentration, whereas interstitial fluid elsewhere in the body is thought to have a concentration one-tenth that of the plasma level. This is due to the fact that the tunica media is highly impermeable to LDLs, so that even when LDLs diffuse slowly across the arterial endothelium, high concentrations are attained in the intima. The high intimal LDL concentration probably explains why pathologic deposits of cholesterol develop regularly with aging in only the arterial intima and nowhere else (Guyton and Gotto, 1992).

Intimal lipid deposits are found both intracellularly and extracellularly at various stages of atherosclerosis. Foam cells commonly are macrophages packed with oily droplets of cholesteryl ester, but smooth muscle cells in the intima sometimes contain cholesteryl ester droplets as well. Lipoprotein uptake via the scavenger receptor or uptake of lipoprotein aggregates by phagocytosis may explain macrophage foam cell formation. In the early core region of small fibrous plaques, extracellular lipid deposits rich in unesterified cholesterol are found. The formation of these deposits is unexplained; their importance is emphasized by an association with disappearance of cells and weakening of tissue in the developing core (Guyton and Klemp, 1993).

Oxidation of LDLs, which can cause widespread chemical alterations in both lipid and protein components, may help explain a number of pathogenic processes in atherosclerosis. Immunostaining for oxidation epitopes suggests that macrophages may be primarily responsible for LDL oxidation, but endothelial and smooth muscle cells could contribute as well (Parthasarathy and Rankin, 1992). Mildly oxidized LDL stimulates endothelial cells to express cell surface adhesion molecules for attachment of monocytes, and several cell types express monocyte chemotactic protein–1 when stimulated by mildly oxidized LDL (Berliner et al., 1990). Highly oxidized LDL is taken up rapidly in macrophages, favoring foam cell formation. Highly oxidized LDL also tends to form aggregates that may produce lipid deposits in the extracellular space. Pharmacologic administration of antioxidants, such as vitamin E and probucol, has been shown to inhibit atherogenesis in rabbits (Steinberg et al., 1989). Epidemiologic data also suggest that vitamin E may help prevent atherosclerotic disease in humans, but clinical trials are needed (Rimm et al., 1993; Stampfer et al., 1993).

## Lipoprotein[a]

*Lipoprotein[a]* (Lp[a]) is a lipoprotein whose structure and role in atherogenesis have been elucidated only recently. Lp[a] is essentially an LDL with an added glycopeptide, apolipoprotein[a] (apo[a]), attached to apoB via a cysteine–cysteine disulfide bond. Lp[a] particles self-aggregate easily, perhaps favoring their deposition in the arterial intima. The amino acid sequence of apo[a] includes multiple repeats of a "kringle" sequence found in plasminogen and in tissue plasminogen activator. The *kringle* (named after a Danish pastry) fosters the attachment of these fibrinolytic enzymes to sites of clot formation. Lp[a] has been shown to interfere competitively with binding of the enzymes and thus with fibrinolysis. In all but a few clinical studies, a strong positive correlation has been found between Lp[a] levels and various manifestations of atherosclerosis, including myocardial infarction and stroke. Lp[a] levels show a strong inheritance pattern and are largely unaffected by diet and medications, except that niacin causes moderate reductions (Rader and Brewer, 1993). Additionally, postmenopausal estrogen replacement in women lowers plasma Lp[a] levels (Soma et al., 1993).

## Opportunities for Lesion Regression and Stabilization

Atherosclerotic regression is often conceived as a diminution in the size of an atherosclerotic lesion, which decreases stenosis. Such regression may occur, but other, more readily achievable, goals should also be considered (Fig. 54–139). For example, hypercholesterolemia can interfere with normal vasorelaxant function of endothelium, and decreases in plasma cholesterol have been shown to normalize endothelium-dependent relaxation (Leung et al., 1993). The presence of macrophages in the fibrous cap of an atherosclerotic lesion predisposes the lesion to rupture (Lendon et al., 1991). Lipid lowering can cause relatively rapid regression of foam cells, which might stabilize the fibrous cap, prevent rupture, and forestall atherothrombotic events.

## APPROACH TO CLINICAL MANAGEMENT

### Brief Summary of Clinical Trials

Medical treatment aimed at atherosclerosis can be classified as primary prevention, secondary prevention, and regression therapy. *Primary prevention* applies to persons who have never had clinical manifestations of atherosclerotic disease. *Secondary prevention* involves lessening the risk of further atherosclerotic events in patients who have already manifested clinical atherosclerotic disease. *Regression therapy,* which represents an extension of secondary prevention, aims to reverse quantifiable parameters of disease such as angiographically determined stenosis. Tables 54–33

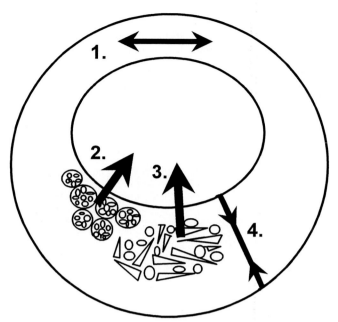

**FIGURE 54–139.** Four ways for risk to improve in an atherosclerotic lesion. (1) Dilatation of a normal segment of the arterial wall. (2) Regression of foam cells in the lesion cap or shoulder. (3) Removal of lipid from the core. (4) Regression of fibrous tissue. Of these potential processes, (1) and (2) seem most feasible.

and 54–34 show some of the clinical trials that have shaped the understanding of the efficacy of therapy. Much of the enthusiasm for lipid-lowering therapy to affect atherosclerosis stems from recent studies in which marked lipoprotein alterations were seen. The risk for the combined end-point of clinical events, including myocardial infarction, unstable angina, and coronary death, has dropped sharply in several of these studies. Although the recently introduced hydroxymethylglutaryl CoA reductase inhibitors are not well represented among the studies listed (see Tables 54–33 and 54–34), early reports suggest that they may be as effective as the regimens shown, or more so (Blankenhorn et al., 1993; Pravastatin Multinational Study Group for Cardiac Risk Patients, 1993).

## Questions About Low Plasma Cholesterol

With regard to primary prevention of atherosclerosis via cholesterol lowering, enthusiasm has been tempered by the consistent epidemiologic observation that persons with total cholesterol levels less than 160 mg/dl have increased noncardiac mortality (Jacobs et al., 1992). Furthermore, the first three trials listed (see Table 54–33) all showed increased noncardiac mortality, although the increase was significant only in the World Health Organization trial of clofibrate. The meaning of these findings is uncertain and requires further study. Since essentially all mammalian species other than humans typically have plasma cholesterol levels of 50 to 75 mg/dl, it is difficult to ascribe a biologic disadvantage to human levels below 160 mg/dl. The epidemiologic observations might be explained by clinically inapparent disease or inadequate nutrition leading to low cholesterol levels and coincidentally to increased mortality. The poor results with clofibrate may be specific for that drug alone, or perhaps may be shared with other fibric acid derivatives such as gemfibrozil.

## Guidelines for Lipid-Lowering Therapy

The guidelines of the United States National Cholesterol Education Program (NCEP), revised in June 1993, provide a well-reasoned approach to the prevention and treatment of atherosclerotic disease via

■ **Table 54–33.** SELECTED TRIALS WITH CLINICAL ENDPOINTS

| Name and Reference | Type of Intervention | Lipid/Lipoprotein Changes Compared with Control Group | Principal Outcomes Compared with Controls |
|---|---|---|---|
| **Primary Prevention** | | | |
| World Health Organization Trial (Committee of Principal Investigators, 1978) | Clofibrate | Total C ↓ 9% | Coronary events ↓ 20% <br> Total mortality ↑ 28% |
| Lipid Research Clinics/Coronary Primary Prevention Trial (1984) | Cholestyramine | Total C ↓ 9% <br> LDLC ↓ 13% | Coronary events ↓ 19% |
| Helsinki Heart Study (Frick et al. 1987) | Gemfibrozil | HDLC ↑ 13%, LDLC ↓ 8% <br> TG ↓ 40% | Coronary events ↓ 34% |
| Physicians' Health Study (1988) | Aspirin | Not determined | Myocardial infarction ↓ 47% |
| **Secondary Prevention** | | | |
| Coronary Drug Project (1975) (Canner et al., 1986) | Niacin | Total ↓ 10%, TG ↓ 26% | Myocardial infarction ↓ 27% at end of trial; total mortality ↓ 11% after additional 9-year follow-up |
| Program on Surgical Control of the Hyperlipidemias (Buchwald et al., 1990) | Partial ileal bypass | LDLC ↓ 38%, HDLC ↓ 4% | Coronary events ↓ 35%; total mortality showed favorable trend; side effects included diarrhea and kidney stones |

*Key*: C = cholesterol; LDLC = LDL cholesterol; HDLC = HDL cholesterol; TG = triglyceride.

■ **Table 54–34.** SELECTED CLINICAL TRIALS AIMED AT REGRESSION OF CORONARY ATHEROSCLEROSIS

| Name and Reference | Type of Intervention | Lipid/Lipoprotein Changes Compared with Control Group | Principal Outcomes Compared with Controls |
|---|---|---|---|
| Cholesterol-Lowering Atherosclerosis Study (Blankenhorn et al., 1987) | Niacin and colestipol | LDLC ↓ 43%, HDLC ↑ 37% | Regression in 16% of treated patients versus 2% of controls |
| Lifestyle Heart Trial (Ornish et al., 1990) | Vegetarian diet, stress reduction, mild exercise | LDLC ↓ 33% No change in HDLC | Angina markedly reduced; average regression of coronary lesions |
| Familial Atherosclerosis Treatment Study (Brown et al., 1990) | Niacin and colestipol Lovastatin and colestipol | LDLC ↓ 25%, HDLC ↓ 38% LDLC ↓ 39%, HDLC ↑ 10% | Both treatment groups had similar outcomes; net regression of coronary stenoses; clinical events reduced by 72% |
| St. Thomas Atherosclerosis Regression Study (Watts et al., 1992) | Diet Diet plus colestipol | LDLC ↓ 14%, HDLC no change LDLC ↓ 34%, HDLC ↓ 3% | Both treatment groups had significantly better outcomes compared with controls; decreased progression and increased regression of stenoses; clinical events reduced by 79% |

lipid-lowering therapy (National Cholesterol Education Program, 1988, 1993). The guidelines use LDL cholesterol as the central criterion for treatment decisions (Table 54–35). Other decision criteria enter the algorithm as "risk factors" (Table 54–36) that modify the LDL cholesterol decision points.

LDL cholesterol (LDLC) is best determined via calculation from the relationship: LDLC = Total C − HDLC − Triglycerides/5, where HDLC = HDL cholesterol. Since postprandial lipoproteins are not included in this calculation, the measurements must be performed on fasting serum or plasma. However, for many patients without atherosclerotic disease, one can simply measure total cholesterol and HDLC in the nonfasting state because these parameters do not change after meals. If the total cholesterol is less than 200 mg/dl, or if it is less than 240 mg/dl in a patient who has one or no risk factors, then the determination of LDLC by fasting lipoprotein analysis is not necessary. However, if HDLC is less than 35 mg/dl, then

fasting lipoprotein analysis is recommended regardless of total cholesterol or other risk factor status.

When LDLC is higher than the desirable level of 130 mg/dl, then dietary recommendations are appropriate. Even when LDLC levels are much higher, indicating a likely need for drug therapy, a period of only dietary change ranging from 6 weeks to several years can be undertaken. The rationale for this approach is twofold: First, diet alone may be sufficient; and second, patient and physician should not make the mistake of depending on drugs alone without dietary effort. The best results in clinical trials with *cardiovascular end-points* often have been obtained in the trials with strong dietary components, with or without pharmacologic intervention (see Table 54–34).

There is a wide range of LDLC levels from approximately 105 to 220 mg/dl, within which a decision to initiate pharmacologic lipid-lowering therapy may or may not be appropriate. Thus, for younger men and premenopausal women, drug therapy can be withheld at LDLC levels up to 220 mg/dl. Aggressive LDLC reduction with drugs can be considered in some patients with severe atherosclerotic disease and LDLC levels as low as 105 mg/dl on diet. At intermediate levels, Table 54–35 or the publications of the NCEP should be consulted. However, it should be noted that the guidelines at lower LDLC levels are

■ **Table 54–35.** LDL CHOLESTEROL DECISION POINTS FROM THE NATIONAL CHOLESTEROL EDUCATION PROGRAM

| | |
|---|---|
| ≤100 mg/dl | Treatment goal if atherosclerotic vascular disease is present |
| <130 mg/dl | Desirable LDLC; treatment goal if 2+ risk factors are present |
| 130–159 mg/dl | Borderline high-risk LDLC; this is the treatment goal if level initially ≥160 and <2 risk factors, but if atherosclerotic disease is present, drug therapy is appropriate at this level after diet trial |
| ≥160 mg/dl | High-risk LDLC; initiate diet, and if LDLC remains high with 2+ risk factors, use drug therapy |
| ≥190 mg/dl | Threshold for drug therapy after sufficient diet trial, if <2 risk factors present (see exception below) |
| 190–219 mg/dl | May withhold drug therapy in younger adults (men aged <35 years and premenopausal women) if otherwise not at risk |

■ **Table 54–36.** ATHEROSCLEROTIC RISK FACTORS (NATIONAL CHOLESTEROL EDUCATION PROGRAM)

| | |
|---|---|
| Male ≥45 years | Low HDL cholesterol (<35 mg/dl) |
| Female ≥55 years or premature menopause without estrogen replacement therapy | Hypertension |
| Family history of premature coronary disease | Diabetes mellitus |
| Current smoker | |

*Negative risk factor:* If HDLC ≥60 mg/dl, then subtract one from the number of risk factors counted above based partly on extrapolation and partly on the increasing understanding of the role of LDL in atherogenesis. No clinical trials have shown solid evidence for benefit of pharmacotherapy in patients with LDLC less than approximately 150 mg/dl.

The emphasis on LDLC in current guidelines has the potential drawback of minimizing the role of HDLC and triglycerides in atherosclerosis development and regression. These other factors are important, but their roles are complex. Moreover, dietary and medical interventions aimed at HDLC and triglycerides are not as straightforward and sometimes not as effective as interventions aimed at LDLC. Thus, only a few recommendations appear warranted at the present time. Patients with triglyceride levels above 500 mg/dl need consideration of treatment to prevent pancreatitis and other complications of severe hypertriglyceridemia. Such treatment does not pertain to atherosclerosis, and is covered in other texts. Triglyceride levels over 200 mg/dl should prompt efforts at dietary management, primarily weight control. The uncommon isolated reduction of HDLC, without other lipoprotein abnormalities, does not require specific treatment. When LDLC levels indicate a need for treatment, and HDLC or triglycerides, or both, are abnormal, then it is appropriate to aim therapy toward triglyceride reduction and HDLC augmentation as well as LDLC reduction. However, the typical drop in plasma levels of HDLC as well as LDLC after the institution of a diet lower in saturated fat seems to be advantageous. Finally, special considerations may apply to patients with high triglyceride levels (over 350 mg/dl). In these patients, triglyceride-lowering therapy often increases LDLC, as VLDLs are converted to LDLs with greater efficiency. This phenomenon is probably not disadvantageous. The opinion of this author is that in such patients, the ratio of total cholesterol to HDLC is the best measure of the anti-atherosclerotic effectiveness of therapy, and changes in LDLC are much less important.

## DIET IN PREVENTION AND TREATMENT

The important areas in dietary management of atherosclerosis concern fatty acids derived from food versus those derived from body stores, quality of fat, fat versus carbohydrate, dietary cholesterol intake versus hepatic cholesterol synthesis, and the special roles of fiber, ethanol, and fish (Grundy and Denke, 1990). Dietary change, especially when it goes beyond the usual recommendations for the population, is one of the most powerful tools by which a patient can change the course of atherosclerotic disease.

### Body Weight

Apart from genetic factors, the most important influence on hepatic production of VLDL triglyceride is the flux of plasma free fatty acids to the liver. The liver removes almost all of the free fatty acids from perfusing blood and mostly reesterifies these into triglycerides destined for export in VLDLs. The most important influence on plasma free fatty acid levels is body fat, or the total mass of triglyceride contained in adipose tissue, and the clinical correlate is simply body weight. Body weight is a strong correlate not only of VLDL triglyceride production, but also production of apoB, which enters the circulation mostly in VLDLs. Since LDL is produced in the plasma from VLDL, it can be rightly stated for many patients that stored body fat drives the production of atherogenic lipoproteins. Furthermore, when VLDL triglyceride levels rise in plasma, HDLC levels decrease, a phenomenon attributed to the transfer of triglyceride into HDL and subsequent removal of triglyceride-enriched HDL from plasma by the liver.

The relationship of body weight to LDLC is complex, although a moderately strong positive correlation is the rule. Short-term weight loss (within 6 to 8 weeks) can cause dramatic reductions in both LDLC and HDLC, but the same degree of weight loss sustained over 6 months generally will produce a more modest reduction of LDLC and a rise in HDLC (Dattilo and Kris-Etherton, 1992). Patients with hypertriglyceridemia or with combined hyperlipidemia appear to respond especially favorably to weight reduction, compared with patients with pure hypercholesterolemia.

To lose weight, or to "get control" of weight, may be the most difficult task that a physician can ask a patient to accomplish. A gradual approach targeting a reduction of weight of 2 to 4 pounds per month and emphasizing behavior modification is best. Since adipose tissue contains 9 calories of energy stored per gram, weight reduction of 2 pounds per month depends on a net reduction of caloric balance of almost 300 calories per day. When the body perceives "depletion" of fat stores, especially after intensive dieting, basal caloric needs may be reduced, making further weight loss difficult. The resistance is not absolute, and a healthy diet producing weight loss can always be prescribed, preferably in collaboration with a dietitian. The patient should understand that basal caloric output is effectively supplemented with exercise, and for many, a long-term exercise program is the key to maintaining weight control. Although it is physiologically possible in essentially every case, ideal weight control is psychologically and practically impossible for many obese patients. It is often the mildly overweight, hyperlipidemic patient who successfully and permanently loses 15 to 20 pounds with excellent lipoprotein changes, simply because this person may be trying to get control of weight for the first time, not having previously experienced multiple cycles of failure.

### Dietary Components

In the ordinary Western diet, saturated fat is the component that can be changed most readily to yield favorable effects on plasma lipoproteins (Grundy and

Denke, 1990). In saturated fat (almost all of which is triglyceride), the fatty acid chains contain maximal numbers of hydrogen atoms and have no carbon–carbon double bonds. Hydrogenation is a food-processing technique that removes double bonds by adding hydrogen atoms, thereby increasing the saturation of fat. Among the saturated fatty acids, palmitic acid (16 carbons, no double bonds, hence 16 : 0) and myristic acid (14 : 0: exert most of the cholesterol-raising effect, whereas stearic acid (18 : 0) may influence lipoprotein levels minimally. Whether this distinction is clinically important is unclear. Older guidelines called for replacing saturated fat with polyunsaturated fat (principally linoleic acid, 18 : 2), but subsequently it was learned that this maneuver reduces HDLC as well as LDLC levels. Monounsaturated fatty acids, particularly oleic acid (18 : 1), when substituted for saturated fatty acids, reduce LDLC but not HDLC in plasma. Knowledge of the roles of polyunsaturated and monounsaturated fat is incomplete. Incorporation of polyunsaturates into LDL lipids increases the susceptibility for LDL oxidation, whereas monounsaturates inhibit oxidation. Nevertheless, clinical studies with cardiovascular end-points suggest that either polyunsaturated or monounsaturated fatty acids may help protect against cardiovascular disease, and there is no evidence from those studies to favor one or the other.

Cholesterol itself in the usual Western diet has less impact than saturated fat, since the liver ordinarily synthesizes approximately 70% of the body's daily cholesterol requirement and can readily increase the synthetic rate several-fold. Changing daily cholesterol consumption from 600 to 400 mg, for example, can be expected to decrease plasma cholesterol by less than 10 mg/dl, if saturated fat intake remains constant (Keys and Parlin, 1966). However, in more restrictive diets, the impact of reducing dietary cholesterol intake along with fat can be considerable. In the Lifestyle Heart Trial, the baseline diet was equivalent to the NCEP Step 2 diet (Table 54–37). The experimental group went on a strict vegetarian diet, essentially eliminating dietary cholesterol (plants do not make cholesterol) and reducing all fat to 7% of total calories. The drop in LDLC was 37%, comparable with that achieved by effective cholesterol-lowering medication (Ornish et al., 1990).

Most people in the world eat a diet high in complex carbohydrates and relatively low in fat and protein, compared with people in Western industrialized society. People on such a diet have very low plasma cholesterol levels, typically 140 to 160 mg/dl, with HDLC also relatively low. In these populations, rates of coronary disease are only a small fraction of the rates among Western nations. Substitution of complex carbohydrates for saturated fat is generally recommended. High-carbohydrate diets can raise plasma triglyceride levels, but usually with little clinical impact.

Moderate intake of alcohol, in the range of one to three drinks per day in men and one-half to two drinks per day in women, can reduce the risk of coronary heart disease by as much as 50% (Kreisberg, 1992). Both $HDL_2$ and $HDL_3$ are increased by ethanol, and direct effects on the arterial wall may be postulated to play a role as well. Risk reduction is not likely to occur in patients with hypertriglyceridemia because ethanol aggravates this condition. Furthermore, the blood pressure–raising effects of ethanol should be kept in mind. Because of the increased rate of motor vehicle accidents and other health and social risks of ethanol, it is not appropriate to counsel persons to drink for cardiovascular health, but ethanol intake can be approved if it is already established as a stable part of their lives.

Nondigestible plant fiber, which tends to form a viscous gel when placed in water—so-called soluble fiber—has been clearly shown to have a modest lowering effect on plasma cholesterol levels (Jenkins et al., 1993). Soluble fiber can be a helpful adjunct in preventing and treating atherosclerosis. Oat and rice bran and bean fiber, but not wheat bran, have this effect. Psyllium, long in use as a bulk-forming laxative agent, and guar gum are particularly effective soluble fibers, but intestinal bloating and flatus limit their usefulness in lowering lipids.

Epidemiologic data show that a high intake of fish in the diet may be particularly beneficial in preventing coronary disease (Connor and Connor, 1990). Omega-3 fatty acids, found in cold-water fatty fish such as salmon and mackerel, have been shown to reduce plasma triglyceride levels in humans, to inhibit platelet clotting modestly in humans, and to inhibit atherogenesis in some but not all animal studies. Because of the equivocal data and the likelihood of increasing LDL oxidation, fish oil capsules are not

■ **Table 54–37.** DIETARY THERAPY OF HIGH BLOOD CHOLESTEROL (NATIONAL CHOLESTEROL EDUCATION PROGRAM)

| Nutrient | Recommended Intake | | |
| --- | --- | --- | --- |
| | Step 1 Diet | | Step 2 Diet |
| Total fat | | 30% or less of total calories | |
|   Saturated fatty acids | 8–10% of total calories | | ≤7% of total calories |
|   Polyunsaturated fatty acids | | ≤10% of total calories | |
|   Monounsaturated fatty acids | | ≤15% of total calories | |
| Carbohydrates | | ≥55% of total calories | |
| Protein | | Approx. 15% of total calories | |
| Cholesterol | <300 mg/day | | <200 mg/day |
| Total calories | | To achieve and maintain desirable weight | |

recommended for preventing and treating atherosclerosis. However, increased ingestion of fish is recommended.

The current American diet contains approximately 36% of calories as fat, including 13% from saturated fat. Average daily intake of cholesterol is about 450 mg for men and 280 mg for women (Fortman et al., 1986). A gradual approach to changing this diet is recommended for somewhat more than half of the United States adult population, who have LDLC levels higher than 130 mg/dl. Step 1 and Step 2 dietary goals, developed by the American Heart Association, are shown in Table 54–33. If a group of men change from the average United States dietary pattern described earlier to the Step 2 diet, then the average reduction in plasma cholesterol will be approximately 20 mg/dl, according to a well-validated predictive equation developed by Keys and colleagues (Keys and Parlin, 1966). Individual cholesterol responses, of course, will vary in both directions from the average. Many patients with symptomatic atherosclerosis are able to make dietary changes that go well beyond the Step 2 diet, and they should be encouraged to do so.

The effect of diet on atherogenesis is imperfectly reflected in its effect of plasma lipoprotein levels. HDLC levels, for example, may not always correlate with the apparent activity of reverse cholesterol transport, which is theoretically of great importance to atherogenesis. The decrease in HDLC that occurs when many patients become serious about dietary change should not be a cause for alarm. In fact, clinical research and anecdotal experience have suggested that intensive dietary intervention can be just as effective as, or more effective than, medication in producing relief of anginal symptoms and reversal of stenosis in patients with coronary artery disease. Institution of a vegetarian or near-vegetarian diet can be an appropriate therapeutic maneuver in patients with advanced atherosclerosis who wish this approach or who develop side effects to medication (Ornish et al., 1990).

## PHARMACOLOGIC PREVENTION AND TREATMENT

Drug therapy for preventing and treating atherosclerosis should begin with consideration of aspirin for every person at risk. Aspirin doses between 30 and 325 mg/day appear to be equivalent in their ability to inhibit arterial thrombosis. In secondary prevention, the risk reduction is 30% for recurrent myocardial infarction and 15% for cardiac death (Antiplatelet Trialists' Collaboration, 1988). Rates in primary prevention are probably similar. Patients with uncontrolled hypertension should not take aspirin regularly because of the risk of hemorrhagic stroke (Physicians' Health Study, 1988). Because aspirin is thought chiefly to affect thrombosis and not to inhibit atherosclerosis development, there is no reason to recommend regular aspirin use until thrombosis risk is substantial—i.e., generally after age 50 years, or earlier if severe or multiple risk factors are present.

Estrogen replacement in postmenopausal women may reduce risk for coronary arterial disease by 35%. This estimate comes from epidemiologic studies of women who mostly took unopposed estrogen, but estrogen-progestin combinations used currently in women with intact uteri are probably also beneficial. Estrogen appears to have direct antiatherogenic effects on the arterial wall. Moderate reduction of LDLC and increase of HDLC can be seen as well. Hypertriglyceridemia can be aggravated by estrogen; hypertriglyceridemic patients should be monitored carefully.

Beyond aspirin and estrogen, drug therapy directed at atherosclerosis is concerned mainly with lowering LDLC. The most effective regimens use, singly or in combination, drugs from three groups: inhibitors of hydroxymethylglutaryl coA reductase (reductase inhibitors), bile acid–sequestering resins, and niacin. Other drugs offer adjunctive benefits or specifically reduce triglyceride levels with little effect on LDLC.

The reductase inhibitors, including lovastatin, pravastatin, simvastatin, and fluvastatin, are the most effective single agents available for lowering LDLC. The safety of these agents, particularly lovastatin, has been confirmed in several tens of thousands of adult patients followed prospectively, the first of whom began taking lovastatin in the early 1980s (Bradford et al., 1991). Reductase inhibitors competitively block the synthesis of mevalonic acid, a precursor in the cholesterol synthetic pathway. Although mevalonic acid leads to several other metabolites as well, the clinically available reductase inhibitors do not ordinarily interfere with crucial cellular functions, nor with the synthesis of steroid and sex hormones that use cholesterol as a precursor. Reductase inhibitors reduce triglycerides and raise HDLC, but both of these effects are modest. Patients should be monitored for hepatic transaminase elevations. Moderate doses of reductase inhibitors should be used initially because high doses cause more side effects while achieving only modest further reductions in LDLC. An interaction of lovastatin with cyclosporine, gemfibrozil, clofibrate, erythromycin, or possibly niacin can lead to myopathy and sometimes rhabdomyolysis (Corpier et al., 1988; Spach et al., 1991). These drugs should be avoided or used with caution in combination with any of the reductase inhibitors. Rarely does the reductase inhibitor alone cause myopathy.

Bile acid–sequestering resins include cholestyramine and colestipol, which are therapeutically very similar. These nonabsorbable resins bind bile acids in the small intestine, preventing their reabsorption in the terminal ileum. The liver detects bile acid depletion and diverts cholesterol stores toward bile acid synthesis, establishing a drain on body stores of cholesterol. The resins reduce LDLC 10 to 30% depending on dose. They have been shown to reduce cardiovascular event rates in primary prevention, but the beneficial effect was much smaller in patients with HDLC levels of 40 mg/dl or less while on treatment (Gordon et al., 1986; Lipid Research Clinics Program, 1984). Triglyceride levels typically increase with resin use; therefore, hypertriglyceridemia is a relative contraindication. Because the resins are not absorbed into the bloodstream, they have excellent theoretical and practical safety, sufficient to recommend them for reducing LDLC in pediatric cases and in women of childbearing potential. The major side effects are constipation (15% of patients) and abdominal bloating. Drug absorption may be inhibited, particularly warfarin, vitamin K (in warfarin-treated patients), digoxin, diuretics, and thyroxine.

Niacin, also known as nicotinic acid, is a form of vitamin $B_3$. Lipid-lowering doses can be 50 to 100 times the vitamin dose. Niacinamide (nicotinamide) also acts as a vitamin, but has no lipid-lowering effect. Niacin acts to inhibit lipolysis and production of free fatty acids from adipose tissue and also to decrease the production of VLDLs from the liver (Guyton and Gotto, 1989). Immediate-release niacin is usually given three or four times per day, always after ingestion of food or skim milk, at a total daily dose beginning as low as 100 mg and increasing over a few weeks to 1000 to 4000 mg. Sustained-released niacin, usually administered twice a day, is more prone to cause hepatotoxicity; the total dose should be limited to 2000 to 2250 mg daily. At 1000 mg per day, increased HDLC is often apparent. Higher doses reduce triglyceride and LDLC levels. Side effects of niacin include flushing (very common, but diminishing markedly with continued regular use), dyspepsia, hyperglycemia, transaminase elevations, atrial arrhythmias, peptic ulcer, gout, skin dryness, and visual disturbances.

Because LDLC of 100 mg/dl or less is the usual target in patients with atherosclerotic disease, combinations of the medications listed previously are often used. In combination therapy, one can often use moderate doses to achieve excellent LDLC reduction. When both cholesterol and triglycerides are elevated, a regimen of weight loss, reductase inhibitor, and niacin (1000 to 2000 mg daily) can be effective, but transaminases must be monitored carefully.

Other agents may be useful in some cases. Gemfibrozil reduced initial coronary events in patients with hypercholesterolemia, especially when a high triglyceride level or low HDLC was also present (Frick et al., 1987). Doubt has been cast on whether this drug should be used in patients with documented atherosclerotic disease. Probucol reduces LDLC modestly, reduces HDLC to a relatively greater degree, inhibits LDL oxidation ex vivo, and inhibits animal atherogenesis (Steinberg et al., 1989). Probucol has not been shown to have any effect on clinical atherosclerotic disease parameters. Fish oil, but not cod liver oil, in doses of at least 9 g daily can be used to treat hypertriglyceridemia, and a few animal studies have suggested additional benefit on atherosclerosis via effects on arterial cells.

## SURGICAL TREATMENT OF HYPERLIPIDEMIA

Partial ileal bypass, performed in half of 838 patients in a randomized clinical trial by Buchwald and associates (1990), reduced LDLC by 38% compared with controls and reduced the combined end-point of coronary death and myocardial infarction by 35% over a 10-year follow-up period. The principal side effect of the procedure was diarrhea. Patients in the surgery group reported an average of 3.0 bowel movements per day compared with 1.5 in controls, and stools in the surgery group were looser. Kidney stones presumably related to increased oxalate absorption occurred at a rate of 4% per year, compared with approximately 0.7% per year in controls. These side effects, plus increased rates of bowel obstruction and gallstone formation, make it difficult to recommend partial ileal bypass as a routine mode of therapy.

## OTHER INTERVENTIONS

### Tobacco

Smoking between one and two packs of cigarettes per day doubles the risk of coronary atherosclerotic events. The most important fact to communicate to patients is that the risk declines rapidly when smoking is stopped, such that coronary risk is almost normal within a few years (Manson et al., 1992). This fact, along with basic research results, suggests that a major effect of smoking is to enhance thrombus formation, perhaps via injurious effects of nicotine or other tobacco components on endothelium. Smoking also promotes atherogenesis, especially in the arterial supply to the lower extremities. Some, but not all, of the chronic atherogenic effects of smoking may be mediated by decreased plasma levels of HDLC. With smoking cessation, an increase in HDLC is commonly seen. Modest weight gain and sometimes plasma triglyceride elevation may accompany smoking cessation, but clinical benefits far outweigh these metabolic consequences.

### Antihypertensive Therapy

Medical therapy for hypertension is highly successful in preventing the complications of stroke and congestive heart failure but is less successful in reducing rates of coronary heart disease. This relative lack of responsiveness of coronary atherogenesis has been ascribed to adverse effects on lipoproteins of the antihypertensive medications used in long-term trials. These trials generally have used diuretics and beta-blockers singly or in combination. Both thiazide and loop diuretics cause, on average, small increases in triglyceride and LDLC levels. Beta-blockers tend to raise triglycerides and reduce HDLC. However, beta-blockers clearly have been shown to reduce mortality after myocardial infarction and thus are often indicated for patients with documented coronary disease.

Calcium channel blockers and angiotensin-converting enzyme inhibitors have almost no effect on plasma lipoprotein levels. Alpha-receptor antagonists (prazosin, doxazosin, and others) modestly decrease LDLC and increase HDLC. All of these drugs might be favored for antihypertensive treatment in patients with atherosclerotic disease (Lardinois and Neumann, 1988; Weidmann et al., 1988). Beta-blockers with intrinsic sympathomimetic activity do not change plasma lipoprotein levels, but these drugs do not reduce cardiac mortality, and it is therefore difficult to recommend them.

The possibility that vasoactive medications may have direct antiatherogenic effects on the arterial wall has been studied mostly in animal experiments. Calcium channel blockers have been shown to inhibit foam cell formation and arterial lipid deposition in rabbits fed atherogenic diets, despite the fact that blood pressure changes were minimal (Henry, 1988). A clinical trial of nifedipine showed a significant decrease in the formation of new lesions in human coronary artery disease, but progression of preexisting stenoses was not altered (Lichtlen et al., 1990). Early results suggest that diltiazem may help inhibit the diffuse arteriosclerotic narrowing that develops in coronary arteries of transplanted hearts (Schroeder et al., 1993). In a few animal experiments, angiotensin-converting enzyme inhibitors blocked smooth muscle proliferation after endothelial injury (Prescott et al., 1991); clinical trials of similar agents thus far have not shown significant inhibition of angioplasty restenosis.

## Exercise

Recent epidemiologic studies have confirmed that unaccustomed moderate to intense exercise acutely raises the risk of myocardial infarction several-fold. However, the same sets of data suggest that a steady pattern of exercise actually reduces risk (Mittleman et al., 1993). Cardiac rehabilitation programs emphasizing dietary management and appropriate medication for high LDLC as well as moderate exercise can be of great value in the treatment of coronary artery disease.

## SUMMARY

Although it is better to prevent atherosclerosis than to treat it, the presence of established disease should no longer be regarded as predictive of inexorable progression. In the treatment of atherosclerosis, smoking cessation is essential. Once this is accomplished, modification of plasma lipoprotein levels, especially LDLC, is the most effective way to change the course of the disease. Strong dietary effort and appropriate medication are often needed together. Control of hypertension and diabetes should be maintained. In most patients, a reasonable goal is more than 50% risk reduction, and highly motivated patients can do substantially better than this.

### SELECTED BIBLIOGRAPHY

Brown, B. G., Zhao, X. Q., Sacco, D. E., and Albers, J. J.: Lipid lowering and plaque regression. Circulation, 87:1781, 1993.

The authors summarize recent trials of lipid lowering for atherosclerosis regression. The conclusion of this review is that a high degree of prevention of clinical cardiovascular events can be achieved, even when arteriographic improvement appears modest.

Connor, W. E., and Connor, S. L.: Diet, atherosclerosis, and fish oil. Adv. Intern. Med., 35:139, 1990.

This is a readable summary of broad dietary knowledge from two of the longtime leaders in the field. A threshhold-and-plateau concept for the effect of dietary cholesterol is presented. Fish oil is a recent research interest of the authors—hence, the emphasis on fish oil—but other topics are also well presented.

Grundy, S. M., and Denke, M. A.: Dietary influences on serum lipids and lipoproteins. J. Lipid Res., 31:1149, 1990.

A comprehensive review of the effects of dietary cholesterol, fat and specific fatty acids, carbohydrates, and overweight on plasma lipoproteins. Insights regarding mechanisms of dietary lipid regulation are provided by these experienced investigators.

Manson, J. E., Tosteson, H., Ridker, P. M., et al.: The primary prevention of myocardial infarction. N. Engl. J. Med., 326: 1406, 1992.

A well-referenced source for information about smoking cessation, lowering of cholesterol, treatment of hypertension, physical activity, weight control, maintenance of normal glucose tolerance, estrogen replacement in postmenopausal women, alcohol, and aspirin as strategies for the prevention of initial myocardial infarction. Quantitative estimates of risk reduction are given for each of these strategies.

National Cholesterol Education Program: Report of the National Cholesterol Education Program (NCEP) Expert Panel on detection, evaluation, and treatment of high blood cholesterol in adults. Arch. Intern. Med., 148:36, 1988.

This is the first report of the NCEP Adult Treatment Panel. Although superseded now in terms of details of guidelines (see later), the first report, published in full in a readily available source, contains a wealth of information regarding dietary and drug therapy of hyperlipidemia. It includes sections on types of hyperlipidemia, strategies for hypertriglyceridemia, and practical suggestions to promote patient adherence to diet and drugs.

National Cholesterol Education Program: Summary of the second report of the National Cholesterol Education Program Expert Panel on detection, evaluation, and treatment of high blood cholesterol in adults (Adult Treatment Panel II). J. A. M. A., 269:3015, 1993.

This is an essential document for the physician treating lipid disorders for the prevention and treatment of atherosclerosis. This second report of the Adult Treatment Panel revises the guidelines of the first report. Although the article referenced here is only a summary of the full report (available from the NCEP), it clearly spells out the new guidelines.

Ornish, D., Brown, S. E., Scherwitz, L. W., et al.: Can lifestyle changes reverse coronary heart disease? The Lifestyle Heart Trial. Lancet, 336:129, 1990.

The results of this study suggest that major changes in lifestyle—principally a vegetarian diet—without addition of any new medications to patients' regimens can achieve striking reductions in frequency and severity of angina pectoris as well as coronary lesion regression documented by quantitative angiography. Although early anecdotal experience tends to support the claims of this report, confirmation by further controlled clinical trials is needed.

Ross, R.: The pathogenesis of atherosclerosis: A perspective for the 1990s. Nature, 362:801, 1993.

The vascular biology of atherosclerosis is reviewed with an emphasis on cytokines and growth factors secreted by or acting on endothelial cells, smooth muscle cells, macrophages, platelets, and T lymphocytes.

### BIBLIOGRAPHY

Antiplatelet Trialists' Collaboration: Secondary prevention of vascular disease by prolonged antiplatelet treatment. Br. Med. J., 296:320, 1988.

Berliner, J. A., Territo, M. C., Sevanian, A., et al.: Minimally modified low density lipoprotein stimulates monocyte endothelial interactions. J. Clin. Invest., 85:1260, 1990.

Blankenhorn, D. H., Azen, S. P., Kramsch, D. M., et al.: Coronary angiographic changes with lovastatin therapy: The Monitored

Atherosclerosis Regression Study (MARS). Ann. Intern. Med., *119*:969, 1993.

Blankenhorn, D. H., Nessim, S. A., Johnson, R. L., et al.: Beneficial effects of combined colestipol-niacin therapy on coronary atherosclerosis and coronary venous bypass grafts. J. A. M. A., *257*:3233, 1987.

Bradford, R. H., Shear, C. L., Chremos, A. N., et al.: Expanded clinical evaluation of lovastatin (EXCEL) study results. Arch. Intern. Med., *151*:43, 1991.

Brown, B. G., Albers, J. J., Fisher, L. D., et al.: Regression of coronary artery disease as a result of intensive lipid-lowering therapy in men with high levels of apolipoprotein B. N. Engl. J. Med., *323*:1289, 1990.

Brown, B. G., Zhao, X. Q., Sacco, D. E., and Albers, J. J.: Lipid lowering and plaque regression. Circulation, *87*:1781, 1993.

Buchwald, H., Varco, R. L., Matts, J. P., et al.: Effect of partial ileal bypass surgery on mortality and morbidity from coronary heart disease in patients with hypercholesterolemia. N. Engl. J. Med., *323*:946, 1990.

Canner, P. L., Berge, K. G., Wenger, N. K., et al.: Fifteen-year mortality in coronary drug project patients: Long-term benefit with niacin. J. Am. Coll. Cardiol., *8*:1245, 1986.

Committee of Principal Investigators: A cooperative trial in the primary prevention of ischaemic heart disease using clofibrate. Br. Heart J., *40*:1069, 1978.

Connor, W. E., and Connor, S. L.: Diet, atherosclerosis, and fish oil. Adv. Intern. Med., *35*:139, 1990.

The Coronary Drug Project Research Group: Clofibrate and niacin in coronary heart disease. J. A. M. A., *231*:360, 1975.

Corpier, C. L., Jones, P. H., Suki, W. N., et al.: Rhabdomyolysis and renal injury with lovastatin use. J. A. M. A., *260*:239, 1988.

Dattilo, A. M., and Kris-Etherton, P. M.: Effects of weight reduction on blood lipids and lipoproteins: A meta-analysis. Am. J. Clin. Nutr., *56*:320, 1992.

Fortman, S. P., Haskell, W. L., and Williams, P. T.: Changes in plasma high density lipoprotein cholesterol after changes in cigarette use. Am. J. Epidemiol., *124*:706, 1986.

Frick, M. H., Elo, O., Haapa, K., et al.: Helsinki Heart Study: Primary-prevention trial with gemfibrozil in middle-aged men with dyslipidemia. Safety of treatment, changes in risk factors, and incidence of coronary heart disease. N. Engl. J. Med., *317*:1237, 1987.

Fuster, V., Stein, B., Ambrose, J. A., et al.: Atherosclerotic plaque rupture and thrombosis. Circulation, *82*(Suppl. II):47, 1990.

Glagov, S., Weisenberg, E., Zarins, C. K., et al.: Compensatory enlargement of human atherosclerotic coronary arteries. N. Engl. J. Med., *316*:1371, 1987.

Goldstein, J. L., and Brown, M. S.: Familial hypercholesterolemia. *In* Scriver, C. R., Beaudet, A. L., Sly, W. S., and Valle, D. (eds): The Metabolic Basis of Inherited Disease. 6th ed. New York, McGraw-Hill, 1989, p. 1215.

Goldstein, J. L., Schrott, H. G., Hazzard, W. R., et al.: Hyperlipidemia in coronary heart disease. J. Clin. Invest., *52*:1544, 1973.

Gordon, D. J., Knoke, J., Probstfield, J. L., et al.: High-density lipoprotein cholesterol and coronary heart disease in hypercholesterolemic men: The Lipid Research Clinics Coronary Primary Prevention Trial. Circulation, *74*:1217, 1986.

Gotto, A. M., Jr., Pownall, H. J., and Havel, R. C.: Introduction to the plasma lipoproteins. Methods Enzymol., *128*:1, 1986.

Grundy, S. M.: Cholesterol metabolism in man. West. J. Med., *128*:13, 1978.

Grundy, S. M., and Denke, M. A.: Dietary influences on serum lipids and lipoproteins. J. Lipid Res., *31*:1149, 1990.

Guyton, J. R.: Mechanical control of smooth-muscle growth. *In* Seidel, C. L., and Weisbrodt, N. W. (eds): Hypertrophic Response in Smooth Muscle. Boca Raton, FL, CRC Press, 1987, p. 121.

Guyton, J. R., and Gotto, A. M., Jr.: Drug therapy of dyslipoproteinemias. *In* Fruchart, J. C., and Shepherd, J. (eds): Clinical Biochemistry: Human Plasma Lipoproteins. Berlin, de Gruyter, 1989, p. 335.

Guyton, J. R., and Gotto, A. M., Jr.: Pathogenesis of atherosclerosis: Lipid metabolism. *In* Loscalzo, J., Creager, M. A., and Dzau, V. J. (eds): Textbook of Vascular Medicine. Boston, Little, Brown, 1992, p. 345.

Guyton, J. R., and Klemp, K. F.: Transitional features in human atherosclerosis: Intimal thickening, cholesterol clefts, and cell loss in human aortic fatty streaks. Am. J. Pathol., *143*:1444, 1993.

Havel, R. C., Goldstein, J. L., and Brown, M. S.: Lipoproteins and lipid transport. *In* Bondy, P. K., and Rosenberg, L. E. (eds): Metabolic Control and Disease. 7th ed. Philadelphia, W. B. Saunders, 1980, p. 393.

Henry, P. D.: Calcium antagonists as antiatherogenic agents. Ann. N. Y. Acad. Sci., *522*:411, 1988.

Innerarity, T. L., Mahley, R. W., Weisgraber, K. H., et al.: Familial defective apolipoprotein B-100: A mutation of apolipoprotein B that causes hypercholesterolemia. J. Lipid Res., *31*:1337, 1990.

Jacobs, D., Blackburn, H., Higgins, M., et al.: Report of the conference on low blood cholesterol: Mortality associations. Circulation, *86*:1046, 1992.

Jenkins, D. J. A., Wolever, T. M. S., Rao, A. V., et al.: Effect on blood lipids of very high intakes of fiber in diets low in saturated fat and cholesterol. N. Engl. J. Med., *329*:21, 1993.

Keys, A., and Parlin, R. W.: Serum cholesterol response to changes in dietary lipids. Am. J. Clin. Nutr., *19*:175, 1966.

Kreisberg, R. A.: A votre sante: Alcohol and coronary artery disease. Arch. Intern. Med., *152*:263, 1992.

Krieger, M., Acton, S., Ashkenas, J., et al.: Molecular flypaper, host defense, and atherosclerosis: Structure, binding properties, and functions of macrophage scavenger receptors. J. Biol. Chem., *268*:4569, 1993.

Lardinois, C. K., and Neumann, S. L.: The effects of antihypertensive agents on serum lipids and lipoproteins. Arch. Intern. Med., *148*:1280, 1988.

Lendon, C. L., Davies, M. J., Born, G. V., and Richardson, P. D.: Atherosclerotic plaque caps are locally weakened when macrophage density is increased. Atherosclerosis, *87*:87, 1991.

Leung, W., Chu, P., and Wong, C.: Beneficial effect of cholesterol-lowering therapy on coronary endothelium-dependent relaxation in hypercholesterolaemic patients. Lancet, *341*:1496, 1993.

Levy, R. I., Brensike, J. F., Epstein, S. E., et al.: The influence of changes in lipid values induced by cholestyramine and diet on progression of coronary artery disease: Results of the NHLBI Type II Coronary Intervention Study. Circulation, *69*:325, 1984.

Lichtlen, P. R., Hugenholtz, P. G., Rafflebeul, W., et al.: Retardation of angiographic progression of coronary artery disease by nifedipine. Lancet, *335*:1109, 1990.

Lipid Research Clinics Program: The Lipid Research Clinics Coronary Primary Prevention Trial results. I. Reduction in incidence of coronary heart disease. J. A. M. A., *251*:351, 1984.

Manson, J. E., Tosteson, H., Ridker, P. M., et al.: The primary prevention of myocardial infarction. N. Engl. J. Med., *326*:1406, 1992.

Mittleman, M. A., Maclure, M., Tofler, G. H., et al.: Triggering of acute myocardial infarction by heavy physical exertion. N. Engl. J. Med., *329*:1677, 1993.

Morrisett, J. D., Guyton, J. R., Gaubatz, J. W., and Gotto, A. M., Jr.: Lipoprotein[a]: Structure, metabolism and epidemiology. *In* Gotto, A. M., Jr. (ed): Plasma Lipoproteins, New Comprehensive Biochemistry. Vol. 14. Amsterdam, Elsevier, 1987, p. 129.

Nachman, R. L.: Thrombosis and atherogenesis: Molecular connections. Blood, *79*:1897, 1992.

National Cholesterol Education Program: Report of the National Cholesterol Education Program NCEP Expert Panel on detection, evaluation, and treatment of high blood cholesterol in adults. Arch. Intern. Med., *148*:36, 1988.

National Cholesterol Education Program: Summary of the second report of the National Cholesterol Education Program NCEP Expert Panel on detection, evaluation, and treatment of high blood cholesterol in adults (Adult Treatment Panel II). J. A. M. A., *269*:3015, 1993.

Ornish, D., Brown, S. E., Scherwitz, L. W., et al.: Can lifestyle changes reverse coronary heart disease? The Lifestyle Heart Trial. Lancet, *336*:129, 1990.

Parthasarathy, S., and Rankin, S. M.: Role of oxidized low density lipoprotein in atherogenesis. Prog. Lipid Res., *31*:127, 1992.

Physicians' Health Study Research Group: Preliminary report: Findings from the aspirin component of the ongoing physicians' health study. N. Engl. J. Med., *318*:262, 1988.

Pravastatin Multinational Study Group for Cardiac Risk Patients: Effects of pravastatin in patients with serum total cholesterol levels from 5.2 to 7.8 mmol/liter (200 to 300 mg/dl) plus two additional atherosclerotic risk factors. Am. J. Cardiol., 72:1031, 1993.

Prescott, M. F., Webb, R. L., and Reidy, M. A.: Angiotensin-converting enzyme inhibitor versus angiotensin II, AT1 receptor antagonist: Effects on smooth-muscle cell migration and proliferation after balloon catheter injury. Am. J. Pathol., 139:1291, 1991.

Rader, D. J., and Brewer, H. B.: Lipoprotein[a]: Clinical approach to unique atherogenic lipoprotein. J. Am. Med. Assoc., 267:1109, 1993.

Reidy, M. A.: Factors controlling smooth-muscle cell proliferation. Arch. Pathol. Lab. Med., 116:1276, 1992.

Rimm, E. B., Stampfer, M. J., Ascherio, A., et al.: Vitamin E consumption and the risk of coronary disease in men. N. Engl. J. Med., 328:1450, 1993.

Ross, R.: The pathogenesis of atherosclerosis: A perspective for the 1990s. Nature, 362:801, 1993.

Schroeder, J. S., Gao, S., Alderman, E. L., et al.: A preliminary study of diltiazem in the prevention of coronary artery disease in heart-transplanted recipients. N. Engl. J. Med., 328:164, 1993.

Smith, L. C., Massey, J. B., Sparrow, J. T., et al.: Structure and dynamics of human plasma lipoproteins. In Pifat, G., and Herak, J. N. (eds): Supramolecular Structure and Function. New York, Plenum Press, 1983, p. 205.

Soma, M. R., Osnago-Gadda, I., Paoletti, R., et al.: The lowering of lipoprotein[a] induced by estrogen plus progesterone replacement therapy in postmenopausal women. Arch. Intern. Med., 153:1462, 1993.

Spach, D. H., Bauwens, J. E., Clark, C. D., and Burke, W. G.: Rhabdomyolysis associated with lovastatin and erythromycin use. West. J. Med., 154:213, 1991.

Stampfer, M. J., Hennekens, C. H., Manson, J. E., et al.: Vitamin E consumption and the risk of coronary disease in women. N. Engl. J. Med., 328:1444, 1993.

Steinberg, D., Parthasarathy, S., Carew, T. E., et al.: Beyond cholesterol. Modifications of low-density lipoprotein that increase its atherogenicity. N. Engl. J. Med., 320:915, 1989.

Sytkowski, P. A., Kannel, W. B., and D'Agostino, R. B.: Changes in risk factors and the decline in mortality from cardiovascular disease. N. Engl. J. Med., 322:1635, 1990.

Watts, G. F., Lewis, B., Bruntt, J. N. H., et al.: Effects on coronary artery disease of lipid-lowering diet, or diet plus cholestyramine, in the St. Thomas' Atherosclerosis Regression Study (STARS). Lancet, 339:563, 1992.

Weidmann, P., Ferrier, C., Saxenhofer, H., et al.: Serum lipoproteins during treatment with antihypertensive drugs. Drugs, 35(Suppl. 6):118, 1988.

Yamamoto, A., Matsuzawa, Y., Yokoyama, S., et al.: Effects of probucol on xanthomata regression in familial hypercholesterolemia. Am. J. Cardiol., 57:29H, 1986.

# 55
## The Surgical Management of Cardiac Arrhythmias

James L. Cox

Since the early 1970s, surgery has played a pivotal role in the elucidation of the anatomic and electrophysiologic abnormalities responsible for supraventricular and ventricular tachyarrhythmias. The development of sophisticated electrophysiologic systems for intraoperative mapping and anatomically precise surgical techniques enabled the ability to cure most medically refractory cardiac arrhythmias. Knowledge gained from the electrophysiologically guided surgical approaches to the Wolff-Parkinson-White (WPW) syndrome and atrioventricular (AV) node reentry tachycardia contributed in large part to the development of endocardial catheter techniques that are capable of curing these specific arrhythmias without the need for surgical intervention (Jackman et al., 1991; Lee et al., 1991). These informational and technologic advances, along with the increasing sophistication and availability of antitachycardia pacemakers and implantable cardioverter-defibrillators (Mirowski, 1985), have narrowed the indications for surgical intervention for refractory cardiac arrhythmias.

Despite this dramatic progress, surgery remains an important therapeutic modality for the treatment of cardiac arrhythmias. Indeed, the development of a surgical technique for the treatment of atrial fibrillation (AF) (Cox, 1991; Cox et al., 1991a, 1991b, 1991c, 1991d) represents perhaps the only means by which this most common of all cardiac arrhythmias can be cured. Moreover, the present results of surgery for ventricular tachycardia (VT), in properly selected patients, are comparable with those once attainable only in patients with supraventricular arrhythmias. Thus, contemporary therapy of cardiac arrhythmias includes a variety of therapeutic options that, when used in a complementary manner, are capable of curing essentially all supraventricular and ventricular tachyarrhythmias.

## BASIC ELECTROPHYSIOLOGIC CONCEPTS

The introduction of the microelectrode by Draper and Weidmann in 1957 led to general acceptance of the theory that normal cardiac cells generate upstrokes by a rapid, voltage-dependent, transient inflow of sodium ions ("rapid channel"). The resultant transmembrane action potential recorded by a microelectrode from normal myocardial cells has five distinctive phases (Fig. 55–1). Phase 0 represents the sharp upstroke recorded during depolarization of the

cell, when sodium ions pass rapidly into the cell. Phases 1 and 2 occur immediately after completion of cellular depolarization, during which time the cell is absolutely refractory to further depolarization. During phase 3, the cell begins to repolarize as sodium ions transfer out of the cell and potassium ions flow inward to reestablish the resting transmembrane potential (phase 4). In 1967, Reuter demonstrated a slow inward current of calcium ions during the plateau (phase 2) of the transmembrane action potential. Because the kinetics of activation, inactivation, and reactivation of sinoatrial (SA) and AV node cells, and of certain abnormal cells with low resting transmembrane potentials are considerably slower than those for the inward sodium current, the "slow channel" of calcium ion influx is considered to be a major factor in the activation of these cells. SA nodal cells probably operate with a mixed dependence on rapid and slow currents (Strauss et al., 1977). Although spontaneous phase 4 depolarization (characteristic of pacemaker cells) is due in part to deactivation of a fast potassium current (McAllister et al., 1975), the sensitivity of SA node cells to slow channel blocking agents (Zipes and Fisher, 1974) suggests that the background inward current may be the slow calcium current rather than

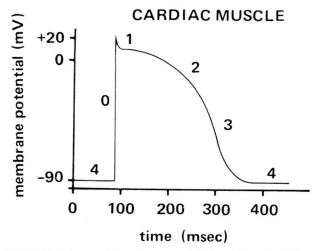

FIGURE 55–1. The cardiac action potential (shown here for Purkinje fiber) lasts for more than 300 msec and consists of five phases, 0 through 4. Spontaneous Phase 4 depolarization is believed to be responsible for automatic arrhythmias. (From Katz, A. M.: The arrhythmias. II: Abnormal impulse formation and reentry, premature systoles, preexcitation. *In* Katz, A. M. [ed]: Physiology of the Heart. New York, Raven Press, 1977, p. 320.)

a sodium current. Although these ionic currents form the basis for normal cardiac impulse generation and conduction, pathologic changes in myocardial cells may lead to a detrimental interplay between the rapid and the slow currents and thereby to the two basic types of cardiac rhythm disturbances—automatic arrhythmias and reentrant arrhythmias.

The appearance of *automaticity* in pathologic myocardial cells is believed to occur on the same electrochemical basis that gives rise to spontaneous activity in normal pacemaker cells. Injured cells exhibit spontaneous phase 4 depolarization, which may cause atrial or ventricular premature systoles or, if repetitive, atrial tachycardia or VT.

The physiologic basis for *reentrant* arrhythmias is somewhat more complex in that several different types of reentry may occur, depending on the type of anatomic-electrophysiologic abnormality present. The simplest type of reentry is that of a "circus movement," first described by Mines in 1914 (Fig. 55–2). In this type of reentrant arrhythmia, it is essential that a unidirectional block develop at some point in a contiguous conducting circuit. If the course of the circuit is sufficiently long (or the refractory period sufficiently short) to allow previously depolarized tissue to repolarize before the electrical wave front traverses the circuit, the wave front will always be preceded by excitable tissue and the arrhythmia may continue indefinitely. This type of reentrant mechanism (usually called *macro-reentry*) is responsible for the reciprocating tachycardia of the WPW syndrome, atrial flutter and fibrillation, and certain types of VT.

Reentrant arrhythmias associated with ischemic heart disease may occur on the basis of macro-reentry or micro-reentry, the latter requiring two conditions for the development of sustained reentry: (1) unidirectional block and (2) slow conduction. Unidirectional block plays the same role in micro-reentry as it does in macro-reentry, that is, it dictates that the wave front of depolarization be propagated in only one direction around the circuit. Although some asymmetry of conduction exists in normal myocardial tissue owing to differences in the passive or active properties of cells, local unidirectional block is an extreme form of asymmetry of conduction. This asymmetry is exaggerated by conditions that depress excitability, such as the high local extracellular potassium concentrations in ischemic myocardium. In addition, myocardial fibrosis, which reduces the ability of an electrical impulse to be propagated by increasing the resistance, can cause unidirectional block when the fibrosis is distributed asymmetrically.

Because of the comparatively long distances traversed by an electrical impulse in macro-reentrant circuits (e.g., in the WPW syndrome), slow conduction in a portion of these circuits is not an absolute requisite for the development of sustained reentry. However, in micro-reentrant circuits, the actual distance traversed by the electrical impulse may be so short (e.g., perhaps involving only a few cells) that sustained reentry cannot occur unless conduction velocity is decreased in some portion of the circuit. Four physiologically interdependent factors influence conduction velocity in myocardial tissue: (1) action potential amplitude, (2) rate of depolarization of the action potential, (3) threshold, and (4) electrical resistance. In regions of ischemia, myocardial cells become partially depolarized because some of the intracellular potassium is replaced with sodium, causing partial inactivation of the rapid sodium channels and, therefore, decreasing both action potential amplitude and the rate of depolarization. Such partially depolarized tissues can conduct a propagated action potential, although extremely slowly and usually with decre-

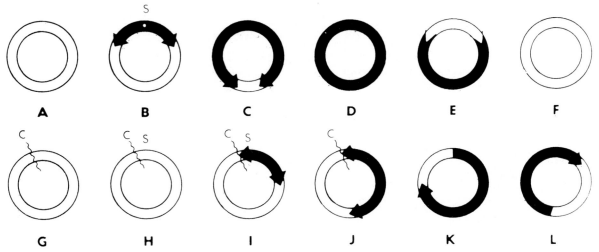

**FIGURE 55–2.** Role of unidirectional block in establishing the circus movement of electrical activity responsible for reentrant arrhythmias. Application of a stimulus (S) to a ring of excitable tissue (*unshaded area*) in the absence of block (*B*) initiates an impulse (*shaded area*) that depolarizes the entire ring (*D*). Mutual cancellation of the impulses moving in opposite directions (*C*) allows the tissue to repolarize completely (*E* and *F*). However, if unidirectional block is established by temporary clamping of the tissue (C in *G–J*), the impulse propagated in the clockwise direction can continue to travel around the ring (*K* and *L*), thus establishing the circus movement. (*A–L*, From Silber, E., and Katz, L.: Heart Disease. New York, McGraw-Hill, 1975. Reproduced with permission of McGraw-Hill, Inc.)

ment. These conductive properties, which give rise to slowly propagated waves of depolarization, exhibit the features of the slow inward current carried mainly by calcium ions. For these reasons, calcium-mediated slow responses are regarded as playing an important, if not exclusive, role in the genesis of micro-reentrant arrhythmias (Katz, 1977). The conditions necessary for the development of sustained microreentrant arrhythmias may occur in an ischemic limb of distal Purkinje's fibers or in an ischemic strand of myocardial muscle.

Clinical differentiation between automatic and reentrant arrhythmias is important in patients who require surgery because automatic arrhythmias are frequently suppressed by general anesthesia. However, the ability to discriminate clinically between these two types of arrhythmias is limited. Current practice involves the use of rapid "burst" pacing or programmed electrical stimulation. With the latter technique, regular pacing stimuli (S1) are introduced at a given cycle length and a premature stimulus (S2) is delivered in late diastole. The S2 is then introduced progressively earlier until it no longer elicits a depolarization, thus delineating the refractory period of the tissue being stimulated. If the arrhythmia is not induced by this single S2 impulse delivered at different intervals throughout electrical diastole, double premature stimuli (S2, S3) are introduced, with S3 being delivered at progressive intervals beginning 50 to 100 msec longer than the effective refractory period of the tissue. This sequence is repeated until the arrhythmia is initiated. The same programmed single, double, and triple stimuli may then be delivered to terminate the arrhythmia. Clinically, arrhythmias that respond to programmed electrical stimulation are considered to be reentrant arrhythmias, and those that do not respond are classified as automatic arrhythmias. Although this clinical classification is strictly empirical, it is useful in that it provides a means of assessing medical management, a rationale for the use of pacemaker devices, and some assurance that the arrhythmia can be invoked for investigative purposes at the time of surgery.

## ANATOMY OF THE CARDIAC CONDUCTION SYSTEM AND RELATED STRUCTURES

The SA node is a small subepicardial group of highly specialized cells located in the sulcus terminalis just lateral to the junction of the superior vena cava and the right atrium (Anderson and Becker, 1978). The cells are arranged around a central SA node artery that may arise from either the right or the left coronary system and may pass either anterior or posterior to the superior vena cava. Studies suggest that the SA node consists of three distinct regions, each responsive to a separate group of neural and circulatory stimuli (Boineau et al., 1977). The interrelationship of these three regions (forming the so-called atrial pacemaker complex) determines the ultimate

output of the SA node. Under normal conditions, these cells are the only ones in the heart capable of spontaneous phase 4 depolarization, thus establishing the SA node as the site of origin of the normal cardiac impulse.

The existence of specialized conduction pathways between the SA node and the AV node has been a subject of controversy for many years. However, most authorities now agree that, although an electrical impulse emanating from the SA node travels to the AV node, preferentially via the crista terminalis and the limbus of the fossa ovalis, these muscle bundles do not represent specialized, insulated conduction tracts comparable with the ventricular bundle branches. Although electrical impulses travel more rapidly through these thick atrial muscle bundles, surgical transection does not block internodal conduction.

The AV junctional area is the most complex anatomic portion of the cardiac conduction system. From a functional standpoint, the AV node should be considered as the area in which a normal delay in AV conduction occurs. This area corresponds anatomically to a group of AV junctional cells that are histologically distinct from working myocardium (Anderson and Becker, 1976). As an atrial impulse approaches the AV node area, it traverses a "transition zone" of specialized cells located anteriorly in the base of the atrial septum slightly to the right of and cephalad to the central fibrous body. This transition zone surrounds the atrial aspect of the *compact AV node*, where the major conduction delay occurs. The lower, longitudinal portion of the compact AV node penetrates the central fibrous body immediately posterior to the membranous portion of the intra-atrial septum to become the bundle of His. The AV node, its transitional zone, and its penetrating bundle are all contained within the triangle of Koch, an anatomically discrete region bounded by the tendon of Tadaro, tricuspid valve annulus, and thebesian valve of the coronary sinus (Fig. 55–3). There is little danger of surgical damage to AV conduction if this triangle is avoided in all procedures.

As mentioned, once the penetrating portion of the AV node traverses the central fibrous body, it becomes the bundle of His. The anatomy in this area is complicated by the fact that the junction of the right-sided heart chambers occupies a different spatial plane from the junction of the left-sided heart chambers, the annulus of the tricuspid valve being situated more toward the ventricular apex than that of the mitral valve (Anderson and Becker, 1979). The bundle of His travels along the posteroinferior rim of the membranous portion of the interventricular septum. The right bundle branch proceeds subendocardially toward the base of the medial papillary muscle and descends toward the ventricular apex, partly crossing the cavity of the ventricle in the moderator band. At the lower level of the membranous interventricular septum, a broad band of fasciculi originates from the His bundle, forming the left bundle branch that extends down the left side of the septum for a distance of 1 to 2 cm, where it divides into a smaller anterior and a larger

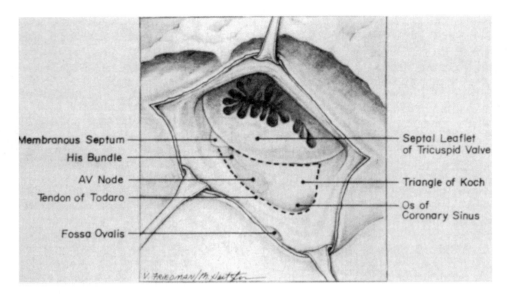

FIGURE 55–3. The right atrial septum viewed through a longitudinal right atriotomy. The patient's head is to the left and the feet to the right. The boundaries of the triangle of Koch are the tendon of Todaro, the tricuspid valve annulus, and a line connecting the two at the level of the os of the coronary sinus. Within the triangle of Koch resides the atrioventricular (AV) node and proximal portion of the His bundle, which enters the ventricular septum immediately posterior to the membranous portion of the interatrial septum. (From Cox, J. L., Holman, S. L., and Cain, M. E.: Cryosurgical treatment of atrioventricular node reentry tachycardia. Circulation, 76:1329–1336, 1987. Reproduced with permission. Copyright 1987 American Heart Association.)

posterior radiation. The medial aspects of each of these radiations usually become intermeshed distally to form three anastomosing nets of fiber—anterior, middle, and posterior. When the left side of the ventricular septum is viewed through the aortic valve, the danger area from the standpoint of the conduction tissue is immediately subjacent to the right coronary-noncoronary commissure.

The distal branches of the conduction system terminate in an intermediate zone between the Purkinje cells and the myocardium, where the cells gradually lose their Purkinje characteristics and take on the characteristics of working ventricular myocardium.

Of particular importance to the cardiac surgeon concerned with conduction abnormalities are the relationships of the various structures and potential spaces composing the junction of the atrial septum, the ventricular septum, the AV grooves, and the fibrous skeleton of the heart. The cardiac skeleton is strongest at the central fibrous body where the annuli of the mitral, tricuspid, and aortic valves meet (Fig. 55–4). Because the tricuspid annulus is more apical in position than the mitral annulus, the anterior part of the central fibrous body extends into the ventricles beneath the attachment of the tricuspid valve and forms the interventricular component of the membranous septum between the aortic outflow tract and the right atrium. Likewise, immediately posterior to the membranous septum, the right atrial wall is in potential communication with the inlet portion of the left ventricle.

The mitral and aortic valve annuli contribute significantly to the structural integrity of the fibrous skeleton and are further strengthened at their left junction to form the left fibrous trigone. The left anterior portion of the central fibrous body is designated as the right fibrous trigone. The AV groove between these two trigones represents the site of continuity between the anterior leaflet of the mitral valve and the aortic valve annulus and is the only area in the AV groove where atrial muscle is not in juxtaposition

to ventricular muscle. For this reason, accessory AV pathways are not found between the left and the right fibrous trigones.

## SURGERY FOR SUPRAVENTRICULAR ARRHYTHMIAS

### Atrial Flutter and Atrial Fibrillation

Atrial fibrillation (AF) is present in 0.4 to 2.0% of the general population (Cameron et al., 1988; Diamantopoulos et al., 1987; Hirosawa et al., 1987; Onundarson et al., 1987; Savage et al., 1983) and in approximately 10% of the population over the age of 60 years (Cobler et al., 1984; Martin et al., 1984; Tammaro et al., 1983; Treseder et al., 1986), making it the most common of all sustained cardiac arrhythmias. Although AF is frequently considered to be an innocuous arrhythmia, it is associated with significant morbidity and mortality because of its three detrimental sequelae: (1) an unusually irregular heartbeat, which

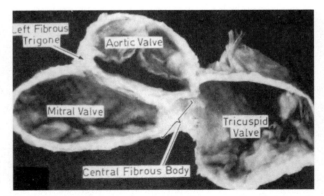

FIGURE 55–4. Dissection showing the fibrous cardiac skeleton after it has been removed from the ventricles. (From Anderson, R. H., and Becker, A. E.: Cardiac anatomy for the surgeon. In Danielson, G. K. [ed]: Lewis' Practice of Surgery. Hagerstown, MD, Harper & Row, 1979.)

causes patient discomfort and anxiety; (2) loss of synchronous AV contraction, which compromises cardiac hemodynamics causing varying levels of congestive heart failure; and (3) stasis of blood flow in the left atrium, which increases the vulnerability to thromboembolism.

### Historical Aspects

Since the early 1980s, several nonmedical techniques have been designed either to ablate the arrhythmia or to ameliorate its attendant detrimental sequelae. In 1980, the author's group first described the *left atrial isolation procedure*, which was capable of confining AF to the left atrium while leaving the remainder of the heart in normal sinus rhythm (Williams et al., 1980) (Fig. 55–5). This procedure was successful in restoring a regular ventricular rhythm without the need for a permanent pacemaker and, unexpectedly, also restored normal cardiac hemodynamics. The reason for the latter is that the right atrium and right ventricle beat in synchrony following the procedure, providing a normal right-sided cardiac output that is then delivered to the left side of the heart. Despite the fact that the left atrium is isolated and therefore cannot beat in synchrony with the left ventricle, the left ventricle adapts instantaneously to the normal right-sided output and delivers a normal forward cardiac output. Thus, the left atrial isolation procedure alleviates two of the three detrimental sequelae of AF, namely, the irregular heartbeat and the compromised hemodynamics. Unfortunately,

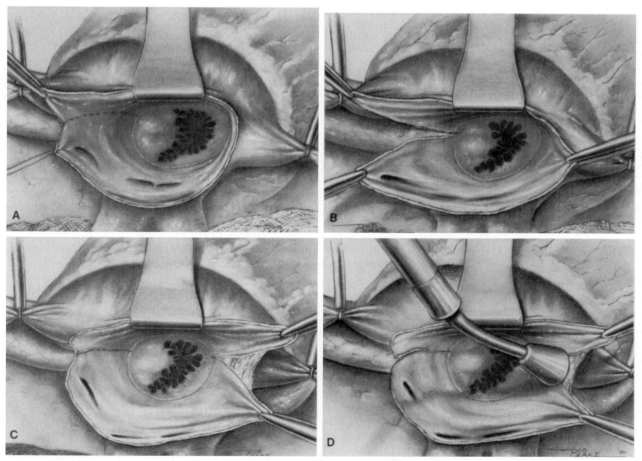

**FIGURE 55–5.** Left atrial isolation procedure. *A,* After a standard left atriotomy incision is made, the interatrial septum is retracted gently, and the atriotomy is extended anteriorly (*dashed line*) across Bachmann's bundle to the level of the mitral valve annulus just to the left of the right fibrous trigone. *B,* The anterior extension of the standard left atriotomy has been completed. The base of the aorta and its juxtaposition with the anterior leaflet of the mitral valve are demonstrated. Note that the anterior atriotomy extends across the mitral valve annulus. The main body of the left atrium has been separated anteriorly from the remainder of the heart. *C,* The transmural left atriotomy is extended posteriorly to the level of the coronary sinus. The remaining portion of the incision is made through the endocardium and extends across the mitral valve annulus posteriorly just to the left of the interatrial septum. At this point, electrical activity continues to be propagated in a 1:1 manner between the right and the left atria because of the presence of interatrial muscular connections accompanying the coronary sinus. *D,* A cryoprobe is positioned over the endocardial aspect of the posterior atriotomy, and its temperature is decreased to −60° C for 2 minutes. This cryolesion ablates the endocardial interatrial fibers accompanying the coronary sinus. A similar cryolesion is created on the epicardial aspect of the AV groove on the opposite side of the coronary sinus to ablate all remaining interatrial epicardial connections. The left atriotomy is closed with a continuous 4–0 nonabsorbable suture. (*A–D,* From Williams, J. M., Ungerleider, R. M., Lofland, G. K., and Cox, J. L.: Left atrial isolation: New technique for the treatment of supraventricular arrhythmias. J. Thorac. Cardiovasc. Surg., *80:*373, 1980.)

because the left atrium may continue to fibrillate, the vulnerability to systemic thromboembolism is unchanged following this procedure.

In 1982, Scheinman and associates introduced *catheter fulguration of the His bundle* as a means of controlling the irregular cardiac rhythm associated with AF and other refractory supraventricular arrhythmias. This procedure is also a type of isolation procedure in that it isolates the supraventricular arrhythmia to the atria and away from the ventricles. Elective ablation of the His bundle dictates the implantation of a permanent ventricular pacemaker, which restores a normal ventricular rhythm. However, the atria continue to fibrillate following ablation of the His bundle; therefore, this technique alleviates only the irregular heartbeat associated with AF. The hemodynamic compromise due to loss of AV synchrony and the vulnerability to thromboembolism are unaffected by ablation of the His bundle.

In 1985, Guiraudon described the *corridor procedure* for the treatment of AF, an open heart technique that does not always require a permanent pacemaker (Guiraudon et al., 1985) (Fig. 55–6). The corridor procedure isolates a strip of atrial septum (the "corridor") harboring both the SA node and the AV node, thereby allowing the SA node to drive the ventricles. This procedure corrects the irregular heartbeat associated with AF, but both atria may continue to fibrillate postoperatively because they are totally isolated from the septal corridor. In addition, both atria are also isolated from their respective ventricles, thereby precluding the possibility of AV synchrony on either side of the heart. Therefore, neither the hemodynamic compromise nor the vulnerability to thromboembo-

lism associated with AF are alleviated by the corridor procedure (Cox, 1992a, 1992b). Indeed, this procedure accomplishes the same physiologic state as does elective ablation of the His bundle, a procedure that can be performed without the need for open heart surgery.

In summary, each of these nonpharmacologic approaches to the treatment of AF provides some advantage over allowing the patient to continue with the arrhythmia, but none of them alleviates all three of the detrimental sequelae of AF.

### Anatomic-Electrophysiologic Basis

Because of the inability of previous surgical procedures to alleviate all three detrimental sequelae of AF, the author's group initiated a series of experimental studies in 1980 with the ultimate aim of achieving a better understanding of the anatomic-electrophysiologic basis of atrial flutter and AF and then developing a surgical cure for both arrhythmias. Subsequent experimental studies (D'Agostino et al., 1987; Smith et al., 1985) using a 256-channel computerized mapping system were performed in parallel with computerized mapping of human AF (156 channels) in patients undergoing surgery for the WPW syndrome (Canavan et al., 1988a, 1988b; Cox et al., 1991b). These experimental and clinical studies documented that a spectrum of arrhythmias occur, from simple atrial flutter to complex AF, that depend on three electrophysiologic components: macro-reentry within the atria; passive conduction in that part of the atrial myocardium not immediately involved in the macro-reentrant circuit(s); and AV conduction. The interaction of these three electrophysiologic components determines the P-wave patterns and the regularity of the QRS complexes recorded on the standard electrocardiogram (ECG) and, consequently, the clinical diagnosis of atrial flutter, "atrial flutter/fibrillation," or AF.

Both the experimental and the clinical electrophysiologic studies documented that atrial flutter and AF occur on the basis of atrial macro-reentry. Equally important from a surgical standpoint was the fact that neither the experimental studies nor the clinical studies revealed any evidence of micro-reentry or automaticity in the cause of this spectrum of arrhythmias. As a result, the author's group sought to develop a surgical technique that would be capable of interrupting *all* of the potential macro-reentrant circuits that could potentially develop in the atria, thereby precluding the ability of the atria to fibrillate. In addition, it was recognized that it was necessary to place the surgical incisions so that the SA node could resume activity postoperatively and "direct" the propagation of the sinus impulse throughout both atria, allowing all of the atrial myocardium to be activated postoperatively, and preserving the atrial transport function that is a prerequisite for the restoration of normal cardiac hemodynamics and the prevention of stasis of blood flow in the left atrium. The resultant surgical procedure is based on the concept

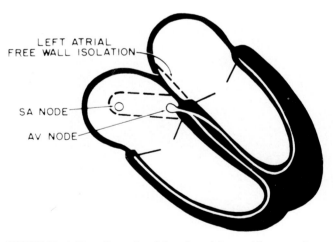

LEFT ATRIAL
FREE WALL ISOLATION

SA NODE

AV NODE

**FIGURE 55–6.** Two-dimensional drawing of the corridor procedure. A strip of atrial septum harboring both the sinoatrial (SA) node and the AV node is isolated from the remainder of the atrial myocardium. This allows the SA node to drive the ventricles, but AV synchrony is precluded because both atria are electrically isolated from their respective ventricles. In addition, both atria may continue to fibrillate postoperatively. (From Guiraudon, G. M., Campbell, C. S., Jones, D. L., et al.: Combined sinoatrial node–atrioventricular node isolation: A surgical alternative to His' bundle ablation in patients with atrial fibrillation. Circulation, 72[Suppl. 3]:220, 1985. Reproduced with permission. Copyright 1985 American Heart Association.)

of a maze and is called the *maze procedure* (Cox et al., 1991d) (Figs. 55–7 and 55–8).

## Surgical Indications and Contraindications

The major indication for surgery is intolerance of the arrhythmia. In many respects, patients with paroxysmal atrial flutter/fibrillation are more symptomatic than those with chronic AF. Major symptoms in the paroxysmal group include dyspnea on exertion, easy fatigability, lethargy, malaise, and a general sense of impending doom during the periods of atrial flutter/fibrillation. The patients with chronic AF are usually better adapted to the sensation of an irregular heartbeat, but most complain of exercise limitations, dypsnea on exertion, and easy fatigability. In addition, they frequently express concern over the possibility of having a stroke.

All patients who are considered for surgery must have failed the maximal amount of tolerable drug therapy preoperatively. In addition, 21% of the patients in the author's group's series had experienced at least one episode of cerebral thromboembolism that caused significant temporary or permanent neurologic deficit. Documented cerebral thromboembolism in a patient with paroxysmal or chronic AF, in the absence of other demonstrable causes, is considered an absolute indication for surgery because anticoagulation does not protect such patients from a *second* stroke (Boston Area Anticoagulation Trial in Atrial Fibrillation Investigators, 1990; Petersen et al., 1989; Stroke Prevention in Atrial Fibrillation Study Group Investigators, 1990). Despite that fact, it should be emphasized that the author's group has not considered the *threat* of thromboembolism to be an indication for surgery in patients who have not previously experienced a transient ischemic attack or frank stroke due to AF. This policy has been pursued because the *incidence* of stroke as a result of AF is low and it would take many years to document that the maze procedure could decrease that incidence.

Contraindications to the maze procedure include the presence of significant left ventricular dysfunction, not attributable to the arrhythmia itself, and concomitant cardiac or noncardiac disease that constitutes an excessive surgical risk.

## Preoperative Electrophysiologic Evaluation

A preoperative endocardial catheter electrophysiology study is routinely performed in all patients with atrial flutter and in patients with *paroxysmal* AF. The primary purpose of this study is to document the function of the SA node, particularly in the AF pa-

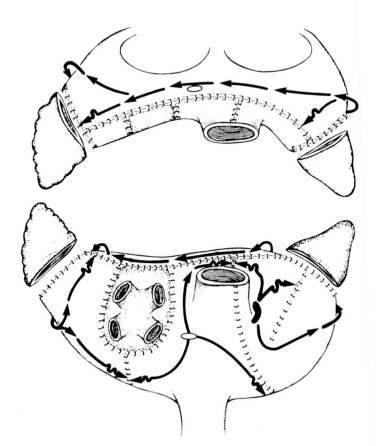
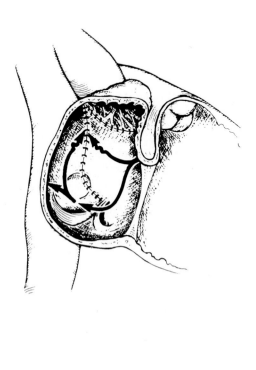

**FIGURE 55–7.** Two-dimensional drawing of the incisions made in the maze procedure. (Modified from Cox, J. L., Schuessler, R. B., D'Agostino, H. J., Jr., et al.: The surgical treatment of atrial fibrillation. III: Development of a definite surgical procedure. J. Thorac. Cardiovasc. Surg., *101*:569–583, 1991.)

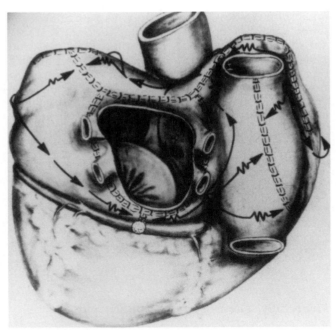

**FIGURE 55–8.** Three-dimensional depiction of the incisions used for performing the maze procedure. Note the presence of the transmural cryolesions (*white dot*) of the coronary sinus at the site of the posterioinferior left atriotomy. Both atrial appendages have been excised. The only completely isolated portions of the atrium are the orifices of the pulmonary veins. The impulse originates from the region of the SA node and can escape from that region only by passing inferiorly and anteriorly around the base of the right atrium. The impulse continues to propagate around the anterior right atrium onto the top of the interatrial septum. There, it bifurcates into two wave fronts, one passing through the septum in an anterior-to-posterior direction to activate the posteromedial right and left atria, and the other continuing around the base of the excised left atrial appendage to activate the posterolateral left atrial wall. In this manner, all atrial myocardium, except the pulmonary vein orifices, is activated. The activation of this atrial myocardium is fundamental to the preservation of atrial transport function postoperatively. (From Cox, J. L., Schuessler, R. B., D'Agostino, H. J., Jr., et al.: The surgical treatment of atrial fibrillation. III: Development of a definite surgical procedure. J. Thorac. Cardiovasc. Surg., *101*:569–583, 1991.)

tients, and to determine both SA node function and the site of the reentrant circuit in patients with atrial flutter. Preoperative electrophysiology studies are not performed in patients with *chronic* AF because the SA node cannot be evaluated without electrical cardioversion, which would introduce too great a risk of thromboembolism.

### Surgical Technique

The first 33 patients in the author's group's series underwent the standard maze procedure (Cox, 1991; Cox et al., 1991a, 1991d). For reasons that are beyond the scope of this chapter, the surgical technique was modified slightly in patients 34 through 48 and again in patients 49 through 87 (Cox, 1993).

Seven of the 87 patients (8%) had undergone previous thoracic surgical procedures that had a potential impact on exactly how the maze procedure could be performed and on the potential operative risk of the

procedure. Because the atriotomies comprising the maze procedure must be placed in precise locations to prevent atrial macro-reentry and to preserve AV synchrony and atrial transport function postoperatively, any previous atriotomy, which necessarily alters the specific placement of the maze atriotomies, has the potential to defeat the effectiveness of the maze procedure (Cox et al., 1993).

Twenty-four of the 87 patients (28%) underwent concomitant cardiac surgical procedures in addition to the maze procedure for AF. In performing the maze procedure, the author's group has routinely employed moderate systemic hypothermia (28° C), and antegrade and retrograde crystalloid or blood cardioplegia with topical hypothermia provided by a cooling jacket.

### Results of Surgery

Since September 25, 1987, 87 patients have undergone the maze procedure for AF, and up to May 25, 1993, 78 patients had been followed for at least 3 months after surgery. AF was cured, AV synchrony was restored, and atrial transport function was preserved in 76 of 78 patients (97%). Surgery was curative without postoperative medication in 71 of 78 patients (91%) and with postoperative medication in 5 of 78 (6%), having failed in combination with postoperative medication in only 2 of 78 patients (3%).

## Wolff-Parkinson-White Syndrome

The introduction of endocardial catheter techniques utilizing radiofrequency energy has had its greatest impact on the treatment of supraventricular arrhythmias due to the WPW syndrome (Jackman et al., 1991). Despite the rather dramatic decrease in the number of patients who now require surgery for this abnormality, a thorough knowledge of the anatomy, electrophysiology, and surgical techniques remains of paramount importance not only to the surgeon but also to the interventional electrophysiologist.

### Historical Aspects

Gaskell was the first to demonstrate that electrical activity propagated from the atrium to the ventricle via myocardial tissue rather than nerves, his studies on the turtle heart being reported in 1883. Kent identified muscular connections between the atria and the ventricles of mammals in 1893, but erroneously concluded that these connections were multiple and that they represented the normal pathways of AV conduction. Despite this misconception, his name serves as the eponym for the accessory AV connections responsible for the WPW syndrome (*Kent bundles*).

Perhaps the most important work delineating the specialized conduction system of the heart was reported in 1906 when Tawara, working in Aschoff's laboratory in Germany, identified and characterized the AV node, His bundle, bundle branches, and the

Purkinje system (Aschoff, 1906). In the same year, Keith and Flack identified the SA node as the heart's normal pacemaker.

During the 1920s, Dr. Paul Dudley White, one of the great teachers and clinical cardiologists of this century, noted that a small group of young, apparently normal patients with ventricular preexcitation on their standard ECGs had frequent bouts of paroxysmal tachycardia. During a trip to London, he discovered that Dr. John Parkinson, an English physician, had collected a similar series of patients. White suggested that Dr. Louis Wolff, one of White's fellows, combine their series of patients and report their observations, which he did in 1930 (Wolff et al., 1930). However, neither the ventricular preexcitation nor the bouts of tachycardia were explained, until Wolferth and Wood reported a patient with the same clinical syndrome in 1933 and suggested that the ECG abnormalities were due to accessory pathways between the atrium and the ventricle similar to those previously described by Kent. Although they accepted Kent's erroneous hypothesis that these accessory pathways were normal and occurred on the right free wall, Wolferth and Wood directed their attention to that region in a patient with the syndrome who died; and fortuitously, they were able to document an accessory pathway histologically at autopsy, which they reported in 1943 (Wood et al., 1943).

Although the basis for the WPW syndrome was suspected, the issue remained controversial for many years. However, the picture became somewhat clearer in 1967 when Dr. Dirk Durrer of Amsterdam, the generally acknowledged father of modern clinical electrophysiology, performed intraoperative mapping in a patient with the WPW syndrome and demonstrated electrical conduction across the AV groove in the region of ventricular preexcitation (Durrer and Roos, 1967). In the same year, Dr. Howard Burchell of the Mayo Clinic performed intraoperative mapping in a patient with the WPW syndrome who was undergoing surgery for closure of an atrial septal defect. After identifying the suspected site of the accessory pathway on the right free wall, he was able to abolish ventricular preexcitation by injecting procainamide into the AV groove at that site (Burchell et al., 1967). Although the preexcitation returned postoperatively, this procedure demonstrated for the first time that a surgical technique might be capable of permanently interrupting conduction across an accessory pathway, thereby curing the WPW syndrome. The first surgical attempt at permanent ablation followed several months later on May 28, 1968, when Dr. Will Sealy of Duke University successfully divided a right free wall accessory pathway in a 31-year-old fisherman (Cobb et al., 1968).

Sixteen years later, Sealy published the following comment, which gives some insight into the role frequently played by serendipity in the advancement of medical science:

Had Kent not published what are now considered to be incorrect observations, Wood and colleagues might never have found the right free wall pathway. Had the fisherman's anomalous pathway been anyplace other than the right free-wall, I would not likely have found it at operation.

**Sealy, 1984**

### Anatomic-Electrophysiologic Basis

The WPW syndrome is characterized by the presence of an abnormal muscular connection between the atrium and the ventricle (accessory AV connection or accessory pathway) that is capable of conducting electrical activity. Because these patients also have a normal His bundle that connects the atria to the ventricles electrically, they have two routes by which an electrical impulse may travel between the atria and the ventricles. When patients with the WPW syndrome are in normal sinus rhythm, the sinus node impulse activates the atria normally. After activating the atria, the electrical wave front propagates to the ventricles across both the His bundle and the accessory pathway. However, this antegrade (atrial-to-ventricular) conduction is delayed before entering the His bundle because of the normal conduction delay that occurs in the AV node. As there is no AV node proximal to the accessory pathway to delay conduction, the electrical activity reaches the ventricle first at the site of insertion of the accessory pathway onto the ventricle. The initial activation of the ventricle at a site remote from the His bundle causes an early deflection off the baseline of the standard ECG, producing a delta wave. As the electrical wave front propagates down the ventricle from the site of ventricular insertion of the accessory pathway, the electrical activity passing through the normal AV node–His bundle complex eventually emerges and passes rapidly down the bundle branches. The fusion of the wave front from the His bundle and the wave front from the accessory pathway causes the QRS complex to be wide. Thus, during normal sinus rhythm, the standard ECG in patients with the WPW syndrome shows: (1) a short P-R interval because of the lack of a delay in conduction from the atrium to the ventricle across the accessory pathway; (2) a delta wave owing to eccentric activation of the ventricle across the accessory pathway; and (3) a wide QRS complex owing to fusion of the electrical activity propagating from the His bundle and that propagating from the accessory pathway. These are the three ECG findings described by Wolff and colleagues in their 1930 paper, which noted that patients with this type of ECG had a high incidence of supraventricular tachycardia (SVT).

Although antegrade conduction across an accessory pathway such as that just described causes an abnormal ECG, it does not produce tachycardia. For tachycardia to occur, antegrade conduction across the accessory pathway must first be blocked. Antegrade block in an accessory pathway may have a variety of causes, including premature atrial or ventricular beats and sudden changes in the autonomic input to the heart. When antegrade block occurs in the accessory pathway with the patient in normal sinus rhythm, the sinus impulse still activates the atria normally. The electrical activity propagates through the AV node–His bundle complex normally and activates the ventricles normally. However, when the electrical activity reaches the AV groove at the base of the heart, it encounters a bundle of muscle, the accessory pathway, that has not yet been depolarized. As a result, the electrical activity simply propagates across the accessory pathway retrogradely (from the ventricle to the atrium) and quickly reactivates the atria. The atrial activation wave front then passes normally through the AV node–His bundle complex again and reactivates the ventricle. In this manner, a macro-reentrant circuit is established around which electrical activity can propagate as fast as 4 times per second or 240 times per minute. Thus, the patient progresses from a normal sinus rhythm at, say, 80 beats per minute (with an abnormal ECG), to a single premature beat, to a SVT ("reciprocating tachycardia") of 240 beats per minute.

### Indications for Surgery

The major contemporary indication for surgical intervention in the WPW syndrome is failure of radiofrequency catheter ablation (RFCA). Between 1980 and 1991, when RFCA became the procedure of choice for the treatment of the WPW syndrome, approximately 500 patients underwent surgery for the WPW syndrome on the author's group's service. The dramatic change from surgical therapy to catheter ablative therapy can be appreciated by noting that during a period of 27 months, the author's group operated on only nine patients for the WPW syndrome, all of whom had failed attempts at RFCA of the accessory pathway(s). Nevertheless, these patients represent a relatively large group in terms of patients who have undergone surgery only after failed RFCA and they are instructive in terms of what surgeons can expect in the future.

Only three patients (33%) were totally free of some type of associated anomaly capable of making RFCA either more difficult or totally impossible to accomplish successfully. Of the other six patients (67%), two had Ebstein's anomaly with thick muscle bands for accessory pathways, one had exercise-induced marked cardiac hypertrophy, one had mitral regurgitation and coronary artery disease, one had catheter perforation of the right ventricle during the electrophysiology study, and one had a small heart owing to age.

At the time of surgery, four patients had insignificant scarring associated with previous attempts at RFCA. Two additional patients had severe scarring in the dissection planes of the AV groove, making surgical dissection both difficult and hazardous because of the proximity of the coronary arteries in the AV groove. One of these patients had Ebstein's anomaly and a posterior septal accessory pathway. A heavy muscle layer encompassing the coronary sinus extended directly down to the posterior ventricular septum as a thick (6 to 8 mm) band of muscle fibers,

representing the accessory pathway. It would have been technically impossible to ablate this accessory pathway with current RFCA technology.

Another patient with Ebstein's anomaly had a much more marked downward displacement of the tricuspid valve leaflets associated with a right free wall pathway. The electrophysiologists had passed a multielectrode catheter into the right coronary artery and another into the right atrium. Once the pathway was localized between these two catheters, radiofrequency current was passed between the two catheters, producing an elevated intimal flap in the coronary artery.

Of the two remaining patients, the surgical dissection was significantly more difficult because of the previous attempts at RFCA. In one of these patients, the right ventricle had been perforated during the attempt at RFCA, causing hemopericardium and marked inflammation of the epicardial surface of the heart. The most serious complication of failed RFCA occurred in the remaining patient, a 7-year-old male who underwent three separate RFCA sessions of 8 hours each in an attempt to ablate his pathways. At surgery, the endocardium of virtually the entire posterior left atrial wall was found to be denuded, swollen, beefy-red, and indurated. A supra-annular incision was placed in the usual position above the posterior mitral valve annulus to expose the underlying AV groove fat pad. However, the tissue was so friable and the circumflex coronary artery so intimately incorporated into the massive destructive process in the groove that the attempt at surgical ablation was abandoned. Even so, it was necessary to place a large pericardial patch over the posterior left atrial wall endocardially to close the supravalvular incision.

This experience suggests that two important principles must be observed regarding how aggressive one should be in attempting RFCA. The first is that if an accessory pathway cannot be ablated in a reasonable period of time, it is highly probable that some type of anatomic abnormality exists. Therefore, electrophysiologists should not consider it a personal failure when they "miss" an accessory pathway. The second principle is that electrophysiologists should exercise common sense in knowing when to terminate their attempts at RFCA, because too much local radiofrequency trauma and injury can render the patient surgically incurable.

### Preoperative Electrophysiologic Evaluation

Patients who are now subjected to surgery for the WPW syndrome have first undergone an endocardial catheter electrophysiologic study in association with their failed attempt at RFCA. The most important information to the surgeon prior to surgery is the location of the accessory pathway, the technique and number of ablative attempts employed by the electrophysiologist during the attempted RFCA, and the associated (if any) anatomic abnormalities to be encountered during surgery.

## Intraoperative Electrophysiologic Mapping

Computerized mapping systems have obviated the need to use cardiopulmonary bypass (CPB) for the intraoperative mapping of patients with the WPW syndrome (Cox et al., 1985b). Epicardial pacing and sensing electrodes are sutured onto the atrium and ventricle near the suspected site of the accessory pathway. A band electrode (Kramer et al., 1985) is placed around the ventricular side of the AV groove, and electrograms are recorded during normal sinus rhythm and atrial pacing. The electrogram recorded from the electrode located nearest the site of the ventricular insertion of the accessory pathway shows the earliest activation. The band electrode is then moved to the atrial side of the AV groove, and reciprocating tachycardia is induced with programmed electrical stimulation. Atrial electrograms are recorded from the bipolar electrodes on the band. This display of the atrial data is especially important because it demonstrates unsuspected concealed accessory pathways that would have gone undetected until this point in the mapping procedure. When reciprocating tachycardia cannot be induced, the retrograde atrial map is performed during ventricular pacing.

These antegrade and retrograde computerized mapping techniques are capable of detecting not only free wall pathways but also anterior septal and posterior septal accessory pathways. However, if either is detected during the computerized mapping procedure, the patient is placed on CPB, a right atriotomy is performed, and endocardial mapping of the right atrium and atrial septum is completed using a hand-held single-point mapping system prior to proceeding with surgical dissection.

## Surgical Technique

Accessory AV connections may be located anywhere around the annulus fibrosus of the heart except between the right and the left fibrous trigones (Fig. 55–9). However, from a surgical standpoint, their locations are classified, in decreasing order of frequency, as (1) left free wall, (2) posterior septal, (3) right free wall, and (4) anterior septal (Cox et al., 1985b). Twenty per cent of the patients in the author's group's series have had multiple (two, three, or four) accessory pathways.

The objective of surgery for the WPW syndrome is to divide the accessory pathway(s) responsible for the syndrome. Physiologically, an accessory pathway is analogous to a wire that conducts electrical activity, and thus, it is unimportant which end of the "wire" is divided, because division at either end permanently interrupts conduction.

Two surgical approaches are commonly employed to divide accessory AV connections (Fig. 55–10). The endocardial technique is designed to divide the ventricular end of the accessory pathway, and the epicardial technique is directed toward division of the atrial end of the pathway. Although some controversy has arisen regarding which approach is preferable (Cox,

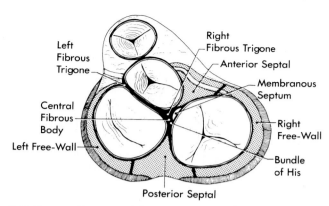

**FIGURE 55–9.** Diagram of the superior view of the heart with the atria cut away demonstrating the boundaries of each of the four anatomic areas where accessory pathways can occur in the Wolff-Parkinson-White (WPW) syndrome. The boundaries of the left free-wall space are the mitral valve annulus and the ventricular epicardial reflection extending from the left fibrous trigone to the posterior septum. The boundaries of the posterior septal space are the tricuspid valve annulus, the mitral valve annulus, the posterior superior process of the left ventricle, and the ventricular epicardial reflection. The boundaries of the right free-wall space are the tricuspid valve annulus and the epicardial reflection extending from the posterior septum to the anterior septum. The boundaries of the anterior septal space are the tricuspid valve annulus, the membranous portion of the interatrial septum, and the ventricular epicardial reflection. All accessory AV connections must insert into the ventricle somewhere within these anatomic boundaries. (From Cox, J. L., Gallagher, J. J., and Cain, M. E.: Experience with 118 consecutive patients undergoing surgery for the Wolff-Parkinson-White syndrome. J. Thorac. Cardiovasc. Surg., 90:490–501, 1985.)

1986; Guiraudon et al., 1986b), excellent results can be obtained with both techniques (Cox et al., 1985b; Guiraudon et al., 1986a; Klein et al., 1984).

**Left Free Wall Accessory Pathways—Endocardial Technique.** Accessory pathways on the left free wall (see Fig. 55–9) are approached through a left atriotomy after the heart has been arrested with cold potassium cardioplegia. After placing a supra-annular incision 2 mm above the posterior mitral valve annulus, a plane of dissection is established between the underlying AV groove fat pad and the top of the left ventricle throughout the length of the supra-annular incision (Fig. 55–11). It is important to carry this plane of dissection all the way to the epicardial reflection off the posterior left ventricle. The two ends of the supra-annular incision are then "squared-off" so that if a juxta-annular pathway is present, the small rim of atrial tissue to which it would be attached is isolated from the remainder of the heart.

**Left Free Wall Accessory Pathways—Epicardial Technique.** The epicardial approach to left free wall accessory pathways incorporates dissection from the atrial side of the AV groove. The epicardial reflection off the atrium is opened, and a plane of dissection is established between the AV groove fat pad and the atrial wall (see Fig. 55–10E). The plane of dissection is extended to the level of the posterior mitral valve annulus and carried slightly onto the top of the posterior left ventricle (see Fig. 55–10F). Although cryosurgery is unnecessary if the pathway has already been divided by the dissection (i.e., ventricular preexcita-

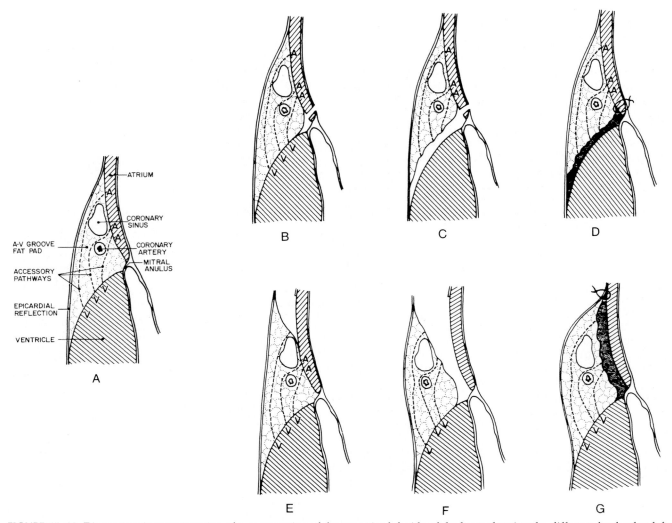

**FIGURE 55–10.** Diagrammatic representation of a cross-section of the posterior left side of the heart showing the different depths that left free-wall pathways can be located in relation to the mitral annulus and epicardial reflection (A). The endocardial surgical technique is depicted in B–D and the epicardial technique in E–G. See text for details.

tion has disappeared), this technique has nevertheless been labelled a *cryosurgical technique* by its advocates (Klein et al., 1984). Moreover, to expose the atrial side of the AV groove on the left side of the heart (the most common site of accessory pathways), it is necessary to elevate the apex of the heart out of the pericardium, a maneuver that causes hypotension in most patients to such an extent that CPB must be instituted to maintain stable hemodynamics. Despite the fact that virtually all of these patients require total CPB, this technique has also been labelled a *closed heart procedure* (Guiraudon et al., 1986a, 1986b).

**Posterior Septal Accessory Pathways.** Accessory pathways located in the posterior septal space (see Fig. 55–9) are divided after normothermic CPB is instituted and a right atriotomy performed to expose the triangle of Koch. The position of the His bundle is identified with a hand-held electrode, and the right atrial endocardium is mapped during induced reciprocating tachycardia to confirm the findings of the computerized epicardial mapping. A supra-annular

incision is placed 2 mm above the posterior medial tricuspid valve annulus beginning well posterior to the His bundle (Fig. 55–12). The supra-annular incision is extended in a counterclockwise direction well onto the free wall of the posterior right atrium. Once the fat pad occupying the posterior septal space has been identified through the supra-annular incision, a plane of dissection is established between the fat pad and the top of the posterior ventricular septum. The junction of the posterior medial mitral and tricuspid valve annuli forms a V at the posterior edge of the central fibrous body, and the fat pad comes to a point at the apex of that V (see Fig. 55–9). The apex of the V is always posterior to the His bundle, although the distance between the apex of the V and the His bundle may vary. However, as long as the dissection in this region remains posterior to the central fibrous body, the His bundle is not damaged. Once the anterior point of the fat pad is gently dissected away from the apex of the V (i.e., away from the posterior edge of the central fibrous body), the mitral valve annulus

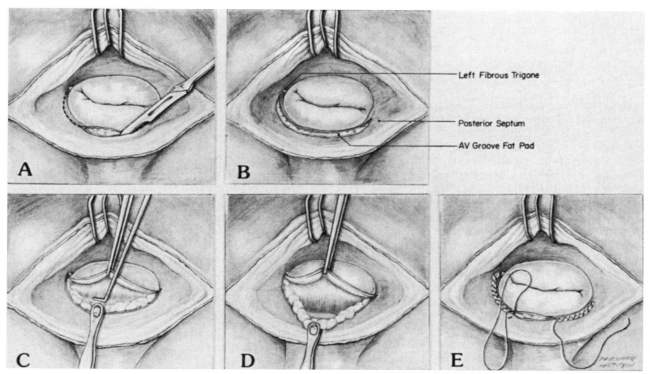

**FIGURE 55–11.** *A–E*, Surgeon's view of the endocardial technique for dividing left free-wall accessory pathways in the WPW syndrome. See text for details. (*A–E*, Modified from Cox, J. L., Gallagher, J. J., and Cain, M. E.: Experience with 118 consecutive patients undergoing surgery for the Wolff-Parkinson-White syndrome. J. Thorac. Cardiovasc. Surg., *90:*490–501, 1985.)

comes into view at the point where it joins the tricuspid valve to form the central fibrous body. The heart is usually arrested with cold potassium cardioplegia at this time, but this is not absolutely necessary. As

the epicardial reflection off of the posterior right ventricle has already been identified (see Fig. 55–12), visualization of the mitral valve annulus in the anterior portion of the posterior septal space completes

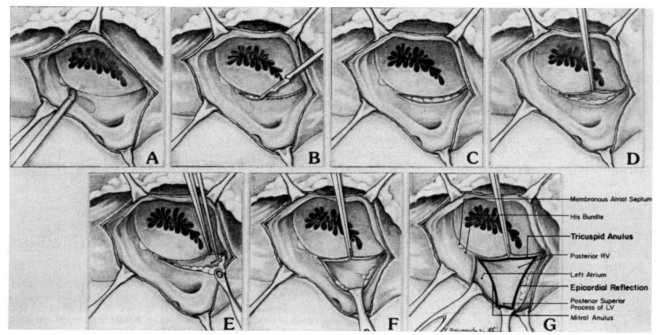

**FIGURE 55–12.** *A–G*, Endocardial technique for surgical division of posterior septal accessory pathways in the WPW syndrome. See text for details. (*A–G*, Modified from Cox, J. L., Gallagher, J. J., and Cain, M. E.: Experience with 118 consecutive patients undergoing surgery for the Wolff-Parkinson-White syndrome. J. Thorac. Cardiovasc. Surg., *90:*490–501, 1985.)

the identification of the boundaries of dissection of the space. The plane of dissection between the fat pad and the top of the posterior ventricular septum is developed completely by following the mitral annulus over to the posterosuperior process of the left ventricle and by following the epicardial reflection from the posterior right ventricle across the posterior crux onto the posterior left ventricle.

It is essential to divide all structures penetrating the posterior ventricular septum in the posterior septal space, including, if necessary, the AV node artery. The author's group has found that the AV node artery does leave the fat pad to enter the posterior ventricular septum within the posterior septal space in approximately 50% of patients with posterior septal accessory pathways. In every case, the author's group has ligated it and has never experienced any AV node dysfunction as a result.

**Right Free Wall Accessory Pathways.** The author's group prefers to open the right atrium to perform endocardial mapping for accessory pathways located in the right free wall space (see Fig. 55–9) because there is frequently a large amount of fat in the AV groove on the right side, making the epicardial mapping less than optimal. After localizing the accessory pathway, the heart is cardioplegically arrested and a supra-annular incision is placed 2 mm above the tricuspid valve annulus around the entire right free wall. A plane of dissection is established between the underlying AV groove fat pad and the top of the right ventricle throughout the length of the supra-annular incision and is developed to the epicardial reflection off of the ventricle so that the entire right ventricular free wall that is in contact with the AV groove fat pad is free of any penetrating fibers from the fat pad.

There are two additional potential problems with right free wall dissections that do not exist on the left side: The plane of dissection between the AV groove fat pad and the heart (atrium or ventricle) is not as well defined on the right, and the atrium and ventricle tend to "fold over" on one another at the tricuspid annulus (Fig. 55–13). To interrupt right free wall accessory pathways that reside too close to the valve annulus to be divided by routine dissection, one of three adjunctive measures must be added to the dissection: (1) mechanical "unfolding" of the atrium and ventricle so that the true valve annulus can be seen and freed of any adjacent fibers connecting the atrium and ventricle (applicable to both the epicardial and the endocardial techniques); (2) application of a cryolesion to the tissues near the valve annulus to destroy the juxta-annular accessory pathway (applicable to both techniques); or (3) "squaring-off" of the supra-annular incision at both ends to isolate the atrial rim of tissue to which a juxta-annular accessory pathway would connect (applicable to the endocardial technique). The "folding over" of the atrium and ventricle at the level of the tricuspid annulus is much more pronounced in patients with Ebstein's anomaly, a condition present in 14% of the patients in the author's group's series.

**Anterior Septal Accessory Pathways.** Epicardial

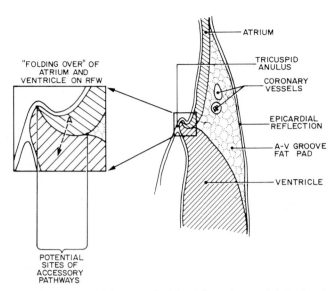

**FIGURE 55–13.** "Folding over" of the right atrium and right ventricle near the tricuspid annulus on the right free wall (RFW). Note that simple dissection of the AV groove fat pad away from the ventricle (endocardial technique) or atrium (epicardial technique) will not divide accessory pathways connecting the atrium and ventricle if they are near the tricuspid annulus. This is a common location for right free-wall accessory pathways, accounting for the erroneous concept that they are "endocardial" pathways.

mapping is excellent for documenting that an anterior septal pathway exists, but it does not localize these pathways very precisely because of the large fat pad covering both the atrium and the ventricle in the anterior septal space (see Fig. 55–9). Therefore, endocardial mapping is especially important in these patients, particularly because these pathways are more frequently located adjacent to the His bundle (anteriorly) than are posterior septal pathways (posteriorly). After retrograde endocardial mapping is performed, a supra-annular incision is placed just anterior to the His bundle 2 mm above the tricuspid annulus and extended in a clockwise direction well onto the right anterior free wall. The initial incision frequently abolishes ventricular preexcitation, but whether or not preexcitation persists, the entire anterior septal space is dissected. After the initial supra-annular incision is completed, a plane of dissection is established between the fat pad occupying the anterior septal space and the top of the right ventricle and is developed completely to the aorta medially and to the epicardial reflection off the ventricle anteriorly. During this dissection, the fat pad must be retracted very gently to avoid injury to the proximal right coronary artery, that courses through the fat pad before entering the AV groove of the anterior right free wall. In addition, when the anteromedial portion of the anterior septal space is being dissected, extreme care should be taken to avoid injury to the aorta.

### Associated Abnormalities

Certain types of congenital heart abnormalities are frequently associated with the WPW syndrome, the most common being Ebstein's anomaly, in which the septal leaflet, and occasionally the posterior leaflet, of the tricuspid valve is displaced downward into the right ventricle (Lev et al., 1970). The position of the AV node and conduction bundles in patients with Ebstein's anomaly is normal, although the right bundle branch may be compressed by thickened endocardium. In the author's group's experience, a distinct association between patients with Ebstein's anomaly and the specific location of the accessory pathways exists. Most commonly, patients with this anomaly have posterior septal accessory pathways. However, in the author's group's series, most patients with Ebstein's anomaly also had a combination of right free wall and posterior septal accessory pathways (Cox et al., 1985b). This correlation is so high that if a patient is found to have this combination of pathways on the preoperative electrophysiologic study, an echocardiogram is indicated to determine the presence or absence of Ebstein's anomaly.

Standard endocardial techniques are used to interrupt these accessory pathways. If valve replacement or placement of an annuloplasty ring is necessary to correct severe Ebstein's anomaly, it should be placed below the coronary sinus by sutures placed through the true tricuspid annulus. Plication of the atrialized ventricle may or may not be necessary.

### Results of Surgery

The incidence of successful surgical correction of the WPW syndrome is near 100% with an operative mortality for elective, uncomplicated cases that ranges from 0 to 0.5% (Cox et al., 1985b; Guiraudon et al., 1986a). There have been no early or late recurrences following surgery utilizing the endocardial technique in the author's group's own series (Cox et al., 1985b), and the recurrence rate following the epicardial technique is small (Guiraudon et al., 1986a). Moreover, the inadvertent creation of heart block is no longer a problem.

## Paroxysmal Supraventricular Tachycardia

*Paroxysmal supraventricular tachycardia* (PSVT) is a contemporary term for what was previously called paroxysmal atrial tachycardia (PAT). PSVT is a clinical condition in which SVT occurs suddenly in a patient who otherwise has a normal ECG. Two abnormalities account for essentially all PSVT: a concealed accessory AV connection and AV node reentry.

### Concealed Accessory Pathway

Accessory AV connections may be *manifest* or *concealed*. If an accessory pathway is capable of conducting in the antegrade (atrial-to-ventricular) direction, thereby causing a delta wave on the standard ECG, it is said to be *manifest* (i.e., its presence is apparent electrocardiographically). The retrograde (ventricular-to-atrial) conduction characteristics of such a pathway

determine the heart rate and frequency of occurrence of the associated reciprocating tachycardia. Some patients harbor accessory AV connections that are capable of conducting in the retrograde direction only. Since antegrade conduction across the accessory pathway does not occur, the ventricles are activated only through the normal AV node–His bundle complex and the standard ECG is normal. Therefore, such accessory pathways are said to be *concealed*. However, because these accessory pathways are capable of conducting in the retrograde direction, reciprocating tachycardia can occur just as it does in the classic WPW syndrome. Thus, from a clinical standpoint, the only difference between patients with manifest accessory pathways and those with concealed accessory pathways is the appearance of the standard ECG during normal sinus rhythm. The former have ECGs characteristic of the WPW syndrome, and the latter have normal ECGs.

In patients with a concealed accessory pathway, the absence of antegrade conduction across the pathway precludes the need to perform antegrade ventricular mapping intraoperatively. Thus, only retrograde atrial mapping is performed, and these maps are recorded during ventricular pacing or during induced reciprocating tachycardia. The surgical technique employed to divide concealed accessory pathways is the same as that for classic WPW syndrome.

### AV Node Reentry Tachycardia

AV node reentry tachycardia is caused by a reentrant circuit that is confined to the AV node or to the perinodal tissues of the lower atrial septum. The anatomic-electrophysiologic basis for this reentrant circuit is the presence of two conduction routes, one slow and one fast, through the AV node, the so-called dual AV node conduction pathways. The *fast* AV nodal pathway manifests rapid conduction but relatively long refractoriness. The *slow* AV nodal pathway exhibits slow conduction but relatively short refractoriness. During SVT, antegrade conduction proceeds through the slow pathway and retrograde conduction through the fast pathway, causing near-simultaneous activation of the ventricles and atria. Whether these functionally distinct dual AV node conduction pathways have an anatomic correlate is a matter of some controversy. Perhaps even more controversial is whether the functionally distinct dual AV nodal pathways of conduction are confined to the anatomic AV node or also involve the perinodal tissues.

Before 1982, the only surgical therapy for medically refractory AV node reentrant tachycardia was surgical division of the His bundle (Sealy et al., 1981). The objective of elective His bundle ablation was to protect the ventricles from the AV node reentry. However, because the procedure caused complete heart block, a permanent ventricular pacemaker was required postoperatively in all patients. In 1982, Scheinman described a technique for ablating the His bundle by introducing an electrical shock through a catheter placed adjacent to the His bundle (Scheinman et al.,

1982). This closed chest procedure immediately replaced the open heart surgical method for interrupting the His bundle. However, because the catheter fulguration technique also created complete heart block, all of those patients also required implantation of permanent pacemaker systems.

Although both the surgical technique and the catheter ablative technique for His bundle interruption ameliorated the unpleasant and detrimental effects of AV node reentry tachycardia, both procedures replaced one type of arrhythmia (tachycardia) with another (heart block). In 1982, the author's group attained the first clinical cure of AV node reentry tachycardia using a discrete cryosurgical technique (Cox, 1983b) (Fig. 55–14). Ross and co-workers (1985) subsequently reported the cure of AV node reentry tachycardia using surgical dissection of the perinodal tissues. Guiraudon and associates reported success with a similar surgical dissection technique (Fujimara et al., 1989).

The surgical techniques designed to cure AV node reentry tachycardia enjoyed excellent results, with no operative deaths in the three major series reported. Following the perinodal cryosurgical procedure, smooth AV node conduction curves through the remaining single conduction pathway were demonstrated in all patients in the author's group's series, and none of the patients had inducible AV node reentry tachycardia postoperatively (Cox et al., 1987). Moreover, all patients maintained normal conduction through the AV node–His bundle complex with no recurrent AV node reentry tachycardia. The surgical dissection techniques were associated with a low incidence of permanent complete heart block and a low incidence of recurrent AV node reentry tachycardia (Fujimara et al., 1989; Ross et al., 1985). At present,

however, radiofrequency catheter techniques have replaced surgery as the procedure of choice for AV node reentry tachycardia (Jackman et al., 1991; Lee et al., 1991)

## Supraventricular Arrhythmias Owing to Mahaim Fibers

Nodofascicular and fasciculoventricular connections, as described by Mahaim, occur between the nodal and fascicular components of the AV node–His bundle complex and the ventricular septum. Classically, these fibers have been depicted as originating from the AV node or its penetrating (His) bundle and then perforating the central fibrous body to insert into the ventricular myocardium. More recently, the appropriateness of depicting these accessory pathways as nodoventricular has been questioned. Tchou and colleagues (1988) suggested that such pathways represent atriofascicular connections with decremental conduction properties without direct anatomic connection to the AV nodal tissue, and Klein and co-workers (1988) suggested that "typical" nodoventricular connections may be atypical accessory pathways with decremental conduction properties and a distal right ventricular insertion site. Whatever the exact substrate, from a surgical point of view, Mahaim fibers may connect the His bundle to the ventricular septum by traversing the posterior septal space or the anterior septal space, in which case the Mahaim fiber is anterior to the His bundle. In addition, right free wall accessory pathways with typical "Mahaim-like" characteristics have been reported (Klein et al., 1988), and left-sided nodoventricular connections have been described as well (Abbott et al., 1987).

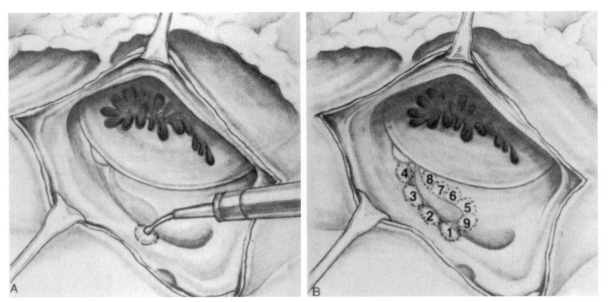

**FIGURE 55–14.** Discrete cryosurgical procedure for the treatment of AV node reentry tachycardia. A 3-mm cryoprobe is employed to place nine cryolesions around the periphery of the AV node (B), beginning at the upper edge of the os of the coronary sinus (A). See text for details. (A and B, Modified from Cox, J. L., Holman, W. L., and Cain, M. E.: Cryosurgical treatment of atrioventricular node reentry tachycardia. Circulation, 76:1329–1336, 1987. Reproduced with permission. Copyright 1987 American Heart Association.)

Depending on the spatial separation of the Mahaim fiber and the His bundle, these accessory connections can be interrupted using standard endocardial surgical dissection techniques that are employed for the WPW syndrome in combination with cryosurgery. The precise surgical approach depends on the location of the accessory pathway as determined by preoperative and intraoperative electrophysiologic mapping. When the posterior septal space is involved, a combination of discrete cryosurgery (Cox et al., 1987) and a posterior septal space dissection is required in some patients, whereas in others cryosurgery alone is sufficient to interrupt the pathway. In still other patients, a combination of cryosurgery with both anterior and posterior septal dissections is necessary. Finally, a subset of patients have what should be classified as "para-Hisian" connections, because despite all maneuvers, the accessory connection is so closely juxtaposed to the His bundle that it cannot be separated surgically. Simultaneous cryosurgical ablation of the His bundle and the accessory pathway is the only therapeutic alternative in such cases.

## Automatic Atrial Tachycardias

Clinical data suggest that derangements in automaticity, not reentry, underlie the genesis of these arrhythmias. These tachycardias appear to have a focal origin and usually originate from the body of the right atrium or left atrium, although they may occasionally arise from the interatrial septum. Accurate preoperative localization is particularly important for patients with automatic atrial tachycardias if surgical ablation of the ectopic focus is contemplated. These tachycardias are frequently suppressed with general anesthesia, and as a result, intraoperative mapping to localize their site of origin may not be possible. In addition, automatic tachycardias are not inducible by standard programmed stimulation techniques. Without accurate intraoperative localization, elective His bundle ablation was once the only surgical alternative. However, alternative surgical techniques that leave the normal AV conduction intact while isolating the arrhythmogenic atrial myocardium from the remainder of the heart have now been developed. If the site of origin of an automatic atrial tachycardia can be localized precisely by intraoperative mapping, the arrhythmogenic focus may be either excised or cryoablated (Gallagher et al., 1984a). Automatic foci located in the free wall of the left atrium or in either of the atrial appendages are ideal for excision or cryoablation. Automatic atrial tachycardias arising near the orifices of the pulmonary veins are best treated either by pulmonary vein isolation or by left atrial isolation (Williams et al., 1980) (see Fig. 55-5).

Theoretically, if intraoperative mapping properly localizes automatic foci in the free wall of the body of the right atrium, those foci can be either excised or cryoablated. However, automatic right atrial tachycardias are frequently multifocal in origin, and the ablation or excision of one automatic focus may be followed by the appearance of another at a later date. Thus, the recurrence rate following local excision or cryoablation of automatic right atrial tachycardias is unacceptably high. As a result, the author's group prefers to perform a right atrial isolation procedure even though the site of origin of the tachycardia may be well defined by intraoperative computerized mapping (Harada et al., 1988a, 1988b) (Fig. 55-15).

## SURGICAL TREATMENT OF VENTRICULAR TACHYARRHYTHMIAS

### Nonischemic VT

The most common tachyarrhythmias arising in the ventricles are those associated with ischemic heart disease, but many types of VT occur in the absence of coronary artery disease. Nonischemic VTs usually arise in the right ventricle, and although they are extremely resistant to medical therapy, newly developed surgical isolation techniques are proving to be most effective in their management. These arrhythmias have been classified into five categories based on their pathologic or clinical characteristics.

#### Idiopathic VT

*Idiopathic VT* refers to an arrhythmia in patients in whom the only clinical manifestation of cardiac disease is the arrhythmia. Both the macroscopic appearance of the heart at operation and the pathologic data acquired at the time of autopsy in such patients fail to show any evidence of primary cardiac disease. The only abnormality noted has been global dilatation of the heart secondary to functional post-tachycardia heart failure. If these patients require surgery, they first undergo intraoperative electrophysiologic mapping during VT in an effort to localize the apparent site of origin of the arrhythmia. Early surgical approaches included simple ventriculotomy, exclusion procedures, and cryoablation, but the results were poor, primarily because many of these arrhythmias arise within the ventricular septum. More recent approaches have included local isolation procedures if the site of origin is in the right ventricular free wall (Cox et al., 1983b, 1985a) and multipoint map-guided cryoablation if the site of origin is in the septum.

#### Nonischemic Cardiomyopathy

A small group of patients has been shown to have VT due to cardiomyopathy unassociated with ischemic heart disease. The patients in this group have angiographic and catheter data indicating some type of abnormal myocardial contractility associated with recurrent VT and usually show a diffuse dilatation of both ventricles with widespread patchy myocardial fibrosis. These tachyarrhythmias frequently arise in the right ventricle, and the author's group's approach

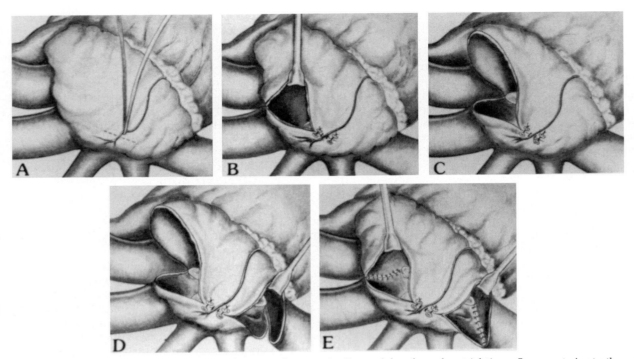

**FIGURE 55–15.** Right atrial isolation. *A*, Initially, the SA node artery is dissected free from the atrial tissue 5 mm anterior to the crista terminalis. A 2-cm incision parallel to the crista terminalis is placed beneath the artery. *B*, The incision beneath the SA node artery is closed with a continuous nonabsorbable 5-0 suture, taking care not to damage the artery. The small pledgets are used above and below the artery to reinforce the incision. The right atriotomy is then extended to a point anterior to the junction of the superior vena cava and the base of the right atrial appendage. *C*, The atriotomy is extended along the anterior limbus of the fossa ovalis to the anteromedial tricuspid valve annulus, just anterior to the membranous interatrial septum. *D*, Caudad extension of the right atriotomy around the posterior right atrial–inferior vena cava junction to the posterolateral tricuspid valve annulus. A cryolesion ($-60°$ C for 2 minutes) is placed at the end of the incision to ensure complete interruption of connecting atrial muscle fibers between the body of the right atrium and the remainder of the heart. *E*, The atriotomy is closed with a continuous 4-0 nonabsorbable suture. (*A–E*, From Harada, A., D'Agostino, H. J., Jr., Boineau, J. P., and Cox, J. L.: Right atrial isolation: A new surgical treatment for supraventricular tachycardia. I: Surgical technique and electrophysiologic effects. J. Thorac. Cardiovasc. Surg., *95*:643, 1988.)

to such patients has been to employ a combination of surgical isolation and cryoablation of the apparent site of origin of the arrhythmia. One of the author's group's patients, a 16-year-old female with coxsackie myocarditis, was documented to have intermittent ventricular tachycardia for 7 years following her initial viral infection. Preoperative electrophysiologic studies indicated that the VT was arising from the pulmonary infundibulum near the level of the pulmonic valve annulus. However, the intraoperative electrophysiologic studies demonstrated the tachycardia to be arising in the high right ventricular septum between the crista supraventricularis and the pulmonic valve annulus. A combination of surgical isolation and cryoablation of the apparent site of origin of the VT caused permanent cessation of the arrhythmia (Fig. 55–16).

### Arrhythmogenic Right Ventricular Dysplasia

Fontaine and associates (1979) described a previously unrecognized form of cardiomyopathy localized to the right ventricle, which they termed *arrhythmogenic right ventricular dysplasia*. This syndrome is a congenital cardiomyopathy characterized by transmural infiltration of adipose tissue causing weakness and aneurysmal bulging of the infundibu-

lum, apex, or posterior basilar region of the right ventricle. The syndrome is characterized clinically by intractable VT originating from one or all of the three pathologic areas of the right ventricle (Fig. 55–17). Because the origin of the tachycardia is in the right ventricle, the standard ECG shows a pattern consistent with left bundle-branch block during the tachycardia. Right ventricular angiography should be performed in all patients who exhibit VT with a left bundle branch-block pattern. In patients with arrhythmogenic right ventricular dysplasia, the right ventricle appears enlarged, ventricular bulges or frank aneurysms are seen in the infundibulum, the apex, or the basal portion of the inferior wall, and right ventricular contractility is usually markedly decreased. Hypertrophic muscular bands in the infundibulum and anterior right ventricular wall produce apparent pseudodiverticula, the so-called feathering appearance of the right ventricular outflow tract.

The author's group's current approach to such patients employs a transmural encircling ventriculotomy that effectively isolates the arrhythmogenic myocardium from the remainder of the heart (Cox et al., 1985a). The operation depicted in Figure 55–18 was performed on a 69-year-old man who was in continuous VT for 28 days prior to his operation. Preoperative electrophysiologic studies revealed the tachycar-

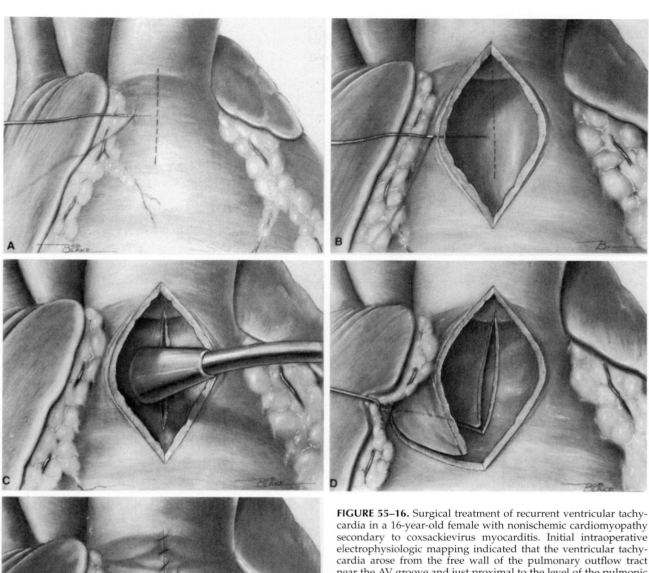

**FIGURE 55–16.** Surgical treatment of recurrent ventricular tachycardia in a 16-year-old female with nonischemic cardiomyopathy secondary to coxsackievirus myocarditis. Initial intraoperative electrophysiologic mapping indicated that the ventricular tachycardia arose from the free wall of the pulmonary outflow tract near the AV groove and just proximal to the level of the pulmonic valve annulus. An intramural needle electrode was inserted at that epicardial site and was passed transmurally so that its tip was positioned in the interventricular septum between the crista supraventricularis and the pulmonic valve annulus. Intramural electrograms were recorded from electrode contacts located every millimeter along the needle shaft. Earliest ventricular activation during ventricular tachycardia occurred at the electrode contact point at the tip of the needle shaft, indicating that the ventricular tachycardia was originating in the supracristal portion of the interventricular septum. *A,* A longitudinal incision was made on the free wall of the pulmonary outflow tract, beginning just distal to the level of the pulmonic valve annulus and extending proximally, as shown by the *broken line.* This free-wall incision did not alter the ventricular tachycardia. *B,* The pulmonary outflow tract has been opened, and the needle electrode is seen intramurally in the supracristal portion of the interventricular septum. A counterincision was made on the posterior wall of the pulmonary outflow tract beginning just distal to the pulmonic valve annulus and extending proximally to the level of the crista supraventricularis (*broken line*). This incision was transmural, and the aortic root could be visualized through this posterior incision. This counterincision did not alter the ventricular tachycardia. *C,* A cryoprobe was positioned over the site of earliest activation during ventricular tachycardia, and the myocardium was frozen at −60° C for 2 minutes. This cryolesion resulted in cessation of the ventricular tachycardia. *D,* The proximal ends of the anterior and posterior ventriculotomies were then connected by a transmural semicircular incision around the left side of the pulmonary outflow tract. This resulted in total isolation of the segment of the pulmonary outflow tract that contained the arrhythmogenic myocardium. *E,* The incisions were closed with a continuous 3-0 nonabsorbable suture. The patient has remained free of ventricular tachycardia for 14 years after this surgical procedure. (*A–E,* From Cox, J. L., Bardy, G. H., Damiano, R. J., et al.: Right ventricular isolation procedures for nonischemic ventricular tachycardia. J. Thorac. Cardiovasc. Surg., *90*:212, 1985.)

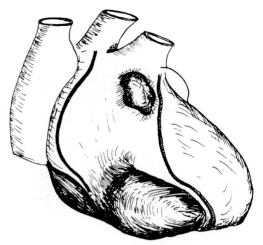

**FIGURE 55–17.** Diagrammatic sketch of the three areas of pathologic involvement in arrhythmogenic right ventricular dysplasia. (Courtesy of Dr. G. Fontaine.)

dia to be originating from the posterior basilar region of the right ventricle. Preoperative right ventricular angiography demonstrated feathering of the right ventricular outflow tract and aneurysmal bulging of the infundibulum, apex, and posterior basilar region of the right ventricle. Intraoperative electrophysiologic studies revealed the tachycardia to be arising in the posterior basilar region of the right ventricle adjacent to an electrically silent area on the anterior right ventricle measuring 2 cm by 3 cm. In such cases, it must be recognized that the actual site of origin of the VT may be in the electrically silent region and that it appears to arise from the border of the silent region only because a certain critical mass of synchronously depolarized myocardium is essential to produce an electrogram large enough to be detected by the exploring electrode. Because the three pathologically abnormal regions of the right ventricle in arrhythmogenic right ventricular dysplasia may exhibit electrical silence on epicardial mapping, every attempt should be made to isolate the entire pathologic area giving rise to the tachycardia from the remainder of the heart. The surgically isolated "pedicle" shown in Figure 55–18*B* is based on a vascular supply originating from the right coronary artery. The incision is begun in the AV groove at the level of the tricuspid annulus, is extended around the arrhythmogenic region of the myocardium, and returned to the level of the tricuspid annulus inferiorly. At both ends of the incision, a cryolesion is placed to ensure complete separation of all ventricular myocardial fibers on either side of the incision. In the operation depicted in Figure 55–18, a separate incision was extended to the right ventricular apex because of the presence of a discrete aneurysm in that location. In making such an incision in the right ventricle, the surgeon takes care to avoid the base of the papillary muscles; but if necessary, the incision can be extended around the base of a papillary muscle. The incision is closed in two layers with a continuous suture.

Although Fontaine's original description of ar-

rhythmogenic right ventricular dysplasia suggested that the cardiomyopathy was confined to three discrete areas of the right ventricle, intraoperative mapping of these patients has suggested that the entire right ventricular free wall may be arrhythmogenic in certain cases. In the author's group's experience, there may be as many as seven different sites of origin of tachycardia in these patients, each site giving rise to a different morphologic type of VT. Computerized intraoperative mapping systems are able to localize these tachycardias only if each of them can be induced at the time of surgery, an unrealistic expectation. As a result of these problems, the author's group has had to resort to surgical isolation of the entire right ventricular free wall on occasion to relieve the life-threatening sequelae of arrhythmogenic dysplasia (Cox et al., 1983b). Isolation of the entire right ventricular free wall (Fig. 55–19) represents a logical extension of the two localized right ventricular isolation procedures described previously, but it should be reserved for only the most dire of circumstances. For example, the procedure depicted in Figure 55–19 was performed on a 16-year-old male in 1982 who had received full cardiopulmonary resuscitation (CPR) over 250 times. In addition, an automatic internal defibrillator had been implanted previously at another institution, one of the first such devices implanted clinically. The patient had continued to require frequent CPR and, as a result, underwent a right ventricular isolation procedure with removal of the automatic defibrillator. Although the follow-up of these patients documents excellent control of their tachycardia (Fig. 55–20), the right ventricle may undergo progressive dilatation postoperatively. Nevertheless, the patients in whom the author's group performed this procedure have remained in excellent functional status for over 11 years.

### Uhl's Syndrome

This is a rare congenital cardiomyopathy that, from the anatomic point of view, may be considered to be a more complete form of arrhythmogenic right ventricular dysplasia. The right ventricle is extremely dilated, but the tricuspid valve remains in a normal position, thus differentiating it from Ebstein's anomaly. The main characteristic of Uhl's syndrome is the complete absence of myocardium in the right ventricular free wall, causing the endocardial and epicardial layers to be in direct contact without interposition of myocardial fibers. Since Uhl's description of this cardiomyopathy in 1952, the descriptive term *parchment heart* has been applied to the abnormality. Although Uhl's syndrome usually leads to rapid cardiac failure in the first months or years of life, an adult form of this condition occurs in which associated VT is the dominant feature.

### The Long Q-T Syndrome and Torsades de Pointes

In 1957, Jervell and Lange-Nielsen described a clinical entity consisting of a long Q-T interval, congenital

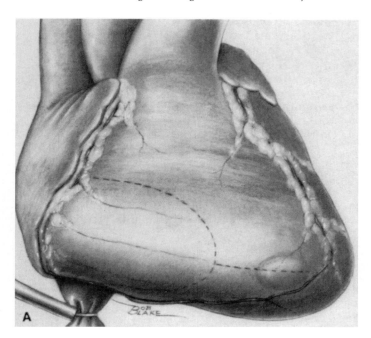

FIGURE 55–18. *A,* Appearance of the right ventricle (RV) in a patient with arrhythmogenic right ventricular dysplasia. Note the three coronary arteries coursing from the AV groove across the surface of the RV. The acute margin of the RV corresponded to the location of the middle coronary artery shown in this drawing. An area approximately 2 × 3-cm near the upper coronary artery was electrically silent. Epicardial mapping during ventricular tachycardia showed the earliest site of activation to be located near the lower edge of this electrically silent region just below the midsegment of the middle coronary region on the posterior basilar region of the RV. A transmural ventriculotomy was placed around the electrically silent area and included the apparent site of origin of the ventricular tachycardia on the posterior basilar region of the heart (*broken line*). The two ends of this incision were based at the AV groove, where cryolesions were applied to ensure isolation of the arrhythmogenic region of myocardium from the remainder of the heart. In addition, a second transmural incision was made from the apex of the semicircular incision to the apex of the RV to include the small saccular aneurysm in that region. *B,* The isolated pedicle of right ventricular myocardium containing the electrically silent area and the apparent site of origin of the ventricular tachycardia has been reflected to show the internal anatomy of the RV. Note the extension of the incision to the right ventricular apex to open the small aneurysm located in that region. *C,* The transmural encircling ventriculotomy around the arrhythmogenic region of the RV and the simple ventriculotomy through the right ventricular apical aneurysm have been closed with a continuous 3-0 nonabsorbable suture. After completion of this procedure for arrhythmogenic right ventricular dysplasia, the isolated pedicle was paced at a rapid rate, but the paced impulses were not conducted to the remainder of the heart. In addition, the remainder of the RV was then paced rapidly, but those paced impulses were not conducted into the isolated pedicle, confirming total isolation of the arrhythmogenic right ventricular myocardium from the remainder of the heart. (*A–C,* From Cox, J. L.: Surgery for cardiac arrhythmias. *In* Harvey, W. P. [ed]: Current Problems in Cardiology. Vol. 8, No. 4. Chicago, Year Book Medical, Copyright 1983. Reproduced with permission.)

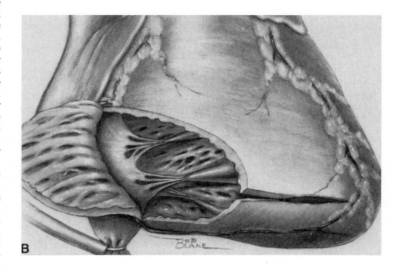

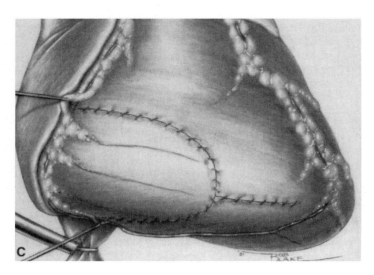

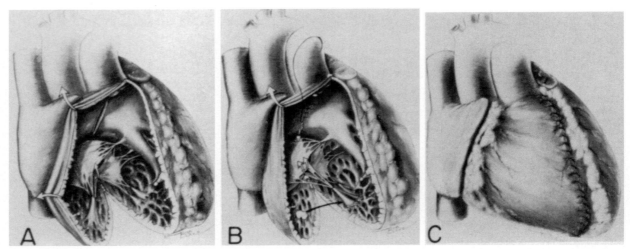

**FIGURE 55–19.** Right ventricular disconnection procedure. *A,* A transmural right ventriculotomy is placed parallel to and 5 mm from the interventricular septum extending from just across the pulmonic valve annulus anteriorly to the tricuspid valve posteriorly. It is necessary to divide several large infundibular muscular bundles and to divide the moderator band of the RV. Although the entire incision is transmural, special care must be taken to avoid injury to the right coronary artery lying in the AV groove at the posterior extent of this incision. After identification of the location of the His bundle and right bundle branch, a second transmural incision is placed from the posterior pulmonic valve annulus to the anterior medial tricuspid valve annulus, exposing the underlying aortic root. If the tricuspid portion of this incision is placed too far anteriorly, the bundle of His may be inadvertently divided. *B,* After completion of the two transmural incisions, the papillary muscle attached to the anterior leaflet of the tricuspid valve is divided at its base and reimplanted on the lower ventricular septum using interrupted 3-0 pledgeted Prolene suture. Cryolesions are placed at each end of the anteroposterior ventriculotomy and at each end of the ventriculotomy between the posterior pulmonic valve annulus and the anterior medial suture followed by closure of the long free-wall ventriculotomy with continuous 3-0 nonabsorbable suture (*C*). (*A–C,* Modified from Cox, J. L.: Surgery for cardiac arrhythmias. *In* Harvey, W. P. [ed]: Current Problems in Cardiology. Vol. 8, No. 4, Chicago, Year Book Medical, 1983.)

deafness, and syncopal attacks owing to ventricular fibrillation following emotional or physical stresses. The absence of congenital deafness characterizes the otherwise identical Romano-Ward syndrome (Romano et al., 1963; Ward, 1964). The prolongation of the Q-T interval in both of these syndromes has been considered to be congenital in origin, and both syndromes are recognized to contribute to sudden death

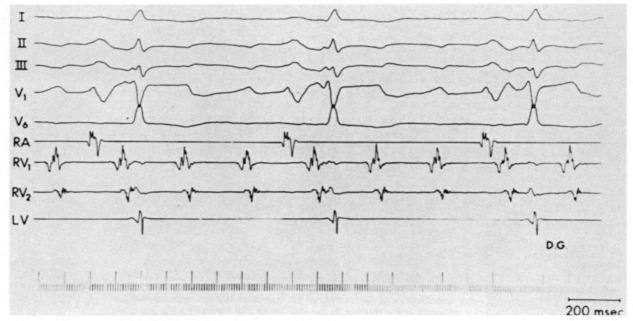

**FIGURE 55–20.** Surface recordings and intracardiac electrograms in a 16-year-old male during an episode of right ventricular (RV) tachycardia following the right ventricular isolation procedure. The limb-lead (I–III) and precordial lead ($V_1$ and $V_6$) electrograms demonstrated normal sinus rhythm in the remainder of the heart documented by right atrial (RA) activity preceding each left ventricular (LV) complex. (From Cox, J. L., Bardy, G. H., Damiano, R. J., et al.: Right ventricular isolation procedures for nonischemic ventricular tachycardia. J. Thorac. Cardiovasc. Surg. *90:*212, 1985.)

in children (Fraser and Froggatt, 1966; Schwartz et al., 1975). Although the pathogenesis of the long Q-T syndrome is poorly understood, James and colleagues (1978) demonstrated the presence of focal neuritis and neural degeneration within the specialized conduction system and the ventricular myocardium. They suggested the possibility that a chronic viral infection or some noninfectious degenerative process of the cardiac nerves might be responsible for the prolongation of the Q-T interval and the associated fatal ventricular arrhythmias.

VT that occurs in association with the long Q-T syndrome is frequently of a distinct type termed *torsades de pointes*, a name derived from the appearance of the VT on a standard ECG, in which the polarity of the tachycardia is inconstant (Fig. 55–21). The electrocardiographic features of torsades de pointes are unique and may be described as follows: (1) the episodes are generally initiated by a ventricular ectopic beat following late after the preceding sinus complex; (2) the successive QRS complexes during tachycardia show an "undulating series of rotations" (Wellens et al., 1975) of the electrical axis; and (3) the episodes most frequently cease spontaneously (Dessertenne, 1966; Krikler and Curry, 1976; Kulbertus, 1978). In addition, the arrhythmia is usually preceded by variations in the T wave during the last several beats prior to development of the tachycardia. One of the most frequent causes of torsades de pointes is the administration of medications that prolong ventricular repolarization, particularly quinidine (Kulbertus, 1980).

These observations support the concept that torsades de pointes represents an abnormality in myocardial *repolarization,* as opposed to most other types of VT, which are thought to be abnormalities in myocardial *depolarization.* As a result, the surgical treatment of recurrent VT associated with long Q-T syndrome has centered around efforts to modify cardiac innervation. The classic studies of Yanowitz and co-workers (1966) showed that unilateral alterations in sympathetic tone altered not only the shape of the T wave but also its duration (Q-T interval). Their study in animals showed that resection of the right stellate ganglion or stimulation of the left stellate ganglion produced prolonged Q-T intervals and increased T-wave amplitude. Conversely, resection of the left stellate ganglion or stimulation of the right stellate ganglion produced increased T-wave negativity without measurable changes in the Q-T interval. Therefore, the hypothesis has been postulated that the electrocar-

diographic changes following unilateral alterations of sympathetic tone provide a functional explanation for the electrocardiographic abnormalities occurring in patients with lesions of the central nervous system as well as in patients with the long Q-T syndrome. Resection of the left stellate ganglion has been reported to abolish symptoms in many patients with the long Q-T syndrome (Malliani et al., 1980; Moss and McDonald, 1971; Schwartz et al., 1975; Smith and Gallagher, 1979). However, the author's group's experience (Benson and Cox, 1982) and that of others (Bhandari et al., 1984) has been characterized by early success and late failure.

## Ischemic VT

Acute myocardial infarction causes the nonuniform juxtaposition of normal and abnormal myocardium, a favorable anatomic substrate for the development of automatic or reentrant arrhythmias. Although ventricular irritability, tachycardia, and fibrillation frequently occur during the initial and early phases of acute myocardial infarction, these manifestations of acute ischemic injury are usually transient and tend to be responsive to medical management. With the subsequent progression of acute ischemic injury to cell death, the substrate for automaticity (primarily cellular membrane instability owing to ischemia) disappears, leaving scar in the place of injured myocardium. The interlacing pattern of the remaining scar and normal myocardium, especially at the periphery of myocardial infarcts or aneurysms, may harbor local areas of slow conduction, unidirectional block, uneven refractoriness, and nonuniform repolarization, the electrophysiologic substrates for the development of reentrant circuits (Boineau and Cox, 1973, 1982; Cox, 1983a). The ventricular tachyarrhythmias that develop as a result of these chronic changes in ischemically injured myocardium are frequently intractable and may be unresponsive to pharmacologic agents. For this reason, a nonpharmacologic solution to these recalcitrant arrhythmias has been sought since the early 1960s.

### Historical Aspects

Sir Thomas Lewis was apparently the first to recognize the relationship between ventricular aneurysm and VT in 1909 when he suggested the need for a

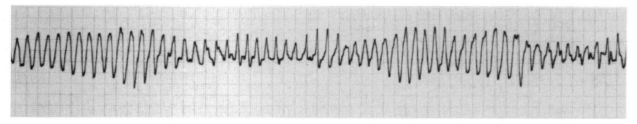

**FIGURE 55–21.** Torsades de pointes. This type of ventricular tachycardia, which is usually associated with the long Q-T syndrome, is characterized by rhythmic changes in the polarity of successive QRS complexes.

controlled method of inducing tachycardia so that it could be studied in a systematic manner (Lewis, 1909). In the absence of such a technique even 50 years later, Couch (1959) performed a simple aneurysmectomy specifically for the treatment of intractable VT. In 1967, Durrer and associates of Amsterdam (Durrer et al., 1967) and Coumel and colleagues of Paris (Coumel et al., 1967) described the technique of programmed electrical stimulation, precisely the tool desired by Lewis to induce and terminate tachycardia in a reproducible manner for purposes of diagnosis and evaluation of interventional therapy.

Experimental studies in the mid- and late 1960s documented the heterogeneity of tissue injury in acute myocardial infarction (Cox et al., 1968), and the reentrant basis of ischemic ventricular tachyarrhythmias was confirmed (Boineau and Cox, 1973; Cox et al., 1969; Durrer et al., 1971; Han et al., 1970; El-Sherif et al., 1977; Scherlag et al., 1974; Waldo and Kaiser, 1973). Thus, with the advent of coronary bypass surgery in the late 1960s, it seemed apparent that ischemic VT would be easily corrected by this new procedure because the basis for the arrhythmia (myocardial ischemia) could be alleviated by myocardial revascularization. However, during the 1970s, it became apparent that neither revascularization nor resection of the injured myocardium produced acceptable cure rates, and in addition, the operative mortality rates reported with these procedures when performed primarily for VT control were prohibitively high (Boineau and Cox, 1982). Although the demonstration that ischemic ventricular tachyarrhythmias occurred on a reentrant basis improved the author's group's concept of the arrhythmia, there remained a profound ignorance of the uncharted interplay among the autonomic nervous system, endogenous humoral stimulants, intracellular electrophysiology, extracellular electrophysiology, the specialized conduction system, coronary artery disease, myocardial ischemia and infarction, and normal myocardial conduction, all of which undoubtedly have a role in the genesis and perpetuation of ischemic ventricular tachyarrhythmias.

Because of the lack of efficacy of myocardial revascularization or resection in controlling ischemic VT, several groups began to approach the problem in a more direct surgical manner. In 1969, Daniel and co-workers and Kaiser and associates independently reported intraoperative mapping in patients with ischemic heart disease to localize the area of ischemic injury. Fontaine and colleagues employed intraoperative mapping prior to performing a standard aneurysmectomy in 1974, but Wittig and Boineau (1975) and Gallagher and co-workers (1975) first reported the use of intraoperative mapping specifically to guide the attempted surgical ablation of ischemic VT. In 1978, Guiraudon and associates described the encircling endocardial ventriculotomy (EEV), a procedure they had successfully employed to ablate VT in five patients. Shortly thereafter, Harken and colleagues (Josephson et al., 1979) described the endocardial resection procedure, modifications of which remain the mainstay of surgery for the treatment of ischemic VT to the present time.

## Preoperative Electrophysiologic Evaluation

All patients who are to undergo surgical therapy for ventricular tachyarrhythmias should first undergo an endocardial catheter electrophysiology study. The objectives of the preoperative study are confirmation that the arrhythmia is ventricular rather than supraventricular in origin; demonstration that the ventricular arrhythmia can be induced and terminated by programmed electrical stimulation techniques (i.e., that it is a reentrant arrhythmia); and localization of the region of origin of the VT by "catheter mapping" when possible. In addition to the preoperative electrophysiology study, patients with ventricular tachyarrhythmias routinely undergo cardiac catheterization and coronary angiography prior to surgical intervention.

The preoperative electrophysiology study may demonstrate the arrhythmia to be VT of a *single morphologic type*, indicating that it is originating from a single region in the left or right ventricle. Following induction, these monomorphic VTs are usually sustained for a sufficient length of time to allow endocardial catheter mapping to determine their site of origin. However, monomorphic VT may be nonsustained, thus precluding adequate mapping during the preoperative electrophysiology study. The preoperative study may also document the arrhythmia to be *polymorphic VT*. This term is applied not only to VT that originates from several different regions of the left ventricle giving rise to different morphologic types of tachycardia but also to tachycardia that originates from one general region of the left ventricle but is characterized electrophysiologically by excessive fragmentation such that individual depolarization complexes may be difficult to identify. Polymorphic VT may also be either sustained or nonsustained, and it commonly deteriorates rather quickly into ventricular fibrillation. Electrophysiologic deterioration to ventricular fibrillation may be the result of primary electrical instability or may occur because of hemodynamic compromise associated with the onset of polymorphic VT. The third type of ventricular tachyarrhythmia that may be identified by the preoperative electrophysiologic study is *primary ventricular fibrillation*. This arrhythmia is characterized by the absence of any type of induced VT prior to the onset of ventricular fibrillation following programmed electrical stimulation.

## Surgical Indications and Contraindications

Decisions regarding surgical intervention for ischemic VT are based on a variety of clinical factors and must be individualized for each patient. Because no surgical technique exists for the ablation of primary ventricular fibrillation, the author's group implants an internal cardioverter-defibrillator (ICD) device in all patients with this unusual problem. It is important to realize, however, that even though ventricular fibrillation may be the primary diagnosis in a given patient who has been resuscitated from an episode of sudden death, an electrophysiology study usually confirms that the episode of fibrillation is preceded by at least a short run of VT, most commonly of the polymorphic type described previously. The author's group considers such patients to have primary VT, not ventricular fibrillation, which the author's group believes to be a secondary problem that is alleviated if the VT can be controlled.

Polymorphic VT was previously considered to be a contraindication to surgical procedure because of its complex nature and the attendant difficulty in mapping it at the time of surgery. However, the availability of computerized intraoperative mapping systems has provided a means of identifying the area or areas of arrhythmogenic myocardium, even with this fleeting, changing type of ventricular tachyarrhythmia.

Perhaps the major contraindication to operation is left ventricular dysfunction so severe that it precludes any reasonable possibility of surviving an operative procedure. Prior to availability of the ICD devices, there was no viable alternative to operation in such patients if their arrhythmia could not be controlled pharmacologically. However, the author's group now prefers to implant an ICD device in such patients because of the lower operative mortality rate associated with this relatively simple procedure. One side benefit of this "selection" of patients who do not undergo VT surgery has been an improvement in the operative mortality rate of the remaining patients who now undergo direct surgery.

Finally, the question of whether the antiarrhythmic agent amiodarone is associated with a higher operative mortality rate or postoperative complication rate is controversial. This question depends in part on how one conducts the operation for VT. For example, in the author's group's experience, amiodarone has caused the low-output syndrome postoperatively only in those patients who require cardioplegic arrest for performance of some portion of the operative procedure. Since the author's group performs all VT procedures in the normothermic beating heart, amiodarone is not a problem unless coronary artery bypass surgery is also necessary, in which case the author's group would employ cardioplegic arrest after completion of the specific tachycardia procedure. In the latter case, the author's group prefers that the amiodarone be discontinued for a minimum of 4 weeks before surgery. If that is not feasible, the author's group performs the coronary bypass procedure during ventricular fibrillation. Only under the most unusual of circumstances is cardioplegic arrest employed in patients on amiodarone.

### Intraoperative Electrophysiologic Mapping

In patients undergoing surgery for ventricular tachyarrhythmias, the first step intraoperatively is to perform detailed electrophysiologic mapping procedures to guide the specific surgical technique to be employed. During the past few years, the author's group has begun using a new method of intraoperative electrophysiologic mapping termed *potential distribution mapping* (Harada et al., 1990; Tweddell et al., 1988, 1989a, 1989b). Form-fitting, molded endocardial electrode arrays (Fig. 55–22) are inserted across the mitral and tricuspid valves to obtain three-dimensional potential distribution electrophysiologic maps of the endocardium (Fig. 55–23). This type of mapping is much more conducive to computerization and, as a result, is quicker and more accurate than the standard activation time mapping.

### Direct Surgical Procedures for the Treatment of Ischemic VT

The *encircling endocardial ventriculotomy* (EEV) was the first technique introduced specifically for the control of refractory ischemic VT (Guiraudon et al., 1978). Guiraudon and associates reasoned that since the reentrant circuits responsible for the tachycardia were suspected to reside at or near the junction of the endocardial fibrosis associated with the infarct or aneurysm and normal myocardium (Fig. 55–24A), and since a standard aneurysmectomy did not remove this area (Fig. 55–24B), one should not expect the latter to be effective in ablating the arrhythmia. They therefore advocated placing an endocardial incision around the entire circumference of the infarct or aneurysm just outside the junction of the fibrosis and normal myocardium (Fig. 55–24C). This incision was a deep one, extending to very near the epicardium on the free wall and 1 cm deep on the septum. The objective of the encircling endocardial incision was either to interrupt the reentrant circuit or to encompass it entirely with the goal of isolating it from the remainder of the ventricle. Although the EEV was extremely effective in controlling VT, its effectiveness stemmed from the fact that the encompassed myocardium was made more ischemic, thus suppressing the reentrant circuit causing the tachycardia (Ungerleider et al., 1982b, 1982c). In addition, because increased ischemia caused by the EEV produced poorer left ventricular function (Ungerleider et al., 1982a), the EEV was associated with an unacceptable incidence of postoperative low-output syndrome and operative mortality (Cox et al., 1982). The EEV as originally described, therefore, is no longer employed for the treatment of VT.

In 1979, Josephson and colleagues introduced the concept of first localizing the site of origin of VT by endocardial mapping and then resecting the endocardial fibrosis in the arrhythmogenic region with the goal of either interrupting or removing the reentrant circuit causing the VT (Fig. 55–24D). This technique, called by a variety of names including the *local endocardial resection procedure* (ERP) and *subendocardial resection* (SER), involved removing approximately 10 cm² of fibrosis from one quadrant of the infarct or aneurysm. Moran and associates (1982) later modified the local ERP so that all of the endocardial fibrosis was removed regardless of the location of the arrhyth-

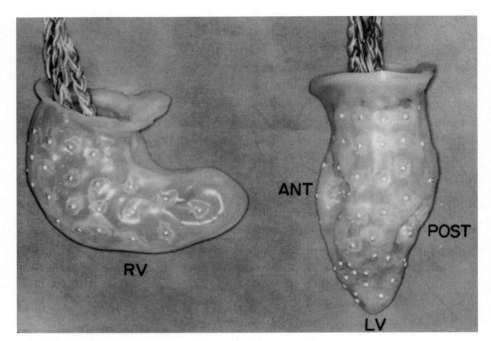

**FIGURE 55–22.** Endocardial electrodes used for recording both activation time maps and potential distribution maps in patients with ventricular tachycardia. The electrode templates are made of Silastic and target-tipped bipolar electrodes are embedded in the wall of the Silastic templates. The templates are constructed over form-fitting molds of the right ventricle (RV) and its outflow tract and of the left ventricle (LV). The indentations of the anterior (ANT) and posterior (POST) papillary muscles can be seen on the left ventricular template. These electrode templates are introduced into the respective ventricles via right and left atriotomies. The flanged portion of each template abuts the respective tricuspid or mitral valve annulus. A low-pressure balloon resides inside each of these templates that, when inflated, ensures excellent electrode contact with the endocardium of each ventricle.

mogenic tissue (the *extended endocardial resection procedure* [EERP]). The author's group advocated using endocardial cryosurgery to ablate arrhythmogenic tissue that was located near the aortic or mitral valve annuli or on the base of the papillary muscles that was not amenable to treatment by the EEV, local ERP, or EERP techniques (Cox et al., 1982) (Fig. 55–24E).

Ostermeyer and co-workers (1984, 1987) have utilized a *partial EEV* technique in which an endocardial incision is placed only in the region of arrhythmogenesis with excellent results. In addition, superior results have been reported with a technique that combines wide endocardial resection with endocardial cryosurgery (Krafchek et al., 1986a, 1986b), the approach that most closely resembles that which the author's group currently employs. The author's group first localizes the site(s) of origin of the VT, as described previously. Then, with the heart in the normothermic beating state, preferably during VT, the ventricle is opened through the infarct or aneurysm and all of the associated endocardial fibrosis is resected except that which extends onto the base of

the papillary muscles (Fig. 55–25). After all visible endocardial fibrosis is resected, endocardial cryolesions are applied to the site(s) of origin of the tachycardia. The cryothermia is applied only after removal of the endocardial scar because, in the author's group's experience, approximately 10% of patients continue to have inducible VT intraoperatively after removal of all visible endocardial fibrosis. This would indicate that the actual site of origin of the tachycardia in these patients is deeper in the myocardium than the visible border of the endocardial fibrosis, and that, therefore, the myocardium underneath the fibrosis must be destroyed to ablate the tachycardia. In those cases in which one site of origin is a scarred papillary muscle, the author's group places one or more cryolesions directly on the base of the involved papillary muscle without removing the scar (Figs. 55–26 and 55–27). The author's group has cryoablated over 100 papillary muscles without a single instance of mitral valve regurgitation, an experience that is consistent with experimental studies showing that cryoablation of papillary muscles does not cause sub-

**FIGURE 55–23.** Three-dimensional potential distribution maps during ventricular tachycardia. This is a left-posterior view of the two ventricular cavities (endocasts) with the LV on the left and the RV on the right. The apex of both ventricles is below and the respective valve annuli are above. The empty space between the two ventricular endocasts is the interventricular septum. *A,* At 6 msec into the first recorded complex of ventricular tachycardia (*upper panel*), the distribution of electrical forces in the ventricles is essentially neutral. *B,* At 15 msec, the earliest site of negative potentials appears on the endocardium of the right side of the ventricular septum (*black area*), representing the "site of origin" of the ventricular tachycardia. This so-called primary potential minima represents the area of the ventricular endocardium where the electrical potentials (or forces) are negative at this particular instant in time. Other areas in the right ventricular septum and a small area on the posterior left ventricle (*gray areas*) are also negative, but less so. They represent the spread of the electrical wave front from the site of the primary potential minima. All other sites in the ventricles are still neutral. *C,* At 24 msec, the primary potential minima has enlarged and the negative forces now involve more of the posterior left ventricle. *D,* At 33 msec, the primary potential minima involves the majority of the endocardial surface of the right side of the ventricular septum. These illustrations of potential distribution maps are single frames of data from a dynamic map (movie) of the electrical events during ventricular tachycardia. The ventricular endocasts can be rotated at will to provide a better view of the site of origin of ventricular tachycardia. These three-dimensional maps of ventricular tachycardia can be obtained within approximately 4 minutes of recording the data.

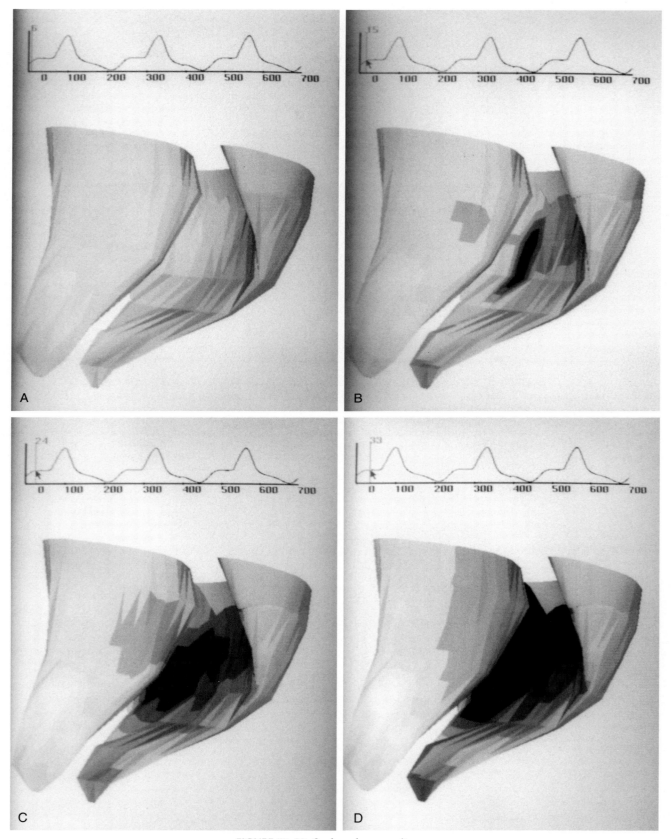

**FIGURE 55–23.** *See legend on opposite page*

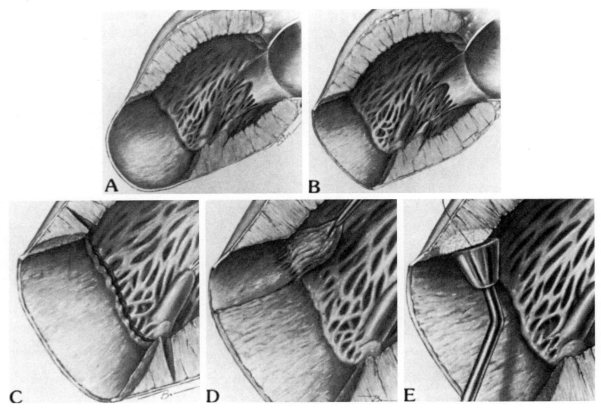

**FIGURE 55–24.** Diagrammatic cross-section of an anterior left ventricular aneurysm showing more proximal extension of the associated fibrosis at the endocardial level than at the epicardial level (*A*). Since the reentrant circuits responsible for ischemic ventricular tachycardia occur most commonly at the junction of this endocardial fibrosis and normal myocardium, a standard left ventricular aneurysm resection (*B*) does not ablate or remove them. The encircling endocardial ventriculotomy (*C*), localized endocardial (or "subendocardial") resection (*D*), and endocardial cryoablation (*E*) were all introduced specifically to ablate ventricular tachycardia associated with left ventricular aneurysms or infarcts. (*A–E*, Modified from Cox, J. L.: Anatomic-electrophysiologic basis for the surgical treatment of refractory ischemic ventricular tachycardia. Ann. Surg., *198*:119, 1983.)

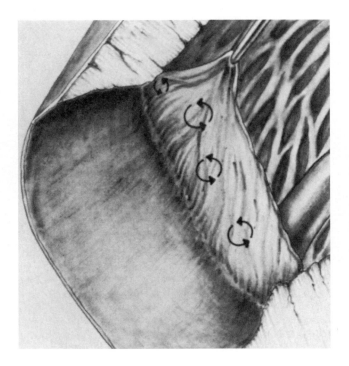

**FIGURE 55–25.** Diagrammatic sketch of an extended endocardial resection procedure (EERP) in an anterior left ventricular aneurysm. The principle involved in this procedure is the same as that for a localized ERP (Fig. 51–24*D*), but in this procedure all of the endocardial fibrosis associated with the aneurysm is resected except that involving the papillary muscles. (From Cox, J. L.: Surgical treatment of ischemic and nonischemic ventricular tachy arrhythmias. *In* Cohn, L. H. [ed]: Modern Technics in Surgery. Mount Kisco, NY, Futura Publishing, 1985.)

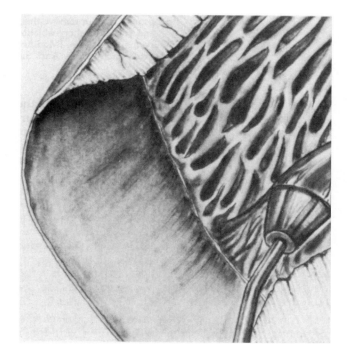

FIGURE 55–26. After all of the endocardial scar is resected as a preliminary measure, endocardial cryolesions are placed at the site or sites of origin of the ventricular tachycardia as determined by intraoperative mapping. In addition, any remaining scar on the papillary muscle is cryoablated. (From Cox, J. L.: Surgical treatment of ischemic and nonischemic ventricular tachyarrhythmias. *In* Cohn, L. H. [ed]: Modern Technics in Surgery. Mount Kisco, NY, Futura Publishing, 1985.)

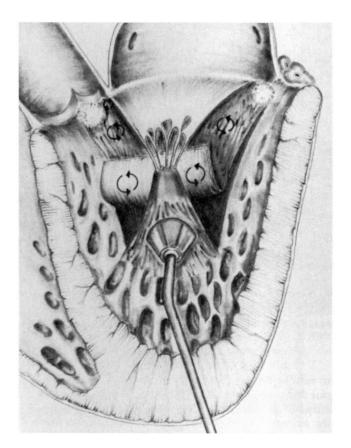

FIGURE 55–27. Extended endocardial resection of the fibrosis associated with a posterior myocardial infarction or aneurysm and cryoablation of the lower two-thirds of the posterior papillary muscle. The endocardial fibrosis is resected to within 5 mm of the aortic and mitral valve annuli. Because the site of origin of ventricular tachycardia is frequently adjacent to the junction of the aortic and mitral valve annuli, endocardial cryolesions (*white circles*) are applied at the base of the aortic and mitral valve annuli to ablate any reentrant circuits that might reside in the remaining endocardial fibrosis immediately beneath the valve annuli. In addition, endocardial cryolesions are applied to the site or sites of origin of ventricular tachycardia as determined by intraoperative mapping, but only after all endocardial scar is removed. (From Cox, J. L.: Surgical treatment of ischemic and nonischemic ventricular tachyarrhythmias. *In* Cohn, L. H. [ed]: Modern Technics in Surgery. Mount Kisco, NY, Futura Publishing, 1985.)

sequent papillary muscle dysfunction. This experience would argue strongly against the practice of resecting papillary muscles for VT, as has been reported in the past (Moran et al., 1983).

Once the author's group has completed the extended endocardial resection and subsequent endocardial cryoablation, programmed electrical stimulation is applied in an attempt to reinduce the arrhythmia. If VT is inducible, it is again mapped and the remaining arrhythmogenic myocardium is cryoablated. If the arrhythmia is no longer inducible, the author's group feels confident that it has been permanently ablated. If other procedures are to be performed, such as coronary bypass grafting, they are carried out with the patient under cardioplegic arrest. However, it is important to note that cardioplegia is absolutely not administered until the author's group is satisfied that the VT has been ablated. The reason for this strict approach is that the cardioplegia itself may temporarily alter the delicate reentry circuits causing the tachycardia. Consequently, if the antitachycardia procedure is performed under cardioplegic arrest, it is impossible to determine intraoperatively whether the surgical procedure has ablated the arrhythmia. This point is often ignored when the factors that predispose to postoperative recurrences are considered, and it emphasizes the importance of the manner in which the operative procedure is conducted. The author's group believes that the practice of performing VT surgery under cardioplegic arrest is the major reason for the high reinducibility rates at the time of the postoperative electrophysiology study reported in most series.

Selle and Svenson have reported promising results using the Nd-YAG laser to ablate arrhythmogenic myocardium following endocardial mapping (Selle et al., 1986; Svenson et al., 1987). A major advantage of this technique is not only that it is easy and quick to perform but that it can also be applied in the normothermic beating heart. As described previously, this allows immediate reapplication of programmed stimulation to determine the efficacy of the procedure without the introduction of any intervening variables. Therefore, it is not surprising that the patients have had no spontaneous or reinducible VT postoperatively.

### Role of ICD Devices

Although various operative techniques have proved to be reasonably effective for the control of ischemic VT, the cumulative experience of the past several years indicates that high operative mortality rates and postoperative reinducibility rates have persisted (Cox, 1989; Miller et al., 1984a, 1984b, 1985).

Because the postoperative reinducibility rate of VT is excessive, some authors have recommended the routine placement of ICD patches at surgery so that, if the arrhythmia is reinducible at the time of the postoperative electrophysiology study, an ICD unit can be implanted without the need for another thoracotomy (Platia et al., 1986). Others have suggested

that because the operative mortality rate for VT surgery is so high, perhaps the map-guided (and nonguided) direct surgical procedures should be abandoned altogether in favor of simple coronary artery bypass grafting and routine implantation of an ICD device (Fonger et al., 1987).

Although both of these suggestions may have some merit, they are based on the assumption that neither the operative mortality rate associated with direct surgical procedures nor the postoperative reinducibility rate can be decreased to acceptable levels. Paradoxically, this assumption overlooks the potential importance of the ICD device in decreasing the operative mortality rate associated with the direct surgical procedures as they are now performed. One of the major reasons for the high operative mortality rate in the past was the lack of a viable therapeutic option in patients with medically refractory VT who had left ventricular dysfunction so severe that there was little hope of their surviving an operation (Cox, 1989). Despite the obvious risk in such patients, if antiarrhythmic drugs were ineffective, there was little choice but to proceed with operation. The results in such patients were considerably different from those attained in patients with more reasonable left ventricular function. ICD devices now provide the previously missing therapeutic option for patients with medically refractory VT who are not surgical candidates. By virtue of the fact that these patients who are prohibitively high operative risks are no longer subjected to surgical treatment, the previous high operative mortality rate for VT surgery is now of historical interest only.

### Role of Intraoperative Mapping

The postoperative reinducibility rate has also been decreased by the increasing availability of multipoint intraoperative mapping systems and by the avoidance of cardioplegic arrest or other variables that prevent the accurate intraoperative assessment of the efficacy of the specific surgical procedure in curing VT (Cox, 1989). Performing an endocardial resection for VT without mapping is analogous to performing coronary artery bypass surgery for angina pectoris without angiography. Approximately 50% of patients with VT can be cured by such "blind" resections (Swerdlow et al., 1986), and it is reasonable to expect that a similar cure rate for angina pectoris could be accomplished by simply bypassing all coronary arteries in every patient. However, if one expects to accomplish optimal cure rates for either condition, the abnormality must be more precisely defined. The cure rates for map-guided VT surgery in some series now exceeds 90% (Ostermeyer et al., 1987; Svenson et al., 1987), an indication that "blind" surgical procedures for this life-threatening arrhythmia should be abandoned except in unusual or emergency situations.

In that multipoint mapping systems are not yet available in all institutions and patients with refractory VT are frequently incapable of being transferred to centers that have them, surgeons must continue to be concerned with how patients are to be selected for VT surgery, which surgical technique should be employed, and how the surgical procedure should be conducted. In the absence of other indications for surgery, the decision regarding surgical intervention for VT should be made only after the patient has failed all medical therapy except amiodarone. Amiodarone therapy is initiated, and an assessment is made of the operative risks and of the likelihood of surgical success. In practical terms, this assessment is based primarily on the status of the patient's left ventricular function, but the morphologic type of tachycardia must also be considered.

If the patient's left ventricular function is considered to be compatible with a reasonable surgical risk, a surgical course should be pursued at this point; but if the ventricular dysfunction poses a prohibitive operative risk, amiodarone therapy should be initiated. The subsequent treatment plan for the latter group of patients is discussed later in this chapter.

Once the decision has been made to pursue surgical therapy, the choices outlined in Figure 55–28 are made at various steps in the procedure. The importance of performing intraoperative mapping and of avoiding cardioplegic arrest is apparent, as this is the only combination that will allow the surgeon to perform *programmed electrical stimulation* (PES) to assess the efficacy of the surgical technique intraoperatively. If such a map-guided procedure is performed in the normothermic beating heart and, on completion, VT cannot be induced, the likelihood of inducing the arrhythmia 7 to 10 days later during the postoperative electrophysiologic study is less than 5% in the author's group's experience. The lack of inducibility

at the time of the postoperative study portends a much better prognosis on long-term follow-up, as noninducible patients are less likely to develop spontaneous recurrence of VT (Kienzle et al., 1983; Swerdlow et al., 1986). In addition, if the tachycardia is noninducible postoperatively, there is no need for further medical therapy.

If nonguided surgery is performed, ICD patches should be placed at the completion of the procedure because of the likelihood that VT will be inducible at the time of the postoperative electrophysiology study (Cox, 1989). If the arrhythmia is inducible, an ICD unit can then be connected to the patches without the need for another thoracotomy. If tachycardia is not inducible, it is not necessary to insert an ICD device unless the patient has a spontaneous recurrence at a later date. Likewise, if map-guided surgery is performed under cardioplegic arrest, PES after completion of the procedure is ineffective in determining whether or not the surgery has ablated the VT, as evidenced by the 30% reinducibility rate postoperatively. The lack of inducibility intraoperatively after completion of the procedure in patients who have inducible tachycardia 7 to 10 days later indicates that even though the surgical procedure was guided by intraoperative mapping, the site of arrhythmogenesis was not ablated. It is reasonable to conclude that the arrhythmia could not be reinduced by PES intraoperatively following the surgical procedure because the cardioplegia temporarily suppressed the offending re-entrant circuit and it had "recovered" by the time of the postoperative study. Thus, if VT surgery is performed under cardioplegic arrest, even though it

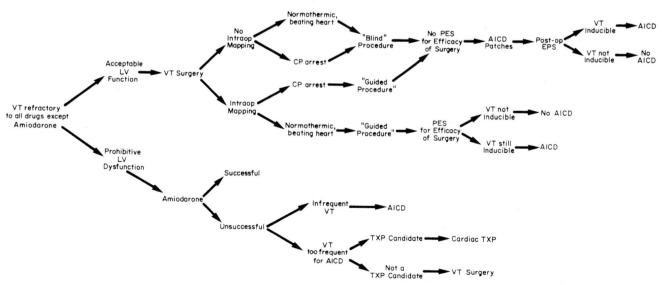

**FIGURE 55–28.** Algorithm for the selection and treatment of patients with ischemic ventricular tachycardia (VT) that is refractory to all antitachycardia drugs except amiodarone. The decision regarding surgery or amiodarone is made at this point because of the increased risk of surgery in patients who are taking amiodarone. See text for further details. (CP = cardioplegic; PES = programmed electrical stimulation; AICD = automatic internal cardioverter-defibrillator; EPS = electrophysiology study; TXP = transplantation.) (From Cox, J. L.: Patient selection criteria and results of surgery for refractory ischemic ventricular tachycardia. Circulation, 79[Suppl. 1]:1163–1177, 1989.)

is map-guided, ICD patches should be placed at the end of the procedure so that an ICD device can be implanted in the 30% of patients who continue to have inducible tachycardia at the time of the postoperative electrophysiology study (Cox, 1989).

As mentioned above, the initial decision to treat ventricular tachycardia with amiodarone should be based primarily on the fact that the patient's left ventricular dysfunction represents a prohibitive operative risk. If amiodarone is unsuccessful in controlling the tachycardia, as is frequently the case (Fogoros et al., 1983; Rasmussen et al., 1982), the next logical step would be to implant an ICD device. However, if the patient has frequent episodes of tachycardia despite amiodarone therapy, the ICD device may not be a viable option because the present units are capable of delivering only 150 total discharges before requiring replacement. In addition, the experience of receiving electrical cardioversions on a frequent basis is not a pleasant one. If such patients are candidates, they should be considered for cardiac transplantation. However, if they are not transplant candidates, there is no alternative but to subject them to ventricular tachycardia surgery. It is this group of patients—who have already been deemed inoperable, have failed Amiodarone therapy, experience tachycardia episodes so frequently that ICDs are of little value, and are not cardiac transplant candidates—that accounts for the inordinately high operative mortality rate associated with ventricular tachycardia surgery. Thus, by keeping this group to a minimum by such measures as earlier surgical intervention, the previous high operative mortality rate reported for ventricular tachycardia has been dramatically decreased.

### Methods of Left Ventricular Aneurysm Repair

During the past few years, two entirely new surgical techniques have been developed for the surgical resection and *repair* of left ventricular aneurysms (Dor et al., 1989; Jatene, 1985). Both of these techniques attempt to restore the normal contour of the left ventricle, eliminate the adverse effects of the septal component of the aneurysm, and realign the myofibrils of the left ventricular free wall to restore their optimal contractile function. The *functional* improvement of the left ventricle following either of these two procedures has been dramatic and remarkable when compared to the old technique of simply resecting the aneurysm and closing the ventricle. Of great interest is the unexpected observation that both of these procedures appear to cure ventricular tachyarrhythmias associated with the aneurysm. The surgical results include an operative mortality rate of 2 to 3% (comparable to that of ICDs), even in higher-risk patients, and a ventricular tachycardia cure rate of approximately 98%. The reason that the operative mortality rate is so much lower, even in higher-risk patients, is threefold: For the first time, a major and immediate improvement in left ventricular function can be attained; the residual postoperative detrimental effects of septal aneurysmal involvement are eliminated; and

CPB time is reduced substantially because the procedures are not only quick and relatively easy to perform, but they require no intraoperative mapping. Because these techniques apparently can eliminate ventricular tachycardia and restore cardiac function with operative mortality and recurrence rates comparable to those attained with ICDs, it is expected that the window of indications for the surgical treatment of VT may again broaden.

## SELECTED BIBLIOGRAPHY

Boineau, J. P., and Cox, J. L.: Slow ventricular activation in acute myocardial infarction. A source of reentrant premature ventricular contractions. Circulation, 48:702, 1973.

This paper is the first to document experimentally that ventricular arrhythmias following a myocardial infarction occur on the basis of a reentrant mechanism.

Cobb, F. R., Blumenschein, S. D., Sealy, W. C., et al.: Successful surgical interruption of the bundle of Kent in a patient with Wolff-Parkinson-White syndrome. Circulation, 38:1018, 1968.

This is the first description of the successful surgical treatment of the Wolff-Parkinson-White syndrome. Although current surgical techniques differ significantly from those described in this original article, this paper represents a milestone in the surgical treatment of cardiac arrhythmias.

Cox, J. L.: Anatomic-electrophysiologic basis for the surgical treatment of refractory ischemic ventricular tachycardia. Ann. Surg., 198:119, 1983.

This article describes the anatomic abnormalities underlying the electrophysiologic derangements that are believed to be responsible for refractory ischemic ventricular tachycardia. The article also describes the rationale for each of the direct surgical procedures used to treat ischemic ventricular tachycardia.

Cox, J. L.: Patient selection criteria and results of surgery from refractory ischemic ventricular tachycardia. Circulation, 79(Suppl. 1):1163, 1989.

This is a comprehensive review of the first ten years' experience with the direct surgical procedures for refractory ischemic ventricular tachycardia. The surgical results are analyzed in detail and the roles of intraoperative mapping, surgical technique, and the automatic internal cardioverter-defibrillator are discussed. An algorithm is then presented for the treatment of these arrhythmias based on the accumulated clinical experience.

Cox, J. L., Boineau, J. P., Schuessler, R. B., et al.: Five-year experience with the maze procedure for atrial fibrillation. Ann. Thorac. Surg., 56:814, 1993.

This paper reports the clinical results and five-year follow-up of the surgical procedure developed to treat atrial fibrillation.

Cox, J. L., McLaughlin, V. W., Flowers, N. C., and Horan, L. G.: The ischemic zone surrounding acute myocardiinfarction. Its morphology as detected by dehydrogenase staining. Am. Heart J., 76:650, 1968.

This is the first anatomic documentation and characterization of the ischemic zone surrounding an acute myocardial infarction. It is believed that most ischemic ventricular tachyarrhythmias originate in this periinfarct zone of heterogeneous tissue injury.

Cox, J. L., Schuessler, R. B., and Boineau, J. P.: The surgical treatment of atrial fibrillation. I: Summary of the current concepts of the mechanisms of atrial flutter and atrial fibrillation. J. Thorac. Cardiovasc. Surg., 101:402, 1991.

Cox, J. L., Canavan, T. E., Schuessler, R. B., et al.: The surgical treatment of atrial fibrillation. II: Intraoperative electrophysiologic mapping and description of the electrophysiologic basis of atrial flutter and atrial fibrillation. J. Thorac. Cardiovasc. Surg., 101:406, 1991.

Cox, J. L., Schuessler, R. B., D'Agostino, H. J., Jr., Stone, C. M., et al.: The surgical treatment of atrial fibrillation. III: Development of a definite surgical procedure., J. Thorac. Cardiovasc. Surg., 101:569, 1991.

Cox, J. L.: The surgical treatment of atrial fibrillation. IV: Surgical technique. J. Thorac. Cardiovasc. Surg., 101:584, 1991.

These four sequential papers describe the electrophysiologic basis of atrial flutter and fibrillation and the surgical technique developed to treat these arrhythmias.

# BIBLIOGRAPHY

Abbott, J. A., Scheinman, M. M., Morady, F., et al.: Coexistent Mahaim and Kent accessory connections: Diagnostic and therapeutic implications. J. Am. Coll. Cardiol., 10:364, 1987.

Anderson, R. H., and Becker, A. E.: Anatomy of conducting tissue revisited. Br. Heart J., 40(Suppl.):2, 1978.

Anderson, R. H., and Becker, A. E.: Cardiac anatomy for the surgeon. In Danielson, G. K. (ed): Lewis' Practice of Surgery. Chap. 16. Hagerstown, MD, Harper & Row, 1979.

Anderson, R. H., and Becker, A. E.: Morphology of the human atrioventricular junction area. In Wellens, H. J. J., Lie, K. I., Janse, M. J., et al. (eds): Conduction System of the Heart: Structure, Function and Clinical Implications. Philadelphia, Lea & Febiger, 1976, p. 264.

Aschoff, K. A. L.: A discussion on some aspects of heart-block. Br. Med. J., 2:1103, 1906.

Benson, D. W., Jr., and Cox, J. L.: Surgical treatment of cardiac arrhythmias. In Roberts, N. K., and Gelband, H. (eds): Cardiac Arrhythmias in the Neonate, Infant and Child. 2nd ed. New York, Appleton-Century Crofts, 1982, pp. 341–366.

Bhandari, A. K., Scheinman, M. M., Morady, F., et al.: Efficacy of left cardiac sympathectomy in the treatment of patients with the long QT syndrome. Circulation, 70:1018, 1984.

Boineau, J. P., and Cox, J. L.: Rationale for a direct surgical approach to control ventricular arrhythmias. Am. J. Cardiol., 49:381, 1982.

Boineau, J. P., and Cox, J. L.: Slow ventricular activation in acute myocardial infarction. A source of reentrant premature ventricular contractions. Circulation, 48:702, 1973.

Boineau, J. P., Mooney, C., Hudson, R., et al.: Observations on reentrant excitation pathways and refractory period distribution in spontaneous and experimental atrial flutter in the dog. In Kulbertus, H. E. (ed): Reentrant Arrhythmias. Baltimore, MD, University Park Press, 1977, pp. 79–98.

Boston Area Anticoagulation Trial in Atrial Fibrillation Investigators: The effect of low-dose warfarin on the risk of stroke in patients with nonrheumatic atrial fibrillation. N. Engl. J. Med., 323:1505, 1990.

Burchell, H. B., Frye, R. L., Anderson, M. W., et al.: Atrial-ventricular and ventricular-atrial excitation in Wolff-Parkinson-White syndrome (type B): Temporary ablation at surgery. Circulation, 36:663, 1967.

Cameron, A., Schwartz, M. J., Kronmal, R. A., and Kosinski, A. S.: Prevalence and significance of atrial fibrillation in coronary artery disease (CASS Registry). Am. J. Cardiol., 61:714, 1988.

Canavan, T. E., Schuessler, R. B., Boineau, J. P., et al.: Computerized global electrophysiological mapping of the atrium in patients with Wolff-Parkinson-White syndrome. Ann. Thorac. Surg., 46:223, 1988a.

Canavan, T. E., Schuessler, R. B., Cain, M. E., et al.: Computerized global electrophysiological mapping of the atrium in a patient with multiple supraventricular tachyarrhythmias. Ann. Thorac. Surg., 46:232, 1988b.

Cobb, F. R., Blumenschein, S. D., Sealy, W. C., et al.: Successful surgical interruption of the bundle of Kent in a patient with Wolff-Parkinson-White syndrome. Circulation, 38:1018, 1968.

Cobler, J. L., Williams, M. E., and Greenland, P.: Thyrotoxicosis in institutionalized elderly patients with atrial fibrillation. Arch. Intern. Med., 144:1758, 1984.

Couch, O. A., Jr.: Cardiac aneurysm with ventricular tachycardia and subsequent excision of aneurysm. Circulation, 20:251, 1959.

Coumel, P., Cabrol, C., Fabiato, A., et al.: Tachycardie permanente par rythme réciproque. Arch. Mal. Coeur, 60:1830, 1967.

Cox, J. L.: Anatomic-electrophysiologic basis for the surgical treatment of refractory ischemic ventricular tachycardia. Ann. Surg., 198:119, 1983a.

Cox, J. L.: Discussion of Defauw, J. J. A. M. T., Guiraudon, G. M., van Hemel, N. M., et al.: Surgical therapy of paroxysmal atrial

fibrillation with the "Corridor" operation. Ann. Thorac. Surg., 53:571, 1992a.

Cox, J. L.: Evolving applications of the maze procedure for atrial fibrillation [Invited Editorial]. Ann. Thorac. Surg., 55:578, 1993.

Cox, J. L.: Manuscript reviewer's comment. J. Thorac. Cardiovasc. Surg., 92:411, 1986.

Cox, J. L.: Patient selection criteria and results of surgery from refractory ischemic ventricular tachycardia. Circulation, 79(Suppl. 1):I163, 1989.

Cox, J. L.: The surgical treatment of atrial fibrillation. IV: Surgical technique. J. Thorac. Cardiovasc. Surg., 101:584, 1991.

Cox, J. L.: Surgical treatment of atrial fibrillation [Letter Reply]. J. Thorac. Cardiovasc. Surg., 104:1492, 1992b.

Cox, J. L.: Surgery for cardiac arrhythmias. Curr. Probl. Cardiol., 8(4):1, 1983b.

Cox, J. L., Bardy, G. H., Damiano, R. J., et al.: Right ventricular isolation procedures for nonischemic ventricular tachycardia. J. Thorac. Cardiovasc. Surg., 90:212, 1985a.

Cox, J. L., Boineau, J. P., Scheussler, R. B., et al.: Five-year experience with the maze procedure for atrial fibrillation. Ann. Thorac. Surg., 56:814, 1993.

Cox, J. L., Boineau, J. P., Schuessler, R. B., et al.: Successful surgical treatment of atrial fibrillation. J. A. M. A., 266:1976, 1991a.

Cox, J. L., Canavan, T. E., Schuessler, R. B., et al.: The surgical treatment of atrial fibrillation. II: Intraoperative electrophysiologic mapping and description of the electrophysiologic basis of atrial flutter and atrial fibrillation. J. Thorac. Cardiovasc. Surg., 101:406, 1991b.

Cox, J. L., Daniel, T. M., Sabiston, D. C., Jr., and Boineau, J.P.: Desynchronized activation in myocardial infarction—A reentry basis for ventricular arrhythmias [Abstract]. Circulation, 39(Suppl. 3):63, 1969.

Cox, J. L., Gallagher, J. J., and Cain, M. E.: Experience with 118 consecutive patients undergoing surgery for the Wolff-Parkinson-White syndrome. J. Thorac. Cardiovasc. Surg., 90:490, 1985b.

Cox, J. L., Gallagher, J. J., and Ungerleider, R. M.: Encircling endocardial ventriculotomy (EEV) for refractory ischemic ventricular tachycardia. IV: Clinical indications, surgical technique, mechanism of action, and results. J. Thorac. Cardiovasc. Surg., 83:865, 1982.

Cox, J. L., Holman, W. L., and Cain, M. E.: Cryosurgical treatment of atrioventricular node reentry tachycardia. Circulation, 76:1329, 1987.

Cox, J. L., McLaughlin, V. W., Flowers, N. C., and Horan, L. G.: The ischemic zone surrounding acute myocardial infarction. Its morphology as detected by dehydrogenase staining. Am. Heart J., 76:650, 1968.

Cox, J. L., Schuessler, R. B., and Boineau, J. P.: The surgical treatment of atrial fibrillation. I: Summary of the current concepts of the mechanisms of atrial flutter and atrial fibrillation. J. Thorac. Cardiovasc. Surg., 101:402, 1991c.

Cox, J. L., Schuessler, R. B., D'Agostino, H. J., Jr., et al.: The surgical treatment of atrial fibrillation. III: Development of a definite surgical procedure. J. Thorac. Cardiovasc. Surg., 101:569, 1991d.

D'Agostino, H. J., Jr., Harada, A., Schuessler, R. B., et al.: Global epicardial mapping of atrial fibrillation in a canine model of chronic mitral regurgitation. Circulation, 76(Suppl. IV):IV-165, 1987.

Daniel, T. M., Cox, J. L., Sabiston, D. C., Jr., and Boineau, J. P.: Epicardial and intramural mapping activation of the human heart. A technique for localizing infarction and ischemia of the myocardium [Abstract]. Circulation, 40(Suppl. III):III-66, 1969.

Dessertenne, F.: La tachycardie ventriculaire à deux foyers opposés variables. Arch. Mal. Coeur, 59:263, 1966.

Diamantopoulos, E. J., Anthopoulos, L., Nanas, S., et al.: Detection of arrhythmias in a representative sample of the Athens population. Eur. Heart J., 8(Suppl. D):17, 1987.

Dor, V., Saab, M., Coste, P., et al.: Left ventricular aneurysm: A new surgical approach. Thorac. Cardiovasc. Surg., 37:11, 1989.

Draper, M. H., and Weidmann, S.: Cardiac resting and action potentials recorded with an intracellular electrode. J. Physiol., 115:74, 1957.

Durrer, D., and Roos, J. P.: Epicardial excitation of the ventricles in a patient with Wolff-Parkinson-White syndrome (type B): Temporary ablation at surgery. Circulation, 35:15, 1967.

Durrer, D., Schoo, L., Schuilenburg, R. M., and Wellens, H. J. J.: The role of premature beats in the initiation and the termination of supraventricular tachycardia in the Wolff-Parkinson-White syndrome. Circulation, 36:644, 1967.

Durrer, D., van Dam, R. T., Freud, G. E., and Janse, M. J.: Reentry and ventricular arrhythmias in local ischemia and infarction of the intact dog heart. Proc. K. Ned. Akad. Wet. (Biol. Med.), 74:321, 1971.

El-Sherif, N., Scherlag, B. J., Lazzara, R., and Hopen, R. R.: Reentrant ventricular arrhythmias in the late myocardial infarction period. I: Conduction characteristics of the infarction zone. Circulation, 55:686, 1977.

Fogoros, R. N., Anderson, K. P., Winkle, R. A., et al.: Amiodarone: Clinical efficacy and toxicity in 96 patients with recurrent, drug-refractory arrhythmias. Circulation, 68:88, 1983.

Fonger, J. D., Guarnieri, T., Griffith, L. S. C., et al.: Impending sudden cardiac death: Treatment with myocardial revascularization and automatic implantable cardioverter defibrillator. Presented at the Twenty-third Annual Meeting of the Society of Thoracic Surgeons, Toronto, Ontario, Canada, September 22, 1987.

Fontaine, G., Frank, R., and Guiraudon, G.: Surgical treatment of resistant reentrant ventricular tachycardia by ventriculotomy: A new application of epicardial mapping [Abstract]. Circulation, 50(Suppl. III):III-182, 1974.

Fontaine, G., Guiraudon, G., and Frank, R.: Management of chronic ventricular tachycardia. In Narula, O. S. (ed): Innovations in Diagnosis and Management of Cardiac Arrhythmias. Baltimore, Williams & Wilkins, 1979.

Fraser, G. R., and Froggatt, P.: Unexpected cot deaths. Lancet, 2:56, 1966.

Fujimara, O., Guiraudon, G. M., Yee, R., et al.: Operative therapy of atrioventricular node reentry and results of an anatomically guided procedure. Am. J. Cardiol., 64:1327, 1989.

Gallagher, J. J., Cox, J. L., German, L. D., and Kasell, J. H.: Nonpharmacologic treatment of supraventricular tachycardia. In Josephson, M. E., and Wellens, H. J. J. (eds): Tachycardias: Mechanisms, Diagnosis, and Treatment. Philadelphia, Lea & Febiger, 1984a, pp. 271–285.

Gallagher, J. J., Oldham, H. N., Jr., Wallace, A. G., et al.: Ventricular aneurysm with ventricular tachycardia. Report of a case with epicardial mapping and successful resection. Am. J. Cardiol., 35:696, 1975.

Gallagher, J. J., Sealy, W. C., Cox, J. L., et al.: Results of surgery for preexcitation caused by accessory atrioventricular pathways in 267 consecutive cases. In Josephson, M. E., and Wellens, H. J. J. (eds): Tachycardias: Mechanisms, Diagnosis, and Treatment. Philadelphia, Lea & Febiger, 1984b, pp. 259–269.

Gaskell, W. H.: On the innervation of the heart, with especial reference to the heart of the tortoise. J. Physiol., 4:43, 1883.

Guiraudon, G. M., Campbell, C. S., Jones, D. L., et al.: Combined sinoatrial node–atrioventricular node isolation: A surgical alternative to His' bundle ablation in patients with atrial fibrillation. Circulation, 72(Suppl. 3):220, 1985.

Guiraudon, G., Fontaine, G., Frank, R., et al.: Encircling endocardial ventriculotomy: A new surgical treatment of life-threatening ventricular tachycardias resistant to medical treatment following myocardial infarction. Ann. Thorac. Surg., 26:438, 1978.

Guiraudon, G. M., Klein, G. J., Sharma, A. D., et al.: Closed-heart technique for Wolff-Parkinson-White syndrome: Further experience and potential limitations. Ann. Thorac. Surg., 42:651, 1986a.

Guiraudon, G. M., Klein, G. J., Sharma, A. D., et al.: Surgical ablation of posterior septal accessory pathways in the Wolff-Parkinson-White syndrome by a closed heart technique. J. Thorac. Cardiovasc. Surg., 92:406, 1986b.

Han, J., Gael, B. G., and Hansen, C. S.: Reentrant beats induced in the ventricle during coronary occlusion. Am. Heart J., 80:778, 1970.

Harada, A., D'Agostino, H. J., Jr., Boineau, J. P., and Cox, J. L.: Right atrial isolation: A new surgical treatment for supraventricular tachycardia. I. Surgical technique and electrophysiologic effects. J. Thorac. Cardiovasc. Surg., 95:643, 1988a.

Harada, A., D'Agostino, H. J., Jr., Boineau, J. P., and Cox, J. L.: Right atrial isolation: A new surgical treatment for supraventricular tachycardia. II. Hemodynamic effects. J. Thorac. Cardiovasc. Surg., 95:651, 1988b.

Harada, A., Tweddell, J., Schuessler, R. B., et al.: Computerized potential distribution mapping: A new intraoperative mapping technique for ventricular tachycardia surgery. Ann. Thorac. Surg., 49:649, 1990.

Hirosawa, K., Sekiguchi, M., Kasanuki, H., et al.: Natural history of atrial fibrillation. Heart Vessels, (Suppl.) 2:14, 1987.

Jackman, W. M., Wang, X. Z., Friday, K. J., et al.: Catheter ablation of accessory atrioventricular pathways (Wolff-Parkinson-White syndrome) by radio frequency current. N. Engl. J. Med., 324:1605, 1991.

James, T. N., Froggatt, P., Atkinson, W. J., Jr., et al.: De subitaneis mortibus. XXX. Observations on the pathophysiology of the long QT syndromes with special reference to the neuropathology of the heart. Circulation, 57:1221, 1978.

Jatene, A. D.: Left ventricular aneurysmectomy: Resection or reconstruction? J. Thorac. Cardiovasc. Surg., 89:321, 1985.

Jervell, A., and Lange-Nielsen, F.: Congenital deaf-mutism, functional heart disease with prolongation of the Q-T interval, and sudden death. Am. Heart J., 54:59, 1957.

Josephson, M. E., Harken, A. H., and Horowitz, L. N.: Endocardial excision—A new surgical technique for the treatment of recurrent ventricular tachycardia. Circulation, 60:1430, 1979.

Kaiser, G. A., Waldo, A. L., Harris, P. D., et al.: New method to delineate myocardial damage at surgery. Circulation, 39(Suppl.):83, 1969.

Katz, A. M.: The arrhythmias. II: Abnormal impulse formation and reentry, premature systoles, preexcitation. In Katz, A. M. (ed): Physiology of the Heart. New York, Raven Press, 1977a.

Kent, A. F. S.: Researches on structure and function of mammalian heart. J. Physiol., 14:233, 1893.

Kienzle, M. G., Doherty, J. U., Roy, D., et al.: Subendocardial resection for refractory ventricular tachycardia: Effects on ambulatory electrocardiogram, programmed stimulation and ejection fraction, and relation to outcome. J. Am. Coll. Cardiol., 2:853, 1983.

Klein, G. J., Guiraudon, G. M., Kerr, C. R., et al.: "Nodoventricular" accessory pathway: Evidence for a distinct accessory atrioventricular pathway with atrioventricular node-like properties., J. Am. Coll. Cardiol., 11:1035, 1988.

Klein, G. J., Guiraudon, G. M., Perkins, D. G., et al.: Surgical correction of the Wolff-Parkinson-White syndrome in the closed heart using cryosurgery: A simplified approach. J. Am. Coll. Cardiol., 3:405, 1984.

Krafchek, J., Lawrei, G. M., Roberts, R., et al.: Surgical ablation of ventricular tachycardia: Improved results with a map-directed regional approach. Circulation, 73:1239, 1986a.

Krafchek, J., Lawrie, G. M., and Wyndham, C. R.: Cryoablation of arrhythmias from the interventricular septum: Initial experience with a new biventricular approach. J. Thorac. Cardiovasc. Surg., 91:419, 1986b.

Kramer, J. B., Corr, P. B., Cox, J. L., et al.: Arrhythmia and conduction disturbances: Simultaneous computer mapping to facilitate intraoperative localization of accessory pathways in patients with Wolff-Parkinson-White syndrome. Am. J. Cardiol., 56:571, 1985.

Krikler, D. M., and Curry, P. V. L.: Torsades de pointes: An atypical ventricular tachycardia. Br. Heart J., 38:117, 1976.

Kulbertus, H. E.: The arrhythmogenic effects of antiarrhythmic agents. In Befeler, B. (ed): Selected Topics in Cardiac Arrhythmias. Mount Kisco, NY, Futura, 1980, p. 113.

Kulbertus, H. E.: La torsades de pointes. Rev. Med. Liege, 33:63, 1978.

Lee, M. A., Morady, F., Kadish, A., et al.: Catheter modification of the atrioventricular junction with radiofrequency energy for control of atrioventricular nodal reentry. Circulation, 83:827, 1991.

Lev, M., Liberthson, R. R., Joseph, R. H., et al.: The pathologic anatomy of Ebstein's disease. Arch. Pathol., 90:334, 1970.

Lewis, T.: The experimental production of paroxysmal tachycardia and the effects of ligation of the coronary arteries. Heart, 1:98, 1909.

Malliani, A., Schwartz, P. J., and Zanchetti, A.: Neural mechanisms and life-threatening arrhythmias. Am. Heart J., *100*:705, 1980.

Martin, A., Benbow, L. J., Butrous, G. S., et al.: Five-year follow-up of 101 elderly subjects by means of long-term ambulatory cardiac monitoring. Eur. Heart J., 5:592, 1984.

McAllister, R. E., Noble, D., and Tsien, R. W.: Reconstruction of the electrical activity of cardiac Purkinje fibers. J. Physiol., *251*:1, 1975.

Miller, J. M., Kienzle, M. G., Harken, A. H., and Josephson, M. E.: Morphologically distinct sustained ventricular tachycardias in coronary artery disease: Significance and surgical results. J. Am. Coll. Cardiol., 4:1073, 1984a.

Miller, J. M., Kienzle, M. G., Harken, A. H., and Josephson, M. E.: Subendocardial resection for ventricular tachycardia: Predictors of surgical success. Circulation, 70:624, 1984b.

Miller, J. M., Marchlinski, F. E., Harken, A. H., et al.: Subendocardial resection for sustained ventricular tachycardia in the early period after acute myocardial infarction. Am. J. Cardiol., 55:980 1985.

Mines, G. R.: On circulating excitations in heart muscle and their possible relation to tachycardia and fibrillation. Trans. R. Soc. Can., 8:43, 1914.

Mirowski, M.: The automatic implantable cardioverter-defibrillator: An overview. J. Am. Coll. Cardiol., 6:461, 1985.

Moran, J. M., Kehoe, R. F., Loeb, J. M., et al.: Extended endocardial resection for the treatment of ventricular tachycardia and ventricular fibrillation. Ann. Thorac. Surg., 34:538, 1982.

Moran, J. M., Kehoe, R. F., Loeb, J. M., et al.: The role of papillary muscle resection and mitral valve replacement in the control of refractory ventricular arrhythmia. Circulation, 68:154, 1983.

Moss, A. J., and McDonald, J.: Unilateral cervicothoracic sympathetic ganglionectomy for the treatment of long Q-T interval syndrome. N. Engl. J. Med., *285*:903, 1971.

Onundarson, P. T., Thorgeirsson, G., Jonmundsson, E., et al.: Chronic atrial fibrillation. Epidemiologic features and 14-year follow-up: A case control study. Eur. Heart J., 8:521, 1987.

Ostermeyer, J., Borggrefe, M., Breithardt, G., et al.: Direct operations for the management of life-threatening ischemic ventricular tachycardia. J. Thorac. Cardiovasc. Surg., 94:848, 1987.

Ostermeyer, J., Breithardt, G., Borggrefe, M., et al.: Surgical treatment of ventricular tachycardias. Complete versus partial encircling endocardial ventriculotomy. J. Thorac. Cardiovasc. Surg., 87:517, 1984.

Petersen, P., Boysen, G., Godtfredsen, J., et al.: Placebo-controlled, randomized trial of warfarin and aspirin for prevention of thromboembolic complications in chronic atrial fibrillation: The Copenhagen AFASAK study. Lancet, 1:175, 1989.

Platia, E. V., Griffith, L. S., Watkins, L., Jr., et al.: Treatment of malignant ventricular arrhythmias with endocardial resection and implantation of the automatic cardioverter-defibrillator. N. Engl. J. Med., *314*:213, 1986.

Rasmussen, K., Winkle, R., Ross, D., et al.: Antiarrhythmic efficacy of amiodarone in recurrent ventricular tachycardia evaluated by multiple electrophysiological and ambulatory ECG recordings. Acta Med. Scand., *212*:367, 1982.

Reuter, H.: The dependence of slow inward current in Purkinje fibers on the extracellular calcium concentration. J. Physiol., *192*:479, 1967.

Romano, C., Gemme, G., and Pongiglione, R.: Aritmie cardiacherare dell'eta pediatrica. Clin. Pediatr., 45:656, 1963.

Ross, D. L., Johnson, D. C., Denniss, A. R., et al.: Curative surgery for atrioventricular junctional ("AV nodal") reentrant tachycardia. J. Am. Coll. Cardiol., 6:1383, 1985.

Savage, D. D., Garrison, R. J., Castelli, W. P., et al.: Prevalence of submitral (anular) calcium and its correlates in a general population-based sample (the Framingham study). Am. J. Cardiol., 51:1375, 1983.

Scheinman, M. M., Morady, F., Hess, D. S., and Gonzalez, R.: Catheter-induced ablation of the atrioventricular junction to control refractory supraventricular arrhythmias. J. A. M. A., *248*:851, 1982.

Scherlag, B. J., El-Sherif, N., Hopen, R. R., and Lazzara, R.: Characterization and localization of ventricular arrhythmias resulting from myocardial ischemia and infarction. Circ. Res., 35:372, 1974.

Schwartz, P. J., Periti, M., and Malliani, A.: The long Q-T syndrome. Fund. Clin. Cardiol., 89:378, 1975.

Sealy, W. C.: The Wolff-Parkinson-White syndrome and the beginnings of direct arrhythmia surgery. Ann. Thorac. Surg., 38:176, 1984.

Sealy, W. C., Gallagher, J. J., and Kasell, J. H.: His bundle interruption for control of inappropriate ventricular responses to atrial arrhythmias. Ann. Thorac. Surg., 32:429, 1981.

Selle, J. G., Svenson, R. H., Sealy, W. C., et al.: Successful clinical laser ablation of ventricular tachycardia: A promising new therapeutic method. Ann. Thorac. Surg., 42:380, 1986.

Smith, P. K., Holman, W. L., and Cox, J. L.: Surgical treatment of supraventricular tachyarrhythmias. Surg. Clin. North Am., 65:553., 1985.

Smith, W., and Gallagher, J. J.: Q-T prolongation syndromes. Practical Cardiol., 5:118, 1979.

Strauss, H. C., Prystowsky, E. N., and Scheinman, N. M.: Sinoatrial and atrial electrogenesis. Prog. Cardiovasc. Dis., 19:385, 1977.

Stroke Prevention in Atrial Fibrillation Study Group Investigators: Preliminary report of the Stroke Prevention in Atrial Fibrillation study. N. Engl. J. Med., *322*:863, 1990.

Svenson, R. H., Gallagher, J. J., Selle, J. G., et al.: Neodymium:YAG laser photocoagulation: A successful new map-guided technique for the intraoperative ablation of ventricular tachycardia. Circulation, 76:1319, 1987.

Swerdlow, C. D., Mason, J. W., Stinson, E. B., et al.: Results of operations for ventricular tachycardia in 105 patients. J. Thorac. Cardiovasc. Surg., 92:105, 1986.

Tammaro, A. E., Ronzoni, D., Bonaccorso, O., et al.: Le aritmie nell'anziano. Minerva Med., 74:1313, 1983.

Tchou, P., Lehmann, M. J., Jazayeri, M., and Akhtar, M.: Atriofascicular connection or a nodoventricular Mahaim fiber? Electrophysiologic elucidation of the pathway and associated reentrant circuit. Circulation, 44:837, 1988.

Treseder, A. S., Sastry, B. S., Thomas, T. P., et al.: Atrial fibrillation and stroke in elderly hospitalized patients. Age Aging, 15:89, 1986.

Tweddell, J. S., Branham, B. H., Harada, A., et al.: Potential mapping in septal tachycardia: Evaluation of a new intraoperative mapping technique. Circulation, 80(Suppl. I):I-97, 1989a.

Tweddell, J. S., Branham, B. H., Stone, C. M., et al.: Focal cryoablation guided solely by intraoperative potential mapping ablates ventricular tachycardia of endocardial origin. Surg. Forum, 40:216, 1989b.

Tweddell, J. S., Harada, A., Schuessler, R. B., et al.: Computerized potential distribution mapping for rapid localization of ventricular tachycardia of septal origin. Surg. Forum, 39:257, 1988.

Uhl, H. S.: A previously undescribed malformation of the heart: Almost total absence of the myocardium of the right ventricle. Bull. Johns Hopkins Hosp., 91:197, 1952.

Ungerleider, R. M., Holman, W. L., Calcagno, D., et al.: Encircling endocardial ventriculotomy (EEV) for refractory ischemic ventricular tachycardia. III. Effects on regional left ventricular function. J. Thorac. Cardiovasc. Surg., 83:857, 1982a.

Ungerleider, R. M., Holman, W. L., Stanley, T. E., III, et al.: Encircling endocardial ventriculotomy (EEV) for refractory ischemic ventricular tachycardia. I. Electrophysiologic effects. J. Thorac. Cardiovasc. Surg., 83:840, 1982b.

Ungerleider, R. M., Holman, W. L., Stanley, T. E., III, et al.: Encircling endocardial ventriculotomy (EEV) for refractory ischemic ventricular tachycardia. II. Effects on regional myocardial blood flow. J. Thorac. Cardiovasc. Surg., 83:850, 1982c.

Waldo, A. L., and Kaiser, G. A.: A study of ventricular arrhythmias associated with acute myocardial infarction in the canine heart. Circulation, 47:1222, 1973.

Ward, O. C.: New familial cardiac syndrome in children. J. Ir. Med. Assoc., 54:103, 1964.

Wellens, H. J. J., Duren, D. R., Liem, K., and Lie, K. I.: Effects of digitalis in patients with paroxysmal atrioventricular nodal tachycardia. Circulation, 52:779, 1975.

Williams, J. M., Ungerleider, R. M., Lofland, G. K., and Cox, J. L.: Left atrial isolation: New technique for the treatment of supraventricular arrhythmias. J. Thorac. Cardiovasc. Surg., 80:373, 1980.

Wittig, J. H., and Boineau, J. P.: Surgical treatment of ventricular arrhythmias using epicardial transmural and endocardial mapping. Ann. Thorac. Surg., 20:117, 1975.

Wolferth, C. C., and Wood, F. C.: The mechanism of production of short P-R intervals and prolonged QRS complexes in patients with presumably undamaged hearts: Hypothesis of an accessory pathway of auriculoventricular conduction (bundle of Kent). Am. Heart J., 8:297, 1933.

Wolff, L., Parkinson, J., and White, P. D.: Bundle branch block with short PR interval in healthy young people prone to paroxysmal tachycardia. Am. Heart J., 5:685, 1930.

Wood, F. C., Wolferth, C. C., and Geckler, G. D.: Histologic demonstration of accessory muscular connections between auricle and ventricle in a case of short P-R interval and prolonged QRS complex. Am. Heart J., 25:454, 1943.

Yanowitz, F., Preston, J. B., and Abildskov, J. A.: Functional distribution of right and left stellate innervation to the ventricles. Circ. Res., 18:416, 1966.

Zipes, D. P., and Fisher, J. C.: Effects of agents which inhibit the slow channel on sinus node automaticity and atrioventricular induction in the dog. Circ. Res., 34:184, 1974.

# 56
## Tumors of the Heart

Peter Van Trigt III and David C. Sabiston, Jr.

Primary neoplasms of the heart are rare forms of cardiac disease. These tumors range in clinical presentation from the more common myxoma, which can usually be cured, to the rare cardiac sarcoma, which is associated with a uniformly poor outcome. These tumors are of great interest because of their low incidence and protean clinical manifestations and because the benign form represents a potentially curable form of serious cardiac disease that can be accurately diagnosed by echocardiography.

Cardiac tumors have been recognized since the report by Columbus from Padua in 1562. In 1934, Barnes and associates made the first antemortem clinical diagnosis of a primary sarcoma of the heart by using electrocardiography and biopsy of a metastatic nodule. In 1936, Beck successfully removed an intrapericardial teratoma (Beck, 1942). In 1945, Mahaim published a classic monograph that described 413 tumors of the heart and pericardium. Angiography was first used clinically to show an intracardiac myxoma (Goldberg et al., 1952); and in 1952, Bahnson and Newman (1953) removed a large right atrial myxoma, but the patient died 24 days later. The first successful resection of a left atrial myxoma was performed in 1954 by Crafoord with use of cardiopulmonary bypass (Crafoord, 1955). The myxoma was diagnosed preoperatively by left-sided heart catheterization in a 40-year-old woman who was referred as having an atypical case of mitral stenosis. The tumor was approached by a left thoracotomy and removed under fibrillatory arrest (Chitwood, 1992). The introduction of echocardiography in 1968 provided a noninvasive technique that allowed accurate diagnosis of cardiac neoplasms (Schattenberg, 1968). Before that time, 90% of tumors were diagnosed at autopsy or as an unexpected finding at cardiac operation.

## INCIDENCE

Primary cardiac tumors are rare; the incidence at autopsy is variously reported between 0.002 and 0.3% (Silverman, 1980). These neoplasms are often difficult to diagnose because of their varied clinical presentation. Approximately 75% of primary tumors of the heart are benign, and 50% of those are myxomas (Table 56–1). The approximately 25% of primary cardiac neoplasms that are malignant are almost always a form of sarcoma (Table 56–2). Malignant neoplasms are most common in adults and constitute less than 10% of primary cardiac tumors in children.

Patients with myxomas have the most favorable

prognosis, with a 90% or greater survival rate after resection. The survival for other benign tumors is lower, and survival rate is less than 10% for primary cardiac malignancies. Reports of several large series reviewed the incidence and the clinical characteristics of cardiac neoplasms (Bloor and O'Rourke, 1984; Goldman et al., 1986; Murphy et al., 1990; Poole et al., 1984; Silverman, 1980); the largest collection was reported from the Armed Forces Institute of Pathology (AFIP), which has more than 500 specimens (McAllister and Fenoglio, 1978). Table 56–3 shows clinical characteristics of 102 patients with benign cardiac tumors resected at the Texas Heart Institute, the largest single series of patients with cardiac tumor treated surgically.

## MYXOMA

Myxoma, the most common primary tumor of the heart, constitutes 27% of all tumors and cysts of the heart in the AFIP series. In adults, 50% of all benign cardiac tumors are myxomas. Myxomas occur less often in children and represent 10% of all pediatric benign tumors (Table 56–4). These lesions are the most significant cardiac tumors, not only because of their relative frequency but also because the potential for total cure after surgical removal is high (Bulkley and Hutchins, 1979). Myxoma arises from the endocardium as a polypoid, often pedunculated, tumor that extends into a cardiac chamber. Cardiac myxomas are derived from multipotential mesenchymal cells of the subendocardial layer and imitate primitive

■ **Table 56–1.** BENIGN CARDIAC NEOPLASMS IN ADULTS

| Tumor | Number | % |
|---|---|---|
| Myxoma | 118 | 49 |
| Lipoma | 45 | 19 |
| Papillary fibroelastoma | 42 | 17 |
| Hemangioma | 11 | 5 |
| Atrioventricular node mesothelioma | 9 | 4 |
| Fibroma | 5 | 2 |
| Teratoma | 3 | 1 |
| Granular cell tumor | 3 | 1 |
| Neurofibroma | 2 | <1 |
| Lymphangioma | 2 | <1 |
| Rhabdomyoma | 1 | <1 |
| Total | 241 | 100 |

From McAllister, H. A., Jr., and Fenoglio, J. J., Jr.: Tumors of the cardiovascular system. *In* Hartman, W. H., and Cowan, W. R. (eds): Atlas of Tumor Pathology. Sec. Series, Fasc. 15. Washington, DC, Armed Forces Institute of Pathology, 1978.

■ **Table 56–2.** PRIMARY MALIGNANT CARDIAC NEOPLASMS IN ADULTS

| Tumor | Number | % |
|---|---|---|
| Angiosarcoma | 39 | 33 |
| Rhabdomyosarcoma | 24 | 21 |
| Mesothelioma | 19 | 16 |
| Fibrosarcoma | 13 | 11 |
| Lymphoma | 7 | 6 |
| Osteosarcoma | 5 | 4 |
| Thymoma | 4 | 3 |
| Neurogenic sarcoma | 3 | 2 |
| Leiomyosarcoma | 1 | <1 |
| Liposarcoma | 1 | <1 |
| Synovial sarcoma | 1 | <1 |
| Total | 117 | 100 |

From McAllister, H. A., Jr., and Fenoglio, J. J., Jr.: Tumors of the cardiovascular system. *In* Hartman, W. H., and Cowan, W. R. (eds): Atlas of Tumor Pathology. Sec. Series, Fasc. 15. Washington, D. C., Armed Forces Institute of Pathology, 1978.

■ **Table 56–4.** BENIGN CARDIAC NEOPLASMS IN CHILDREN

| Tumor | 0–1 Year | | 1–15 Years | |
|---|---|---|---|---|
| | *Number* | *%* | *Number* | *%* |
| Rhabdomyoma | 28 | 62 | 35 | 45.0 |
| Teratoma | 9 | 21 | 11 | 14.0 |
| Fibroma | 6 | 13 | 12 | 15.5 |
| Hemangioma | 1 | 2 | 4 | 5.0 |
| Atrioventricular node mesothelioma | 1 | 2 | 3 | 4.0 |
| Myxoma | — | — | 12 | 15.5 |
| Neurofibroma | — | — | 1 | 1.0 |
| Total | 45 | 100 | 78 | 100 |

From McAllister, H. A., Jr., and Fenoglio, J. J., Jr.: Tumors of the cardiovascular system. *In* Hartman, W. H., Jr., and Cowan, W. R. (eds): Atlas of Tumor Pathology. Sec. Series, Fasc. 15. Washington, DC, Armed Forces Institute of Pathology, 1978.

mesenchyme. In a review of 24 excised atrial myxomas, immunohistochemical techniques identified neuroendocrine markers in 16 tumors, supporting an endocardial nerve tissue origin of the tumor (Krikler et al., 1992). Most experts consider atrial myxomas true neoplasms on the basis of histologic, ultrastructural, electron microscopic, and tissue culture studies, although in the past, some physicians thought that cardiac myxomas developed from organized thrombi and underwent myxomatous degeneration (Salyer et al., 1975). The possibility that at least some myxomas may be reactive rather than neoplastic is supported by one report of a 3- × 2-cm right atrial myxoma developing at the site of transseptal catheterization for balloon mitral valvuloplasty performed 12 months previously (Nolan et al., 1992). Myxomas occur in patients at all ages, but the incidence is greatest in patients in the third to sixth decades of life, and there is a slight predominance in women. A familial tendency for cardiac myxoma has been found and is rarely associated with the constellation of findings that include multiple pigmented skin lesions, myxoid fibroadenoma of the breasts, and pigmented nodular adrenocortical disease (which can produce Cushing's syndrome).

Most myxomas arise singly in the atria, and approximately 75% occur in the left atrium (Sabiston and Hattler, 1983). The remainder usually occur in the right atrium (20%) or in the ventricles (less than 10%). Multiple or multicentric myxoma occurs in 5% of patients. Atrial myxomas are commonly attached to the septum in the region of the fossa ovalis; the next most common site is the posterior atrial wall. Left atrial myxoma has been reported occluding a large secundum atrial septal defect with origin from the atrial free wall at the base of the right inferior pulmonary vein (Jones et al., 1993). Most ventricular myxomas do not arise from the interventricular septum. Rarely, they arise from the mitral or aortic valve leaflet tissue (Gosse et al., 1986; Hajar et al., 1986; Sandrasgra et al., 1979). Right atrial myxoma has been reported to originate from the eustachian valve above the inferior vena cava (Teoh et al., 1993). Bilateral atrial tumors usually arise from corresponding sites on opposite sides of the interatrial septum and represent growth in both directions from a single focus within the atrial septum (Imperio et al., 1980). The growth rate of primary intracardiac myxomas is difficult to estimate, although a few reports document rapid growth on serial echocardiographic studies (Pochis et al., 1991). An analysis by Malekzadeh and

■ **Table 56–3.** PROFILES OF PATIENTS WITH PRIMARY BENIGN TUMORS

| Tumor Type | No. of Patients | Sex | | Age | | Deaths | | Follow-up | | |
|---|---|---|---|---|---|---|---|---|---|---|
| | | *M* | *F* | *Range* | *Mean* | *Early** | *Late* | *No. of Patients* | *Range* | *Mean (yr)* |
| Myxoma | 63 | 24 | 39 | 21–81 yr | 51 yr | 2 | 3 (2†) | 50‡ | 2 mo–25 yr | 7.1 |
| Purkinje cell | 13 | 4 | 9 | 2–20 mo | 12.6 mo | 0 | 1 | 12 | 6 mo–8 yr | 3.8 |
| Rhabdomyoma | 9 | 2 | 7 | 3 days–1 yr | 5.3 mo | 1 | 0 | 8 | 7 mo–8.5 yr | 3.1 |
| Fibroma | 7 | 3 | 4 | 1 mo–12 yr | 3.3 yr | 0 | 0 | 7 | 2–8 yr | 7.3 |
| Lipoma | 4 | 2 | 2 | 21–65 yr | 49 yr | 0 | 0 | 4 | 7–13 yr | 8 |
| Other | 6 | 3 | 3 | 9–55 yr | 39.1 yr | 1 | 1† | 5 | 2–22 yr | 7.1 |
| Total | 102 | 38 | 64 | 3 days–81 yr | 36.17 yr | 4 | 5 (3†) | 86 | 2 mo–25 yr | 6.5 |

From Murphy, M.C., Sweeney, M. S., Putram, J. B., et al.: Surgical treatment of cardiac tumors: A 25-year experience. Reprinted with permission from the Society of Thoracic Surgeons (The Annals of Thoracic Surgery, 1990, Vol. 49, pp. 612–617.)
*Early death is defined as death within the perioperative period or within 30 days of operation.
†These deaths were unrelated to the tumor.
‡Of the 61 patients who lived more than 30 days after operation, 50 were followed-up and data were available.

Roberts (1989) suggested that original atrial myxomas may grow as fast as 5 cm/year.

## Pathology

Although myxomas differ in clinical presentation, most have a similar macroscopic and microscopic character (Wold and Lie, 1980). These tumors are soft, gelatinous, and polypoid clusters, often with a pedunculated attachment to the endocardium (Fig. 56–1). The average diameter is 5 to 6 cm, but they can range from 0.5 to 15 cm. Areas of hemorrhage are often apparent in gross surgical specimens. True sessile myxomas with a wide-based attachment are less common.

Microscopically, these neoplasms consist of a myxoid matrix composed of a basophilic ground substance rich in mucopolysaccharides (Fig. 56–2). Within the myxoid matrix are polygonal cells, which are often stellate and sometimes multinuclear (Ferrans and Roberts, 1973). The cells may be single or occur in clusters and form vascular-like channels that simulate primitive capillaries. Ultrastructurally, these polygonal cells resemble multipotential mesenchymal cells. Other cellular elements include plasma cells, lymphocytes, and mast cells. Foci of calcification are seen in 10% of myxomas (Fig. 56–3).

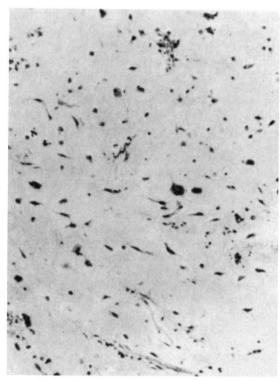

**FIGURE 56–2.** Histologic section of atrial myxoma showing polygonal cells dispensed throughout a lightly staining acid mucopolysaccharide matrix.

## Malignant Potential

Although myxomas are considered to be benign neoplasms, their recurrence and metastatic potential have been noted (Diflo et al.; 1992, Gerbode et al., 1967; Hannah et al., 1982; Markel et al., 1986; McAllister, 1979; Read et al., 1974). McAllister and Fenoglio (1978) thought that cardiac myxomas initially considered malignant were actually examples of sarcomas with extensive areas of myxoid degeneration (liposar-

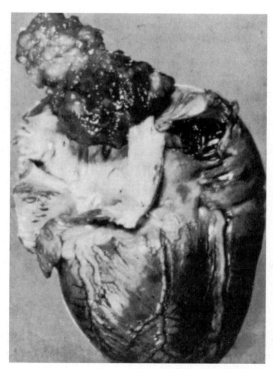

**FIGURE 56–1.** Large, friable, gelatinous myxoma located in the left atrium, attached to the atrial septum. Extreme care must be taken during surgical removal to avoid operative embolization. (From McAllister, H. A., and Fenoglio, J. J., Jr.: Tumors of the cardiovascular system. In Hartman, W. H., and Cowan, W. R. [eds]: Atlas of Tumor Pathology. Sec. Series, Fasc. 15. Washington, DC, Armed Forces Institute of Pathology, 1978.)

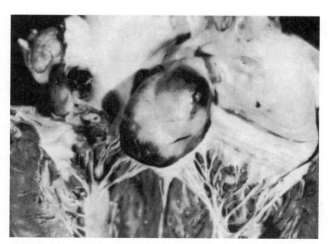

**FIGURE 56–3.** Although most myxomas are polypoid and friable, a significant number are round and smooth, and may be confused with ball thrombi.

coma, rhabdomyosarcoma) and multicentric benign myxomas. Attum and co-workers (1987) reviewed 57 cases of malignant myxomas or "myxoid imitators" documented in the literature between 1933 and 1985. Recurrence of the tumor or metastases occurred in approximately 50% of the patients reviewed. The mortality in this group of patients was 47% and surgical excision was attempted in all except 5 patients. Eight patients had myxoma associated with multiple mycotic cerebral aneurysms that were thought to occur by invasive transgression of arterial walls with replacement of the muscularis by embolic myxomatous tissue. In a separate review of 16 series with a total of 194 patients with atrial myxoma who survived operation, the recurrence rate for "benign" myxoma was 7% (Gray and Williams, 1985). The authors emphasize the importance of follow-up of all patients after resection of cardiac myxoma with serial two-dimensional echocardiography because the tumor may recur. Myxomas that arise from extraseptal locations are thought to be more likely to recur. The interval from first operation to resection of recurrence has ranged from 7 months to 10 years, with a mean time to recurrence of 32 months (Pochis et al., 1991). Second recurrence occurs in 25 to 50% of patients who had a first recurrence. Metastatic myxomas have an affinity for endothelial surfaces and have been located in systemic vessels (femoral artery, radial artery, abdominal aorta, intracerebral arteries) and may present several years following resection of the original cardiac myxoma (Kotani et al., 1991). Right atrial myxomas have been reported to embolize and produce pulmonary hypertension on the basis of obliterative pulmonary vascular obstructive disease. This situation has been successfully managed with resection of the right atrial myxoma and pulmonary thromboendarterectomy (Heck et al., 1992).

The microscopic appearance of the primary tumor has not been considered predictive of the tendency to recur or metastasize (Martin et al., 1987). However, myxomas with aberrant DNA content (aneuploid tumors) determined by flow cytometry are associated with aggressive biologic behavior and are probably more likely to recur (Kotylo et al., 1991).

### Syndrome of "Complex" Cardiac Myxoma

A group of patients from the Mayo Clinic had unusual biologic behavior of cardiac myxomas, including development at an early age, atypical location of the myxomas, and a high risk for recurrence of myxomas (Powers et al., 1979). Of 85 patients evaluated at the Mayo Clinic for cardiac myxoma, 5 had unusual associated findings that included multiple pigmented skin lesions, myxoid fibroadenomas of the breast, skin myxomas, and primary pigmented nodular adrenocortical disease (a cause of Cushing's syndrome) (Carney, 1985). Four of these 5 patients had multiple cardiac myxomas and 3 of the 4 patients who had surgical excision had recurrent myxomas. The occurrence of multiple and recurrent myxomas

in patients with the complex was significantly higher than in the 80 patients with sporadic myxomas (Jones et al., 1986). The authors commented that the myxomas that occur with this complex of findings can be familial (autosomal dominant trait), and because of the high risk of recurrence, screening of patients after resection and screening of asymptomatic family members are indicated (Carney, 1985; Haught et al., 1991; McCarthy et al., 1986; Powers et al., 1979).

### Clinical Presentation

Atrial myxoma produces various clinical presentations that can be categorized into three main types: obstructive manifestations, which are due to tumor occlusion or interference with flow through the atrioventricular valves and simulate mitral and tricuspid valve disease; embolic manifestations; and constitutional manifestations, which simulate a systemic disease.

Before an accurate noninvasive diagnostic modality (two-dimensional echocardiography) was available, most myxomas were diagnosed postmortem. Echocardiography, combined with a higher clinical index of suspicion, has allowed earlier diagnosis and successful surgical removal in most patients (O'Neil et al., 1979; Sutton et al., 1980).

In the AFIP series of 130 cases, 44% of patients with myxomas were seen with signs and symptoms of obstructive valvular disease (McAllister, 1979). In this group, 30% had an initial history of systemic embolization and 12% had no previous symptoms. The clinical features of cardiac myxoma are summarized in Table 56–5 and are particularly relevant to left atrial myxoma. Patients with myxoma may have none, some, or all of the classic manifestations, but the various features are seldom associated and the clinical diagnosis can be difficult to make.

Because the tumor can obstruct flow, left atrial myxomas often mimic mitral stenosis, and the most common symptom is dyspnea or left-sided heart failure (Panidis et al., 1986). If the pedicle of the myxoma is large, the tumor may intermittently obstruct the mitral orifice and cause syncope or sudden death. Careful examination may show positional hemodynamic

■ **Table 56–5.** CLINICAL PRESENTATION OF CARDIAC MYXOMA IN 130 PATIENTS

| | |
|---|---|
| Signs and symptoms of mitral valve disease | 57 |
| Embolic phenomena | 36 |
| No cardiac symptoms—incidental findings | 16 |
| Signs and symptoms of tricuspid valve disease | 6 |
| Sudden unexpected death | 5 |
| Pericarditis | 4 |
| Myocardial infarction | 3 |
| Signs and symptoms of pulmonary valve disease | 2 |
| Fever of undetermined origin | 2 |

From McAllister, H. A., Jr., and Fenoglio, J. J., Jr.: Tumors of the cardiovascular system. *In* Hartman, W. H., and Cowan, W. R. (eds): Atlas of Tumor Pathology, Sec. Series, Fasc. 15. Washington DC, Armed Forces Institute of Pathology, 1978.

alterations that include the classic early diastolic sound or "tumor plop." This sound is best heard at the apex and may be confused with the opening snap of a pliable mitral stenosis, but the tumor plop generally occurs later and has a much lower intensity.

In addition to heart failure and dyspnea, other complaints involve ill-defined chest pain. Hemoptysis is often found in mitral stenosis but is unusual in patients with left atrial myxoma, despite the increase in pulmonary vascular resistance that often occurs with left atrial myxomas (Selzer et al., 1972).

Right atrial myxomas are often larger than left atrial myxomas and may cause obstruction of the tricuspid orifice that produces the clinical presentation of tricuspid stenosis. Alternatively, the tumor may damage the leaflets and cause tricuspid insufficiency. This lesion may also be confused clinically with constrictive pericarditis, pulmonary hypertension, and Ebstein's anomaly (Currey et al., 1967).

Systemic emboli occur in approximately one-third of patients with cardiac myxoma. Embolization is common because of the tumor's friability and the intracavitary location. In many patients, the embolus is the initial clinical presentation, and in most cases, it involves the cerebrovascular circulation (DeSousa et al., 1978). Emboli to lower extremity arteries occur next in frequency, and other sites include the renal arteries, abdominal aorta, and coronary arteries. After embolization of friable myxomatous material, a diagnosis of cardiac myxoma can be made by histologic examination of the surgical specimen removed at thrombectomy. The first antemortem diagnosis of a left atrial myxoma was made by examining peripheral arterial tumor emboli (Goldberg et al., 1952). Embolic episodes in young patients with normal sinus rhythm should arouse suspicion of cardiac myxoma in the absence of active endocarditis. Pulmonary emboli from right atrial myxomas occur similar to emboli in the systemic circulation. Whereas typical pulmonary thromboembolic disease usually resolves after anticoagulation or through the natural fibrinolytic mechanism, tumor defects can remain occlusive for a long time and may create pulmonary hypertension from vascular obstruction. Paradoxical embolism from a right atrial myxoma in association with atrial septal defect has been reported (Powers et al., 1979).

Myxomas can present with unusual constitutional symptoms—most commonly, increased red blood cell sedimentation rate, fever, anemia, weight loss, and protein abnormalities (usually increased serum immunoglobulin levels). The association of fever, anemia, and increased sedimentation rate with myxoma was described by MacGregor and Cullen in 1959. Constitutional manifestations noted since then include leukocytosis, arthralgias, thrombocytopenia, and Raynaud's phenomenon. Most patients have one or more of these symptoms at some stage during the illness and the constitutional symptoms may occur long before obstructive or embolic symptoms. Generally, the constitutional symptoms and serum protein abnormalities vanish after tumor resection (Hattler et al., 1970).

Mechanisms proposed for the constitutional manifestations include hemorrhage and degeneration within the tumor, microembolism, and an immunologic response to the release of tumor fragments that leads to an increase in immunoglobulins (Currey et al., 1967). The probable cause of the increase in sedimentation rate is the hypergammaglobulinemia, but no qualitative abnormalities in globulins have been documented.

Because of the protean clinical manifestations of cardiac myxoma, a high index of suspicion is needed in the clinical approach to diagnosis (Silverman and Sabiston, 1981). The differential diagnosis for a left atrial myxoma includes mitral stenosis, mitral regurgitation, infective endocarditis, acute rheumatic fever, collagen vascular disorders (polyarteritis nodosa), and Wegener's granulomatosis (Leonhardt and Kullenberg, 1977). Right atrial myxoma may be difficult to distinguish clinically from isolated rheumatic tricuspid stenosis or regurgitation, constrictive pericarditis, Ebstein's anomaly, carcinoid syndrome, chronic pulmonary emboli, or pulmonary hypertension.

## DIAGNOSTIC TESTS

The impact of noninvasive screening tests, specifically two-dimensional echocardiography, on the diagnosis and management of cardiac neoplasms is shown in the Mayo Clinic review of 40 patients with atrial myxoma evaluated from 1957 to 1977. Before the introduction of echocardiography in 1968, the diagnosis was made preoperatively or antemortem in only 37% of patients, compared with 90% of patients treated after 1968 (Sutton et al., 1980). Other major diagnostic techniques that help in evaluating cardiac neoplasms before surgical intervention are computed tomography (CT), magnetic resonance imaging (MRI), and cineangiography.

### Echocardiography

Since the use of two-dimensional echocardiography has become routine, almost 100% of atrial myxomas have been diagnosed noninvasively (Goldman et al., 1986). In efficacy and accuracy, preoperative diagnosis by echocardiography is superior to diagnosis by cardiac catheterization and angiography. In the Mayo Clinic review (Sutton et al., 1980), the diagnosis was not made in one-third of the patients who had catheterization. Also, patients with myxomas are at risk of catheter-induced embolization. Most authors agree that the preoperative diagnosis of a myxoma can be based solely on echocardiography and that catheterization is not indicated (Dein et al., 1987; Silverman, 1980).

The M-mode of echocardiography was developed first and it rapidly became helpful in diagnosing atrial myxoma. The characteristic finding from M-mode echocardiography is the presence of a mass of echoes behind the anterior mitral leaflet a few milliseconds

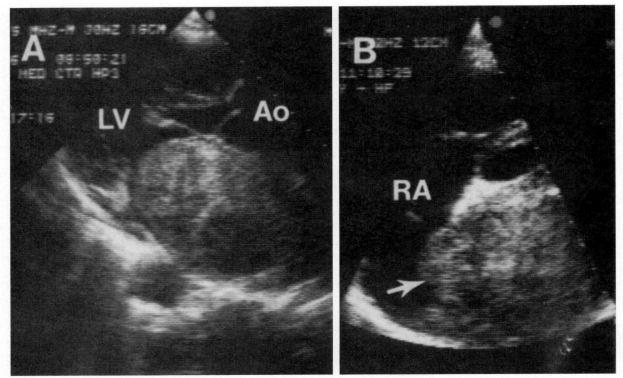

**FIGURE 56–4.** Two-dimensional echocardiographic findings of a large left atrial myxoma, viewed by a parasternal long-axis image (*A*) and parasternal short-axis image (*B*). In *A*, the myxoma is seen to occlude the mitral valve orifice. Almost the entirety of the left ventricle (LV) is filled. In *B*, a portion of the myxoma bulges (*arrow*) through the fossa ovalis. (Ao = aorta; RA = right atrium.) (*A* and *B*, Courtesy of Joseph A. Kisslo, M.D., Duke University Medical Center.)

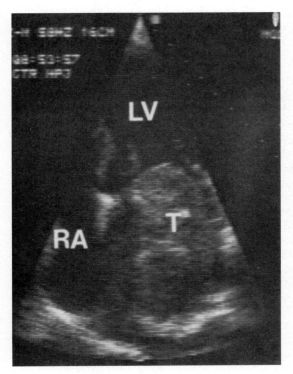

**FIGURE 56–5.** Apical four-chamber view of the patient imaged in Figure 56–4. The myxoma (T) is seen to prolapse through and occlude the mitral valve orifice in diastole. The point of attachment was diffused over the atrial septum, requiring almost complete atrial septectomy and repair with a pericardial patch. (LV = left ventricle; RA = right atrium.) (Courtesy of Joseph A. Kisslo, M.D., Duke University Medical Center.)

after maximal opening. The layered mass of echoes fills the space between the anterior and the posterior mitral leaflets throughout the rest of diastole and then returns to the left atrial cavity during systole.

Two-dimensional echocardiography provides real-time imaging of the entire heart and specifically allows visualization of the entire left atrium, right atrium, interatrial septum, atrioventricular valve, orifices, both ventricles, and the venae cavae (Fig. 56–4). This method is superior to M-mode echocardiography because it provides quantitative information about tumor size, position in the heart, mobility, and effect on valvular and ventricular function (Figs. 56–5 and 56–6). With the resolution and spatial orientation of two-dimensional echocardiography, the attachment site of the tumor and the stalk can be well visualized (DePace et al., 1981). Even very small valvular papillary fibroelastomas (0.5 cm) have been localized accurately (McFadden and Lacy, 1987). Myxoma can be detected in all cardiac chambers, and biatrial and multiple tumors have been detected with this technique (Tway et al., 1981). Two-dimensional echocardiography also provides an excellent means of follow-up to detect late tumor recurrence (Fig. 56–7).

Generally, two-dimensional echocardiographic imaging provides safe and accurate diagnosis and obviates the need for cardiac catheterization for most patients (Dunningham et al., 1981). Other atrial masses that can usually be discriminated from myxoma include thrombi, vegetations, and metastatic tumor (Panidis et al., 1984). Echocardiographic imaging is also useful in the detection of other intramural ventricular lesions, but it cannot be used alone to determine the malignant nature or histologic characteristics of these lesions. Intraoperative transesophageal echocardiography (Fig. 56–8) combined with color-flow Doppler imaging has been used to plan the surgical approach, including selection of the right atrial site for cannulation (Mora et al., 1987).

## Computed Tomography and Magnetic Resonance Imaging

Cardiac tumors including myxomas have been visualized with high resolution by CT and MRI. Although CT scanning times are too long to detect motion of the heart, there is excellent tissue discrimination (based on density or specific gravity of the tissue), and primary or secondary cardiac tumors (such as liposarcomas) can be distinguished from normal cardiac tissue (Chaloupka et al., 1986). CT is of limited use for the diagnosis of myxoma, which is similar in tissue density to normal cardiac tissue, but it gives the best evaluation of the extracardiac mediastinal structures, which are usually not imaged by echocardiography (Shin et al., 1987).

MRI is a newer technique that enables high-resolution tomography in three dimensions. It is nonionizing and provides intravascular and soft tissue contrast without the need for contrast medium. Electrocardiographic gating allows high-resolution imaging of car-

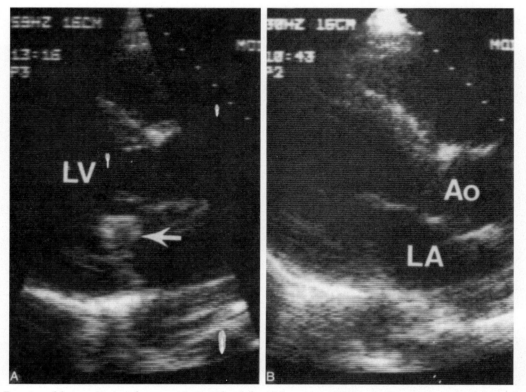

**FIGURE 56–6.** Parasternal long-axis view from a patient with a left atrial myxoma (A) attached to the posterior left atrial wall (arrow). B, The same patient 1 day later following the onset of right lower extremity pain. The tumor was found in the right iliac artery. (LV = left ventricle; LA = left atrium; Ao = aorta.) (A and B, Courtesy of Joseph A. Kisslo, M.D., Duke University Medical Center.)

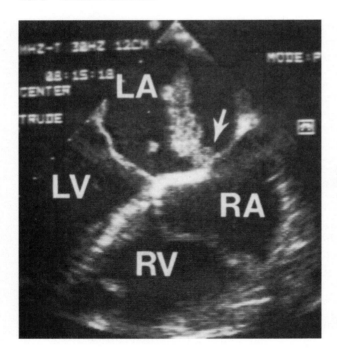

**FIGURE 56–7.** Transesophageal two-dimensional echocardiogram showing a left atrial myxoma attached at the fossa ovalis (*arrow*). (LA = left atrium; LV = left ventricle; RV = right ventricle; RA = right atrium.)

diac morphology (Figs. 56–9 and 56–10) and has made MRI a promising technique for the evaluation of cardiac neoplasms (Camesas et al., 1986). In 14 patients with intracavitary cardiac tumors diagnosed initially by echocardiography who subsequently had MRI, the MRI contributed important additional information about the tumor's relationship to normal intracardiac structures or extension to adjacent vascular and medi-astinal structures (Freedberg et al., 1988). The information was especially helpful for tumors other than myxomas (e.g., angiosarcoma, metastatic melanoma, malignant thymoma, and hypernephroma) (Gindea et al., 1987). In a separate view by Go and colleagues (1985), MRI was found to provide better definition of tumor prolapse, secondary valvular obstruction, and cardiac chamber size than two-dimensional echocar-

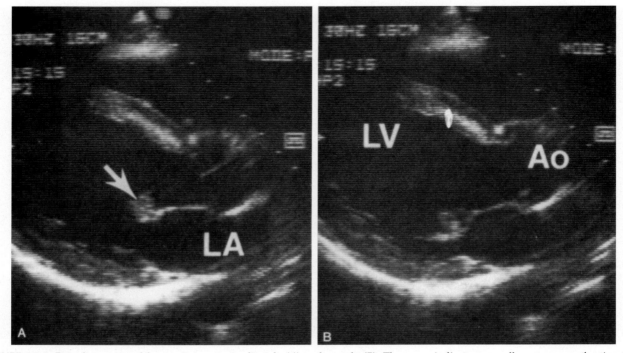

**FIGURE 56–8.** Paired parasternal long-axis images in diastole (*A*) and systole (*B*). The *arrow* indicates a small myxoma on the tip of the anterior mitral valve leaflet. The myxoma was removed with primary excision and repair of the anterior mitral leaflet. (LA = left atrium; LV = left ventricle; Ao = aorta.) (*A* and *B*, Courtesy of Joseph A. Kisslo, M.D., Duke University Medical Center.)

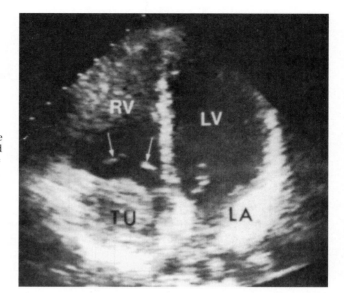

**FIGURE 56–9.** Apical four-chamber echocardiogram showing a large sessile tumor (TU) (angiosarcoma) in the right atrium of a 29-year-old woman who presented with superior vena caval syndrome. (RV = right ventricle; LV = left ventricle; LA = left atrium.)

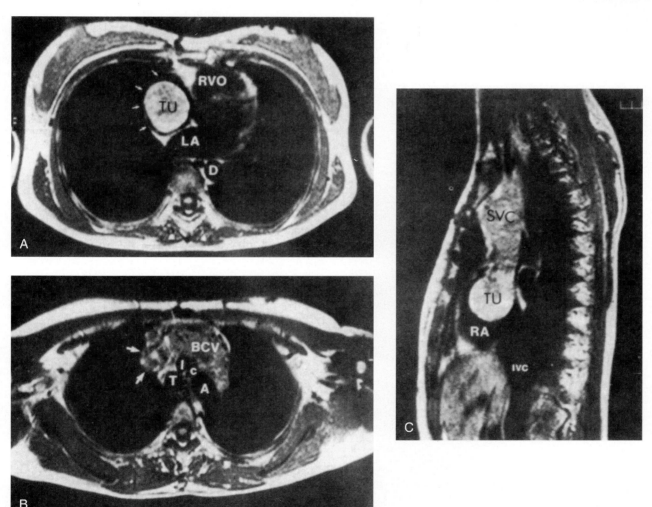

**FIGURE 56–10.** Magnetic resonance tomograms from patient in Figure 56–9, demonstrating the intravenous extension of the tumor (TU). *A,* Axial image through the atria showing a high-signal tumor mass with right atrium (*arrows*). (D = descending aorta; LA = left atrium; RVO = right ventricular outflow tract.) *B,* Axial image at the level of the aortic arch (A) and great vessels showing tumor mass (T) within superior vena cava (*arrows*) and brachiocephalic vein (BCV). (C = left carotid artery; I = innominate artery.) *C,* Sagittal image showing tumor (TU) within the right atrium (RA) extending into the superior vena cava (SVC). (IVC = inferior vena cava.) (*A–C,* From Freedberg, R. S., Kronzon, L., Rumanick, W. M., and Liebeskind, D.: Contribution of magnetic resonance imaging to the evaluation of intracardiac tumors diagnosed by echocardiography. Circulation, *77:*96, 1988. By permission of the American Heart Association, Inc.)

diographic imaging. Although two-dimensional echocardiography is still the technique of choice in the initial evaluation of intracardiac tumors, MRI can be an important adjunct in the diagnostic evaluation of cardiac tumors (Gomes et al., 1987).

## Cineangiography

Before echocardiography, angiocardiography was the standard preoperative test used to confirm the diagnosis of myxoma and other cardiac tumors. Injection of contrast material allows visualization of intracavitary filling defects, and mobile myxomas may be seen to traverse right and left atrioventricular valves during the cardiac cycle (Fig. 56–11). Small atrial ball-thrombi may be mistaken for myxomas, and small intramural tumors may not be visualized. Selective coronary angiography may also show neovascularization of a tumor, but this is not commonly found. With angiography, morbidity and mortality are associated with catheter-induced embolization of the tumor (Seifert et al., 1986). Transseptal injection techniques are not recommended for left atrial myxomas, which most often arise from the fossa ovalis and are best visualized during the levo phase of a pulmonary artery injection. At present, the role of

angiography is small; it should be used if the echocardiogram is normal but the clinical presentation is highly suggestive, or if there is some doubt about the echocardiographic findings.

## Other Diagnostic Tests

Phonocardiography, gated radionuclide cardiac imaging, and plain chest films are sometimes helpful, but the contribution of these screening tests is heavily outweighed by the advantages and accuracy of two-dimensional echocardiography (Come et al., 1981).

## SURGICAL MANAGEMENT OF MYXOMAS

After cardiac myxoma is diagnosed, operation should proceed on an urgent basis; up to 8% of patients with myxoma die while they await operation (Chitwood, 1988). Intracardiac neoplasms are managed best by complete excision under direct vision with use of cardiopulmonary bypass and hypothermic cardioplegic arrest (Castanada and Varco, 1968; Okada et al., 1986) (Figs. 56–12 and 56–13). Recurrence of myxoma, which has been documented (Gerbode et al., 1967; Read et al., 1974), should be pre-

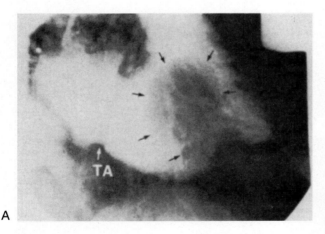

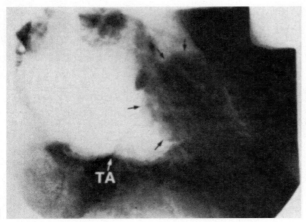

A

B

FIGURE 56–11. Cine angiographic appearance of a large liposarcoma within the right ventricle (*arrows*) after contrast injection in the right atrium. *A,* The large smooth pedunculated tumor is attached to the right ventricular apex. *B,* Systole. The pedunculated tumor virtually fills the right ventricular outflow tract. (TA = tricuspid annulus.) (*A* and *B,* From Godwin, J. D., Axel, L., Adams, J. R., et al.: Computed tomography: A method for diagnosing tumors of the heart. Circulation *63*:448, 1981. By permission of the American Heart Association, Inc.)

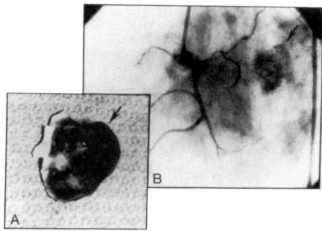

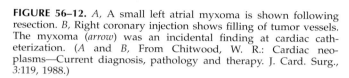

FIGURE 56–12. *A,* A small left atrial myxoma is shown following resection. *B,* Right coronary injection shows filling of tumor vessels. The myxoma *(arrow)* was an incidental finding at cardiac catheterization. (*A* and *B,* From Chitwood, W. R.: Cardiac neoplasms—Current diagnosis, pathology and therapy. J. Card. Surg., 3:119, 1988.)

vented by complete resection with removal of an adequate margin of normal endocardium, atrial septum, or atrial wall. Tumor manipulation should be minimal during cannulation and before aortic cross-clamping and cardioplegic arrest to prevent intraoperative tumor dislodgment and embolization. Most patients do well after resection, and operative mortality is less than 3% (Dein et al., 1987; Hanson et al., 1985). Probably the greatest risk for perioperative mortality and morbidity is tumor embolization to the cerebral or coronary circulation.

The surgical approach for resection of cardiac myxoma is usually a median sternotomy; a right anterolateral thoracotomy through the fourth intercostal space is selected for a better cosmetic result in younger women (Fig. 56–14). The patient is placed on cardiopulmonary bypass with perfusion temperature maintained at 28 to 30° C. Minimal tumor manipulation during cannulation and institution of full cardiopulmonary bypass is required to minimize risk of embolization. The myxoma is then removed through the appropriate atriotomy; right atrial myxomas usually are more easily exposed and more expeditiously resected. A biatrial exposure is recommended by some

centers in order to limit manipulation of the tumor and to allow visualization of all four chambers of the heart (Murphy et al., 1990). For surgical removal of myxomas attached to the atrial septum, part of the atrial septal wall to which the pedicle of the tumor is attached must be removed en bloc with the pedicle of the tumor. The defect is closed either primarily or with a native pericardial patch.

Exposure and resection of left atrial myxomas are usually more difficult. Most surgeons approach these tumors through a left atriotomy made posterior to the interatrial groove in a manner similar to mitral valve exposure (Guiloff et al., 1986). The interatrial septum is positioned anteriorly and exposure is facilitated by use of special atrial retractors. For large myxomas with a broad-based attachment to the atrial septum, the neoplasm is exposed better with a right atriotomy and a transseptal approach. With this method, access is provided to the atrial septum, mitral valve, and free atrial wall, and left atrial myxomas can be readily resected with an adequate button of normal tissue. Removal of a large tumor base usually requires patch closure. Biatrial myxomas generally arise from a common site in the interatrial septum that extends on

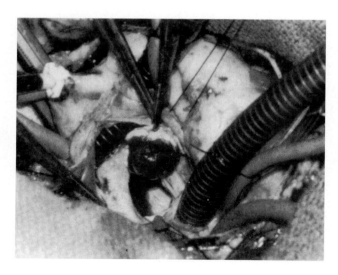

FIGURE 56–13. The left atrial myxoma shown in Figure 56–12 is being removed via a transseptal right atrial approach, with excellent exposure allowed under cardioplegic arrest. (From Chitwood, W. R.: Cardiac neoplasms—Current diagnosis, pathology and therapy. J. Card. Surg., 3:119, 1988.)

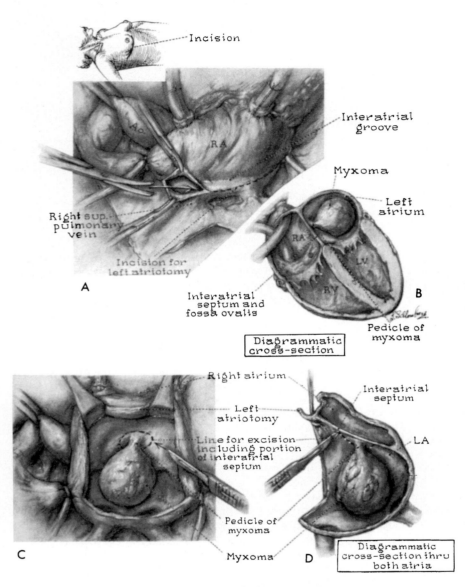

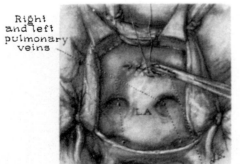

**FIGURE 56–14.** Surgical technique for removal of a left atrial myxoma. *A,* The aorta is clamped and cardioplegic arrest is achieved. The left atrial myxoma is approached through a left atriotomy. *B,* The myxoma arises from the interatrial septum near the fossa ovalis. *C,* The myxoma is exposed and a portion of the atrial septum is excised around the attachment of the pedicle. *D,* If the tumor has a large, broad-based attachment to the atrial septum, the neoplasm is better exposed via a right atrial approach. The fossa ovalis is more easily exposed through a right atriotomy, and the base of the tumor can be readily excised. *E,* The atrial septal defect created by excision of the tumor is closed primarily. With large defects, a patch closure may be required. (*A–E,* From Silverman, N. A., and Sabiston, D. C., Jr.: Cardiac neoplasms. *In* Sabiston, D. C., Jr. [ed]: Textbook of Surgery, 12th ed. Philadelphia, W. B. Saunders, 1981.)

each side. Both myxomas may be removed through separate atrial incisions or through a single atrial incision with a second septal incision.

Prognosis after surgical excision is usually excellent (Hattler et al., 1970; Silverman, 1980). In a review of 54 patients who underwent excision of an intracardiac myxoma, the 20-year actuarial survival was 91% (mean follow-up, 7 years) (Bortolotti et al., 1990). Regression of all preoperative symptoms, including the constitutional symptoms of the myxoma syndrome, has been documented for periods of more than 15 years. Excellent long-term outcome following resection of intracardiac myxoma was documented in a review of 22 patients treated at the University of Iowa and followed for up to 24 years (mean follow-up, 9 years). There were no tumor recurrences in patients without the complex myxoma syndrome, and all patients were New York Heart Association (NYHA) functional Class I or II (Sellke et al., 1990).

Right ventricular myxomas are best excised through a right ventriculotomy because they usually arise from the infundibular wall. Removal of left ventricular myxomas is generally attempted through an aortotomy with retraction of the aortic valve (Palazzuoli et al., 1986). An apical ventriculotomy is sometimes necessary to remove larger tumors. Valvular reconstruction or replacement is sometimes necessary for adequate resection of large tumors.

## RHABDOMYOMA

Rhabdomyoma is the most common cardiac tumor in childhood and the second most common benign tumor at all ages (after myxoma). Ninety per cent occur in children younger than 15 years, and 30 to 50% are associated with tuberous sclerosis (mental retardation, convulsions, speech defects). Up to 90% of these tumors are multiple and occur mainly in the left and right ventricles; 30% involve the atria (Fig. 56–15). These tumors are usually deep within the myocardium and present with recurrent tachyarrhythmias. The tumors can also extend within a cavity and obstruct the cardiac chamber or respective valve orifice (Fig. 56–16). The gross appearance of these tumors is pale yellow to white, with a range in size from 5 mm to 2.5 cm. The lesions are well circumscribed from the surrounding myocardium but are not encapsulated. Microscopically, rhabdomyomas consist of large ovoid, vacuolated cells with abundant glycogen (Kidder, 1950). Classic spider cells are found characteristically, and consist of centrally placed cytoplasmic bodies that contain the nucleus, from which myofibrils project radially to the periphery of the cells (Landing and Farger, 1956). Because of the multicentric pattern and the high incidence in children, rhabdomyomas are thought to be hamartomas rather than true neoplasms, and are probably derived from fetal cardiac myoblasts. Because of the multiple locations, poor encapsulation, and deep myocardial location, surgical resection can be difficult (Corno et al., 1984). The indication for surgery is influenced by the sever-

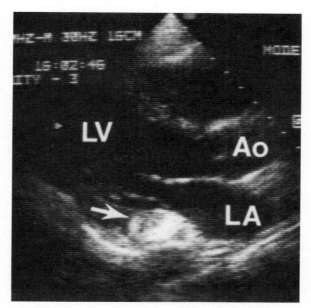

**FIGURE 56–15.** Parasternal long-axis view showing a large rhabdomyoma in the posterior wall of the left ventricle (LV) *(arrow)*. (LA = left atrium; Ao = aorta.)

ity of the clinical presentation, and in young symptomatic patients, there is little chance of survival without surgery. The slow growth and noninvasive ratio of this benign tumor should dictate operative intervention only when the tumor causes clinical hemodynamic impairment and significant symptoms. The primary goal of therapy should be not the total resection of tumor, but rather restoration of best possible heart function (Bertolini et al., 1990). However, because tuberous sclerosis is rare in the symptomatic intracavitary rhabdomyoma and there is evidence that rhabdomyomas do not undergo mitosis after birth, these patients should be considered to be surgical candidates, and reports of small series show acceptable results of surgical treatment in selective cases (Corno

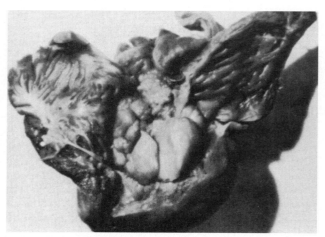

**FIGURE 56–16.** Rhabdomyoma that fills the right ventricle of a newborn infant. The multicentric origin of the tumor is demonstrated. (From Fenoglio, J. J., Jr., McAllister, H. A., Jr., and Ferrans, V. J.: Cardiac rhabdomyoma. Am. J. Cardiol., 28:24, 1976.)

et al., 1984; Reece et al., 1984). The goal of resection is to alleviate the obstructive symptoms, preserve ventricular and valvular function, and prevent injury to the conduction system.

## FIBROMA

Cardiac fibromas almost always occur in a solitary location, usually in the ventricular septum or ventricular myocardium. These tumors are more common in children but have been reported in all age groups (17 patients were reported in the AFIP series). Fibromas are the second most common primary cardiac tumors in the pediatric age group. Grossly, they appear as firm, nonencapsulated masses 3 to 7 cm in diameter. The central part of the tumor consists of hyalinized fibrous tissue with multiple foci of cystic degeneration and calcification. Most fibromas invade the conduction system and patients often die suddenly of arrhythmia. Successful resection of a septal fibroma has been reported (Reece et al., 1983). A 17-year-old patient with an unresectable fibroma was treated successfully with cardiac transplantation (Jamieson et al., 1981).

## LIPOMATOUS HYPERTROPHY OF THE ATRIAL SEPTUM

This lesion, also called interatrial lipoma, is a nonencapsulated mass of adipose tissue in the atrial septum that develops in continuity with the epicardial fat. The condition is thought to be due to hypertrophy of primordial fat rather than true neoplasm. It is most common in patients over 60 years of age and usually appears in obese individuals. The fatty tissue bulges subendocardially into the right atrium and ranges from 1 to 8 cm in diameter. Microscopically, the lesion consists of fat cells that surround separate myocardial cells. The condition is manifested clinically with supraventricular arrhythmias and is occasionally associated with sudden death (Isner et al., 1982). Lipomas other than lipomatous hypertrophy of the atrial septum occur throughout the heart, but are much less common and are generally asymptomatic (McAllister and Fenoglio, 1978).

## MESOTHELIOMA

Primary mesotheliomas occur most commonly in the region of the atrioventricular node. These neoplasms occur usually in adult women and, because of their location, can cause partial or complete heart block. The neoplasm consists of nests of mesothelial cells arranged in a multicystic pattern, and the central portion of the cyst is composed of amorphous colloid material. Grossly, the neoplasms appear as elevated nodules in the atrial septum close to the atrioventricular node. The preferred treatment is with an atrioventricular pacemaker; surgical excision would cause

heart block. Ventricular fibrillation has been reported to develop after cardiac pacing, and a combination of cardiac pacing and antiarrhythmic therapy is indicated for the treatment of this lesion (McAllister and Fenoglio, 1978).

## PAPILLARY FIBROELASTOMA

Papillary fibroelastomas are derived from the endocardium, most commonly valvular endocardium. The neoplasm is most common in adults, is usually asymptomatic clinically, and is an incidental finding at postmortem examination. Occasionally, this tumor embolizes to obstruct a coronary artery or produce a transient ischemic attack (McFadden and Lacy, 1987).

## CARDIAC PHEOCHROMOCYTOMA

Cardiac pheochromocytomas are rare tumors that are commonly located in the roof of the left atrium. These are usually functional tumors and patients present with severe hypertension. In a review of 32 cases of cardiac pheochromocytomas, 3 patients had undergone resection of a previous abdominal pheochromocytoma (Jebara et al., 1992). Coronary arteriography is important in diagnosing this highly vascular tumor because it localizes the lesion as well as the blood supply.

## CARDIAC HEMANGIOMA

These are exceedingly rare cardiac tumors, with 24 cases described in the literature (Brizard et al., 1993). Patients present with symptoms due to compression of cardiac structures or obstruction of outflow tracts. Enhanced contrast CT scan or MRI establishes the diagnosis of a hypervascularized cardiac tumor. Coronary arteriography is important in demonstrating the characteristic tumor blush. Surgical resection is usually curative, although spontaneous regression has been reported.

Other benign tumors reported to arise from the heart are teratoma, chemodectoma, neurilemoma, granular cell myoblastoma, and bronchogenic cysts (Hui et al., 1987; Leithiser et al., 1986; Stowers et al., 1987; Villafane et al., 1987). These neoplasms are rare or have only minor clinical significance.

## MALIGNANT PRIMARY CARDIAC TUMORS

Of all primary cardiac tumors, approximately 25% are malignant. Almost all primary cardiac malignancies are sarcomas; the most common are angiosarcomas (33%) followed by rhabdomyosarcomas (20%), and the remainder are mesotheliomas or malignant fibrous histiocytomas (Laya et al., 1987). Malignant tumors occur usually after the fourth decade of life and, unlike myxomas, occur with approximately the same incidence in men and women. The right atrium is involved most commonly, and patients generally show symptoms of congestive heart failure, arrhythmias, myocardial ischemia, or hemopericardium (Klima et al., 1986). Rapidly progressive congestive heart failure of recent onset refractory to medical therapy is characteristic of a malignant cardiac tumor. By the time the tumor is diagnosed, regional extension or distant metastases have usually occurred and preclude resection (Movahed and Wait, 1986). Most patients die within the first year after diagnosis. The role of surgery is generally to establish the diagnosis and to guide adjunctive therapy. The differentiating features of benign and malignant primary cardiac tumors are shown in Table 56–6.

Clinical and pathologic findings for a large series of malignant primary cardiac tumors were reported from the Cleveland Clinic (Bear and Moodie, 1987). Malignant primary cardiac tumors were found between 1956 and 1986 in 11 patients with a mean age of 44 years and were approximately equally distributed in men and women. No patient was asymptomatic on initial presentation and most patients had respiratory symptoms and chest pain. Angiosarcoma was the most frequent type of tumor (4 patients), followed by malignant fibrous histiocytoma (3 patients), rhabdomyosarcoma (3 patients), mesothelioma (1 patient), and primary lymphoma (1 patient). Of the patients, 70% had surgical biopsy and in 30% surgical excision was attempted. Ten of the patients died within the year after diagnosis; the single long-term survivor had primary lymphoma of the heart, which was treated with radiation. Associated findings

■ **Table 56–6.** CHARACTERISTICS OF BENIGN AND MALIGNANT PRIMARY CARDIAC TUMOR

| Characteristic | Benign | Malignant |
| --- | --- | --- |
| Incidence | 80% | 20% |
| Pathologic type | Mainly myxoma | All are sarcoma |
| Location | Usually left atrial, multiple sites uncommon | Usually right atrial, multiple sites common |
| Age | 30–60 years | 30–70 years, rare less than 30 years |
| Sex (F : M ratio) | 3 : 1 | 1 : 1 |
| Arrhythmias | Uncommon | Common owing to intramyocardial invasion |
| Pericardial effusion | Unusual | Common—usually bloody |
| Diagnosis | Echocardiography | Echocardiography, computed tomography scan, some require open biopsy |
| Prognosis | Excellent following resection | Fatal within 6 mo to 2 yr |
| Management | Surgical excision | Combined approach (excision, chemotherapy, radiation therapy) cardiac transplantation |

in this series were a normochromic, normocytic anemia in 10 patients and cardiac enlargement seen on the chest film in 8 patients. Postsurgical chemotherapy or radiation therapy had little effect on survival except for the patient with a non-Hodgkin lymphoma, who was well 6 years after treatment.

The Texas Heart Institute reported a series of 12 patients with primary malignant cardiac tumors treated between 1964 and 1989 (Murphy et al., 1990). All patients presented with symptoms of congestive heart failure. The most common tumor was angiosarcoma, followed by malignant fibrous histiocytoma. Only 2 of the patients were children. Three of the patients were considered long-term survivors (to 3.5 years postoperatively).

Angiosarcoma is the most common malignant primary cardiac tumor and occurs two to three times more often in men than in women, almost always in the adult age group. The tumor arises from the right atrium in 80% of reported cases and is usually associated with a rapid clinical onset and progressive deterioration (Janigan et al., 1986). In approximately 75% of patients, either right ventricular failure or pericardial disease is found (Chitwood, 1988). Other common symptoms are fever, chest pain, hemoptysis, and malaise. Surgical resection is rarely possible because of distant metastases and frequent pericardial involvement (Percy et al., 1987). Despite adjunctive chemotherapy or radiation therapy, 90% of patients die within 9 to 12 months of diagnosis of the tumor (Dein et al., 1987; Wiske et al., 1986).

Rhabdomyosarcoma, the next most common malignant tumor of the heart, occurs equally in both sexes. There is no predilection for any cardiac chamber and the neoplasm is multicentric in 60% of patients (Becker et al., 1985). These lesions are rare in children and follow malignant teratomas in frequency. Rhabdomyosarcoma is usually seen with intracavitary extension, and most patients have partial or almost complete obstruction of one of the heart valves, most commonly the mitral or pulmonic valves. Unlike benign tumors, these malignant tumors invade the cardiac valves and often destroy them. Pericardial involvement owing to direct tumor extension is common. The histologic diagnosis is based on the presence of rhabdomyoblasts, which may be difficult to locate, and electron microscopy is usually required to identify the muscular origin of the tumor. Most patients die within 1 year after diagnosis of the tumor, but excision of the main tumor mass followed by combined radiation therapy and chemotherapy may be indicated in selected patients.

Fibrosarcoma and malignant fibrous histiocytoma are malignant mesenchymal tumors that are primarily fibroblastic in differentiation. These tumors constitute only 10% of primary cardiac malignancies, although malignant fibrous histiocytoma is one of the more common soft tissue sarcomas. Cardiac involvement occurs commonly in the left atrium (Lee et al., 1987) and the incidence is higher in young women, in whom it may be confused with left atrial myxoma (Smith, 1986). Although radiation and chemotherapy have had minimal success, no therapy has been effective for treating malignant fibroblastic tumors of the heart and the prognosis is uniformly poor, with survival measured in months after appearance of symptoms (Ovcak et al., 1992). Primary lymphoma of the heart has been reported (Chou et al., 1983; Gelman et al., 1986) and associated with AIDS (Constantino et al., 1987), and is best treated by radiation therapy.

In summary, malignant primary cardiac tumors are associated with poor long-term survival because of the advanced local involvement of the tumor at presentation and the fact that most patients already have distal metastases. With two-dimensional echocardiography, noninvasive imaging of these tumors early in their course may allow earlier diagnosis, earlier institution of aggressive surgical resection and advanced chemotherapy, and a potential for better survival. For patients with localized disease but with extensive cardiac involvement, cardiac transplantation may have a role.

## METASTATIC TUMORS OF THE HEART

The most common neoplastic process that involves the heart is metastatic deposits from primary tumors elsewhere in the body. Metastatic tumors of the heart are up to 40 times more frequent than primary tumors of the heart (Fine, 1968; Hallahan et al., 1986; Hanfling, 1960). The incidence of metastatic cardiac disease in patients with known malignancies is approximately 10% (Hanfling, 1960). An increase in cardiac metastases noted in later series may be related to prolonged survival after surgical and adjunctive therapy. Almost every type of malignant tumor from all organs has been reported to spread to the heart and pericardium (Pillai et al., 1986). Up to 50% of patients with leukemia have cardiac involvement (Fine, 1968), and other malignancies that commonly metastasize to the heart include melanoma, carcinoma of the lung, and carcinoma of the breast. In 418 cases of lung carcinoma reported by Strauss and colleagues (1977), the incidence of cardiac metastases was 25%. The parts of the heart affected by metastatic tumors in decreasing order of frequency are pericardium, myocardium, and endocardium. When the heart is affected, metastatic disease is usually found to be widespread throughout the body. The clinical diagnosis of metastatic heart disease is usually not made because only 10% of the patients have symptoms attributable to metastases to the heart. Symptoms that do arise are overshadowed by the primary disease. Symptoms of congestive heart failure not apparently caused by an arrhythmia in a patient with known malignant disease may indicate cardiac involvement of the tumor (Cates et al., 1986). The most frequent clinical expression of secondary cardiac malignancy is pericardial effusion and cardiac tamponade. Also, solid tumor growth may impinge on structures of the heart and cause various symptoms and signs (Cohen et al., 1986).

Metastatic disease usually involves the ventricular chambers more often than the atria and is reported by some authors to be slightly more common on the right side of the heart (Smith, 1986). Malignant involvement of the heart may occur by retrograde invasion from lymphatic channels, by hematogenous routes, or by direct invasion from adjacent mediasti-

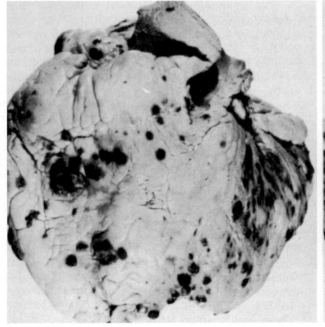
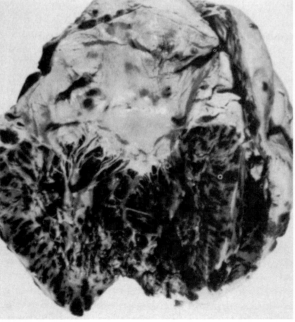

**FIGURE 56–17.** Metastatic melanoma. Dark tumor nodules are clearly seen distributed throughout the myocardium. The mode of metastasis is usually hematogenous spread. (From McAllister, H. A., and Fenoglio, J. J., Jr.: Tumors of the cardiovascular system. *In* Hartman, W. H., and Cowan, W. R. [eds]: Atlas of Tumor Pathology. Sec. Series, Fasc. 15. Washington, D.C., Armed Forces Institute of Pathology, 1978.)

nal structures. Most patients with carcinoma of the breast and lung have cardiac involvement by lymphatic spread rather than by direct extension (McAllister and Fenoglio, 1978). Metastases from sarcomas, leukemias, and melanomas (Fig. 56–17) occur most commonly by hematogenous routes (Ali, 1987). Intrathoracic primary tumors such as esophageal, breast, and lung carcinomas may extend directly into the pericardial and cardiac tissue, and up to 50% of lymphomas involve the heart by direct extension (Armstrong et al., 1986; Balasubramanyam et al., 1986).

Surgical treatment for metastatic cardiac malignancies is indicated for relief of ventricular obstruction caused by isolated lesions or for relief of cardiac tamponade caused by malignant pericardial effusion. Before surgical resection of metastatic disease is considered, primary tumors should be well controlled and the metastatic focus is potentially resectable. Renal cell carcinoma with tumor extension into the right atrium has been treated efficaciously with surgical removal (Novick and Cosgrove, 1980). Patients with moderate to large symptomatic malignant pericardial effusions can be treated effectively with a subxyphoid pericardial window. The procedure can be performed easily with the patient under local anesthesia, has minimal morbidity in these debilitated patients with metastatic disease, and significantly alleviates symptoms of cardiac tamponade. In a review of four series with a total of 100 patients with malignant cardiac tamponade treated with subxyphoid pericardiotomy, Press and Livingston (1987) found that all the patients had relief of tamponade and there were only 3 recurrences and no fatalities. The survival of patients varied from 1 week to more than 8 years, and depended on the progression of malignancy elsewhere in the body. However, of patients with malignant effusions treated with subxyphoid pericardiotomy, approximately 50% die within 3 months from progression of primary heart disease. Left anterior thoracotomy with creation of a pleuropericardial window provides effective decompression of malignant pericardial effusions, but this procedure requires general anesthesia and may be poorly tolerated by debilitated, hemodynamically unstable patients with advanced cancer, and significant morbidity of 10 to 15% can be expected from this procedure (Gregory et al., 1985).

Radiation therapy is beneficial in 60% of patients with malignant pericardial effusion (Cham et al., 1975). In this series, 38 patients with neoplastic effusions were treated with 2500 to 3000 rads of external-beam radiation for 3 to 4 weeks. The median duration of improvement was approximately 4 months. In an alternative approach to delivering radiotherapy, Martini and associates (1977) instilled radioactive chromic phosphate intrapericardially in a series of 28 patients. With this technique of pericardiocentesis followed by pericardial infusion of the radioactive agent, effusions were controlled successfully in 70% of the patients, and the efficacy of this approach has been documented by others (Maher and Buckman, 1986).

## SELECTED BIBLIOGRAPHY

Chitwood, W. R., Jr.: Cardiac neoplasms: Current diagnosis, pathology and therapy. J. Card. Surg., 3:119, 1988.

This well-illustrated review examines almost all diagnostic, pathologic, and therapeutic aspects of benign and malignant cardiac tumors. The various surgical approaches for removal of resectable neoplasms are detailed.

Dein, J. R., Frist, W. N., Stinson, E. B., et al.: Primary cardiac neoplasms. J. Thorac. Cardiovasc. Surg., 93:502, 1987.

This contemporary surgical series reviews 42 patients who had resection of cardiac neoplasms between 1961 and 1986. All 34 patients with benign lesions had resection, with excellent results. All gross tumor was removed in 4 of 8 patients with malignant tumors.

DePace, N. L., Soulen, R. L., Kotler, M. N., and Mink, G. S.: Two-dimensional echocardiographic detection of intra-atrial masses. Am. J. Cardiol., 48:957, 1981.

This paper reviews the role of two-dimensional echocardiographic detection of masses in the left atrium and the distinguishing features of atrial thrombus, myxoma, and malignant tumors as studied by two-dimensional echocardiography.

Harvey, W. P.: Clinical aspects of cardiac tumors. Am. J. Cardiol., 21:328, 1968.

This is a classic description of the signs and symptoms that should alert the clinician to the presence of a cardiac neoplasm. Detailed descriptions of representative cases are especially informative

Jebara, V. A., Uva, M. S., Farge, A., et al.: Cardiac pheochromocytomas. Ann. Thorac. Surg., 53:536, 1992.

The authors report two patients undergoing resection of cardiac pheochromocytoma and review of the literature, which includes 30 additional cases. These tumors are commonly located in the roof of the left atrium and have a characteristic appearance on coronary arteriography, which is important to define its relation to the coronary vessels.

McCallister, H. A., Jr.: Primary tumors and cysts of the heart and pericardium. Curr. Probl. Cardiol., 4:1, 1979.

This article comprehensively reviews the vast experience of the Armed Forces Institute of Pathology with more than 500 primary cardiac tumors. The review is well illustrated and supported by pertinent tables and provides excellent clinical correlations.

Murphy, M. C., Sweeney, M. S., Putram, J. B., et al.: Surgical treatment of cardiac tumors: A 25-year experience. Ann. Thorac. Surg., 49:612, 1990.

The authors review the largest single series of patients with cardiac tumors treated surgically (133), including 19 malignant tumors and 32 tumors in children. The preferred approach for resection of myxomas is biatrial in order to limit manipulation of the mass and potential embolization.

## BIBLIOGRAPHY

Ali, M. K.: Right ventricular metastatic sarcoma. Am. J. Clin. Oncol., 10:270, 1987.
Armstrong, W. F., Buck, J. D., Hoffman, R., and Waller, B. F.: Cardiac involvement by lymphoma: Detection and follow-up by two-dimensional echocardiography. Am. Heart J., 112:627, 1986.
Attum, A. A., Johnson, G. S., Masri, Z., et al.: Malignant clinical behavior of cardiac myxomas and "myxoid imitators." Ann. Thorac. Surg., 44:217, 1987.
Bahnson, H. T., and Newman, E. V.: Diagnosis and surgical removal of intracavitary myxoma of the right atrium. Bull. Johns Hopkins Hosp., 93:150, 1953.
Balasubramanyam, A., Waxman, M., Kazal, H. L., and Lee, M. H.: Malignant lymphoma of the heart in acquired immune deficiency syndrome. Chest, 90:243, 1986.
Barnes, A. R., Beaver, D. C., and Snell, A. M.: Primary sarcoma of the heart: Report of a case with electrocardiographic and pathological studies. Am. Heart J., 9:480, 1934.
Bear, P. A., and Moodie, D. S.: Malignant primary cardiac tumors: The Cleveland Clinic experience, 1956–1986. Chest, 92:860, 1987.
Beck, C. S.: An intrapericardial teratoma and a tumor of the heart: Both removed operatively. Ann. Surg., 116:161, 1942.
Becker, R. C., Hobbs, R. E., and Ratliff, N. B.: Cardiac rhabdomyo-

sarcoma: Case report with review of clinical and pathologic features. Cleve. Clin. Q., 51:83, 1985.

Bertolini, P., Mesner, H., Paek, S. U., and Sebening, F.: Special considerations on primary cardiac tumors in infancy and childhood. Thorac. Cardiovasc. Surg., 38:164, 1990.

Bloor, C. M., and O'Rourke, R. A.: Cardiac tumors: Clinical presentation and pathologic correlations. Curr. Probl. Cardiol., 9:7, 1984.

Bortolotti, U., Maraglino, G., Rubino, M., et al.: Surgical excision of intracardiac myxomas—A 20-year follow-up. Ann. Thorac. Surg., 49:449, 1990.

Brizard, C., Latremouille, C., Jebara, V. A., et al.: Cardiac hemangiomas. Ann. Thorac. Surg., 56:390, 1993.

Bulkley, B. H., and Hutchins, M.: Atrial myxomas: A fifty-year review. Am. Heart J., 97:639, 1979.

Camesas, A. M., Lichstein, E., Kramer, J., et al.: Complementary use of two-dimensional echocardiography and magnetic resonance imaging in the diagnosis of ventricular myxoma. Am. Heart J., 114:440, 1986.

Carney, J. A.: Differences between nonfamilial and familial cardiac myxoma. Am. J. Surg. Pathol., 9:53, 1985.

Carney, J. A., Gordon, H., Carpenter, P. C., et al.: The complex of myxomas, spotty pigmentation, and endocrine overactivity. Medicine, 64:270, 1985.

Castañeda, A. R., and Varco, R. L.: Tumors of the heart: Surgical considerations. Am. J. Cardiol., 21:357, 1968.

Cates, C. U., Virmani, R., Vaughn, W. K., and Robertson, R. M.: Electrocardiographic markers of cardiac metastasis. Am. Heart J., 112:1297, 1986.

Chaloupka, J. D., Fishman, E. K., and Siegelman, S. S.: Use of CT in the evaluation of primary cardiac tumors. Cardiovasc. Intervent. Radiol., 9:132, 1986.

Cham, W. C., Freiman, A. H., Carstens, P. H. B., et al.: Radiation therapy of cardiac and pericardial metastases. Radiology, 114:701, 1975.

Chitwood, W. R., Jr.: Cardiac neoplasms: Current diagnosis, pathology, and therapy. J. Card. Surg., 3:119, 1988.

Chitwood, W. R., Jr.: Clarence Crafoord and the first successful resection of a cardiac myxoma. Ann. Thorac. Surg., 54:997, 1992.

Chou, S. T., Arkles, L. B., Gill, G. D., et al.: Primary lymphoma of the heart: A case report. Cancer, 52:744, 1983.

Cohen, D. E., Mora, C., and Keefe, D. L.: Echocardiographic findings of metastatic chondrosarcoma involving the left atrium. Am. Heart J., 111:993, 1986.

Columbus, M. R.: De Re Anatomica. Libri XV. Paris, 1562.

Come, P. C., Riley, M. F., Markis, J. E., and Malagold, M.: Limitations of echocardiographic techniques in evaluation of left atrial masses. Am. J. Cardiol., 48:947, 1981.

Constantino, A., West, T. E., Gupta, M., and Loghmanee, F.: Primary cardiac lymphoma in a patient with acquired immune deficiency syndrome. Cancer, 60:2801, 1987.

Corno, A., de Simone, G., Catena, G., and Marcelletti, C.: Cardiac rhabdomyoma: Surgical treatment in the neonate. J. Thorac. Cardiovasc. Surg., 87:725, 1984.

Crafoord, C.: Mitral stenosis and mitral insufficiency. In Lam, C. R. (ed): International Symposium on Cardiovascular Surgery. Henry Ford Hospital, Detroit. Philadelphia, W. B. Saunders, 1955, p. 203.

Currey, H. L. F., Matthew, J. A., and Robinson, J.: Right atrial myxoma mimicking a rheumatic disorder. Br. Med. J., 1:547, 1967.

Dein, J. R., Frist, W. H., Stinson, E. B., et al.: Primary cardiac neoplasms: Early and late results of surgical treatment in 42 patients. J. Thorac. Cardiovasc. Surg., 93:502, 1987.

DePace, N. L., Soulen, R. L., Kotler, M. N., and Mintz, G. S.: Two-dimensional echocardiographic detection of intra-atrial masses. Am. J. Cardiol., 48:954, 1981.

DeSousa, A. L., Muller, J., Campbell, R. L., et al.: Atrial myxoma: A review of neurological complications, metastases, and recurrences. J. Neurol. Neurosurg. Psychiatry, 41:1119, 1978.

Diflo, T., Cantelmo, N. L., Haudenechild, C. C., and Watkins, M. T.: Atrial myxoma with remote metastasis: Case report and review of the literature. Surgery, 111:352, 1992.

Dunninghan, A., Oldham, H. N., Serwer, G. A., et al.: Left atrial

myxoma: Is cardiac catheterization essential? Am. J. Dis. Child., 135:420, 1981.

Ferrans, V. J., and Roberts, W. C.: Structural features of cardiac myxomas. Hum. Pathol., 4:111, 1973.

Fine, G.: Neoplasms of the pericardium and heart. In Gould, S. E. (ed): Pathology of the Heart and Blood Vessels. Springfield, IL, Charles C. Thomas, 1968.

Freedberg, R. S., Kronzon, L., Rumanick, W. M., and Liebeskind, D.: The contribution of magnetic resonance imaging to the evaluation of intracardiac tumors diagnosed by echocardiography. Circulation, 77:96, 1988.

Gelman, K. M., Ben-Ezra, J. M., Steinschneider, M., et al.: Lymphoma with primary cardiac manifestations. Am. Heart J., 111:808, 1986.

Gerbode, F., Kerth, W. J., and Hill, J. D.: Surgical management of tumors of the heart. Surgery, 61:94, 1967.

Gindea, A. J., Steele, P., Rumancik, W. M., et al.: Biventricular cavity obliteration by metastatic malignant melanoma: Role of magnetic resonance imaging in the diagnosis. Am. Heart J., 114:1249, 1987.

Go, R. T., O'Donnell, J. K., Underwood, D. A., et al.: Comparison of gated MRI and 2D echocardiography of intracardiac neoplasms. Am. J. Radiol., 145:21, 1985.

Goldberg, H. P., Glenn, F., Dotter, C. T., and Steinberg, I.: Myxoma of the left atrium: Diagnosis made during life with operative and postmortem findings. Circulation, 6:762, 1952.

Goldman, A. P., Kotler, M. N., and Parry, R. A.: Atrial tumors. In Kapoor, A. (ed): Cancer and the Heart. New York, Springer-Verlag, 1986.

Gomes, A. S., Lois, J. F., Child, J. S., et al.: Cardiac tumors and thrombus: Evaluation with MR imaging. Am. J. Roentgenol., 149:895, 1987.

Gosse, P., Herpin, D., Roudaut, R., et al.: Myxoma of the mitral valve diagnosed by echocardiography. Am. Heart J., 111:803, 1986.

Gray, I. R., and Williams, W. G.: Recurring cardiac myxoma. Br. Heart J., 53:645, 1985.

Gregory, J. R., McMurtrey, M. H., and Mountain, C. F.: A surgical approach to the treatment of pericardial effusion in cancer patients. Am. J. Clin. Oncol., 8:317, 1985.

Guiloff, A. K., Flege, J. B., Callard, G. M., et al.: Surgery of left atrial myxomas: Report of eleven cases and review of the literature. J. Cardiovasc. Surg., 27:194, 1986.

Hajar, R., Roberts, W. C., and Folger, G. M., Jr.: Embryonal botryoid rhabdomyosarcoma of the mitral valve. Am. J. Cardiol., 57:376, 1986.

Hallahan, D. E., Vogelzang, N. J., Borow, K. M., et al.: Cardiac metastases from soft-tissue sarcomas. J. Clin. Oncol., 4:1662, 1986.

Hanfling, S. M.: Metastatic cancer to the heart: Review of the literature and report of 127 cases. Circulation, 22:474, 1960.

Hannah, H., III, Eisemann, G., Hiszchnskyj, R., et al.: Invasive atrial myxoma: Documentation of malignant potential of cardiac myxomas. Am. Heart J., 104:881, 1982.

Hanson, E. C., Gill, C. C., Razavi, M., et al.: The surgical treatment of atrial myxomas. J. Thorac. Cardiovasc. Surg., 89:298, 1985.

Hattler, B. G., Fuchs, J. C. A., Coson, R. et al.: Atrial myxomas: An evaluation of clinical and laboratory manifestations. Ann. Thorac. Surg., 10:65, 1970.

Haught, W. N., Alexander, J. A., and Conti, C. R.: Familial recurring cardiomyxomas. Clin. Cardiol., 14:692, 1991.

Heck, H. A., Gross, C. M., and Houghton, J. L.: Long-term severe pulmonary hypertension associated with right atrial myxoma. Chest, 102:301, 1992.

Hui, G., McAllister, H. A., and Angelini, P.: Left atrial paraganglioma: Report of a case and review of the literature. Am. Heart J., 113:1230, 1987.

Imperio, J., Summels, D., Krasnow, N., and Piccone, V. A.: The distribution patterns of biatrial myxomas. Ann. Thorac. Surg., 29:469, 1980.

Isner, J., Swan, C. S., II, Mikus, J. P., and Carter, B. L.: Lipomatous hypertrophy of the interatrial septum: In vivo diagnosis. Circulation, 66:470, 1982.

Jamieson, S. W., Gaudiani, V. A., Reik, B. A., et al.: Operative treatment of an unresectable tumor on the left ventricle. J. Thorac. Cardiovasc. Surg., 81:797, 1981.

Janigan, D. T., Husain, A., and Robinson, N. A.: Cardiac angiosarcomas: A review and a case report. Cancer, 57:852, 1986.

Jebara, V. A., Farge, A., Acar, C., et al.: Cardiac pheochromocytomas. Ann. Thorac. Surg., 53:356, 1992.

Jones, D. R., Hill, R. C., Abbott, A. E., et al.: Unusual location of an atrial myxoma complicated by a secundum atrial septal defect. Ann. Thorac. Surg., 55:1252, 1993.

Jones, K. L., Wolf, P. L., Jensen, P., et al.: The Gorlin syndrome: A genetically determined disorder associated with cardiac tumor. Am. Heart J., 111:1013, 1986.

Kidder, L. A.: Congenital glycogenic tumors of the heart. Arch. Pathol., 49:55, 1950.

Klima, T., Milam, J. D., Bossart, M. L., and Cooley, D. A.: Rare primary sarcomas of the heart. Arch. Pathol. Lab. Med., 110:1155, 1986.

Kotani, K., Matsuzawa, Y., Funabashi, T., et al.: Left atrial myxoma metastasizing to the aorta with intraluminal growth causing renovascular hypertension. Cardiology, 78:72, 1991.

Kotylo, P. K., Kennedy, J. E., Waller, B. F., and Sample, R. B.: DNA analysis of atrial myxomas. Chest, 99:1203, 1991.

Krikler, D. M., Rhode, J., Davis, M. J., et al.: Atrial myxoma: A tumour in search of its origins. Br. Heart J., 67:89, 1992.

Landing, B. H., and Farger, S.: Tumors of the cardiovascular system. In Atlas of Tumor Pathology. Sec. III. Fasc. VII. Washington, DC, United States War Department, 1956.

Laya, M. B., Mailliard, J. A., Bewtra, C., and Levin, H. S.: Malignant fibrous histiocytoma of the heart: A case report and review of the literature. Cancer, 59:1026, 1987.

Lee, J., Cheung, K. L., Wang, R., et al.: Malignant fibrous histiocytoma of left atrium. J. Thorac. Cardiovasc. Surg., 3:450, 1987.

Leithiser, R. E., Jr., Fyfe, D., Weatherby, E., III, et al.: Prenatal sonographic diagnosis of atrial hemangioma. Am. J. Roentgenol., 147:1207, 1986.

Leonhardt, E. T. G., and Kullenberg, K. P. G.: Bilateral atrial myxomas with multiple arterial aneurysms: A syndrome mimicking polyarteritis nodosa. Am. J. Med., 62:792, 1977.

MacGregor, G. A., and Cullen, R. A.: Syndrome of fever, anemia and high sedimentation rate with atrial myxoma. Br. Med. J., 2:991, 1959.

Mahaim, I.: Les tumeurs et les polyps du coeur: Etude anatomoclinique. Paris, Masson, 1945.

Maher, E. R., and Buckman, R.: Intrapericardial instillation of bleomycin in malignant pericardial effusion. Am. Heart J., 111:613, 1986.

Malekzadeh, S., and Roberts, W. C.: Growth rate of left atrial myxoma. Am. J. Cardiol., 64:1075, 1989.

Markel, M. L., Armstrong, W. F., Waller, B. F., and Mahomet, Y.: Left atrial myxoma with multicentric recurrence and evidence of metastases. Am. Heart J., 111:409, 1986.

Martin, L. W., Wasserman, A. G., Goldstein, H., et al.: Multiple cardiac myxomas with multiple recurrences: Unusual presentation of a "benign" tumor. Ann. Thorac. Surg., 44:77, 1987.

Martini, N., Freiman, A. H., Watson, R. C., et al.: Intrapericardial instillation of radioactive chromic phosphate in malignant pericardial effusion. Am. J. Roentgenol., 128:639, 1977.

McAllister, H. A., Jr.: Primary tumors and cysts of the heart and pericardium. Curr. Probl. Cardiol., 4:1, 1979.

McAllister, H. A., Jr., and Fenoglio, J. J., Jr.: Tumors of the cardiovascular system. In Hartman, W. H., and Cowan, W. R. (eds): Atlas of Tumor Pathology. Sec. Series, Fasc. 15. Washington, DC, Armed Forces Institute of Pathology, 1978.

McCarthy, P. M., Piehler, J. M., Schaff, H. V., et al.: The significance of multiple, recurrent, and "complex" cardiac myxomas. J. Thorac. Cardiovasc. Surg., 91:389, 1986.

McFadden, P. M., and Lacy, J. R.: Intracardiac papillary fibroelastoma: An occult cause of embolic neurologic deficit. Ann. Thorac. Surg., 43:667, 1987.

Mora, F., Mindich, B. P., Guarino, T., and Goldman, M. E.: Improved surgical approach to cardiac tumors with intraoperative two-dimensional echocardiography. Chest, 91:142, 1987.

Movahed, A., and Wait, J.: Carcinoma of the heart presenting as myocardial infarction. Am. Heart J., 112:1329, 1986.

Murphy, M. C., Sweeney, M. S., Putram, J. B., et al.: Surgical treatment of cardiac tumors—A 25-year experience. Ann. Thorac. Surg., 49:612, 1990.

Nolan, J., Carder, P. J., and Bloomfield, P.: Atrial myxomas—Tumor or trauma? Br. Heart J., 67:406, 1992.

Novick, A., and Cosgrove, D.: Surgical approach for removal of renal cell carcinoma extending into the vena cava and right atrium. J. Urol., 123:977, 1980.

Okada, M., Ohta, T., Yasuoka, S., et al.: Surgical management of intracavitary cardiac tumors: A review of fifteen patients and current status in Japan. J. Cardiovasc. Surg., 27:641, 1986.

O'Neil, M. B., Grehl, T. M., and Hurley, E. J.: Cardiac myxomas: A clinical diagnostic challenge. Am. J. Surg., 138:68, 1979.

Ovcak, Z., Masera, A., and Lamovic, J.: Malignant fibrous histiocytoma of the heart. Arch. Pathol. Lab. Med., 116:872, 1992.

Palazzuoli, V., Mondillo, S., Angelini, G. D., et al.: Myxoma of the left ventricle. Thorac. Cardiovasc. Surg., 34:271, 1986.

Panidis, I. P., Kotler, M. N., Mink, G. S., and Ross, J.: Clinical and echocardiographic features of right atrial masses. Am. Heart J., 107:745, 1984.

Panidis, I. P., Mink, G. S., and McAllister, M.: Hemodynamic consequences of left atrial myxomas as assessed by Doppler ultrasound. Am. Heart J., 111:927, 1986.

Percy, R. F., Perryman, R. A., Amornmam, E., et al.: Prolonged survival in a patient with primary angiosarcoma of the heart. Am. Heart J., 113:1228, 1987.

Pillai, R., Blauth, C., Peckham, M., et al.: Intracardiac metastases from malignant teratoma of the testis. J. Thorac. Cardiovasc. Surg., 92:118, 1986.

Pochis, W. T., Wingo, M. W., Cinguegrani, M. D., and Sagar, K. B.: Echocardiographic demonstration of rapid growth of left atrial myxomas. Am. Heart J., 122:1781, 1991.

Poole, G. V., Breyer, R. H., Holliday, R. H., et al.: Tumors of the heart: Surgical considerations. J. Cardiovasc. Surg., 25:5, 1984.

Powers, J. C., Falkoff, M., Heinle, R. A., et al.: Familial cardiac myxoma: Emphasis on unusual clinical manifestations. J. Thorac. Cardiovasc. Surg., 77:782, 1979.

Press, O. W., and Livingston, R.: Management of malignant pericardial effusion and tamponade. J. A. M. A., 257:1088, 1987.

Read, R. C., White, J. H., Murphy, M. L., et al.: The malignant potentiality of left atrial myxoma. J. Thorac. Cardiovasc. Surg., 6:857, 1974.

Reece, I. H., Cooley, D. A., Frazier, O. H., et al.: Cardiac tumors: Clinical spectrum and prognosis of lesions other than classical benign myxoma in 20 patients. J. Thorac. Cardiovasc. Surg., 88:439, 1984.

Reece, I. H., Houston, A. B., and Pollick, J. C.: Interventricular fibroma: Echocardiographic diagnosis and successful surgical removal in infancy. Br. Heart J., 50:590, 1983.

Sabiston, D. C., Jr., and Hattler, B. G., Jr.: Tumors of the heart. In Sabiston, D. C., Jr., and Spencer, F. C. (eds): Gibbon's Surgery of the Chest. 4th ed. Philadelphia, W. B. Saunders Company, 1983.

Salyer, W. R., Page, D. L., and Hutchins, G. M.: The development of the cardiac myxoma and the papillary endocardial lesions from mural thrombus. Am. Heart J., 89:4, 1975.

Sandrasagra, F. A., Oliver, W. A., and English, T. A. H.: Myxoma of the mitral valve. Br. Heart J., 42:221, 1979.

Schattenberg, T. T.: Echocardiographic diagnosis of left atrial myxoma. Mayo Clin. Proc., 43:620, 1968.

Seifert, P., Chomka, E. V., Stagl, R., et al.: Application of the cine computed tomographic scan for precise localization of the origin of an atrial myxoma: Surgical implications. Ann. Thorac. Surg., 42:469, 1986.

Sellke, F. W., Lemmon, J. H., Vandenberg, B. F., and Ehrenhaft, J. L.: Surgical treatment of cardiac myxomas—Long-term results. Ann. Thorac. Surg., 50:557, 1990.

Selzer, A., Sakai, E. J., and Popper, R. W.: Protean clinical manifestations of primary tumors of the heart. Am. J. Cardiol., 52:9, 1972.

Shin, M. S., Kirklin, J. K., Cain, J. B., and Ho, K. J.: Primary angiosarcoma of the heart: CT characteristics. Am. J. Roentgenol., 148:267, 1987.

Silverman, N. A.: Primary cardiac tumors. Ann. Surg., 191:127, 1980.

Silverman, N. A., and Sabiston, D. C., Jr.: Cardiac neoplasms. In Sabiston, D. C., Jr. (ed): Textbook of Surgery. 12th ed. Philadelphia, W. B. Saunders Company, 1981.

Smith, C.: Tumors of the heart. Arch. Pathol. Lab. Med., 110:371, 1986.

Stowers, S. A., Gilmore, P., Stirling, M., et al.: Cardiac pheochromo-cytoma involving the left main coronary artery presenting with exertional angina. Am. Heart J., *114*:423, 1987.

Strauss, B. L., Matthews, M. J., Cohen, M. N., et al.: Cardiac metas-tases in lung cancer. Chest, *71*:607, 1977.

Sutton, M. G. St. J., Mercier, L. A., Giuliana, E. R., and Lie, J. T.: Atrial myxomas: A review of clinical experience in 40 patients. Mayo Clin. Proc., *55*:371, 1980.

Teoh, K. H., Amin, M., Tomlinson, C. W., and Lobo, F. V.: Right atrial myxoma originating from the eustachian valve. Can. J. Cardiol., *9*:441, 1993.

Tway, K. P., Shah, A. A., and Rahimtoola, S. H.: Multiple biatrial myxomas demonstrated by two-dimensional echocardiogra-phy. Am. J. Med., *71*:896, 1981.

Villafane, J., Salk, M., Kaiser, G., et al.: A rare right atrial tumor presenting with cyanosis in a newborn. Am. Heart J., *113*:1036, 1987.

Wiske, P. S., Gillam, L. D., Blyden, G., and Weyman, A. E.: Intracar-diac tumor regression documented by two-dimensional echo-cardiography. Am. J. Cardiol., *58*:186, 1986.

Wold, L. E., and Lie, J. T.: Cardiac myxomas: A clinicopathological profile. Am. J. Pathol., *101*:219, 1980.

# 57 Transplantation

## ■ I Clinical Heart-Lung Transplantation

John H. Stevens and Bruce A. Reitz

The conceptual simplicity of replacing the cardio-pulmonary axis has been recognized since the early 1900s. Carrel and, later, Demikhov and Marcus and co-workers mentioned the possibility of heart-lung transplantation to replace diseased organs (Carrel, 1907; Demikhov, 1962; Marcus et al., 1951). The operation requires only a right atrial (inflow) anastomosis and aortic (outflow) anastomoses, with a connection at the trachea (airway). The surgical procedure is easier in some ways than isolated heart replacement, which explains why heart and lung transplantation was attempted before orthotopic heart replacement. However, technical simplicity was offset by the reality of severe difficulties with transplantation of lung tissue.

### HISTORICAL ASPECTS

Almost all of the later developments in cardiovascular surgery were anticipated by the experiments of Alexis Carrel. This French-born American surgeon developed many techniques for vascular surgery, and his life and work provide fascinating reading. Among his studies was the transplantation of both heart and lungs, as described in the following manner:

We attempted also to make the transplantation of the lungs together with the heart. Both lungs, the heart, the aorta, and vena cava of a cat one week old were extirpated and put into the neck of a large adult cat. The aorta was anastomosed to the peripheral end of the carotid and the vena cava to the peripheral end of the jugular vein. The coronary circulation was immediately re-established, and the auricles began to beat. The lungs became red, and, after a few minutes, effective pulsations of the ventricles appeared. But the lungs soon became edematous, and distention of the right part of the heart occurred. This accident seems difficult of prevention. A phlegmon of the neck terminated this observation two days later.

Although this experiment had little success, it and other observations by Carrel anticipated the eventual use of transplantation of organs. For these outstanding accomplishments, Carrel received the Nobel Prize in 1912, the first such award to a scientist working in an American laboratory. Many people have speculated why his work was not applied by other surgeons at the time, but no good answers have been found (Comroe, 1979).

In the mid-1940s in Russia, Demikhov and Sinitsyn began their ingenious experiments that showed the technical feasibility of intrathoracic heterotopic heart transplants. Demikhov was also able to devise a method for transplanting the heart-lung block before the advent of cardiopulmonary bypass and hypothermia techniques.

Demikhov's work was first reported in the West in 1962 with the publication of his book *Experimental Transplantation of Vital Organs,* which documents the work of an extremely innovative surgeon. However, Demikhov thought that the failure of all transplanted organs was secondary to technical factors and that immunology did not have a role. He failed to realize that, because of variations in donor and recipient matching, favorable long-term function can occur occasionally despite immunologic rejection.

Demikhov achieved some remarkable firsts, including the first successful heart-lung transplant. By removing the heart-lung block at normothermia and maintaining a heartbeat, he was able to transfer the heart and both lungs or the heart and one lung into a recipient dog. One variation of this experiment is shown in Figure 57–1. Demikhov accomplished the transfer by alternating one of two venous inflow anastomoses (the superior or inferior vena cava) with one of two outflow anastomoses (the brachiocephalic artery or the transverse aortic arch just distal to the brachiocephalic artery) and then the trachea. Thus, he replaced the heart and lungs of the recipient animal while both the donor and the recipient hearts and lungs continued to function with a circulation. As his surgical technique improved, animal survival increased. In Demikhov's experiment, the animal was removed alive from the operating table. The notes from this experiment relate that after the chest was exposed, "spontaneous respiration was resumed, but respirations were infrequent and deep, 7 per minute. Later, respirations ceased, and the animal died shortly thereafter." Other experiments confirmed that the respiratory pattern was very deep, and the animals used the muscles of the abdominal wall and neck,

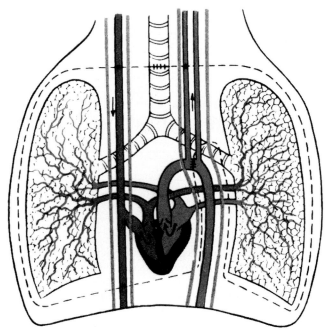

**FIGURE 57–1.** The points of transection and reanastomosis of the heart-lung bloc, as performed by Demikhov in dogs during the late 1940s.

In 1953, Neptune and colleagues from Hahnemann Medical College in Philadelphia and Marcus and associates from the Chicago Medical School presented papers on experimental heart-lung transplantation in the same volume of the *Archives of Surgery*. Neptune and colleagues (1953) reported what they thought was the first successful replacement of the heart and both lungs by using hypothermia and circulatory arrest. In their three experiments, one animal survived as long as 6 hours and had satisfactory blood pressure, spontaneous respiration, and return of reflexes. They concluded that this preparation was an "ideal way of obtaining a completely denervated heart, as well as lungs, for physiologic study."

Marcus and associates (1953) described heterotopic heart-lung transplantation to the intra-abdominal aorta and vena cava of a recipient animal. In eight animals, they sutured the superior and inferior venae cavae of the donor heart and lungs to the distal inferior vena cava of the recipient, the brachiocephalic artery of the donor to the proximal abdominal aorta, and the transverse aortic arch to the distal abdominal aorta. The trachea was then exteriorized and mechanically ventilated. Nitrogen was given to the recipient's own trachea, and circulation was maintained by administering oxygen to the trachea of the donor. The experimental preparation is shown in Figure 57–3.

with their mouths open. These changes in respiratory pattern were later associated with complete cardiopulmonary denervation in the dog.

In all, Demikhov subjected 67 dogs to replacement of the heart and lungs. Although many dogs died on the operating table or within 24 hours after operation, 8 survived more than 48 hours and 2 survived 5 and 6 days, respectively. His experiments proved that the operation was feasible from the point of view of surgical technique. The animal that survived longest is shown in Figure 57–2. In a prophetic statement, Demikhov noted that "In the surgery of the future, when the causes of the complications and failures attending these operations have been studied and overcome, transplantation of the heart, together with the lungs, will find its application in irreversible forms of cardiopulmonary insufficiency."

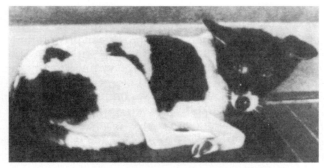

**FIGURE 57–2.** The dog "Damka" in 1951, after heart-lung transplantation by Demikhov. The dog survived for 6 days and died of pulmonary failure, probably as a result of allograft rejection, although this was not appreciated by Demikhov.

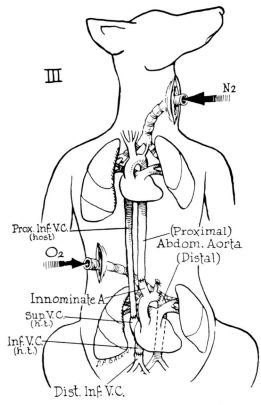

**FIGURE 57–3.** The use of a heterotopic heart-lung transplant to support the host as reported by Marcus and associates. (From Marcus, E., Wong, S. N. T., and Luisada, A. A.: Homologous heart grafts. Arch. Surg., 66:179, 1953. Copyright 1953, American Medical Association.)

The surgeons were able to maintain the recipient for approximately 75 minutes after the heart of the host animal had died.

Marcus and associates described a second experiment. While the heart and lung preparation was functioning in the abdominal position, the chest of the host was entered and the main pulmonary artery was occluded temporarily to empty the left side of the heart. The heart was then opened with an incision in the left atrial appendage, and the mitral valve was manipulated under direct vision. After 7 minutes of intracardiac exposure, the atrium was closed and the heart was allowed to beat again. Thus, these authors had devised a method for open intracardiac surgery with a donor heart and lungs used as the pump oxygenator.

In 1957, Webb and Howard reported the use of a pump oxygenator to do heart-lung transplantation in dogs. They could restore the heart to relatively normal function, and the animals lived from 75 minutes to 22 hours. They anticipated later technical difficulties, because they noted continued bleeding from the extensive raw surfaces that developed during the dissection, and none of the animals returned to spontaneous normal respiration. They also reported four attempts at autotransplantation of the heart and lungs, but although cardiac function was sufficient, the animals were unable to breathe spontaneously. In other experiments where heart transplantation alone was performed, there was an immediate return to spontaneous respiration, which again suggested that cardiopulmonary denervation was not tolerated well by dogs. Webb and Howard concluded that transplantation of the heart and both lungs was not practical because respiratory paralysis would occur. They suggested that transplantation of the heart with one lung would prevent respiratory paralysis by retaining one innervated lung.

The next encouraging report was from Lower and co-workers (1961), who had previously reported the first significant survival after orthotopic heart transplantation in the dog, and who now turned to complete heart-lung replacement. They emphasized the need to preserve the recipient's phrenic and vagus nerves and to carefully ligate bronchial vessels. The donor organs were immersed in cold saline solution at 4° C for topical hypothermia, and anastomoses were performed at the aorta, trachea, and both venae cavae. Six animals resumed spontaneous respiration, although the respiratory pattern showed increased tidal volume and low respiratory rate. This now-familiar pattern is typical of a dog with cardiopulmonary denervation. Two of the animals survived for as long as 4 days postoperatively. These authors concluded that the lung could survive without a bronchial arterial supply, but the question of prolonged survival after pulmonary denervation remained unanswered.

In a study of heart-lung transplantation in dogs, Longmore and colleagues (1969) introduced the concept of a single inflow anastomosis at the right atrium. One dog survived for 25 hours. A co-author,

Cooper (1969), wrote a historical review as part of the study. Clearly, although surgical technique was capable of heart-lung transplantation, cardiopulmonary denervation had to be overcome.

Insight into the breathing difficulties after denervation came from the experiments of Nakae and associates (1967), who performed different types of cardiopulmonary autotransplantation in several species of animals. First, they divided the great vessels, vena cava, and trachea, and divided all other tissue that connected the heart and lungs with the surrounding structures. In dogs who had this type of denervation, the breathing pattern was extremely slow and abnormal, as in dogs who had heart-lung transplantation. When mediastinal denervation was complete but without transection of the great vessels, the breathing pattern was also abnormal. In a third group, complete mediastinal denervation without tracheal transection also caused an abnormal breathing pattern, and the animals died of respiratory failure. In the final group, the major vessels were divided without pulmonary denervation, and these dogs resumed spontaneous respiration with a normal respiratory pattern. The procedure was repeated in cats with the same results. Finally, when the experiments were performed in monkeys, a relatively normal respiratory pattern was resumed despite pulmonary denervation; deaths were caused by technical factors, such as bleeding or air leakage, not by respiratory insufficiency.

Proof of these physiologic experiments came in 1972, with reports by Casteñeda and co-workers at the University of Minnesota. They operated on primates to avoid respiratory difficulties and performed autotransplants to avoid allograft rejection. Among 40 baboons, 6 survived for more than 1 month and several survived for more than 1 year after operation. In addition, these authors examined the pulmonary ventilation and perfusion and circulatory hemodynamics in baboons and found that, in all respects, they were normal (Castañeda et al., 1972a, 1972b). The authors predicted that heart-lung transplantation would be successful in patients.

Primate studies were begun in 1978 by Reitz and associates at Stanford University (Reitz et al., 1980). The initial experiments in small cynomolgus monkeys were with autotransplants. Hypothermia and circulatory arrest was the technique used first; later, cardiopulmonary bypass was found to give better results (Reitz et al., 1981). Animals given autotransplants had normal cardiopulmonary function and long-term survival.

In the late 1970s, cyclosporine was studied in several laboratories, and it was suggested that this immunosuppressive drug could prevent allograft rejection. A small amount of the material was available in the Stanford laboratory, and it was used for the treatment of monkeys after heart-lung allotransplantation; these were the first animals to receive lung transplants with cyclosporine for immunosuppression. The drug prevented allograft rejection without obvious toxicity, and several animals survived for more than 1 year after heart-lung allotransplantation

(Reitz et al., 1980). Several of these animals lived for more than 5 years after allotransplantation (Harjula et al., 1987). The early results suggested that the degree of rejection was similar in the heart and lung and that the clinically useful endomyocardial biopsy might be sufficient after the rejection. Later clinical experience proved that pulmonary rejection could occur without cardiac rejection, but the survival of these animals gave encouragement for a new clinical trial.

Cooley and colleagues made three attempts at human heart-lung transplantation beginning in 1968. The recipient was a 2½-month-old child with atrioventricular canal and severe pulmonary hypertension. The child died 14 hours postoperatively of pulmonary failure (Cooley et al., 1969). In December 1969, Lillehei and associates transplanted the heart and lungs of a 50-year-old woman into a 43-year-old man with end-stage emphysema. He was extubated on the first postoperative day and was ambulatory, but developed bronchopneumonia and died on the eighth postoperative day (Lillehei, 1970). Barnard performed a heart-lung transplant in 1971 in a patient who died of a tracheobronchial fistula and intractable pneumonia 23 days after transplantation (Losman et al., 1982).

A new clinical era of heart-lung transplantation was ushered in at Stanford University in 1981. The first patient was Mary Gohlke, a 45-year-old woman with end-stage pulmonary hypertension. The donor was brought to Stanford to minimize ischemic time, and the heart-lung transplant procedure was identical to that developed in earlier laboratory studies. Figure 57–4 shows the thorax after removal of the heart and lungs. Gohlke was treated with azathioprine and cyclosporine for 14 days, after which time the azathioprine was discontinued and prednisone initiated. An acute rejection episode 10 days after the transplantation required intubation and ventilatory assistance, but she was later discharged from the hospital in

good condition and was very well for more than 5 years after transplantation (Reitz et al., 1982).

Heart-lung transplantation and transplantation in general have experienced continued growth and improvement. Currently, the factors that restrict heart-lung transplantation include the most important, the lack of suitable donors, as well as the shortcomings of available preservation techniques, perioperative hemorrhage, severe and recurrent pulmonary infections, and chronic late rejection manifested as bronchiolitis obliterans. These and other problem areas are addressed later in this chapter.

## RECIPIENT DIAGNOSIS

Many patients with end-stage disease of the heart and lungs can be helped with heart and lung transplantation. The most common indications for heart-lung transplantation include Eisenmenger's complex and primary pulmonary hypertension. Patients with other diseases, such as cystic fibrosis, complex congenital heart disease (including univentricular heart with pulmonary atresia), or pulmonary lymphangioleiomyomatosis, may be best treated with heart-lung transplantation (Kaye, 1992).

Patients with primary pulmonary hypertension, pulmonary fibrosis, emphysema, and alpha-antitrypsin deficiency may also be treated effectively with single-lung or bilateral single-lung transplantation. These indications may also be expanded to include single-lung or bilateral single-lung transplantation with concomitant repair of an atrial septal defect or small ventricular septal defect or closure of a patent ductus arteriosus. With the continuing crisis of severe donor limitation, the optimal use of this scarce resource is yet to be fully defined. Both the lungs and the heart from a single donor may benefit carefully selected recipients (Reitz, 1992). The development of the "domino" procedure, with the recipient of a heart-lung transplant acting as a heart donor, has further improved donor organ allocation (Baumgartner et al., 1989; Yacoub et al., 1988).

## CONSIDERATION FOR SELECTION OF RECIPIENTS

Any patient with severe, end-stage cardiopulmonary disease may be considered for heart-lung transplantation. Suitable candidates should have a life expectancy of less than 1 to 2 years, and generally have marked persistent functional disability. The occurrence of life-threatening complications, such as massive hemoptysis, severe right-sided congestive heart failure, or multiple syncopal episode, suggests the need to list a patient for heart-lung transplantation.

Recipients of heart-lung transplants are generally younger than heart transplant recipients (average age, 30 years versus 45 years) and are more likely to be female (54% versus 19%) (Kaye, 1992). Good candidates must be psychologically stable, have a support-

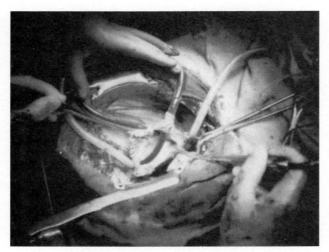

FIGURE 57–4. Appearance of the empty chest of a 45-year-old patient with primary pulmonary hypertension who received a heart-lung transplant in March 1981. The aortic clamp is to the right; the cuff of right atrium is easily seen with the cannulas inserted into the venae cavae.

ive social network, and be willing to comply with a complex and often intrusive medical regimen.

Heart-lung transplantation has become more prevalent as a therapeutic option for cystic fibrosis and complex congenital heart disease in infants and children (Michler and Rose, 1991; Scott et al., 1988; Smyth et al., 1990). These recipients should have an extremely strong family support network in order to cope with the complex and frequent medical follow-up required.

Heart-lung transplantation should be undertaken before multisystem organ failure and severe malnutrition ensue. Many patients, as they await a suitable donor, become increasingly debilitated. Every opportunity to optimize their physical strength and nutritional status should be pursued. Because of the magnitude of the operation and the risk of hemorrhage, patients with significant hepatic dysfunction must be excluded as potential candidates.

In the past, most centers considered a history of previous cardiac and thoracic surgery a contraindication to heart-lung transplantation. Historically, these patients have a marked increase in morbidity and short-term mortality primarily owing to excessive blood loss and concomitant problems associated with massive transfusion. The introduction of aprotinin in thoracic transplantation has provided a tremendous advance for this group of patients. The use of aprotinin has markedly decreased the blood requirements and increased the safety for transplantation (Kemkes, 1993; Roysten, 1993). We now routinely accept patients with previous cardiac or thoracic surgery for transplantation.

In patients selected for transplantation, routine pretransplant screening is done for ABO blood group, the presence of preformed antibodies (by screening against 50 random donors), human leukocyte antigen (HLA) and DR tissue types, and titers of antibodies against cytomegalovirus, herpes simplex virus, and toxoplasmosis. A portable anteroposterior chest film is used to obtain measurements of the transverse and vertical dimensions of the thoracic cavity for comparison with similar measurements of potential donors.

## SELECTION AND MANAGEMENT OF DONORS

There are far fewer suitable donors for lung transplantation than for heart, kidney, or liver transplantation. A wide variety of problems can prohibit the use of many donor lungs. Brain death is occasionally associated with neurogenic pulmonary edema. Blunt trauma frequently causes contusion, aspiration is frequent during resuscitation, and ventilator support predisposes to nosocomial infection. Less than 20% of cadaveric donors have lungs that are suitable for transplantation. In 1992, there were 1849 heart transplants and only 42 heart-lung transplants (Kaye, 1992). These numbers reflect the difficulty in obtaining suitable lungs, as well as the pressure of organ transplant centers to use the heart for critically ill

heart recipients, even if the lungs are acceptable for heart-lung transplantation. This allocation system is unique to the United States. Worldwide, excluding the United States, there were 2695 heart transplants and 129 heart-lung transplants performed in 1992 (Kaye, 1992). The extreme scarcity of heart donors will continue to be a major problem in meeting the clinical need.

The ideal heart-lung donor must meet the criteria for cardiac donation, as well as an arterial oxygen tension of more than 300 mm Hg, with an inspired oxygen concentration of 100%. The chest film must be free of infiltrates, and the sputum should be free of purulence. If a question arises about the suitability of the lungs, bronchoscopy may be useful.

The lung volumes of the donor can be estimated from the anteroposterior portable chest film, as shown in Figure 57–5. Generally, the measurements should not be more than 4 cm greater than the recipient and should preferably be smaller than the measurements of the recipient, although pulmonary stapling techniques have been advocated to accommodate size mismatch with success.

## HEART–LUNG PRESERVATION

Successful uniform preservation of the lung has been elusive. Because it is important to have good lung function immediately following transplantation, little margin is allowed for inadequate preservation. In the initial heart-lung transplants, researchers felt that donor transportation to the transplant center with on-site procurement was essential. As with heart

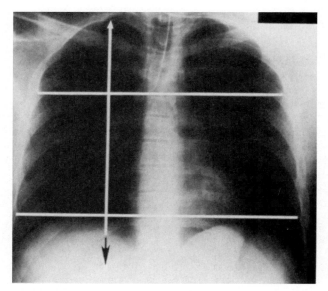

**FIGURE 57–5.** Anteroposterior portable chest radiograph of a potential heart-lung transplant donor. The transverse diameter of the chest is measured at the aortic knob, and the widest portion of the chest is measured at the top of the diaphragm. The vertical dimension from the apex to a line drawn between both costophrenic angles is also measured, and all of these measurements are compared with similar measurements of the potential recipient.

transplantation, adequate preservation techniques would expand the pool of available donors and would make donation simpler for the referring hospitals, as well as for the donor's family. This clinical need produced a variety of creative solutions to the problems of pulmonary ischemia and subsequent reperfusion injury.

The common result of inadequate preservation is an abnormal increase in extravascular pulmonary water. As the alveolar-capillary membrane integrity is lost, the pulmonary interstitium allows passage of high molecular weight proteins. The subsequent passage of fluid causes a progressive exudate of fluid into the interstitium and alveoli. This in turn diminishes airway compliance and gas exchange and increases pulmonary vascular resistance.

The causes of immediate graft dysfunction are most commonly related to direct cellular injury from poor preservation and reperfusion injury. Reperfusion injury is caused by a complex interplay between leukocytes, oxygen free radicals, complement, cytokines, and arachidonic acid metabolites (Hall et al., 1987; McCord, 1983; Pham et al., 1992; Pillai et al., 1990).

Since the early 1980s, various methods have been developed to address the problems associated with inadequate preservation. These have varied from simple graft excision and cold storage to sophisticated autoperfusion with donor blood. Today, only two methods are actively employed. Donor core cooling on cardiopulmonary bypass followed by cold cardioplegia and cold storage has been used with great success (Fraser et al., 1988a; Novick et al., 1992). But because of the simplicity, lower cost, and equivalent clinical result, a single flush perfusion of the lungs has been the most widely adopted method. This perfusion method should include the systemic or local administration of vasodilators, and the pulmonary perfusion solution can be crystalloid or colloid. The preservation techniques of several prominent centers (Baldwin et al., 1987a; Fraser et al., 1988b) are listed in Table 57–1.

## OPERATIVE TECHNIQUE FOR DONOR HEART–LUNG REMOVAL

In the early days of heart-lung transplantation, the donor was transported to the recipient hospital, and in an adjacent operating room, the recipient heart-lung block was excised simultaneously with donor organ preparation. More recently, with improvement in preservation techniques, long-distance procurement is the rule. With numerous procurement teams working together, optimal communication is essential.

Exposure is obtained via a median sternotomy. The pericardium is widely excised anteriorly and laterally to the level of the pulmonary veins. The ascending aorta and aortic arch are dissected free and encircled with tapes. The superior vena cava is dissected to the innominate vein. The azygos vein, innominate vein, and innominate artery are ligated and divided. This allows excellent exposure to the proximal trachea, where it can be looped, keeping dissection of the distal trachea at a minimum to avoid injury to the bronchial vessels.

Gradual weaning of the $F_{IO_2}$ to 21% is accomplished to minimize tissue injury during preservation owing to oxygen free radicals. The patient is given 300 U/kg of intravenous heparin, and an infusion of prostaglandin $E_1$ is initiated, beginning with a dose of 50 ng/kg/min and gradually increasing to 250 ng/kg/min or until systemic hypotension is seen. Inflow occlusion is accomplished by ligating and dividing the superior vena cava proximally to avoid damage to the sinoatrial node. The inferior vena cava is clamped and divided, and the aortic cross-clamp is applied. Crystalloid cardioplegia is administered via the aortic root, and pulmonary perfusate is given through a No. 14 French sump catheter in the main pulmonary artery at 60 ml/kg over 5 minutes. An incision is made in the left atrial appendage to allow a free egress of fluid and to eliminate the possibility of cardiac distention (Fig. 57–6). During the administration of cold cardioplegia and pulmonary perfusate,

■ **Table 57–1.** PRESERVATION METHODS FOR HEART-LUNG AND LUNG TRANSPLANTATION

| Center | Pretreatment | Perfusion Solution | Storage | References |
|---|---|---|---|---|
| Papworth Hospital Cambridge, England | Prostacyclin 10–20 ng/kg/min into pulmonary artery 10–20 min before removal | Ringers 700 ml, 20% salt-poor albumin 200 ml, 20% mannitol 100 ml, donor blood 400 ml, prostacyclin 20 mcg, CPD 63 ml | 4° C Saline | Wheeldon et al., 1988 |
| Stanford University Stanford, California | Systemic PGE₁ 50–250 ng/kg/min 15 min before removal | 60 ml/kg of Collins solution with added 50% dextrose 65 ml/l, magnesium sulfate 12 mEq/l | 4° C Physiosol (Abbott Laboratory) | Baldwin et al., 1987a |
| Harefield Hospital London, England | None | Cold blood by means of CPB | Cold blood from oxygenator | Yacoub et al., 1988 |
| Johns Hopkins Hospital Baltimore, Maryland | Isoproterenol 20 ng/kg/min 10–20 min before bypass | Cold blood by means of CPB | 4° C Collins solution | Fraser et al., 1988a |

*Key:* CPD = citrated phosphate dextrose; CPB = cardiopulmonary bypass.

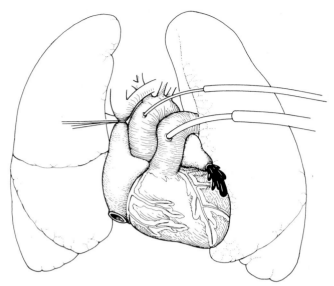

**FIGURE 57–6.** Technique for heart-lung graft procurement. The use of high-volume, low-pressure crystalloid flush for pulmonary preservation, in combination with systemic administration of prostaglandin E, has proved simple and effective in distant graft preservation.

copious amounts of cold topical saline solution are used. The lungs are ventilated with room air with a moderate tidal volume while the dissection is completed, separating the heart-lung block from the posterior mediastinum from inferior to superior. The trachea is stapled with a TA 30-4.8 stapling device and divided during moderate inflation of the lungs. The aorta is divided, and the graft is immersed in Physiosol at 4° C in preparation for transport. Clinically, we have used grafts preserved up to 6 hours with successful implantation and outcome.

## OPERATIVE PROCEDURE

The operative procedure to replace the heart and lungs is one of the most fascinating and challenging procedures for cardiothoracic surgeons. The anatomy that is seen and the areas of the thorax that are dissected are not commonly seen in other procedures. Careful attention to details can simplify the procedure in even the most challenging patients.

Patients with primary pulmonary hypertension are usually the ideal candidates for transplantation. These patients generally have not had previous cardiac or thoracic surgery or large mediastinal collaterals from cyanosis. Patients with congenital heart disease and pulmonary atresia or severe cyanosis owing to Eisenmenger's syndrome may have large mediastinal bronchial collaterals that require careful ligation. The most challenging aspect of the procedure is to remove the heart and lungs without injury to the phrenic, recurrent laryngeal, and vagus nerves. Attention to hemostasis is also necessary because, after implantation of the graft, exposure of many of the areas of dissection is difficult.

The patient is prepared for operation with the usual monitoring lines. After the induction of anesthesia, the chest and both groins are prepared and draped in a sterile manner. A standard median sternotomy incision is made, and both pleural spaces are opened anteriorly. A portion of the pericardium is removed anteriorly, but a large segment of pericardium is left laterally to later support the heart and to protect the phrenic nerves. The ascending aorta and both venae cavae are dissected free and encircled with tapes. If the patient can tolerate further manipulation, the phrenic nerve on the right is then dissected free by incising the pericardium just posterior to the phrenic nerve and anterior to the right pulmonary veins. Alternately, the right phrenic nerve is left in situ and the opening for the right lung is made by opening the left atrium through the orifices of the right superior and inferior pulmonary veins after cardiopulmonary bypass is started and the heart and right lung are removed.

Cannulation is performed routinely in the high ascending aorta, and the superior and inferior venae cavae are cannulated separately. When cardiopulmonary bypass is instituted, the patient is cooled to approximately 30° C. The aorta is cross-clamped, and a small amount of cardioplegia is given to induce cardiac arrest. When the operation was first performed on patients, an effort was made to remove the heart and lungs en bloc. When monkeys were operated on, it was relatively easy to dissect and remove the heart and lungs together. Experience later showed that this was relatively difficult and unnecessary in the human thorax, and the technique of sequential removal of the heart and lungs was used.

The heart is excised at the ascending aorta just above the aortic valve through the main pulmonary artery and the atrioventricular groove along the right atrium and across into the left atrium (Fig. 57–7). This procedure is similar to the standard cardiectomy for cardiac transplantation.

At this point, the left phrenic nerve can be easily dissected free by incising the pericardium anterior to the left pulmonary veins. Both the right and the left phrenic nerves are now freed, and there is good access to both pleural spaces. The pulmonary ligaments are divided inferiorly and the pulmonary artery and vein are divided in each hilum by using electrocautery, which is shown in Figure 57–8. The right and left bronchi are skeletonized, and a stapling device (TA surgical stapler, 30-4.8 mm) is used to occlude them. Cutting the bronchus distally allows the lung to be removed easily and avoids contamination from the open bronchus.

The final step in preparing the recipient is to open the pericardium at the superior part of the pericardial space just anterior to the right and left bronchi, allowing dissection back to the carina. In this area, it is important to stay right on the bronchus, use electrocautery, if possible, and avoid injury to the vagus nerve as it passes posterior to the bronchus and anterior to the esophagus, as shown in Figure

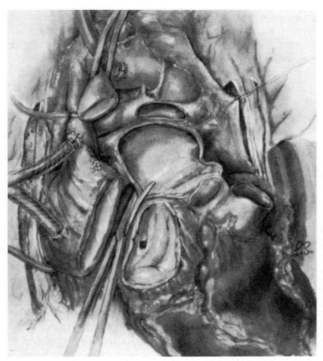

**FIGURE 57–7.** Cannulation for cardiopulmonary bypass is performed in the usual manner: a cannula in the high ascending aorta and a separate vena caval cannula through the right atrium. Cardiectomy is similar to that for standard cardiac transplantation, with an adequate cuff of right atrium left in the recipient for later anastomosis.

57–9. The vascular lymph nodes in this area may be very large, particularly in patients with cystic fibrosis.

A portion of the pulmonary artery is left intact adjacent to the underside of the aorta in the region of the ligamentum arteriosus, which minimizes damage to the recurrent laryngeal nerve. The portion of right pulmonary artery that is left in place can be opened anteriorly and used to wrap the anterior tracheal suture line to separate it from the aorta. The trachea is not opened until just before implantation of the graft, to minimize bronchial spillage into the mediastinum.

The donor heart-and-lung graft is then prepared for implantation. The graft is removed from its sterile container and brought to the operative field in a basin with cold saline solution. The trachea is excised several rings above the carina, and the superior tracheal segment with the clamp attached is then removed from the field. The tracheobronchial tree is aspirated with a sucker that is later discarded. At the same time, a culture is taken directly from the trachea. The trachea is then trimmed back so that only one complete cartilaginous ring is left just above the carina. The authors often use a syringe full of normal saline solution to irrigate the bronchi and visualize them for retained secretions or any foreign body that might have been aspirated by the donor.

Next, the graft is lowered into the chest, with the right lung placed below the right atrial cuff and the right phrenic nerve (Fig. 57–10). Cold saline solution and gauze pads soaked in cold saline solution are

placed over the lung and heart to maintain hypothermia during implantation. The recipient trachea is opened just above the carina, with all the adventitial peritracheal tissue that is adjacent to the superior tracheal segment left in place. Small bronchial vessels may require a Liga clip or suture; use of electrocautery at the cut edge of the trachea should be avoided. The tracheal anastomosis, with a running suture of 3-0 polypropylene is started on the left side of the trachea, and the posterior row is sewn from inside. The same suture is continued anteriorly from outside the trachea. There should be a fairly close size match between donor and recipient, but any disparity can generally be accommodated by the flexible membranous part of the trachea. These bites usually go around at least one cartilaginous ring, and the donor trachea slightly invaginates the recipient trachea in most cases. When the tracheal anastomosis is complete, the chest is irrigated with several liters of ice-cold saline solution to cool the graft and to help remove any contamination from the trachea.

The donor right atrium is opened as in a standard cardiac transplant. The inferior vena cava is opened laterally and then brought up toward the right atrial appendage to make a right atrial cuff that is similar in size to the recipient right atrial opening. The right atria of the donor and recipient should be inspected for the presence of a patent foramen ovale or an atrial septal defect, which is repaired if found. A very long (54-inch) 3-0 polypropylene suture is then used for a continuous anastomosis of the right atrium (Fig. 57–11). The ligation of the superior vena cava, performed

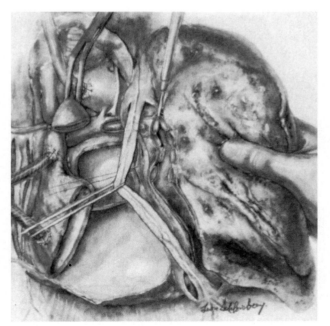

**FIGURE 57–8.** The left phrenic nerve is freed from the hilum of the left lung. The inferior ligament is divided, together with the pulmonary artery and veins, by using the electrocautery. The left bronchus is transected after closure of the proximal segment with a stapling device. A similar maneuver is then performed on the right lung.

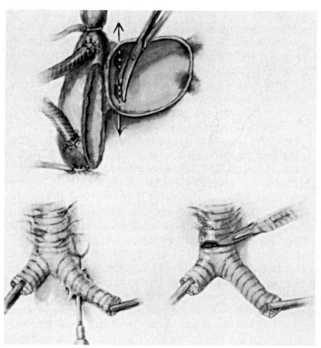

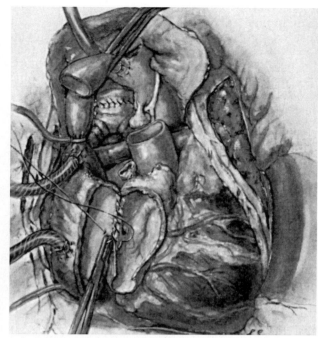

**FIGURE 57–9.** An alternative method of providing access to the right pleural space. The right superior and inferior pulmonary veins can be opened together and the opening is extended by incising the atrial wall superiorly and inferiorly, which creates a space for passing the right lung of the donor into the right thorax. The right and left bronchi are freed by grasping the closed ends of the bronchi and dissecting with an electrocautery. Care must be taken to protect the vagus nerve, which passes just anterior to the esophagus in this area. The recipient's trachea is divided one cartilaginous ring above the tracheal bifurcation.

**FIGURE 57–11.** The donor right atrium is joined to the right atrial cuff of the recipient with a long, running suture of 3-0 polypropylene. The right atrium of the graft has been opened in a manner similar to that for standard cardiac transplantation, with ligation of the superior vena cava and protection of the region of the sinoatrial node (*stippled area*).

earlier, is reinforced with a mattress suture. The patient is then rewarmed to 37° C.

In the case of heart donation from a heart-lung recipient (domino donor), the authors modify the procedure by cannulating the vena cava directly and dividing the vena cava at removal of the heart. The

donor heart-lung is then implanted with separate superior and inferior caval anastomoses, as shown in Figure 57–12.

The donor aorta is trimmed to the appropriate length, and a 4-0 polypropylene suture is used for aortic anastomosis. After the anastomosis, the patient is placed in a slightly head-down position, the ascending aorta and pulmonary artery are aspirated for air, and the caval tapes and aortic clamp are removed. The authors usually begin a slow infusion of isopro-

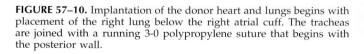

**FIGURE 57–10.** Implantation of the donor heart and lungs begins with placement of the right lung below the right atrial cuff. The tracheas are joined with a running 3-0 polypropylene suture that begins with the posterior wall.

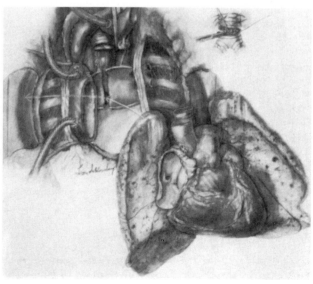

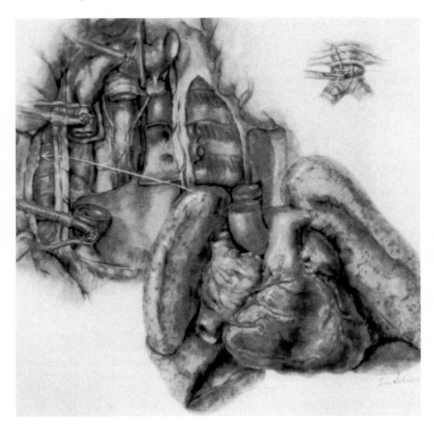

**FIGURE 57–12.** Modification of the heart-lung transplant procedure when the recipient has donated the heart for another heart transplant operation. The venae cavae are cannulated separately, with right-angled cannulas, and separate superior and inferior vena caval anastomoses are required. Otherwise, the implantation is the same as the one described earlier.

terenol (0.02 μm/kg/min) with initial reperfusion, to increase the heart rate slightly and decrease pulmonary vascular resistance. The tracheal tube is aspirated with sterile technique, and ventilation is resumed with an inspired oxygen concentration of 50%. When the patient's body temperature is almost normal and heart and lung function is satisfactory, cardiopulmonary bypass is discontinued and decannulation is done routinely. Temporary pacing wires are applied to the donor right atrium and ventricle and brought out through the skin below the incision. Right-angled chest tubes are left in the right and left pleural spaces, and protamine and any required clotting factors are administered. The appearance of the chest just before closure is shown in Figure 57–13.

By decreasing the tidal volume and using hand ventilation, it is possible to rotate the right or left lung out into the mid-portion of the incision to observe the posterior mediastinum on that side and assess any bleeding from adhesions in either pleural space. The authors use large amounts of saline solution at 37° C to irrigate both pleural spaces and the mediastinum. When hemostasis is satisfactory, the wound is closed routinely with multiple stainless-steel sternal wires.

## POSTOPERATIVE MANAGEMENT

### Intensive Care Unit

The immediate postoperative management of the heart-lung transplant patient is similar to that of any

patient following cardiac surgery. Patients are allowed to awaken early in the postoperative course, and are monitored closely for hemodynamic stability and bleeding. Endotracheal tube suctioning is performed routinely when appropriate, and the patient is weaned from the ventilator in a routine manner. When the patient is appropriately alert and hemodynamically stable and blood gases and ventilatory mechanics are satisfactory, the patient is extubated. Strict attention is paid to fluid balance, and a vigorous diuresis is encouraged in most patients.

As soon as possible, the patient is allowed to sit in a chair and begin ambulation. A physical therapist works with the patient to encourage rapid rehabilitation.

### Immunosuppression

Before transplantation, all patients receive oral cyclosporine at a dose of 10 mg/kg. On release of the aortic cross-clamp, 15 mg/kg of methylprednisolone is administered. No other steroids are given until 2 to 3 weeks postoperatively, when prednisone is begun at 0.2 mg/kg/day. The patient is started on cyclosporine at 10 mg/kg/day in two divided doses, or 2 to 4 mg/kg/day of continuous infusion if the patient is unable to take the oral form. The serum levels of cyclosporine are regulated by adjusting the dose to achieve a serum level of 100 to 200 ng/ml in the first 3 months and 50 to 150 ng/ml thereafter. In addition, patients receive azathioprine as a 4 mg/kg loading dose followed by a maintenance dose of 2 mg/kg/day, which is continued daily if the white blood count remains above 4000/mm$^3$ (Griffith et al., 1992; McCarthy et al., 1990). The most recent addition has been the administration of OKT$_3$ (monoclonal antibodies) at 5 mg/kg/day each day for the first 10 days.

The maintenance regimen then includes cyclosporine, azathioprine, and low-dose prednisone. This has provided effective immunosuppression, with a decreased incidence of renal dysfunction when compared with previous two-drug protocols.

## Complications

### Rejection

The fine balance between adequate immunosuppression and infection or rejection remains one of the most difficult problems facing heart-lung transplantation. The detection of acute rejection is very rare in the first postoperative week. Most rejection episodes are heralded as pulmonary dysfunction with hypoxia, low-grade fever, a decrease in FEV$_1$ and FEF 50%, or diffuse interstitial infiltrate on chest film (Hoeper et al., 1992). In the early postoperative period, pleural effusion is also seen. It has also become clear that simultaneous rejection of the heart and lungs is rare, and endomyocardial biopsy does not help diagnose lung rejection (Baldwin et al., 1987b).

In a study of right ventricular endomyocardial biopsies after heart-lung transplantation, Glanville and colleagues (1987) showed a striking reduction in the frequency of acute rejection after the third postoperative month. A total of 159 biopsies from 35 patients showed an incidence of acute rejection of 1.9% after 4 months. Fully 40% of the transplant recipients had no evidence of acute cardiac rejection. These results are in sharp contrast to those patients who have had a heart transplant alone. Because of these findings, the authors have omitted routine right ventricular endomyocardial biopsy after 6 weeks.

The clinical differentiation between acute allograft rejection or infection can be difficult. The Papworth Hospital group first described the use of histopathologic evaluation of transbronchial biopsy specimens to make the diagnosis of rejection (Stewart et al., 1988). This has become the most important tool in confirming rejection (Starnes et al., 1989; Yousem et al., 1991). The measurement of serum levels of interleukin-6 also shows some promise as a noninvasive test to help diagnose rejection (Yoshida et al., 1993). If rejection is present or highly likely, the authors recommend a 3-day protocol of intravenous methylprednisolone 10 to 15 mg/kg/day. Generally, this therapy reverses the infiltrate and improves compliance as well as oxygenation. The chest film of a 7-year-old patient with the diagnosis of rejection 10 days after heart-lung transplantation is shown in Figure 57–14. The second chest film was taken after 3 days of intravenous methylprednisolone. Resistant

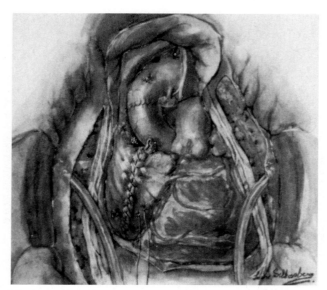

FIGURE 57–13. The completed operation with all cannulas removed. Chest tubes are inserted into both the right and the left pleural space, and temporary pacing wires are applied to the donor right atrium. The sternotomy wound is closed in the usual manner with wire suture.

episodes can be treated with continued high-dose steroids and OKT$_3$ monoclonal antibodies. In refractory cases of rejection, the authors have used total lymphoid irradiation with some success.

### Infection

Infectious complications remain a formidable problem. The spectrum of potential pathogens is extensive, yet some common patterns can be appreciated. In the early postoperative period, bacterial pneumonia is most prevalent, affecting up to 66% of patients (Dummer et al., 1986). Cytomegalovirus (CMV) is a particularly difficult and common problem. It occurs in 50% of patients, and typically is seen in the first 2 months following transplantation. The syndrome of CMV infection can vary from asymptomatic to overwhelming viremia with multisystem organ failure (Maurer et al., 1992). CMV pneumonia is particularly common, and is characterized by fever, cough, hypoxia, and pulmonary infiltrates on chest film (Millet et al., 1989). That the clinical syndrome of pulmonary allograft rejection is identical poses a diagnostic dilemma, and liberal use of transbronchial biopsy has provided essential information. Primary CMV infection has a major impact on mortality and morbidity following heart-lung transplantation (Burke et al., 1986). There is also a strong correlation between early CMV infection and the late development of bronchiolitis obliterans. The authors now routinely treat all seronegative recipients receiving a CMV-positive graft with prophylactic ganciclovir (Duncan et al., 1991; Smyth et al., 1991).

Other common infections include fungi; *Aspergillus* and *Candida* are the most prevalent. *Pneumocystis carinii* and the Epstein-Barr virus are also frequent pathogens. Infectious complications are the cause of

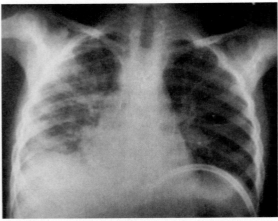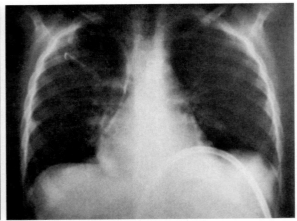

**FIGURE 57–14.** Posteroanterior chest films of a 7-year-old patient after heart-lung transplantation for cystic fibrosis. On the left is the film 10 days after transplantation when the diagnosis of rejection was made. The film on the right shows the patient 3 days later after treatment with intravenous methylprednisolone.

death in 30% of all heart-lung transplant recipients (Kaye, 1992).

### Bronchiolitis Obliterans

The major long-term complication following heart-lung transplantation is the development of chronic lung disease characterized as bronchiolitis obliterans (OB). The disease is histologically identical to OB seen in the nontransplanted individual, which is considered by many to be an immune-mediated disease. This complication develops in over one-third of all patients who survive more than 6 months, and can be seen as early as 2 to 3 months following transplantation. Clinical manifestation of OB includes a cough and progressive dyspnea. Interstitial pulmonary infiltrates are seen on chest film, and an obstructive pattern, primarily a diminished $FEV_1$, is seen in pulmonary function tests (Fig. 57–15). Histologically, the disease is characterized by a diffuse, relatively acellular, fibrosing process, which concentrically narrows the lumina of the terminal bronchioles.

A growing body of evidence suggests that OB is a manifestation of chronic pulmonary allograft rejection. The disease is most commonly found in patients with the greatest degree of HLA mismatch (Harjula et al., 1987), and in the earliest stages, it responds to an increase in immunosuppression (Allen et al., 1986). In addition, histologically confirmed severe, more frequent, and persistent rejection strongly predicts patients who will go on to develop OB (Scott et al., 1990a, 1990b; Yousem et al., 1989a).

It is likely that the cause of OB in lung allograft recipients is multifactorial. Late OB (greater than 6 months) is most commonly an acellular manifestation of chronic rejection. In other patients, OB appears to be related to an infectious process, aspiration, or proximal airway obstruction (Reid et al., 1990), and differs histologically somewhat from "pure" OB associated with chronic rejection (Abernathy et al., 1991). OB is also associated with the development of coronary artery disease in the transplanted heart, which

is thought to arise from chronic cardiac allograft rejection. No patient has been reported with severe coronary artery disease in the heart in the absence of OB.

The best surveillance technique at present is to provide the patient with a portable spirometer, so that expiratory flow can be checked frequently between clinic visits (Otulana et al., 1990). Any deterioration or change in clinical condition is quickly correlated with a chest film and transbronchial biopsy, obtained with fiberoptic bronchoscopy to assess the presence of rejection, infection, or OB (Yousem et al., 1989a). Rejection must be treated aggressively, since this has been the only successful treatment of this relentlessly progressive disease. Despite this approach, patients often go on to severe symptomatic deterioration. At present, OB is the major obstacle to the long-term therapeutic benefit of heart-lung transplantation.

### Complications of Immunosuppression

Several side effects stem from the long-term use of the cyclosporine-based immunosuppressive regimen. Cyclosporine has been associated with renal and hepatic insufficiency, as well as hypertension, hirsutism, and gingival hyperplasia.

The use of corticosteroids is carefully avoided to minimize the risk of tracheal dehiscence in the early postoperative period. Long-term use of steroids causes hirsutism, capillary fragility, and impaired wound healing. One of the more troubling consequences of heart-lung transplantation is the development of post-transplant lymphoproliferative disorder (PTLD) (Yousem et al., 1989b). This is characterized by lymphadenopathy and often a diffuse lymphocytic infiltrate on transbronchial biopsy (Yousem et al., 1991). The treatment is immediate reduction in the intensity of the immunosuppression. The disease has essentially two forms, malignant and nonmalignant. Early onset of PTLD (less than 12 months after transplantation) is typically quite benign and resolves rapidly after reduced immunosuppression. Conversely, late PTLD is associated with a 70 to 80% mortality rate (Armitage et al., 1991) and typically resists a reduction in immunotherapy, as well as traditional chemotherapy.

## PHYSIOLOGY OF THE TRANSPLANTED LUNG

Standard measures of pulmonary function indicate that long-term function of the heart and lungs are well maintained. Integrated cardiopulmonary function with exercise is also largely intact (Theodore et al., 1987, 1991). Some debate has centered around a bronchial hyperresponsiveness to a methacholine challenge (Herve et al., 1992). There does appear to be a decreasing mucociliary clearance, which may be a contributing factor to the serious and repeated infections seen in heart-lung transplant recipients (Herve et al., 1993). In the absence of OB and severe recurrent infection, the function of the transplanted heart and lungs is conducive to an excellent quality of life (Theodore et al., 1991).

## LATE RESULTS

The overall survival of patients who have undergone heart-lung transplantation is lower than that of heart transplant recipients. In the patients reported to the International Society for Heart and Lung Transplantation, actuarial survival at 1 year is 60% in adults and 61% in children (Kaye, 1992).

Individual centers with extensive experience generally have better results, with the Stanford University

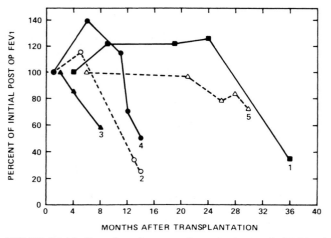

**FIGURE 57–15.** Forced expiratory volume in 1 second (FEV₁) of five patients who developed bronchiolitis obliterans after heart-lung transplantation. The decrease in flow rates occurred between 4 and 36 months after transplantation. The rapid decline in pulmonary function was correlated with symptoms of dyspnea. (From Burke, C. M., Theodore, J., Dawkins, K. D., et al.: Post-transplant obliterative bronchiolitis and other late lung sequelae in human heart-lung transplantation. Chest, 86:824, 1984.)

1-year survival rate at 73% (McCarthy et al., 1990) and the Papworth Hospital group reporting a 1-year survival rate of 75%. Patient selection is important; patients who have pulmonary hypertension do better than patients with congenital heart disease and markedly better than patients who undergo retransplantation (Kaye, 1992). The status of the recipient before transplantation and the quality of donor organs are of paramount importance.

Causes of death after heart-lung transplantation differ over time following operation. Early deaths (less than 1 month) are most often due to multiorgan failure, bleeding, infection, and primary graft failure owing to poor preservation and rejection. The 30-day mortality has varied between 10 and 20% since the late 1980s (Kaye, 1992). The most common cause of death after the immediate postoperative phase is OB. Other late problems include infection, malignancy, and coronary artery disease.

## FUTURE DEVELOPMENTS

Significant improvements in selective immunosuppression and perhaps the development of precise immunotolerance will be required before heart-lung transplantation can restore normal heart and lung function without significant long-term morbidity and mortality. The development of a new generation of immunosuppressive agents, including FK506, rapamycin, and specific monoclonal antibodies to lymphocyte subsets, provides continued hope for an improved outlook for heart-lung transplant recipients. As the problems of precise immunosuppression are solved, the major problem becomes donor availability. Options to solve this problem include a fundamental change in consent laws for organ donation, such as implied consent or xenotransplantation (Sadeghi et al., 1991).

Because of the inherent complexities associated with heart-lung transplantation, it will be reserved for patients who truly have end-stage heart-lung disease.

### SELECTED BIBLIOGRAPHY

Baldwin, J. C., Frist, W. H., Starkey, T. D., et al.: Distant graft procurement for combined heart and lung transplantation using pulmonary artery flush and simple topical hypothermia for graft preservation. Ann. Thorac. Surg., 43:670, 1987.

The simple and transportable technique of pulmonary artery flush was described in this first clinical application. The graft ischemia time was 3 hours and 45 minutes; outstanding early and late graft function was seen. This technique has been adopted by most centers because it is simple, reliable, and effective.

McCarthy, P. M., Starnes, V. A., Theodore, J., et al.: Improved survival after heart-lung transplantation. J. Thorac. Cardiovasc. Surg., 99:54, 1990.

This report details the Stanford University experience through 1985. With increased experience with the technique as well as the aggressive use of transbronchial biopsy to treat infection and rejection at early stages, the survival of patients transplanted since 1986 has been 73% at 1 year, 73% at 2 years, and 65% at 3 years.

Starnes, V. A., Theodore, J., Oyer, P. E., et al.: Evaluation of heart-lung transplant recipients with prospective, serial transbronchial biopsies and pulmonary function studies. J. Thorac. Cardiovasc. Surg., 98:683, 1989.

Transbronchial biopsy is used today as the gold standard for the diagnosis of pulmonary rejection. This report from Stanford University describes 70 serial biopsies in 10 patients during the first 12 weeks after heart-lung transplantation. Forty-eight per cent of the screening lung biopsies were positive for other infection or rejection. Of the biopsies that were performed on clinical grounds, 72.5% were positive for either infection or rejection, and guided the subsequent therapy. The safety and efficacy of this technique have lead to its widespread adoption.

## BIBLIOGRAPHY

Abernathy, E. C., Hruban, R. H., Baumgartner, W. A., et al.: The two forms of bronchiolitis obliterans in heart-lung transplant recipients. Hum. Pathol., 22:1102, 1991.

Allen, M. D., Burke, C. M., McGregor, C. G. A., et al.: Steroid-responsive bronchiolitis after human heart-lung transplantation. J. Thorac. Cardiovasc. Surg., 92:449, 1986.

Armitage, J. M., Kormos, R. L., Stuart, R. S., et al.: Post-transplant lymphoproliferative disease in thoracic organ transplant patients: Ten years of cyclosporine-based immunosuppression. J. Heart Lung Transplant, 10:877–887, 1991.

Baldwin, J. C., Frist, W. H., Starkey, T. D., et al.: Distant graft procurement for combined heart and lung transplantation using pulmonary artery flush and simple topical hypothermia for graft preservation. Ann. Thorac. Surg., 43:670, 1987a.

Baldwin, J. C., Oyer, P. E., Stinson, E. B., et al.: Comparison of cardiac rejection in heart and heart-lung transplantation. J. Heart Transplant., 6:352, 1987b.

Baumgartner, W. A., Traill, T. A., Cameron, D. E., et al.: Unique aspects of heart and lung transplantation exhibited in the "domino-donor" operation. J. A. M. A., 261:3121, 1989.

Burke, C. M., McCormick, S., O'Connell, B. M., et al.: Cytomegalovirus infection in heart-lung transplant recipients. J. Heart Transplant., 5:267, 1986.

Carrel, A.: The surgery of blood vessels. Johns Hopkins Hosp. Bull., 18:18, 1907.

Castañeda, A. R., Arnar, O., Schmidt-Habelmann, P., et al.: Cardiopulmonary autotransplantation in primates (baboons): Late functional results. J. Cardiovasc. Surg., 37:523, 1972a.

Castañeda, A. R., Zamora, R., Schmidt-Habelmann, P., et al.: Cardiopulmonary autotransplantation in primates (baboons): Late functional results. Surgery, 72:1064, 1972b.

Comroe, J. H.: Who was Alexis WHO? Cardiovascular diseases. Bull. Texas Heart Inst., 6:251, 1979.

Cooley, D. A., Bloodwell, R. D., Hallman, G. L., et al.: Organ transplantation for advanced cardiopulmonary disease. Ann. Thorac. Surg., 8:300, 1969.

Cooper, D. K. C.: Transplantation of the heart and both lungs. I: Historical review. Thorax, 24:383, 1969.

Demikhov, V. P.: Experimental Transplantation of Vital Organs. New York, Consultant Bureau, 1962.

Dummer, J. S., Montero, C. G., Griffith, B. P., et al.: Infections in heart-lung transplant recipients. Transplantation, 41:725, 1986.

Duncan, A. J., Dummer, J. S., Paradis, I. L., et al.: Cytomegalovirus infection and survival in lung transplant recipients. J. Heart Lung Transplant., 10:638, 1991.

Fraser, C. D., Tamura, F., Adachi, H., et al.: Donor core-cooling provides improved static preservation for heart-lung transplantation. Ann. Thorac. Surg., 45:235, 1988a.

Fraser, C. D., Tamura, F., Kontos, G. J., et al.: Evaluation of current organ preservation methods for heart-lung transplantation. Transplant. Proc., 20:987, 1988b.

Glanville, A. R., Imoto, E., Baldwin, J. C., et al.: The role of right ventricular endomyocardial biopsy in the long-term management of heart-lung transplant recipients. J. Heart Transplant., 6:357, 1987.

Griffith, B. P., Hardesty, R. L., Armitage, J. M., et al.: Acute rejection of lung allografts with various immunosuppressive protocols. Ann. Thorac. Surg., 54:846, 1992.

Hall, T. S., Breda, M. A., Baumgartner, W. A., et al.: The role of leukocyte depletion in reducing injury to the lung after hypothermic ischemia. Curr. Surg., 44:137, 1987.

Harjula, A., Baldwin, J., Henry, D., et al.: Minimal lung pathology

on long-term primate survivors of heart-lung transplantation. Transplantation, 44:852, 1987.

Herve, P., Picard, N., Ladurie, M. L., et al.: Lack of bronchial hyper-responsiveness to methacholine and to isocapnic dry air hyperventilation in heart-lung and double-lung transplant recipients with normal lung histology. Am. Rev. Respir. Dis., 145:1503, 1992.

Herve, P., Silbert, D., Cerrina, J., et al.: Impairment of bronchial mucociliary clearance in long-term survivors of heart-lung and double-lung transplantation. Chest, 103:59, 1993.

Hoeper, M. M., Hamm, M., Schafers, H. J., et al.: Evaluation of lung function during pulmonary rejection and infection in heart-lung transplant patients. Chest, 102:864, 1992.

Kaye, M. P.: The Registry of the International Society for Heart and Lung Transplantation: Ninth Official Report—1992. J. Heart Lung Transplant., 11(4, Pt. 1):599, 1992.

Kemkes, B. M.: Hemostatic failures and heart-lung transplantation: Assessing the current situation. J. Heart Lung Transplant., 12(1, Pt. 1):S3, 1993.

Lillehei, C. W.: Discussion of Wildevuur, C. R. H., and Benfield, J. R.: A review of 23 human lung transplantations by 20 surgeons. Ann. Thorac. Surg., 9:489, 1970.

Longmore, D. B., Cooper, D. K. C., Hall, R. W., et al.: Transplantation of the heart and both lungs. II: Experimental cardiopulmonary transplantation. Thorax, 241:391, 1969.

Losman, J. G., Campbell, C. D., Replogle, R. L., et al.: Joint transplantation of the heart and lungs. Past experience and present potentials. J. Cardiovasc. Surg., 23:440, 1982.

Lower, R. R., Stofer, R. C., Hurley, E. J., et al.: Complete homograft replacement of the heart and both lungs. Surgery, 50:842, 1961.

Marcus, E., Wong, S. N. T., and Luisada, A. A.: Homologous heart grafts. A. M. A. Arch. Surg., 66:179, 1953.

Marcus, E., Wong, S. N. T., and Luisada, A. A.: Homologous heart grafts: Transplantation of the heart in dogs. Surg. Forum, 2:212, 1951.

Maurer, J. R., Tullis, D. E., Grossman, R. F., et al.: Infectious complications following isolated lung transplantation. Chest 101:1056, 1992.

McCarthy, P. M., Starnes, V. A., Theodore, J., et al.: Improved survival after heart-lung transplantation. J. Thorac. Cardiovasc. Surg., 99:54, 1990.

McCord, J. M.: The biochemistry and pathophysiology of superoxide. Physiologist, 26:156, 1983.

Michler, R. E., and Rose, E. A.: Pediatric heart and heart-lung transplantation. Ann. Thorac. Surg., 52:708, 1991.

Millet, B., Higenbottam, T. W., Flower, C. D. R., et al.: The radiographic appearances of infection and acute rejection of the lung after heart-lung transplantation. Am. Rev. Respir. Dis., 140:62, 1989.

Nakae, S., Webb, W. R., Theodorides, T., et al.: Respiratory function following cardiopulmonary denervation in dog, cat, and monkey. Surg. Gynecol. Obstet., 125:1285, 1967.

Neptune, W. B., Cookson, B. A., Bailey, C. P., et al.: Complete homologous heart transplantation. Arch. Surg., 66:174, 1953.

Novick, R. J., Menkis, A. H., and McKenzie, F. N.: New trends in lung preservation: A collective review. J. Heart. Lung. Transplant., 11:377, 1992.

Otulana, B. A., Higenbottam, T., Ferrari, L., et al.: The use of home spirometry in detecting acute lung rejection and infection following heart-lung transplantation. Chest, 97:353, 1990.

Pham, S. M., Yoshida, Y., Aeba, R., et al.: Interleukin-6, a marker of preservation injury in clinical lung transplantation. J. Heart Lung Transplant., 11:1017, 1992.

Pillai, R., Bando, K., Schueler, S., et al.: Leukocyte depletion results in excellent heart-lung function after 12 hours of storage. Ann. Thorac. Surg., 50:211, 1990.

Reid, K. R., McKenzie, F. N., Menkis, A. H., et al.: Importance of chronic aspiration in recipients of heart-lung transplants. Lancet, 336:206, 1990.

Reitz, B. A.: Adapted indications for lung transplantation: Discussion report. J. Heart Lung Transplant 11(4, Pt. 2):S286, 1992.

Reitz, B. A., Burton, N. A., Jamieson, S. W., et al.: Heart and lung transplantation, autotransplantation, and allotransplantation in primates with extended survival. J. Thorac. Cardiovasc. Surg., 80:360, 1980.

Reitz, B. A., Pennock, J. L., and Shumway, N. E.: Simplified operative method for heart and lung transplantation. J. Surg. Res., 31:1, 1981.

Reitz, B. A., Wallwork, J. L., Hunt, S. A., et al.: Heart-lung transplantation: Successful therapy for patients with pulmonary vascular disease. N. Engl. J. Med., 306:557, 1982.

Royston, D.: Aprotinin therapy in heart and heart-lung transplantation. J. Heart Lung Transplant., 12:S19, 1993.

Sadeghi, A. M., Laks, H., Drinkwater, D. C., et al.: Heart-lung xenotransplantation in primates. J. Heart Lung Transplant., 10:442, 1991.

Scott, J. P., Higenbottam, T. W., Clelland, C. A., et al.: The natural history of chronic rejection in heart-lung transplant recipients: A clinical, pathological, and physiological review of 29 long-term survivors. Transplant. Proc., 22:1474, 1990a.

Scott, J. P., Higenbottam, T. W., Clelland, C. A., et al.: Natural history of chronic rejection in heart-lung transplant recipients. J. Heart Transplant., 9:510, 1990b.

Scott, J., Hutter, J., Stewart, S., et al.: Heart-lung transplantation for cystic fibrosis. Lancet, 2:192, 1988.

Scott, J. P., Sharples, L., Mullins, P., et al.: Further studies on the natural history of obliterative bronchiolitis following heart-lung transplantation. Transplant. Proc., 23:1201, 1991.

Smyth, R. L., Scott, J. P., Borysiewica, L. K., et al.: Cytomegalovirus infection in heart-lung transplant recipients: Risk factors, clinical associations, and response to treatment. J. Infect. Dis., 164:1045, 1991.

Smyth, R. L., Scott, J. P., Whitehead, B., et al.: Heart-lung transplantation in children. Transplant. Proc., 22:1470, 1990.

Starnes, V. A., Theodore, J., Oyer, P. E., et al.: Evaluation of heart-lung transplant recipients with prospective, serial transbronchial biopsies and pulmonary function studies. J. Thorac. Cardiovasc. Surg., 98:683, 1989.

Stewart, S., Higenbottam, T. W., Hutter, J. A., et al.: Histopathology of transbronchial biopsies in heart-lung transplantation. Transplant. Proc., 20:764, 1988.

Theodore, J., Marshall, S., Kramer, M., et al.: The "natural history" of the transplanted lung: Rates of pulmonary functional change in long-term survivors of heart-lung transplantation. Transplant. Proc., 23:1165, 1991.

Theodore, J., Morris, A. J., Burke, C. M., et al.: Cardiopulmonary function at maximum tolerable constant work rate exercise following human heart-lung transplantation. Chest, 92:433, 1987.

Webb, W. R., and Howard, H. S.: Cardiopulmonary transplantation. Surg. Forum, 8:313, 1957.

Wheeldon, D. R., Wallwork, J., Bethune, D. W., and English, T. A.: Storage and transplant of heart and heart-lung donor organs with inflatable cushions and eutectoid cooling. J. Heart Transplant., 7:265, 1988.

Yacoub, M. H., Khaghani, A., Banner, N., et al.: Distant organ procurement for heart-lung transplantation. Presented at the XII International Congress of the Transplantation Society, Sydney, Australia, 1988.

Yoshida, Y., Iwaki, Y., Pham, S., et al.: Benefits of post-transplantation monitoring of interleukin-6 in lung transplantation. Ann. Thorac. Surg., 55:89, 1993.

Yousem, S. A., Dauber, J. A., Keenan, R., et al.: Does histologic acute rejection in lung allografts predict the development of bronchiolitis obliterans? Transplantation, 52:306, 1991.

Yousem, S. A., Paradis, I. L., Dauber, J. H., and Griffith, B. P.: Efficacy of transbronchial lung biopsy in the diagnosis of bronchiolitis obliterans in heart-lung transplant recipients. Transplantation, 47:893, 1989a.

Yousem, S. A., Randhawa, P., Locker, J., et al.: Post-transplant lymphoproliferative disorders in heart-lung transplant recipients: Primary presentation in the allograft. Hum. Pathol., 20:361, 1989b.

# 57 ■ II Cardiac Transplantation

William A. Gay, Jr.

The United States Health Care Finance Administration has concluded that cardiac transplantation is "a medically reasonable and necessary service" for appropriately selected patients with end-stage heart disease (Health Care Finance Administration, 1987). Today, many transplant centers report 1-year survivals of 90% or more and 80% or more at 5 years. (Bolman et al., 1988; Frazier et al., 1988; Renlund et al., 1987a). Since the early 1980s, there has been a dramatic increase in the number of centers performing heart transplantation, although the actual number of transplants being done has levelled off to about 1200 to 1500 per year since about 1990 (Kriett and Kay, 1990). One study concluded that more than 15,000 persons annually could benefit from cardiac transplantation in the United States and that the limiting factor is the number of available donor organs (Evans et al., 1986).

This chapter discusses the important events in the development of cardiac transplantation and the present status of the procedure. Emphasis is placed on the selection and management of recipients, donor evaluation, management and organ recovery, operative techniques, and postoperative management.

## HISTORICAL ASPECTS

Pien Ch'iao, a Chinese physician who lived during the latter years of the Chou dynasty (1121 to 249 B.C.), is said to have exchanged the hearts of two men, Kung Hu and Ch'i Ying, to establish equilibrium between strong and weak forces (yang and yin). The two were later maintained on "supernatural drugs," and except for initial confusion about whose wife and children belonged to whom, they remained well (Wong and Wu, 1936). In 1905, Carrel and Guthrie described a technique for heterotopic transplantation of hearts in experimental animals. Demikov in the

Soviet Union (Demikov, 1962) and Reemtsma in the United States (Reemtsma, 1964) used the heterotopic model to study organ function and to observe the rejection process. Lower and Shumway (1960) reported a method for the orthotopic transplantation of canine hearts. In 1967, Barnard performed the first successful orthotopic human heart transplantation. In the next few years, about 150 human cardiac transplant procedures were performed in centers around the world, but most of the recipients died of rejection or opportunistic infection within the first year after transplantation. Although the technical aspects of cardiac transplantation appeared to have been satisfactorily addressed, the procedure was abandoned in the early 1970s in all but a few centers.

Between 1970 and 1980, the centers that remained active in heart transplants studied the basic principles of organ transplantation in general and cardiac transplantation in particular. The technique of percutaneous endomyocardial biopsy, which allowed surveillance of myocardial histology and facilitated early diagnosis of rejection before deterioration of cardiac function, was developed (Caves et al., 1973). An organized system of grading the histologic manifestations of rejection was described (Billingham, 1979).

In 1959, Schwartz and Dameshek reported that animals given the antimetabolite 6-mercaptopurine were unable to synthesize humoral antibody after an appropriate antigen challenge. Azathioprine, an imidazole derivative of 6-mercaptopurine with a more predictable gastrointestinal absorption pattern, blocks the conversion of inosine monophosphate to adenosine and guanidine monophosphates, and thus inhibits the synthesis of purines. Early immune suppression regimens included azathioprine in addition to corticosteroids (Lower et al., 1965; Reemtsma et al., 1962). In 1976, the polyclonal lymphocytolytic agent antithymocyte globulin (ATG) was introduced (Bieber et al., 1976), and ATG is still a mainstay in early prophylaxis and in the treatment of acute rejection. In some centers, antilymphoblast globulin (ALG), has been used. Cyclosporine, an endecapeptide fungal metabolite, was shown to have immunosuppressive properties (Borel et al., 1976), was studied in the laboratory (Calne et al., 1978; Jamieson et al., 1979; Kostakis et al., 1977), and was then used clinically, first in renal, hepatic, and pancreatic transplantation (Calne et al., 1981). Use of cyclosporine as part of the immune suppression regimen in cardiac transplantation (Bolman et al., 1985; Borel, 1983; Oyer et al., 1982) led to greatly improved survival, an increase in the number of transplant operations, and an increase in the number of centers doing such operations.

## SELECTION AND MANAGEMENT OF RECIPIENTS

Patients with cardiomyopathy and cardiac dilatation originally were considered ideal candidates for cardiac transplantation because of the young age of onset of illness and the poor prognosis of the condition (O'Connell and Gunnar, 1982). Improved management of congestive heart failure (CHF) in these patients, however, may prolong survival by decreasing the incidence of death from progressive cardiac failure without altering the incidence of sudden unexpected death. The prognosis is variable, but 2-year survival of approximately 50% from onset of symptoms is the accepted standard. Poor prognostic indicators include age of onset above 55 years, New York Heart Association (NYHA) Class IV symptoms, marked cardiomegaly detected radiographically and echocardiographically, ejection fraction less than 20%, cardiac index less than 2 $l/min/m^2$, and left ventricular end-diastolic pressure greater than 20 mm Hg. Symptomatic ventricular tachycardia is considered a poor prognostic indicator by most investigators. Even when these poor prognostic indicators are taken into account in considerating risks and benefits, patients deemed too well for transplantation may still have unacceptably high mortality when treated medically (Stevenson et al., 1987). It has been recommended that patients with an ejection fraction less than or equal to 25% be considered a candidate for transplantation, even if their symptoms are relatively mild. Patients with cardiomyopathy and severe ventricular arrhythmia may also be considered for cardiac transplantation.

Generally, cardiac transplantation should be limited to patients with terminal cardiac disease who are unable to do the minimal activity of an acceptable life-style and who cannot achieve palliation or prolongation of life with conventional medical or surgical therapy (Table 57–2). Both uncontrolled and controlled clinical trials (CONSENSUS, 1987; Wilson et al., 1983; Fransiosa et al., 1983; Cohn et al., 1984) have reported that patients with CHF and NYHA Class IV symptoms have 1-year survival rates of less than 60%. These patients, therefore, would achieve maximal survival and symptomatic benefit from cardiac transplantation. Furthermore, although the improvement in survival and symptoms following transplantation may not be as great as for Class IV patients selected, patients with Class III symptoms may be acceptable candidates and should be referred to a transplant center for evaluation. Most recipients have idiopathic cardiomyopathy or end-stage coronary artery disease, but cardiac transplantation is also being offered to selected patients with valvular heart disease and complex forms of congenital heart disease for whom re-

■ **Table 57–2.** ETIOLOGY OF END-STAGE HEART DISEASE IN CARDIAC TRANSPLANT RECIPIENTS

| Disease | Percentage |
|---|---|
| Ischemic heart disease | 49.7 |
| Cardiomyopathy | 40.8 |
| Valvular heart disease | 3.4 |
| Congenital heart disease | 1.4 |
| Rejection of previous transplant | 2.7 |
| Other | 2.0 |
| Total | 100.0 |

pair or palliation is not possible (Addonizio and Rose, 1987; Backer et al., 1992; Bailey et al., 1986; Fricker et al., 1987) (see Table 57–2).

Patients with selected etiologic subtypes of cardiomyopathy have had cardiac transplantation, but little is known about the results. For example, patients with myocarditis proved by biopsy may be considered to be candidates for cardiac transplantation, but it may be advantageous to wait until active myocardial inflammation regresses spontaneously or is modified by immunosuppressive therapy because the myocyte damage is immunologic in origin (O'Connell, 1987). If cardiac transplantation is performed in the presence of active immune-mediated heart disease, early and severe cardiac allograft rejection is possible. Also, because biopsy-proven myocarditis sometimes regresses spontaneously, extended hemodynamic support to ascertain the degree of reversibility of the myocardial dysfunction may be warranted before transplantation is considered. In severe fulminant cases, cardiac transplantation may be required urgently.

The other common condition that requires cardiac transplantation is refractory left ventricular dysfunction secondary to end-stage ischemic heart disease. Patients with angina should be considered only when use of antianginal agents has been maximized and coronary arteriography shows that revascularization is not possible. For patients with symptomatic CHF and coronary artery disease, diagnostic evaluation should include documentation that left ventricular dysfunction is irreversible. Generally, thallium exercise testing should be used to show irreversible perfusion abnormalities or reversible lesions that cannot be revascularized. With these criteria, most patients with coronary artery disease who are considered for transplantation will have had previous coronary artery bypass.

Patients with valvular heart disease who have acceptable pulmonary vascular resistance (PVR) are candidates for transplantation when left ventricular dysfunction becomes refractory. Generally, patients with end-stage valvular heart disease may be more debilitated and have a greater degree of cardiac cachexia because of the chronic nature of their condition. Nutritional factors must be considered before such patients are accepted, and attention to nutrition must be included in perioperative care.

As children with complex forms of congenital heart disease who have successful palliative procedures become older, left ventricular dysfunction may become greater and cardiac transplantation may be considered if they have a protected pulmonary vasculature. The operation must often be tailored to the individual anatomy, and vascular access for biopsy must be considered. Several centers have reported encouraging results in transplantation of neonates with severe forms of congenital heart disease, such as hypoplastic left side of the heart syndrome (Bailey et al., 1986; Mavroudis et al., 1988).

With greater long-term survival, more individuals will require retransplantation for allograft arteriosclerosis. Although cyclosporine and other selective im-

munosuppressive drugs have increased early survival, there is no evidence that the rate of development of graft arteriosclerosis has decreased (Renlund et al., 1989). Coronary artery lesions can be detected by routine coronary angiography in most patients within the first 3 years after cardiac transplantation (Gao et al., 1988). Until the immunology of chronic vascular rejection is better understood, allograft arteriosclerosis will lead to consideration of cardiac transplantation in a greater percentage of patients.

Analysis of the mortality in cardiac transplantation according to the cause of heart disease by the Registry of the International Society for Heart Transplantation (Kriett and Kaye, 1990) showed no difference between patients with cardiomyopathy and those with coronary artery disease. The mortality was higher for patients with congenital heart disease, valvular heart disease, or allograft rejection, but this result may be an artifact because relatively few procedures are performed in patients with these causes.

## Age

In the past, patients over 55 years of age were excluded from cardiac transplantation because of the lack of donor availability and the nonspecific potency of immunosuppression. As potent immunosuppressive agents with corticosteroid-sparing effects were developed and the supply of donor organs increased, patients in the early pediatric population and adults over 55 years of age have been considered to be candidates for cardiac transplantation. The survival of patients between 55 and 65 years of age who have cardiac transplantation is similar to, if not better than, that of younger patients (Carrier et al., 1986; Renlund et al., 1987b), which may be explained by a decreased incidence of acute allograft rejection owing to T-lymphocyte senescence and decreased immunoreactivity to allograft antigens. From a medical perspective, a candidate between 55 and 65 years old who is physiologically youthful should not be excluded from transplantation on the basis of age. However, with age, there is an increased frequency of noncardiac and prostatic complications. Preferential selection of older donors for older recipients has been the practice in some centers.

Cardiac transplantation is also being offered to younger children and neonates with greater frequency. The experience is not as extensive as in the adult population, and definitive statements about survival are not possible. When cardiac transplantation is considered for infants and children, the morbidity associated with immunosuppressive therapy and the difficulties of vascular access for biopsy should be considered.

## Pulmonary Hypertension

As part of the routine evaluation, right-sided heart catheterization must be performed for all potential recipients, and PVR must be calculated (Gay, 1988). Although resting PVR may be above the traditional threshold of 6 to 8 Wood units, the peak pulmonary artery pressure and PVR may be decreased with intensive medical management of CHF and incremental doses of nitroprusside. If the pulmonary artery pressure falls below 60 mm Hg or if the PVR and pulmonary artery pressure are at the upper limits, a donor whose body size is at least equal to that of the recipient is desirable. In some centers, heterotopic cardiac or heart-lung transplantation is considered for recipients with high PVR.

## Other Criteria

If the recipient has had a recent pulmonary embolism or infarction, cardiac transplantation should be delayed until healing occurs. If delay is not possible, the operation is feasible, but pulmonary infection often occurs (Young et al., 1986). The pulmonary infarct can sometimes be resected at the time of transplantation to minimize this complication. Diabetes is a relative contraindication. In some centers, selected insulin-dependent diabetics without evidence of renal, neuropathic, gastrointestinal, or microangiopathic disease are successfully transplanted by using immune-suppression protocols with minimal corticosteroid therapy (Badellino et al., 1988). Intermediate-term (2 to 4 years) survival in selected diabetics has been comparable with that in nondiabetics (Munoz et al., 1991; Ladowsky et al., 1990). Diseases of the liver, kidney, or central nervous system are relative contraindications. Generally, patients with end-stage CHF have abnormalities in glomerular filtration because of decreased renal blood flow. Efforts should be made to ensure that these abnormalities are not due to intrinsic renal disease, because of the additive nephrotoxicity of cyclosporine. Similarly, liver disease should be evaluated, and irreversible changes are considered a contraindication for cardiac transplantation in most centers, although combined heart-liver transplant has been performed. When possible, biopsy of these organs may help resolve these issues. Active peptic ulcer disease is a relative contraindication, and efforts must be made to allow healing of ulcers. If transplantation is necessary in an otherwise ideal candidate, intensive antacid and $H_2$ blocker therapy may allow healing to continue after the procedure. Active systemic infection is a contraindication because of the possibility of dissemination after immunosuppression. Patients with malignancies should not be considered for transplantation because the immunosuppression may inhibit the natural immune system responses that prevent proliferation of such lesions. However, a history of a malignancy cured by medical or surgical management is not an absolute contraindication for cardiac transplantation. The type of tumor, severity, and residual effects must be considered before a decision is made.

## Psychosocial Criteria

Candidates for cardiac transplantation should have strong psychologic support systems and be able to tolerate the stress of living away from their family for long periods, prolonged hospitalizations, and toxicity from immunosuppressive agents (Christopherson, 1987). Candidates must be able to comply with complex medical regimens. All patients should be screened for psychosocial acceptability, but standardized criteria are not available and acceptability is determined on a case-by-case basis. Patients who suffer from alcohol or substance abuse should be evaluated by drug rehabilitation experts and should have a compulsive treatment protocol with which they are compliant. Ideally, compliance should be tested for several weeks to months before the transplant, but when this is not feasible, a frank discussion with the patient is necessary before acceptance. In patients with previous psychiatric histories, psychiatric evaluation is mandatory. Generally, any endogenous psychotic state that could be exacerbated by environmental stress or corticosteroid administration is a contraindication for cardiac transplantation.

## Immunologic Assessment

Immunologic assessment of all patients who have cardiac transplantation should include screening for the presence of lymphocytotoxic antibodies to allograft antigens. In most centers, this is done by mixing serum from the recipient with lymphocytes from a random panel of donors and calculating the percentage of reactive antibody. A cardiac transplant recipient is thought to be sensitized if there is more than 5 to 10% reactive antibody. Some centers require a specific cross-match with the donor if the recipient is sensitized, but this may be unnecessary because the likelihood of a positive cross-match is low (O'Connell et al., 1988a). In the presence of a positive cross-match, alterations of immunosuppression to focus on humoral immune responses have been successful.

The National Heart Transplant Study found that, of more than 1000 patients referred for cardiac transplantation, 350 were accepted; however, 280 never had the procedure. Of this 280, 59% died waiting and 31% refused the procedure (Evans and Maier, 1986). Although there is a trend toward less rigid criteria for cardiac transplantation, the disparity between donor organ availability and recipient need suggests that medically sound guidelines should be developed to produce the most effective use of the donor organ.

## Recipient Management

When a candidate is accepted for transplantation, the major challenge for the medical team is to sustain adequate perfusion until a compatible donor is identified (O'Connell et al., 1987). In general, less use of instrumentation and shorter hospitalization reduce the risk of infection. Hospitalization with intravenous lines should be minimized. In most patients, however, intravenous therapy is needed because of the lack of predictably effective oral agents for inotropic support. Clinical study of a class of orally active phosphodiesterase inhibitors has shown promising early results. One of these agents, enoximone, was effective in providing inotropic support to patients who earlier depended on intravenous inotropes (Weber et al., 1986).

If oral therapy does not sustain adequate perfusion, intravenous inotropes may be required. The drug of choice is dobutamine, which has beta-agonist inotropic properties, without significant peripheral vascular effects. This drug is most effective when infused at doses up to 10 $\mu$g/kg/min and there is no benefit from further increments. If it is difficult to maintain systemic blood pressure, dopamine up to a maximal dose of 5 $\mu$g/kg/min may be added to dobutamine. At higher doses of dopamine, the arrhythmogenic and renal vasoconstrictive effects may predominate and have deleterious effects on organ perfusion. If blood flow is still inadequate with intravenous dobutamine and dopamine, mechanical assistance should be considered.

The use of mechanical assistance devices increases the risk of infectious complications, and these circulatory aids should be used for the shortest time possible. Intra-aortic balloon counterpulsation uses volume displacement to effect afterload reduction and diastolic augmentation. Inotropic agents and other vasoactive drugs are often used with intra-aortic balloon pumping to improve hemodynamics. If left ventricular ejection is severely compromised, because of inadequate ventricular contractility or a rapid or irregular heart rate, intra-aortic balloon pumping will not be effective and some other form of support is needed.

A left or right ventricular assist device diverts blood around the ventricle by removing the blood from the atrium or from the ventricle itself and returning it to the appropriate great vessel. There are two basic types of ventricular assist devices: those that move blood into a sac or diaphragm and then pump it back into the circulation by means of a volume displacement system, usually air or gas, and those that move blood by passing it through a centrifugal pump with electrically driven rotator cones and impellers (Magovern et al., 1987). The pumping mechanism of most ventricular assist devices is external, but prosthetic ventricles have also been placed in the heterotopic internal position and used for circulatory support in patients who await transplantation (Farrar et al., 1988). Neither short-term nor long-term survival after transplantation has been affected by the use of circulatory assist devices; however, cost is dramatically increased (Bolman et al., 1987; Farrar et al., 1988; O'Connell et al., 1988b). Pneumatically powered orthotopically placed total artificial hearts have also been used successfully for circulatory support in patients who await suitable donor organs. The present survival of these patients is approximately 50% and probably reflects the severity of the existing cardiac

disease and some extracardiac organ dysfunction (Olsen, 1988).

## EVALUATION OF CARDIAC DONORS

Acceptable cardiac donors are individuals who sustain a traumatic or medical cerebral insult and are pronounced brain dead by neurologic specialists according to acceptable criteria (Table 57–3) (Emery et al., 1986). A detailed history and physical examination should be obtained, and any history of drug use, cardiac arrhythmia, or previous cardiac symptoms must be considered before acceptance of the donor. Because of the effects of increased intracranial pressure on catecholamine release and subsequent distribution of myocardial blood flow, the ST segments and T waves on the electrocardiogram are often abnormal in donors with normal cardiac function. Tachycardia and arrhythmias do not necessarily indicate intrinsic cardiac abnormalities. Potential donors older than 50 years and younger donors with a suggestive history should undergo coronary arteriography before organ acceptance. There has been a reluctance to accept donors over age 45 years because of the reported increased incidence of allograft arteriosclerosis with older donor hearts (Billingham, 1987), but the medical necessity and the age of the intended recipient should be considered before an older donor is excluded.

Generally, hemodynamic monitoring is done with a radial arterial line and a central venous pressure or a pulmonary artery catheter, and hydration is required in most donors. Because the neurologic injury typically depletes volume from diabetes insipidus and there is a tendency to attempt reduction of cerebral edema when these patients are treated before brain death, early hemodynamic support is achieved primarily with vasopressors, particularly dopamine. After brain death is declared, management of donors should focus on volume replacement and weaning from catecholamines. Prolonged infusion of dopamine at doses of 10 $\mu$g/kg/min or more has been considered a contraindication to acceptance of the heart for cardiac transplantation. When echocardiography is available, allograft function can be assessed noninvasively, and as many as 20% of donors who would have been excluded by conventional criteria are acceptable when normal left ventricular function is evident (Gilbert et al., 1988). If a donor organ is questionable on the basis of noninvasive evaluation, direct visualization of the heart by the harvesting surgical team is essential before acceptance. In that

■ **Table 57–3.** DONOR CRITERIA

1. Meets requirements for brain death
2. Consent from next of kin
3. ABO compatible with recipient
4. Approximately same size as recipient
5. Absence of history of cardiac disease
6. Normal echocardiogram
7. Normal heart by visual inspection at recovery

case, the recipient should be prepared but not under anesthesia until the cardiac surgeon at the donor site has inspected the donor heart.

When the heart is acceptable for transplantation, other systemic conditions must be considered. Systemic infection that has been treated with broad-spectrum antibiotics is not a contraindication for cardiac transplantation, because these infections rarely affect the myocardium. Hepatitis surface antigen positivity and the presence of human immunodeficiency virus (HIV) in the donor are contraindications to acceptance of the organ for transplantation.

## Donor/Recipient Matching

In most cases, a donor within 20% of the recipient's body weight is acceptable. If the recipient's PVR is at the high end of acceptable limits, a larger donor may be preferable. ABO compatibility is required, but ABO-identical organs are preferred because they may be less likely to induce rejection than organs that are merely ABO-compatible. Blood from the donor should be tested for viral titers, particularly for cytomegalovirus (CMV), because the incidence of clinically significant CMV infections approaches 100% when an organ from a CMV-positive donor is procured for a CMV-negative recipient. In such instances, prophylactic treatment with antiviral agents such as gancyclovir has proved useful. Donor lymphocytes should be harvested for a donor-specific cross-match, which should be done for all patients. Recipients with preformed reactive antibody titers (PRA) greater than 5% are at risk for hyperacute rejection and should have prospective cross-match.

## Donor Organ Recovery

There are far more potential recipients for cardiac allografts than donors, and hearts recovered for transplantation must be handled in a way that maximizes their usefulness (Baumgartner, 1990). The logistics of organ retrieval must be carefully coordinated and the technical aspects of the procedure accomplished with dispatch and attention to detail. When the donor and recipient are in the same hospital, the excision of the donor heart and its implantation can take place almost simultaneously, minimizing organ ischemia time. Most often, a suitable organ becomes available at a distant institution, so close coordination of activities that take place simultaneously at two different locations is necessary. Because the heart is usually only one of several transplantable organs that are being recovered, donor cardiectomy must be coordinated with the excision of kidneys, liver, and pancreas, which sometimes involves several transplant surgical teams from distant locations (Brodman et al., 1985; Starzl et al., 1984). Because the final decision about suitability of the organ for transplantation is made at the time of recovery, many institutions have an experienced senior surgeon lead the organ recovery team, usually accompanied by a surgical resident and a transplant coordinator.

Organ ischemic time begins when the aortic cross-clamp is placed in the donor and ends when the aortic clamp is released in the recipient. The upper limit of tolerable ischemia in the transplant setting is not known (Copeland et al., 1973), but most cardiac transplant teams attempt to limit organ ischemic time to 4 hours or less. In the authors' experience with approximately 450 transplants, ischemic time has ranged from 55 to 380 minutes, and no acute organ dysfunction was related to this interval. However, the primary goal of the organ recovery teams should be to excise the transplantable organs in the best possible condition and deliver them to the sites of implantation expeditiously.

Multiple organs are recovered using a midline incision from the sternal notch to the pubis, sometimes with bilateral transverse extensions at or slightly above the level of the umbilicus. The sternum is incised longitudinally, the pericardium opened widely, and the heart inspected for any unsuspected anomalies or injuries, such as contusions. The condition of the heart and its acceptability for transplantation are then reported to the implanting team, with an estimate of the timing of the remaining harvesting procedure to coordinate activities and minimize organ ischemia time. The intrapericardial portions of the superior and inferior venae cavae are dissected free, and encircling transfixion sutures of 2-0 Dacron are placed about the superior vena cava well cephalad to the area of the sinoatrial node. These sutures are not tied until later. Any catheters that enter the heart, such as flow-guided pulmonary artery lines, are removed at this time. The aorta and pulmonary artery are separated, and the pulmonary artery is dissected free to a point distal to its bifurcation. A purse-string suture of 3-0 Dacron is placed in the adventitia of the aorta as far distal as practical, but not so far as to prevent placement of the aortic cross-clamp beyond it.

When all the organ recovery teams have completed preliminary dissection, the donor is completely heparinized and the inferior vena cava is divided slightly above the level of the diaphragm and allowed to bleed into the pericardium. As the arterial pressure of the donor falls with the acute blood loss, the aorta is clamped as far cephalad as possible, and 1000 ml of cold crystalloid potassium cardioplegic solution (Table 57–4) is infused into the aortic root through a 14-gauge catheter inserted through the purse-string suture. Some experimental data indicate that use of University of Wisconsin solution may offer superior preservation (Jeevanandum et al., 1992) (Table 57–5). The superior vena cava is then doubly ligated by

■ **Table 57–4.** CRYSTALLOID CARDIOPLEGIA SOLUTION

1000 ml of 5% dextrose in ¼ normal saline containing
  20 mEq of KCl
  5 mEq of NaHCO₃
Kept iced at 4° C

**■ Table 57–5.** UNIVERSITY OF WISCONSIN SOLUTION

| | |
|---|---|
| Hydroxyethyl starch (Pentafraction) | 50 g/l |
| Lactobionic acid | 100 mmol/l |
| Potassium phosphate | 25 mmol/l |
| Magnesium sulfate | 5 mmol/l |
| Raffinose | 30 mmol/l |
| Adenosine | 5 mmol/l |
| Allopurinol | 1 mmol/l |
| Glutathione | 3 mmol/l |
| Dexamethasone | 16 mg/l |
| Glucose | 0.06 mmol/l |

Potassium = 113 mEq/l
Sodium = 30 mEq/l
Osmolarity = 323
pH = 7.4

tying the previously placed transfixion sutures, and divided between the ligatures. The donor heart is then excised by first dividing the right and then the left pulmonary veins at their entrance into the pericardium and dividing the left and right pulmonary arteries just distal to the bifurcation of the main pulmonary artery. Finally, the aorta is transected distal to the cardioplegic needle but proximal to the aortic cross-clamp. The excised heart is rinsed thoroughly with iced saline solution, placed into two concentric sterile plastic bags, and packed beneath crushed ice in a portable ice chest for transport to the implant team.

## ORGAN IMPLANT

The timing of operation in the cardiac recipient is carefully coordinated with that of the donor. The heart is exposed by a midline sternotomy in most cases. Exposure can be difficult in patients who have had previous cardiac surgery, and the common femoral artery is often used for arterial cannulation in these patients. When the heart is exposed, preparations are made for arterial and bicaval cannulation, heparin is administered, cannulation is performed, and cardiopulmonary bypass is started.

Ideally, bypass is started just before the arrival of the donor heart. Because the heart is to be excised and bypass time is usually short, there is no need for cardioplegia or more than moderate hypothermia; the body temperature is maintained at 30 to 32° C. Cardiectomy is performed by first incising the left and then the right atrium inferiorly and laterally just on the atrial aspect of the atrioventricular groove. The atrial septum is then incised from its most inferior aspect, with a generous remnant left posteriorly. Finally, the great vessels are divided immediately above the commissures of the semilunar valves. The atrial, aortic, and pulmonary arterial cuffs are then appropriately trimmed. The visceral pericardium binding the aortic and pulmonary arterial cuffs is opened for greater mobility.

The donor heart is then prepared by first opening into the left atrium by connecting the orifices of the pulmonary veins and then trimming residual left atrial tissue to facilitate a good fit with the left atrial cuff in the recipient. The anastomoses are shown in Figure 57–16. The left atria are connected with a continuous suture of 3-0 polypropylene, and after the right atrium of the donor heart is opened along its lateral wall, the right atria are joined with a similar suture. The aortic and pulmonary arterial cuffs are trimmed and sized and then joined with continuous sutures of 4-0 polypropylene for each. All air is evacuated from the heart and from the aortic root, the cross-clamp is released, and perfusion of the transplanted heart is resumed. The heart usually develops an effective rhythm spontaneously, but defibrillation is sometimes required. Temporary pacing wires are attached to the right atrium and the right ventricle, to be used for synchronized atrioventricular pacing or as electrocardiographic leads to obtain epicardial electrograms.

Orthotopic placement of the heart is sometimes not possible or practical, in which case heterotopic placement is used. The presence of severely increased PVR is considered by some to be an indication for heterotopic placement (Barnard et al., 1981) because attempts at orthotopic transplantation may cause acute right ventricular failure. The technique for heterotopic transplantation differs significantly from the orthotopic procedure (Fig. 57–17). The inferior vena cava and the right pulmonary veins of the donor heart must be ligated or oversewn at the time of organ recovery. Also, the recovery team should obtain as much length of aorta and superior vena cava as possible. The left atrial anastomosis is performed first; an opening is made in the donor left atrium by connecting the orifices of the two left pulmonary veins and then incising the left atrium of the recipient near the interatrial groove just anterior to the entrance of the right pulmonary veins. The left atria are connected with continuous 3-0 polypropylene. Next, the superior vena cava of the donor heart is anastomosed from end to side to that of the recipient with 5-0 polypropylene. An end-to-side anastomosis is then created between the aortae, and a short length of prosthetic graft or aortic homograft is used to connect the two pulmonary arteries.

## PERIOPERATIVE MONITORING

Because of the risk of infection in the immunosuppressed patient, invasive monitoring techniques are used minimally in cardiac transplantation. Immediately before anesthesia, a radial arterial line is placed. As soon as the patient is asleep, a Foley catheter is placed in the bladder and a large-bore catheter (a triple-lumen device) is inserted in the left internal jugular vein (the right jugular is saved for later percutaneous endomyocardial biopsies). No flow-guided catheter is placed in the pulmonary artery; if one is already in place, it is removed. If indicated on clinical grounds, a pulmonary arterial catheter can be inserted after the donor heart has been implanted.

Most cardiac transplant recipients are anticoagulated with warfarin at the time of transplantation

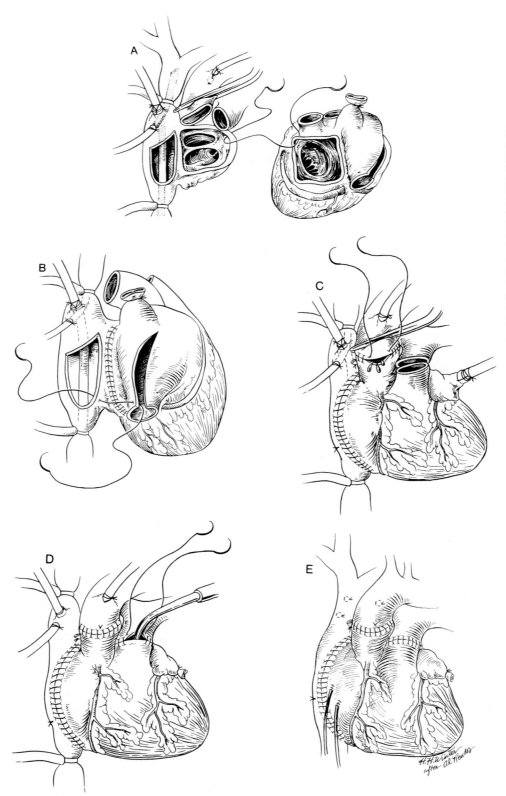

**FIGURE 57–16.** Operative technique for human cardiac transplantation. *A,* Cannulation technique is similar to routine cardiac procedures with central cannulation. Tapes have been placed around the superior and inferior vena cavae, and the aorta has been cross-clamped to exclude the heart from the circulation. The recipient's heart has been excised at the atrioventricular groove. The superior vena cava of the donor's heart has been ligated. The left atrial anastomosis has been started. *B,* The left atrial anastomosis has been completed. The incision in the right atrium of the donor heart is curved away from the superior vena cava and the adjacent sinoatrial node. The right atrial anastomosis is begun at the inferior border of the atrial septum. *C,* The right atrial anastomosis is completed. A perfusion catheter has been inserted into the left atrium through which cold (4°C) normal saline is infused to further cool the left ventricular cavity as well as displace air. The aortic anastomosis is being completed. *D,* The aortic cross-clamp has been released after completion of the aortic anastomosis. The perfusion catheter has been removed from the left atrium, and the pulmonary anastomosis is completed with the heart fibrillating. *E,* The bypass cannulas have been removed. Pacing wires have been inserted on the right atrium of the donor heart. (*A–E,* Reproduced with permission from Baumgartner, W. A., Reitz, B. A., Oyer, P. E., et al.: Cardiac homotransplantation. Curr. Probl. Surg., *16*:1, 1979.)

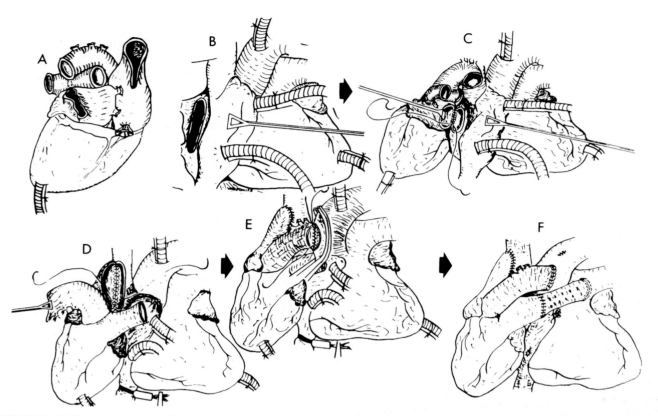

**FIGURE 57–17.** The heterotopic cardiac transplant. *A,* Posterior view of the donor after preparation for anastomosis. *B,* Left atriotomy. *C,* Left atrial anastomosis. *D,* Right atrial anastomosis. *E,* Aortic anastomosis. *F,* Completed anastomosis with a pulmonary-to-pulmonary arterial graft. (*A–E,* Reproduced with permission from Barnard, C. N., and Wolpowitz, A.: Heterotopic versus orthotopic heart transplantation. Transplant. Proc., *11*:309, 1979.)

because of dilated cardiomyopathy, the existence of mural thrombi from prior myocardial infarctions, the presence of atrial fibrillation, or a combination of these. An effort is made to restore a normal coagulation profile preoperatively with vitamin K and fresh frozen plasma, but most patients remain therapeutically anticoagulated at the time of operation. Additional fresh frozen plasma and sometimes platelet transfusions may be required in the early postoperative period. Chest drainage systems that allow reinfusion of mediastinal and pleural drainage after it has been filtered are also useful, because drainage may be considerable for the first few hours. If excessive chest tube drainage continues after the coagulation indices have returned to normal, surgical reexploration for hemostasis is indicated.

## POSTOPERATIVE MANAGEMENT

### Hemodynamic Support

The transplanted heart is a denervated organ and, when appropriately volume loaded, increases its output largely by increases in heart rate (Cannon et al., 1973). Before cardiopulmonary bypass is discontinued, an intravenous drip of isoproterenol is started at 0.1 μg/min and the dosage is increased incremen-

tally until the heart rate reaches 100 to 110 beats per minute. This rate gives satisfactory cardiac output without excessive ventricular irritability. Isoproterenol may also be beneficial because of its bronchodilator action. The drug can usually be discontinued after several days.

Recipients who have PVRs above 3.0 Wood units despite aggressive preoperative treatment, also have an increased risk of acute right ventricular failure in the transplanted heart. The reason is that the donor right ventricle is unaccustomed to pumping blood against high pulmonary resistance. Every effort is made to obtain a heart from a donor of equal or larger body size and to minimize organ ischemic time when it is known that the recipient has increased PVR. Right ventricular failure is seen with elevated venous pressure, dilatation of the right ventricle, and low or normal pulmonary wedge pressure. In this setting, the combination of nitroprusside at 5 to 10 μg/kg/min and the synthetic catecholamine dobutamine at 3 to 10 μg/kg/min has been effective. Prostaglandin $E_1$, a vasoactive product of the enzymatic conversion of cyclooxygenase, has been effective as a selective pulmonary vasodilator (Armitage et al., 1987). It is recommended that a bolus of 25 to 75 μg be administered into a central vein or directly into the pulmonary artery and followed by an intravenous infusion of 0.1 μg/kg/min. Effectiveness of the drug is shown by a decrease in the pulmonary artery pressure with improved cardiac output and systemic oxygenation.

Other agents that are useful immediately after transplantation are dopamine, an L-norepinephrine precursor; the phosphodiesterase inhibitor amrinone; and rarely, the combination of epinephrine and calcium chloride (1 mg epinephrine and 1 g $CaCl_2$ in 500 ml of 5% dextrose and water [D/W]). When enoximone is used intravenously, care should be taken to ensure that the patient has adequate intravascular volume as determined by a left ventricular filling pressure of 15 mm Hg or greater. A loading infusion of amrinone is begun at 75 μg/kg/min for a maximum of 20 minutes, and the infusion is decreased or terminated if the heart rate increases by 15% or more or the systolic blood pressure decreases by 20% or more. The maintenance dose is 7 to 10 μg/kg/min but should not exceed 250 mg in 24 hours.

Except when hyperacute rejection occurs, which is very rare immediately after the operation, mechanical circulatory support is seldom necessary. If the recipient required support by intra-aortic balloon counterpulsation preoperatively, it is probably prudent to continue this support for 12 to 24 hours after transplantation and to remove the balloon electively when coagulation indices are normalized. Rarely, a right or left ventricular assist device is required after transplantation and may be connected in the standard manner with atrial uptake and return to the appropriate great artery. However, external instrumentation should be minimal in these patients, who are soon to be immunocompromised.

## Immunosuppression

The major nonoperative complications are rejection and the predisposition to infection from potent immunosuppression. Although the approach to immunosuppression varies from center to center, the goal of immunosuppression in the early postoperative period is to allow successful wound healing and induce tolerance to the allograft. Cyclosporine is the cornerstone of all immunosuppressive regimens (Cohen et al., 1984; Kahan, 1987). This drug, first approved by the Food and Drug Administration in 1983 for use in transplantation of solid organs, acts primarily by inhibiting the production of interleukin-2 and thus attenuating the recruitment of cytotoxic T lymphocytes. Early use of the this agent produced a high incidence of acute renal failure because large preoperative loading doses were used. Cyclosporine is now given in lower doses (2 to 8 mg/kg/day), and in many protocols, therapy is started only when postoperative hemodynamic stability has been achieved. This approach avoids high peak and trough levels at a time when liver and renal function may not be optimal because of compromised organ perfusion. Early immunoprophylaxis also includes corticosteroids in various doses, and most immunosuppressive regimens prescribe a high early corticosteriod dose that decreases to a maintenance prednisone level of

0.15 to 0.20 mg/kg/day. Cyclosporine and prednisone alone produce 80% survival at 1 year, and addition of azathioprine to this regimen (triple therapy) increases survival to 85 to 90% at 1 year (Bolman et al., 1985). Azathioprine is typically given at 2 mg/kg to maintain the white blood cell count between 4000 and 6000/mm³.

Cytolytic therapy is commonly incorporated in the first 1 to 2 weeks to intensify T-cell immunosuppression. The most common agent for this purpose is equine ATG, but ALGs and rabbit antithymocyte globulin are also used for immunoprophylaxis. These agents are given preoperatively and continued for 1 to 2 weeks. The murine monoclonal antibody against the human CD3 T-cell antigen (OKT3) was shown to decrease the incidence of rejection when compared with a protocol based on equine ATG (Bristow et al., 1988). In addition, significantly more patients were maintained on steroid-free protocols after they received the OKT3-based immunoprophylaxis. The patients who had OKT3 had fewer side effects and infectious complications as well as a decrease in the hypercholesterolemia that accompanies high-dose corticosteriods.

In the patient who has a positive donor-specific cross-match, early immunosuppression is directed toward decreasing humoral antibody load and B-lymphocyte proliferation. Cyclophosphamide may be substituted for azathioprine, and plasmapheresis may be done to decrease antibody load. Because there is little experience with highly sensitized cardiac transplant recipients, no firm recommendations can be given for managing patients with a positive retrospective cross-match.

## Diagnosis of Rejection

Patients with a greater than 5% reactivity to a panel of pooled donor lymphocytes are at risk for hyperacute rejection. Therefore, prospective donor-recipient cross-matching is recommended. Experimental evidence suggests that photochemotherapy may be useful in this setting (Rose et al., 1992).

Cytoimmunologic monitoring with quantitation of lymphocyte subpopulations and interleukin-2 receptors and echocardiographic detection of abnormalities of systolic and diastolic function have been proposed as noninvasive techniques that aid in the diagnosis of rejection, but the endomyocardial biopsy remains the standard (Billingham, 1982). Although pathologic criteria vary, the histologic definition of rejection includes the intensity and characteristics of the inflammatory infiltrate, evidence of myocyte damage, and changes in microvascular integrity. The histologic abnormalities precede left ventricular dysfunction, and surveillance endomyocardial biopsy allows rejection to be diagnosed before end-organ dysfunction occurs. Hence, immunosuppression may be intensified to a lesser degree than is required in other solid-organ allografts, where rejection is diagnosed only after allograft dysfunction is identified. A typical protocol for endomyocardial biopsy recommends weekly procedures for 6 to 8 weeks, with a gradual increase in the interval between biopsies to 3 to 4 months (Table 57–6).

## Treatment of Rejection

When the histologic diagnosis of rejection is established, the degree of intensification of immunosuppression depends on the severity of histologic change and the presence of hemodynamic compromise (Hunt et al., 1991; May et al., 1990; O'Connell and Renlund, 1990; Wahlers et al., 1990). Most episodes of rejection can be managed by increasing the dose of oral corticosteroids or giving a short course of high-dose (pulse) intravenous corticosteroid. With more severe rejection, cytolytic therapy with antithymocyte or ALG or OKT3 may be required. The incidence of rejection is highest in the first 4 to 6 months and then tapers off to a state of relative immune tolerance. At that time, the quantity of immunosuppressive agents may be reduced to decrease the risk of infection. Maintenance immunosuppression usually includes corticosteroid, cyclosporine, and azathioprine in low doses and in various combinations. Aggressive early immunosuppression may make it possible to minimize or eliminate the long-term use of corticosteroids and thus to decrease their side effects (Renlund et al., 1987c; Yacoub et al., 1985).

## Complications of Immunosuppression

The complications of immunosuppressive agents must be assessed to individualize immunosuppression. Corticosteroids may lead to a cushingoid appearance, osteoporosis, cataracts, thinning of the skin and capillary fragility, peptic ulcer disease, and the development of overt diabetes mellitus in previously borderline diabetics. Azathioprine is rarely hepatotoxic and is usually well tolerated. When cyclosporine was introduced in high doses and combined with multiple intensive immunosuppressive agents, a high incidence of lymphoma was identified (Penn, 1987). This unusual lymphoma begins as a polyclonal lymphocyte proliferation stimulated by Epstein-Barr virus

■ **Table 57–6.** SCHEDULE FOR ENDOMYOCARDIAL BIOPSIES

| Biopsy Number | Time |
|---|---|
| 1 | 5–7 days after transplantation |
| 2–6 | Weekly |
| 7–11 | Every 2 weeks |
| 12–14 | Every 4 weeks |
| 15–18 | Every 6 weeks |
| 19–21 | Every 8 weeks |
| 22–23 | Every 12 weeks |

Thereafter, every 6 months
Rejection, 5–7 days after treatment begins
Coronary arteriography done annually

and presents atypically with primary gastrointestinal or cerebral involvement. As the dose of cyclosporine has decreased, the incidence of lymphoma and all malignancies in patients who have cardiac transplants does not differ from that in patients with renal and liver transplant; lymphoma occurs in 6% of transplant patients at any time after operation. Hypertension is so common in patients who receive cyclosporine that it is unusual for a patient who takes the agent not to be hypertensive (Thompson et al., 1986). The hypertension tends to have a reversed diurnal variation, with the highest pressures recorded early in the morning, and is unresponsive to many conventional antihypertensive drugs, although usually responsive to beta-adrenergic and calcium channel blockade. Cyclosporine nephrotoxicity occurs most often when the drug is administered in high loading doses. Most patients who have chronic maintenance cyclosporine have a decrease in glomerular filtration to approximately 50% of normal. Less common side effects are seizures, hirsutism, and gingival hyperplasia.

The most frequent complications of immunosuppressive agents are infections (Andreone et al., 1986). The use of cyclosporine has decreased the incidence of life-threatening bacterial and fungal infections, but viral infections, particularly CMV, are still a major source of morbidity (Hofflin et al., 1987). Pneumocystis may be a common cause of interstitial pneumonia after cardiac transplantation. The treatment for pneumocystis is trimethoprim-sulfamethoxazole, and the antiviral agent ganciclovir is effective in gastrointestinal ulceration and interstitial pneumonia due to CMV infection. An aggressive approach to the treatment of interstitial pneumonia is mandatory for successful recovery of the cardiac transplant recipient.

## Coronary Arteriosclerosis

The major complication that may limit long-term survival after cardiac transplantation is the development of coronary artery disease (Billingham, 1987; Renlund et al., 1989). This form of coronary artery disease is distinct from atherosclerosis in patients who do not have transplants. Allograft coronary artery disease appears to begin in the distal vessels and progress proximally. It is rarely found proximal to the bifurcations of major epicardial vessels, and therefore is not amenable to percutaneous transluminal coronary angioplasty or coronary artery bypass grafting. This form of coronary arteriosclerosis is clinically silent because of the denervated state of the heart, and presents as left ventricular dysfunction or arrhythmia in the absence of chest pain. Annual coronary angiography is performed routinely to screen for this complication. Histologically, these vessels have concentric fibrous narrowing without the classic eccentric atherosclerotic plaque. Most recipients have evidence of coronary artery disease by 3 years. Although the cause of this state is unclear, it probably represents chronic vascular rejection in an atherogenic milieu (e.g., hypertension, hypercholesterolemia). Treatment

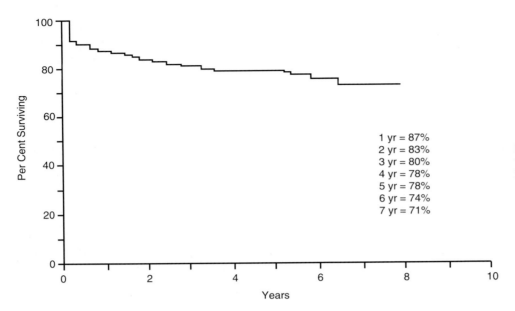

FIGURE 57–18. Actuarial survival in one cardiac transplant program (*n* = 473 patients).

1 yr = 87%
2 yr = 83%
3 yr = 80%
4 yr = 78%
5 yr = 78%
6 yr = 74%
7 yr = 71%

has not prevented the development of this complication and it is the major cause for consideration of retransplantation after the first 6 postoperative months.

## RESULTS AND FUTURE CONSIDERATIONS

Improved immunosuppression and use of surveillance endomyocardial biopsy have resulted in a 1-year survival of more than 85% and comparable 2- and 3-year survivals (Fig. 57–18). The causes of death are essentially unchanged; infection and rejection predominate. Patients who have successful cardiac transplantation are usually functionally rehabilitated without cardiac symptoms. Fewer than 50% return to full-time employment, either because they are unable to reenter the workforce for economic reasons or because society and employers refuse to accept their normal activity level.

Clinical research should be directed toward the development of more specific immunosuppressive protocols to further decrease the incidence of infection and rejection. Monoclonal antibody therapy has improved the management of rejection, with excellent survival in patients who receive this therapy prophylactically. At one center where 147 such operations were performed and an OKT3-based prophylactic protocol was used, in the first 36 months, the actuarial survival rate was 92% at 1 year and 90% at 3 years. As new monoclonal antibodies directed toward lymphocyte receptors (anti-TAC directed toward the interleukin-2 receptor) or blocking antibodies directed toward allograft antigens are developed, the specificity of immunosuppression will increase and the requirement for nonspecific immunosuppression, and thus the risk of infection, will decrease. Clinical trials of newer, more specific, less toxic immunosuppressants such as FK506, mycophenlate mofitil (RS-61443),

and photophoresis have already begun. Despite the possibility of improved management of early postoperative complications, little is known about the pathogenesis of allograft coronary artery disease. When research directed toward the resolution of this problem is fruitful, the long-term prognosis of these patients will be enhanced.

The disparity between the number of organs needed for transplantation and the number available for this purpose requires attention. Progress continues to be made in the specificity of immunosuppressive agents and in tissue typing and cross-matching, but long-term survival in grafts between disparate species has not been reliably achieved (Bailey et al., 1985; Sadeghi et al., 1987). Similarly, experience with the orthotopically placed total artificial heart has been disappointing (DeVries, 1988; Olsen, 1988). With approximately 15,000 patients in need of cardiac replacement in the united States and at most about 2,500 transplantable hearts available, the areas of cardiac xenografting and permanent mechanical replacement deserve further investigation.

## SELECTED BIBLIOGRAPHY

Bolman, R. M., Elick, B., Olivari, M. T., et al.: Improved immunosuppression for heart transplantation. J. Heart Transplant., 4:315, 1985.

Because of the concern about the reported nephrotoxicity of the immune suppressant cyclosporine A, the authors embarked on a trial of triple-drug therapy. The regimen consisted of cyclosporine A, in lower doses than reported earlier, with azathioprine and prednisone. The article describes the initial results of this trial, which were quite good. This regimen has become standard for immunosuppression in many centers.

Gilbert, E. M., Krueger, S. K., Murray, J. L., et al.: Echocardiographic evaluation of potential cardiac transplant donors. J. Thorac. Cardiovasc. Surg., 95:1003, 1988.

By use of echocardiography to evaluate ventricular function in potential heart donors, almost one-third of hearts that were unacceptable by conventional criteria were successfully recovered and transplanted. The authors describe methods for donor evaluation that have proved to be successful. At this time, when the number of donor organs available for transplantation is the critical factor that controls the number of transplants performed, every method possible must be used to recover suitable organs.

Starzl, T. E., Hakala, T. R., Shaw, B. W., Jr., et al.: A flexible procedure for multiple cadaveric organ procurement. Surg. Gynecol. Obstet., 158:223, 1984.

In this beautifully illustrated article, the authors describe in detail a method commonly used for multiple-organ recovery. At present, recovery of multiple transplantable organs from one donor is the best way to provide as many organs as possible to the recipient pool, which is much larger than the donor pool.

Yacoub, M., Alivizatos, P., Hadley-Smith, R., et al.: Cardiac transplantation. Are steroids really necessary? J. Am. Coll. Cardiol., 5:533, 1985.

In this incisive and provocative article, the authors challenge the conventional view that long-term maintenance corticosteroid therapy is necessary for survival after cardiac transplantation. Deletion of maintenance steroids from the immunosuppressive regimen would not only decrease the incidence of infectious complications but also make cardiac transplantation a more realistic option for a wider spectrum of patients (e.g., diabetics and children).

# BIBLIOGRAPHY

Addonizio, L. J., and Rose, E. A.: Cardiac transplantation in children and adolescents. J. Pediatr., 111:1034, 1987.

Andreone, P. A., Olivari, M. T., Elick, B., et al.: Reduction of infectious complications following heart transplantation with triple-drug immunotherapy. J. Heart Transplant., 5:13, 1986.

Armitage, J., Hardesty, R., and Griffith, B.: Prostaglandin E: An effective treatment of right heart failure after orthotopic heart transplantation. J. Heart Transplant., 6:348, 1987.

Backer, C. L., Zales, V. R., Idriss, F. S., et al.: Heart transplantation in neonates and in children. J. Heart Transplant., 11:311, 1992.

Badellino, M., Nairns, B., Fucci, P., et al.: Influence of diabetes mellitus on the course of cardiac transplantation [Abstract]. J. Am. Coll. Cardiol., 11:103A, 1988.

Bailey, L., Concepcion, W., Shattuck, H., and Huang, L.: Method of heart transplantation for treatment of hypoplastic left heart syndrome. J. Thorac. Cardiovasc. Surg., 92:1, 1986.

Bailey, L. L., Jang, J., Johnson, W., and Jolley, W. B.: Orthotopic cardiac xenografting in the newborn goat. J. Thorac. Cardiovasc. Surg., 89:242, 1985.

Barnard, C. N.: The operation. S. Afr. Med. J., 41:1271, 1967.

Barnard, C. N., Barnard, M. S., Cooper, D. K. L., et al.: The present status of heterotopic cardiac transplantation. J. Thorac. Cardiovasc. Surg., 81:433, 1981.

Baumgartner, W. A.: Evaluation and management of the heart donor. In Baumgartner, W. A., Reitz, B., and Achuff, S. C. (eds.): Heart-lung transplantation. Philadelphia, W. B. Saunders, 1990.

Bieber, C. P., Griepp, R. B., Oyer, P. E., et al.: Use of rabbit antithymocyte globulin in cardiac transplantation: Relationship of serum clearance rates to clinical outcome. Transplantation, 22:478, 1976.

Billingham, M. E.: Cardiac transplant atherosclerosis. Transplant. Proc., 19(Suppl. V):19, 1987.

Billingham, M. E.: Diagnosis of cardiac rejection by endomyocardial biopsy. J. Heart Transplant., 1:25, 1982.

Billingham, M. E.: Some recent advances in cardiac pathology. Hum. Pathol., 10:367, 1979.

Bolman, R. M., Cance, C., Spray, T., et al.: The changing face of cardiac transplantation: The Washington University Program, 1985–1987. Ann. Thorac. Surg., 45:192, 1988.

Bolman, R. M., Elick, B., Olivari, M. T., et al.: Improved immunosuppression for heart transplantation. J. Heart Transplant., 4:315, 1985.

Bolman, R. M., III, Spray, T. L., Cox, J. L., et al.: Heart transplantation in patients requiring preoperative mechanical support. J. Heart Transplant., 6:273, 1987.

Borel, J. F.: Cyclosporine: Historical perspectives. Transplant. Proc., 15(Suppl. I):3, 1983.

Borel, J. F., Feurer, C., Gubler, H. U., and Stahelin, H.: Biological effects of cyclosporine A: A new lymphocytic agent. Agents Actions, 6:468, 1976.

Bristow, M. R., Gilbert, E. M., Renlund, D. G., et al.: Use of OKT3

monoclonal antibody in cardiac transplantation: Review of the initial experience. J. Heart Transplant., 7:1, 1988.

Brodman, R. F., Veith, F. J., Goldsmith, J., et al.: Multiple organ procurement from one donor. J. Heart Transplant., 4:254, 1985.

Calne, R. Y., Rolles, K., White, D. J. G., et al.: Cyclosporine A in clinical organ grafting. Transplant. Proc., 13:349, 1981.

Calne, R. Y., White, D. J. G., Rolles, K., et al.: Prolonged survival of pig orthotopic heart grafts treated with cyclosporine A. Lancet, 1:1183, 1978.

Cannon, D. S., Graham, A. F., and Harrison, D. C.: Electrophysiologic studies in the denervated transplanted human heart. Response to atrial pacing and atropine. Circ. Res., 32:268, 1973.

Carrel, A., and Guthrie, C. C.: The transplantation of veins and organs. Am. J. Med., 11:1101, 1905.

Carrier, M., Emery, R. W., Riley, J. E., et al.: Cardiac transplantation in patients over 50 years of age. J. Am. Coll. Cardiol., 8:285, 1986.

Caves, P. K., Stinson, E. B., Billingham, M. E., and Shumway, N. E.: Percutaneous transvenous endomyocardial biopsy in human heart recipients. Ann. Thorac. Surg., 16:325, 1973.

Christopherson, L. K.: Cardiac transplantation: A psychological perspective. Circulation, 75:57, 1987.

Cohen, D. J., Loertscher, R., Rubin, M. F., et al.: Cyclosporine: A new immunosuppressive agent for organ transplantation. Ann. Intern. Med., 101:667, 1984.

Cohn, J. N., Levine, T. B., Olivari, M. T., et al.: Plasma norepinephrine as a guide to prognosis in patients with chronic congestive heart failure. N. Engl. J. Med., 311:819, 1984b.

CONSENSUS: The CONSENSUS Trial Study Group: Effects of enalapril on mortality in severe congestive heart failure. Result of the Cooperative North Scandinavian Enalapril Survival Study. N. Engl. J. Med., 316:1429, 1987.

Copeland, J. G., Jones, M., Spragg, R., and Stinson, E. B.: In vitro preservation of canine hearts for 24 to 48 hours followed by successful orthotopic transplantation. Ann. Surg., 178:687, 1973.

Demikov, V. P.: Experimental Transplantation of Vital Organs. New York, Consultants Bureau, 1962.

DeVries, W. C.: The permanent artificial heart. Four case reports. J. A. M. A., 259:847, 1988.

Emery, R. W., Cork, R. C., Levinson, M. M., et al.: The cardiac donor. A six-year experience. Ann. Thorac. Surg., 41:356, 1986.

Evans, R. W., and Maier, A. M.: Outcome of patients referred for cardiac transplantation. J. Am. Coll. Cardiol., 8:1312, 1986.

Evans, R. W., Mannien, R. L., Garrison, L. P., and Maier, A. M.: Donor availability as the primary determinant of the future of heart transplantation. J. A. M. A., 255:1892, 1986.

Farrar, D. J., Hill, J. D., Gray, L. A., et al.: Heterotopic prosthetic ventricles as a bridge to cardiac transplantation. N. Engl. J. Med., 318:333, 1988.

Fransiosa, J. A., Wilen, M., Ziesche, S. M., et al.: Survival in men with severe chronic left ventricular failure due to either coronary artery disease or idiopathic dilated cardiomyopathy. Am. J. Cardiol., 51:831, 1983.

Frazier, O. H., Macris, M. P., Duncan, J. M., et al.: Cardiac transplantation in patients over 60 years of age. Ann. Thorac. Surg., 45:129,1988.

Fricker, F. J., Griffith, B. P., Hardesty, R. L., et al.: Experience with heart transplantation in children. Pediatrics, 79:138, 1987.

Gao, S. Z., Johnson, D., Schroeder, J. S., et al.: Transplant coronary artery disease: Histopathologic correlations with angiographic morphology [Abstract]. J. Am. Coll. Cardiol., 11:153A, 1988.

Gay, W. A.: Cardiac transplantation—A surgical perspective. J. Cardiothorac. Anesth., 2:513, 1988.

Gilbert, E. M., Krueger, S. K., Murray, J. L., et al.: Echocardiographic evaluation of potential cardiac transplant donors. J. Thorac. Cardiovasc. Surg., 95:1003, 1988.

Health Care Finance Administration (HCFA), Department of Health and Human Services Medicare Program: Criteria for Medicare coverage of heart transplants. Fed. Reg., 52:10935, 1987.

Hofflin, J. M., Potasman, I., Baldwin, J. C., et al.: Infectious complications in heart transplant recipients receiving cyclosporine and corticosteroids. Ann. Intern. Med., 106:209, 1987.

Hunt, S. A., Strober, S., Hoppe, R. T., et al.: Total lymphoid irradiation for treatment of intractable cardiac allograft rejection. J. Heart Transplant., 10:211, 1991.

Jamieson, S. W., Burton, N. A., Bieber, C. P., et al.: Cardiac allograft survival in primates treated with cyclosporine A. Lancet, 1:545, 1979.

Jeevanandum, V., Barr, M. L., Auteri, J. S., et al.: University of Wisconsin solution versus crystalloid cardioplegia for human donor heart preservation. J. Thorac. Cardiovasc. Surg., 103:194, 1992.

Kahan, B. D.: Immunosuppressive therapy with cyclosporine for cardiac transplantation. Circulation, 75:40, 1987.

Kostakis, A. J., White, D. J. G., and Calne, R. Y.: Prolongation of rat heart allograft survival by cyclosporine A. Int. Rev. Cytol., (Suppl.)5:280, 1977.

Kriett, J. M., and Kaye, M. P.: The Registry of the International Society for Heart Transplantation: Seventh Official Report 1990. J. Heart Transplant., 9:232, 1990.

Ladowski, J., Kormos, R. L., Uretsky, B. F., et al.: Heart transplantation in diabetic recipients. Transplantation, 49:303, 1990.

Lower, R. R., Dong, E. J., and Shumway, N. E.: Long-term survival of cardiac homografts. Surgery, 58:110, 1965.

Lower, R. R., and Shumway, N. E.: Studies on orthotopic transplantation of the canine heart. Surg. Forum, 11:18, 1960.

Magovern, G. J., Park, S. B., Magovern, G. J., Jr., et al.: Mechanical circulatory assist devices. Texas Heart Inst. J., 14:276, 1987.

Mavroudis, C., Kline, J. B., Harrison, H. L., et al.: Infant orthotopic heart transplantation. J. Thorac. Cardiovasc. Surg., 96:912, 1988.

May, R. M., Cooper, D. K. C., DuToit, E. D., et al.: Cytoimmunologic monitoring after heart and heart-lung transplantation. J. Heart Transplant., 9:133, 1990.

Munoz, E., Longuist, J., Radovancevic, B., et al.: Long-term results in diabetic patients undergoing cardiac transplantation. J. Heart Transplant., 10:189, 1991.

O'Connell, J. B.: The role of myocarditis in end-stage dilated cardiomyopathy. Texas Heart Inst. J., 14:268, 1987.

O'Connell, J. B., and Gunnar, R. M.: Dilated-congestive cardiomyopathy: Prognostic features and therapy. J. Heart Transplant., 2:7, 1982.

O'Connell, J. B., and Renlund, D. G.: Variations in the diagnosis, treatment and prevention of cardiac allograft rejection: The need for standardization? J. Heart Transplant., 9:269, 1990.

O'Connell, J. B., Renlund, D. G., DeWitt, C. W., and Bristow, M. R.: Cardiac transplantation in sensitized recipients without a prospective crossmatch [Abstract]. J. Heart Transplant., 7:74, 1988a.

O'Connell, J. B., Renlund, D. G., Lee, H. R., et al.: Newer techniques of immunosuppression in cardiac transplantation. In Emery, R. W., and Prizker, M. (eds): Cardiac Surgery: State of the Art Reviews. Vol. 3. Philadelphia, Hanley & Belfus, 1988b, p. 607.

O'Connell, J. B., Renlund, D. G., Robinson, J. A., et al.: Effect of preoperative hemodynamic support on survival following cardiac transplantation. Circulation, 76(Suppl. II):257, 1987.

Olsen, D.: Personal communication, 1988.

Oyer, P. E., Stinson, E. B., Jamieson, S. W., et al.: One-year experience with cyclosporine A in clinical heart transplantation. Heart Transplant., 1:285, 1982.

Penn, I.: Cancers following cyclosporine therapy. Transplantation, 43:32, 1987.

Reemtsma K: The heart as a test organ in transplantation studies. Ann. N. Y. Acad. Sci., 120:778, 1964.

Reemtsma, K., Williamson, W. E., Jr., Iglesias, F., et al.: Studies in homologous canine heart transplantation: Prolongation of survival with a folic acid antagonist. Surgery, 52:127, 1962.

Renlund, D. G., Bristow, M. R., Burton, N. A., et al.: Survival following cardiac transplantation: What are acceptable standards? West. J. Med., 146:627, 1987a.

Renlund, D. G., Bristow, M. R., Crandall, B. G., et al.: Hypercholesterolemia after cardiac transplantation: Amelioration by corticosteroid-free maintenance immunosuppression. J. Heart Transplant., 8:214, 1989.

Renlund, D. G., Gilbert, E. M., O'Connell, J. B., et al.: Age-associated decline in cardiac allograft rejection. Am. J. Med., 83:391, 1987b.

Renlund, D. G., O'Connell, J. B., Gilbert, E. M., et al.: Feasibility of discontinuation of corticosteroid maintenance therapy in heart transplantation. J. Heart Transplant., 6:71, 1987c.

Rose, E. A., Barr, M. L., Xu, H., et al.: Photochemotherapy in human heart transplant recipients at high risk for fatal rejection. J. Heart Transplant., 11:746, 1992.

Sadeghi, A. M., Robbins, R. C., Smith, C. R., et al.: Cardiac xenotransplantation in primates. J. Thorac. Cardiovasc. Surg., 93:809, 1987.

Schwartz, R., and Dameshek N: Drug-induced immunological tolerance. Nature, 183:1682, 1959.

Starzl, T. E., Hakala, T. R., Shaw, B. W., Jr., et al.: A flexible procedure for multiple cadaveric organ procurement. Surg. Gynecol. Obstet., 158:223, 1984.

Stevenson, L. W., Fowler, M. B., Schroeder, J. S., et al.: Poor survival of patients in idiopathic cardiomyopathy considered too well for transplantation. Am. J. Med., 83:871, 1987.

Thompson, M. E., Shapiro, A. P., Johnsen, S. M., et al.: The contrasting effects of cyclosporine A and azathioprine on arterial blood pressure and renal function following cardiac transplantation. Int. J. Cardiol., 11:219, 1986.

Wahlers, T., Heublin, B., Cremer, J., et al.: Treatment of rejection after heart transplantation: What dosage of pulsed steroids is necessary? J. Heart Transplant., 9:568, 1990.

Weber, K. T., Janicki, J. S., and Jain, M. C.: Enoximone (MDL17,043), a phosphodiesterase inhibitor, in the treatment of advanced, unstable chronic heart failure. J. Heart Transplant., 6:105, 1986.

Wilson, J. R., Schwartz, J. S., St. John-Sutton, M., et al.: Prognosis in severe heart failure: Relation to hemodynamic measurements and ventricular ectopic activity. J. Am. Coll. Cardiol., 2:403, 1983.

Wong, K. C., and Wu, L. T.: History of Chinese Medicine. 2nd ed. Shanghai, National Quarantine Service, 1936.

Yacoub, M., Alivizatos, P., Radley-Smith, R., et al.: Cardiac transplantation: Are steroids really necessary? J. Am. Coll. Cardiol., 5:533, 1985.

Young, J. N., Yazbeck, J., Esposito, G., et al.: The influence of acute preoperative pulmonary infarction on the results of heart transplantation. J. Heart Transplant., 5:20, 1986.

# ■ III  Lung Transplantation

Joel D. Cooper and G. Alexander Patterson

Until the early 1980s, attempts at lung transplantation were uniformly fatal, at a time when kidney, liver, and heart transplantation had become clinically well established. However, in the next decade remarkable progress was made, and the success rate with lung transplantation is now similar to that of other organ transplants. For the 183 single and sequential bilateral lung transplants performed at Barnes Hospital, hospital mortality is 7.5%. This progress has been possible because of the solid base of experimental and clinical investigation conducted over many years, the advent of improved immunosuppressive agents, and the rapid accumulation and dissemination of experience obtained with clinical lung transplantation at many centers.

## HISTORICAL ASPECTS

Metras (1950) in France, and Hardin and Kittle (1954) in the United States demonstrated the technical feasibility of lung transplantation in dogs, with a technique that has not changed substantially to this day. Most experimental work has been conducted in dogs using either a reimplantation model, in which the lung is severed and reattached, or allotransplantation, the implantation of a lung from another dog. Reimplantation has been used to eliminate factors relating to rejection and to study those factors associated with the technical aspects of the procedure as well as the effects of lymphatic, neural, and bronchial artery interruption. Early experiments suggested that there was a significant increase in pulmonary vascular resistance in the transplanted lung immediately following implantation. Subsequently, it was demonstrated that, with meticulous anastomotic technique for the pulmonary arterial and venous attachments, the vascular resistance of the transplanted lung was nearly normal (Alican et al., 1971; Benfield and Coon, 1971; Daicoff et al., 1970; Veith and Richards, 1969; Waldhausen et al., 1967). Similarly, it has become apparent that interruption of the lymphatic connections, the vagus nerves, and the bronchial arteries does not cause any significant physiologic derangement. Progress in lung transplantation was impeded in part by the lack of a suitable experimental model that was analogous to the usual clinical situation. With unilateral lung transplantation in the dog, the function of the remaining native lung is sufficient to sustain the animal, and physiologic malfunction of

the transplanted lung may not be apparent. However, unilateral transplantation with immediate ligation of the contralateral pulmonary artery, or contralateral pneumonectomy, requires that the transplanted lung immediately accept the entire cardiac output. This may foster the development of pulmonary edema in the immediate post-transplant period, especially if lung preservation is not optimal.

Early malfunction of a transplanted lung has often been attributed to the *reimplantation response*. This response is attributed variously to the effects of lymphatic, neural, or bronchial artery interruption along with possible effects caused by ischemia and reperfusion. Increasing clinical experience has shown that such a response is not inevitable and that it likely results mainly from ischemic or reperfusion injury, or both.

Accurate diagnosis of lung rejection continues to remain elusive, and in the absence of reliable diagnostic criteria, excessive immunosuppression may be used, increasing the risk of infectious complications. Exposure to bacterial contamination, ischemia of the donor airway caused by interruption of the bronchial circulation, and the adverse effects of immunosuppression combined to cause significant problems with pulmonary sepsis and poor healing of the airway anastomosis.

Finally, the effects of organ ischemia on post-transplant function have been difficult to identify, given the many other factors that may also cause post-transplant malfunction. Thus, the period of safe ischemic time, between extraction of the lung and restoration of its circulation, has been difficult to ascertain.

In summary, early malfunction of the transplanted lung may be attributed to numerous factors and this, together with the lack of a clinically relevant animal model, contributed to the slow pace of progress made with lung transplantation compared with other types of organ transplant.

## HUMAN LUNG TRANSPLANTATION

In 1963, Hardy and co-workers reported the first human lung transplant. The recipient survived for 18 days and died of renal failure. This experience demonstrated the technical feasibility of lung transplantation and stimulated worldwide interest in the field. Over the next 20 years, approximately 40 lung or lobe transplants were performed worldwide with little clinical success. Only 1 recipient survived long enough to be discharged from hospital, a 23-year-old man who underwent right lung transplant for advanced silicosis (Derom et al., 1971). The patient was discharged from hospital 8 months after transplantation and died 2 months later from chronic rejection and pulmonary sepsis.

The report of a successful combined heart-lung transplant by the Stanford University group in 1981 provided an important stimulus for further efforts in lung transplantation (Reitz et al., 1982). This report confirmed that an individual can function satisfactorily solely on transplanted lung tissue, as previously suggested by the 10-month survival of Derom and colleagues' patient (1971). The combined heart-lung transplant had been attempted initially by Cooley and associates (1969) and subsequently by Lillehei (1970) and by Barnard and Cooper (1981), all without success. By using the new immunosuppressant drug cyclosporine, the Stanford group was able to achieve clinical success with the heart-lung transplant procedure in patients with right-sided heart failure and pulmonary hypertension. The present authors' own initial experience with unilateral lung transplant occurred in 1978 when a right lung transplant was performed for a ventilator-dependent patient with inhalation burns (Nelems et al., 1980). The recipient died in the third week, of disruption of the bronchial anastomosis. Review of world experience to that date revealed that only nine patients had survived more than 2 weeks following unilateral lung transplantation, and six of these nine, including the authors' patient, died of bronchial anastomotic disruption within the first month. Following this experience, a laboratory program was initiated to evaluate factors affecting bronchial anastomotic healing following lung transplantation. The initial experiments involved canine lung autotransplantation, with severing and immediate reattachment of the lung (Lima et al., 1981). Half of the animals received no postoperative immunosuppressants, whereas the other half received standard immunosuppression with azathioprine and prednisone. The treated animals exhibited significant bronchial anastomotic complications, including ischemia, necrosis, and disruption of the anastomosis, similar to complications reported following human lung transplantation. The untreated animals exhibited primary healing of the bronchial anastomosis, although narrowing of the bronchus distal to the anastomosis was a frequent occurrence, one that was attributed to ischemia.

Subsequent experiments demonstrated that the adverse effect on wound healing in the immunosuppressed animals related entirely to the prednisone and that the use of azathioprine did not prejudice bronchial healing. Experiments using cyclosporine in place of prednisone indicated that bronchial healing in such animals did not differ from that in untreated animals (Goldberg et al., 1983).

In an attempt to rapidly restore bronchial arterial blood supply following transplantation, the authors employed a pedicle of omentum brought into the

chest with its blood supply intact. This was wrapped around the bronchial anastomosis following its completion. These studies revealed rapid restoration of bronchial blood supply by means of omental collaterals and produced improved anastomotic healing following transplantation (Dubois et al., 1984; Morgan et al., 1983). In 1983, a clinical program of lung transplantation was begun at the University of Toronto based on the principles elucidated in the laboratory: avoidance of routine steroids in the early postoperative period and use of an omental pedicle wrapped around the bronchial anastomosis to improve blood supply and healing and to prevent bronchovascular or bronchopleural fistula in case the anastomosis failed to heal satisfactorily. The result was a series of successful unilateral lung transplants (Toronto Lung Transplant Group, 1986, 1988).

## INDICATIONS FOR SINGLE AND BILATERAL TRANSPLANT

Techniques for single and bilateral lung transplantation have been simplified, and indications for lung transplantation have been correspondingly expanded. Patients with end-stage pulmonary fibrosis initially were considered the ideal candidates for unilateral lung transplantation. The reduced compliance and increased vascular resistance of the native lung ensures that both ventilation and perfusion are preferentially diverted to the transplanted lung. At the outset, the authors were concerned that unilateral transplantation for emphysema might not be ideal because the contralateral native lung might exhibit hyperexpansion and air trapping, causing an unfavorable shift of the mediastinum and restriction of ventilation to the transplant. These concerns proved largely unfounded, and chronic obstructive pulmonary disease is now the single greatest indication for unilateral lung transplantation.

As previously noted, heart-lung transplantation was successfully pioneered by the Stanford University group, for patients with either primary pulmonary hypertension (PPH) or pulmonary hypertension secondary to Eisenmenger's syndrome. It was demonstrated, in a canine model, that the severe right-sided heart failure caused by pressure overload could rapidly recover following restoration of normal right ventricular outflow pressures (Hsieh et al., 1992). Unilateral lung transplant subsequently has been employed, with gratifying results, for patients with either primary or secondary pulmonary hypertension (Pasque et al., 1992). The rationale for using unilateral rather than bilateral transplantation for patients with emphysema and those with pulmonary hypertension is based, among other factors, on the acute shortage of available donor lungs and, thus, the ability to reduce waiting time and transplant more recipients. Technical simplicity is another factor in this choice. However, the choice of single instead of bilateral transplant for patients with emphysema and those with pulmonary hypertension remains controversial. Further experience and long-term follow-up will be required before the issue can be resolved. Unilateral transplant is also used for various other end-stage lung diseases, including sarcoidosis, lymphangioleiomyomatosis, eosinophilic granuloma, and others.

For patients with chronic pulmonary sepsis, such as cystic fibrosis or bronchiectasis, replacement of both lungs is indicated. It is possible to replace one lung and remove the other, but the dangers of bronchial stump fistula, empyema, or infection in the single transplanted lung would pose a considerable risk in such patients. Combined heart-lung transplant initially was employed for such patients, but it soon became obvious that the recipient heart was being replaced simply for technical expedience rather than out of physiologic necessity. Therefore, a procedure was developed for simultaneous en bloc bilateral pulmonary transplantation, a procedure analogous to the combined heart-lung transplant, without the need to transplant the heart.

The concept of simultaneous en bloc bilateral pulmonary transplantation was demonstrated in dogs by Vanderhoeft and co-workers in 1972. That procedure, performed through a right thoracotomy, was not suitable for clinical use. The technique the present authors initially employed used a median sternotomy, bilateral pneumonectomy, and implantation of the double lung en bloc with three anastomoses: the trachea, the common pulmonary artery, and a cuff of donor left atrium containing the pulmonary veins (Dark et al., 1986; Patterson et al., 1988). Initial experience with the procedure was very satisfactory (Cooper et al., 1989), and five of the initial seven recipients are alive and well more than 6 years later. However, further experience showed that airway complications occurred in approximately 25% of cases (Patterson et al., 1990). Use of bilateral bronchial anastomoses rather than the tracheal anastomosis significantly reduced the incidence of ischemic airway complications. Nonetheless, the double-lung transplant, as initially employed, continued to have significant drawbacks. The procedure was complicated and required a prolonged period of cardiopulmonary bypass (CPB) and the need for ischemic arrest of the recipient heart during a portion of the procedure. The excellent success achieved with the unilateral lung transplant prompted the development of a technique for sequential bilateral lung replacement through a transverse thoracosternotomy (Pasque et al., 1990). Exposure afforded by this incision permits each lung to be completely mobilized without CPB. The recipient is maintained on one lung while the opposite lung is replaced using a technique identical to that for single-lung transplantation. The second lung is then replaced with the recipient maintained on the newly implanted lung. In the authors' experience, a brief period of partial CPB has been required in approximately 25% of patients, most commonly during implantation of the second lung. The relative simplicity of this sequential bilateral technique, and improved results, permitted a further widening of indications for the procedure, including patients with cystic fibrosis who have undergone previous thoracic procedures such as pleurodesis or pulmonary resection.

Before 1983, bronchial anastomotic complications were a major source of morbidity and mortality following lung transplantation. Experiments with a canine lung transplant model demonstrated the benefits of a bronchial omentopexy; it rapidly produced collateral circulation to the donor bronchial arteries and protected against bronchovascular and bronchopleural fistula in the case of anastomotic breakdown. Until recently, the authors favored routine use of an omental wrap around the bronchial anastomosis and strict avoidance of perioperative routine steroid administration. The authors no longer feel that either factor is critical. The incidence of fatal airway complications, in the authors' own experience and in that reported to the St. Louis International Lung Transplant Registry (Cooper et al., 1994), is less than 2%. The marked reduction in airway complications is likely due to improved donor lung preservation, better management of infectious complications, and early recognition and prompt treatment of acute rejection. All of these factors have significantly reduced postoperative ventilator dependency, the number of days spent in the intensive care unit, and the overall hospital stay.

## SELECTION OF RECIPIENTS

Various end-stage lung diseases have necessitated transplantation in patients. The most common diagnoses have been chronic obstructive pulmonary disease, alpha$_1$-antitrypsin-deficiency emphysema, pulmonary fibrosis, cystic fibrosis, and PPH. Controversial indications include retransplantation for chronic rejection following previous lung transplantation, patients with systemic diseases with associated pulmonary involvement, and interstitial lung disease caused by chemotherapy or radiotherapy for a previous neoplasm. The relative shortage of usable donor lungs and the desire to obtain the maximal benefit from these lungs have had a major effect on the recipient selection process. Potential recipients should have clinically and physiologically severe lung disease with a poor prognosis for survival despite optimal medical therapy, and should have no other health problems that would either jeopardize the success of the operation or limit life expectancy after transplantation. Prospective transplant recipients undergo psychological testing; any with significant psychosocial problems are excluded because of the considerable stress that the preoperative assessment, long waiting, and postoperative recovery imposes. Furthermore, strict patient compliance and cooperation are essential to ensure a satisfactory long-term result.

General guidelines for recipient selection are listed in Table 57–7. Other considerations include age and steroid dependency. With few exceptions, the authors have limited transplantation to recipients 60 years of age and younger. Steroid requirement of greater than

**■ Table 57–7.** CRITERIA FOR RECIPIENT SELECTION

Clinically and physiologically severe disease with limited
  life expectancy
Medical therapy ineffective or unavailable
Adequate left ventricular function without significant
  coronary artery disease
Ambulatory with potential for rehabilitation
Acceptable nutritional status (80–120% ideal body weight)
Satisfactory psychosocial profile and emotional support
  system

10 mg of prednisone per day continues to be a relative, but not absolute, contraindication. The authors previously considered ventilator dependency a contraindication to transplantation. This restriction was subsequently eliminated for individuals who were found acceptable for lung transplantation but who subsequently deteriorated to the point of ventilator dependency.

In general, transplantation has been reserved for patients whose disability and rate of disease progression suggest that life expectancy is limited to a range of 12 to 24 months. Such individuals are usually oxygen-dependent, show progressive deterioration of pulmonary function and exercise capacity, and have increasing oxygen requirements. For patients with obstructive pulmonary disease, selection has included those with a first-second vital capacity (FEV$_1$) between 15% and 20% of predicted. Recipients with restrictive lung disease have an FEV$_1$ of 50 to 60% of predicted or less, and show arterial oxygen desaturation with mild exercise despite oxygen administration. For patients with cystic fibrosis, no simple algorithm exists to predict life expectancy, although a significant correlation between FEV$_1$ and life expectancy has been demonstrated (Kerem et al., 1992). The need for oxygen administration, a decline in nutritional status, and the need for increasing hospitalization for recurrent pulmonary infection all suggest a limited life expectancy in this disease.

A study of the natural history of patients with PPH indicated a mean life expectancy of 2.8 years from the time of diagnosis (D'Alonzo et al., 1991). Increased right atrial pressure, diminished cardiac output, and increasing right ventricular failure all adversely affect prognosis. Patients with pulmonary hypertension have a high rate of mortality while on the waiting list, in the range of 15 to 25%. The authors employ unilateral lung transplantation for these patients in an attempt to reduce the waiting period and the associated death rate. Table 57–8 lists the indications and the type of transplant used for recipients listed in the St. Louis Lung Transplant Registry.

## SELECTION OF DONORS

The lack of suitable donor lungs is the major obstacle to more widespread application of lung transplantation. Suitable lungs are more difficult to obtain than other donor organs because the lungs are susceptible to infection and edema under the circumstances surrounding brain death. Optimal donor lungs are those in which the chest x-ray is clear, the arterial oxygen tension exceeds 300 mm/Hg with an F$_{IO_2}$ of 1.0 l and 5 cm of positive end-expiratory pressure, and bronchoscopic findings show no grossly purulent secretions or suggestion of aspiration. The authors estimate that no more than 15 to 20% of organ donors have lungs suitable for transplantation. The authors have recently liberalized criteria for donor lungs, and will on occasion use a lung with a small contusion, lungs with a mild infiltrate thought due to pulmonary edema, and lungs from a donor with a suboptimal PO$_2$ when this is thought due to recent development of pulmonary edema. When a single-lung transplant for pulmonary hypertension is performed, however, the strictest criteria are adhered to, including an ischemic time of 6 hours or less. Following single-lung transplant for pulmonary hypertension, the transplanted lung immediately receives more than 90% of the cardiac output because of the very high vascular resistance in the contralateral native lung. This places a unique burden on the transplant.

For purposes of size matching, the vertical and transverse radiologic dimensions of the chest are used. Lateral films are generally not available for the donor, so the dimensions from a portable anteroposterior film must be used. Thus, accurate comparison with the intended recipient is not possible. Together with the x-ray dimensions, the body weight, height, sex, and chest circumference of the donor are compared with those of the recipient in an attempt to assess the suitability of the match.

The predicted lung volumes for the donor and recipient can also be compared using standard tables. Initially, the authors sought a donor lung of approximately the same size as the recipient chest, but subsequently realized that it is more appropriate to select a lung based on the *predicted* normal size of the lung for the height, weight, and sex of the recipient. With restrictive lung disease, the recipient chest is contracted because of the fibrotic lung, but it can expand readily to a more normal configuration when a larger lung is inserted (Fig. 57–19). With emphysema, on the other hand, the recipient chest is grossly overexpanded. The insertion of a normal-sized lung is followed by elevation of the diaphragm to a more normal position and restoration of a more normal

**■ Table 57–8.** INDICATIONS FOR LUNG TRANSPLANTATION

| Diagnosis | n | Single Lung (n = 1459) | Bilateral Lung (n = 709) |
|---|---|---|---|
| COPD | 594 | 493 | 101 |
| A-1 Emphysema | 290 | 206 | 84 |
| Cystic fibrosis | 307 | 5 | 302 |
| PPH/Eisenmenger's | 241 | 180 | 61 |
| IPF | 373 | 346 | 27 |
| Other | 363 | 229 | 134 |

*Key:* COPD = chronic obstructive pulmonary disease; PPH = primary pulmonary hypertension; IPF = idiopathic pulmonary fibrosis.

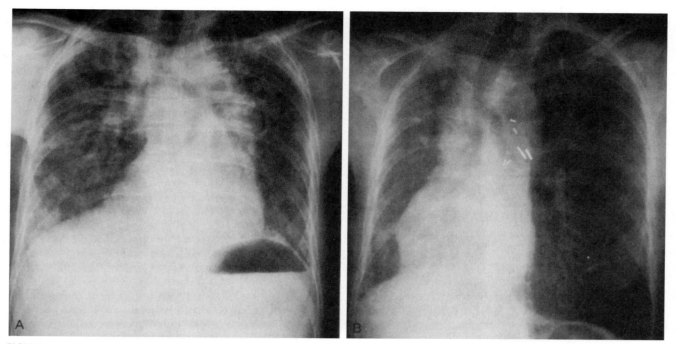

**FIGURE 57–19.** Preoperative (A) and postoperative (B) chest films from a patient who underwent left-sided lung transplantation for end-stage pulmonary fibrosis. An oversized donor lung was used. The postoperative film, taken 2 months after the procedure, shows the diaphragmatic descent and mediastinal shift that allowed accommodation of the transplanted lung.

thoracic configuration (Fig. 57–20). In pulmonary hypertension, the recipient lung is normal in size, and care is taken to avoid oversizing or undersizing the donor lung.

Suitable donors are selected on the basis of ABO blood compatibility. Histocompatibility matching is done only afterward because the effect of such matching remains uncertain and it is currently impractical to delay retrieval until a prospective cross-match has been obtained.

## LUNG PRESERVATION

Various methods for donor lung preservation have been used over the years, but the most common practice is a bolus injection of prostaglandin $E_1$ into the pulmonary artery immediately followed by flushing of the donor lung with a cold electrolyte solution. The heparinized donor is given 500 μg of prostaglandin $E_1$ directly into the pulmonary artery over 10 to 15 seconds. Pulmonary preservation is then achieved by

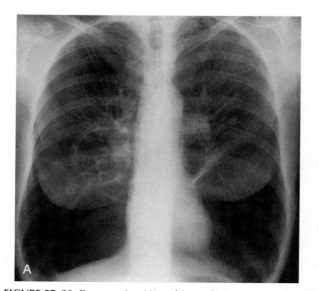
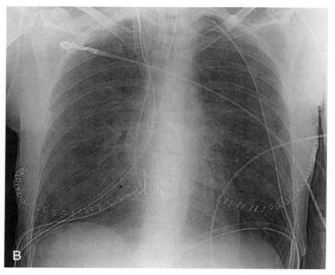

**FIGURE 57–20.** Preoperative (A) and immediate postoperative (B) chest film from a 49-year-old woman with severe emphysema secondary to alpha₁-antitrypsin deficiency. Both the thoracic cage and the diaphragm have assumed a more normal position.

a cold flush through a large-bore catheter in the donor pulmonary artery. The authors use 3 l of ice-cold Euro-Collins solution to which have been added 56 ml of 50% glucose and 8 mEq of magnesium sulfate per liter. In the laboratory, excellent lung preservation can be achieved for periods of 24 hours, but in clinical practice, 10 hours is considered the upper limit, and the authors make every effort to keep ischemic time below 8 hours.

## DONOR LUNG EXTRACTION

Donor lungs are extracted in conjunction with multiple organ retrieval. The method for removing the heart for cardiac transplantation without jeopardizing the use of the lungs has been described by Sundaresan and colleagues (1993). Whenever possible, both lungs are used, either for single-lung transplantation in separate recipients or in combination for a sequential bilateral-lung transplant. The technical aspects of donor lung retrieval are depicted in Figures 57–21 to 57–24.

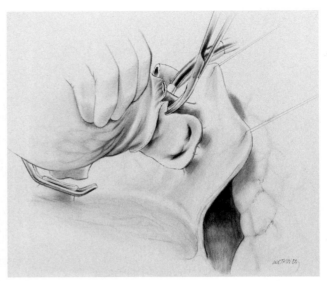

FIGURE 57–22. Cardiac extraction precedes pulmonary extraction. The pulmonary artery is divided at its bifurcation, and the aorta is transected just proximal to the great vessels. The superior vena cava is divided between the previously placed ligatures. The apex of the heart is then rotated upward toward the right shoulder to facilitate left atrial division. Division of the left atrium is begun with a vertical incision just anterior to the left pulmonary veins. The incision in the atrium is then carried transversely superiorly and inferiorly toward the right and is completed just anterior to the orifices of the right pulmonary veins. The heart is then removed from the field.

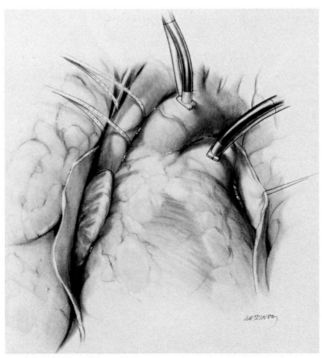

FIGURE 57–21. Preparation for heart and lung extraction. The proximal aorta and pulmonary artery have been dissected free. The superior vena cava has been loosely encircled twice, usually below the level of the azygos vein. The cardioplegia catheter is inserted into the aorta, and a large-bore aortic cannula is inserted through a purse-string in the common pulmonary artery, just proximal to its bifurcation. The inferior vena cava is mobilized just above the diaphragm. Just prior to occlusion of the vena cavae 500 μg of prostaglandin E₁ is injected with a syringe and needle directly into the proximal pulmonary artery. Ten to 15 seconds later, the superior vena cava is ligated and the inferior vena cava is clamped at the level of the diaphragm and transected above the clamp. The cardioplegia solution is then infused. The tip of a lateral atrial appendage is amputated, and the pulmonary artery flush is begun.

Through a median sternotomy, the pericardium is vertically incised, and the superior vena cava, inferior vena cava, ascending aorta, and common pulmonary artery are circumferentially mobilized. A cardioplegia catheter is inserted into the ascending aorta and a large-bore aortic cannula is inserted into the proximal pulmonary artery. The interatrial group is dissected to increase the margin between the right pulmonary veins and the interatrial septum. This helps to provide adequate left atrial cuff in this region for both the heart and the lung specimens. When all retrieval teams are prepared, 500 μg of prostaglandin E₁ is injected directly into the pulmonary artery and 15 seconds later the venae cavae are occluded. Venting for the cardioplegia solution is provided by division of the inferior vena cava, just central to a clamp placed across it at the level of the diaphragm. Venting for the pulmonary flush is provided by excision of the tip of the left atrial appendage. Cardioplegia is then administered through the aortic cannula, and the lungs are flushed with 3 l of cold-modified Euro-Collins solution through the pulmonary artery catheter. Both cavae, the ascending aorta, and the common pulmonary artery (at its bifurcation) are divided. The great vessels from the aortic arch are similarly divided. Careful division of the left atrium is then carried out to leave an adequate cuff on both the cardiac and the pulmonary specimens. Following removal of the heart, the trachea is divided between staple lines at its midpoint, with the lungs held at midinflation. The esophagus is mobilized posterior to the trachea and divided with a linear stapling device. The inferior pulmonary ligaments are divided and the pericardium is divided posteriorly, just above the diaphragm to expose the esophagus and the aorta at the level of the diaphragm. The aorta is transected and the distal esophagus is divided with a linear stapling device. The two lungs are then removed en bloc along with the esophagus and the thoracic aorta. The specimen is placed in a plastic bag containing flushing solution at 4° C. This bag is placed in turn in two additional bags, which are then surrounded by crushed ice and transported. If each of the lungs is to be transported to separate transplant centers, the lungs are separated on a back table at the donor institution. Final preparation of the donor lungs involves removal of the esophagus and the aorta from the specimen, division of the two pulmonary arteries at their common origin, vertical incision of the left atrial cuff midway between the right and the left pulmonary veins, and transection of each bronchus approximately two rings proximal to the origin of the upper lobe bronchus. When donor lungs are separated at the site of retrieval for transportation to separate centers, the left main bronchus is divided between the staple lines just distal to the carina. This maintains a closed airway for both the right and the left lungs, allowing their immersion without flooding the airway. Further trimming of each airway occurs prior to implantation.

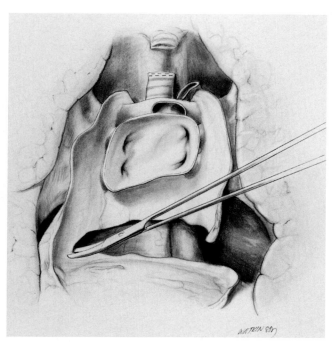

FIGURE 57–24. The pulmonary ligaments are divided, and the inferior pericardium is transversely incised at the level of the diaphragm. The distal esophagus is transected with a linear stapling device just above the diaphragm, and the descending aorta is transected at a similar level. The left lung is rolled forward, out of the chest, and over toward the right side. The double lung block is then released from the prevertebral tissues with sharp dissection posterior to the esophagus to release the double lung block from the chest.

## TECHNIQUE OF SINGLE–LUNG TRANSPLANTATION

For recipient diagnoses other than pulmonary hypertension or Eisenmenger's syndrome, either side generally can be selected with equivalent results. If a preoperative quantitative perfusion scan demonstrates a predominant flow to one lung, then the opposite lung is usually transplanted so as to maintain the recipient on the "best" of the two lungs during the transplant procedure. A previous thoracotomy (other than lung biopsy) or pleurodesis on one side usually dictates selection of the contralateral side for transplantation.

For patients with PPH, or pulmonary hypertension secondary to Eisenmenger's syndrome, CPB is routinely instituted before the recipient lung is extracted. For PPH, either side can be transplanted, although a right lung transplant facilitates the preparation for bypass, using the right atrial appendage and the ascending aorta as the cannulation sites. When transplant is performed through the left chest, cannulation of the left femoral artery and vein may be employed, with the descending aorta and the common pulmonary artery being alternative sites for arterial and venous cannulation, respectively. For patients with Eisenmenger's syndrome, right lung transplant is performed in conjunction with repair of the cardiac defect.

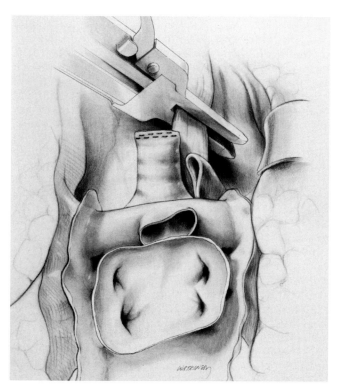

FIGURE 57–23. With the lungs in a semi-inflated state, the mid-trachea is divided between staple lines. The esophagus posterior to this point is divided with a linear stapling device. All mediastinal tissue between the medial surface of the upper lobes and the trachea are incised from front to back, perpendicular to the axis of the phrenic nerve.

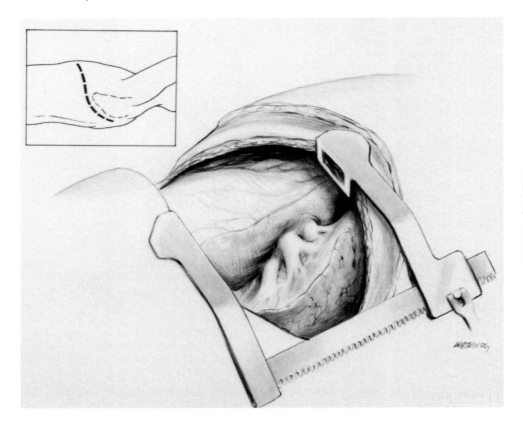

FIGURE 57–25. Technique of left single-lung transplant. A postero-lateral thoracotomy incision *(inset)* is utilized. The fifth rib is excised. The left lung is collapsed, the pulmonary ligament is divided, and hilar structures are mobilized.

Lung transplant has been performed with the aid of one-lung anesthesia administered through a left-sided double-lumen tube, regardless of the side of transplant. CPB is always available on a standby basis and, as previously noted, is routinely performed in cases of pulmonary hypertension. CPB support is almost never required when performing single-lung transplant for emphysema, but occasionally is required with pulmonary fibrosis, especially if there is associated secondary pulmonary hypertension.

The technical aspects of unilateral lung transplanta-

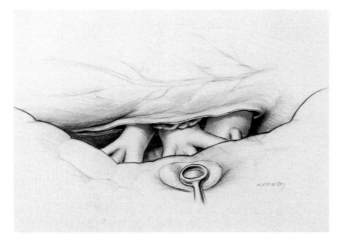

FIGURE 57–26. The pericardium is opened around to the pulmonary artery and the pulmonary veins. The first branch of the pulmonary artery is isolated.

tion are depicted in Figures 57–25 to 57–30. The patient is positioned in the standard lateral thoracotomy position and the chest and ipsilateral groin area are prepared and draped. After the chest is open, the pulmonary artery and its first branch are dissected. The pulmonary veins are mobilized as near as possible to the hilum of the lung. The pulmonary ligament is divided. Temporary occlusion of the pulmonary artery is performed to determine whether or not one-lung anesthesia is well tolerated. The use of trans-esophageal echocardiography is routine for all lung transplants. If the right ventricle maintains its contractility and does not dilate, then the recipient will likely tolerate replacement of the lung without CPB. The first branch of the pulmonary artery is divided between ligatures, and the pulmonary artery distal to this point is divided between staple lines. This exposure may be facilitated by preliminary division of the upper branch of the superior pulmonary vein. The pulmonary veins are divided between ligatures or staple lines close to the hilum of the lung, to leave as long a central stump of pulmonary vein as possible. The bronchus may be divided between staple lines just proximal to the origin of the upper lobe, with subsequent more proximal division after the lung has been removed and hemostasis is secured. Alternatively, the bronchus can be transected with a scalpel, at the proposed site of anastomosis. The authors employ several different techniques for the bronchial anastomosis, none of which seems to influence the result significantly. In each case, the membranous portion of the anastomosis is performed with a continu-

FIGURE 57–27. The first branch of the pulmonary artery is divided between ligatures, and the pulmonary artery distal to that point is divided between staple lines. The pulmonary artery may be decompressed by placing a proximal vascular clamp before the stapler is applied to avoid bleeding into the adventitia through the staple line. The pulmonary veins are divided between ligatures as peripherally as possible. This facilitates subsequent creation of the atrial cuff. The bronchus is divided distal to a staple line placed just proximal to the upper lobe takeoff.

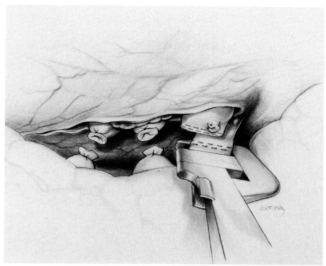

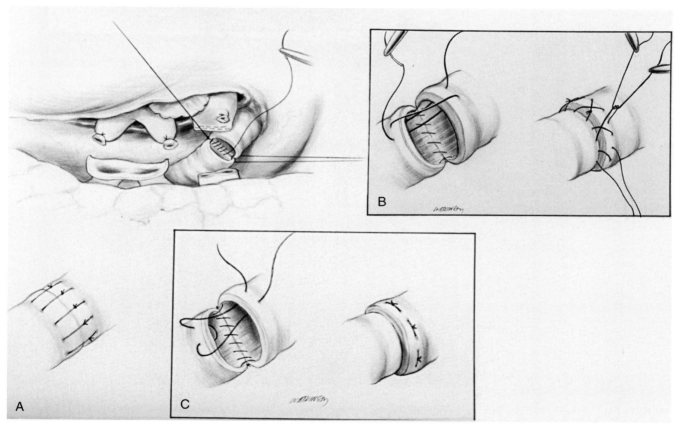

FIGURE 57–28. The main bronchus is retransected just proximal to the staple line. The donor lung, wrapped in a cold moist gauze and surrounded by crushed sterile ice, is placed in the chest. The bronchial anastomosis is then begun. The membranous portion of the anastomosis is performed with running 4-0 absorbable monofilament suture. The cartilaginous portion of the anastomosis is performed with 4-0 absorbable monofilament suture using one of several techniques, which include simple end-to-end anastomosis (A), figure-of-eight sutures with overlapping of the edges of the anastomosis (B), or horizontal mattress sutures to intussuscept either the donor or the recipient bronchus into the opposing bronchus (C). The suture line is then buried with local peribronchial fatty tissue or a pericardial fat pad pedicle.

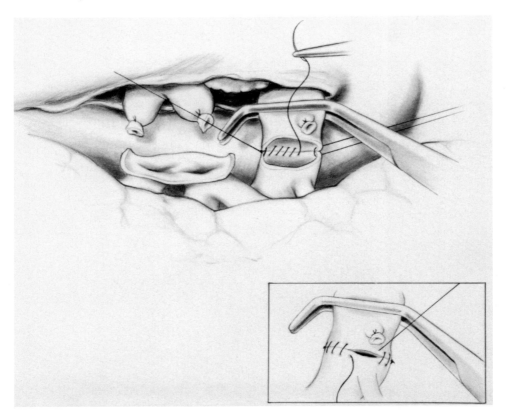

**FIGURE 57–29.** A vascular clamp is placed centrally on the recipient pulmonary artery, and the staple line is trimmed away. Care must be taken to avoid excessive length of either the donor or the recipient pulmonary arteries, because this may lead to kinking of the anastomosis when flow is restored. The posterior wall of the anastomosis is performed with running 5-0 monofilament nonabsorbable suture. This suture line is secured at either end. The anterior portion of the pulmonary artery anastomosis is then performed in similar manner. Just before the suture line is secured, the artery is flushed with saline.

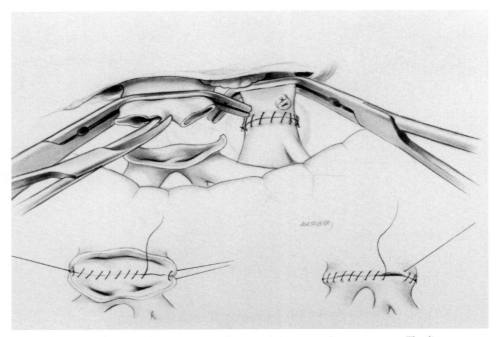

**FIGURE 57–30.** A vascular clamp is placed central to the confluence of the two pulmonary veins. The ligatures are removed from the pulmonary veins, with as much of the venous stumps preserved as possible. The venous stumps are then connected to form the atrial cuff, and this is anastomosed to the donor cuff using running 4-0 monofilament nonabsorbable suture material. As with the pulmonary artery anastomosis, the posterior suture line is performed first and is interrupted at either end to avoid subsequent purse-stringing when the final suture line is secured. Before the completed suture line is secured, the pulmonary artery clamp is momentarily removed with the lung gently inflated to allow flushing of blood through the lung and out the atrial suture line. The arterial clamp is replaced, the venous clamp is removed, and the atrial suture line is secured. The pulmonary artery clamp is then removed, and ventilation to the lung is resumed.

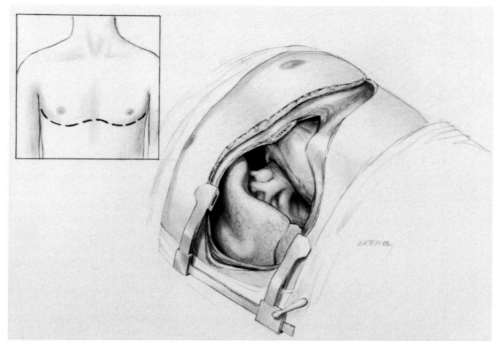

**FIGURE 57–31.** Technique of sequential bilateral lung transplantation. The patient is positioned supine on the table with the arms either along the sides or elevated, and the forearms are wrapped above the patient's face to an ether screen. A fourth- or fifth-interspace incision is made bilaterally with transverse division of the sternum (inset). In the case of bilateral transplant for emphysema, the chest is fully opened on the side to be transplanted first, but the chest is not fully opened on the contralateral side to avoid overdistention of the opposite lung during replacement of the first lung.

ous 4-0 monofilament absorbable suture. For the cartilaginous portion, the authors employ either simple interrupted sutures with an end-to-end anastomosis, figure-of-eight sutures with slight overlapping of the ends of the bronchi, or a telescoping intussusception using horizontal mattress sutures so that either the donor or the recipient bronchus is intussuscepted into the opposing bronchial lumen. Following completion, the bronchial anastomosis is covered either with a pericardial fat pad pedicle or, more commonly, with local tissues that surround the donor and recipient bronchi.

The recipient pulmonary arteries are clamped proximally and trimmed to a point just distal or just proximal to the first branch, depending on the size match with the donor pulmonary artery. The pulmonary artery anastomosis is performed with a continuous 5-0 monofilament, nonabsorbable suture.

A clamp is placed on the left atrium well proximal to the stumps of the pulmonary veins. The ligatures or staple lines are removed from the venous stumps, preserving as much of the vein as possible. The veins are interconnected to produce a suitable atrial cuff, and the atrial anastomosis is then performed with a continuous 4-0 monofilament, nonabsorbable suture. Before the completed left atrial suture line is secured, the lung is gently inflated and the pulmonary artery clamp removed for a brief period to allow brisk bleeding out of the atrial suture line. The pulmonary artery clamp is replaced, the left atrial clamp is temporarily removed, and the suture line is secured. All vascular clamps are then removed and ventilation is restored to the transplanted lung.

## TECHNIQUE OF SEQUENTIAL BILATERAL TRANSPLANTATION

The technique of bilateral transplantation is depicted in Figures 57–31 to 57–34. Anesthesia is provided through a left-sided double-lumen tube. The exposure for sequential bilateral lung transplantation is provided by a transverse thoracosternotomy incision extending from one midaxillary line to the other. The thoracotomy portion of this incision is generally in the fourth or the fifth interspace, depending on the configuration of the chest. This surgical approach, used in the early days of open heart surgery, provides

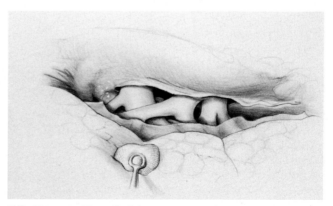

**FIGURE 57–32.** The right hilar structures, including the pulmonary artery and the two pulmonary veins, are mobilized, and the pericardium is opened circumferentially around these structures. The pulmonary ligament is divided.

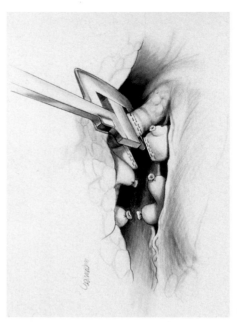

**FIGURE 57–33.** The first branch of the pulmonary artery is divided between ligatures, and the descending branch is divided between staple lines. The pulmonary veins are divided between ligatures or staple lines as close to the lung as possible. The bronchus is transected distal to a staple line placed just at the takeoff of the right upper lobe bronchus. The lung is replaced with a technique identical to that previously illustrated for single-lung transplantation.

excellent exposure of both pleural spaces as well as the mediastinum. If preoperative quantitative perfusion scans demonstrate a predominant flow to one lung, then the opposite lung is the first to be replaced. If there is no major discrepancy in the distribution of pulmonary blood flow between the two lungs, the authors prefer to replace the right lung first and then the left.

The extraction and implantation technique is identical to that required for unilateral lung transplantation. In the authors' experience, a period of partial CPB has been employed in 30% of patients. In most of these instances, bypass was employed during implantation of the second lung, when diversion of the entire cardiac output to the newly implanted lung produced transient pulmonary edema and hypoxemia. Partial CPB was employed via right atrial and ascending aortic cannulation.

## IMMUNOSUPPRESSION

The immunosuppressive regimen used for lung transplantation is similar to that used for other organ transplants. This consists of triple therapy with cyclosporine, azathioprine, and prednisone and perioperative use of an antilymphocyte or antithymocyte antibody. The authors' current regimen is as follows:

Preoperative:
  Azathioprine, 2 mg/kg IV, 1 to 2 hours before induction of anesthesia
Postoperative:

Antithymocyte globulin, 10 to l5 mg/kg/24 hr for 5 days
Azathioprine, 2 mg/kg IV or p.o. daily
Cyclosporine beginning with 3 to 4 mg/hr constant IV infusion; convert to oral dosage as soon as tolerated and adjust IV and oral dose according to serum cyclosporine levels, with target levels of 400 ng/ml by radioimmunoassay on whole blood
Steroids: prednisone, 0.5 mg/kg/day beginning on day 5 (or sooner, according to preference)

Following discharge from hospital, the immunosuppressive protocol is unchanged for the first 3 months. Between the third and the sixth month, the prednisone dose is tapered to a dose of 12.5 to 15 mg/day. By the end of the first year, this is further tapered to an average dose of 12.5 to 15 mg on alternate days. Azathioprine is maintained at 2 mg/kg/ day unless leukopenia develops, in which case, the dose is appropriately adjusted. The cyclosporine level is maintained in the upper therapeutic range for the first year. Thereafter, the cyclosporine dose is tapered to produce a blood level in the midtherapeutic range, unless dose reduction is required by elevated serum creatinine. For proven or presumed episodes of chronic rejection, a boost in the steroid dose has been the primary mode of therapy. This usually takes the form of three bolus doses of methylprednisolone on successive days with or without a concomitant boost and taper of the daily prednisone dose.

## DIAGNOSIS OF ACUTE REJECTION

The diagnosis of postoperative rejection remains imprecise. It is based on a combination of suggestive

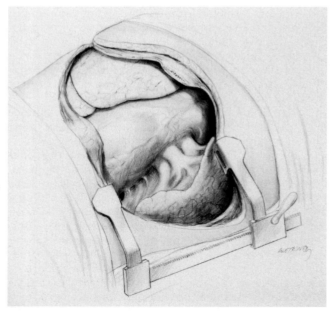

**FIGURE 57–34.** Following completion of the first transplantation, the opposite side of the chest is opened fully, and the lung is collapsed and replaced using the same technique previously illustrated.

signs and symptoms, including deterioration in arterial oxygenation, pyrexia, decreased exercise tolerance or decreased oxygen saturation with exercise, increasing fatigability, or development of a radiologic infiltrate or hilar flare, together with the absence of any alternative cause of deterioration, such as fluid overload or infection. Acute rejection following lung transplantation is virtually the rule, with more than 97% of the authors' recipients having been treated on at least one occasion for acute rejection during the first 3 postoperative weeks. The average number of rejection episodes during this period of time has been between two and three. The single most useful diagnostic sign of rejection has been the response to a pulse dose of intravenous methylprednisolone. Improvement in oxygenation, reduction in temperature, and improvement in exercise tolerance and sense of well-being occurs within hours. Radiologic alterations, if present, generally improve over a 6- to 24-hour period (Fig. 57–35). When rejection is suspected, a bolus dose of 500 to 1000 mg of methylprednisolone is administered intravenously. If, during the next 24 hours, an appropriate response occurs and if, in the interim, a search for other possible causes of pulmonary deterioration is negative, then additional bolus doses of methylprednisolone (250 to 500 mg) are administered 24 and 48 hours after the initial dose.

## BRONCHOSCOPIC SURVEILLANCE AND TRANSBRONCHIAL BIOPSY

Recipients undergo initial fiberoptic bronchoscopic evaluation before leaving the operating room and again on the first postoperative day. Bronchoscopy is also performed just prior to extubation. In the third postoperative week, usually just before discharge from hospital, patients are bronchoscoped under local anesthesia and transbronchial biopsies are performed. Following discharge, bronchoscopy with transbronchial biopsy and bronchoalveolar lavage is performed whenever indicated by clinical parameters such as dyspnea, hypoxemia, decline in $FEV_1$, radiographic infiltrate, or unexplained fever. Routine protocol transbronchial biopsies and bronchoalveolar lavage are obtained at 3, 6, 12, 18, and 24 months, and annually thereafter. Transbronchial biopsies are graded according to the working formulation for the standardization of nomenclature of the diagnosis of the lung rejection reported by the lung rejection study group (Yousem et al., 1990).

## RESULTS OF LUNG TRANSPLANTATION

The outcome of lung transplantation can be measured in terms of survival and in terms of the improvement in lung function, hemodynamics, and exercise capacity. The results may vary according to the nature of the underlying disease and to the type of transplant performed.

To date, over 200 patients have received a single-lung or sequential bilateral transplant at the authors' institution. The hospital mortality rate is 6%. The actuarial survival, depicted in Figure 57–36, is 84 and 81% at 1 and 2 years, respectively.

The authors have maintained a voluntary International Registry for transplant recipients, which to date has received information on over 2300 transplants worldwide. As can be seen from Figure 57–37, most of this experience has been accumulated in recent years; thus, many lung transplant programs remain

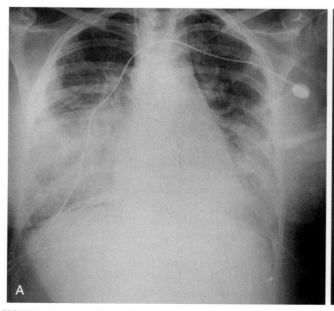
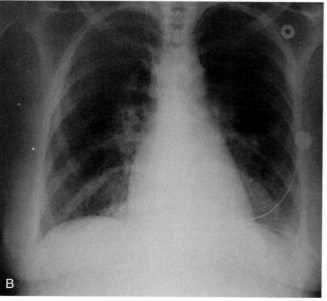

**FIGURE 57–35.** *A,* Chest film 5 days following bilateral lung transplantation. A deterioration in $Po_2$ and an elevation of temperature accompanied the bilateral lower lobe infiltrates. *B,* Six hours following intravenous administration of methylprednisolone, the chest film has significantly cleared. This was associated with defervescence and improved oxygenation.

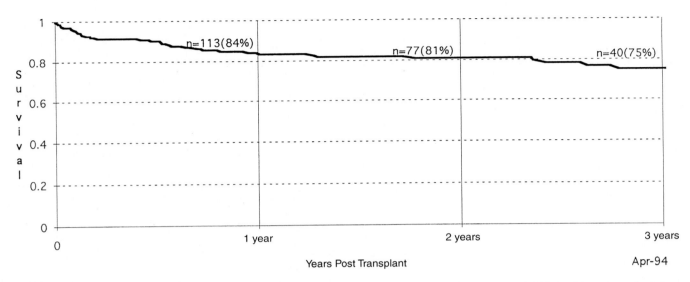

**Washington University Lung Transplant Program**
**(Barnes Hospital)**
**Three Year Actuarial Survival**
**Total Single & Bilateral Transplants**
**n = 204**

**FIGURE 57–36.** Actuarial survival curve for first consecutive 204 recipients undergoing single- or sequential bilateral-lung transplantation at Barnes Hospital.

in the early, learning phase. Considering this, overall results have been very satisfactory, as shown in Figure 57–38.

## CAUSES OF EARLY AND LATE MORTALITY

Tables 57–9 and 57–10 demonstrate the causes of early (less than 3 months) and late (greater than 3 months) mortality, as submitted to the St. Louis International Transplant Registry. The primary causes of early death include sepsis and primary organ failure. The leading causes of death after 3 months are chronic rejection and sepsis, the latter often associated with augmented immunosuppression in an attempt to treat rejection.

## PULMONARY FUNCTION STUDIES

Following lung transplantation, steady improvement in spirometric measurements of lung volumes typically occurs for the first 3 months, followed by a more gradual improvement or plateau. As expected, the degree of improvement in measured lung function is greater for bilateral lung recipients than for single lung recipients. Both groups show a significant increase in the $FEV_1$ and $Pa_{O_2}$ (Fig. 57–39). Comparisons

■ **Table 57–9.** DEATHS OCCURRING LESS THAN OR EQUAL TO 90 DAYS AFTER TRANSPLANT*

| Causes of Death | n | % |
|---|---|---|
| Sepsis | 129 | 27 |
| Primary organ failure | 71 | 15 |
| Heart failure | 38 | 8 |
| Airway dehiscence | 30 | 6 |
| Rejection | 30 | 6 |
| Hemorrhage | 27 | 6 |
| Cytomegalovirus | 24 | 5 |
| Multiorgan failure | 23 | 5 |
| Other | 99 | 21 |

*Transplants = 2330; deaths = 471.

■ **Table 57–10.** DEATHS OCCURRING MORE THAN 90 DAYS AFTER TRANSPLANT*

| Causes of Death | n | % |
|---|---|---|
| Sepsis | 100 | 29 |
| Bronchiolitis obliterans | 54 | 16 |
| Malignancy | 27 | 8 |
| Rejection | 26 | 8 |
| Respiratory failure | 21 | 6 |
| Cytomegalovirus | 19 | 6 |
| Hemorrhage | 10 | 3 |
| Heart failure | 9 | 3 |
| Other | 75 | 22 |

*Transplants = 2330; deaths = 341.

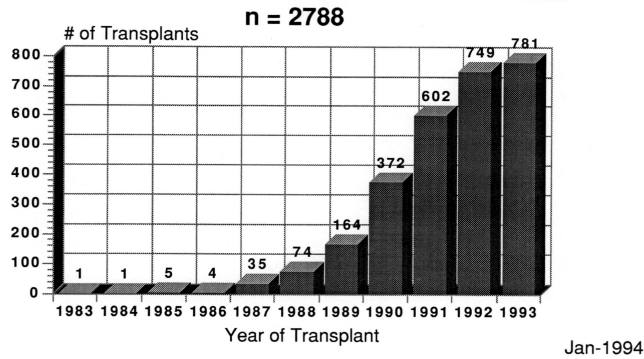

FIGURE 57–37. Annual number of transplants reported to the St. Louis International Lung Transplant Registry. Data reported up to January 1, 1994, are included.

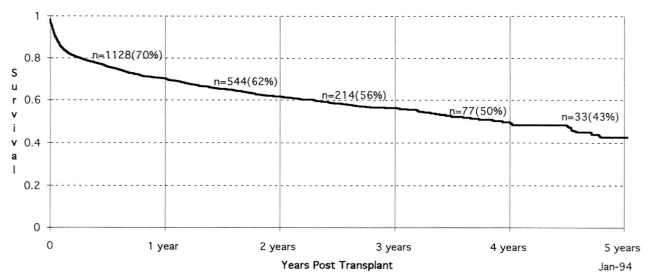

FIGURE 57–38. Three-year actuarial survival curve for Registry patients for whom follow-up data are available.

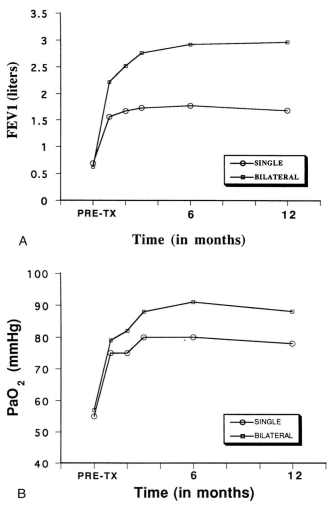

FIGURE 57–39. Improvement in FEV₁ *(A)* and PaO₂ on room air *(B)* following single- (*n* = 47) and bilateral- (*n* = 43) lung transplantation. Patients with pulmonary hypertension were excluded from this analysis. (TX = transplantation.)

Cardiopulmonary exercise performance has been comparable to that of heart-lung transplant recipients. From a clinical standpoint, recipients of a single-lung transplantation have few if any restrictions, and several have skied at altitudes above 10,000 feet without experiencing any limitation or symptoms. However, when such recipients develop chronic rejection, the physiologic consequences are more severe than with other types of transplant. For this reason, many centers favor the use of bilateral transplants for patients with pulmonary hypertension.

## AIRWAY COMPLICATIONS

The bronchial circulation to the donor lung is severed during extraction, and after implantation, the donor bronchus depends on retrograde flow from the pulmonary circulation until systemic collaterals develop. Metras (1950), in his pioneering dog lung-

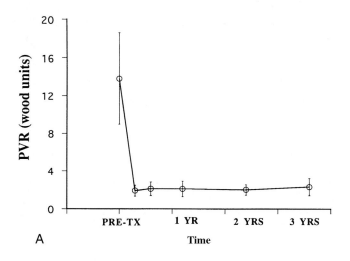

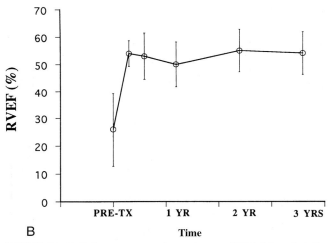

FIGURE 57–40. Pulmonary vascular resistance (PVR) *(A)* and right ventricular ejection fraction (RVEF) *(B)* in seven patients followed 3 or more years after single-lung transplantation for primary pulmonary hypertension. The early, initial improvement has been sustained. (TX = transplantation.)

of exercise capacity, however, have not shown an impressive advantage over the single-lung transplant, and the actuarial survival curves for the two procedures have been similar.

## PPH AND EISENMENGER'S SYNDROME

Until a few years ago, combined heart-lung transplantation was the standard operation for patients with pulmonary vascular disease. However, this type of transplant requires a donor in whom the heart and both lungs are suitable. Because of this and the limited availability of donor hearts for cardiac transplantation, the use of the combined heart-lung transplant has been very limited. The authors have achieved satisfactory results using single-lung transplantation for these patients. Hemodynamic parameters (pulmonary artery pressure, cardiac index, and right ventricular ejection fraction) have returned to the normal range and remained stable for the duration of the authors' current follow-up (Fig. 57–40).

transplant experiments, reattached the origin of the bronchial artery to the recipient aorta. In clinical lung transplantation, a direct reattachment of the bronchial circulation has in general not been incorporated because of technical complexity. Recently, however, several techniques have been developed for direct bronchial artery revascularization at the time of single-lung and bilateral transplantation (Courad et al., 1992; Daly et al., 1993).

In the authors' own experience, healing problems of the airway anastomosis have been identified in 19% of patients. In half, endoscopic evidence of necrosis or partial anastomotic separation, or both, was identified at bronchoscopy, but required no treatment and healed with no complication. In the other half, a significant airway complication resulted, including death (1.5%), stricture or malacia requiring stent (6%) or simple dilatation (1%), or bronchopleural fistula requiring a chest tube (1.5%). At the present time, no correlation has been recognized between technique of anastomosis, length of ischemic time, or type of immunosuppressive regimen and the subsequent development of an airway complication. Death as a result of airway complication has occurred in less than 2% of patients reported to the International Registry.

## BRONCHIOLITIS OBLITERANS AND CHRONIC ALLOGRAFT DYSFUNCTION

It is widely presumed, but is yet unproved, that the pathologic finding of obliterative bronchiolitis reflects chronic allograft rejection. Clinically, this is manifested by progressive reduction in the $FEV_1$, the hallmark of obstructive lung disease. Pathologically, chronic lung rejection may be manifested by chronic vascular rejection as well as by scarring and fibrosis of airways. Bronchiolitis obliterans may also be caused by nonimmunologic conditions such as infection. Both overdiagnosis and underdiagnosis are possible, and may relate to sampling error, to the nonuniformity of the process, or to coexisting pathology. In addition to the pitfalls of histologic assessment, such assessment requires either transbronchial biopsy or open lung biopsy. Furthermore, the clinical manifestations associated with chronic lung rejection may or may not parallel pathologic findings. In some cases, pathologic findings of obliterative bronchiolitis are associated with no apparent clinical or functional deterioration in graft performance, whereas in other cases, severe and progressive deterioration of graft function occurs in the absence of significant pathologic findings. A system for the clinical staging of chronic dysfunction in lung allograft has been proposed (Cooper et al., 1993) based on the ratio of the current $FEV_1$ to the baseline $FEV_1$ value established in the first 3 months following transplantation. According to this proposal, lung allograft dysfunction is referred to as *bronchiolitis obliterans syndrome*. Four stages are described, as demonstrated in Table 57–11. The incidence of the bronchiolitis obliterans syn-

■ Table 57–11. BRONCHIOLITIS OBLITERANS SYNDROME

| Stage | | $FEV_1$—% of Postoperative Baseline Value |
|---|---|---|
| 0 | (no significant abnormality) | 100 |
| I | (mild) | 80 |
| II | (moderate) | 65 |
| III | (severe) | 50 |

drome within the first 2 years following transplantation appears to be in the range of 25 to 30% in most series. The incidence will increase with time. Chronic rejection or complications resulting from the heightened immunosuppression administered to treat rejection are by far the most common causes of late death following lung transplantation.

In some patients, the bronchiolitis obliterans syndrome may reverse even in the presence of biopsy-proven obliterative bronchiolitis, following treatment with augmented immunosuppression. Such patients, unfortunately, are in the minority; the problem of chronic rejection is the most significant obstacle to achievement of long-term success following lung transplantation. A follow-up evaluation of the authors' lung transplant recipients indicated that incidence of chronic allograft dysfunction is unrelated to the type of transplant (single-lung versus bilateral), recipient diagnosis, incidence of acute rejection episodes in the first month, or the matching of donor and recipient cytomegalovirus antibody status (Cooper et al., 1994).

Although the early survival figures following lung transplantation appear optimistic, there is no doubt that the survival curve will steadily decline over time. At this juncture, the authors estimate that the current 5-year survival rate will be between 50 and 60%. There is urgent need for improved immunosuppressive agents and regimens. The induction of specific tolerance, long the dream of transplant surgeons, will, we hope, become a reality. Somewhat further off may be the era of routine xenografting, the ultimate solution to the inadequate supply of donor organs. Until that time, the decisions as to how to distribute the limited and precious supply of donor organs and how best to diagnose and treat chronic rejection will remain among the most difficult problems associated with lung transplantation.

## BIBLIOGRAPHY

Alican, F., Cayirli, M., Isin, E., et al.: Left lung replantation with immediate pulmonary artery ligation. Ann. Surg., *174:*34, 1971.

Barnard, C. N., and Cooper, D. K. C.: Clinical transplantation of the heart: A review of 13 years' personal experience. J. R. Soc. Med., *74:*670, 1981.

Benfield, J. D., and Coon, R.: The role of the left atrial anastomosis in pulmonary reimplantation. J. Thorac. Cardiovasc. Surg., *61:*847, 1971.

Cooley, D. A., Bloodwell, R. D., Hallman, G. L., et al.: Organ transplantation for advanced cardiopulmonary disease. Ann. Thorac. Surg., 8:30, 1969.

Cooper, J. D., Billingham, M., Egan, T., et al.: A working formulation for the standardization of nomenclature and for clinical staging of chronic dysfunction in lung allografts. J. Heart Lung Transplant., 12:713, 1993.

Cooper, J. D., Patterson, G. A., Grosman, R., et al.: Double-lung transplant for advanced chronic obstructive lung disease. Am. Rev. Respir. Dis., 139:303, 1989.

Cooper, J. D., Patterson, G. A., and Trulock, E. P.: Washington University and the Lung Transplant Group. Results of 131 consecutive single and bilateral lung transplant recipients. J. Thorac. Cardiovasc. Surg., 107:460, 1994.

Couraud, L., Baudet, E., Nashef, S. A., et al.: Lung transplantation with bronchial revascularization. Surgical anatomy, operative technique and early results. Eur. J. Cardiothorac. Surg., 6:490, 1992.

Daicoff, G. R., Allen, P. D., and Streck, C. J.: Pulmonary vascular resistance following lung reimplantation and transplantation. Ann. Thorac. Surg., 9:569, 1970.

D'Alonzo, G. E., Barst, R. J., Ayres, S. M., et al.: Survival in patient with primary pulmonary hypertension. Ann. Intern. Med., 5:115, 1991.

Daly, R. D., Tadjkarimi, S., Khaghani, A., et al.: Successful double-lung transplantation with direct bronchial artery revascularization. Ann. Thorac. Surg., 56:885, 1993.

Dark, J. H., Patterson, G. A., Al-Jilaihawi, A. N., et al.: Experimental en bloc double-lung transplantation. Ann. Thorac. Surg., 42:394, 1986.

Derom, F., Barbier, F., Ringoir, S., et al.: Ten-month survival after lung homotransplantation in man. J. Thorac. Cardiovasc. Surg., 61:835, 1971.

Dubois, P., Choiniere, L., and Cooper, J. D.: Bronchial omentopexy in canine lung allotransplantation. Ann. Thorac. Surg., 38:211, 1984.

Goldberg, M., Lima, O., Morgan, E., et al.: A comparison between cyclosporin A and methylprednisolone plus azathioprine on bronchial healing following canine lung allotransplantation. J. Thorac. Cardiovasc. Surg., 85:821, 1983.

Hardin, C. A., and Kittle, C. F.: Experiences with transplantation of the lung. Science, 119:97, 1954.

Hardy, J. D., Webb, W. R., Dalton, M. L., and Walker, G. R.: Lung homotransplantation in man. J. A. M. A., 186:1065, 1963.

Hsieh, C. M., Mishkel, G. J., Cardoso, P. F. G., et al.: Production and reversibility of right ventricular hypertrophy and right heart failure in dogs. Ann. Thorac. Surg., 54:104, 1992.

Kerem, E., Raisman, J., Corey, M., et al.: Prediction of mortality in patients with cystic fibrosis. N. Engl. J. Med., 326:1187, 1992.

Lillehei, C. W.: Discussion of Wildevuur, C. R. H., and Benfield, J.

R.: A review of 23 human lung transplantations by 20 surgeons. Ann. Thorac. Surg., 9:489, 1970.

Lima, O., Cooper, J. D., Peters, W. J., et al.: Effects of methylprednisolone and azathioprine on bronchial healing following lung autotransplantation. J. Thorac. Cardiovasc. Surg., 82:211, 1981.

Metras, H.: Note préliminaire sur la greffe totale du poumon chez le chien. Compt. Rend. Acad. Sci., 231:1176, 1950.

Morgan, W. E., Lima, O., Goldberg, M., et al.: Improved bronchial healing in canine left lung reimplantation using omental pedicle wrap. J. Thorac. Cardiovasc. Surg., 85:139, 1983.

Nelems, J. M., Rebuck, A. S., Cooper, J. D., et al.: Human lung transplantation. Chest, 78:569, 1980.

Pasque, M. K., Cooper, J. D., Kaiser, L. R., et al.: Improved technique for bilateral lung transplantation: Rationale and initial clinical experience. Ann. Thorac. Surg., 49:785, 1990.

Pasque, M. K., Kaiser, L. R., Dresler, C. M., et al.: Single-lung transplantation for pulmonary hypertension. J. Thorac. Cardiovasc. Surg., 1:475, 1992.

Patterson, G. A., Cooper, J. D., Goldman, B., et al.: Technique of successful clinical double-lung transplantation. Ann. Thorac. Surg., 44:626, 1988.

Patterson, G. A., Todd, T. R., Cooper, J. D., et al.: Airway complications following double-lung transplantation. J. Thorac. Cardiovasc. Surg., 99:14, 1990.

Reitz, B. A., Wallwork, J. L., Hunt, S. A., et al.: Heart-lung transplantation: Successful therapy for patients with pulmonary vascular disease. N. Engl. J. Med., 3067:557, 1982.

Sundaresan, S., Gregory, D. T., Aoe, M., et al.: Donor lung procurement: Assessment and operative technique. Ann. Thorac. Surg., 56:1409, 1993.

Toronto Lung Transplant Group (including Cooper, J. D.): Experience with single-lung transplantation for pulmonary fibrosis. J. A. M. A., 259:2258, 1988.

Toronto Lung Transplant Group (including Cooper J. D.): Unilateral lung transplantation for pulmonary fibrosis. N. Engl. J. Med., 314:1140, 1986.

Vanderhoeft, P., Dubois, A., Lauvau, N., et al.: Block allotransplantation of both lungs with pulmonary trunk and left atrium in dogs. Thorax, 27:415, 1972.

Veith, F. J., and Richards, K.: Lung transplantation with simultaneous contralateral pulmonary artery ligation. Surg. Gynecol. Obstet., 129:768, 1969.

Waldhausen, J. A., Daly, W. J., Baez, M., et al.: Physiologic changes associated with autotransplantation of the lung. Ann. Surg., 165:580, 1967.

Yousem, S. A., Berry, G. J., Brunt, E. M., et al.: A working formulation for the standardization of nomenclature in the diagnosis of heart and lung rejection: Lung rejection study group. J. Heart Transplant., 9:593, 1990.

# 58

# The Artificial Heart

William S. Pierce

## HISTORICAL ASPECTS

Having developed the first successful artificial kidney in the early 1940s, Kolff, then Professor of Research Surgery at the Cleveland Clinic, directed attention to the development of an artificial heart. In 1958, 5 years after the successful clinical use of the heart-lung machine for open heart operations, Akutsu and Kolff (1958) reported that two compact vinyl pumps, powered by an external air compressor, had been used to replace the function of the canine heart for a short period. Various ingenious pump designs were later evaluated (Akutsu et al., 1960; Pierce et al., 1965), but problems related to abnormal physiology, thrombus formation, and device failure precluded survival of the animal for more than a few hours. With additional experience, investigators found that the air-powered pumps appeared to be the easiest to control and that the calf, with its large chest and docile nature, was the optimal animal model (Nosé et al., 1965). One decade after the initial studies from Kolff's laboratory, the calf's survival for 3 to 5 days was reported (Klain et al., 1971). This feat, which earlier had seemed impossible, served as a source of further encouragement to investigators. Attention was focused on improved pump designs, use of biocompatible materials for device fabrication, and the construction of more reliable power consoles. Since 1975, several groups in the United States and abroad have maintained calves with implanted pneumatically powered artificial hearts. The calves are able to stand, eat, and do limited treadmill exercise (Honda et al., 1975; Lawson et al., 1975). The longest reported survival time was 100 days; since then, it has gradually increased to 357 days (Pierce, 1986).

In 1969 (Cooley et al., 1969) and again in 1981 (Cooley, 1982), pneumatic artificial hearts were used to support the circulation of patients whose hearts had been removed for 39 and 64 hours, respectively, while suitable donor hearts were identified. In both cases, heart transplantation was performed, but neither patient survived. Clearly, both the artificial hearts and the transplant techniques needed improvement. However, an important concept was proved: A pneumatic artificial heart could provide adequate circulatory support to a critically ill patient awaiting a compatible donor. The use of the artificial heart in these cases is referred to as a *bridge* to transplantation. Important refinements have been made in artificial hearts and in cardiac transplantation techniques since then, and reasonable clinical results have been achieved by using the artificial heart as a bridge in critically ill patients.

In 1982, DeVries and associates, working in Kolff's laboratory at the University of Utah, believed that the pneumatic artificial heart had been developed to a level that could benefit patients with end-stage heart disease when all other conventional methods of treatment had been exhausted. In a historic operation performed on December 2, 1982, Dr. Barney Clark, a 61-year-old dentist with end-stage cardiac disease (DeVries et al., 1984), received a pneumatic artificial heart that was designed at the University of Utah and was referred to as a *Jarvik-7*, named for Robert Jarvik, a co-investigator in Kolff's laboratory. Although the patient's postoperative course was characterized by multiple complications, his condition gradually improved so that he could eat, talk with his family, and walk a few steps with the attached bulky pneumatic power unit. After 112 days, he died of multiple-system failure. At the Humana Heart Institute International, DeVries (1988) later implanted three Jarvik-7 hearts as permanent replacements and one patient survived for almost 2 years. Problems of stroke and infection in addition to the cumbersome percutaneous pneumatic tubes and the external power unit, however, have meant that it is not always advisable to replace hearts with the currently available pneumatic prosthesis.

## PNEUMATIC ARTIFICIAL HEART

### System Components

Pneumatic artificial hearts use a pneumatic pressure console, positioned external to the patient, to generate pulses of air or carbon dioxide that are transmitted by flexible tubing across the chest wall to energize the implanted blood pumps (Atsumi et al., 1981; Bücherl et al., 1985; Hughes et al., 1985; Jarvik et al., 1978; Pierce et al., 1981) (Fig. 58–1). These pumps are modified diaphragm pumps that have rigid outer housings and a flexible inner, or blood-contacting, bladder (Fig. 58–2). Internal tilting disk valves, similar to those used for heart valve replacement, ensure unidirectional blood flow. The internal design of the blood pump is crucial to minimizing hemolysis and preventing thromboemboli. In most blood pumps that are being developed, the blood pump bladder is made of flawlessly smooth-surfaced, seam-free, segmented polyurethane (Boretos and Pierce, 1967). This elastomeric material provides an

2135

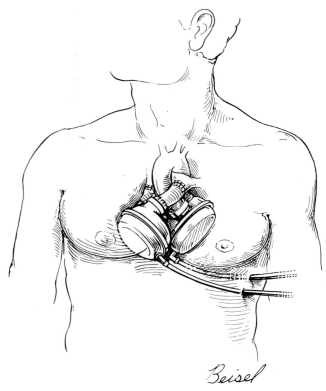

FIGURE 58–1. The pneumatic artificial heart as it is used in clinical application. The ventricles are implanted within the pericardial sac. A separate power line transmits the pressure and vacuum pulses to actuate each ventricle. (From Gaines, W. E., Donachy, J. H., Rosenberg, G., et al.: Studies leading to an artificial heart for clinical application. Contemp. Surg., 24:41, 1984.)

microcomputerized *cardiac output monitor and diagnostic unit* (COMDU) to help to assess pump function based on left air-line flow.

High reliability of the pneumatic power console has been a primary consideration in design. Consoles incorporate a number of safety systems that include a spare power unit, an emergency AC power source, and a series of visible and audible alarms to indicate failure of the console to generate an adequate drive pressure and loss of electrical power. Because of the need for reliability, redundancy, and safety measures, the power consoles are bulky and heavy, and accordingly, severely limit the mobility of experimental animals or patients. To alleviate this problem, Heimes and Klasen (1982) designed a small, portable battery-powered unit able to provide sufficient pneumatic power to maintain an artificial heart for several hours (Fig. 58–6). The unit was small enough that it could be carried by the patient. Unfortunately, the safety systems of the larger console were necessarily minimized.

Control of the output of the blood pumps is required to ensure an adequate left ventricular output, atrial pressures of below 15 mm Hg, and a similar, but not identical, output of both prosthetic ventricles. In the most commonly used control system, each ven-

excellent flexion life and reasonably good thrombus resistance, if attention has been paid to bladder design. Bladder discontinuities must be minimized and adequate surface shear rates must be obtained to wash the surfaces of the bladder surfaces. The left and right pumps are separate entities and have detachable atrial and arterial suture cuffs to facilitate implantation.

A pneumatic power console activates the artificial heart by providing timed pulses of gas that compress the bladder and alternately apply gentle suction to aid in filling the pump (Fig. 58–3). The output of the power console is attached to each ventricle of the artificial heart through a 2- to 3-mm flexible tube that traverses the skin. The power unit provides a controlled systolic pressure of 120 to 250 mm Hg for a preset time, and a diastolic vacuum of 0 to −50 mm Hg for a preset time. In some designs, the pumping frequency and ratio between systolic and diastolic times can be preset. As investigators (Rosenberg et al., 1978) gained experience with this system, they recognized the importance of monitoring left drive unit pressure or gas flow (Fig. 58–4). Complete pump emptying and filling can be detected by the contour of tracings from the air lines. Moreover, abnormal conditions, such as inlet restriction, outlet obstruction, and valve malfunction, can be detected (Fig. 58–5). The Utah group (Nielsen et al., 1983) developed a

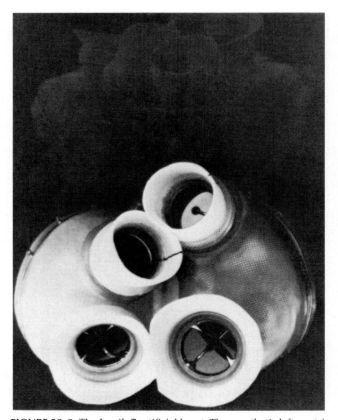

FIGURE 58–2. The Jarvik-7 artificial heart. The prosthetic left ventricle *(left side of photograph)* has a mitral valve *(lower)* and an aortic valve *(upper)*. The prosthetic right ventricle *(right side of photograph)* has a tricuspid inlet valve *(lower)* and a pulmonary valve *(upper)*. The valves are of the tilting-disk, Hall-Medtronic type. The air ports are not seen in this view. (Courtesy of Symbion, Inc.)

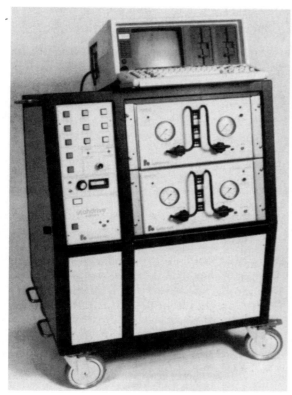

FIGURE 58–3. The power unit designed for the Jarvik-7 artificial heart provides a separate air pulse for the right and the left ventricles. The right side of the console has controls for systolic pressure, diastolic vacuum, and time for each phase that can be set independently for each ventricle. The left side of the console has a monitoring function. The unit contains an emergency power supply and an alarm system. (Courtesy of Symbion, Inc.)

tricle is set at a rate that prevents complete pump filling (Kwan-Gett et al., 1969). The systolic console pressure is set sufficiently high to ensure complete ventricle emptying under all conditions. Any factor that increases venous return, such as exercise, causes

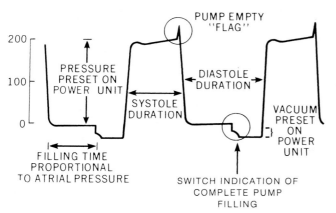

FIGURE 58–4. An idealized pressure tracing from a transducer implanted in the left power line. Visual inspection can detect complete pump filling and emptying and other parameters. The filling time can be related to the atrial pressure. Vertical scale is in millimeters of mercury (mm Hg). (From Pierce, W. S., Myers, J. L., Donachy, J. H., et al.: Approaches to the artificial heart. Surgery, 90:137, 1981.)

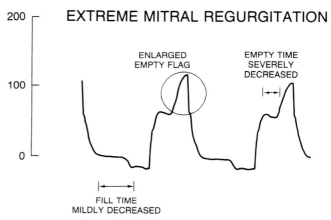

FIGURE 58–5. An idealized pressure tracing from the left power line of an artificial heart with a malfunctioning (regurgitant) mitral valve. Note particularly the large "empty" flag and the short empty time. Urgent reoperation would be required to restore valve function and to improve forward flow. Vertical scale is in mm Hg.

more complete pump filling. In this system, pump output is related to filling pressure and has some of the aspects of output control of the natural heart, often referred to as the *Frank-Starling principle* (Hennig et al., 1978). Although this system works well, the change in output achieved is small, generally in the range of 10 to 20%. Larger increments of output require manual increases in pump rates.

Automatic electronic control of cardiac output has

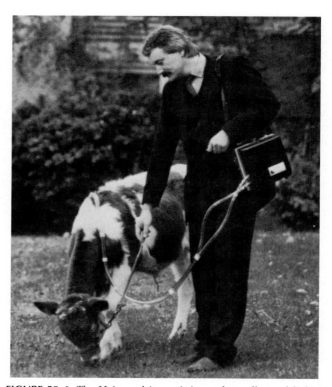

FIGURE 58–6. The Heimes drive unit is much smaller and lighter in weight than the conventional consoles. The unit is shown attached to the calf with an artificial heart through two 3-mm vinyl tubes. (Courtesy of Symbion, Inc.)

been achieved with a system in which each pump is controlled by using a feedback control system (Landis et al., 1977). The pumps always fill and empty completely with this method of control. The left pump rate changes automatically to maintain the arterial blood pressure within a preset normal range. The right pump rate changes automatically to maintain the left atrial pressure within a normal range. This control system provides an automatic increase in output in response to exercise. Some technique is required to measure aortic pressure and left atrial pressure, either directly or indirectly. These measurements are best derived indirectly from the pneumatic power line (Rosenberg et al., 1978) rather than by the use of direct implanted transducers or by indwelling catheters, thus obviating problems associated with the electrical instability of transducers and the risks of sepsis associated with vascular access catheters.

## Animal Studies

A few surgical research laboratories, both in the United States and abroad, have programs to study pneumatic artificial hearts in experimental animals. Most implants are done in calves ranging from 60 to 100 kg, through a right thoracotomy (Olsen et al., 1977). The animals are supported on cardiopulmonary bypass for the 2 hours required for cardiectomy and the implantation of blood pumps. After the operation, they are put into a restraining cage and usually stand within 2 or 3 hours after operation. The calves eat and have a return of normal body function within 12 hours. The animals must be constantly observed to ensure that the pneumatic drive lines are not injured or displaced. Treadmill exercise begins several weeks after operation. The animals remain alert, well, and active, and they gain weight rapidly.

Detailed hemodynamic and clinical chemistry observations have been made in these animals for many months after heart replacement and they show no evidence of organ dysfunction. The animals do, however, have a mild anemia with a hematocrit in the range of 28 to 30% (Hughes et al., 1985; Shaffer et al., 1979), which is most likely to be a result of the four mechanical valves used in the device. Despite satisfactory maintenance of the circulation, animal survival is generally limited to 6 or 7 months, although one calf survived for almost 1 year (Aufiero et al., 1987).

In the 1960s, survival of animals with artificial hearts implanted was limited by mechanical failures and thromboemboli (Klain et al., 1971). During the 1970s, improved design, the use of smooth-surfaced polyurethane pumping bladders, and better understanding of the interactions between the prosthetic device and the host animal increased survival time by several months. Better inlet port design and the use of smooth-surfaced inlet connectors largely eliminated the earlier problems of inlet port pannus growth (Pae et al., 1985). As a result, animals now commonly live for 6 to 7 months after artificial heart implantation. Problems that lead to the termination

of animal studies include infection, elastomer bladder calcification, and relatively inadequate cardiac output as a result of rapid growth.

Bloodstream infection is a serious and sometimes lethal complication in animals with mechanical hearts (Fields et al., 1983; Murray et al., 1983). Infection occurring soon after implantation is due to improper operative technique. The presence of intravascular catheters and percutaneous drive lines poses a constant threat of infection, which can be minimized but not eliminated. Moreover, studies have shown decreased host resistance in animals with implanted pneumatic hearts (Paping et al., 1978). Accordingly, minimal use of vascular access catheters with removal of those used when no longer required is recommended. To reduce the risk of sepsis associated with the percutaneous tubes, considerable research effort has been directed toward developing a bacterial seal between the external environment and the patient. The two best techniques currently available to inhibit bacterial invasion are wrapping the implanted segment of tube with Dacron velour fabric (Hall et al., 1975) and using the Utah skin button (Hastings et al., 1981). The latter device consists of two concentric tubes; the drive line passes through the inner one and the adjacent surfaces are sealed with adhesive. The outer tube is covered with velour and passed through the opening in the skin. Drive line entrance sites must be kept clean, and tension and movement at the skin site must be minimized. Systemic antibiotics are used similar to their use in clinical medicine.

Elastomer bladder calcification was not anticipated, but began to be observed as animal survival lengthened beyond 3 months (Coleman et al., 1981). Dystrophic calcification has been observed on pump bladders made of various materials, including segmented polyurethane, segmented polyurethane-polydimethyl siloxane copolymer, Dacron flock-lined polyurethane, and glutaraldehyde-treated, gelatin-coated polyolefin. Areas of the pump bladder subject to high mechanical stress particularly tended to have calcification (Whalen et al., 1980). The calcific deposits densely adhered to the polymer and caused stiffening, flexion failure, and perforation of the bladder. This dystrophic calcification may have a cause similar to that which occurs in biologic prosthetic valves, most often in young patients (Ferrans et al., 1980). Clinical experience with blood pumps in adults suggests that calcification does not present a major problem, at least during use of the device for several years. Both warfarin sodium, which blocks the formation of gamma-carboxyglutamic acid–containing protein, and diphosphonates, which inhibit crystal formation, have been used in studies on calves and appear to improve, but not eliminate, calcification of the bladder (Hughes et al., 1984; Levy et al., 1983; Pierce et al., 1980).

The first successful uses of implanted artificial hearts were in calves weighing 60 to 100 kg, which continue to serve as the most widely used animal model. Their chest size is ample, and both the cardiac output and the size of their vessels are similar to those of an adult human. The animals are uniform in size, tolerate anesthesia well, and are docile and easy to care for. They grow rapidly, however, gaining 0.4 to 1 kg/day, and quickly outgrow the artificial heart, so that survival is generally limited to less than a year. Moreover, the use of an immature animal appears to increase the likelihood and severity of pump bladder calcification. There is considerable interest among investigators in using an adult animal model whose weight is close to that of the adult human. A subhuman primate might appear to be ideal, but the only species large enough for clinical-sized devices is the baboon, which is dangerous to handle, costly, and an endangered species. Better alternatives to the calf may be the mature goat (Atsumi et al., 1981; Gaines et al., 1985) and sheep (Murray et al., 1985). Successful heart replacement in these species is a formidable undertaking, and the results do not approach those in the calf. Alternatives are an important challenge to research scientists in this field.

## Indications for the Clinical Use of the Pneumatic Artificial Heart

Cardiac transplantation has evolved into an effective, lifesaving procedure for a selected group of patients with end-stage cardiomyopathy. However, a suitable donor heart must be made available as soon as possible to the ill transplant candidate. In 1991, the scarcity of donor hearts created an average waiting period of approximately 2 months, and some patients had to wait much longer. As many as 20% of the candidates die before a compatible heart becomes available. Numerous treatment modalities help maintain the circulation in a transplant candidate who has an inadequate cardiac output, including hospitalization with bed rest, optimized oral drug programs, intravenous infusions of inotropic agents, and the use of the intra-aortic balloon. Even with these regimens, however, a patient may have inadequate hemodynamic indices to support life and may be a candidate for a left ventricular assist pump, biventricular assist pumps, or the artificial heart (Pennock et al., 1986).

Today, most cardiac surgeons believe that the best technique for bridging a patient for cardiac transplantation is univentricular or biventricular assist pumping (Ferrar and Hill, 1993). However, not all surgeons agree with this and a limited number of pneumatic hearts are implanted each year to support the circulation of a critically ill patient awaiting cardiac transplantation (Kawaguchi et al., 1992). Special instances in which an artificial heart may be preferable to the assist pump include a patient who had had a heart transplant with severe rejection where immediate removal of the donor organ may be advantageous. Other such patients may include those with intracardiac shunts (e.g., irreparable acquired ventricular septal defect), those with myocardial infarction with ventricular rupture, and those with aortic regurgitation who also require heart transplantation.

## Clinical Implantation of the Artificial Heart

Before implanting a pneumatic artificial heart in the human chest, the surgeon must be certain that the intrathoracic space is large enough. The former Jarvik-7 100-ml stroke and the Penn State clinical heart are suitable for patients who weigh 70 kg or more and who have enough space between the sternum and the spine to accommodate the device (Jarvik et al., 1986). For slightly smaller males and for females, the former Jarvik-7-70 ml* stroke pump may fit within the available space and certainly would provide an adequate cardiac output index.

Sepsis has been a serious complication following artificial heart implantation (Griffith et al., 1988). Accordingly, before operation, active infection must be eradicated, and extraordinary care must be taken during every step of the procedure to ensure strict asepsis.

The operation is begun with a standard median sternotomy (DeVries and Joyce, 1983; Richenbacher et al., 1986). Ascending aortic and bicaval cannulation is done, and cardiopulmonary bypass is started. The patient's temperature is lowered to 22° C. The ventricles are excised by dividing both great arteries above the valves and dividing the heart at the atrioventricular junction, leaving full atrial remnants. The operation is almost identical to that for heart transplantation (Fig. 58–7). The left atrial cuff is trimmed and double sewn (Fig. 58–8). The prosthetic left ventricle is brought onto the operative field, and the length of the aortic graft is determined. The graft is cut to fit and is sutured to the aorta. Both anastomoses are inspected to ensure that no leaks are present; this step is important because suture lines are difficult to visualize after the ventricles are in place (see Fig. 58–11). Any leaks observed at this early stage are readily controlled by using pledgeted polypropylene mattress sutures.

The left pump is brought onto the operative field. A stab wound is then made in the skin to the left of the umbilicus and a tunnel is created, similar to that used for the placement of a chest tube, from the apex of the pericardium, through the diaphragm, and out through the stab wound. The left drive line is passed through this tunnel and the left pump is positioned within the pericardial sac. The union nuts on the left atrial cuff and on the aortic cuff are aligned and tightened (Fig. 58–9). De-airing of the prosthetic left ventricle is done by passage of a Swan-Ganz catheter through the atrial anastomosis and across the prosthetic mitral valve; the tip is positioned in the highest portion of the pump bladder. Placement of the catheter is facilitated by passage of it through the valve before the threaded atrial connector is seated. When the de-airing catheter is positioned within the blood sac and both connectors are firmly seated, air is withdrawn as the sac fills with blood. After all air has been removed from the blood pump, the catheter

---

*Available for investigational use as C-70 from CardioWest Technology, Inc.

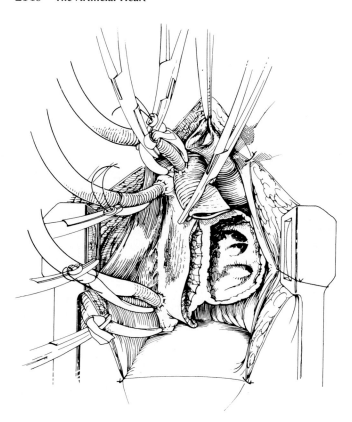

**FIGURE 58–7.** The chest has been opened through a median sternotomy; cardiopulmonary bypass has been initiated, and the heart (ventricles) has been excised. Both venae cavae have been cannulated, and occlusive snares have been placed. The arterial perfusion cannula is positioned in the ascending aorta, distal to an occlusive clamp. (From Richenbacher, W. E., Pennock, J. L., Pae, W. E., Jr., et al.: Artificial heart implantation for end-stage heart disease. J. Card. Surg., *1*:1, 1986.)

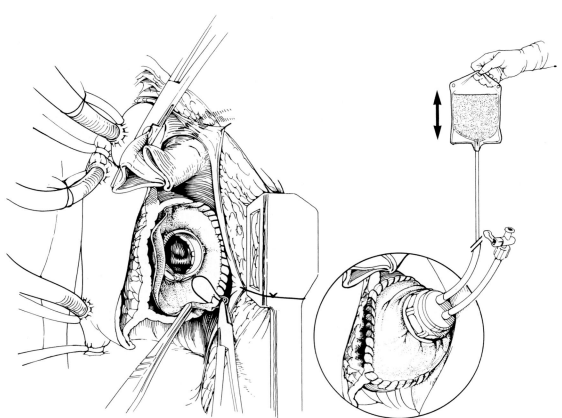

**FIGURE 58–8.** The left atrial connector is trimmed and double-sutured to the left atrial remnant with 4-0 polypropylene suture. This anastomosis is difficult to visualize after both ventricles have been implanted. The *inset* indicates a technique to distend the completed suture line and identify any leaks, which are readily repaired at this stage of the operation. (From Richenbacher, W. E., Pennock, J. L., Pae, W. E., Jr., et al.: Artificial heart implantation for end-stage heart disease. J. Card. Surg., *1*:1, 1986.)

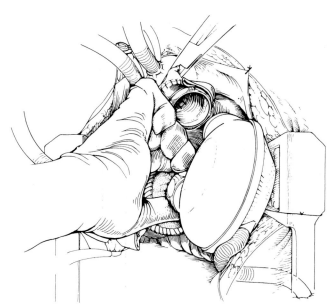

**FIGURE 58–9.** After suturing the left atrial and aortic cuffs, the surgeon passes the left drive line through a skin tunnel. The union nuts on the cuffs facilitate a tight seal to the pump. De-airing is performed and slow pumping of the left ventricle is initiated. (From Richenbacher, W. E., Pennock, J. L., Pae, W. E., Jr., et al.: Artificial heart implantation for end-stage heart disease. J. Card. Surg., 1:1, 1986.)

is withdrawn and the entry site is repaired with a pledgeted polypropylene suture. The aortic cross-clamp is then removed, and the left pump is pulsed slowly. The suture lines are inspected again for bleeding.

The right pump is then brought onto the operative field to determine the proper length for the pulmonary arterial graft. This conduit is cut to length and anastomosed to the pulmonary artery with a continuous suture of 4-0 polypropylene. The right atrial skirt is trimmed and anastomosed to the right atrium remnant by using a double row of 4-0 polypropylene sutures. The right atrial anastomosis is then observed for leaks. At this point, the patient is warmed to 37° C. A second stab wound is created to the left of the umbilicus and a tunnel is formed that leaves the pericardium midway between the left drive line and the inferior vena cava. The drive line is passed through the tunnel, and the right pump is connected (Fig. 58–10). The central venous pressure is raised to 10 mm Hg, the caval snares are loosened, and air is removed from the right blood sac as it was from the left one.

Ventilation of the patient is resumed. Right ventricular pumping is initiated, and cardiopulmonary bypass is gradually discontinued. Again, all anastomoses are inspected carefully for evidence of leaks. When an index of 2.4 l/min/m² has been reached, the atrial cannulae are removed and the insertion sites are oversewn with pledgeted polypropylene mattress sutures (Fig. 58–11). The patient is transfused to a central venous pressure of 10 to 15 mm Hg and the arterial cannula is removed. The previously placed

aortic purse-string sutures are tightened. Mediastinal chest tubes are positioned, and the sternotomy is closed in the usual manner.

The postoperative care of a patient with an implanted artificial heart is similar to the care given to patients who have had open heart surgery. Atrial, pulmonary, arterial, and aortic pressures are readily maintained within narrow limits, which are determined by drive unit pumping parameters. A cardiac output index of between 2.2 and 2.6 l/min/m² is fairly easily maintained. An alpha agent, such as neosynephrine, is sometimes required to maintain an adequate arterial blood pressure. A low-dose infusion of dopamine (3 g/kg/min) to promote adequate renal perfusion and urine output has been helpful.

There is no uniform agreement with regard to the optimal drug program needed to minimize the risk of thromboembolic complications. For a patient with a permanent artificial heart who will not have subsequent cardiac transplantation, an acceptable drug program includes the use of low molecular weight dextran (5%) at 20 ml/hr begun when drainage from the chest tube has decreased to less than 50 ml/hr (Bygdeman and Eliasson, 1967). On the third or fourth postoperative day, warfarin sodium is administered, in much the same manner as it is for patients with a prosthetic heart valve (Harker and Schlicter, 1970). When the prothrombin time is between 20 and 25 seconds, the dextran can be discontinued. The best

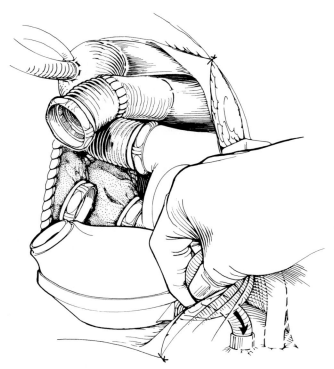

**FIGURE 58–10.** After the right atrial and pulmonary cuffs are sutured to the respective sites, the surgeon passes the right drive line through the preformed skin tunnel. The union nuts on the right cuffs are threaded to the right pump. De-airing is accomplished and right ventricle pumping is begun. (From Richenbacher, W. E., Pennock, J. L., Pae, W. E., Jr., et al.: Artificial heart implantation for end-stage heart disease. J. Card. Surg., 1:1, 1986.)

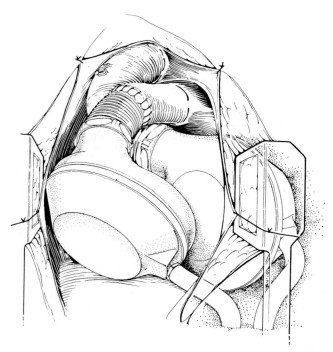

**FIGURE 58–11.** The proper placement of the two pumps within the pericardial sac after removal of the arterial and venous cannulae. (From Richenbacher, W. E., Pennock, J. L., Pae, W. E., Jr., et al.: Artificial heart implantation for end-stage heart disease. J. Card. Surg., 1:1, 1986.)

use of drugs is less clear in the patient in whom the artificial heart has been implanted as a bridge to transplantation. In these patients, adequate coagulation parameters must be restored within a few hours of identifying a suitable donor organ. For this group of patients, a continuous intravenous heparin drip to maintain the activated clotting time between 150 and 250 seconds, combined with dipyridamole 75 mg by mouth every 6 hours, may be a reasonable therapy. Alternatively, warfarin sodium may be employed.

Patients with an artificial heart have a high likelihood of developing septic complications owing to the presence of the large foreign body, percutaneous drive lines, and long operative times. Accordingly, meticulous attention must be directed toward preserving complete asepsis. After operation, these patients are kept in reverse isolation and are given intravenous antibiotics (cefamandole nafate, 1 g every 6 hours). Pulmonary toilet is vigorous and extubation is done when clinically indicated. Strict aseptic technique is observed when handling vascular catheters. Central and peripheral lines are changed every 2 to 3 days, and the urinary catheter is removed as soon as an adequate urine output is maintained. The percutaneous drive lines used are covered with Dacron velour and sutured to the skin at their exit sites; every effort is made to minimize motion at these sites so that fibrous tissue growth into the velour is encouraged. These areas are cleansed with hydrogen peroxide and covered with povidone-iodine ointment daily. Surveillance cultures are obtained and any positive cultures are promptly investigated. Avoiding sepsis in

the bridge patients is the key to subsequent successful cardiac transplantation later (Lonchyna et al., 1992).

### Results

From 1969 to 1993, 242 patients had pneumatic artificial hearts implanted. In most instances, the implanted devices were intended to be temporary and to serve as a bridge to transplantation. Diagnoses included cardiomyopathy, graft failure after heart transplantation, failure to wean after open heart operation, and a miscellaneous group. The average age of the patients was 42 years (range, 13 to 64 years), and the average period of time that the device provided circulatory support was 22 days (range, less than 1 day to 438 days). Most prostheses used (187) were of the Jarvik design, manufactured by Symbion, Inc. This manufacturer is no longer in business. CardioWest Technology has purchased the assets of Symbion, Inc., and recently received Food and Drug Administration approval for sale of a CardioWest prosthesis C-70 for clinical investigation. The remainder were custom-made devices that were developed by physician-engineer teams and were usually used at the same institution in which they were made. The preimplant condition of the patients varied from stable but with severe end-stage heart failure, where a semielective artificial heart implant was performed, to a patient in extremis who had the circulation supported by external cardiac massage. Accordingly, the results might be expected to differ greatly in such a wide spectrum of patients. Many patients have had relatively uncomplicated implantations and have been weaned from the respirator. These patients have been able to eat, converse, and walk around their rooms. If the patient's condition was satisfactory and a suitable donor heart was identified, the prosthesis was removed and transplantation was performed. The length of stay in the hospital has been increased by the use of the bridge device, but the outcome has been excellent. Unfortunately, some patients have had various problems after implantation, including the sequelae of inadequate circulation before implantation generally manifested as multisystem failure. Other problems included bleeding, infection, and thromboembolism and were caused by the interaction between the host and the device (Griffith et al., 1987). Although the timing of transplantation in such a patient is based on the status of organ function and on the availability of a donor organ, experience indicates that the best results are obtained when the artificial heart is kept in place for less than 1 week. However, the difficulty in identifying suitable donor hearts frequently requires that the prosthetic heart remain in place for considerably longer.

The University of Utah Artificial Heart Laboratory maintains a registry of patients who have undergone artificial heart implantation. The world experience with the Jarvik artificial heart is summarized in Table 58–1. One-hundred eighty-seven hearts have been implanted. Of this group, 135 patients were able to be transplanted, with 89 leaving the hospital. The

■ **Table 58–1.** JARVIK ARTIFICIAL HEART AS A BRIDGE FOR TRANSPLANTATION—CLINICAL RESULTS

| | Patients | Number Transplanted (%) | Discharged from Hospital |
|---|---|---|---|
| Jarvik-7* | 41 | 26 (63) | 15 |
| Jarvik-7-70† | 146 | 109 (75) | 74 |
| Total | 187 | 135 (72) | 89 |

Data from Don B. Olsen, D.V.M., University of Utah Artificial Heart Research Laboratory.
*100 ml stroke volume.
†70 ml stroke volume.

smaller Jarvik-7-70 provided an adequate cardiac output for most patients. The largest personal series has come from Cabrol's group at Hôpital de la Pitié, Paris (Kawaguchi et al., 1992). In their series, 58 Jarvik hearts were implanted; 25 of those patients were transplanted, and 17 patients left the hospital. The authors emphasize the importance of patient selection and preoperative condition in achieving a successful outcome. When one considers the novelty of the artificial heart and the magnitude of the staged procedure, these results are certainly acceptable. With additional experience in the selection of patients and improvements in the artificial heart, the results will improve.

A few patients with end-stage heart disease who were not considered to be transplant candidates have had a Jarvik-7 artificial heart permanently implanted (DeVries, 1988). One death occurred 10 days after implantation as a result of cardiac tamponade. Several patients have done reasonably well and were able to eat, sit in a chair, and take walks with the help of someone to move the power unit. The compact Heimes power unit has been used for several hours with the artificial heart functioning well. One patient was able to ride outdoors in a specially equipped van. However, the occurrence of strokes, poor nutrition, or infection led ultimately to their gradual decline and death. Two patients lived for more than 1 year, and the longest survivor lived for 622 days. Most observers believe that pneumatic hearts have not been developed to their fullest potential. Although improvements in their design will reduce the incidence of thromboembolic complications, the problem of infection appears intimately related to the percutaneous power lines, which are intrinsic components of the pneumatic artificial heart. The electric motor–driven artificial heart will overcome most of the problems associated with the pneumatically driven devices and ultimately will replace the pneumatic hearts.

## ELECTRICALLY POWERED ARTIFICIAL HEART FOR PERMANENT HEART REPLACEMENT

Experience with the pneumatically powered heart, both in the laboratory and in the clinical setting, has confirmed the disadvantage of percutaneous passage

of the power lines. A major breakthrough in the transmission of energy in the form of pressurized fluid across the skin does not appear to be imminent. However, investigators (Schuder et al., 1961) have recognized for decades that electrical energy can be transmitted across the intact skin by inductive coupling, a principle widely used in transformers and other commonly used electrical devices. Such a system was used clinically by Glenn and colleagues (1959) to energize pacemakers. However, the low power requirement of a pacemaker and availability of reliable implantable batteries quickly made the inductively coupled pacemaker obsolete. A power requirement of more than a million times that of a pacemaker eliminates from consideration an artificial heart solely dependent on an implantable battery. Accordingly, the permanent artificial heart now under development in several laboratories consists of two implantable blood pumps activated by a miniature electric motor. Energy for the system is supplied continuously to a primary coil on the surface of the skin by either house current or a wearable external battery. The secondary coil, positioned under the skin and energized by the primary coil, actuates the electric motor. An element of safety and comfort is provided by a sophisticated implantable rechargeable battery. This implanted battery powers the heart for only about 30 minutes, which is sufficient time for the external coil to be changed and for minor power interruptions to be rectified. Although the principle of operation and design plans for the electrically powered hearts are well formulated, these plans have only recently resulted in the fabrication of hardware and institution of animal studies.

The electric heart under development at the University of Utah (Rowles et al., 1992) is based on a modification of the Jarvik-7 pneumatically powered ventricle (Jarvik, 1981; Jarvik et al., 1978) (Fig. 58–12). In this design, a high-speed, reversing, brushless DC motor is coupled to an axial flow pump, located between the two ventricles. This motor-pump unit is positioned within a short conduit that joins what were the pneumatic ports of the two ventricles. The system is filled with silicone hydraulic fluid. Axial flow pumping in one direction activates the left blood pump, while axial rotation in reverse activates the right pump. The volume of hydraulic fluid pumped closely approximates the stroke volume of the pump. The maximal output of the pump is 9.2 l/min. A 4.3-mm diameter interatrial shunt is used to balance the output of the two ventricles (Tatsumi et al., 1992). Controllers adjust heart rate and motor speed to maintain normal filling pressures and a full stroke. The heart has now been used in animal studies since 1993. The goal of the Utah program is to develop an integrated system having implanted nickel-cadmium rechargeable batteries, electromagnetic induction energy transfer, and a bidirectional infrared data link. The entire system is being assembled and refined for long-term animal studies. This artificial heart uses a clever design, is compact, and has few moving parts. The requirement of rapidly reversing the high-speed

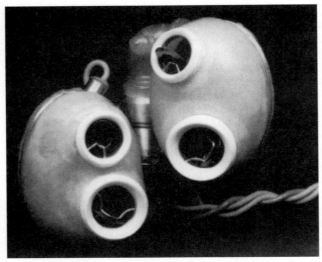

FIGURE 58–12. The electrohydraulic artificial heart being developed at the University of Utah. The axial flow pump, positioned between the two blood pumps, pressurizes the hydraulic fluid and alternately actuates the right and left ventricles. (Courtesy of Donald B. Olsen, D.V.M., University of Utah.)

motor, however, places extreme loads on the miniature bearings, which may limit the functional life of the energy converter.

The Cleveland Clinic Foundation Nimbus electric heart (Fig. 58–13) uses a brushless DC electric motor to power a gear pump that in turn produces hydraulic fluid flow (Himley et al., 1990). This fluid pressure is applied to alternating ends of a hydraulic cylinder. Direction of fluid flow is controlled by the position of spool valves. The unit is magnetically coupled to pusher plates, and the blood pumps eject in an alternating manner. The blood contacting surface is lined

with glutaraldehyde-treated gelatin. Mock circulatory loop and animal testing are currently in progress. The device has been documented to produce flow rates as high as 9.3 l/min with physiologic atrial pressures. Efficiency ranges from 10.5 to 20.4% (hard-wire electrical connection). The longest animal study lasted 120 days. Concerns regarding life of the device center around wear of mechanical components.

The Pennsylvania State University electric heart (Rosenberg et al., 1984, 1985) uses two pusher plate-actuated ventricles (Fig. 58–14). A low-speed, reversing, brushless DC motor with a motion translator is positioned between the two ventricles. The most efficient long-life motion translator available is a roller screw, which functions in a manner similar to a nut rotating on a threaded shaft. In this application, the nut rotates and the shaft moves to and fro for a distance of 25 mm. Again, as in the other electric heart designs, the two ventricles pump alternately. This design requires a larger, heavier motor than does the hydraulic system design. The 2-year functional life design criterion appears to be well within the design specifications for the roller screw and associated bearings.

The output of the electric artificial heart can be varied by changing the stroke or the pumping rate. As with the pneumatic heart, the change in output can occur secondary to change in filling pressure or in response to an electronic control based on atrial or arterial pressures, or their analogs. Electrically powered hearts have lagged behind their pneumatic counterparts, in part because of their complexity of control. In any design of an artificial heart, provisions must be made to prevent atrial collapse in the event that there is inadequate blood to fill the ventricle. In the pneumatic design, a preset low diastolic (filling) vac-

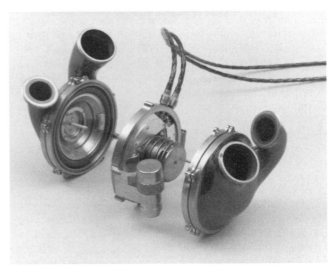

FIGURE 58–13. The Cleveland Clinic Foundation Nimbus artificial heart is shown partially disassembled. The prime mover unit (center) consists of a brushless DC motor–driven gear pump and a spool valve. Hydraulic fluid–actuated pusher plates alternately pump the left and right ventricles. (Photograph courtesy of Cleveland Clinic Foundation.)

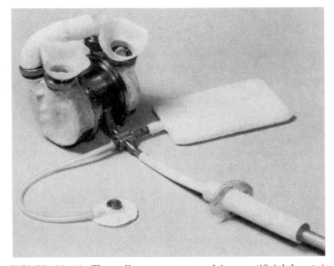

FIGURE 58–14. The roller-screw motor-driven artificial heart is being developed at The Pennsylvania State University. The brushless DC motor and the roller-screw unit are positioned between the two ventricles. The transcutaneous electrical line, compliance chamber, and percutaneous access port are also shown. (From Pierce, W. S.: The artificial heart—1986: Partial fulfillment of a promise. Trans. Am. Soc. Artif. Intern. Organs. 32:5, 1986.)

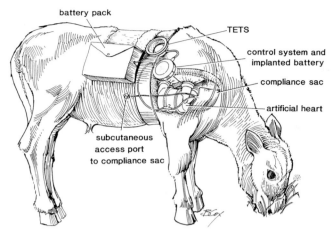

**FIGURE 58–15.** The Pennsylvania State University electric heart is being evaluated in the calf. The placement of the pump is shown within the thorax. The compliance sac and its subcutaneous access port, the location of the transcutaneous energy transmission system (TETS), the control system with the implanted battery, and the external battery pack are also shown. (From Rosenberg, G., Snyder, A. J., Weiss, W. J., et al.: Power requirements for an electric motor-driven total artificial heart. IEEE/Ninth Annual Conference of the Engineering in Medicine and Biology Society. Vol. 1, p. 188. © 1987 IEEE.)

uum prevents atrial collapse; the hydraulic or mechanical types of electric heart must rely on other techniques. In the hydraulic design, a pressure sensor is used in the hydraulic fluid behind each ventricle, which, through appropriate electronic circuitry, promptly slows or stops and reverses axial pump movement when a significant negative pressure is registered. In the pusher plate design (Landis et al., 1980), the bladder is not attached to the pusher plate; this enables the pusher plate to travel a full distance without obligatory bladder filling. Incomplete or slow bladder filling, in turn, provides a signal to the control system that automatically decreases the pump rate to a level at which a full-to-empty cycle will result.

Implanted artificial hearts that are closed to the atmosphere require a volume-displacement device to allow for minor variations in the output of each ventricle and compensation for normal variation in atmospheric pressure (Lee et al., 1984). This is accomplished by the use of a compliance chamber, which consists of a flexible, gas-containing sac that is connected to the gas space of the motor heart (Fig. 58–15). The compliance chamber is covered with Dacron velour, which appears to prevent entrapment by adjacent tissue and resultant loss of function of the chamber.

The *transcutaneous energy transmission system* (TETS) consists of a primary coil of Litz wire energized at 150 kHz. The secondary coil is implanted under the skin and provides energy to power the motor and associated electronics and to recharge the implanted batteries. The energy required for the electric heart can be transmitted, with the coils 5 to 10 mm apart (simulated skin thickness), with a 70% efficiency and no noticeable rise in skin temperature or nutritional effect on the interpositioned skin. Important informa-

tion can be transmitted to and from the implanted electronics by modulation of the 150-kHz power signal, which allows one to assess device function and battery condition and adjust operation modes.

The power input required for the electric heart is between 10 and 20 watts, and is provided easily by conventional house current. For portable function, the heart must be powered by an external, rechargeable battery pack. In addition to the batteries, such a pack must include the electronics required for recharging them and a system to indicate the power remaining and the status of the battery. At present, nickel-cadmium batteries represent the best type of batteries available. Approximately 1 pound of battery is required for each hour of heart function. Development of higher-energy density batteries is a current focus of industrial research; advances in this area should produce a lighter power pack for the patients to carry.

Extensive bench studies now being done with the electric hearts confirm adequate maintenance of pressure and flow during various mock circulatory loop conditions. In vitro fatigue testing is an important part of the evaluation of these hearts. Results generally indicate that failures before the anticipated design life of 2 years frequently occur because of mechanical malfunction or the effect of moisture on electronic circuitry. Minor, but important, design changes continue to remedy these problems.

The Pennsylvania State University electric heart has now functioned in calves for as long as 13 months with hard-wire electrical transmission (Snyder et al., 1992), and for over 4 months with TETS wireless energy transmission (Fig. 58–16). Although premature failures owing to moisture effects on electrical components and mechanical malfunctions continue to occur, thromboembolic complications have been rare, and

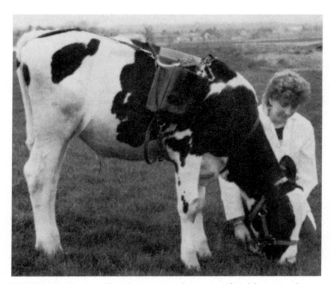

**FIGURE 58–16.** A calf with a motor-driven artificial heart is shown. The implanted components are similar to those shown in Figure 58–15, although the controller is not implanted and electrical energy is supplied through a percutaneous wire. This animal survived for 222 days with the electric heart.

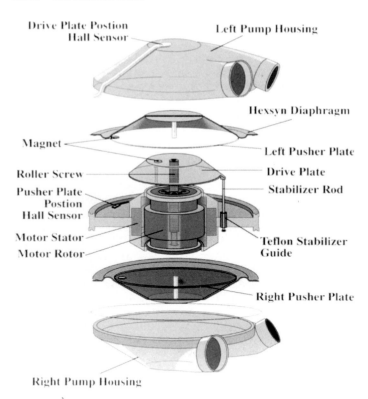

Drive Plate Postion Hall Sensor

Left Pump Housing

Hexsyn Diaphragm

Magnet

Left Pusher Plate

Roller Screw

Drive Plate

Pusher Plate Postion Hall Sensor

Stabilizer Rod

Motor Stator

Motor Rotor

Teflon Stabilizer Guide

Right Pusher Plate

Right Pump Housing

**Electro-mechanical TAH**

**FIGURE 58–17.** The Baylor electric artificial heart uses a DC motor–powered roller screw that alternately compresses the right and the left ventricles. Conical pusher plates are used to achieve a very compact system. (TAH = total artificial heart.) (Photograph courtesy of Y. Nosé, Baylor College of Medicine.)

**FIGURE 58–18.** The implantable electric heart is shown as it is proposed for human use. The artificial heart and associated compliance sac are positioned within the thorax. The compliance sac is accessed through a subcutaneous port. The external battery is carried in a shoulder case. Electrical energy is transferred by using inductive coupling techniques via a belt-located primary and secondary coil. (From Rosenberg, G., Snyder, A. J., Landis, D. L., et al.: An electric motor–driven total artificial heart: Seven months' survival in the calf. Trans. Am. Soc. Artif. Intern. Organs, 30:69, 1984.)

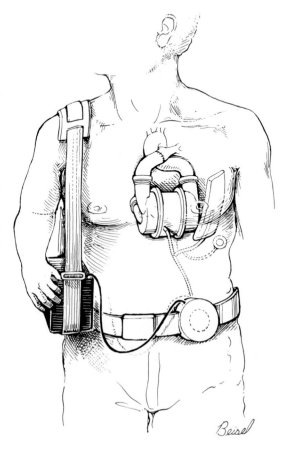

no significant wear has been observed on mechanical components.

The Baylor College of Medicine group has adopted the roller screw concept (Orime et al., 1992) (Fig. 58–17). The electric heart being developed by this group consists of a brushless DC motor and roller screw positioned between conical pusher plates that provides a size advantage. Again, the left and right ventricles pump in an alternate manner. The pump provides up to 8 l/min, with a preload of 15 mm Hg against an afterload of 100 mm Hg. The efficiency with hard-wire electrical transmission ranged from 15 to 18%. Animal implant studies have not yet been performed using this device.

Progress in the development of the electric heart is not limited by lack of basic knowledge or by the unavailability of any particular component. Researchers are particularly receptive to any advances in electronics, batteries, super conductors, ultra-high-strength magnets, and elastomers and to adapting them to the electric heart. Based on current progress, the best estimates suggest that the electric heart will be available for initial clinical application at the end of the 20th century (Fig. 58–18).

## SELECTED BIBLIOGRAPHY

DeVries, W. C.: The permanent artificial heart: Four case reports. J. A. M. A., 259:849, 1988.

This article provides a detailed summary of four patients who had permanent artificial hearts implanted. The blood pumps were able to maintain an adequate circulation for prolonged periods. Most of the problems that have occurred in animal studies with the Jarvik-7 heart have been seen when the device was used in the clinical setting.

Hogness, J. R., and VanAntwerp, M. (eds): The Artificial Heart—Prototypes, Policies and Patients. Institute of Medicine Report. Washington, DC, National Academy Press, 1991.

The Institute of Medicine reviewed the artificial heart program in detail. This fascinating book is their report and provides insight into a broad range of topics, ranging from the complexities of developing an artificial heart to the effect of such advanced technology on ethical and societal issues.

Pierce, W. S., Rosenberg G., Snyder, A. J., et al.: An electric artificial heart for clinical use. Ann. Surg. 212:339, 1990.

In the future, artificial hearts will be "shelf" items, with an availability similar to that of pacemakers and prosthetic valves. This article describes in detail the many components of an electric heart, the problems that remain to be overcome, and the patient population that will benefit from these devices.

## BIBLIOGRAPHY

Akutsu, T., Houston, C. S., and Kolff, W. J.: Artificial hearts inside the chest, using small electro-motors. Trans. Am. Soc. Artif. Intern. Organs, 6:299, 1960.

Akutsu, T., and Kolff, W. J.: Permanent substitutes for valves and hearts. Trans. Am. Soc. Artif. Intern. Organs, 4:230, 1958.

Atsumi, K., Fujimasa, I., Imachi, K., et al.: Three goats survived for 288 days, 243 days, and 232 days with hybrid total artificial heart (HTAH). Trans. Am. Soc. Artif. Intern. Organs, 27:77, 1981.

Aufiero, T. X., Magovern, J. A., Rosenberg, G., et al.: Long-term survival with a pneumatic total artificial heart (pTAH). Trans. Am. Soc. Artif. Intern. Organs, 33:157, 1987.

Boretos, J. W., and Pierce, W. S.: Segmented polyurethane: A new elastomer for biomedical application. Science, 158:1481, 1967.

Bücherl, E. S., Hennig, E., Frank, B. J., et al.: Status of the artificial heart programs in Berlin. World J. Surg., 9:103, 1985.

Bygdeman, S., and Eliasson, R.: Effect of dextrans on platelet adhesiveness and aggregation. Scand. J. Clin. Lab. Invest., 20:17, 1967.

Coleman, D. L., Lim, D., Kessler, T., and Andrade, J. D.: Calcification of nontextured implantable blood pumps. Trans. Am. Soc. Artif. Intern. Organs, 27:97, 1981.

Cooley, D. A.: Staged cardiac transplantation: Report of three cases. Heart Trans., 1:145, 1982.

Cooley, D. A., Liotta, D., Hallman, G. L., et al.: Orthotopic cardiac prosthesis for two-staged cardiac replacement. Am. J. Cardiol., 24:723, 1969.

DeVries, W. C.: The permanent artificial heart: Four case reports. J. A. M. A., 259:849, 1988.

DeVries, W. C., Anderson, J. L., Joyce, L. D., et al.: Clinical use of the total artificial heart. N. Engl. J. Med., 310:273, 1984.

DeVries, W. C., and Joyce, L. D.: The artificial heart. CIBA Clin. Symp., 35:4, 1983.

Ferrans, V. J., Boyce, S. W., Billingham, M. D., et al.: Calcific deposits in porcine bioprostheses—Structure and pathogenesis. Am. J. Cardiol., 46:721, 1980.

Ferrar, D. J., and Hill, J. D.: Univentricular and biventricular thoracic VAD support as a bridge to cardiac transplantation. Ann. Thorac. Surg., 55:276, 1993.

Fields, A., Harasaki, H., Sands, D., and Nosé, Y.: Infection in artificial blood pump implantation. Trans. Am. Soc. Artif. Intern. Organs, 29:532, 1983.

Gaines, W. E., Pierce, W. S., Prophet, G. A., and Holtzman, K. L.: The goat: An animal model for implantable blood pumps. ASAIO J., 8:135, 1985.

Glenn, W. W. L., Mauro, A., Longo, E., et al.: Remote stimulation of the heart by radio frequency transmission. N. Engl. J. Med., 261:948, 1959.

Griffith, B. P., Hardesty, R. L., Kormos, R. L., et al.: Temporary use of the Jarvik-7 total artificial heart before transplantation. N. Engl. J. Med., 316:130, 1987.

Griffith, B. P., Kormos, R. L., Dummer, J. S., and Hardesty, R. L.: The artificial heart: Infection-related morbidity and its effect on transplantation. Ann. Thorac. Surg., 45:409, 1988.

Hall, C. W., Adams, L. M., and Ghidoni, J. J.: Development of skin interfacing cannula. Trans. Am. Soc. Artif. Intern. Organs, 21:281, 1975.

Harker, L. A., and Schlicter, S. J.: Studies of platelet and fibrinogen kinetics in patients with prosthetic heart valves. N. Engl. J. Med., 283:1302, 1970.

Hastings, W. L., Aaron, J. L., Deneris, J., et al.: A retrospective study of nine calves surviving five months on the pneumatic total artificial heart. Trans. Am. Soc. Artif. Intern. Organs, 27:71, 1981.

Heimes, H. P., and Klasen, F.: Completely integrated wearable TAH-drive unit. Int. J. Artif. Organs, 5:157, 1982.

Hennig, E., Grosse-Siestrup, C., Krautzberger, W., et al.: The relationship of cardiac output and venous pressure in long-surviving calves with total artificial hearts. Trans. Am. Soc. Artif. Intern. Organs, 24:616, 1978.

Himley, S. C., Butler, K. C., Massiello, A., et al.: Development of the E4T electrohydraulic total artificial heart. ASAIO Trans. 36:M234, 1990.

Honda, T., Nagai, I., Nitta, S., et al.: Evaluation of cardiac function and venous return curves in awake, unanesthetized calves with an implanted total artificial heart. Trans. Am. Soc. Artif. Intern. Organs, 21:362, 1975.

Hughes, S. D., Butler, M. D., Holmberg, D. L., et al.: Comparative hematological data from animals implanted with a total artificial heart containing different valves. Trans. Am. Soc. Artif. Intern. Organs, 31:224, 1985.

Hughes, S. D., Coleman, D. L., Dew, P. A., et al.: Effects of coumadin on thrombus and mineralization in total artificial hearts. Trans. Am. Soc. Artif. Intern. Organs, 30:75, 1984.

Jarvik, R. K.: The total artificial heart. Sci. Am., 244:74, 1981.

Jarvik, R. K., DeVries, W. C., Semb, B. K. H., et al.: Surgical positioning of the Jarvik-7 artificial heart. J. Heart Transplant., 5:185, 1986.

Jarvik, R. K., Smith, L. M., Lawson, J. H., et al.: Comparison of pneumatic and electrically powered total artificial hearts in vivo. Trans. Am. Soc. Artif. Intern. Organs, 24:593, 1978.

Kawaguchi, A. T., Cabrol, C., Pavie, A., et al.: Survival prediction in staged heart transplantation using Jarvik-7 artificial heart. Circulation, 86:II-311, 1992.

Klain, M., Mrava, G. L., Tajima, K., et al.: Can we achieve over 100 hours' survival with a total mechanical heart? Trans. Am. Soc. Artif. Intern. Organs, 17:437, 1971.

Kwan-Gett, C. S., Wu, Y., Collan, R., et al.: Total replacement artificial heart and driving system with inherent regulation of cardiac output. Trans. Am. Soc. Artif. Intern. Organs, 15:245, 1969.

Landis, D. L., Pierce, W. S., Rosenberg, G., et al.: Long-term in vivo automatic electronic control of the artificial heart. Trans. Am. Soc. Artif. Intern. Organs 23:519, 1977.

Landis, D. L., Rosenberg, G., Donachy, J. H., and Pierce, W. S.: Automatic control for the artificial heart. IEEE 1980 Frontiers of Engineering in Health Care, 1:305, 1980.

Lawson, J. H., Olsen, D. B., Hershgold, E., et al.: A comparison of polyurethane and Silastic artificial hearts in ten long-survival experiments in calves. Trans. Am. Soc. Artif. Intern. Organs, 21:368, 1975.

Lee, S., Rosenberg, G., Donachy, J. H., et al.: The compliance problem: A major obstacle in the development of implantable blood pumps. Artif. Organs, 8:82, 1984.

Levy, R. J., Schoen, F. J., Levy, J. T., et al.: Biologic determinants of dystrophic calcification and osteocalcin deposition in glutaraldehyde-preserved porcine aortic valve leaflets implanted subcutaneously in rats. Am. J. Pathol., 113:143, 1983.

Lonchyna, V. A., Pefarre, R., Sullivan, H., et al.: Successful use of the total artificial heart as a bridge to transplantation with no mediastinitis. J. Heart Lung Transplant., 11:803, 1992.

Murray, K. D., Hughes, S., Bearnson, D., and Olsen, D. B.: Infection in total artificial heart recipients. Trans. Am. Soc. Artif. Intern. Organs, 29:539, 1983.

Murray, K. D., and Olsen, D. B.: The use of calves and sheep as total heart recipients. ASAIO J., 8:128, 1985.

Nielsen, S. D., Willshaw, P., Nanas, J., and Olsen, D. B.: Noninvasive cardiac monitoring and diagnostics for pneumatic pumping ventricles. Trans. Am. Soc. Artif. Intern. Organs, 29:589, 1983.

Nosé, Y., Topaz, S., SenGupta, A., et al.: Artificial hearts inside the pericardial sac in calves. Trans. Am. Soc. Artif. Intern. Organs, 11:255, 1965.

Olsen, D. B., Fukumasu, H., Kolff, J., et al.: Implantation of the total artificial heart by lateral thoracotomy. Artif. Organs, 1:1, 1977.

Orime, Y., Takatani, S., Shiono, M., et al.: Versatile one-piece total artificial heart for bridge to transplantation or permanent heart replacement. Artif. Organs, 16:607, 1992.

Pae, W. E., Rosenberg, G., Donachy, J. H., et al.: A solution to inlet pannus formation in the pneumatic artificial heart. Trans. Am. Soc. Artif. Intern. Organs, 31:12, 1985.

Paping, R., Webster, L. R., Stanley, T. H., et al.: White blood cell phagocytosis after artificial heart implantation. Trans. Am. Soc. Artif. Intern. Organs, 24:578, 1978.

Pennock, J. L., Pierce, W. S., Campbell, D. B., et al.: Mechanical support of the circulation followed by cardiac transplantation. J. Thorac. Cardiovasc. Surg., 92:994, 1986.

Pierce, W. S.: The artificial heart—1986: Partial fulfillment of a promise. Trans. Am. Soc. Artif. Intern. Organs, 32:5, 1986.

Pierce, W. S., Donachy, J. H., Rosenberg, G., and Baier, R. E.: Calcification inside artificial hearts: Inhibition by warfarin-sodium. Science, 208:601, 1980.

Pierce, W. S., Gardner, B. N., Morris, L., et al.: Total heart replacement by a single intrathoracic blood pump. J. Surg. Res., 5:387, 1965.

Pierce, W. S., Myers, J. L., Donachy, J. H., et al.: Approaches to the artificial heart. Surgery, 90:137, 1981.

Richenbacher, W. E., Pennock, J. L., Pae, W. E., Jr., and Pierce, W. S.: Artificial heart implantation for end-stage cardiac disease. J. Card. Surg., 1:1, 1986.

Rosenberg, G., Cleary, T. J., Snyder, A. J., et al.: A totally implantable artificial heart design. Trans. Am. Soc. Mech. Eng., 85-WA/DE-11, 1985.

Rosenberg, G., Landis, D. L., Phillips, W. M., et al.: Determining arterial pressure, left atrial pressure, and cardiac output from the left pneumatic drive line of the left artificial heart. Trans. Am. Soc. Artif. Intern. Organs, 24:341, 1978.

Rosenberg, G., Snyder, A. J., Landis, D. L., et al.: An electric motor-driven total artificial heart: Seven months' survival in the calf. Trans. Am. Soc. Artif. Intern. Organs, 30:69, 1984.

Rowles, J. R., Khanwilkar, P. S., Diegel, P. D., et al.: Development of a totally implantable artificial heart. ASAIO J., 38:M713, 1992.

Schuder, J. C., Stephenson, H. E., Jr., and Townsend, J. F.: Energy transfer into a closed chest by means of stationary coupling coils and a portable high-power oscillator. Trans. Am. Soc. Artif. Intern. Organs, 7:327, 1961.

Shaffer, L. J., Donachy, J. H., Rosenberg, G., et al.: Total artificial heart implantation in calves with pump of an angled port design. Trans. Am. Soc. Artif. Intern. Organs, 25:254, 1979.

Snyder, A. J., Rosenberg, G., Reibson, J., et al.: An electrically powered total artificial heart: Over one year survival in the calf. ASAIO J., 38:M707, 1992.

Tatsumi, E., Diegel, P. D., Holfert, J. W., et al.: A blood pump with an interarterial shunt for use as an electrohydraulic total artificial heart. ASAIO J., 38:M425, 1992.

Whalen, R. L., Snow, J. L., Harasaki, H., and Nosé, Y.: Mechanical strain and calcification in blood pumps. Trans. Am. Soc. Artif. Intern. Organs, 26:487, 1980.

# 59 Thoracoscopic Surgery

James M. Douglas, Jr.

The first clinical use of thoracoscopy was reported by Jacobaeus in 1915 describing endopleural operations by means of a thoracoscope. He developed cautery pneumolysis as an adjunct to collapse therapy for the treatment of pulmonary tuberculosis. In 1928, Cova published the *Atlas Thoracoscopicon*, which contained a number of illustrations of thoracoscopic procedures. However, this technique did not have widespread use until the advent of video-assisted laparoscopic surgery.

## GENERAL APPROACH

Astonishing advances are being made in the refinement of video technology as applied to thoracoscopic surgery. Unlike the abdominal approach in laparoscopic surgery, thoracoscopic procedures have certain constraints. These include a rigid thoracic cavity and the physiologic consequences of intrathoracic operations using single-lung ventilation with collapse of the lung on the operated side to achieve maximal exposure.

The basic equipment includes a fiberoptic light source with an associated video camera system and monitors. In addition, several specific thoracoscopic instruments including endoscopic graspers, clamps, and staplers are used. While both rigid and flexible endoscopes can be used for thoracoscopy, the 0-degree rigid endoscope has proved to be the most useful because it increases the field of view, resolution, and simplicity. Rigid scopes may also have an angled field of vision (usually 30 or 60 degrees away from the in-line angle of incidence). Although these scopes provide views of areas that are at sharp angles from the normal field and can therefore be useful, nevertheless they may be confusing to the untrained observer. Carbon dioxide insufflation into the pleural cavity may occasionally be quite useful because it maximizes visibility by assisting in collapse of the lung. The typical operating room environment, with two video monitors allowing the operator and assistants to easily visualize the procedure, is recommended and shown in Figure 59–1.

## ANESTHESIA

In most instances, a general anesthetic with single-lung ventilation is indicated for *thoracoscopic* procedures. Several alternative techniques are available for individual inflation of the two lungs. For emergency procedures, the rapid placement of an endotracheal tube into the mainstem bronchus of the unoperated side allows the side of the thoracoscopic approach to collapse. Bronchial blockers can be placed on the side of the thoracoscopic procedure, but these tend to become dislodged back into the trachea and cause partial obstruction. However, at times a blocker must be used in children and young adults owing to the small size of the bronchi. The procedure of choice is a double-lumen tube with the use of either right- or left-sided tubes for separate ventilation on each lung. It should be noted that the right-sided tube when applied to collapse the left lung has a risk of obstructing the upper-lobe bronchus. Because of its ease of management, the left-sided double-lumen tube has a lower risk of improper placement and has become the preferred technique for most patients under single-lung anesthesia. It is necessary to be certain of the proper positioning of the tube with a flexible bronchoscope after the patient has been turned to the lateral position.

It should be emphasized that continuous monitoring is essential. The lung should be ventilated with a tidal volume of approximately 10 ml/kg, and the $Pa_{CO_2}$ should be maintained around 40 mm Hg by control of the respiratory rate. When continuous monitoring of the patient's oxygenation indicates hypoxemia, positive end-expiratory pressure or continuous airway pressure, or a combination of both, should be applied. The operation should be interrupted briefly to allow temporary reinflation of the collapsed lung when necessary.

## POSITION

Almost all thoracoscopic procedures can be appropriately performed with the patient in the lateral decubitus position with the arm elevated on the operated side (Fig. 59–2). The intercostal spaces can be widened to increase exposure by flexing the operating table to lower the patient's hips. However, venous pooling of the lower extremities may result and should be noted. The patient should be draped in a manner that would allow a thoracoscopic incision to be made, should it become necessary.

## PROCEDURE

Proper placement of the ports for a thoracoscopic procedure is of maximal importance. This is especially true because the rigidity of the thoracic cavity does

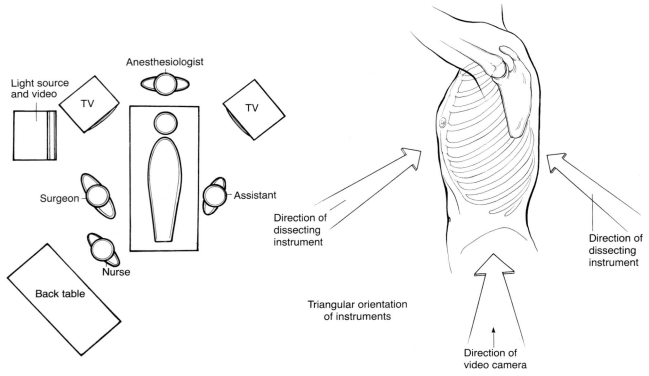

**FIGURE 59–1.** Diagram of typical operating room environment. Two video monitors help the operator and assistants easily visualize the procedure. Also shown is the orientation of instruments and camera during the operation. (From Hanke, I., and Douglas, J. M., Jr.: General approach to video-assisted thoracoscopic surgery. *In* Sabiston, D. C., Jr. [ed]: Atlas of Cardiothoracic Surgery. Philadelphia, W. B. Saunders, 1995.)

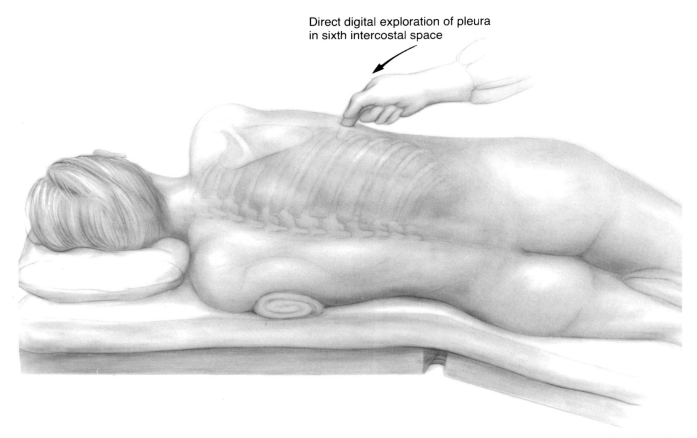

**FIGURE 59–2.** The patient is placed in the lateral decubitus position for video-assisted thoracoscopy. (From Hanke, I., and Douglas, J. M., Jr.: General approach to video-assisted thoracoscopic surgery. *In* Sabiston, D. C., Jr. [ed]: Atlas of Cardiothoracic Surgery. Philadelphia, W. B. Saunders, 1995.)

not afford the flexibility inherent to the abdominal wall or the resulting compensation for imprecise port placement that is possible with laparoscopic procedures.

The endoscopic instruments and the camera should be oriented in the same direction and toward the target of the operative procedure (see Fig. 59–1). It is usually most suitable to place the scope within the fifth to the seventh intercostal space in the anterior-to-posterior axillary line because the intercostal spaces are quite wide in this anatomic area, permitting an easy panoramic view of the thoracic cavity. Positioning can be performed as necessary.

The lungs should be deflated before the trocars are inserted (Fig. 59–3). Because time is required to collapse the alveoli, it is preferable to request lung deflation as soon as the patient is positioned. In most instances, two to four trocars are used to complete the procedure, and the incisions for these trocars should be 1 to 2 cm in length. After the initial trocar is placed, the subcutaneous tissue and underlying muscle are divided by cautery with entry into the pleural space. With the introduction of the finger into the thorax, one can be assured that there are no adhesions and that the lung is indeed collapsed. With this approach, the camera can be inserted safely into the pleural cavity and injury to the pulmonary parenchyma is avoided.

If incomplete collapse of the lung is present, inflation of $CO_2$ into the pleural cavity at a pressure below 10 mm Hg is useful. Under direct endoscopic visualization, the remaining trocars are then inserted and placed above the edge of the lower rib to avoid injury to the intercostal bundle. Some form of thoracoscopic port should be used to allow safe and easy passage of the scopes, but direct passage of instruments through the chest wall can be an acceptable technique. This is especially true when standard thoracic instruments are employed.

On completion of the thoracoscopic procedure, careful hemostasis of the operative sites should be achieved. A chest tube is usually placed through one of the incisions and fixed to the skin with a suture. After removal of the instruments, the incisions are closed in layers and the lung is reexpanded and the intrapleural tube connected to suction. The chest tube is removed later when all air leaks are sealed and drainage is less than 100 ml daily.

## THORACOSCOPIC PULMONARY BIOPSY FOR DIFFUSE LUNG DISEASE

In obtaining a biopsy from patients for diffuse pulmonary disease, the standard approach has been tho-

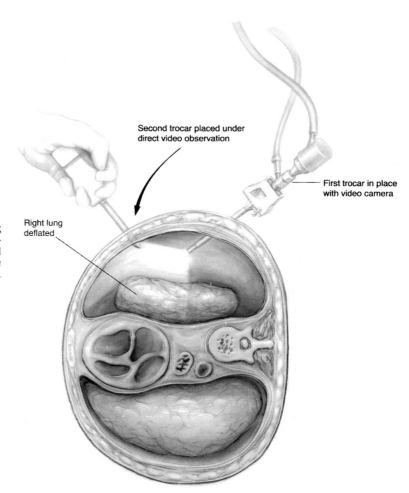

FIGURE 59–3. A cross-section shows the deflated lung with trocars placed for insertion of camera and instruments. (From Hanke, I., and Douglas, J. M., Jr.: General approach to video-assisted thoracoscopic surgery. *In* Sabiston, D. C., Jr. [ed]: Atlas of Cardiothoracic Surgery. Philadelphia, W. B. Saunders, 1995.)

Second trocar placed under direct video observation

First trocar in place with video camera

Right lung deflated

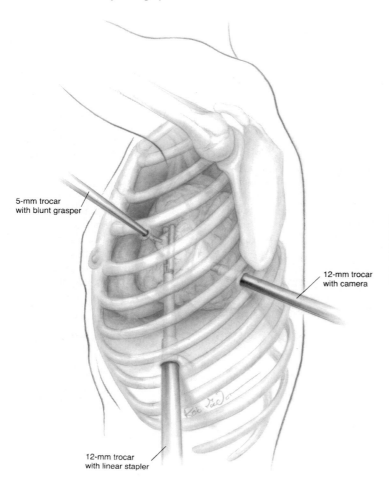

5-mm trocar
with blunt grasper

12-mm trocar
with camera

12-mm trocar
with linear stapler

**FIGURE 59–4.** Three 12-mm trocars are inserted through the ports for introduction of the instruments and camera in the collapsed lung for biopsy. (From Hsu, C.-P., and Douglas, J. M., Jr.: Thoracoscopic pulmonary biopsy for diffuse lung disease. *In* Sabiston, D. C., Jr. [ed]: Atlas of Cardiothoracic Surgery. Philadelphia, W. B. Saunders, 1995.)

racotomy and biopsy. Thoracoscopy is quite appropriate and safe for this procedure and can be easily performed without the discomfort, time, and expense of a formal thoracotomy. It should be emphasized that patients who require mechanical ventilation are not good candidates for this procedure. For these individuals, a standard thoracotomy is generally preferred because it can be done without the need for placement of a new endotracheal tube and one-lung ventilation.

General anesthesia is preferred when thoracoscopy is being performed. Typically, a left-sided double-lumen endobronchial tube is passed and a pulse oximeter is placed for detection of the peripheral oxygen saturation during the procedure. The patient is placed in the lateral decubitus position with a pad beneath the dependent axilla as prophylaxis against neurovascular injury. With the use of one-lung ventilation, the operated lung is collapsed and the thoracoscope is placed in the fifth to seventh intercostal space in the mid- to posterior axillary line (Fig. 59–4). Once the trocar has been introduced and a thorough exploratory thoracoscopy performed, the accessory access sites to obtain the lung biopsy are selected. It is usual to use two additional access sites, and these should be placed at least 10 cm apart in the anterior axillary line and the posterior axillary to mid-scapular line. The margin of the lung is grasped with specially

designed endoscopic lung clamps (ring forceps, lung forceps, or Kelly forceps) through the access site without use of the thoracoscopic port. The endoscopic stapler is introduced via another access site when the biopsy is obtained. Most biopsies can be completed with two or three staplings, and multiple biopsies from different pulmonary lobes can be obtained during the procedure. The biopsy is removed through one of the access sites and used for microbiologic and pathologic studies. Saline solution is instilled to detect any air leakage along the suture line. Adequate hemostasis is essential and a chest tube is inserted into the pleural cavity through the lowest access site attached to water-sealed drainage. The incisions are then closed.

## THORACOSCOPIC WEDGE RESECTION FOR INDETERMINATE PULMONARY NODULE

In the patient with multiple pulmonary nodules requiring a biopsy, the thoracoscopic approach is often ideal. It is especially useful in patients with metastatic disease or infectious or inflammatory disorders. It is also useful in patients with reduced pulmonary function because it can provide resection of a primary carcinoma of the lung that might not be appropriate for open thoracotomy. In these circumstances, obtaining an adequate *margin* is essential. Pulmonary lesions that are located just beneath the surface of the pleura of the lung are the most appropriate for thoracoscopic removal. For lesions less than 1 cm in diameter and located within the pulmonary parenchyma, localization preoperatively may be useful. Pulmonary lesions that are quite small, as well as those in the interlobar fissure or deep within the pulmonary parenchyma and those on the diaphragmatic surface, are less suitable for a thoracoscopic approach.

The procedure is conducted with the patient under general anesthesia with a double-lumen endobronchial tube, and the lateral decubitus position is the most appropriate. If a localization needle has been previously placed, the lung should not be hastily collapsed before the thoracoscope is placed. If the needle is dislodged, the surgeon may be compelled to make a limited thoracotomy for identification and resection of the nodule. The initial incision is made in the fifth to seventh intercostal space in the mid- or posterior axillary line in accordance with the anatomic location of the lesion for introduction of the thoracoscope. Additional incisions for accessory access sites should be made under direct visual control by the thoracoscope. Generally, two more intercostal

space access sites are necessary to complete the pulmonary wedge resection. These sites should be placed at least 10 cm apart to prevent too close contact with the instruments. Before insertion of the trocar, it is always appropriate to employ digital exploration to separate any adhesions. After the lung being biopsied is collapsed, the thoracoscope is introduced through the site of the initial port and a thorough exploratory thoracoscopy is performed. The pulmonary nodule is identified by endoscopic inspection, by instrumental palpation, by digital examination, or occasionally, by ultrasound. The endosurgical Kuttner dissector is particularly useful for instrumental palpation. With the use of one or more of these techniques, the pulmonary nodule can usually be accurately identified. It is only rarely necessary to perform an open thoracotomy for this evaluation.

The pulmonary parenchyma containing the nodule is grasped and the stapler is applied at a 2-cm distance from the nodule for biopsy (Fig. 59–5). The nodule is next grasped and resected with stapling sutures (Fig. 59–6) and the port sites of stapler and grasper are switched to complete the wedge resection. The procedure can usually be performed with two or three staplings and the resected specimen is then extracted through one of the access sites. The specimen should be placed in a specially designed bag or

**FIGURE 59–5.** Three 12-mm trocars are inserted for introduction of camera, grasper, and stapler to resect the tumor. (From Hsu, C.-P., and Douglas, J. M., Jr.: Thoracoscopic wedge resection for indeterminate pulmonary nodule. *In* Sabiston, D. C., Jr. [ed]: Atlas of Cardiothoracic Surgery. Philadelphia, W. B. Saunders, 1995.)

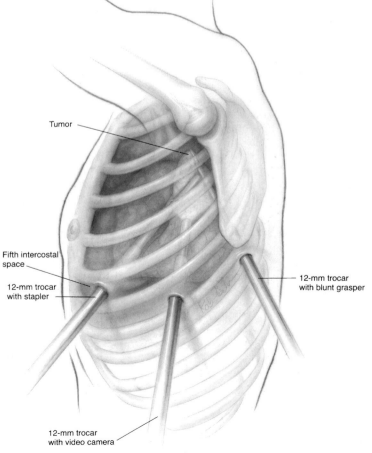

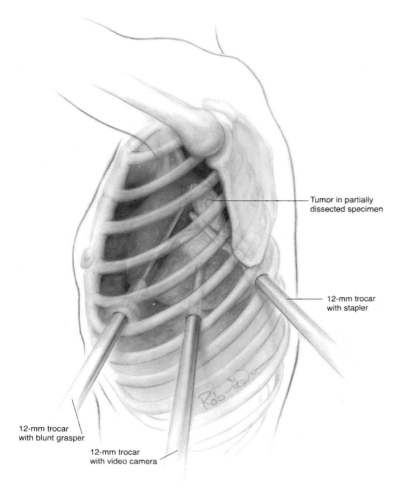

Tumor in partially
dissected specimen

12-mm trocar
with stapler

12-mm trocar
with blunt grasper

12-mm trocar
with video camera

**FIGURE 59–6.** The instruments are switched in the ports to complete the resection. (From Hsu, C.-P., and Douglas, J. M., Jr.: Thoracoscopic wedge resection for indeterminate pulmonary nodule. *In* Sabiston, D. C., Jr. [ed]: Atlas of Cardiothoracic Surgery. Philadelphia, W. B. Saunders, 1995.)

the finger of a sterile surgical glove and removed and sent for pathologic and bacteriologic study. Following complete hemostasis, a chest tube is inserted and attached to underwater drainage with closure of the incisions.

## THORACOSCOPIC RESECTION OF BLEBS AND PLEURODESIS

In some patients with spontaneous pneumothorax, a thoracoscopic approach for the resection of blebs followed by pleurodesis is ideal. Using this approach, one gains complete visualization of the entire thoracic cavity and instrumentation is sufficiently complete to permit the same type of treatment as would be performed during an open thoracotomy. Recovery from a thoracoscopic bleb resection and pleurodesis is much faster than from the open approach and the results appear to be comparable.

The procedure is performed with the patient in the lateral decubitus position with a double-lumen endotracheal tube in place and prepared as for standard thoracotomy. The insertion site for the thoracoscope should ideally be within the fifth to sixth intercostal space in the anterior axillary line. If the patient

has undergone the previous placement of a chest tube in this area, the entry site should be used with excision of the skin incision following extensive sterile preparation of the site. The accessory ports are placed more than 10 cm laterally in the fourth intercostal space and posteriorly in the fourth or fifth intercostal space under direct vision for insertion. Generally, adhesions are present and can be separated with blunt dissection. If the adhesions are fibrous, the electrocautery or scissors may be needed.

Usually, the emphysematous blebs are of sufficient size to be easily seen. If this is not the situation, an air leak can usually be visualized by partial inflation of the lung. Lesions are most common in the apex of the upper lobe and the superior segment of the lower lobe. Pulmonary tissue near the bleb is lifted with an endoscopic grasper (Fig. 59–7). The stapling device is inserted in place with a margin of approximately 1 cm from the bleb on the normal lung tissue. The stapler is fired and the bleb is resected. This can usually be achieved with two or three stapling reloads. Following removal of the specimen from the thorax, the pleural cavity is irrigated with saline solution and the patient is placed in the Trendelenburg position so that the suture line is beneath the water level in the pleural cavity. The lung is inflated to denote any air leak and the irrigation fluid is subsequently removed by suction.

To reduce the probability of recurrent pneumothorax, pleurodesis should be performed (Fig. 59–8). To accomplish this, several techniques can be applied, the simplest being mechanical abrasion using either a Bovie scratch pad on a long Kelly clamp or a sponge on a long ring forceps. Under direct vision, the apical part of the thoracic cavity and the remainder of the parietal pleura are then abraded. On completion of the procedure, a chest tube is inserted through a lower trocar site and attached to water-sealed suction. An additional hole should be made in the tube near the chest wall entry site to allow improved drainage of fluid. This extra perforation should remain within the pleural space and should be comparable in size to those already in the tube.

## THORACOSCOPIC APPROACH TO THE AORTICOPULMONARY WINDOW

The classical cervical mediastinoscopy for pulmonary cancer staging is limited in the aorticopulmonary window and subcarinal regions. The other approach to this area, the Chamberlain incision, served as the standard mediastinoscopic approach to the aorticopulmonary window before the advent of video-assisted thoracoscopy. Although the ultimate usefulness of the thoracoscopic approach for biopsy in this area remains to be established, the advantages include the fact that the entire thoracic cavity can be examined and tumor staging under direct vision made possible as well as identification of the subcarinal and anterior mediastinal lymph nodes that are accessible for biopsy. In all patients undergoing thoracoscopic procedures, consent for possible open thoracotomy should also be obtained before the operation.

Thoracoscopic examination of the aorticopulmonary window is accomplished using a general anesthesia with selected lung-volume ventilation by use of a double-lumen endobronchial tube and intraoperative monitoring. The patient is placed in the left lateral decubitus position with a pad beneath the right axilla for prophylaxis of neurovascular injury. After preparation of the skin, the patient is draped as for a standard thoracotomy and a 1-cm incision is made in the sixth or seventh intercostal space in the midaxillary line for the thoracoscope. An incision is also made in the posterior axillary line an interspace below for introduction of the lung retractor if this be necessary. Generally, two other access sites, one in the

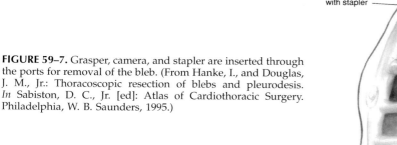

**FIGURE 59–7.** Grasper, camera, and stapler are inserted through the ports for removal of the bleb. (From Hanke, I., and Douglas, J. M., Jr.: Thoracoscopic resection of blebs and pleurodesis. *In* Sabiston, D. C., Jr. [ed]: Atlas of Cardiothoracic Surgery. Philadelphia, W. B. Saunders, 1995.)

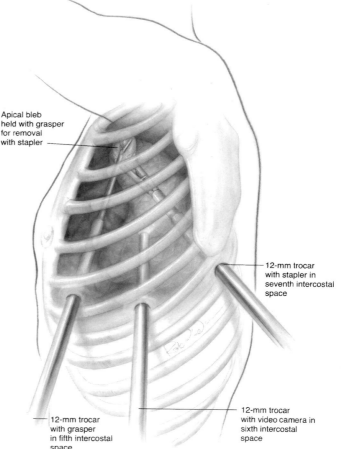

Apical bleb held with grasper for removal with stapler

12-mm trocar with stapler in seventh intercostal space

12-mm trocar with grasper in fifth intercostal space

12-mm trocar with video camera in sixth intercostal space

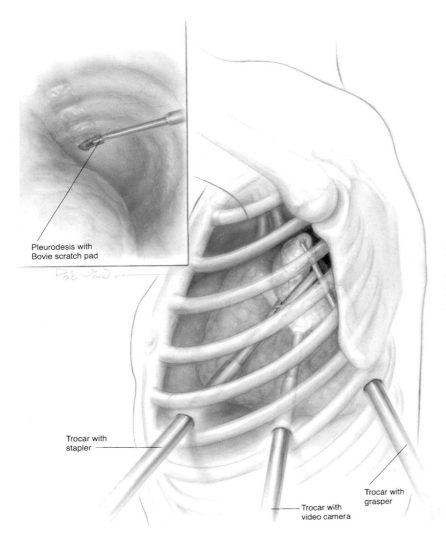

Pleurodesis with
Bovie scratch pad

Trocar with
stapler

Trocar with
video camera

Trocar with
grasper

**FIGURE 59–8.** Pleurodesis is performed with a Bovie scratch pad. (From Hanke, I., and Douglas, J. M., Jr.: Thoracoscopic resection of blebs and pleurodesis. *In* Sabiston, D. C., Jr. [ed]: Atlas of Cardiothoracic Surgery. Philadelphia, W. B. Saunders, 1995.)

fourth intercostal space in the anterior axillary line and the other in the fifth intercostal space posterior to the medial border of the scapula, are made. The phrenic and vagus nerves should be carefully identified before the dissection of the aorticopulmonary window. The lymph nodes are identified and the pleural covering overlying them is opened, and with careful dissection the lymph node is removed. Meticulous dissection is necessary in this area because of the presence of both the pulmonary artery and the aorta as well as the vagus and phrenic nerves. At the end of the procedure, a chest tube is inserted and attached to water-sealed drainage (Fig. 59–9).

## THORACOSCOPIC APPROACH TO POSTERIOR MEDIASTINAL TUMORS

Most posterior mediastinal neoplasms are benign neurogenic tumors. Frequently detected on routine chest film, these tumors are often asymptomatic. A preoperative computed tomography scan should be

obtained to demarcate the limits of the mass and to assess mediastinal invasion and potential involvement of the spinal cord by *dumbbell* tumors. If either of the latter is present, a thoracoscopic approach is not appropriate. However, the vast majority of mediastinal tumors invade neither the mediastinum nor the spinal cord and many are suitable for a thoracoscopic approach and particularly those 5 cm in diameter or less. If the lesion is larger, the potential for malignant change increases, making a standard thoracotomy preferable.

The thoracoscopic approach for a mediastinal mass is performed with the patient under general anesthesia with single-lung ventilation. As in all patients, an oximeter to monitor peripheral $O_2$ saturation is routinely used during collapse of the operated side. It should be remembered that the collapsed lung should be ventilated at least every 30 minutes or the $O_2$ saturation falls below 90%. The patient is placed in the decubitus position with a pad beneath the dependent axilla as prophylaxis against neurovascular injury. The best exposure is obtained by placing the patient in the *jack-knife* position, which spreads the intercostal spaces and permits better manipulation of the various instruments.

A 1-cm incision is made in the fifth intercostal space in the anterior axillary line for introduction of the thoracoscope (Fig. 59–10). A second incision is made in the fourth intercostal space in the anterior axillary line for placement of the lung retractor, and the lung is retracted anteriorly using a fan retractor. Accessory intercostal space access sites should be made anterior to the midaxillary line between the second and the fourth intercostal spaces for upper and middle posterior mediastinal tumors. For neoplasms in the lower posterior mediastinum, the intercostal space access sites should be made at the midaxillary line between the fifth and the seventh intercostal spaces. If the operating table is slightly tilted toward the ventral side, it allows the lung to shift anteriorly and improves the visual field.

Through the accessory intercostal space access sites, the endoscopic dissector, scissors, and grasper are introduced to complete the resection (Fig. 59–11). The tumor is then placed in a plastic bag and withdrawn through one of the access sites with enlargement of the incision, should this be necessary to allow removal of the neoplasm. A chest tube (No. 28 French) is placed in the pleural cavity through the lowest

access site for underwater sealed drainage. The incisions are then closed.

## THORACOSCOPIC APPROACH FOR PERICARDIAL WINDOW

Creation of a pericardial window for pericardial effusion can be ideally performed by the thoracoscopic approach. Either the left or the right side of the pericardium can be exposed. When the effusion is predominant in the left hemithorax, it is most appropriately approached from the right side, whereas moderate to small effusions can be approached from either side. In most surgeons' experience, the left side is found to be preferable.

The patient is placed in the lateral decubitus position and general anesthesia is administered with a double-lumen endotracheal tube. With the usual monitoring, the thorax is draped and an external defibrillator should be available if needed. Following collapse of the lung on the operated side, the trocar for the camera should be placed in the eighth intercostal space in the posterior axillary line with inspection of the pleural space through the scope. The accessory ports should be inserted through the fifth intercostal space in the posterior axillary line and the seventh

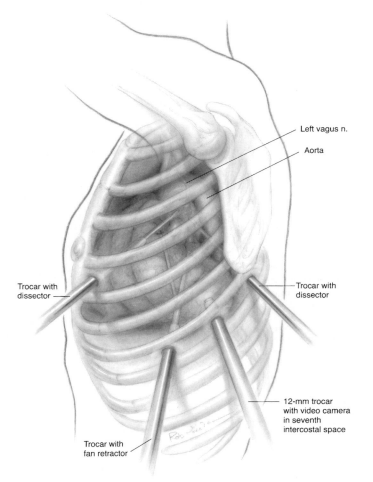

FIGURE 59–9. Dissectors, retractor, and camera are placed for aorticopulmonary window, with care taken to avoid injury to the aorta, pulmonary artery, and vagus and phrenic nerves. (From Hsu, C.-P., and Douglas, J. M., Jr.: Thoracoscopic approach to the aorticopulmonary window. *In* Sabiston, D. C., Jr. [ed]: Atlas of Cardiothoracic Surgery. Philadelphia, W. B. Saunders, 1995.)

Left vagus n.
Aorta
Trocar with dissector
Trocar with dissector
12-mm trocar with video camera in seventh intercostal space
Trocar with fan retractor

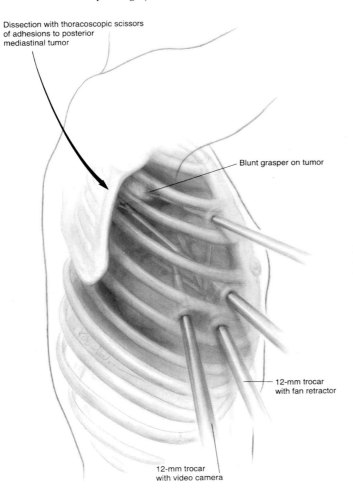

Dissection with thoracoscopic scissors
of adhesions to posterior
mediastinal tumor

Blunt grasper on tumor

12-mm trocar
with fan retractor

12-mm trocar
with video camera

**FIGURE 59–10.** Instruments are placed for excision of posterior mediastinal tumor. (From Hsu, C.-P., and Douglas, J. M., Jr.: VATS for posterior mediastinal tumors. *In* Sabiston, D. C., Jr. [ed]: Atlas of Cardiothoracic Surgery. Philadelphia, W. B. Saunders, 1995.)

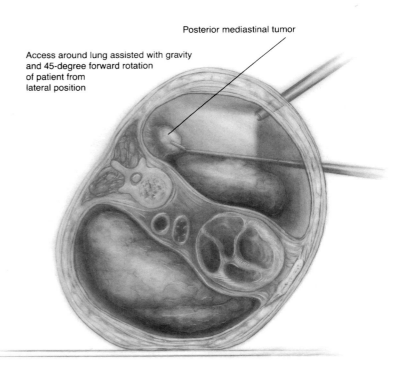

Posterior mediastinal tumor

Access around lung assisted with gravity
and 45-degree forward rotation
of patient from
lateral position

**FIGURE 59–11.** A cross-sectional view shows the mediastinum, tumor, and instruments. The patient is rotated to facilitate access to the tumor. (From Hsu, C.-P., and Douglas, J. M., Jr.: VATS for posterior mediastinal tumors. *In* Sabiston, D. C., Jr. [ed]: Atlas of Cardiothoracic Surgery. Philadelphia, W. B. Saunders, 1995.)

intercostal space in the anterior axillary line. The pericardial window can be created either anterior or posterior to the phrenic nerve, but in most patients, it is usually preferable to initiate the resection posteriorly (Fig. 59–12). At this site, the pericardium is more accessible and allows a larger window to be created. The pericardium is grasped and an incision made with the scissors as the effusion is partly evacuated and the pericardial window is created by excising a 3 × 5 cm segment of pericardium. The anterior border is created by the phrenic nerve, and if the pericardium is quite vascular with thick fatty tissue surrounding it, it is preferable to divide the pericardium using an endoscopic stapler to achieve maximal hemostasis. At times, filmy intrapericardial adhesions are present and can be easily separated with an endosurgical Kuttner dissector. A chest tube is placed at the end and the incisions are closed.

## THORACOSCOPIC APPROACH TO THE ANTERIOR MEDIASTINUM

The anterior mediastinum can be approached by the thoracoscopic route and is being used increasingly for biopsy of anterior mediastinal masses and excision of lymph nodes. Thymectomy can also be performed as well as excision of bronchial and pericardial cysts and other anterior mediastinal masses.

The patient is placed in the lateral decubitus position with the upper extremity being uplifted on the operative side with rotation of the patient somewhat posteriorly. In this position, the mediastinum and lung are more posteriorly located, which facilitates the dissection. A double-lumen endotracheal tube is passed for anesthesia and standard monitoring is performed.

When possible, the anterior mediastinum should be approached from the left side because the heart and pericardium are the anatomic landmarks. The anterior mediastinum extends to the innominate vein superiorly and to the left ventricular prominence inferiorly. The lateral borders of the anterior mediastinum are delineated by the left and right phrenic nerves, and the superior surface is demarcated by the posterior sternum and the floor of the space is the anterior pericardium.

The camera trocar is placed within the mid- to posterior axillary line in the sixth intercostal space (Fig. 59–13). The fifth intercostal space in the anterior axillary line and the third intercostal space in the posterior axillary line are the preferable sites for the other ports. Identification of the innominate vein and its branches as well as the phrenic nerve is essential

FIGURE 59–12. The incision is begun anterior to the phrenic nerve and extended to create the pericardial window. (From Hanke, I., and Douglas, J. M., Jr.: Pericardial window. *In* Sabiston, D. C., Jr. [ed]: Atlas of Cardiothoracic Surgery. Philadelphia, W. B. Saunders, 1995.)

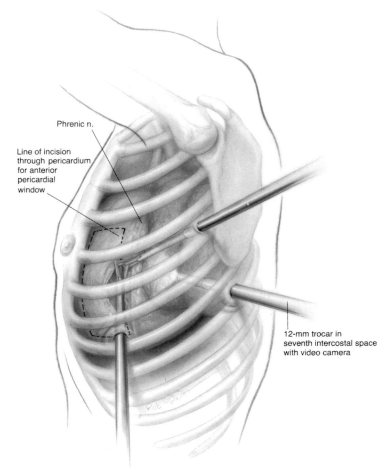

Phrenic n.

Line of incision through pericardium for anterior pericardial window

12-mm trocar in seventh intercostal space with video camera

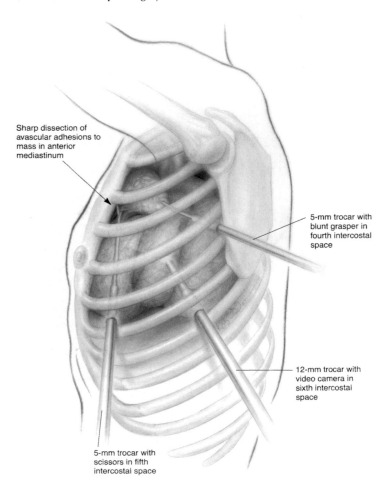

Sharp dissection of
avascular adhesions to
mass in anterior
mediastinum

5-mm trocar with
blunt grasper in
fourth intercostal
space

12-mm trocar with
video camera in
sixth intercostal
space

5-mm trocar with
scissors in fifth
intercostal space

**FIGURE 59–13.** The trocars are placed in a triangular orientation to facilitate dissection. (From Hanke, I., and Douglas, J. M., Jr.: VATS approach to the anterior mediastinum. *In* Sabiston, D. C., Jr. [ed]: Atlas of Cardiothoracic Surgery. Philadelphia, W. B. Saunders, 1995.)

for protection of these structures. With a grasper, the anterior mediastinal tumor is drawn posteriorly and dissected with endoscopic scissors. This dissection is best accomplished by beginning inferiorly and laterally and extending the dissection medially. All blood vessels and tissues suspected of containing blood vessels should be clipped and coagulated and especially the branches of the innominate vein. After removal of the mass, careful hemostasis is achieved and a chest tube is inserted through the lowest port site and connected to underwater sealed drainage.

## THORACOSCOPIC APPROACH FOR THE MODIFIED HELLER ESOPHAGOMYOTOMY FOR ACHALASIA

In most situations, the standard modified Heller esophagomyotomy remains the most effective treatment for patients with achalasia despite the fact that balloon dilatation can be performed. Experience is now being gained with a thoracoscopic approach to the myotomy. The patient is positioned as for a left posterolateral thoracotomy in the event that an open procedure becomes necessary. Anesthesia is induced using single-lung ventilation with the patient in the

right lateral decubitus position. Intraoperative monitoring is routinely used.

It is preferable to have an endoscopist present as part of the team, and a flexible gastroscope should be passed transorally either before or after the patient is placed in the operating position. The thoracoscope is inserted through an incision in the sixth intercostal space in the midscapular line with inspection of the hemithorax (Fig. 59–14). A 10-mm trocar is passed through an incision in the fifth intercostal space in the anterior axillary line and a lung retractor is passed through the trocar as the left lung is retracted superiorly for exposure of the esophageal hiatus. A third trocar is passed through the seventh intercostal space in the anterior axillary line, and this port is used for the placement of suction catheters, grasping instruments, and dissectors. A fourth incision in the seventh intercostal space in the posterior scapular line is used for insertion of scissors and graspers.

An illustration of a cross-section of a chest as viewed from below illustrating these anatomic sites is depicted in Figure 59–15. After the lung is retracted the mediastinal pleura over the lower esophagus is identified and dissected free (Fig. 59–16). The endoscopist then advances the gastroscope, which can be identified by light and improves the visualization of the esophagus. At other times during the dissection,

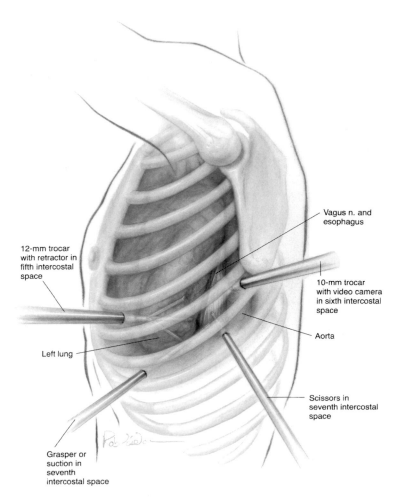

**FIGURE 59–14.** Trocars are inserted into the fifth, sixth, and seventh intercostal spaces to accommodate the thoracoscope, retractor, and catheters, graspers, scissors, and dissectors for the esophageal myotomy. (From Douglas, J. M., Jr.: Modified Heller esophagomyotomy for achalasia. *In* Sabiston, D. C., Jr. [ed]: Atlas of Cardiothoracic Surgery. Philadelphia, W. B. Saunders, 1995.)

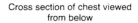

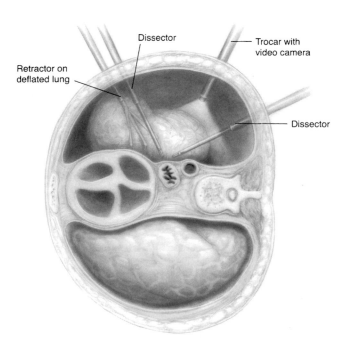

**FIGURE 59–15.** A cross-section of the chest shows the collapsed lung and placement of instruments. (From Douglas, J. M., Jr.: Modified Heller esophagomyotomy for achalasia. *In* Sabiston, D. C., Jr. [ed]: Atlas of Cardiothoracic Surgery. Philadelphia, W. B. Saunders, 1995.)

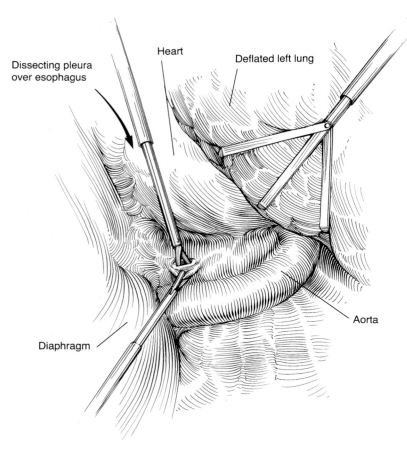

Dissecting pleura over esophagus

Heart

Deflated left lung

Diaphragm

Aorta

**FIGURE 59–16.** The collapsed lung is retracted and the mediastinal pleura is dissected. (From Douglas, J. M., Jr.: Modified Heller esophagomyotomy for achalasia. *In* Sabiston, D. C., Jr. [ed]: Atlas of Cardiothoracic Surgery. Philadelphia, W. B. Saunders, 1995.)

the gastroscope need not be lighted to prevent potential burn of the esophageal mucosa through excessive light use. Attention is then directed toward the lower esophagus, which is dissected laterally and medially from the aorta and pericardium, and the gastroscope

remains in place just distal to the esophagogastric junction. This serves as a stent and aids in the dissection (Figs. 59–17 and 59–18).

With a right-angled instrument, an umbilical tape is passed around the lower esophagus for retraction

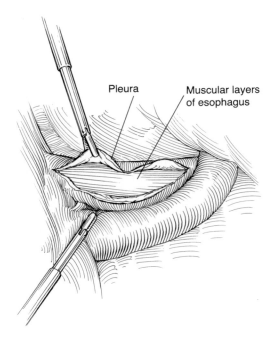

Pleura

Muscular layers of esophagus

**FIGURE 59–17.** Dissection of the pleura reveals the muscular layers of the esophagus. (From Douglas, J. M., Jr.: Modified Heller esophagomyotomy for achalasia. *In* Sabiston, D. C., Jr. [ed]: Atlas of Cardiothoracic Surgery. Philadelphia, W. B. Saunders, 1995.)

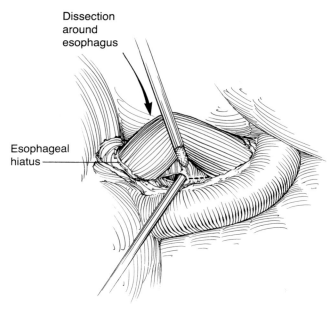

**FIGURE 59–18.** The lower esophagus is dissected laterally and medially away from the aorta and pericardium. (From Douglas, J. M., Jr.: Modified Heller esophagomyotomy for achalasia. *In* Sabiston, D. C., Jr. [ed]: Atlas of Cardiothoracic Surgery. Philadelphia, W. B. Saunders, 1995.)

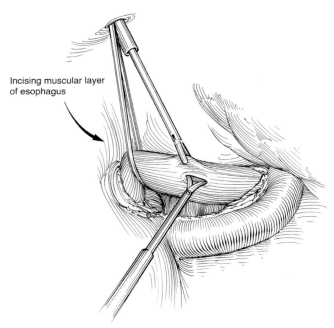

**FIGURE 59–20.** The initial esophagomyotomy is made 3 cm above the esophageal hiatus. (From Douglas, J. M., Jr.: Modified Heller esophagomyotomy for achalasia. *In* Sabiston, D. C., Jr. [ed]: Atlas of Cardiothoracic Surgery. Philadelphia, W. B. Saunders, 1995.)

(Fig. 59–19). With the scissors, the initial esophagomyotomy is made in a longitudinal manner from 3 cm above the diaphragmatic hiatus (Fig. 59–20). The esophagomyotomy is extended, under close visualiza-

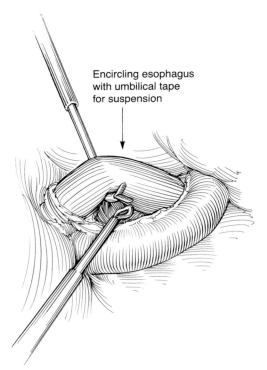

**FIGURE 59–19.** An umbilical tape is passed around the lower esophagus for retraction. (From Douglas, J. M., Jr.: Modified Heller esophagomyotomy for achalasia. *In* Sabiston, D. C., Jr. [ed]: Atlas of Cardiothoracic Surgery. Philadelphia, W. B. Saunders, 1995.)

tion, through the longitudinal and circular muscle until the underlying esophageal mucosa is exposed (Figs. 59–21 and 59–22). The electrocautery should be avoided during this dissection to avoid injury to the esophageal mucosa. Bleeding in this area is usually minimal and can be controlled by intermittent irrigation and passage of time, leaving only the most troublesome of bleeders to be controlled by coagulation and then quite precisely. With careful visualization of the esophagogastric junction, the esophagomyotomy is continued in a caudal direction. It is usually necessary to switch the lung retractor to a lower port to provide downward retraction on the diaphragm and permit improved visualization of the esophagogastric junction (Fig. 59–23). It may be difficult to distinguish the circular muscle and veins that typically identify the area of the lower esophageal sphincter, and the gastroscope is an extremely useful instrument in assessment because, once the lower esophageal sphincter is divided, the endoscopist can readily identify frank relaxation of the constriction at the lower esophageal sphincter.

Following division of the sphincter, the esophagomyotomy is continued in a cephalad direction (Fig. 59–24). Ballooning of the esophageal mucosa can be achieved by insufflation of the esophagus and aids in dissection of the muscular layers from the underlying mucosa. The esophagomyotomy should be continued superiorly to the level of the inferior pulmonary vein. If the decision is made to insert a nasogastric tube, this should be performed under direct visualization by the thoracoscope to avoid injury because the esophageal mucosa is very thin and perforation can occur if the tube is passed blindly. At the end of the

Incision in muscular layer with protection
of submucosa by flexible blunt grasper

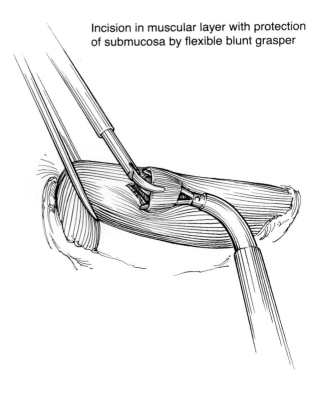

**FIGURE 59–21.** The esophagomyotomy is extended through the longitudinal and circular muscle until the underlying esophageal mucosa is exposed. (From Douglas, J. M., Jr.: Modified Heller esophagomyotomy for achalasia. *In* Sabiston, D. C., Jr. [ed]: Atlas of Cardiothoracic Surgery. Philadelphia, W. B. Saunders, 1995.)

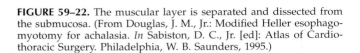

Separation and blunt dissection of
muscular layer from submucosa

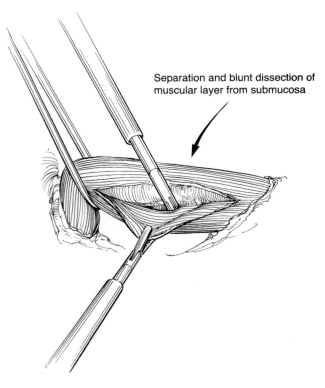

**FIGURE 59–22.** The muscular layer is separated and dissected from the submucosa. (From Douglas, J. M., Jr.: Modified Heller esophagomyotomy for achalasia. *In* Sabiston, D. C., Jr. [ed]: Atlas of Cardiothoracic Surgery. Philadelphia, W. B. Saunders, 1995.)

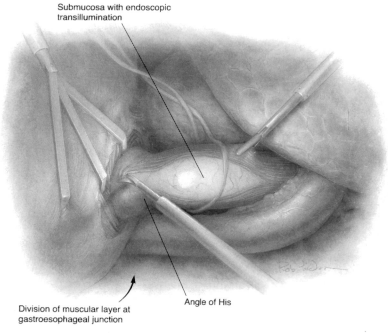

Submucosa with endoscopic
transillumination

Division of muscular layer at
gastroesophageal junction

Angle of His

**FIGURE 59–23.** The esophagomyotomy is continued caudad. The endoscope facilitates visualization of the esophagogastric junction. (From Douglas, J. M., Jr.: Modified Heller esophagomyotomy for achalasia. *In* Sabiston, D. C., Jr. [ed]: Atlas of Cardiothoracic Surgery. Philadelphia, W. B. Saunders, 1995.)

**FIGURE 59–24.** The esophagomyotomy is continued cephalad and completed. (From Douglas, J. M., Jr.: Modified Heller esophagomy-otomy for achalasia. *In* Sabiston, D. C., Jr. [ed]: Atlas of Cardiothoracic Surgery. Philadelphia, W. B. Saunders, 1995.)

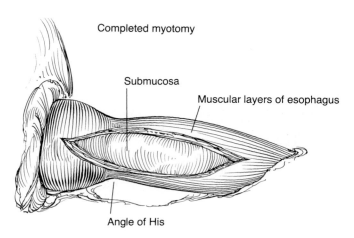

Completed myotomy

Submucosa

Muscular layers of esophagus

Angle of His

procedure, a chest tube is inserted through one of the lower thoracoscopic ports and attached to underwater sealed drainage. The incisions are then closed.

## THORACOSCOPIC APPROACH FOR THORACIC SYMPATHECTOMY

Hyperhidrosis palmaris can be managed by upper thoracic sympathectomy and can be confined to the T2 sympathetic ganglion. Other indications for this procedure include Raynaud's disease, shoulder-hand syndrome, vascular occlusive disease, causalgia, and some types of visceral pain. In each of these, the extent of the sympathectomy should be modified according to the clinical problem.

For the thoracoscopic approach, general anesthesia is recommended and induced through a double-lumen endobronchial tube. The pulse oximeter should be attached for continuous monitoring of peripheral $O_2$ saturation and the skin temperature should be recorded in the arm to reflect peripheral increases in blood flow following the sympathectomy. In quite good-risk patients, a standard endotracheal tube can be employed with temporary collapse of both lungs, with the patient in the apneic condition and rapid performance of the sympathectomy within 3 to 5 minutes. While the patient is apneic, special attention should be directed to the peripheral $O_2$ saturation. If it falls below 90%, the procedure should be temporarily suspended and the lung ventilated with 100% oxygen.

The patient is placed in the supine position and a pad is placed in the interscapular region to hyperextend the upper thoracic spine (Fig. 59–25). Both upper limbs are abducted 90 degrees, and the surface temperature recorder is attached to the tip of the middle finger on the operated side. A 1-cm incision is made on the operated side along the axillary skin fold lateral to the margin of the pectoralis muscle. The anesthesiologist should then collapse the lung on the operated side. With the operated side endobronchial tube open to the atmosphere, the lung usually collapses in several minutes. This can be made more rapid if suction is applied to the endobronchial tube. A Kelly clamp is inserted to dissect the intercostal muscles of the third intercostal space and the pleural cavity is entered with digital exploration before the trocar is inserted. When it is clear that there are no significant intrapleural adhesions at the stab site, a 10-mm trocar is introduced in the pleural cavity and a 10-mm rigid thoracoscope with a 5-mm operating channel is inserted. Following an initial view of the superior cavity and mediastinal structures, the sympathetic chain is

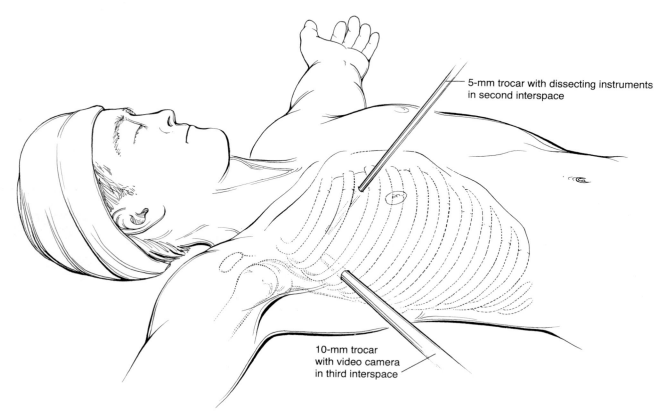

5-mm trocar with dissecting instruments in second interspace

10-mm trocar with video camera in third interspace

**FIGURE 59–25.** The patient is placed in the supine position with trocars placed in the second and third intercostal spaces. (From Hsu, C.-P., and Douglas, J. M., Jr.: Thoracoscopic sympathectomy. *In* Sabiston, D. C., Jr. [ed]: Atlas of Cardiothoracic Surgery. Philadelphia, W. B. Saunders, 1995.)

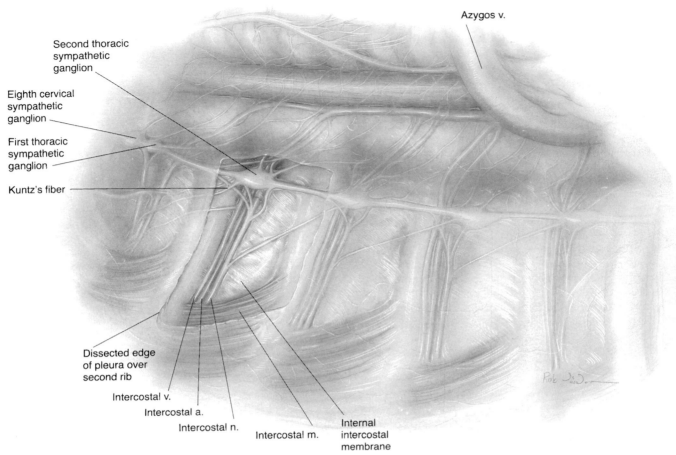

Azygos v.

Second thoracic
sympathetic
ganglion

Eighth cervical
sympathetic
ganglion

First thoracic
sympathetic
ganglion

Kuntz's fiber

Dissected edge
of pleura over
second rib

Intercostal v.

Intercostal a.

Intercostal n.

Intercostal m.

Internal
intercostal
membrane

**FIGURE 59–26.** The pleura is opened over the sympathetic chain to reveal the sympathetic ganglia, Kuntz fiber, vessels, and nerves. (From Hsu, C.-P., and Douglas, J. M., Jr.: Thoracoscopic sympathectomy. *In* Sabiston, D. C., Jr. [ed]: Atlas of Cardiothoracic Surgery. Philadelphia, W. B. Saunders, 1995.)

identified, which lies lateral to the articulation between the ribs and the tranverse processes of the thoracic vertebrae. It is quite important to identify the second rib accurately. This can best be done by visualization of the internal intercostal muscles from the first rib above and terminating at the upper margin of the second rib.

The pleura is then opened overlying the sympathetic chain with the electrocautery, and a segment of the chain between the second and the third ribs including the second thoracic sympathetic ganglion is dissected and freed with the electrocautery (Fig. 59–26). It is preferable to send the ganglion for frozen section for pathologic confirmation as well as to observe the effect on the skin temperature as registered by the recorder on the finger. Usually, the temperature will rise to a plateau within 5 minutes. If necessary, a 5-mm incision can be made at the midclavicular line of the second intercostal space, and the sympathetic chain resected with endoscopic scissors. Finally, a segment about 5 cm in length of the pleura overlying the second and third rib is unroofed for transection of possible existing Kuntz's fibers. At the completion of the procedure, a catheter is passed into the pleural

space through a stab wound previously made for passage of the scope and the anesthesiologist initiates inflation of the lung as the operator moves to the opposite side for the other sympathectomy. The procedure for removal of the left sympathetic ganglion is similar to that on the right except that the dome of the left pleural cavity is lower, and the pleural fat is more prominent. At the end of the procedure, the incisions are closed.

## THORACOSCOPIC APPROACH TO SPLANCHNICECTOMY

Splanchnicectomy has been shown to be effective for control of intractable pain in some patients with pancreatitis, pancreatic cancer, and related conditions. However, use of this procedure has been limited owing to the previous necessity of an abdominal approach to perform the procedure. With the advent of thoracoscopic surgery, this trend is now being reevaluated.

For performance of thoracoscopic splanchnicectomy, general anesthesia with single-lung ventilation is preferable, with the patient in the right lateral decubitus position (Fig. 59–27). The skin incision is made in the sixth intercostal space in the posterior axillary line with collapse of the left lung. The chest is entered and digital palpation is used to confirm a free pleural space. A 10-mm trocar is passed through the entry site, and the laparoscope is inserted and the hemithorax explored. A second trocar is passed through an incision in the anterior axillary line in the seventh intercostal space and a fan retractor is inserted through a 10-mm port. Through two additional ports located in the seventh and eighth intercostal spaces in the posterior scapular line, graspers and scissors are then passed.

The parietal pleura lateral to the aorta is divided and hemostasis is achieved (Fig. 59–28). In its position in the costovertebral angle, the sympathetic chain is identified and the greater splanchnic nerve is observed coursing medially and caudally between the aorta and the sympathetic chain. These nerves should be clipped and divided distally just above the aortic hiatus (Fig. 59–29). The least splanchnic nerve should be identified and divided and the nerve sections are sent for pathologic confirmation. A No. 24 French chest tube is placed and the lung is reexpanded. The incisions are then closed.

## THORACOSCOPIC APPROACH FOR TRUNCAL VAGOTOMY

The thoracoscopic approach to truncal vagotomy can be performed with the patient in the right lateral decubitus position. The procedure can be facilitated by the passage of a No. 36 French esophageal bougie, which aids the dissection of the esophagus from the surrounding tissues (Fig. 59–30). The initial incision is placed in the eighth intercostal space in the posterior axillary line for passage of the laparoscope. A 10-mm trocar is passed to allow standard placement of the scope. With the lung collapsed, examination of the hemithorax is performed and subsequent trocars are inserted in the fourth and eighth intercostal spaces in the anterior axillary line for insertion of retractors.

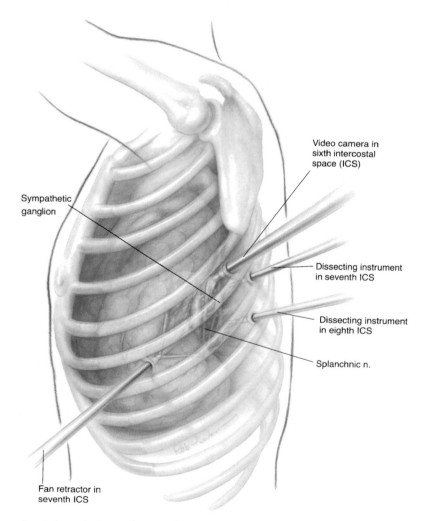

Sympathetic ganglion

Video camera in sixth intercostal space (ICS)

Dissecting instrument in seventh ICS

Dissecting instrument in eighth ICS

Splanchnic n.

Fan retractor in seventh ICS

**FIGURE 59–27.** Trocars are placed through the sixth, seventh, and eighth intercostal spaces for the splanchnicectomy. (From Douglas, J. M., Jr.: Thoracoscopic splanchnicectomy. *In* Sabiston, D. C., Jr. [ed]: Atlas of Cardiothoracic Surgery. Philadelphia, W. B. Saunders, 1995.)

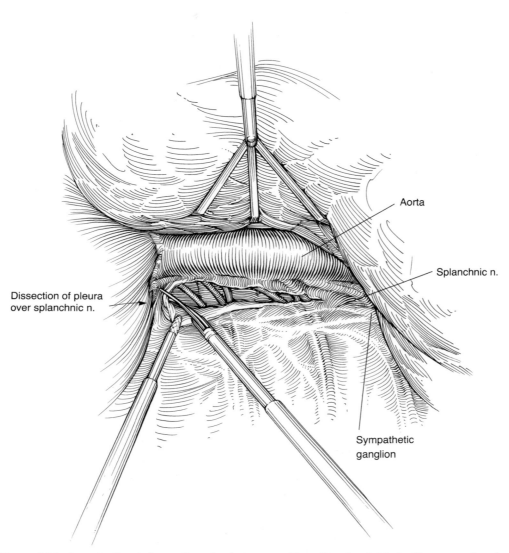

Aorta

Splanchnic n.

Dissection of pleura
over splanchnic n.

Sympathetic
ganglion

**FIGURE 59–28.** The parietal pleura is dissected over the splanchnic nerve. (From Douglas, J. M., Jr.: Thoracoscopic splanchnicectomy. *In* Sabiston, D. C., Jr. [ed]: Atlas of Cardiothoracic Surgery. Philadelphia, W. B. Saunders, 1995.)

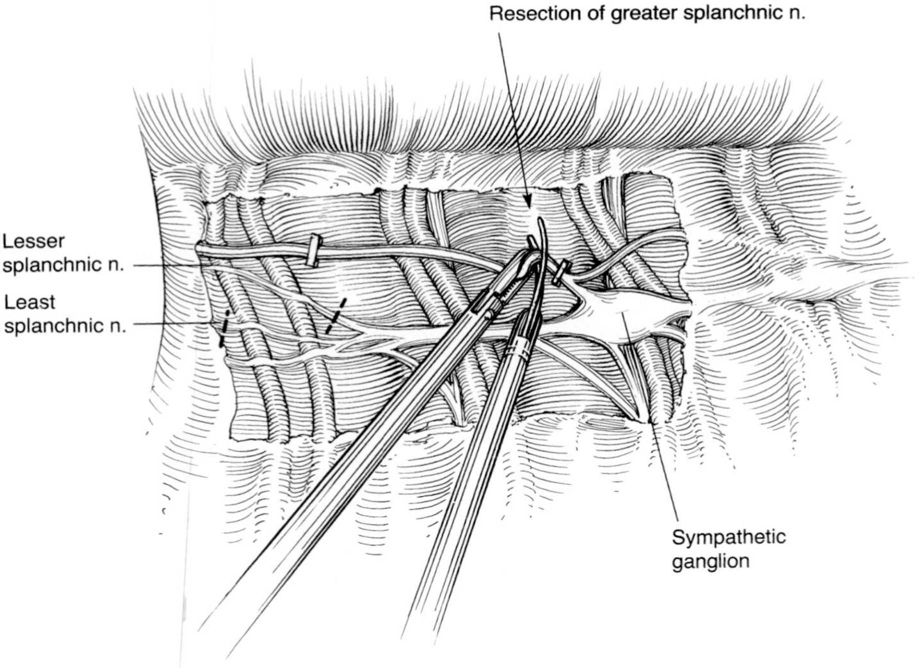

Resection of greater splanchnic n.

Lesser splanchnic n.

Least splanchnic n.

Sympathetic ganglion

**FIGURE 59–29.** The greater splanchnic nerve is dissected. *Dashed lines* indicate the location of dissection of the lesser and least splanchnic nerves. (From Douglas, J. M., Jr.: Thoracoscopic splanchnicectomy. *In* Sabiston, D. C., Jr. [ed]: Atlas of Cardiothoracic Surgery. Philadelphia, W. B. Saunders, 1995.)

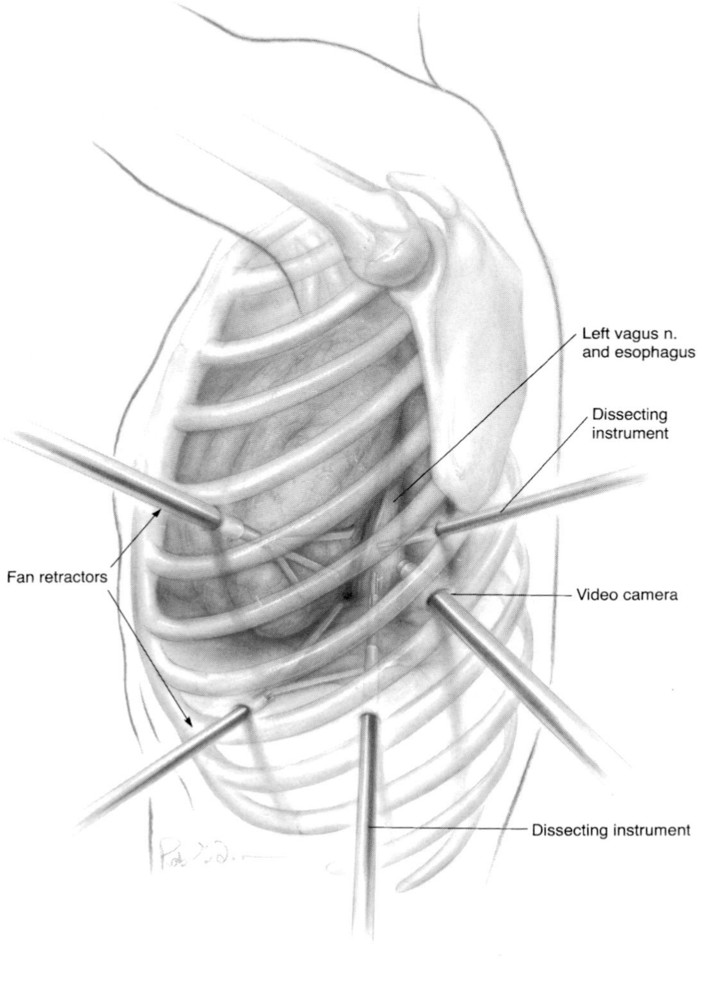

**FIGURE 59–30.** Trocars are placed for insertion of dissectors, retractors, and camera for truncal vagotomy. (From Douglas, J. M., Jr.: Thoracoscopic truncal vagotomy. *In* Sabiston, D. C., Jr. [ed]: Atlas of Cardiothoracic Surgery. Philadelphia, W. B. Saunders, 1995.)

Left vagus n. and esophagus

Dissecting instrument

Fan retractors

Video camera

Dissecting instrument

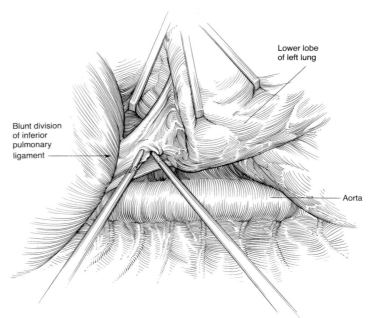

**FIGURE 59–31.** The collapsed lung is retracted and the inferior pulmonary ligament is divided. (From Douglas, J. M., Jr.: Thoracoscopic truncal vagotomy. *In* Sabiston, D. C., Jr. [ed]: Atlas of Cardiothoracic Surgery. Philadelphia, W. B. Saunders, 1995.)

The instruments for dissection are passed through the sixth intercostal space in the midscapular line and the ninth intercostal space in the midaxillary line.

The inferior pulmonary ligament is divided while the lung is retracted medially (Fig. 59–31). It is easy to identify the anterior vagus nerve as it courses along the surface of the esophagus, and it is doubly clipped and a segment removed for pathologic confirmation (Fig. 59–32). The surrounding tissue of the esophagus is then dissected bluntly to localize the posterior vagus nerve (Fig. 59–33). The intraesophageal bougie allows easier manipulation of the esophagus. The posterior vagus nerve will be found within the surrounding tissues immediately adjacent to the esophagus. For this dissection, a cotton-tipped dissector is an appropriate instrument.

When the posterior vagus nerve has been identified, it should be doubly clipped and a segment excised for pathologic evaluation (Fig. 59–34). After hemostasis is assured, a chest tube is passed into the pleural cavity and the lung is inflated. The incisions are then closed.

## THORACOSCOPIC APPROACH FOR LOBECTOMY FOR LUNG CANCER

To perform thoracoscopic lobectomy, a left-sided double-lumen endobronchial tube should be passed and the patient is placed in the right lateral decubitus position (jack-knife). A pad is placed beneath the dependent axilla to serve as prophylaxis for neurovas-

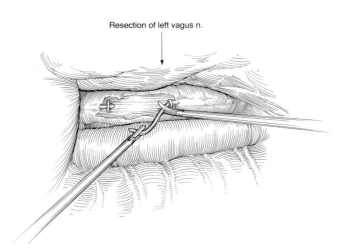

**FIGURE 59–32.** The anterior vagus nerve is resected. (From Douglas, J. M., Jr.: Thoracoscopic truncal vagotomy. *In* Sabiston, D. C., Jr. [ed]: Atlas of Cardiothoracic Surgery. Philadelphia, W. B. Saunders, 1995.)

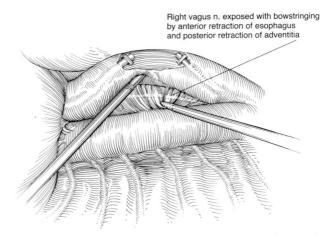

**FIGURE 59–33.** The posterior vagus nerve is identified as the surrounding tissues are retracted. (From Douglas, J. M., Jr.: Thoracoscopic truncal vagotomy. *In* Sabiston, D. C., Jr. [ed]: Atlas of Cardiothoracic Surgery. Philadelphia, W. B. Saunders, 1995.)

Right vagus n. clipped and
resected with scissors

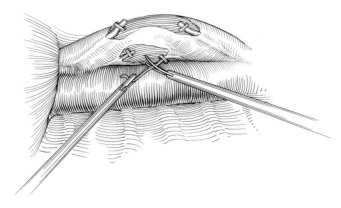

**FIGURE 59–34.** The posterior vagus nerve is clipped and resected. (From Douglas, J. M., Jr.: Thoracoscopic truncal vagotomy. *In* Sabiston, D. C., Jr. [ed]: Atlas of Cardiothoracic Surgery. Philadelphia, W. B. Saunders, 1995.)

cular injury. The patient is prepared and draped such that a standard thoracotomy can be performed should this be necessary. A thoracoscope is inserted through an incision made in the eighth intercostal space in the anterior midaxillary line. Initial thoracoscopic exploration of the pleural cavity is performed, and if there is no evidence of intrapleural spread or $N_2$ lymph node involvement can be identified, an oblique 8- to 10-cm access minithoracotomy just above the major interlobar fissure is performed under direct thoracoscopic guidance (Fig. 59–35). Usually, this incision is made at the fifth intercostal space between the anterior and the posterior axillary lines. A second port is made at the seventh to eighth intercostal space between the anterior and the posterior axillary line to introduce a fan retractor or other instruments. If the

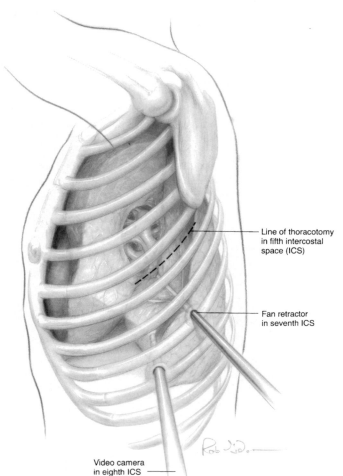

Line of thoracotomy
in fifth intercostal
space (ICS)

Fan retractor
in seventh ICS

Video camera
in eighth ICS

**FIGURE 59–35.** Trocars are placed to facilitate the camera and retractor. The *dashed line* shows the line of thoracotomy. (From Hsu, C.-P., and Douglas, J. M., Jr.: Thoracoscopic pulmonary lobectomy. *In* Sabiston, D. C., Jr. [ed]: Atlas of Cardiothoracic Surgery. Philadelphia, W. B. Saunders, 1995.)

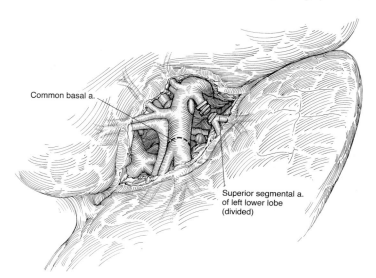

**FIGURE 59–36.** The *dashed line* shows the line of division of the common basal artery. (From Hsu, C.-P., and Douglas, J. M., Jr.: Thoracoscopic pulmonary lobectomy. *In* Sabiston, D. C., Jr. [ed]: Atlas of Cardiothoracic Surgery. Philadelphia, W. B. Saunders, 1995.)

fissure is not complete, the interlobar fusion is opened and the dissection should be performed through the access thoracotomy with long thoracic instruments. Generally, the interlobar pulmonary artery and its branches are identified posterior to the center of the major fissure. After identification of the interlobar pulmonary artery and exclusion of direct tumor inva-

sion or lymph node adhesion, the perivascular space is accessed and the superior segmental artery above the lingular artery is divided with endoscopic clips.

The common basal artery is divided by an endoscopic stapler (Fig. 59–36). The patient is placed in the Trendelenburg position and rotated toward the ventral side. With upward traction of the left lower

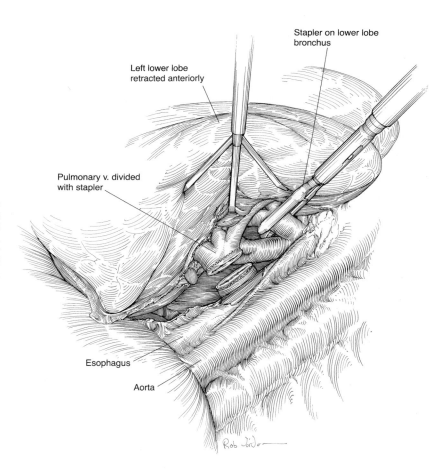

**FIGURE 59–37.** With the left lobe retracted anteriorly, the stapler is inserted through the access thoracotomy to divide the pulmonary vein and then the lower lobe bronchus. (From Hsu, C.-P., and Douglas, J. M., Jr.: Thoracoscopic pulmonary lobectomy. *In* Sabiston, D. C., Jr. [ed]: Atlas of Cardiothoracic Surgery. Philadelphia, W. B. Saunders, 1995.)

lobe, the inferior pulmonary ligament is divided through the second access port and the inferior pulmonary vein is completely freed and stapled. After the pulmonary vessels have been divided, the residual incomplete lobar fissures can be separated, and the mediastinal pleura overlying the lobar bronchus is opened with anterior traction on the lung.

The lung is retracted anteriorly to expose the main and lobar bronchi (Fig. 59–37). With an endoscopic stapler through the access thoracotomy, it is applied to the common basal bronchus proximal to the orifice of the superior segmental bronchus in preparation for transection of the left lower lobe bronchus. The left lower lobe bronchus is carefully dissected and secured with an endoscopic stapler. If the superior seg-

mental bronchus is close to the upper lobe bronchus, it should be transected to prevent compromise of the lumen of the left upper lobe bronchus. The mediastinal nodes are dissected through the minithoracotomy for complete tumor staging. The bronchial stump is then checked with immersion under saline solution to be certain that it is tightly closed. After achieving full hemostasis, a catheter is left in the chest for drainage and the incisions are closed.

## BIBLIOGRAPHY

Cova, F.: Atlas Thoracoscopicon. Milan, Sperling and Kupfer, 1928.
Jacobaeus, H. C.: Endopleural operations by means of a thoracoscope. Beitr. Klin. Tuberk., 35:1, 1915.

# Index

Note: Page numbers in *italics* refer to illustrations; page numbers followed by t refer to tables.

Aortic valve *(Continued)*
  incompetence of, in ventricular septal defect, 1451
  normal orifice area of, 1137
  physiology of, 1733, *1733*
  prosthesis for, 1746–1752, *1746–1752,* 1751t
    assessment of, 1146
  reconstruction of, 1755
    in prosthetic valve endocarditis, 1710, *1711*
  reimplantation of, in aneurysm repair, 1334, *1336,* 1337
  replacement of, antibiotic prophylaxis after, 1757, 1757t
    aortic dissection after, 1345
    cardioplegia in, 1744
    cardiopulmonary bypass in, 1744
    complications of, 1757–1758
    ejection fraction in, 1239
    in abnormally small aortic root, 1753–1754, *1753–1754*
    in aortic aneurysm and insufficiency, 1755
    in aortic dissection and insufficiency, 1755
    in aortic insufficiency, 1740–1741
    in aortic stenosis, 1526–1528, *1526–1531*
    in coronary bypass graft, 1752–1753
    in endocarditis, 1754–1755
    in mitral valve disease, 1755
    in prosthetic valve endocarditis, 1707
    postoperative care in, 1756–1757, 1757t
    repeated, 1754
    results of, 1757–1758
    technique for, 1744–1746, *1745*
    thromboembolism in, 1721–1722
  tricuspid, 1522, *1523*
Aortic valve conduit, thrombosis of, 1725
Aortic valve gradient, calculation of, 1137, *1137*
Aorticopulmonary trunk, common. See *Truncus arteriosus.*
Aorticopulmonary window, 1298–1300, *1299*
  thoracoscopic, 2155–2156, *2157*
Aorticosympathetic paraganglioma, mediastinal, 592–593
Aortitis, aortic regurgitation in, 1737–1738
Aortography, in aortic dissection, *1346,* 1347, *1348*
  in aortic injury, 469–470, *469–470*
  in coronary artery-pulmonary artery connection, 1837, *1837*
  in thoracic aortic aneurysm, 1328–1329, *1330*
Aortopexy, in aortic arch anomalies, 1305, *1305*
Aortoplasty, in thoracic aortic aneurysm, 1337
  subclavian flap, in aortic coarctation, 1288, *1290,* 1294
Aortopulmonary shunt, in tetralogy of Fallot, *1473,* 1476–1477
Aortopulmonary window, 1298–1300, *1299*
  thoracoscopic, 2155–2156, *2157*
Aortoventriculoplasty, in aortic stenosis, 1527, *1528,* 1532, 1534, *1537*
APACHE (Acute Physiology and Chronic Health Evaluation), in shock, 173, 176, *177–178*
Apnea, diaphragmatic pacing in, 1089
  in infants, 446
  intermittent mandatory ventilation in, 60
  mask ventilation in, 290–291
  PEEP in, 60
  sleep, postoperative mechanical ventilation in, 318
Apolipoproteins, 2019, 2020t
Apoplexy, pulmonary, 773, *774*
Aprotinin, 142
  in cardiac surgery, 258
  in cardiopulmonary bypass, 1719, 1723
  in repeated coronary artery bypass, 1936
APUD cells, carcinoid tumor origin in, 604
Arachidonic acid cascade, in cardiopulmonary bypass, 1264–1265, *1265*
Arachidonic acid metabolites. See also *Prostaglandins; Thromboxanes.*

Arachidonic acid metabolites *(Continued)*
  in coronary artery spasm, 1981, *1981*
  in septic shock, 195–196, *196*
Arcuate ligament, median, in Hill repair, 1044, *1045*
Arrhythmia, cardiac. See *Cardiac arrhythmias.*
Arterial oxygen content, 36–37, *37*
  normal range of, 180t
Arterial pressure, mean, calculation of, 1131
Arterial pump, in cardiopulmonary bypass, 1257
Arterial switch operation. See also under *Transposition of great arteries.*
  in univentricular heart, 1621
Arteriovenous fistula, pulmonary, 661, 911–918
  angiography in, 912–913, *913*
  asymptomatic, 912
  bilateral, 911, *913*
  clinical manifestations of, 912
  congenital, 869–871, *869–871*
  embryology of, 911
  etiology of, 911
  hemothorax in, 534–535
  historical aspects of, 911
  internal mammary artery in, 914–915, *915–917*
  large solitary, 914–915
  multiple, 911, 913–915
    surgery in, 914
  pathology of, 911–912
  physiology of, 912
  treatment of, 913–917, *916*
Arteriovenous oxygen difference (A-VO₂), in shock, 179–181
  normal range of, 180t
Arteriovenous ultrafiltration, after cardiac surgery, 265
Arteritis, Takayasu's, 1358, *1359,* 1360–1361
Arthritic disease, aortic regurgitation in, 1738
Artificial heart, 2135–2148
  electrically powered, 2143–2147
  historical aspects of, 2135
  pneumatic, 2135–2143
    animal studies with, 2129–2139
    as permanent replacement, 2143
    bacteremia in, 2138
    before transplantation, 2107
    calcification in, 2138
    components of, 2135–2138, *2136–2137*
    implantation technique for, 2139–2142, *2140–2142*
    indications for, 2139
    postoperative care in, 2141–2142
    results of, 2142–2143, 2143t
    temporary use of, 2135, 2139, 2142, 2143t
    Utah skin buttons in, 2138
  size requirements for, 2139
  thromboembolism of, 1725–1726
Artificial intelligence, in decision making, 393
Asbestos exposure, mesothelioma and, 567
Asbestosis, 710
Ascites, pleural effusion in, 544
Aseptic technique, bacterial contamination during, 98–99
Aspergilloma, *695,* 695–696
Aspergillosis, 695–698
  bronchopulmonary, bronchoscopy in, 80
  fungus ball in, *696–697,* 696–698, 698t
  in chemotherapy, 747
*Aspergillus, 695,* 695–696
Asphyxiating thoracic infantile thoracic-pelvic-phalangeal dystrophy, 511
Asphyxiation, in tracheostomy, 344
Aspiration (needle biopsy), in bronchogenic carcinoma, 79, *79*
Aspiration (pericardial fluid). See *Pericardiocentesis.*
Aspiration (respiratory tract), in achalasia, 977
  in dysphagia, 962, *964–965*
  in gastroesophageal reflux, 1020–1021

Basilic vein, as coronary artery bypass graft, 1896
Baylor College of Medicine artificial heart, *2146, 2147*
Beall's prosthetic valve, assessment of, 1146
Beardmore anastomosis, of esophagus, *889,* 890
Beck's triad, in cardiac tamponade, 483
Beclomethasone, perioperative, 17–18
Belcher's complex aspergillosis, 696
Belscope laryngoscope, *331*
Belsey Mark IV antireflux repair. See *Mark IV antireflux repair.*
Bentall procedure, in thoracic aortic aneurysm, 1332–1334, *1334–1335*
Benzocaine, in tracheal intubation, 302
Benzodiazepines, cardiovascular effects of, 122
  in postoperative psychosis, 266
  pharmacokinetics of, 122
  reversal of, 148
    mechanical ventilation and, 316
Berylliosis, 710
Beta-adrenergic agonists, perioperative, 17, 142–144, *143,* 144t
Beta-adrenergic antagonists, 144–145, 146t
  in coronary artery spasm, 1982
  in hypertrophic cardiomyopathy, 1743
Beta-adrenergic blockers, 142–143, 143t
Beta-adrenergic receptors, 142–143, 143t
Beta-endorphin, in septic shock, 197
Beta-lactam antibiotics, bleeding disorders from, 106
  in coagulase-negative staphylococcal infection, 107–108
Bethanechol, esophageal response to, in achalasia, *979,* 979–980
Bezold-Jarisch reflex, pacing in, 1773–1774
Bicarbonate, carbon dioxide transport and, 10
Bicarbonate buffer system, 12
Bifascicular block, pacing in, 1770–1771
Bile acid-sequestering agents, in lipid lowering, 2027–2028
Bile diversion procedures, in peptic stricture, 999
Bileaflet prosthetic valve, 1146
Biliary disease, after cardiac surgery, 270
Biological sealants, for Dacron aortic graft, 1273
Biopsy, bronchoscopy in, 71, *72, 75–79*
  fine-needle, of mediastinum, 587
  of chest wall, 516–517, *517*
  of esophagus, 959, 959t
    in hiatal hernia, 1021
  of heart, in transplantation rejection, 2112, 2113t
  of lung, after transplantation, 2129
    anterolateral thoracotomy incision in, 215
    in carcinoma, 638
    in diffuse interstitial disease, 706
    in metastasis, 669
    open, 711, *711*
    percutaneous, 711
    pneumothorax in, 534
    technique of, 710–711, *711*
    thoracoscopic, for diffuse lung disease, 2151–2152, *2152*
      with aorticopulmonary window, 2155–2156, *2157*
    transbronchial, 711
  of mediastinum, 587–588
    in lymphoma, 600
    in superior vena cava syndrome, 581–582
    thoracoscopic, 2159–2160, *2160*
  of myocardium, echocardiography in, 1242
    in catheterization, 1147
  of pericardium, 1380
    subxiphoid approach in, 226
  of pleura, 544, 563
    in mesothelioma, 569
    in tuberculosis, 564
  of right ventricle, 1127
  of trachea, 422

Bipolar electrogram, atrial/ventricular, in arrhythmia diagnosis, 247, *247*
Bivona tracheostomy tube, *337*
Bjork disk valve prosthesis. See under *Prosthetic valves.*
Bjork osteoplastic flap thoracoplasty, 555, *556*
Blades, for laryngoscopy, 299–300, *299–300,* 331, *331*
  malposition of, 301, *301–302*
Blalock classification of shock, 175–176
Blalock-Hanlon atrial septectomy, in great artery transposition, 1566–1568
Blalock-Park anastomosis, in aortic arch interruption, 1297
  in aortic coarctation, 1291
Blalock-Taussig procedure, in great artery transposition, 1569
  in tetralogy of Fallot, *1473–1475, 1474–1475*
  in tricuspid atresia, 1633–1634
  modified, in pulmonary atresia with intact ventricular septum, 1497–1499, *1499*
    in tetralogy of Fallot, *1473,* 1475–1476, *1476*
    in tricuspid atresia, 1635
Bland-White-Garland syndrome, 1836
Blastoma, pulmonary, 662
*Blastomyces dermatitidis,* 692–693, *693*
Blastomycosis, 692–693, *693*
  geographic distribution of, 687, *687*
  South American (paracoccidioidomycosis), 699–700, *700*
Blebs, of lung, resection of, 532, *533*
  rupture of, 528–529, *529*
  thoracoscopic resection of, 2154–2155, *2155–2156*
  versus bullous emphysema, 874
Bleeding disorders. See *Coagulation disorders; Hemorrhage.*
Bleomycin, in pleural effusion, 546
Blind nasotracheal intubation, 302
Blood, arterial, oxygen content of, 36–37, *37*
  conservation of, in cardiac surgery, 141–142
    perioperative, 257–258, 258t
  damage of, in cardiopulmonary bypass, 1266t–1267t, 1266–1267, *1266–1267*
  in extracorporeal circulation, 1722
  in cardioplegia, 1824–1825
  in pleural effusion, 543
  loss of, hypovolemic shock in, 182–185, 183t, *184*
  malignancies of, in germ-cell tumors, 598
  reservoirs for, mobilization from, 183
  salvage of, intraoperative, 142
  volume of, versus hemodynamic parameters, *187*
Blood flow, coronary, codominant, *1857, 1858,* 1859
  collaterals in. See *Collateral circulation.*
  crossbridge theory and, 1814, *1815*
  during cardiopulmonary resuscitation, 371, 373, *373*
  insufficient. See *Myocardial infarction; Myocardial ischemia.*
  interruption of. See *Cardioplegia.*
  left dominant (predominant), 1857, *1858*
  maintenance of, in cardiopulmonary bypass, 1822
  myocardial bridging and, 1873
  oxygen delivery rate of, 1814
  pathophysiology of, 1816–1817, *1818–1822,* 1822
  physiology of, 1814, *1815–1817,* 1816
  right dominant, 1857, *1858*
  magnetic resonance imaging appearance of, 1205
  pulmonary, 30–35
    airway geometry and, 34–35, *35*
    alveolar pressure and, *30–31,* 30–33
    alveolar shape and, *35*
    body position and, 31–33, *32–33*
    cardiac dysfunction and, 352–353
    extra-alveolar system in, 34, *34–35*
    gravitational effects on, *30–31,* 30–32
    hypotension and, 32–33, *33*

Carpentier-Edwards annuloplasty ring, 1674
Carpentier-Edwards prosthetic valve. See under
    *Prosthetic valves.*
Caseous lesions, in tuberculosis, 755–756, *756–757*
Castleman's disease, mediastinal, 606, *607*
Catabolism, in septic shock, 194–195
Catamenial pneumothorax, 529–530
Catastrophes, intraoperative, mechanical ventilation
    in, 320
Catecholamines. See also *Dopamine; Epinephrine;*
        *Norepinephrine.*
    action of, 142–143, *143*, 144t
    after anomalous pulmonary vein correction, 1416
    in paraganglioma, 592
    production of, in cardiopulmonary bypass, 1263
    transplanted heart sensitivity to, 133
Catheter(ization) (epidural), for analgesia, 164
Catheter(ization) (intrapleural), for analgesia,
        165–166
Catheter(ization) (pericardial space), 1380
Catheter(ization) (respiratory tract), balloon, in
        bronchoscopy, 83, *84*
    in one-lung ventilation, 135
    in tracheal intubation, 338–339, *339–340*
Catheter(ization) (vascular), balloon. See also *Swan-*
        *Ganz catheter.*
    in cardiogenic shock, 204, 204t
    in pulmonary valve dilatation, 1498
    in patent ductus arteriosus closure, 1280
    infection from, 263
    percutaneous, in pulmonary embolism fragmenta-
        tion, 791
    prosthetic valve endocarditis from, 1705
    thromboembolism of, 1727
Causalgia, dorsal sympathectomy in, 627–629
Caustic substances. See *Corrosive substances.*
Cavernostomy, in aspergillosis, 696
Cavitation, in coccidioidomycosis, *690–691*, 690–692
    in histoplasmosis, 687–688
    in lung abscess, 680, 685
    in paracoccidioidomycosis, 700
Cavopulmonary anastomosis, bidirectional, in
        pulmonary atresia with intact ventricular
        septum, *1610*, 1610–1611
    in tricuspid atresia, 1633–1634, 1638–1639, *1639*
Cc′$_{O2}$ (end-capillary oxygen content), calculation of,
    41
CD4 molecule, HIV tropism for, 733
Cecum, distention of, after cardiac surgery, 269–270
Cefamandole, 112
    bleeding disorders from, 106
    in cardiac surgery, 263
    in mitral valve replacement, 1685
    prophylactic, 101t–102t, 102–103, 104t
Cefazolin, 111–112
    in cardiac surgery, 263
    in mitral valve replacement, 1685
    prophylactic, 102t, 102–103, 104t, 108
    for endocarditis, 1757t
Cefonicid, prophylactic, 102t
Cefoperazone, 113
Ceforanide, prophylactic, 102t
Ceftriaxone, prophylactic, 102t
Cefuroxime, 112
    in cardiac surgery, 263
    prophylactic, 102t, 102–103, 104t
Celestin tube, in esophageal carcinoma, as palliative
        procedure, 930–931, *931*
Cell-mediated immunity, in myasthenia gravis, 1107
Central alveolar hypoventilation, diaphragmatic
        pacing in, 1092–1093
Central nervous system. See also *Brain; Spinal cord.*
    coronary artery spasm and, 1979
Central venous pressure, in cardiac tamponade, 1369
    monitoring of, 232–233
        in shock, 177–179, *178–179*, 186–187

Central venous pressure *(Continued)*
    versus blood volume, *187*
Centrifugal pump, in ventricular assist device, 2004,
    *2004*
Cephalic vein, as coronary artery bypass graft, 1896
    pacemaker electrode insertion in, 1779, *1779–1780*
Cephalosporins, 111–113
    anaphylactic reactions to, 272
    bacterial resistance to, 106
    bleeding disorders from, 106
    first-generation, 111–112
    in coagulase-negative staphylococcal infection,
        105t
    in *Staphylococcus aureus* infection, 108
    pharmacokinetics of, perioperative, 102–103
    prophylactic, 101t–102t, 102–103, 104t, 108
    second-generation, 112
    third-generation, 112–113
Cephalothin, 112
    prophylactic, 101t–102t, 103
    topical use of, 104
Cerebral arteries, implantation of, in aortic
        aneurysm repair, 1337, *1338*
Cerebral blood flow. See under *Brain.*
Cerebral insufficiency, pacing in, 1770, 1774
Cerebrovascular accident. See *Stroke.*
Cervical aortic arch, 1306
Cervical rib syndrome. See *Thoracic outlet syndrome.*
Cervical spine injury, tracheal intubation in, 297
Chagas disease, achalasia in, 976
Chalasia, reflux in, 897
Chalasia chair, for pediatric patients, 1026
Chemical pleurodesis, in pleural effusion, 546
    in pneumothorax, 531
Chemodectoma, of lung, 662
    of mediastinum, 592–593
Chemoreceptors, in hypovolemia, 183, *184*
Chemotherapy, esophagitis from, 747
    for esophageal carcinoma, 927–928
    for germ-cell tumors, 598–599
    for Kaposi's sarcoma, 743, 743t
    for lung carcinoma, metastatic, 672
        non-small-cell, 644–645
        small-cell, 646
    for lymphoma, 600, 603
    for mesothelioma, 570
    for seminoma, 597
    for thymoma, 595–596
    palliative, for lung carcinoma, 645
    pleuropulmonary disease from, 746–747, 747t
    pneumothorax from, 529
Chest. See also *Thoracic* entries.
    compression of, in cardiopulmonary resuscitation,
        371–374, *371–375*
    flail, 461–462, *462*
Chest film. See also specific disorder.
    in cor triatriatum, 1422, *1423*
    in diaphragmatic rupture, 1085–1086, *1086–1087*
    in Ebstein's anomaly, 1650
    in lung carcinoma, 637
    in mediastinal neoplasms, 586
    in mitral valve disease, 1549–1550
    in pericardial disease, 1371
    in pulmonary embolism, 783–784, 804–805, 805t
    in tetralogy of Fallot, 1470, *1470*
    in ventricular septal defect, 1451–1452, *1451–1452*
Chest trauma, 456–493
    blunt, 459–475
        bronchial injury in, 466, *466–467*
        cardiac injury in, 471–473, *472–473*
        chest wall, 459–462, *461*
        diaphragm rupture in, *468–472*, 473–474
        esophageal injury in, 474–475
        flail chest in, *461*, 461–462
        great vessel injury in, 467–471, *468–472*
        hemothorax in, 463–465, *465*

Circulation *(Continued)*
  in newborn, 14, 14t
    normal, *24*
    typical values in, 3t
    unbalanced, in great artery transposition, 1561
    ventilation distribution and, 23–24, *24*
  support of, in cardiopulmonary resuscitation, 370–376, *371–376*
Circulatory collapse. See also *Cardiopulmonary arrest; Shock.*
  after cardiac surgery, cardiopulmonary resuscitation in, 250–253, *251–252*
    causes of, 250, *251*
    diagnosis of, 250, *251*
    management of, 250–253, *252*
Circus movement, 2034, *2034*
Cirrhosis, pleural effusion in, 544
Cisplatin, in germ-cell tumors, 598–599
  in mesothelioma, 570
Cisterna chyli, anatomy of, 535, *536*
Clavicle, fracture of, 460
Clear cell tumor, of lung, 662
Cleveland Clinic Foundation Nimbus electric heart, 2144, *2144*
Clindamycin, in lung abscess, 680–681
  prophylactic, 103–104, 104t
Clinical databases, 380–382, *382–384*
  for microcomputers, 381–382, *382–384*
Clofazamine, in tuberculosis, 762t
Clofibrate, in lipid lowering, 2023t
Closing capacity, ventilation distribution and, 28, *28*
Closing volume, ventilation distribution and, 28–29, *28–29*
  versus expiratory reserve volume, 51, *52*
Clotting disorders. See *Coagulation disorders.*
Clubbing, of digits, in pulmonary arteriovenous malformation, 870
  in tetralogy of Fallot, 1469
Coagulation, activation of, by atherosclerotic plaque, 1183–1184, *1184–1185*
  at artificial surfaces, 1715–1717, *1716*
  opposing mechanism of (fibrinolytic system), 1184–1186, *1185–1186*
  perioperative monitoring of, 121
Coagulation cascade, 1184, *1185*
Coagulation disorders, in adult respiratory distress syndrome, 207
  in antibiotic use, 106
  in anticoagulant therapy, 1720
  in cardiac surgery, 253–255
    diagnosis of, *254,* 254–255
    treatment of, *253,* 253–256, 254t
  in cardiopulmonary bypass, 1263–1264, *1264,* 1722–1724
  in heart transplantation, 2109, 2111
  in septic shock, 196–197
  in tetralogy of Fallot, 1469–1470
  postoperative, 147–148
  pulmonary embolism in, 818
  tracheal intubation in, 298
  venous thrombosis in, 777
Coarctation, of aorta. See *Aortic coarctation.*
Cocaine, as anesthetic, 126
  in bronchoscopy, 74
  in tracheal intubation, 302, 331
*Coccidioides immitis,* 689
Coccidioidomycosis, 689–692
  clinical course of, 690–691, *690–691*
  disseminated, 691
  epidemiology of, 685
  geographic distribution of, 687, *687*
  granuloma in, 690, *690,* 691
  in HIV infection, 739–740
  incidence of, 689–690
  pathology of, 690
  treatment of, 691–692

Coeur en sabot, in tetralogy of Fallot, 1470, *1470*
Cognitive dysfunction, after cardiac surgery, 266
Coils, in arteriovenous fistula embolization, 914–915
  in vascular closure, 1153–1154
Colestipol, in lipid lowering, 2024t, 2027
Colistin, in empyema, 554
Colitis, pseudomembranous, in antibiotic use, 106
Collagen disease, pleural effusion in, 545
Collapse therapy, in tuberculosis, 763–764
Collar incision, in tracheal reconstruction, 425, *427*
Collar of Helvetius, anatomy of, 920
Collateral circulation, of coronary arteries, 1869, *1870–1872*
  in anomalous connection, 1835, 1838
  in atherosclerosis, 1887
Collett and Edwards classification, of truncus arteriosus, 1509, *1509*
Collins solution, in heart-lung transplant preservation, 2094t
Collis gastroplasty, in antireflux repair, 1027
  in peptic stricture treatment, 999, *999*
Collis-Belsey procedure, in peptic stricture, 1067–1069, *1068–1070*
Collis-Nissen procedure, in peptic stricture, 1069, *1070–1073,* 1071–1076, 1074t–1075t
Colloids, in adult respiratory distress syndrome, 56
  in hypovolemic shock, 188
Coloesophagoplasty, *902–904,* 902–905
  in carcinoma, 930
  in esophageal stricture, 1000, *1001,* 1069, 1078
Colon, cancer of, metastasis to lung, 672
  obstruction of, in diaphragmatic rupture, 1084, *1084,* 1086–1087, *1086–1088*
Color-flow Doppler echocardiography, 1238
Commissurotomy, of mitral valve, balloon, 1154–1157, *1156*
  closed technique for, 1680–1681
  historical aspects of, 1673
  open technique for, 1678–1681, *1679,* 1686
  of tricuspid valve, 1669–1670, *1670–1671*
Common data repository, in computer systems, 395, *396*
Common service networks, in computer systems, 395
Communicating bronchopulmonary foregut malformations, 855t, 860, 862, *864*
Communication, computers in, 394
Complement system, in cardiac surgery, 262
  in cardiopulmonary bypass, 1263–1264, *1264–1265*
    versus oxygenator type, 1263–1264, *1264–1265*
  in myasthenia gravis, 1106, *1106*
  in septic shock, 195
Computed tomography, 1194–1202. See also specific disorder.
  advantages of, 1195
  anatomic considerations in, 1195, *1196*
  angiography with, 1201
  applications of, 1195, 1197–1198, *1197–1198*
  in aortic disease, 1199–1200, *1200*
  in aortic dissection, 1347, *1348*
  in aortic injury, 470
  in bronchial atresia, 836, *836*
  in bronchiectasis, 678
  in cardiac neoplasms, 2074–2076
  in congenital heart disease, 1197–1198, *1198*
  in coronary artery bypass graft, 1195
  in intracardiac masses, 1197, *1197–1198*
  in ischemic heart disease, 1197, *1197*
  in lung carcinoma, 637–638
  in lung metastasis, 669
  in mediastinal neoplasms, 586–587
  in pericardial disease, 1198–1199, *1199,* 1371
  in pleural disease, 562–563
  in pneumothorax, 463, *463,* 527, *528*
  in pulmonary artery evaluation, 1200–1201, *1201*
  in thoracic aortic aneurysm, 1329, *1330*

Infant(s) *(Continued)*
  premature, patent ductus arteriosus in, 1276,
    1280–1281
  pulmonary circulation in, 349–351, *349–351*, 352t
  pulmonary function in, 14, 14t
  respiratory distress syndrome in. See *Respiratory*
    *distress syndrome, of newborn.*
  respiratory failure in, causes of, 351, 352t
    types of, 351
    with cardiac surgery, 352–354
  respiratory support in, airway management in,
    355t, 355–356
    equipment for, 354, 354t
    evaluation in, 354–355
    indications for, 351, 352t
    mechanical. See *Infant(s), mechanical ventilation*
      *in.*
    personnel for, 354
    physical plant for, 354
    results of, 363–364
  respiratory system of, anatomy of, 348–349, 349t
    physiology of, 349–351, *349–351*, 350t–351t
  spontaneous pneumothorax in, 529
  tracheal intubation in, 355t, 355–356
  tracheal surgery in, 405–406
  tracheostomy in, 355
Infantile lobar emphysema, 843–846, 844t, *844–846*
Infarct expansion phenomenon, 1187
Infection(s), as aneurysm cause, 1328
  fungal. See *Fungal infection(s).*
  in artificial heart implantation, 2139, 2142
  in blood transfusion, 256
  in cardiac surgery, 261–263, *262*
  in coronary artery bypass, 1900, 1902, 1918, 1920
  in immunosuppressive therapy, 2113
  in intra-aortic balloon pump support, 2002
  in mechanical ventilation, 363
  in median sternotomy, 223–224
  in tracheal intubation, 363
  in transplantation, 743–746, *745*, 746t
    heart-lung, 2099–2100
  in ventricular assist device use, 2009, 2009t
  incubation period in, 100, 100t
  of bronchogenic cyst, 860, *861*
  of donor site, after cardiac surgery, 263
  of lung. See under *Lung(s).*
  of mediastinal teratoma, 596
  of pericardium, *1374*, 1374–1375
  of prosthetic valve. See *Prosthetic valves, infection(s)*
    *of.*
  of trachea, 409–410
  opportunistic. See *Opportunistic infection(s).*
  parasitic. See also *Pneumocystis carinii infection.*
    of lungs, 701–704, *701–704*
  prevention of. See also *Antibiotics, prophylactic.*
    in cardiac surgery, 263
  shock in. See *Shock, septic.*
  viral, pericarditis in, 1373
Inferior vena cava, anomalies of, 1425–1427
  connection of, to left atrium, 1406, 1409–1410,
    *1410*, 1427, *1427*
    to pulmonary vein, 1410–1411
    to right atrium, 1406
  embryology of, 1405–1406, *1409*
  flow from, directing to pulmonary artery, in pul-
    monary atresia with intact ventricular septum,
    1611, *1611*
  interrupted (acquired), in pulmonary embolism,
    791–794, *792–793*, 793t
  interrupted (congenital), 1426–1427
    with azygos continuation, 1406, *1409*
  magnetic resonance imaging of, *1204*
  obstruction of, in great artery transposition repair,
    1576
  pulmonary artery anastomosis to, in pulmonary
    atresia with intact ventricular septum, 1502,
    *1504*

Inferior vena cava *(Continued)*
  pulmonary vein connection with, 1387, *1388*
Inflammation, in cardiopulmonary bypass, 262
Influenza, pericarditis in, 1373
Information systems. See *Computer applications.*
Inhalation anesthetics, pharmacokinetics of, 123–124
Inhalation burns, of trachea, 411
Inhalation scanning, in pulmonary embolism, 785
Initiation function, of mechanical ventilation, 304,
  304t–305t
Injury. See specific anatomic site, e.g., *Chest trauma.*
Innominate artery, anatomy of, 403, *403*
  anomalous origin of, 1304–1305, *1305*
  fistula of. See *Tracheo-innominate artery fistula.*
  graft of, to pulmonary artery, in hypoplastic left
    heart syndrome, 1661
  injury of, penetrating, 478, *479*
  occlusive disease of, 1358, 1359t–1360t, *1361–1362*,
    1362
  protection of, in tracheal reconstruction, 429
  pseudoaneurysm of, in blunt trauma, 467–468, *468*
  pulmonary artery anastomosis to, in tetralogy of
    Fallot, *1473–1475*, 1474–1475
  repair of, 435, *437*, 478, *479*
  suspension of, 1305, *1305*
Innominate vessels, embryology of, 1405, *1408*
  exposure of, in median sternotomy, 223
Inotropic agents, action of, 241–243, 242t–243t
  after cardiac surgery, 236
  after mitral valve repair, 1685
  in cardiac surgery, 240, *240*
  in cardiogenic shock, 203
  in coronary artery bypass, 1900
  in heart transplantation, 2107, 2111
  in pediatric patients, 447, 447t
  in septic shock, 199
  in tetralogy of Fallot, 1487
  nonadrenergic, 143–144, *145*
  types of, 241–243, 242t–243t
Inotropic state, after cardiac surgery, 241, *241*
  measurement of, 233–234, *234–235*
Inoue balloon technique, in mitral commissurotomy,
  1154, 1156, *1156*
Inspiration, mechanical ventilation triggered by, 304
  prolongation of, in inverse ratio ventilation, 310,
    *311*
Inspiratory capacity, definition of, 3
  typical values of, 3t
Inspiratory pause, in mechanical ventilation, 305
Inspiratory reserve volume, definition of, 3
  measurement of, *24*
Insulin, drug interactions with, 272t
  production of, in septic shock, 198
  requirements of, after cardiac surgery, 267, 268t
Intensive care unit, 329
  computerization in, 383–384, 386
  for infants, 354, 354t
  postoperative care in, 146–148
Intercostal arteries, aortic coarctation and, 1284
  laceration of, 476
  preservation of, in thoracic aortic aneurysm repair,
    1341, *1342*
Intercostal nerve block, 165–166
  in incisional pain, 228
  in rib fracture, 460–461
Intercostal veins, embryology of, *1408*
Interferon-alpha, in Kaposi's sarcoma, 743
Interferon-gamma, vaccination with, in lung
  carcinoma, 666–667
Interleukin(s), release of, in cardiopulmonary
  bypass, 1265
  in respiratory distress syndrome, 353
Interleukin-1, antibodies to, in septic shock
  treatment, 201
  in septic shock, 197
Interleukin-2, in lung carcinoma, 666

Intermittent mandatory ventilation, 57–58, *306,* *307–308*
  advantages of, 307–308
  historical aspects of, 288
  in infants, 357t, 357–358
  in ventilator weaning, 325
  synchronous, *306,* 307–308
  weaning from, 308
Intermittent positive-pressure breathing, 58
  historical aspects of, 287
Intermittent spontaneous breathing, in ventilator weaning, 324–325
Internodal pathway, anatomy of, 1768
Interpositional graft, in aortic coarctation, 1288, 1291
Intersociety Commission for Heart Disease Resources, pacemaker codes of, 1784–1785, 1785t
Interstitial pneumonia, 706–707, *707*
  idiopathic diffuse, 706–707, *707–708*
Interstitial pulmonary disease, 850, 853, *854*
  bronchoscopy in, 81
Interventricular veins, anatomy of, *1862*
Intestinal motility, after cardiac surgery, 269–270
Intra-aortic balloon pump, 1999–2003
  anticoagulants for, 1719
  balloon insertion in, 2002
  before cardiac transplantation, 2001–2002
  complications of, 2002–2003
  contraindications to, 2002
  diastolic augmentation with, 1999
  hemodynamic changes with, 1999
  historical aspects of, 1996, *1996*
  in cardiac surgery, 242t, 243
  in cardiogenic shock, 204, 204t, 206, 1999–2000
    postcardiotomy, 2000t, 2000–2001
  in coronary artery bypass, 1893
  in failed coronary angioplasty, 2001
  in heart transplantation, 2107, 2112
  in myocardial infarction, refractory to medical therapy, 2001
    with cardiogenic shock, 1999–2000
    with mechanical complications, 2000
  in septic shock, 2002
  in ventricular arrhythmias, 2002
  in ventricular septal rupture, 1970
  indications for, 1999, 1999t
  inflation-deflation cycle for, 2003
  malfunction of, 2003
  physiologic effects of, *1998*
  thromboembolism of, 1726–1727
  weaning from, 2003
Intrabronchial pressure, 524–525, *525*
Intracranial bleeding, in thrombolytic therapy, 1188, 1190, *1191*
Intracranial pressure, increased, tracheal intubation in, 298
  mechanical ventilation effects on, 312–313
Intraesophageal veins, anatomy of, 943, *944*
Intraluminal graft, aortic, in dissection repair, *1350,* 1350–1351
  sutureless, *1273,* 1273–1274
Intrapericardial pressure, 1368
Intrapleural analgesia, 165–166
Intrapleural pressure, 524–525, *525*
Intrapulmonary shunt. See *Shunt, right-to-left.*
Intrapulmonary tunneling, in coronary artery pulmonary origin, 1840, *1842–1843*
Intrathoracic pressure, in mechanical ventilation, 312
Intravagal paraganglioma, mediastinal, 592–593
Intravascular ultrasound, of coronary arteries, 1173–1174, 1178
Intravenous anesthetics, 122–123, *123,* 123t
Intubation, tracheal. See *Tracheal intubation.*
Inverse ratio ventilation, in hypoxemia, 321–324, *322–323*
  weaning from, 324
Iodine, radioactive, in mediastinal neoplasms, 587

Ionescu-Shiley prosthetic valve. See under *Prosthetic valves.*
  assessment of, 1146
Ipratropium, in tracheal intubation, 297
  perioperative, 18
Irrigation, in mediastinitis, 224, 579
  of chest, in stomach injury, 486
  with antibiotic solutions, 104–105
IRV. See *Inspiratory reserve volume.*
Ischemic heart disease. See also *Myocardial infarction; Myocardial ischemia.*
  anesthesia in, 128, 129t, *130*
  cardiac arrhythmia in, re-entrant, 2034–2035
  cardiopulmonary arrest in, 368
  pathophysiology of, 1183–1184, *1183–1185*
Isoflurane, cardiovascular effects of, 123t, 125
Isoniazid, in tuberculosis, 738, 762t, 762–763
Isoproterenol, as inotrope, *143,* 144t
  in anomalous pulmonary vein correction, 1416
  in cardiac surgery, 241, 242t, 243
  in heart transplantation, 2111
  in heart-lung transplant preservation, 2094t
  in pediatric patients, 447, 447t
  in septic shock, 199
Isovolumic relaxation phase, ventricular pressure-volume relationships in, 232, *232*
Isovolumic systole, ventricular pressure-volume relationships in, 232
Isthmusplastic operation, in aortic coarctation, 1288, 1291, *1291,* 1294
Itraconazole, in fungal infections, 700–701
Ivalon plug, in patent ductus arteriosus closure, 1280

**J**

Jackson bougies, for esophagoscopy, 90, *92*
Jackson dilators, for peptic stricture, *1065*
Jarvik artificial heart, components of, 2135–2138, *2136–2137*
  results with, 2142–2143, 2143t
Jatene circular plication repair, in left ventricular aneurysm, *1952,* 1952–1953
Jaw thrust, in airway clearance, 289, *290*
Jejunum, in esophageal reconstruction, 906
  interposition of, with esophagogastrectomy, in carcinoma, 930
Jet ventilation, in emergency airway establishment, 334
  in infants, 358
Jeune's disease, 511
Jitter measurements, in myasthenia gravis, 1104, *1104*
Jolly test, in myasthenia gravis, 1104
Judkins technique, in cardiac catheterization, 1126–1127
  in coronary angiography, *1874,* 1874–1875
Jugular venous pulse, hemodynamics of, *1368,* 1368–1369
*jun* proto-oncogene, in lung cancer, 665

**K**

Kallidin, in septic shock, 196
Kallikrein, in cardiopulmonary bypass, 1263
  in coagulation, *1716,* 1716–1717
  in septic shock, 196–197
  inhibitors of, in cardiopulmonary bypass, 1723
Kanamycin, 113
  in tuberculosis, 762t
Kaposi's sarcoma, in immunodeficiency, 741–743, *742,* 742t–743t
  in kidney transplantation, 742, 742t
Kartagener's syndrome, bronchiectasis in, 677
  lung anomalies in, 832, *832*

Kawasaki's disease, 1990–1995
  clinical manifestations of, 1990, 1990t
  diagnosis of, 1990–1991, *1991*
  epidemiology of, 1990
  etiology of, 1991–1992
  natural history of, 1992–1993, *1993,* 1993t
  pathology of, 1991–1992
  stages of, 1992
  treatment of, 1993–1994, 1994t
Kay annuloplasty, of tricuspid valve, 1669–1670,
    *1670*
Kay-Egerton annuloplasty, in mitral insufficiency,
    1692
Kent bundles, in Wolff-Parkinson-White syndrome,
    2040
Kerley's lines, in mitral stenosis, 1677
Ketamine, cardiovascular effects of, 122, 123t
Ketoconazole, in blastomycosis, 692–693
  in candidal esophagitis, 741
  in fungal infections, 700–701
  in histoplasmosis, 689
Ketone bodies, in septic shock, 194
Ketorolac, postoperative, 168
Kidney(s), acid-base homeostasis and, 12
  aortic coarctation and, 1286–1287
  blood flow to, postoperative, 236, *237*
  carcinoma of, lung metastasis from, 672–673
    tumor embolism in, 779–780
  dysfunction of, heart transplantation and, 2106
    in adult respiratory distress syndrome, 56
    in multisystem organ failure, 182
    in ventricular assist device use, 2009, 2009t
    pacing in, 1770, 1774
    pericarditis in, 1373–1374, *1398*
  failure of, diagnosis of, 264, 264t
    etiology of, 264–265
    in cardiac surgery, 263–265, 264t
    prevention of, 265
    respiratory insufficiency and, 13
    treatment of, 265
  function of, in mechanical ventilation, 312
    perioperative monitoring of, 121
  injury of, in thoracoabdominal aortic aneurysm re-
    pair, 1342, *1344*
  of pediatric patients, 137, 448–449
  transplantation of, Kaposi's sarcoma in, 742, 742t
Kininogen, in coagulation, *1716,* 1716–1717
Kinins, in septic shock, 196–197
Klinefelter's syndrome, germ-cell tumors in, 598
Koch, triangle of, anatomy of, 2035, *2036*
Koch's phenomenon, in tuberculosis, 753
Kohn, pores of, 829, *830*
Kommerell's diverticulum, *1301,* 1303–1304, 1306
Konno-Rastan procedure, in aortic stenosis, *1527*
Krusen-Caldwell technique, in thoracic outlet
    syndrome, 619–620, *622–623*
Kupffer cell-hepatocyte system, multisystem organ
    failure syndrome and, 181–182

## L

Labetalol, pharmacology of, 145, 146t
Laboratory database, 389, 392
Lactate-pyruvate ratio, in septic shock, 193, 198
Lactic acidosis, in low cardiac output syndrome, 236
Lactic dehydrogenase, in pleural effusion, 540
  in pulmonary embolism, 784
Laks procedure, in pulmonary atresia with intact
    ventricular septum, *1610,* 1610–1611
Laminography, of trachea, 420, *424*
Language, medical, for computer applications, 396
Laparoscopy, in Hill repair, 1047, *1047*
LaPlace's law, ventricular wall tension and,
    1948–1949, 1997
Large-cell carcinoma, of lung, pathology of, 635

Large-cell lymphoma, of mediastinum, 600–601
Larrey's hernia (Morgagni's), 1084, *1084*
Laryngeal mask airway, 291–292, *293,* 303
Laryngeal nerves, injury/preservation of, in tracheal
    surgery, 428
  recurrent, anatomy of, 943
Laryngectomy, in dysphagia, *971*
Laryngoscopy, in cardiopulmonary resuscitation,
    370, *370*
  in esophageal disorders, 963
  in infants, 355
  in tracheal intubation, airway difficulty and, *303*
    blades for, 299–300, *299–300,* 331, *331*
      malposition of, 301, *301–302*
    direct, 302–303
    errors in, 301, *301–302*
    laryngoscope for, 331, *331*
    position for, 288, *289*
    technique for, 298–301, *299–300*
    tongue size versus pharyngeal size and, 295, *296*
Laryngotracheal cleft, with tracheoesophageal
    fistula, 895
Laryngotracheoesophageal cleft, repair of, 406
Laryngotrachiectomy, 431–432, *434*
Larynx, carcinoma of, tracheal extension of, 408
  embryology of, 934, *935*
  endoscopy of. See *Laryngoscopy.*
  fracture of, 410
  injury of, 410, 467
    in tracheal intubation, 411, *412*
  of neonates, 446
  physical examination of, in tracheal intubation,
    295
  release of, in tracheal reconstruction, 426, 428
  ulceration of, in tracheal intubation, 341
Laser therapy, bronchoscopy in, 82
  for coronary angioplasty, 1177–1178
  for esophageal carcinoma, 92, 931
  for lung carcinoma, 646
  for ventricular tachycardia ablation, 2062
  tracheal stenosis in, 411
Lateral decubitus position, for thoracoscopic surgery,
    2149, *2150*
Latissimus dorsi muscle, in bronchopleural fistula
    closure, 557, *557–558*
  in chest wall reconstruction, 219, 518
  in Poland syndrome correction, 507
  sparing of, in thoracotomy incision, 215–217, *216–
    220*
  wrapping around heart, in assisted circulation,
    2010–2011, *2011*
LAV. See *Human immunodeficiency virus.*
Lavage, bronchoalveolar, 77
  tracheal, in tracheal intubation, 339
Leads, for cardioverter-defibrillator, *1802,* 1802–1803,
    *1804,* 1805
  for pacemakers, 1777–1778, *1778*
Lecompte's maneuver, in arterial switch operation,
    1598
Left atrial isolation procedure, in atrial fibrillation,
    *2037,* 2037–2038
Left atrial pressure, in mitral stenosis, 1675–1676
  versus left ventricular pressure, 232
Left ventricular aneurysm. See under *Ventricle(s),
    (left).*
Left ventricular assist devices. See *Ventricular assist
    devices.*
Left ventricular outflow tract obstruction. See also
    *Aortic stenosis; Cardiomyopathy, hypertrophic
    (idiopathic hypertrophic subaortic stenosis).*
  in great artery transposition, 1559–1560, 1565–
    1566, 1599
    treatment of, 1571–1572, *1572,* 1576
  in great artery transposition repair, 1576–1577
Left ventricular pressure, versus left atrial pressure,
    232

Mediastinum *(Continued)*
  subdivisions of, *576,* 576–577
    neoplasm location and, 583t, 583–584
  teratoma of, 595, *596*
  thymic cyst of, 610
  thymoma of. See *Thymoma.*
  widened, in great vessel injury, 468–469, *468–469*
  yolk-sac tumors of, 597–600, *599*
Medical history, in database, 386–387
  in tracheal intubation, 294–295
Medical literature services, 382–383, *385*
The Medical Record (TMR) database, 381
MEDLARS database, 383
MEDLINE database, 383
Medtronic Biomedicus pump, for ventricular assist
    devices, 2004, *2004*
Megaesophagus, in achalasia, *976–978,* 977–979
Meigs' syndrome, pleural effusion in, 544
Meissner's plexus, anatomy of, 946, *948*
Melanoma. See *Malignant melanoma.*
Membrane oxygenation, in cardiopulmonary bypass,
    1257
Meningitis, in coccidioidomycosis, 691
  in cryptococcosis, 695
Menstruation, pneumothorax during, 529–530
Meperidine, characteristics of, 154t
  dosage of, parenteral-oral conversions in, 158t
  in bronchoscopy, 73
  in epidural analgesia, 160t–161t
  in patient-controlled analgesia, 155t, 156
Mephentermine, action of, *143*
Mepivacaine, as local anesthetic, 127t
Mesenchymal patch, in tracheal reconstruction, 406
Mesenchymal tumor, mediastinal, 605
Mesenteric arteries, necrotizing arteritis of, after
    aortic coarctation repair, 1292
Mesocardia, in great artery transposition, 1558–1559
Mesoderm, in esophageal development, 934, *935*
Mesothelioma (cardiac), 2082
Mesothelioma (pleural), 566–570
  benign, 567–568, *568*
  clinical presentation of, 567, 569, *569*
  diffuse, 567–570, *569,* 569t–570t
  epithelial variant of, 567
  forms of, 567
  histology of, 566–567
  localized, 567–568, *568*
  malignant, diffuse, 568–570, *569*
    etiology of, 567
    localized, 568
    metastasis from, 569
    pathology of, 567
    staging of, 569, 569t
    treatment of, 569–570, 570t
  pathology of, 567
  pleural plaques and, 565
Message routes, in computer systems, 395
Metabolic acidosis. See under *Acidosis.*
Metabolic alkalosis. See under *Alkalosis.*
Metabolism, acids formed in, 48
  derangement of, cardiopulmonary arrest in, 369
    in blood transfusion, 256
    in low cardiac output syndrome, 236
    in multisystem organ failure, 199–201
    in septic shock, 194–195, 199–201
  in infants, thermoregulation and, 450, *450*
Metacholine, coronary artery spasm from, 1980
Metaproterenol, perioperative, 17
Metaraminol, action of, *143*
Metastasis, from germ-cell tumors, 598
  from heart, in myxoma, 2072
  from lung. See *Lung carcinoma, metastasis from.*
  from neuroblastoma, 590
  from seminoma, 597
  from thymoma, 595
  pathogenesis of, 669

Metastasis *(Continued)*
  to esophagus, 926–927
  to heart, *2084,* 2084–2085
    computed tomography of, 1197, *1197*
  to lung. See *Lung(s), metastasis to.*
  to mediastinum, 603
  to pericardium, 1375
  to pleura, 570–571
  to trachea, 408–409
Methadone, dosage of, parenteral-oral conversions
    in, 158t
Methicillin, 111
  bacteria resistant to, 108–109
Methotrexate, in lung carcinoma, 646
Methoxamine, action of, 143, *143,* 144t
Methyl methacrylate glue, in chest wall
    reconstruction, 219
Methylprednisolone, in heart-lung transplantation,
    2098–2099
Methylprednisone, in lung transplantation, 2129,
    *2129*
Metoclopramide, in aspiration prevention, 297
Metoprolol, in ventricular arrhythmias, 250t
  pharmacology of, 146t
Metronidazole, in amebiasis, 703
Mexiletine, in ventricular arrhythmias, 250t
Microatelectasis, postoperative, mechanical
    ventilation in, 316
Microbubbles, in echocardiography, 1240–1241, 1249
MicroMeSH literature search aid, 383
Midazolam, cardiovascular effects of, 123t
  in tracheal intubation, 302
  in cardiovascular disease, 297
Middle-lobe syndrome, in histoplasmosis, 689
  lobectomy in, 715, *716–719,* 720
Migraine headache, coronary artery spasm in, 1978
Miliary tuberculosis. See under *Tuberculosis.*
Military antishock trousers, in hypovolemic shock,
    186
Military injury, 456. See also *Chest trauma, blunt.*
Military position, in thoracic outlet syndrome, 617,
    *619*
Miller blade, for laryngoscopy, 299–300, *300*
Milrinone, after cardiac surgery, 242
Minimal effective analgesic concentration, 153–154,
    154t
Minimal inhibitory concentration, in antibiotic
    prophylaxis, 105
Minimum alveolar concentration, of anesthetics, 124
Minute oxygen consumption, pulmonary resection
    risk and, 16
Minute ventilation, calculation of, 24
  spontaneous, in extubation success prediction, 326
Minute volume, in pediatric patients, 14t
  typical values of, 3t
Missile embolism, of pulmonary arteries, 780–781
Mitochondrial function, in septic shock, 195
Mitral arcade (hammock malformation), 1547–1548
Mitral insufficiency, 1688–1699. See also *Ebstein's
    anomaly; Mitral valve, prolapse of.*
  absent papillary muscles in, 1548
  acute, 1144, *1144*
  anatomic considerations in, postinfarction, 1958–
    1959
  anesthesia in, 129t, 132
  annular dilatation in, 1546–1547
  annuloplasty in, 1674, 1691–1692, 1696–1697
  aortic valve disease with, 1755
  asymptomatic, treatment of, 1690–1691
  atrial septal defect with, 1388
  chronic, 1144
  cleft leaflet in, 1551–1552, *1552*
  clinical features of, 132, 1549, 1689
    postinfarction, 1959t, 1959–1961, *1960*
  congenital, morphology of, 1546–1549, 1547t, *1548*
  diagnosis of, 1689–1690, *1690*

Pulmonary function tests *(Continued)*
  guidelines for, 52t–53t, 52–54
  in emphysema, 876–877
  in extubation success prediction, 325–326
  in pulmonary embolism, 784–785
  in respiratory support, 41–42, *43*
  indications for, 1
  interpretation of, 1–2, *2*, 3t
  laboratory report of, 2
  preoperative, 15–17, *16*, 16t–17t, 50–54, 52t–53t
  pressure-volume curve in, 6–7
  temperature corrections for, 2
  typical values in, 3t
Pulmonary hypertension, after cardiopulmonary
      bypass, 262
  balloon occlusion in, 53
  cardiomegaly in, 13
  chronic, 803, *803*
  heart transplantation and, 2105–2106
  heart-lung transplantation in, 2092, *2092*
  in anomalous pulmonary vein connection, 1411–
      1412
  in aortic stenosis, 1736
  in aortopulmonary window, 1299
  in atrial septal defect, 1389, 1391–1392
  in atrioventricular canal defects, 1394, 1435, 1443
  in heart transplantation, 2111
  in mitral stenosis, 1143, 1675
  in mitral valve malformation, 1549
  in patent ductus arteriosus, 1278, 1280
  in pulmonary embolism, 803, *803*
  in pulmonary vein total anomalous connection,
      1399, 1411–1413
  in ventricular septal defect, after surgical treat-
      ment, 1455, 1461
  lung transplantation in, 2118, 2120
  persistent, in infants, 445
Pulmonary insufficiency. See also *Adult respiratory
      distress syndrome; Respiratory failure; Respiratory
      insufficiency.*
  cardiopulmonary arrest in, 368–369
  cardiovascular manifestations of, 13
  in coronary artery bypass, 231, *232*, 1918
  in diaphragmatic hernia, 1082–1083
  in pneumothorax, 530
  in pulmonary artery sling, 1307–1308
  in septic shock, 198
  in ventricular septal defect, 1450–1451
  kidney failure and, 13
Pulmonary obstructive disease. See also *Chronic
      obstructive pulmonary disease; Emphysema
      (pulmonary).*
  air flow rates in, 4–5, *5*
  pulmonary volume in, 4
  surgical risk in, 15
Pulmonary plethora, in tricuspid atresia, 1631
Pulmonary restrictive disease, forced expiratory
      volume in, 4, *5*
  pulmonary volume in, 4
  surgical risk in, 15
Pulmonary sequestration, 855
  communicating, 855t, 860, 862, *864*
  extralobar, 855t, 856–857, *858–859*
  intralobar, 855t, 855–856, *856–857*
Pulmonary stenosis, balloon valvuloplasty in,
      1151–1152, 1152t
  causes of, 1145
  hemodynamics of, 1145
  in tetralogy of Fallot, 1464–1465, *1466*, *1468*
  in tricuspid atresia, *1629*
  infundibular, in ventricular septal defect, 1451
  supravalvular, after arterial switch operation, 1601
  with intact ventricular septum, 1505–1507, *1506*
Pulmonary trunk, right ventricular junction of,
      narrowing of, in tetralogy of Fallot, 1481, *1481*
Pulmonary tuberculosis. See under *Tuberculosis.*

Pulmonary valve, absence of, in tetralogy of Fallot,
      *1468*
  in tricuspid atresia, 1630
  balloon dilatation of, 1498
  diameter of, in children, 1545t
  homograft of, in aortic valve disease, 1750–1751,
      *1750–1751*
  regurgitation at, after tetralogy of Fallot correc-
      tion, *1483*
    causes of, 1145
    hemodynamics of, 1145
  replacement of, thromboembolism in, 1721–1722
  stenosis of. See *Pulmonary stenosis.*
  surgical enlargement of, in tetralogy of Fallot,
      1481, *1481*
  transannular patch in, 1481–1482, *1481–1483*
  transfer of, in aortic stenosis, 1527, *1530*
  tricuspid, in pulmonary atresia with intact ventric-
      ular septum, 1493
  valvotomy of, in pulmonary atresia with intact
      ventricular septum, 1499, *1500–1501*, 1608,
      *1609*
Pulmonary vascular disease, as Fontan operation
      contradiction, 1635–1636
  in arterial switch operation, 1601
  in great artery transposition, 1566
  in univentricular heart, 1617–1618
  in ventricular septal defect, 1448–1450, *1450*
Pulmonary vascular resistance, at birth, 349, *349*
  calculation of, 233
  in diaphragmatic hernia, 1083
  in neonates, *349*, 349–350
  in ventricular septal defect, 1448
  with exercise, pulmonary resection risk and, 16
Pulmonary vein(s), anomalous, 867–869, *868*. See
      also *Atrial septal defect, secundum/sinus venosus
      type of, with partial anomalous pulmonary vein
      drainage.*
  in both lungs, 1388
  in hypoplastic left heart syndrome, 1660
  magnetic resonance imaging of, 1213
  superior vena cava drainage of, 1390–1392
  anomalous connection of. See *Pulmonary vein(s), to-
      tal anomalous connection of.*
  anomalous drainage of, with atrial septal defect.
      See under *Atrial septal defect, secundum/sinus ve-
      nosus type of.*
  arteriovenous malformation of, 869–871, *869–871*
  common, anatomy of, 1405, *1406–1407*
    atresia of. See *Pulmonary vein(s), total anomalous
        connection of.*
    stenosis of. See *Cor triatriatum.*
  connection of, to ductus venosus, 1410–1411, *1411*
    to inferior vena cava, 1410–1411
    to left atrium, 1406, 1409–1410, *1410*
    to right atrium, 1405, 1410, *1410*
  developmental anatomy of, 824, *826*
  embryology of, 1405, *1406–1408*
  location of, in lobectomy, 715, *717–718*, 720
  obstruction of, after correction of anomalies, 1419
    after Senning operation, 1590
    in great artery transposition repair, 1576
    in pulmonary vein total anomalous connection,
        1399
  partial anomalous connections of, embryology of,
      1405, *1407*
  stenosis of, balloon valvuloplasty in, 1153
    in great artery transposition, 1561
  total anomalous connection of, 1398–1402, 1405–
      1429
    anatomy of, 1409–1411, *1410–1411*
    cardiac, 1410, *1410*, 1412t
      surgical treatment of, 1416, *1418*
    cardiac defects with, 1411
    classification of, 1398–1399, 1410–1411, *1410–
        1411*, 1412t

# T

T lymphocytes, in myasthenia gravis, 593
   interactions of, with HIV, *733,* 733–734, 734t
   suppression of, in Kawasaki's disease, 1992
T piece, in ventilator weaning, 324–325
Tachyarrhythmias, pacing in, 1770, 1774
Tachycardia. See also *Ventricular tachycardia.*
   atrial, automatic, 2049
      paroxysmal, after cardiac surgery, 246
   in mitral valve stenosis, 1137
   in pacemaker malfunction, 1795–1796
   in tracheal intubation, 297
   pacemaker-mediated, 1795
   pacing in, 1797–1798, *1798*
   reciprocating, in Wolff-Parkinson-White syn-
      drome, 2042
   re-entry, 1797–1798
   supraventricular. See also *Supraventricular arrhyth-*
      *mias; Wolff-Parkinson-White syndrome.*
      paroxysmal, 2047–2048, *2048*
Tachyphylaxis, in epidural analgesia, 161
Tachypnea, in pulmonary vein total anomalous
     connection, 1399
   in ventilator weaning, 325
*Taenia echinococcus,* 703, *703*
Takayasu's arteritis, 1358, *1359,* 1360–1361
Talc pleurodesis, in pleural effusion, 546
   in pneumothorax, 532
Talcosis, 710
Tamponade, cardiac. See *Cardiac tamponade.*
   mediastinal, 581
Tapeworm, echinococcosis from, 703–704, *703–704*
Technetium scan, 1226
   in mediastinal neoplasms, 587
Teflon, as aortic prosthesis, 1272
Telangiectasia, hereditary hemorrhagic, pulmonary
     arteriovenous fistula in, 869–871, *869–871,* 912
Telescopic attachments, for bronchoscopy, 71, *71–73*
Temperature, correction for, in pulmonary function
     tests, 2
   monitoring of, perioperative, 120–121
   regulation of, in pediatric patients, 449–450, *450*
   versus pH of blood, *1261,* 1261–1262
Tension cyst, of lung, 847, *848*
Tension pneumothorax. See under *Pneumothorax.*
Teratodermoid cyst, of mediastinum, 596, *597*
Teratoma, of bronchus, 662
   of lung, 662
   of mediastinum, 596, *597*
     malignant, 597–600, *599*
Terminal sac, of lung development, 823
Tertiary waves, in esophagus, 953, *954*
"Tet atresia," surgical treatment of, 1485–1486
"Tet" spells, in tetralogy of Fallot, 1465, 1467
   intractable, surgical treatment of, 1486, 1486t
Tetracaine, 127t
   in bronchoscopy, 74
   in tracheal intubation, 331
Tetracycline, in bronchiectasis, 679
   in chemical pleurodesis, 531, 546, 874–875
Tetralogy of Fallot, 1464–1492
   anatomy of, 1464–1465, *1465–1466,* 1467
   boot-shaped heart (coeur en sabot) in, 1470, *1470*
   clinical manifestations of, 1467–1468, *1469*
   coronary artery anomalies in, 1860
   coronary artery spasm in, 1978
   definition of, 1464–1465
   diagnosis of, 1467–1471, *1469, 1471*
   echocardiography in, postoperative, 1487
   historical aspects of, 1464
   laboratory studies in, 1469–1470
   magnetic resonance imaging in, *1213,* 1216
   natural history of, 1467–1468, *1469*
   physical examination in, 1468–1469
   "pink," 1465

Tetralogy of Fallot *(Continued)*
   surgical treatment of, aortopulmonary shunt in,
     *1473,* 1476–1477
     balloon angioplasty in, 1477–1478
     Blalock-Taussig procedure in, *1473–1475,* 1474–
       1475
     cardiac arrhythmia after, 1487–1488
     corrective, *1478–1485,* 1478–1487, 1486t
       versus palliative treatment, 1471–1472
     Glenn anastomosis in, 1473
     hemodynamics after, 1487–1488
     in coronary artery malposition, 1485, *1485*
     in intractable "tet" spells, 1486, 1486t
     in pulmonary atresia, 1485–1486
     in "tet atresia," 1485–1486
     indications for, 1471–1472, *1472*
     mechanical ventilation in, 1487
     modified Blalock-Taussig shunt in, *1473,* 1475–
       1476, *1476*
     mortality in, 1471–1472, 1486, 1486t, 1488
     overview of, 1486–1487
     pacing after, 1482, 1487
     palliative, 1472–1478, *1473–1476*
       versus corrective, 1471–1472
     postoperative management in, 1487–1488
     Potts' anastomosis in, 1473–1474
     pressure measurement after, 1486
     pulmonary artery stenosis relief in, 1481–1483,
       *1483–1484*
     right ventricular outflow tract obstruction relief
       in, 1479–1481, *1480–1483*
     right ventricular outflow tract patch in, *1473,*
       1477
     subclavian-pulmonary anastomosis (Blalock-
       Taussig) in, *1473–1475,* 1474–1475
     sudden death after, 1488
     ventricular septal defect closure in, *1478–1480,*
       1478–1481, *1484*
     Waterston anastomosis in, 1473
TGV (thoracic gas volume), 3–4
Thal fundoplication, in gastroesophageal reflux, 898
   in peptic stricture, *998,* 998–999, *1076,* 1076–1077
Thallium, in radionuclide scans, 1226
   in coronary artery disease, 1229
Theophylline, perioperative, 18
Thermal environment, neutral, for pediatric patients,
     450–451
Thermodilution method, in cardiac output
     measurement, 1133
   in coronary blood flow determination, 1868
Thermogenesis, nonshivering, in infants, 449–450
Thermoregulation, in pediatric patients, 449–450, *450*
Thiocetazone, in tuberculosis, 762t
Thiocyanate formation, in nitroprusside therapy, 239
Thiopental, cardiovascular effects of, 122, 123t
   in bronchoscopy, 74
   pharmacokinetics of, 122
Thoracentesis, in empyema, 549–550
   in pleural disease, imaging techniques in, 563
   in pleural effusion, 545–546
   in pleural tuberculosis, 564
   in pneumothorax, 530
Thoracic. See also *Chest* entries.
Thoracic artery, internal, as coronary artery bypass
     graft, 1926–1927
Thoracic cage, compliance of, typical values of, 3t
   reconstruction of, 518
Thoracic duct, anatomy of, 535–536, *536*
   injury of, 536–537, 537t
   ligation of, in chylothorax, 538
   repair of, in chylothorax, 538
Thoracic dystrophy, 511
Thoracic gas volume, measurement of, 3–4
   typical values of, 3t
Thoracic outlet syndrome, 613–633, 617, *620*
   Adson test in, 617, *618*